BEST PUBLICATIONS OF WILLIAM C. ROBERTS, MD

Collected Reprints (1962-2022)

By

William C. Roberts, MD

and

Colleagues

ISBN: 979-8-88680-082-1
Printed in the United States of America on acid-free paper.

Preface

I think it is useful and educational for authors to pick their best publications near the end of their publishing careers. I would, for example, have loved to see what publications Sir William Osler, William Halsted, Eugene Braunwald, or Michael DeBakey considered their best. Listed herein are publications by William C. Roberts considered by him to be his best. The list is large simply because the author could not separate his best from those not in that category. Also, the list is large because the author did the same thing for 60+ years, not burdened by extensive administrative responsibilities, and worked with many talented investigators. There were few times during those 60+ years when the author (WCR) was not awaiting a letter from an editor indicating whether his manuscript was suitable for publication (with appropriate revision) or not. Having time to write manuscripts is, of course, a privilege but utilizing non-work hours (early mornings or late evenings and weekends or holidays) is essential for success. Nothing in medicine provides the joy of having one's own manuscript accepted for publication!

—William C. Roberts, MD

Table of Contents

Complete Interruption of the Aortic Arch

By William C. Roberts, M.D., Andrew G. Morrow, M.D., and Eugene Braunwald, M.D.

A LOCALIZED NARROWING of the aorta at or distal to the ductus arteriosus (coarctation of the adult type) is one of the most common congenital malformations of the great vessels. A narrowing of the aorta proximal to a patent ductus arteriosus (coarctation of the infantile type) is less common, while complete interruption of the aorta proximal to the ductus is quite rare, and interruption distal to the ductus has not been recorded. Interruption of the aortic arch, also termed absence, interruption, or atresia of the isthmus of the aorta, functionally corresponds to the most severe form of the infantile type of coarctation.

The adult type of coarctation of the aorta is relatively easily recognized by clinical means and the results of surgical treatment are, in general, good. The diagnosis of complete interruption of the aorta, on the other hand, has rarely been made before death or exploratory operation and, although it too is amenable to surgical correction or palliation, few attempts at operative treatment have been made. Three patients with complete interruption of the aortic arch have been studied at the National Heart Institute. In the present report the clinical, hemodynamic, angiographic, and pathologic findings in these patients are described and the information derived from 52 previously reported patients is reviewed.

Embryology

A pathologic classification used by Celoria and Patton[1] of aortic arch interruption, based on the sites of origin of the branches of the aortic arch, has been found applicable in the present study. The embryologic mechanisms by which the various types of aortic arch interruption may occur are illustrated schematically in figure 1. The type A interruption, which occurs immediately distal to the left subclavian artery, appears to result from a regression or atrophy of the segment of left dorsal aorta between the ductus arteriosus and the left subclavian artery (fig. 2A). In the type B deformity, the interruption is just distal to the origin of the left carotid artery and represents a failure of formation of the left fourth arch, since the left subclavian artery arises from the descending aorta (fig. 2B). The pathogenesis of the type C malformation, in which only the right subclavian and right carotid arteries arise from the ascending aorta (fig. 2C), is less clear. Celoria and Patton suggest two possible mechanisms: (1) partial or complete failure of formation of the left third and fourth aortic arches and persistence of the segment of dorsal aorta between these arches as the left common carotid artery, or, (2) a failure of connection of the outgrowth of the aortic sac with the third and fourth arches and fusion of these two arches to form the left common carotid artery.

Four variations of the basic type B interruption have been reported (fig. 3). In two of these (b and d) the ductus persists on the right as well as on the left. Bilateral persistence of the ducti (double ductus arteriosus) occurs when the entire right sixth arch and part of the right dorsal aorta remain. Each ductus connects the subclavian artery with the pulmonary artery on the respective side. According to Wagenvoort et al.,[2] the embryologic basis for the origin of the right pulmonary artery from the ascending aorta (fig. 3C) is the persistence of part of the right dorsal aorta and of the distal part of the right sixth arch.

From the Department of Pathologic Anatomy, Clinical Center, and Clinic of Surgery and Cardiology Branch, National Heart Institute, National Institutes of Health, Bethesda, Maryland.

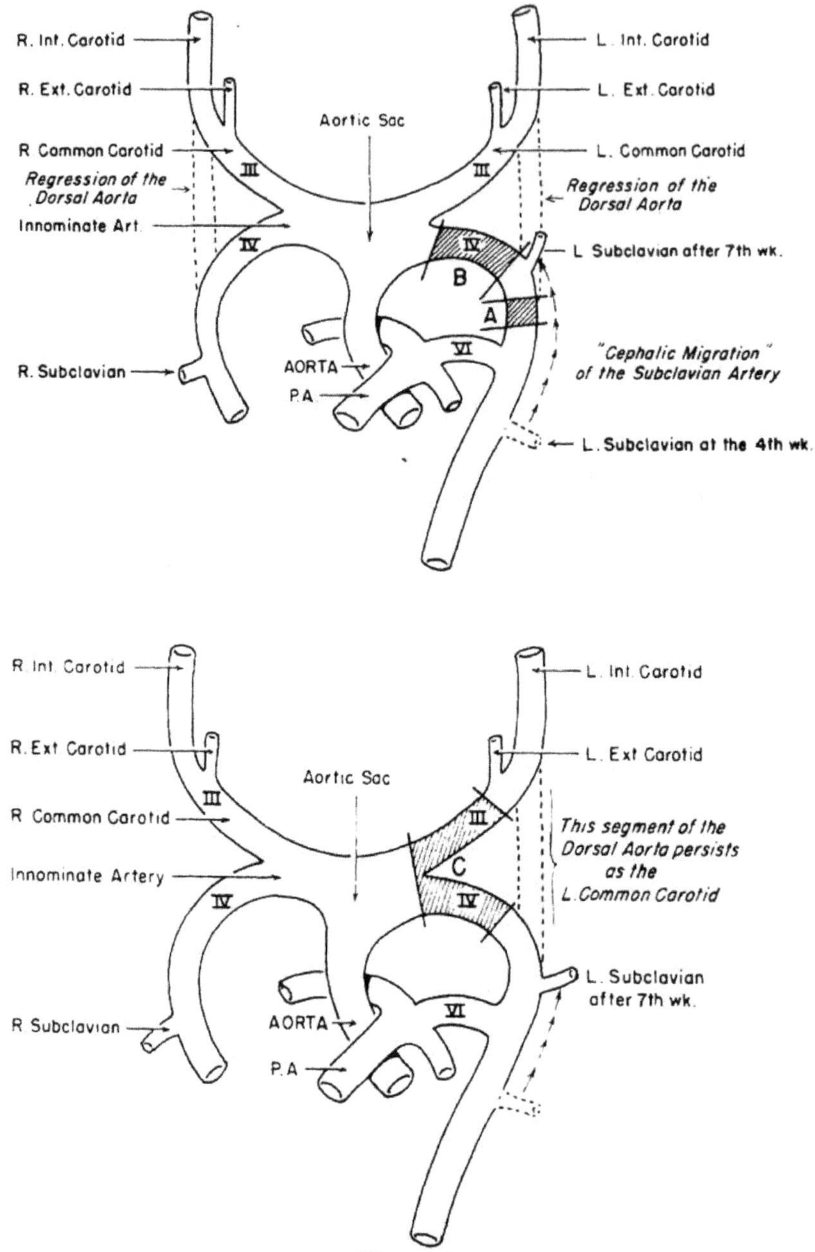

Figure 1

Schematic representation of the great arteries arising from the heart in the fetus. The primitive aortic arches from which the arteries were derived are indicated. Also designated (lined areas) are the sites where defective development produces types A and B complete interruptions of the aortic arch (upper diagram), *and type C* (lower diagram). *(Reproduced with permission of the authors and publisher, C. V. Mosby Co., from Celoria, G. C., and Patton, R. B., Am. Heart J.* **58:** *407, 1959.)*

Clinical Summaries

Case 1

L.N. (no. 01-58-99), a 25-month-old boy, was the product of a full-term normal pregnancy. During the first few months of life he had frequent upper respiratory infections, choking and coughing spells, and occasionally syncope during more severe coughing episodes. At 4 months he was found to have a heart murmur. At 14 months of age cardiac catheterization at another hospital

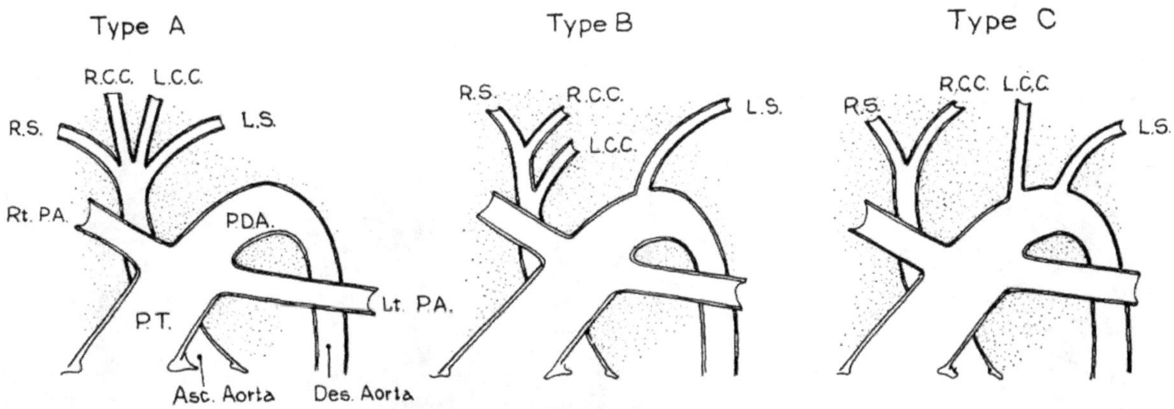

Figure 2

Diagrammatic illustrations of the three principal anatomic types of complete interruption of the aortic arch. P.T., pulmonary trunk; P.D.A., ductus arteriosus; P.A., pulmonary artery; R.S., right subclavian artery; R.C.C., right common carotid artery; L.C.C., left common carotid artery; L.S., left subclavian artery.

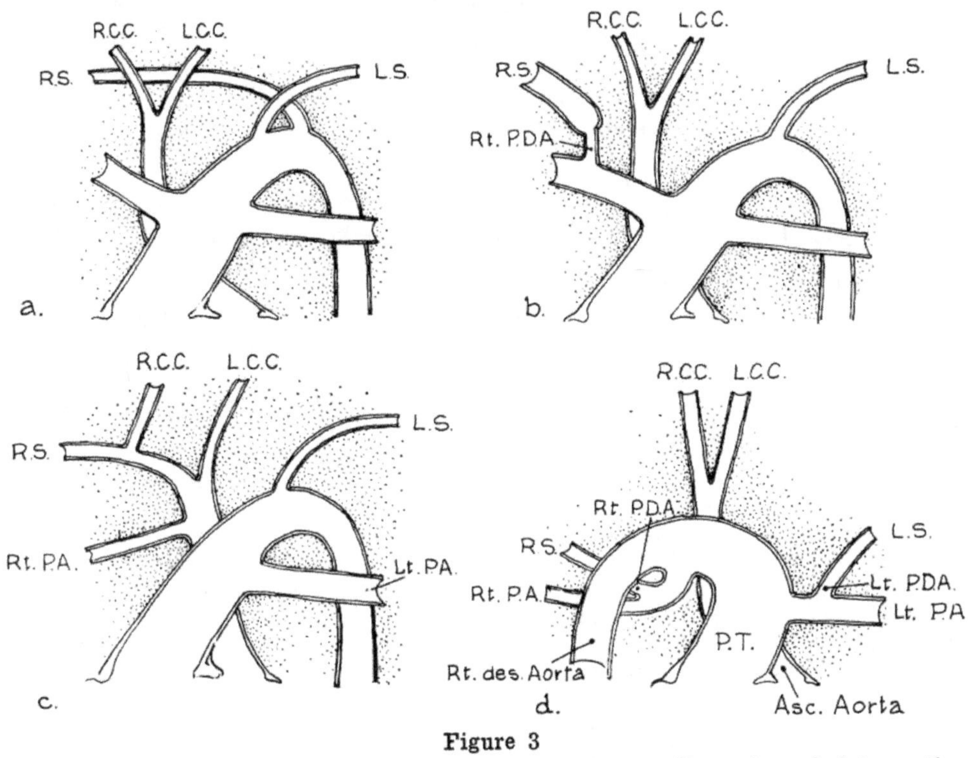

Figure 3

Diagrammatic illustrations of four variations of basic type B aortic arch interruption. In b. and d. the ductus arteriosus persists on the right as well as on the left. Abbreviations as in figure 2.

showed equal systolic pressures (76 mm. Hg) in the right ventricle, pulmonary artery, and left ventricle. A ventricular septal defect was crossed by the catheter. Left-to-right shunts entering both the right atrium and the right ventricle were demonstrated by oximetry. In the ensuing 9 months he grew and developed normally and never evidenced cardiac failure. Two months before admission, however, he had several "spells" of choking and cyanosis and his respiration became progressively more difficult.

On admission the child was normally developed.

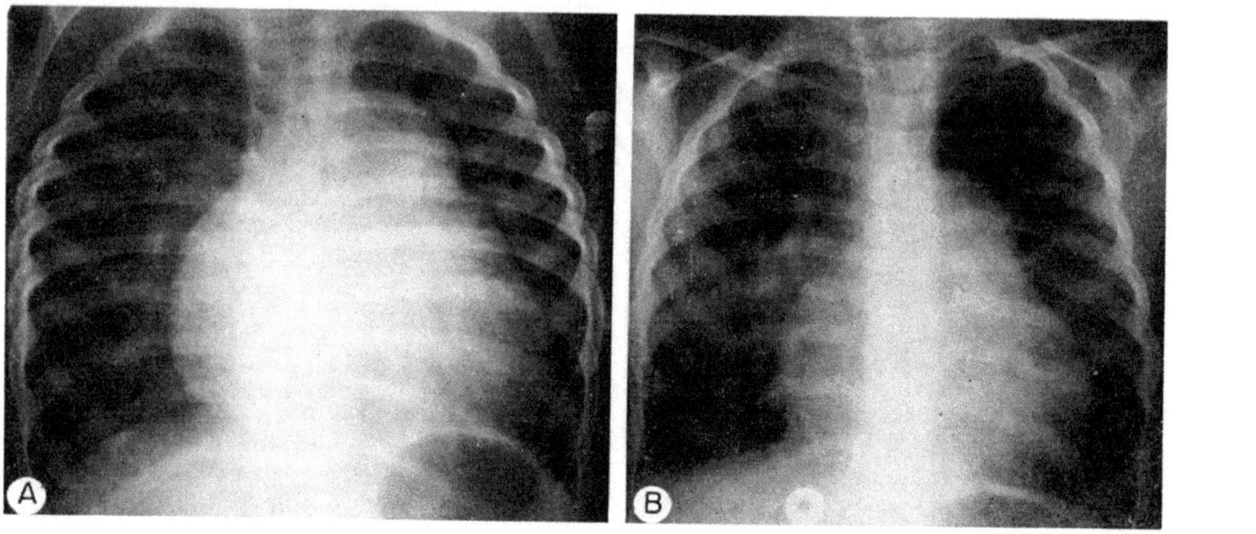

Figure 4
Posteroanterior roentgenograms of chest in patients L. N. (A) and P. S. (B).

The radial and femoral pulses were full and equal. The fingertips of the right hand were redder than those of the left, but the nailbeds of the fingers of both hands, as well as the toes, were cyanotic; there was no clubbing. The left precordium was bulging, and both left and right ventricular lifts and a systolic thrill to the left of the sternum were palpable. The second heart sound was louder in the pulmonic than in the aortic area and a grade 4/6 systolic murmur was audible over the entire precordium, loudest in the fourth and fifth intercostal spaces along the left sternal border.

The hematocrit value was 50 per cent. Fluoroscopic and radiographic examinations (fig. 4A) revealed generalized cardiac enlargement with particular prominence of the right ventricle, left atrium, and main pulmonary artery, and increased pulmonary vascularity. The electrocardiogram (fig. 5A) demonstrated right axis deviation, right ventricular hypertrophy, bi-atrial enlargement, and sinus tachycardia. Right heart catheterization disclosed a mean right atrial pressure of 13 mm. Hg, a right ventricular pressure of 88/16, and a femoral arterial pressure of 90/50 mm. Hg. The pulmonary artery could not be entered. Serial blood samples from both venae cavae, the right atrium, and the right ventricle revealed an increase in oxygen content of 2.2 volumes per cent in the atrium and an additional rise of 1.1 volumes per cent in the ventricle. Blood from the femoral artery had an oxygen saturation of 83.3 per cent.

Shortly following these studies the child became severely dyspneic and cyanotic, and atrial flutter developed. With the administration of digitalis the rhythm became regular. One week later bilateral bronchopneumonia developed and he died in heart failure.

Pathologic Findings

At autopsy, the heart (fig. 6) was greatly enlarged, weighing 125 Gm. (anticipated weight, 65 Gm.). The foramen ovale was closed. The right ventricle was dilated and hypertrophied. A defect, measuring 1.1 cm. in greatest diameter and bordered entirely by myocardium, was present in the basal portion of the ventricular septum, directly beneath the pulmonic valve and a portion of the hypertrophied crista supraventricularis and immediately cephalad to the papillary muscle of the conus. The right ventricular outflow tract, pulmonic valve, and pulmonary trunk and all its branches were greatly dilated. The large pulmonary trunk overrode the ventricular septal defect to take origin in part from the left ventricle. A patent ductus arteriosus, measuring 2.0 cm. in circumference and 1.5 cm. in length, arose from the pulmonary trunk and gave origin to the descending thoracic aorta. The intima of the patent ductus was irregular, in contrast to the smooth linings of the adjacent aorta and pulmonary artery. The left subclavian artery arose from the patent ductus. The pulmonary veins, left atrium, and mitral valve were normal. The left ventricle was dilated and hypertrophied. The outflow tract of the left ventricle was narrowed by a muscular ridge immediately cephalad to the ventricular septal defect. The aortic valve, which was bicuspid, measured only 3.2 cm. in circumference while the pulmonic valve was 6.5 cm. in circumference. The origin and distribution of the coronary arteries

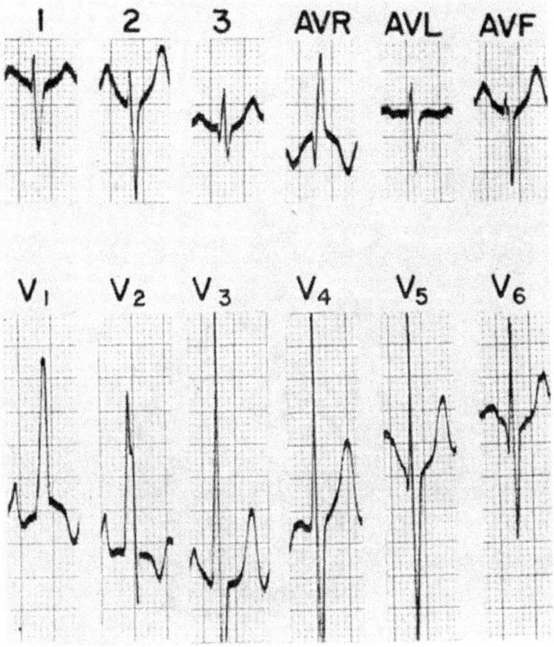

Figure 5A
Electrocardiogram of patient L. N., January 11, 1957.

were normal. The ascending aorta was small and terminated by dividing into the innominate and left common carotid arteries, while the innominate divided normally into right subclavian and common carotid arteries. No structure of any kind connected the ascending to the descending aorta.

Microscopically, there was moderate dilatation of all pulmonary arteries. The walls of the muscular pulmonary arteries were thickened, and a muscular media was present in the arterioles (fig. 7A). There was no intimal proliferation in these vessels. These hypertensive pulmonary vascular changes were grade 1/6, according to the classification of Heath and Edwards.[3] There was also evidence of bilateral bronchopneumonia, pulmonary edema and atelectasis, and chronic passive congestion of the liver.

Case 2

R.S. (no. 03-13-50), a male infant, was admitted to the National Heart Institute at the age of 10 days. He was the product of a full-term normal pregnancy and delivery, but at birth was cyanotic, markedly dyspneic, and had a heart murmur. On his eighth day of life he was digitalized because of evidence of congestive heart failure.

On admission he was well-developed, but undernourished (weight 2,550 Gm.), and in moderate distress. The pulse and respirations were rapid. There was mild cyanosis of the nailbeds, similar

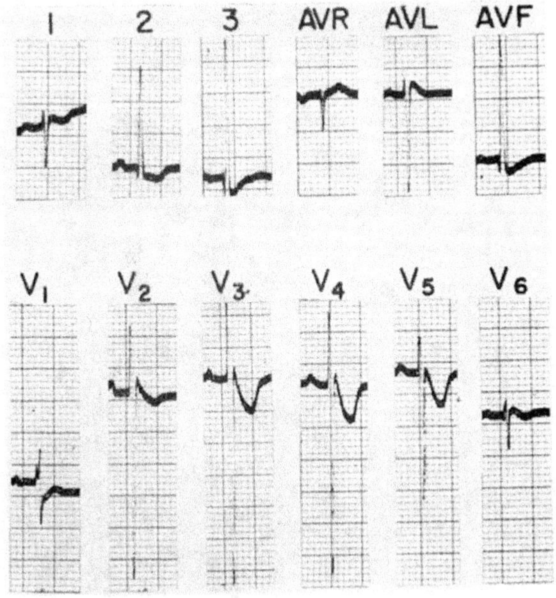

Figure 5B
Electrocardiogram of patient R. S., August 16, 1960.

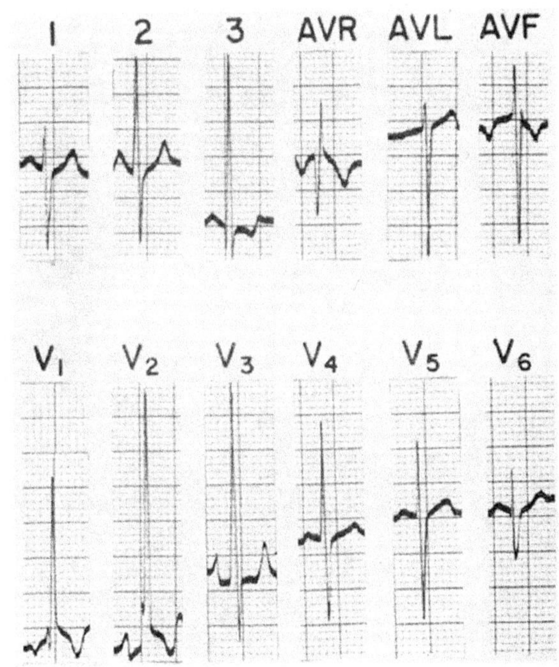

Figure 5C
Electrocardiogram of patient P. S., February 9, 1961.

in the fingers and toes. The brachial pulses were bounding but no femoral pulses could be felt. The systolic blood pressure, recorded by the flush technic, was 100 mm. Hg in each arm and 90

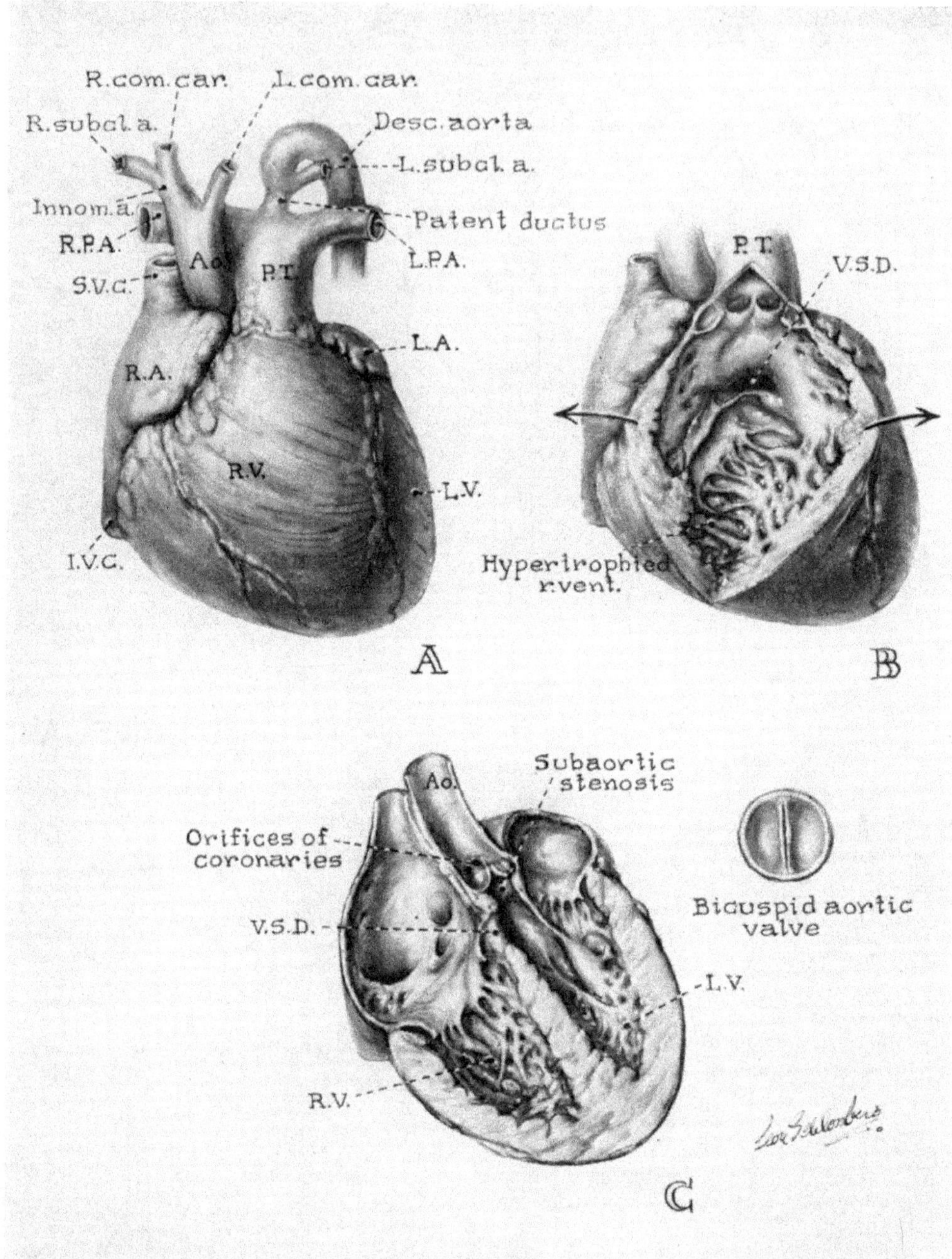

Figure 6

Drawing of heart and great vessels of patient L. N. A. The ascending aorta (Ao.) terminates after giving rise to the left common carotid artery (type B interruption). The descending aorta arises entirely from the pulmonary trunk (P.T.) via the patent ductus arteriosus. The left subclavian artery arises from the "pulmonary-ductus-descending aorta trunk." The pulmonary trunk is markedly dilated and the ascending aorta relatively hypoplastic. The right ventricle is dilated and hypertrophied. B. The right ventricle and pulmonic valve are opened. The ventricular septal defect (V.S.D.) is located below (caudal to) a portion of the crista supraventricularis muscle but above (cephalad to) the papillary muscle of the conus. C. The anterior portion

mm. Hg in the left leg. The left precordium was prominent, a right ventricular lift and a systolic thrill in the suprasternal notch were palpable. The second sound was single at the base and a third heart sound was audible at the apex. A grade 4/6 harsh systolic murmur, maximal in the fourth left intercostal space, was heard over the entire precordium and also in the neck and back. A grade 2/6 early diastolic murmur was audible in the third left interspace.

The hematocrit value was 45 per cent. The chest roentgenogram showed cardiomegaly and increased pulmonary vascularity. The electrocardiogram (fig. 5B) disclosed sinus tachycardia, deviation of the T waves to the right, and digitalis effect.

At cardiac catheterization the mean right atrial pressure was 8 mm. Hg. An interatrial communication was crossed by the catheter and the mean left atrial pressure was 10 mm. Hg. The right ventricular pressure was 132/18 mm. Hg. A vessel considered to be the main pulmonary artery was entered from the right ventricle and a pressure of 132/48 mm. Hg was recorded within it. The oxygen content (volumes per cent) of blood from various sites was: inferior vena cava, 5.3; right atrium, 5.5; right ventricle, 7.0; right pulmonary artery, 9.3; and left atrium, 14.6. The femoral arterial oxygen saturation was 71 per cent. A selective angiocardiogram was performed with injection into the left atrium. The first film showed opacification of the left atrium, left ventricle, right ventricle, and a common arterial trunk arising from both ventricles. The main pulmonary artery appeared to arise from the common trunk. The aorta, originating also from the truncus, terminated by dividing into two innominate arteries, each of which gave rise to carotid and subclavian arteries bilaterally. From these studies diagnoses of ventricular septal defect, persistent common truncus arteriosus, patent ductus arteriosus, and complete interruption of the aortic arch were made. Shortly following the catheterization procedures the infant became severely cyanotic, left heart failure was evident, and he died 2 days later.

Pathologic Findings

At autopsy, both ventricles were dilated and hypertrophied (fig. 8). A single arterial trunk arose from the base of the heart. The semilunar valve at the base of the trunk was composed of only two cusps, the margins of which were corrugated and thickened. The ostia of both coronary arteries were located behind the right cusp but each artery was normally distributed. The common trunk divided into the aorta and main pulmonary artery. The aorta terminated after giving rise to right and left innominate arteries. The main pulmonary artery divided normally and, through a short, "coarcted" ductus arteriosus, communicated with the descending aorta. A ventricular septal defect, measuring 0.9 cm. in largest diameter, was present just beneath the semilunar valve. It involved the entire membranous septum and a portion of the muscular septum. A large, valvular incompetent, foramen ovale was present. Microscopically, there was thickening of the walls of the pulmonary arterioles and muscular arteries without intimal proliferation (Heath and Edwards, grade 1/6) (fig. 7B).

Case 3

P.S. (no. 03-40-87), a 37-month-old girl, was the product of a full-term normal pregnancy. During the first 3 months of life she ate poorly, gained weight slowly, and had episodes of shortness of breath. At 12 weeks of age she had an episode of extreme dyspnea and cyanosis followed by a convulsion. She was hospitalized, found to be in congestive heart failure, and was digitalized. The femoral pulsations were noted to be diminished. At 15 months of age cardiac catheterization was performed at another hospital and a diagnosis of ventricular septal defect and pulmonary hypertension (pulmonary arterial pressure, 62/30 mm. Hg) was made. At 21 months of age, the nailbeds of the toes were noted to be more cyanotic than those of the fingers. Thereafter, until her admission to the Clinical Center 16 months later, she grew poorly, had dyspnea on minimal exertion, and was cyanotic at rest.

On admission she was undernourished and underdeveloped (weight 10 Kg.). The blood pressure was 115/85 in the arms and 100/80 in the legs. There was generalized cyanosis but the nailbeds of the toes were more cyanotic than those of the fingers. There was early clubbing of the distal digits of the toes, but none of the fingertips. Right and left ventricular impulses were palpable, and the second heart sound in the pulmonic area was accentuated. A third heart sound was heard at the lower left sternal border. A grade 2/6

of the heart has been removed. The outflow tract of the left ventricle is narrowed by a muscular ridge immediately cephalad to the ventricular septal defect. The aortic valve is bicuspid and small. L.A., left atrium; L.V., left ventricle; R.A., right atrium; R.V., right ventricle; R.P.A., right pulmonary artery; L.P.A., left pulmonary artery; S.V.C., superior vena cava; I.V.C., inferior vena cava.

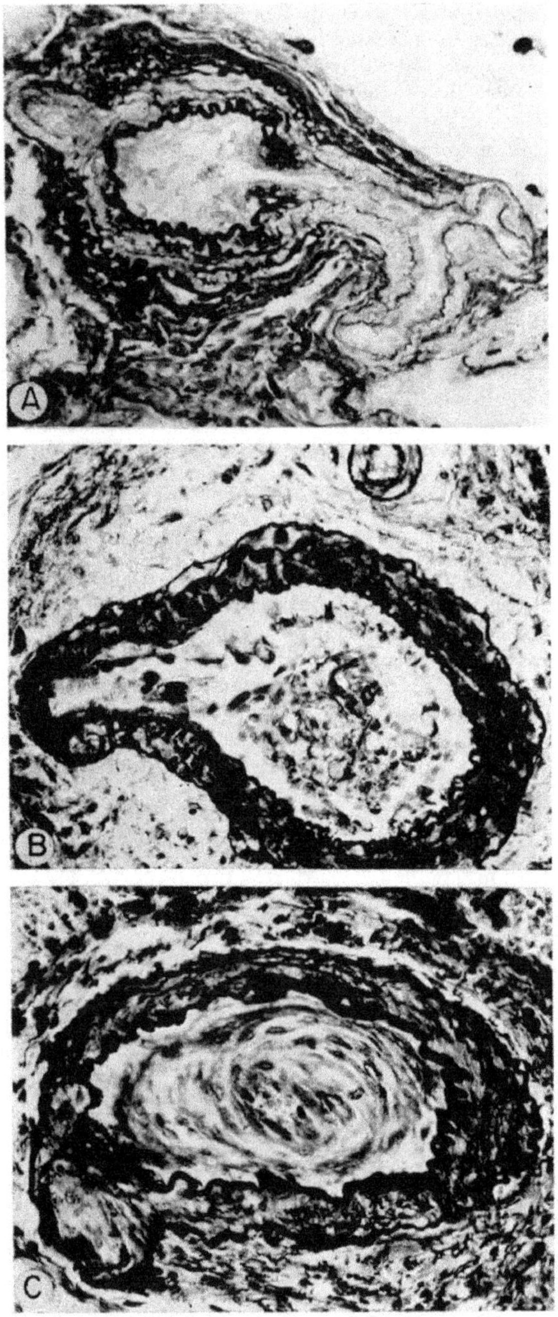

Figure 7

Photomicrographs of representative muscular pulmonary arteries and arterioles from patients L. N. (A), *R. S.* (B), *and P. S.* (C). *Verhoeff-Van Gieson elastic-tissue stains: original magnification of each* × *420.* A. *There is medial hypertrophy in both the muscular pulmonary artery and its branching arterioles. There is slight intimal thickening at the origin of one arteriole.* B. *Medial hypertrophy of the muscular pulmonary artery and of an adjacent arteriole is again evident. There is no intimal proliferation.* C. *The small muscular pulmonary artery is almost totally occluded by fibrocellular intimal proliferation. In the arteriolar branch (lower left) medial hypertrophy is also present.*

short ejection-type systolic murmur was heard along the left sternal border. The hematocrit value was 53 per cent. The electrocardiogram (fig. 5C) showed right axis deviation and right ventricular hypertrophy. Fluoroscopic and radiographic examinations disclosed generalized cardiomegaly, dilatation of the pulmonary trunk, and increased pulmonary vascularity (fig. 4B).

Cardiac catheterization at this time showed equal pressures (100/0 mm. Hg) in the right and left ventricles, and, by oximetry, a left-to-right shunt was shown to be entering the right ventricle. The left atrium was entered through an interatrial communication. Blood from both the left ventricle and outflow tract of the right ventricle had the same oxygen saturation (84 per cent). Selective angiocardiograms with both left and right ventricular injections were performed (figs. 9 and 10). The ascending aorta was small and terminated after giving rise to the innominate, left carotid, and left subclavian arteries. A ventricular septal defect was demonstrated immediately below the semilunar valves. The right ventricular injection showed marked dilatation of the right ventricle and pulmonary trunk, which continued as the descending aorta. The ventricular septal defect was again demonstrated.

Surgical correction of the aortic arch anomaly was carried out on March 1, 1961. A left lateral thoracotomy was made, and the ascending aorta and its branches were dissected free. The descending aorta originated from the main pulmonary artery through a large ductus. The intercostal arteries were of normal size and, when the ductus was temporarily occluded, the pressure in the descending aorta fell to 20 to 30 mm. Hg, indicating that no effective collateral circulation to the distal aorta was present. A partially occluding clamp was placed on the ascending aorta at the origin of the left subclavian artery, and the end of a Teflon vascular graft was sutured to the aorta at this point (fig. 11D). The distal end of the prosthesis was anastomosed to the side of the descending aorta immediately distal to the ductus. When the continuity of the aorta had been restored, the ductus was divided and closed. Postoperatively, bounding femoral pulses were palpable and the child's color was good. The day following operation atelectasis of the right upper lobe was evident by x-ray, and a tracheostomy tube was

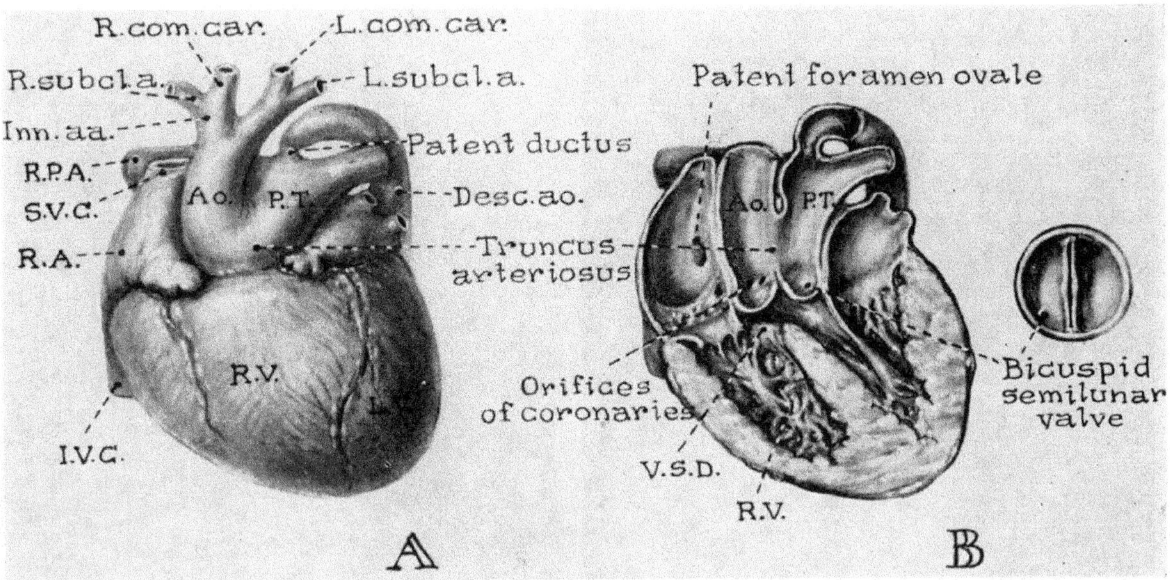

Figure 8

Drawings of heart and great vessels of patient R. S. A. *A single trunk arises from the ventricles and divides into the ascending aorta (Ao) and pulmonary trunk (P.T.). The ascending aorta terminates after giving rise to the left subclavian artery (type A aortic arch interruption). The descending aorta arises entirely from the pulmonary trunk via the ductus arteriosus, which is patent but narrowed or coarcted.* B. *The anterior portion of the heart has been removed. The ventricular septal defect (V.S.D.) is apparent immediately beneath the bicuspid semilunar valve of the common trunk. The valve covering the patent foramen ovale is incompetent. This is the first patient with complete interruption of the aorta to be reported with an associated persistent truncus arteriosus.*

inserted. Respiratory distress became more severe, however, and the child died 48 hours after operation.

Pathologic Findings

At autopsy, acute purulent pericarditis and left empyema were found. Pure cultures of a coagulase-positive hemolytic Staphylococcus aureus were grown from these areas and also from the heart blood. The child's death was clearly attributed to infection.

The heart was greatly enlarged (fig. 11); the walls of each ventricle were markedly hypertrophied. A valvular-incompetent foramen ovale was present. The pulmonary valve and pulmonary trunk were greatly dilated and overrode a ventricular septal defect, which was 1.0 cm. in largest diameter. The defect was in the anterior ventricular septum just beneath the pulmonic valve and a portion of the hypertrophied crista supraventricularis. The membranous ventricular septum was intact. The aortic valve was bicuspid and measured only 2.3 cm. in circumference, while the pulmonic valve was 4.5 cm. in circumference. The ascending aorta was hypoplastic; it terminated after dividing into the innominate, left common carotid, and left subclavian arteries. The prosthetic graft between the ascending and descending aorta was patent and, as observed at operation, there was no evidence of collateral circulation to the descending aorta. The coronary arteries were normal. Microscopically, there were severe medial hypertrophy and fibrocellular intimal proliferation of the smaller muscular pulmonary arteries and arterioles (fig. 7C). These pulmonary vascular changes were of grade 3/6 severity (Heath and Edwards).

Discussion

The first pathologic description of complete interruption of the aortic arch was recorded in the late eighteenth century by Raphael Steidele, Professor of Obstetrics of the University of Vienna and a member of the Royal Council for the Emperor of Austria.[4] Since that time there have been reports of 51 other patients with this malformation.[1, 5–40] A summary of the clinical and pathologic findings

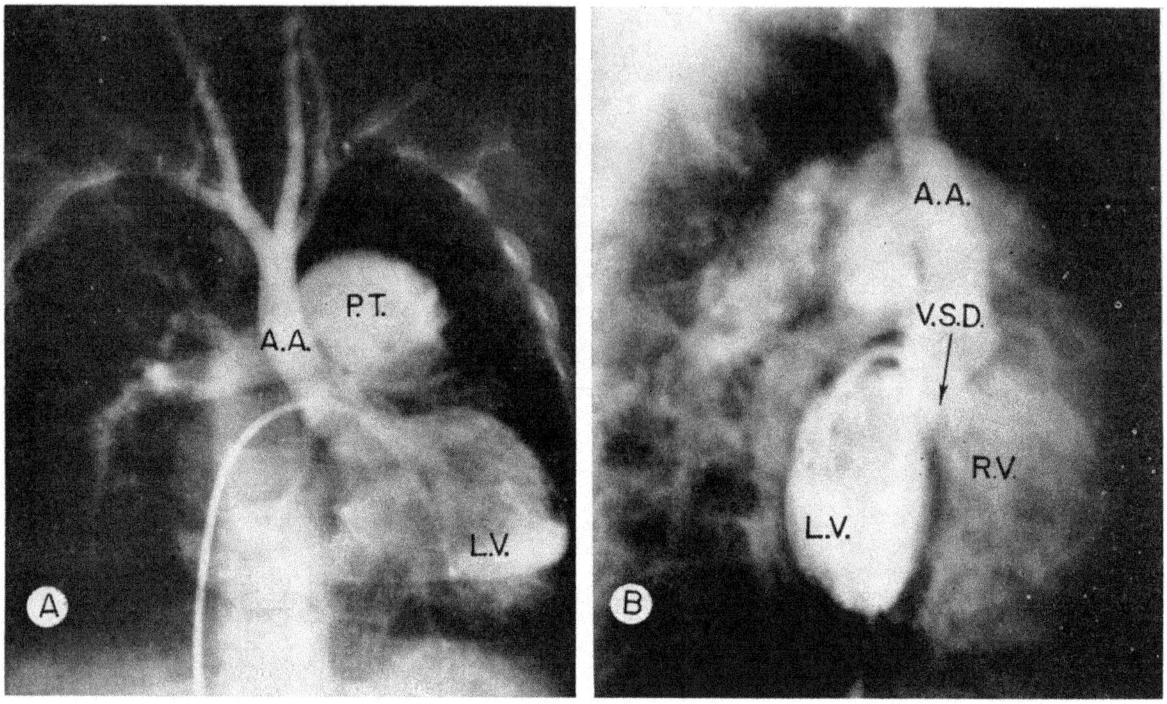

Figure 9

Selective angiocardiogram with left ventricular injection in patient P. S. In the anteroposterior projection (A) *the ascending aorta (A.A.) is seen to terminate with the origin of the left subclavian artery. The pulmonary trunk (P.T.) is opacified also. In the lateral view* (B) *both ventricles are seen as well as the ventricular septal defect through which a large left-to-right shunt occurs.*

in these 52 patients and in the three of the present communication is presented in table 1. The sex was mentioned in 49 of these 55 patients: 23 were male and 26 were female. The age at death was noted in all but one. Forty-one (76 per cent) died in the first month of life or were stillborn, and only six lived for longer than 1 year.

In contrast to coarctation of the aorta, in complete interruption of the aortic arch there is no connection of any kind between the ascending and descending aortas. As an isolated anomaly this malformation is incompatible with life, and the descending aorta always originates from the pulmonary artery through a patent ductus arteriosus. A ventricular septal defect is almost always present as well, having been described in 46 of the 48 patients in which the septum was mentioned. In fact, the association of interruption of the aortic arch, patent ductus arteriosus, and ventricular septal defect is so constant that it has been considered a distinct cardiovascular trilogy by Everts-Suarez and Carson.[33] As pointed out by Becu et al.[24] and Neufeld et al.,[38] the ventricular septal defect in some, and probably in most of the patients with an interrupted aortic arch has an unusual location. These defects seem not to involve the membranous portion of the ventricular septum but lie anterior to it, above the papillary muscle of the conus, but below the pulmonic valve and a portion of the crista supraventricularis. The pulmonary valve is dilated and overrides the defect. The pulmonary trunk is much larger than the ascending aorta.

Another common associated finding is a bicuspid or deformed aortic valve or a narrowed subaortic outflow tract. Becu et al.[24] and more recently Neufeld et al.[38] have each described two patients with subaortic stenosis and biventricular origin of the pulmonary trunk

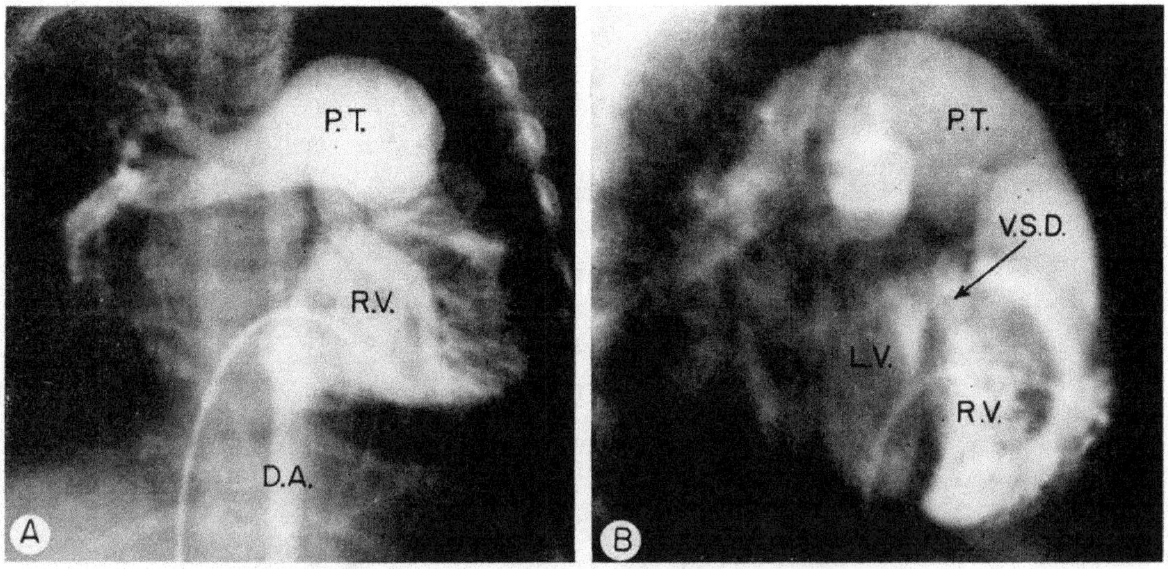

Figure 10

Selective angiocardiogram with right ventricular injection in patient P. S. In the anteroposterior view (A) *the descending aorta (D.A.) is seen to originate from the pulmonary trunk via the patent ductus. In the lateral projection* (B) *the left ventricle (L.V.) is filled from the right (R.V.), indicating right-to-left shunting through the ventricular septal defect (V.S.D.).*

with complete interruption of the aortic arch. The subaortic stenosis was above the ventricular septal defect in each instance. In each of the two patients with two semilunar valves (patients 1 and 3) in the present report, the left ventricular outflow tract above the ventricular septal defect was narrowed by a muscular ridge. In five of the six patients reported by Kleinerman et al.,[29] the aortic valve was bicuspid and in the sixth the valve consisted of one normal and two rudimentary cusps. Two of our patients had bicuspid aortic valves and the third had a bicuspid semilunar valve at the origin of the persistent truncus arteriosus. It seems likely, therefore, that abnormalities of the aortic valve and subaortic stenosis are more frequent than indicated in table 1. Atresia of the mitral valve has also been described in three patients with complete interruption of the aortic arch. The frequent association of obstructive lesions in the left side of the heart with complete interruption of the aortic arch or aortic valvular or subvalvular stenosis or atresia, or mitral stenosis or atresia has prompted Lev[41] and more recently Noonan and Nadas[31] to group these defects under a common term, "the hypoplastic left heart syndrome." There may be justification for this terminology, since in all instances the pulmonary trunk and the right ventricle are disproportionately large. A variety of other intracardiac anomalies has been reported in association with interruption of the aortic arch, and these are listed in table 1.

The site of the interruption of the aortic arch is important from both diagnostic and surgical standpoints. The interruption may occur in one of three sites (fig. 2). In the type A malformation, interruption distal to the left subclavian artery, all branches of the aortic arch are supplied by the left ventricle. The type A anomaly was found in 22 of the 50 patients in whom the site of interruption was precisely stated. In the type B anomaly, interruption immediately distal to the left common carotid artery, the innominate and left carotid arteries are supplied by the left ventricle and the left subclavian artery arises from the "pulmonary-ductus-descend-

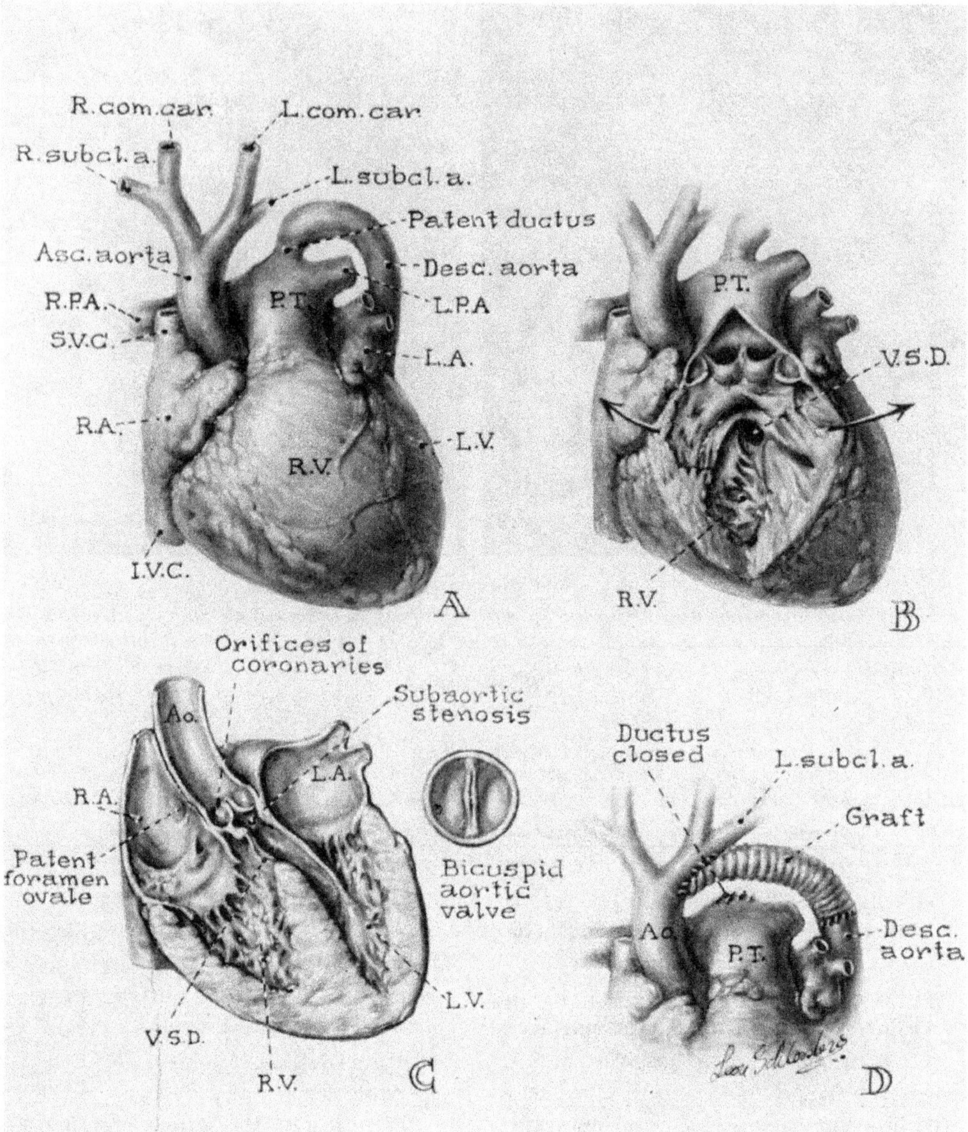

Figure 11

Drawing of heart and great vessels from patient P. S. A. *The ascending aorta terminates after giving rise to the left subclavian artery (type A interruption). The descending aorta arises entirely from the pulmonary trunk (P.T.) via the patent ductus arteriosus. The right ventricle and the pulmonary trunk are markedly dilated and the ascending aorta is relatively hypoplastic.* B. *The right ventricle and pulmonary valve are opened. The ventricular septal defect (V.S.D.) is apparent.* C. *The anterior portion of the heart has been removed. The outflow tract of the left ventricle is compromised by the myocardial ridges immediately below the aortic valve cusps. The root of the aorta overrides the right ventricle. The aortic valve is bicuspid.* D. *The surgical repair is illustrated. The patent ductus is closed, and the ascending aorta is anastomosed to the descending aorta by a graft.*

ing aorta trunk," a term coined by Evans[17] to include the pulmonary trunk, patent ductus arteriosus, and descending thoracic aorta. The type B anomaly occurred in 26 patients. The type C malformation, in which both the left subclavian and left common carotid arteries arise from the pulmonary-ductus-descending aorta trunk, was specifically described in only two patients. Thus in the majority of patients the interruption was distal to the origin of the left common carotid artery. The phrase "absence of the aortic isthmus" has sometimes been applied to these anomalies. Since the isthmus of the aorta is that portion between the left subclavian artery and the ductus arteriosus, this terminology would correctly apply only to the type A interruption and it would seem best to discard it entirely.

In addition to the variation in the site of aortic interruption, there is frequently abnormal origin of the major branches of the ascending aorta and pulmonary trunk. Thus in six patients (table 1) the right subclavian, as well as the left subclavian artery, arose from the pulmonary-ductus-descending aorta trunk (fig. 3A). Bilateral ducti were present in four patients (table 1). In this situation the right subclavian artery arises from the right pulmonary artery via the right ductus (fig. 3B). Kleinerman et al.[29] reported a patient (no. 29, table 1) with complete interruption of the arch and bilateral persistence of the patent ducti who also had a right-sided descending aorta (fig. 3D). The "addendum case" (no. 24, table 1) observed by Becu et al.[24] also had a right-sided descending aorta but in this instance the descending aorta took origin from the right-sided ductus, which in turn arose from the right pulmonary artery. Also rarely, a pulmonary artery arises directly from the ascending aorta (fig. 3C) as in the patient reported by Jew and Gross.[21] Complete transposition of the great vessels has been recorded twice in association with complete interruption of the aortic arch.[18, 35]

Because of the variation in the site of interruption and in the origin of the great vessels, it is not surprising that the diagnosis of aortic arch interruption has rarely been made on the basis of clinical study. Indeed, this malformation was recognized before operation or autopsy in only two[30, 35] of the 52 previously reported patients. In two of the three patients in the present communication, however, the correct diagnosis was established by catheterization and selective angiocardiography.

The symptoms of interruption of the aortic arch are nonspecific and the physical signs are of only limited value. It would seem that differential cyanosis would always be present, but it is apparently the exception rather than the rule. In only 10 of the 38 patients in which the presence or absence of cyanosis was recorded, was differential cyanosis apparent. In seven of these patients cyanosis was evident in the nailbeds of the toes and in the lips. In two patients (nos. 17 and 46, table 1), each of whom also had complete transposition of the great vessels, there was reverse cyanosis, i.e., the nailbeds of the fingers and the lips were cyanotic and the nailbeds of the toes were not. In the tenth patient (no. 26, table 1) there were cyanosis and clubbing of the fingers of the left hand and the toes of both feet, but no cyanosis or clubbing of the fingers of the right hand. This patient, living at the age of 5 years and reported by Dorney et al.,[26] had a type B interruption of the aortic arch. In 10 other patients with various forms of interruption of the aortic arch no cyanosis was evident, and in the remaining 18 it was present but presumably generalized.

The frequent absence of differential cyanosis can, of course, be explained by the presence of a ventricular septal defect, which is invariably present and of large size. Arterialized blood from the left ventricle is shunted through the defect and enters the pulmonary trunk and the lower extremities. As a result, the oxygen saturation of blood in the pulmonary artery, ductus, and descending aorta approaches that in the ascending aorta. Greig,[6] in 1852, clearly appreciated that the left-to-right intracardiac shunt was responsible for the infrequency of differential cyanosis in these patients. In his paper of over 100 years ago he wrote: "The additional

Table 1

Clinical and Pathologic Data from 55 Patients with Complete Interruption of the Aortic Arch Proved at Autopsy or Operation

Patient number	Author year	Sex	Age at death	Heart murmur	Cyanosis D= differential	Location of interruption	Ventricular septal defect	Patent foramen ovale	Associated cardiovascular defects
1	Steidele (1777-1788)		"few hours"			A			
2	Seidel (1818)	M	"infant"			B	+		
3	Greig (1852)		"newborn"			B	+	+	
4	Hicks (1864)	F	3 days		+	A	0	+	
5	Cameron (1871)	M	3 days		+	A or B	+	+	Bicuspid aortic valve
6	Barlow (1876) (Case 1)	M	10 months	0	+	A	+	+	Origin of ascending aorta from R.V.
7	Volbeding (1881) (Case 6)		Stillborn			B	+		Bicuspid aortic valve. Origin of R.S.A. and L.S.A. from "pulmonary-ductus des. aorta trunk"
8	Kohl (1909)	F	"hours"		+	A	+	+ (V.I.)	Aneurysmal dilatation of asc. aorta
9	Dick (1904)		early infancy		+	A			
10	Saltykow (1910)					A	+	+	
11	Letterer (1923)	F	4 days	0		B	+	+	Bicuspid aortic valve
12	Gaspar (1929)	F	6 months	+	+	B	+	+	Aortic valve stenosis
13	Abbott (1932)		15 hours		+	B	+	+	Persistent common atrioventricular canal. Mitral atresia. Bicuspid pulmonic valve
14	Evans (1933) (Case 20)	M	3 days			B	+	+	Origin of both R.S.A. and L.S.A. from "ductus-des. aorta trunk"
15	Evans (1933) (Case 21)	F	11 days			B	+	+	Anomalous drainage of left jugular, axillary, and azygos vein into R.A.
16	Evans (1933) (Case 22)	M	2 days			A	0	+	
17	Hamburger (1937)	M	30 days	+	+(D)*	A	+	+	Complete transposition of great vessels

18	Weisman & Kesten (1948)	M	3 days	0	+	C	+	+ (V.I.)	Bicuspid aortic valve. Origin of L.C.C.A. and L.S.A. from left "ductus-des. aorta trunk"
19	Stewart (1948)	F	2 days	0	+	A	+		
20	Jew & Gross (1952)	M	3 days	+	+	B	+	+	Origin of right P.A. from asc. aorta
21	Kintner (1953)	F	15 hours		+	A	+	0	Mitral atresia, persistent left S.V.C.
22	Barger et al. (1954) Also Becu (Case 3)	F	8 days		+	B	+	+	Biventricular origin of pulmonary trunk. Origin of R.S.A. from right P.A. via right P.D.A. Aneurysm of right aortic sinus. Subaortic stenosis. Bicuspid aortic valve
23	Becu et al. (1955) (Case 2)	F	3 days	+	+	B	+	+	Biventricular origin of pulmonary trunk. Subaortic stenosis-bicuspid aortic valve. Origin of R.S.A. from right P.A. via a right P.D.A.
24	Becu et al. (1955) (Addendum case)	F	14 days			B	+	+	Origin of des. aorta from rt. P.D.A. Origin of R.S.A. from rt. P.A. via rt. P.D.A. Rt. descending aorta. Biventricular origin of pulmonary trunk. Subaortic stenosis.
25	Jew & Gross (1955)	F	3 days	0	+	B	+		Aortic stenosis
26	Dorney et al. (1955)	F	5 years†	+‡	+(D)§	B	? +		
27	Kravtin et al. (1955)	M	11 days	+	+(D)	A	+	0	
28	Merrill et al. (1957)	F	3½ years†	+‡	0	A	? +		
29	Kleinerman et al. (1958)	M	8 days	0	0	B	+	+	Bicuspid aortic valve. Right-sided des. aorta. Origin R.S.A. from right P.A. via right P.D.A.
30	Kleinerman et al. (1958)	M	3 days	+	+(D)	B	+	+	Bicuspid aortic valve
31	Kleinerman et al. (1958)	F	3 days	0	0	B	+	+	Mitral atresia. Bicuspid aortic valve
32	Kleinerman et al. (1958)	M	Stillborn			B	+	+	Cor biloculare. Bicuspid aortic valve
33	Kleinerman et al. (1958)	F	Stillborn			B	+	+	Origin of both R.S.A. and L.S.A. from "ductus-des. aorta trunk." Hypoplastic aortic valve. Quadricusp pulmonic valve

Table 1—Continued

Clinical and Pathologic Data from 55 Patients with Complete Interruption of the Aortic Arch Proved at Autopsy or Operation

Patient number	Author year	Sex	Age at death	Heart murmur	Cyanosis D= differential	Location of interruption	Ventricular septal defect	Patent foramen ovale	Associated cardiovascular defects
34	Kleinerman et al. (1958)	M	2½ hours	0	0	A	+	+ (V.I.)	Bicuspid aortic valve. Single coronary artery
35	Abrams (1958) (Case 7)	F	10 days	+	+	A	+		
36 37 38 39 40 41	Noonan & Nadas (1958)	F=5 M=1	Five lived for less than 20 days. One lived 3½ months	3	+(D)=1	A=2 B or C=4	5		Endocardial fibroelastosis=1
42	Foley (1958)	M	6 days	0	0	A	+	+	"Congenital cyst," tricuspid valve
43	Evarts-Suärez & Carson (1959)	M	3 days	0	0	B	+		
44	Celoria & Patton (1959)	M	12 days	+	0	C	+	+	Origin of L.C.C.A. and L.S.A. from "ductus-des. aorta trunk"
45	Quie et al. (1959) (Case 1)	M	5½ months‖	+	0	B	+		Bicuspid aortic valve
46	Castellanos et al. (1959)‡‡	M	9 years	0	+(D)	A	+††	+ (V.I.)	Complete transposition of the great vessels. Persistent left S.V.C. draining into coronary sinus
47	Fournier & Zaidi (1960)	F	2 months	+	0	A	+	0	"Coarcted" P.D.A., Bicuspid aortic valve
48	Tabakin & Hanson (1960)	F	3 months	+	0	B	+		Persistent left S.V.C. draining directly into R.A. Origin of both R.S.A. and L.S.A. from "ductus-des. aorta trunk"
49	Neufeld et al. (1961) (Case 2)	M	3 days	0	+	B	+		Subaortic stenosis. Biventricular origin of pulmonary trunk. Origin of both R.S.A. and L.S.A. from "ductus-des. aorta trunk"
50	Neufeld et al. (1961)** (Case 3)	F	3 days	+‡	+(D)	B	+		Subaortic stenosis. Biventricular origin of pulmonary trunk. Origin of both R.S.A. and L.S.A. from "ductus-des. aorta trunk"
51	Freedman (1961)	F	2 months	+	+	B	+	+	Probable subaortic or aortic valvular stenosis

52	Ruiz Villalobos et al. (1961)	M	14 years†	+	+(D)	A	? +		
53	Present Authors L.N.	M	25 months	+	+(D)	B	+	0	Bicuspid aortic valve. Subaortic stenosis. Biventricular origin of pulmonary trunk
54	Present Authors R.S.‡‡	M	18 days	+‡	+	A	+	+	Persistent truncus arteriosus. Bicuspid semilunar valve
55	Present Authors P.S.‡‡	F	3 years‖	+‡	+(D)	A	+	+ (V.I.)	Bicuspid aortic valve. Subaortic stenosis. Biventricular origin of pulmonary trunk

*Reverse cyanosis.
†Still living—diagnosis made at thoracotomy.
‡Diastolic murmur in addition to systolic murmur.
§Cyanosis of left hand, both feet; no cyanosis of right hand.
‖Died in early postoperative period following ligation of P.D.A. and anastomotic procedure.
**Cases 49 and 50 are siblings.
††Functionally insignificant V.S.D., but anatomically open.
‡‡Diagnoses made ante mortem (selective angiocardiography).
Abbreviations: V.I.=Valvular incompetent foramen ovale; R.S.A.=Right subclavian artery; L.S.A.=Left subclavian artery; P.A.=Pulmonary artery; P.D.A.=Patent ductus arteriosus; R.A.=Right atrium; L.C.C.A.=Left common carotid artery; S.V.C.=Superior vena cava.

complication, however, of such a large aperture between the ventricles, must have established complete admixture of the blood of the two sides of the heart, before it was sent into the aorta and pulmonary artery, so that, independent of subsequent abnormalities of the vessels, all parts of the body would be supplied with blood of the same quality." There also may, at times, be right-to-left shunting across the ventricular defect, as illustrated by the findings in patient 3 (P. S.), in whom blood from the right ventricular outflow tract had an oxygen content identical to that sampled from the left ventricle. The right-to-left shunt also was demonstrated in the right ventricular selective angiocardiogram. This child, however, was 3 years old, and had severe pulmonary vascular disease, an infrequent finding in younger children.

Although blood in the pulmonary trunk has a higher oxygen content than systemic venous blood, it is unusual, contrary to the examples presented, for the blood in the descending aorta to have an oxygen content equal to that in the ascending aorta. In all four of the previously reported patients with interruption of the aortic arch in whom brachial and femoral arterial blood was sampled, distinct differences in oxygen content were found. Differential cyanosis was clinically apparent, however, in only two of them and no cyanosis was evident in the other two. In summary, differential cyanosis, when present, is an important aid in the diagnosis of interruption of the aortic arch but in the majority of patients with the malformation it will not be apparent on physical examination.

Another sign that might be logically expected in these patients is absence or marked diminution of the femoral pulsations. This is rarely the case, however, because the pressure in the pulmonary trunk and descending aorta is usually similar to that in the ascending aorta. For the same reason, relative hypertension in the arms is infrequent. Patient R. S., however, had absent femoral pulses. In him, this resulted from extreme narrowing or "coarctation" of the patent ductus, the only vessel supplying the descending aorta. In patient 46, table 1, closure of the patent ductus resulting in disappearance of the femoral pulses, was documented by catheterizations and at autopsy. In patient 52, table 1, there was hypertension (220/120 mm. Hg) in the arms, but the blood pressure in the legs was normal. This patient, reported by Ruiz Villalobos et al.,[40] survived operation at the age of 14 years and was doing well 7 months later. Differences in the force of the radial and carotid pulsations, might likewise be expected in type B and C malformations, but this finding has been recorded in only one patient.[31]

Heart murmurs are probably present in all patients with complete interruption of the aortic arch who live for longer than 1 month. A murmur was present in 22 and absent in 15 of the 37 patients in which this finding was mentioned. All 15 patients who had no murmur died within a few days. The murmur, when present, was systolic in all instances; in addition, however, five patients had diastolic murmurs. The ventricular septal defect is probably the source of the systolic murmur, although the aortic valvular or subvalvular stenosis, if present, would contribute. One would not expect a murmur to result from blood flowing through the ductus, since no pressure differential exists between the pulmonary trunk and the descending aorta. A diastolic murmur can be best attributed to pulmonic regurgitation, secondary to pulmonary hypertension. One patient (no. 28, table 1) had a continuous murmur in the left infraclavicular region.[28] Collateral vessels were present in this patient between the ascending and descending aortas. Only one other patient (no. 52, table 1), was described with a definite collateral circulation.

The electrocardiogram in these patients usually shows right axis deviation and right ventricular hypertrophy. Biventricular hypertrophy has been noted occasionally. Right ventricular strain and incomplete right bundle-branch block also have been recorded.

Cardiac catheterization was performed in five patients with interruption of the aortic arch previously reported,[26, 28, 35, 37, 40] and in each of the three described herein. All eight had pulmonary arterial and right ventricular hypertension, the peak pulmonary arterial systolic pressure ranging from 50 to 132 mm. Hg and, in general, equal to peripheral arterial systolic pressure. In each, a left-to-right or bidirectional shunt at the ventricular level was found. It is apparent that these catheterization data are not diagnostic, and selective angiocardiography affords the only means by which the definitive diagnosis of complete interruption of the aortic arch can be made. Abrams,[30] using this method, was the first to diagnose the malformation before operation or autopsy. Selective angiocardiography proved to be the definitive study in Castellanos' patient[35] and in two of the present ones. In patient P. S. (case 3) both right and left ventricular injections were performed (fig. 9) and the nature of the lesion was apparent in both series of films. By selective angiography, one cannot distinguish complete interruption of the aorta from atresia of the aorta in which there is an anatomic connection by a fibrous band between the ascending and descending aortas. This distinction is of little practical consequence, however, since the method of surgical correction for each is similar.

Complete interruption of the arch of the aorta is potentially amenable to surgical correction. The principal limiting factor, to date, appears to be the early recognition of the lesion, since a majority of the patients die before the age of 1 month. In only two patients has a successful repair been reported. Merrill et al.[28] corrected the anomaly of the aortic arch in a patient with a type A interruption. He divided the patent ductus and anastomosed the descending aorta directly to the base of the left subclavian artery in an end-to-side fashion. Recently, Ruiz Villalobos et al.[40] reported the successful closure of the ductus, with anastomosis of the descending aorta to the left subclavian artery by means of a prosthesis, in a 14-year-old boy with a type A interruption. As noted previously, each of these patients was unique in that extensive collateral circulation was present and the descending aorta could be occluded during the repair. Quie et al.[34] reported correction of a type B interruption, but the patient died in the early postoperative period. The ductus, the left subclavian, and the left common carotid arteries were divided, and the left common carotid artery was anastomosed to the descending aorta. In patient P. S. a procedure similar to that employed by Ruiz Villalobos was performed. The absence of collateral vessels, however, necessitated restoration of the continuity of the aorta, by means of a prosthetic graft, before the ductus could be divided. Blake, Manion, and Spencer[42] have reported a successful operation of this type in a child with atresia of the aortic isthmus.

The correction of the rare type C interruption, which has apparently not been attempted, probably would involve division of both the left subclavian and left common carotid arteries and an anastomosis of the descending aorta to the base of the right common carotid artery. It would, of course, be necessary to provide distal perfusion to the left carotid until flow to it from the aorta could be restored.

Restoration of continuity of the aorta is obviously only a first step in the treatment of a patient with interruption of the aortic arch, since a ventricular septal defect remains. All these patients have pulmonary hypertension, and the state of the pulmonary vascular bed, as determined at subsequent study, would indicate whether closure of the defect or palliative constriction of the pulmonary artery would be desirable.

Summary

The clinical, hemodynamic, angiographic, and pathologic findings in three patients with complete interruption of the aortic arch are presented. In addition, data derived from published reports of 52 previous patients are summarized. This malformation is never an isolated one, since a patent ductus arteriosus is always present and a ventricular septal defect is almost invariably found as well. The diagnosis of absence of the aortic arch is difficult, since differential cyanosis is uncommon, relative systolic hypertension of the arms is rare, and the heart murmur, when present, is of a nonspecific nature. At catheterization the pressure in the pulmonary artery, patent ductus arteriosus, and descending aorta is usually similar to that in the ascending aorta and in its branches. Selective angiocardiography has been shown to be the only means of establishing the presence of the malformation prior to operation or autopsy. Since the majority of patients with absence of the aortic arch die within the month following birth, early recognition of the lesion is imperative if surgical correction is to be of benefit.

Addendum

Since this paper was prepared, two additional patients with complete interruption of the aortic arch have been called to our attention. One, a stillborn, reported by Sir William Osler in 1880 (case 4)[43] had a type B interruption and associated ventricular and atrial septal defects, bicuspid aortic and malformed pulmonic valves. Another patient, a 3-year-old girl, reported by Espino-Vela et al.,[44] also had a type B interruption and an associated ventricular septal defect. Shortly after this manuscript was submitted for publication, Newcombe et al.[45] reviewed the surgical and pathologic experiences of the Mayo Clinic in patients with "coarctation" of the aorta, ventricular septal defect, and usually patent ductus arteriosus. The authors used the term "coarctation" in a general sense to include aortic arch interruption as well as aortic narrowing or atresia. The authors mentioned seven examples of aortic arch "coarctation" associated with a distal patent ductus arteriosus, subaortic stenosis, bicuspid aortic valve, and ventricular septal defect. The "coarctation" in at least one of these seven was of the complete interruption form and appears to have already been reported (case 22, tabe 1). In addition, they mentioned a patient with a type B aortic arch interruption who had a persistent truncus arteriosus.

References

1. Celoria, G. C., and Patton, R. B.: Congenital absence of the aortic arch. Am. Heart J. **58**: 407, 1959.
2. Wagenvoort, C. A., Neufeld, H. N., Birge, R. F., Caffrey, J. A., and Edwards, J. E.: Origin of right pulmonary artery from ascending aorta. Circulation **23**: 84, 1961.
3. Heath, D., and Edwards, J. E.: The pathology of hypertensive pulmonary vascular disease,

a description of six grades of structural changes in the pulmonary arteries with special reference to congenital cardiac septal defects. Circulation **18:** 533, 1958.

4. STEIDELE, R. J.: Sammlg. Verschiedener in der chirurg. 'prakt. Lehrschule Gemachten Beobb. Vol. 2, p. 114-116, 1777-88.
5. SEIDEL, J. F.: Index Muse: anatomici Kiliensis, quem praefatus est illustris D. (Joannes Leonardus) Fischer, XIV, 80 pp., Kiliae, C. F. Mohr, 1818.
6. GREIG, D.: Case of malformation of the heart and blood vessels of the fetus: Pulmonary artery giving off descending aorta and left subclavian. Monthly J. M. Soc. Bd. **15:** 28, 1852.
7. HICKS, J. W.: Malformation of aorta and pulmonary artery. Path. Soc. London Transactions **15:** 85, 1864.
8. CAMERON, A. H. F.: Notice of a case of peculiar malformation of the heart and great arteries. J. anat. et physiol. **5:** 339, 1870-71.
9. BARLOW, T.: Congenital heart disease; two cases. Path. Soc. London Transactions **27:** 140, 1876.
10. VOLBEDING, A.: Klinische und pathologisch-anatomische Beiträge zu den tötalen Erkrankungen des Herzens. Inaugural-Dissertation zur Erlangung der Doctorwürde in der Medicin und Chirurgie der vereinigten Friedrichs-Unnersität Halle-Wiltenberg, 1881, p. 155.
11. KOHL: Zentralbl. f. Patholog. **20:** 69, 1909.
12. DICK: Proc. Clin. Path. Society, May 4, 1904. Quoted by Abbott.[1]
13. SALTYKOW (quoted by Herxheimer, G.: Die Morphologen der Missbildungen des Menschen und der Tiere. Hand und Lehrbuch für Morphologen Physiologen Praktische Aertze und Studierende, ed. by Schwalbe. Jena, G. Fisher, 1910, Part 3, No. 3, Section 2, Chapt. 4, p. 461.)
14. LETTERER, E.: Kongenitaler Defekt des Aortenbogens. Zentralbl. f. allg. Path. u. Path. Anat. **33:** 155, 1923.
15. GASPAR, I.: Two of the rarer congenital anomalies of the heart. Am. J. Path. **5:** 285, 1929.
16. ABBOTT, M. E.: Atlas of Congenital Cardiac Disease. New York, The American Heart Association, 1936, p. 50.
17. EVANS, W.: Congenital stenosis (coarctation), atresia, and interruption of the aortic arch (a study of 28 cases). Quart. J. Med. (New Series) **2:** 1, 1933.
18. HAMBURGER, L. P.: Congenital cardiac malformation with complete interruption of isthmus aortae and transposition of great arteries. Bull. Johns Hopkins Hosp. **61:** 421, 1937.
19. WEISMAN, D., KESTEN, H. D., AND PLAINS, W.: Absence of transverse aortic arch with defects of cardiac septums. Am. J. Dis. Child. **76:** 326, 1948.
20. STEWART, M.: Congenital interruption of the aortic arch. Dis. Childhood **23:** 63, 1948.
21. JEW, E. W., JR., AND GROSS, P.: Aortic origin of the right pulmonary artery and absence of the transverse aortic arch associated with patency of interventricular septum and ductus arteriosus. Arch. Path. **53:** 191, 1952.
22. KINTNER, E. P.: Congenital malformation of the heart: Interruption of aortic arch, mitral valve orifice atresia, and persistent left superior vena cava. Lab. Invest. **2:** 388, 1953.
23. BARGER, J. D., CREASMAN, R. W., AND EDWARDS, J. E.: Bilateral ductus arteriosus associated with interruption of the aortic arch. Am. J. Clin. Path. **24:** 441, 1954.
24. BECU, L. M., TAUXE, W. N., DUSHANE, J. W., AND EDWARDS, J. E.: A complex of congenital cardiac anomalies: Ventricular septal defect, biventricular origin of the pulmonary trunk, and subaortic stenosis. Am. Heart J. **50:** 901, 1955.
25. JEW, E. W., JR., AND GROSS, P.: Absence of transverse arch of aorta associated with patency of the interventricular septum and the ductus arteriosus. Lab. Invest. **4:** 304, 1955.
26. DORNEY, E. R., FOWLER, N. O., AND MANNIX, E. P.: Unilateral clubbing of the fingers due to absence of aortic arch. Am. J. Med. **18:** 150, 1955.
27. KRAVTIN, A., SCHLEY, F., AND MONACO, R.: A case of complete interruption of the isthmus aortae. J. M. A. Georgia **44:** 521, 1955.
28. MERRILL, D. L., WEBSTER, C. A., AND SAMSON, P. C.: Congenital absence of the aortic isthmus. J. Thoracic Surg. **33:** 311, 1957.
29. KLEINERMAN, J., YANG, W., HACKEL, D., AND KAUFMAN, N.: Absence of the transverse aortic arch. Arch. Path. **65:** 490, 1958.
30. ABRAMS, H. L.: Persistence of fetal ductus function after birth. Circulation **18:** 206, 1958.
31. NOONAN, J. A., AND NADAS, A. S.: The hypoplastic left heart syndrome. Pediatric Clin. North America **5:** 1029, 1958.
32. FOLEY, B. V.: Congenital interruption of the aortic arch. Arch. Dis. Childhood **33:** 131, 1958.
33. EVERTS-SUÄREZ, E. A., AND CARSON, C. P.: The triad of congenital absence of aortic arch (isthmus aortae), patent ductus arteriosus and interventricular septal defect—a trilogy. Ann. Surg. **150:** 153, 1959.
34. QUIE, P. G., NOVICK, R., ADAMS, P., JR., ANDERSON, R. C., AND VARCO, R. L.: Congenital

interruption of the aortic arch. J. Pediat. **54**: 87, 1959.

35. Castellanos, A., Garcia, O., and Gonzalez, E.: Complete interruption of the aortic arch with transposition of the great vessels. (Report of a case diagnosed in-vivo.) Cardiologia **34**: 53, 1959.
36. Fournier, P., and Zaidi, Z. H.: Congenital absence of the aortic arch. Am. Heart J. **59**: 148, 1960.
37. Tabakin, B. S., and Hanson, J. S.: Congenital absence of the aortic arch associated with patent ductus arteriosus and ventricular septal defect. Am. J. Cardiol. **6**: 689, 1960.
38. Neufeld, H. N., Ongley, P. A., Swan, H. J. C., Burgert, E. O., Jr., and Edwards, J. E.: Biventricular origin of the pulmonary trunk with subaortic stenosis above the ventricular septal defect. Am. Heart J. **61**: 189, 1961.
39. Freedman, H. K.: Congenital absence of the aortic arch. Arch. Path. **72**: 143, 1961.
40. Ruiz Villalobos, M. C., DeBalderrama, D. P., Lopez, J. L. Y., and Castellanos, M.: Complete interruption of the aorta. Am. J. Cardiol. **8**: 664, 1961.
41. Lev, M.: Pathologic anatomy and interrelationship of hypoplasia of the aortic tract complexes. Lab. Invest. **1**: 61, 1952.
42. Blake, H., Manion, W. C., and Spencer, F. C.: Atresia or absence of the aortic isthmus. J. Thoracic and Cardiovasc. Surg. In press.
43. Osler, W.: Cases of cardiac abnormalities. Montreal Gen. Hosp. Rep., Clin. & Path. **1**: 177, 1880.
44. Espino-Vela, J., Acosta, A. R., and De la Cruz, M. V.: Interrupcion del istmo de la aorta: Estudio clinico y analisis embriologico. Arch. Inst. cardiol. México **19**: 53, 1959.
45. Newcombe, C. P., Ongley, P. A., Edwards, J. E., and Wood, E. H.: Clinical, pathologic, and hemodynamic considerations in coarctation of the aorta associated with ventricular septal defect. Circulation **24**: 1356, 1961.

Harvey's monumental discovery was given to the world in 1628 but was very slow in winning adherents, particularly in England. Sydenham himself does not once refer to Harvey, although their lives overlapped, and they lived in the same city for a number of years. This attitude of Sydenham is at first sight difficult to understand, but certain facts help us to solve the riddle. Sydenham had no patience with theories and saw little in the speculations founded on the new physiology but carried to an excess not contemplated by Harvey.—David Riesman, M.D., *Thomas Sydenham, Clinician.* New York, Paul B. Hoeber, Inc., 1926, p. 16.

The Cardiac Disease Associated with the Carcinoid Syndrome (Carcinoid Heart Disease)*

WILLIAM C. ROBERTS, M.D. *and* ALBERT SJOERDSMA, M.D., PH.D.
Bethesda, Maryland

In the early 1930's three patients were described who had metastasizing carcinoid tumors and, in addition, fibrous thickening of the valves on the right side of the heart and reddish discoloration of the skin [*1–4*]. Similar reports followed [*5–8*], and by 1954 three groups independently had recognized what is now referred to as the malignant carcinoid syndrome [*9–11*]. Recently, the clinical and biochemical aspects of this disorder have been emphasized; however, little attention has been given to the morphology of the associated cardiac disease.

The chief purpose of this communication is to describe the pathologic condition of the heart in carcinoid syndrome based on clinical and pathologic studies of seventeen patients with metastatic carcinoid tumors. The present experience and that previously recorded will be discussed in terms of morphology and pathogenesis of the cardiac lesions and clinical features of the patients studied.

PATIENTS STUDIED

Clinical and pathologic features in the seventeen patients are summarized in Table I (nine patients with carcinoid heart disease) and Table II (eight patients without carcinoid heart disease). The nine patients with carcinoid heart disease are described in detail in the appendix. Of the various features listed in the tables, only the presence of a cardiac murmur suggestive of pulmonic stenosis or tricuspid regurgitation served to separate the two groups during life. The cardiac silhouette as seen on chest roentgenogram was of no diagnostic importance. Pathologically, there was no distinguishing feature between the two groups other than the presence of cardiac lesions *per se*. The types of cardiovascular lesions seen in the nine patients with carcinoid heart disease are illustrated in Figures 1 through 11.

SUMMARY OF PATHOLOGIC FINDINGS IN PATIENTS WITH CARCINOID HEART DISEASE

The Carcinoid Tumor. In all nine patients the site of the primary tumor was the small intestine, the ileum in seven and the jejunum in two. Hepatic metastases occurred in all nine patients, and in six the liver weighed more than 1,800 gm. In some patients the hepatic parenchyma was largely replaced by carcinoid implants. The hepatic tissue not involved by tumor showed centrolobular congestion in all but one patient, three to a severe degree, and in seven there was an increase in periportal fibrous tissue which usually contained some chronic inflammatory cells. In five of the nine patients there was fatty change in the liver. Metastases to organs other than the liver occurred in eight of the nine patients. In the one patient without extrahepatic metastases there was recurrence of tumor at the site of intestinal anastomosis (ileum) and at the site of appendectomy. Thus, in all nine patients there was extraportal as well as portal venous drainage of tumor tissue. The regional lymph nodes were involved in all eight patients with extrahepatic metastases. Bone metastases, which occurred in five, were the next most frequent. Metastases to the heart, pancreas and spleen occurred in each of three patients, and metastases to the ovary

* From the Pathologic Anatomy Department, Clinical Center, and Experimental Therapeutics Branch, National Heart Institute, National Institutes of Health, Bethesda, Maryland. Manuscript received December 21, 1962.

Table I

Clinical and Pathologic Data in Nine Patients with Malignant Carcinoid Tumors and Carcinoid Heart Disease

Case No.	Age (yr.) Sex and Race	Length of Illness from Onset of Symptoms (yr.)	Initial Sign and/or Symptom	Diarrhea	Flushing	Bronchoconstriction "Asthma"	Heart Murmur(s)*	Electrocardiogram	Urinary 5-HIAA Excretion† (mg./24 hr.)	Immediate Cause of Death	Site of Primary Tumor	Liver Size (gm.)	Liver Metastases	Other Metastases	Heart Size (gm.)	Location of Carcinoid Fibrous Plaques	Foramen Ovale	Spleen Size (gm.)
I	41,M,W	3	Weight loss, diarrhea	+	+	0	+	Normal	500–700	Hepatic failure	Ileum	7,400	+	Lymph node (regional), lung, pancreas, thyroid gland, bone, heart, pericardium	220	Right atrium, tricuspid valve, pulmonic valve	Closed	120
II	50,F,W	12	Flushing	+	+	+	+	"Metabolic derangement"	1,209–1,270	Hepatic failure	Ileum	4,500	+	Lymph node (regional, supraclavicular, mediastinal), lung, bone, heart, spleen, kidney, ovary, pituitary, adrenal glands	250	Right atrium, coronary sinus, tricuspid valve, right ventricle, pulmonic valve	Closed	100
III	67,M,W	7	Diarrhea, abdominal pain	+	+	+	+	Normal	. . .	Arrhythmia (?)	Ileum	2,500	+	Lymph node (regional, retroperitoneal), appendix	280	Right atrium, tricuspid valve, right ventricle, pulmonic valve	Closed	110
IV	59,M,W	6	Diarrhea	+	+	+	+	Low voltage, right axis deviation	380–580	Congestive heart failure, arrhythmia	Ileum	1,800	+	Recurrence at ileoileal anastomosis and at appendiceal scar	350	Superior vena cava, inferior vena cava, right atrium, tricuspid valve, right ventricle, pulmonic valve	Patent	200
V	57,F,W	4	Diarrhea	+	+	+	+	First degree heart block	161–283	Gastrointestinal hemorrhage	Ileum	2,300	+	Lymph node (regional), bone, thyroid, adrenal glands, kidney, gallbladder	270	Superior vena cava, right atrium, tricuspid valve, right ventricle, pulmonic valve	Closed	400
VI	64,M,W	1.5	Diarrhea, flushing, abdominal pain	+	+	0	+	Low voltage	300–400	Hepatic failure, acute renal shutdown, arrhythmia	Jejunum	1,600	+	Lymph node (regional), bone, pancreas	400	Right atrium, tricuspid valve, right ventricle, pulmonic valve, pulmonary trunk, mitral valve, left ventricle	Closed	160
VII	57,F,W	4	Acute intestinal obstruction	+	+	0	+	Low voltage, vertical axis, prominent P waves	187–274	Electrolyte disturbances	Ileum	1,800	+	Lymph node (regional), pancreas, ovary, spleen, heart	210	Superior vena cava, inferior vena cava, innominate vein, coronary sinus, right atrium, tricuspid valve, right ventricle, pulmonic valve, pulmonary trunk, mitral valve, left ventricle, aorta	Closed	120

Table I (*Continued*)

CLINICAL AND PATHOLOGIC DATA IN NINE PATIENTS WITH MALIGNANT CARCINOID TUMORS AND CARCINOID HEART DISEASE

Case No.	Age (yr.) Sex and Race	Length of Illness from Onset of Symptoms (yr.)	Initial Sign and/or Symptom	Diarrhea	Flushing	Bronchoconstriction "Asthma"	Heart Murmur(s)*	Electrocardiogram	Urinary 5-HIAA Excretion† (mg./24 hr.)	Immediate Cause of Death	Site of Primary Tumor	Liver Size (gm.)	Liver Metastases	Other Metastases	Heart Size (gm.)	Location of Carcinoid Fibrous Plaques	Foramen Ovale	Spleen Size (gm.)
VIII	52,F,W	1.5	Diarrhea, flushing, wheezing, abdominal pain	+	+	+	+	Low voltage	180–220	Hepatic failure	Jejunum	2,800	+	Lymph node (regional), ovary, bone (vertebrae), spleen	200	Inferior vena cava, coronary sinus, right atrium, tricuspid valve, right ventricle, pulmonic valve, pulmonary trunk, mitral valve	Closed	130
IX	69,M,W	1	Abdominal pain, weight loss	+	+	+	+	Left axis deviation, left ventricular ischemia, old anterior myocardial infarct	80–120	Arrhythmia (?)	Ileum	2,600	+	Lymph node (regional)	475	Tricuspid valve, pulmonic valve pulmonary trunk	Closed	475

Note: + = present; 0 = absent.
* Murmur of tricuspid and/or pulmonic valvular disease. † Normal urinary 5-hydroxyindoleacetic acid excretion, 2 to 9 mg. per twenty-four hours.

occurred in three of the four women. Metastases to the kidney, lung, adrenal glands and thyroid glands occurred in each of two patients. There was no apparent correlation between the urinary excretion of 5-hydroxyindoleacetic acid and the number of carcinoid metastases or the size of the liver. (Table I.) The spleen weighed 200 gm. or less in seven patients and was enlarged in only two.

Distribution of Fibrous Lesions in the Heart and Great Vessels. Fibrous plaques of the carcinoid type were present on both tricuspid and pulmonic valves in all nine patients studied. Generally the involvement of each valve was diffuse and uniform. Occasionally, however, involvement of one valve was more extensive than that of the other. For example, in Case I there was severe diffuse fibrosis of the pulmonic valve and only two or three focal minute fibrous plaques on the tricuspid valve. In Case VIII the reverse was true. The tricuspid valve was diffusely involved whereas the pulmonic valve cusps were delicate and contained only small fibrous plaques. In eight patients the right atrium contained carcinoid plaques and the right ventricle in seven of nine patients. The process was always more extensive in the right atrium. Usually the right ventricular involvement was limited to "white capping" of the papillary muscles or only a rare mural plaque. In only one patient (Case V) was the right ventricular plaquing diffuse. Carcinoid plaques were present in the pulmonary trunk in four patients, and in each instance the involvement was limited to that portion lining the sinus of the pulmonic valve or immediately above it. In no case were the pulmonary arteries or veins involved by carcinoid fibrosis.

The systemic veins in several patients contained fibrous plaques. In each of three patients these plaques were seen on the intima of the superior and inferior vena cavae and coronary sinus and in one on the intima of the innominate vein. In Cases I, II and III the great veins were not available for re-examination.

Involvement of the left side of the heart occurred in three of the nine patients, and in none was there an intracardiac communication. The one patient (Case IV) who did have an intracardiac communication (patent foramen ovale) had no cardiac lesions on the left side. The mitral valve was involved by the fibrous process in three, the left ventricle in two and the aorta in one.

Table II

Clinical and Pathologic Data in Eight Patients with Malignant Carcinoid Tumors without Carcinoid Heart Disease

Case No.	Age (yr.) Sex, and Race	Length of Illness from Onset of Symptoms (yr.)	Initial Sign and/or Symptom	Diarrhea	Flushing	Bronchoconstriction "Asthma"	Cardiac Murmur	Electrocardiogram	Urinary 5-HIAA Excretion (mg./24 hr.)	Immediate Cause of Death	Site of Primary Tumor	Liver Size (gm.)	Liver Metastases	Other Metastases	Heart Size (gm.)	Cardiac Valves and Chambers	Foramen Ovale	Spleen Size (gm.)
X	47,M,W	3	Flushing	+	+	0	0	Normal	90–124	Hepatic failure	Caecum	2,100	+	...	300	Normal	Closed	550
XI	69,M,W	9	Diarrhea	+	+	0	0	Normal	717–854	Hepatic failure	Meckel's diverticulum	3,800	+	Lymph node (regional), lungs, bone, spleen, pituitary gland	270	Normal	Patent	150
XII	75,M,W	1	Diarrhea	+	+	0	+*	Suggestion of old anterior myocardial infarct, left axis deviation	40–60	Gastrointestinal hemorrhage	Ileum	1,700	0	Lymph node (regional), lung, bone, heart	320	Arteriosclerotic heart disease	Closed	300
XIII	74,M,W	1.5	Abdominal swelling	+	+	0	+*	Normal	200–400	Hepatic failure	Uncertain, probably small intestine	2,500	+	Lymph node (abdominal and hilar), lung, bone, kidney, spleen, small and large intestine, heart, pancreas, prostate, parathyroid gland	290	Severe arteriosclerotic heart disease, calcification, focal, mitral and aortic valves	Closed	65
XIV	45,M,W	5	Flushing	+	+	+	0	Normal	487–588	Bronchial obstruction by tumor, bronchopneumonia	Uncertain, probably bronchus	6,100	+	Lymph node (abdominal and thoracic), lungs, bone, kidneys, pancreas, gallbladder, heart, adrenal, thyroid, pituitary gland	450†	Hypertensive cardiovascular disease (left ventricular hypertrophy)	Closed	400
XV	67,M,W	8	Abdominal mass	+	+	0	0	Normal	17–43	Hepatic failure	Ileum	2,100	+	Lymph node (regional), spleen, gallbladder, adrenal, stomach, small and large intestine	300	Arteriosclerotic heart disease	Closed	130
XVI	67,M,W	1	Abdominal pain, weakness	0	+	0	+*	Normal	Markedly positive‡	Renal failure (acute pyelonephritis)	Bronchus	1,650	+	Lung	270	Normal	Closed	270
XVII	40,F,W	4	Flushing, intestinal obstruction	+	+	0	0	Low voltage, left ventricular ischemia(?)	30–60	Atelectasis, miliary tuberculosis	Ileum	3,500	+	Lymph node (adnexal), ovary, jejunum, pancreas, pituitary gland	230	Normal	Closed	200

Note: + = present; 0 = absent.
* Murmur not characteristic of tricuspid insufficiency or pulmonic stenosis.
† Intermittent systemic hypertension.
‡ Screening test for urinary 5-HIAA.

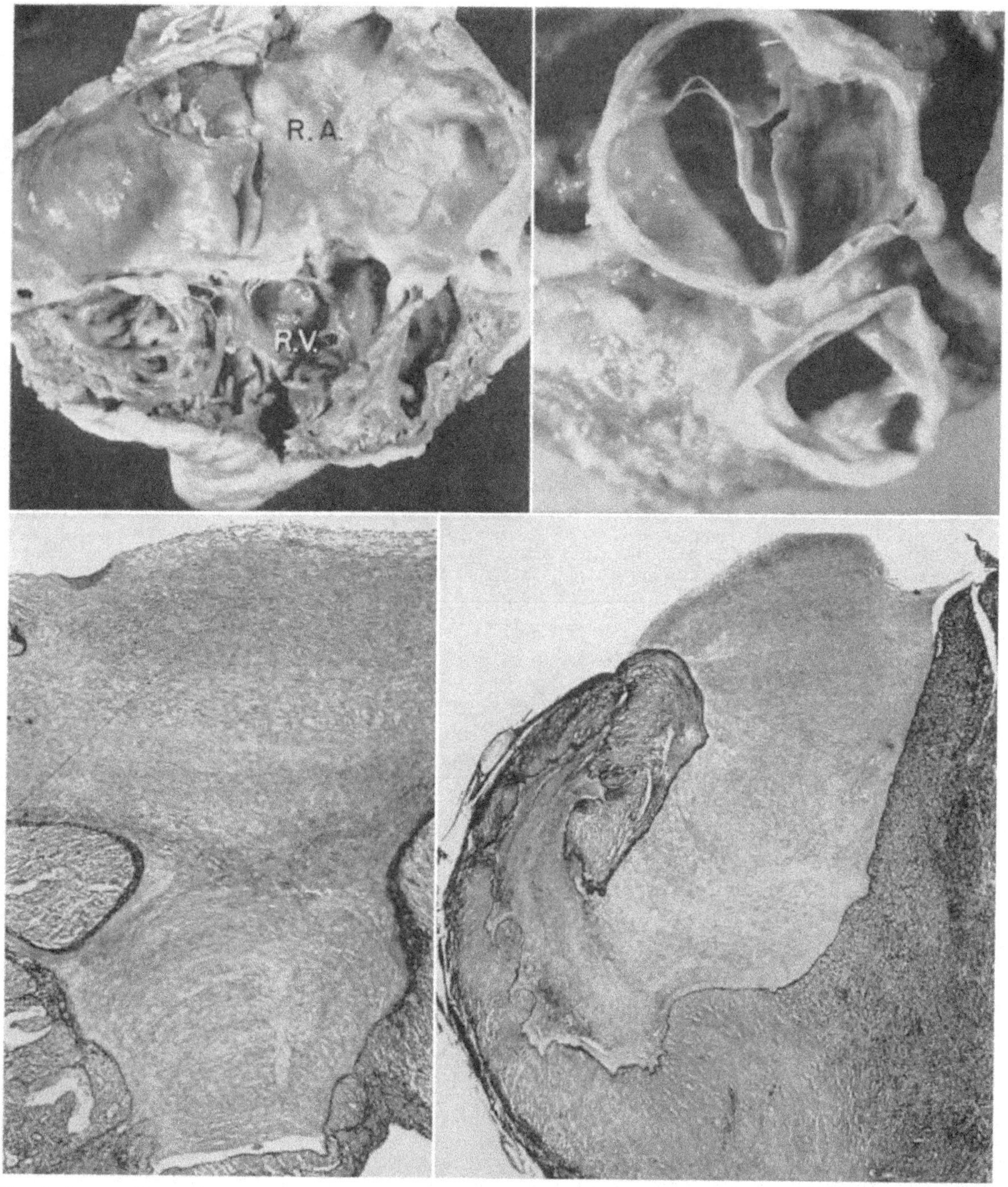

FIG. 1. Case v. *Upper left,* the right atrium (R.A.), tricuspid valve and right ventricle (R.V.) are opened. Each chamber is dilated, but neither is hypertrophied. Diffuse fibrous plaquing covers the endocardium of each chamber. The tricuspid valvular leaflets and chordae are shortened and thickened. *Upper right,* the pulmonic (smaller) and aortic valves (larger) from above. The pulmonic valve cusps are thickened, its commissures mildly interadherent and its opening fixed. The aortic valve cusps, in contrast, are delicate. Normally, in the adult, the aortic valve "ring" is larger than the pulmonic one. The reverse is frequently the case in carcinoid heart disease. *Lower left,* photomicrograph of a section of right atrium showing marked deposition of carcinoid fibrous tissue on the endocardium. The superimposed fibrous plaque is much thicker than is the true right atrial wall. Verhoeff-Van Gieson elastic tissue stain, original magnification × 43. *Lower right,* photomicrograph of a section of pulmonic valve. The valvular cusp is clearly demarcated from the superimposed fibrous tissue by the elastic membrane (black). The distal portion of the cusp is folded inward, and the fibrous deposition takes place almost entirely within the sinus of the valve. The fibrous deposit in this instance completely fills the sinus and contacts the pulmonary trunk. Verhoeff-Van Gieson elastic tissue stain, original magnification × 25.

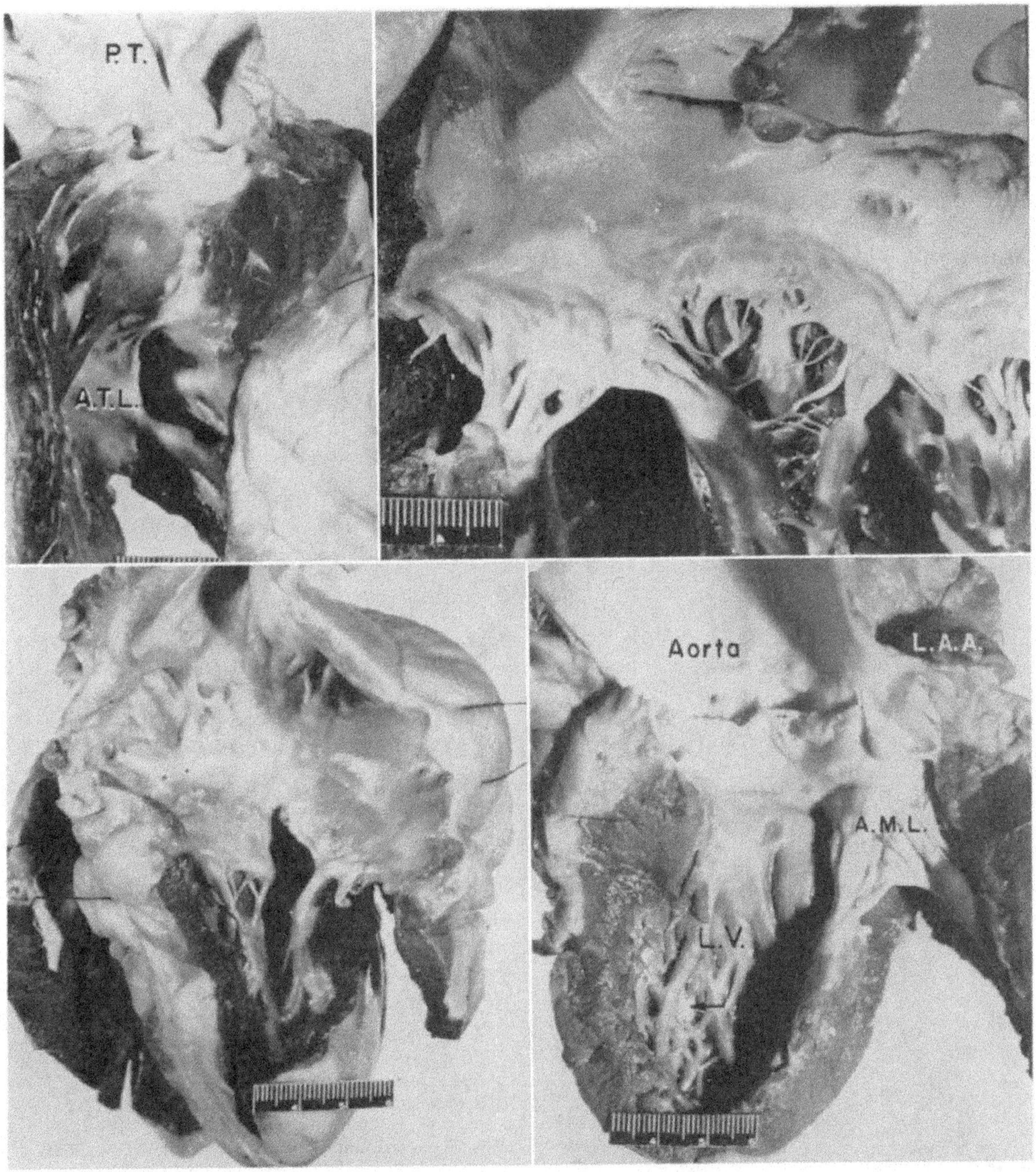

FIG. 2. Case VI. *Upper left,* the pulmonary trunk (P.T.), pulmonic valve and right ventricle are opened. Note the marked contraction of the pulmonic valve. Its cusps are thickened, but the commissures are not fused. The fibrous plaquing of the right ventricle and of the anterior leaflet of the tricuspid valve (A.T.L.) is apparent. *Lower left,* the superior vena cava, right atrium, tricuspid valve and right ventricle are opened. The right atrium is dilated and hypertrophied. Carcinoid plaquing is apparent on the right atrial endocardium, particularly that portion covering the atrial septum. The tricuspid valvular leaflets are shortened, thickened and insert at times directly into the papillary muscles, which also are covered by fibrous plaques ("white capping"). The chordae tendineae are thick and fused. The right ventricle is hypertrophied. *Upper right,* the left atrium, mitral valve and left ventricle are opened. The leaflets and chordae of the mitral valve are thick and white, and there is "white capping" of the papillary muscles. The left atrial endocardium is thicker than normal but free of fibrous plaques. *Lower right,* the ascending aorta, aortic valve and left ventricle (L.V.) are opened. Again note the marked thickening of the anterior mitral leaflet (A.M.L.). The arrow points to a small carcinoid plaque in the left ventricle. A small fibrotic nodule, noncarcinoid in type, is present on the aortic valve. L.A.A. = left atrial appendage.

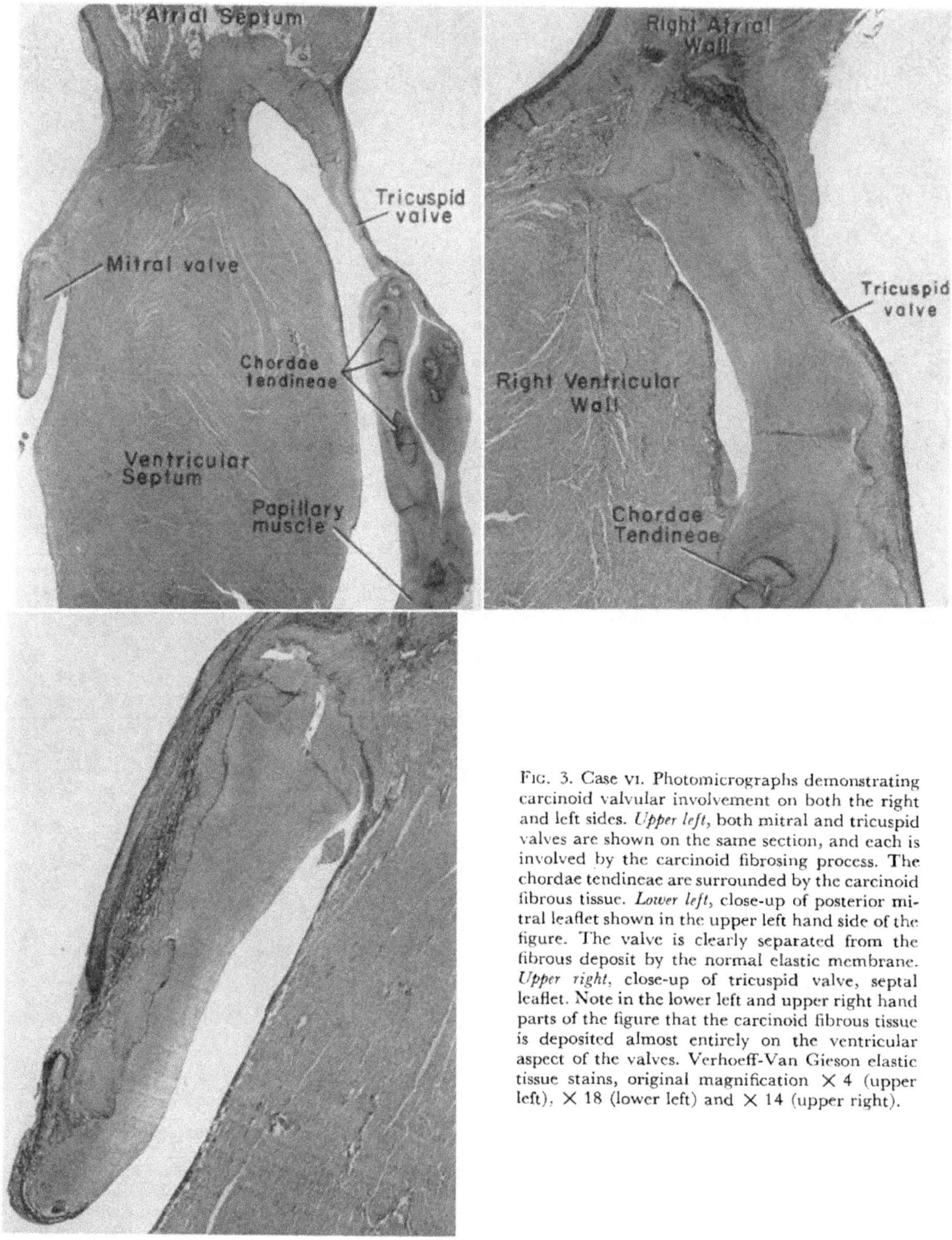

FIG. 3. Case VI. Photomicrographs demonstrating carcinoid valvular involvement on both the right and left sides. *Upper left,* both mitral and tricuspid valves are shown on the same section, and each is involved by the carcinoid fibrosing process. The chordae tendineae are surrounded by the carcinoid fibrous tissue. *Lower left,* close-up of posterior mitral leaflet shown in the upper left hand side of the figure. The valve is clearly separated from the fibrous deposit by the normal elastic membrane. *Upper right,* close-up of tricuspid valve, septal leaflet. Note in the lower left and upper right hand parts of the figure that the carcinoid fibrous tissue is deposited almost entirely on the ventricular aspect of the valves. Verhoeff-Van Gieson elastic tissue stains, original magnification × 4 (upper left), × 18 (lower left) and × 14 (upper right).

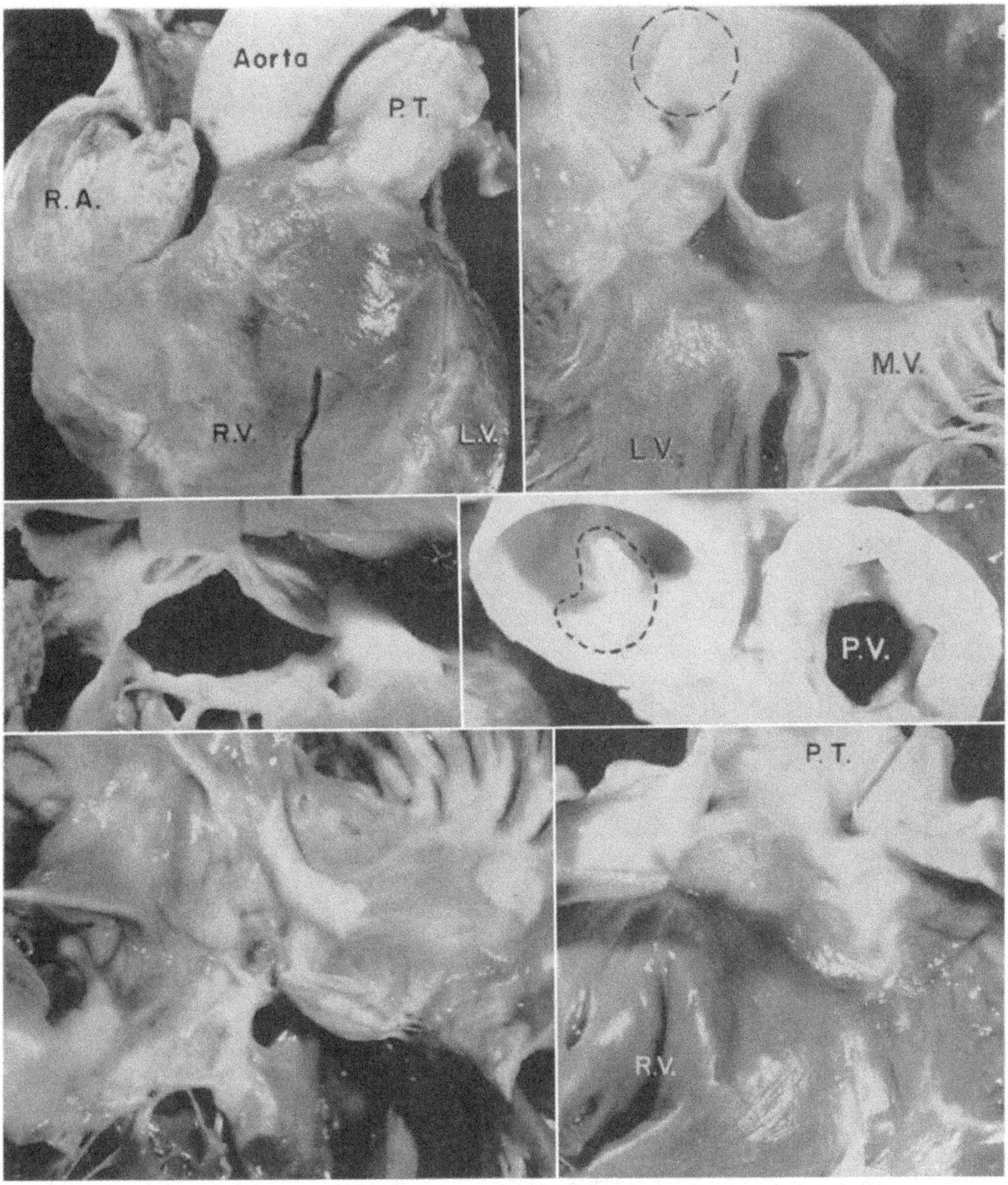

FIG. 4. Case VII. *Upper left*, external view of heart showing dilatation of the right atrium (R.A.) and right ventricle (R.V.) and serous atrophy of the subepicardial adipose tissue. Only a small portion of the left ventricle (L.V.) is visible anteriorly, and the left atrial appendage is almost completely obscured by the pulmonary trunk (P.T.). *Upper right*, the left ventricle (L.V.), aortic valve and ascending aorta are opened. The arrow designates a small carcinoid plaque on the anterior leaflet of the mitral valve (M.V.). The dashed circle encloses another carcinoid plaque in the ascending aorta. *Middle left*, the tricuspid valvular orifice as seen from the right ventricle. The valve orifice is open and consequently regurgitant. *Middle right*, the pulmonic valvular orifice (P.V.) and aorta are seen from above. The pulmonic valvular orifice is fixed and is both stenotic and regurgitant. The carcinoid fibrous plaque in the ascending aorta is again enclosed by the dashed lines. *Lower left*, the right atrium, tricuspid valve and right ventricle. Note the multiple smooth, pearly white fibrous plaques in the right atrium. The tricuspid valvular leaflets and chordae are shortened and thickened. *Lower right*, the pulmonary trunk (P.T.), pulmonic valve and right ventricle (R.V.). The pulmonic valve is diffusely involved by the pearly white fibrosing process.

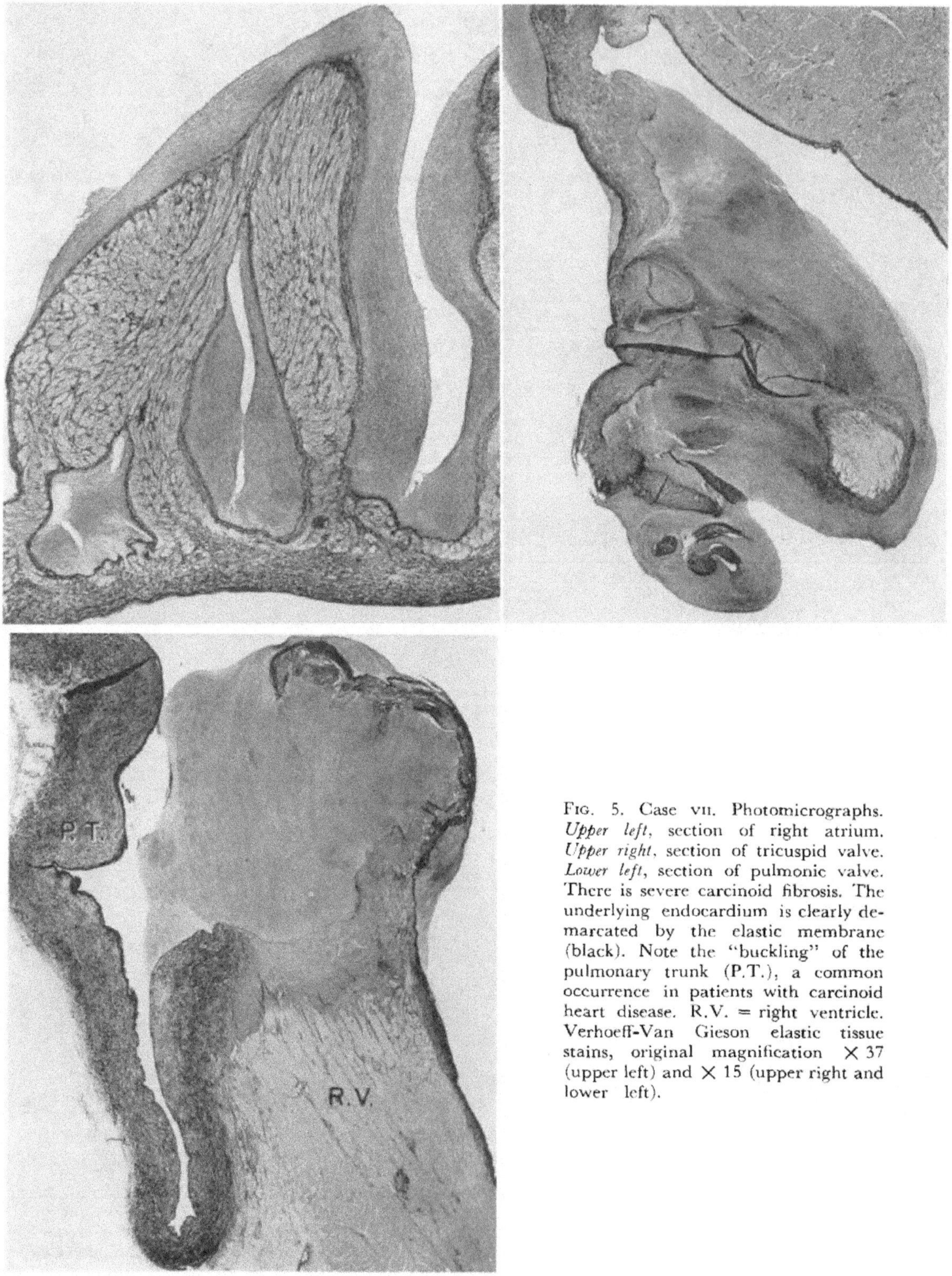

FIG. 5. Case VII. Photomicrographs. *Upper left*, section of right atrium. *Upper right*, section of tricuspid valve. *Lower left*, section of pulmonic valve. There is severe carcinoid fibrosis. The underlying endocardium is clearly demarcated by the elastic membrane (black). Note the "buckling" of the pulmonary trunk (P.T.), a common occurrence in patients with carcinoid heart disease. R.V. = right ventricle. Verhoeff-Van Gieson elastic tissue stains, original magnification × 37 (upper left) and × 15 (upper right and lower left).

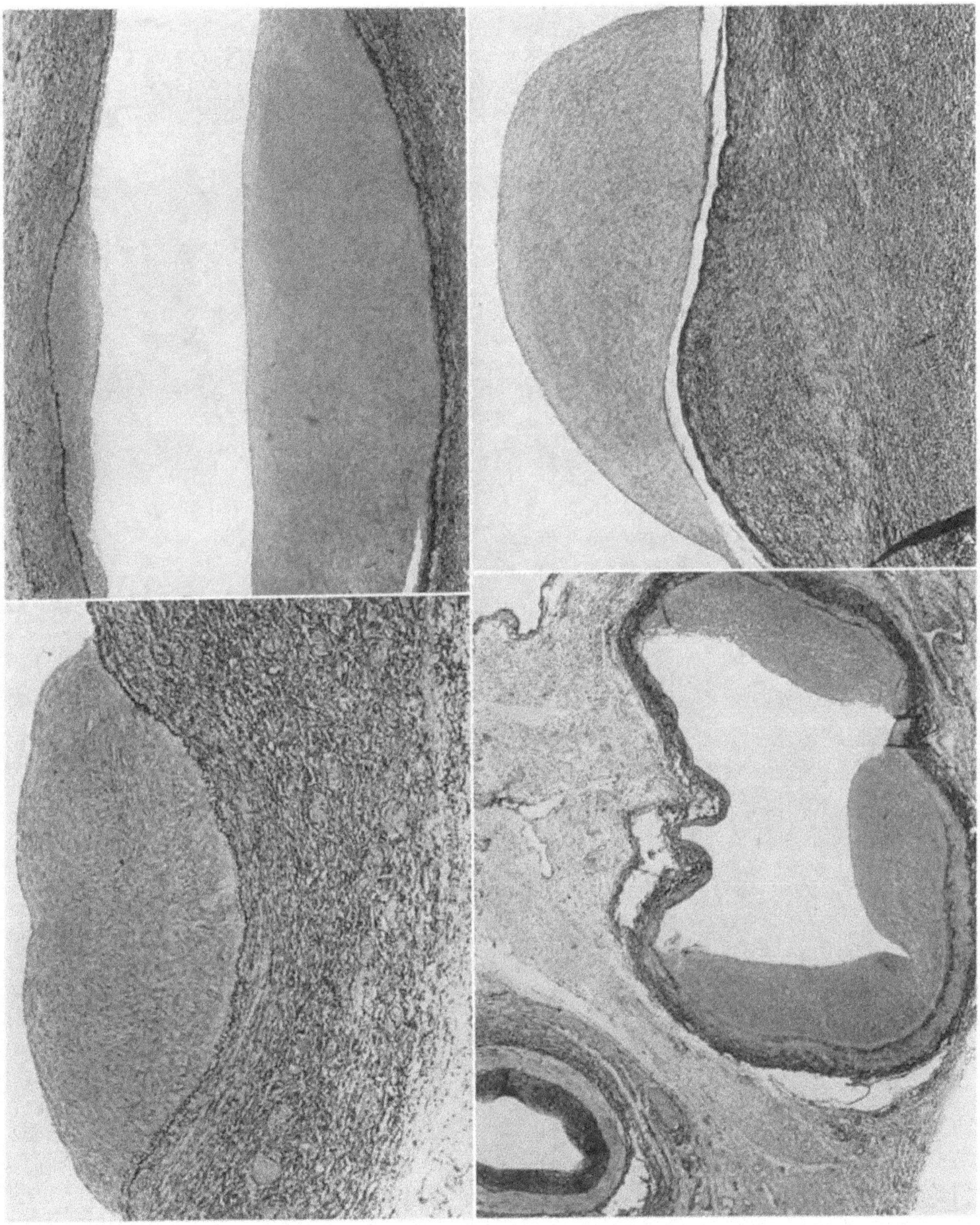

Fig. 6. Case vii. Systemic vessels involved by the carcinoid fibrosing process. *Upper left,* innominate vein. *Lower left,* inferior vena cava. *Upper right,* ascending aorta with a superimposed carcinoid fibrous plaque. The latter became disassociated from the underlying aorta during sectioning. *Lower right,* coronary sinus (large vessel) and coronary artery (small vessel, left lower corner). There is marked carcinoid fibrous plaquing involving the intima of the coronary sinus. The elastic intimal proliferation in the coronary artery, in contrast, is the result of "early" atherosclerosis and bears no resemblance to the process in the coronary sinus which is free of elastic fibrils. Verhoeff-Van Gieson elastic tissue stains; original magnification × 52 (lower left), × 37 (upper left), × 140 (lower right) and × 43 (upper right).

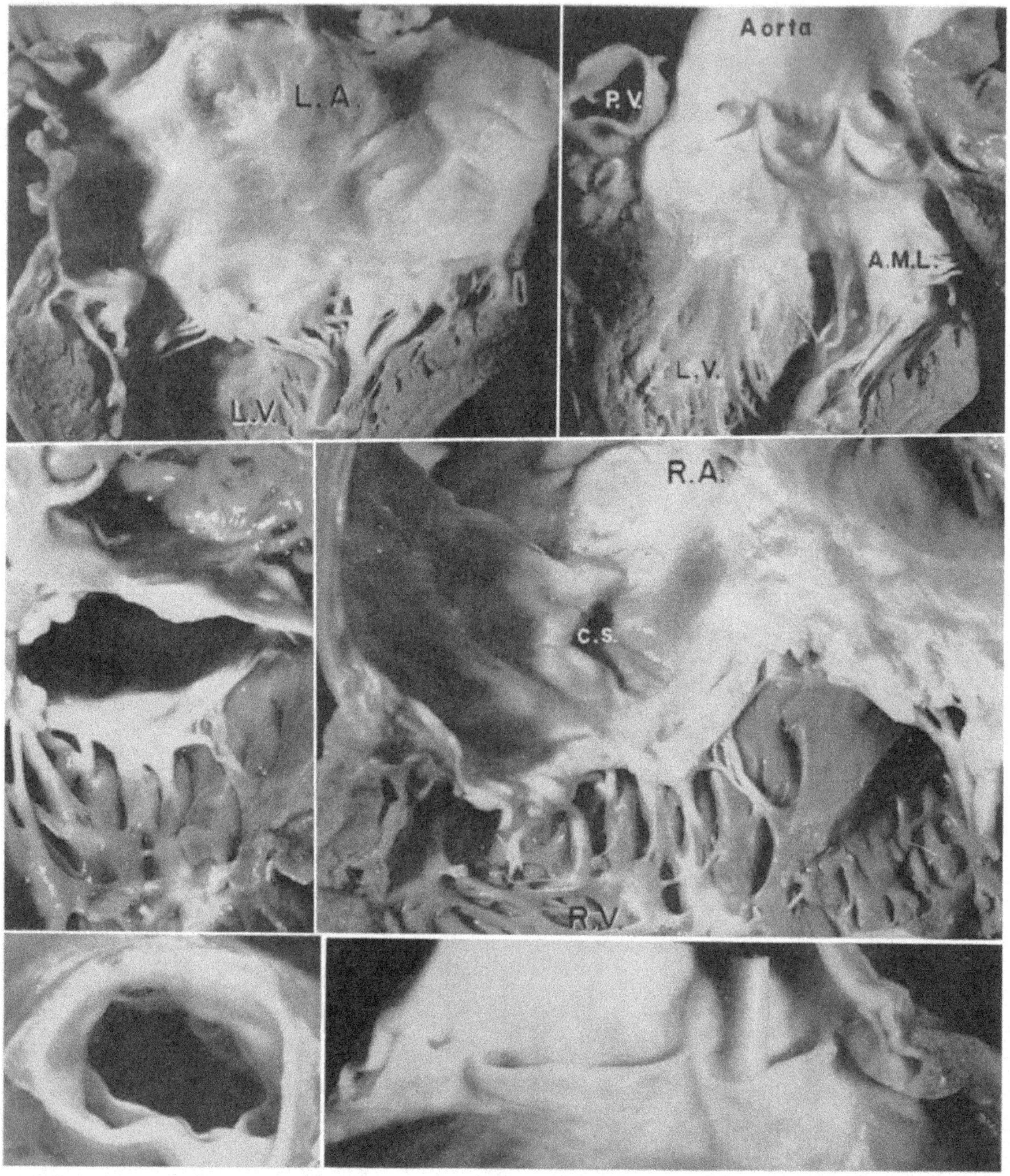

FIG. 7. Case VIII. *Upper left*, the left atrium (L.A.), mitral valve and left ventricle (L.V.). The mitral valvular leaflets and chordae are pearly white and thick. The left atrium is slightly dilated but free of carcinoid fibrous plaques. *Upper right*, the ascending aorta, aortic valve and left ventricle (L.V.) are opened showing the involved anterior leaflet of the mitral valve (A.M.L.) from this view. P.V. = pulmonic valve. *Middle left*, the tricuspid valve as seen from the right ventricle. The orifice is open; the consequence is regurgitation. *Middle right*, right atrium (R.A.) tricuspid valve and right ventricle (R.V.). The right atrium and tricuspid valve are extensively involved by the carcinoid fibrosing process. A single carcinoid plaque is present in the right ventricle. C.S. = ostium of coronary sinus. *Lower left*, the pulmonic valve from above. The appearance of this valve would suggest that it functioned normally. *Lower right*, the pulmonic valve opened. Its cusps are delicate. The lack of gross carcinoid fibrosis of this valve contrasts sharply with the marked involvement of the tricuspid valve.

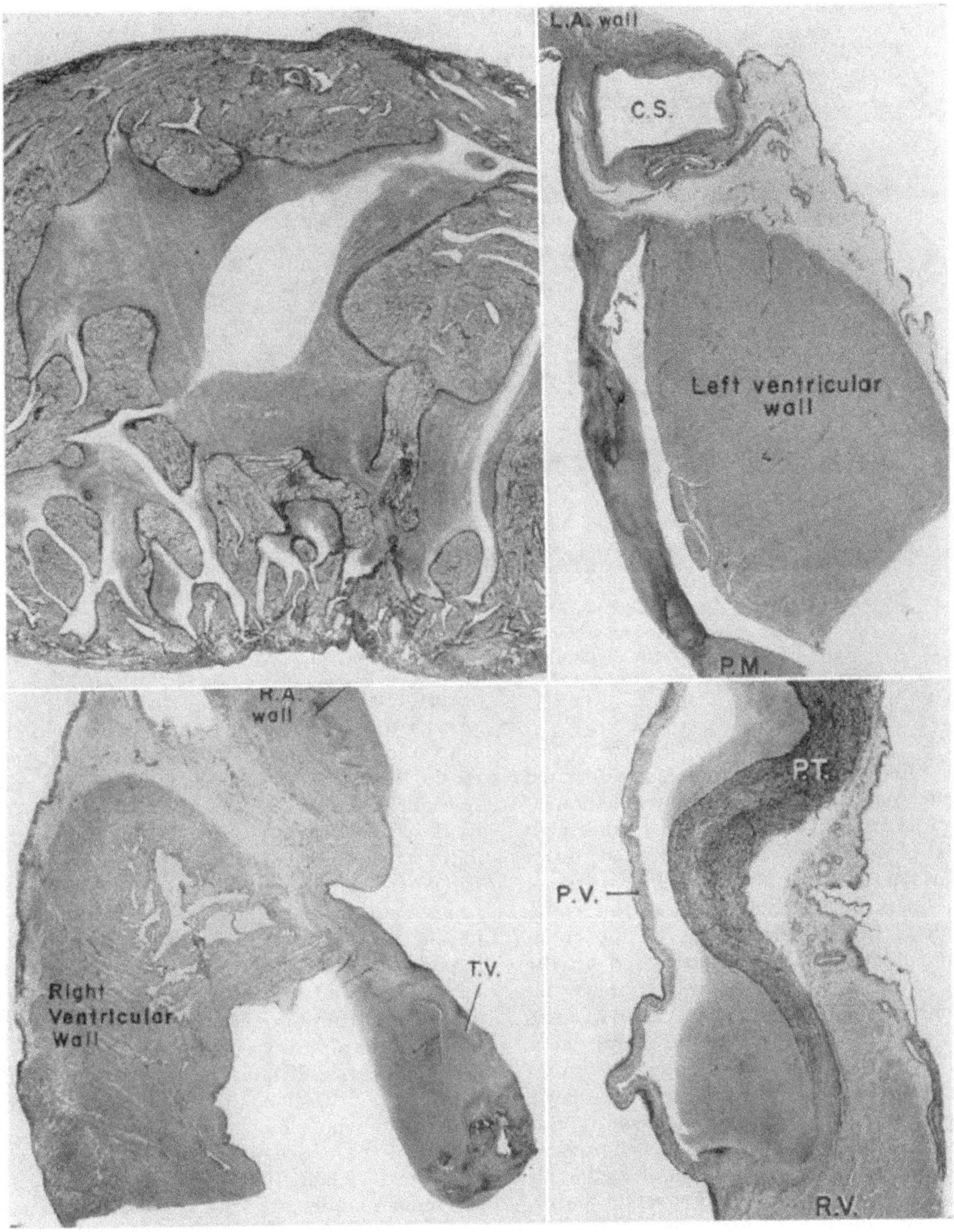

FIG. 8. Case VIII. Photomicrographs of sections demonstrating carcinoid fibrosis of the heart. *Upper left*, cross-section of right atrial appendage. Its lumen is considerably reduced by the widespread carcinoid fibrosis between the pectinate muscles. Note the "blood spaces" in the fibrous tissue. The underlying endocardium is well-demarcated by the black staining elastic membrane. *Upper right*, mitral valve, posterior leaflet. The fibrous process extends down and surrounds the chordae tendineae. Note also the carcinoid plaquing on the intima of the coronary sinus (C.S.). L.A. = left atrium; P.M. = papillary muscle. *Lower left*, tricuspid valve. The deposition of the fibrous stroma occurs on the ventricular aspect of the leaflet. Note also the fibrous plaquing on the right atrial (R.A.) endocardium. T.V. = tricuspid valve. *Lower right*, pulmonic valve. The carcinoid fibrous deposition in this instance occurs only on the intima of the pulmonary trunk (P.T.) causing it to "buckle." The pulmonic-valve (P.V.) cusp is free of fibrous material. R.V. = right ventricle. Verhoeff-Van Gieson elastic tissue stains; original magnification × 18 (upper left), × 7 (lower left), × 10 (lower right) and × 4 (upper right).

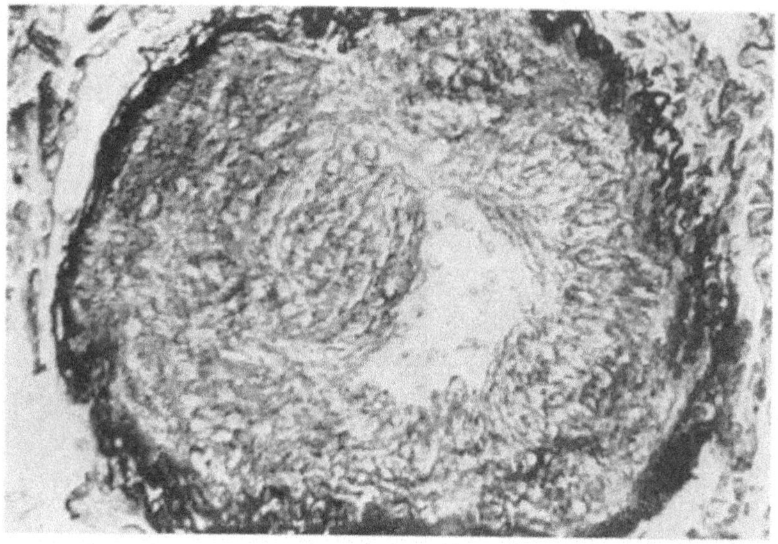

FIG. 9. Case VIII. Small pulmonary vein showing marked intimal fibrous proliferation. Since the fibrous tissue contains elastic fibrils (stained black) the fibrous proliferation is not of the carcinoid type but probably is secondary to increased pulmonary venous pressure, a result of mitral valvular disease. The pulmonary veins in this patient were diffusely and severely involved by this process, but, in addition, there was medial hypertrophy and intimal proliferation, although of only mild degree, of the muscular pulmonary arteries and arterioles. Verhoeff-Van Gieson elastic tissue stain, original magnification × 290.

COMMENTS

Cardiac Pathology. Histology of the fibrous deposits: The cardiovascular disease associated with the metastasizing "clinically functional" carcinoid is pathognomonic. The involvement consists of focal or diffuse collections of a peculiar type of fibrous tissue, which is free of elastic fibers and is deposited on the endocardium of the valvular cusps, on the endocardium of the cardiac chambers and on the intima of the great veins, coronary sinus and occasionally great arteries. The valvular cusps *per se* remain normal as does the mural endocardium, and each is clearly separated from the fibrosing process by the internal elastic membrane. Within the superimposed atypical fibrous tissue there is also a metachromatic ground substance, a few spindle-shaped cells (fibroblasts), blood vessels, oval or round spaces, which frequently contain small hyperchromatic nuclei, usually some lymphocytes, plasmacytes and mast cells, but no fat or fibrin. The oval or round spaces tend to give the fibrous tissue a "cartilage-like" appearance. The borders of these spaces are nicely delineated by the silver stain. The blood vessels, which frequently have thick walls, are located almost exclusively immediately adjacent to the valvular leaflets, usually on the side of the cusp which has initial contact with the stream of blood. The lymphocytes and plasma cells are located almost entirely in the perivascular regions, also immediately adjacent to the cusps. The mast cells, which are considerably increased in number in comparison to hearts of control subjects [*12*], are usually found in the subepicardial adipose tissue, interstitial myocardium, superimposed valvular fibrous tissue and rarely in the mural endocardial fibrous plaques. The ground substance, which is positive for Rinehart stain, lies between the open spaces and the spindle-shaped fibroblasts. These latter cells have elongated densely eosinophilic anisotropic cytoplasm which takes the periodic acid-Schiff and diastase-periodic acid-Schiff stains. Cosh et al. [*13*] described three patients in whom electron microscopic examination of the endocardial fibrous plaques was performed. Their findings indicate that the carcinoid plaques are composed of a material which is consistent in its features with young collagen. To our knowledge the carcinoid fibrous plaques have not been analyzed chemically.

Distribution of the Fibrous Deposits. Right-sided cardiac lesions: The curious atypical fibrous tissue is limited in the majority of instances to the right side of the heart. When the pulmonic valve is involved, the fibrous tissue is deposited almost entirely on the arterial aspect of the pulmonic valve cusps, sometimes contacting the

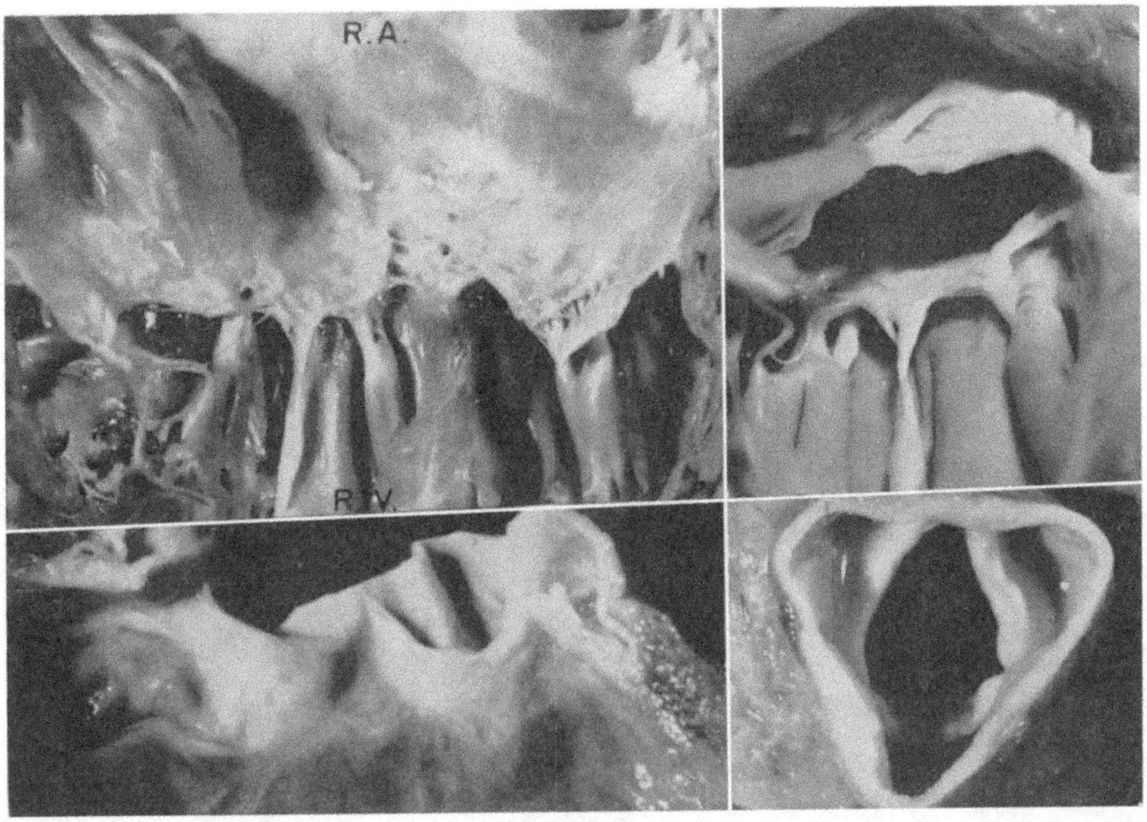

FIG. 10. Case IX. Interior of the heart showing severe carcinoid fibrosis of the tricuspid and pulmonic valves. *Upper left,* the right atrium (R.A.), tricuspid valve, involved by carcinoid fibrosis, and right ventricle (R.V.). The cardiac chambers on the right side are dilated but free of carcinoid plaques. *Upper right,* tricuspid valve as viewed from the right ventricle. The orifice is regurgitant. *Lower left,* pulmonic valve opened. The cusps are thick but the commissures are not fused. *Lower right,* pulmonic valve from above prior to opening. The orifice is rigid. The predominant functional derangement is probably regurgitation although some degree of stenosis is present as well.

intima of the pulmonary trunk. The fibrotic process causes infolding of the distal portion of the valvular cusp toward the sinus of the valve. When the posterior and septal leaflets of the tricuspid valve are involved, the fibrous tissue is located predominately on the ventricular aspect of the leaflets, frequently rigidly adhering the leaflets to the underlying ventricular wall. When the anterior tricuspid leaflet is involved, the fibrous tissue is deposited on the atrial as well as on the ventricular aspects of the leaflet and approximately in equal amounts. The fibrous tissue constricts the pulmonic and tricuspid valves, eventually producing fixed valvular orifices. The pulmonic valve becomes predominantly stenotic, although some regurgitation usually also occurs since the orifice is more or less the same size throughout both phases of the cardiac cycle. Despite the narrowing of its annulus, the tricuspid valve is usually fixed in a wide open position, and thus the predominant functional derangement produced is regurgitation although an element of stenosis generally is present as well. It is apparent that the basic process involving both valves is similar but that the size of the natural orifice of each determines the eventual predominant functional alteration. Thus, since the pulmonic valve orifice is small initially, the contracting process leads to stenosis. The tricuspid valve ring initially is large and, although it becomes contracted, stenosis is usually not the predominant lesion produced. An effective means of producing chronic right-sided cardiac failure in the experimental animal is by making the pulmonic valve stenotic and the tricuspid valve regurgitant [*14*]. It is, therefore, apparent why right-sided congestive failure may be a prominent problem in patients with carcinoid heart diseases.

The atypical fibrous deposits, which we prefer to call "carcinoid fibrous plaques," are commonly seen on the endocardial surface of the right atrium and ventricle as well as on the

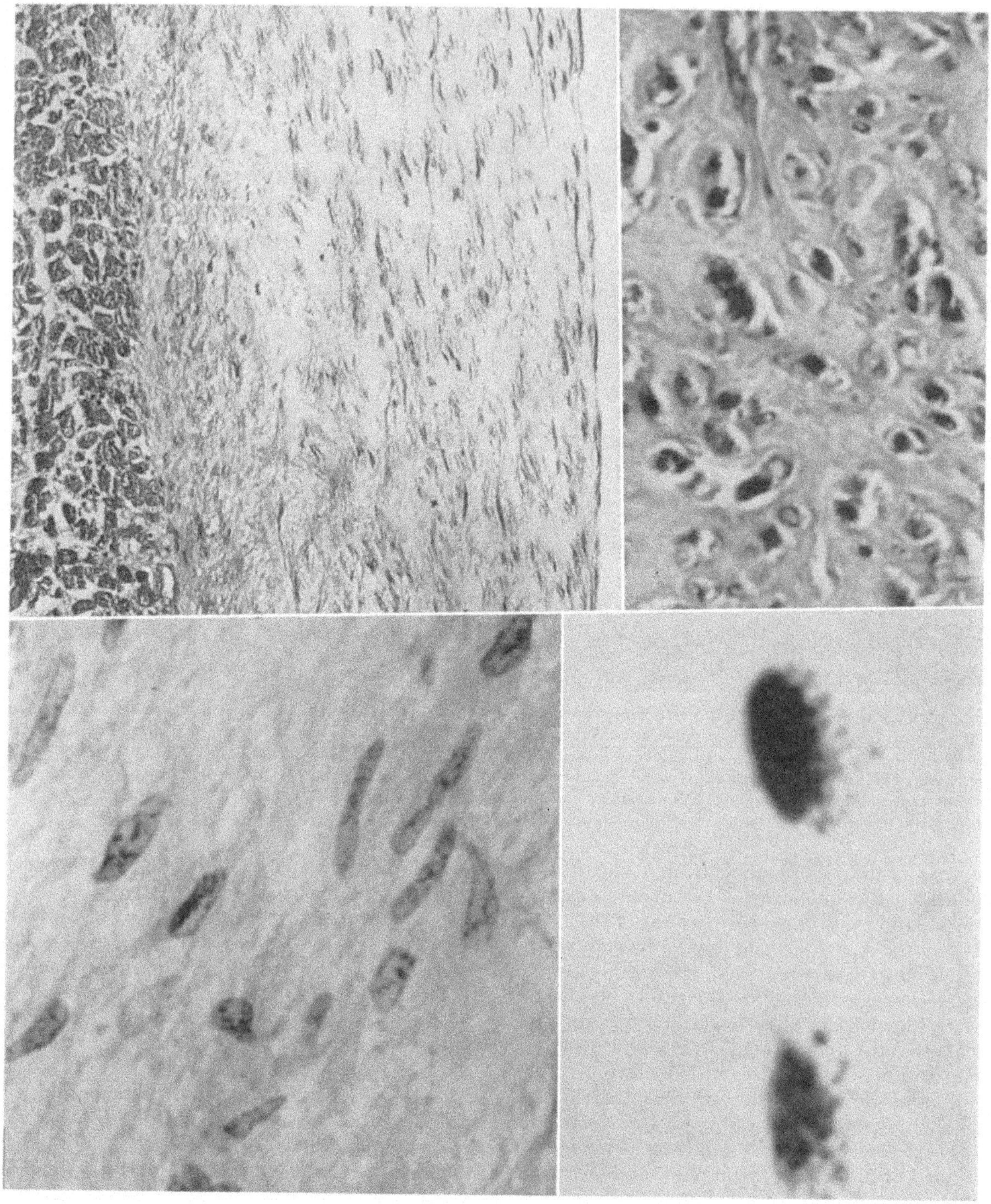

FIG. 11. The carcinoid fibrous plaque. *Upper left*, a mural plaque. The cells are arranged parallel to the surface (on the right), which is covered by cells similar to those in the interior of the plaque. The ground substance between the cells is evident. The underlying myocardium (to the left) is apparent. Hematoxylin and eosin stain, original magnification × 140. *Lower left*, close-up view of the spindle-shaped cells (fibroblasts) within the plaque. Hematoxylin and eosin stain, original magnification × 830. *Upper right*, toluidine blue stain of a plaque showing the "open spaces" which contain hyperchromatic nuclei. Original magnification × 830. *Lower right*, mast cells which are readily seen in the plaques adjacent to the endocardium of the chamber or valve or adjacent to the intima of the vessels. These cells also are present in the underlying myocardium and in the overlying subepicardial adipose tissue. Toluidine blue stain, original magnification × 2,080.

pulmonic and tricuspid valvular leaflets. The plaques are smooth, glistening and whitish gray elevations, which are usually focally distributed, although sometimes diffuse. The plaques appear to be preferentially located in areas of excessive turbulence of blood or in the paths of regurgitant streams. These lesions, therefore, are seen most commonly on the atrial septum immediately above the junction of the septal and anterior tricuspid valvular leaflets and in the right atrial appendage. When the tricuspid valve is involved by carcinoid fibrosis, plaques almost always are present in the right atrium as well.

Fibrous plaques in the right ventricle are less extensive than in the right atrium. Here they frequently are located on the papillary muscles, having extended down the chordae tendineae from the tricuspid valve. In one patient (Case v) the plaquing in the right ventricle was diffuse. Carcinoid fibrous lesions have not been reported in the right atrium or right ventricle unless the tricuspid or pulmonic valves also were involved. In the formalin-fixed hearts the fibrous carcinoid plaques overlying atrial or ventricular endocardium can sometimes be neatly displaced or "plucked" from the underlying endocardium. This procedure is difficult, however, on the fresh specimen. Also, since the involvement of the cardiac valves by this fibrous process is usually diffuse, this technic is not advisable from a therapeutic standpoint during life.

Carcinoid fibrous plaques are found commonly on the intima of the systemic veins. We have seen these characteristic fibrous deposits in the superior and inferior vena cavae, innominate vein and coronary sinus. The lesions in these regions may be attributable to contact with inferior vena caval blood which has been regurgitated through the incompetent tricuspid valve during ventricular systole.

Left-Sided Cardiac Lesions. Carcinoid involvement of the left side of the heart is less common than involvement of the right side but probably more common than generally realized. Many reports have appeared describing various changes in the mitral and aortic valves in patients with the carcinoid syndrome and carcinoid plaquing in the right side of the heart. In probably the first patient described with metastasizing carcinoid syndrome, flushes, diarrhea and endocardial fibrosis, Scholte [*2*] described "irregular, sharply limited, greyish-white, elevated areas" on the endocardium of the anterior mitral leaflet and left ventricle as well as on the endocardium of the pulmonic and tricuspid valves, right atrium and ventricle, and on the intima of the superior vena cava. In one of the patients (Case III) with the malignant carcinoid syndrome described by Isler and Hedinger [*9*] there was "severe fibrosing endocarditis" of the mitral as well as of the tricuspid and pulmonic valves. Of the two patients with the carcinoid syndrome described by Bean and co-workers [*15*], one had "thickening and sclerosis" of all four cardiac valves with "contraction" of the pulmonic and aortic valves, and the other had "valvulitis involving all cardiac valves, most marked in the pulmonic and tricuspid valves." Hand et al. [*16*] mentioned "thickening of the free edge and chordae tendineae of the mitral valve" in addition to typical carcinoid plaques on the pulmonic and tricuspid valves in still another patient with the carcinoid syndrome. These investigators also found changes, similar to those on the endocardium, on the intima of the pulmonary and renal vessels, and in the vessels in the vicinity of the carcinoid tumor. Bean and Funk [*17*] described yet another patient with malignant carcinoid and "lesions on the mitral and, to less degree, the aortic valve similar to" those in the tricuspid and pulmonic valves. Other patients with the syndrome have been described in whom focal thickening or fibrosis occurred on valves on the left side of the heart [*10,18–25*]. In no patient referred to by the authors was a defect in the cardiac septum described. It is probable that in some of these patients the valvular abnormalities on the left side were the result of carcinoid fibrosis, but it is not possible to rule out some other type of cardiac disease, particularly rheumatic, as being responsible.

There remain, to our knowledge, only three described patients in whom there is unequivocal evidence of carcinoid fibrosis on the left side of the heart, and in two others there was probably left-sided carcinoid plaquing. One of the three patients, a sixty-eight year old woman described by McKusick [*21*], had typical focal fibrous deposits on the endocardium of the mitral valve, aortic valve, left ventricle and possibly on the intima of the renal arteries in addition to the more severe ones involving the pulmonic and tricuspid valves, right atrium and ventricle. This patient, whose primary carcinoid tumor was located in the ileum, had a foramen ovale-type atrial septal defect (1.5 cm. in diameter). A similar patient, a seventy year old man, described by Fischer and Lindeneg [26], also had carcinoid plaquing involving the mitral and aortic valves in addition to more extensive deposits on the pulmonic valve, tricuspid valve, right atrium and inferior vena cava. This patient, whose primary carcinoid was situated in the ileum, also had an intracardiac communication, a "slit-like foramen ovale measuring 1 cm. in length." Von Bernheimer and associates [25] described a patient with a nonmetastasizing "clinically active" bronchial carcinoid, in whom there was carcinoid fibrous plaquing of the local pulmonary veins which drained the carcinoid tumor, and of the mitral and aortic valves and coronary arteries, without involvement of the cardiac valves or chambers on the right side. This latter patient thus had isolated left-sided cardiac lesions and appears to be the only one described with this unique distribution. Of all other described patients with clinically active primary bronchial carcinoid tumors proved at autopsy [27–37], none had carcinoid fibrous lesions on the left side, and only three [32,34,37] had endocardial abnormalities on the right side, none of which were unequivocally carcinoid in type. Davies [23] illustrated a mildly thickened mitral valve in a patient with the carcinoid syndrome who also had "capping of the papillary muscle" in the left ventricle, but no information regarding histologic studies was given. A patient with malignant carcinoid recently described by Wolfe et al. [24] had "early thickening of the edges of the mitral valve, and white capping of the papillary muscle" of the left ventricle. This patient had a defect in the atrial septum, a "small" patent foramen ovale.

Three of the nine patients with carcinoid heart disease in the present series had unequivocal carcinoid fibrous plaquing in the left side of the heart in addition to that occurring in the right side. In two patients (Cases vi and viii) the mitral valve was diffusely involved by the carcinoid fibrous process, and in the third (Case vii) a focal carcinoid plaque was present on the ventricular aspect of the anterior mitral leaflet. The leaflets and chordae tendineae of the valve in the two former patients were shortened, thickened and grossly resembled rheumatic mitral disease. On histologic study of sections through this valve in these two patients, however, the characteristic fibrous tissue devoid of elastic fibers was present, being superimposed on the valvular cusps. The deposition was limited to the ventricular aspect of the posterior leaflet but was present in approximately equal amounts on the two surfaces of the anterior mitral leaflet. The primary tumor in each of these three patients was located in the small intestine, and in none was there an intracardiac communication, a pulmonary arteriovenous fistula or a carcinoid tumor in the lung. Thus, these three patients represent the first proved examples of carcinoid heart disease involving the left side of the heart, as well as the right side, in patients with primary intestinal carcinoid tumors without right to left shunts. In one patient (Case vii) there were typical carcinoid plaques in the aorta as well as on the mitral valve. We are not aware of any previous report describing carcinoid plaquing in the aorta. The aortic plaques in this patient were usually superimposed on atheromas, which appeared whitish grey rather than yellow. In no patient in the present series was there carcinoid plaquing of the aortic valve or of the pulmonary arteries or veins. There was minimal carcinoid plaquing of the left atrium in Case vi. These lesions, however, were limited to that portion of the left atrial endocardium immediately above the mitral valvular annulus. We are not aware of any previous report describing carcinoid fibrous lesions in the left atrium, and in only one [21] is aortic valve involvement well described or illustrated, and in this instance it consisted only of "mild change in one aortic cusp." In Case vi the patient had a 0.6 cm. sized nodule on one cusp of the aortic valve, but it bore no resemblance to endocardial fibrosis of the carcinoid type. Nodules of calcium were present on the aortic valvular cusps in Case iii. In two patients (Cases vi and vii) there were focal carcinoid plaques on the endocardium of the left ventricle. In one (Case vii) there was only "white capping" of the left ventricular papillary muscles, and in the other (Case vi) only a rare plaque on the mural endocardium.

Differentiation from other cardiac diseases: Cardiac involvement in malignant carcinoid is specific and bears little resemblance to other types of cardiac disease. MacDonald and Robbins [12] compared the cardiac lesions of carcinoid syndrome to those of rheumatic heart disease, congenital pulmonic stenosis, congenital fibroelastosis, bacterial and nonbacterial thrombotic endocarditis and various collagen diseases. These investigators, and we have confirmed their findings, found the cardiac lesions in the carcinoid syndrome unlike those in any of these other conditions. In rheumatic heart disease the involvement is principally on the left side of the heart, and when the tricuspid and pulmonic valves are involved the mitral or the mitral and aortic valves are almost invariably involved as well. In rheumatic valvular disease the scarring involves the valvular cusp itself, with deposition of densely eosinophilic masses of fibrous tissue within the cusp. There are also strands of elastic fibers within this fibrous stroma. Likewise, in congenital pulmonic stenosis a few elastic fibrils are present within the valvular cusp. Congenital fibroelastosis presents no problem in differentiation since the thickened endocardium in this instance contains a great number of elastic fibers. The African heart disease, namely endomyocardial fibrosis, is readily distinguished from the carcinoid fibrous plaques, in that the structure and location of the lesions are different [*38*]. In this disease the endocardial fibrosis generally begins at the apex of the ventricles, spreads to the atrioventricular valves and spares the semilunar valves. The lesions in the right side of the heart are usually less extensive than those in the left, and isolated right ventricular involvement is unusual. Superimposed thrombi and vegetations are common, and strands of fibrous tissue penetrate the underlying myocardium to varying depths. So called "jet lesions" are distinguished readily from the carcinoid plaques in that these lesions contain a number of elastic fibers and are more frequently present in the left side of the heart except in ventricular septal defect with a left to right shunt. The cardiac lesions of the collagen diseases are generally vascular and myocardial in location and bear no resemblance to the carcinoid plaques. Atypical verrucal endocarditis presents no problem in differentiation from the carcinoid plaque.

Clinical Correlation. Physical findings: The diagnosis of carcinoid heart disease is usually readily established by physical examination. The most characteristic sign of cardiac disease in a patient with the carcinoid syndrome is the presence of a precordial murmur. This was found in all nine patients with endocardial carcinoid fibrosis in the present study. The most frequent murmur in this disease is fairly harsh in quality, grade 1 to 4/6 in intensity, systolic in time and located along the upper left sternal border. This murmur is generally interpreted to represent valvular pulmonic stenosis. The diagnosis of tricuspid valvular disease by clinical examination has proved to be more difficult. A systolic blowing murmur, which became accentuated during inspiration, was audible along the lower left sternal border in only two of the nine patients with carcinoid heart disease described herein. The other patients in this series who were found to have tricuspid insufficiency at autopsy, clinically did not have a precordial murmur which increased in intensity with inspiration. In neither of the two patients with carcinoid mitral involvement was the diagnosis of left-sided valvular disease established prior to autopsy. The cardiac murmurs in the three patients with malignant carcinoid but no heart disease (Table II) were of a nonspecific nature, and none suggested organic valvular involvement. The murmurs in each of these three patients may have been on the basis of anemia (hemoglobin 10 gm. per cent or less in each). It has been noted previously [*39*] that the cardiac murmurs and sounds tend to increase in intensity during the flushing episodes. A rare patient with carcinoid heart disease may have an audible murmur only during cutaneous flushes. The intensity of the cardiac murmur also appears to increase as the disease progresses (Case II). A precordial lift, right ventricular in type, and a systolic thrill often are palpable in these patients.

Supportive evidence for the presence of carcinoid heart disease is obtained by examination of the neck veins and the liver. The superficial jugular veins in the upright position are distended in the majority of these patients, and frequently V waves and occasionally A waves are clearly discernible. A pulsatile liver, confirmative evidence for the presence of tricuspid regurgitation, is present in some patients. However, as pointed out by Thorson [*18*], "cyanosis," hepatomegaly, peripheral edema, ascites, dyspnea and distended systemic veins are not diagnostic of valvular heart disease in patients with the carcinoid syndrome. These signs may result simply from hepatic enlargement secondary to metastatic carcinoid. The intrahepatic metastases may produce portal hypertension which in turn may lead to ascites and peripheral edema, and the large liver may displace the diaphragms, leading to dyspnea. Hypoproteinemia is commonly present in patients with the carcinoid syndrome, and this also may contribute to development of peripheral manifestations of cardiac failure.

Roentgenographic findings: Routine roentgenologic examination of the chest appears to be of little value in determining the presence or absence of carcinoid heart disease. Carcinoid involvement of the heart in itself rarely produces significant thickening of the wall of a cardiac chamber, although histological sections from the right atrium and ventricle usually show hypertrophy of many of the myocardial fibers. If the size of the heart is increased in a patient with the carcinoid syndrome, an associated cardiac disease unrelated to carcinoid should be suspected. The right side of the heart in these patients, however, is frequently dilated to a mild or moderate degree. Poststenotic dilatation of the pulmonary trunk appears not to be a feature of the roentgenogram in patients with carcinoid heart disease.

Electrocardiographic findings: The electrocardiogram is rarely of benefit in determining the presence or absence of carcinoid cardiac disease. The most frequent electrocardiographic abnormality is probably low voltage [*18*], and this was observed in four of our nine patients. Its mechanism is unclear. Pericardial effusion (150 ml.) occurred in only one of four patients with low voltage in the present series, and none had frank pericarditis, although small foci of round cells (primarily lymphocytes) were seen in the subepicardial adipose tissue immediately beneath the visceral pericardium in several patients studied. Prominent P waves suggesting right atrial enlargement occur occasionally. Electrocardiographic evidence of right ventricular hypertrophy was absent in all nine patients with involvement of the heart in this series, and only one had right axis deviation. Right bundle branch block, right ventricular strain, S-T segment depression and flattening of the T waves have been recorded in patients with carcinoid heart disease by others [*18*]. In summary, the electrocardiographic changes in carcinoid heart disease generally are nonspecific.

Hemodynamic findings: Relatively few patients with the carcinoid syndrome have undergone cardiac catheterization [*8,22,40–45*], and studies reported thus far have been limited to the right side of the heart. Tricuspid insufficiency has been the most common hemodynamic alteration reported in patients with carcinoid valvular disease [*8,40,42–44*], followed by pulmonic stenosis [*22,43,44*]. The least common lesion described has been tricuspid stenosis [*22,44*]. V waves up to 34 mm. Hg have been recorded in the right atrium (Case IV). The highest end-diastolic gradient reported across the tricuspid valve was 9 mm. Hg [*22*]. Minimal pulmonary arterial hypertension was found in one patient, described by Charms et al. [*42*], who also had significant valvular disease (tricuspid regurgitation). Arterial oxygen saturation is usually slightly below normal.

An intriguing hemodynamic aspect of the carcinoid syndrome concerns the state of the cardiac output. Recently, Schwaber and Lukas [*45*] reported elevated cardiac outputs in two patients with "metastatic carcinoid and the typical flush syndrome." Neither of these patients had hemodynamic evidence or, in one, necropsy evidence of right-sided valvular cardiac disease. The cardiac outputs were elevated even more during a flush or during exercise than at rest. These authors, in addition, briefly described two further patients with metastatic carcinoid and elevated urinary excretion of 5-hydroxyindoleacetic acid who did "not manifest chronic cutaneous erythema or repeated episodes of flushing." Cardiac outputs in each of these patients, neither of whom had hemodynamic evidence of right-sided valvular heart disease, were low normal. These authors attributed the hyperkinemia in the two patients with chronic cutaneous erythema to the cardiovascular effects of serotonin and concluded that hyperkinemia of itself may contribute to the high incidence of cardiac failure in the carcinoid syndrome. A patient examined earlier with malignant carcinoid, described by Schneckloth et al. [*41*], also was found to have an elevated resting cardiac output. There was no apparent evidence of valvular cardiac disease in this patient. In other reports of patients with carcinoid valvular disease the resting cardiac outputs have not been elevated but, indeed, low [*8,22,42*] or, occasionally, normal [*43*]. In a patient described by Goble et al. [*22*], however, the cardiac output, although low at rest, increased to a normal level during a cutaneous flush, returning to the resting level during an attack of wheezing. Thörson [*39*] noted an increase in the amplitude of the ballistographic waves, as well as an increase in the intensity of the cardiac sounds and murmurs, and in the cardiac rate during episodes of cutaneous flushing in four patients with metastasizing carcinoid.

A word of caution seems advisable in regard to cardiac diagnostic procedures in this disease. A patient with the carcinoid syndrome described by Biörck et al. [*8*] died immediately following angiocardiography, and one patient described by Schwaber and Lukas [*45*] died following routine right heart catheterization.

Pathogenesis of the Cardiac Lesions. The pathogenesis of the endocardial carcinoid plaques remains the subject of controversy. The morphologic appearance of the endocardial lesion would suggest that it was the result of the deposition of a material from the blood. That the underlying endocardium, with its internal elastic membrane, remains intact is evidence that the deposition may come from the blood and not from the underlying endocardium or myocardium. The substance which produces the endocardial fibrosis is unknown, but serotonin (5-hydroxytryptamine) has been implicated to play a major role in the pathogenesis of these lesions. This material is presumed to be liberated in greatest quantity from liver metastases. Unless carcinoid metastases to the liver are present or unless there is drainage of carcinoid tumor by routes other than the portal vein, the endocardial carcinoid lesions do not occur [*18*]. The relative scarcity of left-sided cardiac lesions has been explained by the inactivation of serotonin by monoamine oxidase during its passage through the lungs [*22,46*]. If serotonin does indeed play a role in the production of these endocardial plaques, the occurrence of left-sided cardiac lesions in a third of the patients with carcinoid heart disease in the present series would suggest that plasma serotonin is by no means totally inactivated during its passage through the lungs. This conclusion is in support of the earlier observations of Sjoerdsma and associates [*40*] who were unable to detect significant differences between arterial and venous blood levels of serotonin in patients with the carcinoid syndrome.

Efforts to produce the endocardial carcinoid lesions in experimental animals have been unsuccessful with the possible exception of the work of Spatz [*47*] who made guinea pigs tryptophan-deficient or niacin-deficient and then injected serotonin intraperitoneally for six to eight weeks. The endocardial lesions, mainly on the right side, were described as "early" and bore little resemblance to the typical carcinoid plaques seen in man. Spatz suggested, however, that longer-term experiments might be productive of lesions more similar to those found in man. One of the curious features of the endocardial plaques in man, however, is their uniformity of structure. The histologic appearance of the plaques in the same patient is similar, and there is virtually no variation in this structure from one patient to the next. The concept of an "early" endocardial carcinoid plaque does not appear to apply in man.

Although the inability to produce the carcinoid type of cardiac lesion in animals with serotonin is perhaps not surprising, sufficient work has now been carried out to raise considerable doubt about the role of this substance in the pathogenesis of these lesions. The observations in the present series of patients raise further questions in this regard. The present study, for example, showed no significant difference in the urinary levels of 5-hydroxyindoleacetic acid in those patients with carcinoid heart disease and in those without carcinoid cardiac involvement. (Tables I and II.) It appears that the total serotonin production, by the carcinoid tumor and by its metastases, is similar both in patients with carcinoid heart disease and in those without endocardial lesions. The quantity of hepatic metastases and the distribution of metastases in these two groups also were similar. (Tables I and II.) Why one patient with the carcinoid syndrome has endocardial plaquing and why another one does not is difficult to explain.

Thus, in conclusion, the pathogenesis of the endocardial carcinoid lesions remains obscure. Since no definitive evidence has been obtained that serotonin is responsible for the lesions, investigation should also be directed at mechanisms independent of this substance.

SUMMARY

The clinical and pathologic features of seventeen patients with the carcinoid syndrome are reviewed. Nine had carcinoid heart disease. The only clinical feature which distinguished those patients with carcinoid heart disease from those without was the presence of a precordial systolic murmur suggestive of tricuspid regurgitation or pulmonic stenosis. Urinary excretion of 5-hydroxyindoleacetic acid was similar in the two groups. The chest roentgenogram and the electrocardiogram was of no help in determining presence or absence of carcinoid heart disease. Cardiac catheterization in patients with carcinoid heart disease has shown that tricuspid regurgitation and pulmonic stenosis are the most frequent valvular alterations. Cardiac output appears to be increased in some patients who do not have carcinoid cardiac involvement.

The cardiac lesions associated with the carcinoid syndrome were pathognomonic and bore little resemblance to lesions found in other cardiac diseases. Cardiac involvement in the carcinoid syndrome consisted of focal or diffuse collections of a peculiar type of fibrous tissue, which was free of elastic fibers and which was deposited on the endocardium of the valvular cusps, on the endocardium of the cardiac chambers and on the intima of the great veins, coronary sinus and occasionally great arteries. The valvular cusps *per se* remained normal as did the mural endocardium, and each was clearly separated from the fibrosing process by the elastic membrane which covered its surface. Left-sided cardiac lesions were commoner in the carcinoid syndrome than previously thought and were found in the absence of a right to left shunt or a pulmonary carcinoid tumor.

The pathogenesis of the carcinoid cardiac lesions (carcinoid fibrous plaques) remains unknown. The morphologic appearance of the endocardial lesion suggests that it might be the result of the deposition of a material, possibly collagen, from the blood, but the identity of the substance which either directly or indirectly produced the endocardial fibrosis is unknown. The inability to produce these cardiac lesions in animals with serotonin and the present observation that the urinary excretion of 5-hydroxyindoleacetic acid was similar in the patient with carcinoid heart disease irrespective of the presence or absence of cardiac involvement suggest that mechanisms other than that involving serotonin should be considered.

Acknowledgment: We wish to thank the following: Miss Mary Catherine Bowling for the staining of the histologic sections; Mr. Gebhard Gsell for the photomicrographic work; Mr. Kenzie Edwards for the gross photographic work; and Mrs. Katharine Nichols for the labelling of the photographs.

REFERENCES

1. Cassidy, M. A. Abdominal carcinomatosis with probable adrenal involvement. *Proc. Roy. Soc. Med.*, 24: 139, 1930.
2. Scholte, A. J. Ein Fall von Angioma teleangiectaticum Cutis mit chronischer Endokarditis und malignem Dünndarmcarcinoid. *Beitr. path. Anat.*, 86: 440, 1931.
3. Cassidy, M. A. Postmortem findings in case shown on October 10, 1930, as one of abdominal carcinomatosis with probable adrenal involvement. *Proc. Roy. Soc. Med.*, 24: 920, 1931.
4. Cassidy, M. A. Abdominal carcinomatosis associated with vasomotor disturbances. *Proc. Roy. Soc. Med.*, 27: 220, 1934.
5. Millman, S. Tricuspid stenosis and pulmonary stenosis complicating carcinoid of the intestine with metastases to the liver. *Am. Heart J.*, 25: 391, 1943.
6. Gold, I. R. and Grayzel, D. M. Multiple argentaffinomas in ileum with metastases in lymph nodes and in the liver. *Am. J. Surg.*, 60: 144, 1943.
7. Currens, J. H., Kinney, T. D. and White, P. D. Pulmonary stenosis with intact interventricular septum, report of eleven cases. *Am. Heart J.*, 30: 491, 1945.
8. Biörck, G., Axén, O. and Thörson, Å. Unusual cyanosis in a boy with congenital pulmonary stenosis and tricuspid insufficiency. Fatal outcome after angiocardiography. *Am. Heart J.*, 44: 143, 1952.
9. Isler, P. and Hedinger, C. Metastasierendes Dünndarmcarcinoid mit schweren, vorwiegend das rechte Herz betreffenden Klappenfehlern und Pulmonalstenose—ein eigenartiger Symptomenkomplex? *Schweiz. med. Wchnschr.*, 83: 4, 1953.
10. Rosenbaum, F. F., Santer, D. G. and Claudon, D. B. Essential telangiectasia, pulmonic and tricuspid stenosis, and neoplastic liver disease. A possible new clinical syndrome. (Abstract.) *J. Lab. & Clin. Med.*, 42: 941, 1953.
11. Thörson, Å., Biörck, G., Björkman, G. and Waldenström, J. Malignant carcinoid of the small intestine with metastases to the liver, valvular disease of the heart (pulmonary stenosis and tricuspid regurgitation without septal defects), peripheral vasomotor symptoms, bronchoconstriction, and an unusual type of cyanosis. A clinical and pathologic syndrome. *Am. Heart J.*, 47: 795, 1954.
12. MacDonald, R. A. and Robbins, S. L. Pathology of the heart in the carcinoid syndrome. A comparative study. *Arch. Path.*, 63: 103, 1957.
13. Cosh, J., Cates, J. E. and Pugh, D. W. Carcinoid heart disease. *Brit. Heart J.*, 21: 369, 1959.
14. Barger, A. C., Roe, B. B. and Richardson, G. S. Relation of valvular lesions and of exercise to auricular pressure, work tolerance, and to development of chronic, congestive failure in dogs. *Am. J. Physiol.*, 169: 384, 1952.
15. Bean, W. B., Olch, D. and Weinberg, H. B. The syndrome of carcinoid and acquired valve lesions of the right side of the heart. *Circulation*, 12: 1, 1955.
16. Hand, A. M., McCormick, W. F. and Lumb, G. Malignant carcinoid tumor. A case report with discussion of systemic manifestations. *Am. J. Clin. Path.*, 30: 47, 1958.
17. Bean, W. B. and Funk, D. The vasculocardiac syndrome of metastatic carcinoid. *Arch. Int. Med.*, 103: 189, 1959.
18. Thörson, Å. H. Studies on carcinoid disease. *Acta med. scandinav.*, supp.: 334, 1958.

19. ALTMAN, V. and MANN, N. Metastasizing carcinoid tumor of the appendix and caecum. *Am. J. Surg.*, 76: 434, 1948.
20. RATZENHOFER, M. and LEMBECK, F. Über den Gehalt an 5-Oxytryptamin in Carcinoiden des Darmtraktes. *Ztschr. Krebsforsch.*, 60: 169, 1954.
21. MCKUSICK, V. A. Carcinoid cardiovascular disease. *Bull. Johns Hopkins Hosp.*, 98: 13, 1956.
22. GOBLE, A. J., HAY, D. R., HUDSON, R. and SANDLER, M. Acquired heart disease with argentaffin carcinoma. *Brit. Heart J.*, 18: 544, 1956.
23. DAVIES, A. J. Carcinoid tumors (Argentaffinomata). *Ann. Roy. Coll. Surgeons England*, 25: 277, 1959.
24. WOLFE, H. R. I., DAVIES, A., MATHIAS, A. P. and SCHACHTER, M. Metastatic argentaffinoma secreting 5-hydroxytryptamine in a patient with a patent foramen ovale. *Brit. M. J.*, 5177: 929, 1960.
25. VON BERNHEIMER, H., EHRINGER, H., HEISTRACHER, P., KRAUPP, O., LACHNIT, V., OBIDITSCH-MAYER, I. and WENZL, M. Biologisch aktives, nicht metastasierendes Bronchuscarcinoid mit Linksherzsyndrom. *Wien. klin. Wchnschr.*, 72: 867, 1960.
26. FISCHER, S. and LINDENEG, O. Cardiac changes in argentaffinomatosis. *Acta path. et microbiol. scandinav.*, 44: 128, 1958.
27. WARNER, R. R. P. and SOUTHREN, A. L. Carcinoid syndrome produced by metastasizing bronchial adenoma. *Am. J. Med.*, 24: 903, 1958.
28. SAUER, W. G., DEARING, W. H. and FLOCK, E. V. Diagnosis and clinical management of functioning carcinoids. *J. A. M. A.*, 168: 139, 1958.
29. SCHNECKLOTH, R. E., MCISAAC, W. M. and PAGE, I. H. Serotonin metabolism in carcinoid syndrome with metastatic bronchial adenoma. *J. A. M. A.*, 170: 1143, 1959.
30. JOSEPH, M. and TAYLOR, R. R. Argentaffinoma of the lung with carcinoid syndrome. *Brit. M. J.*, 2: 568, 1960.
31. WILLIAMS, E. D. and AZZOPARDI, J. G. Tumors of the lung and the carcinoid syndrome. *Thorax*, 15: 30, 1960.
32. GRAMLICH, V. F. and WIETHOFF, E. O. Das Carcinoidsyndrom unter Mitteilung eines metastasierenden Bronchialcarcinoids. *Deutsche. med. Wchnschr.*, 85: 1750, 1960.
33. ANLYAN, W. G., HARGROVE, M. D., RUFFIN, J. M., WALLACE, D. K., WEAVER, W. T. and KIRSHNER, N. Metastasizing bronchial adenoma. *J. A. M. A.*, 174: 415, 1960.
34. VON HÜSSELMANN, H. and WENDT, K. H. Metastasierendes Bronchusadenom vom Karzinoidtyp mit atypischem Carcinoid-syndrom. *München. med. Wchnschr.*, 103: 663, 1961.
35. ESCOVITZ, W. E. and REINGOLD, I. M. Functioning malignant bronchial carcinoid with Cushing's syndrome and recurrent sinus arrest. *Ann. Int. Med.*, 54: 1248, 1961.
36. SANDLER, M., SCHEUER, P. J. and WATT, P. J. 5-hydroxytryptophan-secreting bronchial carcinoid tumor. *Lancet*, 2: 1067, 1961.
37. MCCONAGHIE, R. J. The malignant carcinoid syndrome associated with a metastasizing bronchial adenoma. *J. Thoracic & Cardiovasc. Surg.*, 43: 303, 1962.
38. DAVIES, J. N. P. and BALL, J. D. The pathology of endomyocardial fibrosis in Uganda. *Brit. Heart J.*, 17: 337, 1955.
39. THÖRSON, Å. H. Hemodynamic changes during "flush" in carcinoidosis. (The carcinoid syndrome.) *Am. Heart J.*, 52: 444, 1956.
40. SJOERDSMA, A., WEISSBACH, H., TERRY, L. L. and UDENFRIEND, S. Further observations on patients with malignant carcinoid. *Am. J. Med.*, 23: 5, 1957.
41. SCHNECKLOTH, R., PAGE, I. H., DEL GRECO, F. and CORCORAN, A. C. Effects of serotonin antagonists in normal subjects and patients with carcinoid tumors. *Circulation*, 16: 523, 1957.
42. CHARMS, B. L., KOHN, P., APPLEBAUM, H. I. and GELLER, J. Hemodynamic studies in a case of carcinoid cardiovascular syndrome. *Circulation*, 20: 208, 1959.
43. THORSON, Å. and NORDENFELT, O. Development of valvular lesions in metastatic carcinoid disease. *Brit. Heart J.*, 21: 243, 1959.
44. LEVINE, R. J. and FOLSE, R. Hemodynamic observations in a case of carcinoid heart disease associated with an atrial right-to-left shunt. *Am. Heart J.*, 62: 830, 1961.
45. SCHWABER, J. R. and LUKAS, D. S. Hyperkinemia and cardiac failure in the carcinoid syndrome. *Am. J. Med.*, 32: 846, 1962.
46. BRADLEY, T. R., BUTTERWORTH, R. F., REID, G. and TRAUTNER, E. M. Nature of the lung enzyme which inactivates serum vasoconstrictor. *Nature, London*, 166: 911, 1950.
47. SPATZ, M. Carcinoid syndrome in tryptophan- and niacin-deficient guinea pigs. *Univ. Michigan M. Bull.*, 27: 289, 1961.

APPENDIX

Case Reports

CASE I. A forty-one year old white man (D. W., 01-19-90*) died on March 5, 1957. He had been well until June 1954 when he noted the onset of weight loss, easy fatiguability and diarrhea. In October 1955 acute pain in the right upper quadrant associated with fever and leukocytosis led to an exploratory laparotomy. Both the liver and mesenteric lymph nodes were enlarged and contained metastatic carcinoid. A carcinoid tumor 2 cm. in size was resected from the terminal ileum.

He was first seen at the Clinical Center in January 1956 and since operation had gained weight and strength and was asymptomatic. He weighed 68 kg. and measured 154 cm. in height. His blood pressure was 110/70 mm. Hg. There was no skin erythema. The heart was not enlarged. A short, early, grade 2/6 systolic murmur was heard along the upper left sternal border. The liver was greatly enlarged; the spleen was not felt. There was no ascites or peripheral edema. The chest roentgenogram disclosed an elevated right diaphragm. The electrocardiogram was interpreted to be normal. The urinary excretion of

* The clinical aspects of this case were previously reported by Sjoerdsma et al. [*40*], Case VIII.

5-hydroxyindoleacetic acid ranged from 157 to 192 mg. per 24 hours.

During this three week period of hospitalization facial flushing appeared. Following discharge the flushes increased in length and frequency. Diarrhea, easy fatiguability and abdominal fullness recurred, and in August 1956 he was hospitalized again. Physical findings were unchanged except for loss of weight and a more enlarged liver. The urinary excretion of 5-hydroxyindoleacetic acid now averaged 600 mg. per 24 hours. The electrocardiogram and chest roentgenogram were unchanged. His course was progressively downhill and was not significantly altered by therapy with 6-azouracil or 6-mercaptopurine. Terminally, hypotension and hypoglycemia appeared.

At autopsy (A57-49) he was emaciated, weighing 46 kg. The abdomen was greatly distended by a massively enlarged liver (weight, 7,400 gm.) which was largely replaced by a metastatic carcinoid tumor. Many fibrous adhesions bound loops of bowel to one another, to the undersurface of the liver and to the peritoneal surfaces. No residual tumor was seen in the intestinal tract; however, the mesenteric lymph nodes were large and matted together. The peritoneum was thick and gray, and the abdominal cavity contained 200 ml. of serous fluid.

The heart weighed 220 gm. A firm, white carcinoid tumor 1 cm. in size was present in the parietal pericardium. The carcinoid fibrosing process grossly was limited to the pulmonic valve. Its cusps were thickened, contracted and rigid, and the pulmonic valvular orifice was fixed in a more or less open position. A rare fibrous plaque was seen in the right atrium but not in the right ventricle. Grossly, the tricuspid valvular leaflets and chordae appeared normal, but histologically a few focal fibrous plaques were seen on the leaflets. The right ventricle was mildly dilated but not hypertrophied. The cardiac chambers on the left side and valves were normal. Histologically, metastatic tumor was widespread. (Table I.)

Case II. A fifty year old housewife (E. W., 01-14-46) died on November 18, 1957. She had been well until 1945 (age thirty-eight) when she noted the onset of transient episodes of flushing of the face and neck. These "blushing" attacks were not especially bothersome to her, however, until age forty-seven when they became more frequent and lasted longer. Each of three more severe attacks continued for several hours and was associated with wheezing, dyspnea and facial puffiness. In addition, at this time, diarrhea became apparent, and intermittent abdominal pain led to the discovery of an abdominal mass. Exploratory laparotomy was undertaken two and a half years before death, and multiple ileal tumors which histologically proved to be carcinoid were found along with metastatic deposits in the liver.

When first seen at the Clinical Center six months later (November 1955) she appeared healthy. Her blood pressure was 120/80 mm. Hg. There was marked erythema of the face. The heart was not enlarged, and the sounds were of good quality. A grade 1/6 soft blowing systolic murmur was heard in the second left intercostal space. The lungs were clear. The liver was greatly enlarged, nodular and nontender. The spleen was not palpable. There was no ascites or peripheral edema. Heberden's nodes and spindle-shaped deformities of the first interphalangeal joints were noted, but there was no limitation of motion. The electrocardiogram and chest roentgenogram appeared normal. The urinary excretion of 5-hydroxyindoleacetic acid ranged from 294 to 380 mg. per 24 hours.

Following one week in the hospital she returned home and continued to perform her usual household chores without difficulty until a year later (one year before death) when the diarrhea worsened, abdominal pain intermittently recurred and fatiguability, weight loss, low grade fever, pedal edema and anorexia appeared. An increase in the dosages of paregoric and thorazine, and the initiation of salt restriction and periodic injections of mercurial diuretics allowed her to remain comfortable and fairly active until two months before death when these remedies no longer controlled the signs and symptoms. She was rehospitalized and now showed evidence of marked weight loss. The neck veins were distended with the patient sitting up, and a deep systolic jugular pulsation was noted. A massive right pleural effusion was present. The heart was not enlarged, but the previously described murmur had become much louder and harsher, now of grade 4/6 intensity. In addition, a grade 3/6 early and mid-diastolic murmur also was heard along the lower left sternal border. The liver had enlarged, but no ascitic fluid was apparent. There was severe wasting of the extremities and 2 plus pitting edema of the lower part of the legs. The electrocardiogram showed a slight increase in the magnitude of the T waves as compared to the previous tracings. The chest roentgenogram confirmed the presence of a right pleural effusion. The urinary excretion of 5-hydroxyindoleacetic acid averaged approximately 1,250 mg. per 24 hours during her last two months. Treatment with 6-mercaptopurine failed to be of benefit. She became progressively weaker and died in hepatic failure with a "metabolic flap," jaundice and finally coma.

At autopsy (A57-238) she weighed 38 kg. and measured 158 cm. in length. Three discrete carcinoid tumors were found in the ileum with metastases to the regional, mediastinal and supraclavicular lymph nodes, liver (4,500 gm.), spleen (100 gm.), kidneys, ovary, adrenal and pituitary glands, bone marrow and heart. The abdominal cavity contained 200 ml., the right pleural space 1,000 ml., the left pleural space 1,500 ml. and the pericardial sac 100 ml. of serous fluid. Esophageal varices were present, and the stomach contained material the color of coffee grounds.

The heart weighed 250 gm. A metastatic carcinoid tumor was present in the ventricular septum. All chambers were dilated. The endocardium of the right atrium and the leaflets and chordae of the tricuspid valve were irregularly thickened by the deposition of smooth, white, fibrous tissue. This fibrosis extended irregularly over the papillary muscles of the right ventricle. The pulmonic valvular cusps were contracted and thickened by the deposition of similar fibrous material which produced a small, fixed pulmonic orifice. The sinuses of the pulmonic valve were much smaller than normal. The chambers and valves of the left side of the heart were normal. The right ventricle measured 0.3 cm. and the left, 1.2 cm. in thickness. The valve circumference measurements (in centimeters) were: tricuspid, 10.5; mitral, 10.0; pulmonic, 5.5; and aortic, 6.5.

Histologically, sections from the ileal tumors and from the metastatic implants disclosed carcinoid tumor. There was severe fatty change of the liver. In sections from the heart microscopic-sized carcinoid metastases were seen in the right and left atria, in the subepicardial adipose tissue overlying the right ventricle and in the ventricular septum. Sections from the coronary sinus, right atrium, tricuspid and pulmonic valves, and papillary muscles of the right ventricle confirmed typical carcinoid fibrosis in these regions.

Case III. A sixty-seven year old white man (G. M., 03-51-98) died on September 30, 1959. He had been well until 1952 (age sixty) when he noted the onset of periodic severe abdominal pain and diarrhea. An exploratory laparotomy in December 1953 revealed metastatic carcinoid in the mesenteric lymph nodes and in the liver. No search was made for the primary tumor. Following recovery from the operation, he returned to work and did well until January 1957 when he began to feel weak. In July 1958 facial flushing appeared. His liver now was greatly enlarged. He was believed to be in mild congestive cardiac failure and was treated thereafter with digitalis and a low salt diet. His weakness progressively worsened, and in January 1959 he had to discontinue working.

On admission to the Clinical Center June 1959, he was thin and appeared chronically ill. His blood pressure was 110/70 mm. Hg. The skin over the face and neck was thickened, erythematous, "cyanotic" and telangiectatic. The skin over the rest of the body and especially over the legs had a faint purple hue which blanched on pressure. Moderate sized A waves were present in the superficial jugular veins, and a systolic pulse was noted in the deep jugular veins. The anteroposterior diameter of the chest was increased, and occasional wheezes were heard. The heart sounds were distant. A short, high-pitched presystolic murmur, which strikingly increased in intensity with inspiration, was heard along the lower left sternal border. This murmur was discrete and terminated prior to the first sound. In addition, there was a loud systolic murmur in the same area, which began early after the first sound and did not increase with inspiration. After mild exercise a protodiastolic gallop was heard along the left sternal border. The liver was greatly enlarged, nodular and nontender. The spleen was not felt, and there was no ascites or peripheral edema. The electrocardiogram was normal. Chest roentgenogram disclosed a normal-sized heart and normal appearing lungs. His course, unaltered by dichloromethotrexate therapy, was progressively downhill; he became confused, comatose and died.

At autopsy (A59-192) he weighed 66 kg. and measured 183 cm. in length. The skin, particularly over the upper half of the body, was purple. The peritoneal cavity contained 700 ml., the left pleural space, 1000 ml., and the pericardial sac 50 ml. of serous fluid. The ileum, particularly in its distal portion, was matted together and bound to a large retroperitoneal mass which represented matted lymph nodes. Metastatic carcinoid tumor was seen in the mesenteric lymph nodes, as well, and also in the appendix and liver (2,500 gm.). Multiple carcinoid tumors, the largest of which measured 2.0 cm. in diameter, were present in the ileum. The largest ileal tumor burrowed through the bowel wall and was adherent to the omentum, mesentery and to other loops of small intestine and produced a partial intestinal obstruction.

The heart weighed 280 gm. and there was typical carcinoid fibrosis involving the tricuspid and pulmonic valves, right atrium and ventricle. The right atrium was dilated and its endocardium was smooth, thickened and whitish grey in appearance. The tricuspid valve leaflets and its chordae were shortened and thickened. The wall of the right ventricle measured up to 0.3 cm. in thickness, and the chamber was dilated. The three pulmonic valvular cusps were markedly thickened, rigid and contracted and the valve orifice stenotic. The valves and chambers of the left side of the heart were normal. There was moderate atherosclerosis of the coronary arteries.

Case IV. A fifty-nine year old white man (K. W., 01-04-45*) died on November 7, 1959. He had been well except for pulmonary tuberculosis, treated by pneumothorax from 1923 to 1926, until 1953 when he noted the onset of intermittent, explosive diarrhea, increasing fatiguability and weight loss. Erythematous flushes of the face and neck appeared in July 1954 and were noted daily thereafter. Needle biopsy of the liver in November 1954 was thought to show

* The clinical aspects of this case were previously reported by Sjoerdsma et al. [*40*], Case III.

"hepatoma." On exploration the following month, a segment of distal ileum containing two small carcinoid tumors was resected. Extensive metastatic carcinoid was seen in the liver. The flushes and diarrhea continued unabated. During 1955 dependent ankle edema and paroxysmal respiratory distress, characterized by a slightly productive cough, dyspnea and substernal oppression, appeared.

On admission to the Clinical Center April 1955, he weighed 77.1 kg.; his blood pressure was 115/80 mm. Hg. He appeared well but had frequent transient crimson flushes of the face and neck and blotchy erythema of the trunk and extremities. A and V waves were noted in the superficial jugular veins, and systolic pulsations were seen in the deep jugular veins. Wheezes were audible over both lung fields during paroxysms of cough and dyspnea. The heart was not enlarged, and the heart sounds were normal. A soft systolic blowing murmur, which increased in intensity with inspiration, was heard along the lower left sternal border. The upper part of the abdomen was protuberant, the liver extremely large and nodular. Vasomotor episodes were induced repeatedly by manual massage over the liver. The spleen was not felt. There was 2 plus pedal and pretibial pitting edema.

The chest roentgenogram showed extensive pleural and parenchymal changes in the right hemithorax and a slightly enlarged heart. On cardiac fluoroscopy the right atrium was believed to be enlarged. The electrocardiograms were interpreted as normal. Right cardiac catheterization revealed elevated pressures in the right atrium with V waves up to 34 mm. Hg, and a pressure curve typical of tricuspid insufficiency. The A waves were also elevated and tricuspid stenosis was suspected as well, but the catheter could not be passed through the tricuspid valvular orifice. Peripheral arterial oxygen saturation was 95 per cent. The urinary 5-hydroxyindoleacetic acid assays during his seventy-four days in the hospital ranged from 380 to 580 mg. per 24 hours.

In August 1955 the flushes increased in severity, his abdomen increased in size, his ankles and lower legs swelled, and his strength lessened. These signs were improved greatly by diuretic therapy and a single abdominal paracentesis. Thereafter, until his final hospitalization in October 1959, his peripheral edema and abdominal swelling were well controlled by a low salt diet and periodic treatment with diuretics. The diarrhea was well controlled by the administration of paregoric. Physical examination on readmission was unchanged except for a slightly large liver. Electrocardiogram now showed low voltage and right axis deviation. Chest roentgenogram disclosed a left pleural effusion and probably an increase in cardiac size in addition to the changes noted previously. On November 6, 1959, eighteen days following admission, early one morning while sitting on the bedpan, he suddenly collapsed, became hypotensive and comatose. Repeat electrocardiograms showed only bigeminal rhythm and frequent premature ventricular contractions. The following day he died.

At autopsy (A59-223), he weighed 56 kg. and measured 183 cm. in length. The skin over the face, neck and upper anterior chest had a purplish discoloration. The abdomen was protuberant, and there was 2 plus pitting edema of the lower part of the legs. The peritoneal cavity contained excessive fluid. The peritoneum and serosal surface of the bowel were thickened. At the ileoileal anastomosis, two feet proximal to the ileocecal valve, there was a small carcinoid tumor. No other tumor was seen in the intestine except for a small nodule on the serosal surface of the appendix. The liver (1,800 gm.) contained numerous carcinoid implants. No other metastases were seen.

The heart weighed 350 gm. Focal fibrous plaques, carcinoid type, were present on the intima of both the superior and inferior vena cavae. Both the right atrium and ventricle were dilated. The foramen ovale was probe-patent but valvular-competent. The endocardium of the right atrium was thickened, smooth and whitish grey. The tricuspid valvular cusps and chordae were thickened, shortened and fibrotic. This valve measured 15 cm. in circumference and easily admitted three fingers. Only one small endocardial plaque was seen in the right ventricle. Its wall measured 0.4 cm. in thickness. The pulmonary valvular cusps were contracted, shortened and fibrotic, and the orifice, although contracted, was fixed in an open position. The chambers and valves of the left side of the heart were normal. There was severe coronary arterial atherosclerosis.

Case v. A fifty-seven year old white woman (S. W., 09-97-07) died on February 22, 1961. She had been well until 1957 when intermittent diarrhea (eight to ten watery movements daily) and pedal edema appeared. On examination she was found to have cardiomegaly and hepatomegaly. In 1959, one to one and a half years later, she noted periodic wheezing and dyspnea. Nine months thereafter facial flushing and abdominal pain of the right upper quadrant appeared. From 1957 to 1960 her weight decreased from 118 to 82 kg.

On admission to the Clinical Center in May 1960, she was still obese. Her blood pressure was 170/100 mm. Hg. Her face and neck were plethoric and contained telangiectases. No abnormal pulsations were seen in the superficial or deep jugular veins. The anteroposterior diameter of the chest was increased. Breath sounds were distant, but no wheezes were heard. A faint right ventricular lift was felt. The first heart sound at the apex was diminished, but an atrial sound was heard at the lower left sternal border during deep inspiration. A grade 2/6 systolic blowing murmur, which did not increase with inspiration, and an early diastolic rumble without presystolic accentuation, were heard along the lower left sternal border. The liver was markedly enlarged; the spleen was not felt. There was 2 plus pitting edema of the lower part of the legs.

The chest roentgenogram showed the heart to be slightly enlarged and the aorta, tortuous. Electrocardiograms demonstrated normal sinus rhythm, digitalis effect and prolongation of the P-R interval. A gastrointestinal series of the upper part of the gastrointestinal tract disclosed a "markedly irritable" small intestine. The urinary determinations of 5-hydroxyindoleacetic acid varied from 161 to 283 mg. per day during her 117 days in the hospital. She was treated with methyl-dopa, isoniazid and cyproheptidine without detectable benefit.

Following discharge in September 1960 and until her final admission four months later, she noted increasing dyspnea, edema and weight gain despite diuretic and digitalis therapy. The flushes and intermittent abdominal pains persisted. She was readmitted on January 25, 1961, and the physical findings, other than evidence of increased edema and hepatomegaly, were unchanged. On February 21, bronchopneumonia developed, and she died the following day.

At autopsy (A61-68) she was obese (weight 60.6 kg., height 141 cm.). The body cavities contained no excessive fluid. A carcinoid tumor 0.8 cm. in size was present immediately proximal to the ileocecal valve. Other carcinoid nodules were present in the periappendiceal, omental and mesenteric tissues, liver (2300 gm.), kidney and thyroid gland. Carcinoid nodules, microscopically, also were seen in the gallbladder. The lungs were congested and contained foci of bronchopneumonia.

The heart (Fig. 1) weighed 270 gm. The right atrium and ventricle were dilated and their walls "brittle-like" in consistency. The endocardium of the right atrium and right ventricle, tricuspid and pulmonic valves was diffusely involved by the carcinoid fibrosing process. The valves and chambers of the left side of the heart appeared normal.

Case vi. A sixty-four year old white man (B. E., 03-61-20) died on August 12, 1961. He had been well until approximately 1956 when angina pectoris developed which thereafter was present intermittently. In 1958 he noted the onset of weight loss, and during the next three years his weight decreased from 70 to 50 kg. On May 9, 1960, he had an attack of prolonged substernal chest pain not relieved by nitroglycerin treatment and associated with severe weakness and dyspnea, and was hospitalized for two weeks. The following month pedal and sacral edema and occasional paroxysmal nocturnal dyspnea appeared, but these were ameliorated by diuretic therapy. Also, in June 1960, he noted the onset of diarrhea (four to eight bowel movements daily), periodic flushes of the face and upper trunk, intermittent severe abdominal cramps and weakness. In January 1961, on examination at another hospital, he was found to have hepatomegaly and elevated urinary excretion of 5-hydroxyindoleacetic acid.

On admission to the Clinical Center June 13, 1961, he appeared weak and undernourished. The blood pressure was 130/80 mm. Hg. There was a marked reddish blue discoloration of the nose and malar areas of the face, hands, arms, feet and lower part of the legs. V waves were seen in the superficial jugular veins. The lungs were clear. The heart was enlarged, the point of maximal impulse being in the fifth left intercostal space in the left anterior axillary line. Right and left ventricular precordial lifts were palpated. The first heart sound at the apex was normal. The second heart sound over the aortic area was louder than the second heart sound over the pulmonary area and paradoxically split. A protodiastolic gallop was heard at the apex and along the lower left sternal border, and a loud ejection sound was heard at the lower left sternal border. A grade 2/6 short, soft systolic murmur was audible at the base and a grade 3/6 ejection-type systolic murmur, at the apex and along the left sternal border. Also, a grade 2/6 low-pitched diastolic murmur was present at the apex, and a similar but higher pitched diastolic rumble, which increased in intensity with inspiration, along the lower left sternal border. The abdomen was distended. The liver was large, nontender and nodular. There was 3 plus pitting edema of the lower part of the legs. The urinary excretion of 5-hydroxyindoleacetic acid averaged approximately 350 mg. per 24 hours. The electrocardiogram showed only low voltage. Chest roentgenogram revealed slight left ventricular hypertrophy. The gastrointestinal series of the upper part of the gastrointestinal tract and the small bowel series as well as a barium enema were interpreted to be normal.

During his two months in the hospital, the abdominal cramps, diarrhea and flushing episodes continued. He was treated by a salt restricted diet, intermittent diuretics, opiates and two experimental chemotherapeutic agents (methyl-dopa and MK-485) without significant benefit. During the final five weeks his condition rapidly deteriorated. The abdominal pains became severe, and right-sided congestive cardiac failure became evident. He died in hepatic coma.

At autopsy (A61-193) he weighed 50 kg. and measured 138 cm. in length. There was no excessive fluid in the body cavities. The small intestine from the ligament of Treitz to the ileocecal valve, following formalin-fixation, measured 3.1 M. in length. Twelve distinct, firm, white carcinoid tumors were found in the small intestine beginning 147 cm. distal to the ligament of Treitz and ending 75 cm. proximal to the ileocecal valve; the largest measured 2 cm. in diameter, the smallest 0.4 cm. in diameter. Some of the tumors were centrally ulcerated. The serosal surface beneath the tumors was smooth. There was no evidence of bowel obstruction. The liver (1,600 gm.), mesenteric lymph nodes and pancreas contained metastatic carcinoid. The spleen weighed 160 gm., and its surface had a "frost-like" appearance.

The heart weighed 400 gm. All chambers were dilated and hypertrophied. There was severe fibrous involvement, carcinoid type, of the mitral valve as well as of the pulmonic and tricuspid valves and right atrium (Fig. 2 and 3). There was no intracardiac communication. The tricuspid valve appeared incompetent, the pulmonic and mitral valves stenotic. The pulmonic valvular cusps were contracted and thickened. Distinct white fibrous plaques were seen at the base of the pulmonary trunk. The mitral valvular cusps and chordae were thickened and shortened. A fibrous plaque was present on the endocardial surface of the left ventricle. There was severe coronary arterial atherosclerosis.

Histologically, sections from the lungs disclosed proliferation of the intima of the pulmonary veins and, to a lesser extent, of the small muscular pulmonary arteries and arterioles. The media of the muscular pulmonary arteries was thickened. In addition, there was mild fibrous thickening of the alveolar septa, and some of the alveolar spaces contained numerous hemosiderin-laden macrophages. (These changes in the lung are seen commonly in patients with mitral valvular disease.) Also, there was mild focal acute pneumonia. Sections from the pancreas disclosed the presence of acute pancreatitis. Foci of inflammatory cells also were present in the hypothalamus and midbrain. An acute infarct was noted in the spleen. Carcinoid metastases were seen in sections of vertebral bone marrow.

Case vii. A fifty-seven year-old white woman (R. W., 03-85-05) died on November 19, 1961. In 1951 (age forty-seven) she had had a left radical mastectomy for carcinoma of the breast. There had been no evidence of recurrence thereafter, and she had been well until February 1958 when a sudden attack of fecal vomiting prompted the diagnosis of acute intestinal obstruction and a laparotomy was performed. A carcinoid tumor was found in the terminal ileum and was resected along with the ascending colon. Carcinoid metastases were seen in three of twenty-seven mesenteric lymph nodes. Immediately after the operation, the urinary excretion of 5-hydroxyindoleacetic acid was found to be elevated. Shortly thereafter, however, the urinary excretion of 5-hydroxyindoleacetic acid was reported to have dropped to normal levels and remained so until February 1959 when it again became elevated. In June 1960 hepatomegaly was noted. From November 1960 until her death one year later, she was in bed, getting up only to go to the bathroom. During this last year of life, anorexia, watery diarrhea, weight loss and marked weakness appeared. There was no history of asthma or facial blushing.

On admission to the Clinical Center October 4, 1961, she appeared thin and chronically ill. Her blood pressure was 110/65 mm. Hg. There was an atypical symmetric "cyanosis" from the forehead to the umbilicus. Prominent V waves were noted in the superficial jugular veins. A right ventricular precordial lift was felt. A soft, right ventricular diastolic gallop was heard. A grade 2/6 ejection-type systolic murmur was present at the cardiac base, most prominent in the pulmonic area, and a grade 3/6 holosystolic blowing murmur, which increased with inspiration, was heard at the apex. The predominant cardiac lesion was believed to be tricuspid insufficiency. The liver was massively enlarged and pulsatile. The spleen was not felt. There was evidence of a right pleural effusion, otherwise the lungs were clear. There was 1 plus pitting pedal and pretibial edema and 3 plus pitting sacral edema.

Chest roentgenogram disclosed a left pleural effusion but no cardiomegaly. The electrocardiogram showed low voltage, prominent P waves suggestive of right atrial enlargement and a vertical axis. The values for urinary 5-hydroxyindoleacetic acid on two occasions were 187 and 274 mg. per 24 hours. Her final month of life was characterized by multiple electrolyte derangements, azotemia and oliguria. Death came quietly.

At autopsy (A61-266) she was emaciated (weight 50 kg., height 134 cm.). The skin of the face, neck and anterior trunk was "cyanotic" and telangiectatic. There was no evidence of recurrence of tumor in the healed left radical mastectomy incision. Both axillary and supraclavicular regions were free of lymphadenopathy, and no nodules were present in the right breast. The abdomen was protuberant. There was 2 plus pitting pedal, pretibial and sacral edema. Excessive fluid was present in the abdominal cavity (525 ml.), left pleural (300 ml.) and right pleural (450 ml.) spaces. The pericardial cavity contained 15 ml. of watery fluid. The small intestine was matted together by tumorous adhesions but there was no evidence of intestinal obstruction. The ileocolonic anastomosis was intact. No tumor was found in the bowel. The peritoneum was thick, leathery and studded with carcinoid implants. Numerous carcinoid tumors also were seen on the surfaces of the pelvic organs and in the pancreas and liver.

The heart (Fig. 4 and 5) weighed 200 gm. There was serous atrophy of the subepicardial adipose tissue and brown atrophy of the myocardium. The wall of the inferior vena cava was markedly thickened and its intima, white, and a few focal whitish grey elevations were present on the intima of the superior vena cava. (Fig. 6.) The right atrium and ventricle were dilated. The endocardium of the right atrium contained numerous focal greyish white fibrous plaques, most pronounced on the septum.

The foramen ovale was closed. The tricuspid and pulmonic valvular leaflets and the tricuspid chordae were fibrotic, thickened and contracted. Only one fibrous plaque was seen in the right ventricle, and it was located just below the papillary muscle of the conus. The orifice of both the tricuspid and pulmonic valves were fixed. The base of the pulmonary trunk folded double over the pulmonic valve, a result of the fibrous proliferative process within the sinuses of the pulmonic valve. A single fibrous plaque was present on the ventricular aspect of the anterior mitral leaflet and in the ascending aorta. Multiple carcinoid-type plaques also were present throughout the aorta, usually superimposed on atherosclerotic lesions.

Case viii. A fifty-two year old white woman (H. M., 03-41-30) died on January 12, 1962. She had been well until May 1960, when she noted the onset of diarrhea (eight to ten loose bowel movements daily), periodic flushing of the face, neck and upper part of the arm, wheezing, intermittent pain of the right upper part of the abdomen and low grade fever. Because of the persistence of these symptoms she underwent exploratory laparotomy in September 1960, and peritoneal carcinoid implants were found. No search for the site of the primary was undertaken. Following the operation, weight loss and weakness continued unabated.

On admission to the Clinical Center February 14, 1961, she appeared chronically ill (weight 56 kg.). The blood pressure was 120/80 mm. Hg. Numerous telangiectases were noted in the skin over the entire body. No abnormal venous pulsations were seen in the neck. The lungs were clear to auscultation. The heart was not enlarged. The second heart sound was louder at the left than at the right second intercostal space. A grade 2/6 ejection-type systolic murmur was heard along the left sternal border. Also, a grade 2/6 blowing systolic murmur and a grade 1/6 low-pitched diastolic rumble were heard at the apex. The liver was large but nontender. The spleen was not felt. There was no peripheral edema. Urinary excretion of 5-hydroxyindoleacetic acid on numerous occasions averaged approximately 200 mg. per 24 hours. Chest roentgenogram disclosed a normal-sized heart. The electrocardiogram showed generalized diminution in QRS and T wave amplitudes.

During her almost one year period of hospitalization, she was treated with several cancer chemotherapeutic agents without detectable benefit. During the final four months she became extremely cachectic and noted the development persistent peripheral edema and ascites. Her last week of life was characterized by vomiting, extreme weakness and finally coma.

At autopsy (A62-9) she weighed 43 kg. and measured 161 cm. in length. The skin over the anterior chest and neck was plethoric. The abdomen was protuberant. The abdominal cavity contained 4,600 ml. of serous fluid. Portions of the bowel were matted together by multiple adhesions. There also were adhesions of the intestine to the liver, peritoneum and omentum. The liver weighed 2,800 gm. and contained multiple carcinoid metastases, many of which were necrotic. The spleen weighed 130 gm. An annular carcinoid tumor 1 cm. in size was found in the jejunum. No other intestinal tumors were seen. The lungs, pulmonary arteries and veins appeared normal.

The heart weighed 250 gm. There was marked serous atrophy of the subepicardial adipose tissue and brown atrophy of the myocardium. The right atrium and ventricle were dilated. Focal fibrous plaques were present on the intima of the inferior and superior venae cavae, coronary sinus and on the endocardium of the right atrium, tricuspid valve and its chordae, right ventricle, pulmonic valve and mitral valve and its chordae. (Fig. 7 and 8.) Although fibrous plaques were present within the sinuses of the pulmonic valve, its cusps were freely movable, and the appearance of this valve suggested that it had functioned normally. The left atrium was slightly dilated and its endocardium, although uniformly thickened, was free of fibrous plaques. The foramen ovale was closed. The mitral valvular leaflets and chordae were thickened, but the commissures were not fused. The appearance of this valve suggests that it probably was neither significantly stenotic nor regurgitant. No fibrous lesions were seen in the left ventricle. The aortic valve was normal. Histologic study of sections of the lung disclosed marked intimal proliferation in the pulmonary veins. (Fig. 9.)

Case ix. A sixty-nine year old white man (T. M., 04-00-87) died on February 11, 1962. He had been well until March 1961 when he noted anorexia, weight loss and intermittent pain of the lower abdomen. In June 1961 intermittent diarrhea developed (twelve watery bowel movements daily) as well as periodic flushes of the face and neck and, rarely, wheezing respirations. In September 1961 he experienced acute intestinal obstruction and underwent laparotomy. Two carcinoid tumors were found in the ileum. These tumors compressed the mesenteric arteries, producing gangrene of a portion of the small intestine, which was resected. Carcinoid metastases were found in the liver and in the mesenteric lymph nodes. During the six months before operation he had lost 30 kg. During the first four months following operation, he regained 8 kg. Diarrhea did not recur following operation. He had had orthopnea, paroxysmal nocturnal dyspnea and systemic hypertension intermittently for a number of years, but there was no history of angina pectoris.

On admission to the Clinical Center January 8, 1962, he weighed 57.9 kg. and was slightly dyspneic.

His initial blood pressure was 180/110 but thereafter remained in the vicinity of 120/80 mm. Hg. The superficial jugular veins were distended with the patient sitting upright. The anteroposterior diameter of the chest was increased, and inspiratory rales and occasional expiratory wheezes were heard throughout the lung fields. The point of maximum cardiac impulse was in the fifth left intercostal space, just to the right of the left anterior axillary line. The second cardiac sound was louder in the aortic than in the pulmonic area. A grade 2/6 blowing systolic murmur was heard at the apex, and a grade 1/6 low-pitched, ejection-type systolic murmur was heard along the lower left sternal border. No abnormal jugular venous waves and no hepatic pulsations were noted. The liver was enlarged, the spleen not palpable. There was slight pretibial pitting edema.

The chest roentgenogram showed enlargement of the left ventricle and tortuosity of the ascending aorta. The electrocardiogram disclosed normal sinus rhythm, left axis deviation, left ventricular ischemia and absent R waves in leads V_2 and V_3, suggesting an old anterior myocardial infarct. The urinary excretion of 5-hydroxyindoleacetic averaged approximately 100 mg. per 24 hours.

While in the hospital, he had many transient flushes, and occasionally these were associated with hypotension. The number of flushes was decreased considerably during treatment with phenoxybenzamine. On the day of death the patient collapsed while defecating, became cyanotic, complained of left precordial chest pain, had convulsions and died.

At autopsy (A62-34) he was cachectic (weight 51.6 kg., height 177 cm.). The skin of the chest was plethoric and telangiectatic. No excessive fluid was present in the abdominal, pleural or pericardial cavities. Carcinoid metastases were found in the regional lymph nodes and in the liver (2,600 gm.). An intact ileoileostomy was present approximately 60 cm. proximal to the ileocecal valve. No nodules were found in the intestinal tract.

The heart weighed 475 gm. The right atrium, right ventricle and left atrium were dilated. No fibrous plaques were noted on the intima of the vena cavae or on the endocardium of the right atrium. The tricuspid valvular orifice was smaller than normal but fixed in an open position. (Fig. 10.) Its leaflets and chordae were considerably shortened and thickened. The right ventricular wall measured up to 4.5 cm. in thickness. The pulmonic valvular cusps were thickened and pearly white, and the orifice was fixed in an open position. The left atrium and mitral valve were normal. The foramen ovale was closed. The left ventricular wall measured up to 1.0 cm. in thickness. In the apex of the left ventricle and involving the most caudal portion of the ventricular septum there was an old healed myocardial infarct which measured 2 by 4 cm. in size. Foci of calcium were present within each of the aortic sinuses of Valsalva, but there was no fusion of the commissures of the aortic valve. The coronary arteries were markedly tortuous and atherosclerotic.

ADDENDUM

Since this manuscript was submitted for publication, we have studied both clinically and at autopsy two additional patients with the carcinoid syndrome. One, a forty year old Negro man (L. P., 03-10-65), died in April 1963 with widespread carcinoid tumor from a primary tumor in the small intestine. The total length of his illness was three years, during which time he had severe weight loss, diarrhea, flushes, wheezing, exertional dyspnea, hepatomegaly, ascites, peripheral edema and terminally, severe hepatic and renal failure (total serum bilirubin 22 mg. per 100 ml., serum urea nitrogen 199 mg. per 100 ml.). On examination the heart was not enlarged. A blowing pansystolic murmur which increased in intensity with inspiration was audible over the entire precordium, and a rumbling diastolic murmur along the left sternal border. The urinary excretion of 5-hydroxyindoleacetic acid ranged from 296 to 432 mg. per twenty-four hours. Electrocardiogram disclosed low voltage and peaked P waves characteristic of right atrial hypertrophy. At autopsy (A63-96) there was typical carcinoid fibrosis involving the tricuspid, pulmonic and mitral valves and right atrium. There was no intracardiac communication and no carcinoid tumor in the lungs. The mitral valvular fibrosis was less extensive than that of the tricuspid and pulmonic valves. The involvement of the mitral valve, which also included a few of its chordae tendineae, was probably not hemodynamically significant. Carcinoid metastases were present in the peritoneum, appendix, liver (2,900 gm.), pancreas, biliary tree, spleen (200 gm.), prostate gland, testes, bone, abdominal and thoracic lymph nodes, and heart (myocardium of left ventricle and visceral pericardium).

The second patient, a sixty-five year old white woman (L. C., 03-38-59), also died in April 1963 following a three year illness characterized by diarrhea, flushes, partial intestinal obstruction and progressive emaciation. Widespread peritoneal metastases and a primary tumor of the ileum were found at ileotransverse colon anastomosis two years before death. There were no precordial murmurs. Electrocardiogram showed low voltage. The urinary excretion of 5-hydroxyindoleacetic acid before operation ranged from 14 to 23 mg. per twenty-four hours and during the two years after operation was normal (2 to 6 mg. per twenty-four hours). (These are the lowest levels of urinary 5-hydroxyindoleacetic acid recorded at the Clinical Center in a patient with the carcinoid syndrome.) At autopsy (A63-67) the patient weighed only 28 kg. The heart weighed 150 gm., and its valves and chambers were normal. Carcinoid implants were extensive throughout the peritoneal surfaces and abdominal and retroperitoneal lymph nodes. The liver weighed 500 gm. and contained only a few small carcinoid implants, the largest of which measured 1 cm. in diameter. The spleen weighed 30 gm.

Acute Severe Mitral Regurgitation Secondary to Ruptured Chordae Tendineae

Clinical, Hemodynamic, and Pathologic Considerations

By William C. Roberts, M.D., Eugene Braunwald, M.D., and Andrew G. Morrow, M.D.

THE MAJORITY of patients with severe mitral regurgitation have enlarged left atria, atrial fibrillation, a history of acute rheumatic fever, and a gradual onset of symptoms of cardiac decompensation that may persist for many years. This report describes 10 patients with severe mitral regurgitation caused by rupture of one or more chordae tendineae, and contrasts the clinical, radiographic, hemodynamic, and pathologic findings in these patients with those commonly noted in patients with the more usual form of mitral regurgitation. Thus, the majority of the patients with ruptured chordae tendineae had little left atrial enlargement, were in sinus rhythm, and had not had a history of acute rheumatic fever. The symptoms of cardiac decompensation generally appeared abruptly, and were usually present for only several months before they led to the patient's death or necessitated operative treatment. An appreciation of this relatively pure, acute form of mitral regurgitation is important in the understanding of the wide range of physiologic, pathologic, and clinical findings that may accompany this valvular lesion.

Description of Patients

A summary of the clinical, electrocardiographic, hemodynamic and pathologic findings in the individual patients is presented in table 1.

History. The 10 patients ranged in age from 17 to 54 years. Six were women. Only one patient (L. L.) had a history suggestive of acute rheumatic fever, and none had a history of chorea or chest trauma. Six patients had a definite history of bacterial endocarditis, and each had been asymptomatic and fully active prior to the onset of the infection. Pregnancy appeared to have played a role in the appearance of the bacterial endocarditis in three patients; A. L. and A. A. developed the infection shortly after parturition, while patient R. H. developed pyogenic endometritis after an abortion which in turn was followed by bacterial endocarditis. In two patients each *alpha streptococcus* and *staphylococcus aureus* were the organisms responsible for the endocarditis, and in one patient each the causative organisms were *streptococcus faecalis* and *staphylococcus albus.* The onset of cardiac decompensation was abrupt in nine patients and was progressive thereafter, while in patient V. C., who did not have a history of bacterial endocarditis, symptoms developed more slowly. In seven patients the period of time from the onset of symptoms of cardiac failure to autopsy or operation was less than 16 months, while in the other three patients the interval ranged from 5 to 8 years. Seven patients had no knowledge of heart murmurs before the onset of bacterial endocarditis or cardiac failure. Three patients, two of whom had a history of bacterial endocarditis, were known to have had precordial murmurs for periods ranging from 12 to 43 years before operation or death. In one of these patients, the murmur may have resulted from the presence of associated partial anomalous pulmonary venous connection and a small atrial septal defect.

Each of the patients complained of easy fatigability, exertional and nocturnal dyspnea, and all but one had pedal edema. All were treated with digitalis and salt restriction, but despite these measures they were severely disabled and considered to be in functional classes III or IV.

Physical Examination. Each of the 10 patients had prominent right ventricular and less prominent left ventricular lifts as well as easily papable apical systolic thrills. The sound of pulmonic valve closure was accentuated in all patients, and a third heart sound was almost always audible. In every patient, a blowing pansystolic murmur of at least grade IV/VI intensity was heard over the entire precordium, loudest over the cardiac apex, with radiation to the left axilla. In two patients the murmur at the cardiac apex was of whistling or

From the Clinic of Surgery and the Cardiology Branch, National Heart Institute, National Institutes of Health, Bethesda, Maryland.

cooing quality, and in two others the systolic murmur was also audible over the entire vertebral column.[1] In five patients the systolic murmur along the lower left sternal border became louder during inspiration. Seven patients had short, low-pitched, mid-diastolic flow murmurs at the apex, and two patients had high-pitched, blowing, diastolic murmurs along the left sternal border. The liver was palpable and tender in the majority of the patients, and pulsated during systole in three of them.

Electrocardiograms (Fig. 1). Eight patients had sinus rhythm, and two had atrial fibrillation; in one of the latter this arrhythmia appeared shortly before death. Right axis deviation was present in five patients, and left axis deviation in one. Four patients had first-degree atrioventricular block. Right ventricular hypertrophy was present in seven patients and left ventricular hypertrophy as well in three. Seven patients exhibited the peaked P waves characteristic of right atrial enlargement, and one had left atrial enlargement.

Roentgenograms (Fig. 2). Some degree of cardiac enlargement was evident on the chest roentgenograms of all 10 patients. The left atrium was mildly or moderately enlarged in eight patients, and markedly enlarged in only the two patients who had been symptomatic for the longest times, 5 and 8 years. Both ventricles were considered to be enlarged in all 10 patients. Calcification in the region of the mitral valve was detected in only one patient (L. L.). Angiographic studies with left ventricular injection in each of two patients (A. F. and L. S.) showed near-normal sized left atria which expanded strikingly during ventricular systole, but there was no evidence of prolapse of a mitral valve leaflet into the left atrium.

Hemodynamic Findings (Fig. 3). All nine patients who underwent right heart catheterization had markedly elevated pulmonary arterial and right ventricular systolic pressures, ranging from 61 to 110 mm. Hg. The mean left atrial pressures were elevated to between 15 and 32 mm. Hg in eight patients, and within normal limits (11 mm. Hg) in the ninth. The v-wave peaks were abnormally elevated in all nine patients and ranged from 23 to 66 mm. Hg (average, 45 mm. Hg). The left ventricular end-diastolic pressure was normal ($\leqq$ 12 mm. Hg) in six of the eight patients in whom it was measured, and was markedly elevated (20 and 27 mm. Hg) in two. The

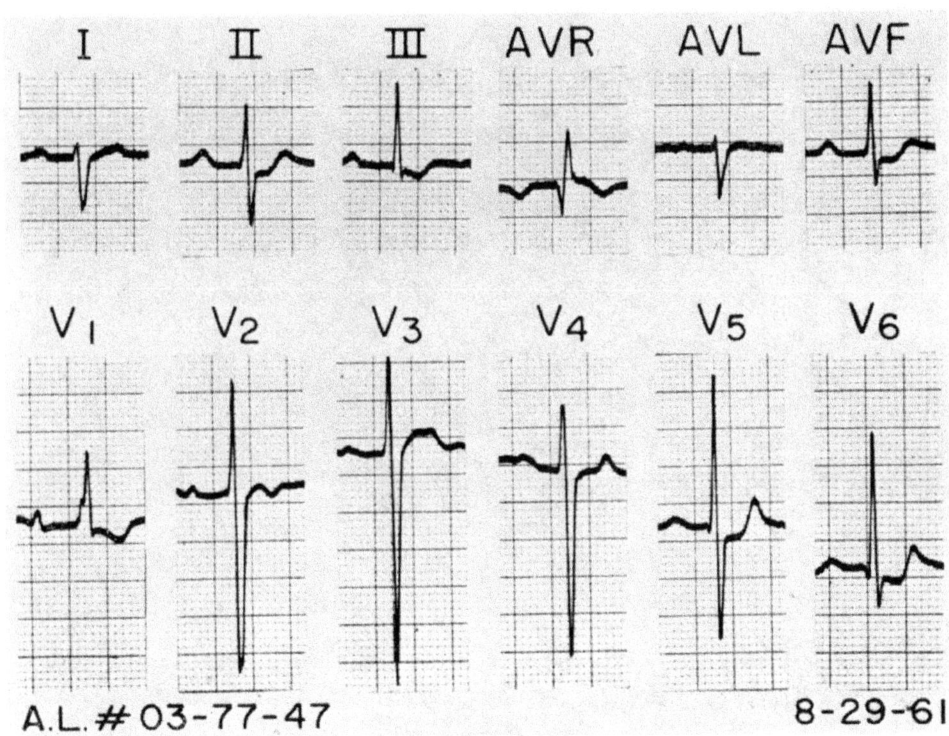

Figure 1

Electrocardiogram of patient A.L. Right axis deviation, right atrial enlargement, right ventricular hypertrophy, and possible left ventricular hypertrophy are present, although mitral regurgitation had been present for only 16 months.

Table 1

Clinical, Electrocardiographic, Hemodynamic, and Pathologic Data from the 10 Patients with Ruptured Mitral Chordae Tendineae

Patient no. (sex)	Age at death or at operation / Length of symptoms	History of bacterial endocarditis (organism)	Electro-cardiogram	Hemodynamic data: PA s/d (mean) (mm. Hg)	LA mean—v wave (mm. Hg)	LV s/d (mm. Hg)	Cardiac index (L./min./M.²)	Pulmonary vascular resistance (dynes sec. cm.⁻⁵)	LA size at operation (O) at autopsy (A)
1. V.C. 01-21-66 (M)	41 yr. / 5 yr.	—	AF, RAD, RAE, RVH, LVH	110/40 (67)	32—39*		1.4	1217	Dilated (A)
2. A.A. 01-71-62 (F)	37 yr. / 7 mo.	—	NSR, RAE, RVH		24—52	92/27			"Normal" (A)
3. A.L. 03-77-47 (F)	19 yr. / 16 mo.	+ Streptococcus Group D	NSR, RAD, RAE, RVH, First-degree HB	70/30 (45)	15—36	100/10	1.7	950	"Normal" (A)
4. R.H. 03-99-19 (F)	24 yr. / 5 mo.	+ Enterococcus	NSR, RAE, First-degree HB	72/32 (54)	27—66	108/11	1.5	1000	"Normal" (A)
5. P.H. 04-94-07 (F)	29 yr. / 5 yr.	+ Staphylococcus albus	NSR, RAD, RAE, RVH, LVH	105/40 (70)	15—35		1.6	2000	"Normal" (A)
6. B.F. 04-85-25 (F)	21 yr. / 13 mo.	+ Staphylococcus aureus	NSR, RAD, RAE, RVH, LVH	65/28† ↓ 32/11 (16)‡	11—23† ↓ 6—11‡	100/9†	1.4† ↓ 3.0‡	1100† ↓ 179‡	"Normal" (O)
7. J.W. 04-87-16 (M)	54 yr. / 8 yr.	+ Alpha strepto-coccus	NSR, RVH, LAE, First-degree HB	70/27 ↓(37)† 44/20 (28)‡	15—32† ↓ 7—10‡	90/11† ↓ 95/5‡	2.8‡	382‡	Dilated (O)
8. L.L. 05-45-40 (M)	53 yr. / 9 mo.	—	AF, LAD	61/25† ↓(39) 29/10 (17)‡	22—56† ↓ 10—21‡	81/9† ↓ 119/9‡	0.9† ↓ 3.2‡	1070† ↓ 94‡	"Normal" (O)
9. A.F. 05-78-22 (M)	48 yr. / 7 mo.	—	NSR, Nonspecific T-wave changes	84/30	25—65	100/20	1.8	609	"Normal" (O)
10. L.S. 05-99-23 (F)	17 yr. / 5 mo.	+ Staphylococcus aureus	NSR, RVH, RAE, RAD, First-degree HB	71/41 (51)	24*	86/12			"Normal" (A)

*Pulmonary arterial wedge pressures.
†Before operation.
‡Several months after operation.

Abbreviations: PA, pulmonary arterial pressure; LA, left atrial pressure; LV, left ventricular pressure; s/d (mean), systolic/diastolic (mean) pressures; AF, atrial fibrillation; RBBB, right bundle-branch block; NSR, normal sinus rhythm; RVH, right ventricular hypertrophy; RAE, right atrial enlargement; LVH, left ventricular hypertrophy; LAE, left atrial enlargement; LAD, left axis deviation; HB, heart block. "Normal," near normal size or only moderately dilated.

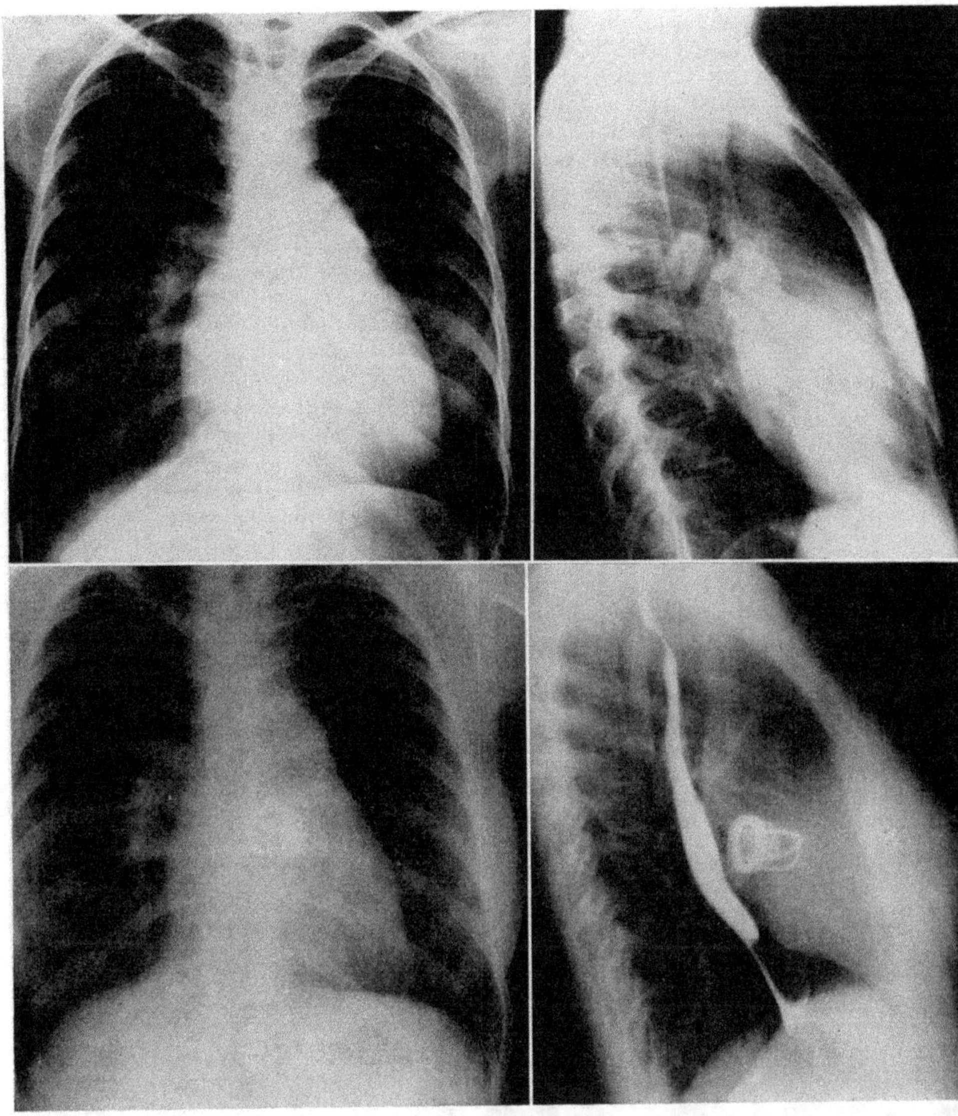

Figure 2

Roentgenograms obtained preoperatively (upper) *and 7 months postoperatively* (lower) *in patient B.F. This patient had had severe mitral regurgitation for 13 months before operation, but there was only minimal left atrial enlargement.*

cardiac output was markedly reduced in each of the seven patients in whom it was measured, and ranged from 0.9 to 1.8 L./min./M.^{2}, with an average of 1.5 L./min./M.^{2}. Pulmonary vascular resistance was calculated in seven patients and ranged from 609 to 2,000 with an average of 1135 dynes sec. cm.$^{-5}$. Indicator-dilution curves recorded from a systemic artery following injection into the left ventricle or left atrium in seven patients showed the prolonged descending limb characteristic of severe mitral regurgitation.

Pathologic Findings (Figs. 4-11). The mitral valves and chordae tendineae were examined in six patients at necropsy. In the other four patients the mitral valve was examined after it had been surgically excised with the chordae tendineae and papillary muscles intact. One patient died of heart failure, one from a complication of cardiac catheterization, three following mitral annuloplasty, and one following Starr-Edwards mitral valve replacement.

Ruptured chordae tendineae were responsible for mitral regurgitation in every patient, and in six of them the rupture was clearly the result of bacterial endocarditis. Active endocarditis was present in two patients (R. H. and L. S.); it involved the posterior half of the aortic leaflet of the mitral valve in one (fig. 6); and both anterior and posterior leaflets in the other patient. All chordae that had inserted into these portions of the valve had been destroyed. Organisms, however, were not found in sections of the valves of either of these patients. In six patients most or all of the chordae to one half of the anterior leaflet of the mitral valve were ruptured, in one patient all of the chordae that had been attached to the posterior leaflet were involved, and in three patients several chordae from both leaflets were destroyed. With the exception of the two patients with active endocarditis, there were no essential differences between the pathologic findings in the patients with and those without a history of bacterial endocarditis. Although some fibrous thickening of the mitral leaflet adjacent to the ruptured chordae was usually evident, the remaining mitral valve leaflets, commissures, and remaining chordae showed no apparent abnormalities. The aortic valve was normal in the six autopsied patients. In the other four patients, no abnormalities of the aortic valve were detected at the time of operation. The tricuspid and pulmonic valves also were normal in the hearts examined at necropsy.

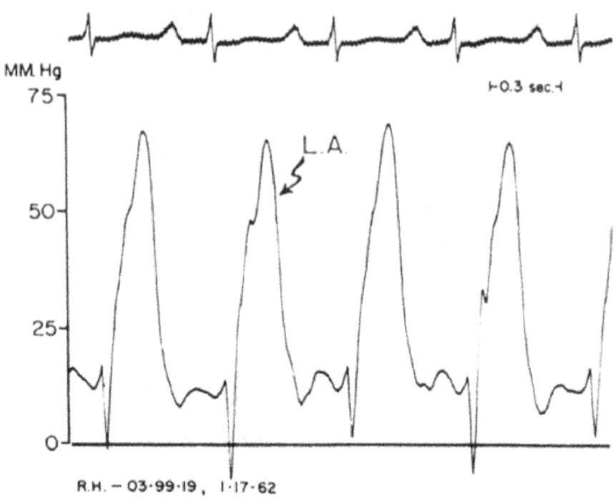

Figure 3

Left atrial pressure tracing in patient R.H., who had had mitral regurgitation for only 5 months.

The left atrial chamber was near normal size, or only moderately enlarged, in the six autopsied patients, and in each of them the left atrial wall was considerably thickened. In two of the patients, who had had symptoms for 5 and 8 years, the left atrium was severely dilated. Jet lesions were present on the endocardial surface of the left atrium in all 10 patients, their location depending upon the position of the ruptured chordae. The right

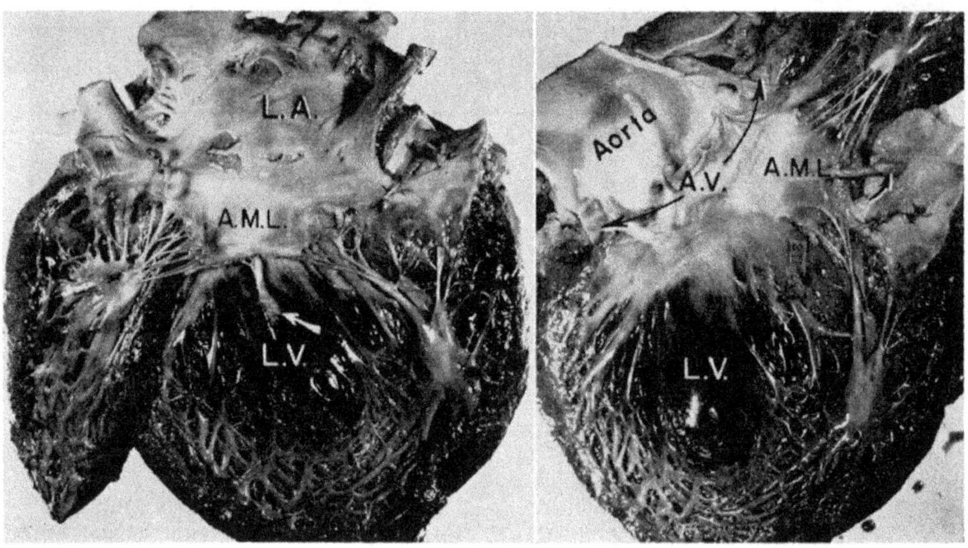

Figure 4

Photographs of heart of patient 2 (A.A.). Left. *The left atrium (L.A.), mitral valve, and left ventricle (L.V.) are seen. The ruptured chorda* (arrow), *which is club-shaped, arises from the midportion of the anterior mitral leaflet (A.M.L.). The nonruptured chordae are normal. The left atrium is not dilated, but the left ventricle is considerably dilated.* Right. *The anterior mitral leaflet (A.M.L.) is now seen from the ventricular aspect. The aortic valve (A.V.) is normal.*

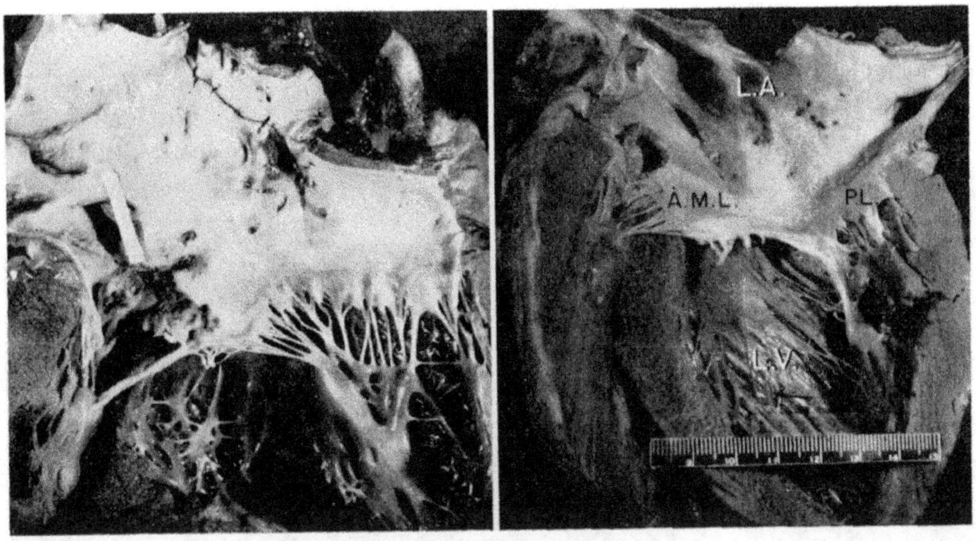

Figure 5

Photographs of opened left atrium (L.A.), mitral valve, and left ventricle (L.V.) of patient 3 (A.L.) left, *and patient 5 (P.H.)* right. *Chordae tendineae that had attached to the anterior (A.M.L.) and posterior (P.L.) mitral leaflets adjacent to the anterolateral commissure are absent in the heart of patient 3* (left). *The arrow points to the site of jet lesion in the left atrium in this patient. All chordae tendineae from the posterior portion of the anterior mitral leaflet (A.M.L.) are severed in patient 5* (right). *The nonruptured chordae in each patient are normal, and in neither is the left atrium dilated.*

ventricle was dilated and hypertrophied in the six patients studied at necropsy.

On microscopic examination, there were no Aschoff bodies in sections of the heart from any of the six autopsied patients, and sections of the left atrial walls disclosed severe hypertrophy of the myocardial fibers and marked thickening of the endocardium (fig. 8). Histologic examination of sections from the lungs of the six autopsied patients disclosed grade 3/6 hypertensive pulmonary vascular changes in each (classification of Heath and Edwards[2]). Three patients had ossific nodules scattered in the lungs. Examples of microscopic changes in the lungs of two patients are shown in figures 9 and 10. The pulmonary vascular changes in patients R. H. and A. A. were particularly noteworthy, since these patients had had clinical evidence of mitral regurgitation for only 5 and 7 months, respectively, before death. There was severe centrolobular hepatic congestion in each of the six autopsied patients, an example of which is shown in figure 11.

Discussion

In the past, the conditions considered to be responsible for ruptured chordae tendineae of the mitral valve included rheumatic fever,[3–5] trauma,[6] so-called spontaneous rupture,[7] and bacterial endocarditis involving either diseased or normal valves.[5, 8–10] Most authors have considered that chordal rupture occurs predominantly in previously diseased valves. In the National Institutes of Health collection of almost 150 hearts with acquired mitral valvular disease, there are only two with ruptured mitral chordae, and in both patients this was clearly of secondary importance in the resultant regurgitation. On the other hand, we have encountered the 10 patients, described in this report, who had ruptured mitral chordae involving a valve that otherwise appeared not to be grossly diseased. Critical review of earlier reports, including published photographs of ruptured mitral chordae, indicated numerous instances of ruptured mitral chordae in valves that also did not appear grossly abnormal,[4, 5, 7, 10–17] although some of the authors had considered that rheumatic heart disease was the underlying process. Although bacterial endocarditis tends to affect obviously malformed or previously diseased valves most often, and chronic rheumatic involvement might thus predispose to chordal rupture, it seems entirely possible that the marked thickening and shortening of the chordae tendineae of a rheumatic valve may actually serve to protect these structures from rupture. On the basis of the experience with the patients described in this report, as well as the many published illustrations of ruptured chordae in valves that do not appear grossly abnormal, it is suggested that bacterial endocarditis occurring in hearts without detectable anatomic valvular abnormalities is an important cause of chordal rupture.

Immediately following rupture of a single chorda in the dog, the left atrial pressure, particularly the v-wave peak, rises abruptly, a systolic thrill and murmur become detectable in this chamber, and the left atrial appendage begins to balloon during each ventricular systole.[18, 19] The animals rapidly develop congestive cardiac failure, and their course is usually one of rapid progression. From the hemodynamic point of view, the

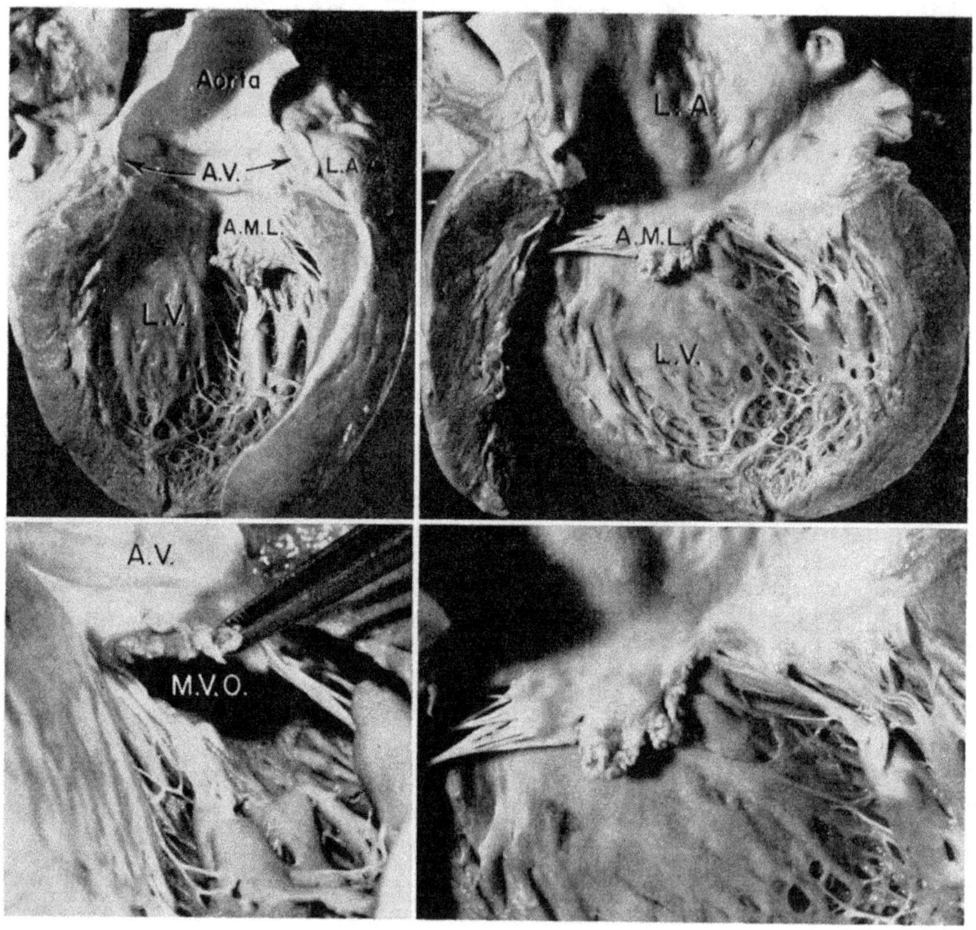

Figure 6

Photographs of heart of patient 4 (R.H.). Upper left. *The mitral valve is exposed by opening the left ventricle (L.V.), aortic valve (A.V.), and aorta. All chordae tendineae that had attached to the posterior portion of the anterior mitral leaflet (A.M.L.) are severed. The endocarditis that ruptured the chordae is active. The aortic valve is normal. L.A.A., left atrial appendage.* Lower left. *The size of the incompetent mitral valve orifice (M.V.O.) is apparent from this view. A.V., aortic valve cusps.* Upper right. *The left atrium (L.A.), mitral valve, and left ventricle (L.V.) are opened. The nonruptured mitral chordae are normal. A.M.L., anterior mitral leaflet.* Lower right. *Close-up of the ruptured mitral chordae of the anterior leaflet.*

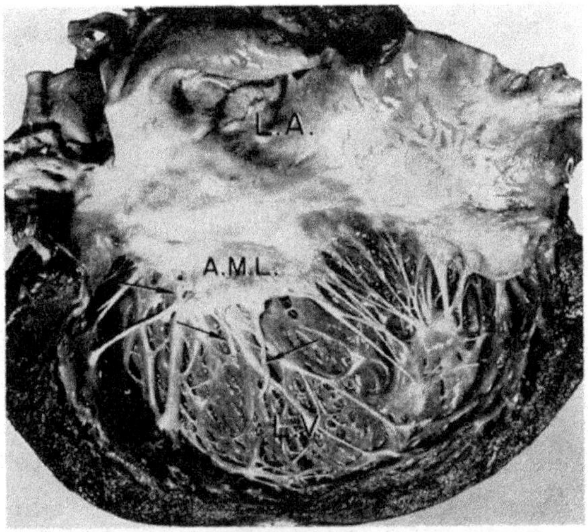

Figure 7

Photograph of heart of patient 1 (V.C.). The left atrium (L.A.), mitral valve, and left ventricle (L.V.) are opened. Both chambers are considerably dilated as is the mitral valve annulus. This patient had known mitral regurgitation for at least 5 years. At least three chordae tendineae (arrows) *from the anterior mitral leaflet (A.M.L.) are severed and each of these is thickened as is a portion of this leaflet. The nonruptured chordae are elongated, but otherwise normal. The posterior leaflet is normal.*

regurgitation produced suddenly in experimental animals more closely resembles the mitral regurgitation that developed acutely in the patients described herein than the regurgitation observed in patients with chronic rheumatic mitral regurgitation. In the latter condition, the regurgitation usually develops gradually, and sufficient time is available for the usual adjustments to this lesion to take place. In addition, the myocardium of the left atrium and of the left ventricle may also be affected by the rheumatic process. In the present group of patients with ruptured mitral chordae tendineae, however, the myocardium and pulmonary vascular bed were presumably normal at the time the chordae ruptured, and the resultant clinical, hemodynamic, and anatomic abnormalities may be attributed entirely or almost entirely to the mechanical defect.

The unusual hemodynamic and clinical features of the majority of patients described herein may be emphasized by comparing them with other groups of patients having severe mitral regurgitation. Patients with se-

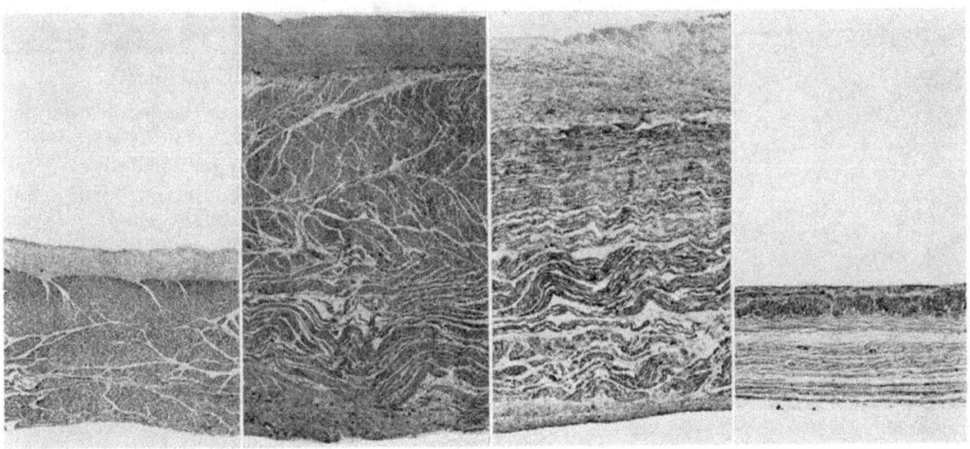

Figure 8

Photomicrographs of sections of posterior wall of left atrium in four patients each taken from a site approximately 3 cm. above the mitral annulus. Left. *Left atrial wall in 30-year-old woman dying of acute leukemia (for control). The endocardium is above, the epicardium, below.* Mid-left. *Left atrial wall in patient 4 (R.H.) showing marked thickening. This patient died 5 months after the onset of cardiac decompensation.* Mid-right. *Left atrial wall in patient 5 (P.H.) who lived for 5 years after the onset of cardiac decompensation. The endocardium is thicker, but the myocardium is thinner than in patient R.H.* Right. *Left atrial wall of a patient with mitral regurgitation, a giant left atrium, and normal left atrial pressures. The myocardial fibers are extremely elongated and thinned. The smooth muscle immediately beneath the endocardium is hypertrophied. Hematoxylin and eosin stains, original magnification in each* $\times$ *20.*

vere mitral regurgitation were previously separated into three major groups on the basis of obvious differences in atrial compliance.[20] I. A group with the sudden development of mitral regurgitation in whom there was mild to moderate enlargement of the left atrium, striking elevation of the mean left atrial pressure, of the left atrial v wave, the pul-

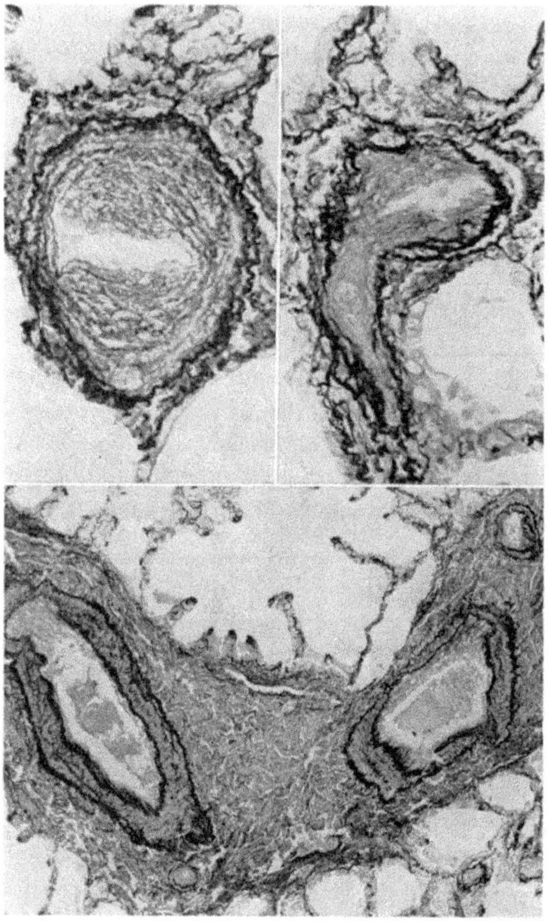

Figure 9

Photomicrographs of sections of pulmonary blood vessels in patient 4 (R.H.) who lived for only 5 months after the onset of mitral regurgitation. Upper left. *Pulmonary vein showing severe intimal proliferation and luminal narrowing.* Upper right. *Small muscular pulmonary artery with arteriolar branch showing severe intimal proliferation in each and luminal obliteration in the arteriole.* Lower. *Larger muscular pulmonary arteries showing medial hypertrophy and mild intimal proliferation. An adjacent small pulmonary artery is markedly narrowed by intimal fibrosis. Elastic tissue stains; original magnification × 340 (two upper), × 125 (lower).*

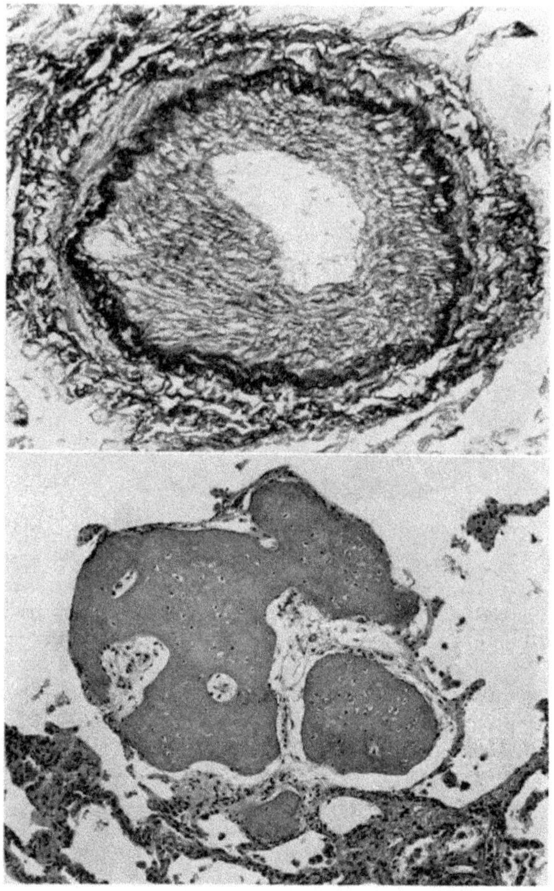

Figure 10

Photomicrographs of sections of lung in patient 2 (A.A.), who survived 7 months after the onset of mitral regurgitation. Upper. *Pulmonary vein showing severe intimal fibrosis.* Lower. *Ossific nodule. These "lung bones" were seen in sections of lungs in three of the six autopsied patients. Elastic tissue stain (upper), hematoxylin and eosin stain (lower); original magnification × 210 (upper), × 135 (lower).*

monary vascular resistance, and in whom severe right heart failure was often present. II. A group who had normal left atrial and pulmonary arterial pressures, normal pulmonary vascular resistance, a low cardiac output, huge left atria, atrial fibrillation, a history of acute rheumatic fever, and a long-standing history of heart failure (the syndrome of severe mitral regurgitation with normal left atrial pressure).[20] III. The largest number of patients with severe mitral regurgitation lies between these two extremes, and they exhibit both gross left atrial enlargement and an

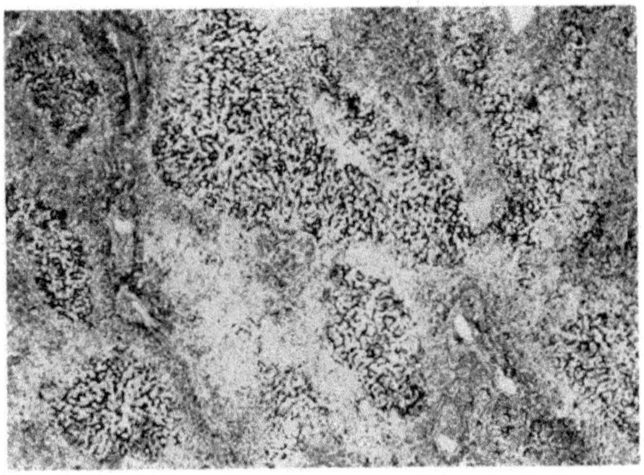

Figure 11

Photomicrograph of section of liver in patient 4 (R.H.), showing massive centrolobular necrosis (dark areas). The few remaining hepatic cells are located adjacent to the portal areas. Similar degrees of hepatic congestion and necrosis were seen in each of the six autopsied patients in this series. Phosphotungstic-acid hematoxylin stain, original magnification × 32.

elevated left atrial pressure. Thus, the patients with the syndrome of severe mitral regurgitation with normal left atrial pressure represent one end of the spectrum of mitral regurgitation, and the seven patients described in this report whose cardiac failure progressed rapidly represent the opposite end.

The severe pulmonary vascular changes observed in these patients with ruptured chordae tendineae are interpreted as anatomic expressions of the markedly elevated left atrial and pulmonary arterial pressures. The advanced pulmonary vascular changes, in association with little or no left atrial enlargement, contrasts sharply with the absence of these changes in patients with huge left atria secondary to long-standing mitral regurgitation.[20] As a consequence of the abnormalities in the pulmonary vascular bed, right ventricular hypertrophy was always present in the patients with acute mitral regurgitation and relatively small left atria, whereas right ventricular hypertrophy is rare in the patients with extremely dilated left atria.[21]

It is likely that the rapidity with which regurgitation develops is the primary determinant of hemodynamic, pathologic, and clinical changes observed in patients with severe mitral insufficiency. It is apparent that the walls of the left atria, and of the pulmonary vessels, were far less compliant in the nine patients with ruptured chordae tendineae who developed heart failure rapidly than in the group of patients with severely dilated left atria and normal left atrial pressures described previously.[20] Long-standing, gradually developing mitral regurgitation would appear, in some instances, to alter the elastic properties of the left atrial wall and, thereby, displace the atrial pressure-volume curve to make this chamber more compliant, so that a normal pressure may exist in a greatly enlarged atrium. Mitral regurgitation was present for only 5 to 16 months in seven of the eight patients in this series with normal or only moderately enlarged left atria. In contrast, symptoms of cardiac decompensation had been present for 5 to 8 years in the two patients with ruptured chordae tendineae who had very large left atria. Additional support for the view that the atrial compliance may increase as a late development in the course of mitral regurgitation was gained from observations in a 9-year-old patient with congenital mitral regurgitation in whom serial catheterization studies were carried out.[22] He was in sinus rhythm and exhibited slight disability at the time his left atrial pressure was grossly elevated (mean, 25; v peak, 45 mm. Hg). Subsequently, the patient developed cardiac failure, atrial fibrillation, and roentgenographic evidence of further increase in size of the left atrium. These changes were accompanied by a decline of left atrial pressure (mean, 15; v peak, 24 mm. Hg). Thus, in this patient a decrease in the mean left atrial pressure and the atrial v-wave peak pressure occurred in the face of an increase in the left atrial size, further substantiating the notion that the elastic properties of the left atrial wall had been altered.

In other reports of patients with ruptured mitral chordae tendineae, the left atrial chamber is usually described as being quite dilated. This finding was present in the six patients with ruptured mitral chordae reported by Menges et al.,[12] and the five described in detail by Osmundson et al.[5] These patients had been symptomatic for a number of years and, in general, the size of the left atrium correlated with the duration of the illness. In contrast, the heart of the first reported patient with ruptured mitral chordae, described by Corvisart in 1812,[23] was not grossly enlarged, but this patient survived for only 10 days after the onset of cardiac symptoms. Similarly, in the patient with ruptured mitral chordae reported by Frothingham and Hass,[7] who had been symptomatic for only 8 months, the left atrium was apparently not enlarged. In the patients described in these reports and others,[4, 10, 11, 13–16] a good correlation existed between left atrial size and the presence or absence of atrial fibrillation. The patients with atrial fibrillation were generally those with symptoms of cardiac disease for several years and very large left atria. The presence of atrial fibrillation in all of the patients with markedly dilated left atrial chambers, but normal atrial pressures,[20] and the absence of this arrhythmia in the patients with ruptured chordae tendineae, as well as in the child with congenital mitral regurgitation discussed above, suggest the possibility that the process that increases atrial compliance may be related to the development of atrial fibrillation.

Operative treatment was undertaken in seven of the 10 patients described herein. Mitral annuloplasty, with or without insertion of artificial chordae, which was originally utilized in this clinic for repair of ruptured chordae, was attempted in two patients, but each of them died in the immediate postoperative period. Mitral valve replacement with a Starr-Edwards prosthesis was carried out in the other five patients, and four have shown considerable improvement. The fifth died 2 weeks after operation of severe pulmonary infection including pulmonary abscess and empyema. Total valve replacement appears to be the most effective operative method for correcting ruptured chordae, although others[12, 15, 16, 17, 24] have reported good results with mitral plication and insertion of artificial chordae tendineae.

Since, with any given magnitude of regurgitant flow, the atrial pressure varies inversely with the compliance of the atrium, the extent to which the atrial pressure can be expected to decline following a corrective operation will also vary inversely with atrial compliance. Accordingly, the clinical and hemodynamic benefits of operation may be expected to be greatest in patients with relatively small left atria and high left atrial pressures. This may be illustrated by two patients in this series who have had postoperative catheterization following mitral valve replacement. B. F., a 21-year-old woman, was completely bedridden immediately before operation, although she had been well until 13 months earlier, when bacterial endocarditis was soon followed by the development of mitral regurgitation. At the time of the operation she weighed only 33 Kg. Preoperatively, the left atrial (mean, 11; v peak, 23 mm. Hg) and pulmonary arterial (65/28, mean 38 mm. Hg) pressures were elevated, roentgenographically the left atrium was only mildly enlarged, and on a standard oral sodium tolerance test she was unable to excrete any sodium.[25] Following replacement of the mitral valve with a Starr-Edwards prosthesis, she has been entirely asymptomatic. Seven months after operation she weighed 50 Kg. and the pulmonary arterial wedge (mean, 6; v peak, 11 mm. Hg) and pulmonary arterial (32/11, mean 16 mm. Hg) pressures were normal, the heart was smaller roentgenographically (fig. 2), and her sodium tolerance had become normal. J. W., a 54-year-old man, also was incapacitated before operation. He was emaciated, in severe cardiac failure, and the mean left atrial pressure was 15 with v waves of 32 mm. Hg, and the pulmonary arterial pressure was 70/27 mm. Hg. Twelve months after replacement of his mitral valve, the left atrial mean pressure had fallen to 7, the v waves to 10 mm. Hg, and the pulmonary arterial pressure to 44/20 mm. Hg. This patient has improved symptomatically, but he continues to accumulate fluid despite diuretic therapy, presumably consequent to persistent "relative" tricuspid regurgitation, and his heart had remained enlarged. Although this man also developed severe mitral regurgitation following rupture of chordae tendineae as a consequence of bacterial endocarditis, 8 years had elapsed from the onset of the valvular regurgitation until the valve was replaced, and the left atrium dilated during this interval. It is suspected that the left atrial pressures were greatly elevated immediately following the mitral chordal rupture, but as the left atrial chamber dilated the left atrial pressures decreased to levels approaching normal.

Summary and Conclusions

This report describes the clinical, radiographic, hemodynamic, and pathologic findings in 10 patients, in each of whom ruptured mitral chordae tendineae were responsible for severe mitral regurgitation. In six patients, the chordal rupture was the result of proved bacterial endocarditis, and in the other four, although the cause was not determined, it is considered that bacterial endocarditis may have been the etiologic factor in them as well. Only one of the patients had a history suggestive of acute rheumatic fever. From examination of the mitral valves at autopsy, or after operative excision, no gross abnormalities of the valves were apparent, other than the ruptured chordae and mild thickening of the adjacent leaflet. The signs and symptoms of mitral regurgitation appeared abruptly in all but one patient and were unrelenting thereafter. Eight patients had sinus rhythm and two had atrial fibrillation. Each of the latter had had symptoms of cardiac decompensation for several years, and their left atria were markedly enlarged. The left atrial chamber in the other eight patients was of near normal size or only moderately enlarged. The interval from the onset of symptoms of mitral regurgitation to operation in the two patients with dilated left atria averaged 6½ years, whereas the interval in the eight patients with near normal or only moderately dilated left atria averaged 15 months. In all patients the pulmonary arterial and the left atrial pressures, particularly the v-wave peak, were elevated. The cardiac index was low, and the calculated pulmonary vascular resistance was elevated in the seven patients in whom it was measured. Mitral annuloplasty was performed in two patients, with insertion of artificial chordae, but both died in the early postoperative period. Replacement of the mitral valve with a Starr-Edwards prosthesis was performed in five patients, with considerable improvement in four. The fifth died of a pulmonary complication 2 weeks after operation.

The distinctive clinical and hemodynamic findings in the majority of these patients, i.e., the rapid progression of heart failure, sinus rhythm, normal-sized or only moderately enlarged left atria, and the greatly elevated pressures in the pulmonary artery and left atrium are attributed to the sudden onset of the mitral regurgitation. These findings are contrasted to those in patients with chronic rheumatic mitral regurgitation, whose disability progresses slowly and who exhibit atrial fibrillation, marked left atrial enlargement, and sometimes normal pulmonary arterial and left atrial pressures. It is proposed that the majority of patients with ruptured chordae cannot sustain the acutely imposed hemodynamic burden for periods of time sufficient to allow the increase in left atrial compliance so frequently observed in patients with chronic rheumatic mitral regurgitation.

References

1. Perloff, J. K., and Harvey, W. P.: Auscultatory and phonocardiographic manifestations of pure mitral regurgitation. Progr. Cardiovas. Dis. **5:** 172, 1962.
2. Heath, D., and Edwards, J. E.: The pathology of hypertensive pulmonary vascular disease. A description of six grades of structural changes in the pulmonary arteries with special reference to congenital cardiac septal defects. Circulation **18:** 533, 1958.
3. Frew, H. W. O.: Rupture of the chordae tendineae following scarlet fever. Glasgow M. J. **115:** 195, 1931.
4. Bailey, O. T., and Hickman, J. B.: Rupture of mitral chordae tendineae. Clinical and pathologic observations on seven cases in which there was no bacterial endocarditis. Am. Heart J. **28:** 578, 1944.
5. Osmundson, P. J., Callahan, J. A., and Edwards, J. E.: Ruptured mitral chordae tendinae. Circulation **23:** 42, 1961.
6. Barber, H.: The effects of trauma, direct and

indirect, on the heart. Quart. J. Med., n.s., **13:** 137, 1944.

7. Frothingham, C., and Hass, G. M.: Rupture of normal chordae tendineae of the mitral valve. Am. Heart J. **9:** 492, 1934.
8. Libman, E., and Friedberg, C. K.: Subacute Bacterial Endocarditis. London, Oxford University Press, 1941, 108 pp.
9. Saphir, O.: Endocarditis. *In* Gould, S. E., Editor: Pathology of the Heart. Springfield, Illinois, Charles C Thomas Publisher, 1953, p. 707.
10. Hepper, N. G. G., Burchell, H. B., and Edwards, J. E.: Cardiac Clinic CXLVI. Mitral insufficiency in healed, unrecognized bacterial endocarditis. Proc. Staff Meet., Mayo Clinic **31:** 659, 1956.
11. Perrin, A., Froment, R., and Pasquier, J.: Insuffisances mitrales par luxation de la petite valve et rupture de cordages. (A propos de 5 observations anatomo-cliniques simulant le retrecissement aortique). Arch. mal. coeur **54:** 82, 1961.
12. Menges, H., Jr., Ankeney, J. L., and Hellerstein, H. K.: The clinical diagnosis and surgical management of ruptured mitral chordae tendineae. Circulation **30:** 8, 1964.
13. Miller, R., Jr., and Pearson, R. J., Jr.: Mitral insufficiency simulating aortic stenosis. Report of an unusual manifestation of Marfan's syndrome. New England. J. Med. **260:** 1210, 1959.
14. Shapiro, H. A., and Weiss, D. R.: Mitral insufficiency due to ruptured chordae tendineae simulating aortic stenosis. New England J. Med. **261:** 272, 1959.
15. January, L. E., Fisher, J. M., and Ehrenhaft, J. L.: Mitral insufficiency resulting from rupture of normal chordae tendineae. Report of a surgically corrected case. Circulation **26:** 1329, 1962.
16. Wolnisty, C., and Freidman, S. L.: Mitral insufficiency secondary to ruptured chordae tendineae. Report of surgically corrected case. J.A.M.A. **188:** 687, 1964.
17. Morris, J. D., Penner, D. A., and Brandt, R. L.: Surgical correction of ruptured chordae tendineae. J. Thor. & Cardiov. Surg. **48:** 772, 1964.
18. Haller, J. A., Jr., and Morrow, A. G.: Experimental mitral insufficiency. An operative method of chronic survival. Ann. Surg. **142:** 37, 1955.
19. Haller, J. A., Jr., and Morrow, A. G.: Experimental mitral insufficiency. Surgery **38:** 518, 1955.
20. Braunwald, E., and Awe, W. C.: The syndrome of severe mitral regurgitation with normal left atrial pressure. Circulation **27:** 29, 1963.
21. Best, P. V., and Heath, D.: The right ventricle and small pulmonary arteries in aneurysmal dilatation of the left atrium. Brit. Heart J. **26:** 312, 1964.
22. Carney, E. K., Braunwald, E., Roberts, W. C., Aygen, M., and Morrow, A. G.: Congenital mitral regurgitation. Clinical, hemodynamic, and angiocardiographic findings in nine patients. Am. J. Med. **33:** 223, 1962.
23. Corvisart, J. N.: An Essay on the Organic Diseases of the Heart and Great Vessels. (Translated by Jacob Gates) Boston, Bradford and Read, 1812, 344 pp.
24. McGoon, D. C.: Repair of mitral insufficiency due to ruptured chordae tendineae. J. Thor. & Cardiov. Surg. **39:** 357, 1960.
25. Braunwald, E., Plauth, W. H., Jr., and Morrow, A. G.: A method for the detection and quantification of impaired sodium excretion: Results of an oral sodium tolerance test in normal subjects and in patients with heart disease. Circulation **32:** 223, 1965.

The Structure of the Aortic Valve in Clinically Isolated Aortic Stenosis

An Autopsy Study of 162 Patients Over 15 Years of Age

By William C. Roberts, M.D.

SUMMARY

The structure of the aortic valve at autopsy is described in 162 patients over 15 years of age with clinically isolated, severe valvular aortic stenosis with or without aortic regurgitation. The valves were congenitally unicuspid, unicommissural in 17 patients, congenitally bicuspid in 67, tricuspid in 71, and in seven the structure was uncertain. Thus, in at least 84 (52%) of the patients the valve was congenitally malformed at birth. It is proposed that minor aortic valvular cuspal inequality, also present from birth, may be an underlying malformation in some of the patients with tricuspid stenotic aortic valves. Degeneration or wear-and-tear from aging almost certainly explains aortic stenosis in most of the elderly patients. Although no patient had clinical evidence of mitral valvular dysfunction, the mitral leaflets were diffusely thickened by fibrous tissue in 26 of the 162 patients. Rheumatic disease is believed to be the cause of the valve involvement in 22 of them (the other four had congenitally bicuspid aortic valves). Rheumatic disease did not appear to be the cause of the aortic stenosis in the other 136 patients with anatomically normal mitral valves.

Additional Indexing Words:

Bicuspid aortic valve | Cardiac calcification | Congenital heart disease

Mitral valvular dysfunction | Rheumatic heart disease | Unicuspid aortic valve

RECENTLY, the aortic valve has been shown to be congenitally bicuspid in a high percentage of patients with valvular aortic stenosis,[1] and other factors[2] have indicated that anatomically isolated aortic valvular disease is usually not rheumatic in origin. In the present postmortem study the hearts of 162 patients who presented clinically with isolated aortic stenosis with or without aortic regurgitation were reviewed. The prime purpose was to determine how often the aortic valve was congenitally malformed and how often the functionally normal mitral valve was anatomically abnormal.

From the Section of Pathology, National Heart and Lung Institute, National Institutes of Health, Bethesda, Maryland.

Received February 27, 1970; accepted for publication March 12, 1970.

Patients Studied

Observations in the 162 patients are summarized in table 1. Clinically, each was in functional class III or IV (New York Heart Association classification). Patients less than age 16 years were excluded. The average age was 52 years; 34 patients were older than 60 years of age and 16 were older than 70 years of age. Aortic valve operation (valvuloplasty or partial or total replacement) was performed in 106 patients; the average age of death in them was 49 years. The average age at death of the 56 patients on whom no cardiac operation was performed was 57 years, but 16 of the 20 who were older than 65 years of age were included in this group. The three patients without grossly visible calcific deposits in the aortic valve were aged 16, 24, and 33 years, and the peak systolic pressure gradients between the left ventricle and a

Table 1

Data in Patients with Clinically Isolated Valvular Aortic Stenosis

Valve structure	No. of patients	Age range (av)	No. of patients older than 65 yr	Sex		History of ARF or chorea	LV-SA PSG (mm Hg)	Aortic valvular calcium (g)	Heart wt. (g) Range (av)
				M	F				
Unicommissural	17	16-62 (44)	0	13	4	1	10-158 (78)*	17	400-880 (616)
Biscuspid	67	16-79 (49)	2	48	19	5	12-165 (93)†	64	295-1000 (600)
Tricuspid	71	21-90 (57)	18	53	18	14	20-160 (84)‡	71	380-1050 (643)
MV normal	49	28-90 (59)	16	34	15	1	20-160 (93)	49	380-1000 (595)
MV leaflets thick; CT normal	16	39-76 (53)	2	14	2	9	25-120 (70)	16	480-900 (717)
MV leaflets and CT thick	6	21-61 (46)	0	5	1	4	20-90 (61)	6	530-1050 (731)
Uncertain	7	41-58 (52)	0	7	0	0	52-105 (81)§	7	400-880 (600)
Total	162	16-90 (52)	20	122 (75%)	41 (25%)	20 (13%)	10-165 (87)	159	295-1050 (619)

*10 patients; PSG < 50 mm Hg in two.
†52 patients; PSG < 50 mm Hg in six.
‡49 patients; PSG < 50 mm Hg in seven.
§5 patients; PSG < 50 mm Hg in none.
Abbreviations: ARF = acute rheumatic fever; CT = chordae tendineae; LV = left ventricle; MV = mitral valve; PSG = peak systolic gradient; SA = systemic artery.

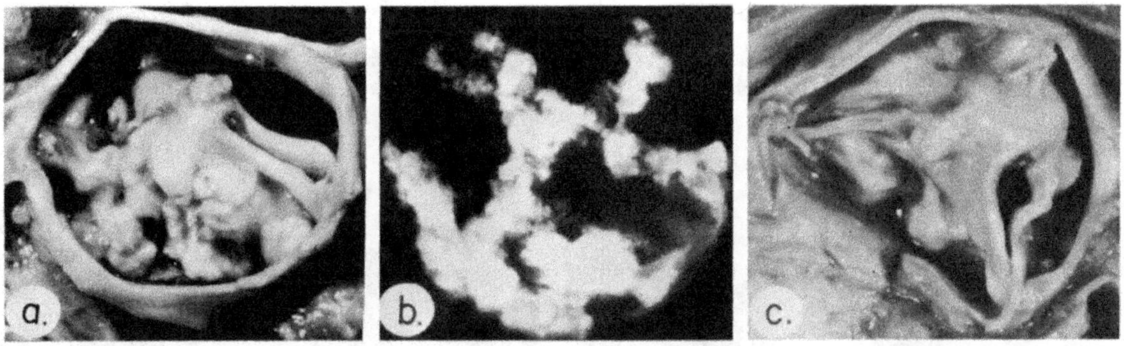

Figure 1

Stenotic unicommissural unicuspid aortic valves from above in two patients. (a) The valve in this 48-year-old man (A68-101) is severely stenotic and heavily calcified. (b) Same patient as a. The heart weighed 750 g. (c) The valve in this 62-year-old man (A69-276) also is severely stenotic, but the heart weighed 400 g. In contrast to the valve shown in a, two false commissures are present in addition to the one true commissure.

systemic artery in them were 80, 150, and 160 mm Hg, respectively.

The 162 patients were divided into four groups depending on the structure of the aortic valve. Representative valves are illustrated in figures 1 to 3. The excised valves in all patients who had undergone valve replacement also were re-examined (most had been removed intact). The prosthetic aortic valve in each, however, was removed so that the number of lateral attachments (commissures) of the cusps to the aorta could be determined.

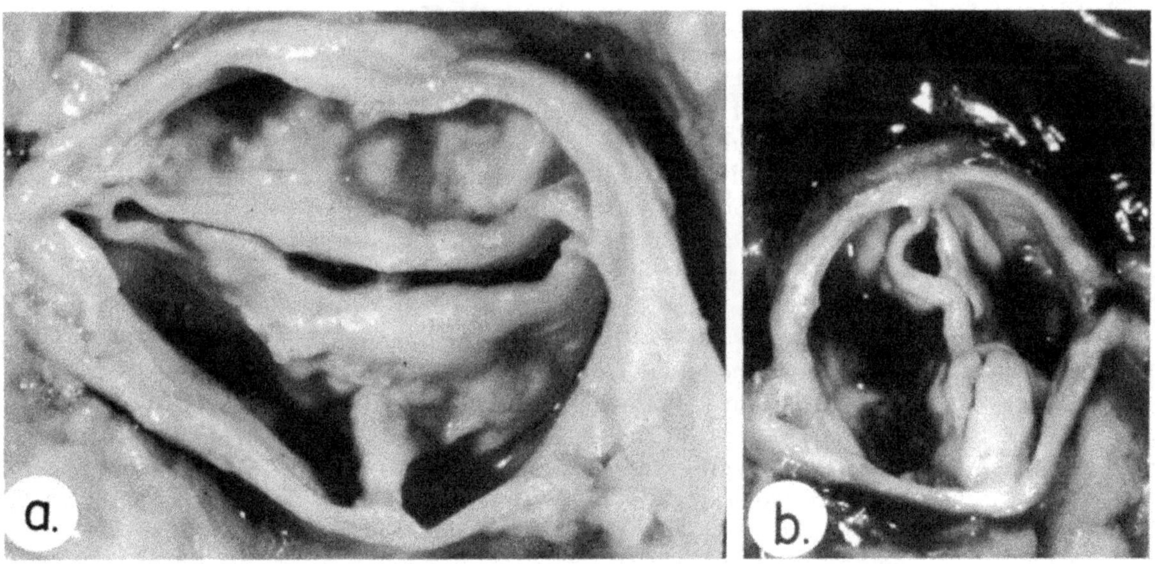

Figure 2

Stenotic congenitally bicuspid aortic valves from above in two patients. (a) The valve in this 61-year-old man (A64-155) contains a raphe in the anterior cusp. The peak systolic left ventricular-to-systemic arterial pressure gradient across this valve 2 years before death was 45 mm Hg. The heart weighed 700 g. (b) The valve in this 56-year-old woman (A70-6) was operatively debrided of calcific deposits a day before death. The peak systolic pressure gradient across the valve preoperatively was 47 mm Hg. The cusps are located on the right and the left, respectively. The heart weighed only 295 g.

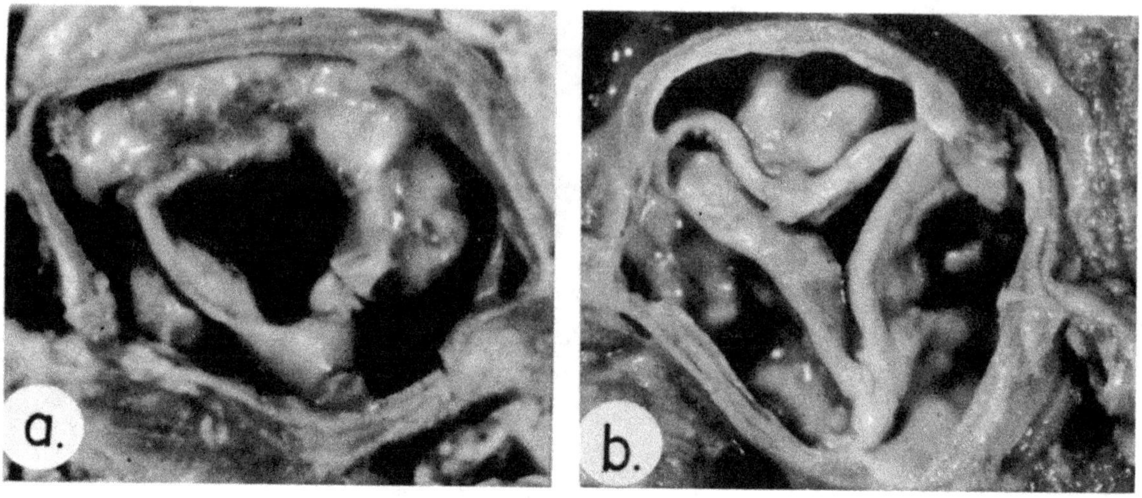

Figure 3

Stenotic three-cuspid aortic valves in two patients. (a) Each of the three commissures are fused in this stenotic and incompetent valve of a 49-year-old man (A58-19). The peak systolic pressure gradient across the valve was 74 mm Hg and the heart weighed 600 g. (b) This valve is from an 80-year-old woman who had clinical features of severe aortic stenosis. One commissure is fused but only minimally. The cusps are made relatively immobile by calcific deposits only. The heart weighed 400 g.

In 17 patients the aortic valve was unicommissural and unicuspid. In a few of the 17, two raphes (false commissures) were visible, but in most no raphe was present.

In 67 patients the aortic valve was congenitally bicuspid. Two basic types of bicuspid valves were seen: (1) In 54% of subjects the two cusps were located right and left, the commissures anteriorly and posteriorly, and a coronary artery arose from behind each cusp. (2) In 46% of the patients the two cusps were located anteriorly and posteriorly, the commissures, on the right and left, and both coronary arteries arose in front of the anterior cusp. Raphes were clearly visible in half the valves. When the cusps were located on the right and the left, the false commissures were always in the right cusp; when the cusps were located anteriorly and posteriorly, the raphe was always in the anterior cusp. In several patients with congenitally bicuspid aortic valves one true commissure was fused, producing in essence an acquired unicommissural aortic valve. The valves were divided, however, according to their original structure.

The 71 patients with tricuspid aortic valves were subdivided according to whether the mitral leaflets and chordae tendineae were normal or thickened by fibrous tissue. In 49 patients (69%), the mitral leaflets and chordae were entirely normal. Sixteen (33%) of these 49 patients were over 65 years of age whereas only four (4%) of the remaining 113 with aortic stenosis were over 65 years of age. In at least three of the 49 patients the aortic valve cusps were unequal in size and one of them also had a congenitally bicuspid pulmonic valve. In 16 of the 71 patients with tricuspid aortic valves the mitral valve leaflets were diffusely although mildly thickened and the mitral chordae tendineae were normal. Nine of these 16 patients had positive histories of acute rheumatic fever or chorea whereas only one of the 49 with tricuspid aortic valves and normal mitral valves had positive histories. In six of the 71 patients with tricuspid aortic valves the mitral chordae tendineae as well as the mitral leaflets were diffusely but mildly thickened, and four of them had positive histories of acute rheumatic fever or chorea. (The mitral valve was normal in each of the 17 patients with unicommissural aortic valves and in 62 of the 66 with congenitally bicuspid valves. In the other four, the leaflets were diffusely but mildly thickened, and the chordae were normal. In each of the seven patients in whom aortic valve structure was uncertain the mitral valve was normal.)

In seven of the 162 patients the underlying structure of the aortic valve was uncertain. Each of these patients had heavily calcified valves, and each had been excised and replaced by a prosthesis. The valves in them were not excised intact, and the number of commissures on the wall of the aortic root was unclear after removing the prosthesis.

At least four histologic sections of myocardium were examined in all 162 patients, and none had Aschoff bodies.

Discussion

The data show that among adults with clinically isolated valvular aortic stenosis with or without aortic regurgitation the aortic valve is congenitally bicuspid in 43%, tricuspid in 46%, and congenitally unicommissural, unicuspid in 11%. Thus, 54% of the patients in whom the aortic valve structure was discernible had congenitally bicuspid or unicuspid aortic valves. The mitral valves were normal in 136 (84%) and thickened in 26 (16%). Of the 136 patients with normal mitral valves, seven (5%) had positive histories of acute rheumatic fever or chorea whereas 13 (50%) of the 26 with thickened mitral valves (including four with congenitally bicuspid aortic valves) had positive histories.

Although the structure of the aortic valves in 96% of the described patients was clear, the cause of the valvular obstruction in most of them is less clear. Without question a congenital malformation was the underlying valve disturbance in the 17 patients with unicommissural valves, in the 67 with bicuspid valves, and probably also in the seven whose valve structure was uncertain. Although the valvular *malformation* was congenital, the valvular *obstruction* may or may not have been present from the time of birth. Edwards[3] has stated that the congenitally unicommissural aortic valve is inherently stenotic and that the unicuspid valve is the only type of valve stenotic at the time of birth. Of the 17 patients with congenitally unicommissural aortic valves described herein, each was stenotic, none was purely incompetent, and only one patient had had a history of infective endocarditis. Edwards[4] has contended that the congenitally bicuspid valve, in contrast to the unicuspid one, is not stenotic at birth but becomes stenotic only as it becomes fibrotic and calcified. In contrast to the congenitally unicommissural aortic valve, however, the congenitally bicuspid aortic valve may be

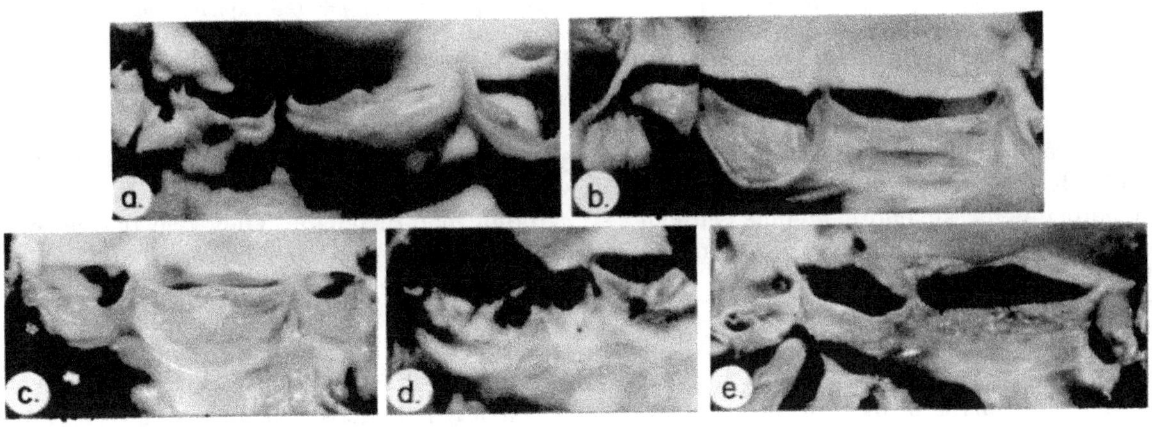

Figure 4

Shown here are opened, functionally normal aortic valves in five patients with unequal-sized cusps. Note the differing distances between the commissures in the patients. (a) Age 4 years. (b) Age 21 years. (c) Age 7 years. (d) Age 36 years. (e) Age 60 years. All five patients died of noncardiac conditions (leukemia [a and c], lymphoma [d and e], and cystic fibrosis of pancreas [b]).

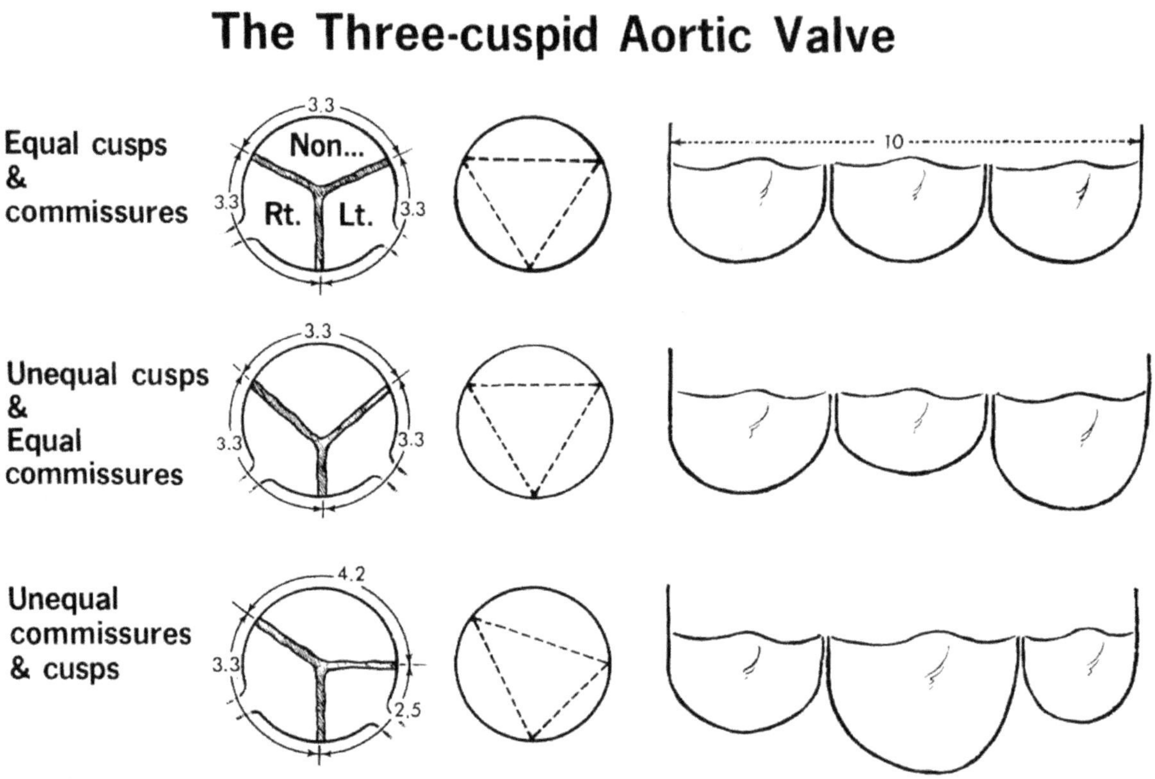

Figure 5

Diagrammatic portrayal of equal and unequal-sized aortic valve cusps. (Top row) *The cusps of the aortic valve are equal in size and the circumferential distances between the commissures are equal. The straight-line distances between the commissures (as indicated by the dashed lines in the center circle) also are equal. On the right the aortic valve is opened.* (Middle row) *Here the cusps are of unequal size, and they are made unequal by differing cephalocaudal lengths of the individual cusps. The distances between the commissures circumferentially around the aorta and the straight-line distances within the lumen of the aorta are similar to the normal shown in the top panel.* (Lower row) *Here not only are the cephalocaudal lengths of the individual cusps different, but the circumferential distances around the aorta and the straight-line distances within the lumen of the aorta between the commissures (lateral attachments) are different.*

purely incompetent, may be more often the site of infective endocarditis, and may function normally for an entire lifetime without developing any complication (stenosis, incompetence, or infection).[1]

The cause of the aortic stenosis in many of the 71 patients with tricuspid aortic valves is speculative. It is reasonable to believe that the etiology is rheumatic in most or all of the 22 patients with associated anatomic disease of the mitral valve. In addition to the anatomic mitral valvular involvement, the incidence of positive histories of acute rheumatic fever in them was high (60%). The cause of the aortic stenosis in the 49 patients with tricuspid aortic valves and normal mitral valves is almost certainly not rheumatic. Only one of the 49 patients had a positive history of acute rheumatic fever or chorea. Healed infective endocarditis likewise seems unlikely from anatomic study of the valves and from the lack of a positive history of infective endocarditis in any patient. No patient had a recorded history of, or anatomic evidence of, brucellosis.[5] Could the aortic valve be tricuspid and still congenitally malformed? At least three of the 49 patients clearly had aortic valve cusps of unequal size. The pulmonic valvular cusps are of slightly unequal size in most normal subjects.[6] Cuspal inequality in the low pressure right side of the heart is obviously of no consequence. Similar inequality of cuspal size in the high pressure left side of the heart, however, may be far more important. Unequal-sized aortic valve cusps are occasionally observed at autopsy in individuals dying of noncardiac conditions (fig. 4). When the cusps become severely fibrotic, nodular, calcified, or focally contracted, however, cuspal inequality probably is difficult to appreciate. This thesis of minor aortic cuspal inequality as an underlying congenital malformation in adults with valvular aortic stenosis is expanded in figure 5.

Fibrosis and calcification of the three aortic valve cusps as a consequence of aging (wear-and-tear) is almost certainly the explanation of the aortic stenosis in a significant percentage of the subjects with three-cuspid aortic valves and intrinsically normal mitral valves. Sixteen of the 49 patients with aortic stenosis, three-cuspid aortic valves, and normal (except for expected age changes) mitral valves were over 65 years of age. In addition to heavy calcific deposits in the aortic valve in these 16 patients, 14 also had calcific deposits in the mitral annulus and subvalvular angle beneath the posterior mitral leaflet, and all 16 had calcific deposits in the walls of one or more of the three major extramural coronary arteries. Commissural fusion in the older patients was unusual. None had positive histories of acute rheumatic fever or chorea. It seems most reasonable to believe that the aortic valvular calcification and stenosis in these 16 patients is on the basis of aging or degeneration.

Acknowledgment

I am enormously indebted to my present and past associates, particularly Dr. Andrew G. Morrow and Dr. Eugene Braunwald, for free access to clinical information on the patients discussed herein.

References

1. Roberts WC: The congenitally bicuspid aortic valve: A study of 85 autopsy patients. Amer J Cardiol. In press
2. Roberts WC: Anatomically-isolated aortic valvular disease: The case against its being of rheumatic etiology. Amer J Med In press
3. Edwards JE: Calcific aortic stenosis: Pathologic features. Proc Mayo Clin 36: 444, 1961
4. Edwards JE: The congenital bicuspid aortic valve. Circulation 23: 485, 1961
5. Peery TM: Brucellosis and heart disease: IV. Etiology of calcific aortic stenosis. JAMA 166: 1123, 1958
6. Roberts WC: Examination of the heart and precordium. Chest In press

The Congenitally Bicuspid Aortic Valve

A Study of 85 Autopsy Cases

WILLIAM C. ROBERTS, MD, FACC

Bethesda, Maryland

Clinical and necropsy observations are described in 85 autopsy cases in which the subjects had congenitally bicuspid aortic valves. Sixty-one subjects had aortic stenosis with or without aortic regurgitation; 11, pure aortic regurgitation; and 13, unexpectedly, had a congenitally bicuspid aortic valve that apparently had functioned normally. The average age at death in patients with stenotic valves was 49 years, and in those with pure regurgitation, 31 years. Aortic valvular calcific deposits occurred in 59 of 61 patients with stenosis but was minimal or absent in the patients with pure regurgitation or normally functioning valves. Infective endocarditis appeared responsible for incompetency in 8 of 11 patients with pure regurgitation. Five of 61 patients with stenosis had had infective endocarditis, but infection occurred on a previously heavily calcified valve in only 1 patient.

Sixty-nine of the 72 patients with functionally abnormal valves were observed in a study of 400 autopsy cases; all subjects were over age 14 years, with severe valvular cardiac disease. The 13 functionally normal valves were found during study of 1,440 necropsy cases in which the subjects were free of other valvular or septal defects. The bicuspid aortic valve is the most frequent congenital malformation of the heart or great vessels. It occurs in over 50 percent of patients with anatomically isolated aortic stenosis and in about 25 percent of patients with clinically pure aortic regurgitation. It is not certain why 1 congenitally bicuspid valve becomes severely scarred, calcified and stenotic, another only mildly scarred and incompetent, another the site of infection, and why another remains free of these complications during life.

In 1844 Paget[1] called attention to the peculiar liability of congenitally bicuspid aortic valves to disease, but their importance as something other than a pathologic curiosity was not appreciated. In 1858 Peacock[2] pointed out that bicuspid aortic valves tended to become "thick . . . ossified . . . inducing first obstruction . . . and then incompetency." Osler[3] in 1886 first described the abnormal liability of the bicuspid aortic valve to develop infective endocarditis. Since that time the tendency of this malformed valve to be the site of infection generally has been recognized, but only in the past 20 years has it become appreciated that the congenitally bicuspid aortic valve is a common cause of isolated calcareous aortic stenosis.[4-6]

The natural history of the congenitally bicuspid aortic valve is unknown. The percentage of individuals born with bicuspid aortic valves in whom stenosis, incompetency or infection develops at this site and the percentage who never have any of these complications

From the Section of Pathology, National Heart and Lung Institute, National Institutes of Health, Bethesda, Md. Manuscript received April 21, 1969, accepted September 23, 1969.

Address for reprints: William C. Roberts, MD, Section of Pathology, National Heart and Lung Institute, National Institutes of Health, Bethesda, Md. 20014.

TABLE I
Eighty-Five Cases of Congenitally Bicuspid Aortic Valve

Patients (no.)	Age (yr) at Death [Range & (Average)]	Sex		Infective Endocarditis	Precordial Murmur		LV-SA PSG [Range & (Average)] (mm Hg)	Aortic Valve Calcium Deposits	Heart Weight (g) [Range & (Average)]
		M	F		Systolic	Diastolic			
Group 1. Aortic Stenosis With or Without Aortic Regurgitation									
61	16–79(49)[a]	45	16	5[c]	61	25	12–165(92)[f]	59[h]	330–1000(605)
Group 2. Pure Aortic Regurgitation									
11	15–55(31)[b]	9	2	8[d]	6	9	0–0 (0)[g]	2[i]	240–950(573)
Group 3. Functionally Normal Valve									
13	23–59(45)	7	6	0	5[e]	0	—	4[i]	200–320(270)[j]
Totals									
85	15–79(46)	61 (72%)	24 (28%)	13 (15%)				65 (76%)	

[a] Average age of death in 21 patients without operation 53 years; in 40 patients with operation 46 years.
[b] Average age of death in 8 patients without operation 34 years; in the 3 patients with operation 26 years.
[c] Healed in each.
[d] Healed in 1; active in 7. Infective endocarditis was the cause of aortic regurgitation in all 8 patients.
[e] In 3 patients the murmur was at the apex; in 2 it was at the base. In 3 patients the murmur was grade 2/6 intensity; in 1, grade 3/6; and 1, grade 1/6. All 5 subjects were over 45 years of age, and 3 were anemic.
[f] Cardiac catheterizations in 48 patients. Only 5 patients had gradients less than 50 mm Hg.
[g] Cardiac catheterizations in 3 patients.
[h] Large in each.
[i] Small focal deposits in each and not roentgenographically visible.
[j] Excludes 3 patients who had systemic hypertension.
LV = left ventricle; SA = systemic artery (aorta, brachial or femoral); PSG = peak systolic gradient.

during an entire lifetime is unknown. To obtain information in this regard, clinical and necropsy findings were reviewed in 85 patients who were found at autopsy to have congenitally bicuspid aortic valves.

Results

Observations in the 85 autopsy cases are summarized in Table I. Subjects 14 years old and under were excluded.

Group 1. Aortic Stenosis With or Without Regurgitation

Sixty-one patients (Fig. 1 to 5) had some degree of aortic stenosis. Accurate heart weights,[7] available in 56 of the 61 patients, ranged from 330 to 1,000 g (average 605 g); in 42 men the heart weights averaged 651 g, and in 14 women, 466 g. The presence of a diastolic precordial murmur typical of aortic regurgitation also altered cardiac weights; in 5 women with murmurs of aortic regurgitation in addition to murmurs of aortic stenosis the heart weights averaged 516 g, whereas in 9 women without murmurs of regurgitation the hearts averaged 438 g; in 20 men with murmurs of aortic regurgitation the hearts averaged 702 g, whereas in 22 men without murmurs of regurgitation the hearts averaged 601 g. Although there was a significant difference in heart weights depending on sex and on the presence or absence of murmurs of aortic regurgitation, neither of these factors tended to alter consistently the peak systolic pressure gradient between the left ventricle and a systemic artery. This gradient in 34 men averaged 91 mm Hg and in 14 women, 97 mm Hg. In 5 women with murmurs of aortic regurgitation the peak systolic gradient averaged 94 mm Hg (the gradient was only 12 mm Hg in 1 patient), and in 7 women without murmurs of regurgitation the gradient averaged 100 mm Hg. Fifteen men with murmurs of aortic regurgitation had a lower peak systolic gradient (average 83 mm Hg) than the 20 men without murmurs of regurgitation (average 97 mm Hg).

Grossly visible deposits of calcium were present on each of the 2 aortic valve cusps in 59 of the 61 patients in Group 1. Of the 2 patients with no aortic valvular calcific deposits 1 was a 16 year old girl with

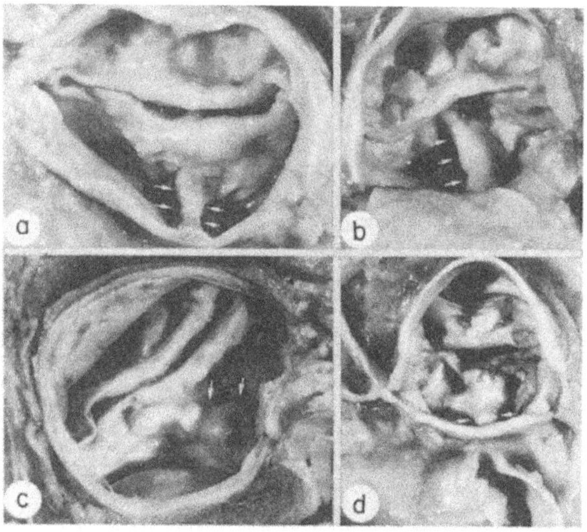

Figure 1. Calcified, stenotic, congenitally bicuspid aortic valves in 4 patients. The cusps in each are situated anteriorly and posteriorly and the commissures right and left, respectively. Each of the valves has a raphe **(white arrows)** in the anterior cusp. **a,** valve of a 61 year old man. At catheterization 2 years before death, the peak systolic gradient across the valve was 45 mm Hg when the cardiac index was 2.6 liters/min per m^2. **b,** valve of a 60 year old man who suddenly collapsed on the street. Electrocardiogram recorded in the emergency room showed left bundle branch block. His only symptom of cardiac dysfunction previously was mild exertional dyspnea. **c,** valve of a 75 year old man who died after resection of an asymptomatic abdominal aortic aneurysm that had been discovered during a routine physical examination. He had no symptoms of cardiac dysfunction. **d,** valve of a 51 year old man. The peak systolic gradient across this valve was 18 mm Hg, but the valve was severely incompetent.

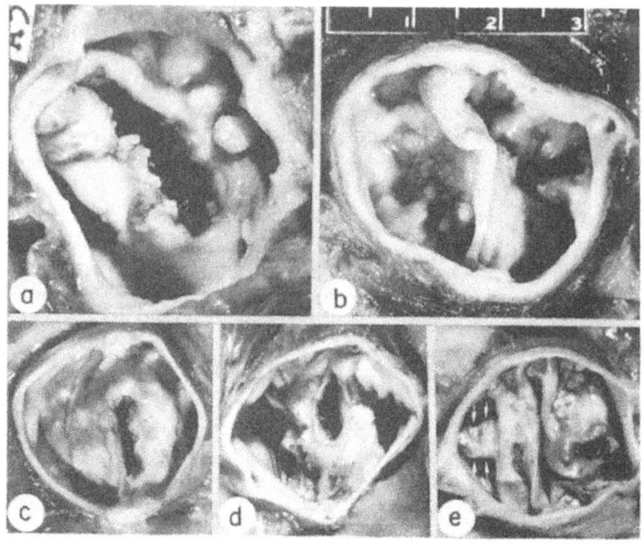

Figure 2. Calcified, stenotic, congenitally bicuspid aortic valves in 5 patients. In each the cusps are located right and left and the commissures, anteriorly and posteriorly. In valve **e** a false commissure is identifiable. In 3 of the 5 patients 1 of the 2 true commissures is partially fused. **a,** valve of a 37 year old man who died of progressive cardiac failure. **b,** valve of a 54 year old man who died during aortic valvuloplasty. The peak systolic gradient across the valve was 70 mm Hg. **c,** valve of a 34 year old man who died of progressive congestive cardiac failure. The peak systolic gradient across the valve was 92 mm Hg. **d,** valve of a 54 year old man who had progressive cardiac failure and, terminally, a massive pulmonary embolus. He had had symptoms of cardiac dysfunction for 6 years. **e,** valve of a 79 year old woman who had been asymptomatic until 2 years earlier when manifestations of cardiac failure appeared. The heart weighed 700 g.

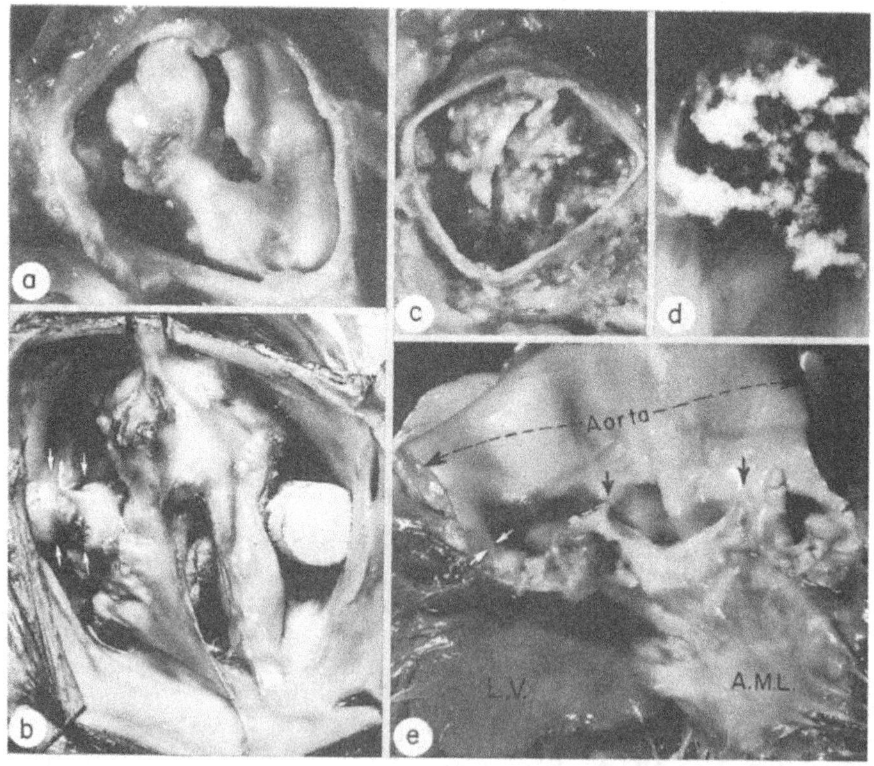

Figure 3. Calcified, stenotic, congenitally bicuspid aortic valves in 4 patients. In 3 the cusps are located right and left, and the commissures anteriorly and posteriorly. One commissure in each is fused. **a,** valve of a 39 year old man who experienced congestive cardiac failure 3 years earlier. He died during thoracotomy. Catheterization disclosed a 75 mm Hg peak systolic gradient across the valve when the cardiac index was 2.2 liters/min per m^2. **b,** valve of a 40 year old woman who died during valvulotomy which caused perforations of the left cusp (stick protruding through the perforation). Preoperatively, the peak systolic gradient across the valve was 70 mm Hg. The heart weighed only 400 g. The raphe is designated by **arrows. c,** valve of a 53 year old man who died suddenly and unexpectedly 77 months after valvuloplasty. Before operation at age 46 the peak systolic gradient across the valve had been 63 mm Hg when the cardiac index was 3.0 liters/min per m^2 and no aortic regurgitation was present. Catheterization 4 months after operation disclosed no systolic gradient, and catheterization 60 months after operation showed a 36 mm Hg peak systolic gradient across the valve when the cardiac index was 2.3 liters/min per m^2. **d,** radiograph of the valve shown in **c** showing large calcific deposits. **e,** opened valve of a 56 year old man who died suddenly and unexpectedly 1 month before scheduled aortic valve replacement. At catheterization 2 months before death the peak systolic gradient across the valve was 87 mm Hg when the cardiac index was 2.6 liters/min per m^2. The 2 commissures are designated by **vertical arrows,** and a small raphe, by **horizontal arrows.** A.M.L. = anterior mitral leaflet, L.V. = left ventricle.

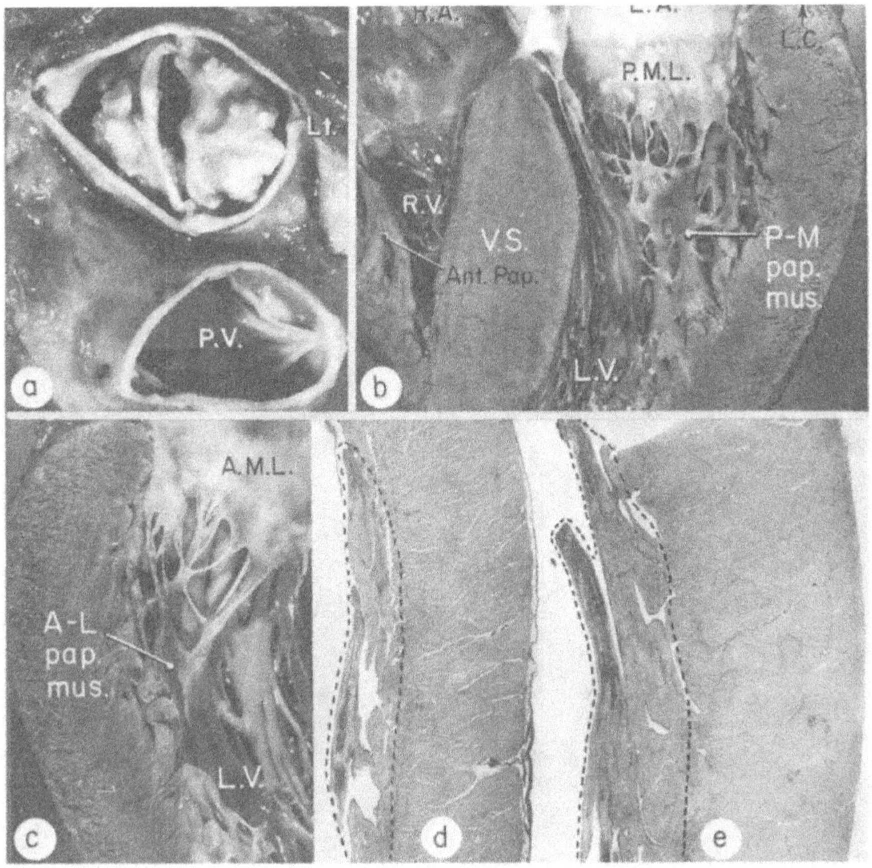

Figure 4. Stenotic, congenitally bicuspid aortic valve and atrophied and scarred papillary muscles in a 52 year old woman. This patient had symptoms of cardiac dysfunction for 3 years and a precordial murmur typical of mitral regurgitation in addition to murmurs of aortic stenosis and regurgitation. At catheterization, the peak systolic gradient across the aortic valve was 130 mm Hg (left ventricle 230/30 and aorta 100/70 mm Hg). The pulmonary arterial wedge mean pressure was 36 with v waves of 46 mm Hg, and the mean diastolic gradient between pulmonary arterial wedge and left ventricle was 12 mm Hg. The pulmonary arterial pressure was 75/40 mm Hg. Cardiac index was 2.1 liters/min per m². Aortic root and left ventricular cineangiocardiograms confirmed aortic regurgitation (3+/4+) and mitral regurgitation (2+/4+). Shortly after catheterization she experienced various atrial arrhythmias and irreversible overt congestive cardiac failure.

a, aortic and pulmonic (P.V.) valves from above showing the heavily calcified bicuspid aortic valve. The anterior commissure is partially fused. Lt. = left coronary artery. All coronary arteries were widely patent. **b,** longitudinal section of heart showing portions of all 4 cardiac chambers. The posteromedial (P-M) left ventricular papillary muscle is atrophied and scarred, and the anterior (ant.) right ventricular papillary (pap.) muscle is focally scarred. The left ventricular cavity is dilated, but the mitral annulus is not dilated. P.M.L. = posterior mitral leaflet; V.S. = ventricular septum; L.C. = left circumflex coronary artery. **c,** section of left ventricle (L.V.) showing severe atrophy of anterolateral (A-L) papillary muscle. The mitral leaflets are normal. A.M.L. = anterior mitral leaflet. **d** and **e,** photomicrographs of section of anterolateral **(d)** and posteromedial **(e)** left ventricular papillary muscles. Both are scarred and the anterolateral papillary muscle is extremely atrophied. The mitral regurgitation in this patient probably resulted from scarring and atrophy of the papillary muscles.

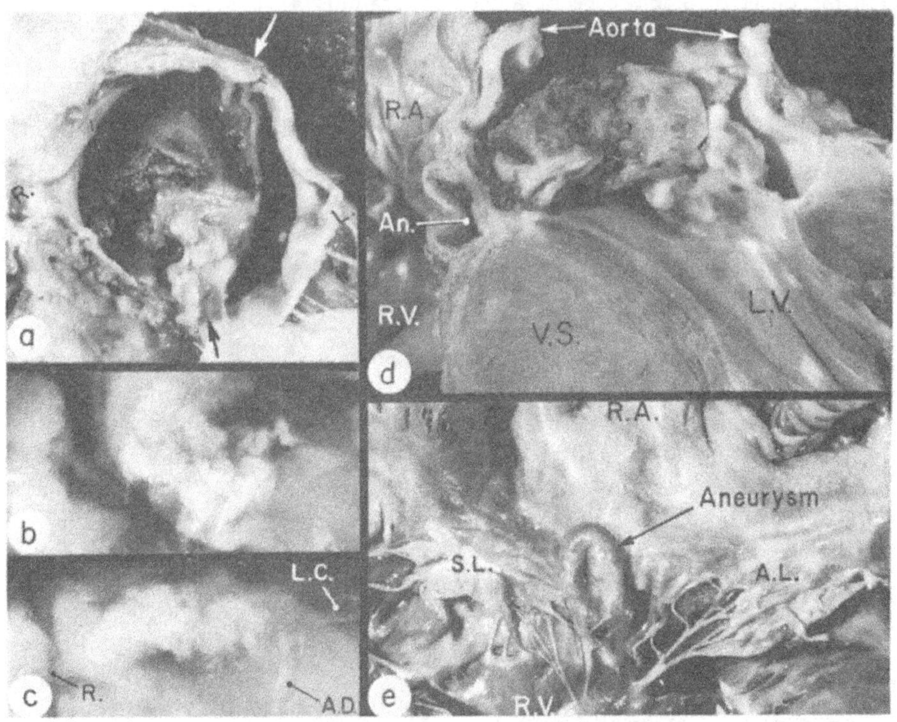

Figure 5. Infective endocarditis in a heavily calcified, congenitally bicuspid, aortic valve of a 63 year old man with features of congestive cardiac failure for at least 3 years. Fever, chills, alteration in intensity of the precordial murmurs, and prolonged P-R interval were noted 3½ months before death and Streptococcus viridans was cultured from the blood. He received penicillin and streptomycin for 1 month, the fever disappeared, and blood cultures became negative. Nevertheless, he fainted twice and complete heart block and atrial fibrillation developed. The congestive cardiac failure worsened, and he died.

The heart weighed 700 g and the aortic valve orifice was tiny **(a).** The anterior commissure **(black arrow)** was fused and only a small posteriorly-located orifice remained. R. = right coronary and L. = left coronary artery. The valve was heavily calcified **(b** and **c).** A radiograph of the valve from above is shown in **b,** and a lateral view, in **c.** All 3 major coronary arteries also are calcified. R. = right, L.C. = left circumflex, and A.D. = anterior descending coronary arteries. **d,** longitudinal section of aortic valve, left ventricular (L.V.) outflow tract, and ventricular septum (V.S.). A large lump of necrotic debris is present in the aortic valve which communicates with an aneurysm (An.) which bulges from the root of the aorta into the right atrium (R.A.), better seen in **e.** The aneurysm is believed to represent a healed "mycotic" aneurysm. No organisms were seen in histologic sections of the valve or aneurysm. S.L. = septal leaflet and A.L. = anterior leaflet of tricuspid valve. This patient thus had infective endocarditis superimposed on a previously heavily calcified valve, a rare circumstance.

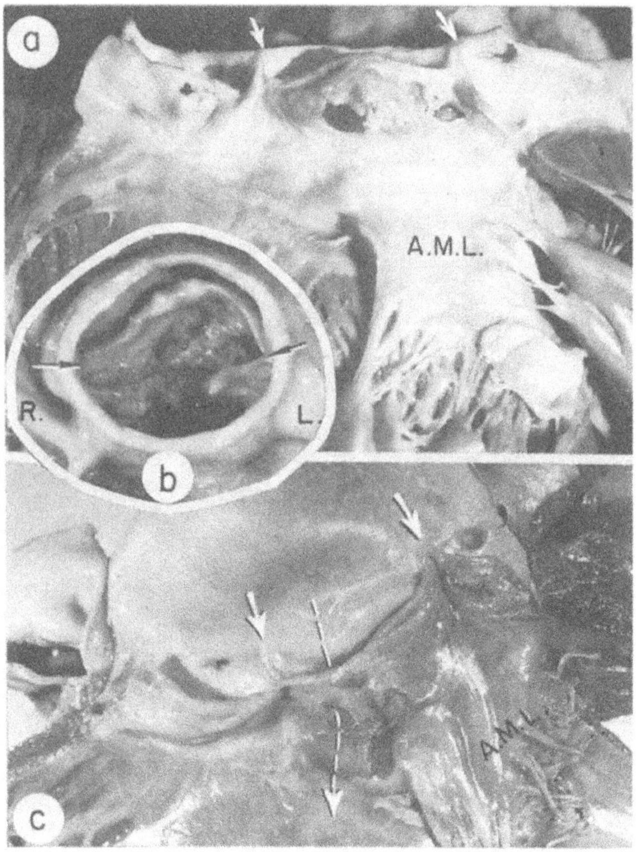

Figure 6. Infective endocarditis on previously functionally normal, congenitally bicuspid aortic valves causing fatal aortic regurgitation. **a,** opened aortic valve of a 55 year old woman. She had no signs or symptoms of cardiac disease until the onset of Staphylococcus aureus endocarditis 4½ months before death. Eradication of the organisms never was successful, the cusps perforated, and massive aortic regurgitation developed. A.M.L. = anterior mitral leaflet. The insert **(b)** shows the valve before it was opened. The **arrows** designate the true commissures. **c,** opened perforated aortic valve of a 33 year old man who developed Streptococcus viridans endocarditis after a tooth extraction and died of heart failure 2 months later. Before the extraction he had had no symptoms or signs of cardiac dysfunction. The **solid arrows** designate the true commissures and the **dashed irregular arrow,** the site of cuspal rupture.

an 80 mm Hg peak systolic gradient between the left ventricle and brachial artery, and the second was a 24 year old man with associated arthrogryposis multiplex congenita and a 150 mm Hg peak systolic gradient across the valve.[8] Two patients, a 53 year old woman and a 25 year old man, had only small focal calcific deposits on their aortic valves, but each had minimal stenosis (peak systolic gradient 12 and 30 mm Hg, respectively). The remaining 57 patients had large calcific deposits on the aortic valve, and all were over 30 years of age.

Group 2. Pure Aortic Regurgitation

In 8 of the 11 patients with pure aortic regurgitation (Fig. 6 and 7) the regurgitation was secondary to infective endocarditis. In 7 of these 8 patients precordial murmurs were absent or not mentioned until the valves became the site of infection. In 7 of the 8 patients with infective endocarditis, 1 or both cusps were perforated and partially destroyed by the inflammatory process. The eighth patient had large vegetations containing Histoplasma capsulatum on his biscuspid aortic valve, but neither cusp was perforated. This 35 year old man had generalized systemic histoplasmosis during his last 20 months of life, but an antemortum diagnosis of histoplasma endocarditis was never established despite 20 blood cultures for fungi. In 2 patients murmurs of the aortic regurgitation type were not heard, but in neither of the patients was infective endocarditis suspected clinically; 1, the 35 year old man just mentioned, had systemic histoplasmosis, and the second was asymptomatic until a day before death when unilateral hemiplegia suddenly appeared. The latter patient had ulcerated aortic cusps at autopsy although the heart weighed only 270 g. In the 3 patients with pure aortic regurgitation without historical or anatomic evidence of infective endocarditis, their aortic valve cusps at necropsy were mildly fibrotic and contracted, and symptoms of cardiac dysfunction had been present for 2 to 7 years before death. Each had associated congenital malformations: patent ductus arteriosus in 1, coarctation of the aorta in 1, and right aortic arch in 1 patient.

Group 3. Functionally Normal Valves

In each of the 13 patients in this group (Fig. 8 and 9) a congenitally bicuspid aortic valve was an incidental finding at necropsy, and in each the valve is believed to have functioned normally during life. Seven died of neoplasms, 1 of coronary heart disease, 1 of chronic parenchymal pulmonary disease, 1 of aplastic anemia, 1 of renal disease and 2 of acute dissecting aortic aneurysms with rupture. The aortic valve cusps in all 13 patients were slightly but focally thickened and in 4 contained small foci of calcium. However, in all patients the aortic valve cusps were freely movable, and in none did the valve orifice appear stenotic or incompetent.

Associated congenital cardiovascular malformations: These occurred in 11 of the 85 patients (13 percent) (Table II).

Positive histories of acute rheumatic fever or chorea: These were present in 5 of the 85 patients. Each had severe aortic stenosis, and 3 were men.

The mitral valves: These valves were normal in 79 of the 85 patients. Of the remaining 6 patients, 4 had mitral valve leaflets that were diffusely thickened by fibrous tissue, but their chordae tendineae

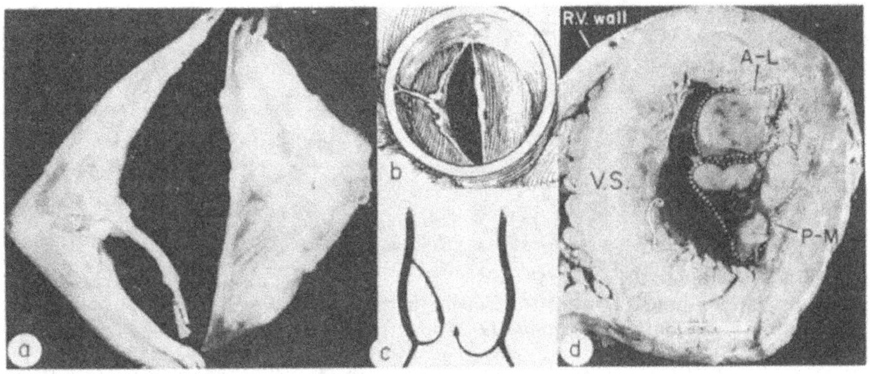

Figure 7. Pure aortic regurgitation complicating a congenitally bicuspid aortic valve without a history of infective endocarditis. The 27 year old man whose aortic valve and portion of left ventricle are illustrated here was found to have aortic regurgitation at age 17, but was asymptomatic until age 25 when moderate exertional dyspnea appeared. At catheterization shortly before valve replacement, the left ventricular pressure was 125/25 and the brachial arterial pressure, 126/54 mm Hg when the cardiac index (Fick method) was 2.2 liters/min per m^2. He died suddenly and unexpectedly 13 months after valve replacement. The heart weighed 800 g. The aortic arch coursed over the right bronchus. **a,** the excised aortic valve. A supporting fibrous band stretched from the margin in the mid portion of one cusp to the aortic wall above the sinuses of Valsalva as shown in **b** and **c. d,** a transverse section across the left ventricle (L.V.) showing atrophy of the posteromedial papillary muscle but no atrophy of the anterolateral papillary muscle. The coronary arteries were widely patent.

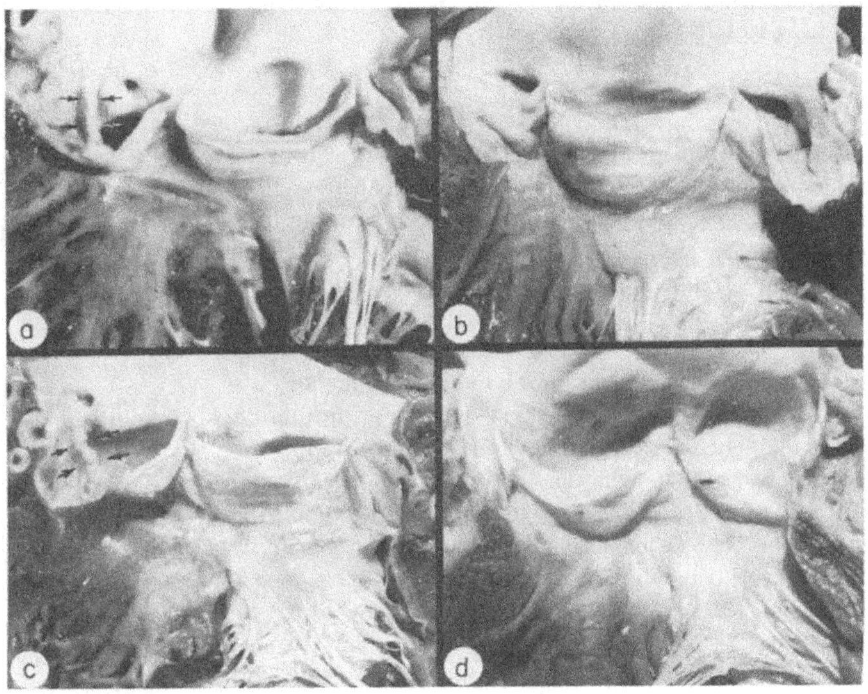

Figure 8. Functionally normal congenitally bicuspid aortic valves in 4 patients. The valve, aorta and left ventricle are opened. Three patients **(a, b, c)** died of leukemia and 1 **(d)** of lymphosarcoma. None of the patients (3 men, 1 woman; ages 23 to 47 years) had signs or symptoms of cardiac disease, and the heart weights ranged from 230 to 290 g. Raphes, designated by **horizontal arrows,** are visible in **a** and **c.**

were normal and there was no clinical evidence of mitral valve dysfunction. A fifth patient, mentioned earlier (Table II), had a congenitally malformed mitral valve. The sixth patient, a 20 year old man who also had the Marfan syndrome, had elongated "floppy" mitral leaflets that contained excessive acid-mucopolysaccharide material and fibrous tissue.

Location of aortic valve cusps: Information regarding the location of each of the 2 aortic valve cusps and the presence or absence of raphes was ascertainable in 59 patients. In some patients who had undergone aortic valve replacement this information was not precise and was therefore omitted. Of the patients who had undergone aortic valve replacement, the valves in most had been excised intact,[9] and each was re-examined. In addition, the prosthetic valves were removed from the hearts at autopsy; this permitted accurate determination of the number of aortic valve cusps and commissures that had been present. In 28 of 59 patients (47.5 percent) 1 cusp was located anteriorly, the second posteriorly and the commissures to the right and left, respectively (Fig. 10). In each of the 28 patients both coronary arteries arose in front of the anterior cusp, and a raphe, present in 16 of the 28 subjects, was always located in the anterior cusp. In 31 of the 59 patients (52.5 percent) the cusps were situated right and left with the 2 commissures situated anteriorly and posteriorly, respectively. When this relation was present the right coronary artery arose from behind the right cusp and the left coronary artery from behind the left cusp. A raphe, present in 14 of the 31 patients, was always located in the right cusp. Raphes were observed in 30 of 59 patients (51 percent). However, their presence in 10 of 13 patients with normally functioning valves, that is, those in

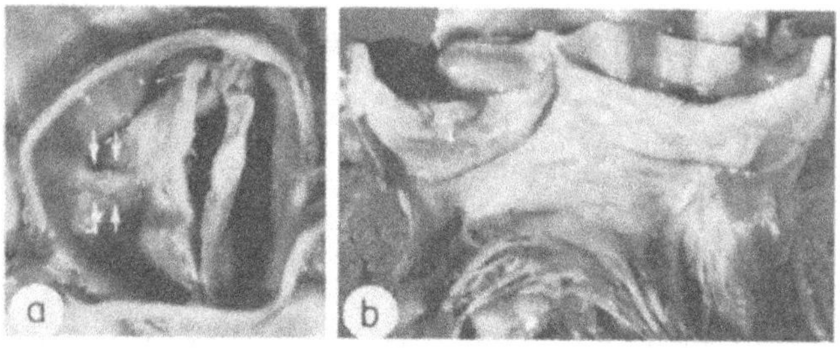

Figure 9. Functionally normal aortic valve with unequal-sized cusps. A raphe (arrows) is present in the right cusp. **a**, valve from above; **b**, valve opened.

whom the valve architecture was best preserved, suggests that some raphes were obscured by heavy deposits of calcium.

Comments

Incidence in general population: The 13 normally functioning congenitally bicuspid aortic valves described were observed by me during examination of the hearts of 1,440 patients who had no other cardiac valvular, septal or great vessel abnormality. The bicuspid condition of the aortic valve was specifically looked for. Since this anomaly otherwise may escape notice, information about its frequency obtained by scanning postmortem records is unreliable. This incidence of 0.90 percent is similar to that reported by others who examined hearts specifically for the presence or absence of congenitally bicuspid aortic valves. Osler[10] found 7 apparently normally functioning congenitally bicuspid aortic valves in 800 autopsies (750 of which were performed by him), an incidence of 1.3 percent. Eight additional patients had infective endocarditis involving congenitally bicuspid aortic valves. Thus, 18 of 800 (2 percent) had either normally functioning or infected congenitally bicuspid aortic valves. Lewis and Grant[11] found 3 apparently normally functioning congenitally bicuspid aortic valves among 215 consecutive autopsies. Grant et al.[12] found apparently normally functioning congenitally bicuspid aortic valves in 12 of 1,350 (0.89 percent) autopsy cases. Neither Osler, Lewis nor Grant et al. appear to have appreciated that the bicuspid condition of this valve may underlie severe stenosis or calcification at this site. Bonnabeau et al.[13] observed at necropsy 5 apparently normally functioning congenitally bicuspid aortic valves in a period during which they also observed 20 severely stenotic congenitally bicuspid aortic valves. The oldest of the 13 patients with normally functioning bicuspid aortic valves described herein was 59 years of age.

TABLE II

Congenital Malformations Associated With Congenitally Bicuspid Aortic Valves Among 85 Patients Over 14 Years of Age

Coarctation of aorta	5
Patent ductus arteriosus	1
Congenital mitral regurgitation	1
Ebstein malformation, tricuspid valve*	1
Right aortic arch*	1
Biscuspid pulmonic valve*	1
Spontaneously-closed ventricular septal defect*	1
TOTAL 11† in 85 patients (13%)	

* Did not cause functional disturbance

† No patient had more than 1 associated congenital anomaly. In addition, 2 men, aged 46 and 57 years, respectively, died of dissecting aortic aneurysms.

Thus, if congenitally bicuspid aortic valves that develop complications (stenosis, incompetency with or without infection) are added to those which function normally during an entire lifetime, the frequency of congenitally bicuspid aortic valves may approach 2 percent of the population. It appears that the bicuspid aortic valve is the most common congenital malformation of the heart or great vessels.

Incidence in patients with aortic valvular disease: Sixty-nine of the 72 patients described herein with abnormally functioning congenitally bicuspid aortic valves were observed during study at necropsy of 400 patients over age 14 years with functionally severe cardiac valvular disease (classes III and IV, New York Heart Association classification).[14] Of the 105 patients with anatomic disease limited to the aortic valve causing stenosis with or without regurgitation, 54 had congenitally bicuspid valves, 13 had congenitally unicommissural, unicuspid valves, 32 had tricuspid valves (3 with distinctly unequal-sized cusps) and 6 had valves so scarred, calcified and deformed that their basic structure was not discernible. It is strongly suspected that these latter 6 patients also had congenitally malformed valves. Thus, over 50 percent of patients studied at autopsy by the author with anatomically isolated aortic stenosis had congenitally bicuspid aortic valves, and over 70 percent had congenitally malformed valves of various types. Campbell,[15] in reviewing a coroner's necropsy records, found bicuspid aortic valves described in 9 of 60 patients (15 percent) with calcific aortic stenosis. Ninety percent of the patients were over 50 years of age. In my necropsy study of 34 patients with clinically pure aortic regurgitation 9 (26.5 percent) had congenitally bicuspid aortic valves. The valves in 7 of the 9 patients were made incompetent by superimposed infective endocarditis. Of the remaining 6 of 69 patients with abnormally functioning congenitally bicuspid aortic valves, 4 had diffuse fibrous thickening of the mitral leaflets but normal chordae tendineae. None of the 4 had evidence of mitral valve dysfunction, and all had aortic stenosis with or without regurgitation. One patient with a congenitally bicuspid stenotic and incompetent aortic valve had a severely incompetent congenitally malformed mitral valve, and another with a congenitally incompetent bicuspid aortic valve had a "floppy" incompetent mitral valve and the Marfan syndrome. Thus, among 173 patients with anatomically abnormal mitral and aortic valves, 6 had congenitally bicuspid aortic valves. However, 4 of the 6 were among 24 patients with fibrous thickening of the mitral leaflets but normal chordae and normal mitral function.

Incidence of valvular stenosis, regurgitation and infection: Valvular stenosis is the most frequent complication of a congenitally bicuspid aortic valve; valvular regurgitation is next, and the latter lesion is most frequently the result of its being the site of infective endocarditis. The reason 1 congenitally bicuspid aortic valve becomes stenotic, another incompetent, and another the site of infective endocarditis is unknown. However, it is clear that stenosis, regurgitation and infection are complications of the bicuspid condition of the aortic valve and none of them are present at birth. It appears likely that a congenitally bicuspid aortic valve becomes stenotic only as its cusps become fibrotic and calcified; neither cusp of a congenitally bicuspid aortic valve is fibrotic or calcified at the time of birth.

The frequency of development of stenosis or incompetency at the site of a congenitally bicuspid aortic valve also is unknown. Lewis and Grant[11] concluded that vegetations develop at these sites in 23 percent of adults (16 of 69) with congenitally bicuspid aortic valves. More information is available regarding the incidence of congenitally bicuspid valves in patients with infective endocarditis involving the aortic valve. Of 31 patients with "subacute infective endocarditis" studied at autopsy by Lewis and Grant,[11] 8 had congenitally bicuspid aortic valves. Four of 13 patients with infective endocarditis involving the aortic valve studied at autopsy by Starling,[16] 2 of 22 patients studied at autopsy by Fulton and Levine[17] and 3 of 20 patients studied at autopsy by Bayles and Lewis[18] had congenitally bicuspid aortic valves. None of these investigators apparently were aware that a congenitally bicuspid aortic valve also could become stenotic.

Valve calcification: Of the 61 patients with congenitally bicuspid stenotic aortic valves, 59 had calcific deposits in the valve. Of the 57 patients over 30 years of age all had large calcific deposits in the valve cusps; of the 4 under 30 years of age 2 had no calcific deposits, and 2 had only small focal ones. None of the 11 patients with pure aortic regurgitation had more than 1 or 2 small focal deposits of calcium in the valves, and most had none. Of the 13 patients with functionally normal aortic valves, 4 had small focal calcific deposits in them. Thus, large calcific deposits on congenitally bicuspid aortic valves are unusual before the age of 30 years, and stenotic congenitally bicuspid aortic valves without calcific deposits are rare in persons over 30 years of age. Heavy deposits of calcium do not occur in purely incompetent congenitally bicuspid aortic valves; valvular stenosis appears to be prerequisite for the development of heavy deposits of calcium at this site. Development of infective endocarditis on a heavily calcified valve also is rare. Of 5 patients with stenotic congenitally bicuspid aortic valves only 1 had heavy deposits of calcium on his valve before the onset of the infection. Of the 11 patients with pure aortic regurgitation, infective endocarditis was the cause of the valvular incompetency in 8, and none had significant valvular calcific deposits.

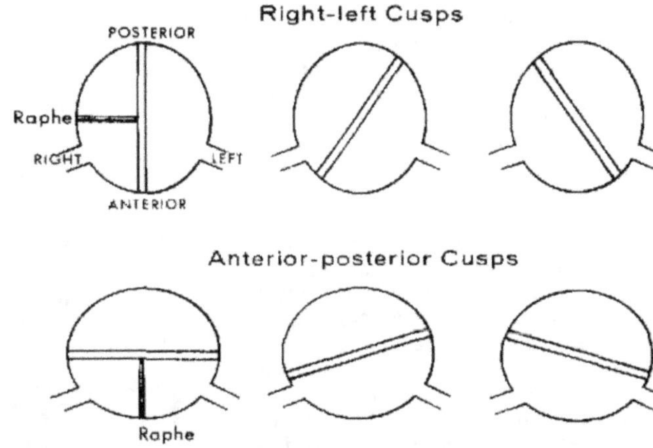

Figure 10. Diagram showing the 2 basic types of congenitally bicuspid aortic valves. See text for explanation.

Mechanism of valvular stenosis and regurgitation: The mechanism by which a congenitally bicuspid aortic valve becomes stenotic or incompetent is uncertain. There is no evidence to indicate that the valve is stenotic or incompetent at birth. Likewise, there is no evidence to indicate that superimposed rheumatic fever or rheumatic heart disease is the cause of the stenosis or incompetency. Five of the 85 patients (6 percent) described herein had histories of acute rheumatic fever or chorea. However, it is suspected that their illness had been inaccurately diagnosed as acute rheumatic fever. All 5 patients had aortic stenosis, and many patients with this valvular lesion have precordial murmurs during childhood. The presence of a febrile illness in a child with a precordial murmur tends to be diagnosed as acute rheumatic fever when this may not be the case. In contrast to its low incidence in the patients with anatomically isolated aortic valvular disease, a his-

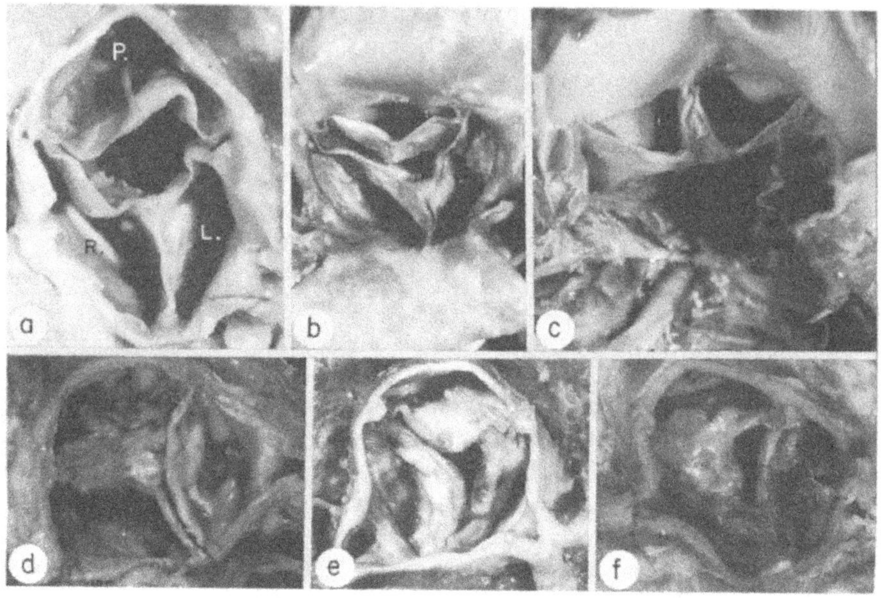

Figure 11. Acquired bicuspid aortic valves (viewed from above) in 6 patients. **a,** valve of a 54 year old man who died of bronchogenic carcinoma. Unexpected findings at necropsy were a left atrial myxoma and fibrous fusion of 1 of 3 commissures of the aortic valve. This valve caused no known cardiac dysfunction during life. The mitral valve leaflets were focally thickened. **b,** valve of a 76 year old man who had systemic hypertension but no other evidence of cardiac dysfunction. The mitral valve was normal. **c,** opened valve in a 30 year old man with Fallot's tetrad. Fusion of the commissure between the left and posterior cusps was an incidental necropsy finding.[24] The mitral valve was normal. **d,** valve in a 68 year old man who had shown clinical features of acute rheumatic fever 1 month before death and at autopsy had numerous myocardial Aschoff bodies. The commissure between the right and posterior cusps is completely fused. The mitral leaflets were diffusely thickened and focally calcified. **e,** valve of a 70 year old woman who died of gastric carcinoma but during life was believed to have mitral regurgitation. The mitral leaflets and chordae were anatomically normal, but the aortic cusps were fibrotic, calcified and rigid and the commissure between the left and posterior cusps was fused. **f,** valve of a 50 year old woman who had a history of acute rheumatic fever at age 7 years and on examination shortly before death was believed to have mitral and tricuspid regurgitation. The tricuspid valve leaflets were mildly thickened, the mitral leaflets were diffusely fibrotic and calcified, and the aortic cusps were diffusely fibrotic, focally calcified, and the commissure between the right and posterior cusps was completely fused.

Fusion occurred in 1 of the 3 commissures of the aortic valve in each of these 6 patients. The circumferential distances between a fused and a nonfused commissure were similar to the distances between the 2 nonfused commissures in all patients. The most cephalad margin of the fused commissures in each patient was on the same horizontal level as the most cephalad margins of the nonfused commissures. In 2 patients **(d and f)** the cause of the commissural fusion was rheumatic since both had extensive mitral valvular scarring. The cause of the commissural fusion in the other 4 subjects is unknown, but in only 1 **(e)** of them did the commissural fusion cause functional disturbance. Histologic sections of the fused commissures illustrated showed that they were devoid of elastic fibrils, evidence that the fusion was acquired.

tory of acute rheumatic fever or chorea was present in nearly 70 percent of 256 patients with anatomic disease of the mitral valve with or without anatomic involvement of the aortic valve studied at autopsy by me.[19] Further evidence supporting the theory that superimposed rheumatic heart disease is not the cause of stenosis or incompetency of the congenitally bicuspid aortic valve is that no patient with anatomically isolated aortic valvular disease had Aschoff bodies in the heart at necropsy. These lesions were found in the hearts of 11 of the 256 patients over 14 years of age with anatomic mitral valvular disease, and 10 of them had anatomic involvement of other valves as well.

Since superimposed rheumatic heart disease is clearly not the cause of the stenosis or incompetence of a congenitally bicuspid aortic valve, a search for other causes is necessary. The explanation advanced by Edwards[20] is attractive. He proposed that it is not mechanically possible for a congenitally bicuspid aortic valve to open and close properly. The distances between lateral attachments of normal aortic valvular cusps along their free margins are curved lines. The extra lengths allow the cusps to move freely during opening and closing of the valves. In contrast, the distances between lateral attachments of congenitally bicuspid aortic valves along their free margins approach straight lines. If these distances were exactly straight lines, the valves could not open during ventricular systole. Consequently, at least 1 cusp is larger than the other. The excessive length of 1 or both cusps of a congenitally bicuspid aortic valve produces abnormal contact between the cusps. This abnormal contact, in turn, causes focal fibrous thickening that with time becomes diffuse, and dystrophic calcification thereafter occurs. Thus, stenosis of a congenitally bicuspid aortic valve may be the result of trauma to these cusps produced by their abnormal contact with each other. Although this explanation is appealing, it does not explain why 1 congenitally bicuspid valve becomes stenotic, another becomes entirely incompetent, and another remains free of complications.

Differentiation of congenital and acquired bicuspid valve: Criteria for differentiating a bicuspid valve of congenital origin from a bicuspid valve of acquired origin (Fig. 11) have been debated. No controversy has arisen in distinguishing a congenitally bicuspid aortic valve devoid of a raphe (false commissure or ridge) and of complications (stenosis, incompetency or infection) from a tricuspid aortic valve also devoid of similar complications. Controversy has existed about the means of differentiating a congenitally bicuspid aortic valve with a raphe from an acquired bicuspid aortic valve resulting from fusion of 2 cusps at 1 true commissure.* Osler,[3] from the study of 18 hearts (15 adults), listed the following characteristics, all recognizable by gross observation, of the congenitally bicuspid aortic valve: (1) The raphe is located where normally the true commissure would be, between the right and left anterior aortic valve cusps; (2) the length of the free margin of the cusp containing no raphe is slightly shorter (by an average of 12 percent in his measurements on 7 hearts) than the length of the margin of the cusp containing a raphe, the "conjoint" cusp; (3) the free border of the conjoint cusp is straight or curled and free of nodular thickenings indicative of corpus Arantii; (4) the border of attachment of the conjoint cusp, as viewed from the ventricular aspect, presents either the contour of a single semilunar cusp or a shallow groove, indicative of the junction of 2 cusps; (5) the raphe may be located on the aortic wall alone or may extend onto the cusp for variable distances, but in either case it usually divides the sinus of Valsalva into equal-sized units.

In 1923 Lewis and Grant[11] clarified several gross features of unequivocally congenitally bicuspid aortic valves and presented histologic criteria for differentiating bicuspid valves of "congenital" origin from those of "inflammatory" origin. In contrast to Osler, these authors found that fusion could occur not only between right and left anterior cusps but also between right anterior and posterior cusps. A raphe, dividing one of the 2 cusps, was observed "in about half the cases." The 2 cusps could be equal or unequal in size, but usually the conjoined cusp was larger, but not twice the size of the undivided cusp. Or, "the subdivided cusp is larger than 1 normal cusp but

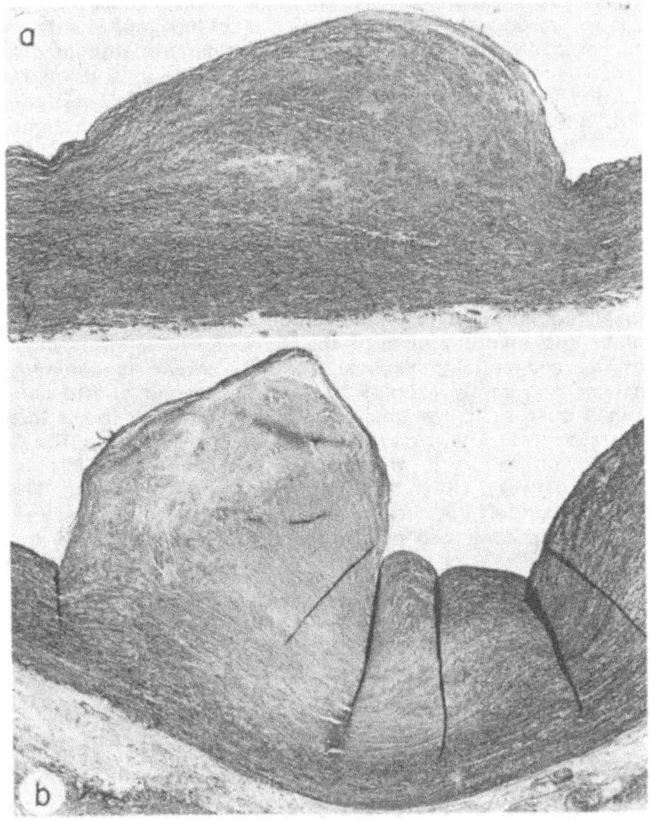

Figure 12. Photomicrographs of transverse sections of raphes in 2 patients with congenitally bicuspid aortic valves, each stained for elastic fibers (elastic Van Gieson method). **a**, characteristic appearance of raphe showing many elastic fibers, similar to aortic media. **b**, raphe from patient whose valve is illustrated in Figure 2d. The raphe is devoid of elastic fibers, but the valve grossly is unequivocally congenitally bicuspid. The raphe, although difficult to see in Figure 2d, is in the right cusp. Original magnification × 27 (a), × 24 (b); reduced by 25 percent.

smaller than 2 normal cusps." However, Lewis and Grant considered gross distinction between congenital and acquired bicuspid aortic valves unreliable. Elastic tissue stains of transverse sections of congenital raphes disclosed them to consist mainly of elastic fibers; thus the raphe histologically was similar to the media of the aorta. In contrast, transverse sections of 2 fused cusps at a true commissure disclosed that the fused commissure was devoid of elastic fibers and consisted of fibrous valvular tissue. Other investigators[21,22] confirmed these histologic criteria. Koletsky[22] also pointed out that congenital raphes were devoid of vascular channels and of inflammatory cells whereas both were seen in acquired, fused commissures. Since Lewis and Grant described these histologic features, many pathologists have been reluctant to distinguish between congenital and acquired bicuspid aortic valves without microscopic examination of raphes. However, these histologic criteria are helpful but not specific (Fig. 12).

* The definition of a commissure differs depending on whether a semilunar or an atrioventricular (A–V) cardiac valve is under consideration. The aortic valve commissure is the space between 2 lateral attachments on the aortic wall. Normally each aortic valve cusp is an independent similar-sized unit and adherence of one cusp with another at the narrow space (commissure) between the 2 cusps is abnormal. In contrast to a semilunar valve, the leaflets of an atrioventricular valve are continuous one with another. Thus, the commissures of the A–V valves are the sites of attachment between the unequal-sized leaflets, not the spaces between the cusps as in the case of the semilunar valves.

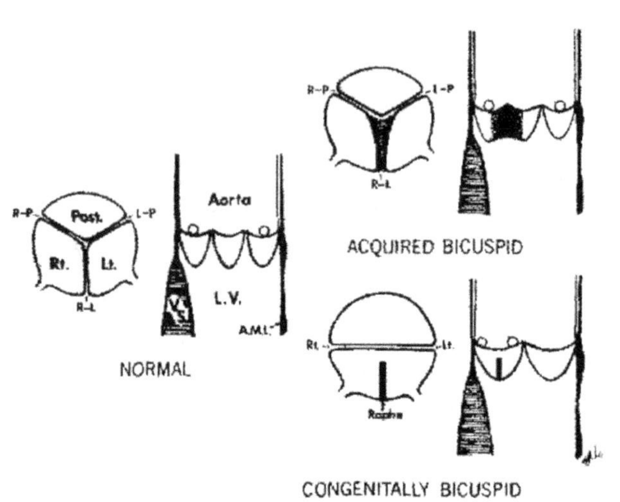

Figure 13. Diagram illustrating differences between bicuspid aortic valves of acquired and of congenital origins as compared to the normal valve. The circumferential distances between each of the 3 commissures in a normally formed valve are similar. L-P = left-posterior, R-L = right-left, and R-P = right-posterior commissures; Rt. = right, Lt. = left, and Post. = posterior cusps; V.S. = ventricular septum; L.V. = left ventricular outflow tract; and A.M.L. = anterior mitral leaflet. **In the acquired bicuspid valve** the circumferential distance between the commissures remains equal, as in the normal. The fused commissure is wide, the distal margins of each of the 2 fused cusps are still usually visible, and the most cephalad margin of the fused commissure is on the same horizontal level as the most cephalad margins of the 2 nonfused commissures. **In the congenitally bicuspid valve** the raphe is generally narrow and rarely extends to the free margin of the conjoined cusp or to the cephalad level reached by the 2 true commissures. The circumferential distance between the 2 true commissures is greater than the circumferential distances between either true commissure and the raphe. The circumferential distance between the true commissures around the conjoined cusp, that is, the cusp that has the raphe, is equal to or slightly greater than the circumferential distance between the true commissures around the cusp devoid of the raphe.

In patients in whom some sections of a raphe show a structure like that of the aortic media, other sections of the same raphe may show only fibrous tissue. Also, the congenital raphe may lose its elastic fibers as the valvular cusps become fibrotic and calcified. The raphe may be the first portion of a congenitally bicuspid aortic valve to calcify, and these deposits destroy existing elastic fibers. Interestingly, Lewis and Grant and others who emphasized the importance of histologic distinction between congenital raphes and fused true commissures were unaware that calcific stenosis was a consequence of a congenitally bicuspid aortic valve. Once the valve is extensively scarred and calcified, histologic examination of the raphe is often fruitless. Furthermore, as Edwards[24] pointed out, in an occasional patient with a bicuspid aortic valve that must be assumed to be congenital, as in infants with aortic coarctation, the raphe not only may be fibrous, but may grossly display features suggesting fusion of 2 distinguishable, separate cusps.

Useful features to distinguish between bicuspid aortic valves of acquired and of congenital origin are summarized in Figure 13. Emphasis is placed on obvious gross differences between fused true commissures and raphes.

Acknowledgment

I am indebted to my past and present colleagues, particularly Drs. Andrew G. Morrow and Eugene Braunwald, for free access to the clinical data on the patients described in this study.

References

1. **Paget J:** On obstructions of the branches of the pulmonary artery. Med-Chir Trans 27:162–188, 1844
2. **Peacock TB:** On Malformations of the Human Heart, second edition. London, Churchill, 1866, p 204
3. **Osler W:** The bicuspid condition of the aortic valves. Trans Ass Amer Physicians 2:185–192, 1886
4. **Campbell M, Kauntze R:** Congenital aortic valvular stenosis. Brit Heart J 15:179–194, 1953
5. **Smith DE, Matthews MB:** Aortic valvular stenosis with coarctation of the aorta. With special reference to the development of aortic stenosis upon congenital bicuspid valves. Brit Heart J 17:198–206, 1955
6. **Bacon APC, Matthews MB:** Congenital bicuspid aortic valves and the aetiology of isolated aortic valvular stenosis. Quart J Med 28:545–560, 1959
7. **Roberts, WC:** Examining the precordium and the heart. Chest, in press
8. **Friedman WF, Mason DT, Braunwald E:** Arthrogryposis multiplex congenita associated with congenital aortic stenosis. J Pediat 67:682–685, 1965
9. **Roberts WC, Morrow AG:** Cardiac valves and the surgical pathologist. Arch Path (Chicago) 82:309–313, 1966
10. **Osler W:** On the condition of fusion of two segments of the semilunar valves. Montreal Gen Hosp Reports 1:233, 1880
11. **Lewis T, Grant RT:** Observations relating to subacute infective endocarditis. Heart 10:21–99, 1923
12. **Grant RT, Wood JE Jr, Jones TD:** Heart valve irregularities in relation to subacute bacterial endocarditis. Heart 14:247–255, 1928
13. **Bonnabeau RC Jr, Lillehei CW, Edwards JE:** Relationship of the congenital bicuspid aortic valve to calcific aortic stenosis (abstr). Circulation 29, 30: Suppl III:51, 1964
14. **Roberts WC:** Severe valvular cardiac disease. A study

of 400 autopsy patients over 14 years of age. In preparation
15. **Campbell M:** Calcific aortic stenosis and congenital bicuspid aortic valves. Brit Heart J 30:606–616, 1968
16. **Starling HJ:** Endocarditis lenta. Quart J Med 16:263–281, 1923
17. **Fulton MN, Levine SA:** Subacute bacterial endocarditis, with special reference to the valvular lesions and previous history. Amer J Med Sci 183:60–77, 1932
18. **Bayles TB, Lewis WH Jr:** Subacute bacterial endocarditis in older people. Ann Intern Med 13:2154–2163, 1940
19. **Roberts WC:** Anatomically isolated aortic valve disease. The case against its being of rheumatic etiology. Amer J Med, in press.
20. **Edwards JE:** The congenital bicuspid aortic valve. Circulation 23:485–488, 1961
21. **Bishop LF Jr, Trubek M:** Bicuspid aortic valve: a differential study between inflammatory and congenital origin. J Tech Meth 15:111–131, 1936
22. **Koletsky S:** Congenital bicuspid aortic valves. Arch Intern Med (Chicago) 67:129–176, 1941
23. **Edwards JE:** Congenital malformations of the heart and great vessels. C. Malformations of the valves. In, Pathology of the Heart and Blood Vessels, third edition (Gould SE, ed). Springfield, Ill., Charles C Thomas, 1968 p 341
24. **Glancy DL, Morrow AG, Roberts WC:** Malformations of the aortic valve in patients with the tetralogy of Fallot. Amer Heart J 76:755–759, 1968

Anatomically Isolated Aortic Valvular Disease

The Case Against Its Being of Rheumatic Etiology

WILLIAM C. ROBERTS, M.D.
Bethesda, Maryland

Data are presented in 400 autopsy patients, each over fourteen years of age (average age, forty-five years) with functionally severe valvular cardiac disease. Of 139 patients with anatomically isolated aortic valvular disease (aortic stenosis [AS] in 105 and pure aortic regurgitation [AR] in thirty-four), 6 per cent had positive histories of acute rheumatic fever (ARF) or chorea, none had Aschoff bodies, nearly all had histologically normal atrial walls, and 72 per cent of the 105 patients with AS and 26.5 per cent of the thirty-four patients with pure AR had congenitally malformed aortic valves. In contrast, of 235 patients with anatomic mitral disease with or without anatomic involvement of other valves, 68 per cent had positive histories of ARF or chorea, twelve (5 per cent) had Aschoff bodies, nearly all had histologically abnormal left atrial walls, and only two patients (<1 per cent) had congenitally malformed valves. It is concluded that anatomically isolated aortic valve disease is of nonrheumatic etiology and most frequently the consequence of a congenital malformation.

Considerable evidence indicates that isolated mitral stenosis is nearly always of rheumatic etiology. Likewise, combined anatomic disease of both mitral and aortic valves is generally rheumatic in origin. Anatomically isolated aortic valvular disease causing stenosis or regurgitation or both also has been considered by numerous investigators generally to be of rheumatic etiology. Study of 400 autopsy patients with various forms of functionally severe valvular cardiac disease, however, has convinced me that anatomically isolated aortic valvular disease is not rheumatic in origin. Observations on these 400 patients which allowed this conclusion are described.

PATIENTS STUDIED AND RESULTS

Data in the 400 patients studied at necropsy are summarized in Table I. Each patient died between 1953 and 1968 inclusive: 331 had been studied clinically at the National Heart Institute, and sixty-nine were studied clinically at other institutions and their hearts submitted to me for examination. Clinical data were available in all patients. Cardiac catheterization had been performed in 315 patients, and cardiac valvular operation (commissurotomy, valvuloplasty or replacement) had been performed in 280 patients, a few of whom had never undergone cardiac catheterization. Each of the 400 patients was over fourteen years of age (range fifteen to eighty-eight years; average forty-five years); twelve were over seventy and thirty-seven were under thirty years of age at death. Each had been considered to be in functional classes III or IV (New York Heart Association Classification). Patients with carcinoid heart disease [1,2] and left ventricular papillary muscle dysfunction, fibrosis or necrosis [3] were excluded. The hospital charts of all 400 patients

From the Section of Pathology, National Heart and Lung Institute, National Institutes of Health, Bethesda, Maryland 20014. Requests for reprints should be addressed to Dr. William C. Roberts. Manuscript received September 11, 1969.

TABLE I Data in 400 Autopsy Patients Over Fourteen Years of Age with Valvular Cardiac Disease

Group	Valve Involved Anatomically	No. Patients	% of Total	Age (yr) Range	Age (yr) Average	Sex (No.) Male	Sex (No.) Female	Sex (%) Male	Sex (%) Female	Nonrheumatic Etiology No.	Nonrheumatic Etiology %	Rheumatic Etiology No.	Rheumatic Etiology %	History of ARF or Chorea (No.)	Rheumatic Subjects with History of ARF or Chorea (%)	Total with History of ARF or Chorea (%)
I	Aortic only	163	41	15–88	48	134	29	82	18	141	87	?22	?13	21	. . .	13
	a. AS with or without AR	105	26	16–88	50	80	25	76	24	105	100	0	0	6*	0	6
	b. Pure AR	34	9	15–69	40	31	3	91	9	32	89	?4	11	2†	0	6
	c. Clinically AS or pure AR but thickened mitral leaflets and normal chordae tendineae	24‡	6	34–74	50	23	1	96	4	4§	17	20	83	13	65	54
II	Mitral + aortic	116	29	20–85	45	75	41	65	35	4	3	112	97	87	78	75
III	Mitral only	75	19	15–78	42	27	48	36	64	18¶	24	57#	76	40	70	53
IV	Mitral + aortic + tricuspid‖	38	9	18–65	41	16	22	42	58	1	3	37	97	27	73	71
V	Mitral + tricuspid	6	1.5	30–57	47	1	5	17	83	0	0	6	100	5	83	83
VI	Tricuspid only	2¶	0.5	31–65	48	1	1	50	50	2	100	0	0	0	0	0
	Totals	400	100	15–88	45	254	146	63.5	36.5	166	41.5	234	58.5	180	77**	45

* Five had congenitally bicuspid aortic valves.
† One had ankylosing spondylitis.
‡ Five patients had pure AR; nineteen had some degree of AS.
§ Each had congenitally bicuspid aortic valves; none had a positive history of ARF.
¶ Each had pure mitral regurgitation.
# Each had mitral stenosis with or without regurgitation.
‖ Two also had focally thickened but functionally normal pulmonic valve cusps.
** If group I were excluded this percentage would be 75 instead of 77.

were reviewed. A history of acute rheumatic fever (ARF) was considered positive if the patient stated that he had been told that he had ARF in the past or if he described a febrile illness during childhood characterized by signs or symptoms of arthritis necessitating rest in bed. Most of the latter patients were told that they had heart murmurs during their febrile illnesses. Electrocardiographic, roentgenographic, hemodynamic and autopsy observations were recorded. The heart of each patient was examined on at least two occasions by me. The patients were divided according to which cardiac valve or valves were involved anatomically (Table I).

The aortic valve only was involved in 163 patients. (group I). Aortic stenosis (AS) with or without aortic regurgitation (AR) (group Ia) occurred in 105 of them: eighty (76 per cent) were male, twenty-five (24 per cent) female; six (6 per cent) had a history of acute rheumatic fever (ARF) or chorea, but five of the six had congenitally bicuspid aortic valves. The diagnosis of ARF in these five therefore is probably fallacious. Left heart catheterization was performed in seventy-four of the 105 patients with isolated AS. The peak systolic pressure gradients between the left ventricle and a systemic artery ranged from 18 to 165 mm Hg (average 97 mm Hg). In only three patients were these pressure gradients less than 50 mm Hg. Of the thirty-four patients with pure AR, thirty-one (91 per cent) were male, and two (6 per cent) had a history of ARF or chorea. The various causes of AR in these thirty-four patients are summarized in Table II. Cardiac catheterization in nineteen patients with pure AR showed zero or negative systolic pressure gradients between the left ventricle and a systemic artery in each. In addition to the 105 patients with AS and the thirty-four with pure AR, twenty-four other subjects are included in the "aortic only" group since they also had AS or AR or both. In contrast to the other 139 patients in group I, however, their mitral leaflets also were diffusely thickened (Fig. 1). Their mitral chordae tendineae, however, were normal, and the valves functioned normally. It is suspected that thickening of the mitral leaflets in some of them resulted from the elevated left ventricular pressures, but others probably belong in the mitral plus aortic category (group II), especially since thirteen (54 per cent) had a positive history of ARF or chorea. If the four patients with congenitally bicuspid aortic valves, none of whom had a positive history of ARF, are excluded, this percentage rises to 65 per cent. Cardiac catheterization was performed in twenty of the twenty-four patients in group Ic. Of the fifteen with AS, the peak systolic pressure gradients between the left ventricle and a systemic artery ranged from 18 to 120 mm Hg (average 65 mm Hg). No pressure gradient between the left ventricle and a systemic artery occurred in any of the five patients with pure AR.

Accurate heart weights were available in 146 of the 163 patients in group I. The heart weight ranged from 330 to 1,100 gm (average 650 gm). The heart weight of ninety-two patients with isolated AS ranged from 330 to 1,000 gm (average 608 gm). The weight depended more on the sex than the degree of obstruction across the aortic valve: in the twenty women the heart weight averaged 477 gm (range 330 to 700 gm) and in the seventy-two men 645 gm (range 400 to 1,000 gm). In ten (all women) of the ninety-two patients with accurately weighed hearts in group I, the heart weight was 400 gm or less; and in the six in whom cardiac catheterization was performed, the peak systolic pressure gradients between the left ventricle and a systemic artery ranged from 70 to 145 mm Hg (average 98 mm Hg). Of thirty-one patients with pure AR the heart weight ranged from 390 to 1,100 gm (average 691 gm). Of thirty-three patients in group Ic (Table I) the heart weight ranged from 530 to 1,050 gm (average 754 gm). In none of the patients in group Ic did the heart weigh 400 gm or less, but in one man in group Ib in whom infective endocarditis caused acute fatal AR, the heart weighed 390 gm.

In contrast to its low incidence (6 per cent) in the 139 patients with anatomically isolated AS (group Ia) and pure AR (group Ib), the incidence of a positive history of ARF or chorea in the 235 patients with anatomic mitral valvular involvement (groups II through V, Table I) ranged from 53 to 83 per cent (average 68 per cent). The latter average rises to 74 per cent if the twenty-three patients with clearly nonrheumatic valvular disease in groups II through V are eliminated. Although male subjects predominated (65 per cent) in the 116 patients with anatomic disease of both mitral and aortic valves (group II), female subjects predominated (63 per cent) in the other 119 patients with involvement in the mitral valve, whether alone (group III), in combination with both aortic and tricuspid valves (group IV) or in combination with the tricuspid valve (group V). In twenty-three of the 235 patients with mitral valvular disease the etiology was clearly nonrheumatic. Eighteen had isolated mitral involvement with pure regurgitation resulting from rupture of chordae tendineae (infective endocarditis) in previously normal valves [4] (ten patients), "floppy" mitral leaflets [5] (four patients), congenital malformations (two patients), probably secondary to mitral annular calcification (one patient) and uncertain etiology [6] (one patient). Each of the four patients with combined mitral and aortic involvement of nonrheumatic etiology had severe mitral and aortic regurgitation, and one had mild (30 mm Hg peak systolic pressure gradient) AS in addition. The latter patient had a congenitally bicuspid aortic valve and a congenitally malformed mitral valve. Two of the other patients had the Marfan syndrome, and the third had Marfan-type diseased valves without the clinical syndrome **(forme fruste).** The only patient with three-valve involvement of nonrheumatic nature had rheumatoid heart disease [7]. Anatomically isolated tricuspid valve disease is nonrheumatic; each of the two patients (group VI, Table I) studied by me was a heroin addict with infective endocarditis superimposed on previously normal valves [8].

The structure of the aortic valve in the 163 patients with anatomically isolated aortic valvular disease is summarized in Table III. Of the 105 patients with

TABLE II Etiology of Pure Aortic Regurgitation. Thirty-Four Patients > Age Fourteen Years with Anatomically Isolated Aortic Valve Disease*

Etiology	No. of Patients
Infective endocarditis	9†
Syphilis	9‡
Medial cystic necrosis of aorta	5§
Ankylosing spondylitis	5
Congenital	2#
Trauma	1
Juvenile rheumatoid arthritis	1
Chronic dissecting aortic aneurysm	1
Etiology undetermined	1¶
	34

* Eight other patients among the 400 studied also had clinically pure aortic regurgitation (AR), but the mitral valve was anatomically abnormal in each, although three were in class 1c. The etiology in each is considered rheumatic.

† Seven and possibly eight had congenitally bicuspid aortic valves, and none had evidence of AR until manifestations of the cardiac infection appeared.

‡ Serologic test for syphilis positive in only three patients; histologic changes in ascending aorta consistent with syphilis in each.

§ Four had the Marfan syndrome.

\# Each had congenitally bicuspid aortic valves which were intrinsically incompetent and neither patient ever had clinical or anatomic evidence of infective endocarditis.

¶ Patient was stated to have "had acute rheumatic fever at age ten years."

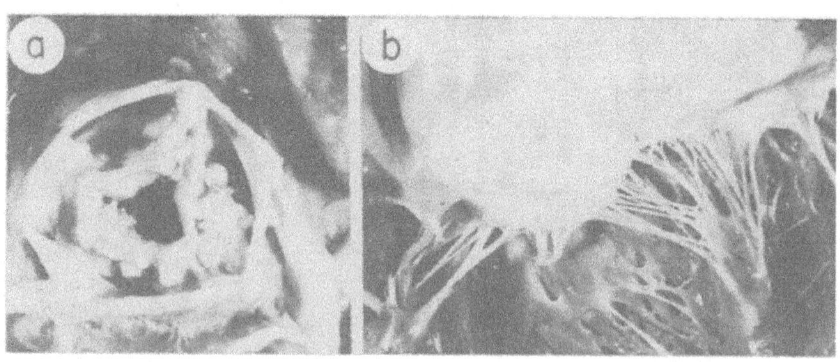

Fig. 1. *Aortic valve from above (a) and opened mitral valve (b) in a forty-one year old man (A66-136) with a positive history of acute rheumatic fever and severe aortic stenosis and regurgitation. The aortic valve is three-cuspid but each of the three commissures is partially fused, producing a central triangular shaped orifice. The two mitral leaflets are diffusely thickened but the chordae tendineae are normal. Thus, this case is in group Ic (Table I).*

TABLE III Valve Structure in Anatomically Isolated Aortic Valvular Disease. Summary of 163 Autopsy Patients Over Age Fourteen

Group	Functional Lesion	No. Patients	Unicuspid	Bicuspid	Tricuspid	Structure Uncertain	Per Cent Congenitally Malformed
1a	AS with or without AR	105	13	54	32*	6	64†
1b	Pure AR	34	0	9‡	25	0	26.5
1c	Clinically AS or AR but thickened mitral leaflets and normal chordae tendineae	24	0	4§	20#	0	17
	Totals	163	13	67	77	. . .	49

* In three patients the cusps were of unequal size, and one of them also had a congenitally bicuspid pulmonic valve.
† This percentage rises to 72 per cent if the "uncertain" category is either included in or excluded from the congenitally malformed group and if the three patients with unequal sized three-cuspid aortic valves are included in the congenitally malformed group.
‡ In seven of the nine patients infective endocarditis caused the valve to be incompetent.
§ In two patients the valvular orifice was severely stenotic, and in two it was only mildly stenotic (18 and 24 mm Hg peak systolic pressure gradients, respectively) but severely incompetent.
\# In fourteen patients the valve orifice was severely stenotic, in one patient mildly stenotic and severely incompetent, and in five subjects purely incompetent.

AS with or without AR, thirteen had congenitally unicuspid unicommissural aortic valves [9,10] (Fig. 2), fifty-four had congenitally bicuspid valves [11] (Fig. 3), thirty-two had three-cuspid valves (Fig. 4), and in six the valves were so deformed, scarred and calcified that the structure was not discernible. Thus, 64 per cent had congenitally malformed valves. It is likely that the six patients in whom the valve structure was uncertain also had congenitally malformed valves (either bicuspid or unicommissural) since tricuspid aortic valves are relatively easily delineated. In three of the thirty-two patients with tricuspid aortic valves the cusps were clearly unequal in size. Thus, if the "structure-uncertain" group (Table III) and the three subjects with unequal sized three-cuspid valves were included with the sixty-seven patients with congenitally unicommissural or bicuspid valves, the number of patients with congenitally malformed valves rises to seventy-six (72 per cent). Of the thirty-four patients with pure AR, nine (26.5 per cent) had malformed valves, and each was congenitally bicuspid.

In each of the 400 patients studied at least one section from the wall of each cardiac chamber was examined histologically. An average of seven histologic sections of heart were studied in each patient; Aschoff bodies were found in twelve patients. In only five of the twelve patients, however, were Aschoff bodies plentiful and unequivocal; Aschoff bodies were rare and equivocal in the other seven. None was found in the 163 patients with anatomically isolated aortic valve disease. All twelve patients had anatomic involvement of the mitral valve, eleven also had aortic valve involvement, and five also had tricuspid valve involvement.

Histologic sections of the walls of the right and left atria were examined in all patients. Some myocardial fiber degeneration or atrophy with or without interstitial myocardial fibrosis was observed in the sections of left atrial walls and often also of right atrial wall in nearly all patients with anatomic mitral valvular disease (groups II through V) (Fig. 5). In contrast, myocardial fiber degeneration or interstitial fibrosis was nearly always absent in sections of left and right atrial walls in the patients with anatomically isolated aortic valvular disease. In both groups, however, the myocardial fibers of the atrial walls and the smooth muscle fibers of

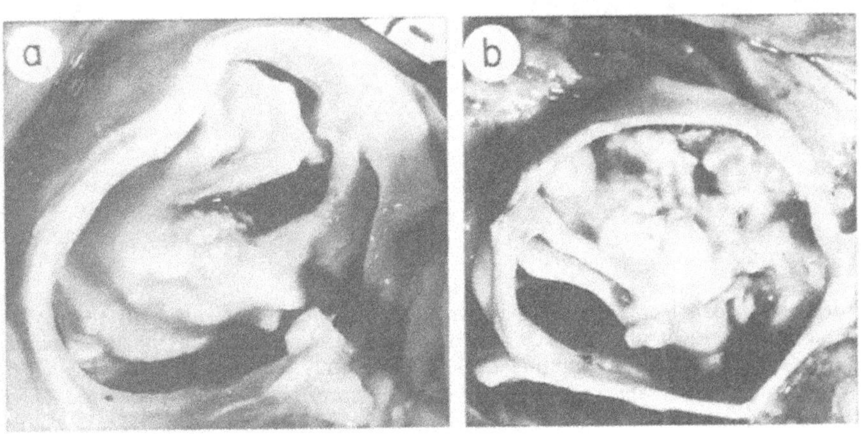

Fig. 2. *Congenitally unicuspid, unicommissural aortic valves from above in two men (A57-59 and A68-109), aged twenty-eight (a) and aged forty-eight years (b). Congenitally unicommissural aortic valves are always stenotic.*

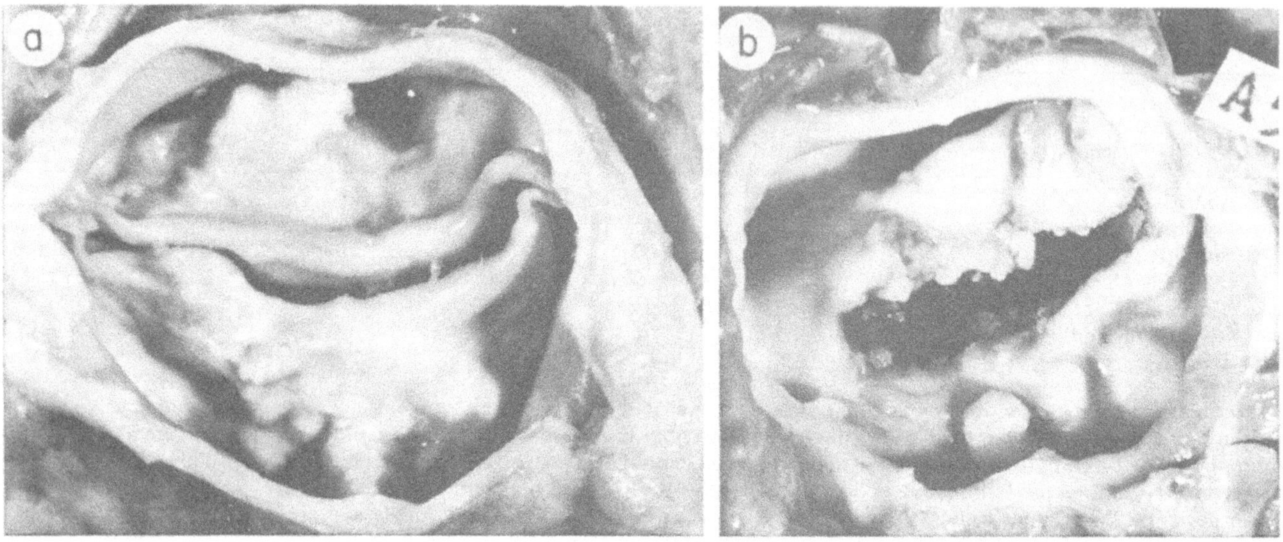

Fig. 3. *Congenitally bicuspid aortic valves in two men (A64-155 and A58-219), aged sixty-one (a) and thirty-seven years (b), respectively. Each is severely stenotic.*

the left atrial endocardium were nearly always hypertrophied.

COMMENTS

These findings in 400 autopsy patients with functionally severe valvular cardiac disease indicate that anatomically isolated aortic valvular disease is nonrheumatic in etiology. Four factors allow this conclusion: (1) the low incidence (6 per cent) of a history of ARF or chorea in the subjects with anatomically isolated aortic valvular disease (groups Ia and Ib, Table I) compared to the high incidence (68 per cent) of a positive history in the patients with anatomic mitral valvular disease with or without involvement of other cardiac valves; (2) the absence of Aschoff bodies in any of the 163 patients with anatomically isolated aortic valvular disease compared to the presence of the pathognomonic bodies in twelve of 235 patients (5 per cent) with mitral valvular disease; (3) the absence of interstitial fibrosis and myocardial fiber degeneration in the left atrial walls of patients with anatomically isolated aortic valvular disease compared to the nearly universal presence of these lesions in patients with mitral valvular disease; (4) the high incidence (72 per cent) of congenitally malformed valves in the patients with anatomically isolated aortic valvular disease causing stenosis compared to a zero incidence in the patients with anatomically isolated mitral valvular disease causing stenosis.

Although a similar incidence has been reported [12–15] in patients with isolated aortic valvular disease and in patients with mitral valvular disease with and without other valvular involvement, positive histories of ARF or chorea have been found by most observers infrequently in patients with isolated aortic valvular disease or at least far less frequently than in subjects with mitral or multivalvular disease. Of forty-two autopsy patients with "calcareous aortic valvular disease" described by Margolis and associates [16], three (7 per cent) had a history of ARF or chorea. Nineteen of seventy-three autopsy patients (26 per cent) with isolated aortic stenosis and thirty-seven of fifty autopsy patients (74 per cent) with combined mitral and aortic stenosis reported by McGinn and White [17] had a posi-

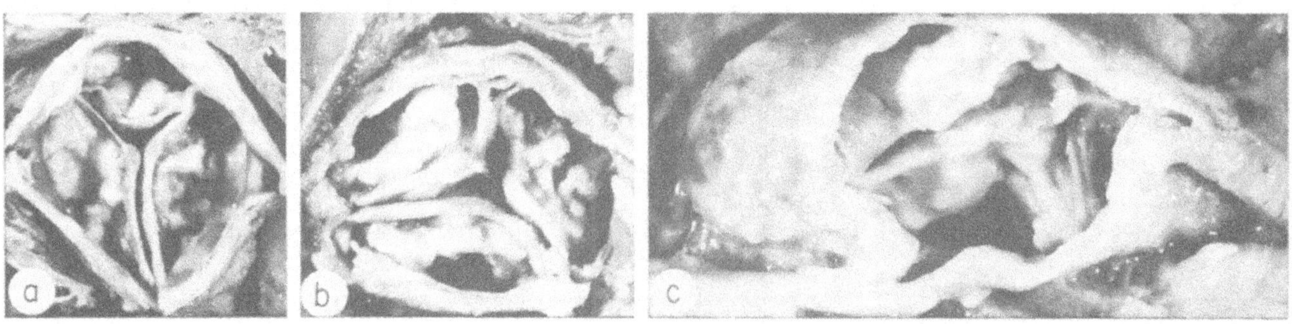

Fig. 4. *Heavily calcified, stenotic tricuspid aortic valves seen from above, in three patients. The mitral valves in each were normal except for focal aging changes. a, the three cusps are of unequal size in this eighty year old man. b, the three cusps are of similar size in this eighty-five year old man. c, one of the three commissures is completely fused in the aortic valve of this fifty-two year old man. The peak systolic pressure gradient across this valve was 85 mm Hg and the calculated valve area was 0.35 cu cm.*

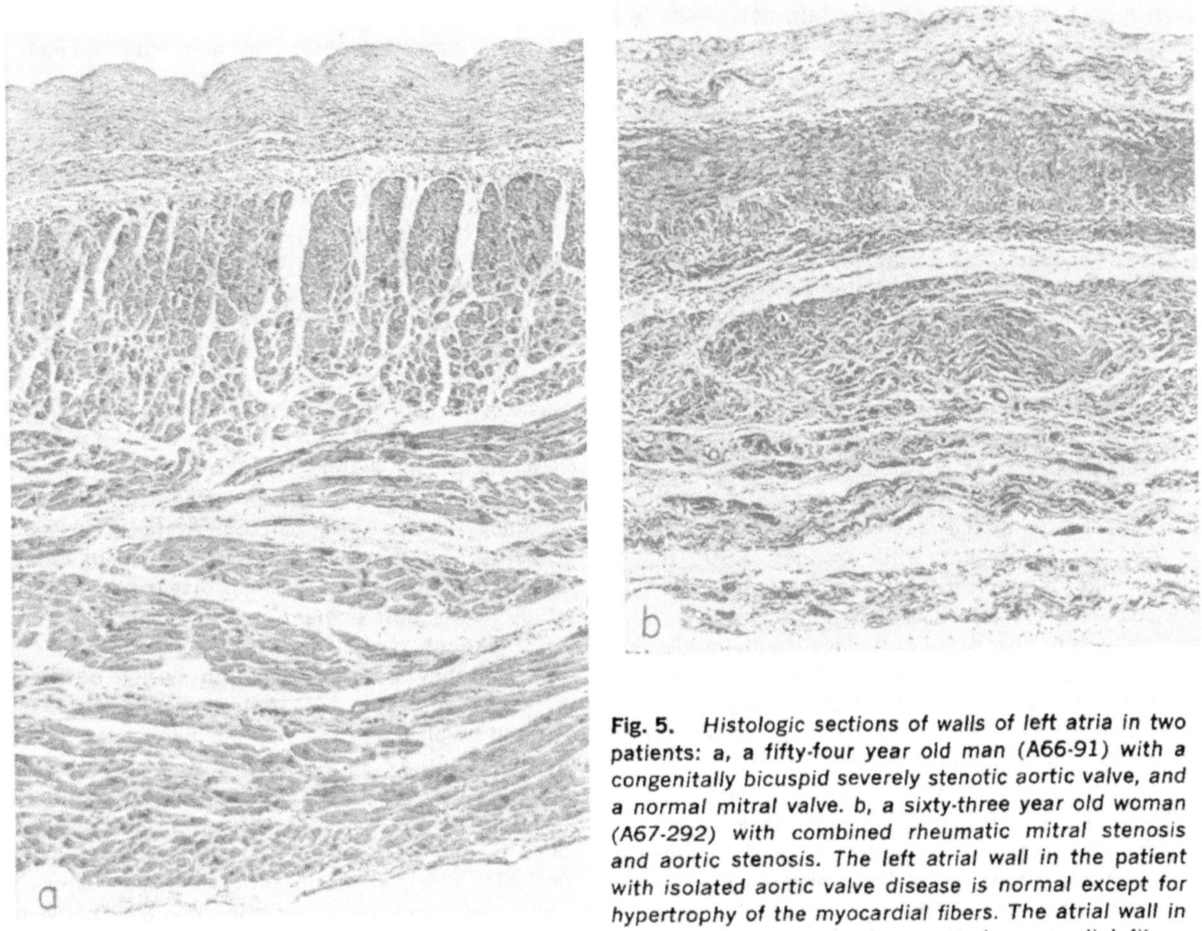

Fig. 5. *Histologic sections of walls of left atria in two patients: a, a fifty-four year old man (A66-91) with a congenitally bicuspid severely stenotic aortic valve, and a normal mitral valve. b, a sixty-three year old woman (A67-292) with combined rheumatic mitral stenosis and aortic stenosis. The left atrial wall in the patient with isolated aortic valve disease is normal except for hypertrophy of the myocardial fibers. The atrial wall in the patient with combined mitral and aortic valve disease contains severely degenerated myocardial fibers and extensive interstitial and replacement myocardial fibrosis. Hematoxylin and eosin stains; original magnification* $\times$ *55 (a) and* $\times$ *60 (b).*

tive history of ARF. Of 200 autopsy patients with "the calcified nodular deformity of the aortic valve" studied by Clawson and associates [18] seventy (35 per cent) had a positive history of ARF but eighty-nine of the 200 patients had associated mitral valvular disease. Of 106 autopsy patients with calcified aortic valves studied by Dry and Willius [19], sixteen (15 per cent) had a history of ARF; thirty-two of the 106 patients, however, had associated mitral valvular disease, and fifteen of the sixteen patients with a positive history were among these thirty-two subjects. Thus, only one of the seventy-four patients with isolated calcific aortic valvular disease had a history of ARF, and in this patient it is not clear whether it was isolated or associated with mitral involvement. In contrast, of 106 autopsy patients with mitral stenosis studied by the same investigators, sixty-seven (63 per cent) had a positive history of ARF. None of the nine autopsy patients reported by Cohen et al. [20], five of twenty-two autopsy patients (23 per cent) studied by Reich [21], twenty-one of 100 autopsy patients (21 per cent) studied by Horan and Barnes [22] and thirteen of forty-nine autopsy patients (27 per cent) studied by Anderson and associates [23] with calcific aortic "stenosis" had a positive history of ARF or chorea. Among 200 autopsy patients with "calcific disease of the aortic valve" studied by Karsner and Koletsky [24] thirty-five (18 per cent) had a positive history of migratory polyarthritis or chorea. Of the 109 patients with isolated aortic valvular disease, however, only three (2.8 per cent) had a history of ARF or chorea, whereas thirty-two of ninety-one patients (35 per cent) with multivalvular disease (aortic plus mitral with or without involvement of the tricuspid or pulmonic valve) had a positive history.

Thus, the reported incidences of a positive history of ARF or chorea in patients with presumed isolated aortic valvular disease has varied from possibly zero [19] to 67 per cent [15]. The wide spread between these percentages probably results from lack of discrimination between isolated aortic valve disease and that complicated by mitral disease. Willius and Dry [19], and later Anderson and associates [23], emphasized that separating patients with isolated aortic valve disease from those with mitral or multivalvular involvement could lead to missing a rheumatic etiology in the former group. As early as 1909, however, Allbutt [25] stated: "to understand [cardiac valvular] stenosis we must study it in its unmixed form." Kumpe and

Bean [15] in 1948 again emphasized this point. Another cause of disagreement in reported incidences of a positive history of ARF or chorea in patients with various cardiac valvular diseases is that the anatomic data in nearly all previous studies has been obtained by review of autopsy protocols and not by re-examination of hearts by an investigator seeking preplanned specific information. The latter method, however, is the only reliable one. The heart of each of the 400 patients included in the present study was examined by me on at least two occasions, the second without knowledge of how the heart had been classified on the initial examination.

The relatively low incidences of a positive history of ARF or chorea in patients with anatomically isolated aortic valvular disease have not deterred most investigators from attributing this valvular lesion to a rheumatic etiology. Their reasoning has been as follows: The episodes of ARF in the patients with isolated aortic disease were so **mild** or **atypical** that their true nature went unrecognized. Since the attack of ARF in them was mild, the mitral value and myocardium escaped with minimal or no injury. Or, since the patients with isolated aortic valvular disease are **older** than the subjects with mitral disease, the episode of ARF was forgotten or occurred in an era when ARF was not well recognized.

Although some investigators recorded a similar incidence of histories of ARF or chorea in patients with apparently isolated aortic valvular disease and in those with isolated mitral disease, a striking difference in **sex** and **age** among those two groups was universally recognized. Cabot [12] explained the age difference by reasoning that the "heart and circulatory system accommodates itself more easily to a pure aortic lesion than to any of the other valve lesions or combinations of such," and as a result the patients live into old age. Cabot found no explanation for the sex difference but Willius and Dry [26] reasoned that "although the incidence of rheumatic fever is about the same in the two sexes, women apparently do not have the same **relative immunity** to serious and widespread cardiac involvement by the disease as men."

Koletsky [27] and others have listed several gross and histologic "unequivocal stigmas of rheumatic heart disease," but none of them is specific except the Aschoff body. It is present in the heart of two-thirds of the patients who die of ARF or chorea [28]. Of 190 autopsy patients with ARF or chorea collected by Clawson by combining studies of several investigators, 127 (67 per cent) had Aschoff bodies in their heart [28]. Aschoff bodies also are reported to occur frequently in operatively excised atrial appendages, the incidence ranging from 18 to 74 per cent (average 33 per cent) in 1,180 patients tabulated by Tedeschi, Wagner and Pani [29]. In contrast, the incidence of Aschoff bodies in autopsy patients with rheumatic heart disease is relatively low. Clawson [18] found myocardial Aschoff nodules in seven of fifty-four patients (13 per cent) with isolated calcareous aortic "stenosis," and in nine of sixty-eight autopsy patients (13 per cent) in whom "other" valves were involved. Hall and Ichioka [14] reported Aschoff bodies in nine of nineteen autopsy patients (47 per cent) with isolated aortic valvular disease, and in seven of twelve autopsy patients (58 per cent) with mitral plus aortic valvular disease. It is apparent, however, that they used loose histologic criteria for diagnosing Aschoff bodies. Interestingly, eight of their nineteen patients with isolated aortic valvular disease had bicuspid valves, whereas none of their twelve patients with combined valvular disease had bicuspid valves. Karsner and Koletsky [24] reported myocardial Aschoff bodies in only three of 119 autopsy patients (2.5 per cent) with isolated "calcific disease of the aortic valve" and in seventeen of ninety-one autopsy patients (19 per cent) with mitral and aortic disease with or without associated tricuspid or pulmonic valvular involvement. These investigators explained the frequent absence of cardiac Aschoff bodies in their patients "by the fact that the specimens all represent chronic or healed stages of disease." In the present study no Aschoff bodies were found in the hearts of the 163 patients with isolated aortic valvular disease, whereas they were observed in twelve of the 235 patients (5 per cent) with mitral valvular disease with or without involvement of other cardiac valves. The criteria I use for defining an Aschoff body are those initially described by Aschoff and summarized by Saphir [30].

Study of the walls of the atria, particularly the left one, is useful in arriving at an etiologic diagnosis in patients with valvular cardiac disease. Gross [31] in 1935 described histologic abnormalities in the left atrial walls in each of eighty-seven patients with rheumatic disease: sixty-seven had active rheumatic fever with Aschoff bodies, and twenty had chronic valvular scarring and no Aschoff bodies. The atrial histologic changes observed other than Aschoff bodies included small lymphocytic infiltrates, distorted, concentrated and reduplicated elastica, increased and irregular smooth muscle in the endocardium and thickened, fibrotic and abnormally vascularized subendocardium; marked fiber hypertrophy, lymphocytic infiltrates and fibrosis in the myocardium; and inflammation and/or fibrosis in the pericardium. Gross considered these atrial changes to be evidence of rheumatic disease, and a year later he and Sohval [32] reported their presence in thirteen autopsy patients with multivalvular heart disease and their absence in nineteen patients with isolated calcific sclerosis of the aortic valve. In the present study a difference also was noted in the histologic, and often also in the gross appearance of the left atrial walls in patients with anatomically isolated aortic valvular stenosis or regurgitation or both and in patients with isolated mitral or combined mitral and aortic disease. The histologic changes in the left atrial wall appear to result at least in part from rheumatic involvement of the wall itself and not entirely from altered left atrial hemodynamics produced by the mitral valve lesion. In subjects with anatomic (rheumatic) involvement of both mitral and aortic valves causing dysfunction of only the aortic valve, these histologic changes occur. Furthermore, in subjects with severe mitral regurgitation secondary to ruptured chordae tendineae in otherwise normal valves, i.e., nonrheumatic etiology, no changes have been noted in the left atria histologically other than hypertrophy of the myocardial fibers [4]. Virtually none of the 163 patients with anatomically isolated aortic valvular disease had degeneration or distortion of myocardial fibers, interstitial myocardial fibrosis or abnormal fibrous thickening of the endocardium or subendocardium. In contrast, these lesions were observed histologically in the sections of atria of nearly all subjects studied with isolated rheumatic mitral or combined mitral and aortic disease.

The factor most against a rheumatic etiology of anatomically isolated aortic valvular disease causing stenosis is the high incidence of congenital malformations of this valve. In the present study fifty-four of the 105 patients with isolated aortic stenosis with or without regurgitation had congenitally bicuspid valves [11], thirteen had congenitally unicommissural unicuspid valves, six had probable congenitally malformed valves, and thirty-two had three-cuspid valves. Nine of the thirty-four patients with pure aortic regurgitation had congenitally bicuspid valves, and in seven the regurgitation was secondary to infective endocarditis partially destroying one or both of its cusps. Although it has been appreciated for nearly ninety years that congenitally bicuspid aortic valves are frequently the site of infective endocarditis, only during the past few years has it become widely recognized that congenitally bicuspid aortic valves become stenotic [11,33–38]. Paget [39], however, in 1844 had suggested that bicuspid aortic valves. because of their defective development, peculiar shape and imperfect tissue were "very liable to disease," and Peacock [40] fourteen years later had pointed out that bicuspid aortic valves could become thick, rigid, ossified, obstructed and finally incompetent. Although he emphasized their frequency and their liability to subacute infective endocarditis, Osler apparently was unaware that a congenitally bicuspid aortic valve could become the site of stenosis [41]. Likewise, Lewis and Grant [42], who in 1923 reviewed all cases of congenitally bicuspid aortic valves reported up to that time and established histologic criteria for distinguishing between congenital and acquired aortic valve deformities, were apparently unaware that this malformed valve could become stenotic although they mentioned "calcific sclerosis" in one of their eleven personally studied cases. Of twenty-eight autopsy patients with calcific aortic stenosis described by Cabot [12] in 1926, no mention is made of the possibility of congenital malformation of this valve although one of two valves illustrated (Fig. 39, p. 224) almost surely is congenitally bicuspid. Christian [13] in 1931 did not consider the possibility of a congenital origin of aortic stenosis. Libman [43], however, the same year stated that calcareous deposits may be superimposed on a congenitally bicuspid aortic valve. McGinn and White [17] in 1934 mentioned congenitally bicuspid aortic valves in four of 123 autopsy patients with aortic stenosis (fifty also had mitral stenosis), but in none of the 123 patients did they consider the stenosis to be of congenital origin. Four of their fifty patients (8 per cent) with combined mitral and aortic disease and twenty-six of seventy-three patients (36 per cent) with presumably isolated aortic stenosis, however, had "fusion of two aortic cusps giving a bicuspid arrangement." One of nine autopsy patients described by Cohen and associates [20] and nine of nineteen autopsy subjects with isolated calcific aortic stenosis reported by Hall and Ichioka [14] had bicuspid aortic valves. Twenty-three of the 200 patients with calcareous disease of the aortic valve reported by Karsner and Koletsky [24] in 1947 had bicuspid aortic valves. The latter investigators considered only two of the twenty-three to be congenitally malformed. This view is debatable. The aortic valve illustrated in their Figure 7 is labeled "acquired bicuspid aortic valve with stenosis" but to me it is a classic congenitally bicuspid valve.

Nearly one third of the 105 patients with anatomically isolated aortic stenosis had three-cuspid aortic valves. The cause of the valvular stenosis in them is uncertain but probably variable. Congenital malformation may be possible in a few. In at least three of the thirty-two patients with isolated aortic stenosis and three-cuspid valves, the circumferential distances between the lateral attachments of the cusps were variable. In the other twenty-nine patients the circumferential distances between the lateral cuspal attachments appeared similar. The cusps, however, may vary in size even though the distances, measured along the aortic root at the most cephalad margins of the commissures between the lateral attachments, are identical. One or more cusps may be elongated. In this case the distances along the cuspal margins vary. When the cusps are fibrotic and calcified, however, it is usually difficult to appreciate inequality of cuspal·size. Unequal sized cusps are common in the pulmonic valve but cause no cuspal scarring or apparent hemodynamic consequence in this low pressure circuit. But when aortic valve cusps are of unequal size it is possible that the usual wear and tear on these cusps in this high pressure circuit may be exaggerated. Congenitally unequally sized cusps almost certainly do not contact one another properly during ventricular diastole and the prolonged abnormal contact or trauma in the systemic circulation may lead to fibrous thickening of the cusps and eventually to calcification and valvular stenosis.

Calcific deposits on aortic valve cusps are extremely common in elderly persons. Although these aortic valve calcific deposits may produce murmurs characteristic of "aortic stenosis," true obstruction is usually not present as judged by the lack of left ventricular hypertrophy either at autopsy or on the electrocardiogram. Of the 105 patients described with isolated aortic stenosis (group Ia), five were over seventy years of age; three had tricuspid and two had bicuspid aortic valves. Thus, this degenerative process is probably not the explanation for the stenosis in the patients with three-cuspid aortic valves described here.

REFERENCES

1. Roberts WC, Sjoerdsma A: The cardiac disease associated with the carcinoid syndrome (carcinoid heart disease). Amer J Med 36: 5, 1964.
2. Roberts WC, Mason DT, Wright LD Jr: The nondistensible right atrium of carcinoid disease of the heart. Amer J Clin Path 44: 627, 1965.
3. Cohen LS, Roberts WC: The clinical and pathologic spectrum of mitral regurgitation caused by malformation of the papillary muscles of fibrosis of the left ventricular free wall. Circulation 37, 38 (supp): VI-57, 1968.
4. Roberts WC, Braunwald E, Morrow AG: Acute severe mitral regurgitation secondary to ruptured chordae tendineae. Clinical, hemodynamic, and pathologic considerations. Circulation 33: 58, 1966.
5. Read RC, Thal AP, Wendt VE: Symptomatic valvular myxomatous transformation (the floppy valve syndrome). A possible forme fruste of the Marfan syndrome. Circulation 32: 897, 1965.
6. Roberts WC, Ross RC, Eggleston JC, Massumi RA: Chronic mitral regurgitation of unresolved etiology in the elderly. A clinico-pathologic study of two patients. Johns Hopkins Med J 122: 26, 1968.
7. Carpenter DF, Golden A, Roberts WC: Quadrivalvular rheumatoid heart disease associated with left bundle branch block. Amer J Med 43: 922, 1967.
8. Glancy DL, Marcus FI, Cuadra M, Ewy GA, Roberts WC: Isolated organic tricuspid valvular regurgitation: causes and consequences. Amer J Med 46: 989, 1969.
9. Edwards JE: Pathologic aspects of cardiac valvular insufficiencies. Arch Surg 77: 634, 1958.
10. Roberts WC, Morrow AG: Congenital aortic stenosis produced by a unicommissural valve. Brit Heart J 27: 505, 1965.
11. Roberts WC: The congenitally bicuspid aortic valve. A study of 85 autopsy patients. Amer J Cardiol (in press).
12. Cabot RC: Facts on Heart Disease, Philadelphia, W. B. Saunders Company, 1926, p 205.
13. Christian HA: Aortic stenosis with calcification of the cusps. JAMA 97: 158, 1931.
14. Hall EM, Ichioka T: Etiology of calcified nodular aortic stenosis. Amer J Path 16: 761, 1940.
15. Kumpe CW, Bean WB: Aortic stenosis: a study of the clinical and pathologic aspects of 107 proved cases. Medicine 27: 139, 1948.
16. Margolis HM, Ziellessen FO, Barnes AR: Calcareous aortic valvular disease. Amer Heart J 6: 349, 1931.
17. McGinn S, White PD: Clinical observations on aortic stenosis. Amer J Med Sci 188: 1, 1934.
18. Clawson BJ, Noble JF, Lufkin NH: The calcified nodular deformity of the aortic valve. Amer Heart J 15: 58, 1938.
19. Dry TJ, Willius FA: Calcareous disease of the aortic valve. A study of two hundred twenty-eight cases. Amer Heart J 17: 138, 1939.
20. Cohen L, Gray I, Nash PI, Fink H: Calcareous aortic stenosis; report of nine cases with autopsy findings. Ann Intern Med 13: 2091, 1940.
21. Reich NE: Calcific aortic valve stenosis: a clinico-pathologic correlation of 22 cases. Ann Intern Med 22: 234, 1945.
22. Horan MJ, Barnes AR: Calcareous aortic stenosis and coronary artery disease. Amer J Med Sci 215: 451, 1948.
23. Anderson MW, Kelsey JR Jr, Edwards JE: Clinical and pathological considerations in cases of calcific aortic stenosis. JAMA 149: 9, 1952.
24. Karsner HT, Koletsky S: Calcific Disease of the Aortic Valve, Philadelphia, J. B. Lippincott Company, 1947.
25. Allbutt C: Diseases of the aortic area of the heart, A System of Medicine by Many Writers, vol 6. Diseases of the Heart and Blood Vessels. (Allbutt C, Rolleston HD, eds) London, MacMillan & Company, Ltd., 1909, p 444.
26. Willius FA, Dry TJ: Cardiac clinics. LVIII. A talk on the etiology of calcareous stenosis of the aortic valve. Proc Staff Meet Mayo Clinic 14: 245, 1939.
27. Koletsky S: Bicuspid aortic valves and endocarditis. Amer Heart J 26: 343, 1943.
28. Clawson BJ: The Aschoff nodule. Arch Path 8: 664, 1929.
29. Tedeschi CG, Wagner BM, Pani KC: Studies in rheumatic fever. I. The clinical significance of the Aschoff body based on morphologic observations. Arch Path 60: 408, 1955.
30. Saphir O: The Aschoff nodule. Amer J Clin Path 31: 534, 1959.
31. Gross L: Lesions of the left auricle in rheumatic fever. Amer J Path 11: 711, 1935.
32. Sohval AR, Gross L: Calcific sclerosis of the aortic valve (Mönckeberg type). Arch Path 22: 477, 1936.
33. Campbell M, Kauntze R: Congenital aortic valvular stenosis. Brit Heart J 15: 179, 1953.
34. Smith DE, Matthews MB: Aortic valvular stenosis with coarctation of the aorta. With special reference to the development of aortic stenosis upon congenital bicuspid valves. Brit Heart J 17: 198, 1955.
35. Bacon APC, Matthews MB: Congenital bicuspid aortic valves and the aetiology of isolated aortic valvular stenosis. Quart J Med 28 (n.s.): 545, 1959.
36. Edwards JE: Calcific aortic stenosis: pathologic features. Proc Staff Meet Mayo Clinic 36: 444, 1961.
37. Morrow AG, Goldblatt A, Braunwald E: Congenital aortic stenosis. II. Surgical treatment and results of operation. Circulation 37: 450, 1963.
38. Campbell M: Calcific aortic stenosis and congenital bicuspid aortic valves. Brit Heart J 30: 606, 1968.
39. Paget J: On obstructions of the branches of the pulmonary artery. Trans Royal Med Chir Soc, London 27: 162, 1844.
40. Peacock TB: On Malformations of the Human Heart, 2nd ed, London, J Churchill & Sons, 1866.
41. Osler W: The bicuspid condition of the aortic valves. Trans Ass Amer Physicians 2: 185, 1886.
42. Lewis T, Grant RT: Observations relating to subacute infective endocarditis. Heart 10: 21, 1923.
43. Libman E: Discussion of paper by Christian, H. A. Trans Ass Amer Physicians 46: 103, 1931.

Severe Valvular Aortic Stenosis in Patients Over 65 Years of Age

A Clinicopathologic Study

WILLIAM C. ROBERTS, MD, FACC
JOSEPH K. PERLOFF, MD, FACC
THOMAS COSTANTINO, MD

Bethesda, Maryland
Washington, D. C.

Clinical and anatomic data are presented in 21 autopsy cases of patients over 65 years of age with severe valvular aortic stenosis. Attention is called to the unusual nature of the valvular lesion in the elderly compared to its manifestations in younger adults. The degree of aortic stenosis even in the very elderly may be extreme. The aortic valve in 2 patients was congenitally bicuspid, and in 19, tricuspid. The latter valves usually were characterized by the uniform distribution of nodular calcific deposits on the aortic aspects of the cusps and by the lack or near lack of commissural fusion. Calcification of the mitral annulus occurred in 16 of the 21 patients. Clinically, aortic stenosis in the elderly is characterized by several features that are either absent or more prominent than in younger subjects with this valvular lesion: The systemic arterial pulse pressure may be increased due to systolic hypertension; a harsh right basal systolic murmur may be relatively inconspicuous, whereas a pure musical systolic murmur may be prominent at the apex; a coexisting apical systolic murmur of mitral regurgitation may be related to mitral annular calcification and not to left ventricular failure; and systemic systolic hypertension can result in a comparatively small pressure gradient despite severe left ventricular outflow obstruction.

It has long been appreciated that aortic systolic murmurs and aortic valvular calcific deposits are common in older people. Although these murmurs in older patients may be prominent, they are usually not considered indicative of significant aortic valvular obstruction.[1] Indeed, Hancock et al.[2] referred to this condition as "aortic stenosis of no physiologic significance." It is less well known that the same pathologic process can result in extensive valvular calcification and severe aortic stenosis.[3] The true incidence of valvular aortic stenosis in elderly persons is unknown for several reasons. The lesion may be missed since its clinical signs are not necessarily those occurring in younger individuals with valvular aortic stenosis; relatively few hemodynamic studies have been performed; and mild degrees of obstruction may be overlooked at necropsy. During the past 4 years we have assembled clinical and necropsy information on 21 patients over 65 years of age with severe valvular aortic stenosis. Five underwent left heart catheterization. This report summarizes clinical, hemodynamic and autopsy observations in these patients and provides evidence that the valvular lesion in the elderly is unique, often severe, and amenable to operative repair.

From the Section of Pathology, National Heart and Lung Institute, National Institutes of Health, Bethesda, Md., and the Department of Medicine, Georgetown University School of Medicine, Division of Cardiology, Georgetown University Hospital, Washington, D. C. This study was supported in part by U. S. Public Health Service Research Career Program Award HE 14009 and the Eric T. Paglin Memorial Fund for Cardiovascular Teaching and Research. Manuscript received April 27, 1970, accepted July 28, 1970.
Address for reprints: William C. Roberts, MD, Section of Pathology, National Heart and Lung Institute, National Institutes of Health, Bethesda, Md. 20014.

Observations in Patients Studied

Clinical and autopsy data from the 21 patients are summarized in Table I. Their ages ranged from 66 to 90 years (average 78); 12

TABLE I
Valvular Aortic Stenosis in Patients More than 65 Years of Age

Case no.	Age (yr) & Sex	Chronic CHF	Angina Pectoris	Syncope	Murmurs: Basal Systolic	Murmurs: Apical Systolic	Murmurs: Basal Diastolic	AF by ECG	LVH by ECG	Aortic Stenosis Diagnosed During Life	Aortic Valve: no. of Cusps	Aortic Valve: Commissural Fusion	Mitral Valve Annular Calcium	Coronary Artery Calcium	Coronary Artery Luminal Narrowing (%)	Left Ventricle: Dilation	Left Ventricle: Scarring	Left Ventricle: Necrosis	Heart Weight (g)
1	79F	+	0	0	+	+	0	0	0	+	2	0	0	0	<25	+	+	0	700
2	75M	+	0	0	+	+	0	0	+	0	2	0	0	+	>75	+	+	0	600
3	69M	+	0	0	+	0	0	+	+	+	3	0	+	0	<25	0	+	0	510
4	70M	0	0	0	+	0	0	0	+	0	3	0	0	+	<50	+	0	0	480
5	80M	+	0	0	+	+	+	0	0	0	3	0	+	+	<50	+	0	0	660
6	89M	0	+	0	+	0	0	+	0	0	3	0	0	+	<50	0	0	0	440
7	85F	+	0	0	+	+	0	0	+	0	3	0	+	+	>75	+	+	+	...
8	80M	+	0	0	+	+	0	0	0	0	3	0	+	+	>75	+	+	?	400
9	66M	+	0	0	+	0	0	+	0	0	3	+	+	+	<50	+	+	0	800
10	70F	+	0	0	+	+	0	0	0	0	3	+	+	+	<50	+	+	0	550
11	76F	0	+	+	+	0	+	0	+	+	3	0	+	+	<25	0	+	0	480
12	82M	+	+	+	+	0	0	0	+	+	3	+	+	+	>75	+	+	0	450
13	71M	+	0	0	+	+	0	0	+	0	3	+	+	+	>75	+	+	+	650
14	75F	0	+	+	+	0	+	0	+	+	3	+	+	+	>75	0	+	...	390
15	90F	+	0	+	+	+	0	+	+	+	3	0	+	+	>75	+	0	+	550
16	83F	0	0	+	+	+	0	+	0	+	3	0	+	+	>75	0	0	+	380
17	80F	0	0	0	+	+	0	0	0	0	3	+	+	+	>50	0	+	+	390
18	81F	0	+	0	+	+	0	0	+	+	3	0	+	+	>75	0	0	+	400
19	74F	+	0	0	+	+	+	+	0	+	3	0	+	0	<25	+	0	0	530
20	76F	+	0	0	+	0	+	+	0	+	3	+	+	+	<25	+	0	0	480
21	73F	+	0	0	+	0	0	0	+	0	3	0	+	+	<50	+	0	0	530

AF = atrial fibrillation; CHF = congestive heart failure; LVH = left ventricular hypertrophy.

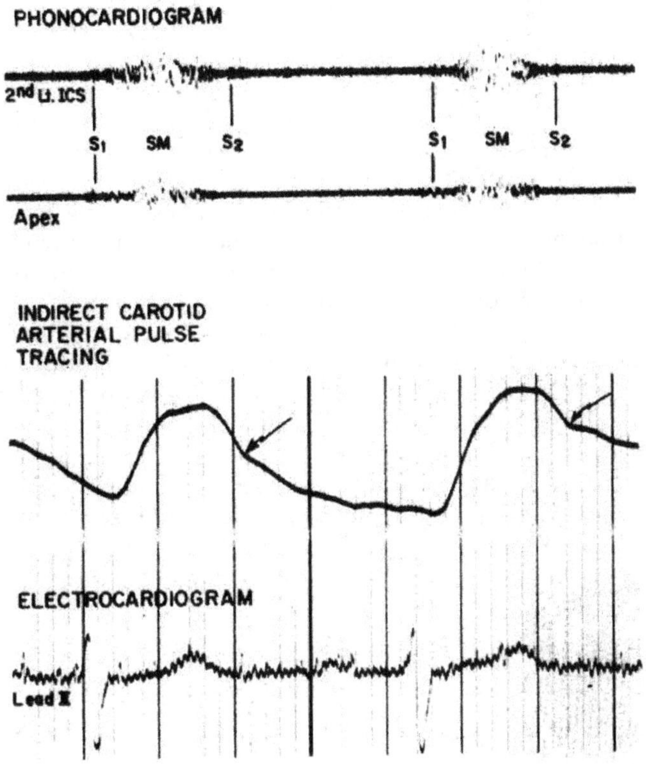

Figure 1. Case 16. Chest wall phonocardiogram with indirect carotid arterial pulse tracing and lead II of the electrocardiogram. A crescendo-decrescendo systolic murmur (SM) is equally well recorded at both base and apex. The indirect carotid arterial pulse tracing shows marked retardation of the rate of rise and slurred dicrotic notch (**arrow**).

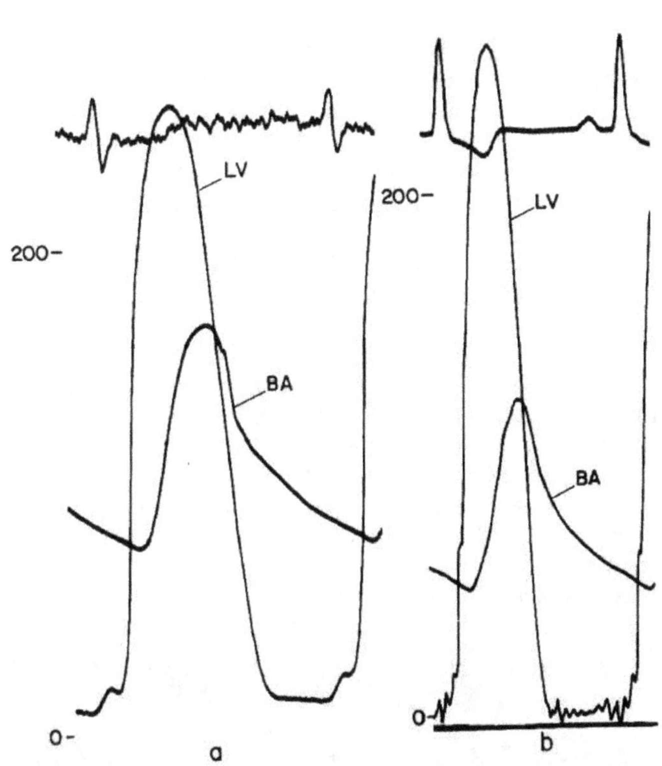

Figure 2. Simultaneous left ventricular (LV) and brachial arterial (BA) pressure tracings of 2 patients. **a,** Case 18, age 81 years. Although the LV systolic pressure is 265 mm Hg, the peak systolic pressure gradient across the aortic valve is only 93 mm Hg since the BA systolic pressure is elevated (172 mm Hg). **b,** Case 11, age 76 years. The LV systolic pressure in this patient is 256 mm Hg, slightly lower than that of Patient 18, but the peak systolic pressure gradient is much higher (160 mm Hg) since the BA systolic pressure is much lower (126 mm Hg).

were women and 9 were men. None had a history of rheumatic fever, chorea, brucellosis or infective endocarditis. All patients had evidence of cardiac dysfunction for various periods: 14 manifested chronic congestive cardiac failure, 5 angina pectoris, and 5 syncope. In addition, 3 patients had had myocardial infarcts, 4 had a history of systemic hypertension, and 3, mild diabetes mellitus.

Clinical findings: All patients had precordial systolic murmurs ranging from grade 2/6 to 4/6 (Fig. 1). Harsh midsystolic murmurs of varying intensity were uniformly present at the right base. In 11 patients high frequency, occasionally musical cooing, apical systolic murmurs of equal or greater intensity were present (Fig. 1). The apical murmurs were usually midsystolic but occasionally holosystolic. Five patients had high frequency early diastolic murmurs considered to represent aortic incompetence, minimal in 3, and moderate in 2.

TABLE II

Hemodynamic Findings in 5 Patients

Case no.	Pressures (mm Hg)			Gradient (mm Hg) LV-BA		CO	CI	Aortic Valve Area (cm²)
	RV	LV	BA	Peak Systolic	Mean			
11	30/8	256/12	126/55	130	102	2.0	1.4	0.2
14	...	280/8	120/50	160	...	2.2	1.7	0.2
16	23/4	180/4	115/40	65	55	3.6	...	0.5
18	48/9	265/25	172/78	93	59	...	...	...
19	...	205/20	135/44	70	55	1.8	1.1	0.3

BA = brachial artery; CI = cardiac index (liters/min per m²); CO = cardiac output (liters/min); LV = left ventricle; RV = right ventricle.

Chest roentgenograms showed evidence of left ventricular enlargement in 15 patients, but the heart was of normal size in the posteroanterior projection in 6 patients. Aortic valve calcific deposits were identified in 15 patients. Electrocardiograms showed left ventricular hypertrophy in 11 patients, atrial fibrillation in 7, complete left bundle branch block in 1, complete right bundle branch block in 1, and transient complete heart block in 3.

Catheterization of the left side of the heart was performed in 5 patients. The hemodynamic data are summarized in Table II, and a pressure tracing from 2 patients is shown in Figure 2.

Clinical diagnoses of aortic stenosis were made in 10 of the 21 patients; correct clinical diagnoses were achieved in only 3 of the first 10 patients studied.

An operation on the aortic valve was carried out in 3 patients. The 2 patients (Cases 11 and 19) with an aortic prosthesis (Hufnagel discoid type) survived 2 and 15 months, respectively, after operation; 1 patient died of infection at the site of the prosthesis, and the second, of aortic regurgitation secondary to a peribasilar leak. The third patient (Case 14) underwent aortic valve debridement but during this procedure 1 cusp was inadvertently perforated and she died 6 months later of severe, operatively induced aortic regurgitation.

The 18 patients unoperated on died of various causes: 5 of acute myocardial infarction; 7 of acute (2 patients) or progressive (5 patients) congestive cardiac failure; 4 of noncardiac conditions (gastric carcinoma in 2, complications of portal cirrhosis in 1, and immediately after operative resection of an abdominal aortic aneurysm in 1; each of these patients, however, had evidence of congestive cardiac failure); 1 died suddenly of un-

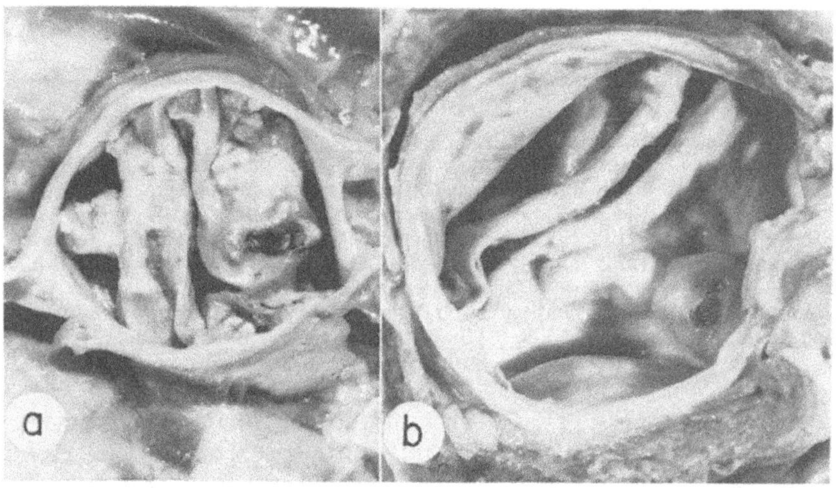

Figure 3. Congenitally bicuspid aortic valves in 2 patients. **a,** Case 1; **b,** Case 2. In both, the valves are heavily calcified and severely stenotic. In neither are the commissures fused. Calcified raphes (false commissures) are present in 1 cusp of each valve.

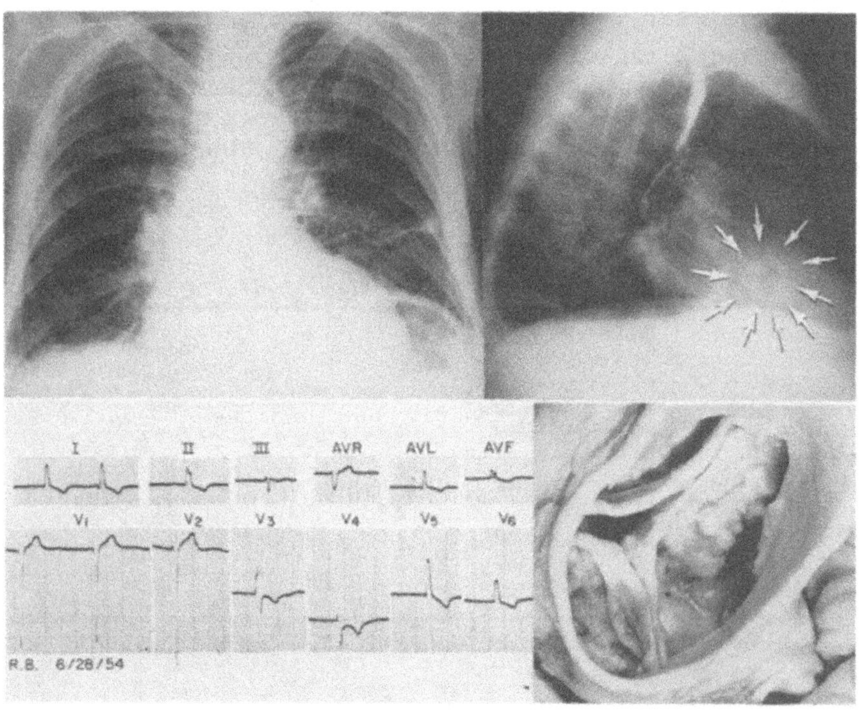

Figure 4. Case 3. Chest roentgenograms, electrocardiogram and aortic valve. The heart is enlarged on X-ray. On the lateral view a heavy ring of calcium (**arrows**) is present in the aortic valve. The electrocardiogram shows left ventricular hypertrophy with strain. Heavy deposits of calcium are present on the aortic aspects of each aortic valve cusp. None of the 3 aortic valve commissures is fused.

determined cause; and 1 died of cardiac tamponade shortly after cardiac catheterization performed by left ventricular puncture.

Autopsy findings: The left ventricular wall in all 21 patients was hypertrophied (greater than 1.5 cm thick). The left ventricular cavity was considered normal in size in 7 patients and mildly to moderately dilated in 14. The hearts weighed from 380 to 800 g (average 524). Two of the 3 patients whose hearts weighed less than 400 g had undergone cardiac catheterization; the peak left ventricular to systemic arterial systolic pressure gradient in 1 was 65 and in the second, 160 mm Hg. The aortic valves in all 21 patients (including the excised valves in 2 patients who had undergone aortic valve replacement) were severely stenotic,

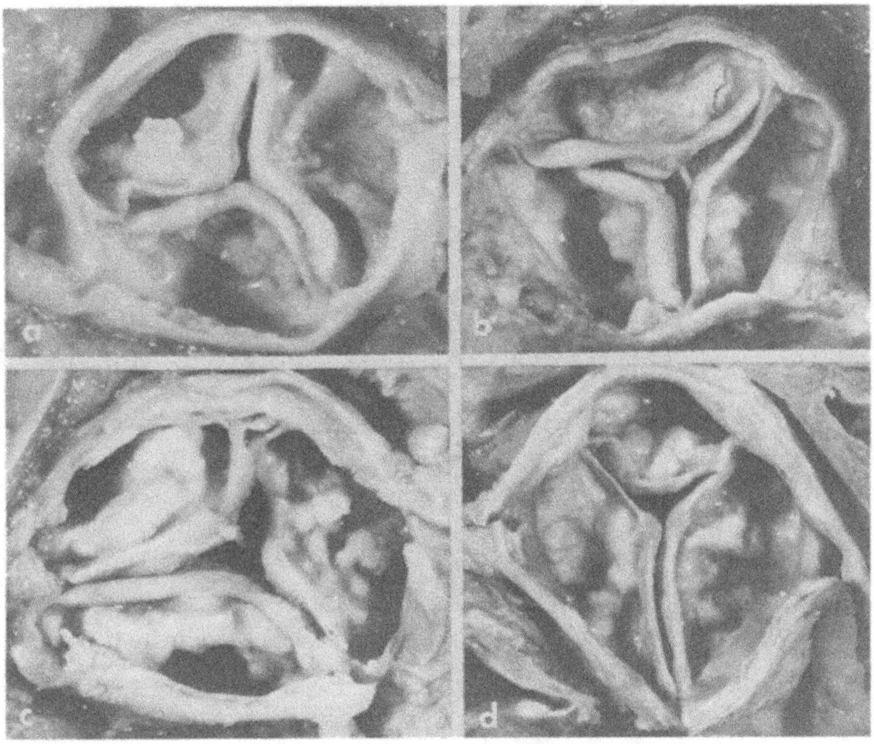

Figure 5. Aortic valves in 4 patients. **a**, Case 16; **b**, Case 18; **c**, Case 7; **d**, Case 8. One commissure in the valves shown in **c** and **d** is slightly fused. All other commissures are open. The cusps in **d** are of unequal size.

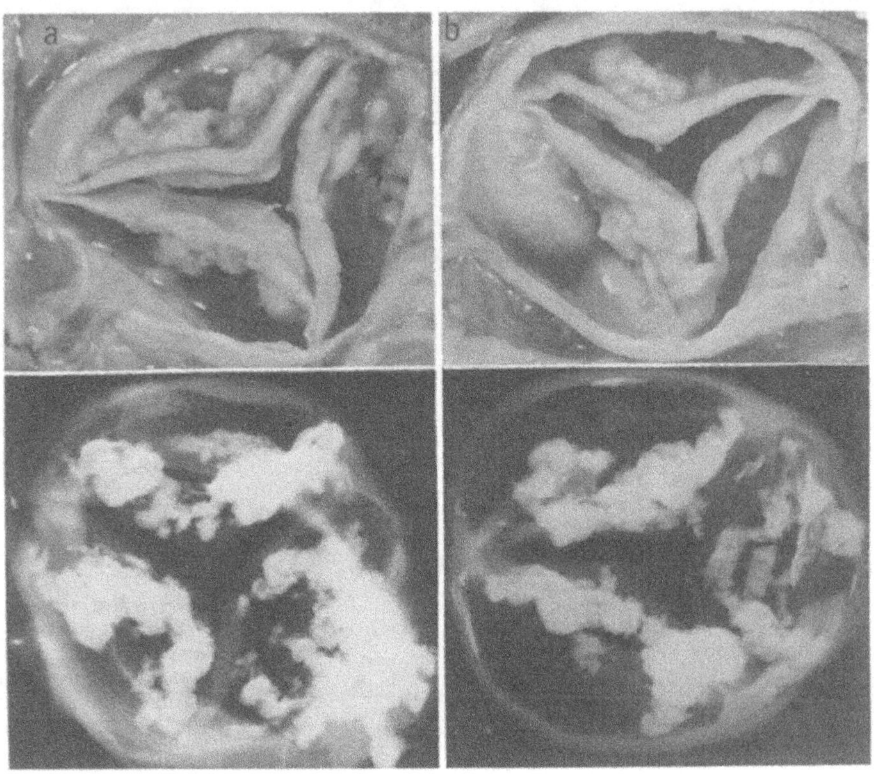

Figure 6. Aortic valves with radiographs below in 2 patients. **a**, Case 15; **b**, Case 21. The cusps of both valves are heavily calcified. One of the 3 commissures in **b** is fused.

and in 5 patients aortic regurgitation of mild degree also was present. In 2 patients the aortic valve was congenitally bicuspid (Fig. 3) and in the other 19 patients the valve was tricuspid (Fig. 4 to 10). No commissural fusion occurred in 12 of the 19 patients with tricuspid aortic valves or in the 2 patients with congenitally bicuspid valves; in 4 others the commissural fusion was minimal and involved only 1 of 3 commissures; and in 3 patients commissural fusion was significant, involving 1

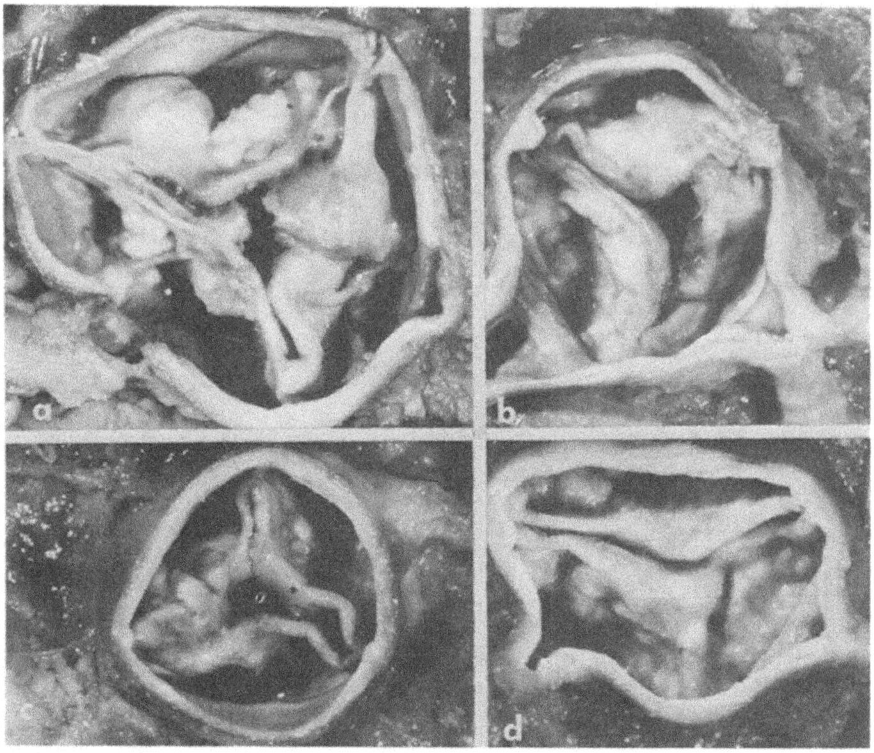

Figure 7. Aortic valves in 4 patients. In 3 (**b** to **d**) 1 commissure is fused, and in 1 (**a**) 2 commissures are fused. Each valve is severely stenotic and heavily calcified. **a,** Case 9; **b,** Case 10; **c,** Case 20; **d,** Case 12.

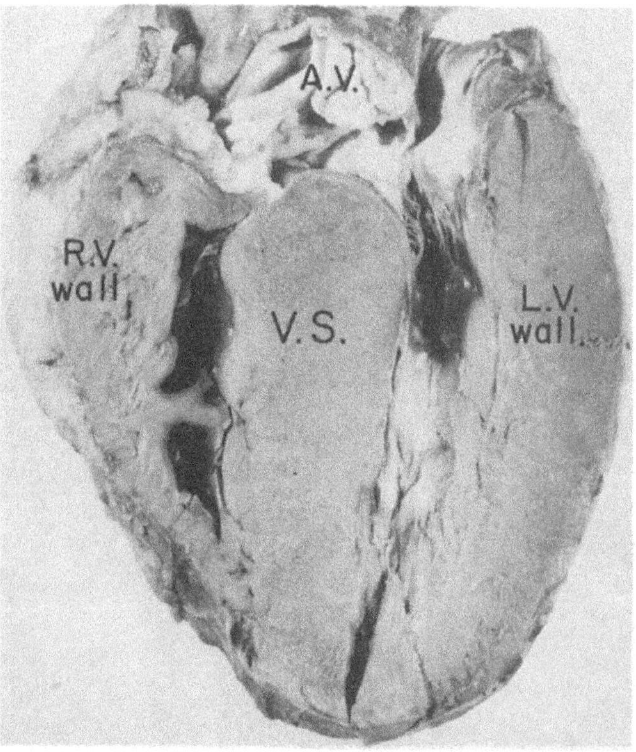

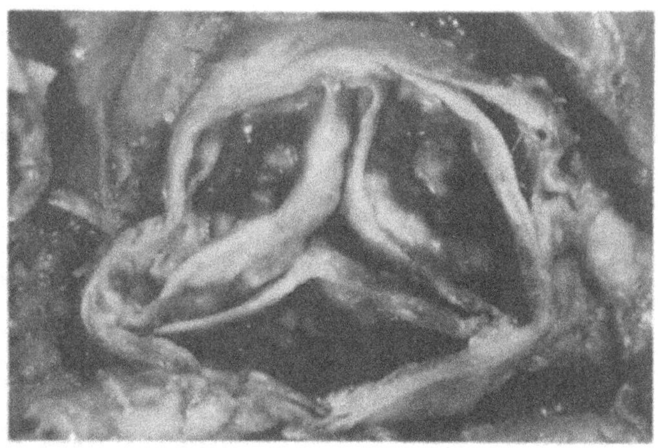

Figure 8. Case 6. Aortic valve (A.V.) **(left)** and longitudinal section of heart **(right)**. The valve is heavily calcified, severely stenotic, but free of commissural fusion. The longitudinal section shows that the cephalad portion of the ventricular septum (V.S.) is thicker than the free wall of the left ventricle (L.V.). The septum beneath the aortic valve bulges toward the mitral valve, giving the septum a sigmoid shape. This sigmoid configuration commonly occurs in persons over age 50 years but is rare in hearts weighing over 400 g.[16] The heart shown weighed 440 g. The sigmoid septum also is unusual in hearts with a dilated left ventricular cavity[4], and the chamber of the heart shown here is of normal size or small. R.V. = right ventricular.

commissure in 2 patients and 2 commissures in 1 patient. In all 21 patients the aortic valves were heavily calcified. The calcific deposits were located on the aortic aspects of the cusps in all patients, but in 3 the calcified deposits also extended a short distance down the ventricular aspect of the anterior mitral leaflets. The cusps were made rigid by the calcific deposits, and the stenoses were attributable to the rigidity of the cusps which contacted or nearly contacted one another when the valves were viewed from either above or below.

In addition to the calcific deposits in the aortic valves of all 21 patients, calcific deposits were present in the coronary arteries in 18 patients and in the annulus and subleaflet area of the posterior mitral leaflet in 17 patients. The deposits in the

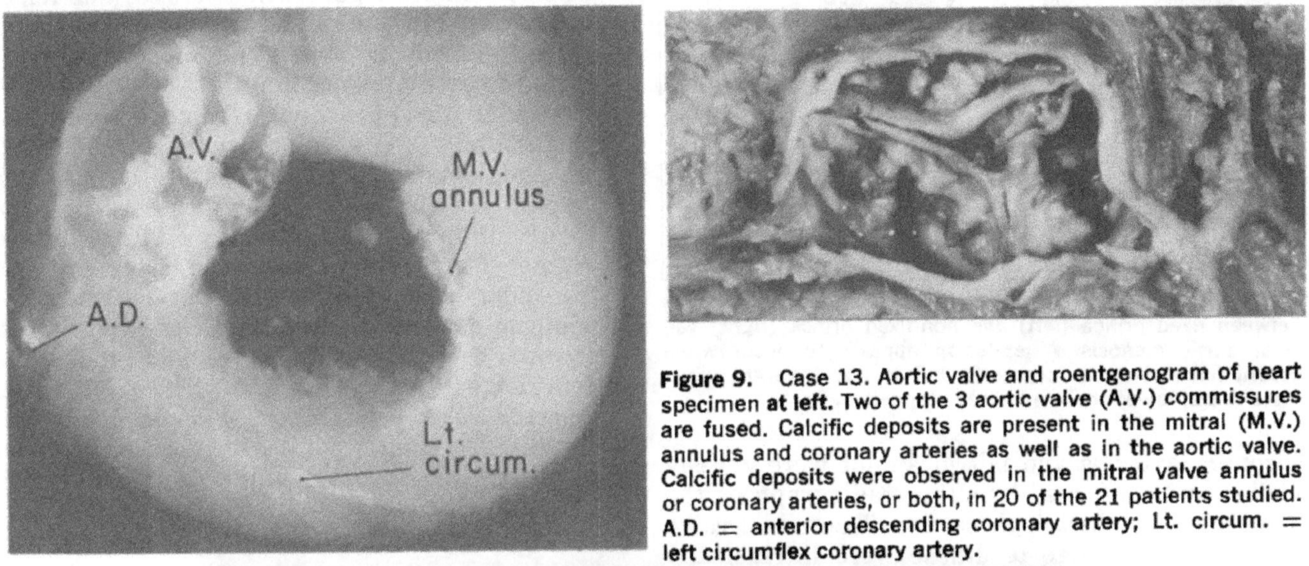

Figure 9. Case 13. Aortic valve and roentgenogram of heart specimen **at left.** Two of the 3 aortic valve (A.V.) commissures are fused. Calcific deposits are present in the mitral (M.V.) annulus and coronary arteries as well as in the aortic valve. Calcific deposits were observed in the mitral valve annulus or coronary arteries, or both, in 20 of the 21 patients studied. A.D. = anterior descending coronary artery; Lt. circum. = left circumflex coronary artery.

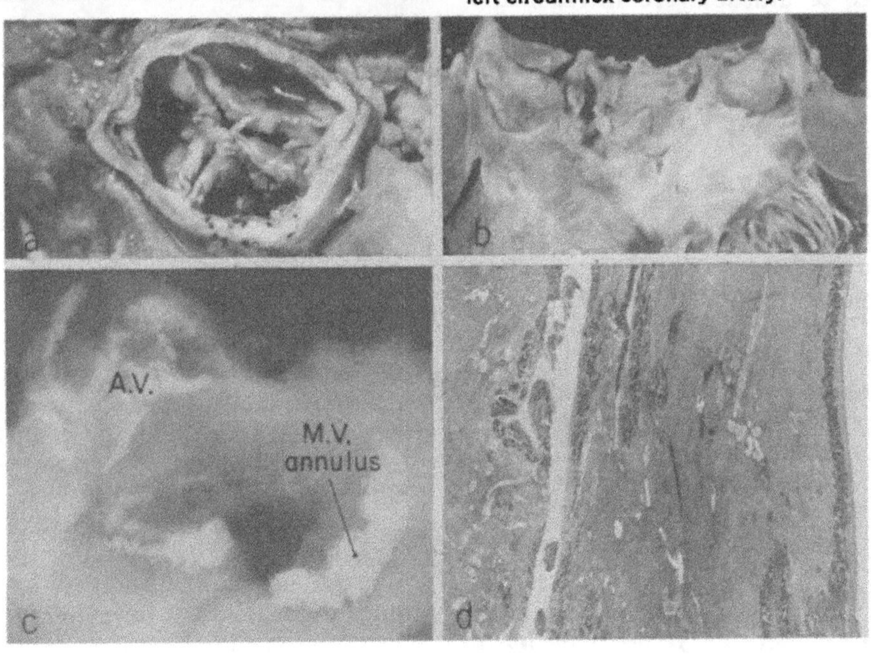

Figure 10. Case 14. Aortic valve, radiograph of heart, and portion of left ventricular papillary muscle. A 160 mm Hg peak systolic pressure gradient was recorded between the left ventricle and the brachial artery before aortic valve debridement 6 months before death. None of the 3 valve commissures is fused. The opened valve (**b**) shows no calcific deposits on the ventricular aspects of the cusps. The radiograph (**c**) shows heavy calcific deposits in the aortic valve cusps despite the absence of nodules of calcium on either the aortic (**a**) or ventricular (**b**) aspects of the cusps. Also, large deposits of calcium are present in the mitral annulus and submitral area (**c**) and in the coronary arteries. Both papillary muscles and left ventricular free walls beneath their bases were severely scarred. A portion of one is shown in **d.** Mitral annular calcification and left ventricular papillary muscle scarring, both of which are common lesions in elderly people, may present auscultatory features simulating those produced in older patients by valvular aortic stenosis alone.

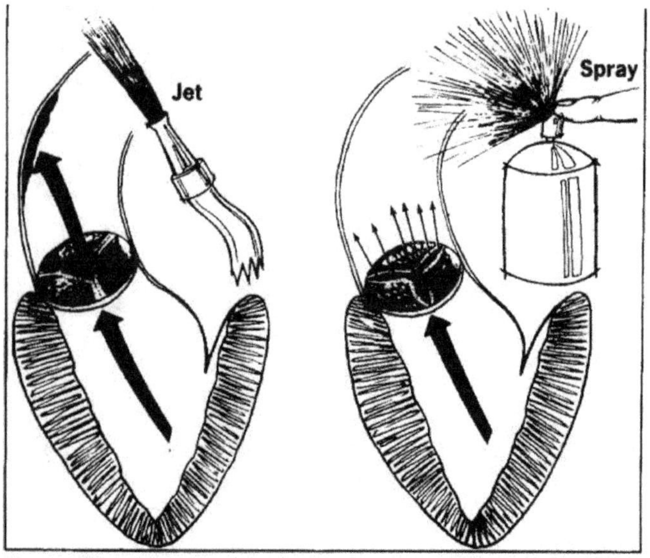

Figure 11. Diagram illustrating the auscultatory differences between fixed orifice (left) and non-fixed orifice (right) valvular aortic stenosis. A jet lesion appears to occur when severe fixed stenosis is present but is not apparent when there is a spray effect in non-fixed stenosis.

coronary arteries and mitral annuli were grossly visible and confirmed by either radiograph of the specimen or by histologic section. The mitral valve leaflets and chordae tendineae were intrinsically normal in 19 patients and thickened by fibrous tissue in 2; however, all mitral valves showed mild aging changes.[5] The tricuspid and pulmonic valves were normal in all 21 patients. The lumens of 1 or more of the 3 major extramural coronary arteries were narrowed by more than 50 percent in 10 patients and by less than 50 percent in 11 patients. Eleven patients had foci of myocardial fibrosis involving the left ventricular free wall with or without papillary muscle scarring, and 4 others had papillary muscle scarring only. Unequivocal atrophy of the left ventricular papillary muscles occurred in 2 patients. Five subjects had anatomic evidence of acute myocardial infarction (necrosis). At least 1 histologic section from the wall of each cardiac chamber was examined, and no Aschoff bodies were found in the sections from any of the 21 patients.

Comments

Differences between older and younger patients with aortic stenosis: Comparison of certain clinical and anatomic features in these 21 autopsy patients over 65 years of age with 119 autopsy patients between 16 and 65 years of age who had clinically isolated severe valvular aortic stenosis (described in detail elsewhere[6]) discloses several striking differences. First, the aortic valve *structure* is often different. It was tricuspid in approximately 90 percent and congenitally bicuspid in 10 percent of the 21 elderly patients; in contrast, the aortic valve was tricuspid in 45 percent, congenitally bicuspid in 45 percent, congenitally unicommissural unicuspid in 10 percent of the 119 younger patients. In addition to differences in basic valvular configuration, *commissural fusion* was unusual in older patients but common in the younger subjects. Second, the *origin* of the valvular lesion was different in the 2 age groups. Congenital malformations were the commonest causes of isolated aortic stenosis in the younger age group,[6–8] whereas simple degeneration or wear and tear was believed to be the most frequent cause in the older patient. Third, the *clinical diagnosis* of aortic stenosis in older patients may be overlooked because of peculiarities of the intensity and frequency composition of the systolic murmurs and because the systemic arterial pulse is likely to have a normal rate of rise and a normal or increased pulse pressure.[9,10] Fourth, *sex* in the 2 groups is different: Women were more frequent (57 percent) among the older patients, whereas 80 percent of the younger patients were men. Fifth, the *method of operative repair* may differ in the 2 groups: Valve debridement may prove useful in older patients, whereas valve replacement will usually be necessary in the younger adult. However, valve debridement was carried out in only 9 of 70 older surgical patients with aortic stenosis (age range 57 to 80 years, average 64) studied by Finegan and associates.[3]

Auscultatory signs: Certain auscultatory signs that accompany aortic stenosis in the elderly require explanation. Ejection sounds are characteristically absent, presumably because the cusps remain as individual units (since commissural fusion is absent) and the valve does not move abruptly as a single unit. Atrial sounds (fourth heart sounds), useful for judging the severity of aortic stenosis in the younger adult, are of little diagnostic help in the elderly since these sounds occur in elderly persons without aortic stenosis due to the decreased left ventricular compliance with age. Ordinarily, the murmur of valvular aortic stenosis is harsh, rough, grunting and loudest at the right base with radiation upward and to the right. In elderly patients with aortic stenosis, the harsh murmur at the right base may persist but with appreciably less intensity, and auscultation may be dominated instead by a loud, pure frequency musical systolic murmur maximal at or near the cardiac apex. At least 3 reasons account for these patterns: (1) Older persons tend to have increased upper thoracic chest dimensions which soften the basal murmurs.[10] (2) The morphology of the stenotic aortic valve differs in the 2 age groups. A rigid, calcified valve *with* commissural fusion provides a suitable mechanism for a high velocity jet into the ascending aorta (Fig. 11); the noisy murmur at the right base appears to originate within the ascending aorta because of turbulence caused by the high velocity jet.[10] A calcified, stenotic trileaflet aortic valve *without* commissural fusion, the most common type in the elderly, appears to behave differently. Ejection into the ascending aorta may take the form of a "spray" instead of a jet (Fig. 11), so that the harsh murmur at the right base may be comparatively inconspicuous. Since the cusps are not fused, each may vibrate during ventricular ejection. The accompanying pure frequency, musical cooing murmur probably results from these periodic vibrations.[10] Such murmurs are recordable within the left ventricular cavity and therefore are transmitted best to the chest wall overlying the left ventricle, that is, the cardiac apex. (3) Calcification of the mitral annulus, itself a producer of precordial murmurs, frequently accompanies calcification of the aortic valve in elderly patients. Mitral regurgitation can result from inability of the calcified annulus to decrease its circumference during ventricular contraction.[11] Accordingly, the holosystolic murmur of mitral regurgitation may be present at the apex and may be difficult to distinguish from the coexisting pure frequency aortic stenotic apical murmur. Seventeen of the 21 elderly patients described herein had calcified mitral annuli, and in 10 of them the deposits were "massive." These large deposits at the annulus and beneath the posterior mitral leaflet may well have prevented this valve from closing completely during ventricular systole. Although mitral annular calcification tends to complicate the auscultatory diagnosis of aortic stenosis, its radiologic identification is useful since it implies that coexisting aortic stenosis is likely to be caused by calcific deposits on a trileaflet valve without commissural fusion.

Systolic hypertension: The degree of left ventricular systolic hypertension in elderly patients may be considerably higher than that occurring in younger subjects with similar degrees of aortic stenosis since the peripheral systolic systemic pressure usually increases with age.[12] The degree of systolic hypertension which the left ventricle in the elderly is capable of achieving can be astonishingly high, particularly since this chamber seldom maintains a systolic pressure in excess of 250 mm Hg even in younger subjects.[13] In Patient 18 (Table II) the left ventricular systolic pressure was 265 mm Hg, but the peak systolic pressure gradient across the valve was only 93 mm Hg since the peripheral systemic systolic pressure was elevated (172 mm Hg) (Fig. 2). Thus, systemic hypertension may reduce the aortic gradient, and the degree of obstruction may be underestimated in these elderly patients if the systolic pressure difference is taken as the only index of severity. As the gradient diminishes in the presence of systemic systolic hypertension, the murmur at the right base may soften and shorten. Even if this auscultatory change does not occur with systemic hypertension, the modification of the systemic arterial pulse may be misleading since the rate of rise can be relatively normal and the pulse pressure increased despite severe obstruction to left ventricular outflow.

Atrial fibrillation: Another important clinical feature was the presence of atrial fibrillation in 7 of the 21 patients presented. It is recognized that this arrhythmia is common in elderly persons without valvular cardiac disease. The left atrial cavities were mildly dilated in all 21 patients, but left atrial dilatation commonly accompanies old age in the absence of functionally significant valvular lesions. It is also appreciated that the left ventricular wall becomes less compliant with age and that the superimposed left ventricular hypertrophy (without left ventricular dilatation) of aortic stenosis may further impede left atrial emptying. In addition, the mitral orifice may be narrowed by annular or subleaflet calcific deposits that might slow left atrial emptying and result in left atrial dilatation. The only common anatomic feature in elderly patients with atrial fibrillation is left atrial dilatation.[14] The combination of atrial fibrillation, a long apical systolic murmur and left atrial dilatation can obscure the diagnosis of aortic stenosis and lead to a mistaken diagnosis of isolated mitral regurgitation. Furthermore, atrial fibrillation is especially undesirable in aortic stenosis since the left ventricle requires the help of augmented left atrial contraction which increases end-diastolic fiber length and permits the left ventricle to contract with greater force.

Etiology: The cause of the aortic stenosis in elderly patients is uncertain, but simple wear and tear or degeneration appears to be the most reasonable explanation.[15] The presence in the same hearts of other wear and tear lesions such as calcified mitral annuli, calcified coronary arteries and focal thickening of other valve leaflets supports this contention. Certainly there is nothing to support a rheumatic origin—none of the patients had a history of acute rheumatic fever or chorea, none had Aschoff bodies, and all but 2 had intrinsically normal mitral valves.[7]

Addendum

During the 10 month interval from submission of this manuscript to receipt of the galleys severe valvular aortic stenosis was seen at necropsy by us in 11 additional patients aged 68 to 87 years (average 76). Seven were men, 4 women. All 11 patients had precordial systolic murmurs and evidence of congestive cardiac failure. Only 1 patient underwent cardiac catheterization, and she had a peak systolic pressure gradient of 100 mm Hg between the left ventricle and a systemic artery. At necropsy, the heart weight in the 11 patients ranged from 400 to 770 g (average 536). Ten patients had tricuspid aortic valves. In 8 no commissural fusion was present, and in 2 patients, 1 of 3 commissures was slightly fused. The eleventh patient had a congenitally bicuspid aortic valve.

References

1. **Bruns DL, Van der Hauwaert LG:** The aortic systolic murmur developing with increasing age. Brit Heart J 20:370–378, 1958
2. **Hancock EW, Madison WM Jr, Proctor MH, et al:** Aortic stenosis of no physiologic significance. New Eng J Med 258:305–312, 1958
3. **Finegan RE, Gianelly RE, Harrison DC:** Aortic stenosis in the elderly: relevance of age to diagnosis and treatment. New Eng J Med 281:1261–1264, 1969
4. **Goor D, Lillehei CW, Edwards JE:** The "sigmoid septum." Variation in the contour of the left ventricular outlet. Amer J Roentgen 107:366–376, 1969
5. **Sell S, Scully RE:** Aging changes in the aortic and mitral valves. Histologic and histochemical studies, with observations on the pathogenesis of calcific aortic stenosis and calcification of the mitral annulus. Amer J Path 46: 345–365, 1965
6. **Roberts WC:** The structure of the aortic valve in clinically isolated aortic stenosis. An autopsy study of 162 patients over 15 years of age. Circulation 42:91–97, 1970
7. **Roberts WC:** Anatomically isolated aortic valvular disease. The case against its being of rheumatic etiology. Amer J Med 151–159, 1970
8. **Roberts WC:** The congenitally bicuspid aortic valve. A study of 85 autopsy cases. Amer J Cardiol 26:72–83, 1970
9. **Perloff JK, Binnion PF, Caulfield WH, et al:** The use of angiotensin in the assessment of left ventricular function in fixed orifice aortic stenosis. Circulation 35:347–357, 1967
10. **Perloff JK:** Clinical recognition of aortic stenosis. The physical signs and differential diagnoses of the various forms of obstruction to left ventricular outflow. Progr Cardiovasc Dis 10:323–348, 1968
11. **Korn D, DeSanctis RW, Sell S:** Massive calcification of the mitral annulus. A clinicopathological study of fourteen cases. New Eng J Med 267:900–909, 1962
12. **Colandrea MA, Friedman GD, Nichaman MZ, et al:** Systolic hypertension in the elderly. An epidemiologic assessment. Circulation 41:239–245, 1970
13. **Gorlin R, McMillan IKR, Medd WE, et al:** Dynamics of the circulation in aortic valvular disease. Amer J Med 18:855–870, 1955
14. **Neufeld HN, Wagenvoort CA, Burchell HB, et al:** Idiopathic atrial fibrillation. Amer J Cardiol 8:193–197, 1961
15. **Hultgren HN:** Calcific disease of the aortic valve. Arch Path (Chicago) 45:694–706, 1948

Congenital Aortic Stenosis Resulting From a Unicommissural Valve

Clinical and Anatomic Features in Twenty-one Adult Patients

By M. Wayne Falcone, M.D., William C. Roberts, M.D., Andrew G. Morrow, M.D., and Joseph K. Perloff, M.D.

SUMMARY

Clinical, electrocardiographic, phonocardiographic, radiographic, hemodynamic, and anatomic findings are presented in 21 adult patients with stenotic unicommissural aortic valves. Distinction between congenitally unicuspid and bicuspid aortic valves before operation or autopsy was not possible. Although the basic structure of the valve may render it inherently stenotic, the age at which a murmur was first noted (average, 19 years), the duration of a known murmur (average, 25 years), and the age of onset of first symptoms of left ventricular outflow obstruction (average, 41 years) strongly suggest that stenosis at least in part is acquired. The relationship of the true and false commissures to the coronary arterial ostia could be determined with certainty in 12 patients. The basic division of the aortic valve into left, right, and noncoronary cusps is maintained, but the raphes do not extend to the valve orifice. Because the aortic valve is attached to the ascending aorta at only one point (the true commissure), which is at the level of the orifice, valvotomy is hazardous, and valve replacement appears indicated when operative treatment becomes necessary in the adult patient with a stenotic unicommissural aortic valve.

Additional Indexing Words:

Aortic regurgitation — Aortic valve surgery — Bicuspid aortic valve
Infective endocarditis — Papillary muscle dysfunction

A CONGENITAL malformation of the aortic valve is the most common cause of anatomically isolated aortic stenosis.[1, 2] Usually the stenotic valve is found to be congenital-

From the Section of Pathology and Clinic of Surgery, National Heart and Lung Institute, National Institutes of Health, Bethesda, Maryland, and the Departments of Medicine and Pediatrics, Georgetown University School of Medicine, Division of Cardiology, Georgetown University Hospital, Washington, D. C.

Address for reprints: William C. Roberts, M.D., Section of Pathology, National Heart and Lung Institute, National Institutes of Health, Bethesda, Maryland 20014.

Received February 11, 1971; accepted for publication March 23, 1971.

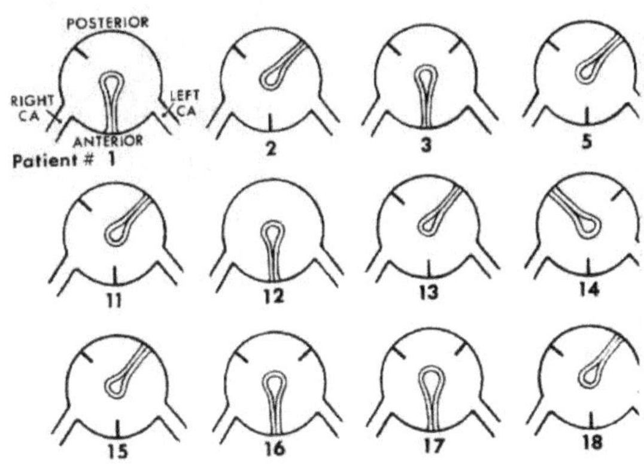

Figure 1

Schematic representation of the positions of the tr commissure and raphes in 12 patients with congenit ly unicommissural aortic valves. CA = coronary arte ly bicuspid,[3] but not infrequently stenosis may result from a congenitally unicuspid aortic valve, two forms of which are recognized.[4] Both have a dome shape: one has no commissures or lateral attachments to the aorta at the level of the orifice (*acommissural*); the second has one lateral attachment to the aorta at the level of the orifice (*unicommissural*). The dome-shaped valves are reported to be stenotic from birth,[4] and constitute the major cause of symptomatic valvular aortic stenosis in the first year of life.[5] Unicommissural aortic valves are known to cause severe aortic stenosis in childhood, but relatively little attention has been paid to the occurrence of this aortic valvular malformation in adults. This report describes the clinical, hemodynamic, and anatomic findings in 21 adult patients in whom isolated aortic stenosis resulted from a unicommissural valve.

Patients Studied

Among 543 patients over 14 years of age with severe (functional classes III and IV, New York Heart Association classification) valvular cardiac disease, studied at autopsy, 182 or 34% had isolated aortic stenosis, with or without associated aortic regurgitation. Of these 182 patients, 27

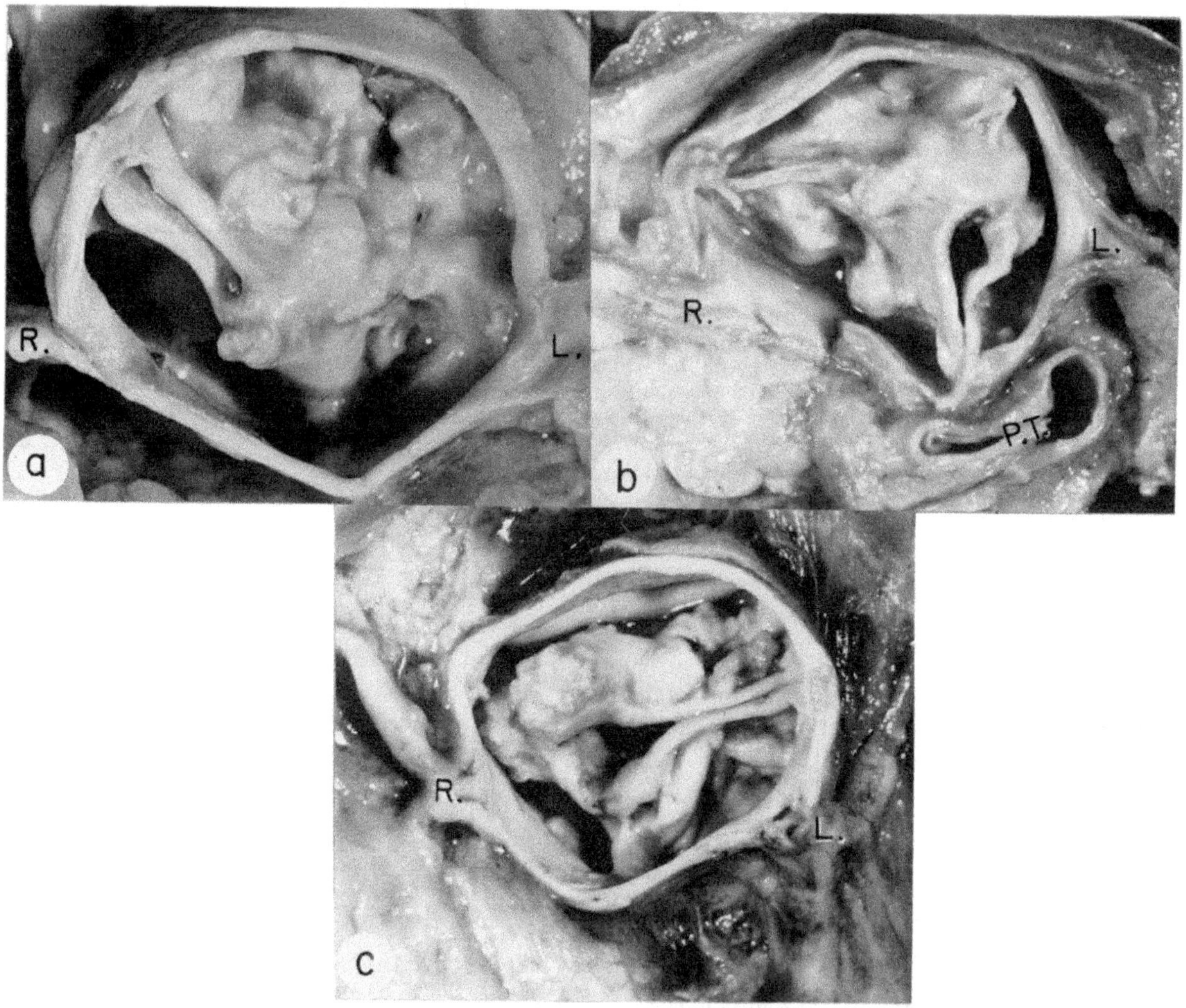

Figure 2

Photographs of in situ congenitally unicommissural aortic valves in three patients. (a) Patient No. 14. (b) Patient No. 17. (c) Patient No. 15. L. = left coronary artery; P.T. = pulmonary trunk; R. = right coronary artery.

Table 1

Clinical and Morphologic Data in Twenty-One Adult Patients with Stenotic Congenitally Unicommissural Aortic Valves

Pt.	Age at death (yr)	Sex	Age murmur first heard (yr)	Hx of ARF	Duration of CHF (yr)	Angina	Syncope	AR
1	47	F	32	0	2	+	0	+
2	16	M	Birth	0	7	+	0	0
3	40	F	Infancy	0	6/12	+	+	+
4	32	F	5	0	6/12	+	0	0
5	57	M	35	0	3	0	0	0
6	50	M	47	0	8/12	+	0	+
7	19	F	17	0	2	+	+	+
8	37	M	7	0	6	+	0	+
9	55	M	12	+	0	0	0	+
10	61	M	13	+	2	0	0	+
11	31	M	5	0	3/12	0	0	+†
12	28	M	16	0	1 6/12	0	0	+
13	57	M	55	0	1	+	0	+
14	48	M	10	0	11	0	0	0
15	59	M	58	+	1	0	+	+
16	52	M	13	+	2	0	0	+
17	62	M	6	0	1	+	0	+
18	35	M	18	+	1/12	0	0	+
19	41	M	4	0	4	+	+	+
20	53	M	12	0	6	+	0	+
21	47	M	27	0	1	+	+	0
Total no. of patients		17 M 4 F		5		12	5	16
Range	16–62		Birth–58		1½–11			
Average	44		19		2 ½			

*Cardiac catheterization in each patient was performed within 1 month of death.

†The predominant functional lesion was AR. AR was mild in 12 of the 16 patients wih AR murmurs.

Abbreviations: ARF = acute rheumatic fever; AR = aortic regurgitation; AV = aortic valve; CHF = congestive heart failure; CI = cardiac index; ECG = electrocardiogram; F = female; Hx = history; IE = infective endocarditis; IPO = immediate postoperative period; LAD = left axis deviation; LBBB = left bundle-branch block; LPO = late postoperative period (> 2 years postop.); LVH = left ventricular hypertrophy; LVI = left ventricular ischemia; LV PAP fibrosis = left ventricular papillary muscle fibrosis; LV-SA PSG = left ventricle-systemic arterial peak systolic gradient; M = male; NC = noncardiac; op. = operation; SUD = sudden, unexpected death.

were older than age 65 (average, 78 years), and 25 had tricuspid and two had bicuspid aortic valves. Of the remaining 155 patients, aged 15 to 65 years (average, 46 years), 18 (12%) had congenitally unicommissural valves, 72 (46%) had congenitally bicuspid valves, 57 (37%) had tricuspid aortic valves, and in eight (5%) the basic structure of the stenotic aortic valve was not discernible.

In addition to the 18 patients with congenitally unicommissural aortic valves studied at autopsy, congenitally unicommissural aortic valves were excised at operation in three additional living patients. Table 1 summarizes the clinical and necropsy findings in these 21 patients. In each, only one aortic valve commissure was attached to the aortic wall at the level of the valve orifice, which, when viewed from above, had an exclamation-point configuration (figs. 1–3). Raphes (false commissures), extending only part way from the base of the valve toward its free edge, also were present in most patients. All had midsystolic murmurs characteristic of aortic stenosis, and 16 also had murmurs of aortic regurgitation (fig. 4). Three patients (nos. 10, 11, and 15) had holosystolic, blowing apical murmurs indicating mitral regurgitation; each patient was in terminal congestive cardiac failure, and two (nos. 11 and 15) also had murmurs of tricuspid regurgitation. Two patients (nos. 4 and 18) had histories of infective endocarditis. Of 13 patients in whom phonocardiograms were ob-

ECG	LV-SA* PSG (mm Hg)	CI* (liters/min/m²)	AV op.	Cause of death	Heart weight (g)	Calcium AV (0–4+)	LV PAP fibrosis (0–4+)
LVH	150	3.0	+	IPO	400	4+	1+
LVH	90	—	0	SUD	600	2+	1+
LVH	158	2.8	+	IPO	550	4+	1+
LVH	90	—	0	CHF	500	4+	0
LAD; LVI	82	2.4	0	CHF	630	4+	—
LVH	80	3.2	+	LPO	700	4+	3+
LVH; LBBB	105	2.9	+	IPO	500	4+	4+
LBBB	29	3.0	+	LPO	860	4+	4+
LVH	104	2.3	+	NC	400	4+	3+
LAD; LVH	18	2.0	+	IPO	620	2+	3+
LAD; LVH	15†	—	0	CHF	880	3+	1+
LAD; LBBB	—	—	0	SUD	640	4+	0
LAD; LVH	—	—	0	CHF	760	3+	1+
LVH	—	—	0	SUD	750	4+	1+
LAD; LBBB	—	—	0	SUD	650	3+	1+
LVH	—	—	0	CHF	640	2+	—
LVH	—	—	0	NC	400	4+	2+
LVH	—	—	0	IE	550	2+	1+
LVH	150	—	+	(Living)	—	4+	—
LVH	—	—	+	(Living)	—	4+	—
LVH	65	—	+	(Living)	—	4+	—
17 LVH 6 LAD 4 LBBB			10			21/21	14/16
	15–158 87	2.0–3.2 2.7			400–800 590		

tained, unequivocal ejection sounds were present in two (nos. 7 and 15), and questionable ones in two others (nos. 2 and 4) (fig. 4). Representative electrocardiograms and chest roentgenograms are illustrated in figures 5 and 6, respectively, and atrophied left ventricular papillary muscles are shown in figure 7.

Comments

It is apparently impossible to determine before operation or autopsy the presence of a stenotic unicommissural unicuspid aortic valve in an adult. The frequency of congestive cardiac failure, angina pectoris, syncope, left ventricular hypertrophy, aortic regurgitation, aortic valvular calcification, aortic ejection sound, and infective endocarditis are similar among patients with stenotic congenitally unicuspid and bicuspid aortic valves.

Edwards[4] believes that the unicuspid aortic valve is intrinsically stenotic from birth, and Moller and associates[5] found congenitally unicommissural aortic valves in nine of 11 children less than 1 year of age who had symptomatic aortic stenosis. Their patients exhibited gross enlargement of all four cardiac chambers. Left ventricular endocardial fibroelastosis also was present in eight of these 11 patients. In all five patients in whom left ventricular angiocardiograms were obtained mitral regurgitation was evident and presumed to be the result of papillary muscle infarction.[5]

Of our 21 patients, a precordial murmur was discovered in infancy in two, by age 7 in five, between ages 7 and 30 in nine, and after 30 years of age in five. The duration of a known murmur ranged from birth to 56 years (average, 25 years), and the age at onset of symptoms referable to left ventricular outflow

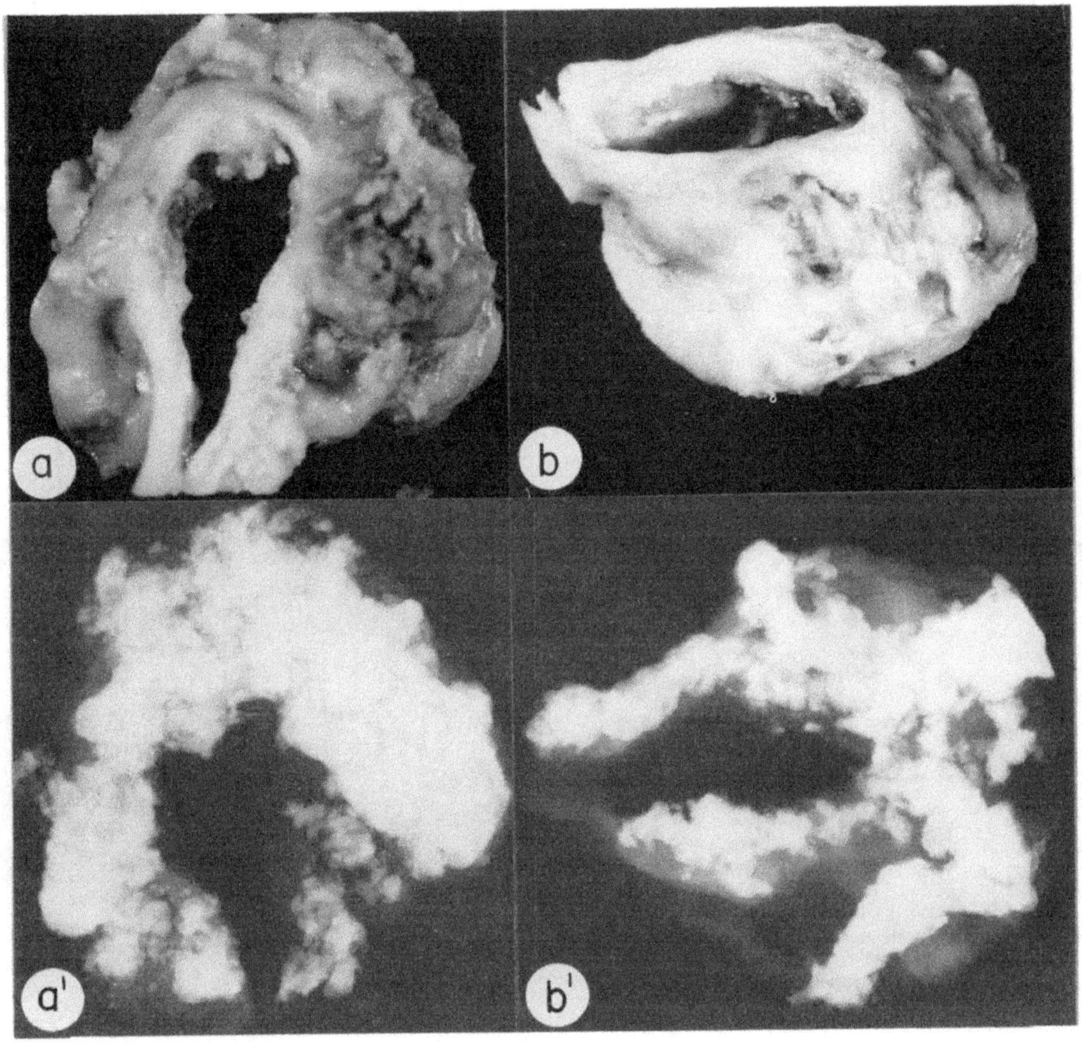

Figure 3

Photographs (a and b) and radiographs (a^1 and b^1) of congenitally unicommissural aortic valves excised at operation in patient No. 20 (a and a^1) and patient No 19 (b and b^1). Both valves are heavily calcified.

Figure 4

Phonocardiograms in four patients. (a) Patient No. 10. Crescendo-decrescendo systolic murmur (SM) with delayed upstroke of carotid pulse tracing. (b) Patient No. 7. Aortic ejection sound (E) timing with onset of carotid upstroke. (c) Patient No. 15. Severe delay of carotid upstroke accompanied by left bundle-branch block. Left axis deviation and paradoxical splitting of S_2. (d) Patient No. 11. Crescendo-decrescendo systolic murmur with high frequency early diastolic murmur (EDM), low frequency middiastolic murmur (MDM) (Austin-Flint murmur), and third heart sound (S_3). Abbreviations: 2 RICS = second right intercostal space; A_2 = aortic component of second heart sound; P_2 = pulmonic component of second heart sound; S_1 = first heart sound; S_2 = second heart sound; 2 LICS and 4 LICS = second and fourth left intercostal spaces, respectively.

obstruction ranged from 9–61 years (average, 41 years). Apparently some patients with congenitally unicommissural aortic valves have evidence of left ventricular outflow obstruction at birth, while in others obstruction does not appear until adulthood. It seems likely that in the latter patients stenosis is gradually acquired as the result of fibrosis and

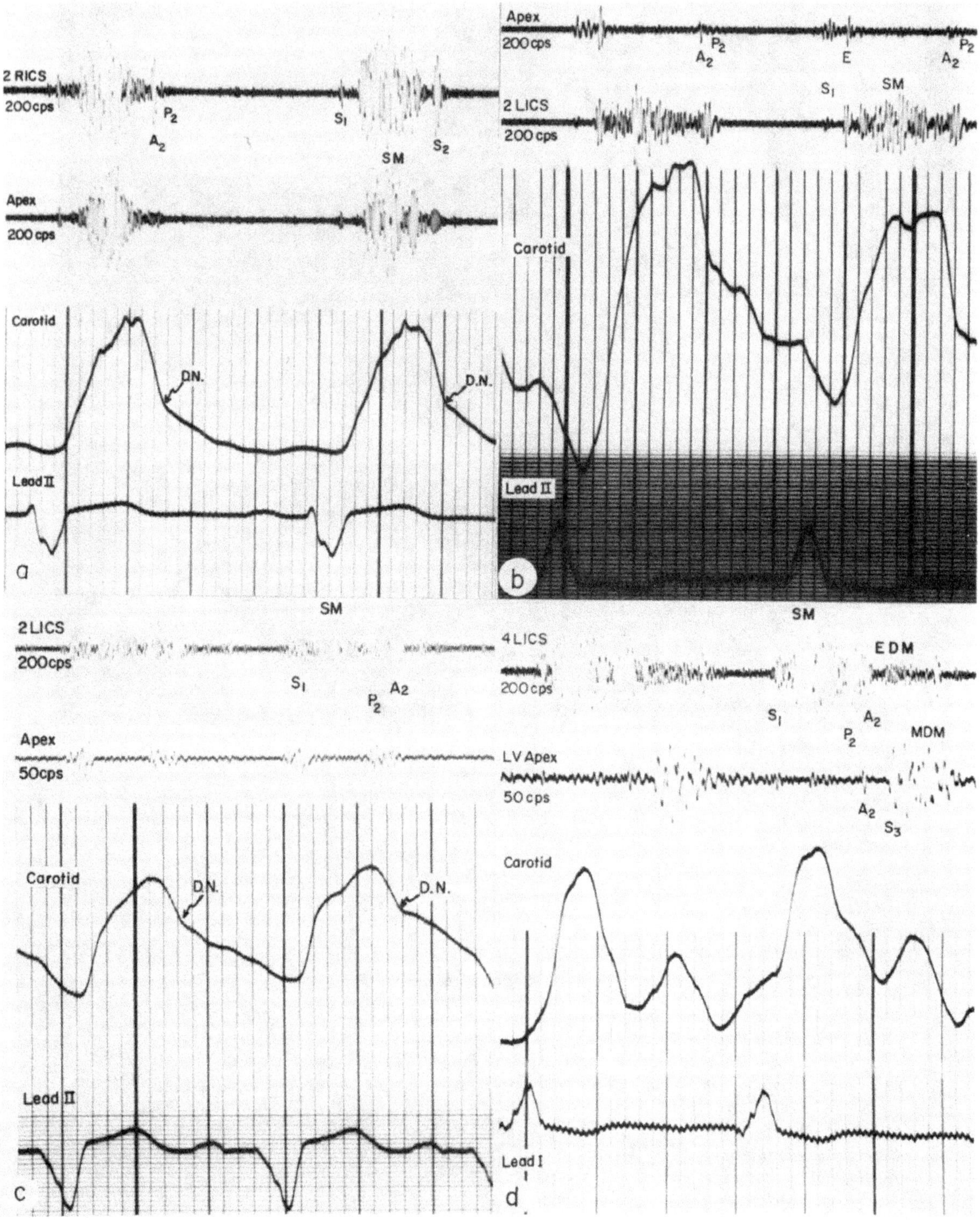

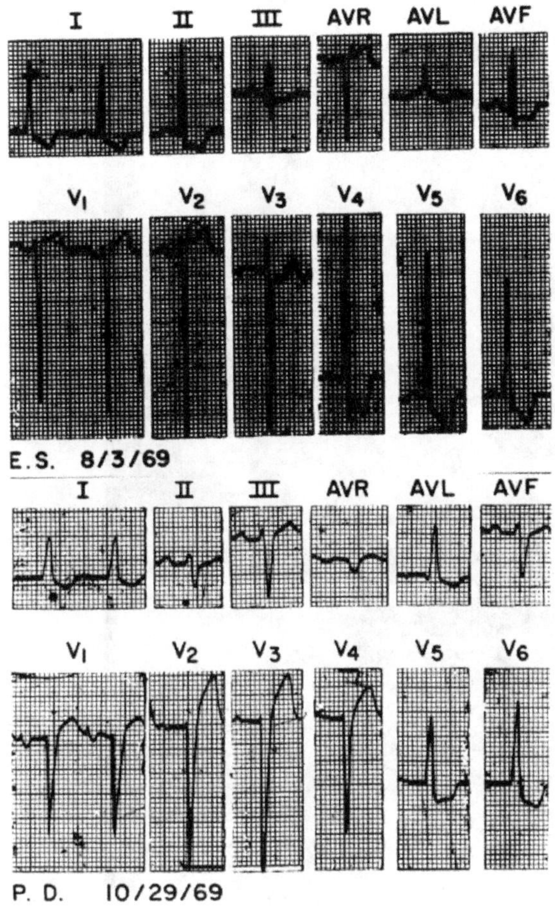

Figure 5

Electrocardiograms in patient No. 17 (top) and patient No. 11 (bottom). Both show left ventricular hypertrophy with repolarization abnormalities. In addition, patient No. 11 (P.D.) has left axis deviation and an intraventricular conduction delay.

calcification of the valve rather than from the inherent structure of the valve.

The location of the single commissure was noted in 12 hearts in which it was possible to determine the anatomic relations with certainty (fig. 1). Two raphes were present in ten patients, one in one patient, and none in one patient. The distances between the true and false commissures, when present, were essentially equal, dividing the valve into thirds, and maintaining the normal anatomic division of the aortic valve into right, left, and posterior (noncoronary) cusps. There was no separation of the "cusps," however, and none of the raphes reached the free edges of the cusps. The one true commissure was located at the junction of the normal left and right coronary cusps in five hearts, at the junction of the left coronary and noncoronary (posterior) cusps in six, and at the junction of the right coronary and noncoronary cusps in one.

Despite left ventricular hypertrophy in all 18 autopsied patients, the posteromedial papillary muscle was atrophied in 11 hearts and severely fibrotic in five (fig. 7). No patient had hypertrophied papillary muscles. Four patients had focal thickening of the free edge of the anterior mitral leaflet, but in each of these four patients aortic regurgitation also had been present.

Only one patient (no. 2) had an aortic valvotomy, and he developed aortic regurgitation postoperatively; nine other patients had aortic valve replacement. Aortic valvotomy is hazardous in patients with congenitally unicommissural aortic valves because the valve has a lateral attachment at only one point.[7] Of seven infants undergoing valvotomy reported by Moller et al.,[5] four died during operation or in the immediate postoperative period. Of the three who survived from 2 to 6 years, all retained loud systolic murmurs, and all developed grade 2/6 diastolic murmurs of aortic regurgitation. One patient with no systolic pressure gradient across the aortic valve postoperatively had angiographic evidence of aortic regurgitation.

Figure 6

Chest roentgenograms in four patients. (a and a¹) Patient No. 7. (b and b¹) Patient No. 17. Large calcific deposits (arrows) are present in the aortic valve of both patients. (c) Patient No. 15. (d) Patient No. 11. Both latter patients have very large hearts and pulmonary venous congestion. When the (c) and (d) roentgenograms were taken both patients were in terminal congestive cardiac failure and had the murmurs of mitral and tricuspid regurgitation also.

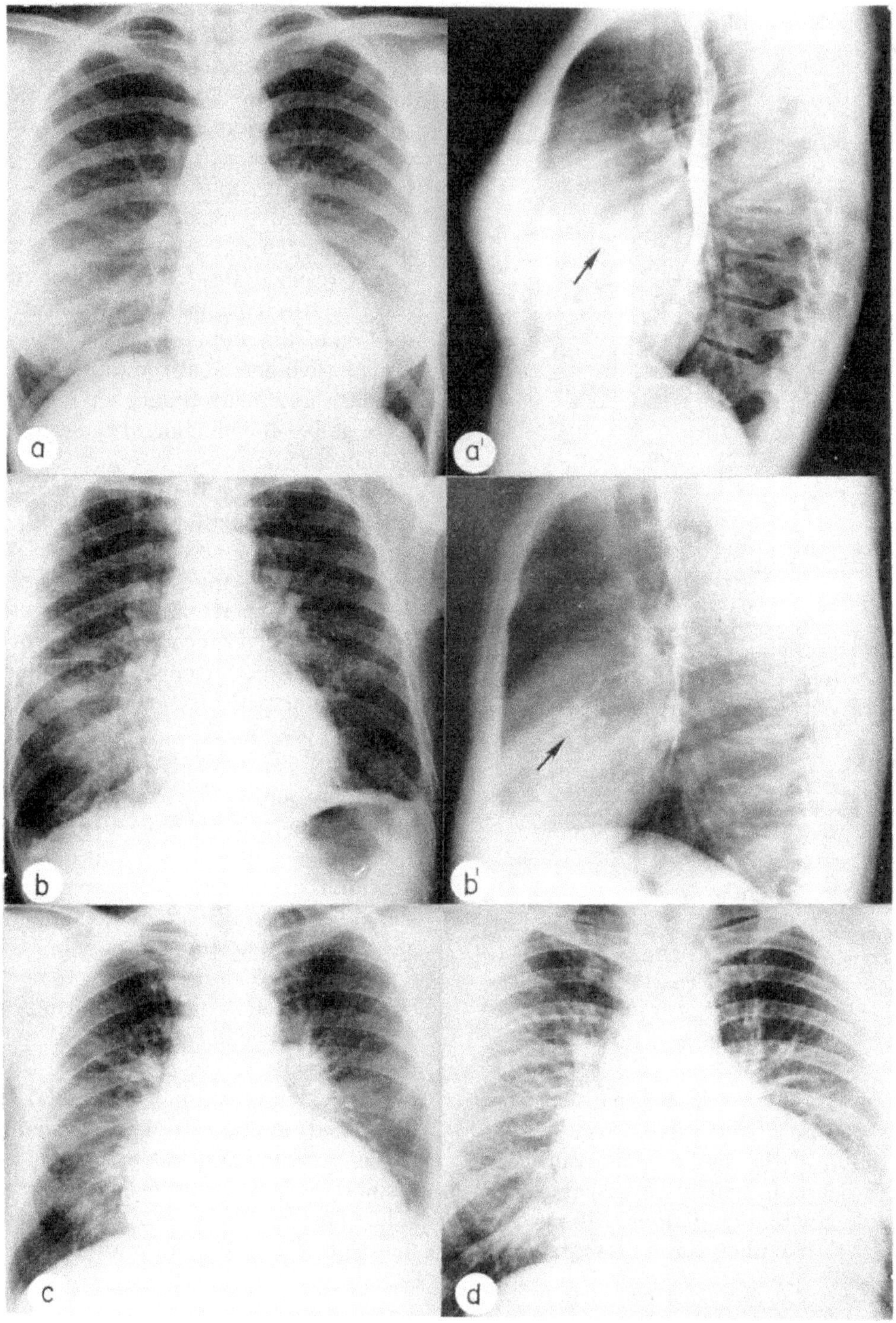
a
a'
b
b'
c
d

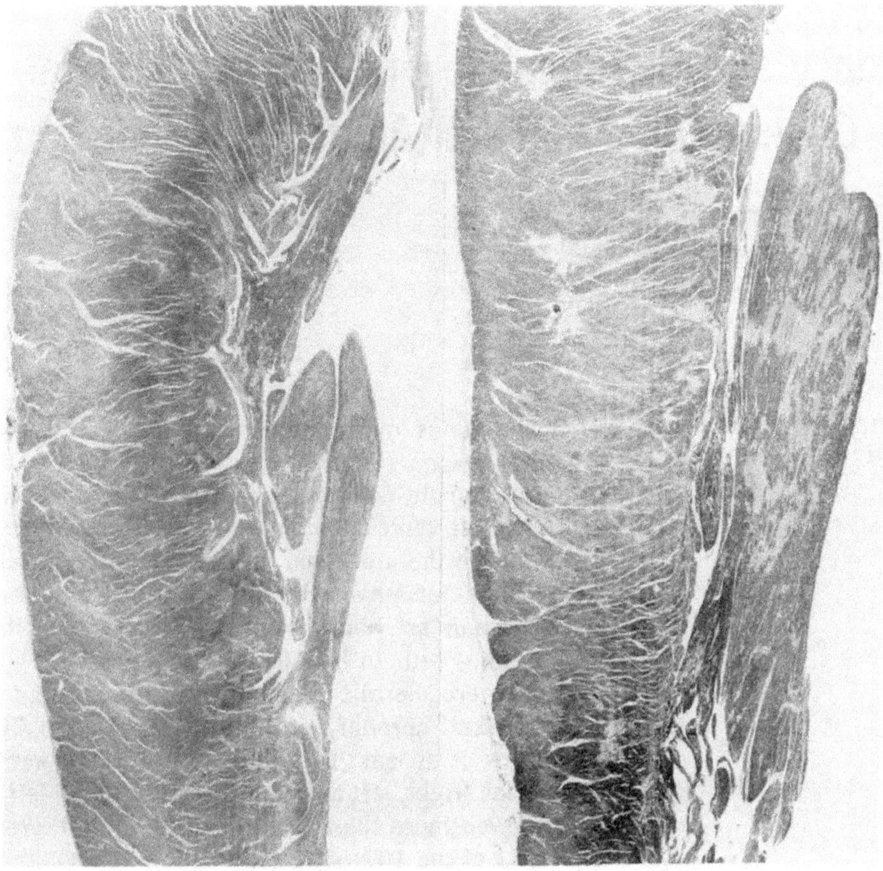

Figure 7

Longitudinal sections of posteromedial left ventricular papillary muscles in two patients with congenitally unicommissural aortic valves. (Left) Patient No. 7. The papillary muscle is severely scarred and atrophied. (Right) Patient No. 6. The papillary muscle is focally fibrotic and only minimally atrophied. Hematoxylin and eosin stains; each × 2.

References

1. Roberts WC: The structure of the aortic valve in clinically-isolated aortic stenosis. A study of 162 autopsy patients over 15 years of age. Circulation **42**: 91, 1970
2. Roberts WC: Anatomically isolated aortic valvular disease. The case against its being of rheumatic etiology. Amer J Med **49**: 151, 1970
3. Roberts WC: The congenitally bicuspid aortic valve. A study of 85 autopsy patients. Amer J Cardiol **26**: 72, 1970
4. Edwards JE: Pathologic aspects of cardiac valvular insufficiencies. Arch Surg (Chicago) **77**: 634, 1958
5. Moller JH, Nakib A, Eliot RS, Edwards JE: Symptomatic congenital aortic stenosis in the first year of life. J Pediat **69**: 728, 1966
6. Moller JH, Nakib A, Edwards JE: Infarction of papillary muscles and mitral insufficiency in association with congenital aortic stenosis. Circulation **34**: 87, 1966
7. Roberts WC, Morrow AG: Congenital aortic stenosis produced by a unicommissural valve. Brit Heart J **27**: 505, 1965

The Frequency and Significance of Coronary Arterial Thrombi and Other Observations in Fatal Acute Myocardial Infarction

A Study of 107 Necropsy Patients

WILLIAM C. ROBERTS, M.D.
L. MAXIMILIAN BUJA, M.D.
Bethesda, Maryland

Observations made from histologic study of the entire extramural coronary arterial tree are described in 107 patients who died of acute ischemic heart disease: seventy-four had transmural left ventricular myocardial infarction, nine had necrosis limited to the inner one half of the left ventricular myocardium (acute subendocardial infarcts) and twenty-four died suddenly (less than six hours from onset of symptoms of myocardial ischemia) without histologically detectable myocardial necrosis. Old atherosclerotic plaquing was diffuse and extensive in the extramural coronary arteries in 104 of the 107 patients. The lumens of at least two of the three major extramural coronary arteries (right, left anterior descending and left circumflex) were narrowed more than 75 per cent by old atherosclerotic plaques in 101 of the 107 patients.

Coronary arterial thrombi were found in forty (54 per cent) of the seventy-four patients with transmural necrosis, in none of the nine with only subendocardial necrosis and in two (8 per cent) of the twenty-four who died suddenly. In thirty-seven of the forty-two patients with antemortem coronary arterial clots the lumen of the vessel containing the thrombus was already narrowed more than 75 per cent by old atherosclerotic plaques at or distal to the thrombus. The infrequency of coronary thrombi in patients who died of acute cardiovascular collapse without myocardial necrosis, in those in whom necrosis was limited to the subendocardium, in those who died without cardiogenic shock or congestive cardiac failure, and their occurrence at, or proximal to, sites already severely narrowed by old atherosclerotic plaques suggest that coronary thrombi are consequences rather than causes of acute myocardial infarction. The occurrence of components of thrombi, i.e., fibrin and platelets, in old atherosclerotic plaques and the finding of components of old atherosclerotic plaques, i.e., foam cells, cholesterol clefts, pultaceous debris and calcific deposits, in known thrombi (for example, those located in the left atrium of patients with mitral stenosis) strongly suggest, however, that old atherosclerotic plaques are derived, at least in part, from organization of thrombi.

From the Section of Pathology, National Heart and Lung Institute, National Institutes of Health, Bethesda, Maryland 20014. Requests for reprints should be addressed to Dr. William C. Roberts. Manuscript received August 31, 1971.

TABLE I Clinical and Necropsy Data in Fatal Acute Myocardial Infarction (AMI)

Data	Transmural AMI	Subendocardial AMI	Sudden Death	Totals
No. of patients	74	9	24	107
Age range (yr)	26–90	49–83	28–85	26–90
Average	60	69	54	59
Men:Women	52(70%):22(30%)	6(67%):3(33%)	20(83%):4(17%)	78(73%):29(27%)
Old MI*	41 (55%)	7 (78%)	15 (62%)	63 (59%)
Hypertension†	33 (45%)	3 (33%)	11 (46%)	47 (44%)
"Diabetes"‡	26 (35%)	3 (33%)	3 (13%)	32 (30%)
Total no. of major coronary arteries§	222	27	72	327
No. of major coronary arteries narrowed >75% by old plaques	168 (76%) (2.3 per patient)	20 (74%) (2.2 per patient)	56 (78%) (2.3 per patient)	244 (75%) (2.3 per patient)
3	41 (55%)	5 (56%)	11 (46%)	57 (53%)
2	17 (23%)	2 (22%)	10 (42%)	29 (27%)
1	11 (15%)	1 (11%)	3 (12%)	15 (14%)
0	5 (7%)	1 (11%)	0	6 (6%)
Coronary artery thrombi	40 (54%)	0	2 (8%)	42 (39%)
Coronary artery hemorrhages	20 (27%)	1 (11%)	5 (21%)	26 (24%)
Heart weight >400 gm	56 (76%)	9 (100%)	15 (63%)	80 (75%)

* Either transmural or subendocardial fibrosis observed at autopsy. This number does not include microscopic-sized microinfarcts.

† Systemic diastolic blood pressure >90 mm Hg.

‡ Includes patients with abnormal fasting blood glucose levels and/or abnormal glucose tolerance tests in addition to patients being treated (by either diet or oral agents or both) for adult onset diabetes mellitus. None of the patients was treated with insulin.

§ Number derived by multiplying number of patients by 3—the number of major coronary arteries (right, anterior descending and left circumflex) per patient.

Acute myocardial infarction (AMI) is generally considered to be the result of thrombotic occlusion of a major extramural coronary artery. Indeed, coronary thrombosis was the name used for years to describe AMI both clinically and pathologically. The inability to find thrombi in major extramural coronary arteries in many patients who died of AMI stimulated us to study the coronary arterial tree systematically in consecutive patients who died from results of extensive myocardial necrosis or from acute cardiovascular collapse in the absence of myocardial necrosis (sudden death). Described here are our observations resulting from the histologic study of the major extramural coronary arteries in 107 such consecutive patients.

TABLE II Relationship Between Coronary Arterial Thrombosis and Duration of Survival After AMI

Survival Time	Patients (no.)	Thrombi No.	Thrombi %
Less than 6 hours	24	2	8
6 hours–3 days	36	18	50
4 days–14 days	31	15	48
15 days–45 days	16	7	44
Totals	107	42	39*

* If the nine patients with subendocardial necrosis and the twenty-four patients who died suddenly (less than six hours) were excluded this percentage would be 54 per cent.

PATIENTS STUDIED AND METHODS

The 107 patients (Table I) ranged in age from twenty-six to ninety years (average fifty-nine years); the seventy-eight men ranged in age from twenty-eight to eighty-five years (average fifty-seven years) and the twenty-nine women, twenty-six to ninety years (average sixty-four years). Five patients (four male, one female) were less than forty years old; four had transmural and one had subendocardial infarcts. Of the twenty-six patients (fifteen male, eleven female) more than sixty-nine years of age, nineteen had transmural and five had subendocardial infarcts; two died suddenly. The diagnosis of AMI was established or strongly suggested during life in sixty-six of the seventy-four patients with transmural infarcts and in five of the nine with subendocardial infarcts by history of prolonged substernal chest pain and/or electrocardiographic changes, and usually also elevations in serum enzyme levels. Of the twenty-four patients who died suddenly (less than six hours after onset of symptoms; no myocardial necrosis), fifteen died before and the remainder within three hours after their arrival at the hospital. Of the twelve patients with myocardial necrosis in whom the diagnosis of AMI was not established or strongly suggested during life, five had a sudden worsening of chronic congestive cardiac failure without chest pain (three had complete left bundle branch block) and four had sudden cerebrovascular accidents without chest pain (electrocardiograms were not recorded in two of the four patients).

The interval between the onset of symptoms of AMI and death varied from minutes to forty-five days; the interval was less than six hours in twenty-four patients and more than twenty-one days in six patients (Table II). Each of the latter six patients had clinical evidence of continuing myocardial infarction.

At necropsy, with the exception of the twenty-four patients in whom the interval between onset and death was less than six hours, all had myocardial coagulation necrosis. The infarcts, which involved the left ventricular free wall or ventricular septum or both, were transmural or nearly transmural in seventy-four patients and subendocardial (limited to inner one half of wall) in nine patients (Table I). Patients in whom myocardial necrosis was limited to left ventricular papillary muscles were excluded. At least three sections for histologic study of left ventricular wall were examined in every patient. In ten patients (all with transmural infarcts) the infarcted myocardial wall was aneurysmally dilated at autopsy. In ten other patients a necrotic wall (either left ventricular free wall or ventricular septum) was perforated. In addition to the acute infarcts sixty-three patients had old scars in the left ventricular free walls or ventricular septums, and thirty-five of them had had previous histories of AMI.

Excluding thirteen patients with valvular heart disease (heart weights from 370 to 1,050 gm [average 590 gm]) and one with congenital ventricular septal defect (VSD) (heart weight 730 gm), the hearts in the remaining ninety-three patients weighed from 300 to 800 gm [1] (average 472 gm); in the sixty-nine men without associated valvular heart disease or congenital VSD the average weight was 480 gm and in the twenty-four women, 438 gm. Of the total 107 patients the heart weighed more than 400 gm in eighty (75 per cent). Excluding the fourteen patients with valvular heart disease or congenital VSD, the hearts weighed more than 400 gm in thirty-seven (86 per cent) of forty-three patients with and in twenty-five (64 per cent) of thirty-nine patients without known histories of systemic diastolic hypertension (more than 90 mm Hg). Of thirty men without associated valvular heart disease, congenital VSD or systemic hypertension, the hearts weighed from 300 to 610 gm (average 439 gm) and of nine women, from 300 to 530 gm (average 403 gm). Of thirty men without associated heart disease except for systemic hypertension, the hearts weighed from 360 to 850 gm (average 544 gm) and of thirteen women from 375 to 610 gm (average 459 gm).

The major extramural coronary arteries were sectioned in their entirety in the following manner (Figure 1). Usually before the ventricles or coronary arteries were opened, the right, left main, left circumflex, left anterior descending and posterior descending coronary arteries were excised intact. Each was placed in a separate appropriately labeled container and fixed in 10 per cent buffered formalin. After fixation, each coronary artery was decalcified, its length measured and diagrammatically sketched, and cut transversely at 0.5 cm intervals. Four 0.5 cm segments were placed in a single plastic cricket and decalcified lightly again. The tissues were then dehydrated (alcohols), cleared (xylene), imbedded in paraffin and cut. At least two histologic sections, one stained by hematoxylin and eosin and the other by either Movat's method or elastic Van Gieson or both, were prepared from each 0.5 cm segment. Later, each section was examined by light

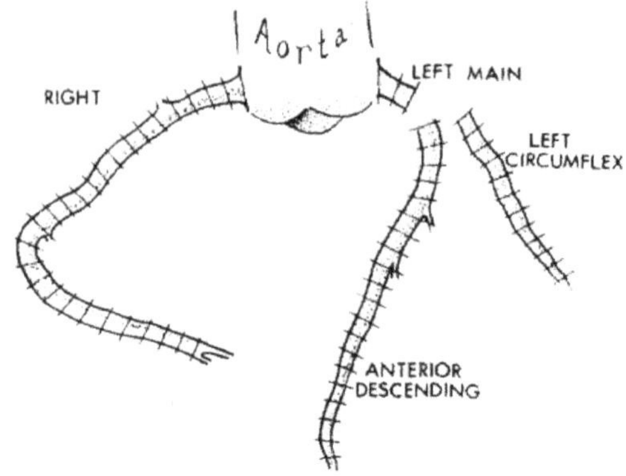

Figure 1. *Method of cutting coronary arteries. Often the left diagonal or marginal vessel also was examined in similar fashion.*

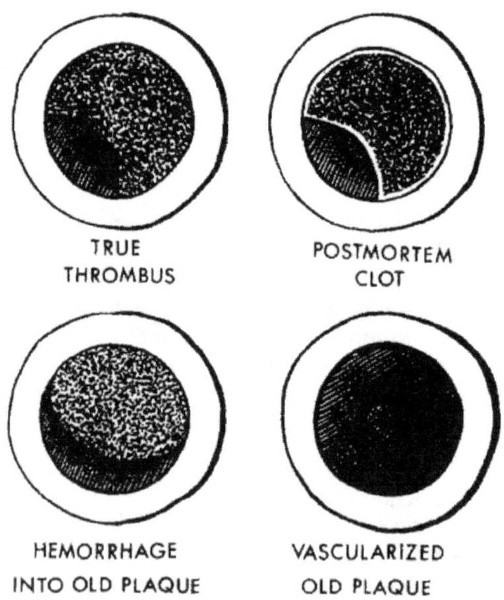

Figure 2. *Diagram illustrating four causes of red lesions in coronary arteries. By gross examination these lesions may be confused with one another. For this reason, histologic examination is essential, and judgments made purely by gross examination are fraught with error.*

microscopy, and the maximal degree of luminal narrowing caused by old atherosclerotic plaques in each vessel was recorded as follows: 0 or none; less than 25 per cent; 26 to 50 per cent; 51 to 75 per cent; and more than 75 per cent. The presence or absence of thrombi, hemorrhage into old atherosclerotic plaques and calcific deposits (graded 0 to 4) were recorded. If thrombus was found, the vessel thrombosed was recorded; the status of the coronary artery at the site of thrombosis was noted, i.e., whether or not the lumen at the site of thrombosis was already narrowed, and to what degree, by old atherosclerotic plaques; the degree of luminal narrowing by old atherosclerotic plaques distal to the thrombus was carefully observed and the components of the thrombus, i.e., erythrocytes, fibrin, platelets and leukocytes, were noted and graded 0 to 4. A

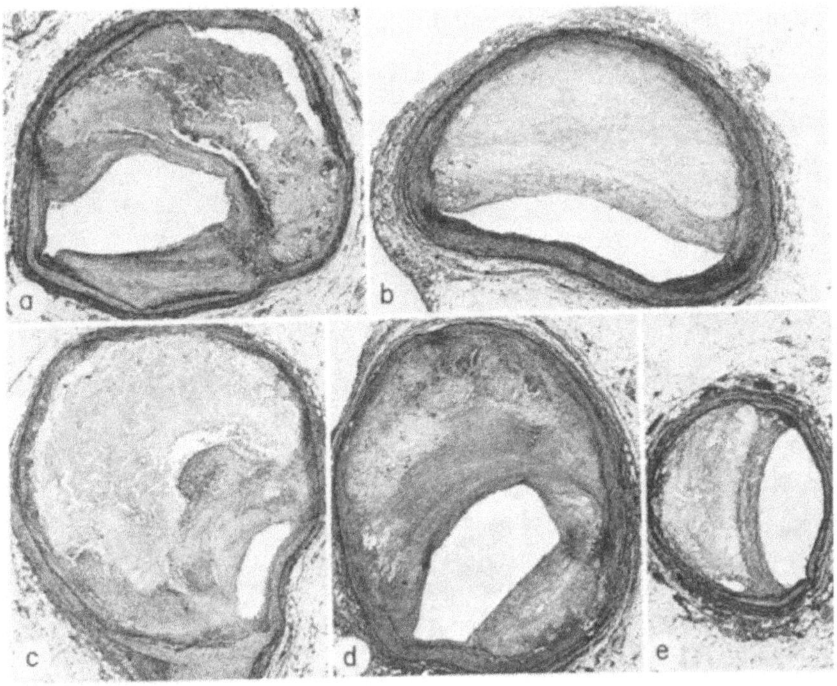

Figure 3. *Major extramural coronary arteries in a sixty-three year old woman (A69-262) who died of acute* **transmural** *myocardial necrosis* **eight** *days after onset of symptoms. Death was sudden without antecedent shock or congestive cardiac failure. At necropsy, a large anteroseptal transmural AMI was present, and blood was present in the pericardial space although no discrete focus of myocardial rupture was seen. The heart weighed 375 gm, and no foci of myocardial fibrosis were seen. All extramural coronary arteries were narrowed by old atherosclerotic plaques, and no thrombi or hemorrhages were found in them.* ***a,*** *right coronary artery 3 cm from aortic ostium.* ***b,*** *left main coronary artery.* ***c,*** *left circumflex artery in first 1 cm.* ***d,*** *left anterior descending artery in first 1 cm.* ***e,*** *left marginal artery. Movat stains; original magnification, each × 16.*

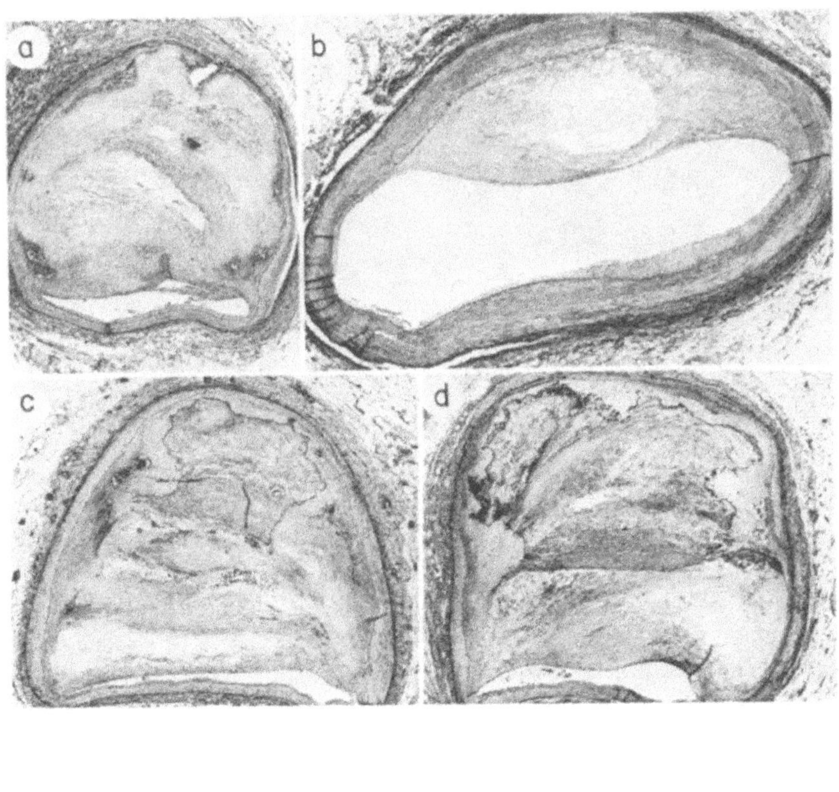

Figure 4. *Major extramural coronary arteries at sites of maximal narrowing in a fifty-four year old man (SH No. A4705) who died of acute* **subendocardial** *myocardial necrosis twelve hours after onset of chest pain. The patient had angina pectoris and adult onset diabetes mellitus but never congestive heart failure or shock. The heart (weight = 430 gm) was severely scarred; left ventricular fibrosis was mainly subendocardial and virtually circumferential from apex to base; rarely, a focus of transmural fibrosis was present. No thrombi or hemorrhages were present in the coronary arteries.* ***a,*** *right artery.* ***b,*** *left main artery.* ***c,*** *left circumflex artery.* ***d,*** *left anterior descending artery. All three of the major coronary arteries were narrowed more than 75 per cent by old atherosclerotic plaques. The coronary arteries were heavily calcified, a common observation in patients with diabetes mellitus. Movat stains; original magnification, each × 21.*

section of thrombus usually was stained with phosphotungsten-acid hematoxylin to aid in roughly quantitating its various components.

RESULTS

The findings are summarized in Table I and illustrated in Figures 2 to 21. The lumens of one or more of the three major extramural coronary arteries (right, left anterior descending and left circumflex) were narrowed more than 75 per cent by old atherosclerotic plaques in 101 of the 107 patients: in fifteen patients only one of three vessels was narrowed more than 75 per cent; in twenty-nine patients, two vessels; and in fifty-seven patients, the lumens of all three major coronary arteries were narrowed more than 75 per cent (Figures 3 to 6). Excluding three patients with coronary embolism, of the several thousand sec-

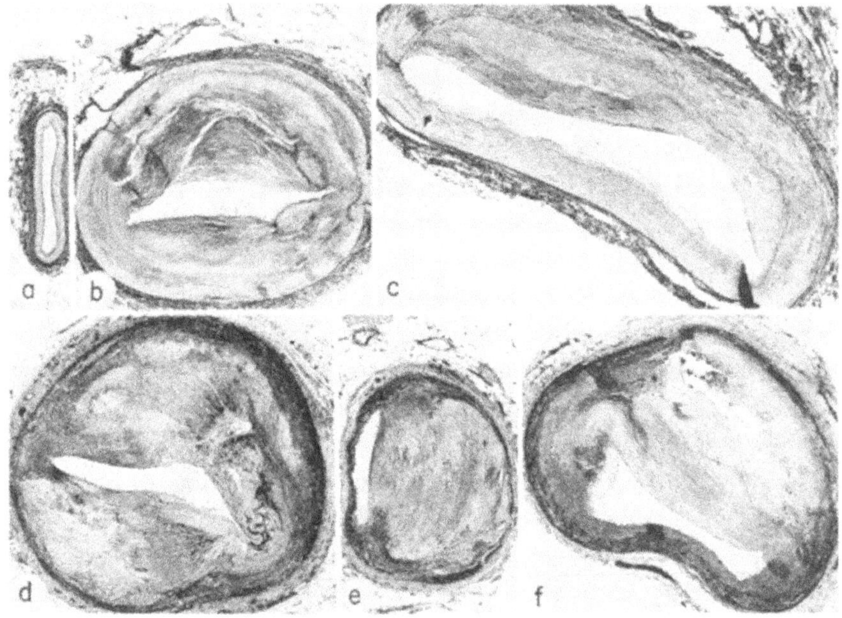

*Figure 5. Extramural coronary arteries in a forty-one year old man (SH No. A4570) who died suddenly and unexpectedly at home (**sudden death**). He apparently had no previous symptoms of cardiac disease. At necropsy, the heart weighed 430 gm and all three major coronary arteries were narrowed more than 75 per cent by old atherosclerotic plaques. No coronary thrombi or hemorrhages were observed. **a,** right posterior descending branch. It is unusual to find a branch of a major coronary artery normal, and this one is, when the major vessels are severely diseased. **b,** right main coronary artery. **c,** left main coronary artery. **d,** left circumflex artery. **e,** left marginal artery. **f,** left anterior descending artery. Movat stains; original magnification, each × 20.*

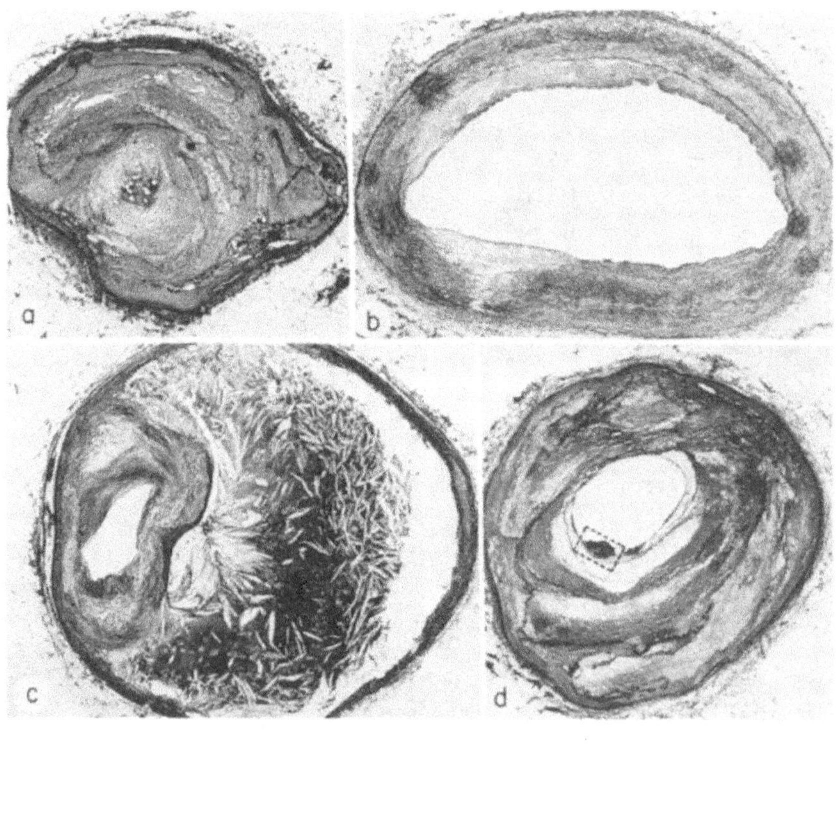

*Figure 6. Major coronary arteries at sites of maximal narrowing in a sixty-five year old man (A71-6) who died three hours after suddenly collapsing while standing. During the final three hours he had multiple arrhythmias, severe shock and congestive cardiac failure. Until this episode he had been asymptomatic, although he was known to have systemic hypertension. At necropsy, the heart weighed 540 gm. The lumens of the right (**a**), left circumflex (**c**) and anterior descending (**d**) arteries were more than 75 per cent narrowed by old plaques. In addition, extravasated blood was present in a plaque in the left circumflex artery (**c**) and a small mural (nonocclusive) platelet thrombus (better seen in Figure 7) was present in the anterior descending branch (**d**). The right artery (**a**) was occluded except for a few recanalized channels. The left main artery (**b**) was wide open. Movat stain (**a**), elastic van Gieson stain (**b**), hematoxylin and eosin stains (**c** and **d**); original magnification, each × 20.*

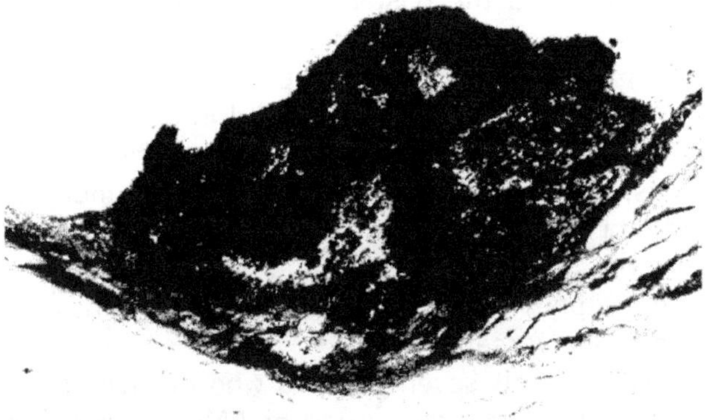

Figure 7. Platelet thrombus shown in brackets in left anterior descending coronary artery of patient described in Figure 6. This is probably the appearance of an early thrombus and it consists almost entirely of platelets. Hematoxylin and eosin stain, original magnification × 250.

tions examined only four sections were totally free of old atherosclerotic plaques.

Thrombi or emboli were observed in one of the three major extramural coronary arteries in forty-two (39 per cent) of the 107 patients; thirty-nine had thrombi and three had emboli (Figures 6 to 16). The thrombi in all thirty-nine patients were superimposed on old atherosclerotic plaques, but the emboli in all three patients were not superimposed on old plaques (Figures 18 and 19). The lumens of the coronary arteries distal to antemortem clots were more than 75 per cent narrowed by old atherosclerotic plaques in thirty-seven of the thirty-nine patients with thrombi but in none of the three with emboli. One coronary

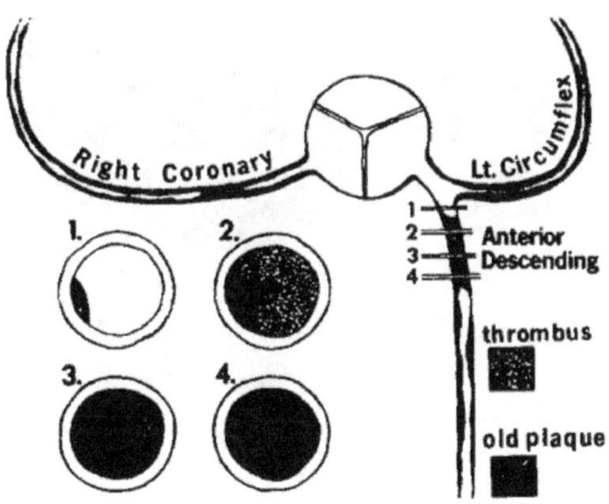

Figure 8. Diagram illustrating the diffuse nature of coronary atherosclerosis and the usual status of a vessel at and distal to a thrombus. At level 2 in the anterior descending artery the lumen is obstructed primarily by a thrombus. At level 3, however, the major per cent of narrowing is the result of old atherosclerotic plaquing and just distal to the thrombus, the lumen is severely narrowed (more than 75 per cent) or totally obstructed by old plaque only.

arterial clot was found in thirty-seven of the thirty-nine patients with thrombosis and in each of the three with embolism. The site of myocardial necrosis in each corresponded properly with the artery containing the thrombus or embolus; all patients with antemortem clots in the anterior descending vessel, for example, had anterior wall infarcts. The location of the antemortem clots in the forty patients with single vessel involvement was left anterior descending artery, eighteen patients; right, twelve patients; and left circumflex, ten patients. In the other two patients, each of two coronary arteries contained thrombus. In twenty-nine of the thirty-seven patients with thrombi in a single coronary artery, the lumen was completely closed at the site of thrombosis by combined old arteriosclerotic plaques and recent thrombus. In the other eight patients the lumen was only partially occluded by the recent thrombus. In each of the two patients with thrombi in two coronary arteries the lumen of one artery was completely occluded by thrombus, and the lumen of the second artery was only partially occluded by thrombus. The lumens were completely closed by clot in each of the three patients with embolism. The interval from death to autopsy ranged from two to twenty-three hours (average twelve hours) in the forty-two patients with antemortem clots, and from two to twenty-six hours (average eleven hours) in the sixty-five patients without antemortem clots. There was no sex difference among patients with and without coronary arterial clots; of forty-two with thrombi or emboli, twelve (28 per cent) were women and thirty (72 per cent) were men; of sixty-five patients without thrombi or emboli, seventeen (26 per cent) were women and forty-eight (74 per cent) were men.

None of the three patients with coronary arterial emboli had previous narrowing at the site of embolism by old plaques or luminal narrowing by old plaques distal to the embolus (Figures 18 and 19). Furthermore, none of these three patients had luminal narrowing by old plaques more than 25 per cent in any of the three major coronary arteries. The embolus in each was located in the more distal portion of the coronary artery (left anterior descending in two; right in one) whereas the thrombi in the other thirty-nine patients occurred in the more proximal portions of the coronary arteries. Embolic material in each of these three patients also was present in the small epicardial and in the intramural branches of the coronary arteries. In none of the thirty-nine patients with coronary thrombi was thrombus found in an intramural coronary artery. In one patient with presumed coronary arterial embolism, a thirty-seven year old man with a large congenital VSD, rapid atrial fibrillation suddenly developed, was converted to normal sinus rhythm by electroshock, and was followed four hours later by cardiac arrest. He was resuscitated but never regained consciousness and died three days later. Necropsy disclosed massive necrosis of the caudal portion of the ventricular septum and anterior free wall of left ventricle. The second patient with presumed coronary embolism, a sixty-three year old woman, had rheumatic mitral and aortic valvular stenosis and atrial fibrillation. In this patient severe chest pain suddenly developed and an electrocardiogram showed typical changes of AMI. Necropsy showed extensive necrosis of the anterior portion of the left ventricular free wall and ventricular septum. In the third patient with presumed coronary embolism electrocardiographic features of acute posterior wall myocardial infarction suddenly developed during cardiac catheterization. These changes appeared immediately after flushing the cardiac catheter which lay in the right coronary artery. At necropsy, thirty-one days later, a large embolus was found in the distal right coronary artery and its posterior descending branches, and the posterior wall of the left ventricle was massively necrotic.

Hemorrhages into old atherosclerotic plaques (Figures 6 and 12) were observed in one or more extramural coronary arteries in twenty-six patients, sixteen of whom also had superimposed thrombi. In only one of the twenty-six patients, however, did the extravascular blood in the old plaque appear to actually further narrow the lumen of the vessel.

Of the twenty-seven patients who received anticoagulants during the period of AMI, at necropsy eight had thrombi in a major coronary artery. Three of them also had hemorrhage into an old plaque and two other patients had hemorrhages into plaques unassociated with thrombosis. Six of the twenty-seven patients receiving anticoagulants had subendocardial infarcts (three patients) or died within six hours (sudden death, three patients).

The intramural coronary arteries (Figures 20 and 21) in the left ventricular free walls and ventricular septums were free of significant luminal narrowing in all 107 patients. Foam cells, cholesterol clefts, calcific deposits or fibrin-platelet thrombi were not observed in any intramural coronary artery, and at least three histologic sections of left ventricular wall were examined in each patient.

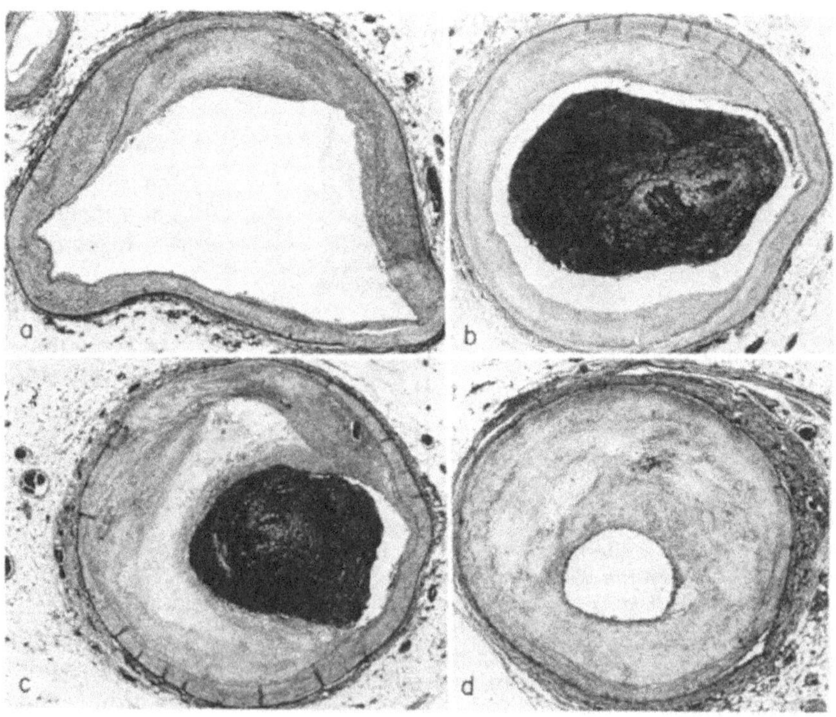

Figure 9. *Left circumflex coronary artery in a fifty-seven year old woman (A69-131) who died four days after the onset of transmural AMI. Four levels in the area of the thrombus, as shown in Figure 8, are shown.* ***a,*** *proximal to thrombus (level 1).* ***b,*** *at this point thrombus is present but it is not attached to the interior lining of the artery (level 2).* ***c,*** *now the thrombus is firmly attached. The retraction of the thrombus on one side is an artefact (level 3).* ***d,*** *distal to the thrombus (level 4). The lumen is more than 75 per cent narrowed by old plaque. Movat stains; original magnification, each × 21.*

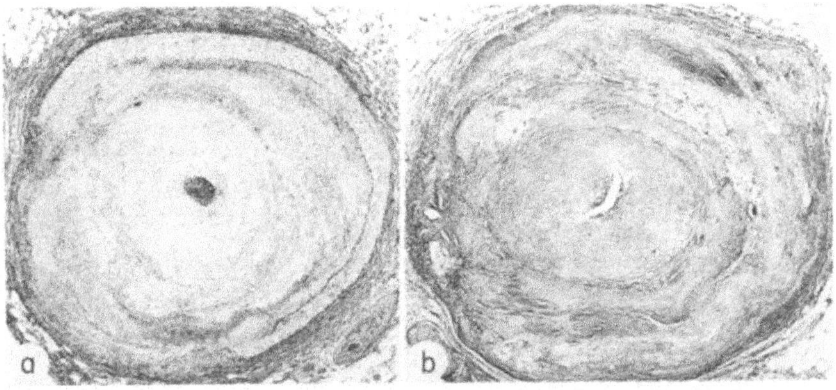

Figure 10. *Anterior descending coronary artery 6 to 7 cm from aortic ostium in a fifty-nine year old woman (A68-285) who had the onset of transmural AMI forty-eight hours before death. She began to have intermittent chest pain two months earlier and had had systemic hypertension for ten years. Her final two days were characterized by shock, pulmonary edema and bradycardia. At necropsy, a "massive" anterior wall infarct, which was aneurysmally dilated, was present. The lumens of all three major coronary arteries were more than 75 per cent narrowed by old plaques. In addition, a small occluding thrombus was present in the left anterior descending vessel (**a**). The per cent of narrowing caused by the thrombus is small, however, compared to the per cent of narrowing resulting from old atherosclerotic plaques. The lumen both proximal and distal (**b**) to the thrombus is already severely narrowed by old plaque. Movat stains (**a**); hematoxylin and eosin stain (**b**), original magnification, each × 25.*

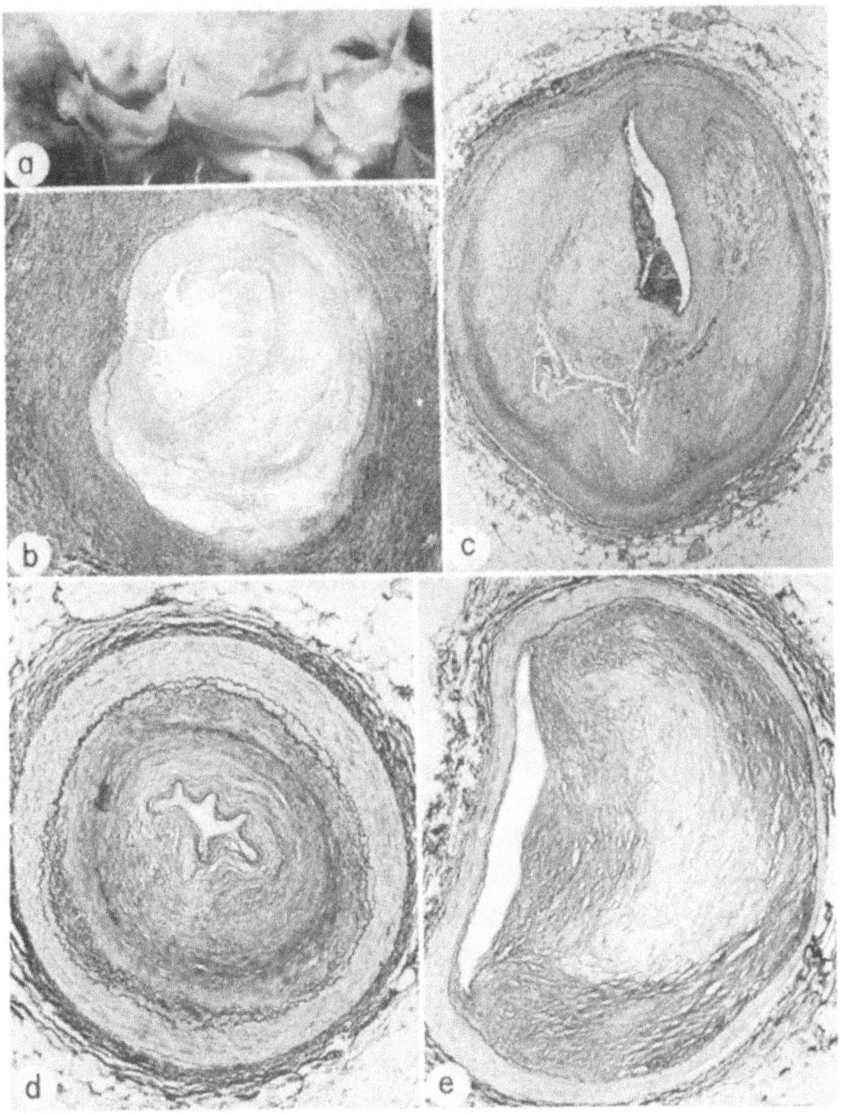

Figure 11. *Major coronary arteries in a forty-seven year old man (A69-179) who died of an arrhythmia twelve hours after the onset of cardiac ischemic pain. He never had shock or congestive heart failure. He did have systemic hypertension. At necropsy, transmural necrosis was present in the posterolateral left ventricular wall and the aortic ostium of the right coronary artery was severely narrowed (**a**). A histologic section of the right coronary artery as it arises from the aorta is shown in **b**. The lumen of the left circumflex just as it arises from the left main coronary artery is shown in **c**. Its lumen contains a nonoccluding thrombus. The thrombus contains several cholesterol clefts indicating that a plaque may have ruptured upstream. Immediately distal to the thrombus, this artery divided into two branches (**d** and **e**) both of which were more than 75 per cent narrowed by old plaques. Movat stains (**b** and **c**) and elastic van Gieson stains (**d** and **e**); original magnification × 15 (**b**), × 25 (**c**), × 60 (**d**) and × 50 (**e**).*

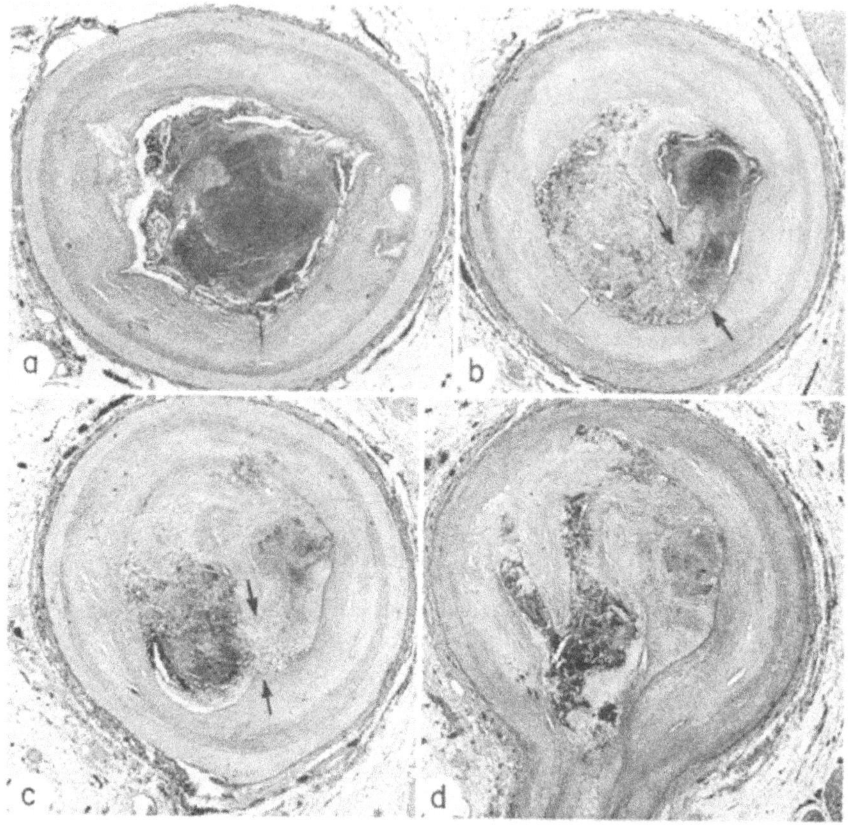

Figure 12. Four sections of anterior descending coronary artery in a forty-seven year old woman (A68-129) who had recurring AMI over a forty-two day period. The sections show a thrombus which is located over a ruptured plaque (between the arrows). Extravasated erythrocytes also are present in the plaque. Serial sections were cut of the area of thrombosis. The four sections shown here were from a segment 360 μ long; **a,** at 12 μ. **b,** at 120 μ. **c,** at 240 μ. **d,** at 360 μ. Movat stains; original magnification, each $\times$ 14.

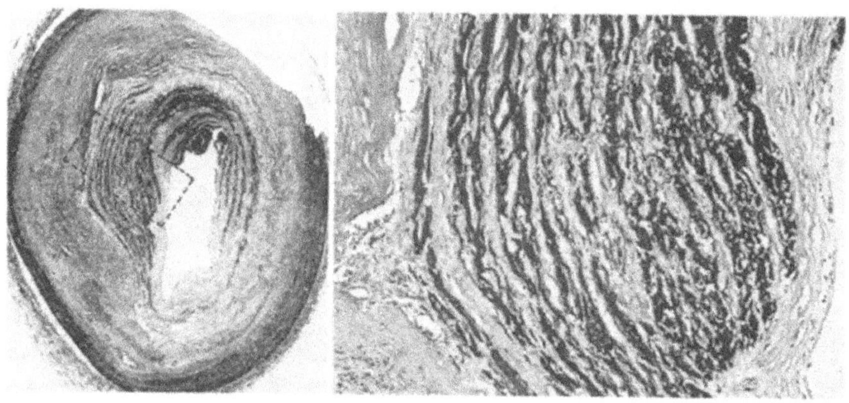

Figure 13. Right coronary artery in a forty-seven year old man (A70-72) with healed posterior wall left ventricular transmural infarct and rheumatic mitral stenosis. The lumen of the right coronary artery was narrowed more than 75 per cent primarily by fibrous plaques interspersed with fibrin as shown here. The fibrin is dark and the organized fibrous tissue is lighter. A close-up view of the deposits located in the bracket is shown at right. The occurrence of fibrin in atherosclerotic plaques is evidence that thrombosis and atherosclerosis are in some way closely related. Phosphotungstic acid-hematoxylin stain, original magnification $\times$ 23 (**left**) and $\times$ 120 (**right**).

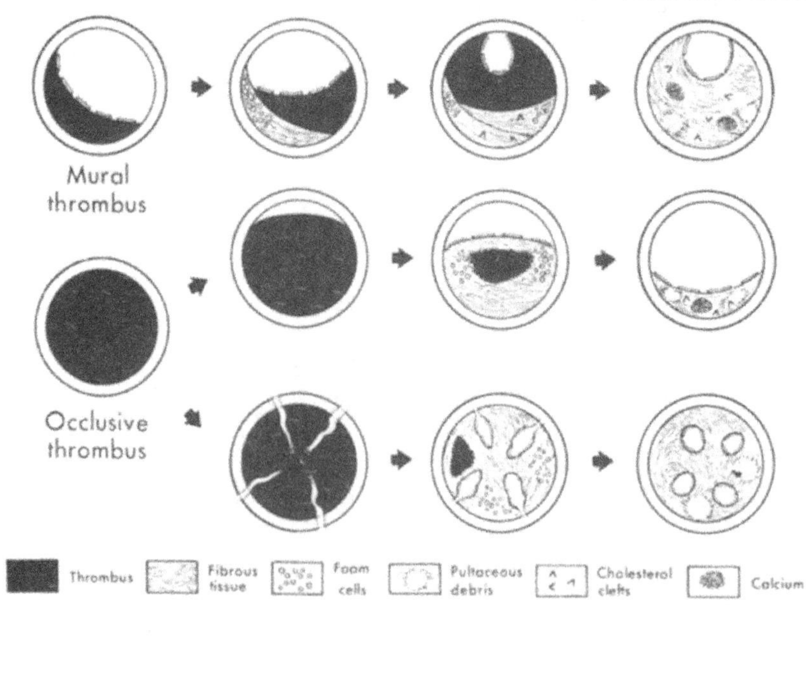

Figure 14. Diagram depicting formation of coronary arterial atherosclerotic plaques from mural and occlusive thrombi. The mural thrombus initially contacts only a portion of the intimal lining. The fibrin-platelet thrombus is covered by endothelial cells and retraction occurs as it organizes into fibrous tissue. Foam cells appear. Another mural thrombus follows, the process of organization is repeated. The lines of demarcation between the separate thrombi gradually fade so that at the final stage histologic study makes recognition of previous components of thrombus difficult. Organization of an occlusive thrombus may occur in two ways. In one, the thrombus retracts from one intimal surface to form a single channel. As it organizes the surface of the thrombus exposed to the lumen is covered by endothelial cells. Organization takes place from the overlying newly grown endothelium and from preexisting intima to encase in fibrous tissue the residual thrombus which may undergo fatty degeneration. Alternatively, organization may occur by capillaries growing into the thrombus at its base. The capillaries may dilate as the thrombus retracts during organization finally leading to the plaque with recanalized channels.

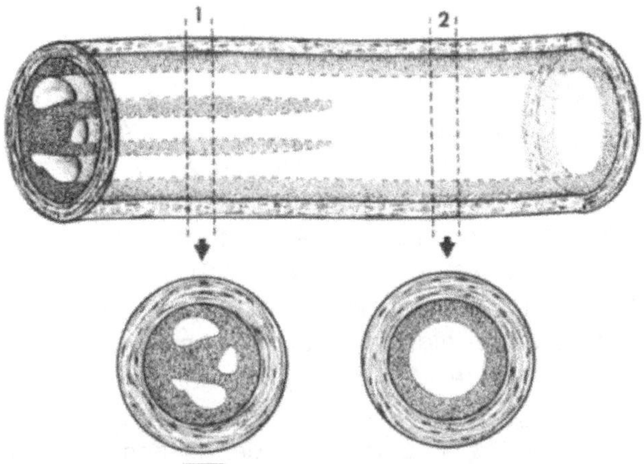

Figure 15. The multi- and the unichanneled coronary arterial atherosclerotic plaque. Duguid, when studying serial sections of an "organized thrombus," noted that the tissue present between channels in an artery containing multiple revascularized channels was similar to that found in arteries with only one channel. Since the multichannel artery had been recognized as the hallmark of an organized thrombus and since the tissue in both multi- and unichanneled arteries was similar, he reasoned that the causative process also was similar.

COMMENTS

Although many clinicians and pathologists apparently consider coronary arterial thrombosis the cause of fatal acute myocardial infarction (AMI), the reported frequency of such thrombosis has varied from 21 to 91 per cent [2–22]. Inclusion of cases of subendocardial infarction and sudden death ("acute cardiovascular collapse in the absence of myocardial necrosis") [23] with cases of transmural necrosis is probably the major cause for the variation in frequency.

Coronary arterial thrombi are infrequent in patients who die suddenly with or without previous histories of cardiac disease and in those in whom necrosis is limited to the inner half of the left ventricular wall (subendocardium). Among our twenty-four patients who died suddenly (less than six hours from onset of symptoms), two (8 per cent) had a thrombus in a coronary artery, and of our nine patients with only subendocardial necrosis, none had a coronary arterial thrombus. In contrast, of our seventy-four patients with transmural myocardial necrosis, forty (54 per cent) had a thrombus in a coronary artery.

Although the type of myocardial infarct is probably the most important factor, differing technics of examining coronary arteries at necropsy and differing definitions of what constitutes a true thrombus also may contribute to the varied reported incidence of coronary thrombosis in fatal AMI. Studies utilizing only gross inspection of these vessels without confirmation of the presence or absence of thrombus by histologic study are inadequate. Postmortem clots, hemorrhage into old atherosclerotic plaques and even highly vascularized old plaques may be confused with antemortem thrombi (Figure 2). True (antemortem) thrombi are adherent to the luminal surfaces of the arteries and are composed of platelets or fibrin or both, and usually also of erythrocytes and leukocytes. Coronary arterial thrombi are usually about 1 cm in length, and although they are adherent distally they may not be adherent proximally. The composition of a thrombus at varying levels may differ. Distally it is more likely to consist of platelets or fibrin or both (white thrombus), and more proximally it may be composed of erythrocytes, lesser quantities of fibrin, few platelets and some leukocytes (red thrombus). Early thrombi may be composed purely of platelets and are often small and nonocclusive (Figures 6 and 7). The postmortem or false thrombus, in contrast to the true one, is nonadherent and composed mainly of erythrocytes.

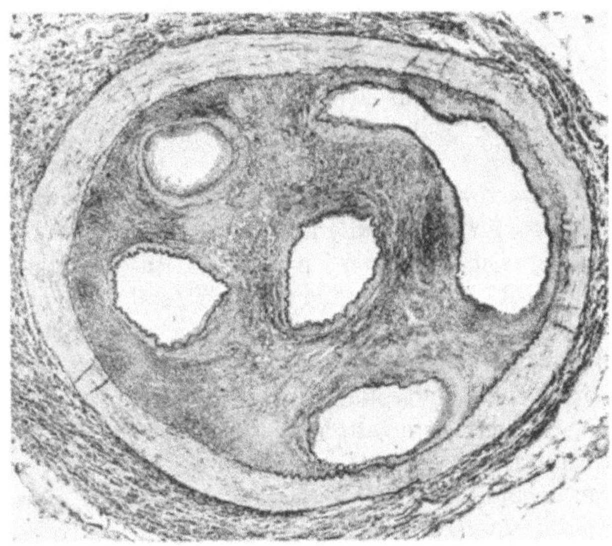

Figure 16. Recanalized embolus in distal anterior descending coronary artery of a twenty-six year old man (A63-170) in whom a massive anterior wall AMI developed three years before when he had infective endocarditis of the aortic valve. This process clearly resulted from organization of fibrin-platelet-erythrocyte-leukocyte clot, almost surely embolus, and similar lesions are found in patients with extensive coronary arterial atherosclerosis. Note that each recanalized channel has developed its own internal elastic membrane and smooth muscle medial wall. Elastic van Gieson stain, original magnification × 46.

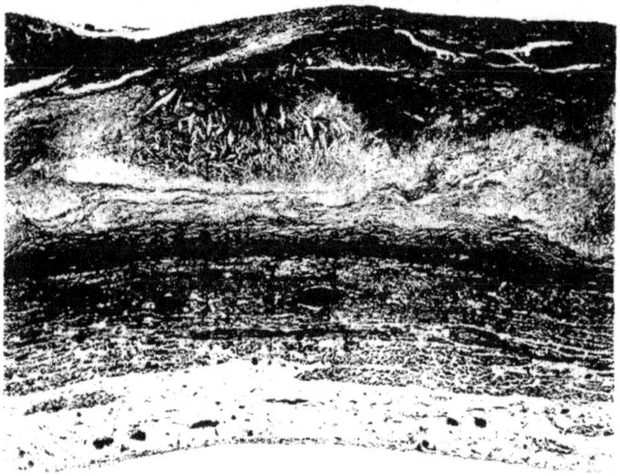

Figure 17. Left atrial thrombus in a patient with mitral stenosis. Organization of a thrombus may result in plaques which look identical to complicated atherosclerotic plaques. Shown here is a section of left atrial wall from a fifty year old woman (A67-210) with a huge thrombus. Organization of portions of the thrombus led to development of numerous cholesterol clefts, pultaceous debris, calcific deposits as well as fibrous tissue—components of arterial atherosclerotic plaques. Hematoxylin and eosin stain, original magnification × 20.

Thrombi occurring in patients who died of AMI are, except in cases of embolism, superimposed on old atherosclerotic plaques. Usually the artery containing the thrombus is more than 50 per cent narrowed already by old atherosclerotic plaques, and frequently the degree of luminal narrowing is more than 75 per cent at the distal attachment. In most patients with fatal AMI and coronary arterial thrombi the lumen of the artery distal to the thrombus is more than 75 per cent narrowed by old plaques. In thirty-seven of our forty-two patients with antemortem coronary clots (thrombi in thirty-nine, emboli in three), thrombus was located at or proximal to a site already more than 75 per cent narrowed by old plaque. To reemphasize; in only five of our forty-two patients with coronary arterial thromboembolic material was the vessel containing the clot not narrowed more than 75 per cent by old atherosclerotic plaques, and three of these five had coronary emboli. In a few patients the thrombus occurred in a segment of artery between two sites of extreme narrowing by old plaques. The observation of severe narrowing by old plaques of the coronary artery distal to a thrombus has not been commented on in previous reports to our knowledge. Experimentally, the site of predilection of a thrombus has been within a "dilated" segment or at the poststenotic luminal expansion [24].

Why fresh thrombi are located at or proximal to sites of narrowing is unclear. Several investigators [4,25–33] have observed thrombi covering cracks in old atherosclerotic plaques, and some [29–31,33] have considered rupture of the innermost layer of plaques the most important precipitating cause of coronary arterial thrombosis. Ruptures occur particularly in fibrous tissue covering deposits of pultaceous debris and lead to discharge of necrotic debris into the arterial lumens or to bleeding into plaques. The break in the plaque exposes collagen to the flowing blood, and this site is said to be a strong stimulus for platelet accumulation [34]. The sudden change in volume of the plaque by discharge of plaque material into the lumen or from hemorrhage into the plaque via the rupture also creates alterations in flow patterns which favor platelet thrombosis [29]. Jørgensen et al. [25] suggested that the pathogenesis of coronary thrombi associated with ruptures of necrotic plaques is different from that unassociated with rupture. That coronary arterial thrombi are related to rupture of necrotic plaques, however, is far from a proved observation. Serial sections are usually necessary to observe cracks in plaques (Figure 12) and even by this means interpretation is often difficult. Cracks in plaques were infrequently observed beneath thrombi in the patients studied by us, and prob-

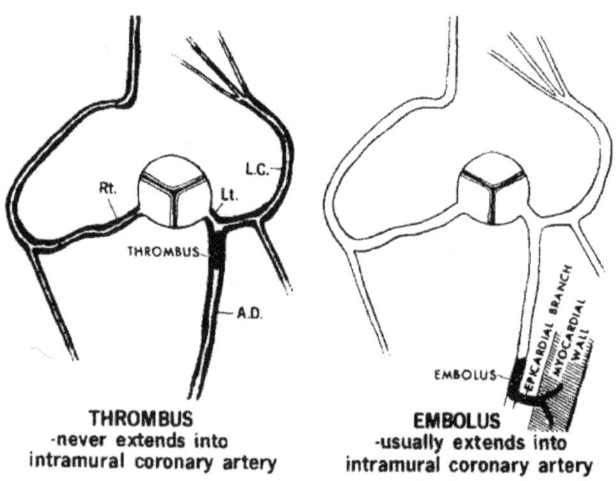

Figure 18. Diagram depicting differences between coronary arterial embolism and thrombosis. The thrombus is usually proximal and is superimposed on an old plaque. The thrombus does not extend into intramural coronary arteries. The embolus is distal and extends into intramural arteries. The embolus usually occurs in a coronary tree devoid of significant old atherosclerotic plaquing.

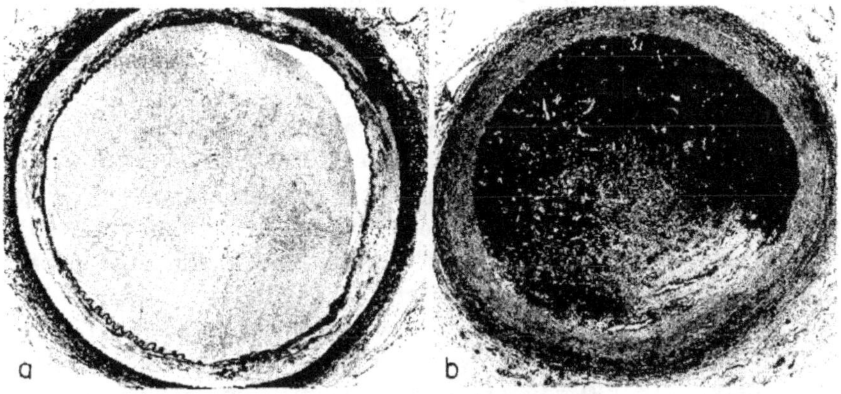

Figure 19. *Embolus to right coronary artery in a fifty-six year old man (A70-244). It occurred during cardiac catheterization thirty-one days before death and caused transmural necrosis of the posterior left ventricular wall. Note that the clot has formed in an artery which was previously free of atherosclerotic plaquing. The embolus is showing some evidence of organization distally (**b**). Elastic van Gieson stain, original magnification × 22 (**a**); hematoxylin and eosin stain, original magnification × 25 (**b**).*

ably most thrombi form over plaques with intact surfaces [35,36]. Rupture of a plaque may result at times from fixing and cutting an artery without providing prior support of its wall by injection. Fulton [36] injected coronary arteries with a solid supporting medium before sectioning, and in few the intima produced convexity of the lining. In none of his twenty-five patients who died of coronary heart disease (fourteen with AMI) was ulceration of a plaque observed. Interpretation of whether a plaque is cracked or if present, an artefact or real, is fraught with too much difficulty in our opinion to give this possible mechanism of thrombosis undue weight.

The thrombus in fatal AMI is practically always located in the coronary artery which supplies the infarcted myocardium; if the infarct involves the anterior wall of the left ventricle, and if a thrombus occurs, it will be located in the anterior descending coronary artery. Thrombi in either the left anterior descending or circumflex coronary artery generally are located within 2 cm of the bifurcation of the left main coronary artery (or within 4 cm of the left aortic ostium). The left main coronary artery is rarely the site of thrombosis. The proximal portion of the right coronary artery, in contrast, does not appear to be a more frequent site of thrombus formation than does the mid or distal portions. Thrombi are infrequently seen in the small epicardial branches of the major extramural coronary arteries and never occur, other than as platelet aggregates, in intramural coronary arteries.

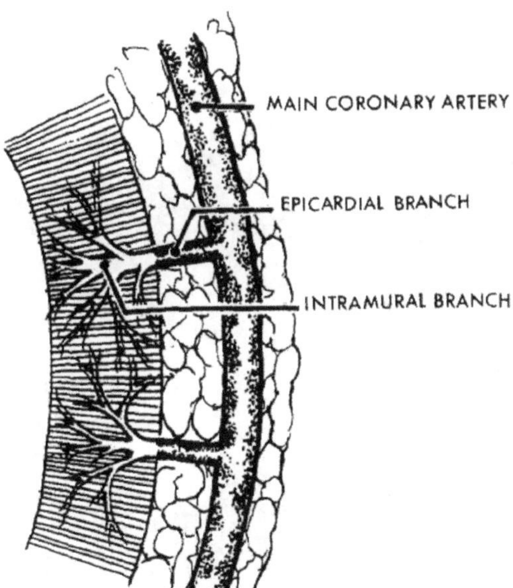

Figure 20. *Diagram of a major extramural coronary artery and its epicardial and intramural branches in atherosclerosis. The main artery and its epicardial branches are extensively involved by the atherosclerotic process but the intramural vessels are spared.*

Not all coronary arterial thrombi produce total luminal occlusion. (The term "occlusion" is not synonymous with "thrombosis" as implied in many reports, since occlusion may be partial as well as complete and since the vessel may be occluded by material other than that which forms a thrombus.) Partially occluding ("mural" or nonocclusive) thrombi were found in seven (18 per cent) and totally occluding (occlusive) thrombi in thirty-three (82 per cent) of our forty patients with thrombi and fatal transmural myocardial necrosis. Pure platelet thrombi, as mentioned earlier, are usually small and infrequently totally occlude lumens. Nonocclusive thrombi, since they are small, may have little functional significance. Even totally occluding thrombi when formed in arteries already more than 90 per cent occluded by old atherosclerotic plaques also may have little functional significance. Thus, it is not enough to know whether or not a coronary artery contains a thrombus. The degree of luminal narrowing by old atherosclerotic plaques at the site of, and distal to, the thrombus, and whether the thrombus is totally or only partially occlusive must also be known before the significance of a coronary arterial thrombus can be judged.

The role of coronary thrombosis in AMI is unclear. For several decades coronary thrombosis was considered the cause of AMI. Clinically, AMI represents a sudden change for the patient compared to his preinfarction status. This often dramatic clinical event has been equated at necropsy with the finding of a "fresh" thrombus in a coronary artery. But, only about 50 per cent of the patients with transmural myocardial necrosis and about 10 per cent of the patients with subendocardial necrosis or "sudden cardiovascular collapse without myocardial necrosis" have a thrombus in a coronary artery at necropsy. Thus, nothing new is found in the coronary arteries in the majority of patients who die of cardiac disease. The virtual absence of coronary arterial thrombi in patients who die suddenly of cardiac disease and their presence in only about half of those with myocardial necrosis has given rise to the concept that coronary arterial thrombi are consequences rather than causes of AMI. Comparison of histologic ages of coronary arterial thrombi and of acute myocardial infarcts has indicated to some observers [12] that thrombosis follows rather than precedes myocardial necrosis. Judging the age of a coronary thrombus, however, is difficult and probably inaccurate, and therefore this comparison is unreliable.

An examination of the clinical events during the period of myocardial infarction has provided a possible explanation for the occurrence of coronary arterial thrombi in some patients with AMI and their absence in others. Spain and Bradess [9,20] have shown that the frequency of finding coronary thrombi rises with increasing intervals between the onset of symptoms of myocardial ischemia and death. In their study in 1960 [9] the frequency rose from 16 per cent of 303 patients who survived for less than one hour to 37 per cent of sixty-five patients who survived from one to twenty-four hours, and to 54 per cent of 200 patients who survived for more than twenty-four hours; in their study in 1970 [20] of other patients the frequency rose from 17 per cent of eighty patients who survived for less than one hour to 36 per cent of twenty-two patients who survived from one to eight hours, and to 57 per cent of 100 patients who survived for more than eight hours. Thus, a certain but variable period of survival after the onset of infarction is usually necessary for a thrombus to form.

The presence of coronary arterial thrombi in AMI also has been found to correlate with the presence of the power failure syndrome—a form of shock resulting in "an inability of the myocardium to maintain the level of cardiac output necessary for adequate organ perfusion. There is evidence of underperfusion of one or more organ systems" [22]. In a clinicopathologic study of thirty-seven patients who died of AMI Walston and associates [22] found thrombi in seventeen (71

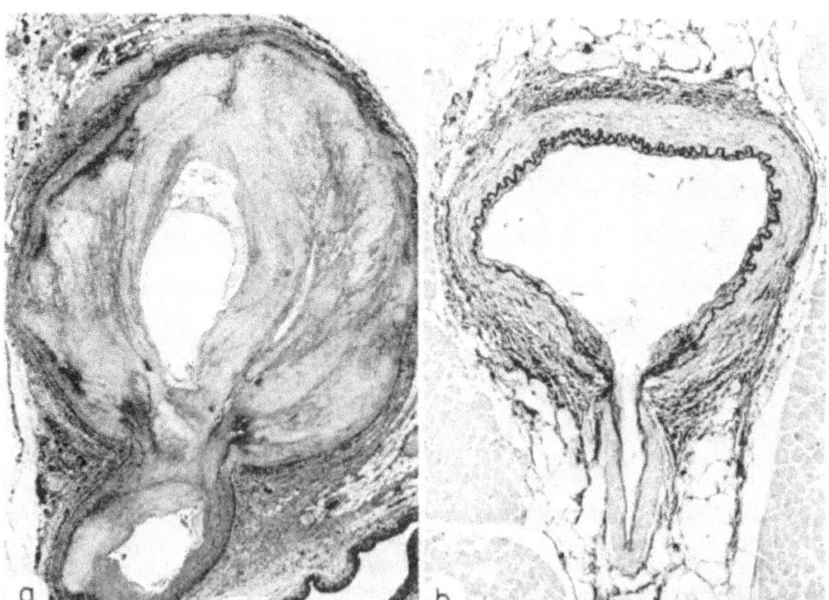

Figure 21. *Major coronary artery and its branches in atherosclerosis.* ***a,*** *left anterior descending artery and an epicardial branch from it are severely atherosclerotic in a fifty-four year old man (A70-116) in whom AMI developed eight hours before death. Movat stain, original magnification × 20.* ***b,*** *intramural coronary artery and one of its branches in a fifty-eight year old man (SH No. A4703) with known severe systemic hypertension and angina pectoris. He died three hours after the development of severe chest pain (sudden death). The lumens of the extramural right, left anterior descending, left circumflex and left main coronary arteries were all more than 75 per cent narrowed by old plaque. Despite the severe narrowing of the extramural coronary arteries, the intramural coronary arteries were normal, one of which is seen here. Elastic van Gieson stain, original magnification × 100.*

TABLE III Types of Activity at Onset of AMI*

Activity	Attacks	
	No.	%
Sleep	198	22†
Rest (lying or sitting)	277	31†
Mild activity	180	20†
Moderate activity (excludes walking)	76	9†
Walking	141	16†
Unusual or severe exertion	18	2†
Totals	890	100

* Adapted from Master, Dack, Jaffe, Amer Heart J 18:434, 1939 [38].

† The percentages for these six activities are very similar to those occurring in the daily lives of most subjects.

per cent) of twenty-four patients with and in only two (15 per cent) of thirteen patients without the power failure syndrome. Of their thirty-seven patients, nineteen had coronary arterial thrombi and seventeen (90 per cent) of these had the power failure syndrome; of their eighteen patients without coronary arterial thrombi, seven (39 per cent) had had the power failure syndrome. Thus a severely diminished cardiac output and consequently slowed coronary arterial blood flow are usually required for a thrombus to form in a coronary artery. It has also been observed at necropsy that the larger the area of myocardial necrosis, the more likely will a thrombus be present in a coronary artery. Of course, the larger the infarct, the more likely will pump failure occur [37].

The type activity experienced by patients at the time of onset of AMI also may reflect slowed blood flow. Master, Dack and Jaffe [38] interviewed 890 patients with AMI and found that symptoms of myocardial infarction appeared in 73 per cent of them during sleep, rest or mild activity (Table III). For myocardial necrosis to begin during inactivity is in direct contrast to angina pectoris, which appears during activity, but is associated with similar degrees of luminal narrowing of the coronary arteries [39–42]. It would appear that decreased coronary arterial blood flow, i.e., relative stasis, is necessary for thrombus to form in a coronary artery and that shock, congestive cardiac failure and inactivity all decrease coronary blood flow. The slow flow concept, however, does not explain the occurrence of coronary arterial thrombi at sites of, and proximal to, severe stenoses caused by old atherosclerotic plaques. Luminal narrowing, however, does introduce points of high velocity gradients which appear to favor platelet aggregation [43]. A high shearing stress also may damage erythrocytes [44], followed by release of adenosine diphosphate [45] and platelet damage.

Several explanations have been offered for the absence of coronary arterial thrombi in patients who die of AMI or of "acute cardiovascular collapse without myocardial necrosis." Lysis of thrombi before or after death as a result of excessive production of fibrinolysins has not been proved or disproved, although several observations tend to discount the role of postmortem lysis. In fatal AMI or sudden death the major coronary arteries in patients without thrombi are frequently free of blood or blood products. If fresh thrombi had been lysed immediately after death, partially liquefied blood or a remnant of thrombus within the lumen would be expected; this may not be the case. Necropsies performed within fifteen minutes on patients with coronary heart disease who died suddenly have not disclosed evidence of partially lysed thrombi [20]. It is unlikely that postmortem lysis of thrombi could be so selective as to liquefy only those thrombi which allegedly might have been present in patients with subendocardial necrosis and not those associated with transmural necrosis. It is unlikely that postmortem lysis, an artefact, which in a sense occurs by chance, could account for the occurrence of identical percentages of thrombi being present in separate but similar studies carried out a decade apart by the same investigators [9,20].

Inadequate examination of the coronary tree so that thrombi, although actually present, were not observed, is highly unlikely. At least two histologic sections of every 5 mm segment of the entire extramural coronary arterial tree were examined in this study of 107 patients. The chance of missing a thrombus by this technic is unlikely.

The absence of thrombi in coronary arteries of many patients with AMI may partially explain the lack of clear-cut benefits provided to patients with AMI treated with anticoagulants. After twenty years of using these drugs, controversy still continues as to whether or not they are beneficial to patients with AMI. Of factors favoring the use of anticoagulants in patients with AMI, the ability of these drugs to reduce the body's ability to form or extend a thrombus in a coronary artery has been high on the list. This factor, however, has been based on the supposition that AMI is usually caused by coronary thrombosis. The incidence of coronary arterial thrombi in patients with fatal

AMI treated with anticoagulants is similar to that in patients not receiving anticoagulants [25].

Although it may not be the precipitating cause of AMI, thrombosis may still play a major role in causing the underlying coronary atherosclerosis. Indeed, there is little doubt that organization of thrombi contributes to the development of the complicated atherosclerotic plaque. The presence of fibrin and platelets in atherosclerotic plaques strongly connects atherosclerosis with thrombosis. Each has been found in plaques by immunofluorescent technics [46,47], and fibrin is commonly found in plaques by histologic (Figure 13) and electron microscopic examination. Histologic evidence that a plaque is derived from thrombus, however, is frequently obscured [48]. As a thrombus is covered by new endothelium, the underlying endothelium is replaced by connective tissue from the intima with resultant obliteration of the original line of demarcation (Figure 14). Thrombi appear to organize by ingrowth of overlying endothelial cells and by connective tissue from the intima [49]. Modified smooth muscle cells [50–52], which are capable of synthesizing collagen, elastin and probably mucopolysaccharides [50,53], and which are present in connective tissue of arterial intima (they also may be derived from endothelium [50]), invade the bases of attached thrombi. Small mural thrombi organize by an avascular process [48,54] whereas larger thrombi become vascularized [55] (Figures 14–16). Capillaries extend from the new overlying endothelium to provide a direct blood supply from the lumen and from vasa vasora to penetrate thrombi at their bases [55,56]. Vascularization is considered the hallmark of an organized thrombus [55]. Capillaries growing into a thrombus have fibrinolytic activity [57] which contributes to resolution of a thrombus as it organizes. These capillaries, which may later atrophy, can be a source of hemorrhage into plaques. Occlusive thrombi, like mural thrombi, may be incorporated into the intima of arteries as atherosclerotic plaques [48]. Occlusive thrombi may retract before endothelioization is complete and thereby appear later as mural or nonocclusive plaques (Figure 14).

The source of lipids in atherosclerotic plaques is unclear. Fatty degeneration may occur in any thrombus or hematoma; organization of a left atrial thrombus in mitral stenosis, for example, may look identical to an atherosclerotic plaque (Figure 17). Platelets, erythrocytes and plasma all may provide lipids to plaques. When whole blood clots are injected into systemic veins of rabbits, fibrous intimal plaques (containing little lipid) form in pulmonary arteries [58]. Even though the emboli are occlusive they organize by retracting into eccentric plaques. The conversion of thromboemboli to plaques is important evidence for the thrombotic origin of atherosclerosis. When platelet-rich thrombi rather than whole blood clots are injected, typical fatty atherosclerotic plaques containing many foam cells and foci of calcium develop [59]. Erythrocytes contain less lipid than do platelets, but repeated small hemorrhages may lead to accumulation of large amounts of lipid, especially cholesterol [60]. The plasma supplies lipoproteins which are found in both recent and organizing thrombi [61] as well as in old plaques [62].

Atherosclerotic plaques are like fingerprints. No two are alike. In this study of the entire extramural coronary tree of 107 patients with fatal AMI, tremendous variation in the composition of adjacent plaques was noted. Some plaques contained lipid and large quantities of pultaceous debris, whereas others were composed primarily of fibrous tissue. Differences in composition of original thrombi may explain differences in composition of atherosclerotic plaques. Mixed white and red thrombi form plaques that contain some foam cells [63] but not in the quantity found in plaques derived from platelet-rich or white thrombi [59]. The type thrombus, whether mural (nonocclusive) or occlusive, also may affect the composition of a plaque. Occlusive platelet thrombi usually do not accumulate fibrin while undergoing transformation to fibrofatty plaques [59]. Mural platelet thrombi, in contrast, appear to be partially or totally replaced by fibrin before undergoing organization; consequently the plaques that form are mainly fibromuscular [64–66].

Hemorrhages into old atherosclerotic plaques are common, occurring in twenty-six (24 per cent) of our 107 patients. They probably are of little functional significance. In only one of our twenty-six patients with hemorrhages into plaques did the lumen of the artery appear to have been compromised by the extravasated blood. In contrast to thrombi in coronary arteries in fatal AMI, hemorrhages often occur in coronary arteries unrelated to the areas of necrosis, and they may occur in more than one artery or in multiple sites in the same artery. Hemorrhages appear to form from either breaks in the fibrous capsule covering a plaque or from rupture of a small vascular channel within a plaque. Each of these mechanisms is difficult to prove in the individual patient. Possibly small hemorrhages into old plaques occur chronically and have little to do with AMI. It is possible that some hemorrhages into old plaques may be produced artifactually during cutting and processing of coronary arteries for histologic study. A possible detrimental effect of hemorrhages into plaques is the occurrence of superimposed thrombi. This association, however, may not be as frequent as once supposed. The two may occur together, presumably when a crack in a plaque is the responsible mechanism. Fulton [36] and Jørgensen et al. [25] did not find an association between hemorrhages into plaques and coronary thrombosis, probably because the majority of thrombi were observed over plaques which consisted predominately of fibrous tissue [36]. The incidence of hemorrhages into plaques does not appear to be increased by the use of anticoagulants [25,36].

It is essential to recall that fatal AMI, indeed, nearly all symptomatic ischemic heart disease, is associated with diffuse and severe coronary arterial atherosclerosis. Examination of several thousand histologic sections of coronary arteries in these 107 patients with fatal AMI disclosed atherosclerotic plaquing in all but four sections (excluding those in the three patients with coronary embolism). The degree of luminal narrowing varied, but some plaquing was present on virtually every millimeter of major coronary artery. The lumen of at least one of the three major extramural coronary arteries was narrowed more than 75 per cent by old atherosclerotic plaques in 101 of our 107 patients, and three of the six without this degree of narrowing had coronary emboli. A coronary artery, however, may contain a considerable amount of atherosclerosis and yet be capable of transporting considerable quantities of blood to myocardium. When the degree of coronary narrowing decreases the original lumen by more than 75 per cent, the flow in the vessel is significantly decreased. In the carotid artery, a detectable reduction in flow and pressure does not occur until the degree of luminal narrowing is more than 80 per cent [67]. Among our 107 necropsy patients, the average number of major coronary arteries (three per patient; excludes the left main coronary artery) narrowed more than 75 per cent by old atherosclerotic plaques were: 2.4 in seventy-four patients with transmural necrosis; 2.3 in nine patients with only subendocardial necrosis; and 2.4 in twenty-four patients who died suddenly. Similar observations had been made by Saphir and associates [4], Blumgart et al. [39] and Yater et al. [68] who found "complete occlusions" of usually two major coronary arteries in patients who died with angina pectoris or of AMI. The degree of luminal narrowing of coronary arteries by old atherosclerotic plaques is identical in patients with fatal AMI who have coronary thrombi and in those without coronary thrombi [25].

The sites of maximum narrowing of major extramural coronary arteries are highly variable in a particular patient but certain patterns emerge when large groups of patients with fatal AMI are examined. The lumen of the left main coronary artery is rarely narrowed more than 75 per cent by old atherosclerotic plaques. Maximum narrowing of the left anterior descending and left circumflex coronary arteries is usually within 2 cm of the bifurcation of the left main. The proximal and mid-portions of the right coronary artery are not predisposed to greater degrees of luminal narrowing by old plaques than is the distal portion. The right coronary artery's main function is to supply the posterior wall of the left ventricle via its posterior descending branches. Thus, narrowing of the right coronary artery at any site promixal to the origins of the posterior descending branches might have similar functional significance. Or, in other words, the left coronary arterial tree begins supplying the left ventricle with oxygen about 2 cm from its origin from the aorta; the right coronary artery does not begin perfusing the left ventricle until it has travelled in the right atrioventricular sulcus for about 12 cm. Thus, severe narrowing of the right coronary artery 11 cm from its aortic ostium might be as significant a lesion as a similar narrowing 2 cm from its ostium. In contrast, severe narrowing of the left anterior descending coronary artery 11 cm downstream without significant proximal narrowing may have less myocardial consequences.

Atherosclerotic lesions generally have been classified into three types [69]: (1) yellow (fatty) streaks or dots, (2) fibrous plaques and (3) complicated plaques. The latter plaques contain calcific deposits, cholesterol clefts, thrombus or all three, and they may ulcerate (into the arterial lumen) or weaken the vessel wall so that it dilates. The atherosclerotic plaques observed in extramural coronary arteries in fatal AMI are of the complicated type. Significant degrees of luminal narrowing of the coronary arteries only by foam cell lesions do not occur with the possible exception of patients with type III hyperlipoproteinemia [70].

In most complicated plaques few foam cells are present, and the luminal narrowing is caused primarily by fibrous tissue, with or without calcific deposits, and pultaceous debris (presumably the end result of the breakdown of foam cells). Why calcific deposits are absent in coronary arteries of some patients with fatal AMI and extensive in others is unknown. Intimal calcific deposits in these vessels increase with age (more than 95 per cent of patients in the United States over eighty years of age have coronary arterial calcific deposits [71] and are more frequent and extensive in patients with systemic hypertension than in normotensive patients [71]. Patients with diabetes mellitus also appear to have larger and more extensive coronary calcific deposits than patients without diabetes.

The occurrence of a clot in the distal portion of a major extramural coronary artery suggests that the cause is embolism rather than thrombosis. This situation occurred in three of our 107 patients. Coronary arterial embolism differs from thrombosis in the following manner (Figure 18): (1) the clot is located distally, not proximally, and is usually in the anterior descending coronary artery; (2) the clot extends into intramural coronary arteries and into the epicardial branches of the major extramural vessel (in thrombosis, no clot is found in intramural coronary arteries and uncommonly in the small epicardial branches of major vessels); and (3) the entire extramural coronary arterial tree is relatively free of old atherosclerotic plaques. (It is difficult to make the diagnosis of embolism anatomically if the lumens of the coronary arteries are more than 50 per cent narrowed by old plaque.) Also, patients with emboli are usually relatively young and have certain predisposing conditions (arrhythmia, infective endocarditis, intracardiac mural thrombosis, etc.) [72–76].

Much has been written about disease of the small coronary arteries. That intramural coronary arteries are narrowed in certain conditions, particularly the neurogenic heart diseases (Friedrich's ataxia, progressive muscular dystrophy, myotonic dystrophy), is now a well established fact [77]. Conditions involving extramural coronary arteries, in our view, have not been shown also to involve the intramural coronary arteries. There are dissenting views, however, on this point [78–81]. Likewise, conditions which clearly involve intramural coronary arteries tend to spare the extramural coronary arteries. With the exception of the small arteries in the left ventricular papillary muscles, which are subjected to maximal systolic intraventricular pressure over the entire circumference of their surfaces, diseases which affect the intramural coronary arteries do not affect the extramural coronary arteries and vice versa. Other than insignificant minimal fibrous intimal proliferation in a rare intramural coronary artery, and that usually in the left ventricular papillary muscles, no abnormality was observed in the intramural coronary arteries in any of our 107 patients. Indeed, the intramural vessels in the heart appear to be protected from intimal proliferation and luminal narrowing by the contracting adjacent myocardium. In coronary atherosclerosis, plaques occur routinely in epicardial branches of major extramural arteries, but as soon as these branches penetrate myocardium, the lumen is suddenly wide open again (Figures 20 and 21). Even in systemic hypertension, the intramural coronary arteries are not affected as are other small systemic arteries in this condition. The coronary arteries are not exposed to the high systolic pressure because they are perfused mainly in diastole. The contracting ventricular myocardium may further lower the intraluminal pressure in these small vessels. Although patients with diabetes mellitus have been reported to have disease of intramural coronary arteries [79], this finding has not been observed by us. Foam cells, cholesterol clefts and pultaceous debris, components of plaques in extramural coronary arteries, are virtually never found in intramural vessels. Thus, significant involvement of intramural coronary arteries does not occur in patients with significant luminal narrowing of extramural coronary arteries.

ACKNOWLEDGMENT

We sincerely thank Dr. Abner Golden, Professor and Chairman, Department of Pathology, Georgetown University, Washington, D.C., Dr. Joseph O'Connell, Pathologist, Suburban Hospital, Bethesda, Maryland, and Dr. Michael Cuadra, Chief of Pathology, District of Columbia General Hospital, Washington, D.C. who allowed us to study the hearts of many patients who had died of acute ischemic heart disease at their respective hospitals. Also, we thank Mrs. Sandra Lewis, Mrs. Louise Holthaus, and Miss Margaret Burk, Section of Pathology, National Heart and Lung Institute, for the several thousand beautifully prepared histologic sections of coronary arteries examined in this study. The photomicrographs were taken by Mr. Walter G. P. Seewald and Mr. Robert W. Nye.

REFERENCES

1. Fortuin NJ, Roberts WC: Congenital atresia of the left main coronary artery. Amer J Med 50: 385, 1971.
2. Barnes AR, Ball RG: The incidence and situation of myocardial infarction in one thousand consecutive postmortem examinations. Amer J Med Sci 183: 215, 1932.
3. Lisa JR, Ring A: Myocardial infarction or gross fibrosis: analysis of 100 necropsies. Arch Intern Med (Chicago) 50: 131, 1932.
4. Saphir O, Priest WS, Hamburger WW, Katz LN: Coronary arteriosclerosis, coronary thrombosis and the resulting myocardial changes. An evaluation of their respective clinical pictures including the electrocardiographic records, based on the anatomical findings. Amer Heart J 10: 567, 1935.
5. Friedberg CK, Horn H: Acute myocardial infarction not due to coronary artery occlusion. JAMA 112: 1675, 1939.
6. Foord AG: Embolism and thrombosis in coronary heart disease. JAMA 138: 1009, 1948.
7. Miller RD, Burchell HB, Edwards JE: Myocardial infarction with and without acute coronary occlusion. A pathologic study. Arch Intern Med (Chicago) 88: 597, 1951.
8. Branwood AW, Montgomery GL: Observations on the morbid anatomy of coronary artery disease. Scot Med J 1: 367, 1956.
9. Spain DM, Bradess VA: The relationship of coronary thrombosis to coronary atherosclerosis and ischemic heart disease. (A necropsy study covering a period of 25 years.) Amer J Med Sci 240: 701, 1960.
10. Kurland GS, Weingarten C, Pitt B: The relation between the location of coronary occlusions and the occurrence of shock in acute myocardial infarction. Circulation 31: 646, 1965.
11. Meadows R: Coronary thrombosis and myocardial infarction. Med J Aust 2: 409, 1965.
12. Ehrlich JC, Shinohara Y: Low incidence of coronary thrombosis in myocardial infarction. A restudy by serial block technique. Arch Path 78: 432, 1964.
13. Mitchell JRA, Schwartz CJ: Arterial Disease, Philadelphia, F.A. Davis, 1965.
14. Baroldi G: Acute coronary occlusion as a cause of myocardial infarct and sudden coronary heart death. Amer J Cardiol 16: 859, 1965.
15. Harland WA, Holburn AM: Coronary thrombosis and myocardial infarction. Lancet 2: 1158, 1966.
16. Kagan A, Livsic AM, Sternby N, Vihert AM: Coronary-artery thrombosis and the acute attack of coronary heart-disease. Lancet 2: 1199, 1968.
17. Chapman I: Relationships of recent coronary artery occlusion and acute myocardial infarction. J Mount Sinai Hosp 35: 149, 1968.
18. Jørgensen L, Hoerem JW, Chandler AB, Borchgrevink CF: The pathology of acute coronary death. Acta Anaesth Scand 29 (suppl): 193, 1968.
19. Hackel DB, Estes EH, Walston A, Koff S, Day E: Some problems concerning coronary artery occlusion and acute myocardial infarction. Circulation 39,40 (suppl): IV-31, 1969.
20. Spain DM, Bradess VA: Sudden death from coronary heart disease. Survival time, frequency of thrombi, and cigarette smoking. Chest 58: 107, 1970.
21. Bouch DC, Montgomery GL: Cardiac lesions in fatal cases of recent myocardial ischemia from a coronary care unit. Brit Heart J 32: 795, 1970.
22. Walston A, Hackel DB, Estes EH: Acute coronary occlusion and the "power failure" syndrome. Amer Heart J 79: 613, 1970.
23. Edwards JE: What is myocardial infarction? Circulation 39,40 (suppl): IV-5, 1969.
24. Jørgensen L: Experimental platelet and coagulation thrombi. A histological study of arterial and venous thrombi of varying age in untreated and heparinized rabbits. Acta Path Microbiol Scand 62: 189, 1964.
25. Jørgensen L, Chandler AB, Borchgrevink CF: Acute lesions of coronary arteries in anticoagulant-treated and in untreated patients. Atherosclerosis 13: 21, 1971.
26. Leary T: Coronary spasm as a possible factor in producing sudden death. Amer Heart J 10: 338, 1935.
27. Clark E, Graef I, Chasis H: Thrombosis of the aorta and coronary arteries with special reference to the "fibrinoid" lesions. Arch Path 22: 183, 1936.
28. Osborn GR: The Incubation Period of Coronary Thrombosis, London, Butterworth & Co., Ltd., 1963.
29. Chapman I: Morphogenesis of occluding coronary artery thrombosis. Arch Path 80: 256, 1965.
30. Constantinides P: Plaque fissures in human coronary thrombosis. J Atheroscler Res 6: 1, 1966.
31. Friedman M, Van den Boverkamp GJ: The pathogenesis of a coronary thrombus. Amer J Path 48: 19, 1966.
32. Jørgensen L: Thrombosis and the complications of atherosclerosis, Atherosclerosis, Proceedings of the Second International Symposium (Jones RJ, ed), New York, Springer-Verlag, 1970, p 94.
33. Friedman M: The coronary thrombus. Its origin and fate. Human Path 2: 81, 1971.
34. Hovig T, Jørgensen L, Packham MA, Mustard JF: Platelet adherence to fibrin and collagen. J Lab Clin Med 71: 29, 1968.
35. Anitschkow N: Morphodynamik der Koronarsklerose des Herzens. Acta Path Microbiol Scand 49: 426, 1960.
36. Fulton WFM: The Coronary Arteries. Arteriography, Microanatomy, and Pathogenesis of Obliterative Coronary Artery Disease, Springfield, Ill., Charles C Thomas, 1965.
37. Page DL, Caulfield JB, Kastor JA, DeSanctis RW, Sanders CA: Myocardial changes associated with cardiogenic shock. New Eng J Med 285: 133, 1971.
38. Master AM, Dack S, Jaffe HL: Activities associated with the onset of acute coronary artery occlusion. Amer Heart J 18: 434, 1939.
39. Blumgart HL, Schlesinger MJ, Davis D: Studies on the relation of the clinical manifestations of angina pectoris, coronary thrombosis, and myocardial infarction to the pathologic findings with particular reference to the significance of the collateral circulation. Amer Heart J 19: 1, 1940.
40. Zoll PM, Wessler S, Blumgart HL: Angina pectoris. A clinical and pathologic correlation. Amer J Med 11: 331, 1951.
41. Lenegre J, Himbert J: Critical study of the relationship between angina pectoris and coronary atherosclerosis. Amer Heart J 58: 539, 1959.

42. Allison RB, Rodriguez FL, Higgins EA Jr, Leddy JP, Abelman WH, Ellis LB, Robbins SL: Clinicopathologic correlations in coronary atherosclerosis. Four hundred thirty patients studied with postmortem coronary angiography. Circulation 27: 170, 1963.
43. Dintenfass L, Rozenberg MC: The influence of the velocity gradient on *in vitro* blood coagulation and artificial thrombosis. J Atheroscler Res 5: 276, 1965.
44. Nevaril CG, Lynch EC, Alfrey CP Jr, Hellums JD: Erythrocyte damage and destruction induced by shearing stress. J Lab Clin Med 71: 784, 1968.
45. Harrison MJG, Mitchell JRA: The influence of red blood cells on platelet adhesiveness. Lancet 2: 1163, 1966.
46. Woolf N, Crawford T: Fatty streaks in the aortic intima studied by an immuno-histochemical technique. J Path Bact 80:405, 1960.
47. Woolf N, Carstairs KC: Infiltration and thrombosis in atherosclerosis. A study using immunofluorescent techniques. Amer J Path 51: 373, 1967.
48. Duguid JB: Thrombosis as a factor in the pathogenesis of coronary atherosclerosis. J Path Bact 58: 207, 1946.
49. Crawford T, Levene CI: Incorporation of fibrin in the aortic intima. J Path Bact 64: 523, 1952.
50. Haust DM, More RH, Movat HZ: The role of smooth muscle cells in the fibrogenesis of arteriosclerosis. Amer J Path 37: 377, 1960.
51. Geer JC, McGill HC Jr, Strong JP: The fine structure of the human atherosclerotic lesions. Amer J Path 31: 263, 1961.
52. Wissler RW: The arterial medial cell, smooth muscle or multifunctional mesenchyme? J Atheroscler Res 8: 201, 1968.
53. Getz GS, Vesselinovitch D, Wissler RW: A dynamic pathology of atherosclerosis. Amer J Med 46: 657, 1969.
54. Haust MD, More RH, Movat HZ: The mechanism of fibrosis in arteriosclerosis. Amer J Path 35: 265, 1959.
55. Geiringer E: Intimal vascularization and atherosclerosis. J Path Bact 63: 201, 1951.
56. Morgan AD: The Pathogenesis of Coronary Occlusion, Springfield, Ill., Charles C Thomas, 1956.
57. Todd AS: Localization of fibrinolytic activity in tissues. Brit Med Bull 20: 210, 1964.
58. Harrison CV: Experimental pulmonary atherosclerosis. J Path Bact 60: 289, 1948.
59. Hand RA, Chandler AB: Atherosclerotic metamorphosis of autologous pulmonary thromboemboli in the rabbit. Amer J Path 40: 469, 1962.
60. Hartroft WS: Ceroid-like pigments, hemoceroid and hyaloceroid, in atheromatous lesions of human subjects. Amer J Path 28: 526, 1952.
61. Woolf N, Pilkington TRE, Carstairs KC: The occurrence of lipoproteins in thrombi. J Path Bact 91: 383, 1966.
62. Kao VCY, Wissler RW: A study of the immunohistochemical localization of serum lipoproteins and other plasma proteins in human atherosclerotic lesions. Exp Molec Path 4: 457, 1965.
63. Filshie I, Scott GBD: The organization of experimental venous thrombi. J Path Bact 76: 71, 1958.
64. Jørgensen L, Rowsell HC, Hovig T, Mustard JF: Resolution and organization of platelet-rich mural thrombi in carotid arteries of swine. Amer J Path 51: 681, 1967.
65. Woolf N, Bradley JWP, Crawford T, Carstairs KC: Experimental mural thrombi in the pig aorta. The early natural history. Brit J Exp Path 49: 257, 1968.
66. Woolf N, Carstairs KC: The survival time of platelets in experimental mural thrombi. J Path 97: 595, 1969.
67. Brice JG, Dowsett DJ, Lowe RD: The effect of constriction on carotid bloodflow and pressure gradient. Lancet 1:84, 1964.
68. Yater WM, Traum AH, Brown WG, Fitzgerald RP, Geisler MA, Wilcox BB: Coronary artery disease in men eighteen to thirty-nine years of age. Report of eight hundred sixty-six cases; four hundred fifty with necropsy examination. Amer Heart J 36: 334; 481; 683, 1948.
69. Classification of atherosclerotic lesions. Report of a study group. WHO Techn Rep Ser (No. 143), 1958.
70. Roberts WC, Levy RI, Fredrickson DS: Hyperlipoproteinemia. A review of the five types with first report of necropsy findings in type 3. Arch Path 90: 46, 1970.
71. Frink RJ, Achor RWP, Brown AL Jr, Kincaid OW, Brandenburg RO: Significance of calcification of the coronary arteries. Amer J Cardiol 26: 241, 1970.
72. Saphir O: Coronary embolism. Amer Heart J 8: 312, 1933.
73. Hamman L: Coronary embolism. Amer J Med 21: 401, 1941.
74. Shrader EL, Bawell MB, Moragues V: Coronary embolism. Circulation 14: 1159, 1956.
75. Wenger NK, Bauer S: Coronary embolism. Review of the literature and report of fifteen cases. Amer J Med 25: 549, 1958.
76. Oakley C, Yusuf R, Hollman A: Coronary embolism and angina in mitral stenosis. Brit Heart J 23: 357, 1961.
77. James TN: Etiologic concept concerning the obscure myocardiopathies. Progr Cardiovasc Dis 7: 43, 1964.
78. Saphir O, Ohringer L, Wong R: Changes in the intramural coronary branches in coronary arteriosclerosis. Arch Path 62: 159, 1956.
79. Blumenthal HT, Alex M, Goldenberg S: A study of lesions of the intramural coronary artery branches in diabetes mellitus. Arch Path 70: 13, 1960.
80. Donomae I, Matsumoto Y, Kokubu T, Koide R, Kobayashi R, Ikegami H, Ueda E, Fujisawa T, Fujimoto S: Pathological studies of coronary atherosclerosis: especially of sclerosis of intramuscular coronary arteries. Jap Heart J 3: 423, 1962.
81. More BM, Sommers SC: The status of the myocardial arterioles in angina pectoris. Amer Heart J 64: 323, 1962.

Right-Sided Valvular Infective Endocarditis

A Clinicopathologic Study of Twelve Necropsy Patients

WILLIAM C. ROBERTS, M.D.
NEIL A BUCHBINDER, M.D.
Bethesda, Maryland

Clinical and necropsy features are described in twelve patients with infective endocarditis involving right-sided cardiac valves. In six patients infective endocarditis was limited to the tricuspid valve; in the other six vegetations also were present on one left-sided cardiac valve, but in only one of them was the infective endocarditis definitely primary on the left side of the heart. The tricuspid valve was the site of infective endocarditis in eleven patients and the pulmonic valve in one. The organisms responsible for the infective endocarditis were Staphylococcus aureus in six patients, Diplococcus pneumoniae in four, alpha Streptococcus in one and Aspergillus flavus in one. Five patients were alcoholics, four were heroin addicts, two had blood dyscrasias, and one had congenital cardiac disease (ventricular septal defect). The infective endocarditis in each of the nine patients with alcoholism or heroin addiction and in the one with congenital heart disease was primary in the heart; in the remaining two patients, it was secondary to generalized infection affecting many body organs.

Acute pneumonia was a dominant clinical feature in ten of the twelve patients and appeared to be secondary to dislodgment of material from the right-sided cardiac vegetations. Six patients also had acute meningitis. Although the vegetations caused considerable damage to the right-sided cardiac valves, evidence of cardiac dysfunction was either absent or attributable to acute cor pulmonale secondary to the acute pneumonia. Attention is called to the common tetrad of chronic alcoholism, acute pneumonia, acute meningitis and infective endocarditis. In nine of the twelve patients the right-sided vegetations did not extend to involve the basal attachments of the leaflets to the annuli. Thus, in these nine patients total excision of the valve leaflets would have eradicated their valvular endocarditis.

With the striking increase in heroin addiction in recent years, right-sided infective endocarditis has received considerable attention. Emphasis has been placed on the clinical features of right-sided infective endocarditis, and little attention has been given to the morphologic findings in infective endocarditis involving the tricuspid or pulmonic valves. We attempt to fill in this void by describing cardiac necropsy observations and relating them to clinical findings in twelve fatal cases of infective endocarditis involving right-sided cardiac valves.

From the Section of Pathology, National Heart and Lung Institute, National Institutes of Health, Bethesda, Maryland 20014. Requests for reprints should be addressed to Dr. William C. Roberts, Section of Pathology, National Heart and Lung Institute, Bethesda, Maryland 20014. Manuscript received November 4, 1971; revised January 18, 1972

TABLE I Clinical and Necropsy Data in Twelve Patients with Right-Sided Infective Endocarditis (IE)

Case	Age (yr) and Sex	Valve(s) Involved	Causative Organism	Predisposing Factor	Acute Pneumonia	Acute Meningitis	Systolic Precordial Murmur and Intensity (0–6)	Diagnosis of IE During Life	Valve Dysfunction	Heart Failure: Right-sided	Heart Failure: Left-sided
1	64,M	TV	Staph. aureus*	Lymphoma	0	0	0	0	0	0	0
2	31,F	TV	Staph. aureus	H	+	0	+ (3/6)	+	TR	+	0
3	65,M	TV	D. pneumoniae	A	+	+	+ (3/6)	+	TR	+	0
4	33,M	TV	Staph. aureus	H	+	0	0	0	0	0	0
5	35,F	TV	Staph. aureus	H	+	+	+ (2/6)	0	?TS	+	0
6	22,F	TV	Staph. aureus	H	+	0	+ (2/6)	+	TR	+	0
7	62,M	AV,TV	D. pneumoniae	A	0	+	+ (2/6)	0	0	0	0
8	10 mo,M	MV,TV	A. flavus*	Thymic dysplasia‖	+	0	0	0	0	0	0
9	55,M	MV,PV	Staph. aureus	A	+	0	+ (1/6)	0	PR	0	0
10	58,M	AV,MV,TV	D. pneumoniae	A	+	+	+ (3/6)¶	0	AR	+	+
11	55,M	AV,TV	D.pneumoniae	A	+	+	+ (3/6)¶	+	TR,AR	+	+
12	5,F	AV,MV,TV	Strep. viridans	0	+	0	+ (5/6)¶	+	AR	+	+

NOTE: A = alcoholism; AR = aortic regurgitation; AV = aortic valve; CA = coronary artery; CHF = congestive heart failure; GN = glomerulonephritis; H = heroin addiction; IE = infective endocarditis; MV = mitral valve; PR = pulmonic regurgitation; PV = pulmonic valve; TR = tricuspid regurgitation; TS = tricuspid stenosis; TV = tricuspid valve.

* IE secondary to generalized sepsis.

† Represent minimum duration.

PATIENTS STUDIED

Among fifty-seven patients with fatal active valvular infective endocarditis studied at necropsy by us, forty-five had vegetations limited to the left side of the heart [1], and twelve had vegetations involving one right-sided cardiac valve. Certain clinical and necropsy observations in the latter twelve patients are summarized in Table I. Their ages ranged from ten months to sixty-five years; eight were male, and four were female. In six, vegetations were confined to the tricuspid valve; in the other six, vegetations involved one left-sided cardiac valve in addition to the tricuspid (five patients) or pulmonic valve (one patient). Blood cultures, obtained in eleven patients, were positive in each: Staph. aureus in six, D. pneumoniae in three, alpha Streptococcus in one and Aspergillus flavus in one. Culture of cerebrospinal fluid in the twelfth patient yielded D. pneumoniae, and histologic study of his vegetations at necropsy showed gram-positive diplococci. Nine patients were either alcoholics (five patients) or heroin addicts (4 patients), two others had altered defense mechanisms (Hodgkin's disease in one and thymic dysplasia in one) and one had congenital cardiac disease (ventricular septal defect). Four of the five alcoholics had pneumococcal endocarditis, and all four heroin addicts had staphylococcal endocarditis. The infective endocarditis in each of the nine patients with alcoholism or heroin addiction and in the patient with congenital heart disease was primary in the heart; in the remaining two patients (Cases 1 and 8), the infective endocarditis appeared secondary to generalized infection affecting many body organs.

The clinical features in all twelve patients were dominated by symptoms clearly attributable to extracardiac foci of infection. In eleven of the twelve patients, either acute pneumonia (six patients), acute meningitis (two patients) or both (four patients) were the major initial presentations and remained the dominant clinical feature in ten. Although evidence of congestive cardiac failure (cardiomegaly, distended neck veins, hepatomegaly or ventricular gallop sounds) developed in seven patients, in four the "failure" could be attributed to acute cor pulmonale from the acute pneumonia; each of the other three patients (Cases 10, 11 and 12) had both right- and left-sided congestive cardiac failure secondary to endocarditis, causing regurgitation of one left-sided cardiac valve in two patients and a left ventricular-right atrial shunt in one (Case 11).

Precordial murmurs were heard in nine of the twelve patients. All nine had systolic murmurs, and three of them (Cases 10, 11 and 12) had diastolic murmurs (from destruction of aortic valves by infection). Four of six patients with endocarditis limited to the tricuspid valve had systolic murmurs, but in only one did the murmur get louder with inspiration. In one patient (Case 11) whose membranous ventricular septum was ruptured by the infective process, a continuous precordial murmur developed several days before his death, and clinically a diagnosis of acquired ventricular septal defect was made. All twelve patients had fever (oral temperature more than 100°F). The spleen was palpated in three patients, fundal hemorrhages were observed in two, and one had dermal petechiae. The diagnosis of infective endocarditis was made during life in only three of the six patients with isolated tricuspid valve endocarditis and in only two of six with

Duration of IE (days)	Principal Causes of Death	Heart Weight (gm)	Ruptured TV Chordae Tendineae	Bacteria in TV or PV	Papillary Muscle Necrosis	Myocarditis: Abscess	Myocarditis: Non-suppurating	Renal Abnormalities	Spleen Weight (gm)
56†	Generalized infection	325	0	+	0	+	0	GN	960‡
35	Renal failure	340	+	+	0	0	0	GN	300
112	Meningitis	450§	+	0	0	0	0	Healed infarcts	350
28	Pneumonia	260	+	+	0	0	0	GN	350
	Meningitis	290	+	+	0	0	0	GN	400
49	Pneumonia	340	+	+	0	0	0	Chronic pyelonephritis	180
35	Meningitis	230	0	0	0	0	0	0	...
42	Generalized infection	40	0	+	+	+	+	Abscesses	35‡
4	Pneumonia + renal failure	410	0	0	+	+	+	Abscesses	200
2	CHF	300	0	+	0	0	0	GN	100
21	CHF	420	+	0	0	0	+	0	...#
120	CHF	150	0	0	+	0	0	Septic infarcts	120

‡ Spleen palpated clinically.
§ Patient had systemic hypertension.
‖ Agammaglobulinemia and lymphocytopenia.
¶ Diastolic murmur of aortic regurgitation present also.
\# Operatively excised in distant past.

combined right- and left-sided endocarditis. Eleven patients received antibiotics: eight received a drug appropriate for the causative organism, three a questionably appropriate antibiotic and one an inappropriate drug

All valves were functionally normal before they became the sites of active infective endocarditis. Infective endocarditis caused valve dysfunction in seven patients regurgitation in six (tricuspid valve three, aortic valve three) and possible tricuspid stenosis in one Each of these seven patients had right- (four patients) or left-sided (three patients) cardiac failure. Congestive heart failure was the principal cause of death, however, in only three patients, and each of them had aortic regurgitation. In the remaining nine patients in whom congestive cardiac failure was either not present (five patients) or of secondary importance (four patients), the principal cause of death was related to extracardiac abnormalities: acute pneumonia, acute meningitis, generalized infection, renal failure or combinations of these. Acute pneumonia was the most common factor, occurring in ten of the twelve patients, and the two without pneumonia had either single or small flat tricuspid valve vegetations.

NECROPSY FINDINGS

Certain necropsy findings are summarized in Table I and illustrated in Figures 1 through 12. Vegetations were present on twenty of the forty-eight cardiac valves of the twelve patients. The tricuspid valve was involved in eleven, pulmonic valve in one, mitral valve in four and aortic valve in four. With the exception of the aortic valve in one patient (Case 12) each of the twenty valves containing vegetations appeared to be anatomically normal at sites not involved by the infection. The aortic valve in this patient (Case 12), who also had a small ventricular septal defect, consisted of three distinctly unequal sized cusps, but none was thickened, and the valve almost certainly functioned normally before it became infected. Thus, the infective endocarditis in eleven of the twelve patients involved previously anatomically normal valves.

Of the eleven patients with infective endocarditis involving the tricuspid valve vegetations were present on twenty-four of the thirty-three tricuspid valve leaflets; five patients had vegetations on all three leaflets, three on two leaflets and three on only one leaflet. Each of the three patients with only one tricuspid valve leaflet involved also had infective endocarditis involving one or both left-sided cardiac valves. Six of the eight patients with vegetations on two or more tricuspid valve cusps had infective endocarditis limited to the right side of the heart; the seventh patient (Case 11) had left-sided involvement only because of extension of the tricuspid valve infection through the membranous ventricular septum to the base of one aortic valve cusp; the eighth patient had vegetations on all three tricuspid valve cusps and only a minute vegetation on one of the three aortic valve cusps. In the latter patient, therefore, the left-sided infection is considered secondary to the

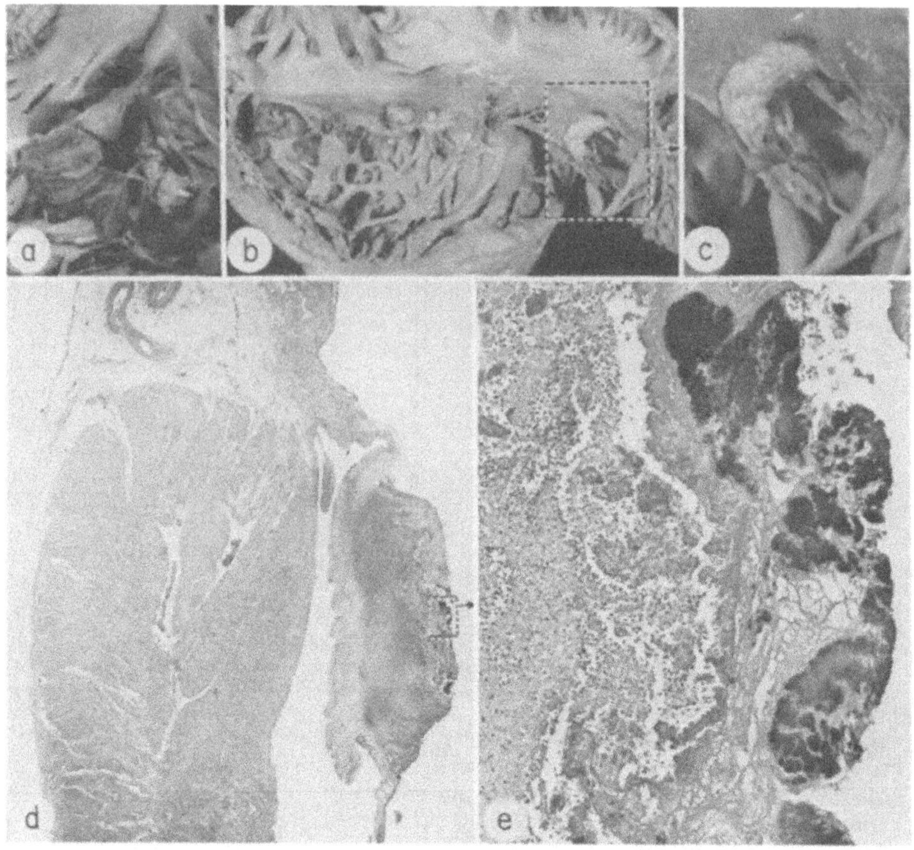

Figure 1. Case 2. Staphylococcus aureus endocarditis of tricuspid valve in a thirty-one year old female heroin addict (A67-257). Acute pneumonia developed, probably from septic emboli, about thirty-five days before death. Pulmonary abscesses were seen on the chest roentgenogram when she was hospitalized thirteen days before death. A grade 3/6 blowing precordial systolic murmur was audible and the liver was pulsatile. She died of congestive heart failure and renal failure. "Focal embolic" glomerulonephritis was found at necropsy. **a,** tricuspid valve viewed from right ventricle showing vegetations on each leaflet. **b,** opened right heart showing vegetations on each tricuspid valve cusp. **c,** close-up of bracketed area in **b** showing several ruptured chordae tendineae. **d,** photomicrograph of section through right atrium, right ventricle and tricuspid valve leaflet. Hematoxylin and eosin stain; original magnification × 5, reduced by 28 per cent. **e,** high power view of bracketed area in **d.** Vegetation consists of numerous polymorphonuclear leukocytes enmeshed in a fibrin network. Darkly stained areas are colonies of gram-positive cocci. Hematoxylin and eosin stain; original magnification × 108, reduced by 28 per cent.

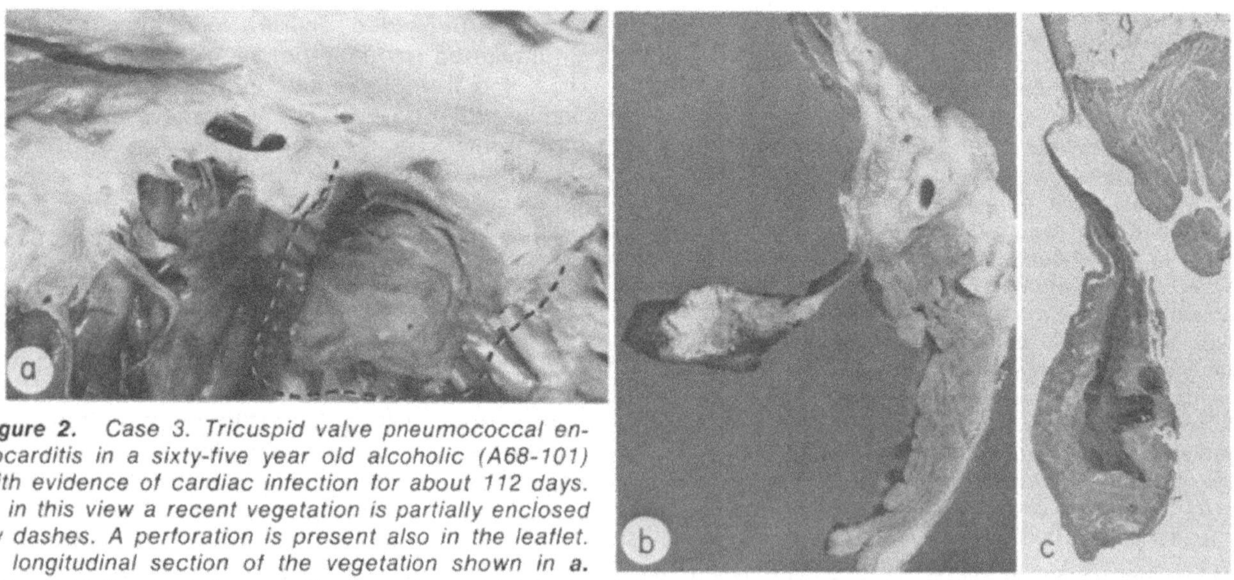

Figure 2. Case 3. Tricuspid valve pneumococcal endocarditis in a sixty-five year old alcoholic (A68-101) with evidence of cardiac infection for about 112 days. **a,** in this view a recent vegetation is partially enclosed by dashes. A perforation is present also in the leaflet. **b,** longitudinal section of the vegetation shown in **a.** The vegetation contains calcific deposits. **c,** histologic section of vegetation which contained fibrin and inflammatory cells but no stainable organisms. Elastic van Gieson stain; original magnification × 3, reduced by 25 per cent.

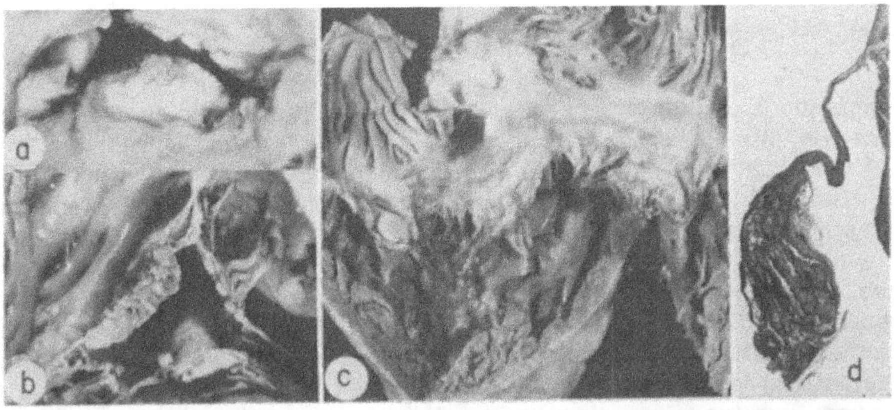

Figure 3. Case 4. Staphylococcus aureus endocarditis of tricuspid valve (A70-140). **a,** tricuspid valve viewed from right atrium. **b,** same valve viewed from right ventricle. **c,** view of opened right atrium, tricuspid valve and right ventricle. **d,** histologic section of vegetation which involves the distal half of the anterior tricuspid leaflet. Movat stain; original magnification × 4, reduced by 30 per cent.

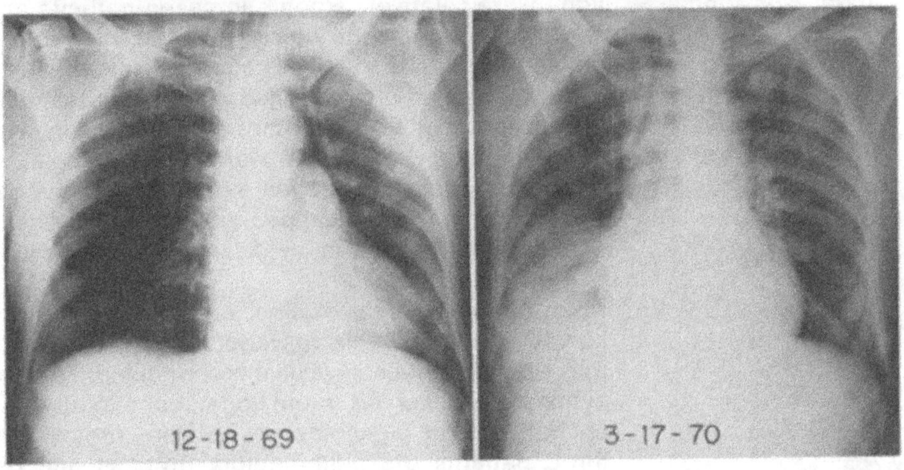

Figure 4. Case 5. Chest roentgenograms taken on dates shown (A70-87). Patient died of pulmonary infection on March 17, 1970.

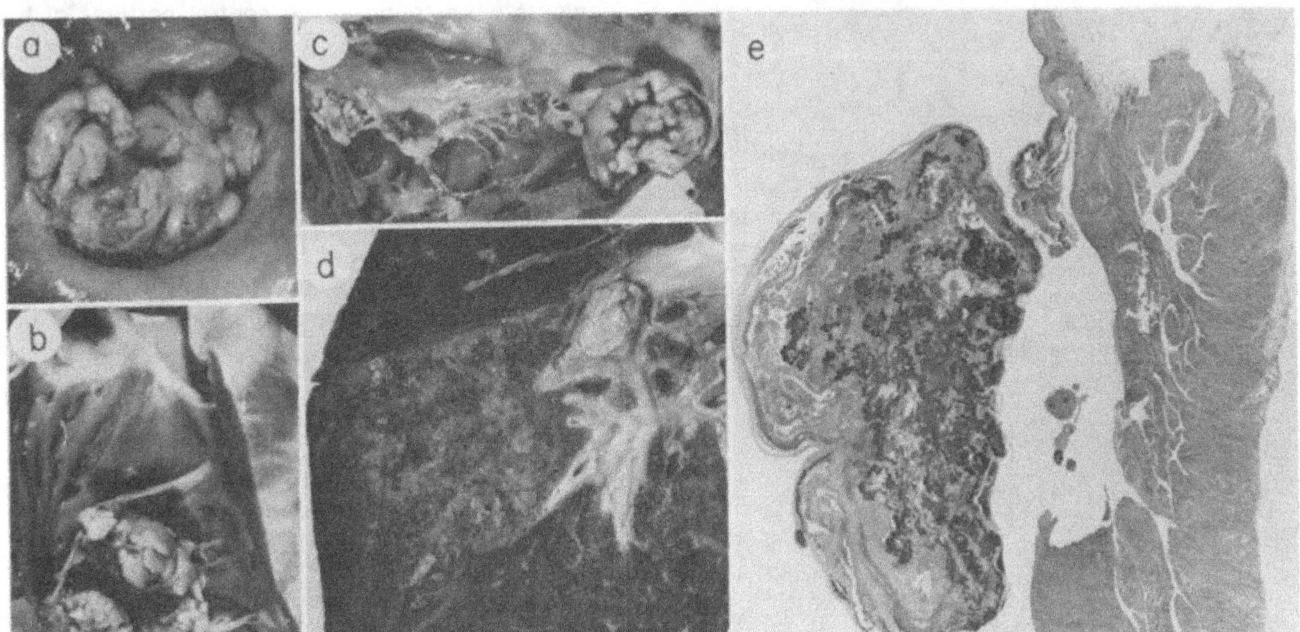

Figure 5. Case 5. Staphylococcus aureus endocarditis of tricuspid valve in a thirty-five year old female heroin addict whose chest roentgenograms are shown in Figure 4. She had been well until about one week before death when "acute pneumonia" developed. About three days before death, she suffered from headache and stiff neck. When hospitalized several hours before death, in addition to evidence of acute pneumonia, probably from septic emboli, and acute meningitis, she had a grade 2/6 precordial systolic murmur, which increased with inspiration, and a pulsatile liver. **a,** tricuspid valve viewed from right atrium. The orifice appears to be narrowed by the vegetation. **b,** tricuspid valve viewed from right ventricle. **c,** view of opened tricuspid valve. **d,** section of right lung showing infarct caused by septic embolus in right pulmonary artery. **e,** photomicrograph of portion of tricuspid valve vegetation. Dark staining areas in the leaflet represent gram-positive cocci. The surface of the vegetation is relatively smooth. Movat stain; original magnification × 5, reduced by 17 per cent.

right-sided one. The number of vegetations on the tricuspid leaflets varied from one (in three patients) to innumerable (in Case 5). The number of vegetations on the tricuspid valve leaflets in the remaining seven patients varied from two to five. The individual vegetations on the tricuspid valve varied from 0.1 to 5 cm in largest diameter. The largest single vegetation occurred in Case 5, and although it appeared to obstruct the valvular orifice it was attached entirely to the anterior leaflet. The next largest occurred in a patient with fungal endocarditis (Case 8). The tricuspid valve vegetations involved the basal attachments of the leaflets, i.e., the annulus, in three patients, but in only one of them (Case 11) did it actually extend into the annulus and cause a ring abscess. Thus, excision of the leaflets would have totally removed the tricuspid valve vegetations in eight of the eleven patients. The shapes of the tricuspid valve vegetations in six patients were relatively flat and in the other five fungating. The surfaces of most vegetations were relatively smooth in seven patients and relatively rough in the other four. The vegetations caused rupture of several chordae tendineae in five patients, all of whom had multiple and usually large vegetations; in the other six without ruptured chordae the vegetations were either single or small. In none of the eleven patients did the vegetations cause gross disappearance of leaflet tissue either by perforation or by dissolution of a portion of tricuspid leaflet.

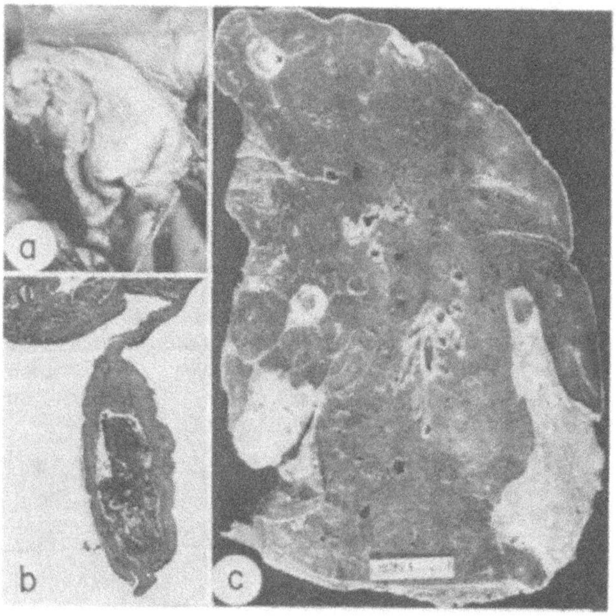

Figure 6. *Case 6. Staphylococcus aureus endocarditis of tricuspid valve with septic pulmonary emboli (A70-42).* ***a,*** *view of portion of friable vegetation on tricuspid valve.* ***b,*** *longitudinal section of vegetation involving distal two thirds of the leaflet. Movat stain; original magnification × 4, reduced by 18 per cent.* ***c,*** *section of lung showing multiple septic infarcts with abscess formation.*

On histologic examination, organisms were observed in tricuspid valve vegetations in seven of the eleven patients. Polymorphonuclear leukocytes were observed in the vegetations in all eleven patients; in eight abscesses were present. In three patients the inflammatory process and organisms were found in the central portions of the leaflets with preservation of cuspal tissue peripherally. In four other patients, distal portions of leaflet were completely destroyed, being incorporated into the inflammatory process; in three other patients the inflammatory process was superimposed on the surface of the tricuspid leaflets with good preservation of the underlying cusp. Calcific deposits were present in one tricuspid valve (Case 3), but this patient had had clinical evidence of infective endocarditis for at least 112 days.

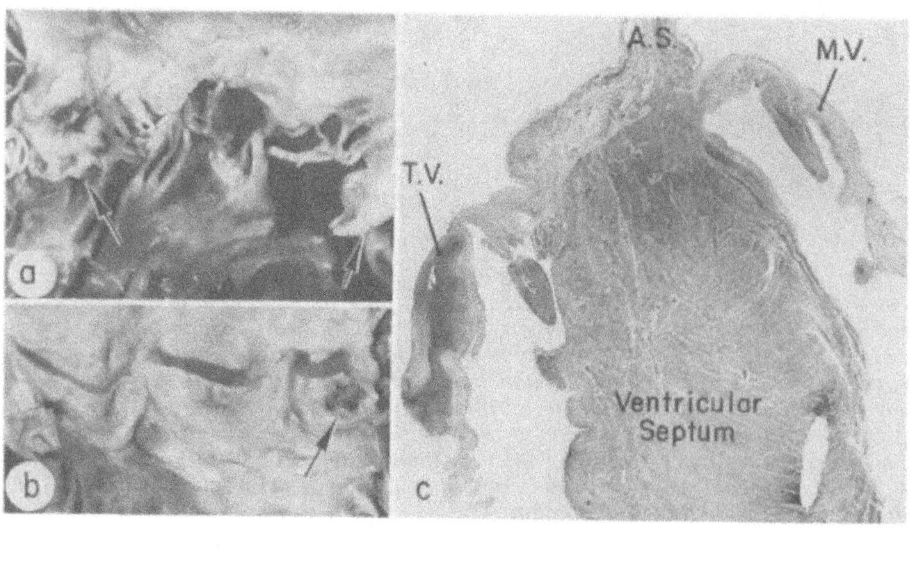

Figure 7. *Case 7. Pneumococcal endocarditis involving tricuspid* ***(a)*** *and aortic* ***(b)*** *valves (A69-155). That the vegetations are larger and involve all three tricuspid valve cusps as compared to their being smaller and involving only one aortic valve cusp is evidence that the infection originated on the right side of the heart.* ***c,*** *histologic section showing vegetations in middle two thirds of a tricuspid valve (T.V.) cusp. M.V. = mitral valve leaflet; A.S. = atrial septum. Hematoxylin and eosin stain; original magnification × 3, reduced by 24 per cent.*

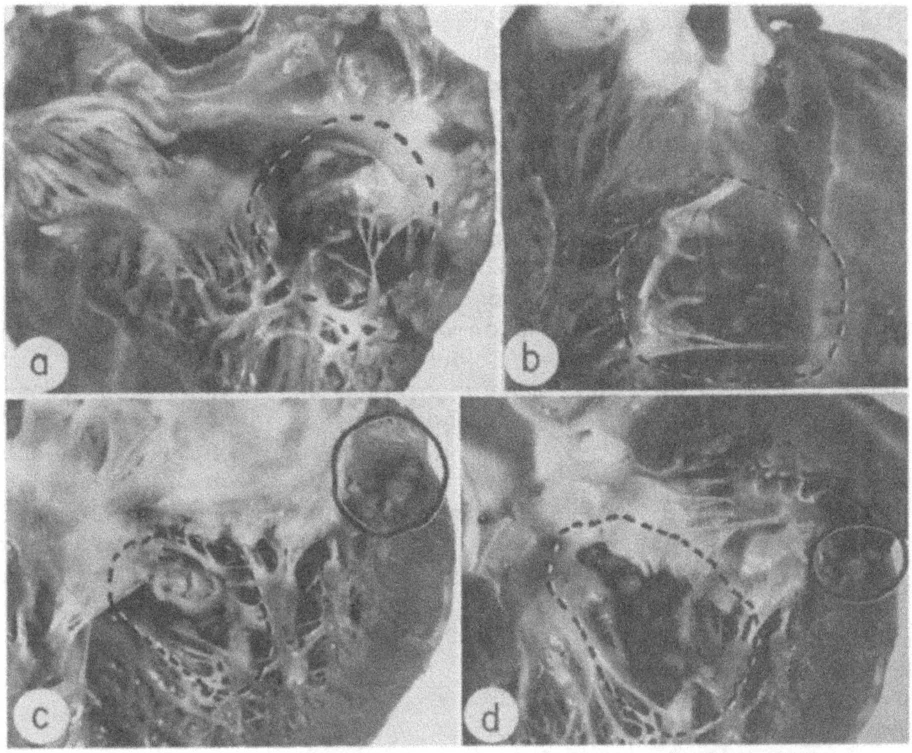

Figure 8. Case 8. Fungal endocarditis in a ten month old boy with a generalized infection involving many body organs (A70-78). Single large vegetations (dashed circles) were present on the tricuspid (**a** and **b**) and mitral (**c** and **d**) valves. A large myocardial abscess is designated by the closed circle in **c** and **d**.

The infection involving the pulmonic valve in one patient consisted of a single flat, relatively rough-surfaced vegetation involving two cusps and the intervening commissure. The vegetation produced a large tear in one cusp, almost surely producing pulmonic regurgitation. The infective process extended to the margin of attachment of one cusp. On histologic study, the involved pulmonic cusps contained large collections of polymorphonuclear leukocytes, and both surfaces were covered by fibrin. Organisms were not found in the involved pulmonic cusps.

Mural vegetations were present in three patients. In two they were located on the right ventricular endocardium: in one (Case 3) from contact with the free swinging anterior tricuspid leaflet (since its chordae were ruptured), and in one (Case 12) on a mural jet lesion produced earlier by congenital ventricular septal defect. In the third patient (Case 5) vegetative material was located on the right atrial endocardium and was due to contact of a large tricuspid valve vegetation.

On gross examination, distinct lesions were observed in myocardial walls in only two of the twelve patients: one (Case 8) had well circumscribed abscesses in the left ventricular free wall; the other (Case 9) had extensive, less well circumscribed foci of inflammatory necrosis in both left ventricular papillary muscles and a focus of acellular necrosis in the left ventricular free wall. On examination of 100 separate histologic sec-

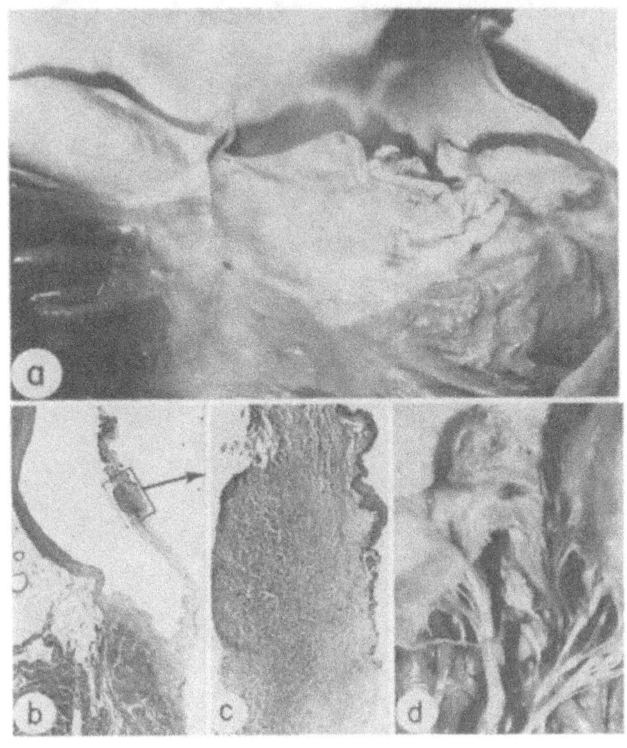

Figure 9. Case 9. Staphylococcus aureus endocarditis involving pulmonic (**a**, **b** and **c**) and mitral (**d**) valves in a fifty-five year old alcoholic who died of pneumonia (A70-141). The vegetation on the pulmonic valve caused tearing of one leaflet. **b**, histologic section through portion of pulmonic valve cusp. **c**, close-up view of portion of inflamed cusp. Hematoxylin and eosin stain; original magnification × 4 (**b**) and × 27 (**c**), reduced by 33 per cent.

tions of cardiac wall (five to fourteen per patient [average 9]) including sections of at least two of the three major papillary muscles of each heart, focal myocardial lesions were observed in the hearts of four patients. Three patients (Cases 1, 8 and 9) had myocardial abscesses. In the latter two patients (Cases 8 and 9), as already mentioned, they were large enough to be visible grossly; in the third (Case 1) only one minute myocardial abscess, containing colonies of bacteria, was observed on examination of eight large [2] sections of myocardial wall. Colonies of organisms also were observed in the myocardial abscesses in two patients (Cases 8 and 9), in both of whom septic emboli were observed in one or more coronary arteries (extramural in Case 9, intramural in Case 8). A minute focus of acute inflammatory cells also was observed in one patient (Case 11), but the cells were present in fibrous tissue, not in myocardium, in the distal portion of one papillary muscle. Only three patients had foci of myocardial necrosis, and two of them had coronary arterial emboli. The foci of necrosis in all three were located in both left ventricular papillary muscles, and two also had foci of necrosis in the left ventricular free wall. None of the other nine patients had papillary muscle necrosis, and none of the twelve had necrosis of the anterior papillary muscle of the right ventricle. The necrosis in one patient (Case 8) was associated with extensive dystrophic calcification of individual myocardial fibers. In another patient (Case 11) calcific deposits also were found in several individual myocardial fibers. Except for microscopic-sized foci in the apices of the left ventricular papillary muscles in several patients, no interstitial or replacement myocardial fibrosis was observed.

At necropsy, acute pneumonia with pulmonary infarcts was found in ten of the twelve patients, and seven had pulmonary abscesses. Material similar to that forming the right-sided cardiac vegetations was found in pulmonary arteries in

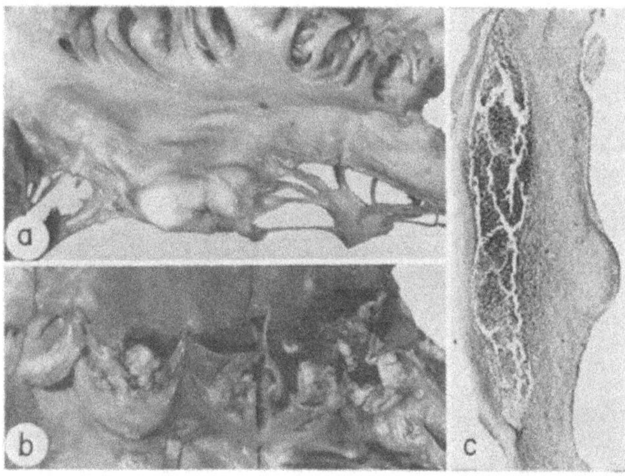

Figure 10. *Case 10. Pneumococcal endocarditis involving tricuspid (**a**) and aortic (**b**) valves in a fifty-eight year old alcoholic (DCGH No. 71A-14). The vegetation on the tricuspid valve is small, whereas the vegetations on the aortic valve are large and cause extensive destruction of the cusps. **c,** histologic section of a portion of tricuspid leaflet showing abscess formation. Hematoxylin and eosin stain; original magnification × 16, reduced by 33 per cent.*

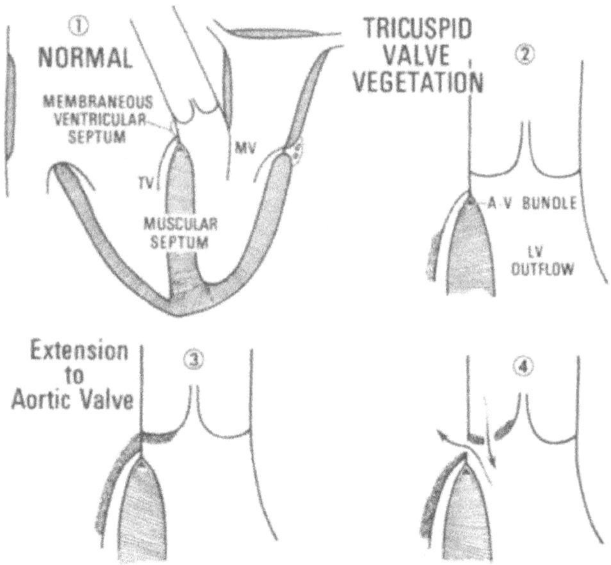

Figure 11. *Diagrammatic representation of development of aortic regurgitation and left to right shunt in a fifty-five year old man (WHC No. A70-155) with pneumococcal endocarditis and alcoholism. He noted fever, cough, and neck and knee pain twenty-six days before death. Overt signs of acute meningitis were present at the time of hospitalization nineteen days before death. Subsequently a murmur and signs of aortic regurgitation developed, and after that a "continuous murmur" due to the aortico-right atrial fistula. Death was due to intractable heart failure. (1) Normal cardiac anatomy. (2) Initial nidus of infection on tricuspid valve leaflet. (3) Extension of tricuspid vegetation through membranous portion of ventricular septum onto one of three aortic valve cusps. (4) Consequent perforation of aortic valve cusp causing aortic regurgitation and rupture of the membranous ventricular septum causing a left ventricular-right atrial fistula.*

seven of the ten patients with pneumonia, strongly suggesting that the pneumonia was secondary to dislodgment of vegetative material into the pulmonary circulation.

COMMENTS

Certain facts regarding right-sided infective endocarditis have emerged from review of previous reports on this subject and from study of our patients: (1) Its frequency is far less than left-sided infective endocarditis. It composes about 10 per cent of all cases of infective endocarditis. (2) It is usually caused by highly virulent or unusual organisms, the Staphylococcus being the most common. (3) The involved right-sided valve is, with rare exception, anatomically and functionally normal before the onset of infective endocarditis. (4) A predisposing factor is nearly always apparent. The most frequent ones are opiate addiction; alcoholism; generalized infections in patients with immunologic deficiencies, particularly lymphoma; congenital cardiac disease and dermal infections, particularly in young children or infants, with subsequent septicemia. (5) Diagnosis is difficult since the predominant clinical features are extracardiac, mainly, acute pneumonia; precordial murmurs are frequently absent or if present are soft and atypically located, and evidences of congestive cardiac failure are absent or if present rarely prominent.

The infrequency of right-sided infective endocarditis compared to the relative frequency of left-sided infective endocarditis has been explained by the lower pressure in the right side of the heart [3]. If the difference in pressure on the two sides of the heart is the major factor, the ratio between the frequency of right-sided to left-sided infective endocarditis might be expected to approximate the ratio between the peak systolic pressure in the right ventricle and that in the left ventricle,

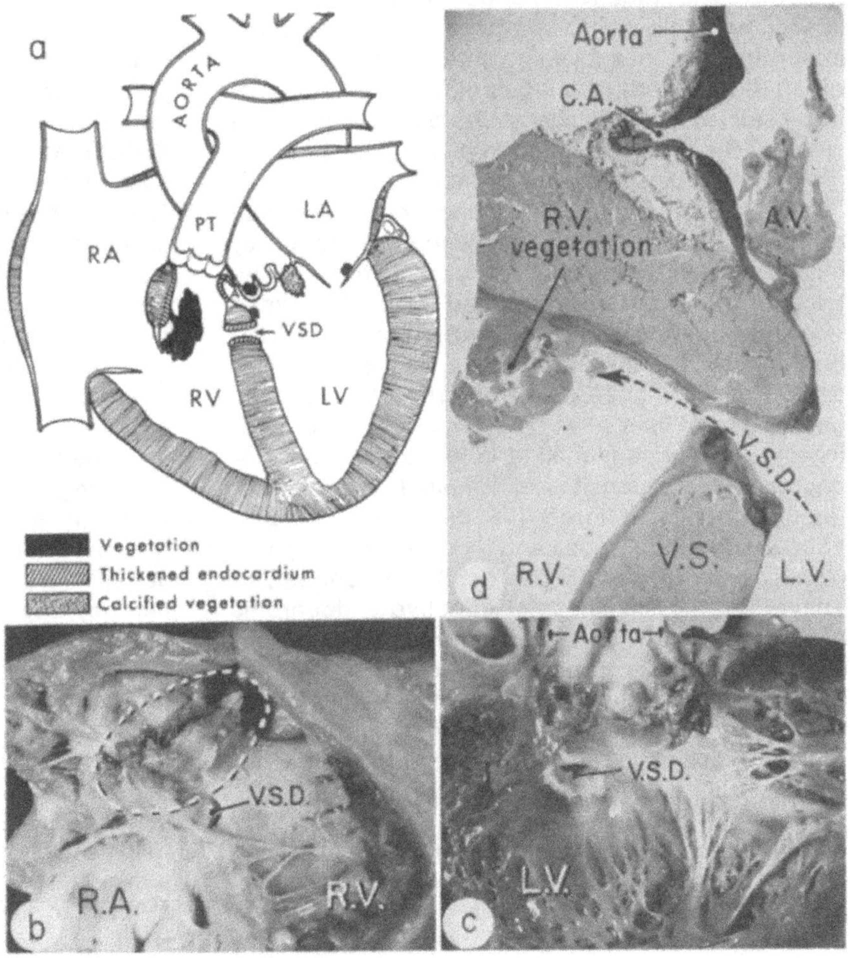

__Figure 12.__ Alpha hemolytic Streptococcus endocarditis in a five year old girl (A68-260) with congenital ventricular septal defect (VSD). Pneumonia and anemia developed four months before death, and two months later a grade 2/6 murmur of aortic regurgitation was noted for the first time. Death resulted from a large brain embolus. Vegetation probably formed initially on the jet lesion in the right ventricular outflow tract. Dislodgment of portions of right ventricular vegetation produced septic pulmonary emboli which presented clinically as "acute pneumonia." The exact mechanism of involvement of the aortic valve by the infective process is uncertain. __a,__ diagrammatic representation of location of vegetative material. Calcific deposits developed in aortic valve vegetation during the four month course. RA = right atrium; RV = right ventricle; PT = pulmonary trunk; LA = left atrium; A = aneurysm with orifice just below aortic valve. __b,__ view of opened right atrium, tricuspid valve and right ventricle showing the large vegetation (enclosed by dashed line) in the right ventricular outflow tract adjacent to the small ventricular septal defect. __c,__ view of opened left ventricle, aortic valve and aorta showing partial but extensive destruction of aortic valve cusps by vegetative material. The borders of the ventricular septal defect are free of vegetation. __d,__ photomicrograph of section through the ventricular septal defect including a portion of aorta, aortic valve (A.V.) cusp and ventricular septum (V.S.). The endocardium bordering the ventricular septal defect and that in the right ventricular outflow tract is very thick. C.A.-coronary artery. Elastic van Gieson stain; original magnification × 8, reduced by 15 per cent.

and indeed this is the case. The peak ventricular systolic pressure normally is about one sixth or 17 per cent of the peak left ventricular systolic pressure, and in at least 10 per cent of all cases of infective endocarditis the right-sided valves are involved. Thus, these figures of 10 and 17 per cent are sufficiently close to one another to allow this pressure explanation to be extremely plausible. Another factor mentioned as explaining the much lower frequency of right-sided infective endocarditis is lack of underlying disease of the right-sided cardiac valves compared to that involving the left-sided valves. In our study [1] of forty-five necropsy patients with active valvular infective endocarditis limited to the left side of the heart, there was evidence that the valve had been anatomically abnormal before the onset of infective endocarditis in 47 per cent whereas there was no evidence of previous right-sided valvular disease in any of our patients with right-sided infective endocarditis. The increased susceptibility of previously abnormal valves to infective endocarditis is well established, and this factor may be the second most important one in explaining the higher frequency of left-sided infective endocarditis. Whether or not the lower oxygen tension of the blood in the right side of the heart is important (by discouraging growth of aerobic bacteria) is uncertain.

Most studies [4–18], including ours, show that right-sided cardiac valves are usually attacked by highly virulent and unusual organisms. Of the twenty-three necropsy patients with right-sided (two had pulmonary arterial endarteritis from patent ductus arteriosus) infective endocarditis observed at the Mayo Clinic from 1910 to 1955 and described by Bain et al. [11] in 1958, the offending organism was identified in nineteen: Staphylococcus was responsible in eleven (58 per cent), Pneumococcus in three (16 per cent), Streptococcus in four (21 per cent) (viridans in two) and Gonococcus in one (5 per cent). In contrast, of Thayer's total 536 cases of infective endocarditis described in 1931 [5], Staph. aureus was responsible in only 7 per cent, Pneumococcus in 15 per cent, Streptococcus in 63 per cent and Gonococcus in 11 per cent. Of 100 patients with infective endocarditis acquired outside the hospital between 1956 and 1965 [19], Staphylococcus was responsible in twenty-three, Streptococcus in fifty-six (viridans in twenty-seven), miscellaneous in seven (but none had Pneumococcus or Gonococcus) and negative in fourteen. Studies in opiate addicts [7–10,13–18] have shown an even greater propensity for the Staphylococcus to be the cause of right-sided infective endocarditis. A review of forty-eight cases (69 per cent fatal) of infective endocarditis in opiate addicts by Louria et al. [14] disclosed that the offending organism was Staphylococcus (aureus in thirteen, epidermidis in two) in fifteen of the sixteen patients with right-sided endocarditis (tricuspid valve in each). Among sixty-two fatal cases of infective endocarditis in opiate addicts reviewed by Sapira [16] in 1968, Staph. aureus was the offending organism in nine of thirteen with isolated right-sided cardiac vegetations, whereas it was responsible in only six of forty-six patients with isolated left-sided infective endocarditis (organism unknown in thirteen). Of sixteen opiate addicts with infective endocarditis described in 1970 by Ramsey et al. [18], Staph. aureus was the cause in three of the four patients with right-sided (tricuspid) infective endocarditis in whom the organism was known but in only one of twelve patients with isolated left-sided infective endocarditis. Staph. aureus also was the cause of the right-sided infective endocarditis in each of four heroin addicts described herein but was responsible for infective endocarditis in only one of the remaining eight patients. Although it usually attacks previously normal right-sided cardiac valves, Staphylococcus is commonly the offending organism in patients with infective endocarditis complicating congenital cardiovascular malformations. Of thirty-eight patients with infective endocarditis and congenital heart disease (twenty-three had ventricular septal defect) described by Vogler and Dorney [20], Staphylococcus was responsible for the infection in thirteen (41 per cent) and alpha Streptococcus in nine (28 per cent) of the thirty-two patients in whom the organism was known.

In none of the multiple papers concerning right- or left-sided infective endocarditis in opiate addicts has Pneumococcus been mentioned as the offending organism. In four of our twelve patients with right-sided infective endocarditis, D. pneumoniae was the offending bacterium. Each of these patients was a chronic alcoholic and three also had meningitis. In the pre-heroin-addiction era, however, Pneumococcus was recognized as a frequent cause of right-sided infective endocarditis. Of twenty cases of infective endocarditis involving the tricuspid valve reported before 1940 [6], nine (45 per cent) were caused by Pneumococcus. Of a total of 584 patients with infective endocarditis subjected to necropsy at the Philadelphia General Hospital from 1920 to 1940, only eleven (2 per cent) had infective endocarditis restricted to the tricuspid valve, but of the sixty-two with pneumococcal endocarditis the tricuspid valve alone was involved in nine (15 per cent) [6]. Even earlier, in 1904, Preble [4] in reviewing 141 cases of pneumococcal endocarditis showed that in 18 per cent there were vegetations on right-sided cardiac valves, whereas infective endocarditis due to organisms other than Pneumococcus caused right-sided vegetations in only 7 per cent of the cases. Preble also mentioned alcoholism, as well as malnutrition, as a predisposing factor to pneumococcal endocarditis, and he also stressed the frequent association of pneumococcal infective endocarditis with meningitis and pneumonia. He found that 60 per cent of patients with pneumococcal endocarditis had meningitis and that 30 per cent of patients with pneumococcal meningitis had endocarditis. Goldburgh et al. [6] found pneumococcal endocarditis in 5 per cent of the patients who died with lobar pneumonia. Although Pneumococcus was the offending organism in 15 per cent of Thayer's 536 patients with infective endocarditis described before 1931 [5], since the introduction of antibiotics it has caused less than 3 per cent of the cases of infective endocarditis [21]. Of fifteen patients (ten fatal) with pneumococcal endocarditis studied at the Cincinnati General Hospital from 1945 to 1965, three had vegetations limited to the tricuspid valve (the other twelve had either mitral or aortic vegetations) [21]. Thirteen of the fifteen patients also had meningitis.

Although heroin addiction is now a well recognized predisposing factor to infective endocarditis on either side of the heart, the frequency of alcoholism as a predisposing factor to right-sided infective endocarditis apparently is not well appreciated. Congenital cardiac disease is a well recognized predisposing factor to infective endocarditis [20,22–24]. In this circumstance the right-sided vegetations are most frequently observed in patients with small ventricular septal defects and left to right shunts through them as in our Case 12. The resulting vegetations, however, most often occur on the thickened right ventricular mural endocardium rather than on valvular (tricuspid) endocardium, but both were involved in our patient. Persistent patent ductus arteriosus also may be complicated by vegetations occurring on the pulmonary arterial side of the left to right shunt. Strictly speaking, however, vegetations involving the ductus or pulmonary artery represent endarteritis and not endocarditis. Infective endocarditis complicating previously stenotic tricuspid or pulmonic valves is uncommon. Rheumatic tricuspid valve disease is always accompanied by rheumatic mitral stenosis and frequently also by aortic valvular involvement [25]. Infective endocarditis involving hearts with previously diseased left- and right-sided valves nearly always attacks only one or both left-sided valves and spares the right-sided valves. Infective endocarditis, however, rarely attacks hearts with previous three- or four-valve involvement anyway, possibly because the left-sided valves in this circumstance are usually heavily calcified and stenotic, and superimposition of infective endocarditis on heavily calcified valves is uncommon. Furthermore, involvement of congenitally malformed, particularly stenotic, pulmonic valves is infrequent, although several patients with congenital pulmonic stenosis and infective endocarditis have been described [20,22–24].

Although the diagnosis of left-sided infective endocarditis is usually established during life, the diagnosis of right-sided infective endocarditis is far more difficult to make and often is not even suspected during life. The major reason is because the latter illness is dominated by extracardiac signs and symptoms. Acute pneumonia is the usual presenting feature of right-sided infective endocarditis, occurring in ten of our twelve patients, and it dominates the clinical course. The pneumonia is usually embolic in origin, resulting from dislodgment of vegetative material from the right-sided cardiac vegetations. Acute meningitis also may occur and be the dominant feature. Signs of right-sided congestive cardiac failure may be absent or minimal or, if present, readily explainable as secondary to acute cor pulmonale from the acute pneumonia. Precordial murmurs may be absent entirely and, if present, may be soft, atypically located and may not increase in intensity with inspiration. Since fever and anemia are common, the precordial murmurs may be dismissed as being "hemic" in origin. Cardiomegaly, distention of jugular veins and pulsation of the liver are often not observed in patients with right-sided infective endocarditis. Death in patients with isolated right-sided infective endocarditis usually can be attributed to the extracardiac manifestations, usually pneumonia. In none of our six patients with isolated right-sided infective endocarditis was congestive cardiac failure an important factor. Furthermore, in only two of the six patients with infective endocarditis involving both right- and left-sided cardiac valves was congestive cardiac failure a major manifestation of the illness, and in both infective endocarditis caused severe aortic regurgitation.

A number of papers have been published on right-sided infective endocarditis, but none have emphasized the cardiac-pathologic features of this condition, and few have even illustrated its morphologic aspects. Of our twelve patients, infective endocarditis was definitely primary on the right side of the heart in nine; in six of these no left-sided vegetations were present, and in the other three the right-sided vegetations were large or extensive, and the left-sided vegetations were minute or smaller. Dislodgment of organisms from the inflamed lungs into the pulmonary veins may be the mechanism responsible for the left-sided vegetations. In two other patients single similar-sized vegetations were located on both tricuspid and mitral valves and therefore which one came first is uncertain; both patients had generalized infection involving several body organs. In one of the twelve patients large vegetations destroyed the aortic valve, and only one small vegetation was present on the right side of the heart. Thus, this patient (Case 10) appears to be the only one in whom the right-sided infective endocarditis was definitely secondary to left-sided infective endocarditis.

Vegetations on the tricuspid valve may be similar in appearance to those involving the mitral valve. Rupture of chordae tendineae is common, occurring in five of our eleven patients with tricuspid valve vegetations. Unlike rupture of chordae tendineae of the mitral valve, which virtually always leads to severe mitral regurgitation [26], rupture of tricuspid valvular chordae may produce no clinical evidence of tricuspid regurgitation since normally the pressures in the right ventricle and right atrium are low and not markedly different. When evidence of tricuspid regurgitation is present in patients with infective endocarditis involving this valve, it is probable that the elevation in right ventricular pressure is a consequence of extensive acute pneumonia and acute cor pulmonale. Perforation or disappearance of tricuspid leaflet tissue occurred in none of our eleven patients despite highly virulent organisms. Again, this difference may be explained by the lower pressure on the right side of the heart which may decrease the rate of valve destruction by the infective process. Another factor may be the duration of illness which is shorter in patients with right-sided infective endocarditis as compared to patients with isolated left-sided infective endocarditis. Possibly the former patients die of widespread pneumonia before the right-sided vegetations have had time to destroy the valves more extensively.

From study of our twelve patients and from reports of others of right-sided infective endocarditis [4–18,20–24,27–30], it appears that the tricuspid valve is far more prone to be the site of vegetations than is the pulmonic valve. Only one of our twelve patients had pulmonic valve vegetations, and he also had mitral valve infective endocarditis. Pulmonic valve vegetations were present in only one of the twelve fatal cases of isolated right-sided infective endocarditis reported by Sapira [16]. In contrast, infective endocarditis on the left side involves the semilunar (aortic) valve more frequently than the atrioventricular (mitral) valve [1]. Fungating vegetations on the pulmonic valve also appear to be infrequent as contrasted to their frequency on the aortic valve. In none of our twelve patients with infective endocarditis were both right-sided cardiac valves involved, whereas involvement of both left-sided cardiac valves by infective endocarditis is common. This difference results from several factors. Although pulmonic regurgitation may result from infective endocarditis involving this valve, the amount of regurgitation is usually small since the valve usually is not extensively damaged and the pulmonary pressure is relatively low. In contrast, vegetations on the aortic valve are usually larger and frequently severely damage the cusps with resultant marked regurgitation. Also, the higher aortic diastolic pressure may dislodge the aortic vegetations and cause them to attach to mitral leaflets or chordae. The pulmonary arterial pressure may not be high enough to dislodge the pulmonic valve vegetations retrogradely. Also, the pulmonic valve is separated from the tricuspid valve by myocardium (crista supraventricularis), whereas the anterior mitral leaflet is continuous with the aortic valve.

Although myocardial lesions are frequent in patients with infective endocarditis involving one or both left-sided cardiac valves, they are usually absent in patients with isolated right-sided infective endocarditis. Only one of our six patients with isolated right-sided infective endocarditis had myocardial lesions and he had widespread abscesses in many body organs. Two of our six patients with combined right- and left-sided infective endocarditis had myocardial foci of inflammation, and in each coronary arterial septic emboli were the explanation.

Recently, total valve excision has been employed as therapy for patients with right-sided infective endocarditis unresponsive to antibiotic therapy [31]. In nine of our eleven patients with tricuspid valve infective endocarditis, the vegetations did not extend to the basal attachments of the leaflets. Therefore, total excision of the tricuspid valves would have eradicated the right-sided infective endocarditis. In only one of the two patients in whom the infective process extended to the level of the basal attachment of a tricuspid leaflet did it actually burrow into the annulus to cause a ring abscess. Even though the infective endocarditis may have extended to the level of the valve annulus, this would not necessarily preclude total valve excision and successful outcome because valve excision may serve simply to eradicate the source of septic emboli to the lungs which cause infarction, pneumonia and abscesses, and the pulmonary infection is the major cause of death in these patients. Although man may tolerate total excision of either the tricuspid or pulmonic valve without symptomatic evidence of cardiac dysfunction, if both valves become incompetent, or if one becomes stenotic and the other incompetent, cardiac decompensation is the result. An ideal way to produce severe congestive heart failure in animals is to incise or excise the tricuspid valve causing incompetency and banding the pulmonary trunk causing stenosis [32].

ACKNOWLEDGMENT

Eight patients described herein were studied clinically at Washington, D.C., hospitals. We are, therefore, indebted to Doctors Frank I. Marcus, Gordon A. Ewy, Ross D. Fletcher, Lucia Gomez, Rashid A. Massumi, Tazewell Banks and Michael Cuadra at the D.C. General Hospital, and to Doctors James Bocus, Sander H. Mendelsohn and Chester Emmonds at the Washington Hospital Center for allowing us to include their patients in this study.

REFERENCES

1. Buchbinder NA, Roberts WC: Left-sided valvular active infective endocarditis ·A study of 45 necropsy patients. Amer J Med 53: 000, 1972
2 Ent LD, Roberts WC: The processing of large blocks of tissue. Amer J Clin Path 50: 726, 1968.
3. Lepeschkin E: On the relation between the site of valvular involvement in endocarditis and the blood pressure resting on the valve Amer J Med Sci 224 318, 1952.
4 Preble HB. Pneumococcus endocarditis. Amer J Med Sci 128: 782, 1904.
5 Thayer WS· Bacterial or infective endocarditis. Edinburgh Med J 38: 237, 307, 1931
6 Goldburgh HL, Baer S, Lieber MM: Acute bacterial endocarditis of the tricuspid valve. Amer J Med Sci 204 319, 1942
7. Hussey HH, Keliher TF, Schaefer BF, Walsh BJ: Septicemia and bacterial endocarditis resulting from heroin addiction. Report of five cases. JAMA 126. 535, 1944
8 Hussey HH, Katz S: Septic pulmonary infarction. Report of 8 cases Ann Intern Med 22 526, 1945.
9 Luttgens WF Endocarditis in "main line" opium addicts Report on eleven cases. Arch Intern Med (Chicago) 83 653, 1949
10 Dowling HF, Lepper M, Caldwell ER, Spies HW: Staphylococcic endocarditis. an analysis of 25 cases treated with antibiotics, together with a review of the recent literature. Medicine 31 155, 1952.
11 Bain RC, Edwards JE, Scheifley CH, Geraci JE· Right-sided bacterial endocarditis and endarteritis Amer J Med 24 98, 1958.
12 Bain RC, Edwards JE, Scheifley CH, Geraci JE· Right-sided bacterial endocarditis and endarteritis. Staff Meet Mayo Clin 33. 182, 1958.
13 Olsson RA, Romansky MJ· Staphylococcal tricuspid endocarditis in heroin addicts Ann Intern Med 57· 755, 1962.
14 Louria DB, Hensle T, Rose J. The major medical complications of heroin addiction. Ann Intern Med 67· 1, 1967
15 Massumi RA, Just H, Twawkkol A: Pulmonary valve regurgitation secondary to bacterial endocarditis in heroin addicts Amer Heart J 73· 308, 1967.
16. Sapira JD: The narcotic addict as a medical patient. Amer J Med 45· 555, 1968
17 Cherubin CE, Baden M, Kavaler F, Lerner S, Cline W. Infective endocarditis in narcotic addicts. Ann Intern Med 69 1091, 1968.
18 Ramsey RG, Gunnar RM, Tobin JR Jr· Endocarditis in the drug addict. Amer J Cardiol 25. 608, 1970.
19. Lerner PI, Weinstein L: Infective endocarditis in the antibiotic era. New Eng J Med 274: 199, 259, 323, 388, 1966.
20. Vogler WR, Dorney ER: Bacterial endocarditis in congenital heart disease. Amer Heart J 64 198, 1962.
21 Straus AL, Hamburger M: Pneumococcal endocarditis in the penicillin era. Arch Intern Med (Chicago) 118 190, 1966
22. Gelfman R, Levine SA The incidence of acute and subacute bacterial endocarditis in congenital heart disease. Amer J Med Sci 204: 324, 1942.
23. Barker PS: A clinical study of subacute bacterial infection confined to the right side of the heart or the pulmonary artery. Amer Heart J 37: 1054, 1949.
24 Bashour FA, Winchell CP: Right-sided bacterial endocarditis. Amer J Med Sci 240: 411, 1960.
25 Roberts WC. Valvular heart disease. A look at 1000 necropsied patients (In preparation)
26. Roberts WC, Braunwald E, Morrow AG: Acute severe mitral regurgitation secondary to ruptured chordae tendineae. Clinical, hemodynamic, and pathologic considerations. Circulation 33: 58, 1966.
27. Olesen KH, Fabricius J: Pulmonic valvular regurgitation during twenty-seven years after gonorrheal endocarditis Report of a case with catheterization data Amer Heart J 52: 791, 1956.
28 Levin HS, Runco V, Wooley CF, Ryan JM. Pulmonic regurgitation following staphylococcal endocarditis. An intracardiac phonocardiographic study Circulation 30: 411, 1964
29 Garcia R, Taber RE: Bacterial endocarditis of the pulmonic valve Association with atrial septal defect of the ostium secundum type Amer J Cardiol 18: 275, 1966
30. Laniado S, Frater RWM, Jordan A, Kafka EC, Kadish AS, Zelefsky M. Endocarditis of the pulmonic valve simulating cardiac tumor. Chest 59: 464, 1971.
31. Arbulu A, Thoms NW, Chiscano A, Wilson RF. Total tricuspid valvulectomy without replacement in the treatment of Pseudomonas endocarditis Surg Forum 22: 162, 1971.
32 Barger AC, Roe BB, Richardson GS· Relation of valvular lesions and of exercise to auricular pressure, work tolerance, and to development of chronic, congestive failure. in dogs. Amer J Physiol 169· 384, 1952

Left-Sided Valvular Active Infective Endocarditis

A Study of Forty-Five Necropsy Patients

NEIL A. BUCHBINDER, M.D.
WILLIAM C. ROBERTS, M.D.
Bethesda, Maryland

Clinical and anatomic features are described in forty-five necropsy patients with left-sided valvular active infective endocarditis. Vegetations in 53 per cent of the patients involved previously anatomically normal valves, and 76 per cent of all patients had previously functionally normal valves. Predisposing factors allowing entrance of virulent or unusual organisms or alterations of host defense mechanisms appear to account for the frequency of infective endocarditis on normal valves. Valvular dysfunction resulting from infective endocarditis occurred in at least 59 per cent and possibly as high as 74 per cent of the forty-five patients causing congestive heart failure in all. Myocardial lesions were present in 87 per cent of the thirty-eight patients in whom multiple histologic sections were examined, but in none did heart failure appear to result from these lesions. Papillary muscle necrosis was present in 58 per cent, but in none did it appear to cause mitral regurgitation. Congestive heart failure could not be attributed in any patient to myocardial lesions. Pericarditis occurred in eight patients (20 per cent), and in each a site of direct extension of the inflammation into the pericardium was apparent. Ring abscesses occurred in twelve of thirty-one patients with aortic valve vegetations and in none of twenty-six with mitral valve vegetations. Ring abscesses indicate severe destruction of valvular cusps and severe valvular dysfunction.

Infective endocarditis before the advent of antibiotics was virtually always a fatal disease and consequently received particular attention from many pathologists. With the introduction of antibiotics and therefore definitive therapy for the first time, the pathologic features of infective endocarditis became less important, and attention was focused on proper diagnosis and choice of antibiotic(s). It became increasingly evident, however, that antibiotic therapy often was not curative. During recent years cardiac valve replacement or rarely cuspal repair has afforded another form of therapy for infective endocarditis, and now surgery is being increasingly used in treatment of both active and healed infective endocarditis. Relatively few morphologic studies on infective endocarditis have appeared since the introduction of antibiotics or open cardiac surgery, thus a review of the autopsy data on patients with this entity primarily from the anatomic viewpoint seemed appropriate.

From the Section of Pathology, National Heart and Lung Institute, National Institutes of Health, Bethesda, Maryland 20014. Requests for reprints should be addressed to Dr. William C. Roberts, Bldg 10A, Room 3E-30, Section of Pathology, National Heart and Lung Institute, National Institutes of Health.
Manuscript received November 4, 1971; revised January 18, 1972

Summarized here are clinicopathologic observations in forty-five patients with left-sided infective endocarditis who died between 1955 and 1971

PATIENTS STUDIED AND METHODS

Clinical and necropsy records of all patients were reviewed: twenty-three patients were studied clinically and at necropsy at the Clinical Center of the National Institutes of Health; the remaining twenty-two were studied clinically elsewhere, and their hearts were submitted to the Section of Pathology, National Heart and Lung Institute, for examination Patients with endocarditis after cardiac valve replacement [1-3] and patients with vegetations occurring exclusively on mural endocardium were excluded [4] Three of the forty-five patients had histories of successful therapy for previous episodes of infective endocarditis The heart of every patient was studied originally by one of us (W C.R.) and forty were reexamined by both of us At reexamination, additional histologic sections were cut in thirty-eight patients, and old histologic sections of heart were reviewed in forty-two patients At least four hematoxylin and eosin stained histologic sections of heart were examined in every patient including at least one special stain for bacteria (Brown and Brenn) or fungi (methenamine silver)

The forty-five patients ranged in age from seventeen to seventy years (average thirty-nine years) (Figure 1), thirty-two were men, and thirteen were women One patient was less than twenty years of age and two were more than sixty-five years of age.

RESULTS

The sites of the cardiac vegetations are shown in Table I. Of 180 cardiac valves present in the forty-five patients, fifty-seven (32 per cent) contained vegetations: the aortic valve was involved alone or in combination with other valves in thirty-one (69 per cent) and the mitral valve in twenty-six (58 per cent)

The status of the infected valve before infective endocarditis is shown in Table II. Of forty-five patients with vegetations on cardiac valves, twenty-four (53 per cent) had anatomically normal valves before infective endocarditis and twenty-one (47 per cent) had anatomically abnormal valves. The abnormality was rheumatic in ten, congenital in eight (bicuspid aortic valves in six) and of uncertain etiology in three. Of the twenty-one anatomically abnormal valves, ten functioned normally before the onset of infective endocarditis as judged by the absence of signs or symptoms of cardiac dysfunction before the onset of infective endocarditis, and by necropsy evaluation of the involved valve Thus, infective endocarditis occurred on functionally abnormal cardiac valves in only eleven (24 per cent) of the forty-five patients: seven valves were stenotic with or without an element of incompetency and four were purely incompetent. Of the seven patients with stenotic valves, operative commissurotomies (mitral in three, aortic in one) were performed just before the appearance of infective endocarditis in four of them; the fifth patient had systemic crytococcosis and at necropsy fungal vegetations were present on both mitral

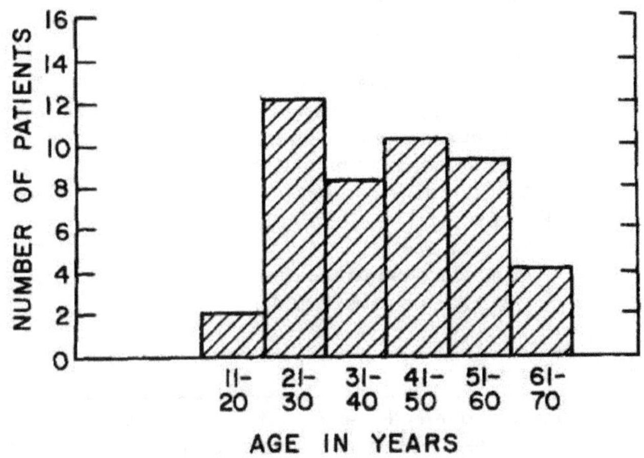

Figure 1. Age distribution of the forty-five patients with active valvular infective endocarditis

TABLE I Valves Involved in Left-Sided Infective Endocarditis (45 Necropsy Patients)

Sites of Vegetations	Patients No.	%
Aortic valve	19	42
Mitral valve	14	31
Aortic and mitral valves	12	27
Totals	45	100

TABLE II Status of Left-Sided Cardiac Valve Before Onset of Infective Endocarditis (45 Necropsy Patients)

Status		Patients No.	%
Valve anatomically normal		24	53
Valve anatomically abnormal		21	47
Functionally normal	10		
Functionally abnormal	11		
Aortic stenosis* (AS) 3			
Pure aortic regurgitation . . . 3			
Mitral stenosis* (MS) 3			
Pure mitral regurgitation . . . 1			
AS + MS 1			

* With or without associated valvular regurgitation.

TABLE III **Organism Causing Left-Sided Infective Endocarditis (IE) and Status of Valve Before Infection (45 Necropsy Patients)**

Causative Organism		No. Patients	Status of Valve Before IE: Anatomically Normal	Anatomically Abnormal: Functionally Normal	Anatomically Abnormal: Functionally Abnormal
Bacterium					
Staphylococcus aureus	31	10	5	3	2*
Staphylococcus epidermidis		2	1		1
Alpha Streptococcus		4	1	1	2
Beta Streptococcus		2		2	
Streptococcus faecalis		3	1	2	
Diplococcus pneumonia		4	4		
L forms corynebacterium and Streptobacillus moniliformis		1	1		
Gram positive coccus†		5	3		2*
Fungus					
Candida species	7	5	2		3‡
Cryptococcus neoformans		1			1
Histoplasma capsulatum		1	1		
Unknown		7	5	1	1
Totals		45	24	9	12

* One developed infective endocarditis after cardiac surgery.
† Organisms identified only on histologic sections of vegetations.
‡ Each developed infective endocarditis after cardiac surgery.

and aortic valves, each of which had been stenotic previously [5,6]; the remaining two patients had infective endocarditis superimposed on stenotic, heavily calcified aortic valves. One of the latter had a congenitally unicommissural valve [7], and the other, a seventy year old man, had degenerative type of aortic stenosis on a three-cuspid valve [8]. Of the four purely incompetent valves, none of which was calcified, before the occurrence of infective endocarditis, two aortic valves were congenitally bicuspid; the third was rheumatically deformed and three-cuspid; the one scarred mitral valve was rheumatic in origin.

The organisms causing infective endocarditis and the relationship of the causative organisms to the underlying status of the valves are summarized in Table III. Of the thirty-one with infective endocarditis caused by bacteria, twelve (39 per cent), and possibly as many as seventeen (55 per cent), were due to Staphylococcus species and only four (13 per cent) to alpha hemolytic Streptococcus. Blood cultures, performed in thirty-six patients, were positive in twenty-nine (81 per cent) and negative in seven (19 per cent). No organisms were cultured from blood or observed on histologic examination of vegetations in three patients, but each had been treated with antibiotics and each otherwise had typical clinical and necropsy findings of infective endocarditis. The valves were normal in five of ten patients with infective endocarditis caused by Staph. aureus and in all four with infective endocarditis caused by Diplococcus pneumoniae. In contrast, three of the four patients with infective endocarditis caused by alpha hemolytic Streptococcus had anatomically abnormal valves before the appearance of infective endocarditis. In forty-three patients the infection was primary in the heart; in the other two the cardiac infection was secondary to infection primary in other organs of tissues, and fungi were the cause in both of them.

Predisposing factors (Table IV) were found in thirty patients (67 per cent). Heroin addiction, alcoholism, malignancy and cardiac surgery accounted for more than 75 per cent of the predisposing factors. A predisposing factor was found in six of twelve patients with infective endocarditis caused by either Staph. aureus or Staph. epidermidis, in four of seven caused by fungi and in all four caused by Pneumococcus. All four patients with pneumococcal endocarditis were alcoholics. Of six heroin addicts the aortic valve alone was involved in four patients, the mitral valve alone in one and both the aortic and mitral valves in one; the causative organism was Staph. aureus in two patients, Staph. epidermidis in one, gram-positive coccus in one, Candida species in one and unknown in one. Three of the four patients with infective endocarditis due to alpha hemolytic Streptococcus had infection on aortic valves which previously had been anatomically abnormal: one had been made incompetent by jet lesions from discrete subaortic stenosis [9], the second had an incompetent rheumatically-deformed three-cuspid aortic valve and the third had an incompetent congenitally bicuspid aortic valve.

The functional status of the cardiac valves after infection is summarized in Table V. Valvular dysfunction occurred in thirty-three patients, twenty-six of whom had dysfunction in whole or in part from infective endocarditis. Further dysfunction from superimposed infective endocarditis in the other seven patients with already abnormally functioning valves due to underlying disease could not be clearly demonstrated. All thirty-three patients with valvular dysfunction had congestive cardiac failure. Of the twelve patients without valvular dysfunction only two had congestive cardiac failure and each of them had coronary heart disease. The principal causes of death in the forty-five patients are summarized in Table VI. Although congestive cardiac failure occurred in thirty-five patients, it appeared to be the principal cause of death in only twenty-one; in the other fourteen, it was a contributing factor. The type valve damage resulting from infective endocarditis and the mechanism of the resulting valve dysfunction are summarized in Table VII. Infective endocarditis caused thirty valves to function abnormally in twenty-six patients: twenty-eight valves were made incompetent, and two valves appeared to have been made stenotic by large vegetations. One of the latter was an aortic valve infected by Candida parapsilosis [10], the other was a mitral valve infected by beta hemolytic Streptococcus (group B) [10].

The physical signs are summarized in Table VIII Six patients presented with acute meningitis and one with cerebrovascular accident. Of forty-one patients with electrocardiograms, thirty-three had sinus rhythm, seven had atrial fibrillation, and one had atrial flutter. Three patients had P-R intervals of more than 0.20 second; one other had second degree atrioventricular block. In the latter patient the inflammatory process extended into the area of the atrioventricular bundle. The clinical diagnosis of active infective endocarditis was established before death in twenty-four patients, strongly suspected in twelve and never considered in nine. Embolic episodes were diagnosed clinically in nineteen patients. The duration of illness (onset of symptoms to death) was known in thirty-two patients: it was less than six weeks in ten (31 per cent) and more than six weeks in twenty-two (69 per cent). Antibiotics were given to forty-one of the forty-five patients although the diagnosis of infective endocarditis had been suspected clinically in only thirty-six: thirty patients received the proper dosage of the proper antibiotic recommended for active infective endocarditis but not necessarily for a sufficient duration, five received a questionably appropriate antibiotic, and six definitely received an improper antibiotic.

Necropsy Findings. Various necropsy findings are illustrated in Figures 2 through 15. Colonies of organisms were found in thirty-five (87 per cent) of forty patients in whom histologic sections of vegetations were available. Organisms were observed histologically in twenty-two of twenty-five patients with positive blood cultures and in four of seven patients with negative blood cultures. The types and frequencies of acute myocardial lesions (Fig-

TABLE IV Predisposing Factors in Left-Sided Infective Endocarditis (IE) and Status of Valve Before Infection

Factor	No. Patients	Status of Valve Before IE: Normal	Abnormal
None	15	7	8
Malignancy*	7	7	0
Heroin addiction	6	3	3
Alcoholism	5	4	1
Cardiac operation	5	0	5
Dental procedure	2	1	1
Genitourinary procedure	2	1	1
Skin infection	1	0	1
Intravenous catheter	1	1	0
Septic abortion	1	0	1
Totals	45	24	21

* Six patients received chemotherapy.

TABLE V Valve Function in Left-Sided Infective Endocarditis (IE) (45 Necropsy Patients)

Valve Function		Patients No.	%
Valve dysfunction		33	74
From IE	22 (50%)		
From IE worsening underlying valve dysfunction	4 (9%)		
From underlying valve dysfunction alone	7 (15%)		
No valve dysfunction		12	26
Totals		45	100

ures 4–6, 10, 14 and 15) are summarized in Table IX and the gross anatomic cardiac findings in Table X. Acute myocardial lesions were observed in thirty-three of thirty-eight (87 per cent) patients in whom histologic sections of walls of each cardiac chamber and of both left ventricular papillary muscles were examined. Foci of myocardial necrosis were found in twenty-three patients (61 per cent) but limited to papillary muscle in eighteen. The papillary muscles in twenty-two patients (58 per cent) were focally (eleven patients) or diffusely (eleven patients) necrotic. Papillary muscle necrosis (Figure 13) occurred in ten (62 per cent) of sixteen patients with infective endocarditis in-

TABLE VI Principal Cause of Death in Left-Sided Infective Endocarditis (45 Necropsy Patients)

Type		Patients No.	Patients %
Cardiovascular		24	53
Congestive heart failure . . .	21		
Arrhythmia	1		
Cardiac tamponade	1		
Pulmonary embolus	1		
Central nervous system		9	20
Embolus	6		
Meningitis	3		
Generalized infection		3	7
Acute pneumonia		1	2
Unknown		8	18
Totals		45	100

TABLE VII Valve Dysfunction Resulting from Left-Sided Infective Endocarditis (30 Valves)

Dysfunction	Valve (no.) Aortic	Valve (no.) Mitral
Pure regurgitation	19	9
Cuspal perforation	14	3
Cuspal destruction	5	0
Ruptured chordae tendineae	0	6
Stenosis	1	1

TABLE VIII Physical Signs in Left-Sided Infective Endocarditis (45 Necropsy Patients)

Signs	% of Patients*
Fever (>100°F)	95
Precordial murmur	91
Dermal petechiae	38
Splenomegaly	33
Retinal lesions	5
Janeway lesions	5
Subungual hemorrhages	2
Clubbing	2
Osler's nodes	2

* Percentages based only on cases in which clinical information was sufficient to allow evaluation regarding presence or absence of the particular physical sign.

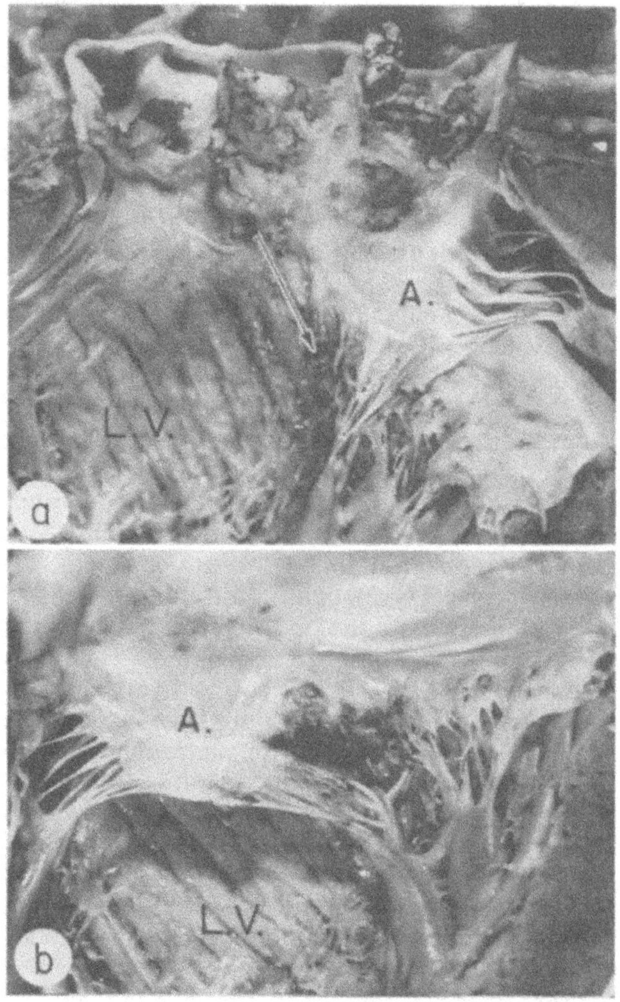

Figure 2. *Strep. faecalis endocarditis involving both aortic and mitral valves in a sixty-one year old man (DCGH No. 71A-120). Symptoms and signs of infective endocarditis appeared three weeks after catheterization of his urinary bladder. Both aortic and mitral valves were probably normal before they became sites of infection.* ***a,*** *opened left ventricle (L.V.) and aortic valve. The vegetations have partially destroyed each cusp causing severe aortic regurgitation. Vegetation on the left ventricular outflow endocardium and mitral leaflet and chordae tendineae almost certainly resulted from retrograde spread of the aortic vegetations by the aortic regurgitant stream* ***(arrow)****. A. = anterior mitral leaflet.* ***b,*** *opened mitral valve showing vegetations at the posteromedial commissure. A number of chordae tendineae are ruptured.*

volving only the aortic valve and in five (42 per cent) of twelve patients with infective endocarditis limited to the mitral valve. Papillary muscle necrosis was present in twenty (67 per cent) of thirty patients with valvular dysfunction and in one (12 per cent) of eight patients without valvular dysfunction ($p < 0.02$). Three patients with papillary muscle necrosis had coronary heart disease; one had more than 50 per cent luminal narrowing of the three major extramural coronary arteries by atherosclerosis as well as by an embolus to one extramural coronary artery; two patients had coronary arterial emboli to intramural coronary arteries located in a papillary muscle in one patient and in left ventricular free wall in the other. Nine patients without papillary muscle necrosis had coronary arterial disease: one due to atherosclerosis, eight due to emboli. The latter involved extramural coronary arteries in two and intramural vessels in six. Myocardial inflammation was observed histologically in twenty-three patients, nine of whom had abscesses. Myocardial inflammation was extensive in only one patient who had an eosinophilic myocarditis possibly due to a drug reaction. Interstitial myocardial fibrosis, observed in twenty-two of thirty-nine patients, was patchy and mild or minimal in all. One other patient had a healed transmural myocardial infarct. With the exception of papillary muscle necrosis, the presence or absence of other myocardial lesions (necrosis of ventricular free walls, inflammation, or fibrosis) did not correlate with the presence or absence of congestive heart failure.

Aortic valve cusps were perforated (fifteen patients) or otherwise partially destroyed (four patients) (Figures 2–6 and 12) in nineteen (65 per cent) of thirty-one patients with aortic valve vegetations, and all nineteen had aortic regurgitation and congestive heart failure. Mitral valve leaflets were perforated in three (12 per cent) of twenty-six patients with mitral vegetations. Ruptured chordae tendineae (Figure 2) were found in nine (35 per cent) of twenty-six patients with mitral valve vegetations.

Valve ring abscesses (Figures 3–6) were found in twelve patients, and each had aortic valve vegetations. The infective endocarditis in these patients was caused by D. pneumoniae in three, Staph. aureus in two, Staph. epidermidis in one, beta Streptococcus in one, Strep. faecalis in one, gram-positive coccus in two and was unknown in two. In only two patients were organisms seen in histologic sections of the ring abscesses. Of twenty patients with aortic regurgitation resulting from infective endocarditis, eleven had ring abscesses. Of twelve patients with aortic valve ring abscesses, eleven had severe regurgitation, and one had a previously stenotic valve. Two patients

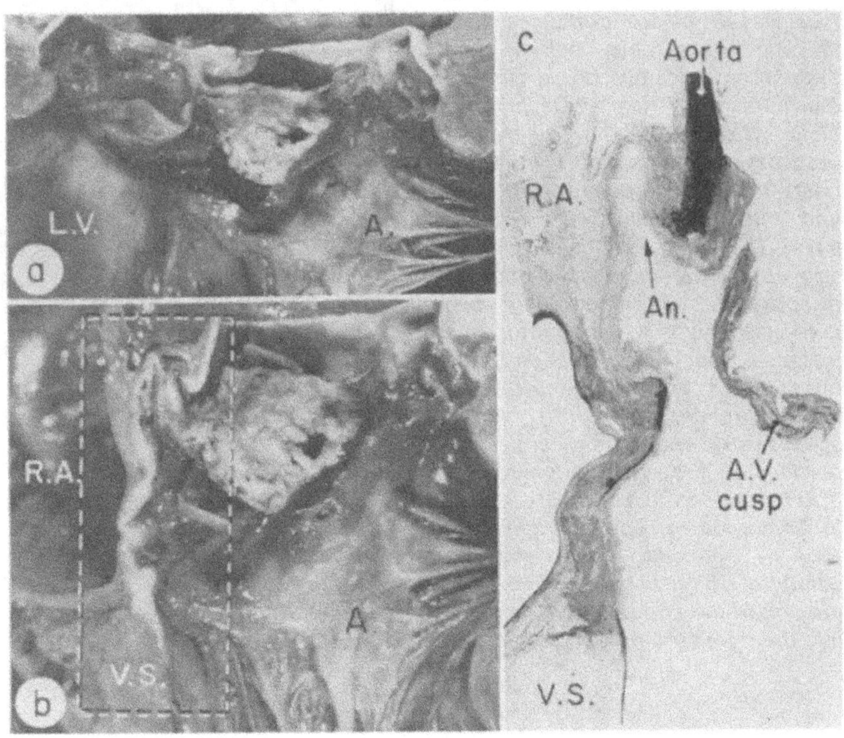

Figure 3. *Staph. epidermidis endocarditis in a twenty-two year old heroin addict (A69-313). The infection was on a congenitally bicuspid aortic valve which, although mildly incompetent before becoming infected, produced no symptoms.* ***a,*** *opened bicuspid aortic valve. L.V. = left ventricle; A. = anterior mitral leaflet.* ***b,*** *longitudinal section showing a huge perforation in one cusp and a subcuspal aneurysm, resulting from partial healing of a "ring" abscess. R.A. = right atrium; V.S. = ventricular septum. A photomicrograph of the area in brackets is shown in* ***c.*** *An. = aneurysm; A.V. = aortic valve. Elastic van Gieson stain; original magnification × 2, reduced by 19 per cent. A pericardial friction rub developed during hospitalization. Progressive aortic regurgitation and heart failure caused death twenty-one days after initiation of antibiotic therapy.*

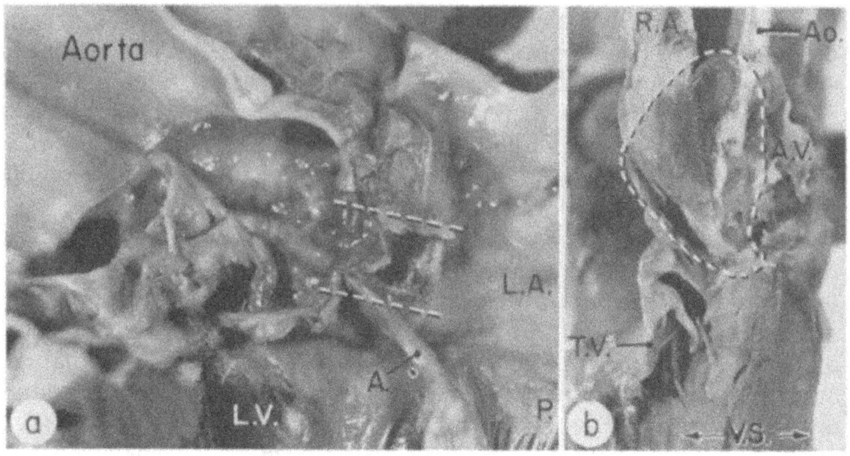

Figure 4. *Aortico-left atrial fistula caused by pneumococcal endocarditis in a fifty-four year old man with alcoholism (SH No. A71-28). After a one month history of cough and weakness he was hospitalized with overt signs of acute pneumonia, acute meningitis and congestive heart failure; he died within twenty-four hours. His blood pressure was 120/0 mm Hg.* ***a,*** *longitudinal section through aorta, aortic valve, anterior mitral leaflet (A.), left ventricle (L.V.) and left atrium (L.A.). The fistula, outlined by the dashed lines, presumably resulted from rupture of a "ring" abscess. The aortic valve is virtually destroyed by the infection. It was normal before the infection appeared. P. = posterior mitral leaflet.* ***b,*** *longitudinal section through aorta (Ao.), aortic valve (A.V.), ventricular septum (V.S.) and right atrial wall (R.A.). The infective process has extended into the right atrial and right ventricular walls. The area of the "ring" abscess is enclosed by the dashed lines. T.V. = septal tricuspid leaflet.*

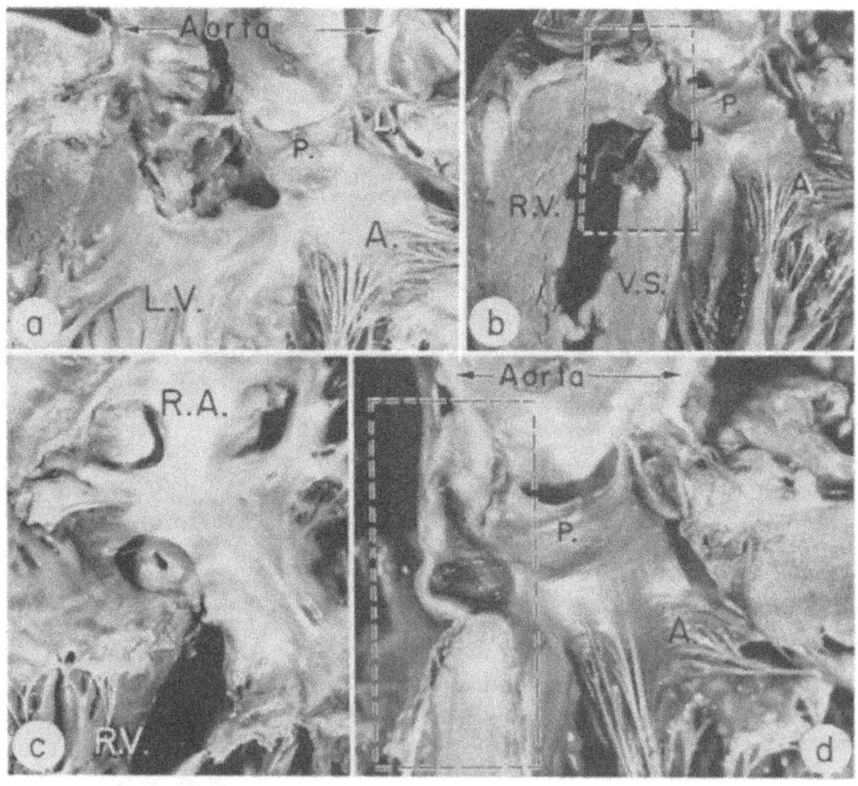

Figure 5. *Staph. epidermidis endocarditis in a seventeen year old boy with an aneurysm of the membranous ventricular septum (A69-42), possibly congenital in origin. Fever and exertional dyspnea developed four weeks before death. At hospitalization, ten days before death, systolic and diastolic precordial basal murmurs were heard. Despite antibiotic therapy, aortic regurgitation progressed, and he died of intractable heart failure.* ***a,*** *opened aortic valve and left ventricular (L.V.) outflow tract. The right cusp is virtually destroyed by the infective process. P. = posterior or noncoronary cusp; L. = left cusp; A. = anterior mitral leaflet.* ***b,*** *longitudinal section through right (R.V.) and left ventricles and ventricular septum (V.S.). An abscess is present in the most cephalad portion of the V.S. A photomicrograph of the area in brackets is shown in Figure 6a.* ***c,*** *opened right atrium (R.A.), tricuspid valve and right ventricle (R.V.) showing extension of the aneurysm of the membranous V.S. into the right atrium. A perforation is present in the aneurysm.* ***d,*** *longitudinal section through aorta and ventricular septum showing protrusion of aneurysm into the right atrium. A photomicrograph of the area in brackets is shown in Figure 6b.*

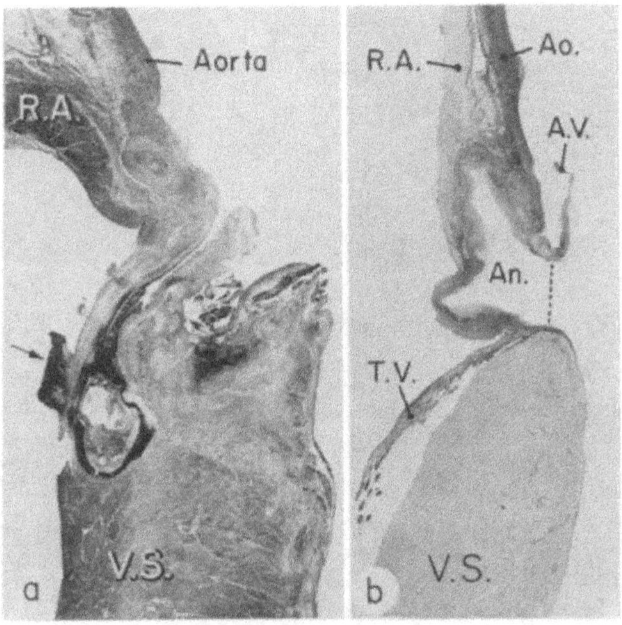

Figure 6. *Photomicrographs of longitudinal sections of ventricular septum (V.S.) at two levels in the patient described in Figure 5.* ***a,*** *section showing extension of the infective process through the entire thickness of the muscular V.S. A small vegetation (arrow) is apparent on the endocardium of the right side of the heart. R.A. = right atrium.* ***b,*** *section includes aneurysm (An.) of membranous portion of V.S. The dashed line represents the normal site of the membranous V.S. T.V. = tricuspid valve leaflet; A.V. = aortic valve cusp; Ao. = aorta. Phosphotungstic acid-hematoxylin stains; original magnification each × 2.9, reduced by 19 per cent.*

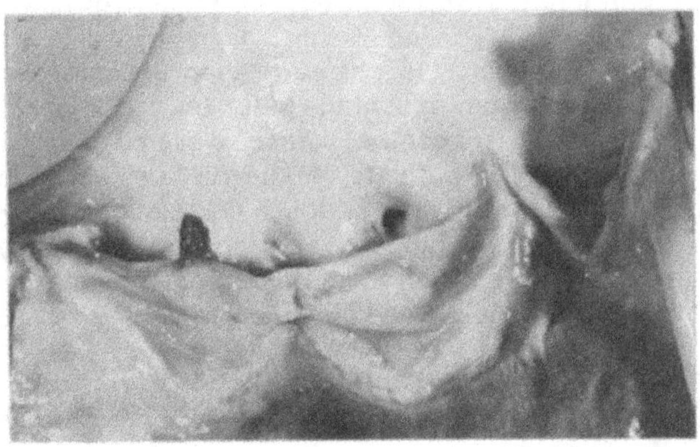

Figure 7. *Small vegetation on one aortic valve cusp in a fifty-three year old man with carcinoma of the prostate (A56-119). Endocarditis was not primary but occurred as part of a generalized staphylococcal septicemia. Organisms were present in this vegetation on histologic examination. Small vegetations like this one cause no cardiac dysfunction.*

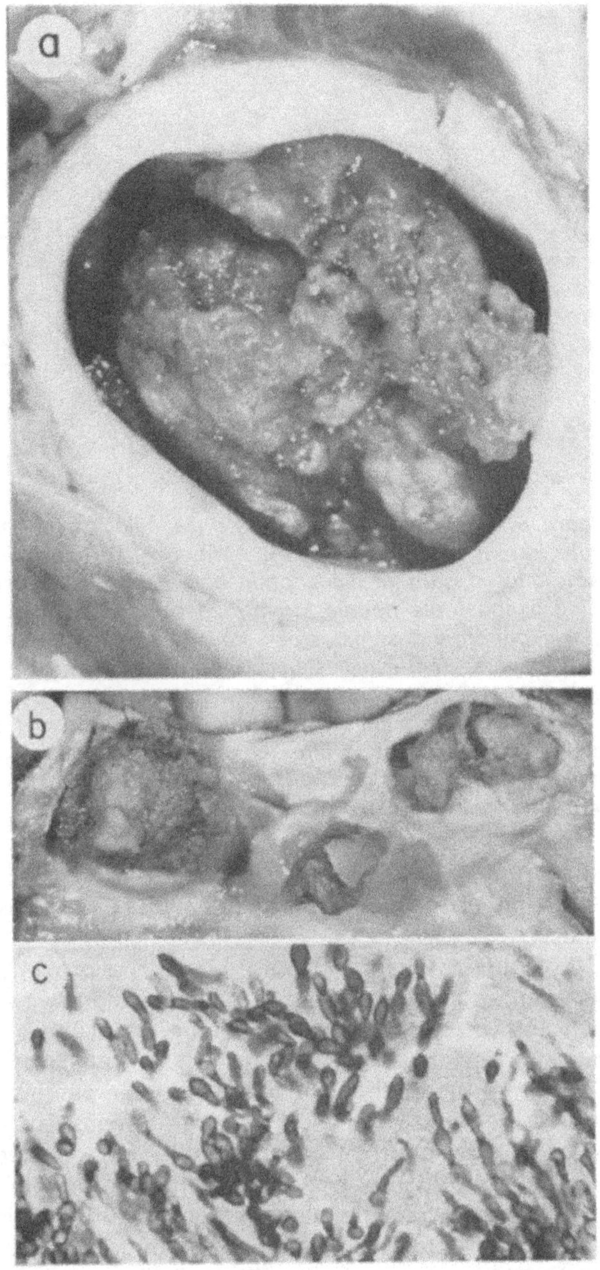

Figure 8. *C. parapsilosis endocarditis involving aortic valve of a twenty-six year old male heroin addict (A60-36). This patient, who was described elsewhere [56], lived for eight months after initial symptoms and signs of infective endocarditis appeared. He had an embolus to the left anterior descending coronary artery with a huge transmural acute myocardial infarct two months before death.* ***a,*** *aortic valve viewed from above. The large vegetations appear to obstruct the valve orifice.* ***b,*** *opened valve showing vegetations on each cusp.* ***c,*** *photomicrograph of vegetation showing pseudomycelia of C. parapsilosis. Methenamine silver stain; original magnification × 775, reduced by 9 per cent.*

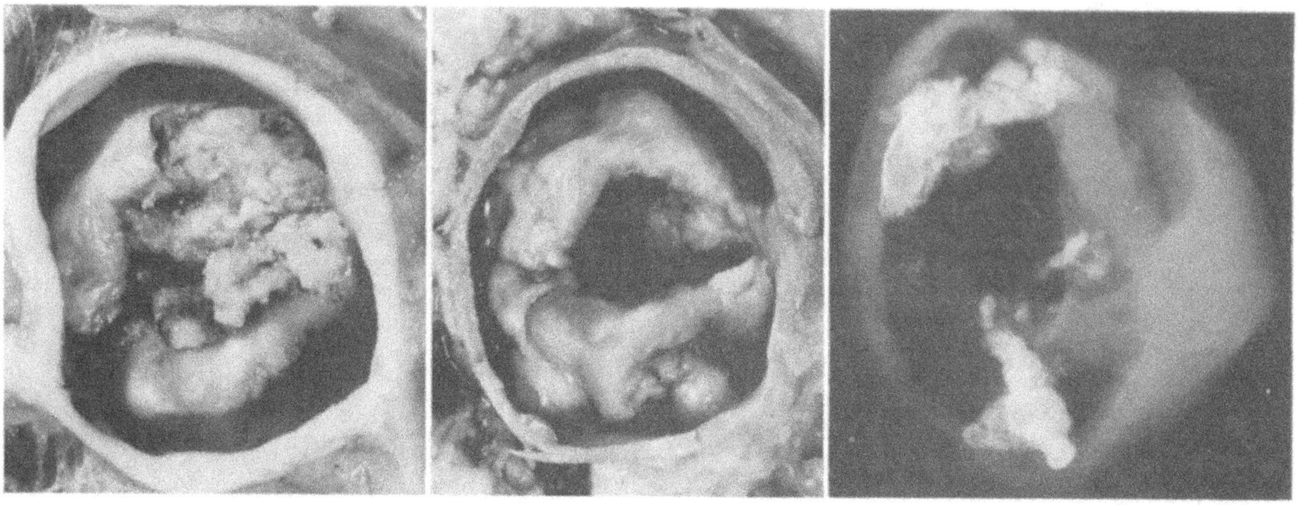

Figure 9. *Infective endocarditis on a calcified congenitally unicommissural aortic valve in a thirty-five year old male heroin addict (A70-181). Although a precordial murmur was present at age eighteen years he never had symptoms of cardiac dysfunction before endocarditis occurred. Ten weeks before death his left arm swelled after using a nonsterile needle for intravenous heroin injections. Seven weeks before death he noted painful red spots on his palms and soles. When hospitalized, six weeks before death, he had dermal and conjunctival petechiae, Roth's spots, Janeway lesions, a grade 5/6 systolic precordial murmur in the aortic area, a grade 2/6 diastolic blow of aortic regurgitation and a grade 3/6 apical systolic murmur; he was semistuporous. Electrocardiogram showed left ventricular hypertrophy. Numerous blood cultures were negative. Death resulted from congestive heart failure which developed after admission.* ***a,*** *aortic valve from above showing vegetations.* ***b,*** *aortic valve after removal of vegetations showing the densely fibrotic cusp with only one commissure (located at 3 o'clock).* ***c,*** *roentgenogram of aortic valve showing calcific deposits.*

with ring abscesses also had fistulas (Figures 4 and 5).

Mycotic aneurysm (Figure 12) of the proximal ascending aorta occurred in twelve patients, two of whom also had a mycotic aneurysm of the anterior mitral leaflet.

Acute pericarditis occurred in fourteen patients: in six of them it resulted from operation. Thus, eight (20 per cent) of the thirty-nine nonoperated patients had acute pericarditis. In none of the eight were organisms demonstrable in histologic sections of epicardium. All eight had fibrinofibrous pericarditis. One patient with a 1,200 ml serosanguineous pericardial effusion died of cardiac tamponade. The pericarditis in these eight patients resulted from extension of the inflammatory process into pericardium from ring abscesses (seven patients) or from a septic embolus to an extramural coronary artery (one patient).

Coronary arterial emboli (Figure 15) were seen in twelve patients: in three the embolus occluded an extramural coronary artery with resultant acute transmural myocardial infarct in two; in the other nine emboli were found on histologic examination only and in intramural coronary arteries.

Gross infarcts in various body organs occurred in twenty-nine (65 per cent) of the forty-five patients (Table XI), and, in addition, five patients had emboli to systemic arteries without infarcts. Multiple organs contained infarcts in twenty patients. Only nineteen of the thirty patients with organ infarcts were suspected clinically of having emboli.

Splenomegaly (weight more than 300 gm) was present in 52 per cent of the patients.

Histologic sections of kidney were reexamined in thirty-seven patients. Abnormalities were observed in twenty-nine patients (78 per cent); five had clinically significant renal disease. Acute pyelonephritis or interstitial inflammation was the most common renal lesion observed.

COMMENTS

Active infective endocarditis occurring on previously normal valves has been considered unusual. Of 1,056 necropsy patients with infective endocarditis summarized from several studies [11–22] in Table XII, 26 per cent had previously normal valves. In the present study of forty-five patients, 53 per cent had anatomically normal valves before the infection, and almost half of the remaining 47 per cent with anatomically abnormal valves had functionally normal valves. Thus, 76 per cent of our forty-five patients had functionally normal

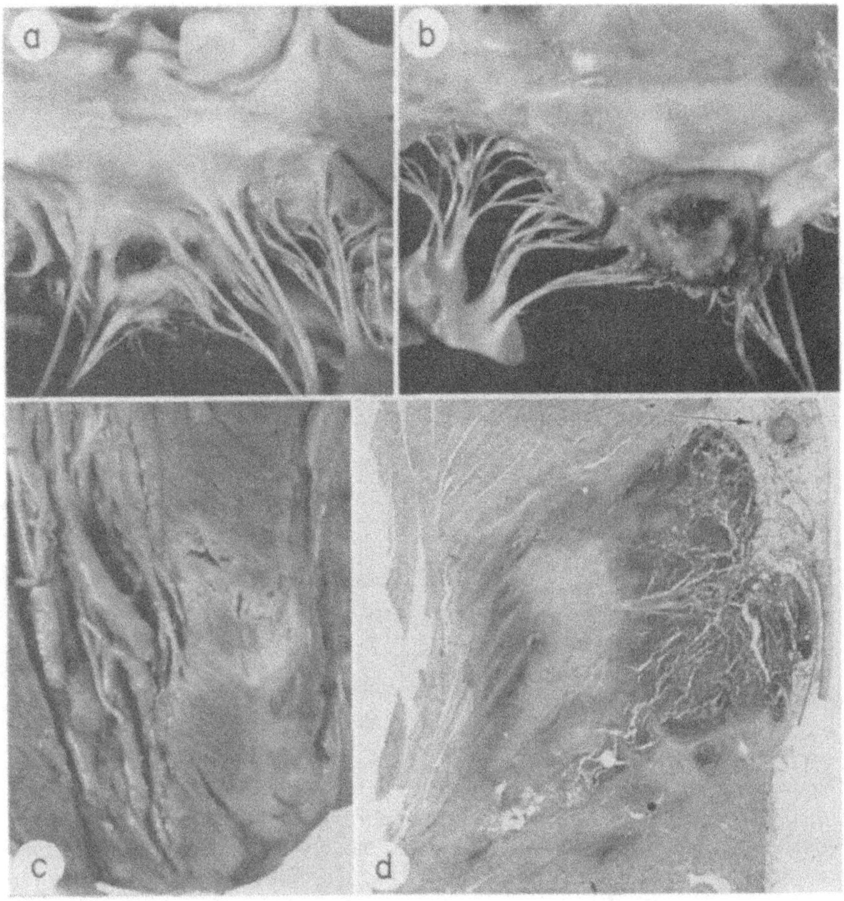

Figure 10. *Pneumococcal endocarditis on the mitral valve of a forty-three year old man with alcoholism (DCGH No. 71A-70). Two weeks before death he noted nausea, vomiting and diarrhea, and six days before death he was hospitalized for acute pneumonia and acute meningitis. He never had signs of cardiac dysfunction and died of gastrointestinal hemorrhage.* ***a,*** *opened left ventricle showing small amount of vegetative material on the ventricular surface of the anterior mitral leaflet.* ***b,*** *atrial aspect of anterior mitral leaflet showing one vegetation. The valve cusps otherwise are normal.* ***c,*** *longitudinal section through the apical portion of the left ventricular wall showing an area of transmural necrosis.* ***d,*** *photomicrograph of area in* ***c*** *showing extensive myocardial necrosis. An extramural coronary artery* ***(arrow)*** *is occluded by vegetative material. Hematoxylin and eosin stain; original magnification × 2.5, reduced by 21 per cent.*

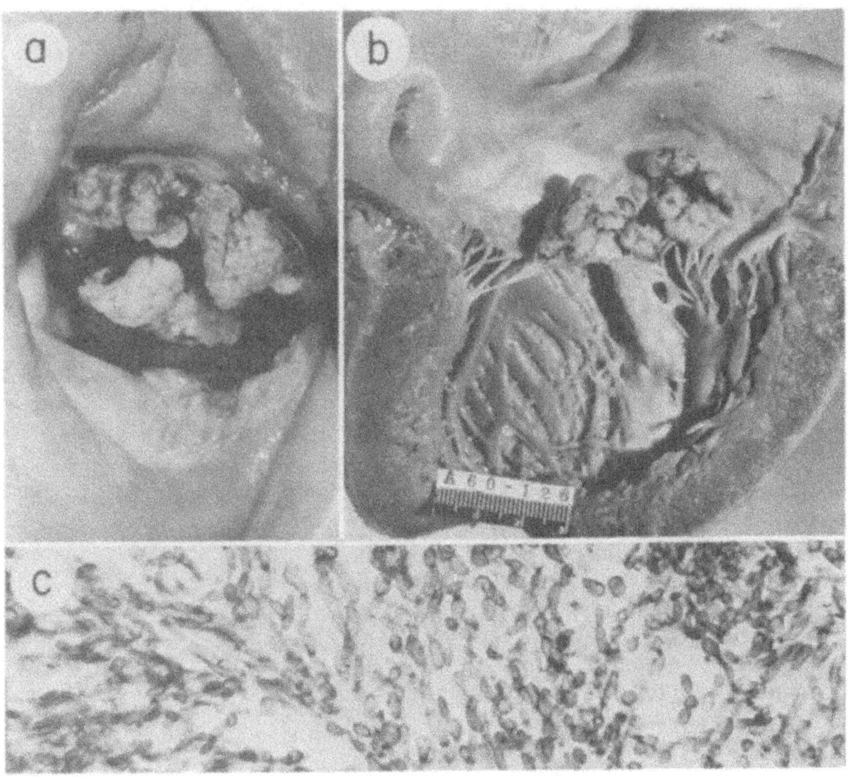

Figure 11. *C. parapsilosis endocarditis on a previously normal mitral valve of a sixty-eight year old man with chronic lung disease and coronary heart disease (A60-126). Five months before death he had fever, and forty-five days later he was hospitalized. A grade 2/6 apical systolic murmur was present. Despite amphotericin B therapy, blood cultures remained positive, and he died of congestive heart failure. A large embolus to the left common iliac artery occurred during hospitalization.* ***a,*** *mitral valve viewed from left atrium showing huge vegetations on both leaflets.* ***b,*** *opened left heart showing large vegetations on both mitral leaflets.* ***c,*** *photomicrograph of portion of vegetation showing spores and pseudomycelia of Candida species. Methenamine silver stain; original magnification × 500, reduced by 25 per cent.*

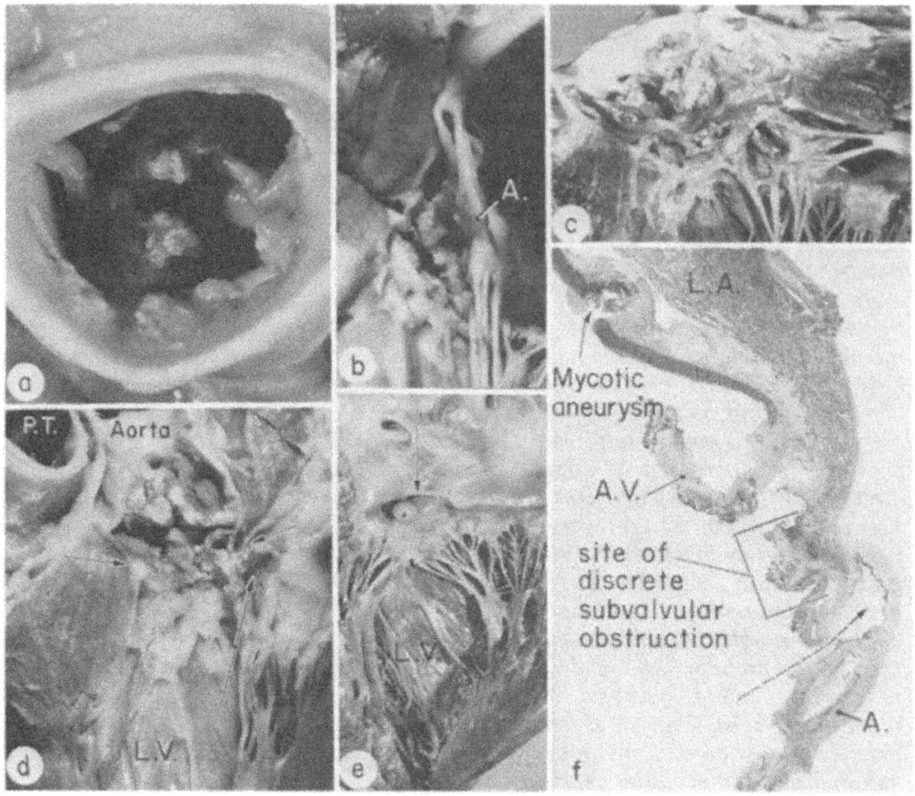

Figure 12. *Alpha hemolytic streptococcus endocarditis complicating congenitally discrete subaortic stenosis in a twenty-eight year old man (A64-20). The infection, which appeared about nine months before death, produced severe valvular aortic regurgitation. This patient was described previously [9].* ***a,*** *aortic valve as viewed from above.* ***b,*** *left ventricular outflow tract viewed from below showing vegetative material on the subvalvular "membrane" adjacent to the anterior mitral leaflet (A).* ***c,*** *opened left ventricular outflow tract showing vegetations on each aortic cusp and on the subvalvular "membrane" and ventricular surface of anterior mitral leaflet.* ***d,*** *longitudinal section showing the left ventricular outflow tract. The area of subaortic stenosis is well seen (between the solid arrows), and a mycotic aneurysm (dashed arrow) is seen in the anterior mitral leaflet. The mitral aneurysm is in the high pressure portion of the left ventricle (L.V.), i.e., below the discrete subvalvular obstruction. P.T. = pulmonary trunk.* ***e,*** *opened mitral valve showing atrial aspect of the mycotic aneurysm (dashed arrow) on the anterior leaflet.* ***f,*** *photomicrograph of section through aorta, left atrium (L.A.), aortic valve (A.V.) cusp, subvalvular "membrane," and anterior mitral leaflet (A.). A mycotic aneurysm is present in the ascending aorta as well as in the anterior mitral leaflet (dashed arrow). Vegetations are present on the aortic valve cusp and on the subvalvular membrane. Hematoxylin and eosin stain; original magnification × 3.2, reduced by 39 per cent.*

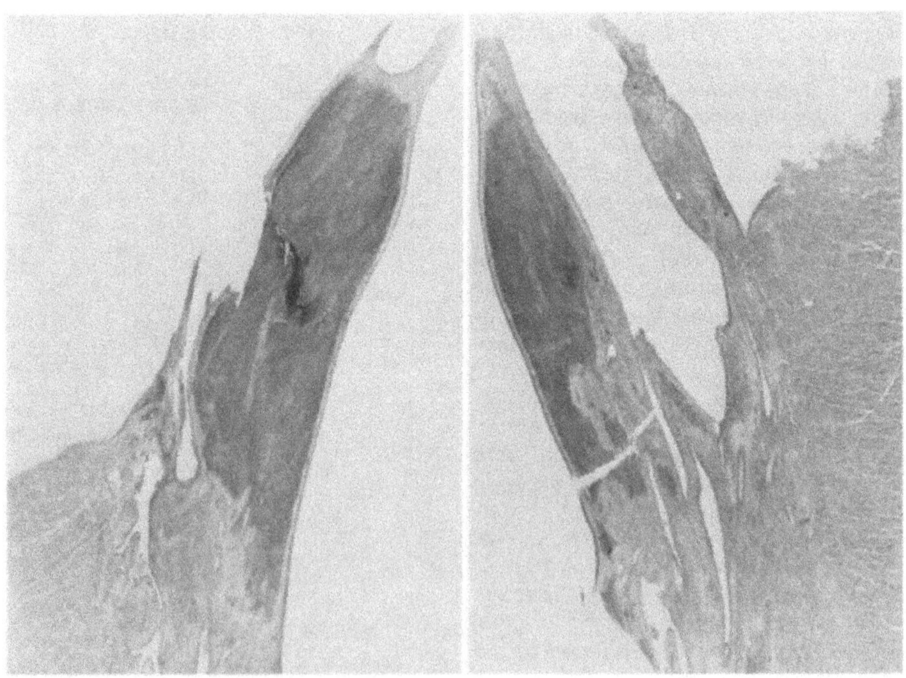

Figure 13. *Photomicrographs of both left ventricular papillary muscles of the patient described in Figure 3. Extensive necrosis is present in each papillary muscle while the left ventricular free wall is normal. Hematoxylin and eosin stain; original magnification × 4, reduced by 16 per cent.*

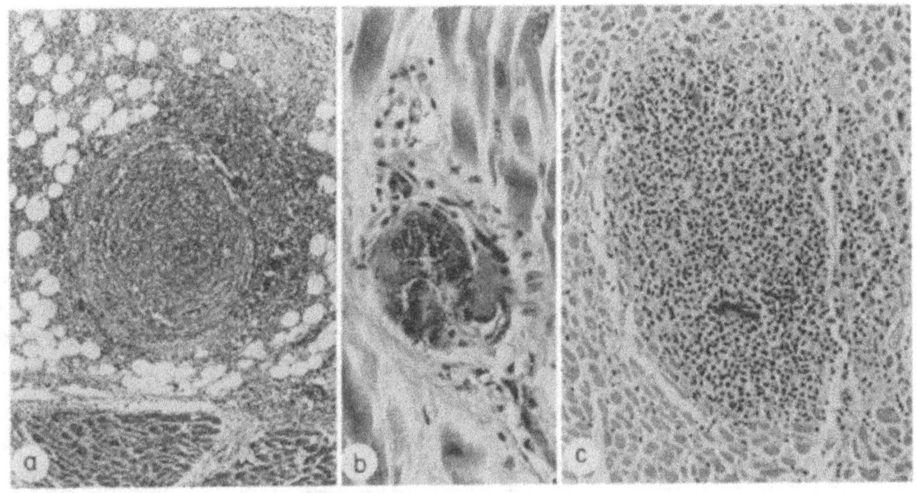

Figure 14. *Photomicrographs of acute inflammatory lesions in the heart in active infective endocarditis.* ***a,*** *extramural coronary artery occluded by vegetative material with resultant extension of the acute inflammation through the vessel wall and into epicardium and myocardium. Hematoxylin and eosin stain; original magnification × 80, reduced by 39 per cent.* ***b,*** *intramural coronary artery occluded by vegetative material containing numerous organisms. This thirty-six year old man (A65-8) had mycosis fungoides and generalized staphylococcal septicemia. Hematoxylin and eosin stain; original magnification × 400, reduced by 39 per cent.* ***c,*** *myocardial abscess with organisms in same patient described in* ***a.*** *Patient died of overwhelming pneumonia and renal failure without signs of cardiac dysfunction. Hematoxylin and eosin stain; original magnification × 220, reduced by 39 per cent.*

valves before the onset of infective endocarditis. When an anatomically normal cardiac valve is the site of infection, the organism is usually a highly virulent one (Staph. species, Pneumococcus) or a very unusual one (fungus, for example). When an anatomically abnormal valve is the site of infection, the organism tends to be a less virulent one (alpha hemolytic Streptococcus, for example). Thayer [12] noted infective endocarditis on previously normal valves in 63 per cent of seventy patients with pneumococcal or staphylococcal endocarditis but in only 20 per cent of patients with infective endocarditis caused by alpha hemolytic Streptococcus. Finland and Barnes [23] found clinically normal valves in 185 (68 per cent) of 271 episodes of infective endocarditis caused by an organism other than alpha hemolytic Streptococcus or Staph. epidermidis.

Infective endocarditis involving previously anatomically normal valves would appear to have a higher mortality than infective endocarditis involving previously anatomically and/or functionally abnormal valves [24]. In a study by Rabinovich et al. [25] ten (83 per cent) of twelve patients with

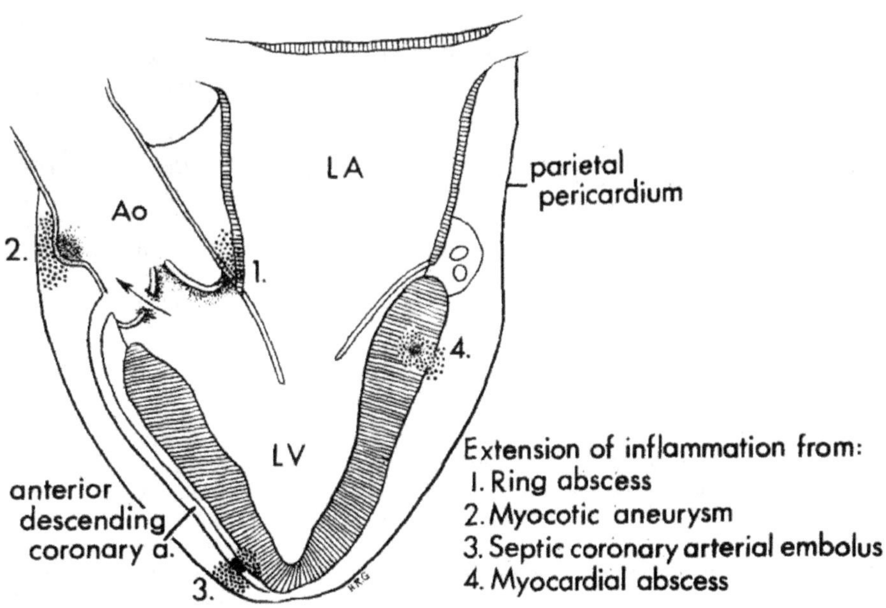

Figure 15. *Schematic portrayal of the pathogenesis of pericarditis in infective endocarditis. Ao = aorta; LV = left ventricle; LA = left atrium.*

infective endocarditis on normal valves died, whereas sixty-one (48 per cent) of 129 patients with infective endocarditis on previously abnormal valves died.

Predisposing factors were apparent in seventeen (71 per cent) of our twenty-four patients with infective endocarditis on previously normal valves and in thirteen (62 per cent) of twenty-one patients with infective endocarditis on previously abnormal valves. Of the thirty patients with predisposing factors eighteen were alcoholics, heroin addicts or had a malignancy, and fourteen (78 per cent) had previously anatomically normal valves before the onset of infective endocarditis. The presence of these various predisposing factors increases the likelihood that infective endocarditis will occur on previously normal valves, that it will be caused by an unusual or virulent organism and that it will carry a high mortality.

Myocardial lesions are frequent in patients with active infective endocarditis [11,12,16,17,21, 26–36] (Table XIII). Clawson [27], Buch-

TABLE IX Acute Myocardial Lesions in Left-Sided Infective Endocarditis (33* of 38† Patients = 87%)

Myocardial Lesion		Patients No.	Patients %
Necrosis‡		23	61
Papillary muscle only	18		
Papillary muscle + LV free wall	4		
Left ventricular free wall only	1		
Myocytolysis		21	55
Inflammation		23	61
Interstitial and perivascular (nonsuppurating myocarditis)	14		
Abscesses	2		
Both	7		

* Eleven patients with one or more of the three myocardial lesions listed had coronary arterial emboli and one other patient had severe coronary atherosclerosis.
† Includes only those subjects in whom sections of both left ventricular papillary muscles as well as left ventricular free wall or septum were available for examination.
‡ Unassociated with myocardial abscesses.

TABLE X Cardiac Findings in Left-Sided Infective Endocarditis (45 Necropsy Patients)

Lesion		Patients No.	Patients %
Perforated or partially destroyed cusp*		22	49
Aortic	19		
Mitral	3		
Mycotic aneurysm		12	27
Ascending aorta	12		
Anterior mitral leaflet	2†		
Ring abscess		12	27
Ruptured chordae tendineae		9	20
Mitral	9		
Pericarditis‡		8	20

* One patient each had a perforated aortic and mitral valve cusp as a result of a previous episode of IE.
† Each patient also had mycotic aneurysms of the ascending aorta.
‡ Six patients with operatively-induced pericarditis were excluded.

TABLE XI Gross Embolic Infarcts* in Left-Sided Infective Endocarditis (29 Patients = 65% of Total of 45)

Site	Patients No.	Patients %
Kidney	19	42
Spleen	17	38
Brain	15	33
Liver	3	7
Heart	2	4
Lung	1	2
Pancreas	1	2

* Total infarcts = fifty-eight of possible 203 organs of twenty-nine patients. In addition, five patients had emboli to systemic arteries without infarction.

TABLE XII Necropsy Incidence of Infective Endocarditis on Normal Valves

Source	Patients Total No.	With Normal Valves No.	With Normal Valves %
Clawson [11] 1924	132	47	36
Thayer [12,13] 1926, 1931	306*	92	30
Seabury [14] 1947	58	10	17
Traut et al. [15] 1949	94†	18	19
Cates, Christie [16] 1951	86	0	0
Perry et al. [17] 1952	52	19*	37
Morgan, Bland [18] 1959	56	8	14
Kalman et al. [19] 1962	80	34*	42
Wilson [20] 1963	103	16	16
Guze, Pearce [21] 1963	64	17	27
Lerner, Weinstein [22] 1966	25	8	32
Totals	1,056‡	269	26
Present series	45	24	53

* Refers to absence of congenital or rheumatic heart disease.
† Only patients more than sixty years old were included.
‡ At least 116 of these 1,056 patients had vegetations on right-sided cardiac valves [11,13,15–17,20,21]. Thus, if they could be excluded the number with normal valves would probably be about 20 per cent rather than 26 per cent.

binder and Saphir [29], Saphir [28] and Perry et al. [17] each observed myocardial lesions in 88 to 100 per cent of 187 patients studied by them at necropsy. Acute myocardial lesions were observed in thirty-three (87 per cent) of our thirty-eight necropsy patients in whom numerous histologic sections of myocardium were examined. The significance of the myocardial lesions observed in patients with infective endocarditis has been debated. Clawson [27] and Correll et al. [34] considered the lesions to be a major cause of congestive heart failure in patients with active infective endocarditis. de Navasquez [30] and Perry et al. [17], however, believed that congestive heart failure in patients with infective endocarditis was rarely the result of myocardial lesions. In none of our patients could we attribute congestive cardiac failure to the acute myocardial lesions. With the exception of two patients with severe coronary heart disease, congestive cardiac failure occurred in our patients only when valvular dysfunction was also present.

The location in the left ventricular wall of acute myocardial lesions in patients with active infective endocarditis has, to our knowledge, not been commented on previously. Although it has been described in infective endocarditis as the result of coronary arterial emboli [37,38], papillary muscle necrosis has not been commented on previously in patients with infective endocarditis in whom coronary narrowing was not present. Foci of necrosis were observed in left ventricular papillary muscles in twenty-two of our thirty-eight patients with active infective endocarditis, and in eleven they were diffusely necrotic. Only three of the twenty-two patients had coronary arterial narrowing: by emboli to intramural coronary arteries in two and by severe (more than 50 per cent luminal narrowing) atherosclerosis in one. The significant ($p < 0.02$) correlation between papillary muscle necrosis and valve dysfunction resulting in congestive heart failure suggests that the necrosis results from poor arterial perfusion associated with the heart failure since the papillary muscles are the last to be supplied by arterial blood [39]. Despite papillary muscle necrosis, no patient had mitral regurgitation in the absence of destruction of mitral leaflets or ruptured chordae tendineae. No patient with papillary muscle necrosis, however, had necrosis in the free wall beneath the papillary muscles.

Valvular dysfunction is the leading cause of congestive cardiac failure in patients with infective endocarditis. Of our forty-five patients with infec-

TABLE XIII Myocardial Lesions in Active Infective Endocarditis (IE)

Source	No. Necropsy Patients*	% Necrosis	% Fibrosis	Inflammation: % Nonsuppurating	Inflammation: % Suppurative	% Coronary Emboli	Total % With Lesions
Blumer [26] 1923	150	3	...	7	2	...	20†
Clawson [11] 1924	103	...	...	24	...	...	...
Thayer‡ [12] 1926	92	...	...	53§ 42#	23	...	...
Clawson [27] 1928	60	...	64	>74	22	...	88
Saphir [28] 1935	35	83¶	43	32	27‖	51	100
Buchbinder, Saphir [29] 1939	40	68	58	48	35‖	50	98
de Navasquez [30] 1939	20	...	...	95	...	80**	...
Middleton, Burke [31] 1939	49	14	47	10	4	...	...
Flaxman [32] 1943	252	...	...	...	3	...	...
Hildebrand, Priest [33] 1947	10	...	...	100	10	...	...
Correll et al. [34] 1951	44	...	...	80	...	...	...
Cates, Christie [16] 1951	442	...	...	..	...	4	...
Perry et al. [17] 1952	52	90‖	40	>51	>8	...	98
Pankey [35] 1961	60	...	...	...	...	8	...
Pankey [36] 1962	48	...	...	22	35	10	...
Guze, Pearce [21] 1963	64	...	...	74	...	...	...

* A few had IE involving right-sided cardiac valves but the exact number is uncertain.
† Includes 12 patients with "cloudy swelling."
‡ Includes patients with staphylococcal, pneumococcal, and streptococcal IE.
§ Acute inflammatory cells.
# Chronic inflammatory cells.
¶ Abscess used synonymously with focal necrosis.
‖ Refers to miliary infarcts.
** Refers to inflammation in areas with vessels; does not specify actual presence of emboli.

TABLE XIV Necropsy Evidence of Pericarditis

Source	Patients No.	With Pericarditis No.	%
Blumer [26] 1923	150	16	11
Clawson [11] 1924	132	24	21
Thayer [12] 1926	166*	16	10
Thayer [40] 1931–32	186	7	4
Middleton, Burke [31] 1939	49	12	24
Beck [41] 1942	43	8	16
Traut et al. [15] 1949	94	13	14
Pankey [35] 1961	60	9	15
Pankey [36] 1962	48	13	27
Robinson, Ruedy [42] 1962	267	37	14
Guze, Pearce [21] 1963	50	9	18
Totals	1,245	164	14
Present series	39†	8†	20

* Patients with pneumococcal, streptococcal and staphylococcal endocarditis only.
† Excludes six patients with operatively-induced pericarditis.

tive endocarditis, thirty-five had congestive cardiac failure, and thirty-three of them had severe valvular dysfunction. The remaining two had severe coronary heart disease. Although it is well appreciated that destruction of valvular cusps and chordae tendineae causes regurgitation, it is less well appreciated that vegetations may be large enough to actually obstruct a valve orifice. Valvular stenosis from large vegetations appears to have occurred in two of our patients [10].

The frequency of pericarditis in infective endocarditis is presented in Table XIV [11,12,15,21,26,31,35,36,40–42]. Middleton and Burke [31] reported pericardial rubs in 6 per cent of eighty-eight patients with active infective endocarditis. Even when recognized, pericarditis usually has been attributed to factors other than infective endocarditis, such as uremia [43], active rheumatic carditis [11] or myocardial infarction [44]. Pericarditis has been described in association with myocardial abscesses in the area of valve rings [41,45–47] and in association with mycotic aneurysms [41,48,49]. A site of extension of inflammation into the pericardium was found in each of our eight patients with pericarditis. The mechanisms of pericarditis resulting from infective endocarditis are shown in Figure 15.

Sheldon and Golden [50] called attention to the occurrence of ring abscesses in acute bacterial endocarditis. Infective endocarditis in their twelve patients was caused by Staph. aureus and D. pneumoniae. They did not find abscesses in eleven patients with subacute bacterial endocarditis. Ring abscesses were found in twelve of our forty-five patients. They occurred in patients with clinical courses longer than six weeks and in whom the causative organism was Strep. faecalis and Staph. epidermidis as well as Staph. aureus and D. pneumoniae. Aortic valve ring abscesses occurred in twelve of our thirty-one patients with aortic vegetations, eleven had severe aortic regurgitation and one had previous aortic stenosis. Several investigators have commented on the problem of valve replacement when the infection has extended into the "annulus." Wallace et al. [51] considered ring abscesses to probably preclude successful valve replacement. Stason et al. [52] postulated that annular involvement may contribute to postoperative paraprosthetic leaks. Several workers [53–55] have noted good operative results in the presence of ring abscesses.

REFERENCES

1 Cohn LH, Roberts WC, Rockoff SD, Morrow AG: Bacterial endocarditis following aortic valve replacement. Clinical and pathologic correlations. Circulation 33: 209, 1966.
2. Archard HO, Roberts WC· Bacterial endocarditis after dental procedures in patients with aortic valve prostheses. J Amer Dent Ass 72: 648, 1966.
3 Roberts WC, Morrow AG: Bacterial endocarditis involving prosthetic mitral valves. Clinical and pathologic observations. Arch Path (Chicago) 82: 164, 1966.
4. Buchbinder NA, Roberts WC: Active infective endocarditis confined to mural endocardium. A study of 6 necropsy patients. Arch Path (Chicago) (in press).
5 Lombardo TA, Rabson AS, Dodge HT· Mycotic endocarditis Amer J Med 22. 664, 1957.
6. Merchant RK, Louria DB, Geisler PH, Edgcomb JH, Utz JP. Fungal endocarditis. review of the literature and report of three cases. Ann Intern Med 48. 242, 1958.
7 Falcone MW, Roberts WC, Morrow AG, Perloff JG: Congenital aortic stenosis resulting from a unicommissural valve: clinical and anatomic features in 21 adult patients Circulation 44: 272, 1971
8. Roberts WC, Perloff JK, Constantino T: Severe valvular aortic stenosis in patients over 65 years of age A clinicopathologic study. Amer J Cardiol 27: 499, 1971.
9. Morrow AG, Fort L III, Roberts WC, Braunwald E: Discrete subaortic stenosis complicated by aortic valvular regurgitation Clinical, hemodynamic, and pathologic studies and results of operative treatment. Circulation 31· 163, 1965.
10. Roberts WC, Ewy GA, Glancy DL, Marcus FI· Valvular stenosis produced by active infective endocarditis. Circulation 36: 449, 1967.
11. Clawson BJ· An analysis of two hundred and twenty cases of endocarditis with special reference to the subacute bacterial type. Arch Intern Med (Chicago) 33: 157, 1924.

12. Thayer WS Studies on bacterial (infective) endocarditis. Johns Hopkins Hosp Rep 22. 1, 1926.
13. Thayer WS: Bacterial or infective endocarditis Edinburgh Med J 38. 237, 1931.
14. Seaburg JH. Subacute bacterial endocarditis: experiences during the past decade Arch Intern Med (Chicago) 79. 1, 1947.
15. Traut EF, Carter JB, Gumbiner SH, Hench RN. Bacterial endocarditis in the elderly. Geriatrics 4· 205, 1949
16. Cates JE, Christie RV. Subacute bacterial endocarditis A review of 442 patients treated in 14 centers appointed by the Penicillin Trials Committee of the Medical Research Council. Quart J Med 20. 93, 1951.
17 Perry EL, Fleming RG, Edwards JE. Myocardial lesions in bacterial endocarditis Ann Intern Med 36 126, 1952
18. Morgan WL, Bland EF: Bacterial endocarditis in the antibiotic era. Circulation 19 753, 1959.
19. Kalman C, Thomison JB, Shapiro JL Bacterial endocarditis. autopsy experience over a thirty year period. Southern Med J 55: 1208, 1962
20 Wilson LM: Pathology of fatal bacterial endocarditis before and since the introduction of antibiotics. Ann Intern Med 58: 84, 1963.
21 Guze LB, Pearce ML. Hospital-acquired bacterial endocarditis Arch Intern Med (Chicago) 112: 102, 1963.
22 Lerner PI, Weinstein L: Infective endocarditis in the antibiotic era. New Eng J Med 274. 199;259;388, 1966.
23. Finland M, Barnes MW Changing etiology of bacterial endocarditis in the antibacterial era Ann Intern Med 72: 341, 1970
24 Kerr A Jr· Subacute Bacterial Endocarditis, Springfield, Ill., Charles C Thomas, 1955, p 225.
25. Rabinovich S, Evans J, Smith IM, January LE: A long term view of bacterial endocarditis. Ann Intern Med 63. 185, 1965
26. Blumer G Subacute bacterial endocarditis. Medicine 2 105, 1923.
27 Clawson BJ: Myocarditis. Amer Heart J 4: 1, 1928.
28. Saphir O Myocardial lesions in subacute bacterial endocarditis Amer J Path 11· 143, 1935.
29. Buchbinder WC, Saphir O: Heart failure in subacute bacterial endocarditis. Arch Intern Med (Chicago) 64 336, 1939.
30. de Navasquez S· The incidence and pathogenesis of myocardial lesions in subacute bacterial endocarditis J Path 49. 33, 1939
31 Middleton WS, Burke M: Streptococcus viridans endocarditis lenta Amer J Med Sci 198: 301, 1939
32 Flaxman N. Myocardial abscess. JAMA 122: 804, 1943.
33. Hildebrand E, Priest W. Cardiac lesions in subacute bacterial endocarditis treated with penicillin Amer J Clin Path 17· 345, 1947.
34. Correll HL, Lubitz JM, Lindert MCF: Bacterial endocarditis: clinicopathologic studies of untreated, treated and cured patients. Ann Intern Med 35: 45, 1951.
35 Pankey GA· Subacute bacterial endocarditis at the University of Minnesota Hospital, 1939 through 1959 Ann Intern Med 55· 550, 1961
36. Pankey GA: Acute bacterial endocarditis at the University of Minnesota Hospital, 1939 through 1959 Amer Heart J 64. 583, 1962.
37 Case records of the Massachusetts General Hospital. Weekly clinicopathological exercises New Eng J Med 284 1084, 1971
38 Edwards JE Mitral insufficiency resulting from "overshooting" of leaflets Circulation 43 606, 1971
39 Estes EH, Dalton FM, Entman ML, Dixon HB III, Hackel DB The anatomy and blood supply of the papillary muscles of the left ventricle Amer Heart J 71, 356, 1966.
40 Tahyer WS Observations on rheumatic pericarditis and infective endocarditis. Ann Intern Med 5: 247, 1931–32
41. Beck D: Pericarditis and subacute bacterial endocarditis J Mount Sinai Hosp NY 8: 364, 1942
42 Robinson MJ, Ruedy J Sequelae of bacterial endocarditis. Amer J Med 32: 922, 1962.
43 Friedberg CK Diseases of the Heart, Philadelphia, W. B. Saunders, 1966, p 1384
44 Libman E Subacute bacterial endocarditis Brit Med J 2· 301, 1920
45. Gross L, Kugel MA: Topographic anatomy and histology of the valves of the human heart Amer J Path 7 445, 1931
46 Ryon DS, Pastor BH, Myerson RM. Abscess of the myocardium Amer J Med Sci 251: 698, 1966.
47 Berger HR, Kossmann CE: Solitary myocardial abscess in subacute bacterial endocarditis. Ann Intern Med 35 1125, 1951.
48. Pirani CL· Erosive (mycotic) aneurysm of the heart with rupture Arch Path (Chicago) 36· 579, 1943.
49 Bristow JD, Parker BM, Hang WA: Hemopericardium following rupture of a bacterial aortic sinus aneurysm Amer J Cardiol 6: 355, 1960.
50 Sheldon WH, Golden A: Abscesses of the valve rings of the heart, a frequent but not well recognized complication of acute bacterial endocarditis. Circulation 4: 1, 1951.
51. Wallace AG, Young WG Jr, Osterhout S Treatment of acute bacterial endocarditis by valve excision and replacement. Circulation 31: 450, 1965.
52. Stason WB, DeSanctis RW, Weinberg AN, Austen WG: Cardiac surgery in bacterial endocarditis. J Thorac Cardiovasc Surg 54: 491, 1967
53. Krutschmer KP, Lawrence GH. Valve replacement in patients with bacterial endocarditis. Amer J Surg 118 273, 1969
54 Symbas PN, Parr JA. Early surgical treatment for acute pneumococcal aortic valvulitis with aortic insufficiency, acquired ventricular septal defect, and aortico-right ventricular shunt. Ann Surg 167 580, 1968
55 Hurley EJ, Eldridge FL, Hultgren HN. Emergency replacement of valves in endocarditis. Amer Heart J 73 798, 1967.
56 Andriole VT, Kravetz M, Roberts WC, Utz JP Candida endocarditis. Clinical and pathologic studies. Amer J Med 32 251, 1962.

Left Ventricular Papillary Muscles

Description of the Normal and a Survey of Conditions Causing them to be Abnormal

By WILLIAM C. ROBERTS, M.D., AND LAWRENCE S. COHEN, M.D.

SUMMARY

The left ventricular papillary muscles appear to be the last portions of the heart to be perfused by coronary arterial blood. As a consequence they are sensitive anatomic markers of myocardial ischemia. Foci of necrosis or fibrosis therefore are commonly seen in these structures, particularly the posteromedial papillary muscle, which has a poorer blood supply than does the anterolateral muscle. Coronary arterial luminal narrowing is the most common cause of necrosis or fibrosis of the left ventricular papillary muscles. Other conditions, all associated with inadequate cardiac output, which may produce these lesions include left ventricular outflow tract obstruction, especially that resulting from congenitally malformed aortic valves, acute valvular regurgitation (infective endocarditis), various cardiomyopathies, and primary endocardial fibroelastosis with or without anomalous origin of one or both coronary arteries from the pulmonary trunk. Various infiltrative diseases, including inflammation (Aschoff bodies, sarcoid, abscesses), amyloid, iron, and neoplasms, also may involve the papillary muscles. Their most common congenital malformation is the parachute or single papillary muscle. Fibrosis or necrosis of adjacent left ventricle free wall without involvement of the papillary muscles themselves may simulate clinically "papillary muscle dysfunction." The anterior papillary muscle of the right ventricle is frequently affected by conditions which also affect the left ventricular papillary muscles. Whether or not necrosis or fibrosis of the right ventricular papillary muscle causes tricuspid regurgitation, however, is unknown at present.

Additional Indexing Words:
Coronary heart disease · Congenital heart disease · Myocardial infarction
Aortic stenosis · Idiopathic cardiomegaly · Cardiac surgery

ONE OF THE MOST significant advances in clinical cardiology during the decade of the 1960's was the appreciation of the importance of the left ventricular papillary muscles to closure of the mitral orifice during ventricular systole. It is now a well-recognized fact that hypoxia, necrosis, or fibrosis of the left ventricular papillary muscles may be associated with varying degrees of mitral regurgitation. Although coronary atherosclerosis is the most common cause of papillary muscle disease, scarred or necrotic papillary muscles have been observed in a number of conditions in which the coronary arteries were normal. Despite our increased awareness of disorders of the papillary muscles, a number of discrepancies have appeared which indicate that our knowledge about these structures is incomplete. For example, a number of patients without precordial murmurs during life have been observed at necropsy to have severe necrosis or fibrosis or both of one or both left ventricular papillary muscles; severe mitral regurgitation during or after acute myocardial infarction has been found at necropsy to be

From the Section of Pathology and the Cardiology Branch, National Heart and Lung Institute, National Institutes of Health, Bethesda, Maryland.

Address for reprints: Dr. William C. Roberts, Section of Pathology, National Heart and Lung Institute, National Institutes of Health, Bethesda, Maryland 20014.

Received January 10, 1972; revision accepted for publication February 7, 1972.

associated with normal papillary muscles, normal mitral leaflets and chordae tendineae, and normal-sized mitral annulae. This report attempts to clarify some of these discrepancies by reviewing some necropsy observations on the cardiac papillary muscles and correlating them with clinical findings.

Normal Left Ventricular Papillary Muscles

Each of the two left ventricular papillary muscles receives chordae tendineae from each mitral valve leaflet (fig. 1). Thus, damage to either papillary muscle may affect both leaflets. Each papillary muscle may be viewed as consisting of a major trunk from which an average of six heads or fingers project (fig. 2). Each papillary muscle has an average of 12 chordae tendineae per head. Each primary or first-order chorda tendinea divides into an average of two secondary or second-order chordae tendineae. Each second-order chorda divides into two or three tertiary or third-order chordae tendineae which attach to the mitral leaflet. Thus, for each primary chorda an average of five tertiary chordae result, and each head of a papillary muscle anchors two first-order and 10 third-order chordae. Consequently, each papillary muscle supports an average of 62 chordae actually attached to mitral leaflets, or both papillary muscles support about 124 third-order chordae or 24 first-order chordae. There is considerable variation, however, in the number of chordae tendineae attached to either papillary muscle or to either mitral leaflet.

Generally in a normal heart the thickness of either papillary muscle is about the same as is that of the left ventricular free wall or ventricular septum. The anterolateral (A-L) papillary muscle normally is slightly larger than the posteromedial (P-M) one. Just as the

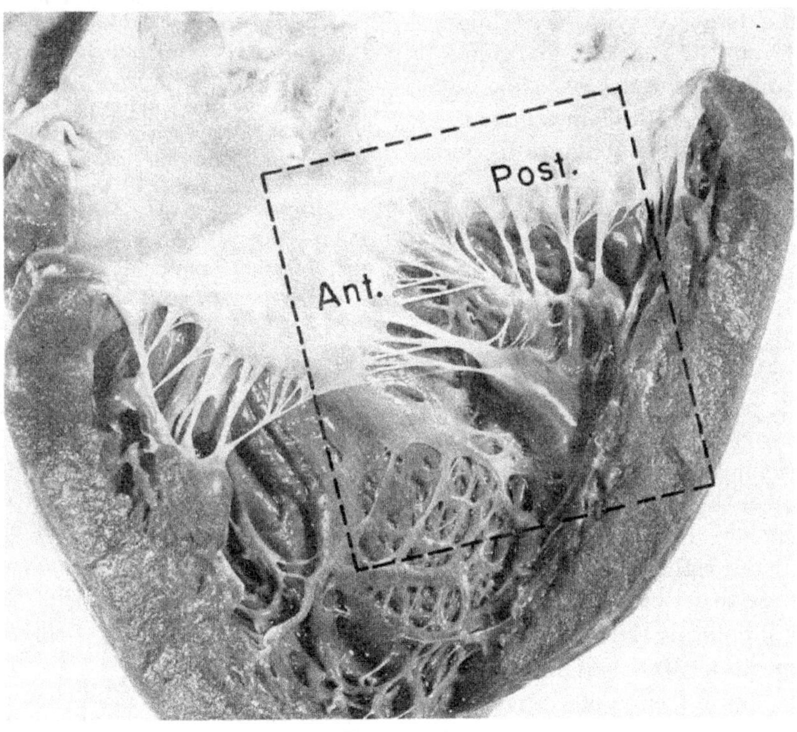

Figure 1

Normal left ventricular papillary muscles. The posteromedial (P-M) papillary muscle, its chordae tendineae, and portions of anterior (Ant.) *and posterior* (Post.) *mitral leaflets attached to it are enclosed by dotted lines. Each papillary muscle receives chordae from both mitral leaflets. Thus, rupture of one head or of the entire trunk of a papillary muscle alters support to both leaflets.*

P-M and A-L papillary muscles can differ from each other in the same heart, considerable morphologic variation is observed in comparing either or both muscles from one heart with those of another. The A-L papillary muscle usually (75%) consists of a single major muscle group, whereas the P-M papillary muscle often (65%) consists of two or three major muscle groups.[1] The basal to apex lengths of the papillary muscles also vary considerably. In most individuals the papillary muscles are attached to the left ventricular free walls over a large base and often by several trabecular bridges. Sometimes the site of attachment or anchorage is only slightly larger than the widest circumference of the papillary muscle. Ranganathan and Burch[2] called the former type of papillary muscle *tethered,* in contrast to the *fingerlike* type which protrudes freely into the left ventricular cavity with few or no trabecular attachments. Mixtures of these two types also exist. It is probable that the tethered type has a more abundant blood supply. The axis of orientation of the papillary muscles is generally parallel to the long axis of the left ventricular cavity which is nearly perpendicular to the left atrioventricular valve annulus.[3]

The A-L papillary muscle appears to have a richer blood supply than does the P-M one.[2, 3] Myocardial infarction involving the posterior left ventricular wall usually results in necrosis of the P-M papillary muscle, whereas anterior-wall infarction may spare the A-L papillary muscle.[4] The A-L papillary muscle is supplied by branches from both left anterior descending and left circumflex coronary arteries.[2, 3] The major supply of the P-M papillary muscle is dependent on which coronary artery is dominant. When the right coronary is dominant, and this is the situation in 90% of human hearts, its major supplier is the right coronary artery, and when the left one is dominant the major supplier is the left circumflex. The left circumflex contributes some blood, however, to the P-M papillary muscle no matter which coronary is dominant. The arrangement of the intramural coronary arteries supplying the papillary muscles appears to depend to some

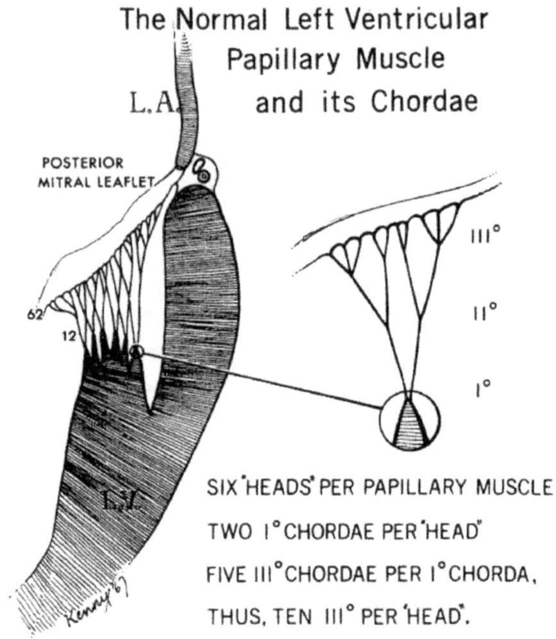

Figure 2

Diagram of a single normal left ventricular papillary muscle and its attached chordae tendineae. Each left ventricular papillary muscle contains an average of six "heads," each of which contains two primary or first-order chordae tendineae. Each primary cord subdivides into two secondary chordae, each of which divides into two or three tertiary or third-order chordae. The number of chordae attached to each left ventricular papillary muscle thus averages 12, and the number of chordae inserting directly into the mitral leaflets from a single papillary muscle averages 62. (These numbers resulted from counting chordae and papillary muscle heads in 12 normal hearts.) Thus, rupture of one papillary muscle head, which contains usually two primary chordae, causes loss of function of at least 10 tertiary chordae.

extent on their gross structure. When they have a fingerlike configuration one or several major intramural vessels (class B arteries of Estes et al.[3, 5]) arise from the epicardial branch, extend through the left ventricular free wall to the bases of the papillary muscles, turn uphill, so to speak, coursing to the apices of the muscles giving off branches along the way. When this artery is single it has been called the "central artery."[2] Papillary muscles or portions of them receiving the central artery usually have few or no anastomotic connections with the extrapapillary subendocardial plexus. The tethered papillary muscles usually do not have a single central artery but many small ones (class A arteries of Estes et al.[3, 5]) with rich anastomotic connections among themselves as well as with the extrapapillary subendocardial plexus.[2, 3]

Although their major blood supply is from intramural coronary arteries, the most peripheral portions of the left ventricular papillary muscles are perfused by intracavitary blood. The actual mechanism by which oxygen diffuses into the immediate subendocardial regions is uncertain. Possibly endocardial pores provide the means.

Abnormal Left Ventricular Papillary Muscles

Types of papillary muscle damage and the causes of the various types are outlined in table 1.

Anatomically Normal Papillary Muscles but Papillary Muscle Dysfunction

Transient ischemia of the papillary muscles is believed to be extremely common and probably results in varying degrees of mitral regurgitation.[6–8] A murmur of mitral regurgitation may occur during an attack of angina pectoris and be absent during pain-free periods.[6–10] Transient systolic murmurs during and after myocardial infarction probably result from papillary muscle ischemia. Arterial perfusion of the left ventricular papillary muscles may be influenced by body position. Brody and Criley[9, 10] documented severe mitral regurgitation and interscapular back pain in a man when he lay supine but both disappeared when he assumed an upright position. Possibly, transient ischemia of the papillary muscles may occur during emotional stress in individuals with normal or nearly normal coronary arteries in a manner similar to that which leads to constriction of the peripheral vascular beds during anxiety or during cigarette smoking.

Left ventricular dilatation of any origin is a frequent cause of papillary muscle dysfunction.[6–8] Under such circumstances the papillary muscles may contract normally, but the spatial relationships between the papillary muscles, the chordae tendineae, and the orifice are altered by the caudal and lateral migration of the left ventricular wall away from the mitral annulus. The valve leaflets are thus pulled downward into the left ventricle, and consequently the mitral orifice becomes incompetent. Also, the axes of the papillary muscles become more oblique with respect to the mitral annulus.

Although it may accompany left ventricular dilatation, mitral annular dilatation is probably a rare cause of mitral regurgitation, and most patients in the past with mitral regurgitation believed to be the result of mitral annular dilatation probably had papillary muscle dysfunction instead. Mitral annular dilatation to the degree capable of causing mitral regurgitation probably does not occur because the surface area of the mitral leaflets is about two times the area of the mitral orifice,[11] and the annulus contracts during ventricular systole.[12] Indeed, the mitral ring has a sphincter-like action since the mitral orifice is smaller during systole than during diastole.[12] In patients with dilated left ventricles, the widest diameter occurs not at the left ventricular base, the area which includes the mitral annulus, but in the midportion of the chamber between apex and base. Indeed, the base of the left ventricle is prevented from dilating freely because the "fibrous skeleton" is attached to it whereas the midportion of the left ventricle is not thus inhibited. Severe left ventricular dilatation may occur without any dilatation of the mitral annulus.

Although it is now well appreciated that mitral regurgitation may occur in patients with dilated left ventricles from any cause without associated left ventricular necrosis or fibrosis, it is less well recognized that necrosis or fibrosis of the left ventricular free wall unassociated with left ventricular dilatation or papillary muscle or mitral tissue lesions also may be associated with mitral regurgitation (fig. 3). Generally, the scarring or necrosis of the myocardium adjacent to the papillary muscles fails to move or moves paradoxically during ventricular systole and the abnormal ventricular contraction may lead to abnormal papillary muscle anchoring with resultant

Table 1

Spectrum of Left Ventricular Papillary Muscle Disease

I. Anatomically normal papillary muscles but papillary muscle dysfunction:
  - A. Transient ischemia
  - B. Left ventricular dilatation from any cause
    - 1. Generalized
    - 2. Localized
  - C. Necrosis or fibrosis in adjacent left ventricular free wall
    - 1. With coronary arterial narrowing
    - 2. Without coronary arterial narrowing
  - D. Small left ventricular cavity (hypertrophic cardiomyopathy)

II. Necrosis or fibrosis of papillary muscle(s) without rupture:
  - A. With coronary arterial narrowing
    - 1. Acute myocardial infarction
    - 2. Healed myocardial infarction
  - B. Without coronary arterial narrowing
    - 1. Acute
      - a. Shock
      - b. Acute valvular regurgitation (infective endocarditis)
    - 2. Chronic
      - a. Anemia
      - b. Left ventricular outflow obstruction
        - (1) Valvular aortic stenosis
        - (2) Discrete and diffuse subaortic stenosis
        - (3) Supravalvular aortic stenosis
      - c. Systemic hypertension
      - d. Origin of left coronary artery or of both coronary arteries from pulmonary trunk
      - e. Primary endocardial fibroelastosis of left ventricle
      - f. Endomyocardial disease and eosinophilia
        - (1) Löffler's fibroplastic parietal endocarditis
        - (2) Endomyocardial fibrosis of Davies
      - g. Idiopathic cardiomegaly (primary or diffuse myocardial disease)
      - h. Focal myocardial disease
        - (1) Idiopathic
        - (2) "Neurogenic" heart disease
          - (a) Progressive muscular dystrophy
          - (b) Friedreich's ataxia
          - (c) Myotonic muscular dystrophy

III. Necrosis or fibrosis of papillary muscle(s) with rupture:
  - A. Acute myocardial infarction from coronary heart disease
  - B. Trauma
  - C. Miscellaneous

  Types of papillary muscle rupture
    - 1. Total ("belly or trunk") → rapid death
    - 2. Partial ("head")
      - a. Rapid death
      - b. Survival but chronic congestive heart failure

IV. Infiltrative diseases of papillary muscles:
  - A. Pyogenic abscess
  - B. Granulomas
    - 1. Aschoff bodies
    - 2. Sarcoid
  - C. Amyloid
  - D. Neoplasm
  - E. Calcium

(Continued on next page)

F. Iron
G. Other

V. Congenital malformations of papillary muscle(s):
A. Single papillary muscle (parachute mitral valve syndrome)
B. Accessory papillary muscle
C. Abnormally large and malpositioned papillary muscles
D. Abnormally small and malpositioned papillary muscle
E. Insertion of papillary muscle directly into mitral leaflet

VI. Miscellaneous afflictions of papillary muscle(s):
A. Excision, partial or complete, during mitral valve replacement
1. Atrophy of nonexcised portion of papillary muscle after valve replacement
2. Left ventricular aneurysm at site of papillary muscle excision
B. Disuse atrophy after excision of mitral leaflets and chordae without excision of papillary muscle(s)

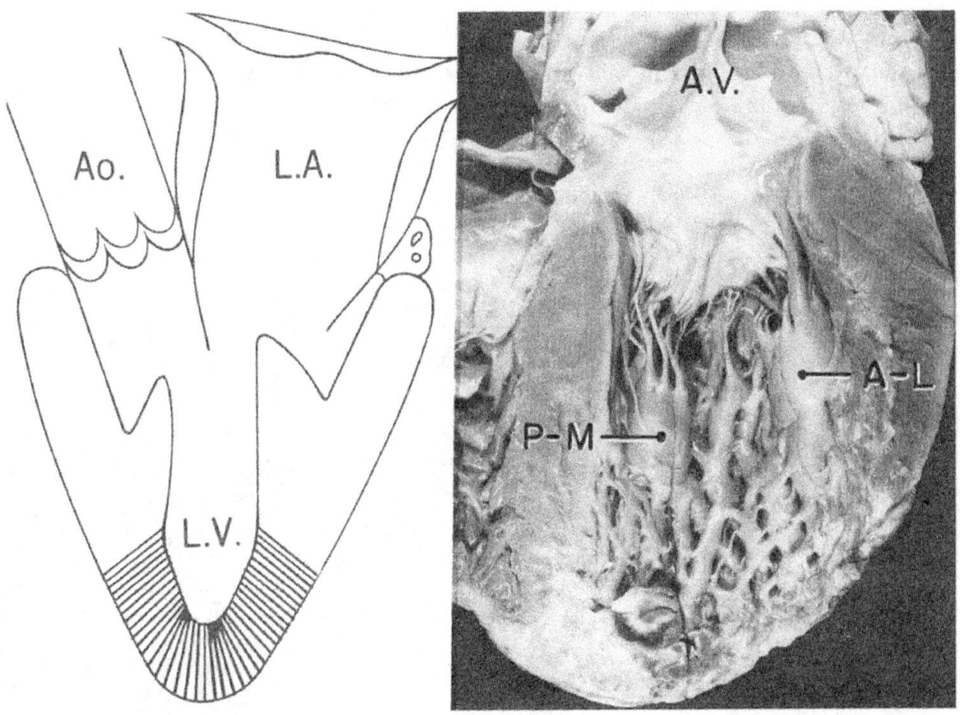

Figure 3

Mitral regurgitation from scarring of the left ventricular free walls but not of the papillary muscles. The heart shows severe scarring of the left ventricular wall from the base of the papillary muscles to the cardiac apex, but the posteromedial (P-M) and anterolateral (A-L) muscles are spared from significant scarring. This 72-year-old man (A68-83) had an acute myocardial infarct at age 60 years. He was well thereafter until age 69 (3 years before death) when mild congestive cardiac failure appeared, but no precordial murmur was heard. On examination 9 months before death a grade I/VI pansystolic apical murmur was heard. Five months later severe congestive heart failure appeared, and cardiac catheterization was performed. The left atrial v waves ranged from 60 to 75 mm Hg and left ventricular cineangiocardiogram disclosed 3+/4+ mitral regurgitation. Despite this angiographic documentation of mitral regurgitation the precordial murmur was never louder than grade I/VI intensity and located in early and midsystole only. Cardiotomy was performed 3 months before death. The anterior mitral leaflet was found to herniate into the left atrium during ventricular systole but the mitral leaflets and chordae appeared normal. The mitral valve was plicated but congestive cardiac failure, which ultimately was fatal, persisted postoperatively.

mitral regurgitation.[8, 13] Anatomic left ventricular aneurysms unassociated with papillary muscle necrosis or fibrosis may cause mitral regurgitation by the same mechanism (fig. 4).

Abnormal pulling on the papillary muscles unassociated with left ventricular necrosis or fibrosis or with cavity dilatation may occur in patients with hypertrophic cardiomyopathy, and this mechanism may account for the mitral regurgitation in them.[14] The huge thickening of the ventricular septum—the thickest portion is midway between left ventricular base and apex[15]—may distort or bend the anterolateral papillary muscle and prevent proper contraction of this structure during ventricular systole.

Necrosis or Fibrosis of Papillary Muscle(s) without Rupture

Necrosis and fibrosis of one or both left ventricular papillary muscles is extremely common. The necrosis or fibrosis may be either focal or diffuse, involving only one papillary muscle or both, and auscultatory mitral regurgitation may or may not be present. When they are focal, the papillary muscle lesions are generally of two types: (1) involve nearly all the distal or apical portion of the papillary muscle, or (2) involve many areas throughout the entire papillary muscle. The latter lesions usually are small and spare areas adjacent to intramural coronary arteries.[16] When only one papillary muscle contains foci of necrosis or fibrosis it is virtually always

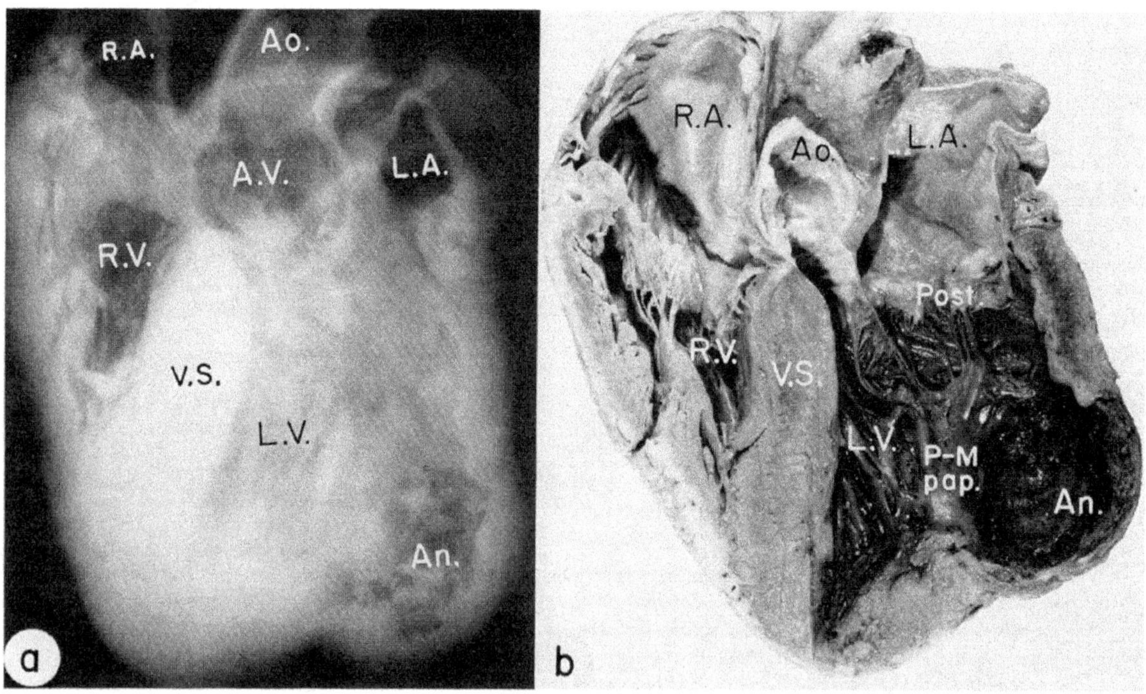

Figure 4

Radiograph of heart specimen (a) *and longitudinal section of heart* (b) *in a 65-year-old man (A67-71) who had an acute myocardial infarct 2 months before death with subsequent development of a left ventricular* (L.V.) *aneurysm* (An.) *located in the lateral wall. He developed a murmur consistent with mitral regurgitation. Both left ventricular papillary* (pap.) *muscles grossly appeared normal but their bases were adjacent to the aneurysm. The mitral regurgitation can probably be attributed to the poor anchorage of the papillary muscles as a result of the aneurysm.* R.A. = *right atrium;* R.V. = *right ventricle;* V.S. = *ventricular septum;* L.A. = *left atrium;* A.V. = *aortic valve;* Ao. = *aorta.*

the P-M muscle, since this one has the poorer blood supply.

It is now clear from experimental studies[17–19] that mitral regurgitation is not a consequence of fibrosis involving only papillary muscles themselves. If one or both left ventricular papillary muscles are made fibrotic in the dog, either by injection of formalin or by ligating the base of the muscle, no regurgitation of contrast material from left ventricle to left atrium later occurred on angiographic studies. If, however, the free wall beneath the papillary muscle was made fibrotic at the same time so that ventricular contraction was impaired, mitral regurgitation did result. We have observed a number of patients at necropsy with extensive fibrosis or necrosis of one or both left ventricular papillary muscles, and no precordial murmur had been audible during life. Fibrosis or necrosis of the left ventricular papillary muscles and of the free walls beneath them, however, does not necessarily assure the appearance of a precordial murmur of mitral regurgitation during life. Several patients with silent mitral regurgitation by auscutation have been shown to have mitral regurgitation when left ventricular injection of contrast material also was performed.[20, 21] Necrosis or fibrosis has been observed at necropsy in these patients to involve the papillary muscles extensively and the entire thickness (transmural) of the left ventricular free wall.[21] Silent mitral regurgitation during acute myocardial infarction has been attributed to a diminished flow velocity across the mitral valve secondary to diminished myocardial contractility.[20]

The most common cause of papillary muscle necrosis or fibrosis is narrowing of the coronary arterial lumen by atherosclerosis.[4, 22, 23] The P-M papillary muscle is usually involved in acute posterior myocardial infarction. In anterior-wall infarction, however, the A-L papillary muscle may be spared, presumably because its blood supply is better than that of the P-M muscle. Since infarction limited to the ventricular septum or to the lateral portion of the left ventricular free wall (i.e. the portions of the left ventricular wall unassociated with papillary muscles) is rare, the papillary muscles are usually involved when myocardial infarction occurs. It, therefore, is surprising that papillary muscle dysfunction is not more frequently observed during or after acute myocardial infarction.

Necrosis or fibrosis of one or both left ventricular papillary muscles is frequent in a number of conditions unassociated with luminal narrowing of the extramural coronary arteries. Inadequate oxygenation of the papillary muscles may occur if the amount of oxygen in the blood is low (i.e., anemia) or if the cardiac output for any reason is inadequate. It is well to keep in mind that the left ventricular papillary muscles are the last portions of the heart to be perfused with coronary arterial blood. To perfuse the apices of the papillary muscles the coronary artery must extend through the entire thickness of the myocardial free wall, turn up hill, and ascend a distance of at least one and often two thicknesses of the free wall. Consequently, it is of little wonder that these structures often show evidences of inadequate oxygenation. Furthermore, the papillary muscles serve as the most sensitive markers of inadequate myocardial oxygenation. Since the P-M papillary muscle is less well perfused than the A-L one, if only one shows foci of necrosis or fibrosis it will nearly always be the P-M muscle. We have observed foci of necrosis in these papillary muscles in patients with anemia from a variety of causes, particularly chronic anemias like sickle-cell disease (fig. 5).

In patients with left ventricular outflow obstruction, lesions are often observed in the papillary muscles. [24–28] Valvular aortic stenosis, whether in infants [24, 25] or in adults, [26–28] when superimposed on a congenitally malformed valve, either unicuspid or bicuspid, is nearly always associated with fibrosis and atrophy of at least the P-M papillary muscle. Rheumatic valvular aortic stenosis combined with organic mitral stenosis or regurgitation, however, infrequently is associated with papillary muscle fibrosis or

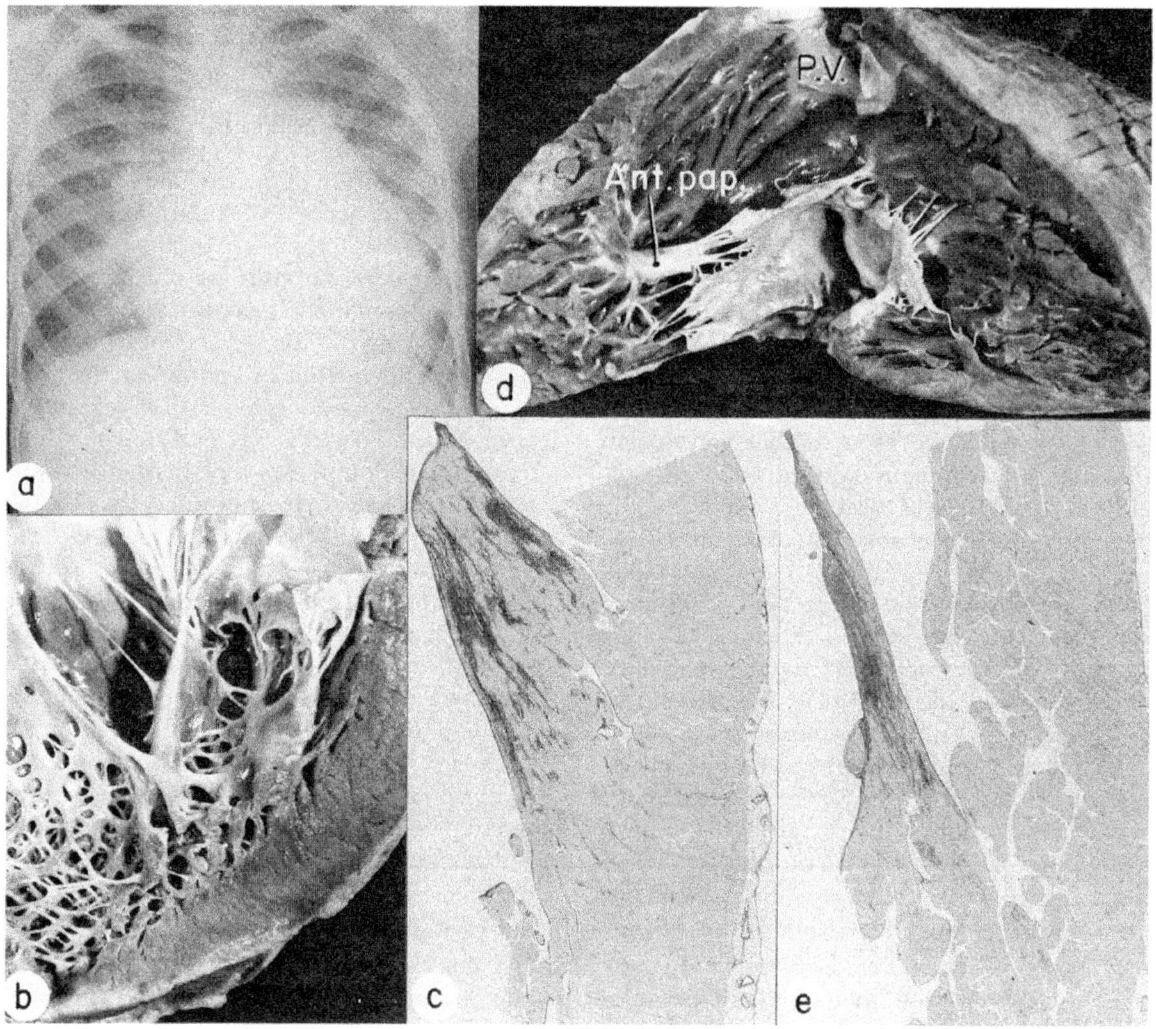

Figure 5

The heart in a 14-year-old girl (A69-13) with sickle-cell disease diagnosed by hemoglobin electrophoresis when she was 4 years old. She had multiple sickle-cell crises and at age 12 years developed congestive cardiac failure. During her last 6 months she had nightly paroxysmal dyspnea and multiple episodes of exertional syncope. She had a grade II/VI systolic murmur over the pulmonic area. Electrocardiogram showed right-axis deviation, right ventricular hypertrophy, and P-pulmonale. The pulmonary arterial pressure was 47/13 mm Hg, and the cardiac output was 6.5 liters/min. (a) *Chest roentgenogram.* (b) *Posteromedial (P-M) left ventricular papillary muscle.* (c) *Section of P-M papillary muscle showing focal fibrosis.* (d) *Opened right ventricle showing fibrosis of the anterior* (Ant.) *papillary* (pap.) *muscle.* P.V. = *pulmonic valve.* (e) *Section of scarred anterior right ventricular papillary muscle. The papillary muscle fibrosis is presumably related to the chronic anemia.*

atrophy. Nearly all adult patients with discrete subaortic stenosis or hypertrophic cardiomyopathy with or without diffuse subaortic stenosis have small fibrous scars in both left ventricular papillary muscles, but severe atrophy of one or both muscles is uncommon.

Foci of necrosis also are common in patients with fatal severe valvular regurgitation of recent onset. Among 47 patients dying of active valvular infective endocarditis, 34 (72%) had necrotic lesions in one or both left ventricular papillary muscles, and none had

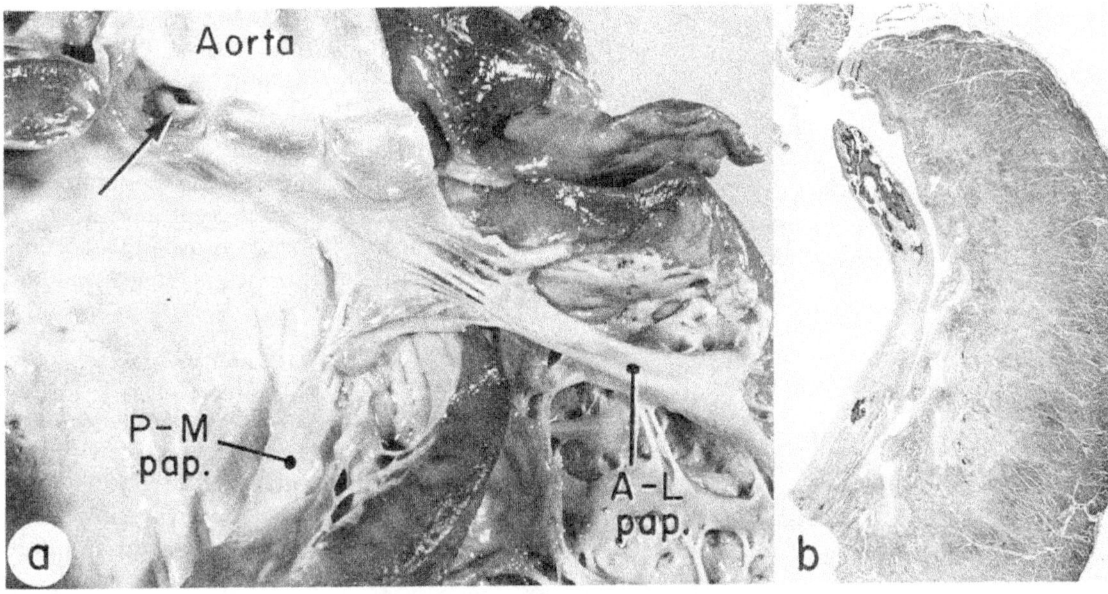

Figure 6

Severe diffuse fibrosis and calcification of the anterolateral left ventricular papillary muscle in a 9-month-old girl (A56-14) in whom the left coronary artery arose anomalously from the pulmonary trunk. She had a grade III/VI systolic precordial murmur. Diffuse endocardial fibroelastosis of the left ventricle and left atrium also was present. **(a)** *Opened left ventricle, aortic valve, and aorta. The ostium of the right coronary artery is designated by the arrow. No left ostium is observed. The distal half of the A-L papillary muscle is severely scarred and calcified.* **(b)** *Section of the fibrotic, atrophied, and calcified A-L papillary muscle. (Hematoxylin and eosin stain, × 4.)*

significant narrowing of the extramural coronary arteries.[29] Most patients had pure aortic regurgitation, but some had pure mitral regurgitation secondary to the active infective endocarditis. Severely diminished cardiac output with resultant poor myocardial perfusion was believed to be the cause of the papillary muscle necrosis in them.

Small fibrous scars in the papillary muscles are common in patients with systemic hypertension but atrophy of these structures in this condition, unless coronary heart disease also is present, is infrequent. When left ventricular hypertrophy occurs from any cause, the hypertrophy of the papillary muscles probably should be proportional to that of the left ventricular free wall or ventricular septum. This proportional hypertrophy usually exists in cases of systemic hypertension, but infrequently in patients with left ventricular outflow obstruction.

Fibrosis with atrophy of the papillary muscles is to be expected in patients with primary endocardial fibroelastosis of the left ventricle.[30] Histologically, the thickened endocardium in this condition is similar to the media of the aorta, being characterized by the presence of elastic fibrils running parallel to one another and to the surface. Primary left ventricular endocardial fibroelastosis may represent simply an anatomic expression of chronically inadequate coronary arterial perfusion of the left ventricle, and, since the P-M papillary muscle is the least well-perfused portion of the heart, this structure is affected the most. In the congenital condition, origin of the left[31] or both[32] coronary arteries from the pulmonary trunk, diffuse endocardial fibroelastosis of the left ventricle is nearly always an associated lesion. Fibrosis and atrophy of the left ventricular papillary muscles is to be expected in this anomaly, and these patients may present clinically with features of pure mitral regurgitation[33] (fig. 6).

PAPILLARY-MUSCLE RUPTURE

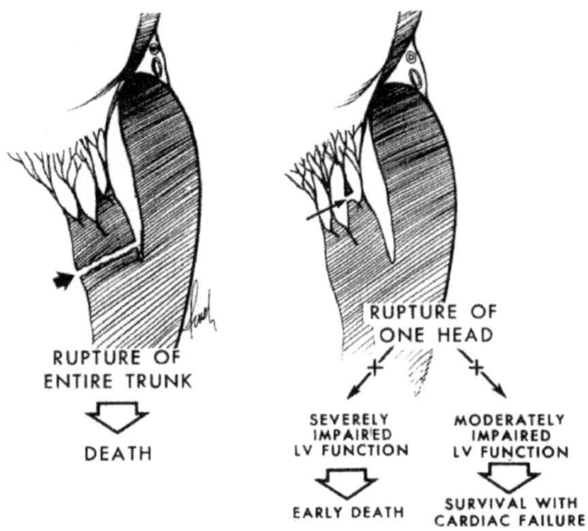

Figure 7

Diagram depicting two major types of papillary muscle rupture. It is likely that rupture of the entire trunk (acute myocardial infarction or trauma) **(left)** *is incompatible with survival since a major portion of the support to both valve leaflets is destroyed. With rupture of an apical head* **(right)**, *survival would appear to depend upon the extent to which the function of the left ventricle has been impaired by necrosis. With severely impaired ventricular function, the additional burden of even modest mitral regurgitation may be intolerable, and death is quick. If the left ventricle is less severely compromised, survival is possible for weeks or months, but congestive cardiac failure will almost invariably develop.*

Foci of fibrosis or necrosis in the left ventricular papillary muscles are infrequent in patients with the congestive or dilated type of cardiomyopathy. Severe scarring of one papillary muscle and of the free wall beneath it was responsible for severe mitral regurgitation in a patient with primary myocardial disease studied by Marcus et al.[34] Generally, however, left ventricular cavity dilatation alone is the cause of mitral regurgitation in these patients. Rarely, myocarditis may be localized to papillary muscle and adjacent left ventricular free wall.[35] Patients with the neurogenic heart diseases (Friedreich's ataxia, progressive muscular dystrophy, and myotonic muscular distrophy)[36] generally have scarred left ventricular papillary muscles, especially the P-M one. The African cardiomyopathy—endomyocardial fibrosis—may be associated with extensive scarring of the papillary muscles.[37] Usually the P-M one in this condition is covered by a thrombus or by dense fibrous tissue which may represent organization of thrombus. Likewise, Löffler's fibroplastic parietal endocarditis, which may represent one stage of endomyocardial fibrosis,[38] is usually associated with extensive scarring of one or both papillary muscles.[39]

Necrosis or Fibrosis of Papillary Muscle with Rupture

In contrast to necrosis of a papillary muscle which occurs in over 50% of patients with fatal acute myocardial infarction,[4] rupture of a papillary muscle is rare, occurring in < 1% of patients with fatal acute myocardial infarction. The rupture may be of two types (fig. 7). One involves the entire central muscle belly of the papillary muscle and this type rupture is incompatible with survival since half the support to each valve leaflet is destroyed and mitral regurgitation of overwhelming severity results. The second type of rupture involves only one or two apical heads of a papillary muscle. The resulting mitral regurgitation is of lesser magnitude, and immediate survival is then dependent upon the degree to which the function of the left ventricle has been impaired by the infarct. In patients who survive after papillary muscle rupture, the functional capacity of the left ventricle also will govern the extent of clinical and hemodynamic improvement after mitral valve replacement.[40]

Although the entire papillary muscle is usually necrotic, the mitral regurgitation resulting from rupture of an entire trunk of a papillary muscle may justifiably be attributed entirely to the rupture. In contrast, the mitral regurgitation following rupture of only one head of a left ventricular papillary muscle cannot necessarily be attributed entirely to the rupture since the remainder of the papillary muscle is nearly always also necrotic. What percentage of the regurgitant volume is due to the rupture of a single head and what percentage to the associated papillary muscle necrosis is uncertain. Rupture of a single

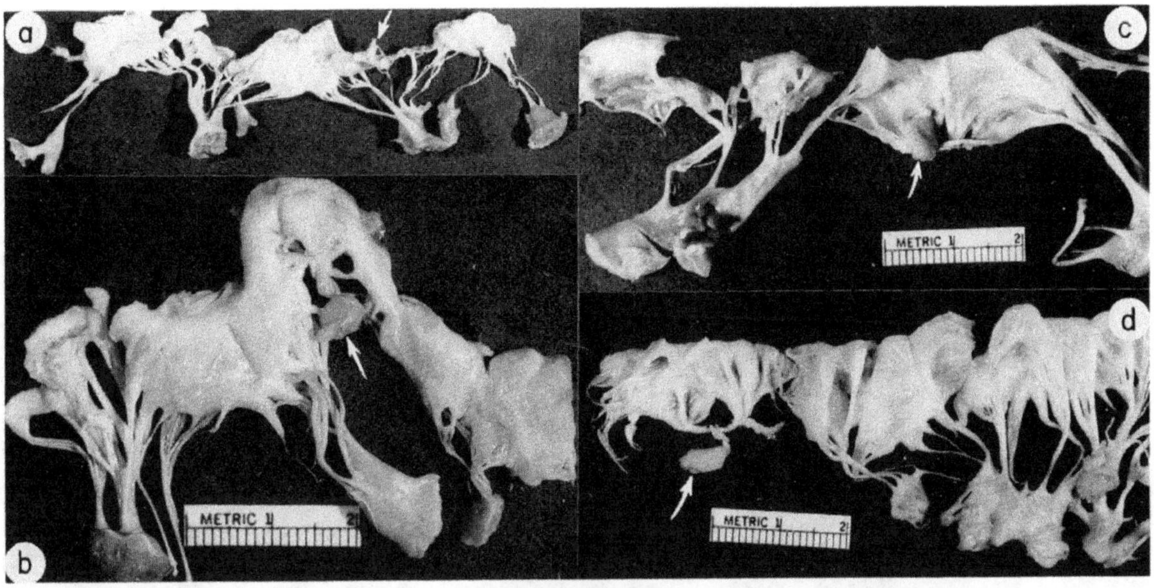

Figure 8

Operatively excised mitral valves in four patients demonstrating rupture of a papillary muscle head in each. Acute myocardial infarction (AMI) had occurred in each 15 months (**a**), *13 months* (**b**), *3 months* (**c**), *and 14 months* (**d**) *earlier. All four patients were men, aged 51 to 69 years at the time of operation, and all developed loud (grade III-IV/VI) systolic murmurs typical of mitral regurgitation at the time of AMI. Congestive cardiac failure persisted after AMI. The arrows designate the ruptured papillary muscle heads. All four patients died within 3 years of operation. (The valve replacements were performed by Dr. Andrew G. Morrow.)*

primary chorda tendinea in the dog, however, produces immediate severe mitral regurgitation;[41] consequently, rupture of a head, which is equivalent to rupturing two primary chordae tendineae, must in itself be severe. Ruptured papillary muscle heads in four patients are illustrated in figure 8. Each patient was described in detail elsewhere.[40]

Although coronary arterial luminal narrowing by atherosclerosis accounts for most cases of ruptured papillary muscle, trauma may cause either partial or complete rupture of these structures. Blunt trauma, however, when severe enough to cause papillary muscle rupture, is also usually severe enough to rupture the left ventricular free wall. Brock[42] described total rupture of a papillary muscle during mitral commissurotomy, and death ensued in two days.

Infiltrative Diseases of Papillary Muscles

The papillary muscles are subject to various infiltrative processes just like any other portion of myocardium. Pyogenic abscesses, Aschoff bodies, granulomas (fig. 9),[43] neoplasms, amyloid,[44] and iron[45] have all been observed in these structures. Congestive heart failure from severe mitral regurgitation may be the initial symptom of sarcoidosis (fig. 9).

Congenital Malformations of the Left Ventricular Papillary Muscles

The most frequent congenital malformation of these structures is the occurrence of only one papillary muscle (fig. 10). This condition, described as the parachute mitral valve, consists of only one left ventricular papillary muscle to which all mitral chordae tendineae are attached.[46] The resulting mitral valve is usually stenotic,[46] but it may be purely incompetent[47] or it may function normally.[47] The single papillary muscle is usually associated with other malformations including a supramitral valve ring, diffuse subaortic stenosis, and coarctation of the aorta.[46] Other malformations, including valvular aortic stenosis, ventricular septal defect, and valvular

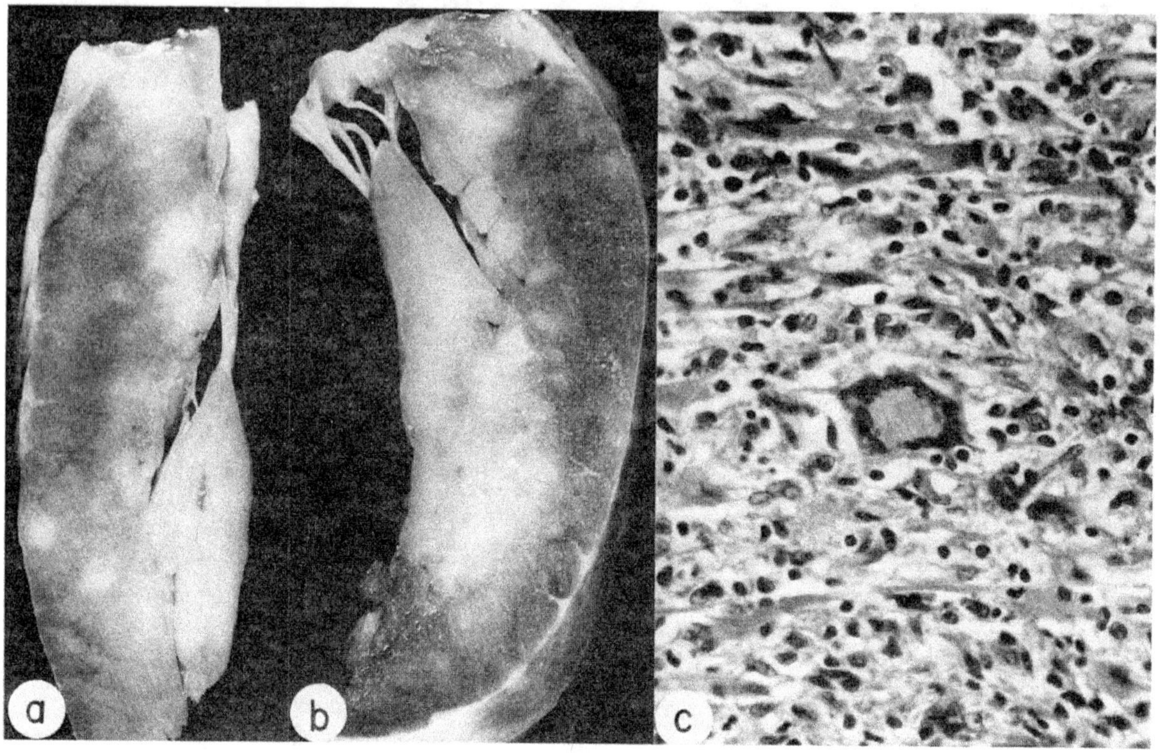

Figure 9

Anterolateral (a) *and posteromedial* (b) *left ventricular papillary muscles in a 26-year-old woman (PGGH A-70-541) who was asymptomatic until 10 days before death when dyspnea appeared. The dyspnea rapidly worsened, and when hospitalized on the day of death she was in acute pulmonary edema. The blood pressure was 80/70 mm Hg, heart rate 160 beats/min, and a grade III–IV/VI pansystolic blowing apical murmur, which radiated into the axilla, was audible. Chest roentgenogram showed congested lungs, cardiomegaly, and prominent hilar adenopathy. Electrocardiogram showed nonspecific ST-T wave changes and atrial hypertrophy. Several hours after admission ventricular fibrillation occurred, she was resuscitated, but complete heart block appeared. A transvenous pacemaker was inserted, but asystole occurred shortly thereafter. At necropsy, large firm white deposits were present in the walls of all four cardiac chambers and completely replaced both left ventricular papillary muscles* (a *and* b). *On histologic section, the firm white areas represented hard granulomas typical of* **sarcoidosis** *as seen in* (c). *(Hematoxylin and eosin stain, × 400.) Similar hard granulomas were present in lymph nodes, liver, spleen, and lung. Stains for acid-fast organisms, other bacteria, and fungi were negative. (Specimen was kindly provided by Dr. James Hutchinson.)*

pulmonic stenosis also may occur in association with the single left ventricular papillary muscle.[47] The single papillary muscle malformation may be the most common cause of congenital mitral stenosis.[48]

Not only may one too few papillary muscles occur, but one too many also may occur. An accessory papillary muscle is usually of no functional significance but it has been seen in association with congenital mitral regurgitation.[49] Two papillary muscles may be present and yet one or both still be congenitally malformed. Each of the two papillary muscles may be abnormally large and malpositioned so that the primary orifice of the valve is narrowed.[48, 50] The malpositioning consists of origin of the papillary muscles at sites higher in the left ventricle than normal. Both papillary muscles also may be poorly developed and small. This finding is particularly characteristic of origin of the left coronary artery from the pulmonary trunk. In the latter

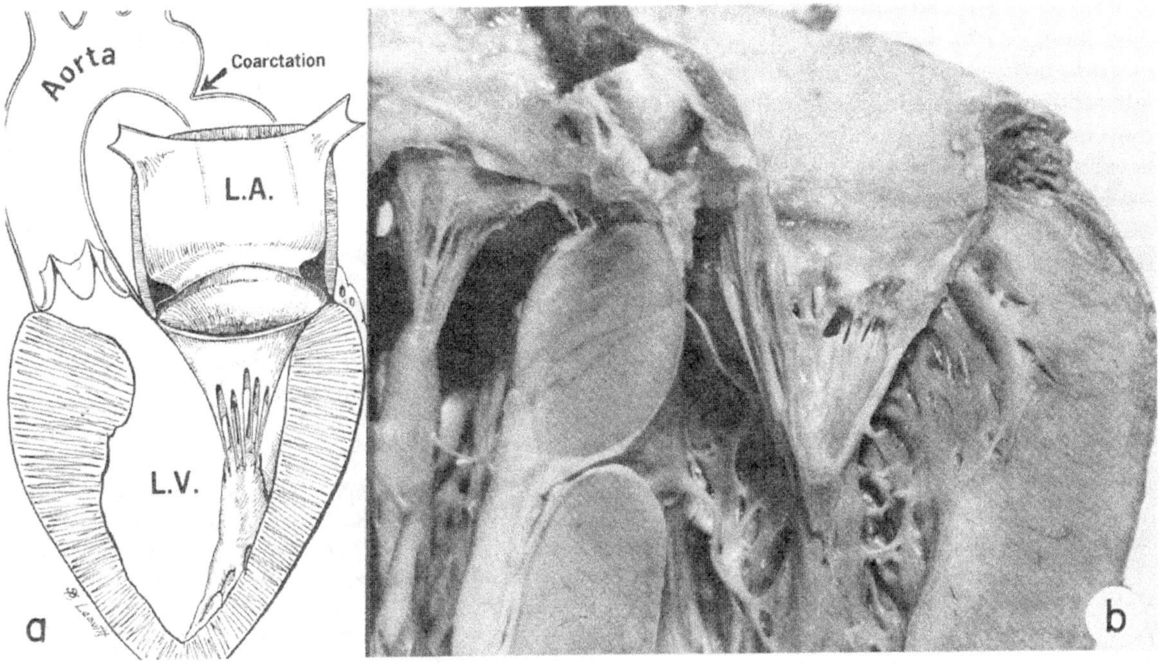

Figure 10

Single left ventricular papillary muscle or parachute mitral valve syndrome. Most patients with a single left ventricular papillary muscle also have a partial or completely circumscribing ring just above the mitral valve or at its annulus, subaortic stenosis, and aortic isthmic coarctation **(a)**. *Other anomalies, particularly ventricular septal defect and valvular aortic stenosis, as shown here* **(b)**, *are also common. A single left ventricular papillary muscle with a parachute mitral valve from a 14-year-old boy (GT#71A-215) is shown in* **(b)**. *In addition, this child had severe valvular and discrete subvalvular aortic stenosis as well as spontaneous closure of a ventricular septal defect. The aortic valve was congenitally bicuspid. The peak systolic pressure gradient between left ventricle and systemic artery was 80 mm Hg. He died in acute pulmonary edema. He had been asymptomatic until 1 year before death. No abnormality of the mitral apparatus was apparent clinically. (This child was cared for by Dr. Joseph K. Perloff.)*

condition the papillary muscles also arise high on the left ventricular wall.[48] Contrasted to the normal heart wherein the papillary muscles arise at the junction of the middle and lower thirds of the left ventricle, in this condition they arise from the upper third of the ventricular wall. Minor functionally insignificant abnormalities of the papillary muscles may occur. A not uncommon one consists of insertion of one papillary muscle directly into one or both mitral leaflets. In acquired rheumatic mitral stenosis, fusion and shortening of the chordae tendineae may be so extensive that it appears that both papillary muscles insert directly into the mitral leaflets.

Consequences of Operative-Excision of the Papillary Muscles at the time of Mitral Valve Replacement

Both left ventricular papillary muscles are excised by most surgeons at the time of mitral valve replacement. The myocardium of the free wall at the sites of excision of these muscles is always infiltrated by inflammatory cells if this area is examined in the early postoperative period.[51] If the papillary muscles are not excised when the mitral leaflets and chordae tendineae are excised during mitral valve replacement, the papillary muscles atrophy and are focally replaced by fibrous tissue.[52]

When the papillary muscles are excised at operation, each is grasped by a clamp extending through the mitral orifice from the left atrium. If the papillary muscles are pulled too vigorously by the clamp when the muscle is excised a portion of left ventricular free wall beneath the left ventricular papillary muscle also may be excised. This may result in perforation of the left ventricular wall, or it may cause severe thinning of the wall at this point with formation of a functioning or anatomic aneurysm or both.

Anterior Papillary Muscle of the Right Ventricle

This structure appears to be susceptible to all the afflictions which affect the left ventricular papillary muscles. This structure in length is usually equivalent to several thicknesses of right ventricular wall, and blood also is required to course "up hill" to perfuse this papillary muscle. This muscle is also most frequently made necrotic or fibrotic by myocardial infarction from coronary arterial atherosclerosis. Its involvement usually indicates "massive" anterior-wall myocardial infarction. Whether or not tricuspid regurgitation is a consequence of necrosis or fibrosis or of infiltrative disease of the right ventricular papillary muscle is uncertain. Necrosis of the distal portion of this papillary muscle is common in coronary heart disease, acute valvular dysfunction as in infective endocarditis, and in chronic anemias (fig. 5).

References

1. Rusted IE, Scheifley CH, Edwards JE, Kirklin JW: Guides to the commissures in operations upon the mitral valve. Mayo Clin Proc **26**: 297, 1951
2. Ranganathan N, Burch GE: Gross morphology and arterial supply of the papillary muscles of the left ventricle of man. Amer Heart J **77**: 506, 1969
3. Estes EH Jr, Dalton FM, Entman ML, Dixon HB II, Hackel DB: The anatomy and blood supply of the papillary muscles of the left ventricle. Amer Heart J **71**: 356, 1966
4. Heikkilä J: Mitral incompetence as a complication of acute myocardial infarction. Acta Med Scand **182** (suppl 475): 1, 1967
5. Estes EH Jr, Entman ML, Dixon HB II, Hackel DB: The vascular supply of the left ventricular wall: Anatomic observations, plus a hypothesis regarding acute events in coronary artery disease. Amer Heart J **71**: 58, 1966
6. Burch GE, De Pasquale NP, Phillips JH: Clinical manifestations of papillary muscle dysfunction. Arch Intern Med (Chicago) **112**: 112, 1963
7. Phillips JH, Burch GE, De Pasquale NP: The syndrome of papillary muscle dysfunction: Its clinical recognition. Ann Intern Med **59**: 508, 1963
8. Burch GE, De Pasquale NP, Phillips JH: The syndrome of papillary muscle dysfunction. Amer Heart J **75**: 399, 1968
9. Brody W, Criley JM: Functional mitral regurgitation. New Eng J Med **279**: 1058, 1968
10. Brody W, Criley JM: Intermittent severe mitral regurgitation: Hemodynamic studies in a patient with recurrent acute left-sided heart failure. New Eng J Med **283**: 673, 1970
11. Brock RC: The surgical and pathological anatomy of the mitral valve. Brit Heart J **14**: 489, 1952
12. Smith HL, Essex HE, Baldes, EJ: A study of the movements of heart valves and of heart sounds. Ann Intern Med **33**: 1357, 1950
13. Shelburne JC, Rubinstein D, Gorlin R: A reappraisal of papillary muscle dysfunction: Correlative clinical and angiographic study. Amer J Med **46**: 862, 1969
14. Simon AL, Ross J Jr, Gault JH: Angiographic anatomy of the left ventricle and mitral valve in idiopathic hypertrophic subaortic stenosis. Circulation **36**: 852, 1967
15. Roberts WC, Ferrans VJ: Pathologic aspects of hypertrophic cardiomyopathy: A study of 30 necropsy patients. In preparation
16. Brand FR, Brown AL, Berge KG: Histology of papillary muscles of the left ventricle in myocardial infarction. Amer Heart J **77**: 26, 1969
17. Miller GE Jr, Cohn KE, Kerth WI, Selzer A, Gerbode F: Experimental papillary muscle infarction. J Thorac Cardiovasc Surg **56**: 611, 1968
18. Tsakiris AG, Rastelli GC, Amorim DD, Titus JL, Wood EH: Effect of experimental papillary muscle damage on mitral valve closure in intact anesthetized dogs. Mayo Clin Proc **45**: 275, 1970
19. Mittal AK, Langston M Jr, Cohn KE, Selzer A, Kerth WJ: Combined papillary muscle and left ventricular wall dysfunction as a cause of mitral regurgitation: An experimental study. Circulation **44**: 174, 1971
20. Forrester JS, Diamond G, Freeman S, Allen HN, Parmley WW, Matloff J, Swan HJC:

Silent mitral insufficiency in acute myocardial infarction. Circulation **44**: 877, 1971

21. Falcone MW, Ronan JA Jr, Roberts WC: Silent mitral regurgitation complicating silent myocardial infarction: Hemodynamic and morphologic documentation. Chest. In press
22. Cederqvist L, Söderström J: Papillary muscle rupture in myocardial infarction: A study based upon an autopsy material. Acta Med Scand **176**: 287, 1964
23. Roberts WC, Buja LM: The frequency and significance of coronary arterial thrombi and other observations in fatal acute myocardial infarction: A study of 107 necropsy patients. Amer J Med **52**: 425, 1972
24. Moller JH, Nakib A, Edwards JE: Infarction of papillary muscles and mitral insufficiency associated with congenital aortic stenosis. Circulation **34**: 87, 1966
25. Arosemena E, Moller JH, Edwards JE: Scarring of the papillary muscles in left ventricular hypertrophy. Amer Heart J **74**: 446, 1967
26. Roberts WC: The congenitally bicuspid aortic valve: A study of 85 autopsy cases. Amer J Cardiol **26**: 72, 1970
27. Roberts WC, Perloff JK, Costantino T: Severe valvular aortic stenosis in patients over 65 years of age: A clinicopathologic study. Amer J Cardiol **27**: 497, 1971
28. Falcone MW, Roberts WC, Morrow AG, Perloff JK: Congenital aortic stenosis resulting from a unicommissural valve: Clinical and anatomic features in twenty-one adult patients. Circulation **44**: 272, 1971
29. Buchbinder NA, Roberts WC: Active left-sided valvular infective endocarditis: A study of 45 necropsy patients. Amer J Med. In press
30. Moller JH, Lucas RV Jr, Adams P Jr, Anderson RC, Jorgens J, Edwards JE: Endocardial fibroelastosis: A clinical and anatomic study of 47 patients with emphasis on its relationship to mitral insufficiency. Circulation **30**: 759, 1964
31. Noren GR, Raghib G, Moller JH, Amplatz K, Adams P Jr, Edwards JE: Anomalous origin of the left coronary artery from the pulmonary trunk with special reference to the occurrence of mitral insufficiency. Circulation **30**: 171, 1964
32 Roberts WC: Anomalous origin of both coronary arteries from the pulmonary artery. Amer J Cardiol **10**: 595, 1962
33. Burchell HB, Brown AL Jr: Anomalous origin of coronary artery from pulmonary artery masquerading as mitral insufficiency. Amer Heart J **63**: 388, 1962
34. Marcus FI, Gomez L, Glancy DL, Ewy GA, Roberts WC: Papillary muscle fibrosis in primary myocardial disease. Amer Heart J **77**: 681, 1969
35. Roberts WC, Ross RS, Eggleston JC, Massumi, RA: Chronic mitral regurgitation of unresolved etiology in the elderly: A clinicopathologic study of two patients. Johns Hopkins Med J **122**: 26, 1968
36. Perloff JK: Cardiomyopathy associated with heredofamilial neuromyopathic diseases. Mod Conc Cardiovasc Dis **40**: 23, 1971
37. Davies JNP, Ball JD: The pathology of endomyocardial fibrosis in Uganda. Brit Heart J **17**: 337, 1955
38. Roberts WC, Buja LM, Ferrans VJ: Löffler's fibroplastic parietal endocarditis, eosinophilic leukemia, and Davies' endomyocardial fibrosis: The same disease at different stages? Path Microbiol **35**: 90, 1970
39. Roberts WC, Liegler DG, Carbone PP: Endomyocardial disease and eosinophilia: A clinical and pathologic spectrum. Amer J Med **46**: 28, 1969
40. Morrow AG, Cohen LS, Roberts WC, Braunwald NS, Braunwald E: Severe mitral regurgitation following acute myocardial infarction and ruptured papillary muscle: Hemodynamic findings and results of operative treatment in four patients. Circulation **38** (suppl II): II-124, II-132, 1968
41. Haller JA Jr, Morrow AG: Experimental mitral insufficiency: An operative method of chronic survival. Ann Surg **142**: 37, 1955
42. Brock RC: Arterial route to aortic and pulmonary valves: Mitral route to aortic valves. Guy Hosp Rep **99**: 236, 1950
43. Chisholm JC Jr: Sarcoid cardiomyopathy. J Nat Med Ass **58**: 265, 1966
44. Buja LM, Khoi NB, Roberts WC: Clinically significant cardiac amyloidosis: Clinicopathologic findings in 15 patients. Amer J Cardiol **26**: 394, 1970
45. Buja LM, Roberts WC: Iron in the heart: Etiology and clinical significance. Amer J Med **51**: 209, 1971
46. Shone JD, Seller RD, Anderson RC, Adams P Jr, Lillehei CW, Edwards JE: The developmental complex of "parachute mitral valve," supravalvular ring of left atrium, subaortic stenosis, and coarctation of aorta. Amer J Cardiol **11**: 714, 1963
47. Glancy DL, Chang MY, Dorney ER, Roberts WC: Parachute mitral valve. Further observations and associated lesions. Amer J Cardiol **27**: 309, 1971
48. Davachi F, Moller JH, Edwards JE: Diseases of the mitral valve in infancy: An anatomic

analysis of 55 cases. Circulation **43**: 565, 1971

49. Carney EK, Braunwald E, Roberts WC, Aygen M, Morrow AG: Congenital mitral regurgitation: Clinical, hemodynamic and angiocardiographic findings in nine patients. Amer J Med **33**: 223, 1962
50. Castaneda AR, Anderson RC, Edwards JE: Congenital mitral stenosis resulting from anomalous arcade and obstructing papillary muscles: Report of correction by use of ball valve prosthesis. Amer J Cardiol **24**: 237, 1969
51. Roberts WC, Morrow AG: Causes of death and other anatomic observations after cardiac valve replacement: *In* Long-Term Prognosis following Valve Replacement; Advances in Cardiology. Basel, S. Karger, 1972, vol 7, p 226
52. Rastelli GC, Kirklin JW, Titus JL: Fate of papillary muscles after prosthetic replacement of mitral valve. Mayo Clin Proc **42**: 210, 1967

Mitral Valvular Disease

A Clinicopathologic Survey of the Conditions Causing the Mitral Valve To Function Abnormally

WILLIAM C. ROBERTS, M.D., and JOSEPH K. PERLOFF, M.D., Bethesda, Maryland

The mitral valve is the most complex of the cardiac valves. Its leaflets are unequal in size: one is continuous with the left atrial endocardium and the other with the aorta. The valve contains about 120 chordae tendineae connecting the leaflets to myocardial pillars (papillary muscles), which in turn are continuous with the left ventricular free wall. It has only a partial anulus fibrosis (only at the base of the posterior mitral leaflet). Since the mitral valve connects with the left atrial wall via the mural endocardium, conditions affecting this chamber also may affect mitral function. This review surveys conditions involving the mitral anulus, leaflets, chordae tendineae, papillary muscles, and left ventricular free wall that may cause this valvular orifice to be either stenotic or incompetent, or both.

DR. WILLIAM C. ROBERTS*: This conference concerns the mitral apparatus or complex. Dr. Joseph K. Perloff will discuss clinical features. I shall present pathologic features of several conditions affecting mitral leaflets, chordae tendineae, papillary muscles, anulus, and free walls of both the left atrium and left ventricle. But first a note on the origin of the term (Figure 1) and some comments on the structure of the normal mitral valve.

* Chief, Section of Pathology, National Heart and Lung Institute.

► An edited transcription of a Combined Clinical Staff Conference at the Clinical Center, Bethesda, Md., by the National Heart and Lung Institute, National Institutes of Health, U.S. Department of Health, Education, and Welfare.

The mitral valve is, in comparison with the semilunar valves, a complex structure consisting of four major components: leaflets, chordae tendineae, papillary muscles, and anulus (Figure 2). Unlike the other three cardiac valves, each of which has three cusps, the mitral valve consists of only two leaflets. The anterior leaflet has a much longer basal-to-margin length than does the posterior leaflet, but the length of anular attachment of the posterior leaflet is about twice that of the anterior leaflet (Figure 3). The posterior leaflet is attached for about 6 cm, and the anterior leaflet, approximately 3 cm. Although the basal-to-margin lengths and the lengths of the basal attachments of each mitral leaflet are quite different, the surface area of each leaflet is virtually identical. The posterior leaflet has a true bundle of fibrous tissue (the anulus) separating the myocardium of left atrium from the myocardium of left ventricle. The posterior leaflet, in a large sense, is simply an extension of mural endocardium from the posterior and lateral walls of the left atrium (Figure 3). In contrast to the posterior mitral leaflet, the anterior leaflet does not have a true anulus but is continuous with the wall of the ascending aorta, aortic valve, and membraneous ventricular septum (Figure 3). The area of the leaflets is approximately 2.5 times that of the area of the primary mitral orifice—that is, the area at the level of the mitral anulus (1). The mitral leaflets are connected with each other at the commissures. In contrast to the semilunar cusps, which are independent or discontinuous of each other, the two mitral leaflets are continuous with

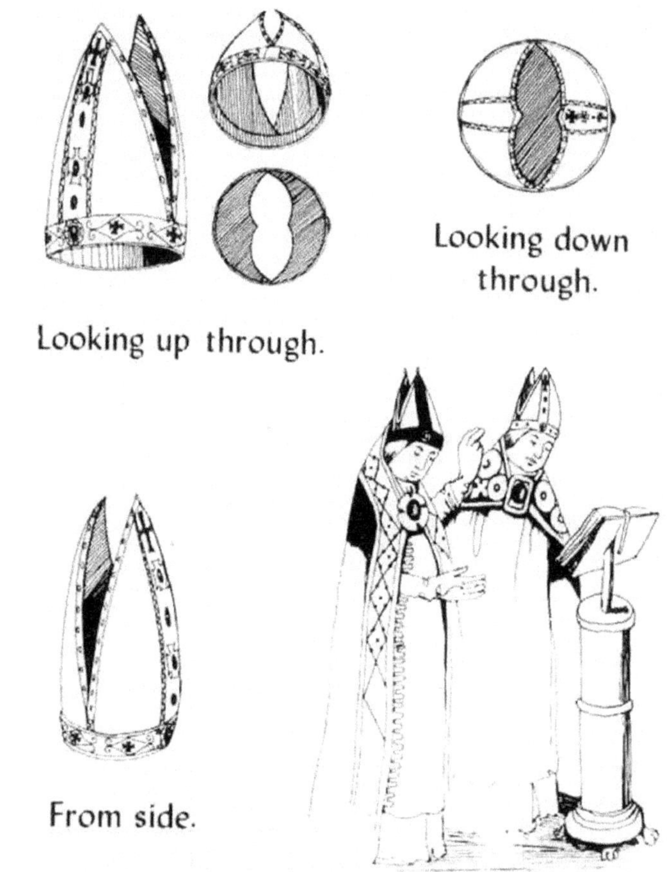

Figure 1. The miter of the mitral valve. The term "mitral" is derived from the Latin term "mitra," meaning cap, which in turn was derived from the Greek word "mitra," meaning turban or headdress. Bishops of the Christian Church wore headdresses, which they called "miters," fashioned after those of ancient Hebrew high priests. Vesalius is recorded as having compared the shape of the bishop's miter with that of the mitral valve. Disease of this valve, namely mitral stenosis, was first recorded by John Mayow in 1969.

each other.

The chordae tendineae of the mitral valve are even more complex than its leaflets. Chordae from each leaflet insert into both papillary muscles (Figure 2). About five times as many chordae are attached to leaflets as to papillary muscles (2). On an average, 24 chordae tendineae are attached to the papillary muscles (12 to each), and 120 chordae are attached to mitral leaflets (2) (Figure 4). The chordae insert onto the undersurfaces—that is, the ventricular surfaces—of both leaflets. The chordae subdivide as they progress from papillary muscle to leaflet. The subdivisions may be viewed as primary (first order), secondary (second order), and tertiary (third order) chordae. The spaces between the chordae serve as secondary orifices between left atrium and left ventricle. Obviously, the major orifice is the area between the leaflets, but much blood passes between the interchordal spaces (Figure 5). Therefore, fusion of chordae tendineae narrows the mitral inlet.

The two left ventricular papillary muscles are preferably designated anterolateral and posteromedial. There is considerable variation in the appearances of these two structures in the same person. When corresponding structures are compared in different persons, considerable variation is apparent (2). The anterolateral papillary muscle is generally the more uniform of the two. It usually consists of a single trunk that protrudes more into the cavity than the posteromedial one. The posteromedial papillary muscle is generally smaller than the anterolateral structure and often consists of two or three smaller pillars

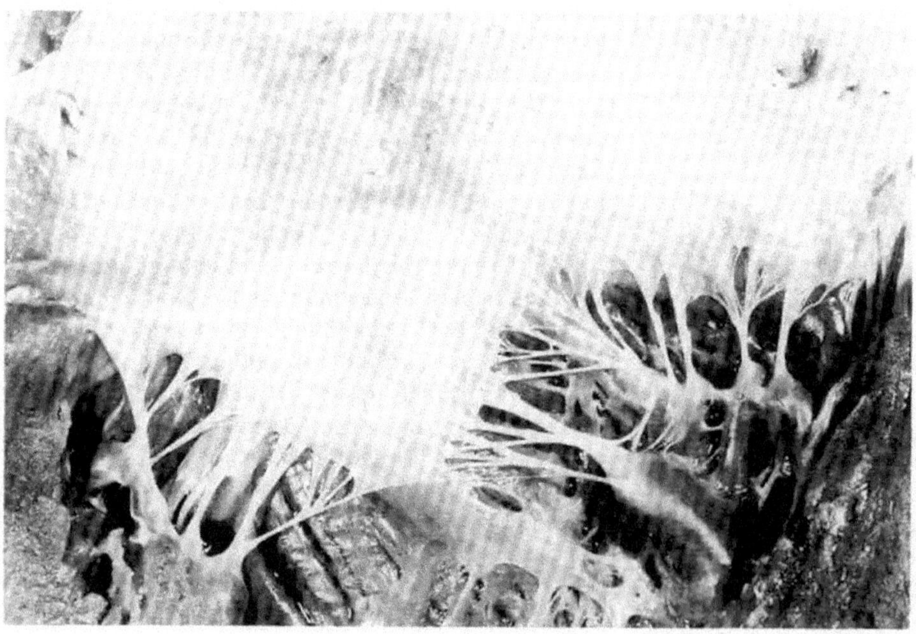

Figure 2. Opened normal mitral valve. Each papillary muscle receives chordae tendineae from both leaflets. The chordae insert on the ventricular or under-surface of the leaflets. The leaflets are continuous with one another, in contrast to the semilunar valve cusps, each of which is a separate independent unit. The mural endocardium of left atrium above the posterior leaflet is similar in appearance to the posterior leaflet; this is to be expected, since one presumably is derived from the other. The mural endocardium above the anterior leaflet, however, is not as white as this leaflet, and the leaflet is not an extension of left artrial endocardium, as is the posterior leaflet.

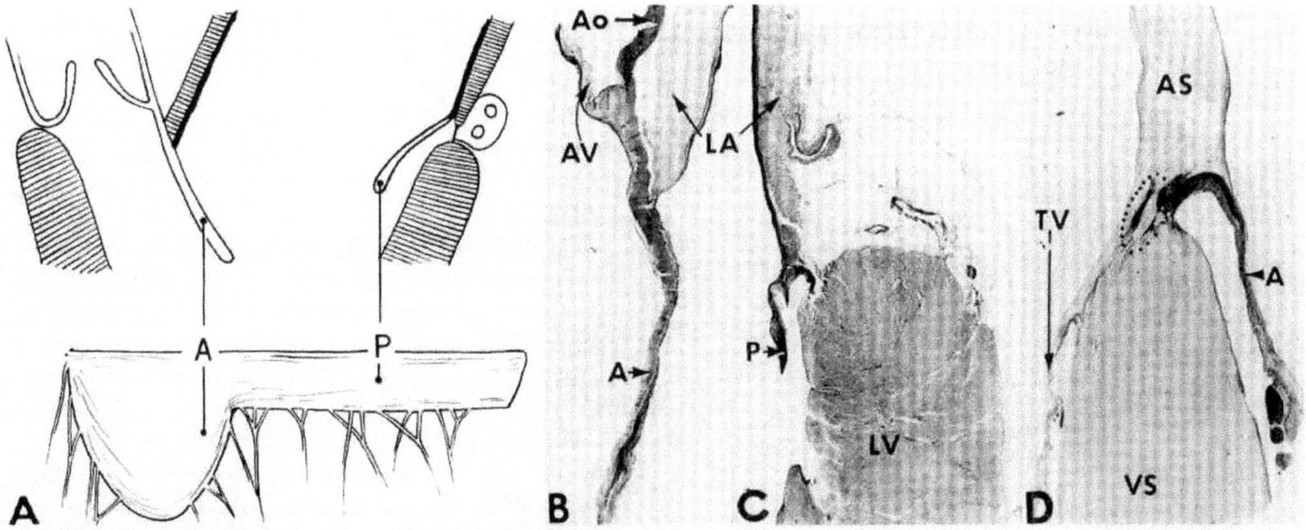

Figure 3A. Diagram of mitral valve showing that the anterior (*A*) leaflet is continuous with the ascending aorta and aortic valve and that the posterior (*P*) leaflet is continuous with left atrial endocardium. The inflow and outflow tracts of the left ventricle are divided by the anterior leaflet. The basal attachment of the posterior leaflet is twice as long as that of the anterior leaflet, although the basal-to-margin length of the anterior leaflet is twice that of the posterior leaflet. **B-D.** Histologic sections of mitral valve confirming the observations depicted in Figure 3A. **B.** This section includes anterior (*A*) mitral leaflet, aortic valve cusp (*AV*), wall of aorta (*Ao*), and left atrial (*LA*) wall. **C.** This section includes posterior (*P*) mitral leaflet and walls of left atrium and left ventricle (*LV*). **D.** This section extends through atrial septum (*AS*) and ventricular septum (*VS*) and includes portions of anterior (*A*) mitral leaflet and septal tricuspid leaflet (*TV*). Between the bases of these two leaflets is the penetrating portion of the atrioventricular bundle (*outlined by dots*). Thus, it is easy to see how calcific deposits from the mitral valve might extend into the conduction system and cause heart block. (Elastic van Gieson; Original magnifications: **B.** × 4.5; **C** and **D**, × 3.)

rather than a single pillar. The posteromedial muscle usually has several connections to the left ventricular wall in addition to the base of the major trunk. Both papillary muscles are attached to the lower or caudal third of the left ventricular free wall. Both papillary muscles have relatively poor blood supplies, and both are located at considerable distances from the orifices of the coronary arteries. The major supplier of the anterolateral muscle is the left anterior descending coronary artery, and the major supplier of the posteromedial muscle is the right coronary artery (3). The left circumflex contributes blood to both. To oxygenate the apexes of the papillary muscles, blood from the epicardial coronary arteries must penetrate the entire thickness of the left ventricular free wall, turn uphill, so to speak, and ascend a distance equivalent to about two more full thicknesses of left ventricular wall. Thus, it is no mystery that the papillary muscles, and particularly their apical portions, are sensitive indicators of minor deficiencies of myocardial oxygenation.

The Mitral Valve and Aging

With aging, this valve, like other tissues, may show wear and tear changes, mainly in leaflet and chordal thickening (4). The left ventricular cavity gets smaller, presumably because the cardiac output decreases as we grow older (Figure 6, *Top*). As the cavity gets smaller, less area is available in the left ventricle to accommodate the leaflets and chordae. As a consequence, the leaflets contact one another abnormally during ventricular systole and focal fibrous thickening results. Since the left ventricular cavity diminishes with age, the mitral anulus does also (Figure 6, *Bottom*). The latter change further increases the abnormal contact of the mitral leaflets with each other and furthers the leaflet scarring.

Functions of Normal Mitral Apparatus

Dr. Joseph K. Perloff*: The mitral apparatus is a complex, finely coordinated mechanism that can be deranged by a multiplicity of acquired and congenital disorders; its competency depends on the functional integrity of six anatomic components acting in delicate concert. These are posterior and lateral left atrial wall, anulus, leaflets, chordae tendineae, papillary muscles, and left ventricular free wall (5).

The exact mode of closure of the normal mitral valve is still uncertain (6-7). Left ventricular systole begins with contraction of the papillary muscles. The vertical forces exerted by this contraction move the leaflets into apposition. As the intraventricular pressure rises, the edges of the cusps coapt and mutually support each other along a comfortable margin of their atrial surfaces, firmly sealing the orifice. The

* Chief, Section of Cardiology, University of Pennsylvania School of Medicine, Philadelphia, Pa.

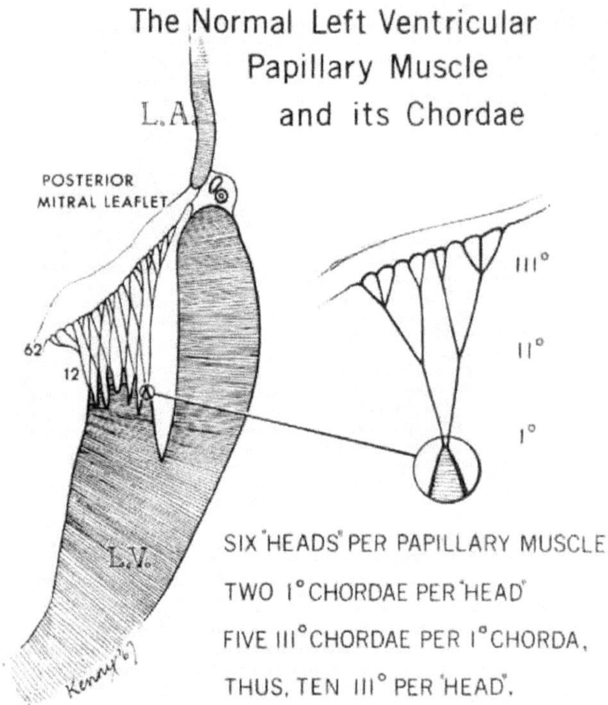

Figure 4. Diagram of the average number of chordae tendineae normally originating from each left ventricular papillary muscle. Although great variation exists, each left ventricular papillary muscle contains about six "heads," each of which contains two primary or first-order chordae tendineae. Each primary cord subdivides into two secondary chordae, each of which divides into two or three tertiary or third-order chordae. The number of chordae attached to each left ventricular papillary muscle thus averages 12, and the number of chordae inserting directly into the mitral leaflets from a single papillary muscle averages 62. (These numbers were found by counting chordae and papillary muscle heads in 12 normal hearts.) L.A. = left atrium; L.V. = left ventricle.

free edges do not merely touch; they coapt along a considerable area of their atrial surfaces. The rest of each leaflet bulges like a parachute toward the left atrium (8).

The anulus, long considered inert, not only serves as a fulcrum on which the leaflets move but also, during ventricular systole, decreases its circumference, reducing the area that the leaflets are required to seal (9, 10). As the left ventricle ejects, its apex and base approach each other. The shortening of the vertical axis of the left ventricle is accompanied by synergistic contraction of the papillary muscles and contiguous portions of left ventricular free wall, so that an appropriate vertical anchoring force is applied to the chordae tendineae, preventing eversion of the leaflets into the left atrium.

When any of its six anatomic components are faulty, the harmony of the mitral mechanism may be altered. Because of coordinated interplay among these elements, which are interdependent, more than one are usually disturbed at any given time, although with various degrees of significance. Regurgitation or stenosis, or both, is the functional consequence of derangement of the mitral complex; stenosis is the simpler of the two.

Obstruction at the mitral orifice can either be acquired (commonest), congenital, or caused by the interposition of nonleaflet tissue within the left atrial cavity.

The essential hemodynamic fault caused by obstruction at the mitral orifice is the inability of the left atrium to empty normally (11). In sinus rhythm an increased force of left atrial contraction serves to augment its emptying. This mechanical advantage is lost in atrial fibrillation, causing the mean left atrial pressure to rise or the mitral flow (and cardiac output) to fall. The obstruction, represented by a pressure gradient across the valve, is the basic mechanical disturbance of rheumatic (common) (12) or congenital (rare) (13) mitral stenosis. The consequences of obstruction at the mitral orifice can be seen most graphically in plain films of the chest (14). The posteroanterior X ray shows vascular redistribution to the upper lobes—that is, prominent upper lobe pulmonary veins, loss of the normal angle between the right upper pulmonary vein and the right pulmo-

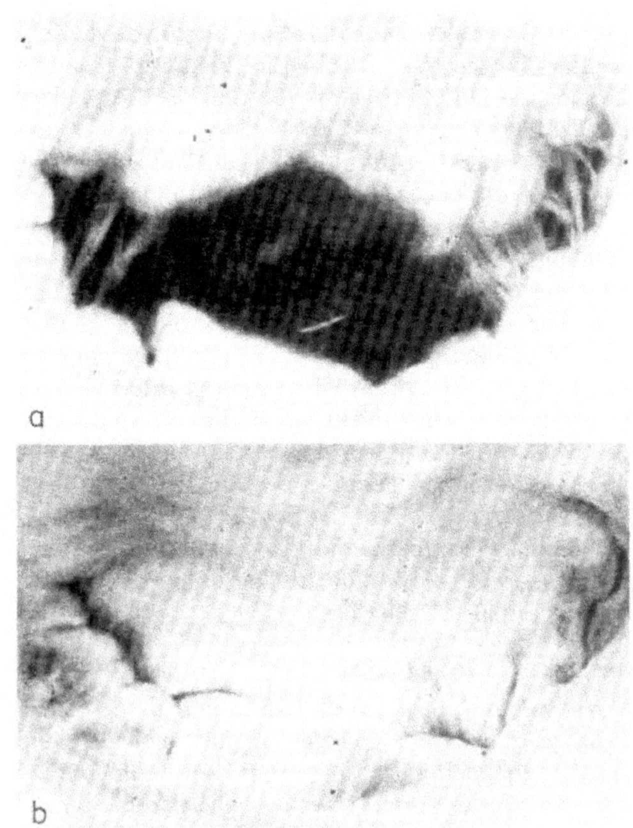

Figure 5. Normally functioning mitral valve during ventricular diastole (*a*) and systole (*b*). The valve closes over a large surface area (*b*) and not just at its margins.

nary artery, costrophrenic Kerley B lines (thickened interlobular septae), peribronchial cuffing (best seen end-on), and a general haze of interstitial pulmonary edema.

Thus, stenosis of the mitral orifice due to rheumatic endocarditis is conceptually a relatively simple anatomic fault that is translated into the mechanical problem of pulmonary venous obstruction.

Dr. Roberts: Of the nine single or combined cardiac valve lesions (excluding tricuspid regurgitation and papillary muscle dysfunction) severe enough to be fatal, mitral stenosis, in my experience, ranks second (15-17) (Table 1). Of 543 patients over age 14 years with functionally severe (classes III or IV) valvular cardiac disease whom I studied at necropsy, 206 (37%) had mitral stenosis. Only valvular aortic stenosis was commoner. Mitral stenosis occurred alone in 94 patients and in combination with other functional valvular lesions in the other 112 patients. Mitral stenosis was rheumatic in origin in all 206 patients.

Although a functional classification of valvular heart disease, as shown in Table 1, is most useful from physiologic and therapeutic standpoints, an anatomic classification is most helpful from an etiologic standpoint. Five anatomic categories have proved useful (15): isolated mitral, isolated aortic, combined mitral and aortic, combined tricuspid and mitral with or without aortic, and tricuspid with or without pulmonic. Isolated aortic valve disease is virtually never rheumatic in origin (15). Isolated mitral disease causing stenosis is, with rare exception, rheumatic in origin, but isolated mitral disease causing pure regurgitation is nonrheumatic nearly as often as it is rheumatic (Table 2). Combined valve disease is usually rheumatic in origin. Isolated anatomic disease of the tricuspid or pulmonic valves, or both, is usually congenital in origin or is associated with the carcinoid syndrome (17).

A valve may function normally and yet be anatomically abnormal. Only 57% of the 94 patients with isolated mitral stenosis (with or without mitral regurgitation) had anatomic involvement limited to the mitral valve. In contrast, 87% of the 182 patients with clinically isolated aortic stenosis (with or without regurgitation) had anatomic disease of the aortic valve only.

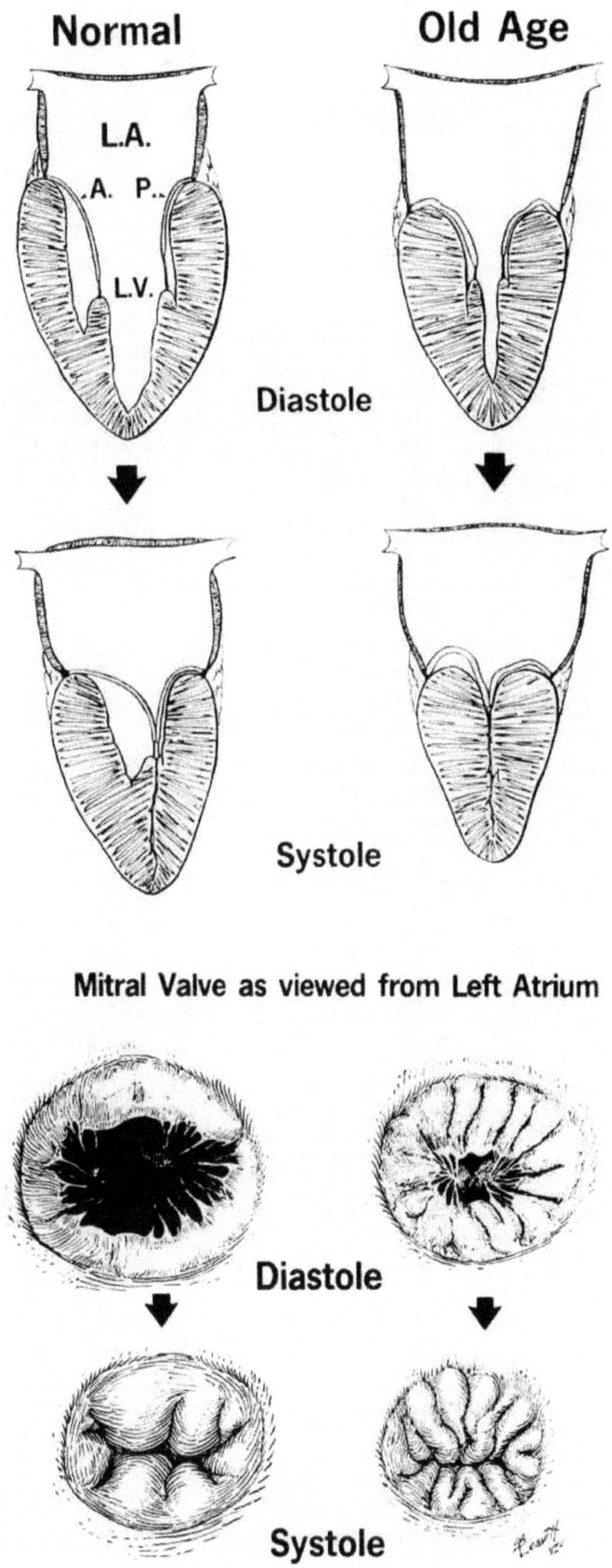

Figure 6 Top. Changes in left atrium (*LA*), anterior (*A*) and posterior (*P*) mitral leaflets, and left ventricle (*LV*) with aging. Because the left ventricular cavity is smaller, the left ventricular wall appears thicker and is probably less compliant. As a result, the left atrium has to work harder to fill the left ventricle; because of this increased effort the atrium dilates, and its wall becomes thinner. Finally, when it reaches a certain degree of dilation, atrial fibrillation occurs (idiopathic atrial fibrillation of the elderly). **Bottom.** Mitral valve viewed from left atrium in youth, compared with in the elderly. In the older person the left ventricular cavity is smaller, and since the mitral leaflets do not become smaller, there is now relatively more leaflet than cavity. The leaflets consequently contact one another abnormally and thicken. In the elderly the mitral valve during ventricular systole has the appearance of dilated hemorrhoids.

Table 1. Functional Classification of Valvular Heart Disease Data on 543 Autopsy Patients More Than 14 Years of Age

Functional Valve Lesion	Number of Patients
	(%)
Aortic stenosis (AS)	182 (34)
Mitral stenosis (MS)	94 (17)
Aortic and mitral stenosis	66 (12)
Pure aortic regurgitation (AR)	60 (11)
Pure mitral regurgitation (MR)	55 (10)
MS + AR	34 (6)
MR + AR	24 (5)
AS + MR	16 (3)
Tricuspid stenosis + MS ± AS	12 (2)
Total	543 (100)

Rheumatic heart disease may be viewed as a disease of the mitral valve; other valves may also be involved both anatomically and functionally, but anatomically the mitral valve is always involved. To my knowledge, Aschoff bodies have never been found in hearts without anatomic disease of the mitral valve. Twelve of the 543 patients with severe valvular heart disease whom I studied at necropsy had Aschoff bodies, and all had mitral valve disease both anatomically and functionally.

Rheumatic heart disease not only is a disorder of the cardiac valves but also affects mural endocardium, pericardium, and myocardium. Histologically, the atrial walls virtually always show interstitial myocardial fibrosis, atrophy of some myocardial cells, and hypertrophy of the smooth muscle cells of the mural endocardium (15).

Anatomic Features of Rheumatic Mitral Stenosis

The anatomic features of rheumatic mitral stenosis are illustrated in Figure 7. In all patients with rheumatic mitral stenosis the leaflets are diffusely thickened, either by fibrous tissue or calcific deposits, or both; the commissures are usually fused, and the chordae tendineae are shortened and usually fused to some degree. The greatest obstruction to this funnel-shaped valve occurs at its apex, which is within the left ventricular cavity. The primary orifice, located at the level of the anulus, is far less narrowed. Fusion may involve one or both commissures. When only one is fused or one is fused more than the other, the stenotic orifice is eccentrically located. A centrally located orifice indicates symmetrical commissural fusion. In rheumatic mitral stenosis the chordae tendineae are occasionally so retracted that the leaflets appear to insert directly into the papillary muscles. When this occurs, the stenosis is always severe because the interchordal spaces are virtually entirely obliterated. Sometimes chordae inserting into one papillary muscle are well preserved, whereas those inserting into the other papillary muscle are completely fused. Mitral commissurotomy on a valve in which the leaflets insert almost directly into the papillary muscle(s) usually must include a splitting of the papillary muscle(s) as well as the leaflet commissure(s). If there are normally about 120 third-order chordae and about 24 first-order chordae, in mitral stenosis these numbers are usually halved and, on occasion, even reduced to just 1, for practical purposes.

The amount of calcium in the leaflets of stenotic mitral valves varies considerably. Generally, men have more calcium than women, and older patients have more calcium than younger patients. The rapidity with which calcification progresses also varies considerably. Figure 7, for example, shows a heavily calcified stenotic mitral valve excised from a 26-year-old man who had had acute rheumatic fever at age 12 years. The same figure shows another stenotic mitral valve from a 62-year-old woman who also had had acute rheumatic fever when she was 12 years old. Virtually no calcific deposits are present in her valve despite a mitral commissurotomy 14 years earlier. Gross calcific deposits generally preclude mitral commissurotomy and necessitate valve replacement. Previous commissurotomy, however, does not necessarily preclude a second commissurotomy, since the first procedure does not necessarily predispose the leaflets to the deposition of calcium.

A new, acquired cause of mitral stenosis, the rigid-frame prosthetic valve, was introduced in 1960. Since the natural mitral valve is within the left ventricle, a prosthetic mitral valve is also located within this cavity. The prosthesis must be small enough for the contracting left ventricular wall not to interfere with the prosthetic poppet or disk. When the prosthesis is too large for the cavity into which it was inserted, the poppet may be prevented from moving adequately and may therefore obstruct left atrial emptying (Figure 8) (18). The latter state is far commoner than obstruction to left ventricular emptying by the prosthesis (19). Thrombus formation on a mitral prosthesis also may obstruct left atrial emptying (19).

Some Congenital Causes of Mitral Obstruction

Dr. Perloff: Congenital obstruction to left atrial flow falls into three categories (13): [1] congenital mitral stenosis (obstruction at valvular level caused by congenitally abnormal leaflets and chordae), the parachute mitral valve, or supravalvular stenosing ring; [2] cor triatriatum; and [3] congenital pulmonary-vein stenosis. Congenital mitral stenosis means that the obstruction is at the orifice itself—that is, within the leaflets or their chordal support. Cor

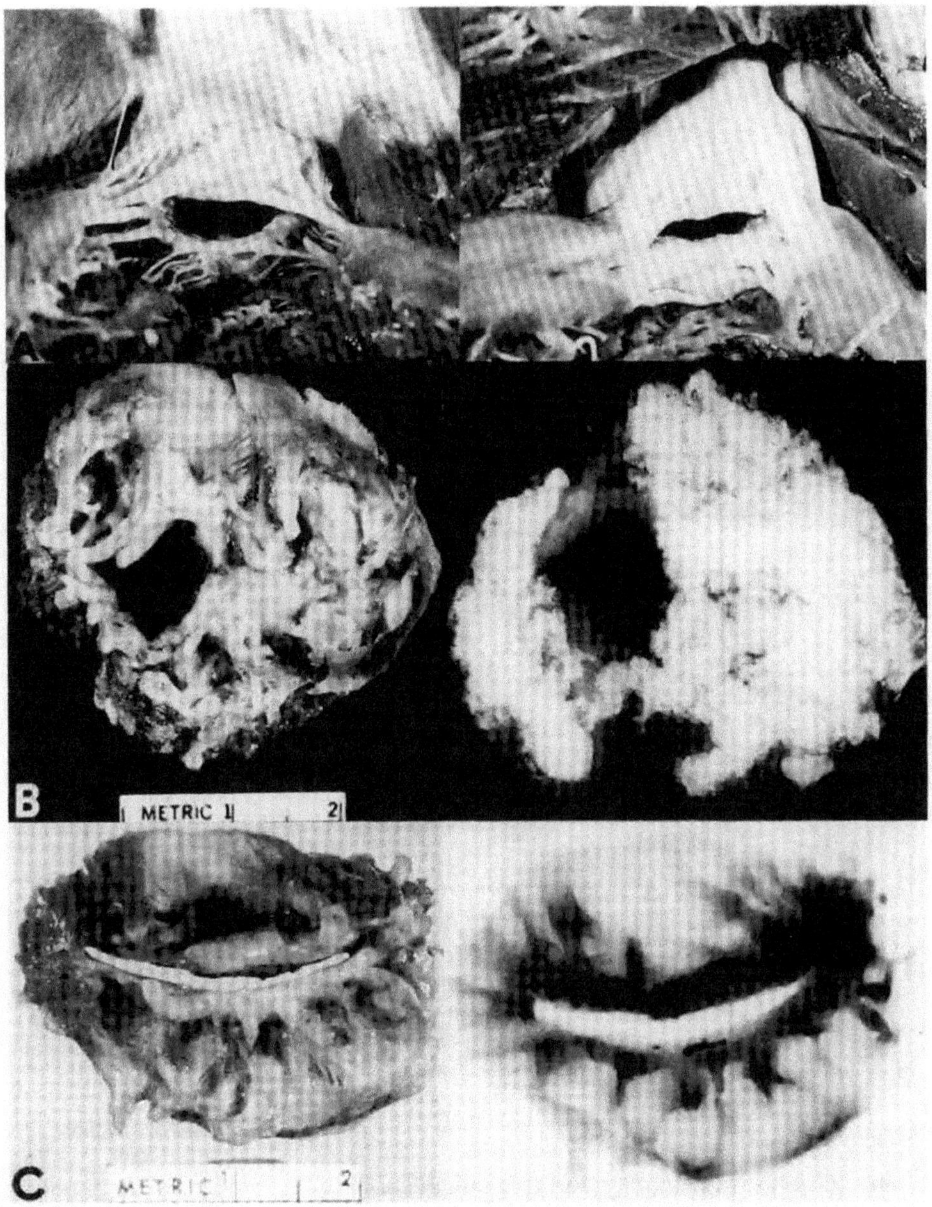

Figure 7A. Mitral valves viewed from left ventricle in two patients with mitral stenosis. **Left.** Valve in a 41-year-old woman who died of mesenteric vascular insufficiency 3 years after mitral commissurotomy (98). This orifice has the typical so-called "fish-mouth" appearance. The leaflets are separated from the papillary muscles by chordae that are thicker than normal. **Right.** Valve in a 39-year-old woman who died during induction of anesthesia for mitral commissurotomy. At catheterization several days earlier the left atrial-left ventricular mean diastolic gradient was 23 mm Hg. The left atrial pressures were mean, 35 and V wave, 43 mm Hg, and left ventricular pressure, 110/7 mm Hg. In this valve, as contrasted to the one on the left, the leaflets appear to insert directly into the papillary muscles. In other words, all chordae have fused, and commissurotomy, if carried out, probably would have required splitting of the papillary muscles as well as of the mitral commissures. **B** and **C.** Operatively excised mitral valves from two patients with mitral stenosis, showing striking differences in degrees of leaflet calcification. On the left are the valves as they would have appeared from the left ventricle, and on the right are roentgenograms of the excised valves. **B.** Valve from a 26-year-old man who died 3 days after mitral replacement. This patient, who had had acute rheumatic fever at age 12 years, preoperatively had a 15 mm Hg mean diastolic gradient between left atrium and left ventricle. This valve is massively calcified 14 years after the presumed initial attack of rheumatic fever. **C.** Valve from a 62-year-old woman who had had acute rheumatic fever at age 12 years and a mitral commissurotomy at age 48. Fourteen years later there was still only a trace of calcium in the valve.

triatriatum is caused by a partition within the left atrial cavity; the mitral valve and its chordal apparatus are normal. Pulmonary vein stenosis (very rare) is remote from the mitral orifice and left atrium.

Congenital mitral stenosis has a characteristic phonocardiogram. No opening snap is present because the mitral leaflets, even though not calcified, are not pliant. Nevertheless, a mid-diastolic or presystolic murmur may occur. With severe pulmonary hypertension murmurs may be absent (silent congenital mitral stenosis), principally because the hypertrophied right ventricle displaces the left ventricle from the apex (20, 21).

PARACHUTE MITRAL VALVE

Dr. Roberts: The commonest cause of congenital mitral stenosis is the parachute mitral valve, or single papillary muscle syndrome (22) (Figure 9). In addition to mitral stenosis, these patients usually have other cardiovascular anomalies: supravalvular mitral ring, which in itself may cause stenosis; subaortic stenosis; valvular aortic stenosis, usually superimposed on a congenitally malformed valve; and coarctation of the aortic isthmus. Other anomalies are also frequent (23).

Congenital mitral stenosis also may occur in individuals with two well-formed left ventricular papillary muscles. Probably the most frequent valve observed is one with an arcade configuration (24, 25). In this situation the chordae tendineae are extremely short.

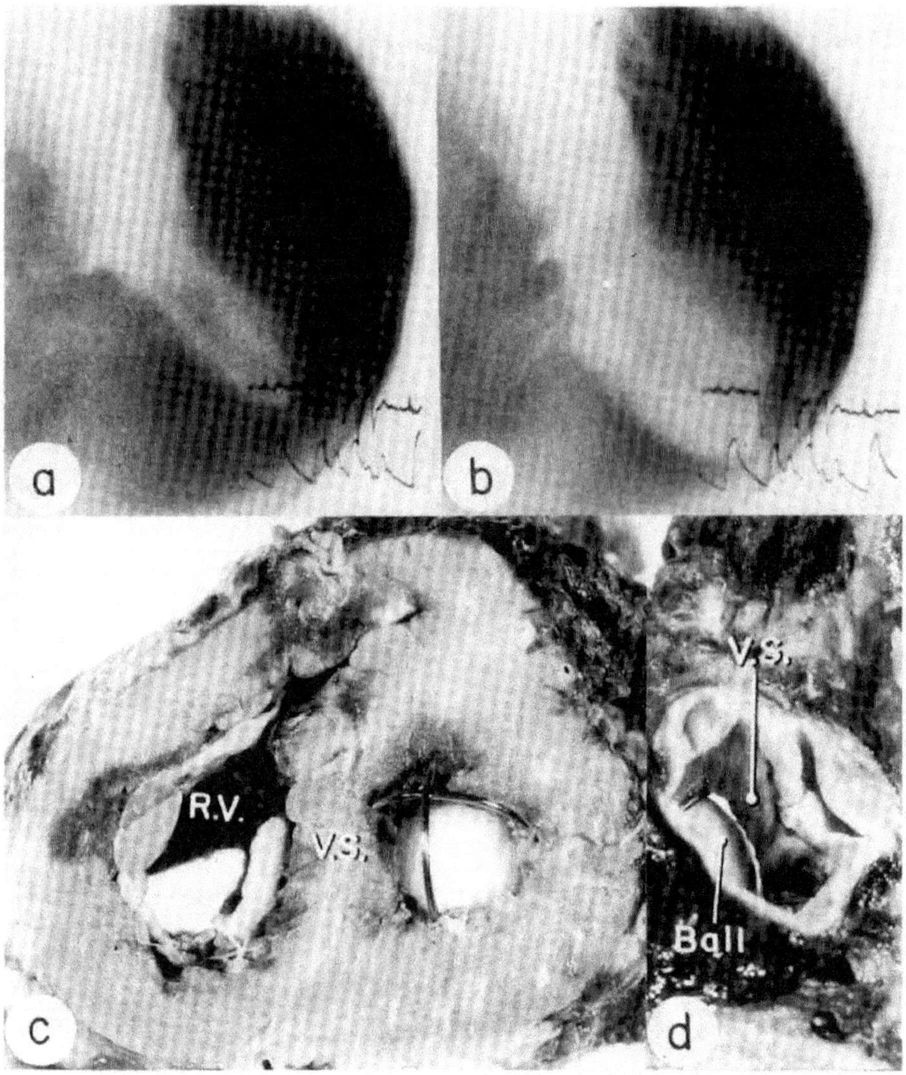

Figure 8. Stenosis of a prosthetic mitral valve in a 57-year-old man who had a small left ventricular cavity that was evident preoperatively on the cineangiocardiogram. **a.** Angiographic appearance of the left ventricular cavity at peak systole. **b.** At end-diastole. The diameter of the left ventricular outflow tract, even during diastole, is smaller than the diameter of the ascending aorta. In both angiographic frames the electrocardiogram and brachial arterial pressure pulse, recorded simultaneously, also are shown. **c.** Valve replacement was performed, but, after insertion of the prosthesis, bleeding from the right ventricular (*R.V.*) cannulation site occurred, and he died. At necropsy it was clear that the mitral poppet was immobile, because the prosthesis was too large for the left ventricular cavity into which it was inserted. Poppet immobility was caused by protrusion of the ventricular septum (*V.S.*) into the cage. Thus, there was no outlet for left atrial blood, and this led to severe elevation of pulmonary arterial and right ventricular pressures with rupture at the cannulation site. **d.** The poppet also caused narrowing of the left ventricular outflow tract.

Myxomas

Dr. Perloff: Still another form of obstruction to left atrial flow is the left atrial myoxma. A cineangiocardiogram (retrograde catheter in the left ventricle) will show a radiolucent area (negative contrast), typical of left atrial myxoma. Left atrial myxoma may present as a systemic (noncardiac) disease before symptoms of obstruction at the mitral orifice become evident (26). Some patients have systemic emboli, fever, anemia, and high erythrocyte sedimentation rates. The sex distribution is the same as it is with other forms of mitral obstruction—that is, the female predominates 2 or 3 to 1. In myxoma of the left atrium the mitral orifice is not only obstructed by the intracavitary mass, but, as a rule, the valve is also incompetent. Accordingly, it is diagnostically useful to inject contrast material into the left atrium to outline the myoxoma.

Dr. Roberts: Two left atrial myxomas are illustrated in Figure 10 (27). These myxomas may be small, thus not interfering with left atrial emptying, and may be found incidentally at necropsy. On the other hand, they may completely obstruct left atrial outflow, causing sudden death or a variety of other symptoms. Tumors of similar sizes may cause symptoms in some patients and none in others, depending on the location of the stalk. Small tumors may cause symptoms in some patients, and large tumors may not in others, again depending on the location of the stalk. The key is the site of attachment of the tumor to the atrial wall. If the left atrial tumor contacts the mitral leaflets too vigorously for too long, the leaflets may become thickened.

Although some early writers described difficulties in distinguishing left atrial myxoma from left atrial thrombus, the differences between them are great; there are many more differences than similarities between the two (27). The myxoma is attached to the atrial wall by a pedicle, the diameter of which

Figure 9. Parachute mitral valve (single papillary muscle) in a 14-year-old boy who presented clinically with left ventricular outflow tract obstruction. The peak systolic gradient between left ventricle and a systemic artery was 80 mm Hg. Obstruction was caused by a small aortic "anulus" with a bicuspid aortic valve and by discrete obstruction just below the aortic valve (*b*). At necropsy the mitral valve showed a parachute configuration, and all of its chordae inserted into a single left ventricular papillary muscle (*a*). Preoperatively, the left atrial mean pressure was 30 mm Hg, and the pulmonary arterial systolic pressure was 50 mm Hg. It was not realized while he was alive, however, that the mitral valve was stenotic. In addition, a functionally insignificant coarctation of the aorta was present. A ventricular septal defect had closed spontaneously (*a*).

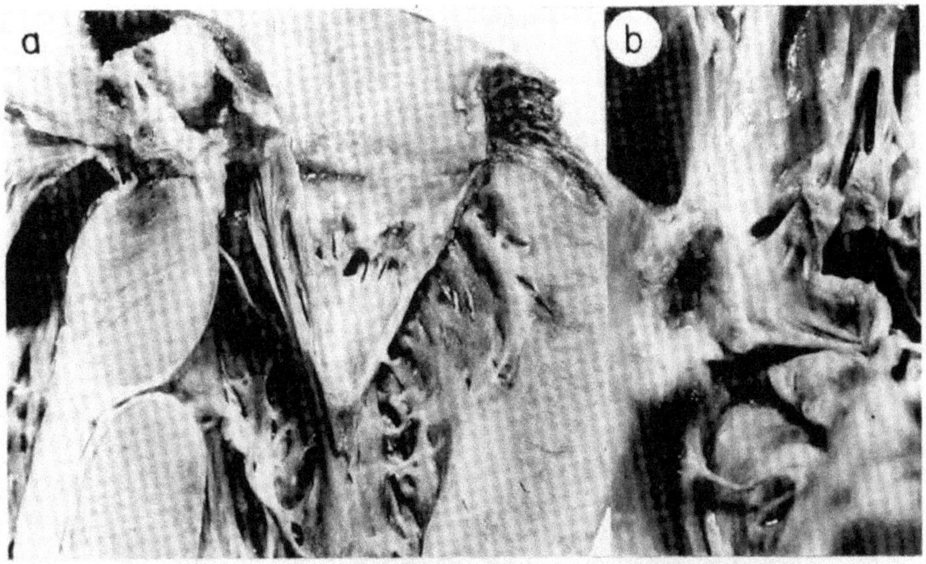

is far smaller than the largest diameter of the myxoma. A thrombus is virtually never attached by a pedicle but is instead attached to atrial endocardium over a large area. The myxoma resembles a ping-pong ball floating in a glass of water; as the water level drops (blood descending from left atrium to left ventricle), the ping-pong ball descends. Since the myxoma more or less floats in the atrial cavity, injection of contrast material into the cavity "lights up" the entire surface of the tumor. Contrast material in a left atrial cavity containing a thrombus in its body shows an area of no filling, and the borders of the thrombus are usually not well outlined. The surface of the myxoma is smooth and shiny; that of the thrombus is often ragged. With rare exception, neither thrombus nor myxoma in left atrium interferes

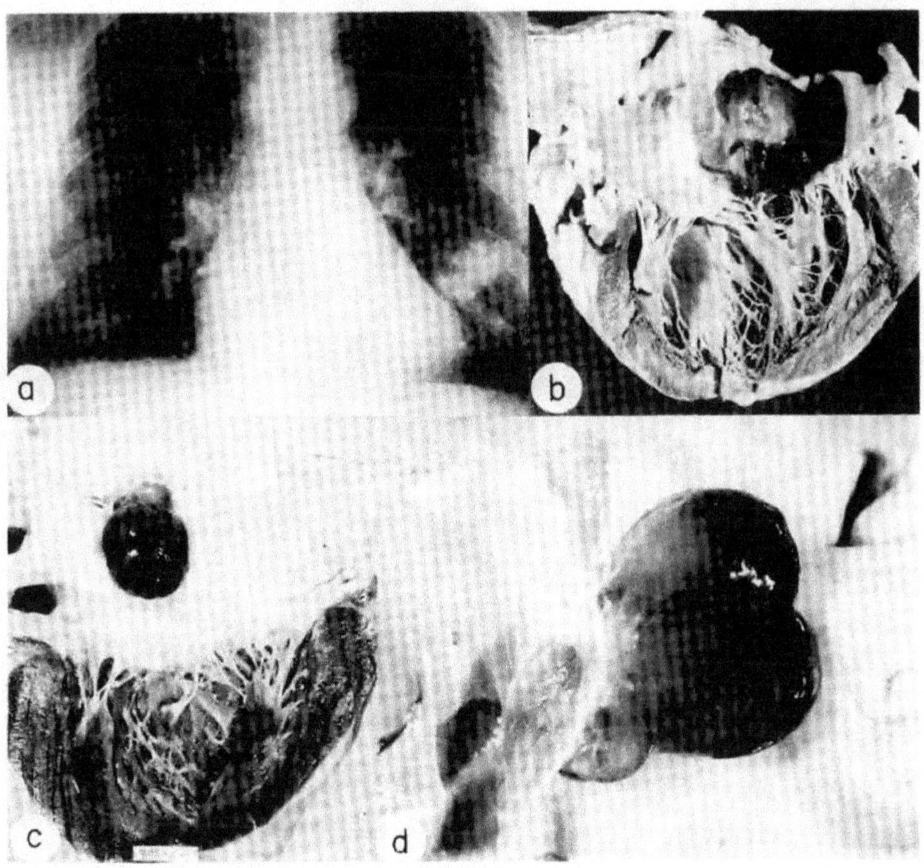

Figure 10. Left atrial myxomas in two patients. a and b. Chest radiograph and opened left atrium and ventricle in a 54-year-old man who died suddenly 2 weeks after lobectomy for carcinoma of the bronchus. Myxoma was an unexpected necropsy finding, but he had had evidence of congestive cardiac failure for 48 months before death. The myxoma (*b*) weighed 95 g and clearly partially obstructed left atrial outflow. c and d. Two views of a left atrial myxoma in a 60-year-old man who died of the carcinoid syndrome. This tumor weighed only 30 g and did not prolapse into the mitral orifice. Thus, this patient never had evidence of cardiac dysfunction. The tumor arises from the atrial septum (*d*).

with pulmonary venous drainage. Although thrombi occur in left atrial appendages in a variety of conditions (usually those associated with severely depressed cardiac output), thrombi occur in the body of the atrium only in patients with mitral stenosis. In other words, relatively severe stasis of blood is required for thrombus formation in the atrial body. Thrombi virtually never occur in the bodies of left atria in patients with pure mitral regurgitation, presumably because their atrial cavities are constantly being "washed out" during both phases of the cardiac cycle, thus preventing stasis. In contrast, myxomas occur entirely within the bodies of atria, never in atrial appendages, and the "valvular obstruction" totally disappears after excision of the neoplasm. Both thrombi and myxomas tend to form in atria that are of normal size or, at most, are moderately dilated. The huge left atrium rarely contains a thrombus.

Although thrombi and myxomas are the common-

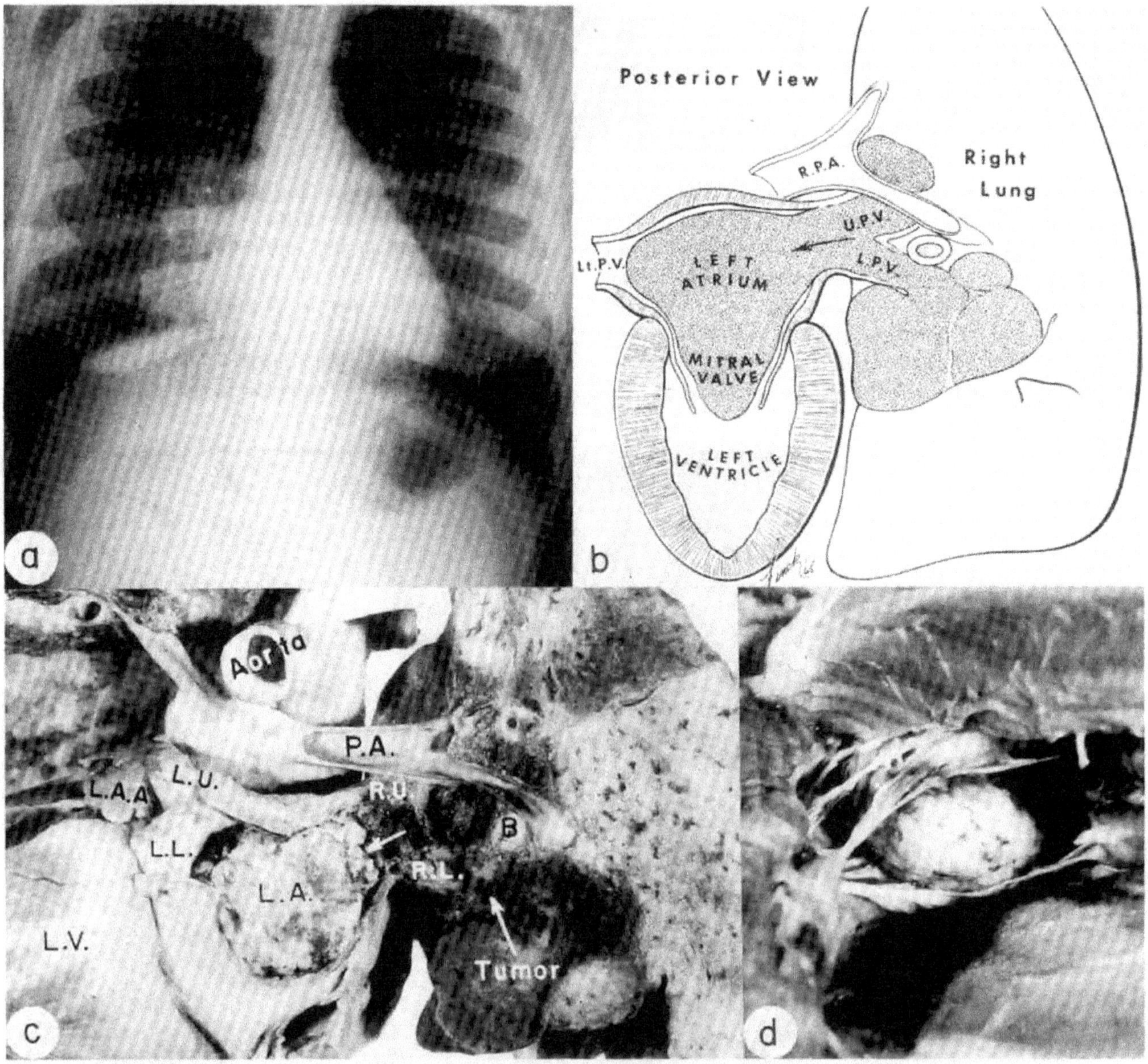

Figure 11. Neoplasm from right lung extending via pulmonary veins into left atrium to partially obstruct the mitral valve (*a-d*). This 28-year-old woman died from complications of intracranial metastases from uterine choriocarcinoma. At no time was a precordial murmur heard, nor could any of her symptoms be attributed to cardiopulmonary disease. At necropsy, tumor from the right lung was found to have extended into the left atrium (*b* and *c*) to partially obstruct the mitral orifice (*d*). Chest roentgenogram (*a*) showed a density just to the right of the heart. R.P.A. = right pulmonary artery; U.P.V. = upper pulmonary vein; L.P.V. = lower pulmonary vein; Lt.P.V. = left pulmonary vein; P.A. = pulmonary artery; L.V. = left ventricle; L.A. = left atrium; L.A.A. = left atrial appendage; B = bronchus; R.U. and L.U. = right and left upper pulmonary veins; R.L. and L.L. = right and left lower pulmonary veins.

est cause of filling defects in the left atrium, neoplasms (28, 29) and infected masses (30) may occur in this chamber and interfere with left atrial emptying (Figure 11). In contrast to thrombus and myxoma, however, the other filling defects also usually interfere with pulmonary venous return.

Mitral Regurgitation

Dr. Perloff: Remember that normal coordinated function of the left atrial wall, mitral anulus, leaflets, chordae tendineae, papillary muscles, and left ventricular free wall is required for competence of the mitral orifice.

First, we will consider the leaflets and chordae tendineae. The leaflets in mitral regurgitation may function abnormally because they are too small or too large or because they are tethered or immobilized by short chordae. A common cause of inadequate leaflet tissue is the scarring and contracture after rheumatic endocarditis. A rare but interesting feature in some patients with recurrent active rheumatic fever is Jaccoud's arthritis (Figure 12) (31). Appreciable mitral regurgitation generally coexists.

Now let us contrast two types of severe mitral regurgitation, one chronic and the other acute. In severe chronic (rheumatic) mitral regurgitation, the left atrium can be immense. Despite the large volume of regurgitant flow, the left atrial pressure may rise little, if at all, because the large left atrium is remarkably compliant (32). Accordingly, this form of severe mitral regurgitation occurs with normal or nearly normal left atrial pressure, without pulmonary hypertension, and with typical physical signs—namely, atrial fibrillation, an apical holosystolic murmur with axillary radiation, a prominent third heart sound, an apical left ventricular impulse, and anterior displacement of the heart due to systolic expansion of the large left atrium (33). In chronic severe mitral regurgitation the posterior wall of the large left atrium is displaced downward and posteriorly (8). Because of the continuity between left atrial endocardium and posterior mitral leaflet, the posterior cusp is pulled across its anulus, so that the cusp functionally shortens as the left atrium enlarges. Thus mitral regurgitation is augmented by atrial enlargement, or, as Edwards and Burchell (34) said, "mitral incompetence begets mitral incompetence."

In contrast to the chronic variety, acute severe regurgitation enlarges the left atrium hardly at all (35, 36). As a rule, the cause of the sudden regurgitation is rupture of chordae tendineae. Patients have normal sinus rhythm, as opposed to atrial fibrillation in those with chronic severe mitral regurgitation (32). Their history shows the recent onset of a systolic murmur and congestive heart failure. The apical murmur tends to be decrescendo and often radiates to the left sternal edge and base. The third heart sound of mitral regurgitation is present, but there is also a prominent fourth heart sound (37), which is not a feature of chronic mitral regurgitation. The fourth heart sound is accompanied by presystolic distention of the left ventricle. Physical signs of pulmonary hypertension develop rapidly because there is a large volume of regurgitant flow into a small, noncompliant left atrium in which the pressure

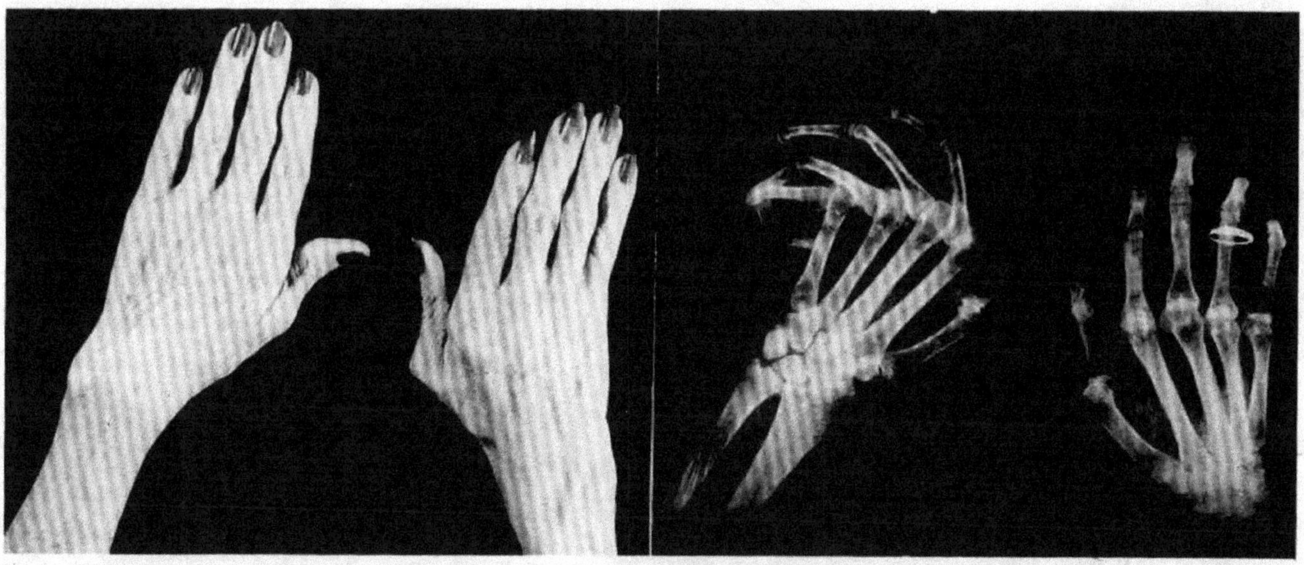

Figure 12. Hands of two patients with Jaccoud's arthritis. The inner photograph and X ray show deformities caused by subluxation of metacarpophalangeal joints. The outer photographs (hand and X ray) show that the patient can voluntarily "correct" the deformity. (With kind permission of Dr. Nathan T. Zvaifles, University of California, San Diego.)

Table 2. Cause of Clinically Isolated Fatal Pure Mitral Regurgitation in 55 Necropsy Patients More Than 14 Years of Age

Cause	Number of Patients	
Rheumatic	30	
Rupture of chordae tendineae in previously normal valve	15	
Floppy valve	4	
Congenital	4	
Corrected transposition		1
Partial A-V canal		1
Endocardial fibroelastosis		1
Parachute valve		1
Possible anular calcification	1	
Uncertain	1	
Total (20 males, 35 females)	55	

rises steeply, in striking contrast to chronic severe mitral regurgitation with a large compliant left atrium and a normal or near-normal left atrial pressure. The decrescendo systolic murmur is a useful feature in the clinical recognition of acute severe mitral regurgitation. The proposed mechanism is as follows: the left ventricular and left atrial pressure pulses and a phonocardiogram will show tall left atrial V waves and a decline in the left ventricular pressure pulse at the end of ejection; the steeply rising left atrial V wave approaches the left ventricular pressure in later systole, with the result that there is a late systolic decline in regurgitant flow and in murmur intensity (holosystolic but decrescendo). Occasionally, the decrescendo murmur ends before the second heart sound (early systolic).

An increased force of left atrial contraction accompanies acute severe mitral regurgitation. Palpation of the cardiac apex detects presystolic distention of the left ventricle, and on auscultation an accompanying fourth heart sound is heard. These two physical signs distinguish acute severe from chronic severe mitral regurgitation. The reason is evident. The previously normal left atrium in acute severe mitral regurgitation responds to an increase in volume and pressure by increasing its wall thickness and its contractile force. This force is delivered into the left ventricular cavity, resulting in presystolic distension and a fourth heart sound.

Dr. Roberts: In contrast to mitral stenosis, which has mainly one cause (rheumatic), pure mitral regurgitation has numerous causes (Table 2). Of the 543 patients with functionally severe valvular heart disease whom I studied at necropsy, 55 had pure mitral regurgitation. Cases of papillary muscle dysfunction were excluded. Rheumatic heart disease accounted for over half the cases.

Why the mitral valve affected by acute rheumatic fever becomes stenotic in some patients and why it becomes purely incompetent in others is unknown. Although the cause may be similar (rheumatic), the structural alterations in the purely incompetent mitral valve are quite different from those in the stenotic valve. The purely incompetent rheumatic valve infrequently contains calcific deposits; its commissures are virtually never fused; its chordae tendineae are only mildly thickened, if at all; and chordal fusion

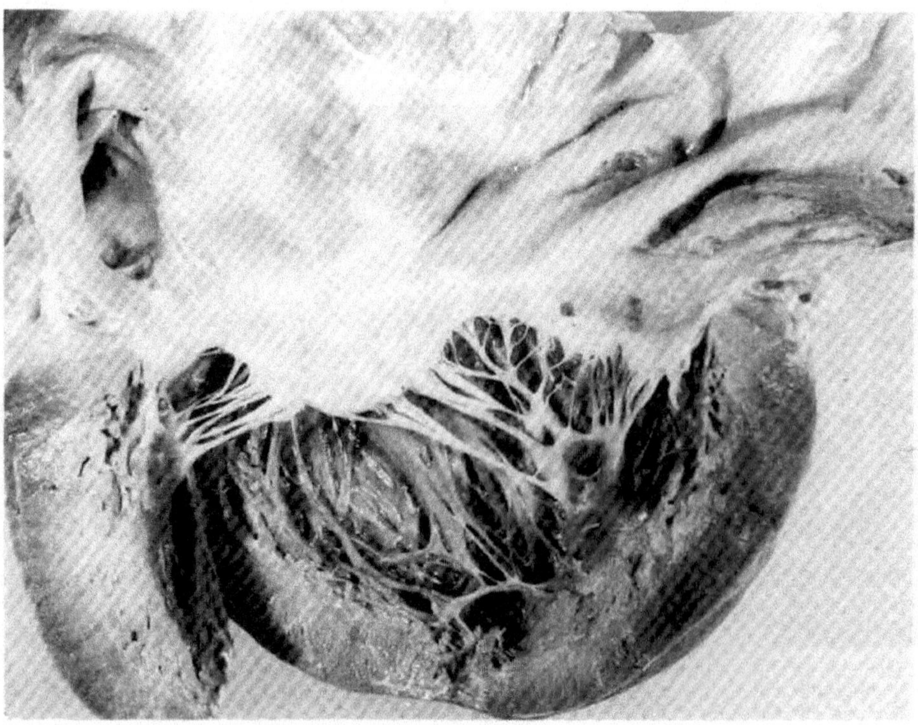

Figure 13. Pure mitral regurgitation of rheumatic cause. This 42-year-old man was said to have had acute rheumatic fever at age 7 years, with a precordial murmur since then. At age 39 years he developed congestive cardiac failure, and a grade 4/6 systolic murmur typical of mitral regurgitation was heard. Catheterization at age 40 years showed the following pressures (in mm Hg): pulmonary artery, 44/19; left atrium—V wave, 28 and mean, 16; left ventricle, 148/13; and brachial artery, 150/84. Left ventricular cineangiogram showed 4+/4+ mitral regurgitation, and aortic root cine showed no aortic regurgitation. He died of progressive congestive cardiac failure 2 years after the catheterization. At necropsy the mitral valve leaflets were diffusely but mildly thickened; the chordae were not shortened, and only a few were thickened; neither commissure was fused. The left atrium was severely dilated. This is the type of valve that is purely incompetent, presumably from damage initiated by rheumatic fever.

is infrequent (Figure 13). It is often difficult to explain the mechanism of mitral regurgitation in a valve made purely incompetent by consequences of rheumatic fever. The mitral anuli in these patients are also usually dilated, but this mechanism in and of itself rarely appears to be an adequate explanation for the regurgitation.

Rheumatic disease is never limited to endocardium. Inflammatory cells are always found in atrial walls of patients dying with acute rheumatic fever (38). The inflammation appears to weaken the walls, and superimposed mitral regurgitation tends to dilate the chamber out of proportion to the dilation that would occur with similar degrees of mitral regurgitation into a left atrium with previously normal walls. What causes the left atrium to dilate enormously in some patients with rheumatic mitral regurgitation is uncertain. Possibly, the patients with so-called giant atria have had more frequent or more severe attacks of acute rheumatic fever, with particularly severe destruction of atrial myocardial fibers. When the left atrium in pure mitral regurgitation is giant in size, intimal proliferation is rarely found in the pulmonary veins or arteries, and the right ventricular walls are not hypertrophied (39) (Figure 14). The anatomy of pure mitral regurgitation in this context thus follows the physiologic alterations outlined by Dr. Perloff. The larger the left atrial cavity in pure mitral regurgitation, the lower its intracavity pressure. Since the right ventricular walls in these patients are

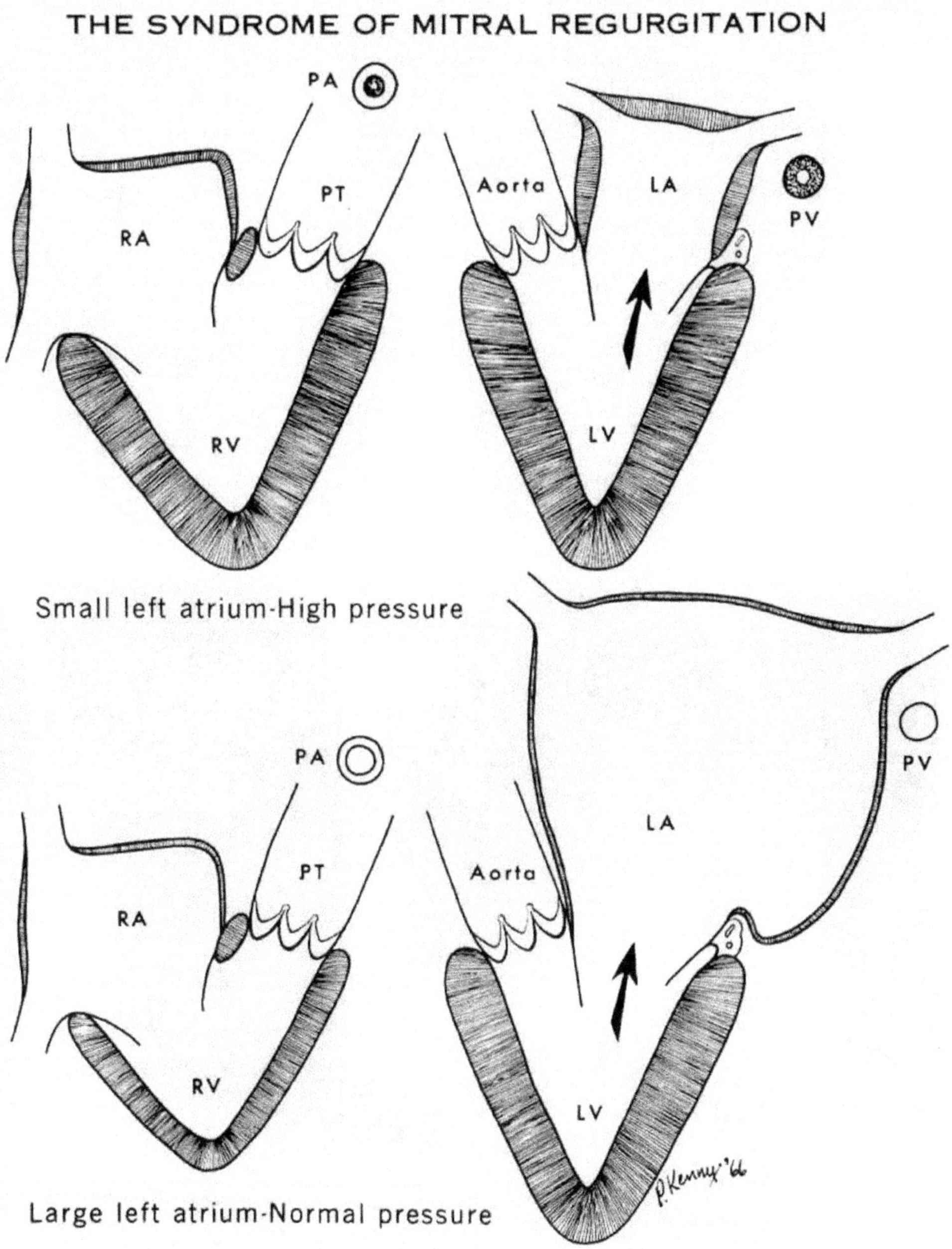

Figure 14. The two extremes of the spectrum of pure mitral regurgitation. When severe mitral regurgitation appears suddenly in individuals with previously normal or near-normal hearts, the left atrium (*LA*) is relatively small, and the high pressure within it is reflected back into the pulmonary vessels and right ventricle (*RV*). The anatomic indicator of this latter physiologic event is severe hypertrophy of the left atrial and right ventricular walls and marked intimal proliferation and medial hypertrophy of the pulmonary arteries (*PA*), arterioles, and veins (*PV*). In the other extreme, the left atrial cavity is of giant size, and its wall is thin. It is thus able to "absorb" the left ventricular (*LV*) pressure without reflecting it back into the pulmonary vessels or right ventricle. As a consequence, the pulmonary vessels remain normal, and the right ventricular wall does not thicken. PT = pulmonary trunk; RA = right atrium.

usually not hypertrophied (because the right ventricular systolic pressures are normal or near normal), tricuspid regurgitation is infrequent. In contrast, patients with large left atria from mitral stenosis or combined mitral stenosis and regurgitation have elevated left atrial, pulmonary venous, pulmonary arterial, and right ventricular pressures, and the right ventricular walls are therefore hypertrophied. Thus, tricuspid regurgitation is a common consequence.

Rupture of mitral chordae tendineae is the second commonest cause of fatal pure mitral regurgitation in patients studied by me at necropsy (35) (Table 2). The normal chordae tendineae are the ones most likely to rupture, not the previously thickened ones. Thus, rupture of one or several thick chordae tendineae in patients with mitral stenosis is extremely rare. The cause of the rupture varies. Infective endocarditis is the commonest cause of acute rupture. However, of 42 patients with healed ruptured mitral chordae tendineae studied by Buchbinder, Roberts, and Morrow (40), only 14 had had infective endocarditis. Infective endocarditis causes acute severe mitral regurgitation by chordal rupture and not, with rare exception, by leaflet perforation (41). The syndrome of acute severe mitral regurgitation associated with normal- or near-normal-sized left atria and severe elevations of left atrial, pulmonary venous, pulmonary arterial, and right ventricular pressures is usually the result of rupture of chordae tendineae by infective endocarditis involving previously normal valves (35). The left atrial myocardial fibers in these patients, as contrasted to those in patients with chronic rheumatic mitral regurgitation, have not been previously damaged by rheumatic fever, and therefore the left atrial wall is capable of responding to the sudden elevation of left atrial pressure by vigorous contractions, leading to fiber hypertrophy. The ventricular systolic pressures in these patients are reflected quickly into the vasculature of the lungs, and severe medial hypertrophy and intimal proliferation of the pulmonary arteries and veins progress rapidly. The already diseased left atrium, in contrast, appears to respond to volume load by dilating, not by contracting. Thus, the smaller the left atrial cavity in pure mitral regurgitation, the thicker the right ventricular wall, and, conversely, the larger the left atrial cavity, the thinner the right ventricular wall.

How many mitral chordae tendineae must rupture for severe regurgitation to occur? Haller and Morrow (42) ruptured only one or two primary chordae in dogs, by inserting fishhooks into left ventricles, and severe mitral regurgitation developed immediately, as evidenced by prominent expansions of the left atria during each ventricular systole.

A newly discovered cause of acquired pure mitral regurgitation is fistulas around bases of prosthetic valves (19). Small peribasilar leaks around mitral prostheses are difficult to diagnose clinically without injecting contrast material into left ventricle (43).

Dr. Perloff: The chordae, like the leaflets, can be too short, too long, or partially destroyed (ruptured) (44). First, we will discuss the chordae that are too long and the leaflets that are too long for their mitral orifices. Mid- to late-systolic clicks, single or multiple,

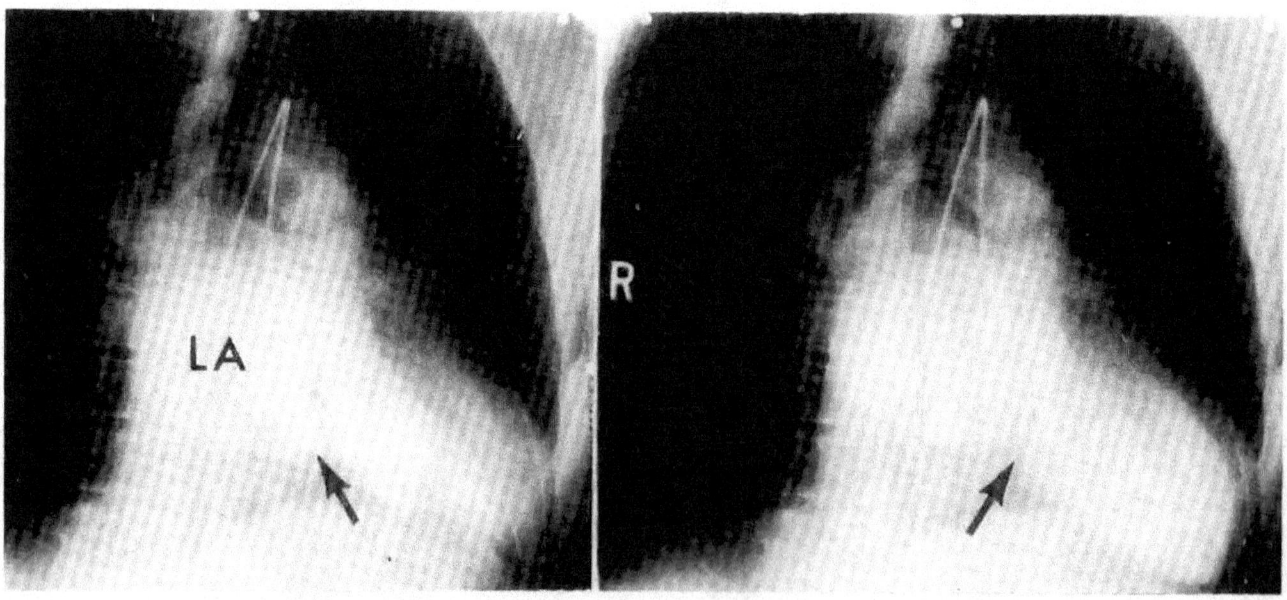

Figure 15. Right anterior oblique left ventricular angiocardiograms from a 49-year-old asymptomatic man with clicks and a late systolic murmur. **Left.** Systolic frame shows lip-like prolapse of the posterior leaflet (*arrow*). **Right.** Diastolic frame shows absence of prolapse (*arrow*). Note opacification of left atrium (*LA*) caused by late systolic mitral regurgitation.

alone or introducing a late systolic murmur, have been recognized for many years. Formerly, these auscultatory signs were believed to be extracardiac (pericardial), especially the clicks alone. Let us examine the evidence that clicks and late systolic murmurs can—and generally do—originate in the mitral apparatus, specifically in redundant posterior cusps and elongated chordae (45-47). When systemic pressure is acutely elevated (pharmacologically) in a patient with a click and a late systolic murmur, the left atrial V wave promptly rises, and the late systolic murmur becomes much louder (48). The converse effect is seen during an acute decrease in systemic pressure induced by inhalation of amyl nitrite (48). Both responses are similar to those in mitral regurgitation (33). Occasionally, during the postamyl nitrite inhalation period, the murmur becomes holosystolic, resembling that of typical mitral regurgitation (48). We can get still closer by examining the intracardiac source of clicks and late systolic murmurs. If an intracardiac phonocardiogram is recorded from the left atrium, systolic clicks and late systolic murmurs can be recovered from just above the mitral valve, a site appropriate for mitral regurgitation (48).

The best clinical evidence of mitral valve origin is the angiocardiogram, as shown in Figure 15, a right oblique left ventricular angiocardiogram. In the systolic frame the arrow points to a lip-like herniation of the redundant posterior cusp into the left atrium, which is opacified because of mitral regurgitation.

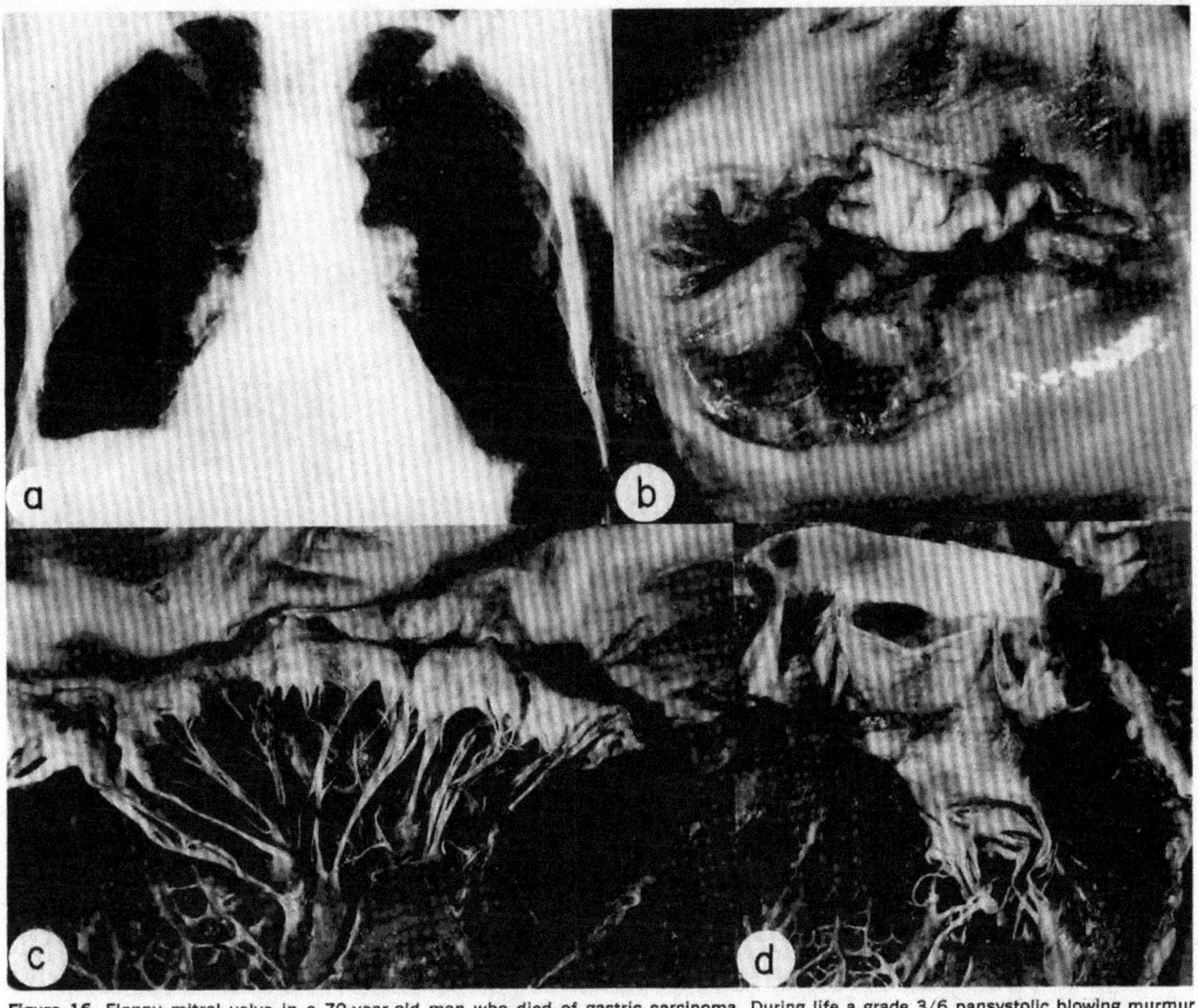

Figure 16. Floppy mitral valve in a 70-year-old man who died of gastric carcinoma. During life a grade 3/6 pansystolic blowing murmur was heard, loudest over the apex, with radiation to the left axilla. The rhythm was atrial fibrillation. He never had symptoms of cardiac dysfunction. Radiograph showed that the heart was enlarged (*a*), but at necropsy it weighed only 310 g. Both atria were quite dilated. The mitral leaflets protruded toward the left atrium (*b*) because the chordae tendineae were too long. A portion of opened mitral valve showing the elongated chordae is shown in c. The opened left ventricle and aortic valve are shown in *d*, again showing excessively long chordae. It is possible that the chordal elongation in the older patients, particularly those with debilitating diseases, results from shortening or atrophy of the ventricles.

In the diastolic frame the posterior cusp falls back into the left ventricular cavity and is not seen. Systolic prolapse of the posterior cusp is a common accompaniment of clicks and late systolic murmurs (45-47, 49). In later systole, as the apex of the left ventricle approaches the mitral anulus, the redundant chordae and posterior leaflet are too long to prevent cuspal eversion. Early in systole the leaflets coapt and seal the mitral orifice; in later systole they give way to late systolic regurgitation. The clicks are believed to

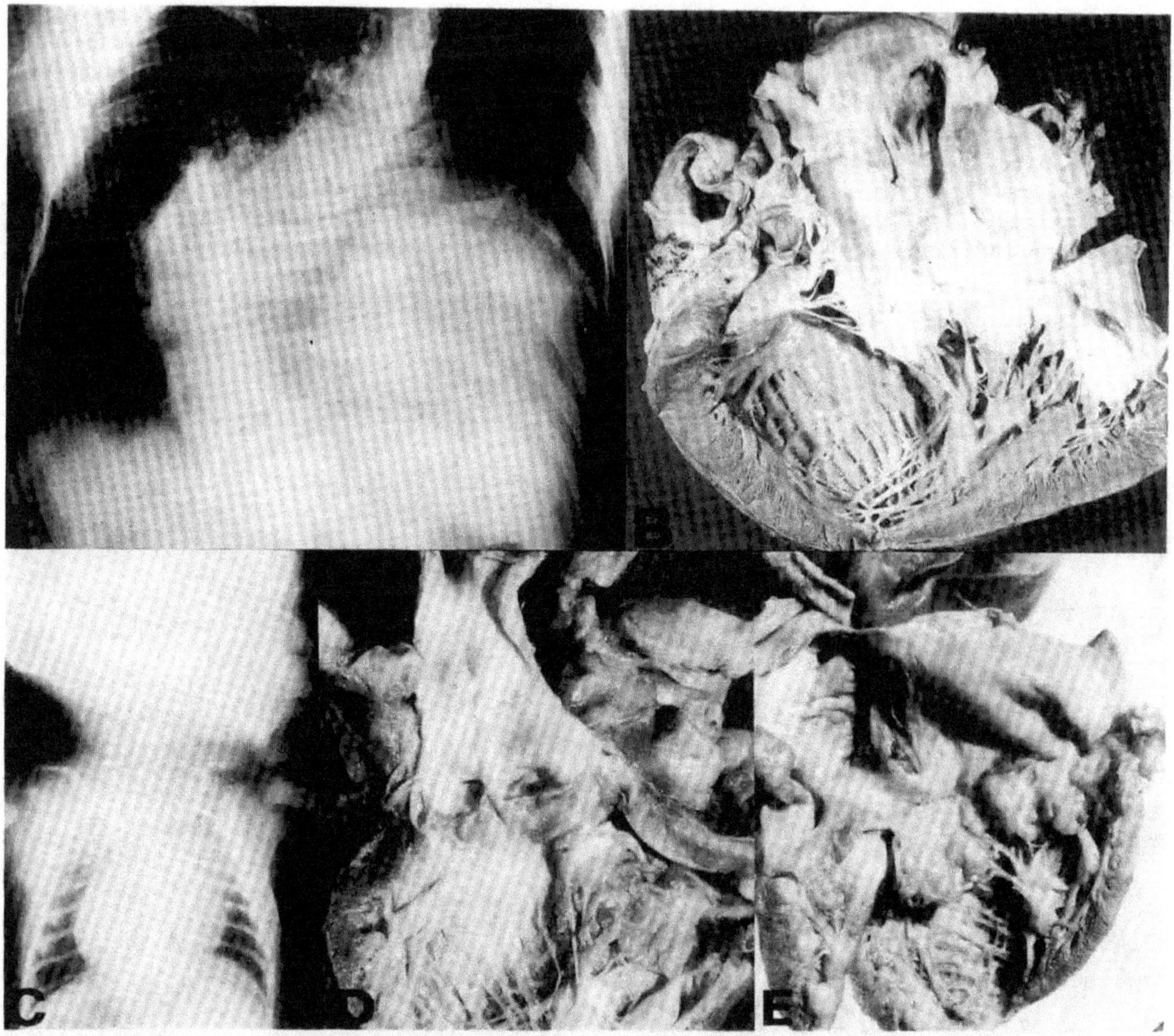

Figure 17A and B. Chest roentgenogram and opened left atrium, mitral valve, and left ventricle in a 28-year-old man with typical (arachnodactyly, myopia, kyphoscoliosis, high-arched palate and arch, and pectus excavatum) features of Marfan's syndrome and severe mitral regurgitation. He had been well until age 24 years, when he developed exertional dyspnea and hemoptysis and was found to have cardiomegaly. Catheterization was performed at age 25 years, and the pressures (in mm Hg) were as follows: pulmonary artery, 19/10; right ventricle, 19/5; right atrial mean, 5; pulmonary arterial wedge mean, 10; and systemic artery, 130/80. The cardiac output was 2.3 litres/min. He remained functionally class II for the next 3 years, but during his last year of life the congestive heart failure worsened, and he became class IV. On examination (7 days before death) he was quite ill. A grade 5/6 pansystolic precordial murmur, loudest over the apex, was audible. No diastolic murmur was present. The chest radiograph showed a big heart and severe kyphoscoliosis (*A*). Electrocardiogram showed sinus rhythm and left ventricular hypertrophy. He died of progressive heart failure. At necropsy, the heart was large (weight, 850 g). The mitral leaflets were mildly thickened and elongated, and the mitral anulus was severely dilated (15 cm) (*B*). Calcific deposits were present in the anulus behind the posterior mitral leaflet. The left atrium was quite dilated, as was the left ventricle. The aortic valve and ascending aorta were normal on both gross and histologic examinations. Thus, this patient represents pure mitral regurgitation without aortic disease in Marfan's syndrome. **C-E.** Floppy mitral valve in a 2-day-old boy who had long toes and fingers, a high-arched palate, and a grade 3/6 precordial systolic murmur typical of mitral regurgitation. The heart was enlarged (*C*). He died of congestive cardiac failure. At necropsy the intima of the ascending aorta was wrinkled (*D*), suggesting that the underlying media was abnormal at this early stage. Shown here is the opened aorta, aortic valve, and left ventricle. **E.** The opened left atrium, mitral valve, and left ventricle. The mitral leaflets are considerably elongated in both longitudinal and transverse dimensions. The left atrium is dilated. This case is particularly important because it shows that the floppy mitral valve and abnormalities in the aorta may be present from birth.

result from abrupt tautening of the chordae tendineae or the redundant leaflet and have been called "chordal snaps" (45).

Another interesting concept regarding clicks and late systolic murmurs concerns abnormal movement of the wall of the left ventricle at the site of origin of the posterior papillary muscle (50). This movement takes the form of a rather striking ventricular contraction band that is believed to prevent proper tautening of posterior leaflet support. Accordingly, during later systole the posterior papillary muscle and its supporting chordae tendineae are thrown into a slack position, and mitral regurgitation follows (50). We thus have three points of view regarding the origin of clicks and late systolic murmurs: redundant leaflet tissue, elongated chordae, and abnormal left ventricular free wall.

In 1880 William Osler published an article (51) with the engaging title "On a Remarkable Heart Murmur Heard at a Distance from the Chest Wall." He described what is now known as systolic whoops or honks (52). These very loud honking or whooping systolic events occur intermittently in some patients who have isolated clicks and late systolic murmurs (53). Redundant leaflets, elongated chordae tendineae, left ventricular contraction bands, systolic clicks, late systolic murmurs, and occasional high-frequency whoops or honks may all be variations of the same theme.

Another interesting feature in such patients—generally healthy young women—are abnormal electrocardiograms (T-wave inversions in diaphragmatic or left chest leads [50], and ectopic rhythms [54]). Sudden death has occurred in such patients, but the frequency of this complication—probably small—is unknown.

One other point regarding systolic clicks and late systolic murmurs. Patients with Marfan's syndrome are traditionally regarded as having aortic root disease. Three causes of mitral regurgitation in Marfan's syndrome are recognized, two of which we shall touch on later. In passing, I mention the third, the long redundant chordae and leaflets.

Dr. Roberts: Fortunately, patients with systolic clicks and late systolic murmurs infrequently have mitral regurgitation severe enough in itself to be fatal. As a consequence, relatively few mitral valves have been examined at necropsy in patients known to have systolic clicks and late systolic murmurs unequivocally documented during life. Several "floppy" mitral valves, the type believed responsible for the ausculatory syndrome, are illustrated in Figures 16 and 17. The posterior mitral leaflet unassociated with ruptured chordae tendineae or necrotic or fibrotic papillary muscles may prolapse abnormally toward the left atrium during ventricular systole because the chordae or the leaflets, or both, are too long. What causes the chordae to elongate in the absence of severe left ventricular dilation is unknown. Prolapsed posterior mitral leaflets are nearly always thickened, but they are nearly always devoid of calcific deposits. Despite their thickening, the leaflets are usually elongated in their basal-to-margin lengths, and usually the amount of leaflet tissue also is increased transversely. The accordion-like buckling of the posterior leaflet causes the floppy mitral valve to appear as dilated hemorrhoids when viewed intact from the left atrium (Figure 16). All floppy mitral valves have increased amounts of acid mucopolysaccharide material in them. Although normally present in all cardiac valves, the amount of acid mucopolysaccharide is greatly increased when the valve has the "floppy" appearance. Most patients with Marfan's syndrome have floppy mitral (Figure 17) and tricuspid valves. Pure mitral regurgitation without aortic regurgitation in them, however, is unusual. The floppy atrioventricular valves seen in Marfan's syndrome are almost certainly present at birth, not something acquired later in life. Evidence for this is the occurrence of floppy mitral and tricuspid valves in a 2-day-old boy studied clinically by Dr. Perloff several years ago (Figure 17*C-E*).

Various cardiovascular findings in Marfan's syndrome are summarized in Figure 18. The major lesion in the aorta in this condition is great loss of elastic fibers. Acid mucopolysaccharide is increased in the aorta in patients with Marfan's syndrome, but the accumulation of this material is not the explanation for weakening of the aortic wall. The latter results from degeneration of its elastic fibers. The smooth muscle cells in the aortic media also show evidence of degeneration by electron-microscopic examination, but this may be a secondary rather than a primary event.

Dr. Perloff: We have discussed chordae tendineae that are too long and leaflets that are too mobile. Now to mitral regurgitation caused by restricted leaflet mobility—namely, abnormally short or ectopically inserted chordae tendineae, as in endocardial cushion defect and congenitally corrected transposition of the great arteries.

Patients with endocardial cushion defects characteristically have cleft anterior mitral cusps and abnormal chordal arrangements (13). The anterior leaflet is almost invariably anatomically faulty but not always functionally incompetent. Mitral regurgitation in partial endocardial cushion defect probably depends more on the abnormally inserting chordae than on the cleft anterior leaflet. When contrast material is injected into the left ventricle in such patients, a peculiar "swan's neck" or "gooseneck" deformity of the outflow tract is seen in diastole (55). The deformity results from a combination of cleft anterior leaflet and abnormally inserting chordae and is present whether the mitral valve is functionally competent or not. The chordae arise from the margins of the cleft and insert directly into the crest of the ventricular septum just below the aortic valve. Such chordae have no counterpart in the normal heart.

A second form of congenital "mitral" regurgitation due to restricted leaflet mobility is congenitally corrected levo-type transposition of the great vessels or ventricular inversion (Figure 19). Normally, right atrial blood crosses a tricuspid valve, enters an anatomic right ventricle, and is ejected into the pulmonary trunk. Left atrial blood crosses a mitral valve, enters an anatomic left ventricle, and flows into the aorta. The pulmonary trunk is anterior to the aortic root. In congenitally corrected transposition the ventricles and their respective atrioventricular (A-V) valves are inverted—that is, right to left interchange (Figure 19). Right atrial blood crosses an anatomic mitral valve and enters an anatomic left ventricle that communicates with a pulmonary trunk. Left atrial blood crosses an anatomic tricuspid valve and enters an anatomic right ventricle that connects with the aorta. Because of this arrangement, the left A-V valve is "tricuspid" and has a relatively

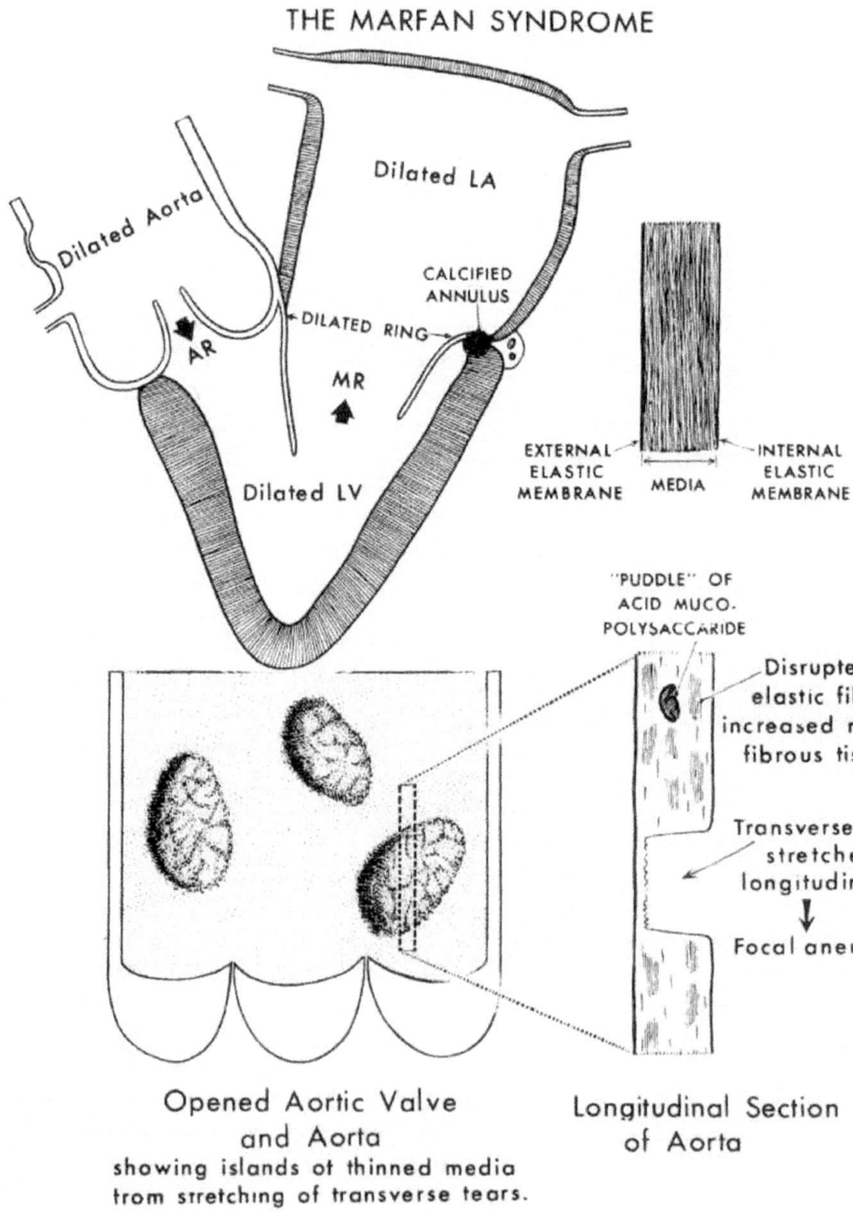

Figure 18. The various cardiovascular abnormalities in Marfan's syndrome. The aortic regurgitation (*AR*) appears to be related primarily to dilation of the aorta. The mitral regurgitation (*MR*) probably results from a combination of factors: dilation of the left ventricular cavity (*LV*) altering the papillary muscle-mitral leaflet angle; dilation of the mitral anulus; calcification of the mitral anulus; and elongation of the mitral leaflets and chordae, allowing prolapse of the leaflets into left atrium during ventricular systole. At top right is a longitudinal section of normal aorta. At bottom right is a longitudinal section in a patient with Marfan's syndrome. There is marked loss of elastic fibers, deposition of abnormal amounts of acid mucopolysaccharide material, and tears in the wall, which later expand to cause the islands of thinning noted in the view of the opened aortic valve and aorta.

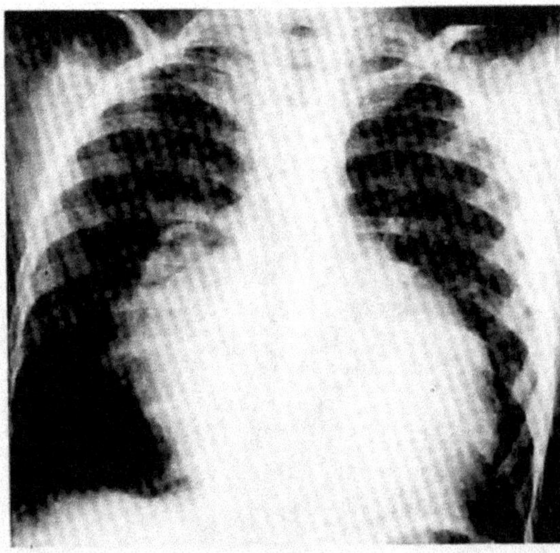

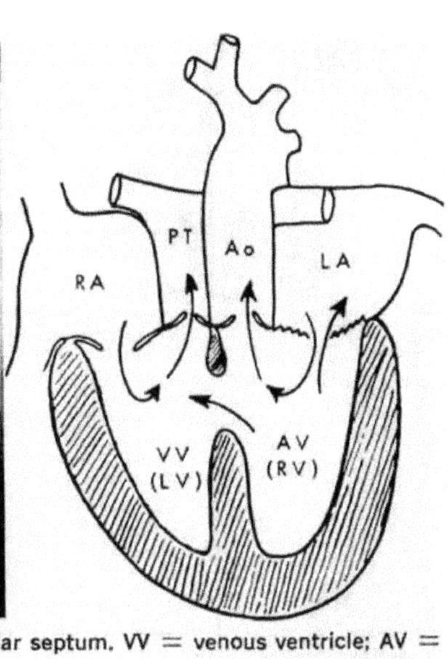

Figure 19 Left. X ray from a 2-year-old girl with congenitally corrected transposition and marked "mitral" regurgitation due to Ebstein's anomaly of the left atrioventricular valve, which was anatomically tricuspid. The vascular pedicle is narrow because the aorta courses vertically upward. A double density of left atrial enlargement is seen to the right of the vertebral column. **Right.** The aorta (*Ao*) and pulmonary trunk (*PT*) arise parallel to each other and do not cross as in the normal heart. Right atrial (*RA*) blood flows across a morphologic mitral valve into an anatomic left ventricle (*LV*) and into the pulmonary trunk. Left atrial (*LA*) blood flows across a morphologic tricuspid valve into an anatomic right ventricle (*RV*) and into the aorta. The left atrioventrioventricular valve may be incompetent (*reversed arrows*) because of an Ebstein-like deformity, and there is often a defect in the ventricular septum. *VV* = venous ventricle; *AV* = arterial ventricle. From Perloff (13); reproduced by permission of W. B. Saunders Co.

high frequency of an Ebstein-type anomaly—that is, leaflet tissue is tethered directly to ventricular endocardium below the anulus (56). Ebstein's anomaly of the tricuspid valve in its normal location causes right A-V valve incompetence; Ebstein's anomaly of a left-sided tricuspid valve (ventricular inversion) causes incompetence of the left A-V valve that may be mistaken for "mitral" regurgitation (57).

Dr. Roberts: Congenital mitral regurgitation is usually associated with other anomalies (58). "Isolated" congenital mitral regurgitation is usually accompanied by endocardial fibroelastosis of the left ventricle (Figure 20). However, it is sometimes difficult to determine what causes the mitral valve to be incompetent in this circumstance.

Neither is it always clear why the mitral valve is frequently incompetent in partial atrioventricular canal (endocardial cushion defect). As Dr. Perloff indicated, nearly all patients with partial A-V canal have a cleft, either partial or complete, in the anterior mitral leaflet. It would be easy to attribute the regurgitation to this cleft, but the regurgitation usually disappears after operative closure of the associated defect in the lowermost portion of the atrial septum (ostium primum defect), irrespective of whether the cleft in the anterior mitral leaflet is closed by suture (59). For the same reason, it is unlikely that the anomalous chordae tendineae that insert onto the crest of the ventricular septum play a significant role in the production of mitral regurgitation. It is well to think of a partial A-V canal as a syndrome consisting of five components: [1] defect in the lowermost portion of atrial septum; [2] cleft in the anterior mitral leaflet; [3] absence of tissue, either partial or complete, in the septal tricuspid valve leaflet; [4] anomalous chordae tendineae from the anterior mitral leaflet to the crest of ventricular septum; and [5] ventricular septal defect. The syndrome may include all five components or may have as few as two; most commonly, the first four components are present. A cleft in the anterior mitral leaflet may occur, however, in the absence of a defect in the lowermost portion of the atrial septum. These individuals usually present with evidence of isolated mitral regurgitation or with features of isolated ventricular septal defect. Occasionally, the ostium primum defect may be so small that the shunt through it is missed or is only trivial, and these patients also may present with essentially pure mitral regurgitation (60, 61) (Figure 21).

Corrected transposition is an entity that has produced much confusion. Corrected transposition and complete transposition are quite different; the only thing they have in common is the word "transposition." Complete transposition is essentially one defect: the great arteries are transposed, so that the aorta arises from the right ventricle and the pulmonary trunk from the left ventricle. In corrected transposition also the great arteries are transposed, but, in addition, the ventricles, atrioventricular valves, coronary arteries, and conduction system are inverted. Patients with complete transposition die because they have inadequate communications between the two circuits. Patients with corrected transposition theoretically should be able to live a full life-span, but usually this is not the case because associated defects—namely, ventricular septal defect or incompetency of the left-sided A-V valve, or both—cause the heart to function abnormally. Abnormalities of the left-sided A-V valve, a systemic valve but

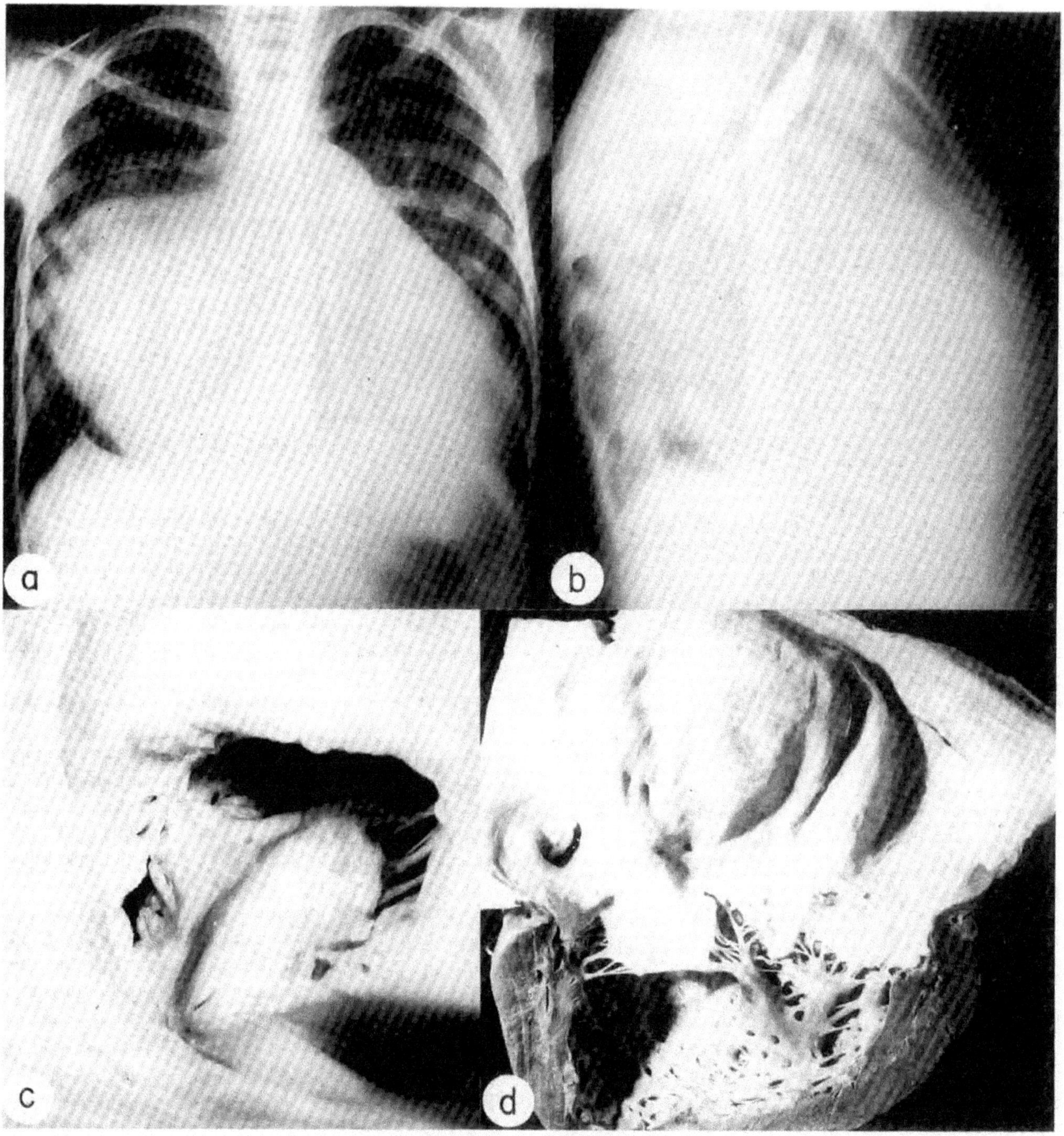

Figure 20. Congenital mitral regurgitation associated with diffuse fibroelastosis of the left ventricle in a 9-year-old boy. He was believed to be normal at birth. At age 3 years peripheral edema was noted, and examination showed generalized cardiomegaly and a grade 3/6 systolic murmur of mitral regurgitation. Electrocardiogram showed sinus rhythm and left ventricular hypertrophy. Catheterization at age 4 years showed the pulmonary arterial pressure to be 42/24 and pulmonary arterial wedge pressure mean to be 24 mm Hg. He had progressive congestive failure over the next 4 years. Examination 5 months before death showed severe cardiomegaly (*a* and *b*), atrial fibrillation, and a grade 5/6 systolic precordial murmur. On repeat catheterization the pressures (in mm Hg) were as follows: pulmonary artery, 66/36; right ventricle, 66/8; right atrium, mean 9; left atrium, mean 9; left atrium—mean, 21 and V wave, 32; left ventricle, 102/12; and brachial artery, 116/72. At operation (4 months before death) severe mitral regurgitation was found. Mitral valvuloplasty and anuloplasty was carried out. During his entire 4-month postoperative period he had evidence of progressive congestive cardiac failure. At necropsy the mitral valve orifice was severely incompetent, as viewed from the left atrium (*c*). Both left atrium and left ventricle were severely dilated, and the endocardium of both chambers (*d*) was diffusely thickened by fibroelastosis. The mitral anulus was also considerably dilated.

anatomically a tricuspid valve, are the commonest associated anomalies in corrected transposition (56). Of the anomalies the most frequent is the Ebstein-type malformation (Figure 22). These valves are intrinsically incompetent because the chordae are short and the leaflets are closely adherent to the ventricular endocardium.

A mitral valve may be abnormal anatomically and yet function entirely normally. A congenital malformation illustrating this point is the entity "double-orifice mitral valve" (62) (Figure 23), which looks like a double-barreled shotgun. Generally, both orifices are totally competent, and the patient should be asymptomatic.

PAPILLARY MUSCLE DYSFUNCTION

Dr. Perloff: Now to the muscular apparatus of the mitral valve, namely, the papillary muscles and left

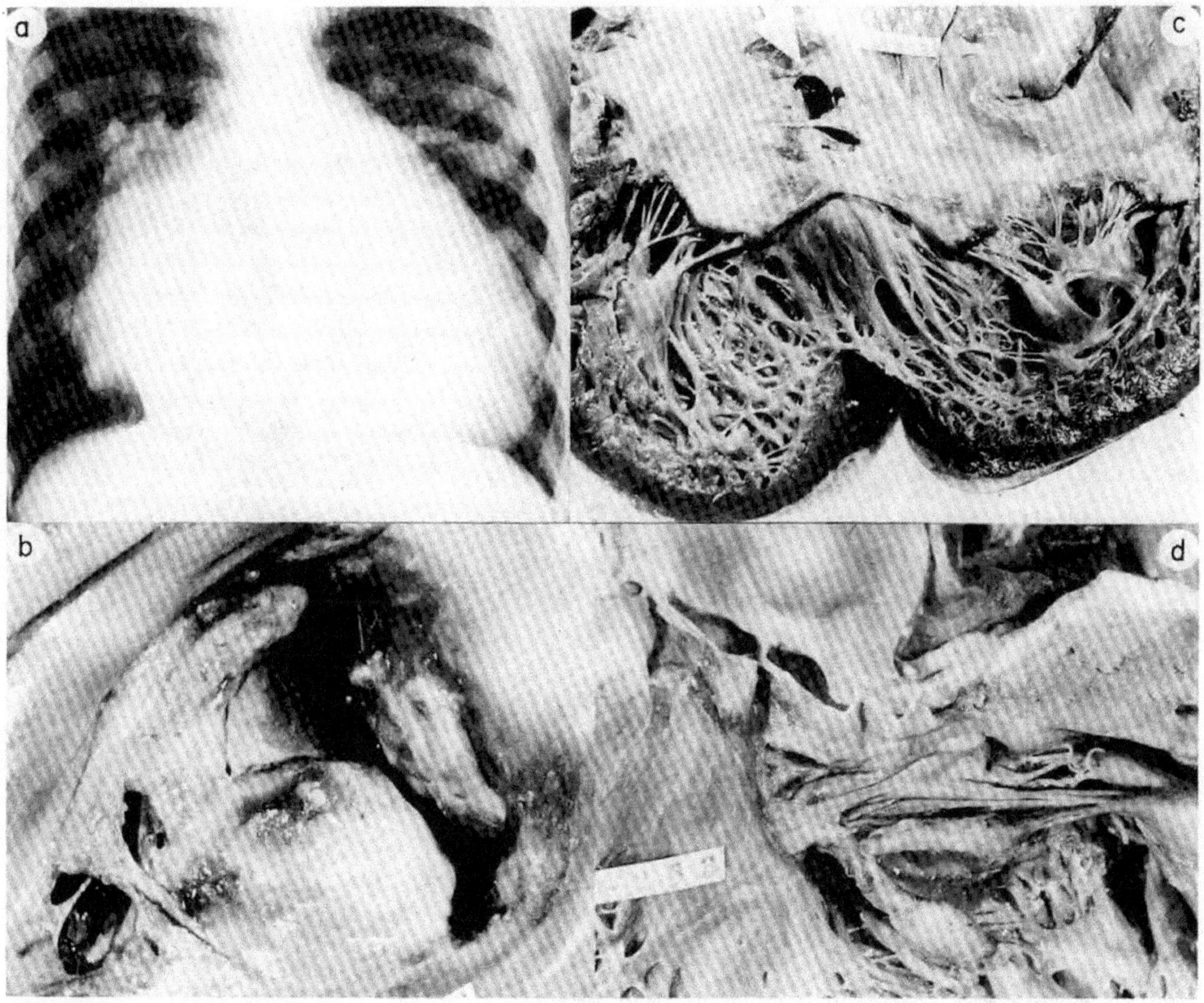

Figure 21. Congenital mitral regurgitation secondary to partial atrioventricular canal (endocardial cushion defect) in a 13-year-old boy. At age 6 years he was found to have a systolic precordial murmur and mitral regurgitation. He limited his activities because of fatigue but at age 11 years developed overt right- and left-sided congestive cardiac failure. At age 12 years atrial fibrillation appeared. On examination during his last month of life he was cachetic. A grade 3/6 pansystolic precordial murmur, loudest over the apex, and a grade 3/6 mid-diastolic rumble at the apex were audible. Electrocardiogram showed atrial fibrillation, left axis deviation, and left ventricular hypertrophy, and chest radiograph showed a large heart (*a*). At catheterization the pressures (in mm Hg) were as follows: right ventricle, 55/15; right atrium—mean, 13 and V wave, 17; and left atrium—mean, 15 and V wave, 27. Surprisingly, the catheter passed into the left atrium via an atrial septal defect. The calculated pulmonary to systemic flow ratio was 1.4/1.0. The child died 1 day after operative closure of a cleft in the anterior mitral leaflet and of a small, 1.0-cm defect in the lowermost portion of the atrial septum. At necropsy, a large cleft was found in the anterior mitral leaflet (*b* and *c*), and at the apex of the cleft there was a tiny atrial septal defect. **c.** The cleft and defect with the mitral valve, left atrium, and left ventricle opened. The left atrium is quite dilated. **d.** The opened aorta, aortic valve, and left ventricular outflow tracts, showing anomalous chordae tendineae extending from the apex of the anterior mitral leaflet to the crest of the ventricular septum. These anomalous chordae tendineae are universally found in partial atrioventricular canal and are responsible for the gooseneck deformity seen on the left ventricular angiography.

ventricular wall. First, there is papillary muscle dysfunction with loss in continuity, that is, rupture (63). The cause is almost always myocardial infarction. Rupture of chordae is unrelated to myocardial infarction. The clinical picture of ruptured papillary muscle is acute overwhelming mitral regurgitation (*see* above), although the consequences depend in part on just where in the papillary muscle structure the discontinuity occurs.

Dr. Roberts: Rupture of a portion of a papillary muscle is really an old entity, but it was not appreciated until less than 5 years ago (63). The original concept of papillary muscle rupture was rupture of its entire trunk, caused either by myocardial infarction from coronary narrowing or by trauma. Complete transsection of a left ventricular papillary muscle is incompatible with life because about 60 chordae tendineae are thus disrupted (2) (Figure

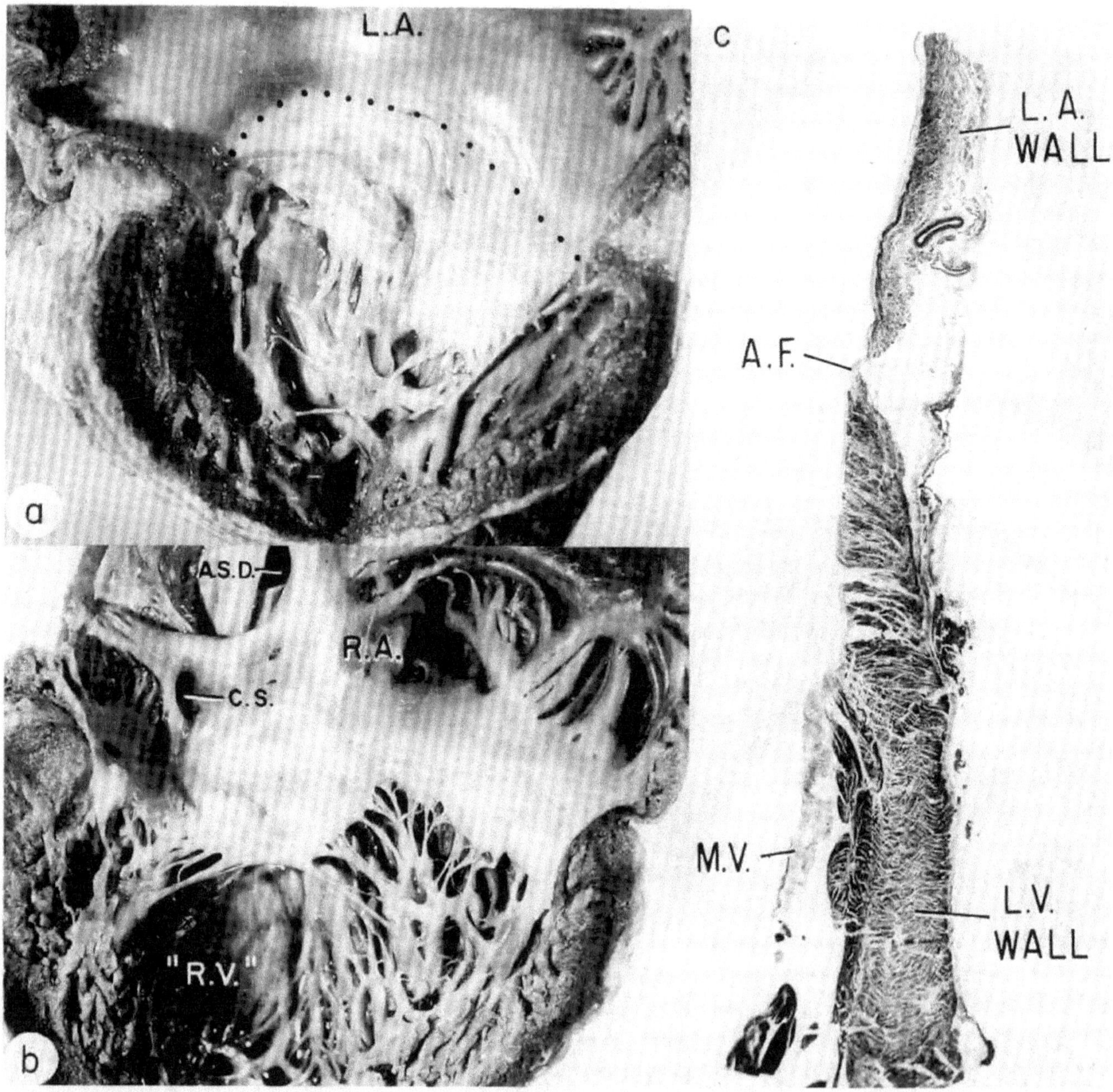

Figure 22. Congenital "mitral" regurgitation in corrected transposition of the great vessels with Ebstein-type malformation. **a.** The opened left atrium (*L.A.*), "tricuspid" valve—showing an Ebstein-type malformation—and left ventricle in a 38-year-old man who also had subvalvular pulmonic stenosis and a small atrial septal defect (*A.S.D.*). Ebstein's malformation is a downward displacement of the left-sided (anatomic tricuspid) valve. **c.** A longitudinal histologic section of the anulus fibrosis (*A.F.*), left ventricle (*L.V.*), and mitral valve (*M.V.*) (anatomically the tricuspid valve). The valve leaflet normally arises from the left ventricular wall below the anulus. The true anulus is shown by dots in *a*. **b.** The opened right atrium (*R.A.*), right-sided atrioventricular valve (anatomically the mitral valve), and the right-sided ventricle ("*R.V.*", anatomically a left ventricle). C.S. = ostium of the coronary sinus.

24*A*). More frequent is rupture of a portion of a papillary muscle (Figure 24*A*). In this situation the largest amount of regurgitation is probably caused by the rupture, but all these patients have severe necrosis of the remaining portion of the papillary muscle, and the latter probably contributes to the regurgitation (Figure 24*B*). When 1 head of a papillary muscle is ruptured, about 10 third-order chordae tendineae are disrupted (Figure 4).

Dr. Perloff: Rupture of a papillary muscle can be considered papillary muscle dysfunction with loss in continuity (44). Burch, DePasquale, and Phillips (64-66) popularized the idea that the papillary muscles may function abnormally without loss in continuity, and we now know that this is clinically the commoner form of papillary muscle dysfunction. Contraction of the papillary muscles initiates ventricular systole, pulling the two leaflets into apposition. As the left ventricle continues to contract, there must be synergistic contraction of the papillary muscles so that the mitral leaflets do not evert into the left atrium as the apex of the left ventricle approaches the anulus. If a papillary muscle cannot perform that function, the mitral leaflets evert, and regurgitation occurs.

I shall now comment briefly on certain current

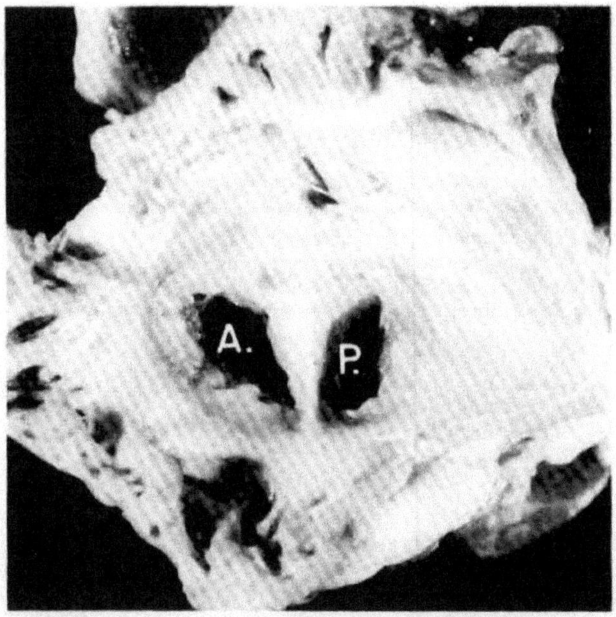

Figure 23. Congenital malformation of the mitral valve, namely, double orifice, causing no cardiac dysfunction. The two orifices, anterior (*A.*) and posterior (*P.*), have the appearance, from the left atrium, of a double-barrelled shotgun. This heart belonged to a cow killed for other reasons, but similar valves have been observed in humans.

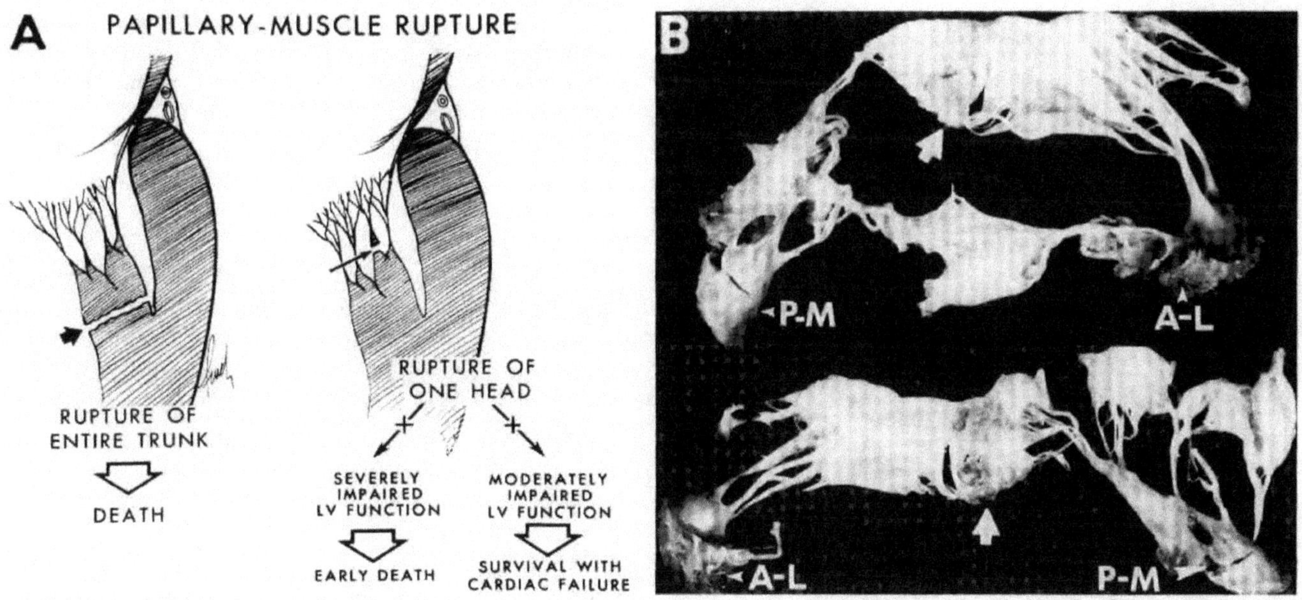

Figure 24A. Diagrammatic representation of the types, and possible consequences, of papillary muscle rupture during acute myocardial infarction. Rupture of the entire trunk (*left*) is probably incompatible with survival in any patient, since a major portion of the support to both valve leaflets is destroyed. With rupture of an apical head (*right*), survival would appear to depend on the extent to which the function of the left ventricle has been impaired by the infarct. With severely impaired ventricular function the additional burden of even modest mitral regurgitation may be intolerable, and death will ensue. If the left ventricle is less severely compromised, survival is possible for weeks or months, but congestive cardiac failure will almost invariably develop. **B.** Rupture of a portion of one papillary muscle during acute myocardial infarction in a 51-year-old man who underwent mitral valve replacement 3 months after the onset of the infarction. Preoperatively, the pulmonary arterial pressure was 60/28 mm Hg (mean, 40 mm Hg); pulmonary arterial wedge pressure —mean, 28 and V wave, 42 mm Hg; left ventricular pressure, 74/17 mm Hg; and cardiac index, 1.7 litres/min·m^2 body surface area. Shown is the excised (by Dr. Andrew G. Morrow) mitral valve. The leaflets are normal but the posteromedial (*P-M*) papillary muscle is necrotic and fibrotic, and a portion (*arrow*) of it is intwined in chordae tendineae at the margin of the anterior mitral leaflet. **Top.** Ventricular aspects of the leaflets. **Bottom.** Opened valve, showing the atrial aspects of the leaflets. A-L = anterolateral papillary muscle.

Table 3. Spectrum of Left Ventricular Papillary Muscle Disease

- Anatomically normal papillary muscles but papillary muscle dysfunction
  - Transient ischemia
  - Left ventricular dilation from any cause
    - Generalized
    - Localized
  - Necrosis or fibrosis in adjacent left ventricular free wall
    - With coronary arterial narrowing
    - Without coronary arterial narrowing
  - "Small" left ventricular cavity (hypertrophic cardiomyopathy)
- Necrosis or fibrosis of papillary muscle(s) without rupture
  - With coronary arterial narrowing
    - Acute myocardial infarction
    - Healed myocardial infarction
  - Without coronary arterial narrowing
    - Acute
      - Shock
      - Acute valvular regurgitation (infective endocarditis)
    - Chronic
      - Anemia
      - Left ventricular outflow obstruction
        - Valvular aortic stenosis
        - Discrete and diffuse subaortic stenosis
        - Supravalvular aortic stenosis
      - Systemic hypertension
      - Origin of left coronary artery or of both coronary arteries from pulmonary trunk
      - Primary endocardial fibroelastosis of left ventricle
      - Endomyocardial disease and eosinophilia
        - Löffler's fibroplastic parietal endocarditis
        - Endomyocardial fibrosis of Davies
      - Idiopathic cardiomegaly (primary or diffuse myocardial disease)
      - Focal myocardial disease
        - Idiopathic
        - "Neurogenic" heart disease
          - Progressive muscular dystrophy
          - Friedreich's ataxia
          - Myotonic muscular dystrophy
- Necrosis or fibrosis of papillary muscle(s) with rupture
  - Acute myocardial infarction from coronary heart disease
  - Trauma
  - Miscellaneous
- Infiltrative diseases of papillary muscles
  - Pyogenic abscess
  - Granulomas
    - Aschoff's bodies
    - Sarcoid
  - Amyloid
  - Neoplasm
  - Calcium
  - Iron
  - Other
- Congenital malformations of papillary muscle(s)
  - Single papillary muscle (parachute mitral valve syndrome)
  - Accessory papillary muscle
  - Abnormally large and malpositioned papillary muscles
  - Abnormally small and malpositioned papillary muscle
  - Insertion of papillary muscle directly into mitral leaflet
- Miscellaneous afflictions of papillary muscle(s)
  - Excision, partial or complete, during mitral valve replacement
    - Atrophy of nonexcised portion of papillary muscle after valve replacement
    - Left ventricular aneurysm at site of papillary muscle excision
  - Disuse atrophy after excision of mitral leaflets and chordae without excision of papillary muscle(s)

concepts of papillary muscle dysfunction without loss in continuity. In the early 1950s the murmur of mitral regurgitation was considered holosystolic. It is now well established that regurgitant flow across the mitral orifice can be accompanied not only by a holosystolic murmur but also by midsystolic, late systolic, or early systolic murmurs. I have already mentioned the click and the late systolic murmur. In papillary muscle dysfunction, lack of synergistic control of the chordae and leaflets may allow regurgitation early in systole, late in systole, throughout systole, or chiefly in midsystole. All variations occur, and all may be related to dysfunction of papillary muscle without loss in continuity (6, 64, 67).

An interesting variety of papillary muscle dysfunction gives rise to severe intermittent mitral regurgitation (68). It is well known that during angina, mild mitral regurgitation may transiently appear because of ischemic papillary muscle dysfunction without infarction. It has now been shown that transient severe regurgitation occasionally occurs during bouts of ischemic pain (68). Such an event can be looked on as the transient counterpart of acute severe persistent mitral regurgitation after chordal or papillary muscle rupture.

Ischemic papillary muscle dysfunction also occurs in congenital coronary arterial disease, namely, anomalous origin of the left coronary artery from the pulmonary trunk (69). In this disorder mitral regurgitation is common in patients surviving infancy.

Papillary muscle dysfunction without loss of continuity has, since first described by Burch, DePasquale, and Phillips (64), been related to the papillary muscle per se. More recent information indicates that the contiguous portion of left ventricular free wall—that is, the segment of left ventricle from which papillary muscle springs—is functionally a part of the papillary muscle (70-72). In experimentally induced infarction confined to a canine papillary muscle, the mitral valve is not necessarily rendered incompetent (70-72). However, if the base of the papillary muscle—the segment of left ventricle from which the papillary muscle springs—is infarcted, then the valve becomes incompetent (70-72).

Dr. Roberts: Necrosis or fibrosis of a papillary muscle without rupture is far commoner than rupture. Table 3 lists conditions frequently associated with papillary muscle dysfunction, particularly necrosis or fibrosis (2). Although coronary arterial luminal narrowing is the most frequent cause of papillary muscle necrosis or fibrosis, many other conditions may be accompanied by papillary muscle lesions. The papillary muscles are fibrotic or necrotic in so many conditions because they are the last structures in the heart to be perfused by arterial blood (73). Of the two left ventricular papillary muscles, the posteromedial one has the poorer blood supply, and, consequently, lesions are more frequent in it than in the anterolateral muscle. The posteromedial muscle receives its oxygen mainly from blood passing through the right coronary artery. The mouth of this artery may be more than 15 cm from the apex of the posteromedial muscle. To perfuse it, blood must pass through the entire thickness of left ventricular wall, turn uphill, and ascend a distance equivalent to two more full thicknesses of left ventricular wall. Thus, the apexes of the papillary muscles are the sites furthest from the coronary ostia, and they receive oxygen only after the other myocardium has had an opportunity to extract its oxygen needs. Although the entire surfaces of the papillary muscles are bathed by intracavitary ventricular blood, only a small amount of oxygen diffuses into these structures from the intracavitary blood (Figure 25).

The commonest cause of papillary muscle necrosis or fibrosis is narrowing of the coronary arterial lumen by atherosclerosis (Figure 26). The posteromedial papillary muscle is usually involved in acute posterior myocardial infarction. In anterior wall infarction, however, the anterolateral papillary muscle may be spared, presumably because its blood supply is better than that of the posteromedial muscle. Since infarction limited to the ventricular septum or to the lateral portion of the left ventricular free wall (that is, the portions of the left ventricular wall unassociated with papillary muscles) is rare, the papillary muscles are usually involved when myocardial infarction occurs. It is, therefore, surprising that papillary muscle dysfunction is not more frequent during or after acute myocardial infarction (74).

In patients with left ventricular outflow obstruction, lesions often occur in the papillary muscles. Valvular aortic stenosis, whether in infants or in adults, when superimposed on a congenitally malformed valve, either unicuspid or bicuspid, is nearly always associated with fibrosis and atrophy of at least the posteromedial papillary muscle (75-79) (Figure 27). Rheumatic valvular aortic stenosis combined with organic mitral stenosis or regurgitation, however, infrequently is associated with papillary muscle fibrosis or atrophy. Nearly all adult patients with discrete subaortic stenosis or hypertrophic cardiomyopathy with or without diffuse subaortic stenosis have small fibrous scars in both left ventricular papillary muscles, but atrophy of one or both muscles is uncommon (80).

Foci of necrosis are also common in patients with fatal severe valvular regurgitation of recent onset. Among 47 patients dying of active valvular infective endocarditis, 34 (72%) had necrotic lesions in one or both left ventricular papillary muscles, and none had significant narrowing of the extramural coronary arteries (41, 81). Most patients had pure aortic regurgitation, but some had pure mitral regurgitation secondary to the active infective endocarditis. Severely diminished cardiac output resulting in poor myocardial perfusion was believed to be the cause of the papillary muscle necrosis in these patients.

Small fibrous scars in the papillary muscles are common in patients with systemic hypertension, but atrophy of these muscles is infrequent in this condition, unless coronary heart disease also is present. In left ventricular hypertrophy of any cause, the hypertrophy of the papillary muscles should probably be proportional to that of the left ventricular free wall or ventricular septum. This proportional hypertrophy usually exists in patients with systemic hypertension but is infrequent in patients with left ventricular outflow obstruction.

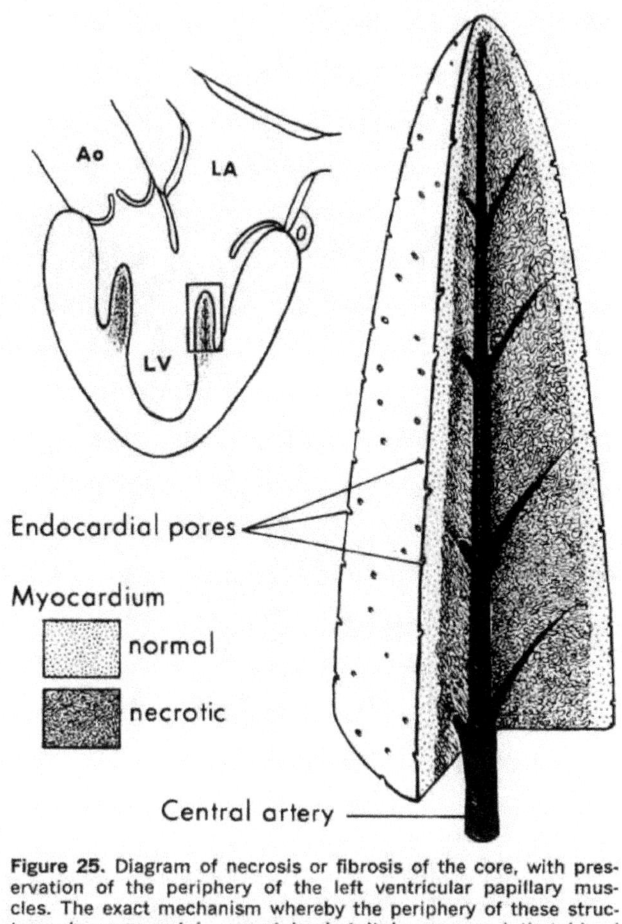

Figure 25. Diagram of necrosis or fibrosis of the core, with preservation of the periphery of the left ventricular papillary muscles. The exact mechanism whereby the periphery of these structures is preserved is uncertain, but it is presumed that blood from the left ventricular (*LV*) cavity diffuses, possibly via endocardial pores, into their outer portions. The central artery appears to supply only the inner portion of the papillary muscle with arterial blood. Ao = aorta; LA = left artery.

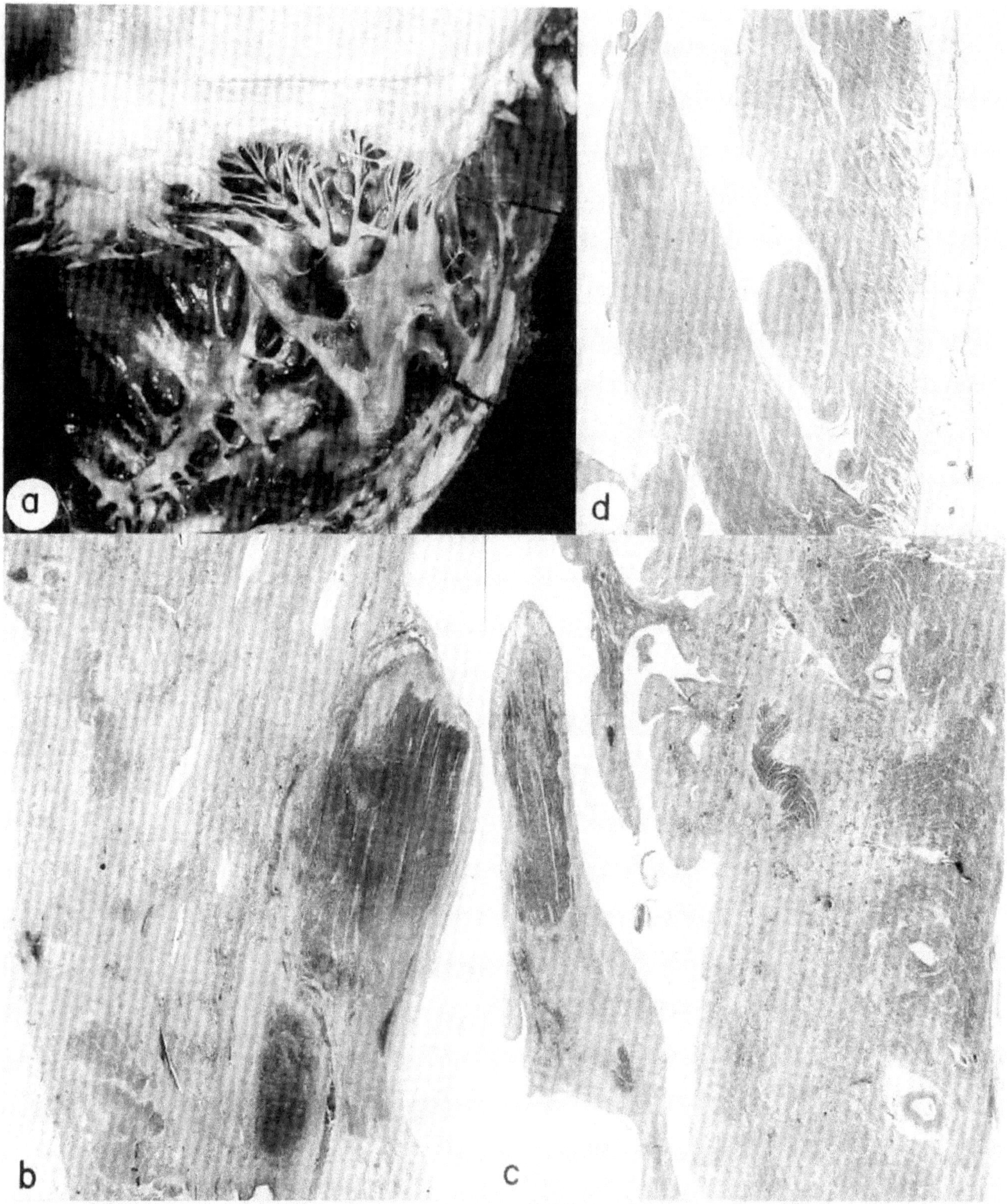

Figure 26. Papillary muscle necrosis without rupture during silent acute myocardial infarction in a 71-year-old man who developed congestive cardiac failure 2 months before death and a grade 4/6 systolic murmur of mitral regurgitation 2 weeks before death. Electrocardiograms did show an evolving acute myocardial infarction. **a.** Opened left ventricle, showing extensive necrosis of the posteromedial papillary muscle and of the left ventricular free wall beneath it. **b.** Histologic section, showing diffuse necrosis of the entire posteromedial papillary muscle and extensive fibrosis with patchy necrosis of the free wall beneath it. **c.** Anterolateral papillary muscle that is also necrotic and fibrotic. **d.** Anterior papillary muscle of right ventricle showing focal necrosis in its apical third. (Hematoxylin and eosin. Original magnification: **b** and **c**, × 6; **d**, × 3.)

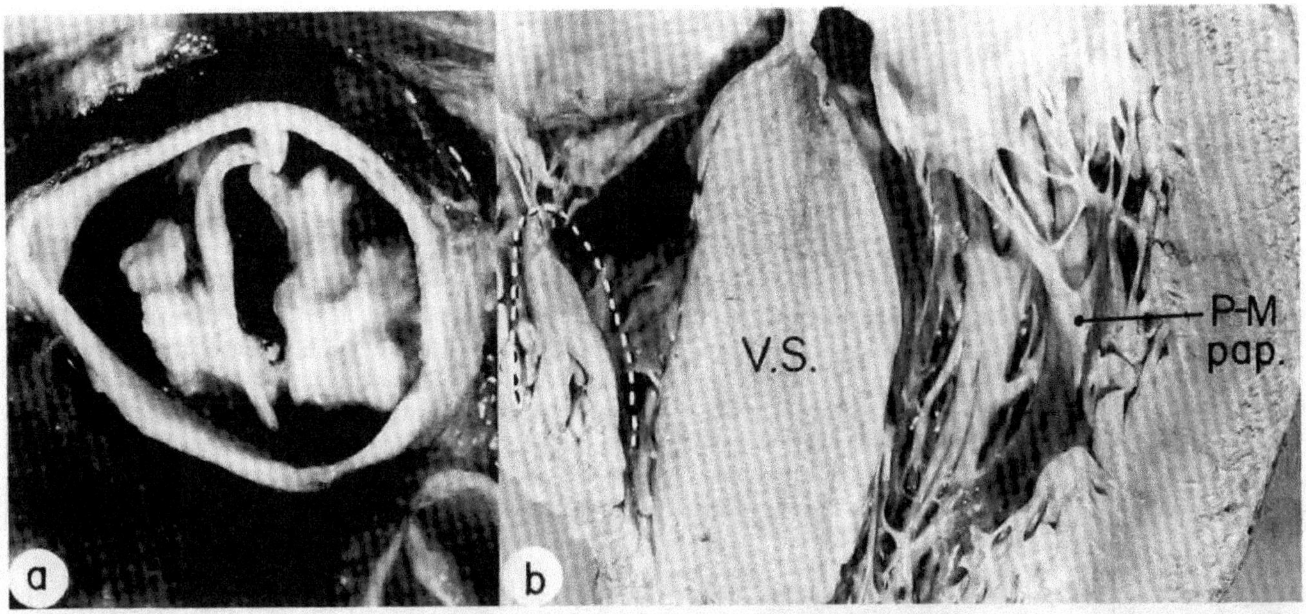

Figure 27. Papillary muscle fibrosis and atrophy associated with aortic stenosis involving a congenitally bicuspid aortic valve and unassociated with coronary arterial luminal narrowing. This 52-year-old woman had symptoms of cardiac dysfunction for 3 years and a precordial murmur typical of mitral regurgitation in addition to murmurs of aortic stenosis and regurgitation. The peak systolic gradient across the valve was 130 mm Hg. **a.** Stenotic aortic valve from above. **b.** Longitudinal section, showing portions of all four chambers. The posteromedial papillary muscle (*P-M pap.*) is severely atrophied (it hardly protrudes into the left ventricular cavity) and scarred. The apical portion of the anterior papillary muscle of the right ventricle is also scarred (*dots*). The reason for papillary muscle scarring and atrophy in patients with aortic stenosis superimposed on congenitally malformed valves is unknown. VS = ventricular septum.

Fibrosis with atrophy of the papillary muscles is to be expected in patients with primary endocardial fibroelastosis of the left ventricle (82). Histologically, the thickened endocardium in this condition is similar to the media of the aorta, being characterized by elastic fibrils running parallel to one another and to the surface. Primary left ventricular endocardial fibroelastosis may be an anatomic expression of chronically inadequate coronary arterial perfusion of the left ventricle; since the posteromedial papillary muscle is the least well perfused portion of the heart, this structure is affected the most. In the congenital anomaly, origin of the left (69) or both (83) coronary arteries from the pulmonary trunk, diffuse endocardial fibroelastosis of the left ventricle is nearly always an associated lesion. Fibrosis and atrophy of the left ventricular papillary muscles are to be expected in this anomaly, and these patients may present clinically with features of pure mitral regurgitation (84) (Figure 28).

Foci of fibrosis or necrosis in the left ventricular papillary muscles are infrequent in patients with the congestive or dilated type of cardiomyopathy (85) (Figure 29). Severe scarring of one papillary muscle and of the free wall beneath it was responsible for severe mitral regurgitation in a patient with primary myocardial disease studied by Marcus and coworkers (86). Generally, however, left ventricular cavity dilation alone is the cause of mitral regurgitation in these patients. Rarely, myocarditis may be localized to papillary muscle and adjacent left ventricular free wall (39). Patients with the neurogenic heart diseases (Friedreich's ataxia, progressive musculary dystrophy, and myotonic muscular dystrophy) (87) generally have scarred left ventricular papillary muscles, especially posteromedial ones. The African cardiomyopathy, endomyocardial fibrosis, may be associated with extensive scarring of the papillary muscles (2). In this condition the posteromedial muscle is usually covered by a thrombus or by dense fibrous tissue that may be organization of thrombus. Likewise, Löffler's fibroplastic parietal endocarditis (Figure 30), which may be one stage of endomyocardial fibrosis (88), is usually associated with extensive scarring of one or both papillary muscles (89).

The papillary muscles are subject to various infiltrative processes, just like any other portion of myocardium. Pyogenic abscesses, Aschoff bodies (Figure 31), granulomas (85), neoplasms, amyloid (90), and iron (91) have all been observed in these structures. Congestive heart failure from severe mitral regurgitation may be the initial symptom of sarcoidosis (2).

The most frequent congenital malformation of papillary muscles is the occurrence of only one such muscle in the left ventricle (22) (Figure 9). In this condition, described as the parachute mitral valve, all mitral chordae tendineae are attached to the one left ventricular papillary muscle. The resulting mitral valve is usually stenotic (22), but it may be purely incompetent (23), or it may function normally (23). The single papillary muscle is usually associated with other malformations, including a supramitral valve ring, diffuse subaortic stenosis, and coarctation of the aorta. Other malformations, including valvular aortic stenosis, ventricular septal defect, and valvular pulmonic stenosis may also occur.

There may be not only one too few papillary muscles but also one too many. An accessory papillary muscle is usually of no functional significance, but it has been seen in association with congenital mitral regurgitation (58). When two papillary muscles are present, one or both may still be congenitally malformed. Each of the papillary muscles may be abnormally large and malpositioned, so that the primary orifice of the valve is narrowed (24, 25). Both papillary muscles also may be poorly developed and small. This finding is particularly characteristic with origin of the left coronary artery from the pulmonary trunk. In the latter anomaly the papillary muscles also arise high on the left ventricular wall (24), in contrast to the normal heart, in which the papillary muscles arise at the junction of the middle and lower thirds of the left ventricle. Minor, functionally insignificant, abnormalities of the papillary muscles may occur. A not uncommon one consists of insertion of one papillary muscle directly into one or both mitral leaflets. In acquired rheumatic mitral stenosis,

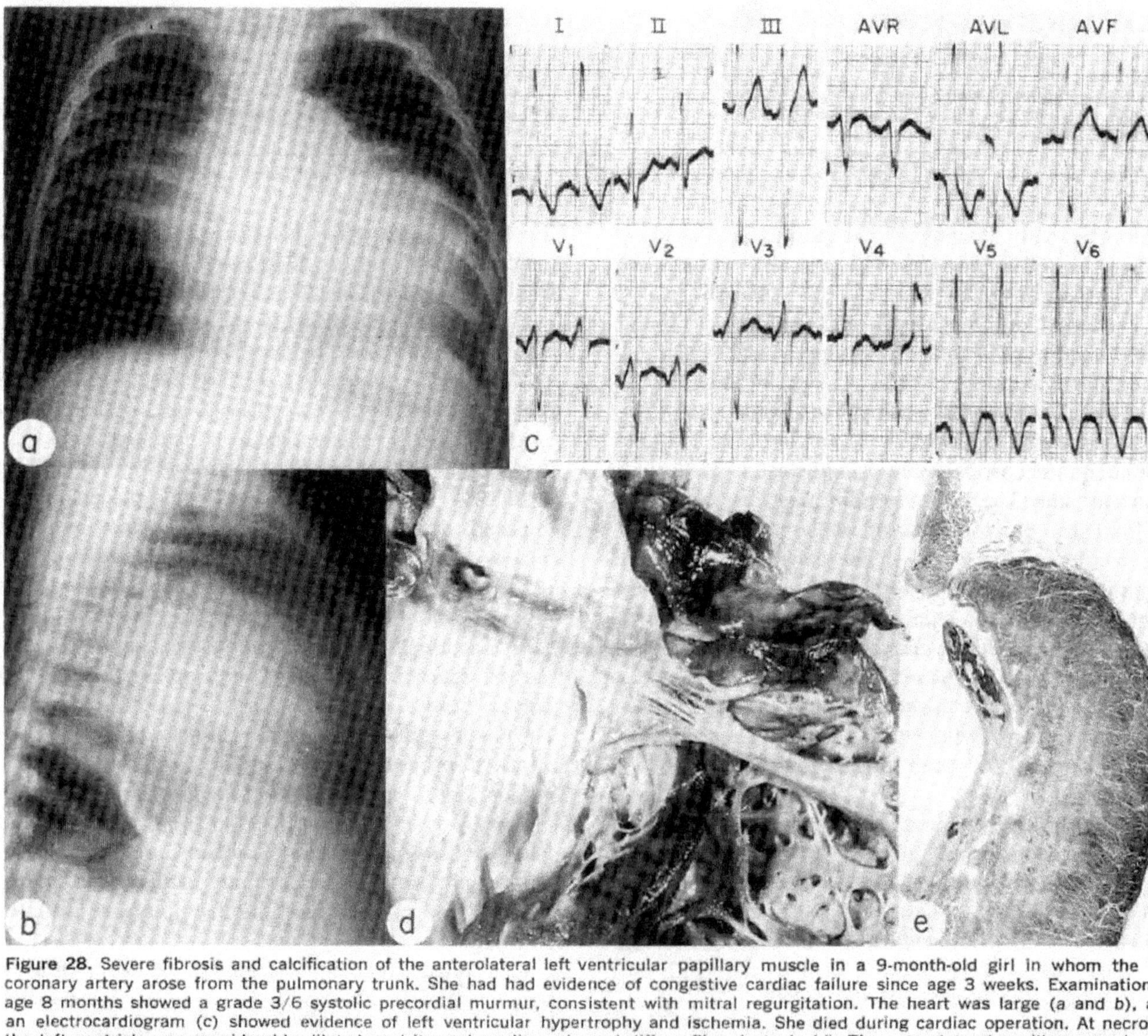

Figure 28. Severe fibrosis and calcification of the anterolateral left ventricular papillary muscle in a 9-month-old girl in whom the left coronary artery arose from the pulmonary trunk. She had had evidence of congestive cardiac failure since age 3 weeks. Examination at age 8 months showed a grade 3/6 systolic precordial murmur, consistent with mitral regurgitation. The heart was large (*a* and *b*), and an electrocardiogram (c) showed evidence of left ventricular hypertrophy and ischemia. She died during cardiac operation. At necropsy the left ventricle was considerably dilated, and its endocardium showed diffuse fibroelastosis (*d*). The anterolateral papillary muscle was severely thinned, scarred, and calcified (e). (Hematoxylin and eosin; original magnification, × 4.)

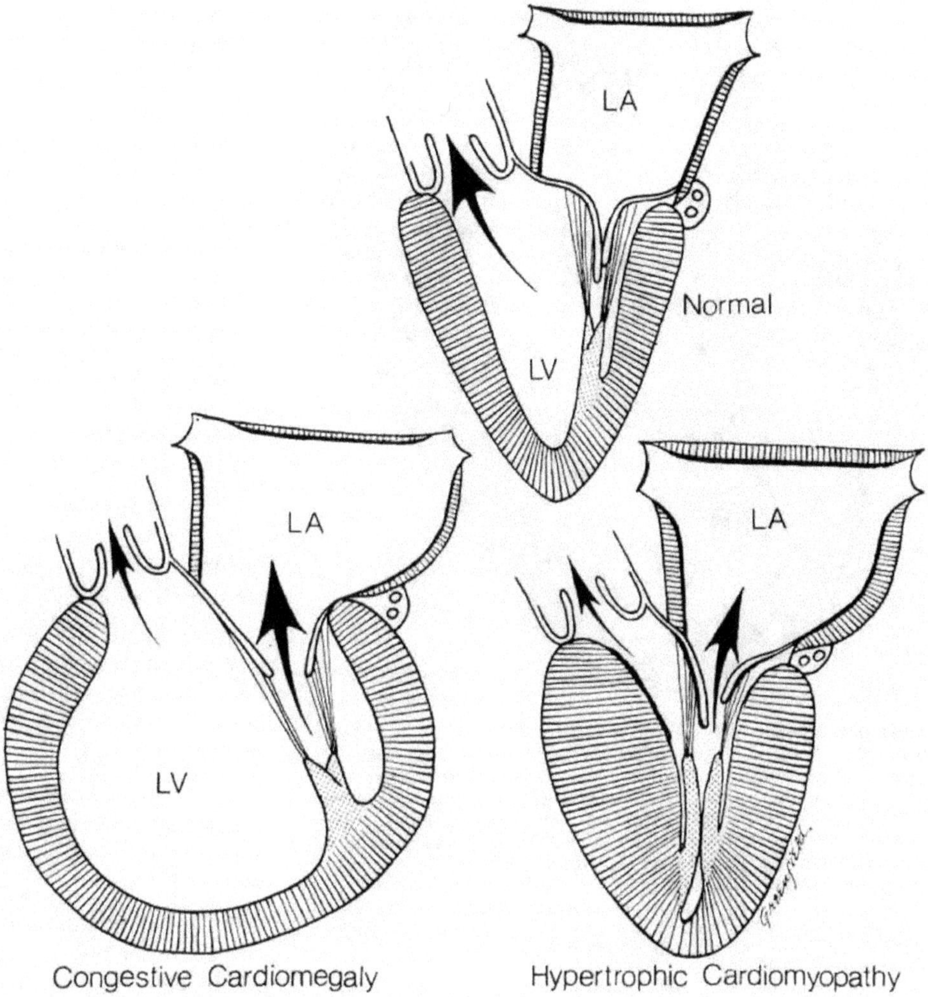

Figure 29. Diagram of how a dilated left ventricle (*LV*) (congestive cardiomyopathy) may lead to mitral regurgitation by pulling the papillary muscles laterally and caudally, and how a small left ventricular cavity, produced mainly by severe disproportional hypertrophy of the ventricular septum (hypertrophic [asymmetric] cardiomyopathy) may lead to mitral regurgitation by distorting or bending the papillary muscles and thus preventing their proper contraction during ventricular systole. The normal left ventricle is shown for comparison. Normally, the axes of the papillary muscles are more or less parallel to the major axes of the left ventricular walls. LA = left artery.

fusion and shortening of the chordae tendineae may be so extensive that both papillary muscles appear to insert directly into the mitral leaflets.

Both left ventricular papillary muscles are excised by most surgeons at the time of mitral valve replacement. The myocardium of the free wall at the sites of excision of these muscles is always infiltrated by inflammatory cells when this area is examined in the early postoperative period (19). With time these areas are covered by dense fibroelastic tissue simulating the composition of the media of the aorta (19). If the papillary muscles are not excised when the mitral leaflets and chordae tendineae are excised during mitral valve replacement, the papillary muscles atrophy and are focally replaced by fibrous tissue (92). When the papillary muscles are excised at operation, each is grasped by a clamp extending through the mitral orifice from the left atrium. If the papillary muscles are pulled too vigorously by the clamp when the muscle is excised, a portion of left ventricular papillary muscle also may be excised. This may result in perforation of the left ventricular wall or in severe thinning of the wall, with formation of a functioning or anatomic aneurysm, or both.

LEFT VENTRICULAR WALL AND MITRAL ANULUS

Dr. Perloff: I shall complete this discussion by commenting on the left ventricular wall and mitral anulus as important components of the mitral apparatus.

Regurgitation may have no other effect on a normal mitral apparatus except for changing the shape of the left ventricle. Such is the case in patients with ordinary heart failure, left ventricular dilation, and mitral regurgitation. It has often been assumed that under these circumstances the mitral anulus dilates, thus accounting for the incompetence. This explanation is an oversimplification (8). Left ventricular dilation—an undoubted cause of mitral regurgitation—may exert its effects independently of dilation of the mitral anulus. Nevertheless, the size of the anulus does play a role in preserving competence of the mitral orifice—albeit a role that relates less to dilation than to failure to decrease its circumference dur-

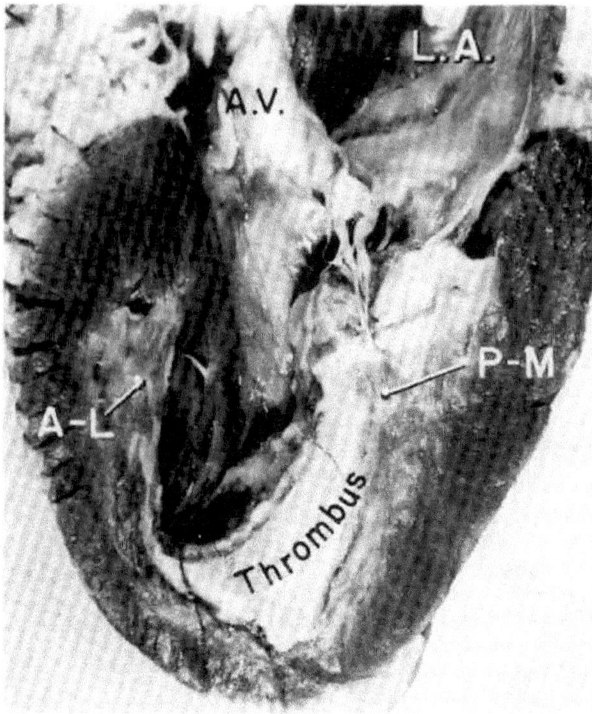

Figure 30. Opened left ventricle, aortic valve (*A.V.*) and left atrium (*L.A.*) in a 47-year-old man with Löffler's fibroplastic parietal endocarditis. This patient had been well until 13 months before death, when congestive cardiac failure associated with leukocytosis (62 000 leukocytes/mm^3) and eosinophilia (33%) appeared. He died of heart failure. At necropsy a large thrombus filled the inflow portion of the left ventricle, completely encasing the posteromedial (*P-M*) papillary muscle. In addition, both papillary muscles and portions of the left ventricular free wall subendocardium were fibrotic. No precordial murmur had been present during life. A-L = anterolateral papillary muscle.

ing systole. In the presence of ventricular dilation there are many stresses on the mitral apparatus that precede dilation of the anulus. Normally, the contracting papillary muscles exert vertical tension on the mitral leaflets, pulling them into apposition. As the left ventricle becomes globular, there is lateral migration of the papillary muscles, so that the normal vertical axis of tension is replaced by lateral tension, which tends to keep the leaflets apart (58). Accordingly, the average person with heart failure and a dilated globular left ventricle has lateral migration of the papillary muscles, lateral pull of these muscles on the chordae tendineae and leaflets, and mitral regurgitation because of that mechanism. In other patients, for example those with aortic regurgitation, the left ventricle becomes principally elongated rather than globular. Under these circumstances the papillary muscles elongate with the ventricle, and the interval between apex and anulus is too long for closure of the leaflets. The anulus still may not dilate significantly.

One final comment on the shape of the left ventricle as a cause of mitral regurgitation in idiopathic hypertrophic subaortic stenosis. In this disorder the following mechanism has been proposed for mitral regurgitation, based on a change in the shape of the left ventricle at the site of attachment of the anterolateral papillary muscle (93, 94). Early in systole there is rapid ejection. Then, as obstruction to outflow develops, the anterior mitral leaflet is pulled away from its closed position as the septum angulates at the site of origin of the anterolateral papillary muscle. The anterior mitral leaflet is pulled across the left ventricular outflow tract as late systolic mitral regurgitation develops.

Dr. Roberts: Although it may accompany left ventricular dilation, mitral anular dilation is probably a rare cause of mitral regurgitation, and in the past most patients with mitral regurgitation that was believed to be the result of mitral anular dilation probably had papillary muscle dysfunction. Mitral anular dilation to a degree capable of causing mitral regurgitation probably does not occur, because the surface area of the mitral leaflets is more than twice the area of the mitral orifice (1), and the anulus contracts during ventricular systole (9, 10). Indeed, as Dr. Perloff has pointed out, the mitral ring has a sphincter-like action, since the mitral orifice is smaller during systole than during diastole. In patients with dilated left ventricles the widest diameter does not occur at the left ventricular base, the area that includes the mitral anulus, but in the midportion of the chamber between apex and base. In fact, the base of the left ventricle is prevented from dilating freely because the "fibrous skeleton" is attached to it, whereas the midportion of the left ventricle is not so restricted. Severe left ventricular dilation may occur without any dilation of the mitral anulus.

Although it is now well known that mitral regurgitation may occur in patients with dilated left ventricles from any cause without associated left ventricular necrosis or fibrosis, it is less well recognized that necrosis or fibrosis of the left ventricular free wall, unassociated with left ventricular dilation or papillary muscle or mitral tissue lesions, also may be associated with mitral regurgitation (2). Generally, the scarring or necrosis of the myocardium adjacent to the papillary muscles fails to move or moves paradoxically during ventricular systole, and the abnormal ventricular contraction may lead to abnormal papillary muscle anchoring, resulting in mitral regurgitation. Anatomic left ventricular aneurysms unassociated with papillary muscle necrosis or fibrosis may cause mitral regurgitation by the same mechanism.

Abnormal pulling on the papillary muscles unassociated with left ventricular necrosis or fibrosis or

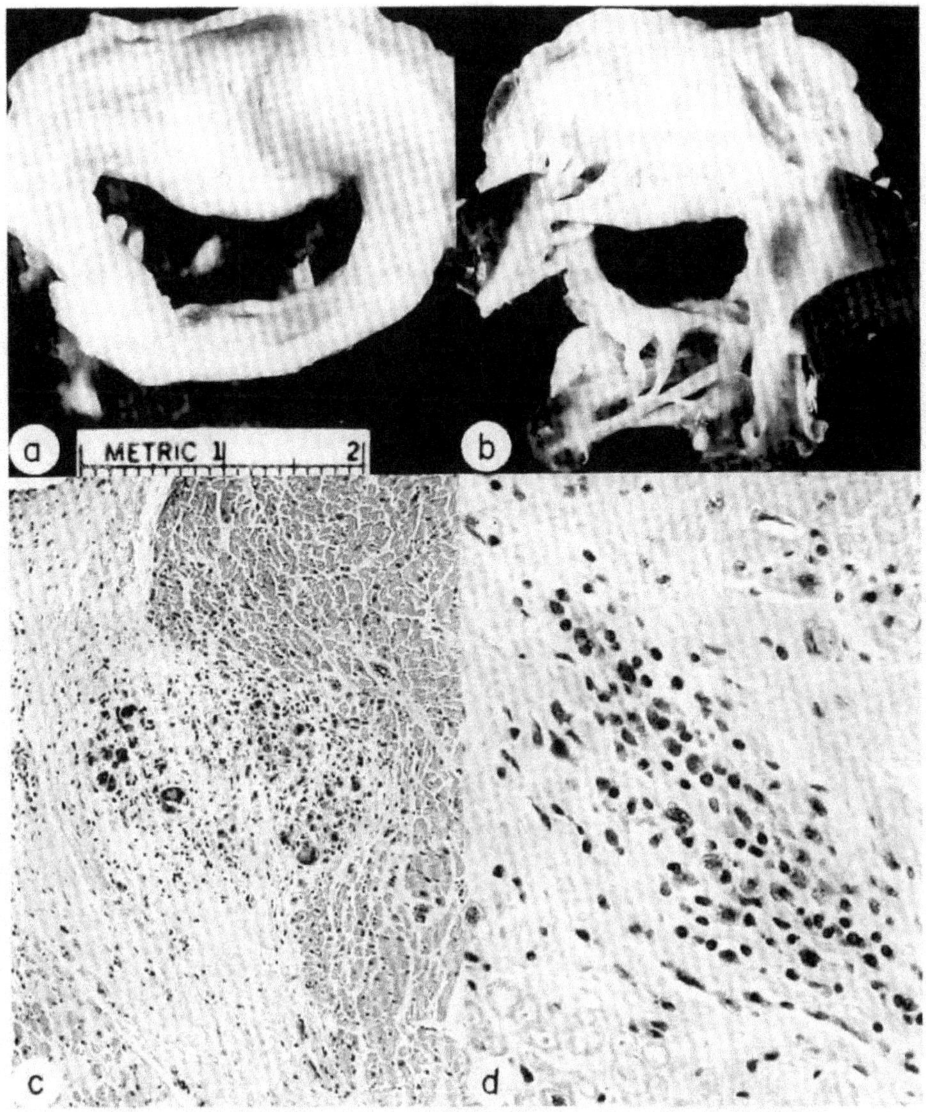

Figure 31. Excised mitral valve in a 23-year-old Indian woman with mitral stenosis (13 mm Hg mean diastolic pressure gradient between pulmonary artery wedge and left ventricle) and regurgitation. This patient had had acute rheumatic fever initially at age 7 and recurrence of migratory polyarthritis at age 22 years (14 months before operation). During the early postoperative period after mitral replacement she had swelling and pain in one knee and one ankle and erythema about two joints. When heard from 9 months postoperatively, she was much improved, although a murmur of tricuspid regurgitation was heard, and the liver pulsated. At operation earlier, mild (1+/4+) tricuspid regurgitation had been palpated, but the tricuspid leaflets and chordae were normal by palpation. Shown are the excised valve viewed from the left atrium (*a*) and from left ventricle (*b*) and Aschoff bodies (*c* and *d*), which were numerous in both excised left ventricular papillary muscles. (Hematoxylin and eosin. Original magnification: **c**, × 110; **d**, × 400.)

cavity dilation may occur in patients with hypertrophic (asymmetric) cardiomyopathy, and this mechanism may account for their mitral regurgitation (80). The huge thickening of the ventricular septum —the thickest portion is midway between left ventricular base and apex—may distort or bend the anterolateral papillary muscle and prevent proper contraction of this structure during ventricular systole. In addition to actual bending of the anterolateral left ventricular papillary muscle, however, the mitral leaflets in adults with hypertrophic cardiomyopathy are always thickened (80). It is easy to explain the thickening of the anterior mitral leaflet as being caused by its contraction of the mural endocardium in the left ventricular outflow tract during ventricular systole. But the posterior mitral leaflet also is thickened, probably as a result of its contacting itself abnormally during ventricular systole. It must be remembered that the mitral leaflets and chordae tendineae are within the left ventricular cavity. A major abnormality in hypertrophic cardiomyopathy is the small size of the left ventricular cavity. As a consequence, there is not enough room in the left ventricle to accommodate the mitral leaflets and chordae freely, and with vigorous contractions portions of the posterior leaflets contact other portions abnormally. Fibrous thickening is the consequence. I have been shown a mitral valve, excised because of incompetence, with the question, "Is the thickening rheumatic in origin?" The leaflets and chordae were focally thickened, and other features in retrospect clearly showed that the patient had had hypertrophic (asymmetric) cardiomyopathy presenting as mitral regurgitation. Of the 32 patients with hypertrophic cardiomyopathy studied by me at necropsy, 1 presented initially with pure mitral regurgitation associated with aneurysmal dilation of the pulmonary trunk (Figure 32). The mitral regurgitation in hypertrophic cardiomyopathy usually disappears after operative excision or incision of myocardium in the left ventricular outflow tract (95).

Calcification of the Mitral Anulus

Dr. Perloff: Now to the sixth element in the mitral apparatus, the anulus. As indicated, the anulus provides systolic sphincteric action, decreasing the area that the leaflets must seal. We have all seen calcified mitral anuli on roentgenograms. The J- or U-shaped appearance of a calcified anulus in an elderly person is typical. The calcific deposits assume J or U shapes because they are located nearly always only behind the posterior leaflet; they are rarely circumferential because the anulus is not circumferential. The anterior leaflet has no anulus because it is continuous with the aorta. A thick calcified anulus cannot act as a sphincter, cannot decrease the size of the mitral orifice during systole, and, accordingly, may be responsible for mitral regurgitation, generally only mild to moderate. Mitral anular calcification may occur in Marfan's syndrome and is an additional cause of mitral regurgitation in that disorder (96).

Dr. Roberts: Calcification of the mitral anulus is one of the more frequent abnormalities of the heart. Mitral anular calcification is generally considered to be a disease of elderly women. Indeed, of 14 patients with "massive" mitral anular calcification reported by Korn, DeSanctis, and Sell (97) in 1962, all were women and all were over 65 years of age. It is incorrect, however, to believe that this entity is reserved for a particular sex at a particular time in life. During

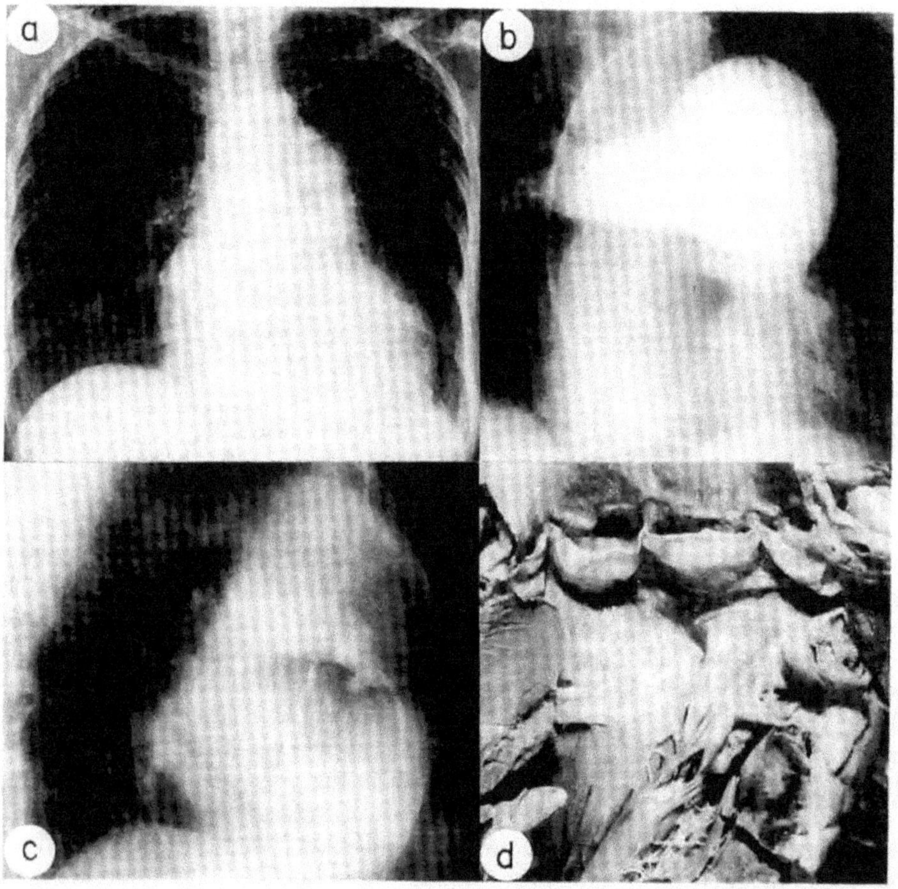

Figure 32. Hypertrophic (asymmetric) cardiomyopathy (idiopathic hypertrophic subaortic stenosis) presenting as pure mitral regurgitation. This 41-year-old woman had a precordial murmur and cardiomegaly on insurance examination at age 33 years, and overt right- and left-sided congestive cardiac failure, which progressed, appeared at age 38 years. When examined a month before death, she was severely ill, functionally class IV. A grade 4/6 blowing pansystolic precordial murmur, loudest along the lower left sternal border, was audible. Electrocardiogram showed atrial fibrillation and a marked clockwise rotation. By X ray (*a, b, c*) the heart was enlarged, and the pulmonary trunk was aneurysmally dilated. The total serum protein level was 5.3 g/100 ml, with an albumin level of 1.9 g/100 ml, and 2.2 g of protein were measured in the urine in a 24-hour period. The total serum cholesterol was 318 mg/100 ml. At catheterization the pressures (in mm Hg) were as follows: pulmonary artery, 34/7; right ventricle, 34/5; right atrial mean, 4; pulmonary arterial wedge—mean, 11 and V wave, 14; left ventricle, 112/11; and femoral artery, 122/65. The cardiac output (Fick method) was 1.6 litre/min·m^2 body surface area. Left ventricular cineangiogram showed 4+/4+ mitral regurgitation. (Retrospective examination showed this angiogram to be strongly suggestive of hypertrophic cardiomyopathy.) Aortic root injection of contrast material showed no aortic regurgitation. A day before death cardiotomy was performed, to replace the severely incompetent mitral valve. At operation, however, no systolic thrill was palpable over the left atrium, which expanded hardly at all during ventricular systole. Examination of the mitral valve after cardiopulmonary bypass had been instituted showed that the mitral leaflets and chordae were "normal" and that the left ventricular cavity was not dilated. Therefore, valve replacement was not carried out. The patient died the next day because of inadequate cardiac output. Necropsy showed a large transmural acute myocardial infarct involving the posterior left ventricular free wall. Histologic study indicated that the infarct was about 14 days old. The mitral leaflets and chordae were focally thickened, but the anulus was not dilated, and the left ventricular cavity was of normal size. In the outflow tract of the left ventricle a mural endocardial plaque was in direct apposition to the anterior mitral leaflet (*d*). Since the aortic valve cusps were normal, it was clear that this endocardial plaque indicated that hypertrophic cardiomyopathy was the proper diagnosis. The ventricular septum was nearly twice as thick as was the left ventricular free wall. Thus, this patient shows how idiopathic hypertrophic subaortic stenosis may present as pure mitral regurgitation. The cause of the aneurysmal dilation of the pulmonary trunk is uncertain. (At operation, a diastolic thrill had been palpated over this artery, indicating the presence of pulmonic regurgitation.)

the past 4 years I have examined at necropsy the hearts of 87 patients in whom various amounts of calcium involved the mitral anulus. Of the 87 patients, 44 were male and 43 were female. Sixty-one patients (26 male, 35 female) were age 65 years or greater, and 26 patients (18 male, 8 female) were less than 65 years of age. Of the latter 26 patients, 8 were less than 40 years of age: 3 of them had Marfan's syndrome, 2 had Hurler's syndrome, and 3 had metabolic disturbances with hypercalcemia.

The extent of mitral anular calcification was graded 1+ to 4+ (Figure 33); 45 patients (28 male, 17 female) had 1+ or 2+ deposits, and 42 (16 male, 26 female) had 3+ or 4+ deposits. Thus, this condition is slightly more frequent in the male, but the larger deposits (those likely to be seen on chest roentgenogram) are more frequent in the female. The smaller deposits (grades 1+ and 2+) almost surely have no functional importance. The larger deposits (grades 3+ and 4+), in contrast, may produce mitral regurgitation by the mechanism discussed by Dr. Perloff. Although stenosis has been mentioned as a possible complication of "massive" mitral anular calcification, obstruction has never been shown either anatomically or functionally to be caused by this mechanism. Wide-open severe mitral regurgitation, likewise, is probably never caused by mitral anular calcification.

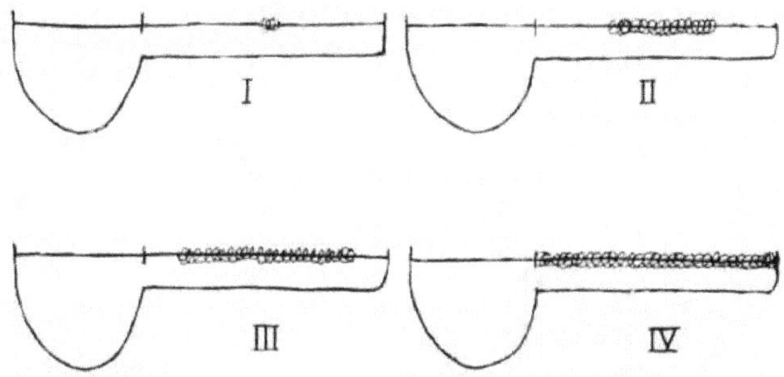

Figure 33. Method of grading mitral anular calcification. Grade I indicates only a single small deposit; grade II, a large single, or more than one small, deposit. Grade III and IV represent extensive deposits. The entire anulus behind the posterior leaflet is involved in grade IV, and, on rare occasion, calcific deposits also may extend across the anterior leaflet.

In patients with calcific deposits in the mitral

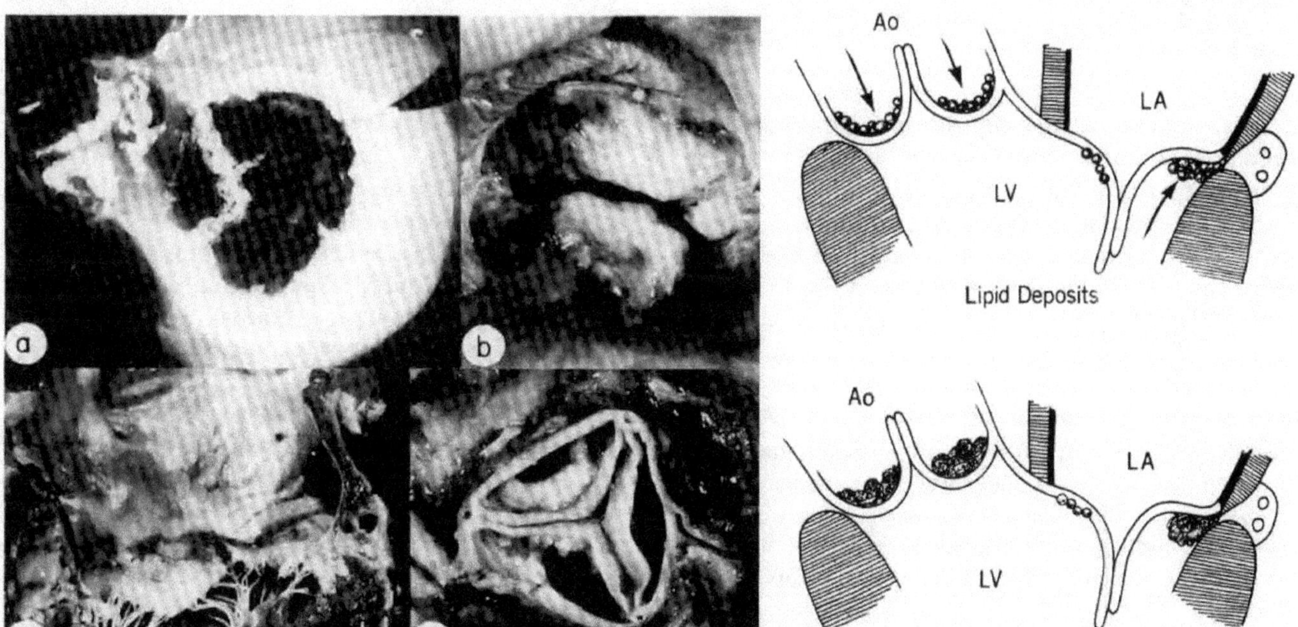

Figure 34 A-D. Massive mitral anular calcification associated with aortic valvular and coronary arterial calcification in an 82-year-old woman who died of volvulus of the caecum. She never had symptoms of cardiac dysfunction. **a.** Radiograph of heart at necropsy, showing circumferential mitral anular calcification. Most of the calcium is located behind the posterior mitral leaflet. Calcific deposits are also present in the aortic valve, root of aorta, and coronary arteries. **b.** Mitral valve as viewed from left atrium. The valve orifice appears to be only slightly incompetent. **c.** Opened dilated left atrium, mitral valve, and left ventricle. Calcium is apparent beneath the posterior leaflet. **d.** Aortic valve from above. Calcific deposits are present on the aortic aspects of each cusp, and none of the three commissures are fused. This valve is stenotic, as evidenced by left ventricular hypertrophy and by decreased mobility of the cusps. The heart weighed 440 g. **e.** The cause of calcification of the mitral anulus is uncertain. Since most patients with mitral anular calcific deposits also have calcific deposits in the aortic valve cusps and coronary arteries, it seems reasonable to believe that the cause of the calcification in each of these sites is similar. In young adults, yellow deposits are nearly always seen on the ventricular surface of both mitral leaflets and on the aortic surface of the aortic valve cusps. The lipid may be both intra- and extra-cellular in location. Degeneration of the lipid appears to lead to the calcification. The latter occurs behind the posterior mitral leaflet and on the aortic aspects of the cusps, since these are sites of high pressure, and there is nowhere else for the blood to go—it is, in effect, pushed into the valve leaflets. In contrast, the high pressure on the anterior leaflets is reflected off into the aorta. In other words, the impact of pressure contacts the posterior mitral leaflet and aortic valve cusps at right angles to the cusps, whereas the angle of contact with the anterior leaflet approaches a 180-deg angle.

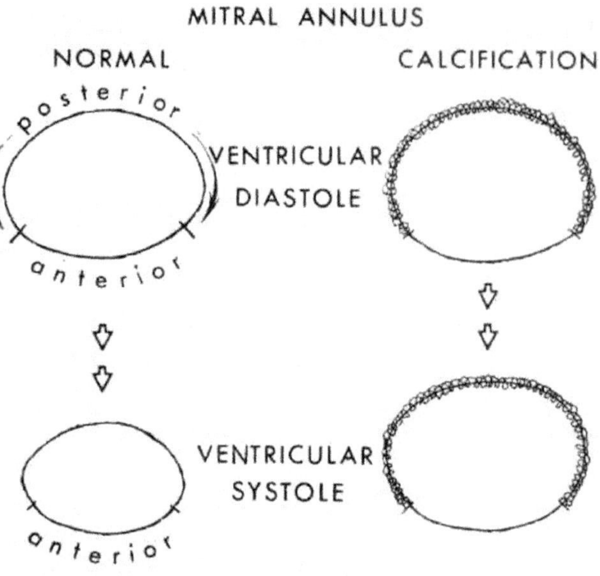

Figure 35. The mechanism of mitral regurgitation in patients with calcification of the mitral anulus. During ventricular systole the base of the left ventricle contracts like a sphincter. Included in the base of the left ventricle is the anulus behind the posterior mitral leaflet. Thus, this circumference decreases during systole. If, however, the anulus behind the posterior mitral leaflet is calcified, the sphincter-like contraction of the left ventricular base no longer occurs. The area of the mitral orifice thus is not decreased, and mild degrees of mitral regurgitation may result.

anulus, similar calcific deposits are often also observed in the aortic valve cusps and in the extramural or epicardial coronary arteries (Figure 34 *A-D*). Of the 87 patients with mitral anular calcification, 64 (74%) also had calcific deposits in the aortic valve, and in 35 of them the deposits were so extensive that the aortic valve orifice appeared stenotic. In several of them large peak systolic pressure gradients were recorded across the aortic valve (78). In this situation the aortic valve usually contains calcific deposits only on its aortic surfaces, the commissures are not fused, and there is no associated incompetence (78). Calcific deposits were observed grossly in the coronary arteries in 76 (87%) of the 87 patients. Of the 11 patients without deposits, 8 were less than age 53 years, and only 3 were more than age 65 years. Thus, of the 61 patients with mitral anular calcification aged 65 years or more, 58 (85%) had calcific deposits in the coronary arteries, and 47 (77%) had calcific deposits in the aortic valve cusps. Calcification in these three locations—mitral anulus, aortic valve, and coronary arteries—therefore is extremely common in the elderly population and suggests that the cause of the deposits in each location is similar. The deposits occur on the undersurface, that is, the ventricular surface, of the posterior mitral leaflet at or below the anulus and on the aortic surfaces of the aortic valve cusps. Foam cells are common in these locations in younger adults. Breakdown of these lipid deposits is probably responsible for the calcification at these sites (Figure 34*E*).

Calcification in the mitral anular area appears to be accelerated by conditions that elevate left ventricular pressure—namely, systemic hypertension, aortic valvular stenosis, and hypertrophic cardiomyopathy—and by conditions that accelerate atherosclerosis—for example, diabetes mellitus. The former conditions increase the mitral closing pressure, and the latter conditions increase the supply of lipids. An intrinsic defect of the fibrous skeleton of the heart appears to be the explanation for early mitral anular calcification in Marfan's and Hurler's syndromes. The mechanism by which mitral regurgitation is produced in patients with calcified mitral anuli is illustrated in Figure 35.

Conclusion

In closing, I refer you to Figure 36. Until the last 20 years or so, valvular cardiac disease in adults was considered rheumatic in origin. A major purpose of this review has been to call attention to many conditions other than rheumatic heart disease that may cause the mitral valve to function abnormally. One of the major contributions to cardiology in the 1960s was the realization that the left ventricular papillary muscles played an important role in closing the mitral orifice during ventricular systole and that ischemia, necrosis, or fibrosis of these structures could be the cause of severe mitral regurgitation even when the leaflets and chordae were normal. With the introduction of the concept of papillary muscle dysfunction, the role played by the mitral anulus in causing regurgitation has been deemphasized. With few exceptions it no longer seems reasonable to attribute mitral regurgitation to anular dilation. Papillary muscle dysfunction usually is a better explanation. Although numerous conditions can affect the mitral leaflets and cause regurgitation (far fewer conditions produce stenosis), myocardial disease with or without coronary arterial luminal narrowing now is recognized as the commonest cause of mitral regurgitation, even though the conditions that affect primarily the leaflets and chordae lead to the more severe degrees of regurgitation.

ACKNOWLEDGMENTS: Received 14 September 1972; accepted 2 October 1972.

► Requests for reprints should be addressed to William C. Roberts, M.D., Chief, Section of Pathology, National Heart and Lung Institute, Bldg. 10A, Room 3E-30, National Institutes of Health, Bethesda, Md. 20014.

References

1. Brock RC: The surgical and pathological anatomy of the

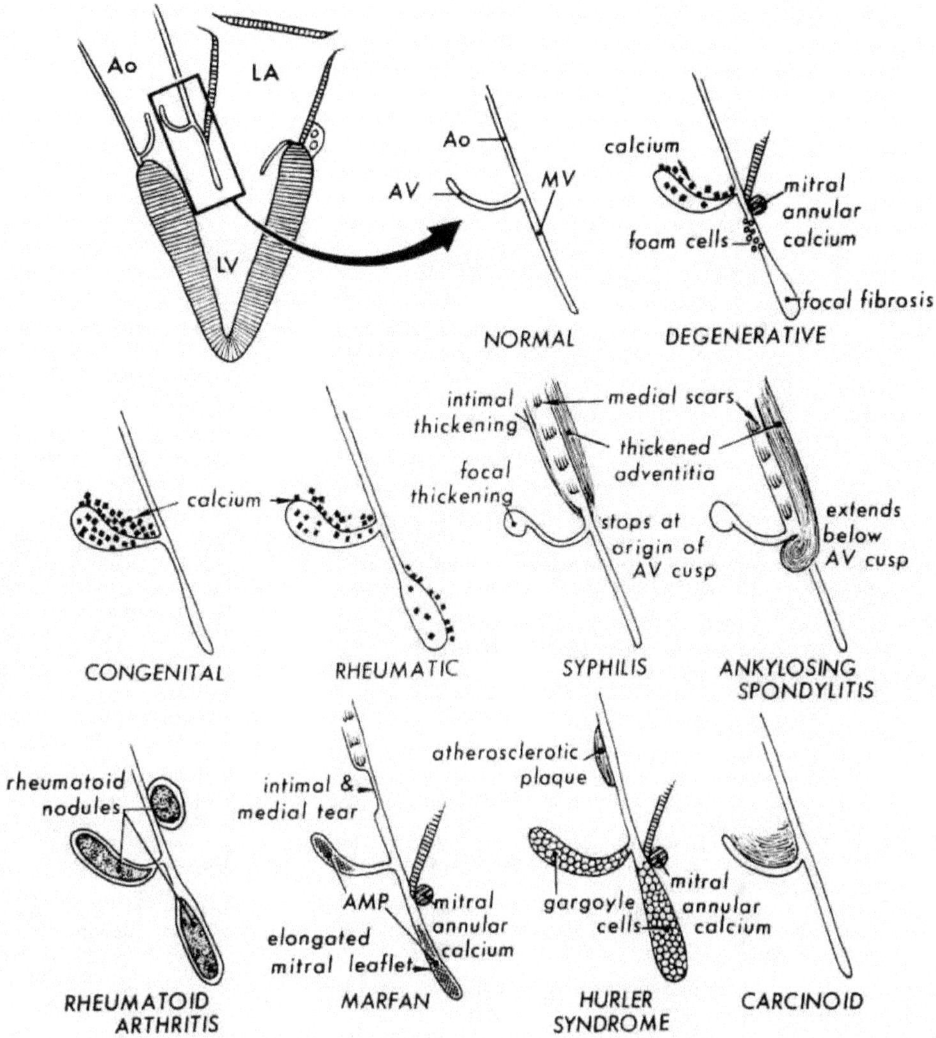

Figure 36. Diagram of some of the conditions affecting the mitral leaflets, most of which also affect the aortic valve. Degenerative, congenital, and rheumatic conditions frequently are associated with some degree of valvular stenosis. Syphilis never affects the mitral leaflets, but ankylosing spondylitis extends below the aortic valve and may lead to some degree of mitral regurgitation. Rheumatoid arthritis, floppy valves with or without Marfan's syndrome, and the Hurler syndrome produce purely incompetent lesions. Carcinoid usually affects, or more severely affects, the right-sided cardiac valves, but carcinoid plaques also have been observed on the mitral and aortic leaflets. Ao = aorta; LV = left ventricle; LA = left atrium; AV = aortic valve; MV = mitral valve; AMP = acid mucopolysaccharide material.

mitral valve. *Br Heart J* 14:489-513, 1952

2. Roberts WC, Cohen LS: Left ventricular papillary muscles. Description of the normal and a survey of conditions causing them to be abnormal. *Circulation* 46:138-154, 1972
3. Estes EH Jr, Dalton FM, Entman ML, et al: The anatomy and blood supply of the papillary muscles of the left ventricle. *Am Heart J* 71:356-362, 1966
4. Sell S, Scully RE: Aging changes in the aortic and mitral valves. Histologic and histochemical studies, with observations on the pathogenesis of calcific aortic stenosis and calcification of the mitral annulus. *Am J Pathol* 46:345-365, 1965
5. Perloff JK, Roberts WC: The mitral apparatus. Functional anatomy of mitral regurgitation. *Circulation* 46:227-239, 1972
6. Cheng TO: Some new observations on the syndrome of papillary muscle dysfunction. *Am J Med* 47:924-945, 1969
7. Rushmer RF, Finlayson BL, Nash AA: Movements of the mitral valve. *Circ Res* 4:337-342, 1956
8. Levy MJ, Edwards JE: Anatomy of mitral insufficiency. *Prog Cardiovasc Dis* 5:119-144, 1962
9. Davis PKB, Kinmonth JB: The movements of the annulus of the mitral valve. *J Cardiovasc Surg (Torino)* 4:427-431, 1963
10. Brolin I: The mitral orifice. *Acta Radiol [Diagn] (Stockh)* 6:273-295, 1967
11. Selzer A, Cohn KE: Natural history of mitral stenosis. A review. *Circulation* 45:878-890, 1972
12. Blackmon JR, Murray JA: Valvular heart disease, in *Cardiovascular Hemodynamics*, edited by Rushmer RF. Philadelphia, W. B. Saunders Co., 1970, p. 469
13. Perloff JK: *The Clinical Recognition of Congenital Heart Disease*. Philadelphia, W. B. Saunders Co., 1970, pp. 116-120
14. Short DS: Radiology of the lung in severe mitral stenosis. *Br Heart J* 17:33-40, 1955
15. Roberts WC: Anatomically isolated aortic valvular disease. The case against its being of rheumatic etiology. *Am J Med* 49:151-159, 1970
16. Roberts WC: Pathologic aspects of valvular and subvalvular (discrete and diffuse) aortic stenosis, in *The Natural History and Progress in Treatment of Congenital Heart Disease*, edited by Kidd BSL, Keith JD. Springfield, Ill., Charles C Thomas, Publisher, 1971, pp. 221-244
17. Roberts WC, Sjoerdsma A: The cardiac disease associated with the carcinoid syndrome (carcinoid heart disease). *Am J Med* 36:5-34, 1964
18. Roberts WC, Morrow AG: Mechanisms of acute left atrial thrombosis after mitral valve replacement. Pathologic findings indicating obstruction to left atrial emptying. *Am J Cardiol* 18:497-503, 1966
19. Roberts WC, Morrow AG: Causes of death and other anatomic observations after cardiac valve replacement. *Adv Cardiol* 7:226-247, 1972
20. Perloff JK: Auscultatory and phonocardiographic manifestations of pulmonary hypertension. *Prog Cardiovasc Dis* 9:303-340, 1967
21. Wood P: An appreciation of mitral stenosis. *Br Med J* 1: 1051-1063, 1113-1124, 1954
22. Shone JD, Sellers RD, Anderson RC, et al: The developmental complex of "parachute mitral valve," supravalvular ring of left atrium, subaortic stenosis, and coarctation of aorta. *Am J Cardiol* 11:714-725, 1963
23. Glancy DL, Chang MY, Dorney ER, et al: Parachute

mitral valve. Further observations and associated lesions. *Am J Cardiol* 27:309-313, 1971
24. Castaneda AR, Anderson RC, Edwards JE: Congenital mitral stenosis resulting from anomalous arcade and obstructing papillary muscles. Report of correction by use of ball valve prosthesis. *Am J Cardiol* 24:237-240, 1969
25. Davachi F, Moller JH, Edwards JE: Diseases of the mitral valve in infancy. An anatomic analysis of 55 cases. *Circulation* 43:565-579, 1971
26. Nasser WK, Davis RH, Dillon JC, et al: Atrial myxoma. I. Clinical and pathologic features in nine cases. *Am Heart J* 83:694-704, 1972
27. Ferrans VJ, Roberts WC: Structural features of cardiac myxomas. Histology, histochemistry and electronmicroscopy. *Hum Pathol*. In press
28. MaClowery JD, Roberts WC: Metastatic choriocarcinoma of the lung. Invasion of pulmonary veins with extension into left atrium and mitral orifice. *Am J Cardiol* 18:938-941, 1966
29. Sterns LP, Eliot RS, Varco RL, et al: Intracavitary cardiac neoplasms. A review of fifteen cases. *Br Heart J* 28:75-83, 1966
30. Buchbinder NA, Roberts WC: Active infective endocarditis confined to mural endocardium. A study of six necropsy patients. *Arch Pathol* 93:435-440, 1972
31. Zvaifler N: Chronic postrheumatic-fever (Jaccoud's) arthritis. *N Engl J Med* 267:10-14, 1962
32. Braunwald E, Awe WC: The syndrome of severe mitral regurgitation with normal left atrial pressure. *Circulation* 27:29-35, 1963
33. Perloff JK, Harvey WP: Auscultatory and phonocardiographic manifestations of pure mitral regurgitation. *Prog Cardiovasc Dis* 5:172-194, 1962
34. Edwards JE, Burchell HB: Endocardial and intimal lesions (jet impact) as possible sites of origin of murmurs. *Circulation* 18:946-960, 1958
35. Roberts WC, Braunwald E, Morrow AG: Acute severe mitral regurgitation secondary to ruptured chordae tendineae. Clinical, hemodynamic, and pathologic considerations. *Circulation* 33:58-70, 1966
36. Ronan JA Jr, Steelman RB, DeLeon AC, et al: The clinical diagnosis of acute severe mitral insufficiency. *Am J Cardiol* 27:284-290, 1971
37. Cohen LS, Mason DT, Braunwald E: Significance of an atrial gallop sound in mitral regurgitation. A clue to the diagnosis of ruptured chordae tendineae. *Circulation* 35:112-118, 1967
38. Gross L: Lesions of the left auricle in rheumatic fever. *Am J Pathol* 11:711-735, 1935
39. Roberts WC, Ross RS, Eggleston JC, et al: Chronic mitral regurgitation of unresolved etiology in the elderly. A clinico-pathologic study of two patients. *Johns Hopkins Med J* 122:26-36, 1968
40. Buchbinder NA, Roberts WC, Morrow AG: The pathology of healed infective endocarditis. Unpublished
41. Buchbinder NA, Roberts WC: Left-sided valvular active infective endocarditis. A study of forty-five necropsy patients. *Am J Med* 53:20-35, 1972
42. Haller JA Jr, Morrow AG: Experimental mitral insufficiency. An operative method of chronic survival. *Ann Surg* 142:37-51, 1955
43. Rockoff SD, Ross J Jr, Oldham NN Jr, et al: Ventriculoatrial regurgitation following prosthetic replacement of the mitral valve. Angiocardiographic and hemodynamic findings. *Am J Cardiol* 17:817-824, 1966
44. Edwards JE: Mitral insufficiency resulting from overshooting of leaflets. *Circulation* 43:606-612, 1971
45. Barlow JB, Bosman CK, Pocock WA, et al: Late systolic murmurs and non-ejection ("mid-late") systolic clicks. An analysis of 90 patients. *Br Heart J* 30:203-218, 1968
46. Bittar N, Sosa JA: The billowing mitral valve leaflet. *Circulation* 38:763-770, 1968
47. Dillon JC, Haine CL, Chang S, et al: Use of echocardiography in patients with prolapse mitral valve. *Circulation* 43:503-507, 1971
48. Ronan JA, Perloff JK, Harvey WP: Systolic clicks and the late systolic murmur. Intercardiac phonocardiographic evidence of their mitral valve origin. *Am Heart J* 70:319-325, 1965
49. Jeresaty RM: The syndrome associated with mid-systolic click and/or late systolic murmur. Analysis of 32 cases. *Chest* 59:643-647, 1971
50. Ehlers KH, Engle MA, Levin AR, et al: Left ventricular abnormality with late mitral insufficiency and abnormal electrocardiogram. *Am J Cardiol* 26:333-340, 1970
51. Osler W: On a remarkable heart murmur heard at a distance from the chest wall. *Med Times Gazette* 2:432, 1880
52. Rizzon P, Biasco G, Maselli-Campagna G: The precordial honk. *Br Heart J* 33:707-715, 1971
53. Leon DF, Leonard JJ, Kroetz FW, et al: Late systolic murmurs, clicks, and whoops arising from the mitral valve. A transseptal intracardiac phonocardiographic analysis. *Am Heart J* 72:325-336, 1966
54. Gooch AS, Vicencio F, Maranhao V, et al: Arrhythmias and left ventricular asynergy in the prolapsing mitral leaflet syndrome. *Am J Cardiol* 29:611-620, 1972
55. Baron MG: Abnormalities of the mitral valve in endocardial cushion defects. *Circulation* 45:672-680, 1972
56. Berry WB, Roberts WC, Morrow AG, et al: Corrected transposition of the aorta and pulmonary trunk. Clinical, hemodynamic and pathologic findings. *Am J Med* 36:35-53, 1964
57. Roberts WC, Ross RS, Davis FW Jr: Congenital corrected transposition of the great vessels in adulthood simulating rheumatic valvular disease. *Bull Johns Hopkins Hosp* 144:157-172, 1964
58. Carney EK, Braunwald E, Roberts WC, et al: Congenital mitral regurgitation. Clinical, hemodynamic and angiographic findings in nine patients. *Am J Med* 33:223-235, 1962
59. Cohn LH, Morrow AG, Braunwald E: Operative treatment of atrial septal defect: clinical and haemodynamic assessments in 175 patients. *Br Heart J* 29:725-734, 1967
60. Braunwald E, Ross RS, Morrow AG, et al: Differential diagnosis of mitral regurgitation in childhood: clinical pathological conference at the National Institutes of Health. *Ann Intern Med* 54:1223-1242, 1961
61. Brockenbrough EC, Braunwald E, Roberts WC, et al: Partial persistent atrioventricular canal simulating pure mitral regurgitation. *Am Heart J* 63:9-17, 1962
62. Rosenberg J, Roberts WC: Double orifice mitral valve. Study of the anomaly in two calves and a summary of the literature in humans. *Arch Pathol* 86:77-80, 1968
63. Morrow AG, Cohen LS, Roberts WC, et al: Severe mitral regurgitation following acute myocardial infarction and ruptured papillary muscle. Hemodynamic findings and results of operative treatment in four patients. *Circulation* 37 and 38 (suppl II):124-132, 1968
64. Burch GE, DePasquale NP, Phillips JH: Clinical manifestations of papillary muscle dysfunction. *Arch Intern Med* 112:112-117, 1963
65. Phillips JH, Burch GE, DePasquale NP: The syndrome of papillary muscle dysfunction. Its clinical recognition. *Ann Intern Med* 59:508-520, 1963
66. Burch GE, DePasquale NP, Phillips JH: The syndrome of papillary muscle dysfunction. *Am Heart J* 75:399-415, 1968
67. Shelburne JC, Rubinstein D, Gorlin R: A reappraisal of papillary muscle dysfunction. Correlative clinical and angiographic study. *Am J Med* 46:862-871, 1969
68. Brody W, Criley JM: Intermittent severe mitral regurgitation. Hemodynamic studies in a patient with recurrent acute left-sided heart failure. *N Engl J Med* 283:673-676, 1970
69. Noren GR, Raghib G, Moller JH, et al: Anomalous origin of the left coronary artery from the pulmonary trunk with special reference to the occurrence of mitral insufficiency. *Circulation* 30:171-179, 1964
70. Miller GE Jr, Cohn KE, Kerth WJ, et al: Experimental papillary muscle infarction. *J Thorac Cardiovasc Surg* 56:611-616, 1968
71. Tsakiris AG, Rastelli GC, Amorim D deS, et al: Effect of experimental papillary muscle damage on mitral valve closure in intact anesthetized dogs. *Mayo Clin Proc* 45:275-285, 1970
72. Mittal AK, Langston M Jr, Cohn KE, et al: Combined papillary muscle and left ventricular wall dysfunction as a cause of mitral regurgitation. An experimental study. *Circulation* 44:174-180, 1971
73. Estes EH Jr, Entman ML, Dixon HB II, et al: The vascular supply of the left ventricular wall. Anatomic observations, plus a hypothesis regarding acute events in coronary artery disease. *Am Heart J* 71:58-67, 1966
74. Heikkilä J: Mitral incompetence as a complication of acute myocardial infarction. *Acta Med Scand* 182 (suppl 475):1-

149, 1967
75. MOLLER JH, NAKIB A, EDWARDS JE: Infarction of papillary muscles and mitral insufficiency associated with congenital aortic stenosis. *Circulation* 34:87-91, 1966
76. AROSEMENA E, MOLLER JH, EDWARDS JE: Scarring of the papillary muscles in left ventricular hypertrophy. *Am Heart J* 74:446-452, 1967
77. ROBERTS WC: The congenitally bicuspid aortic valve. A study of 85 autopsy cases. *Am J Cardiol* 26:72-83, 1970
78. ROBERTS WC, PERLOFF JK, COSTANTINO T: Severe valvular aortic stenosis in patients over 65 years of age. A clinicopathologic study. *Am J Cardiol* 27:497-506, 1971
79. FALCONE MW, ROBERTS WC, MORROW AG, et al: Congenital aortic stenosis resulting from a unicommissural valve. Clinical and anatomic features in twenty-one adult patients. *Circulation* 44:272-280, 1971
80. ROBERTS WC: Valvular, subvalvular, and supravalvular aortic stenosis. Morphologic features. *Cardiovasc Clin*. In press
81. ROBERTS WC, BUCHBINDER NA: Papillary muscle necrosis in active valvular infective endocarditis (abstract). *Am J Cardiol* 29:287, 1972
82. MOLLER JH, LUCAS RV JR, ADAMS P JR, et al: Endocardial fibroelastosis. A clinical and anatomic study of 47 patients with emphasis on its relationship to mitral insufficiency. *Circulation* 30:759-782, 1964
83. ROBERTS WC: Anomalous origin of both coronary arteries from the pulmonary artery. *Am J Cardiol* 10:595-600, 1962
84. BURCHELL HB, BROWN AL JR: Anomalous origin of coronary artery from pulmonary artery masquerading as mitral insufficiency. *Am Heart J* 63:388-393, 1962
85. ROBERTS WC, FERRANS VJ: Morphologic observations in the cardiomyopathies, in *The Cardiomyopathies*, edited by FOWLER NO. New York, Grune & Stratton. In press, 1973
86. MARCUS FI, GOMEZ L, GLANCY DL, et al: Papillary muscle fibrosis in primary myocardial disease. *Am Heart J* 77:681-685, 1969
87. PERLOFF JK, ROBERTS WC, DELEON AC, et al: The distinctive electrocardiogram of Duchenne's progressive muscular dystrophy. An electrocardiographic-pathologic correlative study. *Am J Med* 42:179-188, 1967
88. ROBERTS WC, BUJA LM, FERRANS VJ: Löffler's fibroplastic parietal endocarditis, eosinophilic leukemia, and Davies' endomyocardial fibrosis: the same disease at different stages? *Pathol Microbiol (Basel)* 35:90-95, 1970
89. ROBERTS WC, LIEGLER DG, CARBONE PP: Endomyocardial disease and eosinophilia. A clinical and pathologic spectrum. *Am J Med* 46:28-42, 1969
90. BUJA LM, KHOI NB, ROBERTS WC: Clinically significant cardiac amyloidosis. Clinicopathologic findings in 15 patients. *Am J Cardiol* 26:394-405, 1970
91. BUJA LM, ROBERTS WC: Iron in the heart. Etiology and clinical significance. *Am J Med* 51:209-221, 1971
92. RASTELLI GC, KIRKLIN JW, TITUS JL: Fate of papillary muscles after prosthetic replacement of mitral valve. *Mayo Clin Proc* 42:210-217, 1967
93. ADELMAN AG, MCLOUGHLIN MJ, MARQUIS Y, et al: Left ventricular cineangiographic observations in muscular subaortic stenosis. *Am J Cardiol* 24:689-697, 1969
94. OAKLEY CM: Hypertrophic obstructive cardiomyopathy—patterns of progression, in *Hypertrophic Obstructive Cardiomyopathy*, edited by WOLSTENHOLME GEW, O'CONNOR M. London, J. & A. Churchill, Ltd., 1971, p. 9
95. MORROW AG: Hypertrophic subaortic stenosis. Some physiologic concepts and the role of operative treatment. *Arch Surg* 99:677-683, 1969
96. GROSSMAN M, KNOTT AP JR, JACOBY WJ JR: Calcified annulus fibrosis with mitral insufficiency with Marfan's syndrome. *Arch Intern Med* 121:561-563, 1968
97. KORN D, DESANCTIS RW, SELL S: Massive calcification of the mitral annulus. A clinicopathological study of fourteen cases. *N Engl J Med* 267:900-909, 1962
98. BRAWLEY RK, ROBERTS WC, MORROW AG: Intestinal infarction resulting from nonobstructive mesenteric arterial insufficiency. With a note on hepatic hypoglycemia as a possible aid in diagnosis. *Arch Surg* 92:374-378, 1966

Cardiovascular Pathology in Hyperlipoproteinemia

Anatomic Observations in 42 Necropsy Patients with Normal or Abnormal Serum Lipoprotein Patterns

WILLIAM C. ROBERTS, MD, FACC
VICTOR J. FERRANS, MD, PhD
ROBERT I. LEVY, MD, FACC
DONALD S. FREDRICKSON, MD, FACC

Bethesda, Maryland

Certain clinical and cardiovascular necropsy findings are described in 28 patients with known hyperlipoproteinemia and 14 patients known to have a normal lipoprotein pattern. Of the 42 patients, 28 had symptomatic ischemic heart disease: 20 of these had hyperlipoproteinemia (9 type II, 2 type III, and 9 type IV), and 8 had a normal lipoprotein pattern. The average age at death in the 20 patients with hyperlipoproteinemia and symptomatic ischemic heart disease was 48 years, and in the 8 with a normal lipoprotein pattern and ischemic heart disease, 46 years. The degree of coronary arterial luminal narrowing was severe in all patients with ischemic heart disease whether their lipoprotein pattern was normal or abnormal. In all 28 patients with symptomatic ischemic heart disease, the lumen of at least 1 of the 3 major coronary arteries was narrowed more than 75 percent by old atherosclerotic plaques, and in 25 of these all 3 major coronary arteries were narrowed to this extent. With the exception of 1 of the 2 patients with a type III pattern, the composition of the coronary atherosclerotic plaques was similar among patients with type II, III and IV hyperlipoproteinemia and among those with a normal lipoprotein pattern. Attention is called to the unique type of valvular aortic stenosis that frequently develops in the homozygote with a type II pattern and also to the reversed distribution of the aortic atherosclerotic plaquing in the homozygote with a type II pattern. In these patients the amount of plaquing appears to be greater in the ascending than in the abdominal portion of the aorta. Lipid plaques were observed on left atrial endocardium in 2 patients: One had type I hyperlipoproteinemia without associated coronary or aortic atherosclerosis; the second had a type III pattern with extensive coronary and aortic atherosclerosis. These left atrial endocardial lipid deposits may be unique to these hyperlipoproteinemias. In conclusion, it appears clear that atherosclerosis is accelerated or occurs prematurely in patients with type II, III and IV hyperlipoproteinemia, but that hyperlipoproteinemia is not a prerequisite for premature development of severe atherosclerosis.

In 1965 Fredrickson and Lees [1] introduced a system for partial phenotyping of hyperlipoproteinemias. Subsequently, numerous reports on this subject have appeared, but relatively few have focused on the morphologic aspects of the hyperlipoproteinemias. This communication describes certain cardiovascular observations in 28 necropsy patients with known hyperlipoproteinemia and 14 necropsy patients known to have normal lipoprotein patterns.

From the Section of Pathology and the Molecular Disease Branch, National Heart and Lung Institute, National Institutes of Health, Bethesda, Md.
Address for reprints: William C. Roberts, MD, Section of Pathology, National Heart and Lung Institute, National Institutes of Health, Bethesda, Md. 20014.

Patients Studied and Methods

For 9 years serum cholesterol and triglyceride determinations and lipoprotein phenotyping have been performed, by methods described elsewhere,[2-5] in the Molecular Disease Branch of the National Heart and Lung Insti-

TABLE I

Clinical and Cardiac Necropsy Data

Case no.	Age (yr) & Sex	Symp-toms of of IHS	Duration of Symptoms (yr)	Age at Onset of Symptoms (yr)	Angina Pectoris	History of AMI	CHF	HT*	DM	FH of HD	TC†	TG‡
						A. Type II Hyperlipoproteinemia						
1§	28M	+	11	17	+	+	0	0	0	++‖	588	100
2§	29F	+	4	25	+	0	0	0	0	++	430	86
3	36M	+	2.5	33	+	+	0	0	0	0	482	224
4§	42M	+	<1 hr	42	0	0	0	+	+	0	364	142
5§	47M	+	2	45	+	0	0	0	0	0	572	253
6§	49M	+	18	31	+	0	0	+	0	++	591	388
7§	51M	+	10	41	0	+	0	0	0	+‖	388	134
8§	51M	+	9	42	+	0	0	+	0	++	460	220
9	55M	+	4	51	+	+	0	0	0	+	282	76
10	16F	0	...	...	0	0	0	+	0	0	302	356
11	21F	0	...	...	0	0	0	0	0	0	422	320

* Systemic systolic blood pressure >150 or diastolic pressure >90 mm Hg.
† Normal values 150 to 310 mg/100 ml.
‡ Normal values 10 to 160 mg/100 ml.
§ These patients had multiple xanthomas.
¶ Both parents also had type II hyperlipoproteinemia. This is the only homozygote among these fatal cases. The aortic valve cusps contained foam cells and cholesterol clefts indicating that the origin of the aortic stenosis was "atherosclerosis."
♯ This patient had been asymptomatic since left ventricular outflow myotomy and myectomy for idiopathic hypertrophic subaortic stenosis 3 years before death. He died about 1 hour after onset of chest pain typical of acute myocardial infarction.
‖ Two pluses indicate that hyperlipoproteinemia was documented in other family members. One plus indicates a history of heart disease in other family members before age 55 years but no confirmation of hyperlipoproteinemia or hypercholesterolemia in other family members.

Case no.	Age (yr) & Sex	Symp-toms of of IHS	Duration of Symptoms (yr)	Age at Onset of Symptoms (yr)	Angina Pectoris	History of AMI	CHF	HT*	DM	FH of HD	TC†	TG‡
						B. Type III Hyperlipoproteinemia						
12*	52F	+	18	34	+	+	+	+	+	+	338	429
13*,†	57F	+	11	46	+	+	0	0	+	++	700	1100

* Each had intermittent claudication of both legs.

Case no.	Age (yr) & Sex	Symp-toms of of IHS	Duration of Symptoms (yr)	Age at Onset of Symptoms (yr)	Angina Pectoris	History of AMI	CHF	HT*	DM	FH of HD	TC†	TG‡
						C. Type IV Hyperlipoproteinemia						
14	31F	+	10	21	+	0	0	+	0	0	212	216
15	43M	+	4	39	+	+	0	+	0	+	239	266
16	44M	+	8 mo	44	0	+	+	0	0	0	140	264
17	50M	+	17	33	+	+	0	0	0	+	246	600
18	54M	+	10	44	+	+	0	0	+	0	188	520
19	56M	+	17	38	+	+	0	0	0	0	400	1500
20	56M	+	5	51	+	+	0	0	+	+	735	2820
21	59M	+	17	42	+	0	0	+	+	+	183	228
22	65M	+	3 hr	65	0	0	0	+	0	0	193	210
23	22M	0	...	...	0	0	0	+	0	0	282	250
24	28F	0	...	...	0	0	0	+	0	0	314	372
25	46F	0	...	...	+‖	0	+‖	0	0	+	256	208
26	54F	0	...	...	0	0	+	+	0	0	262	456

* Patient severely hypertensive before nephrectomy for hypoplastic kidney at age 18.
† Died of acute myocardial infarction several hours after insertion of carotid sinus stimulator.
‡ Died of acute myocardial infarction 5 days after Vineberg procedure (internal mammary implants into left ventricular wall).
§ Cerebral arterial embolism during cardiac catheterization. Died in coma 3 days later.
¶ Died 3 days after aortocoronary arterial saphenous vein bypass grafts implanted.

Case no.	Age (yr) & Sex	Symp-toms of of IHS	Duration of Symptoms (yr)	Age at Onset of Symptoms (yr)	Angina Pectoris	History of AMI	CHF	HT*	DM	FH of HD	TC†	TG‡
						D. Normal Lipoprotein Pattern						
27	34M	+	7	27	+	+	0	0	+	+	258	158
28	40M	+	4	36	+	0	0	0	0	+	233	112
29	41M	+	7	35	+	0	+	0	+	0	214	150
30	43M	+	2	41	+	0	0	0	0	0	195	86

Case no.	Other Disease	Cause of Death	Heart Weight (g)	% Luminal Narrowing of Coronary Arteries by Old Atherosclerotic Plaques			Myocardial Necrosis	Myocardial Fibrosis
				LAD	LC	Rt		
A. Type II Hyperlipoproteinemia								
1§	AS¶	Sudden	370	>75	>75	>75	0	+(TM)
2§	0	Sudden	300	51–75	51–75	>75	0	0
3	0	AMI	370	>75	>75	>75	+	+(patchy)
4§	IHSS#	Sudden	590	>75	>75	>75	0	+(patchy)
5§	Gout	Sudden	330	>75	>75	>75	0	+(patchy)
6§	0	AMI	400	>75	>75	>75	+	+(TM)
7§	0	Sudden	350	>75	>75	>75	0	+(SE)
8§	Neuromuscular disorder**	Sudden	380	51–75	>75	>75	0	+(SE)
9	AS	Operation††	440	>75	>75	>75	+	+(patchy)
10	SLE	SLE	300	<25	<25	<25	0	0
11	CESD,AS	AS‡‡	340	26–50	51–75	51–75	0	0

** Several family members had similar neuromuscular disorders and a type II pattern. This patient is described elsewhere.[8]

†† Aortic valve replacement for severe aortic stenosis (70 mm Hg peak systolic pressure gradient between the left ventricle and a systemic artery). None of the 3 valve cusps contained foam cells or cholesterol clefts.

‡‡ Congenitally bicuspid aortic valve that was severely stenotic despite valvulotomy 6 years earlier. However, lipid material was present in each aortic valve cusp and in the wall of the ascending aorta.

AMI = acute myocardial infarction; AS = valvular aortic stenosis; CESD = cholesteryl ester storage disease; CHF = congestive heart failure; DM = diabetes mellitus; FH = family history; HD = heart disease; HT = hypertension; IHS = ischemic heart disease; IHSS = idiopathic hypertrophic subaortic stenosis; LAD = left anterior descending; LC = left circumflex; Rt = right; SE = subendocardium only; SLE = systemic lupus erythematosus; TC = total serum cholesterol (mg/100 ml); TG = serum triglyceride (mg/100 ml); TM = transmural.

B. Type III Hyperlipoproteinemia								
12*	0	AMI	480	>75	>75	>75	+	+(TM)
13*,†	0	Sudden	330	>75	>75	>75	0	+(SE)

† This patient, described in detail elsewhere,[9] had yellow (lipid) deposits on the palms and fingers and in many other areas.

C. Type IV Hyperlipoproteinemia								
14	Renal*	Sudden	300	>75	>75	>75	0	+(SE)
15	0	Operation†	350	>75	>75	>75	0	+(TM)
16	Polyneuropathy	AMI	500	>75	>75	>75	+(TM)	+(TM)
17	0	Operation‡	450	>75	>75	>75	+(TM)	+(TM)
18	0	Catheterization§	505	>75	>75	>75	+(SE)	+(TM)
19	0	Sudden	460	>75	>75	>75	0	+(patchy)
20	0	AMI	450	>75	>75	>75	+(SE)	+(TM)
21	0	Operation¶	640	>75	>75	>75	0	+(TM)
22	0	Sudden	540	>75	>75	>75	0	+(SE)
23	Pheochromocytoma#		420	<25	<25	<25	0	0
24	SLE	SLE	400	>75	51–75	>75	0	0
25	IHSS	IHSS	420	51–75	51–75	>75	0	+(TM)‖
26	MR, AR	Operation**	510	26–50	51–75	51–75	0	0

Malignant-widespread metastases.

** Aortic and mitral valve replacements for mitral regurgitation (MR) and aortic regurgitation (AR).

‖ Probably secondary to the associated idiopathic hypertrophic subaortic stenosis, or at least not solely the result of coronary heart disease.

D. Normal Lipoprotein Pattern								
27	0	Operation*	390	>75	>75	>75	+(TM)	+(TM)
28	0	Catheterization†	370	>75	>75	>75	+(TM)	+(SE)
29	0	Sudden	450	>75	>75	>75	0	+(SE)
30	0	Operation‡	475	>75	>75	>75	+(TM)	+(TM)

continued

TABLE I (continued)

Case no.	Age (yr) & Sex	Symptoms of IHS	Duration of Symptoms (yr)	Age at Onset of Symptoms (yr)	Angina Pectoris	History of AMI	CHF	HT*	DM	FH of HD	TC†	TG‡
31	46M	+	13	33	+	+	0	0	0	0	230	169
32	47M	+	2	45	+	+	0	+	0	0	136	76
33	57M	+	6	51	+	+	0	0	0	+	178	124
34	59F	+	7	52	+	0	0	+	0	+	236	79
35	33M	0	...	...	+¶	0	+	0	0	+	214	68
36	33M	0	...	...	0	0	0	0	0	0	196	66
37	47M	0	...	...	+¶	0	+	+	0	0	204	146
38	47M	0	...	...	0	0	0	0	+	0	256	114
39	50M	0	...	...	0	0	0	+	0	0	176	118
40	62M	0	...	...	0	0	+	+	0	0	134	87

* Acute myocardial infarction during Vineberg procedure.
† Fatal coronary arterial embolism during cardiac catheterization.
‡ Fatal acute myocardial infarction immediately after insertion of coronary sinus stimulator.
§ Died 1 day after aortocoronary bypass grafts inserted.

tute on patients admitted to the Clinical Center with positive or suspected clinical evidence of ischemic heart disease or hyperlipidemia. During most of this time these same determinations were performed for screening purposes on patients admitted to certain wards of the Clinical Center. Thus, 2 pools of typed subjects were available. Within these 2 groups, 42 patients died and underwent necropsy. The clinical and necropsy records of all 42 patients were reviewed. In addition, the heart of each subject was reexamined, and the histologic sections of it were reviewed. The major extramural coronary arteries of each patient were examined in their entirety, by methods described elsewhere,[6,7] if they had not been examined in this manner at the time of necropsy. In essence, the right, left main, left anterior descending and left circumflex coronary arteries were excised intact, decalcified, cut at 0.5 cm intervals, embedded as a whole and processed, and 3 histologic sections from each 0.5 cm segment were cut, stained and examined. The maximal percent of luminal narrowing of each artery was recorded.

Histologic sections of spleen, stained by hematoxylin-eosin and by the periodic acid-Schiff methods, were examined in each of the 42 necropsy patients.

Results

Clinical Features

Pertinent clinical and morphologic data in 40 of the 42 necropsy patients are summarized in Table I; data from 2 patients, 1 with type I and 1 with type V disease, are not included. Some morphologic observations are illustrated in Figures 1 to 15. Of the 28 patients with hyperlipoproteinemia, 23 had the primary variety, heritable in at least 13, and 5 had the secondary variety; that is, the hyperlipoproteinemia was caused by another known disease. Of the 42 patients, 28 had clinical evidence of ischemic heart disease, namely, angina pectoris, acute myocardial infarction or sudden death, or a combination of these findings. Among these 28 patients, 23 of whom were men and 5 women, 9 had type II, 2 type III, 9 type IV, and 8, normal lipoprotein patterns. Their ages ranged from 28 to 65 years (average age 47); patients with a type II pattern averaged 43 years, those with type IV 47 years, and those with a normal lipoprotein pattern 46 years. The 2 patients with a type III pattern were 52 and 57 years of age, respectively. Of the 14 patients without clinical evidence of ischemic heart disease, 2 had asymmetric septal hypertrophy (idiopathic hypertrophic subaortic stenosis) (type IV in 1, normal lipoprotein pattern in 1), 2 had valvular heart disease (type II in 1, normal lipoprotein pattern in 1), 2 systemic lupus erythematosus (type II in 1, type IV in 1), 1 scleroderma (normal lipoprotein pattern), 1 metastatic pheochromocytoma (type IV), 1 cholesteryl ester storage disease (type II),[10] 1 fatal pancreatitis (type I), and 1 glycogen storage disease (type V). Of the 14 patients without clinical evidence of ischemic heart disease, 9 were male and 5 were female. Excluding the 9 month old boy with glycogen storage disease, their ages ranged from 16 to 62 years (average 38); the single patient with a type I pattern was 30 years old, the 2 patients with a type II pattern were 16 and 21 years old, respectively; the 3 with a type IV pattern averaged 35 years; and the 7 with a normal lipoprotein pattern averaged 45 years.

Of the 28 patients with symptomatic ischemic heart disease, all died from consequences of severe coronary arterial luminal narrowing: 12 died suddenly (less than 6 hours after the onset of chest pain) (acute cardiovascular collapse without myocardial necrosis), 6 from acute myocardial infarction, 8 from cardiac operations to improve myocardial oxygenation, and 2 from complications of coronary arteriography. The average age at death of the 18 patients who died from natural consequences of ischemic heart disease was 46 years; the average age in the 10 patients who died from diagnostic or surgical cardiac procedures was 49 years.

Pathologic Findings

The hearts in 28 patients with symptomatic ischemic heart disease weighed 330 to 640 g (average

Case no.	Other Disease	Cause of Death	Heart Weight (g)	% Luminal Narrowing of Coronary Arteries by Old Atherosclerotic Plaques			Myocardial Necrosis	Myocardial Fibrosis
				LAD	LC	Rt		
31	0	Sudden	400	>75	>75	>75	0	+(SE)
32	0	AMI	460	26–50	>75	>75	+(TM)	+(SE)
33	0	Operation§	420	>75	>75	>75	+(TM)	+(TM)
34	0	Operation*	320	>75	>75	>75	0	+(SE)
35	IHSS	IHSS	1020	<25	<25	26–50	0	0
36	Leukemia	Leukemia	380	<25	<25	<25	0	0
37	MR, AR	Operation‡	770	51–75	51–75	51–75	0	+(SE)
38	Leukemia	Leukemia	270	26–50	26–50	26–50	0	0
39	Scleroderma	Scleroderma	450	26–50	26–50	51–75	0	0
40	MR, AR	Operation**	1230	51–75	51–75	>75	0	+(TM)

¶ Probably secondary to the associated heart disease (idiopathic hypertrophic subaortic stenosis or combined mitral regurgitation [MR] and aortic regurgitation [AR]) or at least not the result solely of coronary heart disease.

‡ Died 57 days after mitral and aortic valve replacements and aortocoronary arterial bypass graft insertions.

** Died 2 days after mitral and aortic valve replacements.

weight 422): the hearts of the 23 men averaged 439 g and those of the 5 women 346 g. In 14 of the 28 patients, the hearts weighed more than 400 g; 6 of the 14 had systemic hypertension (4 patients), hypertrophic (asymmetric) cardiomyopathy (1 patient) or valvular aortic stenosis (1 patient). Chronic myocardial ischemia probably was a factor in producing cardiomegaly in the other 8 patients.

Focal myocardial fibrosis (subendocardial, transmural or patchy) was present in 27 of the 28 patients with symptomatic ischemic heart disease, and in only 3 of the 14 patients without it.

Severe coronary arterial luminal narrowing was present in all 28 patients with symptomatic ischemic heart disease. In 25 of the 28 patients the lumens of each of the 3 major extramural coronary arteries (right, left anterior descending, left circumflex) was narrowed more than 75 percent by old atherosclerotic plaques; in 2 others, the lumens of 2 of the 3 arteries were narrowed more than 75 percent; and in the remaining patient, the lumen of 1 of the 3 vessels was narrowed to this extent. No significant difference in degrees of luminal narrowing of the coronary arteries was observed among patients with a type II, III, IV or normal lipoprotein pattern and ischemic heart disease.

The degree of coronary arterial luminal narrowing was much less among the 14 patients without symptomatic ischemic heart disease: Only 3 had more than 75 percent luminal narrowing of any coronary vessel, and 5 had normal coronary arteries on gross inspection. Several patients without ischemic heart disease but with type II or IV hyperlipidemia had considerable coronary atherosclerosis for their age, but the luminal narrowing was not great enough to cause clinically apparent myocardial disease.

Atherosclerotic plaques: No obvious differences in composition of the atherosclerotic plaques were noted among patients with type II or IV or with a normal lipoprotein pattern. The major component of the plaques in these patients was fibrous tissue. Deposits of pultaceous debris containing cholesterol clefts and strongly oil red O positive material (indicating mainly cholesteryl esters or glycerides) were present in many arteries; these deposits were covered by fibrous capsules. Calcific deposits also were frequent in patients with type II and IV disorders and in those with a normal lipoprotein pattern. These deposits were definitely larger in the older patients. Relatively few foam cells were present in most plaques. The exception occurred in 1 of the 2 patients with a type III disorder who had severe degrees of luminal narrowing at some sites resulting primarily from large collections of foam cells.[9] However, in the second patient with type III disease, the coronary plaques looked no different from those observed in the patients with type II or IV or a normal lipoprotein pattern and symptomatic ischemic heart disease.

With the exception of the patient with a type I pattern, atherosclerotic plaques were present diffusely in the coronary arteries of all 40 adult patients—not just the 28 with symptomatic ischemic heart disease—and similar, complicated atherosclerotic plaques were present in the aorta as well. The plaquing was most severe in the abdominal portion of the aorta except in the patient with a homozygous type II pattern[4] (Fig. 1 to 3) whose plaquing was more severe in the ascending than in the abdominal portion of the aorta. Both coronary ostia also were considerably narrowed by calcified plaques. In addition, this patient had diffuse fibrous thickening of the 3 aortic valve cusps, each of which contained a few foam cells and cholesterol clefts. The rigidity imparted to the cusps caused the orifice to be stenotic. This patient had typical clinical features of valvular aortic stenosis including left ventricular hypertrophy. Foam cell plaques were observed in the left atrial endocardium in 2 patients: One, a 57 year old woman, had a type III pattern with associated severe atherosclerosis of

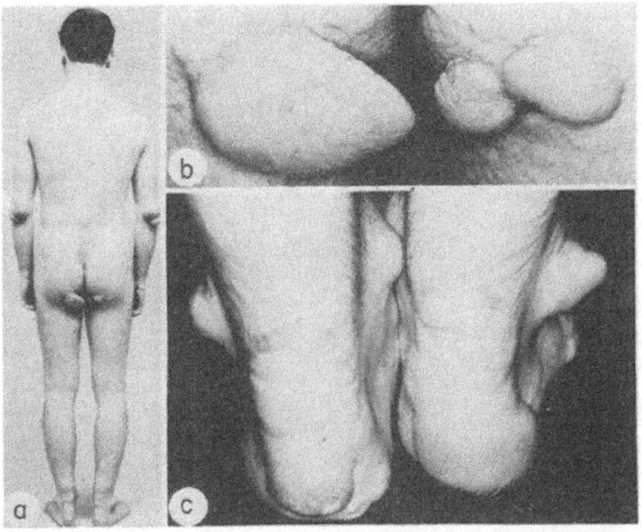

FIGURE 1. Case 1 (Table IA). Photograph of patient with *homozygous type II* hyperlipoproteinemia. **a,** from the back showing large xanthomas on the elbows, buttocks and ankles. Close-up view of buttocks in **b,** and ankles in **c.** This man, who died suddenly at age 28 on December 20, 1969, had xanthomas noted at age 2 years. The left eye was enucleated at age 2 for suspected melanoma, but the tumor histologically was a xanthoma. He ate low-fat foods most of his life. He was asymptomatic until age 17 years when angina pectoris appeared. At age 23, the first of several episodes of syncope occurred, and at age 26 he had an episode of acute pulmonary edema without evidence of acute myocardial infarction. When admitted a month later (April 1968) to the National Institutes of Health, he had mild exertional dyspnea and angina. He slept flat in bed. Several family members, including both parents, had type II hyperlipoproteinemia. In addition to the large widespread tuberotendinous xanthomas, he had a sustained left ventricular impulse and a grade 3/6 mid-systolic, ejection-type murmur over the left sternal border with radiation into the neck. He had no signs of congestive cardiac failure. The blood pressure was 115/65 mm Hg. The heart was of normal size on chest roentgenogram. The electrocardiogram showed old anterior and inferior myocardial infarction and left ventricular hypertrophy. The initial serum total cholesterol level was 588 mg with beta, alpha and very low density lipoprotein fractions of 529, 31 and 28 mg/100 ml, respectively. The total serum triglyceride level was 100 mg/100 ml. Protein electrophoresis showed a bifid peak in the beta region with a quantitation of 1.3 g/100 ml. During his last 2 years, the patient was treated with a low cholesterol diet and large doses (48 g daily) of cholestyramine. With this therapy the total serum cholesterol decreased to a low value of 340 mg/100 ml, the xanthomas softened slightly and became less yellow. He died suddenly at home. The immediate cause of death was not determined at necropsy.

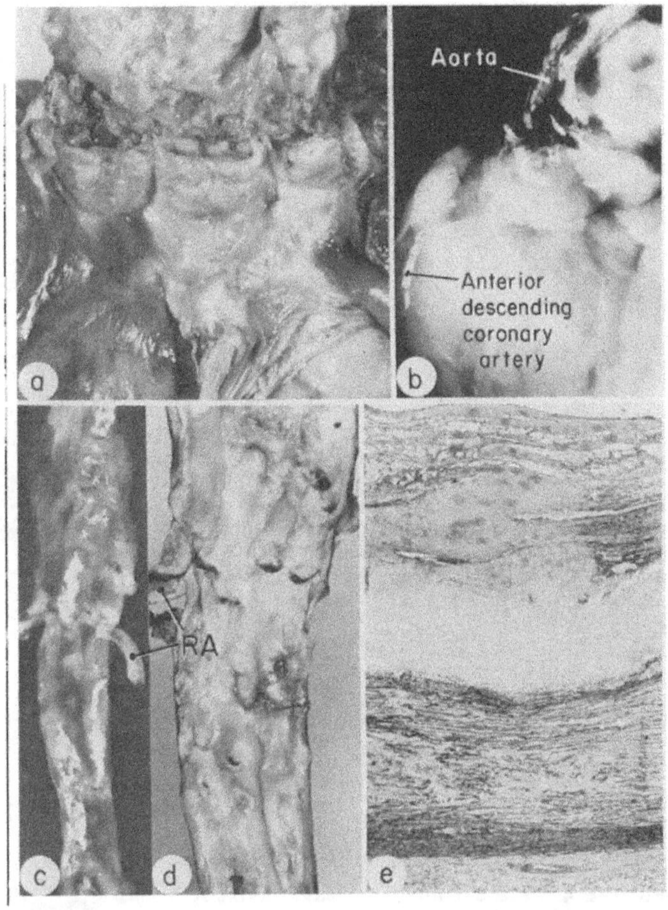

FIGURE 2. Case 1. **a,** close-up view of opened aortic root, aortic valve and left ventricular outflow tract. The intimal surface of the entire ascending aorta is 100 percent involved by complicated atherosclerotic plaques. The ostia of the coronary arteries are narrowed by the heavy calcific deposits in the aortic root. The aortic valve cusps are thickened, and their mobility is considerably diminished. Relatively few calcific deposits were present in the cusps compared to the extensive deposits in the ascending aorta. The aortic valve orifice appeared moderately stenotic but competent. The commissures are not fused. A calcific deposit also is present on the anterior mitral leaflet near its posteromedial commissure. **b,** radiograph of heart showing heavy calcific deposits in the ascending aorta and anterior descending coronary artery and a few deposits in the aortic valve cusps. **c,** radiograph of abdominal aorta showing fewer calcific plaques than in the ascending aorta. **d,** opened abdominal aorta. RA = renal arteries. **e,** photomicrograph of portion of abdominal aorta. Foam cells, similar in size to those present in the aortic valve cusps and in the anterior mitral leaflet, are present in the atherosclerotic plaque near the lumen. (Movat stain ×36, reduced by 31 percent.)

the coronary arteries and aorta[9]; the second, a 30 year old man, had a type I pattern but, in contrast, his coronary arteries and aorta were free of atherosclerotic plaques on gross inspection.

Sections of spleen: Foam cells were not observed in the spleen of any of the 24 patients with type II or IV hyperlipoproteinemia or in any of the 14 with a normal lipoprotein pattern in preparations stained with hematoxylin-eosin. By autofluorescent techniques, however, a few small scattered, weakly autofluorescent cells were observed in the spleen of patients with type II and IV disorders and in those with a normal lipoprotein pattern. In contrast, easily identifiable foam cells were observed in the spleen of the 1 patient with a type I pattern, in the 2 patients with type III, and in the 1 patient who had glycogen storage disease with a type V lipoprotein pattern.

Comments

Observations in these patients clearly indicate that extensive atherosclerosis of the coronary arteries and aorta is definitely accelerated and extensive in

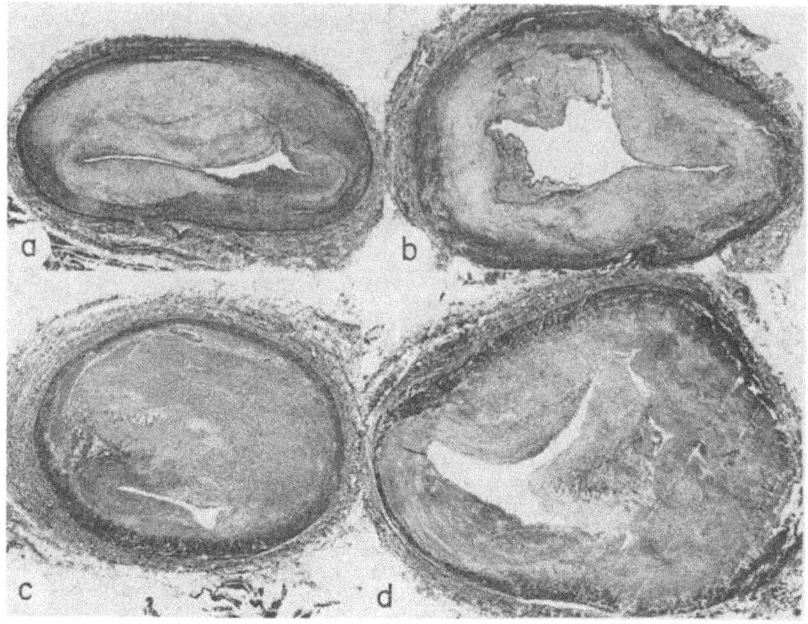

FIGURE 3. Case 1. Histologic sections of coronary arteries at sites of maximal narrowing. The lumens of each of the right (**a**), left circumflex (**c**) and anterior descending (**d**) arteries are more than 75 percent narrowed by atherosclerotic plaques, composed mainly of fibrous tissue. **b,** left main coronary artery. (Movat stains [**a** and **b**], hematoxylin-eosin stains [**c** and **d**]; each ×22, reduced by 36 percent.)

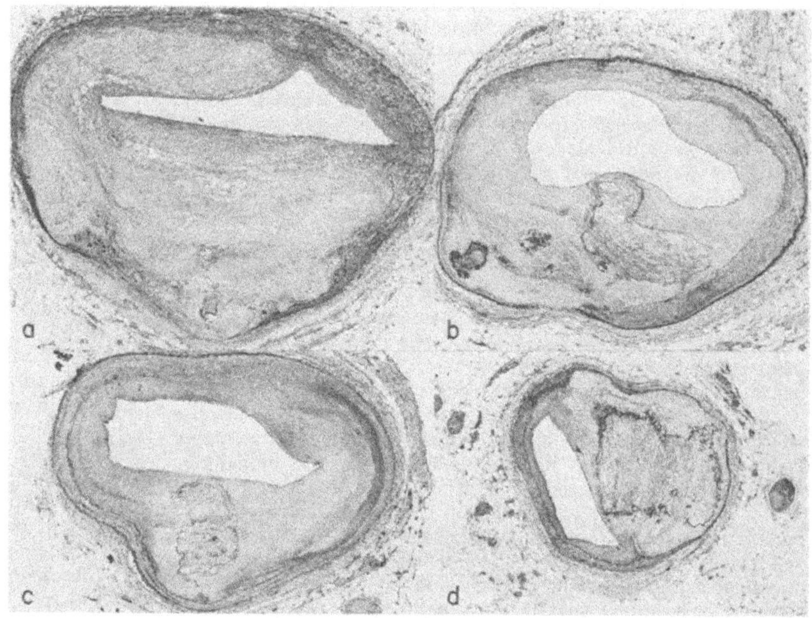

FIGURE 4. Case 8 (Table IA). Major coronary arteries at sites of maximal narrowing in a 51 year old man with type II hyperlipoproteinemia.[43] This patient had noted xanthomas at age 35 years, and angina pectoris appeared at age 42. He also had a neuromuscular disease of unknown type due to degeneration of the anterior horn cells of the spinal cord during his last 5 years.[43] Four brothers had a type II pattern as did 2 children. The lipoprotein pattern of his parents is unknown. He died suddenly after worsening of his angina. Shown here are histologic sections of his major coronary arteries at sites of maximal narrowing. **a,** right coronary artery (3 cm from ostium). **b,** left anterior descending coronary artery (first 1 cm). **c,** left circumflex coronary artery (first 1 cm). **d,** left marginal coronary artery (first 1 cm). (Movat stains; each ×25, reduced by 42 percent.)

patients with type II, III and IV hyperlipoproteinemia and symptomatic ischemic heart disease. It also is clear that hyperlipoproteinemia is not a prerequisite for the premature development of severe atherosclerosis. Among our 28 patients with symptomatic ischemic heart disease, 20 had an abnormal (type II in 9, type III in 2, and type IV in 9) and 8 a normal lipoprotein pattern. The average age at death in the 20 patients with an abnormal lipoprotein pattern and ischemic heart disease was 48 years, and in the 8 with a normal lipoprotein pattern and ischemic heart disease, 46 years. The degree of luminal narrowing among all our patients with symptomatic ischemic heart disease, whether they had normal or abnormal lipoprotein patterns, was severe: In all 28 patients at least 1 of the 3 major coronary arteries was narrowed more than 75 percent by old atherosclerotic plaques, and in 25 each of the 3 major vessels was narrowed to this extent.

With the exception of 1 patient with a type III pattern, the composition of the coronary atherosclerotic plaques was similar among patients with type II and IV hyperlipoproteinemia and those with a normal lipoprotein pattern. In 1 of the 2 patients with a type III disorder several areas of the coronary tree were narrowed by plaques consisting primarily of foam cells.[9] In contrast, the latter cells were sparse in the plaques of patients with type II and IV and

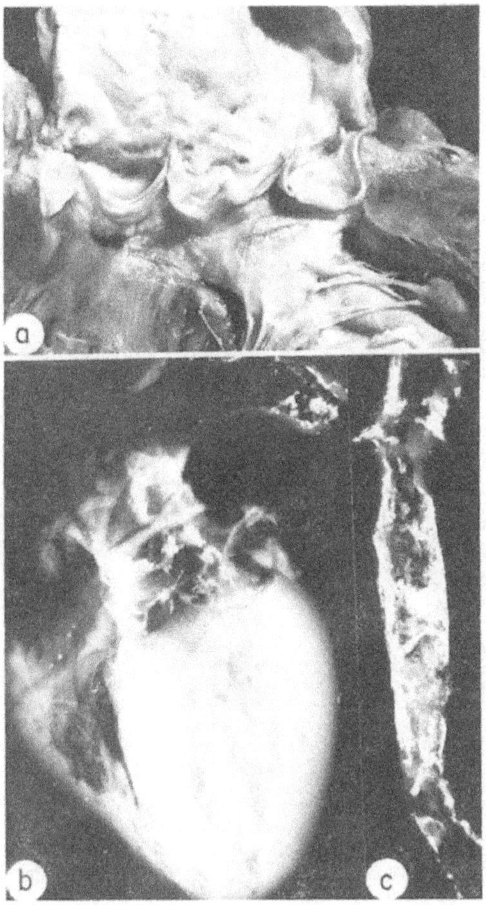

FIGURE 5. Case 8. Heart and aorta. During life the patient had a grade 2/6 systolic ejection murmur interpreted as evidence of "aortic stenosis." At necropsy, small calcific deposits were present on the aortic aspects of each cusp, but the cusps were freely mobile and the valve orifice was not stenotic. **a,** opened ascending aorta, aortic valve and left ventricle. Although extensive atherosclerotic plaquing is present in the ascending aorta, the degree is far less than that observed in the patient in Case 1 (Table IA), who had homozygous type II hyperlipoproteinemia. This patient almost certainly had a heterozygous type II pattern. **b,** radiograph of heart specimen disclosing calcific deposits in the aortic valve, root of aorta, and coronary arteries. **c,** radiograph of abdominal aorta showing more extensive calcific deposits than in the ascending aorta.

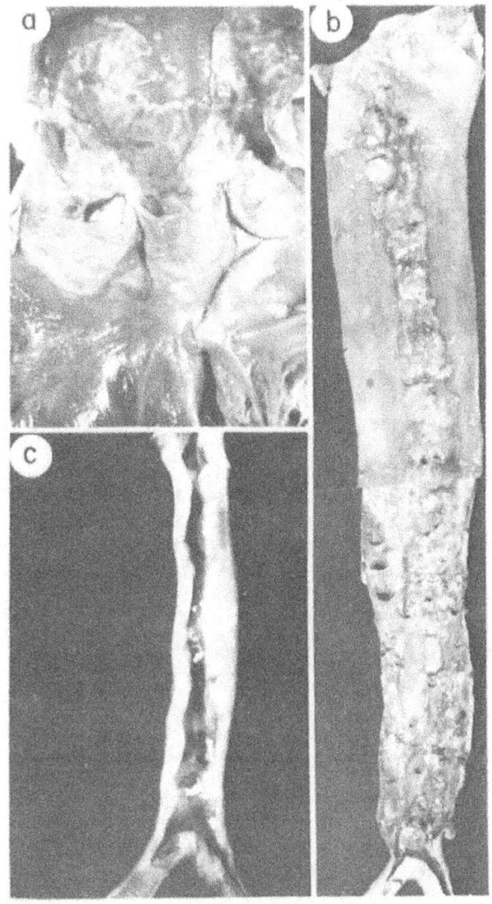

FIGURE 6. Case 2 (Table IA). Extensive atherosclerotic plaquing of aorta in a 29 year old woman with type II disease. Her father died of acute myocardial infarction at age 28, and 2 of her children have type II disease and xanthomas of the Achilles tendons. She died suddenly after 4 years of angina pectoris. **a,** opened ascending aorta, aortic valve and left ventricle. **b,** opened descending thoracic and abdominal aorta. **c,** radiograph of unopened abdominal aorta disclosing some calcific deposits.

normal lipoprotein pattern with symptomatic ischemic heart disease. However, a number of foam cells were present in the patients with hyperlipoproteinemia who did not have symptomatic ischemic heart disease. These latter patients were relatively young adults. The response of lipids to therapy in patients with a type III disorder is prompt and usually more dramatic than in those with a type II or IV disorder. Plaques formed mainly of foam cells, as may be the case in some[9] but not all[11] patients with a type III pattern, might be expected to disappear with good therapy, whereas those consisting primarily of fibrous tissue with some calcific deposits and cholesterol clefts, as in patients with type II and IV disorders and a normal lipoprotein pattern, would appear to be much less reversible.

Lipoprotein Patterns and Premature Vascular Disease

Type I: Although little anatomic information on the cardiovascular system is available in type I hyperlipoproteinemia, there is no clinical evidence that premature atherosclerosis is a feature of this disorder. Patients with this disorder, however, are few and, as a group, young. Our 1 necropsy patient with type I disease was a 30 year old man who died of pancreatitis. Although he did have lipid deposits on the endocardium of his left atrium, his coronary arteries and aorta were free of atherosclerotic plaques on gross examination.

Type II: It is now well established that vascular disease occurs prematurely in patients with a type II pattern. In the heterozygote the vascular complications—namely, angina pectoris, acute myocardial infarction, sudden death and probably also stroke and intermittent leg claudication—usually do not occur until adulthood, most commonly between the ages of 40 to 55 years.[12-17] Likewise, xanthomas in the

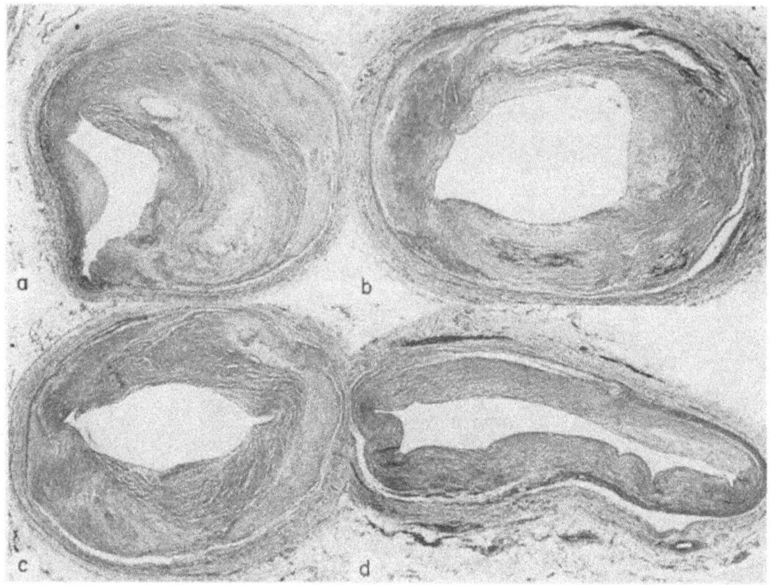

FIGURE 7. Case 2. Coronary arteries at sites of maximal narrowing: **a**, right; **b**, left main; **c**, left circumflex; **d**, left anterior descending coronary arteries, (Hematoxylin-eosin stains; each ×33, reduced by 49 percent.)

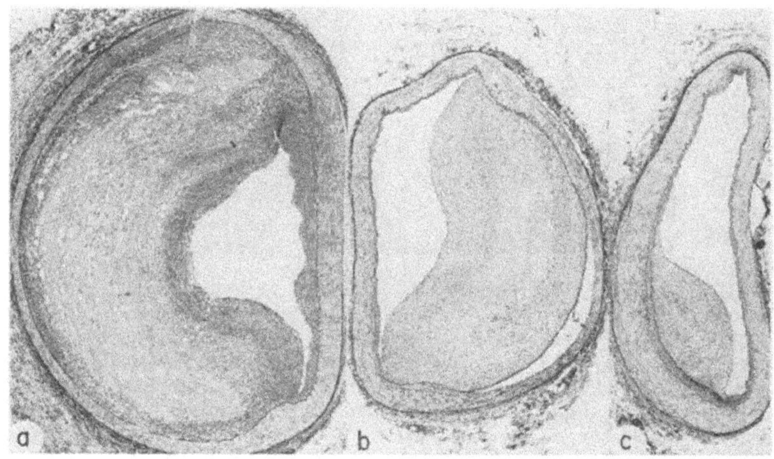

FIGURE 8. Case 11 (Table IA). Coronary arteries in a 21 year old woman with a type II disorder but no symptoms of ischemic heart disease. She died suddenly from severe aortic stenosis superimposed on a congenitally bicuspid aortic valve. **a**, right; **b**, left circumflex; **c**, left anterior descending coronary arteries. (Movat stains; each ×34, reduced by 40 percent.)

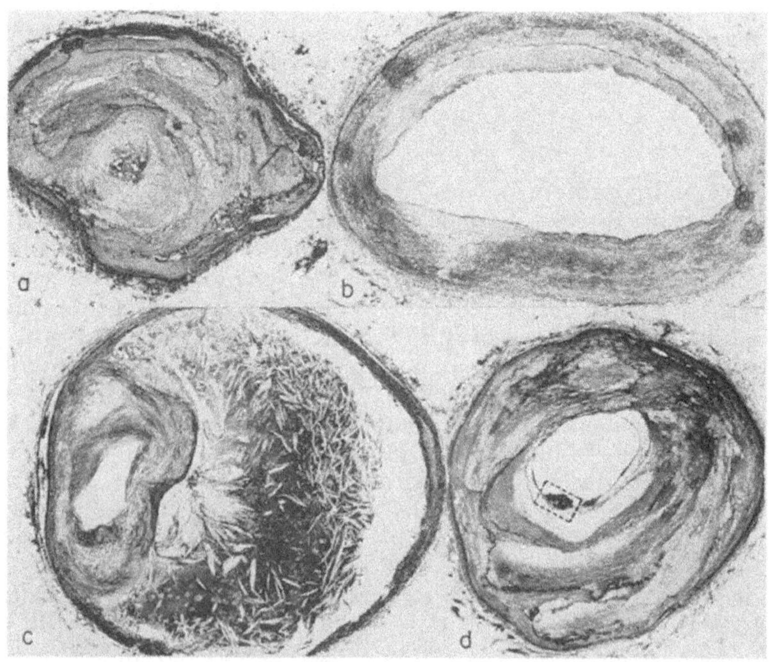

FIGURE 9. Case 22 (Table IC). Coronary arteries, at sites of maximal narrowing in a 65 year old man with a type IV disorder. He died suddenly without previous symptomatic evidence of ischemic heart disease. **a**, right; **b**, left main; **c**, left circumflex; **d**, left anterior descending coronary arteries. The luminal narrowing in 3 of the vessels is severe and due to various types of complicated atherosclerotic plaques. The area in brackets in **d** is a small platelet thrombus. (Movat stain [**a**], elastic-van Gieson stain [**b**], hematoxylin-eosin stain [**c** and **d**]; each ×20, reduced by 58 percent.)

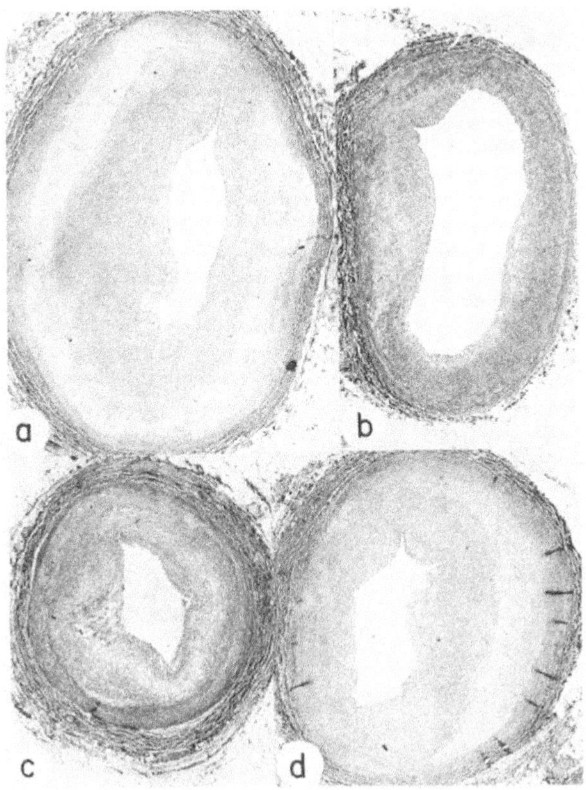

FIGURE 10. Case 24 (Table IC). Major coronary arteries at sites of maximal narrowing in a 28 year old woman with a type IV disorder and systemic lupus erythematosus. She never had symptoms of ischemic heart disease. **a,** right; **b,** left main; **c,** left circumflex; **d,** left anterior descending coronary arteries. The luminal narrowing is mainly by fibrous tissue but much intra- and extracellular lipid is present. (Hematoxylin-eosin stains; each ×16, reduced by 25 percent.)

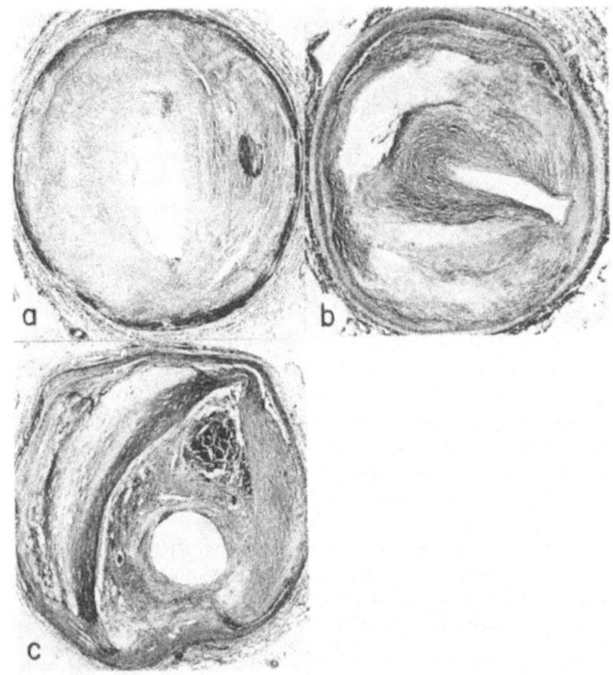

FIGURE 11. Case 27 (Table ID). Right (**a**), left anterior descending (**b**) and left circumflex (**c**) coronary arteries at sites of maximal narrowing in a 34 year old man who had symptoms of ischemic heart disease for 7 years and a normal lipoprotein pattern. He died suddenly. (Elastic tissue stains [**a** and **d**] and hematoxylin-eosin stain [**b**]; each ×25, reduced by 30 percent.)

heterozygote with type II pattern usually do not appear until adulthood. Ischemic heart disease, by far the major vascular complication, occurs in both male and female heterozygotes at much higher rates than would be expected in the general population.[12-16]

All vascular complications seen in the heteroxygote with a type II pattern also occur in the homozygote with this pattern, but in the latter the complications, as well as the xanthomas, occur at a much younger age, often before 10 years. Few homozygotes actually reach the fourth decade of life. The extensiveness of the atherosclerosis in the homozygote with a type II disorder, as illustrated by Case 1 (Table I, Fig. 1 to 3), is usually striking, and many reports have described vascular death or disability in youth from atherosclerosis.[4,18-32] The atherosclerotic plaquing in the homozygote appears to be particularly severe in the ascending aorta. Here the entire intimal surface is often involved, and frequently the ostia of the coronary arteries are considerably narrowed by the plaques. Atherosclerosis in adults, except when superimposed on syphilitic aortitis, is nearly always worse in the abdominal portion than in the ascending portion of the aorta. This usual distribution appears to be reversed in the homozygote with a type II pattern, although the transverse, descending thoracic and abdominal portions of the aorta, and even the major pulmonary arteries, also may contain considerable atherosclerotic plaquing. Narrowing of the coronary ostia in the type II homozygote may cause sudden death or acute myocardial infarction without much luminal narrowing of the coronary arteries themselves. Usually, however, the amount of coronary luminal narrowing also is severe.

A unique feature of the homozygote with a type II pattern, not found in the heterozygote with this pattern or in patients with other forms of hyperlipoproteinemia, is the occurrence of a peculiar type of valvular aortic stenosis.[18-29,32] The cusps are often thickened and relatively immobile, and histologic study has disclosed foam cells, cholesterol clefts and calcific deposits within the leaflets. The occurrence of intracellular lipid and cholesterol clefts within the cusps is distinctive and not seen in other forms of valvular aortic stenosis.[33-36] Similar lesions in the aorta and aortic valve suggest that the origin of both is similar. The aortic valve in these patients may become quite stenotic. Stanley et al.[25] described a peak systolic pressure gradient of 108 mm Hg between the left ventricle and systemic artery in a 12 year old girl with xanthomatosis and hypercholesterolemia. She underwent successful aortic valvulotomy and excision of many atherosclerotic plaques in the aortic root, particularly about the coronary ostia. In these patients, the considerable plaquing in the aortic root may cause obstruction just above the valve

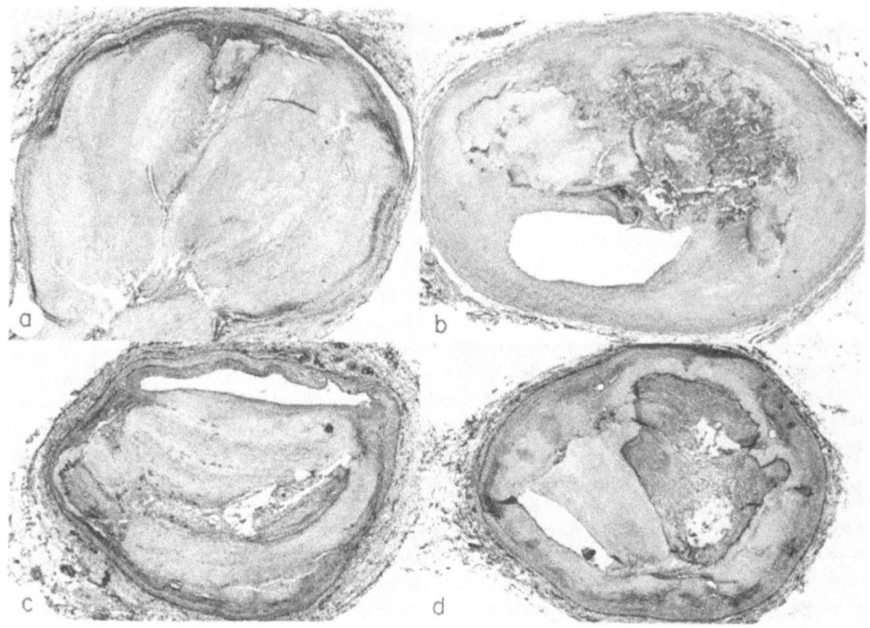

FIGURE 12. Case 29 (Table ID). Right (a), left main (b), left circumflex (c) and left anterior descending (d) coronary arteries, at sites of maximal narrowing, in a 42 year old man who had symptoms of ischemic heart disease for 7 years and a normal lipoprotein pattern. He died suddenly. (Elastic tissue stains [a, c, d] and hematoxylin-eosin stain [d]; each ×25, reduced by 41 percent.)

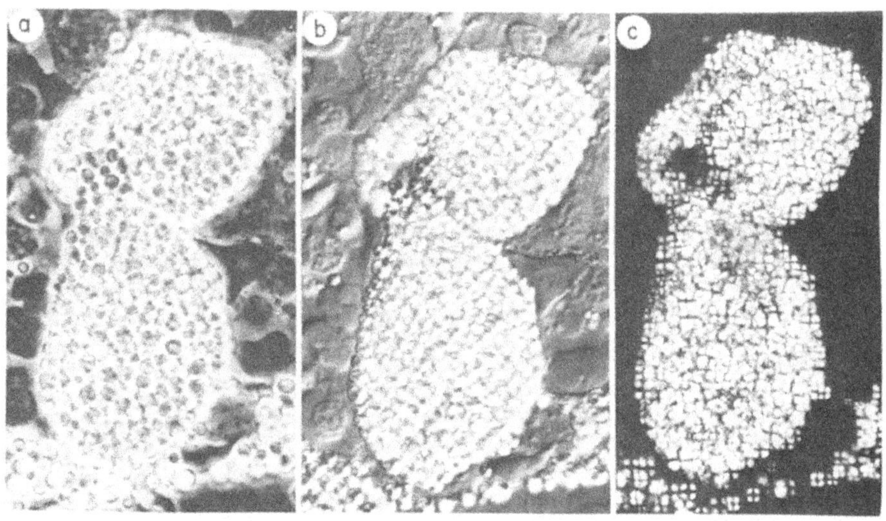

FIGURE 13. Unstained foam cells in bone marrow aspirate from a 35 year old man with a type I pattern are shown as seen by phase-contrast (a), Nomarski interference-contrast (b) and polarization (c) microscopy. These cells are large (up to 100μ in diameter) and strongly birefringent. (Each ×625, reduced by 46 percent.)

(supravalvular) rather than at the valve itself.[32] The aortic valvular stenosis observed in the homozygote patient with a type II pattern has been produced experimentally in squirrel monkeys fed a high cholesterol diet which are offspring of parents shown to be hyperresponders to such a diet.[37] The offspring were even more sensitive to dietary cholesterol than their parents, and their serum showed a type II pattern.

Although yellow plaques occur on the mitral valve in nearly all persons over 10 years of age, the amount of plaquing on this valve appears to be decidedly increased in patients with a homozygous type II pattern. These plaques, which appear to occur initially on the ventricular surfaces of both leaflets, do not seem to cause valvular dysfunction. However, if these patients lived longer, the deposits underneath the posterior leaflet probably would lead to "calcifi-

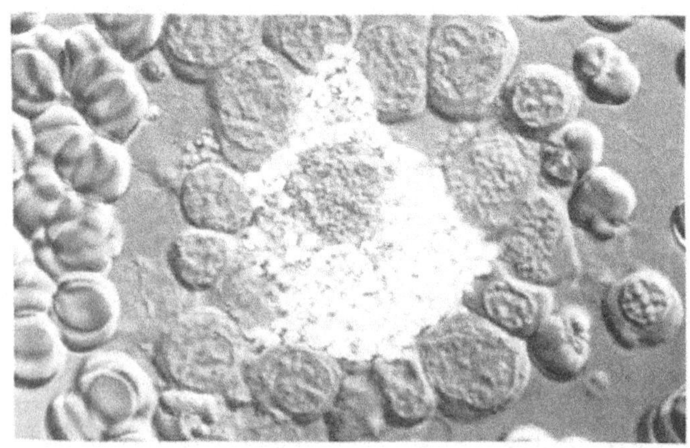

FIGURE 14. Foam cell in bone marrow of a 39 year old man with type III disease. Unstained specimen, Nomarski interference-contrast microscopy. (×550, reduced by 36 percent.)

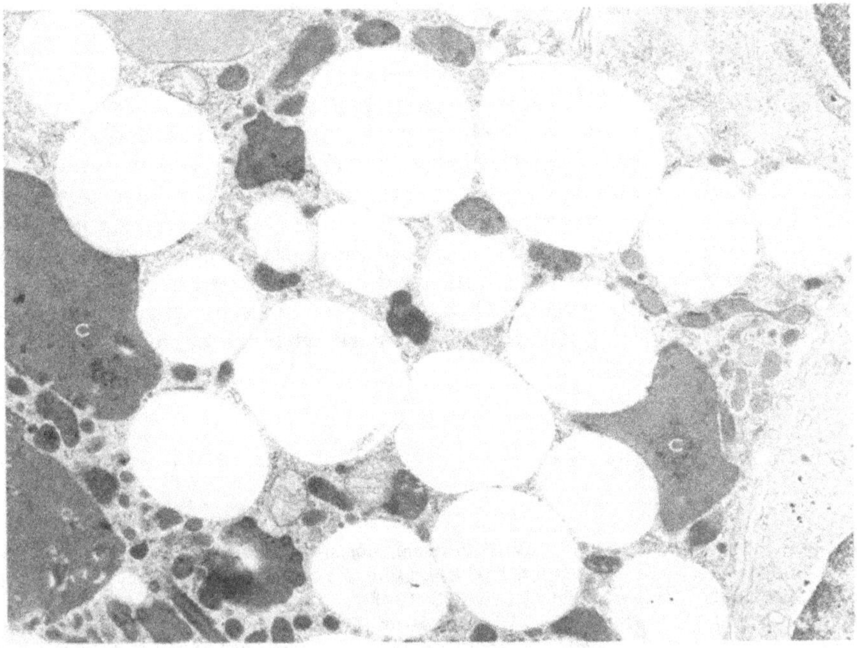

FIGURE 15. Same case. Electron micrograph of foam cell. The cell contains large lipid droplets and ceroid deposits (C). (×14,500, reduced by 25 percent.)

cation of the mitral annulus." Foam cells also have been observed in mural endocardium of the left ventricular outflow tract of these patients.[23]

Type III: Although the prevalence of premature vascular disease in patients with a type III pattern unquestionably seems to be high,[4] the exact figure remains to be established. Of 51 patients with a type III pattern studied clinically by 2 of us,[4] 27 (53 percent) had a history or signs of ischemic heart disease and 49 percent had peripheral vascular disease, as indicated by decreased pulses in the femoral, popliteal or smaller leg arteries. In the aggregate, more than 80 percent of the men and about 25 percent of the women under age 50 years with a type III pattern had evidence of vascular disease. Peripheral vascular disease appears to have a particularly high frequency in the type III disorder, and a history of intermittent claudication in a patient with hyperlipidemia should suggest this phenotype. Peripheral arterial blood flow in patients with a type III pattern has been demonstrated to increase, sometimes strikingly, after the blood lipid levels have been lowered by therapy.[38] Deposits of foam cells have been observed on left atrial endocardial tissue in the type III disorder.[9] These superficial lipid deposits on the endocardium were reminiscent of the cutaneous xanthomas seen in the type III disorder, thereby leading to speculation as to whether such changes in the vascular system might respond as quickly and as completely to therapy as do the skin lesions.

Type IV: Premature vascular disease also appears very probable in the type IV disorder but the risk cannot yet be estimated accurately. A history of angina pectoris or of acute myocardial infarction was present in 38 percent of 78 patients with a type IV pattern studied clinically by Fredrickson and Levy,[4] and of 54 questioned specifically, 17 percent had intermittent claudication of the legs. A type IV pattern is commonly found in patients with myocardial infarction.[39] A combined metabolic and coronary angiographic study by the National Heart and Lung Institute and the Peter Bent Brigham Hospital disclosed that 68 (54 percent) of 126 patients with ischemic heart disease and angiographically demonstrated narrowed coronary arteries had an abnormal lipoprotein pattern.[40] Among the 126 patients with angiographically demonstrated narrowed coronary arteries, 36 had a type II and 32 a type IV pattern.

Type V: Although nearly 50 patients with a familial type V pattern have been studied clinically by us,[4] none have died. Morphologic cardiovascular data in other patients with a type V pattern also are lacking. This complex lipoprotein abnormality has only recently been separated from other examples of familial hyperlipemia. In retrospect, the patient reported by Martt and Connor[41] in 1956 may have had a type V disorder. Their patient died at age 39 years of a second acute myocardial infarction which was preceded by angina pectoris. At necropsy, each of the 3 major coronary arteries was severely narrowed by complicated plaques. Of 10 patients with "essential hyperlipemia" ("chylomicrons and increased beta peak on lipoprotein electrophoresis") studied clinically by Malmros et al.[42] in 1954, 6 had angina pectoris, and 3 of these had had acute myocardial infarcts.

Foam cells in various lipoprotein types: Foam cells occur in the spleen, bone marrow, lymph nodes and liver of patients with hypertriglyceridemia. In our experience, they have been observed in hematoxylin-eosin stained tissue sections only in patients with type I, III, and V and not in those with type II and IV patterns.[9] This may be because triglyceride levels are usually higher in type I, III and V disorders, but it may also be that chylomicrons provoke a greater foam cell reaction than very low-density lipoproteins (VLDL) at a given triglyceride level. Hepatomegaly and splenomegaly may accompany extensive infiltration of organs by foam cells.

The foam cells in type I, III and V patterns appear similar by examination of hematoxylin-eosin stained sections.[43] They are macrophages (as shown by their high content of acid phosphatase and esterase), and at least in types I and III they also contain ceroid (identified on the basis of its autofluorescence, acid-fastness, sudanophilia, positivity to periodic acid-Schiff and insolubility in organic solvents).[43] The foam cells in type V seem to lack the birefringence seen in those in patients with type I and III disorders.

Although macrophages in normal spleen, lymph node and bone marrow may contain autofluorescent granules, the large foam cells observed in type I, III and V hyperlipoproteinemia have not been observed in patients with a type II or IV disorder or in those with a normal lipoprotein pattern. However, a few scattered, small, weakly autofluorescent cells may be observed in these organs in patients with a type II or IV pattern and in those with a normal lipoprotein pattern.

References

1. **Fredrickson DS, Lees RS:** A system for phenotyping hyperlipoproteinemia. Circulation 31:321–327, 1965
2. **Lees RS, Hatch FT:** Sharper separation of lipoprotein species by paper electrophoresis in albumin-containing buffer. J Lab Clin Med 61:518–528, 1963
3. **Fredrickson DS, Levy RI, Lees RS:** Fat transport in lipoproteins—an integrated approach to mechanisms and disorders. N Eng J Med 276:32–44, 94–103, 148–156, 215–226, 273–281, 1967
4. **Fredrickson DS, Levy RI:** Familial hyperlipoproteinemia. In, The Metabolic Basis of Inherited Disease, third edition (Stanbury JB, Wyngaarden JB, Fredrickson DS, ed). New York, McGraw-Hill, 1972, p 554–614
5. **Masket BH, Levy RI, Fredrickson DS:** The use of polyacrylamide gel electrophoresis in differentiating type III hyperlipoproteinemia. J Clin Lab Med, in press
6. **Roberts WC:** Examining the precordium and the heart. Chest 57:567–571, 1970
7. **Roberts WC, Buja LM:** The frequency and significance of coronary arterial thrombi and other observations in fatal acute myocardial infarction. A study of 107 necropsy patients. Amer J Med 52:425–443, 1972
8. **Quarfordt SH, DeVivo DC, Engel WK, et al:** Familial adult-onset proximal spinal muscular atrophy. Report of a family with type II hyperlipoproteinemia. Arch Neurol 22:541–549, 1970
9. **Roberts WC, Levy RI, Fredrickson DS:** Hyperlipoproteinemia. A review of the five types with first report of necropsy findings in type 3. Arch Path (Chicago) 90:46–56, 1970
10. **Sloan HR, Fredrickson DS:** Rare familial diseases with neutral lipid storage: Wolman's disease, cholesteryl ester storage disease, and cerebrotendinous xanthomatosis. In Ref 4, p 817–824
11. **Hollmon JL, Wasserman AJ:** Autopsy findings in type 3 hyperlipoproteinemia. Arch Path 92:415–417, 1971
12. **Epstein FH, Block WD, Hand EA, et al:** Familial hypercholesterolemia, xanthomatosis and coronary heart disease. Amer J Med 26:39–53, 1959
13. **Harlan WR Jr, Graham JB, Estes EH:** Familial hypercholesterolemia: a genetic and metabolic study. Medicine 45:77–110, 1966
14. **Jensen J, Blakenhorn DH, Kornerup V:** Coronary disease in familial hypercholesterolemia. Circulation 36:77–82, 1967
15. **Hould F, Leclerc R, Marcoux J:** Essential familial hypercholesterolemia with xanthomatosis. Pediatrics 43:455–459, 1969
16. **Slack J:** Risks of ischaemic heart-disease in familial hyperlipoproteinaemic states. Lancet 2:1380–1382, 1969.
17. **deGennes J-L, Rouffy J, Chain F:** Complications vasculaires cérébrales des xanthomatoses tendineuses hypercholestérolémiques familiales. Soc Med Hop Paris 119:569–575, 1968
18. **Cook CD, Smith HL, Geisen CW, et al:** Xanthoma tuberosum, aortic stenosis, coronary sclerosis, and angina pectoris: report of a case in a boy 13 years of age. Amer J Dis Child 73:326–333, 1947
19. **Rigdon RH, Willeford G:** Sudden death during childhood with xanthoma tuberosum: review of literature and report of a case. JAMA 142:1268–1271, 1950
20. **Barr DP, Rothbard S, Eder HA:** Atherosclerosis and aortic stenosis in hypercholesteremic xanthomatosis. JAMA 156:943–947, 1954
21. **Boas EP, Elster SK, Adlersberg D:** Calcific aortic stenosis: study of serum cholesterol with observations on calcific aortic stenosis in familial xanthomatosis and hypercholesteremia. Amer Heart J 48:485–496, 1954
22. **Harris-Jones JN, Jones EG, Wells PG:** Xanthomatosis and essential hypercholesterolaemia. Lancet 1:855–857, 1957
23. **Maher JA, Epstein FH, Hand EA:** Xanthomatosis and coronary heart disease: necropsy studies of two affected siblings. Arch Intern Med 102:437–442, 1958
24. **Khachadurian AK:** The inheritance of essential familial hypercholesterolemia. Amer J Med 37:402–407, 1964
25. **Stanley P, Chartrand C, Davignon A:** Acquired aortic stenosis in a twelve-year-old girl with xanthomatosis. Successful surgical correction. New Eng J Med 273:1378–1380, 1965
26. **Kumbhani AP, Daftary VG, Yawalkar SJ, et al:** Xanthomatous aortic stenosis in familial hypercholesterolaemia. Indian Heart J 19:171–177, 1967
27. **Rothbard S, Hagstrom JWC, Smith JP:** Aortic stenosis and myocardial infarction in hypercholesterolemic xanthomatosis. Amer Heart J 73:687–692, 1967
28. **Miettinen M:** Familial hypercholesterolaemic xanthomatosis and coronary heart disease in a ten-year-old girl. Ann Paediat Fenn 13:35–38, 1967
29. **Buchwald H, Lee GB, Amplatz K, et al:** Severe atherosclerotic cardiovascular disease in a 14-year-old homozygous familial hypercholesterolemic. Minn Med 51:477–481, 1968
30. **Polano MK, Baes H, Lemmens HEF, et al:** Heredity in primary hyper-B-lipoproteinemia with concomitant xanthomata. Report on three kindreds with presumably six homozygotes. Acta Med Scand 188:397–401, 1970
31. **Watanabe T, Tanaka K, Yanai N:** Essential familial hypercholesteremic xanthomatosis—an autopsy case with special reference to the pathogenesis of its cardiovascular lipidosis. Acta Path Jap 18:319–331, 1968
32. **Wennevold A, Jacobsen JG:** Acquired supravalvular aortic stenosis in familial hypercholesterolemia. A hemodynamic and angiographic study. Amer J Med 50:823–827, 1971
33. **Roberts WC:** The structure of the aortic valve in clinically isolated aortic stenosis. An autopsy study of 162 patients over 15 years of age. Circulation 42:91–17, 1970
34. **Roberts WC:** The congenitally bicuspid aortic valve. A study of 85 autopsy cases. Amer J Cardiol 26:72–83, 1970
35. **Roberts WC:** Anatomically isolated aortic valvular disease. The case against its being of rheumatic etiology. Amer J Med 49:151–159, 1970

36. **Roberts WC, Perloff JK, Constantino T:** Severe valvular aortic stenosis in patients over 65 years of age. A clinicopathologic study. Amer J Cardiol 27:497–506, 1971
37. **Clarkson TB, Lofland HB Jr, Bullock BC, et al:** Genetic control of plasma cholesterol. Studies on squirrel monkeys. Arch Path (Chicago) 92:37–45, 1971
38. **Zelis R, Mason DT, Braunwald E, et al:** Effects of hyperlipoproteinemias and their treatment on the peripheral circulation. J Clin Invest 49:1007–1015, 1970
39. **Brown DF:** Blood lipids and lipoproteins in atherogenesis. Amer J Med 46:691–704, 1969
40. **Heinle RA, Levy RI, Fredrickson DS, et al:** Lipid and carbohydrate abnormalities in patients with angiographically documented coronary artery disease. Amer J Cardiol 24:178–186, 1969
41. **Martt JM, Connor WE:** Idiopathic hyperlipemia associated with coronary atherosclerosis. Arch Intern Med 97:492–496, 1956
42. **Malmros H, Swahn B, Truedsson E:** Essential hyperlipaemia. Acta Med Scand 149:91–108, 1954
43. **Ferrans VJ, Buja LM, Roberts WC, et al:** The spleen in type I hyperlipoproteinemia. Histolochemical, biochemical, microfluoricetric and electron microscopic observations. Amer J Path 64:67–96, 1971

Pathologic Anatomy of Cardiac Valve Replacement: A Study of 224 Necropsy Patients

William C. Roberts, Bernadine H. Bulkley, and Andrew G. Morrow

DURING THE PAST 12 YR numerous reports have described the use of prostheses of various types to replace malfunctioning cardiac valves. Most valvular prostheses have been evaluated in terms of clinical and hemodynamic improvement, and less attention has been given to alterations observed at necropsy. This report focuses attention on findings at necropsy in 224 patients who died after replacement of one or more cardiac valves at the National Heart and Lung Institute from 1963 through October 1972.

PATIENTS STUDIED

The 224 patients were divided into two groups: (1) 128 patients dying within 2 mo of operation (early deaths), and (2) 96 patients dying at later periods up to 116 mo (late deaths). Not included among the 224 patients were three who died during operation before valve replacement could be carried out: One had cardiac arrest during thoracotomy and two had acute dissection of the entire aorta with compression-occlusion of the coronary arteries immediately after cardiopulmonary bypass was instituted. The cardiac valves replaced in the 224 patients are listed in Table 1.* All patients were in functional classes III or IV (New York Heart Association Classification) before operation. The ages and sexes of the patients are summarized in Table 2. Of the 224 patients, 141 (63%) were males and 83 (37%) were females; their ages ranged from 4–69 yr (average 46). The functional valve lesions necessitating valve replacement are summarized in Table

---

From the Section of Pathology and the Clinic of Surgery, National Heart and Lung Institute, National Institutes of Health, Bethesda, Md.

William C. Roberts, M.D.: *Chief, Section of Pathology, National Heart and Lung Institute, National Institutes of Health, Bethesda, Md.; Associate Professor of Pathology and Medicine (Cardiology), Georgetown University School of Medicine, Washington, D.C.* Bernadine H. Bulkley, M.D.: *Staff Associate, Section of Pathology, National Heart and Lung Institute, National Institutes of Health, Bethesda, Md.* Andrew G. Morrow, M.D.: *Chief, Clinic of Surgery, National Heart and Lung Institute, National Institutes of Health, Bethesda, Md.*

Reprint requests should be addressed to William C. Roberts, M.D., Building 10A, Room 3E-30, National Heart and Lung Institute, National Institutes of Health, Bethesda, Md. 20014.

*Tables 1–23 are compiled in the appendix at the end of this paper, pp. 575–585.

3. All 224 patients had undergone cardiac catheterization preoperatively. Of 281 valves replaced, stenosis of some degree occurred in 194 valves (69%), and the remaining 87 valves (31%) were purely incompetent. There was no correlation between the functional valve lesion and the incidence of early or late death. Most stenotic valves also were incompetent, and in some the predominant hemodynamic lesion was regurgitation rather than stenosis. All purely regurgitant valves had no pressure gradients across them.

The *etiology of the valvular lesions* was variable. Most patients undergoing isolated aortic valve replacement for either stenosis or pure regurgitation had nonrheumatic lesions:[1-3] Congenitally malformed valves, particularly the bicuspid condition, was the most common cause of isolated aortic stenosis. Of 29 patients undergoing valve replacement for isolated pure aortic regurgitation, the etiology was rheumatic in ten (each also had anatomic disease of the mitral valve), "cystic medial necrosis" of aorta in four (three had the Marfan syndrome), healed infective endocarditis in five (on congenitally malformed valves in three and on previously normally formed valves in two), congenitally bicuspid valve (never the site of infection) in one, prolapsed aortic cusp associated with ventricular septal defect in three, unknown in three, and syphilis, arteriosclerosis, and ankylosing spondylitis, one each. Combined mitral and aortic disease and combined mitral, aortic, and tricuspid disease was nearly always rheumatic in origin. Mitral stenosis was of rheumatic origin in all subjects. Sixteen of 17 patients in whom the tricuspid valve was replaced also had mitral stenosis; the seventeenth had tricuspid valve was replaced also had mitral stenosis; the seventeenth had tricuspid valve replacement only after he was unable to come off cardiac bypass after aortic valve replacement. Of the 24 patients undergoing replacement for isolated pure mitral regurgitation, the etiology was rheumatic or probably rheumatic in 12, congenital endocardial fibroelastosis in two, ruptured chordae tendineae on previously normal valves (secondary to healed infective endocarditis,[4]) in five, floppy mitral valve in one, cleft mitral valve associated with ostium primum defect in one, papillary muscle fibrosis secondary to coronary heart disease in one, hypertrophic (asymmetric) cardiomyopathy in one, and unknown in one. Both patients with primary muscle disease, hypertrophic cardiomyopathy or papillary muscle dysfunction, died early.

The 281 prosthetic valves used in the 224 patients are shown in Table 4. The sizes of the 250 Starr-Edwards prostheses employed are summarized in Table 5. There was no correlation between the size of the prosthetic valve utilized and the incidence of early or late death. In addition to one or more valve replacements in the 224 patients, valve annuloplasty or commissurotomy also was performed in 13 patients, 12 of whom died early. Four other patients, each of whom had pure aortic regurgitation had their ascending aortas replaced with grafts: Two died early and two died late; three had aortic "cystic medial necrosis," and the fourth had syphilis.

Accurate[5] weights of the hearts in the 224 patients are summarized in Table 6. No significant difference was noted between the weights of hearts of those patients dying early and those dying late when corresponding sexes and similarly replaced valves were compared.

Significant extramural coronary arterial luminal narrowing occurred in 36 (16%) of the 224 patients (Table 7). At least one of the three major extramural coronary arteries (right, anterior descending and left circumflex) was narrowed > 75% by old plaques in each of the 36 patients. The per cent of patients with this degree of narrowing in both early and late death groups were similar: 15% in the former and 18% in the latter. The average age of these 36 patients was 52 yr; 30 were men and six were women. Only one was < 40 yr of age, and he was a 26-yr-old man who had coronary arterial narrowing secondary to an embolus dislodged from vegetations on the aortic valve; the embolus subsequently organized. Only 10 of the 36 patients with severe coronary arterial luminal narrowing by old lesions had healed transmural infarcts; nine others had subendocardial free wall scars.

Embolic material was found in *intramural coronary arteries* on histologic sections* in 12 of 128 patients (9%) dying early and in 9 of 96 patients (9%) dying late after valve replacement. The embolic material consisted of *calcium* in seven patients, *foreign particle* (refractile anisotropic material), probably silicone,[6] in seven, *fibrin-platelets* in five, both calcium and foreign particle in one, and *bone marrow* in one. Excision of the cardiac valves *intact* at operation may lower the frequency of calcific emboli.[7] The most common site of emboli to intramural coronary arteries was left ventricular papillary muscle. The myocardium adjacent to the occluded artery often was focally necrotic or fibrotic.

Aschoff bodies were observed on histologic section in only two of the 224 patients. Each died early and each had anatomic disease of both mitral and aortic valves.

Various findings in patients dying early are illustrated in Figs. 1–19 and in those dying late, in Figs. 20–40.

ANALYSIS OF THE EARLY POSTOPERATIVE DEATHS

The intervals between operation and death (prosthetic valve implantation periods) in the 128 patients dying within 2 mo of operation are summarized in Table 8. Seventy-eight patients (61%) died within 1 wk, and 93 of the 128 patients (72%), within 2 wk of operation. The prime causes of death (one principal cause per patient) are shown in Table 9. The per cent of patients dying from *prosthetic dysfunction* was 28%. In the early experience with cardiac valve replacement with rigid frame prostheses, relatively large-sized prostheses were employed, and not infrequently the prostheses utilized were too large for either the left ventricle or aortic root into which they were inserted[8–12] (Figs. 1–4). The motion of the poppets in these circumstances was limited. Beginning about 1965, efforts were made to use smaller protheses, and the mortality rate, particularly after mitral replacement, dropped. With the introduction of Starr-Edwards prostheses with fully cloth-covered struts and bases in 1967, (models 6300 and 2300), it became apparent[13,14] that the smaller mitral and aortic prostheses were inherently stenotic, and that stenosis probably worsened as tissue grew into the cloth bordering the orifice and also into the struts. By late 1968 the manufacturer had widened the orifice areas of these prostheses (models 6310 and 2310). Prosthetic

*A total of 1310 histologic sections of myocardium were reexamined in the 224 patients. This averaged 5.9 sections of heart in each patient. In most patients at least one section from the wall of each cardiac chamber was examined; in all patients at least one section of left ventricular wall was studied.

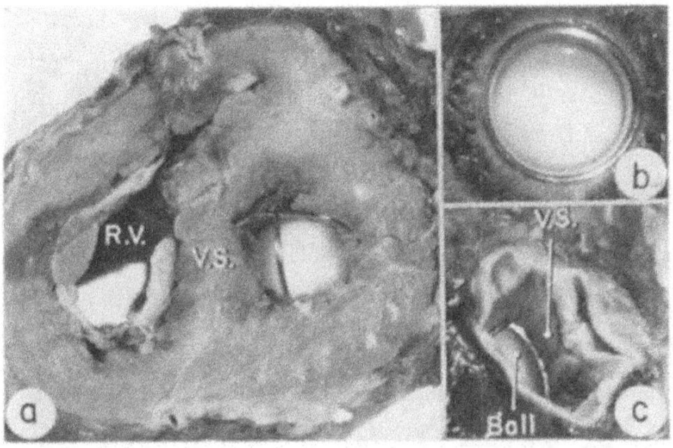

Fig. 1. Prosthetic dysfunction. Heart (weight = 360 g) of a cachectic, functionally class IV, 57-yr-old man with severe mitral stenosis preoperatively. Following replacement of mitral valve with size 3M Starr-Edwards prosthesis, patient was unable to come off cardiopulmonary bypass and died in operating room. At autopsy (A65-170), the mitral prosthesis was shown after transverse sectioning of ventricles (A) to be too large for left ventricular cavity. Ventricular septum (V.S.) protruded into mitral cage almost totally blocking motion of ball. In this patient there also appeared to be obstruction to left ventricular emptying. With the mitral ball in the closed position simulating ventricular systole (B), the photograph in C was taken. Following excision of the three aortic valve cusps, the mitral ball is seen almost to contact the muscular ventricular septum and obstruct the outflow tract. (By permission.[12])

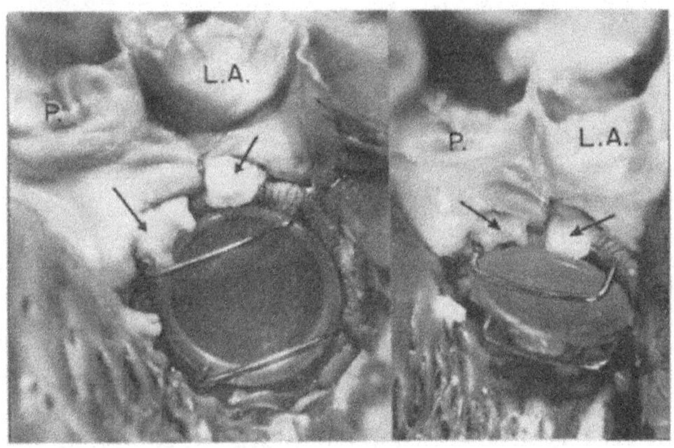

Fig. 2. Prosthetic dysfunction. Opened left ventricle and aortic valve in a 51-yr-old woman in whom the stenotic mitral valve was replaced with Kay-Shiley disc prosthesis. Her 3-day postoperative period was characterized by features of low cardiac output syndrome. At necropsy (A70-200), two fragments (arrows) of unexcised anterior mitral leaflet prevented complete seating of disc during ventricular systole. Regurgitation, therefore, must have occurred, and this mechanical interference appears to be prime explanation for low cardiac output syndrome postoperatively. P. and L.A., posterior (non-coronary) and left anterior aortic valve cusps.

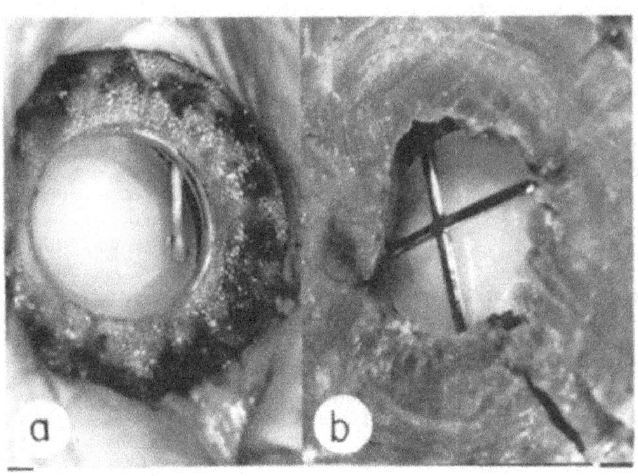

Fig. 3. Prosthetic dysfunction. Starr-Edwards mitral prostheses (model 6520, size 3M) implanted in this 38-yr-old man (A72-47) 48 hr before death. (A) Mitral valve as viewed from left atrium. A small chorda tendinea not excised at operation protrudes between disc and metallic base, causing incomplete closure. (B) Same valve viewed from left ventricle. Margins of the disc contact endocardium of left ventricle at most points. Death in this patient appears to be related to the prosthesis being too large for the left ventricle, causing obstruction to left atrial emptying.

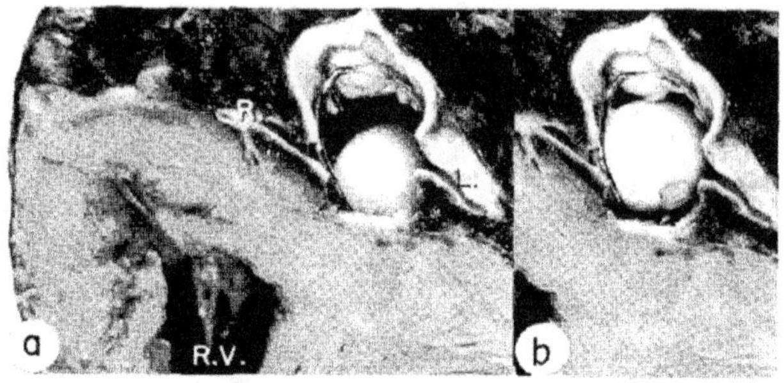

Fig. 4. Prosthetic dysfunction. Opened aortic valve in a 25-yr-old man (A65-133) with congenitally malformed mitral and aortic valves, causing severe mitral and aortic regurgitation and slight aortic stenosis. The aortic prosthesis, even though it is a small-sized one (8A Starr-Edwards), is too large for the aortic root. During simulated ventricular diastole (A) ball is seated, but during simulated ventricular systole (B) ball is prevented from ascending completely to apex of cage by wall of the aorta, which protrudes between two metallic struts, restricting ball movement in cage. A match head projects from the residual prosthetic orifice. R.V., right ventricle; R. and L., right and left coronary arteries.

dysfunction reappeared dramatically in mid-1970, however, when the manufacturer decreased the third-strut clearances (between the surface of the prosthetic aortic balls and the inner margins of the cloth-covered struts) from 0.040–0.070 to 0.008–0.020 inches (Figs. 5–8). Five deaths listed under "prosthetic dysfunction" in Table 9 resulted from this manufacturing error, which was corrected in late 1970. The current Starr-Edwards aortic valve (model 2320) has a third-strut clearance of 0.050–0.060 inches, except at its base, which has a smaller clearance. The cloth on this newer model also has been altered; polypropylene has been added to the Teflon on the struts and on the sewing ring. It is hoped that the polypropylene will decrease the frequency of strut cloth wear. The current Starr-Edwards mitral prosthesis (model 6320) has a uniform radial cage-to-ball clearance of 0.017–0.021 inches, and this clearance is maintained constant from base to dome. Polypropylene also has been added to its Teflon cloth. The metal struts have now been united at the domes of both new prostheses; in previous models the struts were held together at their domes only by cloth.

It is hazardous to implant a large-sized prosthesis into a relatively small-sized

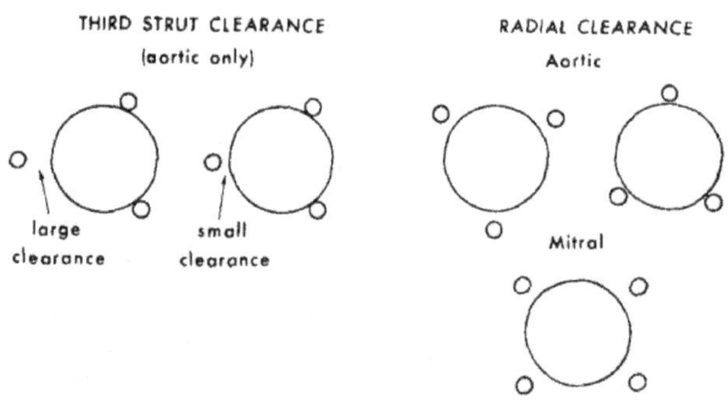

Fig. 5. Diagram to illustrate the concepts of third strut and radial clearance of caged-ball prostheses. With development of cloth-covered aortic prostheses, it was believed that large ball-to-cage third-strut clearance (distance between the surface of the prosthetic aortic ball and inner margin of strut) of earlier models would allow excessive lateral motion of ball and lead to cloth wear and chattering of metal ball within cage. Hence, to "guide" the poppet, the third-strut clearance of the model 2310 aortic prosthesis was decreased from 0.04–0.07 to 0.008–0.02 in. Growth of tissue over the cloth of the strut reduced third-strut clearance even further, causing the ball to stick in the mid-portion of the cage. In the model 2320, third-strut clearance was increased to 0.05–0.06 in, except at the base, where close-clearance was initially retained. Radial-cage-to-ball clearance of mitral valve also was decreased in some model 6310 cloth-covered prostheses, but current model 6320 has uniform radial-cage-to-ball clearance of 0.017–0.021 in.

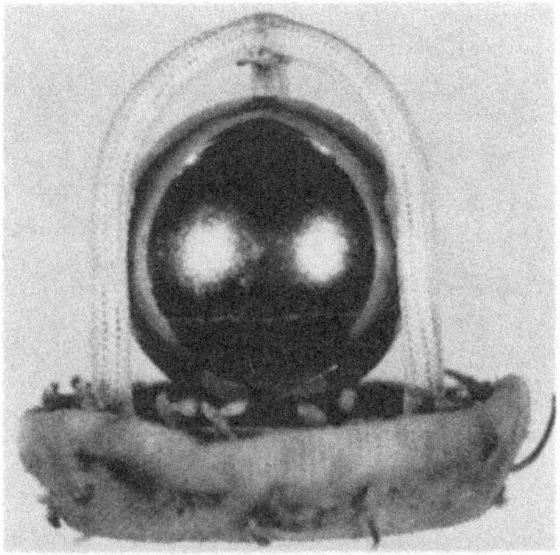

Fig. 6. Prosthetic dysfunction from close-clearance Starr-Edwards aortic prostheses, Aortic prosthesis (size 10A) in which the ball stuck in the mid-portion of cage. This 45-yr-old man died suddenly five days postoperatively. At necropsy (A70-227), ball was immobile as shown and a small thrombus was present on inner aspects of each of the three struts about midway between base and apex. The clearance between the surface of the ball and one strut when ball was pushed against the other two struts (so-called third-strut clearance) was only 4 mils when this prosthesis was manufactured.

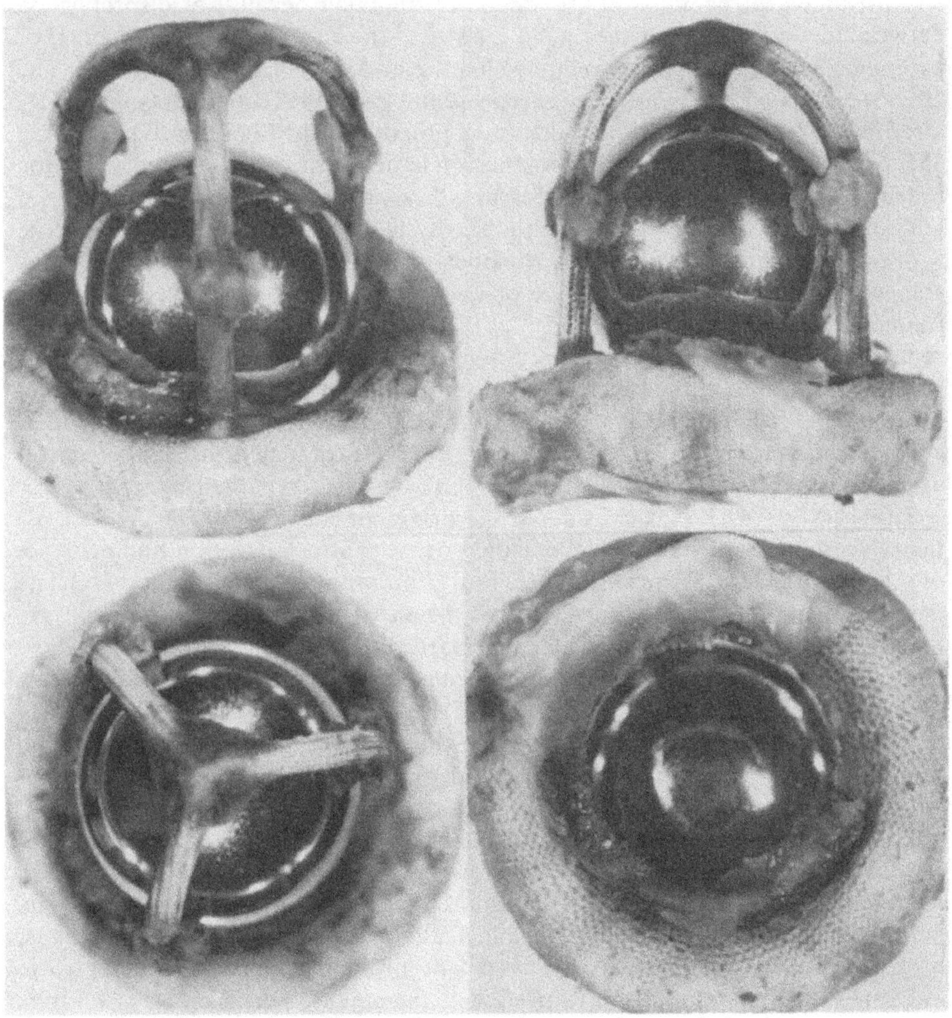

Fig. 7. Prosthetic stenosis due to thrombi on close-clearance Starr-Edwards aortic valve. This 29-yr-old man (A71-197) died suddenly 12 mo after replacement with a close-clearance Starr-Edwards cloth-covered aortic prosthesis (site 11A, Model 2310). Thrombi formed near junctions of the vertical and curved portions of strut, causing ball to stick in mid-position. He developed these prosthetic thrombi and renal embolism despite warfarin therapy.

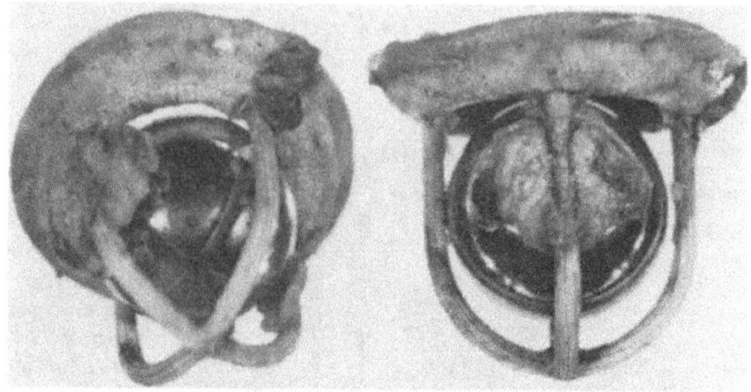

Fig. 8. Mitral prosthesis (size 3M) that developed thrombi on three of the four struts, causing immobility of the ball. This 56-yr-old man (A70-244) died 20 days postoperatively as a result of the ball's sticking. The exact clearance between the surface of the ball and the inner margins of the struts in this four-strut prosthesis is uncertain, but it is reduced. Thrombi *on mid-struts* unassociated with thrombi on bases of prostheses occur, in our experience, only in the close-clearance prosthesis manufactured in 1970.

left ventricle or ascending aorta. In 28 (Table 9) patients who died early, death was attributed at necropsy to prosthetic dysfunction because of disproportion between the size of the prosthesis and the size of the left ventricle (20 patients) or ascending aorta (eight patients) into which the prosthesis had been inserted. The 20 dysfunctioning mitral prostheses represent 24% of the 83 patients dying early after mitral replacement with rigid-framed prostheses. In 12 of the 20 patients, a 3M- or 4M-sized Starr-Edwards prosthesis had been utilized to replace a stenotic mitral valve. (The 3M Starr-Edwards prosthesis is too large for a normal-sized left ventricular cavity, and because this cavity is often of normal size in patients with isolated mitral stenosis, this prosthesis may be too large in this circumstance.) Disproportion between size of cavity and size of prosthesis was a less frequent cause of death among patients with aortic valve prostheses, representing 12% of 65 early deaths. Small-sized (7A, 8A or 2M) Starr-Edwards prostheses were used, however, in eight patients, and Kay-Shiley prostheses in two patients with prosthetic stenosis. Thus, it appears that some left ventricles and aortas are simply not large enough for rigid-framed prostheses. Central orifice prostheses are presently preferred in these selected patients.

Table 10 lists what was considered the principal cause of death in each patient. Nearly all patients dying several days or more after operation had evidence of "hepatic failure," "renal failure," or "pulmonary insufficiency." These manifestations do not represent failure of the particular organ, however, but are manifestations of that organ's inadequate arterial perfusion because of cardiac pump failure from known or unknown causes. With the exception of a few patients dying suddenly, presumably from arrhythmias, most patients dying early from the causes listed in Table 10 had evidence of *inadequate cardiac output* sometime in the postoperative period. Inadequate arterial perfusion to the lungs is usually manifested by *alveolar hemorrhage,*[15] (Fig. 19) and acute pneumonia is often superimposed. Inadequate arterial perfusion of the *liver* leads to *centrolobular hemorrhage, with or without necrosis* (Fig. 19), an anatomic picture identical to acute hepatic venous congestion. Inadequate arterial perfusion of the *kidneys* usually does not lead to histologically visible anatomic renal changes, probably because oliguria or anuria is not prolonged. True *hemoglobinuric nephrosis* (tubular necrosis) was infrequent. Inadequate perfusion of bowel may cause mucosal and submucosal hemorrhages (Fig. 19). Focal *left ventricular subendocardial and papillary muscle necrosis* (Fig. 19) occurred in many patients

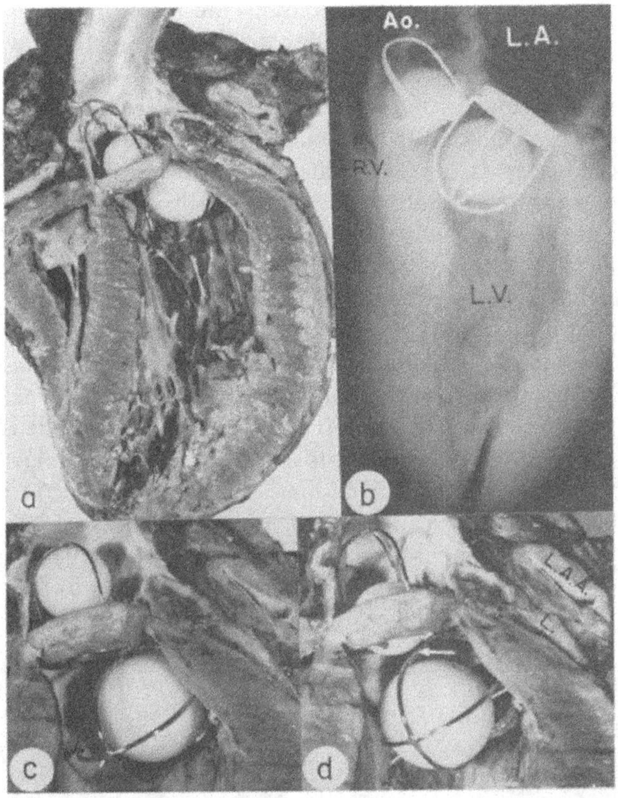

Fig. 9. Prosthetic dysfunction from contact of two prostheses. This 45-yr-old man underwent mitral and aortic valve replacement with Starr-Edwards prostheses for severe mitral and aortic regurgitation. After both valves had been inserted, there was evidence of regurgitation through or around the aortic prosthesis. A blowing diastolic murmur was audible along left sternal border postoperatively. Four days after the initial operation, thoracotomy was performed because of possibility of atrial thrombosis. No thrombus was found after left atriotomy, but there was massive regurgitation of blood from aorta into left ventricle. Refractory cardiac arrest occurred during procedure. Necropsy (A65-121) disclosed that both prostheses were securely sutured, and no peribasilar communications were present. The aortic regurgitation resulted from incomplete seating of the ball of the aortic prosthesis, which contacted one of the metallic struts of the mitral prosthesis during ventricular diastole. (A) Longitudinal section of the cardiac ventricles and aorta; (B) radiograph of the heart, again demonstrating the close proximity of the two prostheses to one another; (C and D) close-up views of the left ventricular outflow tract during simulated ventricular systole (C) and diastole (D). Arrow points to metallic strut of mitral cage, which contacted the aortic ball during ventricular diastole. Pressure in the aorta at beginning of ventricular diastole not only returned ball toward its seating position but, almost certainly, also caused movement of entire aortic prosthesis toward the left ventricle. Consequently, the aortic ball was prevented from seating by the mitral strut and aortic regurgitation resulted. Ao., aorta; R.V., right ventricle; L.V., left ventricle; L.A., left atrium; L.A.A., left atrial appendage; and L., left coronary artery. (By permission.[11])

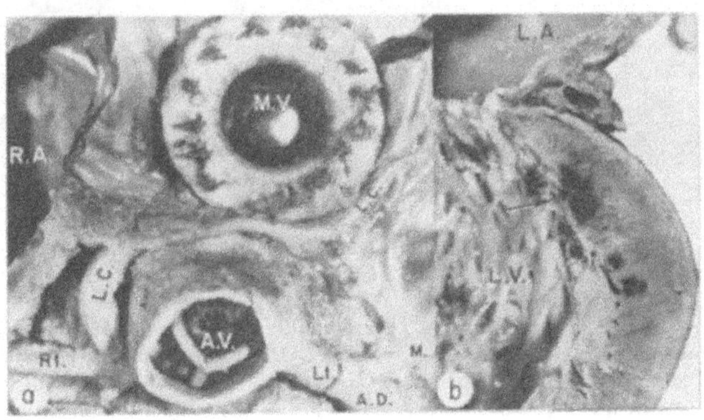

Fig. 10. Prosthetic dysfunction from compression of anomalous left circumflex (L.C.) coronary artery by rings of mitral (size 3M) (M.V.) and aortic (size 8A) (A.V.) Starr-Edwards prostheses. This 45-yr-old man with severe mitral and aortic regurgitation underwent double valve replacement 10 days before death. The entire postoperative period was characterized by features of low cardiac output syndrome. At necropsy (A68-22), the left circumflex (L.C.) coronary artery was found to arise from first portion of the right (Rt.) coronary artery and to course in groove between aortic root and base of the left atrium (L.A.) (A). This anomalously arising artery was compressed between rings of the two rigid-frame caged-ball prostheses. As a result, the lumen of the left circumflex coronary artery was occluded by this external compression leading to necrosis of the lateral wall of the left ventricle (L.V.) (B). R.A., right atrium; Lt., left main coronary artery; A.D., anterior descending coronary artery; and M., marginal coronary artery. (By permission.[9])

with the low cardiac output syndrome (Table 11). This necrosis may be simply the anatomic consequence of poor myocardial oxygenation, the result of inadequate coronary perfusion, although others[16–18] consider it the cause of the low cardiac output syndrome. Subendocardial and papillary muscle necrosis, in our view, is infrequently the cause of the low cardiac output syndrome, because it was seen as frequently in subjects having known anatomic causes of death, e.g., prosthetic dysfunction or bleeding, or associated uncorrected valve disease, etc. (see Table 8 or 10) as in those without an anatomic cause of death.

Focal myocardial necrosis of the *stumps of the amputated left ventricular* or right ventricular papillary muscles is to be expected after mitral and tricuspid valve replacements, respectively. The only exceptions occurred in patients dying very early (usually in the operating room) or who survived long enough for healing to occur. Also, nearly all patients had a drain inserted into the left ventricular cavity from its apex at operation. Consequently, nearly all patients dying early had transmural necrosis at the apex of the left ventricle, or, if they died late, transmural fibrosis, at this site. Necrosis or fibrosis at the left ventricular apex, therefore, was not included in the tabulations shown in Table 11. *Contraction bands*[19] appear to be the earliest lesion of myocardial necrosis in these patients. Calcification of individual necrotic myocardial fibers (Fig. 17) occurred in 12 patients. The cause of this *myocardial dystrophic calcification* is uncertain, but it probably results from myocardial ischemia because a similar lesion

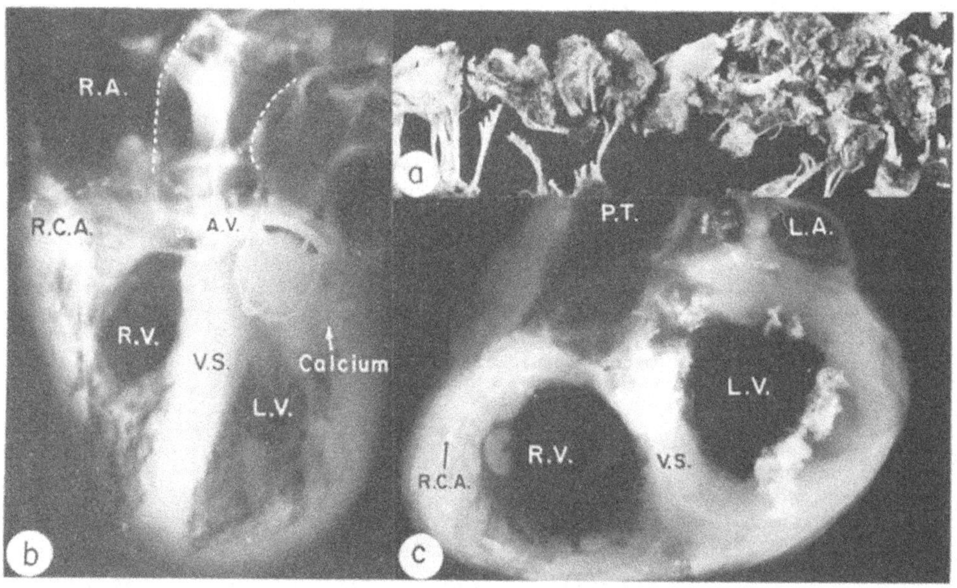

Fig. 11. Cerebral embolus after replacement of an extremely calcified, stenotic, and incompetent mitral valve, a complication of removing too little cardiac calcium. This 51-yr-old man (A66-150) never awakened postoperatively, and roentgenograms of the skull suggested a calcific embolus in the right middle cerebral artery; the embolus was found at necropsy 5 days after operation. Mitral valve was excised in numerous fragments (A), and presumably at least one escaped into the systemic circulation. (B) Radiograph shows considerable residual calcium in the mitral anulus and adjacent left ventricular myocardium, as well as in the aortic valve (A.V.) and right coronary artery (R.C.A.). The prosthesis is size 3M. (C) Radiograph of cephalad portions of cardiac ventricles and of both atria and great vessels. Amount of mitral calcific deposits remaining is very large. (By permission.[8])

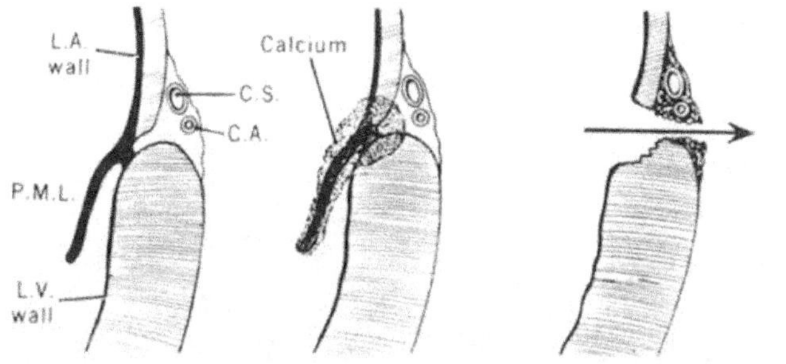

Fig. 12. Rupture of the heart at the left atrioventricular sulcus, a complication of removing too much mitral valvular calcium. If mitral leaflet calcium extends into the anulus, the surgeon will be unable to remove the deposit completely. If all mitral anular calcium is removed, as attempted in one patient, the left atrial wall may be separated from the left ventricular wall with massive bleeding. This diagram also depicts how the left atrial (L.A.) myocardium normally is totally separated from the left ventricular (L.V.) wall. The posterior mitral leaflet (P.M.L.) is formed by the junction of endocardium from the left atrium and left ventricle. C.S., coronary sinus; C.A., coronary artery.

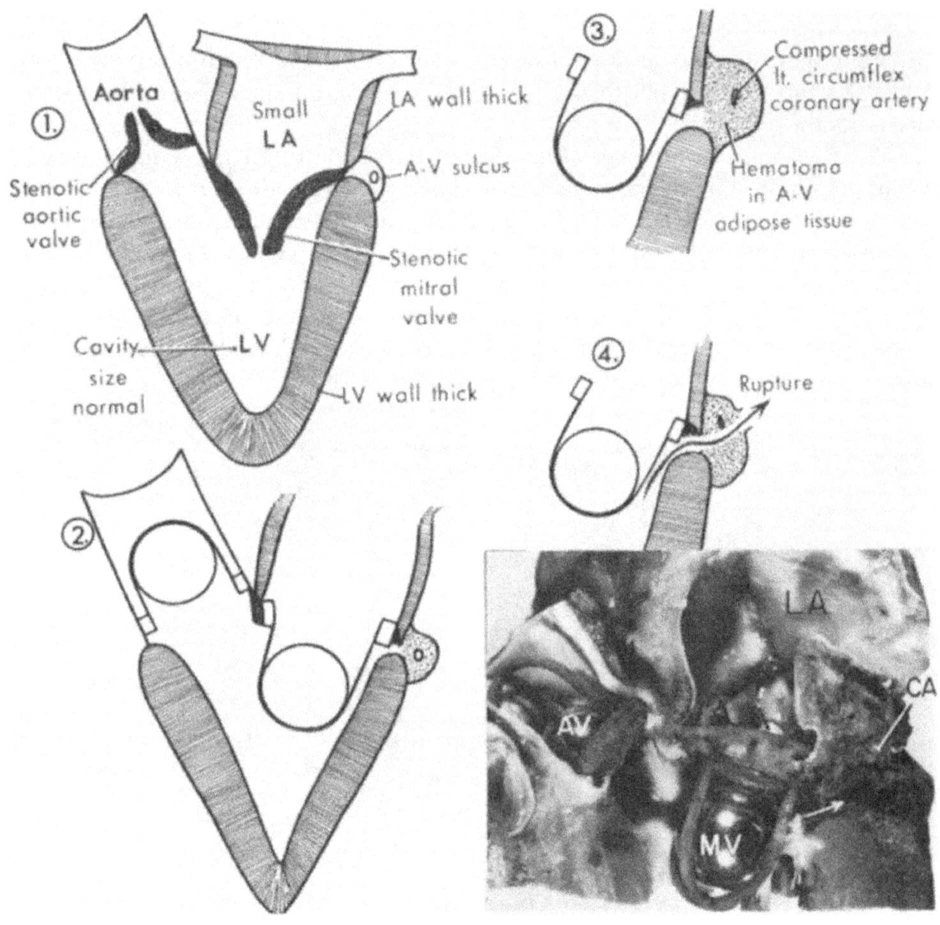

Fig. 13. Rupture of left atrioventricular (AV) sulcus during excision of mitral valve in a 57-yr-old woman (A72-124) with combined mitral and aortic stenosis. She died of "low cardiac output syndrome" 2 days after replacement of both valves (9A and 2M Starr-Edwards prostheses). The normal size of the left atrium prevented good exposure of the mitral valve from the interatrial groove incision and a portion of anulus was excised during excision of the valve leading to disruption of the left AV sulcus.

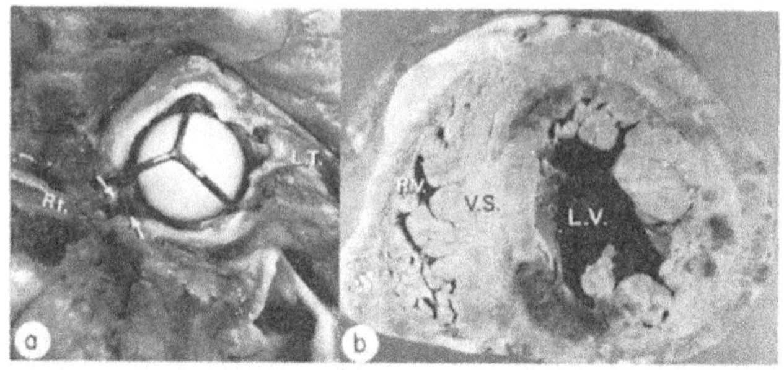

Fig. 14. Thrombotic occlusion of the proximal right coronary artery after replacement of mitral (size 2M) and aortic (size 8A) valves with Starr-Edwards prostheses. This patient's entire 6-day postoperative period was characterized by features of the low *cardiac output syndrome*. At necropsy (A67-207), a thrombus (between the arrows) was present in the mouth of the right (Rt.) coronary artery, having extended cephalad from the base of the prosthetic aortic valve (A). Several foci of necrosis were present in the left ventricular (L.V.) wall, and the largest one was in the posteroseptal wall (B). Many necrotic myocardial fibers were calcified (see Fig. 17). Lt., left coronary artery; R.V., right ventricle; and V.S., ventricular septum.

can be produced in myocardium of dogs by anoxia.[20] Determinations postoperatively of serum calcium, phosphorus, and magnesium in four of these 12 patients were normal.

Intramyocardial hemorrhage (Fig. 18) occurred in all patients dying within 7 days of operation. Intramyocardial hemorrhage occurred adjacent to all incisions in the walls of cardiac chambers. In all subjects in whom the atrium was entered via a dissection into the interatrial groove, bleeding of considerable extent occurred in the atrial septum. The extravasated blood not infrequently extended caudally into the area of the atrioventricular (AV) node or bundle or both. Extravasated blood usually occurred in the area of the AV node or bundle after aortic valve replacement because of the proximity of the valve and the conduction

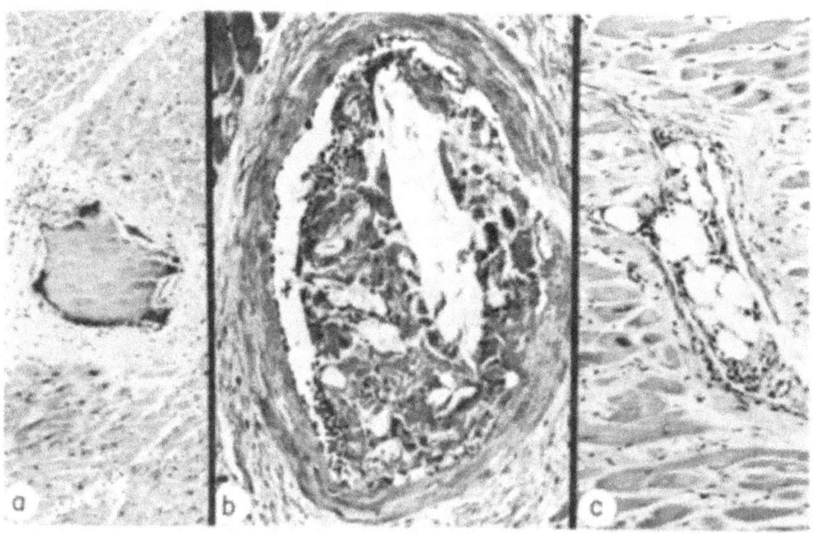

Fig. 15. Emboli to intramural coronary arteries. The emboli were of various types and probably most occurred at or shortly after valve replacement. (A) Calcific embolus in 60-yr-old woman (A64-225) in whom a heavily calcified, bicuspid, stenotic, aortic valve was replaced 20 mo earlier. (B) Foreign particle embolus in a 46-yr-old man (A69-33) in whom a heavily calcified predominantly incompetent mitral valve was excised 6 days before death. (C) Bone marrow embolus in a 41-yr-old man (A65-102) who underwent aortic valve replacement 7 days before death because of pure aortic regurgitation. Hematoxylin and eosin stains. (A) × 99, (B) × 250, (C) × 160.

tissue. Petechiae occurred also on endocardium and epicardium of nearly all patients dying early. Epicardial, myocardial, and endocardial hemorrhages were more frequent and extensive after cardiac massage.

ANALYSIS OF THE LATE POSTOPERATIVE DEATHS

The pertinent clinical and pathologic data in the 96 patients dying later than 2 mo after valve replacement are summarized in Tables 12 and 13.[21,22]

Causes of Death

These are listed (one principal cause per patient) in Table 13. *Forty patients died suddenly* and unexpectedly without preceding periods of congestive cardiac failure postoperatively. The aortic valve had been replaced in 30 of the 40 patients (six also had had mitral replacement), nine had had isolated mitral replacement, and one had had both mitral and tricuspid valves replaced. Either swelling and impaction (seven patients) or dislodgment (six patients) of aortic silicone rubber balls caused death in 13 patients. Five patients had coronary arterial emboli. No recent anatomic cardiac lesion was observed in the remaining 22 patients: Two of them, however, had severely narrowed coronary arterial ostia, and six others had severe (>75%) luminal narrowing by old plaques of one or more of the three major coronary arteries; two others had cloth-covered prosthetic aortic valves known to be moderately stenotic (50 mm Hg peak systolic pressure gradients), and one had a porcine valve known to be stenotic (35 mm Hg peak systolic gradient). The coronary arteries were free of luminal narrowing in the remaining 11 patients, but three had transmural left ventricular scars with aneurysm formation at sites of excision of left ventricular papillary muscles.

Forty-two patients died after periods of congestive cardiac failure. Five were not improved by operation, and their deaths are attributed to underlying cardiac disease. The other 37 patients were improved by operation, but heart failure

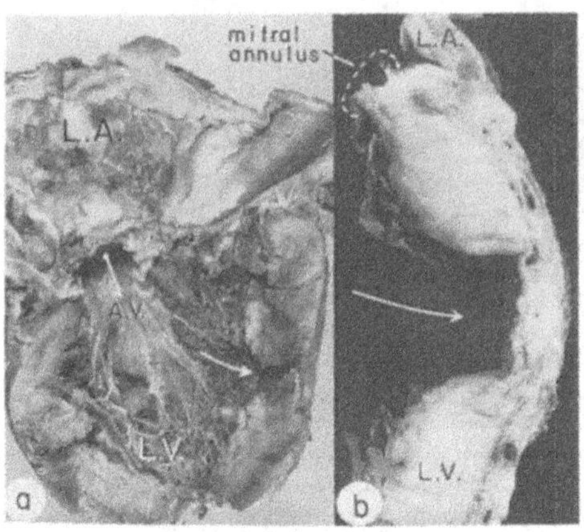

Fig. 16. Rupture and aneurysm formation at site of excision of left ventricular papillary muscles during or after mitral valve replacement. When the left ventricular papillary muscles are excised at operation, these structures are grasped with a clamp and pulled toward the left atrium. If they are pulled too vigorously before excision, a portion of the left ventricular free wall beneath the papillary muscles may also be excised. In both (A) and (B) too much left ventricular (L.V.) free wall beneath the papillary muscles (arrows) was excised, producing probable functional aneurysms in each. The 42-yr-old man (A64-147) whose heart is illustrated in (A) died 5 hr after mitral replacement. He had clinical features of the low cardiac output syndrome. The 58-yr-old woman (A68-14), a portion of whose heart is shown in (B), died suddenly of unknown cause 3 mo after mitral replacement. This is a gross longitudinal section of left atrial (L.A.) wall, mitral anulus, and left ventricular wall. Left ventricular wall beneath excised papillary muscle consisted entirely of fibrous tissue. A.V., aortic valve.

reappeared and progressed in each. Problems with the prosthetic valve accounted for death in 22 of the 37 patients: swelling with impaction of the aortic (seven patients) or mitral (one patient) silicone rubber poppets; infection at the site of attachment of the prosthesis (five patients); parabasilar prosthetic leaks (three); extensive secondary endocardial fibrosis of the left ventricle (two); prosthetic thrombosis (three); and obstruction of the prosthetic orifice due to faulty design and to overgrowth of tissue (one). In only four patients could death

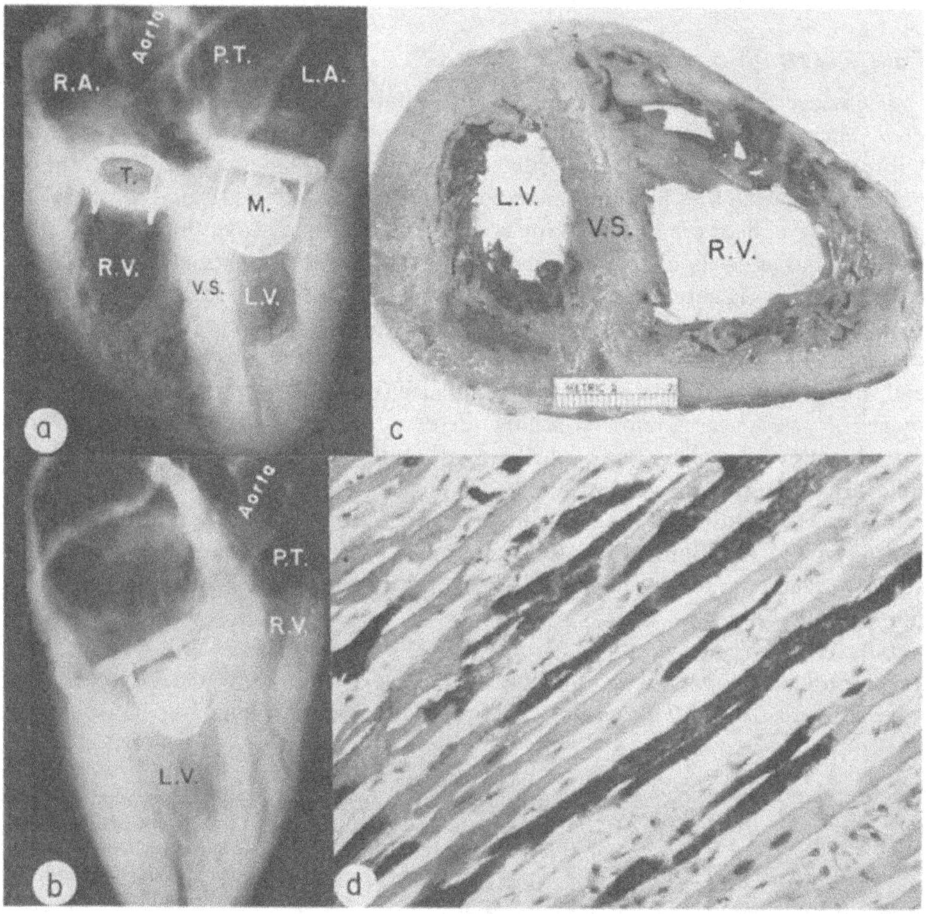

Fig. 17. Dystrophic calcification in cardiac and skeletal (pharyngeal) muscle fibers and in lung in a 46-yr-old woman who died 20 days after replacement of the mitral valve with a Starr-Edwards prosthesis (M.) and of the tricuspid valve with a Kay-Shiley prosthesis (T.). This patient's entire postoperative period was characterized by the low cardiac output syndrome. Radiographs of the excised heart at necropsy (A66-146) disclosed focal calcific deposits in the walls of both left (L.V.) and right (R.V.) ventricles (A and B). R.A., right atrium; L.A., left atrium; P.T., pulmonary trunk; and V.S., ventricular septum. A transverse section of cardiac ventricles (C) shows focal lesions in walls of both chambers. *Since the patient was severely jaundiced these myocardial lesions had a greenish color.* Histologic section of several myocardial lesions disclosed that they consisted of necrotic myocardial fibers, many of which contained calcific deposits (D). Hematoxylin and eosin stain. × 200. The cause of the focal calcific deposits in individual myocardial and skeletal muscle fibers and in alveolar septal walls and pulmonary arteries in the above patient is unknown. Determinations of serum calcium, phosphorus, and magnesium were made on 2 days during the week before operation and 5 days after operation; each was normal.

be attributed to myocardial fibrosis, in four others to associated uncorrected valve disease, and in seven the cause was never determined.

None of the remaining 14 patients had evidence of congestive cardiac failure postoperatively. They died of noncardiac causes (six patients), central nervous system catastrophies (seven patients), or hepatitis (one patient).[23]

Necropsy Observations

Prosthetic valve thrombi (Figs. 6–8, 14, 22). Thrombi were found on prosthetic valves at necropsy in 71 (80%) of the 96 patients dying later than 2 mo after operation, and 49 of them had received warfarin (Table 12). Of the 118 prosthetic valves utilized in these 96 patients, 81 (69%) had antemortum thrombi. In 21 (30%) of the 71 patients with thrombi, the thrombus appeared to have rendered the prosthesis incompetent, stenotic, or both, but in four of them the thrombus was infected. In the other 50 patients valve function was not impaired

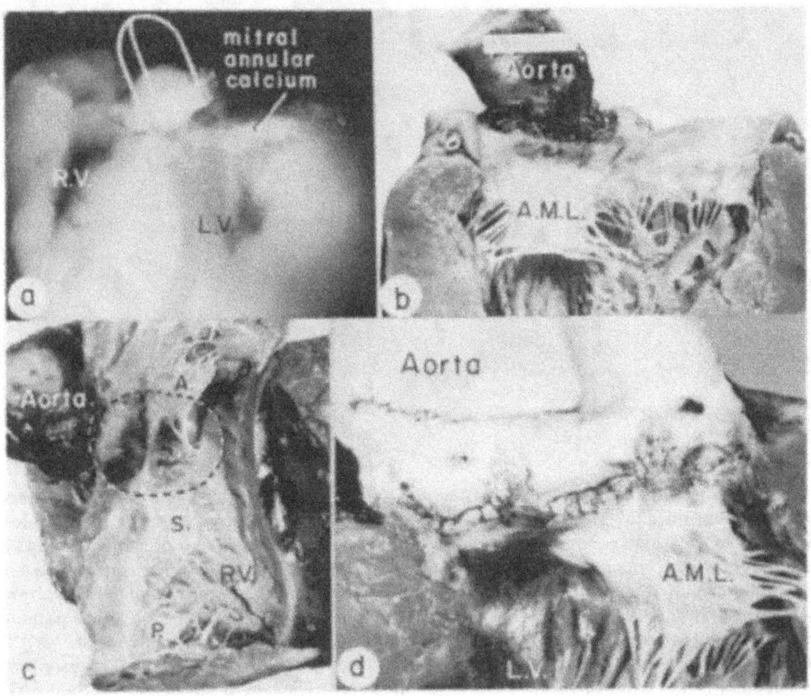

Fig. 18. Extensive myocardial and endocardial hemorrhages after aortic valve replacement. This 64-yr-old man had his stenotic aortic valve replaced with a size 9A Starr-Edwards prosthesis. During cardiopulmonary bypass he had progressive myocardial deterioration evidenced on electrocardiogram even though the coronary arteries were being perfused. Immediately after coming off cardiopulmonary bypass, the heart rate slowed and nodal rhythm was present. Ventricular fibrillation occurred several minutes later and he died. At necropsy (A66-109), radiograph of the specimen (A) disclosed extensive calcification of the mitral anulus, although the mitral leaflets and chordae tendineae were normal (B). The interstitial myocardium adjacent to the aortic root contained numerous extravasated erythrocytes. Their presence in the area of the atrioventricular node (C) (broken circle) and bundle (D), both of which are hemorrhagic, may have accounted for the severe bradycardia. Subendocardial hemorrhages in the left ventricular (L.V.) outflow tract are apparent. Entire membraneous ventricular septum is hemorrhagic. R.V., right ventricle; A.M.L., anterior mitral leaflet; and A., S., and P., anterior, septal and posterior tricuspid leaflets.

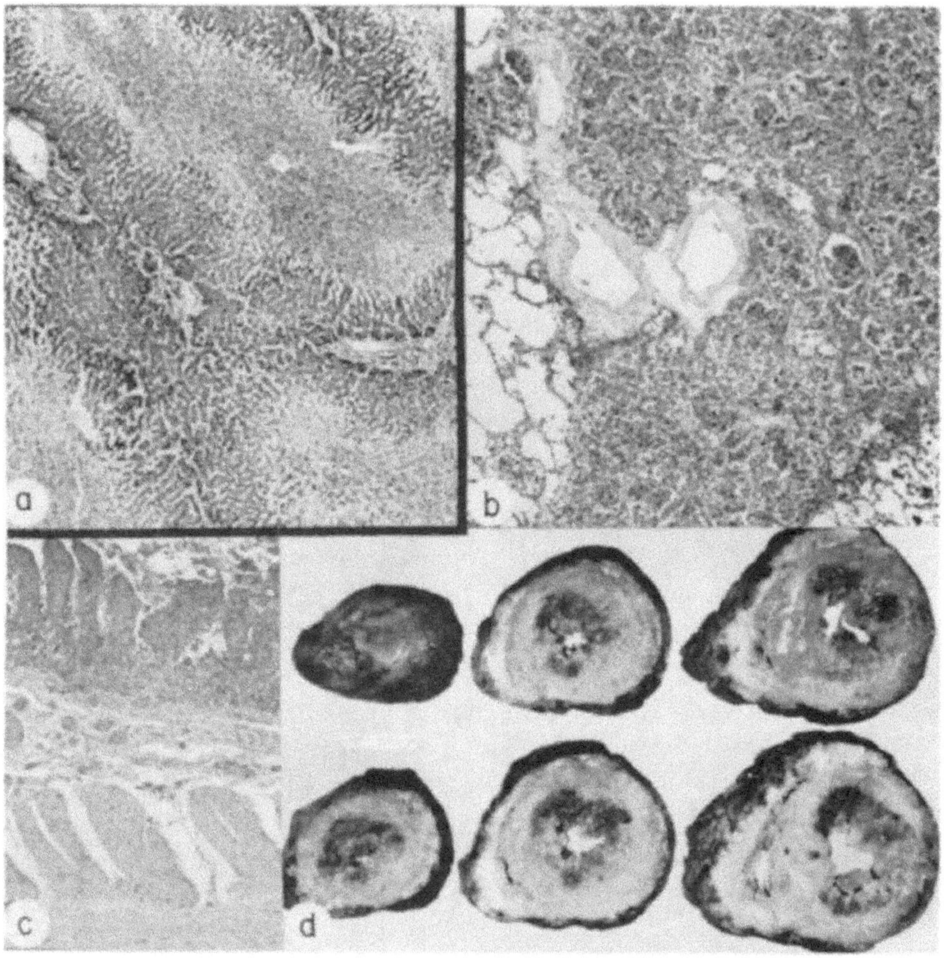

Fig. 19. Lesions in liver (A), lung (B), bowel (C), and heart (D) resulting from inadequate oxygenation of these organs after cardiac valve replacement. These lesions are the pathologic consequences of the low cardiac output syndrome. Inadequate arterial perfusion of the liver leads to centrolobular hemorrhage and necrosis (A), a lesion identical to that resulting from passive venous congestion of the liver. This 30-yr-old woman (A69-33) died 2 days after mitral valve replacement. The liver weighed 1640 g. (B) Pulmonary alveolar hemorrhage ("shock lung") in the same patient (A69-33). This lesion was more common than alveolar edema following valve replacement.[15] (C) Hemorrhage into the bowel mucosa occuring in a 31-yr-old man (A69-53) who died 6 days after mitral valve replacement. (D) Transverse sections of cardiac ventricles in a 57-yr-old woman (A72-124) who died 2 days after aortic and mitral valve replacement. Several foci of subendocardial necrosis are present in left ventricle. These foci of myocardial necrosis are considered consequences not causes of low cardiac output syndrome. Hematoxylin and eosin stains. × 40 (A, B and C).

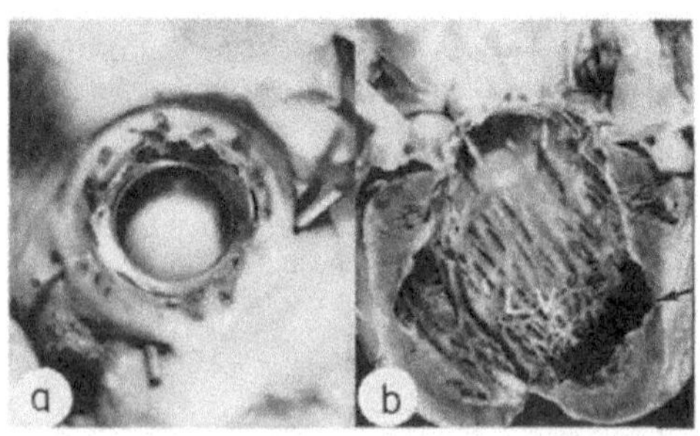

Fig. 20. *Prosthetic peribasilar communications.* (A) Mitral prosthesis implanted 6 mo earlier in a 47-yr-old man (A64-90). Small wooden sticks are inserted into each of the three peribasilar leaks. Small communications as shown here apparently may cause severe regurgitation during life. (B) Opened left atrium, mitral anulus and left ventricle (L.V.) in the same patient. Wooden sticks again designate the sites of the peribasilar leaks. Excessive left ventricular muscle (arrow) was excised when the papillary muscles were removed at the time of mitral replacement. This excessive removal of left ventricular wall probably resulted in a functional aneurysm during life. This patient died of severe congestive cardiac failure, but a murmur of mitral regurgitation was not audible postoperatively.

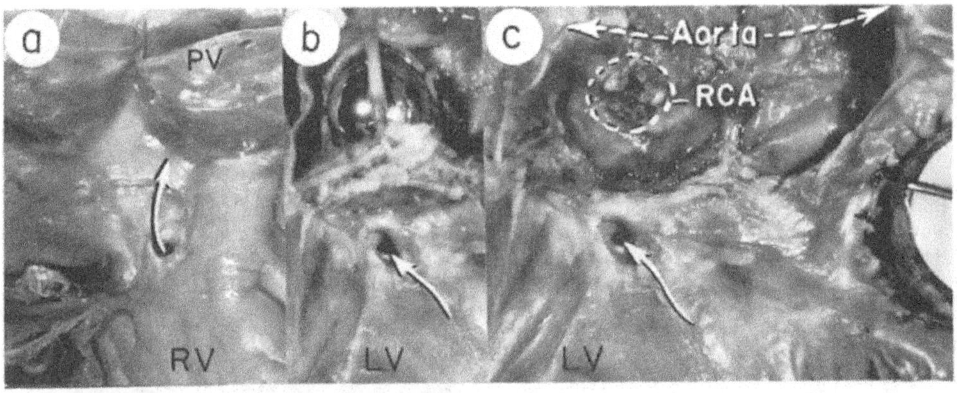

Fig. 21. Operatively induced ventricular septal defect during aortic valve replacement with Starr-Edwards prosthesis (size 10A, 2320) implanted 52 mo earlier in a 62-yr-old man (A72-36) who died of associated uncorrected valve disease. His aortic valve prosthesis apparently had functioned well. (A) Opened right ventricular (RV) outflow tract and pulmonic valve (PV) showing defect (arrow). (B) View of left ventricular (LV) outflow tract showing defect (arrow) just below base of aortic prosthesis. (C) View of left ventricle and ascending aorta after removal of aortic prostheses. Complete occlusion of ostium of right coronary artery (RCA) also was present.

by the thrombus. Although 71 patients had prosthetic thrombi at necropsy, only 16 (23% of those with thrombi; 18% of the total of 96 patients) had clinical evidence of systemic embolism during life. The thrombi on noncloth-covered struts typically were located at the junction of the prosthetic struts with the metallic rings, extending up the aortic struts and down the mitral struts for variable distances, occasionally completely covering the metallic rings. In the close-clearance aortic prostheses, however, thrombi formed in the mid-portion of the struts, sparing both apex and base (Figs. 6–8). In nonclose-clearance cloth-covered struts, thrombi formed initially at the apices, not at the bases (Fig. 22). Histologic study of several thrombi disclosed that they consisted mainly of fibrin and platelets and were devoid of bacteria or fungi, except in the subjects with documented septicemia.

Fistulae around prosthetic valve rings (Fig. 20). Peribasilar communications occurred in 11 patients (11%) (excluding those with infective endocarditis). Five

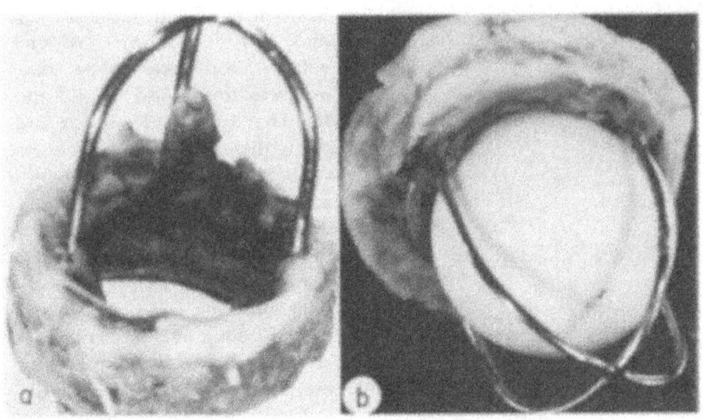

Fig. 22. Prosthetic thrombus on Starr-Edwards aortic (A) and mitral (B) prostheses. (A) This prosthesis had been implanted for 37 mo. The patient (A67-176) died suddenly and unexpectedly from dislodgement of the ball from the aortic cage (see Fig. 24C). Thrombus encircles the inner lining of the prosthetic ring and the caudal half of one of the three metallic struts. (B) The implantation period of this mitral prosthesis was 7 mo. She (A65-43) also died suddenly and unexpectedly. Thrombus encircles most of the metallic ring and descends slightly onto each of the four metallic struts. Neither patient had clinical evidence of a systemic embolus during life.

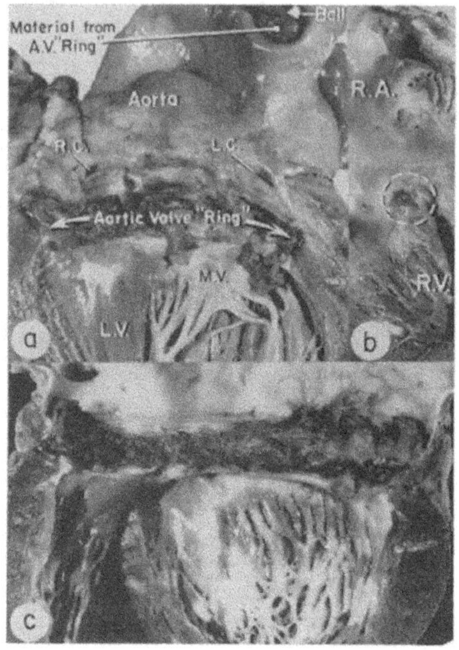

Fig. 23. Infection at the site of attachment of aortic (A and B) and mitral (C) prostheses. (A) Patient A64-189 (see Table 14). Opened left ventricle (L.V.), aortic valve (A.V.) "ring" and ascending aorta. The infection in this patient totally dislodged the aortic Starr-Edwards prosthesis, which migrated to the tranverse aorta. The prosthetic ball is visible. R.C., right coronary ostium; L.C., left coronary ostium; and M.V., anterior mitral valve leaflet. (B) Opened right atrium (R.A.), tricuspid valve, and right ventricle (R.V.) in same patient. Circled lesion is a ring abscess, having extended through from the necrotic prosthetic "ring." (C) Opened left atrium, mitral anulus, and left ventricle in patient A65-221 (see Table 14). The anulus is totally necrotic. The necrotizing nature of infections at sites of attachment of prosthetic valves appears to preclude successful reoperation once infection is established.

had isolated aortic valve replacement; three had isolated mitral replacement, but reoperation in two closed the peribasilar communications; and in three, both mitral and aortic valves had been replaced. In the three patients with two valves, fistulae were present around mitral rings only. The presence of an accessory communication was established before death in each of the 4 patients with periaortic ring leaks, but in only two of the five patients with paramitral ring leaks.[24] The mitral peribasilar communications were considered the cause of death in two patients (Table 13). The frequency of peribasilar prosthetic fistulae appears to be decreasing.

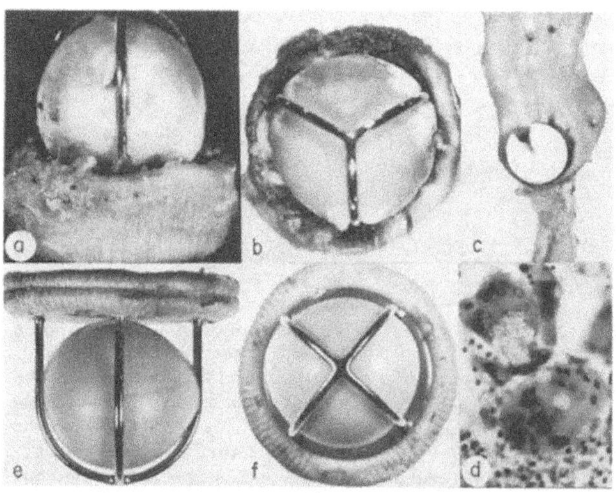

Fig. 24. Degeneration of silicone rubber poppets of Starr-Edwards prostheses. (A and B) Swollen, grooved, yellow, impacted aortic valve poppets implanted for 60 mo. (C) This fractured poppet suddenly dislodged from the aortic valve cage and migrated to the abdominal aorta. He died suddenly (A67-176). Particles of probably silicone rubber within giant cells were found in the liver, spleen, and in several lymph nodes in this patient (D) suggesting that small fragments of silicone rubber dislodged periodically for some time before total ball dislodgement occurred. (E and F) Swollen, deformed, yellow, impacted mitral poppet, which had been implanted 78 mo earlier. This patient died as a result of the swelling of this ball.

In addition to peribasilar leaks, defects in the cardiac septa below valve annuli may develop. Such was the case in the patient described in Fig. 21. He had a small ventricular septal defect created at the time of operation.

Infection at the site of attachment of a prosthetic cardiac valve (Fig. 23). Pertinent clinicopathologic observations in the eight patients who died of this complication are summarized in Table 14.[25,26] Three died within 2 mo of valve replacement, two precipitated by operative wound infections, and the third had infection before operation. The other five patients developed valve infection later, after periods of time sufficient to allow healing of the operative wounds. Precipitating events were clear in three of them and unknown in two. *Staphylococcus epidermidis* was the offending bacterium in five patients, *Staphylococcus aureus* in one, *Proteus mirabilis* in one, and *Serratia marcescens* in one. The intervals from the onset of symptoms or signs consistent with infective endocarditis to death ranged from 16–90 days. Five patients developed conduction disturbances, heart block or bundle-branch block during the period of cardiac infection. Death in four of the five patients with infected aortic prostheses resulted from partial or complete detachment of the prosthesis with production of massive aortic regurgitation, heart failure, and death. Prosthetic detachment, which was partial, occurred in only one of the three patients with infection at sites of attachment of mitral prostheses. All three patients with infected mitral prostheses developed large infected left atrial thrombi, which partially obstructed the mitral orifices.

Infection at sites of attachment of rigid-frame prosthetic valves, particularly in the case of the aortic prostheses, tends to extend deeply into adjacent structures. In four of the five patients with infected aortic prostheses, the inflammatory process extended through the atrial septum to the area of the atrioventricular node and caused a high degree of atrioventricular block. Although prosthetic infective endocarditis cured by antibiotics has been reported, considerable doubt exists as to whether the patients described actually had infection on or at the site of attachment of the prosthesis, or whether they had septicemia without endocarditis; the latter appears more likely. The extent of the infection and the character of the tissue beneath the prosthetic anuli in our patients clearly indicate that an attempt at secondary operative intervention in them at this late stage would have been fruitless. If reoperation has a place in the therapy of prosthetic infective endocarditis, the operative intervention must come early, because once the infection beneath the prosthetic ring is well established, the outcome is fatal regardless of the mode of therapy. Thus, since neither presently available antibiotics or operative methods are effective in eradicating infection at sites of attachment of prosthetic cardiac valves, the infection must be prevented. The value of administering penicillin to patients with rheumatic heart disease before they undergo dental or other operative procedures is well established, but an even more vigorous prophylactic regimen is probably necessary in patients with prosthetic cardiac valves who must undergo similar procedures.

Degeneration (variance) of the silicone rubber prosthetic ball (Fig. 24). Of the 118 prosthetic valves used in the 96 patients who died late, 87 contained silicone rubber poppets, 23 had hollow metal balls, and 4 had silicone rubber discs. Four other patients had porcine aortic valves. Damage to the poppets occurred in none of the patients in whom metal balls or discs were used, but the implantation periods were relatively short (range, 3–52 mo; average, 16) in these 23 patients.

Of the 87 silicone rubber poppets, 45 had been implanted for periods <24 mo, and all appeared normal at necropsy. Of the 42 silicone rubber poppets implanted for 24 mo or longer, 20 were normal, and 22 showed evidence of degeneration or variation consisting of gross alteration in ball color, shape, consistency, volume, and/or surface damage, abrasion, or fracture (Table 15). Only five of the 17

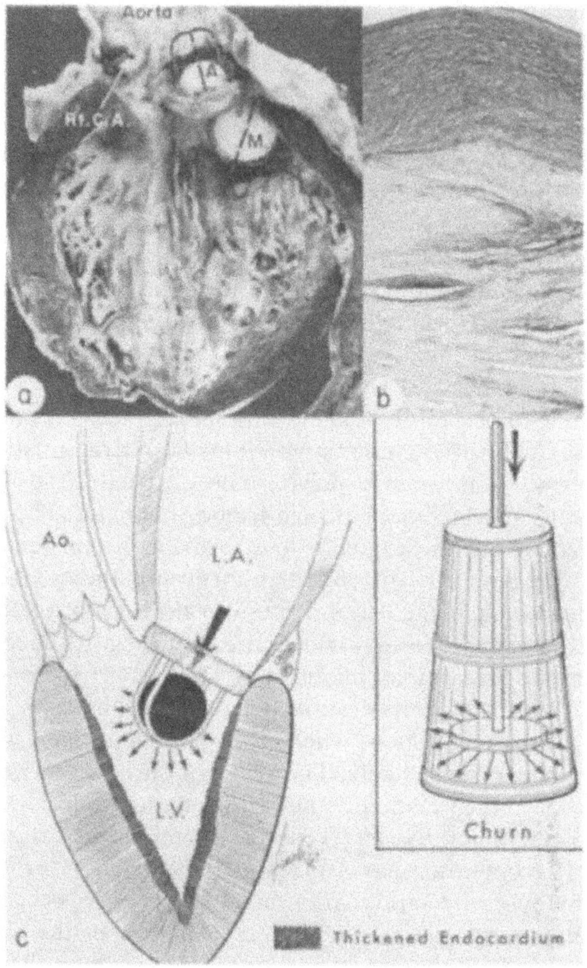

Fig. 25. **Secondary left ventricular endocardial fibroelastosis after mitral valve replacement. (A) Opened left ventricle and aorta in a 56-yr-old man who had undergone both mitral (M.) and aortic (A.) valve replacements 11 mo before death. Although he was improved in the early postoperative period, congestive cardiac failure returned 4 mo after valve replacements. Cause of the recurrence of failure was not determined clinically. At necropsy (A67-50), the endocardium of the left ventricle was diffusely thickened and the underlying myocardium was free of gross scars. Histologically, the thickened endocardium consisted primarily of elastic fibers (B). Elastic van Gieson stain. × 25. Since the endocardium of the papillary muscles excised at the time of valve replacement were not thickened, it is clear that the endocardial thickening was acquired postoperatively. (C) Diagrammatic representation of the possible mechanism of the secondary left ventricular (L.V.) endocardial fibroelastosis after replacement of the mitral valve with a caged-ball prosthesis. The cage and ball of the mitral prosthesis are located within the left ventricular cavity. Thus, when the ball moves, either descends or ascends, it pushes blood laterally, producing turbulence. This effect may be compared to the turbulence produced by the butter churn. The anatomic indicator of turbulent flow is proliferation of connective tissue on the surface in contact with that flow; in this case, endocardium. Ao., aorta; L.A., left atrium. (By permission.[31])**

mitral silicone rubber balls implanted for <24 mo showed evidence of degeneration: In three the poppets were discolored but functioned normally; in two the poppets were discolored, swollen and impacted.[27] All five had been implanted for 78 mo or more, and had an average implantation time of nearly twice that of the normal poppets (100 and 58 mo, respectively). Of the 25 silicone rubber aortic poppets implanted for 24 mo or longer, 17 showed evidence of degeneration: In ten the poppets were swollen (usually about 10% increase in volume compared to the poppet volume at the time of implantation), grooved, and impacted in the cage; in six the balls had fractured and embolized from the cage (in five patients the dislodged poppets were found in the aortic bifurcation; in one it had fallen back into the left ventricular cavity).[28] In 16 patients ball variance was the cause of death. The seventeenth variant aortic poppet showed only mild discoloration, and this change did not cause the prosthesis to function abnormally. The average implantation periods for the eight normal and 17 abnormal poppets were similar, 45 and 41 mo, respectively.

All six patients in whom the aortic ball had dislodged from the cage underwent aortic valve replacement in 1964 and all died in 1967. We have not observed silicone rubber ball embolism in any prosthetic valve implanted after 1964. Some manufacturers of silicone rubber balls for cardiac valve prostheses altered the processing of these poppets in 1965 in an attempt to decrease their propensity to absorb lipids. Possibly the "post-curing" of the silicone rubber will have a beneficial effect on the frequency of ball variance, but insufficient data presently are available on poppets manufactured since 1965 to be certain.

Not only can the entire aortic silicone rubber ball embolize, but so may portions of it.[28,29] In two of the six patients with dislodged aortic balls, fragments of silicone rubber had embolized earlier, as evidenced by the presence of particles of refractile material in and about large foreign body giant cells in liver, spleen, and lymph nodes.

The frequency of prosthetic peribasilar fistulae or thrombi was not significantly increased in the 22 patients with variant silicone rubber poppets as compared with the 20 without variant balls but also implanted for 24 mo or longer. Three peribasilar fistulae and 17 thrombi were encountered among the 22 prosthetic valves with varied or degenerated silicone rubber balls, whereas two fistulae and 16 thrombi were found among the 20 prostheses with normal silicone rubber balls.

It is clear that degeneration of the aortic silicone rubber ball is far more common at this time than is degeneration of a mitral silicone rubber ball, and, to our knowledge, variance of a tricuspid prosthetic poppet has not been reported. That the total number of Starr-Edwards mitral prostheses and aortic prostheses supplied to surgeons is approximately equal further emphasizes this difference in frequency. Differences in pressure and flow across aortic and mitral prostheses are probably the explanation. Typically, the orifice diameters of aortic prostheses are smaller than those of mitral prostheses, and the time of ventricular systole is approximately half that of ventricular diastole for a patient at rest. The velocity of flow through the orifice of the average aortic prosthesis is at least three times greater than the velocity through the orifice of the average mitral prosthesis. Also, the aortic ball contacts both the valve ring and the apex of the cage under

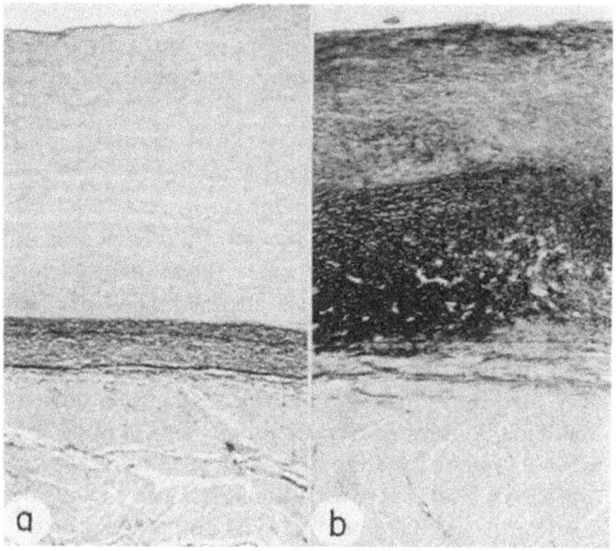

Fig. 26. Secondary endocardial fibrosis of left atrium in addition to secondary endocardial fibroelastosis of left ventricle after mitral valve replacement. Shown are sections of left atrial (A) and left ventricular walls (B), each stained for elastic fibers (Elastic van Gieson stains, each × 32), in a 53-yr-old woman (A65-43) who died suddenly and unexpectedly 7 mo after replacement of the mitral valve with a Starr-Edwards prosthesis without recurrence of symptoms of cardiac dysfunction postoperatively. Endocardial thickening of the left atrium is always found in patients dying late after mitral replacement. In contrast to that occurring in the left ventricle, however, the secondary left atrial endocardial thickening is uncertain but may be the result of local trauma at the time of operation. (By permission.[21])

high pressure, whereas the mitral ball contacts only the ring under high pressure, since the ball passes to the apex of the cage during ventricular diastole.

It is unclear why one aortic or mitral silicone rubber poppet degenerates and why another aortic or mitral poppet implanted for a similar period shows no evidence of degeneration. Table 15 showed that 17 (72%) of 25 aortic silicone rubber poppets implanted for an average of 41 mo showed degeneration, whereas 8 other

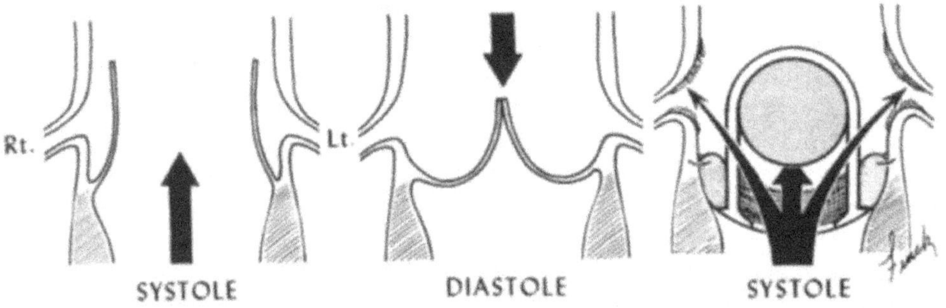

Fig. 27. Diagrammatic representation of the aortic valve region in the normal heart (left and center) and after replacement with a caged-ball prosthesis. Flow of blood during systole across the normal aortic valve is laminar, and the coronary arteries fill mainly by retrograde flow during diastole. Following caged-ball prosthetic replacement, the flow of blood across the aortic valve area is no longer laminar. The force of left ventricular ejection is directed centrally, as in the normal, but the ball prevents central flow, producing severe turbulence in the area. Thus, during ventricular systole blood between surface of the ball and intima of the aortic root is flowing in a turbulent fashion. The anatomic indicator of turbulent flow under high pressure is intimal proliferation, which has been observed in the proximal aorta of each subject dying in the late postoperative period after aortic valve replacement. Since the coronary ostia are no longer "guarded," so to speak, by the aortic cusps during ventricular systole and, much more importantly, since they are in the area of turbulent flow, they also are subject to intimal proliferation, which has been observed in them in several subjects (see text). (By permission.[10])

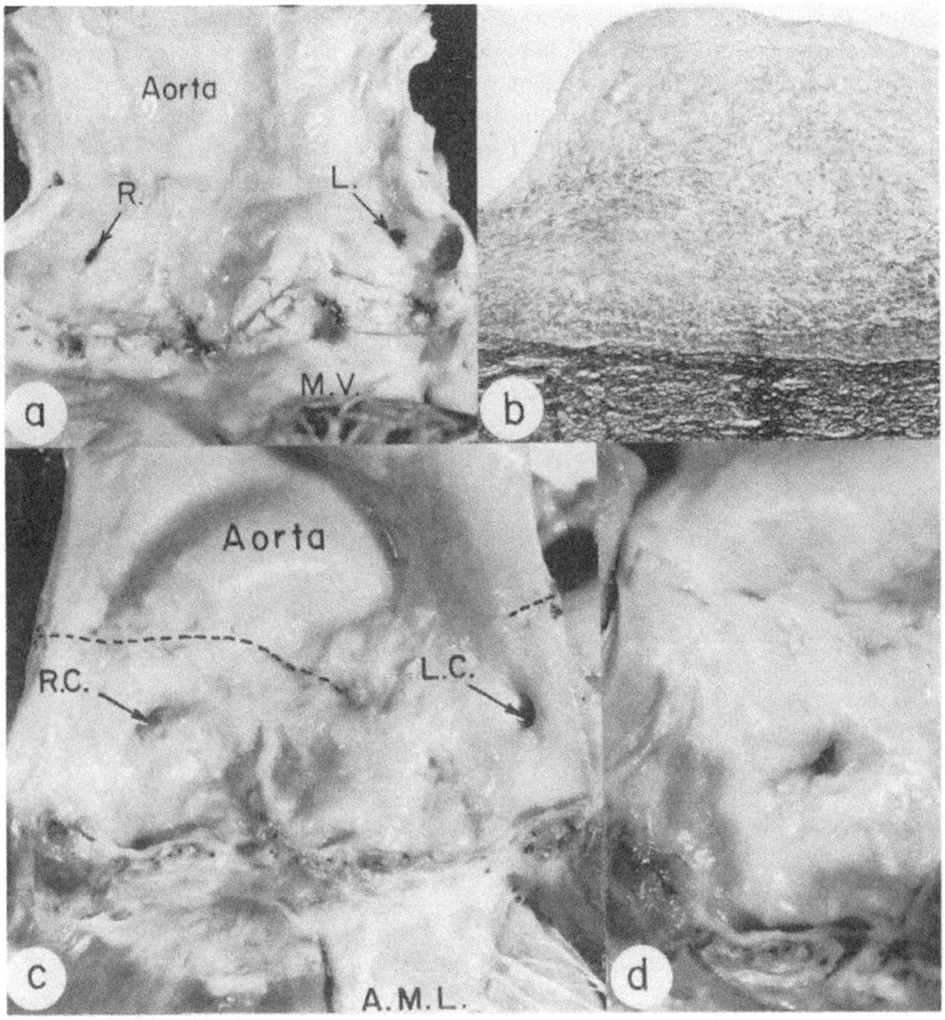

Fig. 28. Intimal proliferation in ascending aorta late after aortic valve replacement. Opened aorta and left ventricular outflow tract (A) in a 48-yr-old man who underwent aortic valve replacement with a Starr-Edwards prosthesis 4 mo earlier. Before operation he had no chest pain but 2 mo postoperatively he developed angina pectoris and died during one of the attacks. At operation, both right (R.) and left (L.) coronary arteries were cannulated without difficulty, but at necropsy (A64-163) cannulae could not be inserted. (A) Considerable intimal proliferation is apparent and both coronary ostia are small. The aortotomy incision is completely obscured by fibrous tissue. (B) Section of ascending aorta showing that the thickening is due to proliferation of fibrous tissue devoid of elastic fibers. The underlying media is normal. Elastic van Gieson stain. × 25. Sections of the coronary arteries in this patient are shown in Fig. 23. This patient had severe renal hemosiderosis, the result of trauma to erythrocytes traversing the aortic prosthesis. (C) Opened aorta and left ventricular outflow tract in a 50-yr-old man (A65-143) who died suddenly 24 mo after aortic valve replacement. Again, there is intimal proliferation in the aorta but it is focal. There is no intimal proliferation about the left coronary (L.C.) ostium as contrasted to its presence about the right (R.C.) one. The broken line designates the previous aortotomy incision. A.M.L., anterior mitral leaflet. (D) Close-up of the narrowed right coronary arterial ostium in this patient.

aortic poppets implanted for an average of 45 mo showed no degeneration. Could it be that the trauma to the poppet produced by the force of left ventricular ejection was greater in the patients with variant aortic balls? A possible quantification of this trauma might be obtained by determining the amount of intravascular hemolysis caused by the turbulent flow of blood across the valvular prosthesis. The anatomic indicator of intravascular hemolysis is renal hemosiderosis.[29,30] Although the per cent of patients with renal hemosiderosis was similar, the amount of iron present in the kidneys of the patients with degenerated silicone rubber poppets was greater than in those without degeneration but with similarly long implantation periods. Kidneys were available for examination in 17 patients in whom Starr-Edwards prostheses with silicone poppets had been im-

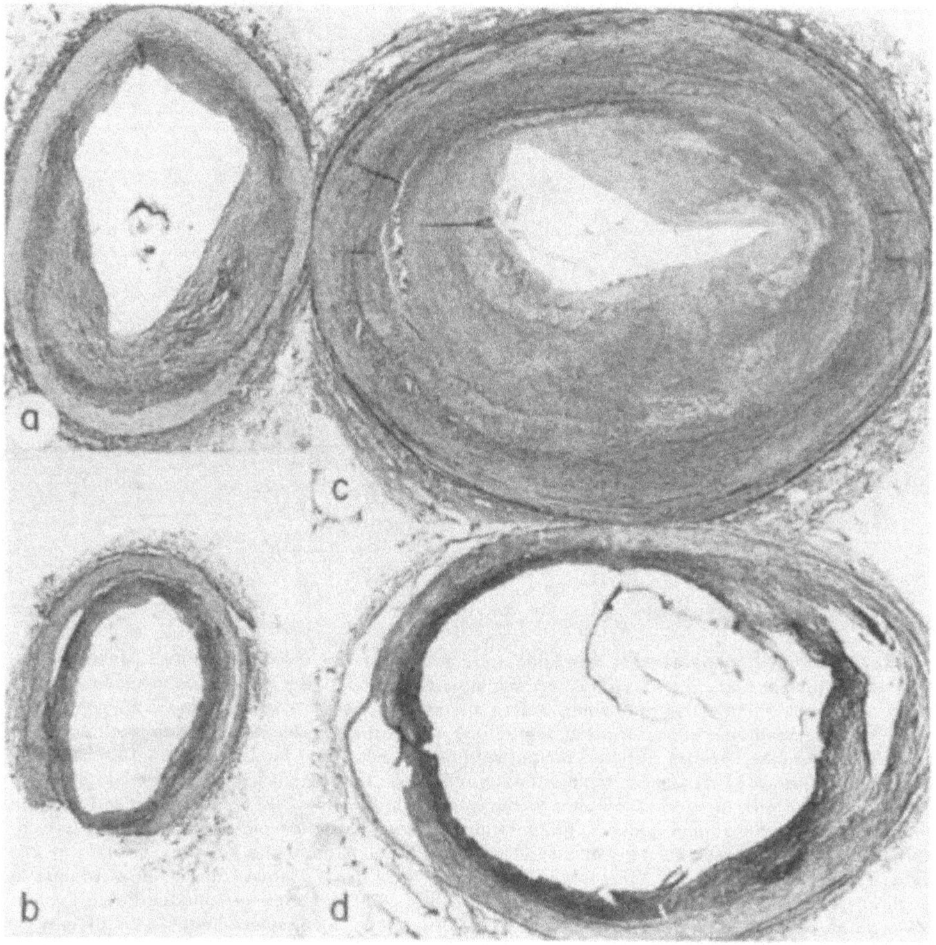

Fig. 29. Photomicrographs of the coronary arteries in the patient whose aortic root is illustrated in Fig. 22 A and B. (A) Right coronary artery at its ostium showing considerable intimal proliferation. This artery is hypoplastic. (B) Right coronary artery 1.5 cm from its ostium. At this point, and distally, the lumen is widely patent. (C) Left coronary artery at its ostium. The lumen is severely narrowed, the result of intimal proliferation. (D) Left coronary artery immediately proximal to its bifurcation into anterior descending and left circumflex branches; both branches were widely patent. Elastic van Gieson stains, all × 20. (By permission.[21])

planted for 24 mo or longer. Thirteen of the seventeen had iron deposits (Prussian blue stains) in the cytoplasm of proximal renal tubular cells: Of the ten with ball variance eight had renal iron deposits; of the seven with normal poppets, five had renal hemosiderosis. Among the aortics without ring leak, however, none of two without ball variance had renal hemosiderosis, and seven of nine *with* ball variance had renal hemosiderosis.

Clinical features of *aortic* ball variance are variable, but this diagnosis must be suspected in any patient in whom a prosthesis containing a silicone rubber poppet has been in place 24 mo or longer. When the aortic ball swells, death may occur suddenly, or may be preceded by congestive cardiac failure. Alterations of prosthetic sounds are often apparent. Dislodgement of the aortic ball from the cage was not preceded by symptoms of cardiac dysfunction in any of our six patients. The clinical features resulting from severe degeneration of the silicone rubber *mitral* poppet also are variable, and consist of syncope or near syncope, congestive heart failure, and alterations in prosthetic sounds. Aortic ball degeneration should be considered in any patient doing poorly 2 yr or more after aortic valve replacement with a prostheses containing a silicone rubber ball. Mitral poppet degeneration should be considered in any patient doing poorly 5 yr

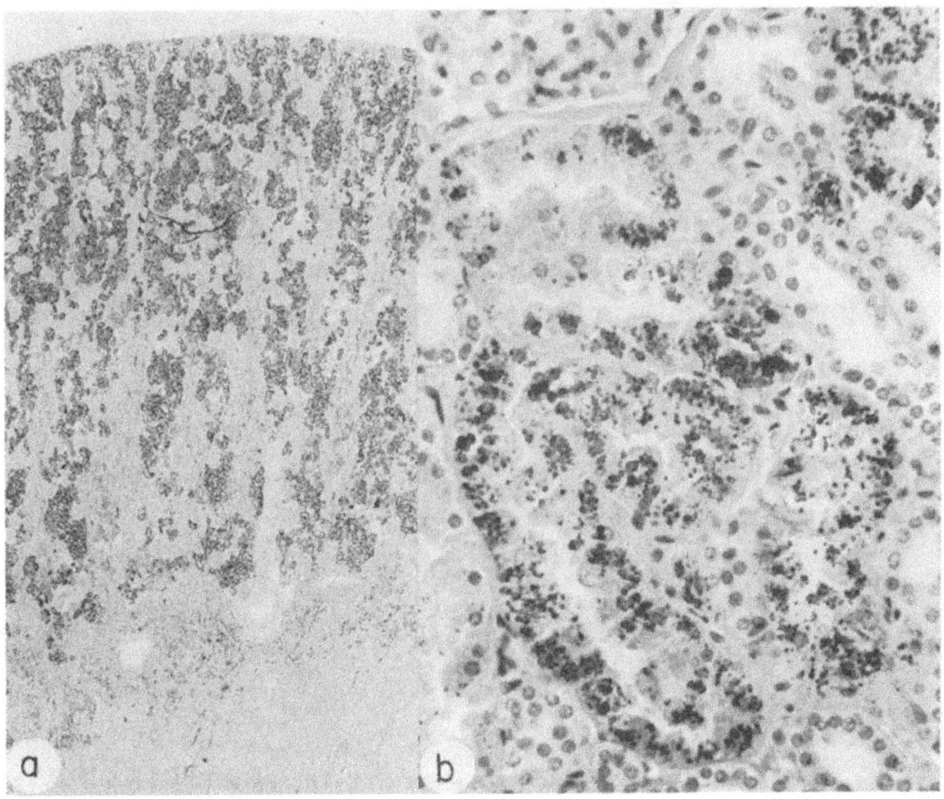

Fig. 30. Renal hemosiderosis late after aortic valve replacement (A64-10). (A) Section of kidney stained for iron (Prussian blue) disclosing numerous deposits of iron in renal tubules. × 16. (B) Close-up view showing deposits of iron in the cytoplasm of the proximal tubules. Hematoxylin and eosin stains. × 290.

or more after mitral valve replacement with a prosthesis containing a silicone rubber poppet. It is hoped that the hollow metal ball made of Stellite 21 alloy (Table 16) in Starr-Edwards prostheses of current design will not degenerate. This newer prosthesis, introduced in 1967, as yet has shown no evidence of wear.

Secondary left ventricular endocardial fibroelastosis after mitral valve replacement (Figs. 25 and 26). In each of the 49 patients who died late after mitral replacement, some degree of left ventricular endocardial thickening was found at necropsy.[31] In each of these patients, the stumps of the amputated left ventricular papillary muscles and the left ventricular apex, the site of drain insertion at operation, were covered by fibrous tissue, but in 35 of the 49 patients the fibrous process extended to involve other areas of left ventricular endocardium as well.

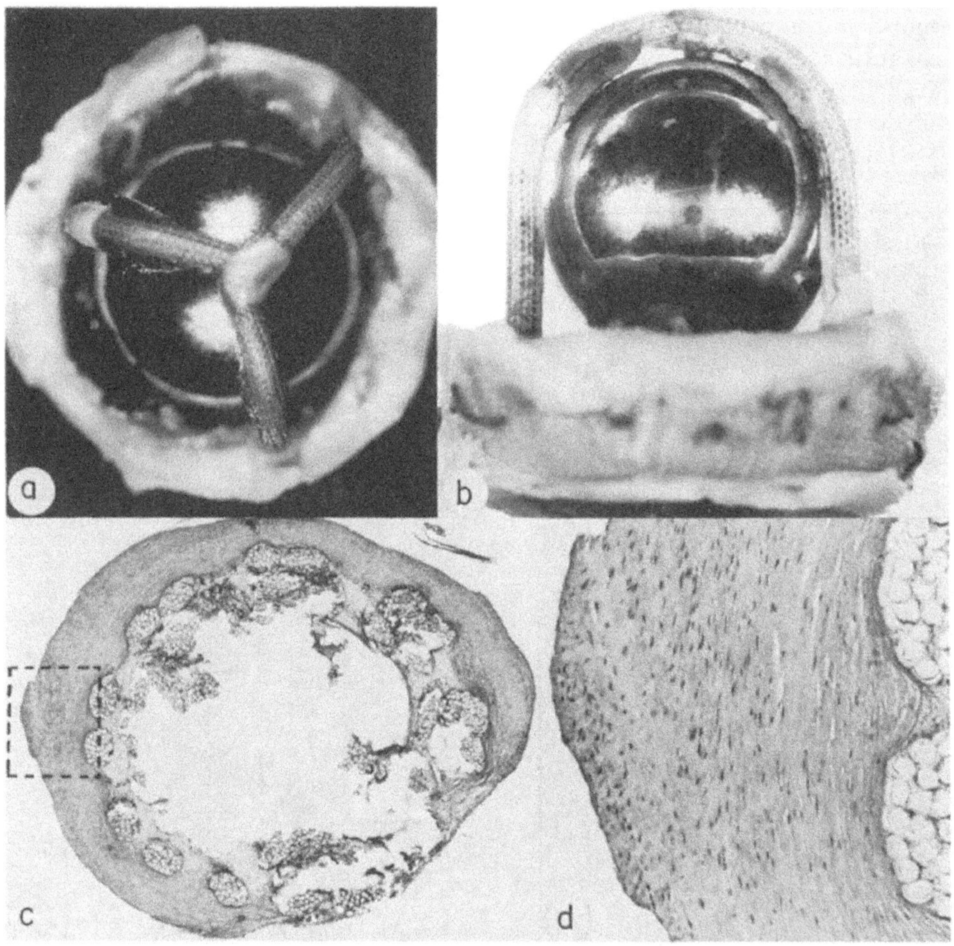

Fig. 31. Collagen deposits on cloth-covered struts of Starr-Edwards prosthesis implanted in a 53-yr-old man (A70-54) for 12 mo. (A) Prosthesis as viewed from above showing a collagen plaque at the apex of the cage. (B) Same prosthesis viewed laterally showing both collagen plaques and fibrin platelet thrombi on the Teflon-covered struts. (C) Section of collagen plaque after removal of the cloth from the metallic strut. (D) Close-up of the area shown in C, showing that fibrous tissue, containing many fibroblasts, covers the cloth. Hematoxylin and eosin stains. (C) × 34, (D) × 160.

The absence of endocardial thickening of the papillary muscles excised at the time of mitral valve replacement (except in one patient, a 15-yr-old girl who had primary endocardial fibroelastosis) and the presence of extensive left ventricular endocardial fibrous tissue containing numerous elastic fibers at necropsy indicates that the endocardial fibroelastosis was acquired postoperatively. The most extensive secondary left ventricular endocardial fibrosis was observed in two patients who had had aortic as well as mitral valve replacements. In these patients the left ventricular endocardial thickening was believed to have been of functional significance. Both had severe, intractable cardiac failure several mo postoperatively without other anatomic explanation. In the other patients with significant, although less severe, left ventricular endocardial fibrosis, death was attributable to other causes. Left ventricular endocardial thickening did not occur in patients with isolated aortic valve replacement, unless there had been a previous myocardial infarct.

The endocardium of the left atrium also was focally but extensively thickened in all 49 patients who had had mitral valve replacement. In contrast to the left ventricular endocardial fibrosis, which contained numerous elastic fibers, that which occurred in the left atrium, with rare exception, was devoid of elastic fibers. The left atrial endocardial thickening almost certainly appeared postoperatively also, probably the result of operative trauma to the interior lining of this chamber.

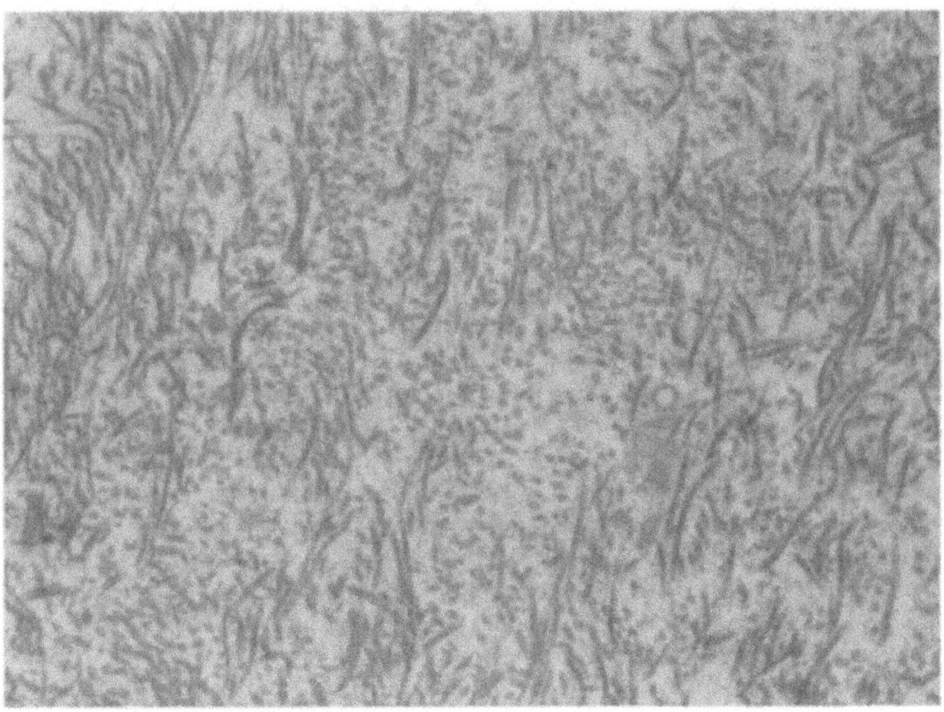

Fig. 32. Electronmicrograph of fragment of fibrous tissue covering a cloth-covered strut in a prosthesis inserted about 1 yr earlier. Tissue covering the strut consists entirely of collagen fibrils with a few fibroblasts. × 37,755. (Electronmicrograph taken by Dr. Victor J. Ferrans.)

The endocardial thickening, which occurs over the stumps of the amputated papillary muscles after mitral replacement, may be regarded as simple healing. The cause of the more widespread left ventricular endocardial thickening observed in these patients is uncertain, but it may be the result of turbulent blood flow in this chamber. The leaflets and chordae tendineae of the natural mitral valve are within the left ventricular cavity, but these structures are thin and readily movable, and the blood flows centrally, between the two leaflets. In contrast, after insertion of a caged-ball mitral prosthesis, blood flows peripherally, or around the caged ball, and the endocardial lining of the left ventricle is not protected from blood flowing across the mitral prosthesis. Also, the ball in the prosthetic mitral valve moves up and down, imparting a churning turbulence to the blood within the left ventricular cavity. The anatomic indicator of turbulent flow is fibrous proliferation, and in this case its site is the left ventricular endocardium. Similar fibrous proliferation occurs in the aortic root after replacement of the aortic valve with a caged-ball prosthesis.

Intimal thickening of the aortic root and proximal coronary arteries after aortic valve replacement (Figs. 27–29). In each of the 66 patients with prosthetic aortic valves, there was intimal thickening in the aortic root. This thickening appears to have been produced by the deposition of fibrous tissue, devoid of foam cells, on the internal elastic membrane of the proximal portion of the ascending aorta. The degree of intimal proliferation varied from minimal to severe; in some patients it was diffuse, and in others, focal.

In addition to the changes in the aortic root in all 66 patients, 37 also had intimal proliferation, with or without actual narrowing, of one or both coronary arterial ostia or proximal coronary arteries. One of the difficulties encountered in evaluating coronary ostial narrowing in these patients was inherent differences in the sizes of the ostia. In most subjects with aortic valvular disease, the left coronary arterial ostium is larger than the right; often the difference is striking. Thus, if the right coronary ostium is smaller than the left one, postoperative narrowing can be assumed to have occurred only if there is extensive intimal proliferation about the origin of the vessel. In 18 patients, there was intimal proliferation about the right ostium; it caused severe narrowing in 4 patients. The other 19 patients had narrowing of varying degree of both coronary ostia. In 14 of the latter 19 subjects, the narrowing was mild and functionally insignificant, and in the other 5, there was considerable narrowing of each ostium and of the proximal main left and right coronary arteries as well. Two of the latter 5 patients, however, had had replacement of the ascending aorta by a graft at the time of valve replacement, and the proximity of the suture line to the coronary ostia may have been a factor in the production of ostial narrowing. The third patient had severe narrowing, not only of the ostia but of the entire coronary arterial tree, secondary to atherosclerosis. The fourth patient had severe intimal thickening in the proximal 1-cm segments of the right and left coronary arteries, but the coronary vessels distal to this point were widely patent. In this patient, coronary arterial perfusion cannulae could not be inserted into the ostia at the time of necropsy, although such cannulae had been utilized without difficulty at the time of valve replacement only 4 mo earlier. This man, who was 48 yr old, had not had chest pain before operation, but 2 mo postoperatively began to have angina pectoris and thereafter had numerous anginal attacks. This patient also had mild anemia postoperatively, and at necropsy the presence of large amounts of iron in his kidneys indicated that the anemia was secondary to intravascular hemolysis. The presence of the anemia in this patient may be interpreted as indicating an excessive turbulence of blood in the area of the valvular prostheses. The fifth patient died suddenly; both coronary arterial ostia were severely narrowed.

The thickening of the intima of the aortic root appears to have occurred in these patients during the postoperative period. It was clear from necropsy examination that the healing of the aortotomy incision was not the responsible factor, since intimal thickening also was present at some distance from it. In only 2 of the 66 patients was coronary ostial narrowing evident at the time of aortic valve replacement. It is unlikely that any functional disturbances are produced by intimal thickening in the ascending aorta itself. When this process involves the ostia and proximal coronary arteries, however, the effects, when severe, may be compared to those of syphilitic aortitis.

The flow of blood through a normal aortic valve and ascending aorta is laminar, but when a ball-valve prosthesis is present, flow in these areas is grossly turbulent. The anatomic indicator of localized turbulent flow is intimal proliferation.

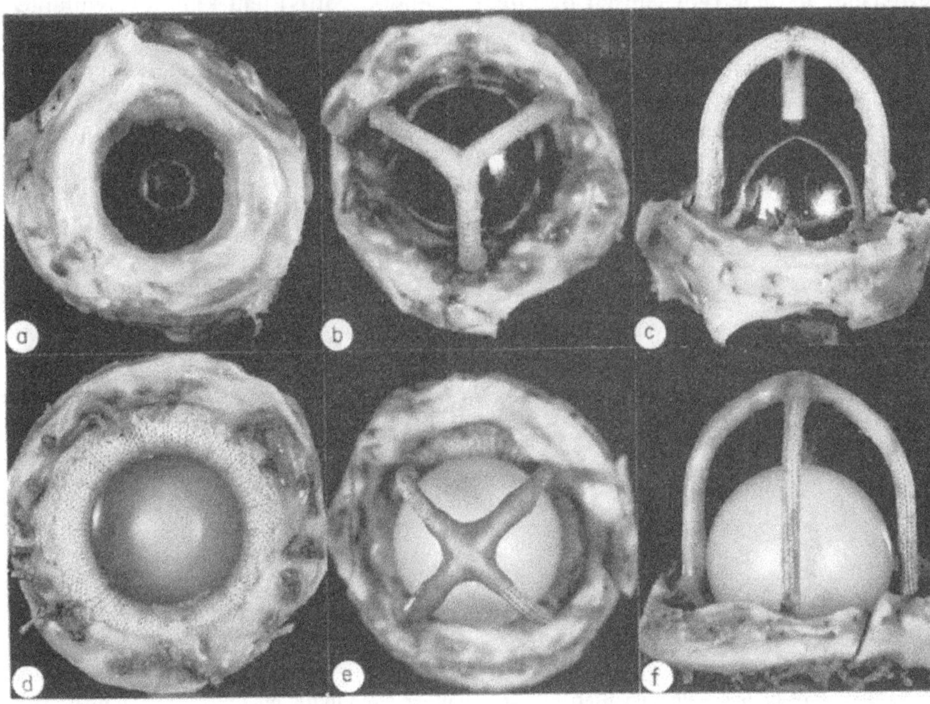

Fig. 33. Starr-Edwards prostheses. (A, B, and C) Aortic prosthesis (size 9A, model 2300). (D, E, and F) Mitral prosthesis (size 3M, model 6300). Each was implanted for 44 mo in a 58-yr-old man (A71-162). He died 8 hr after the onset of severe chest pain. Note the heavy deposition of fibrous tissue (collagen) on the ventricular aspect of the aortic prosthesis (A) and the relatively light deposition on the atrial aspect of the mitral prosthesis (D). Furthermore, the deposits of collagen on the aortic struts are thin and the Teflon is easily visible (B and C). In contrast, heavy deposits of collagen are present at the apices of each of the four struts of the mitral prosthesis (E) and on the vertical portions of two of the four struts of the mitral prosthesis (F).

Although the changes in the coronary ostia and proximal coronary arteries were relatively unimpressive in most of the 66 patients, their average survival time after valve replacement was relatively short. It is possible that intimal proliferation in these areas will become more extensive with time.

Traumatic intravascular hemolysis (Fig. 30). It is now well appreciated that intravascular hemolysis occurred in virtually all patients with malfunctioning flexible Teflon aortic valves,[29] and in a few patients with incompetent and stenotic aortic valves that have not been operated upon.[30] The intravascular hemolysis in these subjects is the result of trauma to erythrocytes traversing the malfunctioning natural or artificial aortic valve. The anatomic indicator of intravascular hemolysis is renal hemosiderosis, the so-called blue kidney. The mechanisms by which iron is deposited in the kidneys have been described elsewhere.[29]

The kidneys were available for examination in 51 of the 96 subjects dying late (Table 17). In 36 (71%) of the 51 patients, histologic sections stained by the Prussian blue reaction, disclosed iron in the kidneys. The amount of iron deposited in the kidneys, almost all of it in the cytoplasm of the proximal tubules, was heavy in 27 patients and in 9 it was minimal or mild. The valves replaced in the patients with renal hemosiderosis are shown in Table 17. Eight patients with peribasilar fistulae (not caused by infective endocarditis) had kidneys available for examination, and all eight had renal hemosiderosis. All but one of the eight had aortic prostheses. The degree of intimal proliferation in the aortic root was striking in all 28 patients with heavy deposits of renal iron after aortic replacement. As mentioned earlier, it would appear that both aortic root intimal

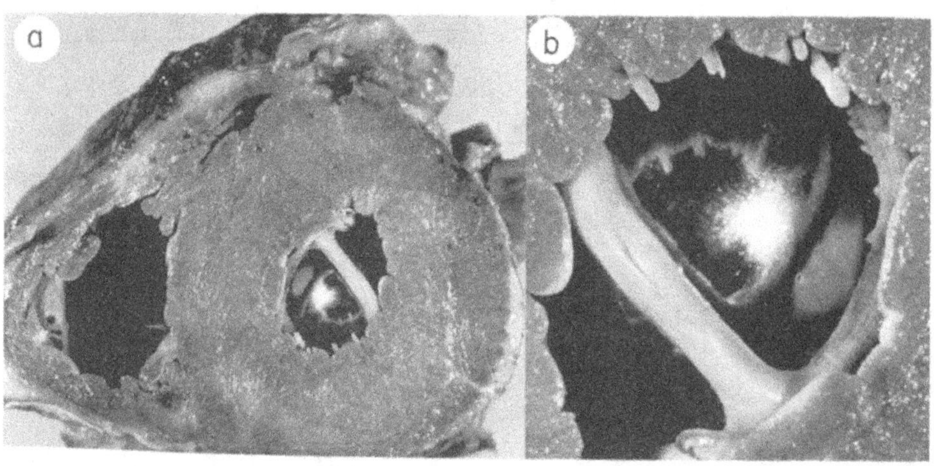

Fig. 34. Prosthetic dysfunction. Starr-Edwards cloth-covered mitral prosthesis (model 6320, size 4M) implanted in a 58-yr-old man (A72-31) 6.5 mo before death. His preoperative lesion was aortic stenosis and mitral stenosis, and left ventricular cavity was of normal size. (A) Mitral prosthesis as viewed from left ventricle. (B) Close-up of same valve. Each of the four struts of the mitral prosthesis contacts endocardium of left ventricle and the ventricular septum bulges into the mitral cage, preventing the metal poppet from descending completely to apex of cage. Cloth-covered struts show considerable collagen overgrowth. Mean diastolic pressure gradient between left atrium and left ventricle before valve replacement was 7 mm Hg, and at catheterization 6 mo postoperatively this gradient was 11 mm Hg. Thus, this case is an example of prosthetic stenosis confirmed by hemodynamic study. If a smaller sized prosthesis had been utilized, for example a 2M rather than a 4M, obstruction may not have resulted. (By permission.[40])

proliferation and renal hemosiderosis are indicators of excessive trauma to blood as it is ejected against the aortic poppet and aortic wall.

Although deposits of iron in kidneys produce striking anatomic lesions, no significant renal damage or impairment of renal function appears to occur as a result of this deposition. The bone marrow is usually able to compensate for the increased red blood cell destruction. The hematocrit values in the late post-operative period were available in 25 of the 36 patients with renal hemosiderosis: In 12 the hematocrit was normal ($\geqq$ 40%) and in 13 it was low (32%–37%).

Fatal central nervous system hemorrhage associated with hypoprothrombinemia after cardiac valve replacement. Of 67 patients on warfarin dying > two months after operation, five died of complications of anticoagulation (Table 18). Three of the five had developed serum hepatitis in the early postoperative period with striking elevations of prothrombin times. The other two patients also developed severe hypoprothrombinemia, but neither had hepatitis.

Systemic emboli from prostheses were a cause of late death in ten of the 96 patients and prosthetic thrombosis the cause in one. All but two of these 11 patients had been on warfarin. Of the 29 patients not on warfarin, two died as a result of emboli. Thus, *the hazards of long-term anticoagulants may outweigh their clinical benefit.*

Aneurysm formation at sites of excised left ventricular papillary muscles after mitral valve replacement (Figs. 16 and 20). In three patients who had had

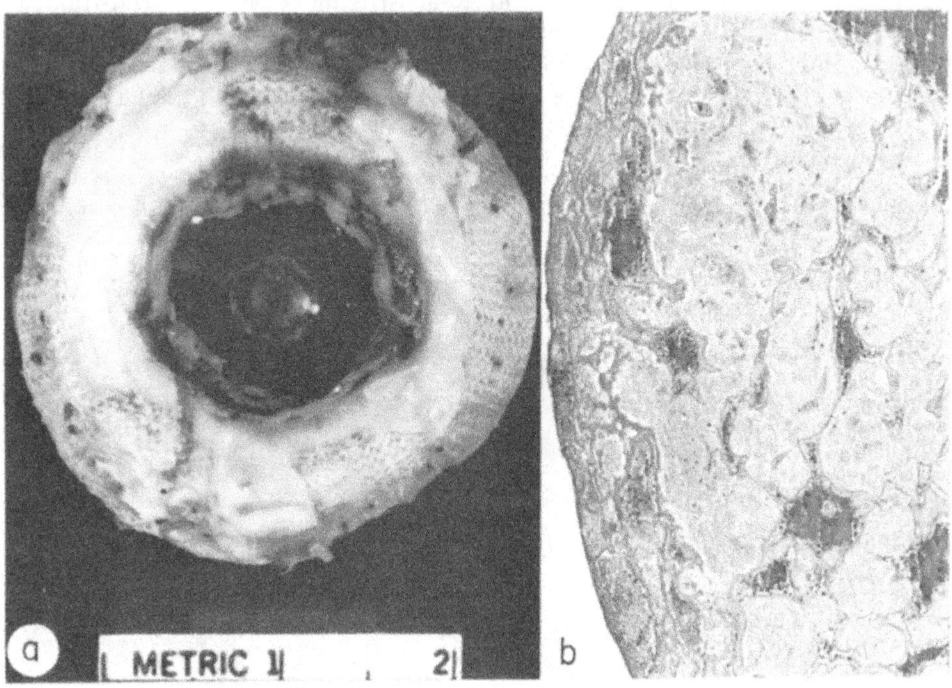

Fig. 35. Starr-Edwards aortic valve as viewed from the ventricular aspect in a 45-yr-old man (A69-281) who had valve replacement 23 mo earlier. This patient had a model 2300 prosthesis (the present one is model 2320), which was made stenotic by the manufacturer. The inlet orifice was further narrowed in this patient by a rim of fibrin-platelet thrombus (B). This patient had a 50 mm Hg peak systolic pressure gradient between left ventricle and aorta and the entire gradient appears to be at the inlet of the prosthesis. Hematoxylin and eosin stain. × 80 (B).

mitral valve replacements 3, 6, and 9 mo, respectively, before death, necropsy disclosed fibrosis of the entire left ventricular free wall beneath the site of amputation of one of the papillary muscles.[22] The thinness of the left ventricular walls at these sites indicates that functional aneurysms had been present during life. Left ventricular saccular aneurysms are almost certainly the result of excision of a portion of left ventricular free wall beneath the papillary muscles at the time of mitral valve excision. This complication may be prevented by not pulling the papillary muscle toward the left atrium at the time it is severed at operation. No known clinical consequences resulted from the left ventricular aneurysms in any of the three patients, although two died suddenly without other anatomic explanation. One patient died in the operating room from perforation of the left ventricular wall at the site of excision of one of the papillary muscles.

Calcification of mitral anulus. A previously undescribed late complication of valve replacement with rigid-framed caged-ball prostheses is calcification at the site of attachment of the prosthesis. Six (Table 19) patients dying 44–116 mo (average, 88) after mitral replacement for pure regurgitation had calcific deposits in prosthetic anuli. None of the six had valvular or anular calcification preoperatively or at operation. The anular calcific deposits at necropsy varied from focal to diffuse. The most extensive deposits occurred in two patients in whom the implantation periods exceeded 100 mo.

The mechanism of calcification of the mitral anuli in these patients is uncertain, but it is likely that constant to-and-fro movement of rigid-framed prostheses accelerates wear of the tissues beneath the site of attachment. A danger of prosthetic ring calcification is obvious in the event of reoperation to replace a faulty prosthesis. Because prostheses appear to be held in place by su-

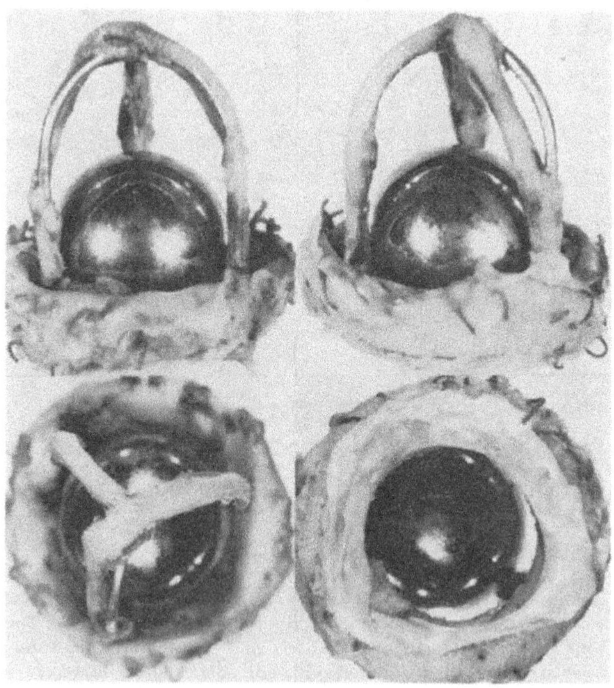

Fig. 36. Wear of cloth on struts of Starr-Edwards prosthesis (size 11A, model 2310) implanted 24 mo earlier in a 50-yr-old man who died of cancer. Upper: Lateral views of prosthesis. Lower left: Prosthesis as viewed from above. Lower right: Prosthesis as viewed from left ventricle. Collagen has covered the seat of the prosthesis but there has been little ingrowth of tissue on the cloth of the struts. Severe through-and-through wear of cloth exposed two of the three metallic struts. Although evidence of increased red cell destruction was present, the valve apparently functioned well.

tures and not by ingrowth of tissue, it is also possible that calcific deposits at prosthetic rings might tear sutures and cause peribasilar leaks.

Status of cloth-covered struts of Starr-Edwards prosthetic valves in patients dying later than 2 mo after cardiac valve replacement (Figs. 7, 31–36). Twenty-five cloth-covered prostheses implanted in 20 patients from 3–52 mo (average, 18) were examined (Table 20). Of 15 aortic prostheses, eight were model 2300, five, model 2310, and two, model 2320. Of nine mitral prostheses, four were model 6300, four, model 6310, and one, model 6320. One prosthesis implanted in the tricuspid position was model 6300. On gross examination some struts appeared free of tissue covering; however, on histologic examination, each of the 25 prostheses showed some degree of tissue growth over the cloth of the struts and bases. The initial deposit, as learned from histologic study of a number of cloth-covered prostheses in patients dying early (< 2 mo after operation), appears to be a fibrin-platelet thrombus. This material organized into dense fibrous tissue containing fibroblasts, and rarely exhibited vascular channels and mononuclear cells. Electron microscopic examination of the fibrous tissue covering the struts and bases in two patients dying late disclosed that it consisted of collagen fibrils and an occasional fibroblast[32,33] (Fig. 32). Thus, the dense fibrous tissue covering the cloth should be referred to as collagen. In several patients dying late (> 2 mo after operation), fibrin-platelet deposits were observed on the struts or bases, or both, adjacent to dense collagen.

The collagen deposits appear to form first at the apex of the cage, except in the close clearance prostheses where the deposits form on the vertical portions of the struts just before they bend to form the apex. The deposits cover some struts in their entirety; in others they are focal on one strut and grossly absent on another of the same prosthesis.

The amount of tissue growing over the struts is not proportional to the length of the implantation period, and in patients with two prostheses, it did not consistently favor a prosthesis in one position. Collagen deposition on the cloth struts was fairly heavy in some prostheses implanted for less than 6 mo, but in each of two patients in whom prostheses had been implanted for 35 and 40 mo, respectively, virtually no tissue overgrowth was observed on the struts on gross examination.

Cloth wear on the struts was observed in two of the 25 prostheses examined. Both were aortic valves: One had been implanted for 24 mo, and the other for 25 mo (Fig. 36). Fibrin platelet thrombi also were present on the struts. Two aortic valves with longer implantation periods (35 and 52 mo) were free of cloth wear and thrombi.

In addition to wear of cloth covering the struts, disruptions also may occur in the Teflon cloth in the orifice of the model 6310–6320 mitral valves. These cloth disruptions may be minor, or they may produce significant regurgitation and require reoperation. Significant cloth disruption has been observed as soon as 2 mo following valve replacement. These periorifice cloth disruptions may in part result from damage at the time of valve replacement by the prosthesis holder. Nevertheless, the use of polypropylene orifice cloth instead of Teflon is currently being evaluated. It may be less susceptible to damage from the valve holder, less apt to migrate over the stud edges, and less liable to unravel or run should a break in the yarn occur. Interestingly, disruption of orifice cloth in the composite seat of the aortic prostheses (models 2310–2320) has been far less frequent, and at this time of no clinical significance.

Although thrombo-embolism is less with cloth-covered prostheses,[34,35] compared to similar noncloth-covered prostheses, hemolysis is increased. As mentioned earlier, renal hemosiderosis is an anatomic indicator of intravascular hemolysis. Kidneys were available for histologic examination in 49 of the 92 patients dying late with rigid-framed ball valve prostheses (Table 21). Cloth-covered prostheses had been used in 14 of the 49 patients; renal iron was present in 12 patients (86%) and heavy in 10 (71%). Of the 35 patients with noncloth-covered struts, 24 (69%) had renal hemosiderosis and 18 (51%) had heavy deposits of renal iron. Excluding ten patients with peribasilar leaks (which in

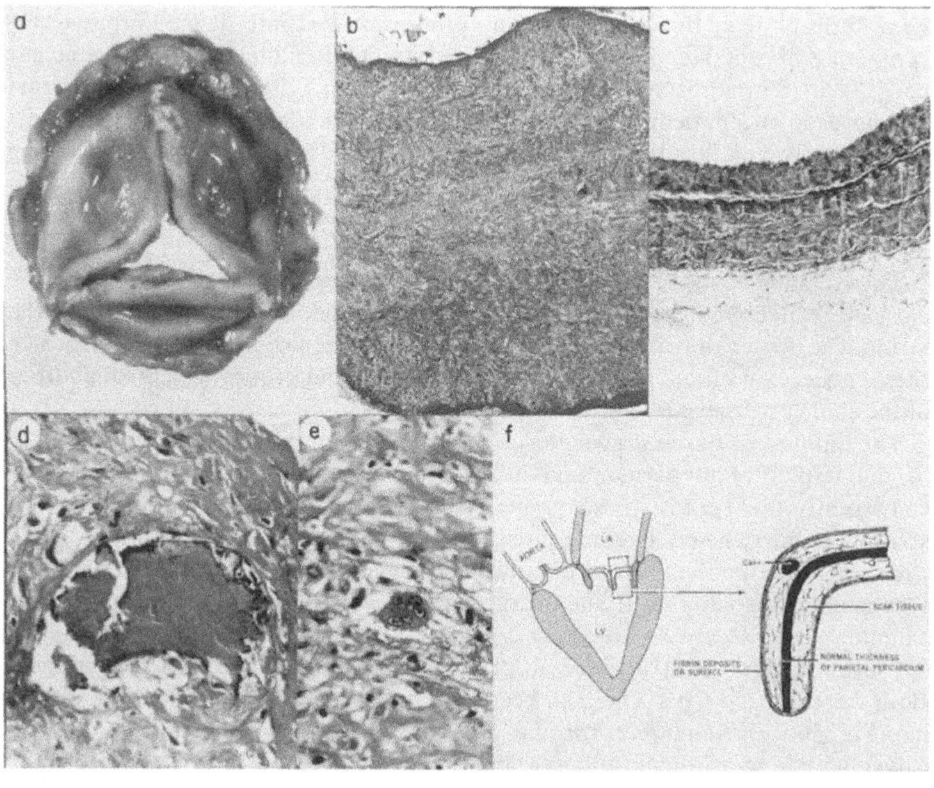

Fig. 37. Fresh autogenous pericardial valve implanted in mitral position in a 50-yr-old woman (A71-61) 39 days before death. There was no evidence of dysfunction of this tissue valve during the postoperative period. (A) View of pericardial valve from above. The "cusps" are thickened and one is retracted. The valve orifice was competent when water was injected under pressure into the left ventricle at necropsy. (B) Photomicrograph of section through one "cusp." The surfaces of the "cusp" are lined by fibrin. The cusp is about four times thicker than normal. The implanted parietal pericardium may be compared to its thickness at time of implantation, a portion of which is shown in C. Both B and C were taken at the same magnification. Thickening of the implanted pericardium is due mainly to proliferation of fibrous tissue, which probably resulted from organization of surface fibrin. (D) Deposit of calcium in the implanted valve. (E) Close-up of portion of implanted valve showing multinucleated cell of uncertain significance. (F) Schematic diagram of changes (seen in B), which occurred in the implanted autogenous pericardial valve. Hematoxylin and eosin stains. C and D, × 70. E and F, × 400.

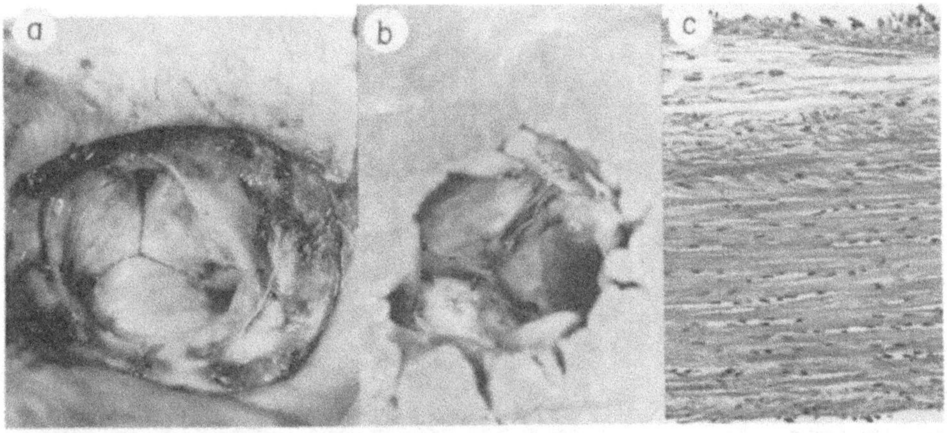

Fig. 38. Glutaraldehyde-fixed porcine aortic valve implanted in the mitral portion in a 60-yr-old man (A70–280) for pure mitral regurgitation. He died 50 days after operation but never awoke after operation. The implanted tissue valve functioned normally. (A) Implanted valve, which is competent, viewed from left atrium. (B) Same valve viewed from left ventricle. The leaflets are freely mobile. (C) Photomicrograph of a portion of one cusp. The cuspal tissue appears well preserved. Hematoxylin and eosin stain. × 160.

themselves may cause intravascular hemolysis), heavy deposits of renal iron were present in 10 of 26 (39%) patients without cloth-covered prostheses and in 9 of 13 (69%) patients with cloth-covered prostheses. Although hemolysis may initially be increased by the cloth covering of the prosthesis and lead to increased intravascular hemolysis, trauma to erythrocytes may then diminish as tissue overgrowth on the struts and bases smooths the rough cloth surfaces.

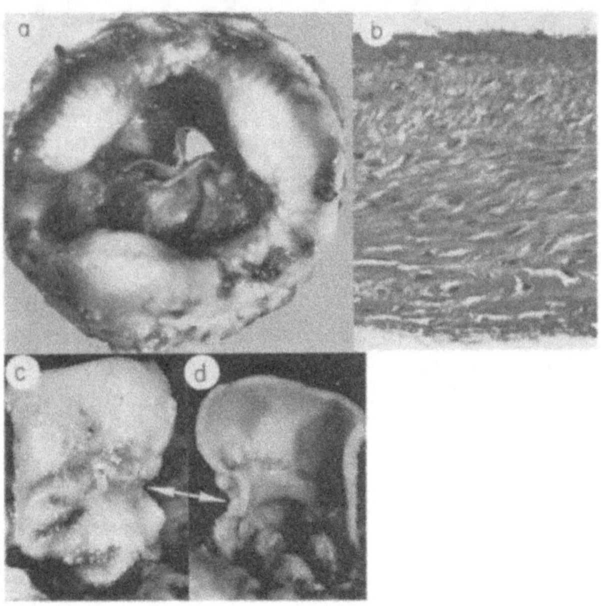

Fig. 39. Glutaraldehyde fixed porcine aortic valve implanted in aortic position in a 51-yr-old man (A71–78) 150 days before death. He died suddenly at home of uncertain cause after a previously asymptomatic postoperative course. (A) Porcine valve as viewed from above showing thrombi in two of three sinuses of Valsalva. One week before death a 35 mm Hg peak systolic pressure gradient between left ventricle and brachial artery was demonstrated, and the gradient may have been due to the thrombi causing poor leaflet mobility and to the small orifice of the tissue involved. (B) Photomicrograph of section of implanted valve cusp. The cuspal tissue appears well preserved and free of inflammation or necrosis. Hematoxylin and eosin stain. × 400. (C and D) Views of ascending aorta anteriorly (C) and of porcine valve from above (D). Arrow designates the healed aortotomy incision, which appears to cause some narrowing anatomically. Note close apposition of the struts of the porcine valve at the central orifice (suggesting inherent stenosis).

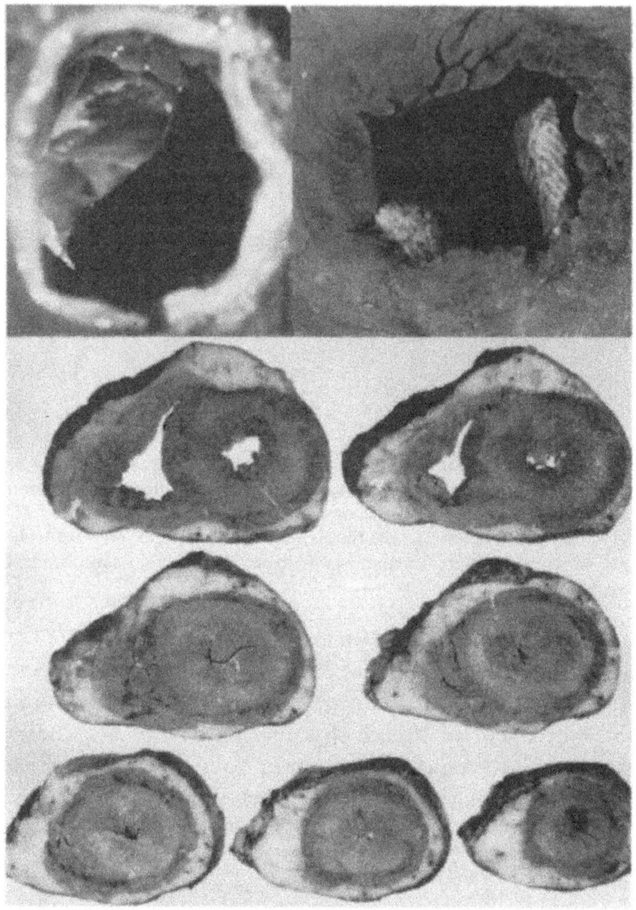

Fig. 40. Porcine aortic heterograft, fixed in stabilized glutaraldehyde, implanted in the mitral position for stenosis in a 44-yr-old man (A71–101) 14 days before death. He had a smooth early postoperative course and was discharged 12 days after operation. Two days later he died suddenly. Upper left: View from aorta showing stint of mitral prosthesis partially obstructing left ventricular outflow. Upper right: View of porcine valve from left ventricle showing two of three stints of the tissue valve frame contacting left ventricular endocardium. Left ventricular cavity is smaller than normal, and cavity obliteration in systole had been demonstrated by left ventricular cineangiography before operation. The lower photograph shows transverse cuts of the ventricles disclosing a very small left ventricular cavity.

Myocardial necrosis and fibrosis in patients dying late after cardiac valve replacement. The incidence and location of myocardial necrosis and fibrosis in these patients are summarized in Table 22. In contrast to the frequency of its occurrence in the patients who died early (Table 11), myocardial necrosis was rare in the patients dying late, occurring in only five patients, and in three of them it was limited to papillary muscle. Myocardial fibrosis, in contrast, occurred in 72 of the 96 patients: In 30 it was limited to papillary muscle; in 15 it occurred in the subendocardium of the left ventricular free wall or ventricular septum, or both, in addition to papillary muscle; and in 27 patients, it was transmural. Transmural fibrosis in three patients was located in the free walls beneath sites where left ventricular papillary muscles had been excised.

Tissue valves (Figs. 37–40). Porcine aortic valve heterografts fixed in stabilized glutaraldehyde were utilized in seven of the 224 patients (Table 23): Five were placed in the mitral position, one in the aortic, and one in the tricuspid. No patient had clinical evidence of systemic emboli and none received warfarin. Three patients died early and four died late (4–14 mo) after operation. Of the patients dying early, one never awoke postoperatively; one, who also had a parietal pericardial mitral valve, died of upper gastrointestinal bleeding; and one was unable to maintain adequate blood pressure for unknown reasons after mitral replacement. All three valves appeared to function well postoperatively. Of the four patients dying > 2 mo after valve replacement, the cause was uncertain in each: Two died of progressive congestive cardiac failure and two died suddenly. Clinically, none had evidence of valvular dysfunction, and necropsy did not provide explanations for death. In one patient dying suddenly with a porcine heterograft in the aortic position, a systolic pressure gradient of 35 mm Hg between left ventricle and brachial artery was documented 1 wk before death. At necropsy, thrombus was present within the sinuses of Valsalva of two of the three cusps. This was the only porcine valve to contain thrombus.

At necropsy, all seven porcine valves appeared in good condition: The leaflets were freely mobile, not thickened, and not calcified; the orifices were neither stenotic nor incompetent. On histologic section, the cusps were not inflammed or necrotic. Renal hemosiderosis was absent in all seven patients, and none had significant left ventricular endocardial thickening or ascending aortic intimal thickening.

The fresh autogenous pericardial valve fared less well. After only 39 days, it was approximately four times thicker than when inserted (Fig. 37). The thickening of the implanted pericardium resulted from proliferation of fibrous tissue organized from fibrin.

Tissue valves have certain advantages over caged-ball or disc prostheses: A central nonobstructive orifice causes less trauma to blood constituents and to adjacent vascular linings; thrombi are infrequent and, therefore, anticoagulants are unnecessary. Hemolysis is decreased, although significant hemolysis has been reported in fascia lata grafts that have become incompetent.[36] The long-term fate of these grafts, however, is as yet undetermined. A variety of tissue valves have been tried. Parietal pericardium is not a good valve substitute because it thickens rapidly and loses its mobility.[37,38] It also appears highly susceptible to infective endocarditis. Fascia lata is poor as a valve substitute because it is inherently too stiff and rapidly becomes even more stiff from fibrosis and calcification.[37,39]

The porcine aortic valve, when fixed in stabilized glutaraldehyde, appears to be a good valve substitute. Similar valves fixed in formalin, however, have rapidly degenerated.[37] The porcine valves in our seven patients were well preserved, and each appeared to have functioned normally, up to 14 mo after implantation in one patient. From clinical and morphologic standpoints, death in all seven appeared unrelated to the tissue valves *per se*. The porcine heterografts fixed in stabilized glutaraldehyde are promising, and deserve thorough and continuing clinical evaluation.

SUMMARY

Necropsy observations are described in 224 patients who died from 1963 through October 1972 after replacement of one or more cardiac valves by prostheses: 128 patients died within 2 mo of operation, and 96 patients at later periods up to 116 mo. Of the 281 valves replaced, Starr-Edwards prostheses were used in 250. Prosthetic dysfunction continues to be the most common cause of death (approximately 30%) in patients dying either early or late after valve replacement. It is hoped that the metal balls and cloth-covered struts will decrease the late frequency of prosthetic dysfunction, but not enough time has elapsed for this altered prosthesis to be tested adequately. Present data indicate that the frequency of clinical embolism and prosthetic thrombosis after use of the cloth-covered prostheses is less than that observed in the noncloth-covered prostheses. Cloth wear with possible dislodgement and increased intravascular hemolysis, however, remains of concern. The frequencies of peribasilar fistulae, infection at sites of attachment of prostheses, and aneurysm formation at sites of excision of left ventricular papillary muscles are decreasing. It appears that secondary left ventricular endocardial fibroelastosis after mitral replacement, aortic root and coronary ostial intimal proliferation after aortic valve replacement and calcification of valve anuli will only increase with time after valve replacement. The latter changes may prove to be major long-term problems.

It is clear after a decade of cardiac valve replacement that the ideal valve prosthesis is not yet available, or if available, not adequately tested. Thus, valve replacement at this time must be reserved for the patient severely disabled by cardiac valve disease.

APPENDIX

Table 1. Patients Studied at Necropsy After Cardiac Valve Replacement

Valve Replaced	Early Death (<2 mo)	Late Death (>2 mo)	Totals
Aortic (A)	42	47	89
Mitral (M)	52	28	80
A + M	20	18	38
Tricuspid (T)	2	0	2
T + A	1	0	1
T + M	8	2	10
T + M + A	3	1	4
Totals	128	96	224

Table 2. Age and Sex in 224 Necropsy Patients Dying After Cardiac Valve Replacement

	Early (<2 Mo) Deaths					Late (>2 Mo) Deaths				
Valve Replacement	No. Males	No. Females	Total Patients	Age Range	Average (Yr)	No. Males	No. Females	Total Patients	Age Range	Average (Yr)
Aortic (A)	29	13	42	5–65	45	44	3	47	21–69	46
Mitral (M)	25	27	52	4–63	43	11	17	28	15–65	48
A + M	12	8	20	25–27	46	16	2	18	23–63	49
Tricuspid (T)	0	2	2	42 & 57	49	0	0	0	—	—
T + A	1	0	1	20	20	0	0	0	—	—
T + M	1	7	8	32–57	45	0	2	2	49 & 51	50
T + M + A	2	1	3	33–54	45	0	1	1	52	52
Totals	70 (54%)	58 (46%)	128	4–67	(45)	71 (74%)	25 (26%)	96	15–69	(47)

Table 3. Types of Functional Valve Lesions Requiring Valve Replacement

Valve Replaced	Early Deaths: Stenosis	Early Deaths: Pure Regurgitation	Early Deaths: Totals	Late Deaths: Stenosis	Late Deaths: Pure Regurgitation	Late Deaths: Totals
Aortic (A)						
A only	26	16	42	34	13	47
A + M	12	8	20	14	4	18
A + M + T	2	1	3	1	0	1
A + T	0	1	1			
Mitral (M)						
M only	38	14	52	18	10	28
M + A	14	6	20	16	2	18
M + T	8	0	8	1	1	2
M + T + A	3	0	3	1	0	1
Tricuspid (T)						
T only	1	1	2	0	0	0
T + M	3	5	8	0	2	2
T + A	0	1	1	0	0	0
T + M + A	2	1	3	0	1	1
Totals	109	54	163	85	33	118
	(67%)	(33%)	(100%)	(72%)	(28%)	(100%)

Table 4. Prosthetic Valves Used in the 224 Necropsy Patients

Valve Replaced	Type Prosthesis: Starr-Edwards	Kay-Shiley	Magovern	Porcine Heterograft	Pericardial Valve	Totals
Aortic	127	0	4	1	0	132
Mitral	116	10	0	5	1	132
Tricuspid	7	9	0	1	0	17
Totals	250	19	4	7	1	281

Table 5. Sizes of Starr-Edwards Prostheses Employed

Valve Replaced	Valve Sizes							
Aortic	7A	8A	9A	10A	11A	12A	13A	Totals
Early deaths								
No.	3	22	17	12	7	2	1	64
(%)	(4)	(34)	(27)	(19)	(11)	(3)	(2)	(100)
Late deaths								
No.	2	17	9	15	16	2	2	63
(%)	(3)	(27)	(15)	(24)	(25)	(3)	(3)	(100)
Mitral	1M	2M	3M	4M				Totals
Early deaths								
No.	1	21	42	8				72
(%)	(1)	(29)	(59)	(11)				(100)
Late deaths								
No.		9	20	15				44
(%)		(21)	(45)	(34)				(100)
Tricuspid	2M	3M	4M					Totals
Early deaths								
No.	0	3	3					6
Late deaths								
No.	0	1	0					1
								250

Table 6. Weight (Range [Avg.]) of Hearts in Patients With Prosthetic Cardiac Valves

	Early (< 2 Mo) Deaths			Late (> 2 Mo) Deaths		
Valve Replaced	Males	Females	All	Males	Females	All
Aortic (A)	440–1250 (735)	450–800 (588)	440–1250 (694)	440–1350 (707)	330–340 (330)	330–1350 (699)
Mitral (M)	350– 850 (595)	300–600 (464)	300– 850 (517)	400– 870 (669)	370–800 (525)	370– 800 (610)
A + M	450–1090 (730)	440–550 (530)	440–1090 (657)	450– 960 (718)	420–530 (475)	420– 850 (688)
Tricuspid (T)	—	670 & 760 (715)	670 & 760 (700)	—	—	—
T + A	700 (700)		700 (700)			
T + M	390 (390)	350–680 (530)	350– 680 (530)	—	570 & 610 (590)	570 & 610 (590)
T + M + A	660 & 750 (705)	690	660 & 690 (700)	—	540	540 (540)

Table 7. Extramural Coronary Arterial Luminal Narrowing > 75% by Old Atheroscerotic Plaques in Patients With Prosthetic Cardiac Valves

	Early	Late
Aortic (A)	7 of 42	10 of 47
Mitral (M)	9 of 52	6 of 28
M + A	3 of 10	1 of 18
Tricuspid ± M ± A	0 of 14	0 of 3
	19 of 128 (15%)	17 of 96 (18%)

Table 8. Period of Time Between Valve Replacement and Death in the 128 Patients Dying Early

	Day of Death After Operation							
Valve Replaced	Zero	1–3	4–7	8–14	15–21	22–30	31–60	Totals
Aortic (A)	10	11	6	5	4	2	4	42
Mitral (M)	6	15	15	3	7	3	3	52
A + M	5	3	1	5	1	0	5	20
Tricuspid (T)	0	1	0	1	0	0	0	2
T + A	0	1	0	0	0	0	0	1
T + M	1	1	2	1	1	0	2	8
T + M + A	0	0	0	0	1	2	0	3
Totals	22*	32	24	15	14	7	14	128

*Sixteen patients died in the operating room.

Table 9. Prosthetic Stenosis* as a Cause of Early Death (<2 Mo)

	Total No. of Patients	Patients With Prosthetic Dysfunction	Prosthesis Size				
			SE 2M	SE 3M	SE 4M	K-S	Magovern
Mitral Valve	83	20 (24%)					
MS		18	4	11	1	2	0
MR		2	0	2	0	0	0
			SE 7A	SE 8A	SE 9A	SE 11A	
Aortic Valve	65	8 (12%)					
AS		2	0	1	0	0	1
AR		6	1	2	2	1	0

*Prosthetic stenosis caused by prostheses' being too big for ventricular cavity or aortic root.

Abbreviations: AS, aortic stenosis; AR, aortic regurgitation; K-S, Kay Shiley prosthesis; MR, mitral regurgitation; MS, mitral stenosis; SE, Starr-Edwards prosthesis.

Table 10. Causes of Death Early (<2 Mo) After Cardiac Valve Replacement (128 Necropsy Patients)

	Valves Replaced					
	Aortic (A)	Mitral (M)	M + A	Tricuspid (T)	T + M + A	Totals No. (%)
1. Prosthetic dysfunction	9	19	4	1	4	37(28)
Prosthesis too big for ventricular cavity or aortic root (prosthetic stenosis)	5	18	2	1	2	28
Prosthetic ball prevented from seating completely (prosthetic regurgitation)	2	0	0	0	2	4
Manufacturing error: low clearance with sticking of poppet	2	1	2	0	0	5
2. No anatomic cause	14	15	4	0	7	40(31)
Low cardiac output syndrome	7	13	3	0	7	30
Sudden (? arrhythmia)	4	2	1	0	0	7
Pump failure (in operating room)	3	0	0	0	0	3
3. Bleeding	7	2	2	0	1	12(10)
4. Technical mishap	5	3	4	0	0	12(10)
5. Central nervous system catastrophe	3	6	1	0	0	10(8)
6. Associated undiagnosed or uncorrected valve disease	1	4	1	1	0	7(5)
7. Infection	2	1	1	0	0	4(3)
At site of attachment of prosthesis	1	1	1	0	0	3
Other	1	0				1
8. Miscellaneous	1	2	3	0	0	6(5)
Totals	42	52	20	2	12	128(100)

Table 11. Myocardial Necrosis and Fibrosis in 128 Patients Dying *Early* After Cardiac Valve Replacement

	Aortic (A) (42 Patients)	Mitral (M) (52 Patients)	A + M (20 Patients)	Tricuspid ± M ± A (14 Patients)	Totals 128 Patients (%)
Myocardial necrosis, LV					
Papillary muscles only	6	26	3	7	42 (33)
Subendocardium*	6	10	3	1	20 (16)
Transmural†	4	10	4	3	21 (16)
Myocardial fibrosis, LV‡					
Papillary muscles only	4	10	0	2	16 (13)
Subendocardium*	14	5	5	2	26 (20)
Transmural†	4	3	0	1	8 (6)

*Inner half of wall of left ventricle (LV) or ventricular septum; papillary muscles usually also involved.

† Excludes patients with necrosis or fibrosis in the papillary muscle and subendocardial regions, although necrosis or fibrosis at these sites also usually are present.

‡ Replacement fibrosis only. Excludes interstitial and perivascular fibrosis, visible histologically, which occurred to varying degrees in most patients. Six patients with myocardial necrosis (four transmural) and 13 patients with myocardial fibrosis (four transmural) had luminal narrowing > 75% by old plaques of one or more of the three major extramural coronary arteries. In three patients, transmural necrosis involved only the free wall of the left ventricle at sites where excision of papillary muscles had occurred.

Table 12. Deaths Late (>2 Mo) After Cardiac Valve Replacement

			Prosthetic Thrombus				
Valve(s) Replaced	No. Patients	Implantation Periods (Mo) Range (Average)	No. Patients With Thrombi (No. Prostheses)	Patients With Thrombi on Warfarin	Thrombi Causing Dysfunction	*Clinical* Emboli	Ring* Leak
Aortic (A)	47	2.5–67 (26)	35 (35)	17	10	7	5
Mitral (M)	28	3–116 (38)	21 (21)	17	7	6	3
A + M	18	2.1–70 (20)	13 (21)	13	2	3	3
M + Tricuspid (T)	2	9 and 29 (19)	2 (4)	2	2	0	0
M + T + A	1	40	0	0	0	0	0
118 valves	96	2.1–116 (28)	71 (81)	49	21	16	11

*Patients with infective endocarditis at site of prosthesis were excluded.

Table 13. Causes of Death Late (>2 Mo) After Cardiac Valve Replacement (96 Necropsy Patients)

Cause	Valves Replaced				Totals
	Aortic (A)	Mitral (M)	M + A	Tricuspid + M	No. (%)
1. Prosthetic dysfunction	19	6	6	1	32 (33)
Degeneration, *silicone rubber ball*	13	2	3	0	18
Peribasilar leak	0	1	1	0	2
Prosthetic stenosis	4	0	1	1	6
Prosthetic thrombosis	0	1	0	0	1
Infective endocarditis	2	2	1	0	5
2. Factors *secondarily related* to prosthesis	6	9	5	0	20 (21)
Systemic embolism (acute)					
Myocardial infarction	2	2	1	0	5
Cerebral infarction	0	4	0	0	4
Bowel infarction	0	1	0	0	1
CNS hemorrhage from hypoprothrombinemia	2	2	1	0	5
Secondary endocardial fibrosis, LV *	0	0	2	0	2
Secondary intimal fibrosis, ascending aorta	2	0	0	0	2
Hepatitis	0	0	1	0	1
3. Sudden, cause uncertain	10	5	2	1	18 (19)
4. Underlying cardiac disease	9	6	3	1	19 (20)
Chronic CHF, cause uncertain	4	4	2	1	11
Extensive myocardial fibrosis, LV	1	0	1	0	2
Complications of Marfan Syndrome	2	0	0	0	2
Associated uncorrected valve disease	2	2	0	0	4
5. Noncardiac	3	2	2	0	7 (7)
Totals	47	28	18	3	96 (100)

Abbreviations: *CHF, congestive heart failure; CNS, central nervous system; LV, left ventricle.*

Table 14. Infection at Sites of Attachment of Starr-Edwards Prostheses

Patient	Age/Sex	Valve Replaced	Valve Infected	Interval Op→Death	Length of Infection	Precipitating Cause	Organism	Conduction Disturbance	Cause of Death
Early Deaths									
A63-176	55/M	Aortic	Aortic	45 days	45 days	Unknown	*Staphylococcus epidermidis*	1°HB, 2°HB LBBB	AR
A68-57	60/F	Mitral	Mitral	38 days	30 days	Wound infection	*Proteus mirabilis*	0	MS
A70-144	36/M	Aortic Mitral	Aortic	35 days	23 days	Wound infection	*Staphylococcus epidermidis*	0	Stroke AR
Late Deaths									
A64-189	51/M	Aortic	Aortic	13 mo	45 days	Teeth extractions	*Staphylococcus epidermidis*	LBBB	AR
A65-186	47/M	Mitral	Mitral	4 mo	30 days	Skin graft	*Staphylococcus aureus*	0	MS
A65-221	46/M	Mitral	Mitral	4 mo	25 days	Unknown	*Staphylococcus epidermidis*	0	MS
A67-22	48/M	Aortic	Aortic	3 mo	16 days	Unknown	*Staphylococcus epidermidis*	1°HB_N 2°HB, Nodal	AR
A68-33	57/M	Aortic Mitral	Aortic	7 mo	90 days	Wound infection	*Serratia marcescens*	1°HB LBBB	AR

Abbreviations: AR, aortic regurgitation; 1° HB, *PR interval* > 0.20 sec; 2° HB, second degree heart block; LBBB, left bundle branch block; MS, mitral stenosis.

Table 15. Status of Silicone Rubber Poppets Implanted 24 Mo or Longer

Valve	Total	Normal	Abnormal	Discolored but Functioned Normally	Discolored, Swollen and Impacted	Discolored, Fractured, Dislodged
Aortic						
No. Poppets	25	8	17	1	10	6
Implantation						
period (mo)		27–70	24–67	65	24–67	28–37
Range (average)		(45)	(41)		(43)	(33)
Mitral						
No. Poppets	17	12	5	3	2	0
Implantation						
period (mo)		28–116	78–114	105–114	78 and 94	0
Range (average)		(58)	(100)	(100)	(86)	
Totals	42	20	22	4	12	6

Table 16. Composition of Stellite 21

Chemical Element	Nominal Composition	Atomic Number	Atomic Weight
Cobalt (Co)	58%–69%	27	58.94
Chromium (Cr)	25%–30%	24	52.01
Molybdenum (Mo)	4.5%–6.5%	42	95.95
Nickel (Ni)	1.5%–3.5%	28	58.69
Iron (Fe)	Up to 2%	26	55.85
Carbon (C)	0.2%–0.4%	6	12.01

Table 17. Renal Hemosiderosis in Patients Dying Later After Cardiac Valve Replacement

Valve	No. Patients	Renal Iron			
		Absent	Present	3+ or 4+	1+ or 2+
Aortic	30	8	22	17	5
Aortic + mitral	8	2	6	5	1
Mitral	12	5	7	5	2
Mitral + tricuspid	1	0	1	0	1
Totals	51	15	36	27	9
		(29%)	(71%)		

Table 18. Fatal CNS Hemorrhage Associated With Hypoprothrombinemia After Cardiac Valve Replacement

Patient	Age/Sex	Interval (Mo) Op→Death	Hepatitis	Warfarin
S63-2617	23/M	2	+	+
A69-27	53/M	3	+	+
A69-292	44/F	4	+	+
A65-81	65/F	8	0	+
A67-29	69/M	14	0	+

Table 19. Calcification of Anulus After Mitral Valve Replacement

Patient	Age/Sex	Pre-op Mitral Lesion	Calcium MV Pre-op	Prosthetic Implantation Period (mos)	Calcium Prosthetic Anulus	Peribasilar Ring Leak
A67-118	47/M	Pure MR	0	44	+	0
A72-30	63/M	Pure MR	0	70	+	+
A70-123	49/F	Pure MR	0	79	+	0
A72-107	49/F	Pure MR	0	105	+	0
A72-44	45/F	Pure MR	0	111	+	0
A72-88	29/F	Pure MR	0	116	+	0

Abbreviations: MR, mitral regurgitation; MV, mitral valve.

Table 20. Necropsy Study of Cloth-covered Starr-Edwards Prostheses Implanted > 2 Mo (25 Prostheses in 20 Patients)

	No. Patients	Implantation Period Range (Average) (Mo)	Valve Model Numbers 2300/2310/2320			6300/6310/6320		
Aortic (A)	11	3–52 (23)	5	5	1	—	—	—
Mitral (M)	5	3–7 (5)	—	—	—	1	4	0
A + M	3	3–44 (18)	2	0	1	2	0	1
A + M + T	1	40	1	0	0	2	0	0
Totals	20	3–52 (18)	8	5	2	5	4	1

Table 21. Renal Hemosiderosis: Cloth-covered vs. Noncloth-covered Struts

	Rigid-framed Prosthesis in Patients Dying Late: Cloth-covered Struts	Noncloth-covered Struts
No. patients	14	35
No. aortics	10 (72%)	28 (80%)
No. with renal iron	12 (86%)	24 (69%)
No. with heavy deposits	10 (71%)	18 (51%)

Table 22. Myocardial Necrosis and Fibrosis in 96 Patients Dying Late After Cardiac Valve Replacement

	Aortic (A) 47 Patients	Mitral (M) 28 Patients	A + M 18 Patients	Tricuspid + Mitral 3 Patients	Totals 96 Patients (%)
Myocardial necrosis, LV					
Papillary muscles only	1	0	0	2	3(3)
Subendocardium*	0	0	1	0	1(1)
Transmural†	0	1	0	0	1(1)
Myocardial fibrosis, LV‡					
Papillary muscles only	14	5	7	4	30(31)
Subendocardium*	8	2	4	1	15(16)
Transmural†	14	10	3	0	27(28)

*Inner half of LV (left ventricular) free wall or ventricular septum. Papillary muscle also usually involved.

† Excludes patients with papillary muscle and subendocardial necrosis or fibrosis, although necrosis or fibrosis at these sites also was present in most of these patients.

‡ Replacement fibrosis only. Excludes interstitial and perivascular fibrosis, visible histologically, which occurred to varying degrees in most patients.

Table 23. Porcine Aortic Valve Heterografts

Patient	Age	Sex	Valve Replaced	Valve Size (mm)	Implantation Period (mo)	Cause of Death	Thrombus on Prosthesis	Renal Iron
Early (<2 mo)								
A70-280	60	M	MV	34	1.7	CNS catastrophe	0	0
A71-61	50	F	TV†	30	1.3	Bleeding	0	0
A71-101	44	M	MV	29	0.5	Unknown*	0	0
Late (>2 mo)								
A71-78	51	M	AV	25	5	Sudden	+	0
A71-113	55	F	MV	25	4	Unknown*	0	0
A71-181	64	F	MV	29	6	Unknown*	0	0
A72-190	50	F	MV	29	14	Sudden	0	0

*Inadequate cardiac output of uncertain etiology

† Mitral valve also replaced with tissue valve made of parietal pericardium.

Abbreviations: MV, mitral valve; TV, tricuspid valve; AV, aortic valve; CNS, central nervous system.

REFERENCES

1. Roberts WC: The structure of the aortic valve in clinically isolated aortic stenosis. An autopsy study of 162 patients over 15 years of age. Circulation 42:91, 1970

2. —: The congenitally bicuspid aortic valve. A study of 85 autopsy cases. Am J Cardiol 26:72, 1970

3. —: Anatomically isolated aortic valvular disease. The case against its being of rheumatic etiology. Am J Med 49:151, 1970

4. —, Braunwald E, Morrow AG: Acute severe mitral regurgitation secondary to ruptured chordae tendineae. Clinical hemodynamic and pathologic considerations. Circulation 33:58, 1966

5. —: Examining the precordium and the heart. Chest 57:567, 1970

6. Helmsworth JA, Gall EA, Perrin EV, et al: Occurrence of emboli during perfusion with an oxygenator pump. Surgery 53:177, 1963

7. Roberts WC, Morrow AG: Cardiac valves and the surgical pathologist. Arch Pathol 82:309, 1966

8. —, —: Causes of early postoperative death following cardiac valve replacement. J Thorac Cardiovasc Surg 54:422, 1967

9. —, —: Compression of anomalous left circumflex coronary arteries by prosthetic valve fixation rings. J Thorac Cardiovasc Surg 57:834, 1969

10. —, —: Anatomic studies of hearts containing caged-ball prosthetic valves. Johns Hopkins Med J 121:271, 1967

11. —, Lambird PA, Gott VL et al: Fatal aortic regurgitation following replacement of the mitral and aortic valves. A mechanical complication of double valve replacement. J Thorac Cardiovasc Surg 52:189, 1966

12. —, Morrow AG: Mechanisms of acute left atrial thrombosis after mitral valve replacement. Am J Cardiol 18:497, 1966

13. Glancy DL, O'Brien KP, Reis RL, et al: Hemodynamic studies in patients with 2M and 3M Starr-Edwards prostheses: Evidence of obstruction to the left atrial emptying. Circulation 39 and 40 (Suppl. I): I/113, 1969

14. Reis RL, Glancy DL, O'Brien K, et al: Clinical and hemodynamic assessments of fabric-covered Starr-Edwards prosthetic valves. J Thorac Cardiovasc Surg 59:84, 1970

15. Buja LM, Freed TA, Berman MA, et al: Pulmonary alveolar hemorrhage. A common finding in patients with severe cardiac disease. Am J Cardiol 27:168, 1971

16. Taber RE, Morales AR, Fine G: Myocardial necrosis and the postoperative low-cardiac-output syndrome. Ann Thorac Surg 4:12, 1967

17. Morales AR, Fine G, Taber RE: Cardiac surgery and myocardial necrosis. Arch Pathol 83:71, 1967

18. Niles NR, Sandilands JR: Pathology of heart valve replacement surgery: Autopsies of 62 patients with Starr-Edwards prostheses. Dis Chest 56:373, 1969

19. Reichenbach DD, Benditt EP: Myofibrillar degeneration. A response of the myocardial cell to injury. Arch Pathol 85:189, 1968

20. Buja LM, Levitsky S, Ferrans VJ, et al: Acute and chronic effects of normothermic anoxia on canine hearts: Light and electron microscopic evaluation. Circulation 43 and 44 (Suppl. I): I/44, 1971

21. Roberts WC, Morrow AG: Late postoperative pathological findings after cardiac valve replacement. Circulation 35 and 36 (Suppl. I): I/48, 1967

22. —, —: Later postoperative pathologic findings following cardiac valve replacement with Starr-Edwards prostheses, in Brewer LA III (ed): Prosthetic Heart Valves. Springfield, Ill, Thomas, 1969

23. —, Berard CW, Braunwald NS: Roentgenogram of the month. Dis Chest 51:439, 1967

24. Rockoff SD, Ross J Jr, Oldham NN Jr, et al: Ventriculo-atrial regurgitation following prosthetic replacement of the mitral valve. Angiocardiographic and hemodynamic findings. Am J Cardiol 17:817, 1966

25. Cohn LH, Roberts WC, Rockoff SD, et al: Bacterial endocarditis following aortic valve replacement. Clinical and pathologic correlations. Circulation 33:209, 1966

26. Roberts WC, Morrow AG: Bacterial endocarditis involving prosthetic mitral valves. Clinical and pathologic observation. Arch Pathol 82:164, 1966

27. —, Levinson GE, Morrow AG: Lethal ball variance in the Starr-Edwards prosthetic *mitral* valve. Arch Intern Med 126:517, 1970

28. —, Morrow AG: Fatal degeneration of the silicone rubber ball of the Starr-Edwards prosthetic aortic valve. Am J Cardiol 22:614, 1968

29. —, —: Renal hemosiderosis in patients with prosthetic aortic valves. Circulation 33:390, 1966

30. —: Renal hemosiderosis (blue kidney) in patients with valvular heart disease. Am J Path 38:409, 1966

31. —, Morrow AG: Secondary left ventricular endocardial fibroelastosis following mitral valve replacement. Cause of cardiac failure in the late postoperative period. Circulation 37 and 38 (Suppl. II): II/101, 1968

32. —, Reis RL, Ferrans VJ, et al: Anatomic studies on cloth-covered Starr-Edwards prosthetic valves implanted for longer than two months (abstract). Am J Cardiol 29:287, 1972

33. Winter TQ, Reis RL, Glancy DL, et al: Current status of the Starr-Edwards cloth-covered prosthetic cardiac valves. Circulation 45 and 46 (Suppl I):I/14, 1972

34. Isom OW, Williams CD, Falk EA, and et al: Long-term evaluation of cloth-covered metallic ball prostheses. J Thorac Cardiovasc Surg 64:354, 1972

35. Hodam R, Anderson R, Starr A, et al: Further evaluation of the composite seat cloth-covered aortic prosthesis. Ann Thorac Surg 12:621, 1971

36. Dave KS, Madan CK, Pakrashi BC, et al: Chronic hemolysis following fascia lata and Starr-Edwards aortic valve replacement. Circulation 46:240, 1972

37. Yarbrough JW, Roberts WC, Reis RL: Structural alterations in tissue cardiac valves implanted in humans and calves. J Thorac Cardiovasc Surg, in press

38. Suzuki A, Mackrell J, Kay EB: Mitral valve replacement with transplant valves. J Thorac Cardiovasc Surg 60:13, 1970

39. McEnany MT, Ross DN, Yates AK: Valve failure in seventy-two frame-supported autologous fascia lata mitral valves. Two-year follow-up. J Thorac Cardiovasc Surg 63:199, 1972

40. Shepherd RL, Glancy DL, Stinson EB, et al: Hemodynamic confirmation of obstruction to left ventricular inflow by a caged-ball prosthetic mitral valve. J Thorac Cardiovasc Surg 65:252, 1973

Operative Treatment of Hypertrophic Obstructive Cardiomyopathy

The Case Against Mitral Valve Replacement

WILLIAM C. ROBERTS, MD, FACC
Bethesda, Maryland

In the January 1973 issue of this Journal, Cooley et al.[1] proposed that "mitral valve replacement should be considered the surgical procedure of choice in patients with advanced hypertrophic stenosis." This conclusion was based on "excellent" operative results from mitral valve replacement in nine patients, two of whom died, with hypertrophic obstructive cardiomyopathy. Cooley and associates switched from partial resection of the ventricular septum in this condition to mitral valve replacement because (1) valve replacement relieved both the left ventricular outflow systolic pressure gradient and the mitral regurgitation; (2) postoperative conduction disturbances were reduced; (3) the septectomy procedure failed "to obtain complete or even acceptable relief of the stenotic gradient;" and (4) "many of the patients who initially obtained an adequate result [from septectomy] later experienced gradual recurrence of the obstructive hypertrophy." Because Cooley et al. did not discuss or reference results of others using the partial septectomy technique, it seemed appropriate to summarize reported results from the septectomy procedure and to discuss the advantages and disadvantages of partial septectomy versus mitral valve replacement for hypertrophic obstructive cardiomyopathy in light of these results.

Results of septectomy performed by five different surgeons are summarized in Table I.[2-6] Results in 26 patients operated on by Cooley using the septectomy technique also are included. The mortality rate for the 167 patients was 19 percent. Ninety-five of the 126 survivors (75 percent) of the operative procedure were in functional class III or IV (New York Heart Association classification) preoperatively and only 6 (5 percent) were in class III or IV postoperatively. Thus, *clinical improvement by septectomy is usually excellent.*

Septectomy usually completely alleviates the left ventricular outflow tract gradient. In 68 of the tabulated 167 patients, left ventricular and systemic arterial pressures were measured both pre- and postoperatively (Table II). In 80 percent (54 patients) no left ventricular outflow tract pressure gradient at rest was present postoperatively; in another 16 percent the pressure gradient was ≤20 mm Hg, and only 4 percent had a gradient >20 mm Hg postoperatively. Small (<25 mm Hg) gradients could be provoked postoperatively in most patients.[2,4,5] Resting gradients have been observed at catheterization during the first year postoperatively when no gradients were evident at later studies.[2,4] In no reported cases has there been any recurrence or exacerbation of outflow obstruction at any time after operation.

The left ventricular end-diastolic pressure usually decreases after septectomy. Left ventricular end-diastolic pressure decreased in 55 of 76 patients (72 percent) in whom it was measured both before and after septectomy (Table III). Preoperatively, it was increased (>12 mm Hg) in 54 patients (71 percent), and postoperatively in 36 patients (47 percent). The left ventricular end-diastolic pressure in the 76 patients averaged 19 mm Hg preoperatively and 13 mm Hg postoperatively.

Mitral regurgitation, a well recognized accompaniment of hypertrophic obstructive cardiomyopathy, usually disappears after septectomy. In 14 patients operated on by Morrow et al.[2] in whom adequate left ventricular contrast studies were obtained both pre- and postoperatively, mitral regurgitation was evident before operation in 13, and postoperatively in 2 (mild in each). Of 21 patients operated on by Barratt-Boyes[4] in whom postoperative angiographic studies were performed, 18 had no mitral regurgitation, 2 had mild and 1 had moderate regurgitation.

Cooley et al. also were among those (Table I) describing favorable results with partial ventricular septectomy: "with two exceptions, striking clinical inprovement followed septal myocardiectomy in nearly every surviving patient who was symptomatic before operation."[6] Septectomy was carried out from a right ventricular approach in 10 of their 26 patients, in part because this approach prevented "damage to the mitral valve suspension."[6] Cooley et al. subsequently abandoned septectomy, however,

Address for reprints: William C. Roberts, MD, Section of Pathology, National Heart and Lung Institute, National Institutes of Health, Bethesda, Md. 20014.

TABLE I

Results of Septectomy

Authors	Patients (total no.)	Preoperative Functional Class of Survivors I	II	III	IV	Postoperative Functional Class of Survivors I	II	III	IV	Deaths
Morrow et al.[2]	43	0*	1*	17*	13*	22*	9*	0*	0*	6
Tajik et al.[3]	43	2*	3*	23*	0*	12*	13*	2*	1*	11
Barratt-Boyes and O'Brien[4]	30	1	12	7	7	24	2	1	0	3
Adelman et al.[5]	25	2	3	14		8	11	0	0	6
Cooley et al.[6]	26	2	5	14	0	19		2	0	5
Totals	167	31 (25%)		95 (75%)		120 (95%)		6 (5%)		31
		126				126				(19%)

* Includes only those patients followed up more than 12 months after septectomy.

and now consider mitral valve replacement the operative procedure of choice for hypertrophic obstructive cardiomyopathy. This conclusion is based on early (up to 18 month follow-up) results in only nine patients, two of whom died; results in the other seven are described as "excellent." A "low profile disc valve with full orifice design" was employed (Biork-Shiley tilting disc valve or the Cooley-Cutter disc valve). Cardiac catheterization (performed 2 weeks to 8 months postoperatively) in eight of the nine patients disclosed small (5 to 15 mm Hg) left ventricular to systemic arterial peak systolic pressure gradients in eight and no gradient in one. Left ventricular end-diastolic pressure averaged 21 mm Hg preoperatively, and 12 mm Hg postoperatively.

A major reason given by Cooley et al. for advocating mitral valve replacement rather than septectomy was that valve replacement alleviated both the left ventricular outflow obstruction and, at the same time, the accompanying mitral regurgitation. But septectomy also relieves both disorders and it relieves the outflow gradient more completely. In only 1 of the 7 surviving patients of Cooley et al. was the left ventricular outflow gradient in fact totally relieved by mitral valve replacement, whereas in 80 percent of 68 patients treated by septectomy (Table II), the left ventricular outflow gradient was totally obliterated. Moreover, mitral regurgitation (as proved by left ventricular angiography) is infrequent after septectomy.[2,4] It is assumed that mitral regurgitation was also obliterated in the patients of Cooley et al., but left ventricular angiography was not performed postoperatively in any of them, and the clinical diagnosis of mitral regurgitation after mitral valve replacement may be difficult without left ventricular angiography.[7]

Cooley et al. also stressed that the mitral valve leaflets are anatomically abnormal and that their chordal attachments are bizarre in hypertrophic cardiomyopathy. Fibrous thickening of these leaflets and chordae, well recognized in this condition,[8-13] is not the cause of the regurgitation because the latter

TABLE II

Effect of Septectomy on Left Ventricular Outflow Tract Obstruction

Author	Patients Undergoing Septectomy (no.)	Patients with Both Pre- and Postop Catheterization Data (no.)	Postoperative: Patients with No PSG (no.)	Patients with PSG ≤20 mm Hg (no.)	Patients with PSG >20 mm Hg (no.)
Morrow et al.[2]	43	29	27	2	0
Tajik et al.[3]	43	0	...	...	...
Barratt-Boyes and O'Brien[4]	30	22	18	2	2
Adelman et al.[5]	25	11	8	3	0
Cooley et al.[6]	26	6	1	4	1
Totals	167	68	54 (80%)	11 (16%)	3 (4%)

Postop = postoperative; PSG = peak systolic pressure gradient at rest between left ventricle and systemic artery.

TABLE III

Effect of Septectomy on Left-Ventricular End-Diastolic Pressure (LVEDP)

		Preoperative				Postoperative			
Author	Patients (total (no.)	Patients with Pre- and Postop LVEDP Recorded (no.)	Patients with LVEDP >12 mm Hg (no.)	Patients with LVEDP ≤12 mm Hg (no.)	Average LVEDP (mm Hg)	Patients with LVEDP >12 mm Hg (no.)	Patients with LVEDP ≤12 mm Hg (no.)	Patients with Reduced LVEDP ↓ (no.)	Average LVEDP (mm Hg)
Morrow et al.[2]	43	29	21	8	20	17	12	24	12
Tajik et al.[3]	43	...	...	...	...	...	...	...	...
Barratt-Boyes and O'Brien[4]	30	22	12	10	13	4	18	13	8
Adelman et al.[5]	25	19	16	3	21	12	7	14	16
Cooley et al.[6]	26	6	5	1	21	3	3	4	17
Totals	167	76	54 (71%)	22 (29%)	19	36 (47%)	40 (53%)	55 (72%)	13

disappears after septectomy.[2,4] Rather, the regurgitation appears to result from malalignment of the left ventricular papillary muscles,[14] particularly the anterolateral one. The bending of these structures by the disproportionally thickened ventricular septum is relieved by septectomy, but it is uncertain whether it is relieved by mitral valve replacement.

Another advantage of mitral valve replacement over septectomy according to Cooley et al. is that there are fewer postoperative conduction disturbances. In nearly all patients undergoing septectomy from the left ventricular side left bundle branch block or hemiblock develops, and in nearly all undergoing septectomy from the right side right bundle branch block develops. Complete heart block is infrequent. It appears unlikely, however, that left bundle branch block produced by septectomy has the same prognostic significance as that produced by its more common cause, coronary atherosclerosis. But if the patient has right bundle branch block preoperatively—and this occurs in about 3 percent of patients with hypertrophic obstructive cardiomyopathy[15]—septectomy, at least from the left side, should not be performed. Thus, conduction disturbances are consequences of septectomy, but they infrequently cause major complications, and these complications do not compare to those associated with prosthetic cardiac valves.

Cooley's major criticism of the septectomy procedure was that it failed "to obtain complete or even acceptable relief of the stenotic gradient," and that "many of the patients who initially obtained an adequate result [from septectomy] later experienced gradual recurrence of the obstructive hypertrophy." Both claims are incorrect. Hemodynamic data (Table II) show that the outflow gradient is usually completely abolished by septectomy. Furthermore, left ventricular outflow obstruction has never been reported to develop after septectomy in any patient during long postoperative follow-up periods. Symptomatic improvement also has been long-lasting.[2-4]

Thus, mitral valve replacement has few advantages and several disadvantages compared to septectomy as the operative procedure of choice for patients with hypertrophic obstructive cardiomyopathy. Because complications inherent to prosthetic valves are so common, results of valve replacement for this condition must be unequivocally better than those from the other procedure (septectomy) to justify this radical approach. To conclude, as did Cooley et al., that "mitral valve replacement should be considered the surgical procedure of choice in patients with advanced hypertrophic stenosis"[1] on the basis of their preliminary and incomplete data in nine patients is unjustified and dangerous. No information, for example, regarding the hemodynamic status of the mitral valve prostheses was presented. That mitral regurgitation was eliminated has not been documented and, of more concern, there is no evidence that mitral stenosis has not been added. Some degree of prosthetic obstruction occurs after every mitral valve replacement utilizing a low-profile prosthesis.[16] When replacement is carried out in patients with a small left ventricular cavity, as is the case with hypertrophic obstructive cardiomyopathy, the likelihood of considerable prosthetic obstruction is much greater. The left ventricle in hypertrophic obstructive cardiomyopathy is too small to accommodate a caged-ball type mitral prosthesis—indeed, its insertion in this condition has proved disastrous—and low-profile valves even of "smaller than usual diameter"[1] and of the central flow type do not assure against prosthetic dysfunction. Impairment to left ventricular filling occurs naturally in hypertrophic obstructive cardiomyopathy,[17] and this impairment may well be increased after mitral valve replacement. The need for anticoagulant agents in patients with a prosthetic mitral valve adds another serious long-term disadvantage to this procedure.

The most dangerous aspect of valve replacement for hypertrophic obstructive cardiomyopathy, however, is that a new disease—namely, "prosthetic cardiac valve"—is introduced and *it has a higher 5 year mortality rate than does symptomatic hypertrophic obstructive cardiomyopathy,* whether or not septectomy is performed. Of 100 patients who underwent mitral valve replacement for stenosis or regurgitation, or both, by Morrow,[18] only 63 percent are alive 5 years after operation and only 51 percent after 8 years, and these long-term results are as good as any reported. There have been several changes in prostheses subsequently but there is no proof that the presently employed prostheses, including the Cooley-Cutter disc valve, will provide better long-term results than those obtained by Levine et al.[18] The survival rate for symptomatic hypertrophic obstructive cardiomyopathy even without septectomy is better.[19] Of 56 patients followed up at the National Heart and Lung Institute for up to 12 years (average 32 months) with hypertrophic obstructive cardiomyopathy, 47 (84 percent) are alive and all were in functional class II, III or IV (New York Heart Association) when initially examined.

Mitral valve replacement cannot be justified by the facts presented here or by any theoretical considerations. Mitral replacement for hypertrophic obstructive cardiomyopathy is not directed at the primary fault, namely, disproportional hypertrophy of the ventricular septum; that is, the septum is considerably thicker than the left ventricular free wall.[8,10-13,20,21] Ultrastructural[22] and histologic studies[21] have shown that the myocardial fibers in the ventricular septum are bizarre in appearance and have abnormal orientations one to another. In contrast, the orientations of the myocardial fibers in the free walls are normal. The left ventricular outflow obstruction is produced by contact of the anterior mitral leaflet and the thickened ventricular septum during systole. Fibrous thickening of the mitral valve leaflets and chordae results from this contact, which is alleviated by septectomy. Mitral valve replacement also nearly obliterates the left ventricular outflow gradient, as Cooley et al. have nicely shown, but the vigorous contractions of the ventricular septum may remain. After septectomy, the left ventricular cavity dilates to near normal proportions,[21] that is, similar to those of the left ventricular free wall. In contrast, there is no indication that the septum gets thinner or that the left ventricular cavity increases to normal size after valve replacement. Because the cavity is still small and the septum still disproportionally hypertrophied, the septum may contact the inserted prosthetic mitral valve during ventricular systole as it does the anterior mitral leaflet before replacement. This contact could produce prosthetic dysfunction.

In an occasional patient with hypertrophic obstructive cardiomyopathy the ascending aorta is too small to allow septectomy by way of the aorta alone. An alternate surgical procedure, therefore, is necessary in these patients. Septectomy by way of the right ventricle rather than mitral valve replacement may still be the more reasonable procedure because of complications inherent to valvular prostheses, and because left ventricular incisions may lead to incisional aneurysms.

In summary, the conclusion of Cooley et al. that mitral valve replacement is "the surgical procedure of choice" for patients with hypertrophic obstructive cardiomypathy is at best premature and potentially dangerous. The mortality rate from the prosthesis alone is greater than that for the underlying disease, hypertrophic obstructive cardiomyopathy. Furthermore, everything that can be accomplished by mitral valve replacement can be better accomplished by septectomy. Septectomy more completely abolishes the left ventricular outflow tract pressure gradient and at the same time alleviates the associated mitral regurgitation. Moreover, septectomy, by attacking the primary fault, abolishes the disproportional hypertrophy of the ventricular septum, and in so doing allows the left ventricular cavity to dilate to normal dimensions. There is no evidence at this time that the disproportional ventricular septal hypertrophy is relieved or that the left ventricle dilates after mitral valve replacement. And, finally, there is no evidence that the mitral prosthesis, inserted in the small left ventricle, functions normally.

References

1. **Cooley DA, Leachman RD, Wukasch DC:** Diffuse muscular subaortic stenosis: surgical treatment. Amer J Cardiol 31:1-6, 1973.
2. **Morrow AG, Epstein SE, Rodgers BM, et al:** Idiopathic hypertrophic subaortic stenosis: a current assessment of the results of operative treatment. In, Hypertrophic Obstructive Cardiomyopathy (Wolstenholme GEW, O'Connor M, ed). London, J & A Churchill, 1971, p 140–149
3. **Tajik AJ, Giuliani ER, Frye RL, et al:** Idiopathic hypertrophic subaortic stenosis (IHSS); results of long-term surgical follow-up (abstr). Amer J Cardiol 31:161, 1973
4. **Barratt-Boyes BG, O'Brien KP:** Surgical treatment of idiopathic hypertrophic subaortic stenosis using a combined left ventricular-aortic approach. In Ref 2, p 150–159
5. **Adelman AG, Wigle ED, Ranganathan N, et al:** The clinical course in muscular subaortic stenosis. A retrospective and prospective study of 60 hemodynamically proved cases. Ann Intern Med 77:515–525, 1972
6. **Cooley DA, Bloodwell RD, Hallman GL, et al:** Surgical treatment of muscular subaortic stenosis. Results from septectomy in twenty-six patients. Circulation 35 & 36: suppl I: I-124–I-132, 1967
7. **Rockoff SD, Ross J Jr, Oldham NN Jr, et al:** Ventriculo-atrial regurgitation following prosthetic replacement of the mitral valve. Angiocardiographic and hemodynamic findings. Amer J Cardiol 17:817–824, 1966
8. **Morrow AG, Roberts WC, Ross J Jr, et al:** Obstruction to left ventricular outflow. Current concepts of management and operative treatment. Ann Intern Med 69:1255–1286, 1968
9. **Ewy GA, Marcus FI, Bohajalian O, et al:** Muscular subaortic stenosis. Clinical and pathologic observations in an elderly patient. Amer J Cardiol 22:126–132, 1968
10. **Roberts WC:** Pathologic aspects of valvular and subvalvular (discrete and diffuse) aortic stenosis. In, The Natural History and Progress in Treatment of Congenital Heart Defects. An International Symposium Sponsored by the Ontario Heart Foundation in Cooperation with the Hospital for Sick Children and the University of Toronto (Kidd BSL, Keith JD, ed). Springfield, Ill, Charles C Thomas, 1971, p 221
11. **Roberts WC, Perloff JK:** Mitral valvular disease. A clini-

copathologic survey of the conditions causing the mitral valve to function abnormally. Ann Intern Med 77:939–975, 1972

12. **Roberts WC:** Valvular, subvalvular, and supravalvular aortic stenosis: morphologic features. Cardiovasc Clin 7:140–121, 1973
13. **Roberts WC, Dangel JC, Bulkley BH:** Non-rheumatic valvular cardiac disease. A clinico-pathologic survey of 27 different conditions causing valvular dysfunction. Cardiovasc Clin 5:332–446, 1973
14. **Adelman, AG, McLoughlin MJ, Marquis Y, et al:** Left ventricular cineangiographic observations in muscular subaortic stenosis. Amer J Cardiol 24:689–697, 1969
15. **Braunwald E, Lambrew CT, Rockoff SD, et al:** Idiopathic hypertrophic subaortic stenosis: I. A description of the disease based upon an analysis of 64 patients. Suppl. to Circulation 29 & 30: suppl IV: IV-3–IV-119, 1964
16. **Hawe A, Frye RL, Ellis FH Jr:** Late hemodynamic studies after mitral valve surgery. J Thorac Cardiovasc Surg 65:351–358, 1973
17. **Stewart S, Mason DT, Braunwald E:** Impaired rate of left ventricular filling in idiopathic hypertrophic subaortic stenosis and valvular aortic stenosis. Circulation 37:8–14, 1968
18. **Levine FH, Copeland JG, Morrow AG:** Prosthetic replacement of the mitral valve: continuing assessments of the 100 patients operated upon during 1961–1965. Circulation 47:518–526, 1973
19. **Frank S, Braunwald E:** Idiopathic hypertrophic subaortic stenosis. Clinical analysis of 126 patients with emphasis on the natural history. Circulation 37:759–788, 1968
20. **Henry WL, Clark CE, Epstein SE:** Asymmetric septal hypertrophy. Echocardiographic identification of the pathognomonic anatomic abnormality of IHSS. Circulation 47:225–233, 1973
21. **Roberts WC, Ferrans VJ:** The pathologic anatomy of the cardiomyopathies (idiopathic dilated and hypertrophic types, infiltrative types and endomyocardial disease with and without eosinophilia). Circ Res: suppl: in press
22. **Ferrans VJ, Morrow AG, Roberts WC:** Myocardial ultrastructure in idiopathic hypertrophic subaortic stenosis. A study of operatively excised left ventricular tract muscle in 14 patients. Circulation 45:769–792, 1972

Ankylosing Spondylitis and Aortic Regurgitation

Description of the Characteristic Cardiovascular Lesion From Study of Eight Necropsy Patients

By BERNADINE H. BULKLEY, M.D., AND WILLIAM C. ROBERTS, M.D.

SUMMARY

Clinical and cardiovascular necropsy findings are described in eight patients with combined ankylosing spondylitis and aortic regurgitation. All were men (aged 34-55 years), each had peripheral arthritis in addition to spondylitis, all had severe congestive failure, and six had conduction disturbances. In three patients aortic regurgitation was present before distinctive radiologic changes of ankylosing spondylitis were apparent and only two patients had advanced arthritic changes of ankylosing spondylitis. Thus, cardiac dysfunction may be present before signs of spondylitis are apparent, and aortic regurgitation may be severe when signs of spondylitis are minimal. A characteristic cardiovascular morphologic abnormality was present in each patient. The aortic valve cusps and the aorta behind and immediately above the sinuses of Valsalva were thickened, the latter by dense adventitial scar tissue and by intimal fibrous proliferation. In each patient the scar tissue in the root of aorta extended below the base of aortic valve to produce a subaortic fibrous ridge. The subaortic bump involves the base of anterior mitral leaflet and may cause mitral regurgitation. Extension of the fibrous scar into ventricular septum may cause heart block. The distinctive cardiovascular morphologic findings in patients with ankylosing spondylitis clearly separate this condition from syphilis and other entities associated with aortic regurgitation.

Additional Indexing Words:
Valvular heart disease   Syphilis   Rheumatoid arthritis

ANKYLOSING SPONDYLITIS and rheumatoid arthritis were recognized as distinct entities about 15 years ago.[1-5] Subsequently, aortic regurgitation was recognized as a fairly frequent accompaniment of ankylosing spondylitis, but as an extremely rare accompaniment of rheumatoid arthritis. Despite several reports on lesions of aortic valve and aorta in ankylosing spondylitis, the distinctive features of the cardiovascular lesions have not been defined. Study of eight necropsy patients with combined ankylosing spondylitis and aortic regurgitation disclosed distinctive cardiovascular abnormalities in each. This report describes the cardiovascular findings in these eight patients, and calls attention to the unique features of the cardiovascular lesions.

From the Section of Pathology, National Heart and Lung Institute, National Institutes of Health, Bethesda, Maryland.

Address for reprints: William C. Roberts, M.D., Section of Pathology, National Heart and Lung Institute, National Institutes of Health, Bethesda, Maryland 20014.

Received May 21, 1973; revision accepted for publication June 28, 1973.

Methods

The clinical records, heart specimens and histologic sections were reexamined in all eight patients. At least two sections of ascending aorta, two of left ventricle, one of aortic valve, and two of mitral valve were examined in each patient. Radiographs, gross specimens and histologic sections of involved joints were examined in seven of eight patients. The morphologic cardiovascular findings in these eight patients were compared with the necropsy findings associated with aortic regurgitation in 20 patients with cardiovascular syphilis, three with rheumatoid arthritis, and 11 with the Marfan syndrome.

Results

Clinical Findings

Pertinent findings in the eight patients are summarized in tables 1 and 2. The patients ranged in age from 34–57 years (average 46) and all were men. In addition to spondylitis, all eight patients had peripheral arthritis. One patient also had Reiter's syndrome. Symptoms of arthritis developed at an average age of 26 years, precordial murmurs at 32 and congestive cardiac failure at 41. The duration of arthritic symptoms averaged 21 years, valvular dysfunction 16 years, and congestive

Table 1

Clinical and Necropsy Observations in Eight Patients

Patient	Age at death (yrs.)	Age at onset arthritis (yrs.)	Clinical: Age onset in years, Murmur	Age onset in years, CHF	Duration in years, Arthritis	Duration in years, Murmur	Duration in years, CHF	ECG: Conduction disturbances	Hemodynamics: Pressures (mm Hg), LV	Pressures (mm Hg), SA	Heart weight (gms)	Cardiovascular pathology: Thick AV cusps	Sub-AV fibrosis	Thickening of aorta limited to sinuses
1 A61-99	52*	24	37	43	28*	15*	9	1° HB RBBB	160/18	168/30	850	+	+	+
2 A61-262	55	45	45	53	15	15	2	1° HB	114/40	124/40	680	+	+	+
3 A61-274	34*	18	31	31	16*	3*	3	1° HB	100/22	120/25	700	+	+	+
4 A64-17	35*	6	6	29	29*	29*	6	0	170/12	170/50	840	+	+	+
5 A66-127	57	42	41	55	16	17	2	0	—	180/40	520	+	+	+
6 A68-142	38*	13	14	32	25*	24*	6	1° HB	170/16	190/20	1100	+	+	+
7 A68-300	54	40	40	48	14	14	6	CHB	170/50	170/50	620	+	+	+
8 A68-350	46*	18	38	38	28*	8y*	8	LBBB	128/32	128/32	610	+	+	+
Average	46	26	32	41	21	16	6				740			

*Each underwent aortic valve replacement: 3 died within a month of operation and the other 2 at 18 and 19 months, respectively, after operation.

Abbreviations: AR = aortic regurgitation; AV = aortic valve; CHB = complete heart block; CHF = congestive cardiac failure; 1° HB = first degree heart block (P-R interval > 0.20 sec); LBBB = left bundle branch block; LV = left ventricle; RBBB = right bundle branch block; SA = systemic artery.

failure six years. Conduction disturbances were present in six patients: prolonged (> 0.20 sec) P-R intervals in four, complete left bundle branch block in one, complete right bundle branch block in one, and complete heart block in one. In four patients precordial murmurs were noted at the same time or within one year of onset of joint symptoms. In three patients aortic regurgitation was diagnosed before distinctive radiologic changes of ankylosing spondylitis were present, and a clinical explanation for valvular dysfunction was initially uncertain. All patients had severe congestive cardiac failure and each was in functional class III or IV (New York Heart Association classification). One patient had mild mitral regurgitation documented by left ventricular angiogram. Aortic valve replacement was carried out in five patients; four died within two months, the fifth 12 months later. Each of the three non-operated patients died of congestive cardiac failure.

Necropsy Findings

Cardiovascular necropsy findings in several patients are illustrated in figures 1–7. The hearts weighed 520 to 1100 gms (avg. 740). The ascending aortas including the sinuses of Valsalva were mildly dilated in all eight patients. The aortic walls behind and immediately above the sinuses of Valsalva, especially that portion behind the comissures, were thickened, up to five times normal. The thickening of aorta resulted primarily from adventitial scarring and intimal proliferation. Although focally scarred, the media was not thickened. Many vasa vasora were surrounded by collections of plasma cells and lymphocytes and their lumens often were narrowed. In all eight patients the adventitial scarring was present in the groove between aortic valve cusps and anterior mitral leaflet producing a ridge beneath aortic valve, especially the basal portion of anterior mitral leaflet. The adventitial scarring in each patient also was continuous with similar scarring in membranous ventricular septum. The aortic valves in all eight patients appeared incompetent. Both basal and distal portions of the cusps were shortened and thickened by fibrous tissue. The fibrous thickening of aortic wall behind the commissures caused the cusps to sag toward left ventricle. The commissures, however, were neither widened nor fused. The coronary ostia were widely patent. The parietal and viseral pericardia were diffusely adherent to one another in the five patients with previous thoracotomies but the pericardium was normal in the

Table 2

Arthritic Features of Eight Patients with Ankylosing Spondylitis and Aortic Regurgitation

		No. patients
I. *Clinical abnormalities*		8/8
Back pain		8
Restricted spinal movement		8
Dorsal kyphosis		4
Peripheral arthritis		8
Urethritis alone		2
Urethritis + iritis (Reiter's)		1
Negative rheumatoid factor		8
Negative STS		8
II. *Radiologic abnormalities*		7/7
Sacroiliac joints		7
Blurred	(7)	
Fused	(3)	
Vertebral bodies		6
Squared	(6)	
Narrowing IV space	(6)	
Calcification, discs	(4)	
Calcification, ligaments	(2)	
Peripheral joints		1
Ankylosis	(1)	
III. *Morphologic abnormalities*		7/7
Sacroiliac joints		7
Vertebral bodies		7
Peripheral joints		4

three nonoperated patients. Amyloid deposits were not observed in any patient.

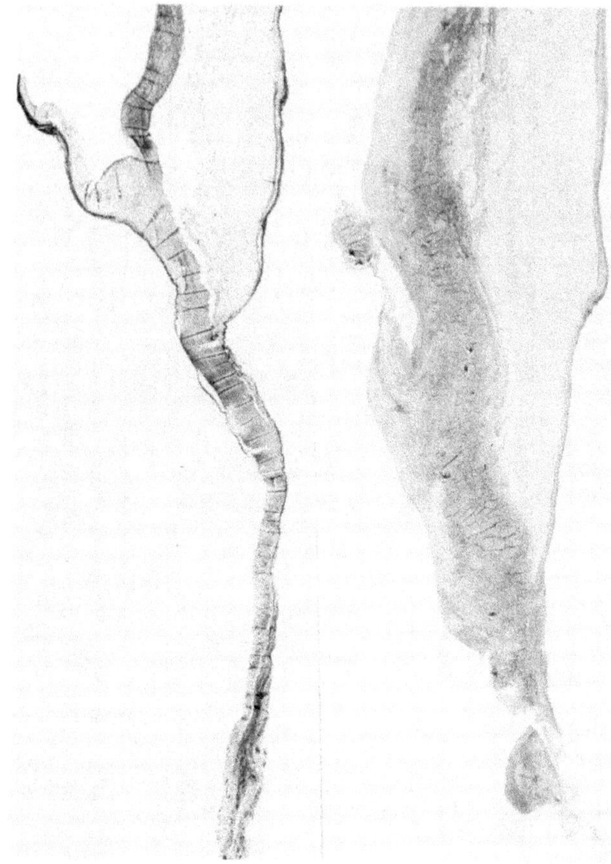

Figure 1

Heart of patient with ankylosing spondylitis compared to the normal. (**left**) *Histologic section through aorta, aortic valve and anterior mitral leaflet from a normal heart and* (**right**) *a section from the same area from the heart of a patient (A68-300) with ankylosing spondylitis and severe aortic regurgitation. In ankylosing spondylitis the aortic wall is thickened by dense adventitial scar and less dense intimal scar. Inflammatory tissue also thickens the base of the aortic valve cusp and anterior mitral leaflet. (Elastic van Gieson stain: (left) ×4, (right) ×2.5.)*

Discussion

Although described briefly in previous reports, the cardiovascular lesions of ankylosing spondylitis have been poorly defined and their distinctive nature not appreciated. In 1936, Mallory[6] described cardiovascular necropsy findings in two young men with combined aortic regurgitation and arthritis of both peripheral joints and spine. He described a "pannus-like overgrowth" or a "queer fibrous growth over the intima and the first portion of ascending aorta [which] . . . extended only a centimeter up the aorta but balanced this by extending about the same distance down below the aortic valve." The aortic wall lesion histologically was identical to syphilis. Twenty years later, Clark, Kulka and Bauer[7] reviewed these two patients along with eight other necropsy patients with combined aortic regurgitation and "rheumatoid arthritis with spinal involvement." These authors did not distinguish between ankylosing spondylitis and rheumatoid arthritis and, therefore, considered the aortic regurgitation to be an unusual manifestation of rheumatoid arthritis. The cardiac findings at necropsy were "strikingly similar to those of luetic heart disease." Although the subvalvular region was not described, the involvement of aorta was limited to the root area: "intimal plaques, centered about each valve commissure . . . , blended with the valvular lesion. These plaques reached into the sinuses of Valsalva and extended . . . up to 2.5 cm distally into ascending aorta." In retrospect, it appears that their patients had ankylosing spondylitis rather than rheumatoid arthritis, and that the cardiac necropsy findings were those of ankylosing spondylitis. Descriptions of the cardiovascular lesion in at least eight more necropsy patients with ankylosing spondylitis appeared subsequently,[8–13] and findings in the 16 previously reported patients

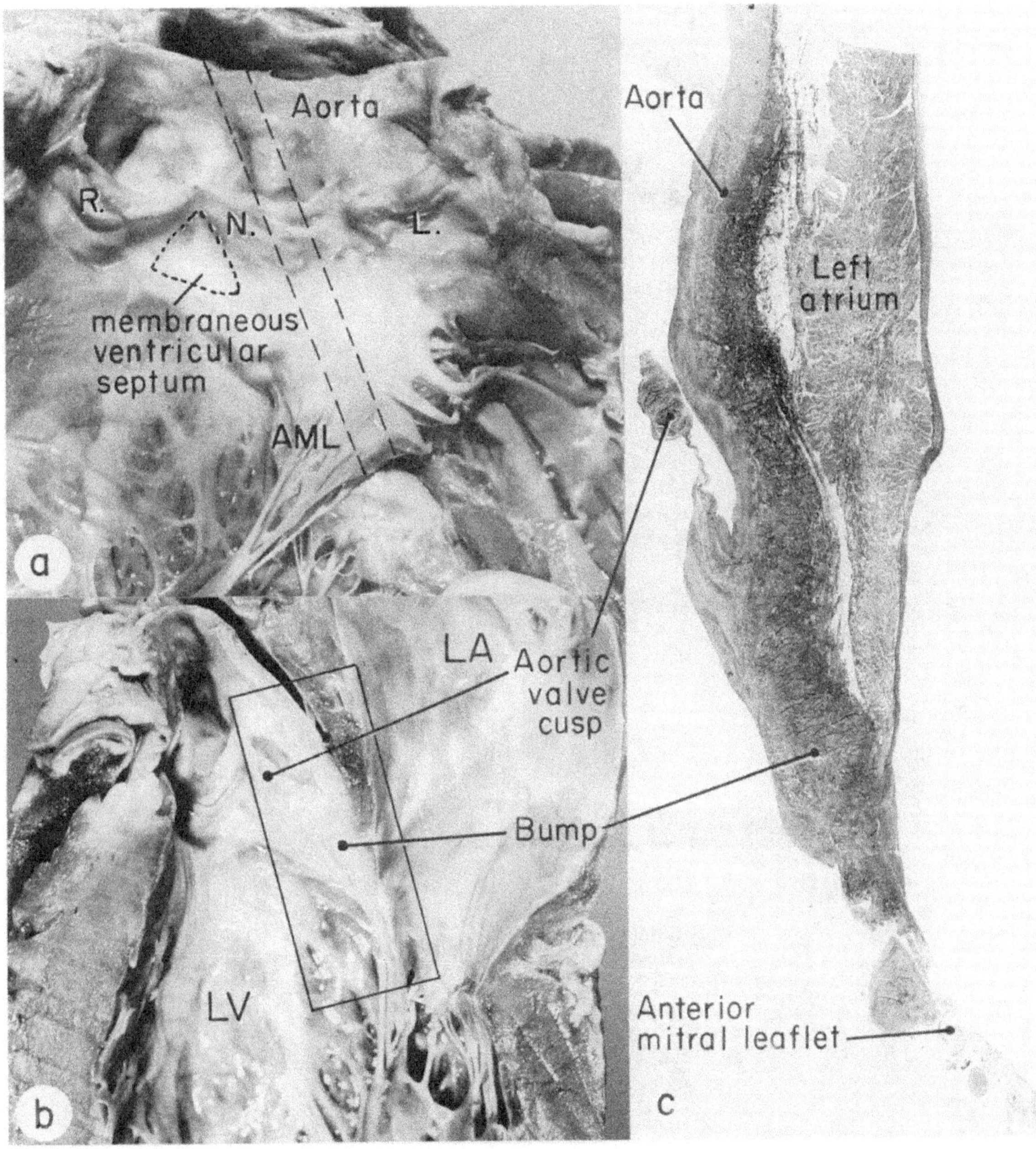

Figure 2

The heart of a 54-year-old man (A68-300) who presented with aortic regurgitation and left bundle branch block six years before death. Four years later the diagnosis of ankylosing spondylitis was made by retrospective examination of serial "spinal" roentgenograms and by a story of longstanding low back pain. The characteristic features of the cardiovascular lesion are shown. (**a**) *Opened left ventricle, aorta, aortic valve right coronary cusp* (R), *non-coronary cusp* (N) *and left coronary cusp, and anterior mitral leaflet. The aortic wall thickening is limited to wall immediately behind and above the sinuses of Valsalva, especially behind the commissures. The basal portion of anterior mitral leaflet* (AML) *and the membranous septum are thickened by fibrous tissue. The dotted lines indicate the longitudinal cut through non-coronary (N) cusp of aortic valve, left atrium* (LA) *and ventricle* (LV) *which is shown in* **b** *and* **c**. *The subvalvular fibrous bump beneath aortic valve is best shown in histologic section* (**c**). *(Phosphotungstic acid-hematoxylin stain;* ×3.*)*

are summarized in table 3. The occurrence of fibrous scarring below the aortic valve was commented upon in four of the 16 patients. Necropsy cardiovascular observations consistent with ankylos-

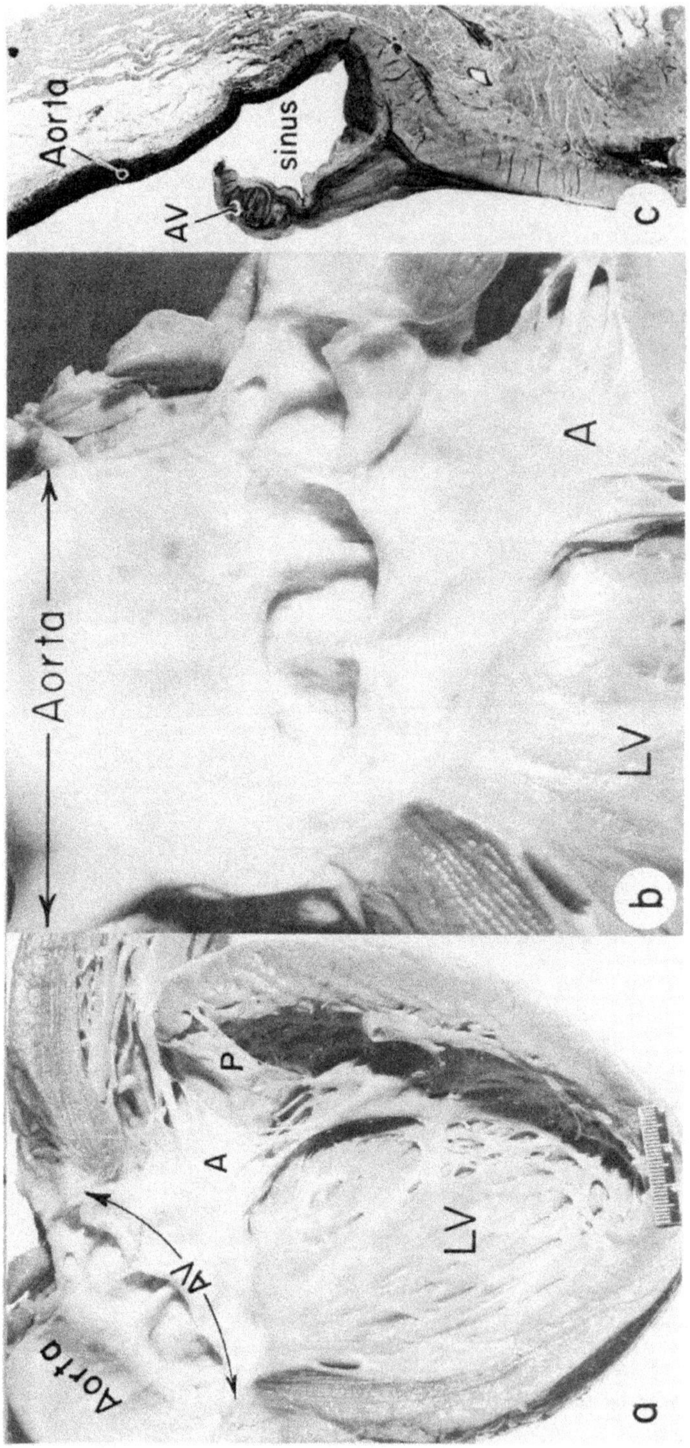

Figure 3

The heart of a 55-year-old man (A61-262) with ankylosing spondylitis who died of intractable congestive cardiac failure due to aortic valvular regurgitation. Left ventricle (LV) is opened in **a** *and* **b** *showing aorta, aortic valve (AV) and anterior (A) and posterior (P) mitral leaflets. The scarring process of aortic wall is limited to the region of the sinuses, which are dilated. Fibrous tissue extends below the aortic valve (AV) cusps, which are thickened* (**b** *and* **c**). *(Elastic-van Gieson stain;* ×3 (**c**).)

ing spondylitis have been described in ten other patients[1, 14] with ankylosing spondylitis, but specific information about individual cases was lacking. The mitral valve was abnormal, however, in four of these ten patients, one of whom had mitral regurgitation.

The cardiovascular lesion of ankylosing spondylitis is morphologically unique. The aortic inflammatory process is limited to aortic wall behind and immediately above the sinuses of Valsalva, particularly behind and adjacent to the commissures. The dense adventitial scar extends *below* the base of aortic valve to form a characteristic subvalvular ridge. The fibrous tissue

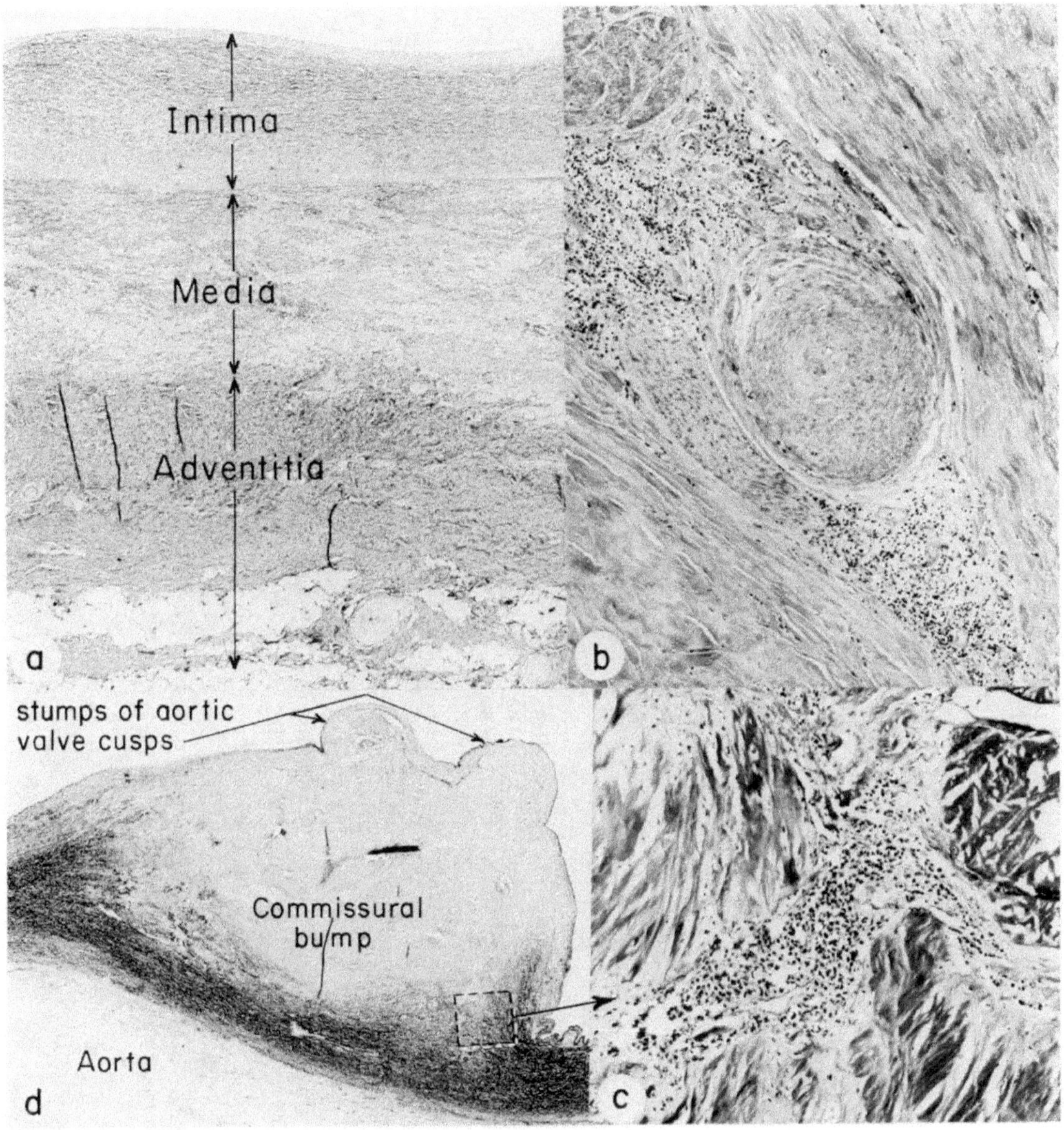

Figure 4

Aorta in ankylosing spondylitis. Aortic wall in ankylosing spondylitis is histologically similar to that in syphilis. **(a)** *The aorta is thickened by adventitial scarring, and intimal proliferation. The media is scarred and the vasa vasora* **(b)** *are narrowed and surrounded by plasma cells and lymphocytes. The adventitial scarring* **(c)** *extends into and below the base of aortic valve. The aortic wall thickening is particularly prominent behind the commisures of aortic valve cusp* **(d)** *forming a fibrous commissural bump which causes malalignment of the cusps and their sagging toward left ventricle. (Hematoxylin and eosin stains;* $\times 25$ **(a)**, $\times 88$ **(b)**, $\times 100$ **(c)**; *Elastic van Gieson stain,* $\times 16$ **(d)**.*)*

also extends into the base of anterior mitral leaflet to form a bump which may be associated with mitral regurgitation, usually of mild degree. Extension of fibrous tissue into the most cephalad portion of muscular ventricular septum is also characteristic, and it explains the associated conduction disturbances, which are frequent. The aortic valve cusps are shortened, and usually diffusely thickened. Occasionally, however, the midportion of a cusp was not thickened.

The cardiovascular lesion of ankylosing spondylitis is readily distinguished from other conditions also associated with aortic regurgitation (table 4, fig. 8). *Rheumatic disease* spares the aorta and

Table 3

Clinical and Necropsy Observations in Previously Reported Cases

Age Sex	Clinical: Peripheral arthritis	Urethritis	Iritis	Age at onset arthritis (yrs.)	Age at onset cardiac disease (yrs.)	Duration of heart disease (yrs.)	CHF	ECG: Conduction disturbances	Cardiovascular pathology: Heart weight (gms)	Thick AV cusps	Sub-AV fibrosis	Thickening of aorta limited to sinuses	Pericarditis	Refs.
39 M	+	–	+	9	26	13	+	0	785	+	–	+	0	(7)
40 M	+	–	+	23	39	1½	+	–	550	+	–	+	foca	(7)
27 M	+	+	0	19	27	< 1	+	LBBB	580	+	+	+	foca	(7)
36 M	+	–	0	16	20	16	+	LBBB	900	+	–	+	foca	(7)
51 M	+	–	+	30	42	9	+	–	–	+	–	+	0	(7)
43 M	+	–	0	24	–	–	+	–	–	+	–	+	0	(7)
45 M	0	–	+	26	–	–	0	0	–	+	–	+	0	(7)
35 M	+	–	0	31	35	< 1	+	LBBB	–	+	–	+	0	(7)
52 M	+	+	0	11	50	2	+	1° HB	930	+	–	–	0	(8)
48 M	0	–	0	28	42	6	+	1° HB	770	+	–	+	foca	(8)
38 M	+	–	–	27	29	9	+	1° HB	700	+	–	+	0	(8)
35 M	+	–	+	27	33	2	+	RBBB	515	+	–	0	–	(10)
54 M	+	+	+	51	51	3	+	1° HB 1° HB LBBB	650	+	–	0	diffuse	(11)
50 M	+	0	0	30	50	< 1	0	1° HB	550	+	+	+	0	(11)
57 M	+	+	0	30	54	3	+	CHB	850	+	+	+	diffuse	(12)
59 M	+	–	–	39	58	1	0	CHB	550	+	+	–	0	(13)
Average 44 M	14	4	6	27	39	5	13		700					

Abbreviations: AV = aortic valve; CHB = complete heart block; CHF = congestive heart failure; 1 HB = first degree heart block (P-R interval > 0.20 sec); LBBB = left bundle branch block; RBBB = right bundle branch block.

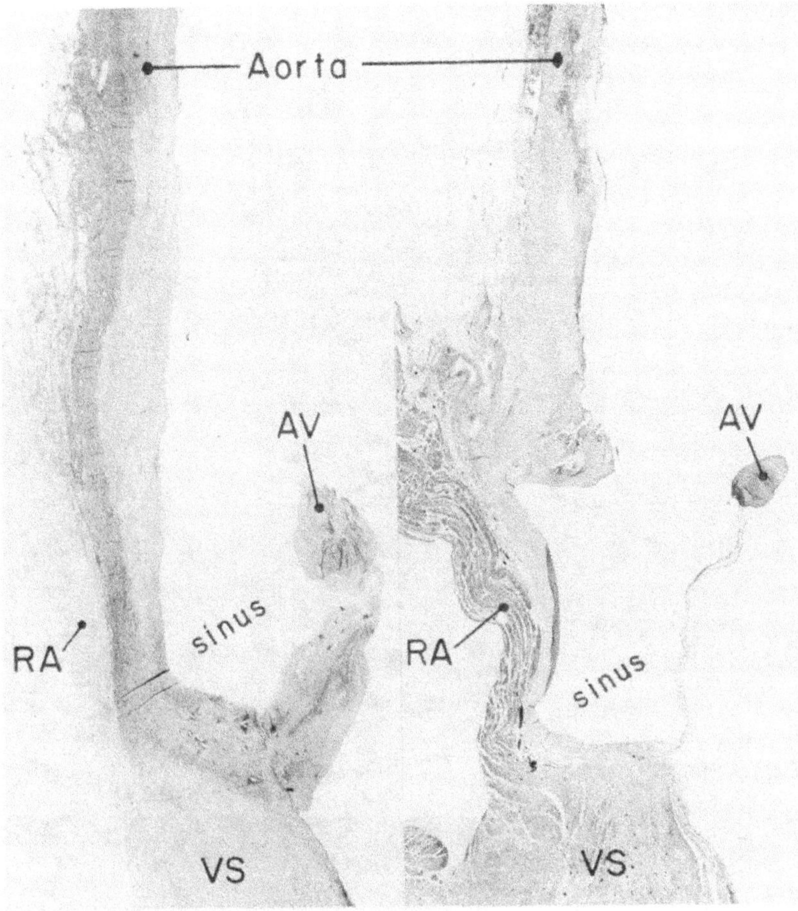

Figure 5

Longitudinal sections through wall of aorta, aortic valve (AV) cusps and ventricular septum (VS) from two patients: one **(left)** *was a 54-year-old man (A68-300) with aortic regurgitation and ankylosing spondylitis, and the other* **(right)**, *a 69-year-old man (A67-43), had aortic regurgitation from syphilis. In ankylosing spondylitis the aortic wall behind the sinuses is involved by the scarring process, whereas in syphilis a similar proces frequently begins* distal *to the sinus of Valsalva. Only the distal margin of aortic valve is thickened in syphilis whereas the proximal portions of valve are thickened as well in ankylosing spondylitis.* RA = *right atrial wall. (Elastic-van Gieson stain;* ×3.5.*)*

always anatomically involves mitral valve.[15-16] The aortic wall lesion of cardiovascular *syphilis* is histologically identical to that of ankylosing spondylitis. The former, however, may spare the aortic wall behind the sinuses of Valsalva (fig. 6) and the adventitial scar tissue does not extend below the aortic valve or involve mitral valve or ventricular septum. Only the distal margins of the aortic valve cusps are thickened in syphilis, not the proximal portions which are always involved as well in ankylosing spondylitis. In *rheumatoid arthritis*, distinctive nodules similar to subcutaneous nodules, may infiltrate pericardium, myocardium and mural and valvular endocardium.[16-18] If valvular tissue is involved, regurgitation usually of only mild degree results. Aortic regurgitation in the *Marfan syndrome* is a consequence of disease of aortic wall, not of aortic valve; the aorta is thinner than normal, and usually contains medial and intimal tears. The ascending aorta is diffusely involved and dilatation of the aortic root causes the aortic regurgitation, which is usually severe. The mitral, and rarely the aortic valve, cusps may be redundant ("floppy") in patients with the Marfan syndrome.

The valular regurgitation and conduction disturbances of ankylosing spondylitis have anatomic explanations. Aortic regurgitation appears to result from a combination of three factors: 1) thickening and shortening of the cusps; 2) displacement of the cusps caudally by the fibrous tissue bump located behind the commissures; and 3) dilatation of aortic root. Mitral regurgitation, although rare, appears to

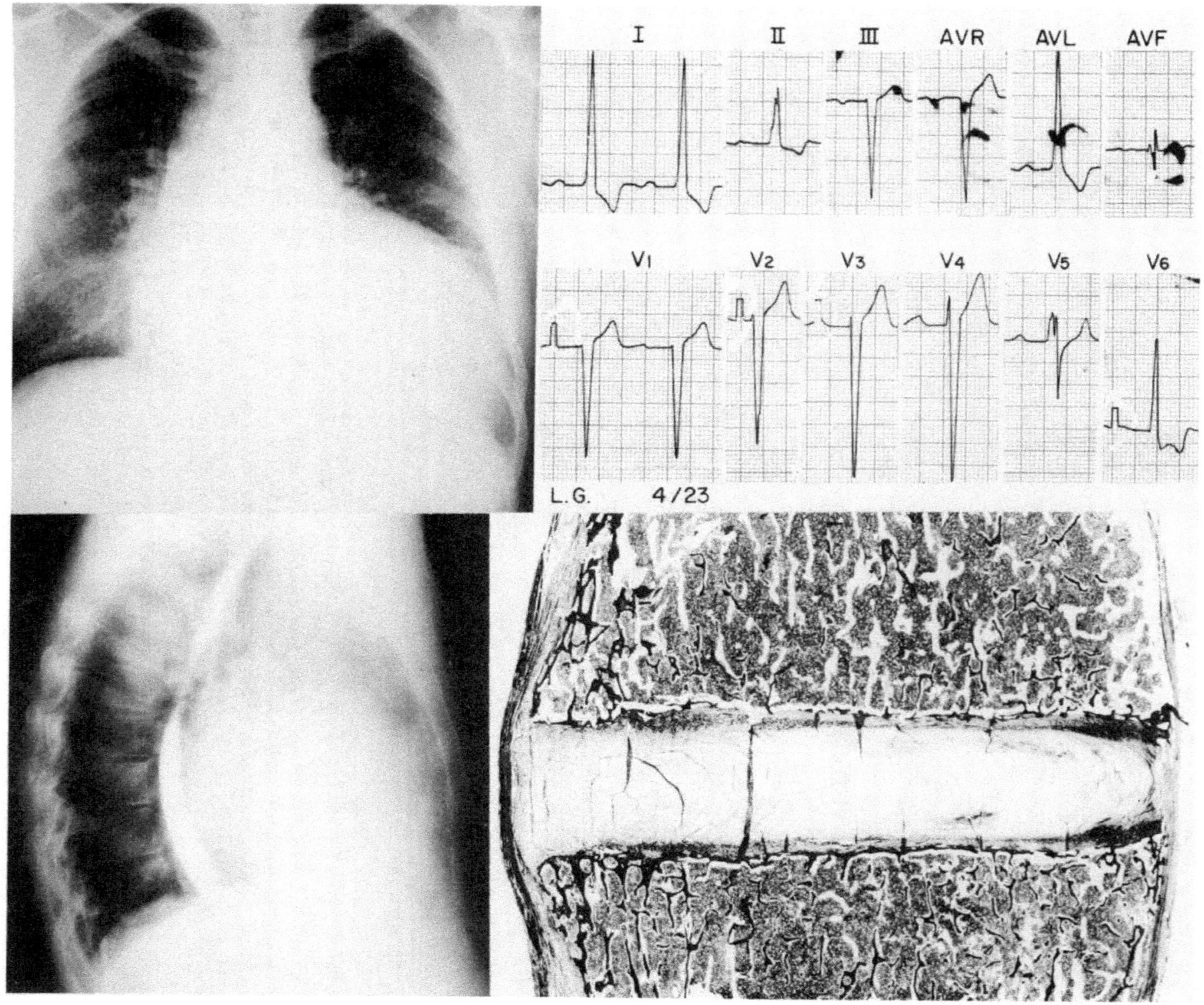

Figure 6

This 38-year-old man (A68-142) had congestive heart failure associated with a murmur of aortic regurgitation two years before the diagnosis of ankylosing spondylitis was suspected clinically. Chest roentgenograms **(left)**, *and electrocardiogram* **(upper right)**, *were taken two years before death. The latter shows a prolonged P-R interval and an interventricular conduction delay. Although at necropsy early morphologic changes of ankylosing spondylitis were present in the sacroiliac joints and intervertebral spaces* **(lower right)** *the cardiac lesion had progressed to wide open lethal aortic regurgitation. (Masson stains, ×4* **(d)**.*)*

Table 4

Causes of Aortic Regurgitation

	Ankylosing Spondylitis	Syphilis	Marfans	Rheumatic	Rheumatoid Arthritis
Average age	45	50	30	45	70
Usual sex	Men	Men	Men	Men	Women
Aortic regurgitation	++++	++++	++++	+++	+
Mitral regurgitation	+	0	+++	++++	+
Conduction disturbances	++++	+	0	0	++
Aorta:					
Adventitial scarring	+++	+++	0	0	0
Medial degeneration	+++	+++	++++	0	0
Intimal proliferation	++	++	0	0	0
Limited to sinuses	+	0	0	0	0
Subaortic lump	+	0	0	0	0
Aortic cuspal thickening	Diffuse	Focal	Focal	Diffuse	Focal
Anterior mitral leaflet thickening	++	0	+	++++	+

result from two factors: 1) dilatation of the left ventricle (from aortic regurgitation) with resulting malalignment of the papillary muscles, and 2) fibrous thickening at the basal portion of anterior mitral leaflet. Bundle branch block and complete heart block in patients with ankylosing spondylitis appear to result from extension of the fibrous process from the membranous ventricular septum into the muscular septum to interrupt or destroy the conduction fibers in the atrioventricular bundle or proximal bundle branches.

The underlying cause of pure aortic regurgitation, severe enough to be fatal, is usually readily determined. The usual etiologies include rheumatic, infective endocarditis,[19] congenitally malformed valves with and without superimposed infection,[20] "floppy" valves with and without the Marfan syndrome,[16] trauma,[16] dissecting aortic aneurysm and a few miscellaneous conditions. Among patients with pure aortic regurgitation, the etiology in a few is usually unclear. Among the latter, ankylosing spondylitis must be considered as an underlying condition. Diagnosis of ankylosing spondylitis, however, is often difficult because few patients with combined ankylosing spondylitis and aortic regurgitation have advanced and readily diagnosable skeletal deformities. Only two of our eight patients had bony ankylosis with bamboo spine, classic late arthritic changes of ankylosing spondylitis. Two others had evidence of cardiac dysfunction years before the diagnosis of ankylosing spondylitis could be made. Thus, in them and in other reported patients,[9, 11, 21, 22] aortic regurgitation clinically may exist as a forme fruste of ankylosing spondylitis. A possible reason why signs of ankylosing spondylitis may be absent or minimal in a patient with combined ankylosing spondylitis and severe aortic regurgitation is that the latter condition when severe may cause death before there has been time to develop severe arthritic signs. The average life span of patients with ankylosing spondylitis unassociated with aortic regurgitation is normal (about 70 years)[23, 24] whereas the life span of patients with ankylosing spondylitis associated with wide open and therefore fatal aortic regurgitation is much shorter (about 45 years).[7] Hence, cardiac dysfunction may appear before joint signs are definite, and the aortic regurgitation may be severe when the joint signs are minimal or absent.

The spectrum of cardiovascular disease in patients with ankylosing spontylitis is presumably wide (figure 9). Our patients represent one end of this spectrum, those with wide open fatal aortic regurgitation. Little information is available about the patients at the other end of the spectrum, i.e., those with anatomic involvement of the aortic root area but without any evidence of cardiac dysfunction. Furthermore, there is little information about patients with combined ankylosing spondylitis and minimal, mild or moderate aortic regurgitation. Of 25 necropsy patients with ankylosing spondylitis studied by Davidson et al.[14] five (20%) had anatomically abnormal aortic valves but only two of them had clinically detectable aortic regurgitation.

Although its frequency in patients with ankylosing spondylitis is unclear, aortic regurgitation does appear to increase with increasing duration of arthritis. Aortic regurgitation appears to occur in about 12% of patients with signs of ankylosing

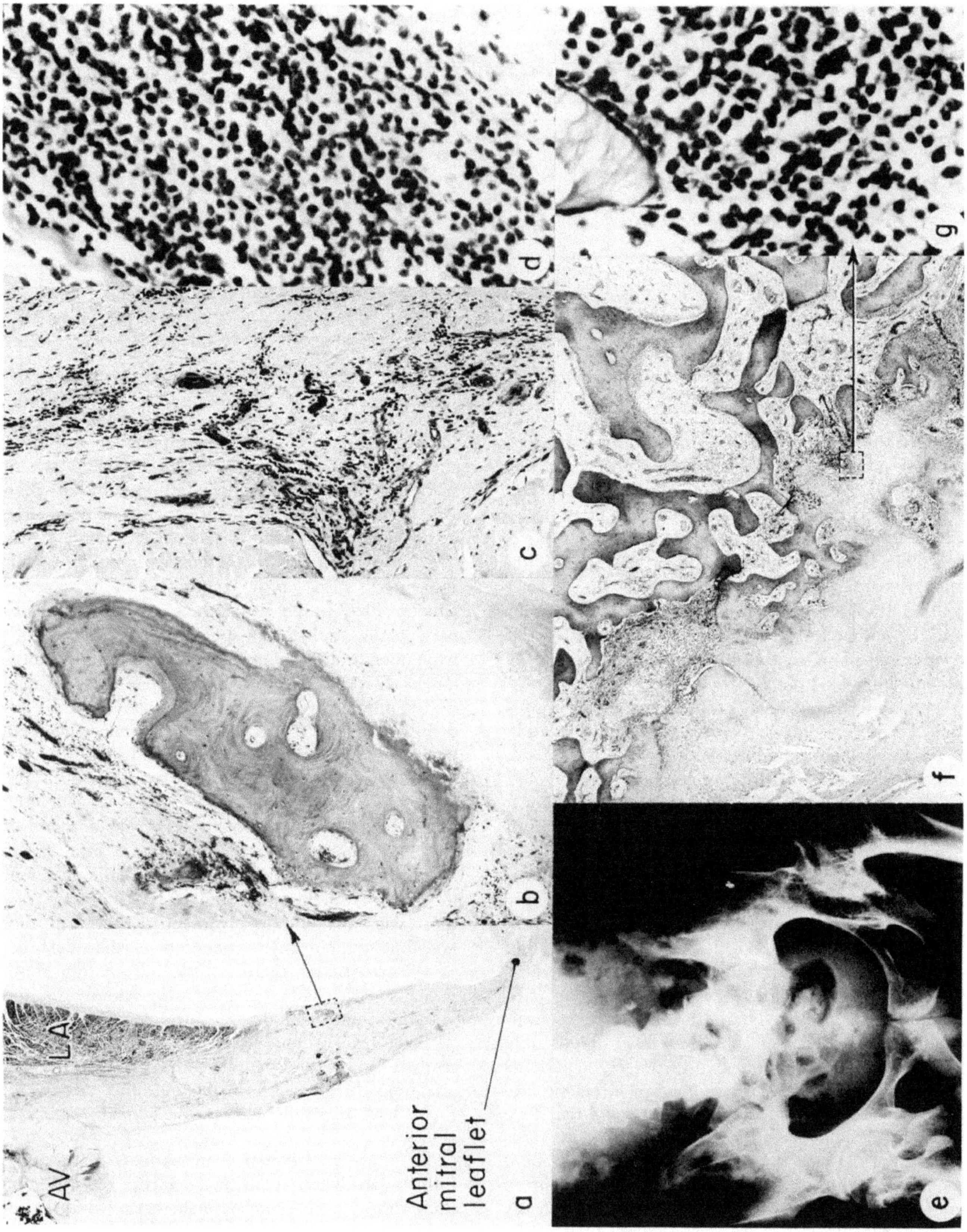
AV
LA
Anterior mitral leaflet
a
b
c
d
e
f
g

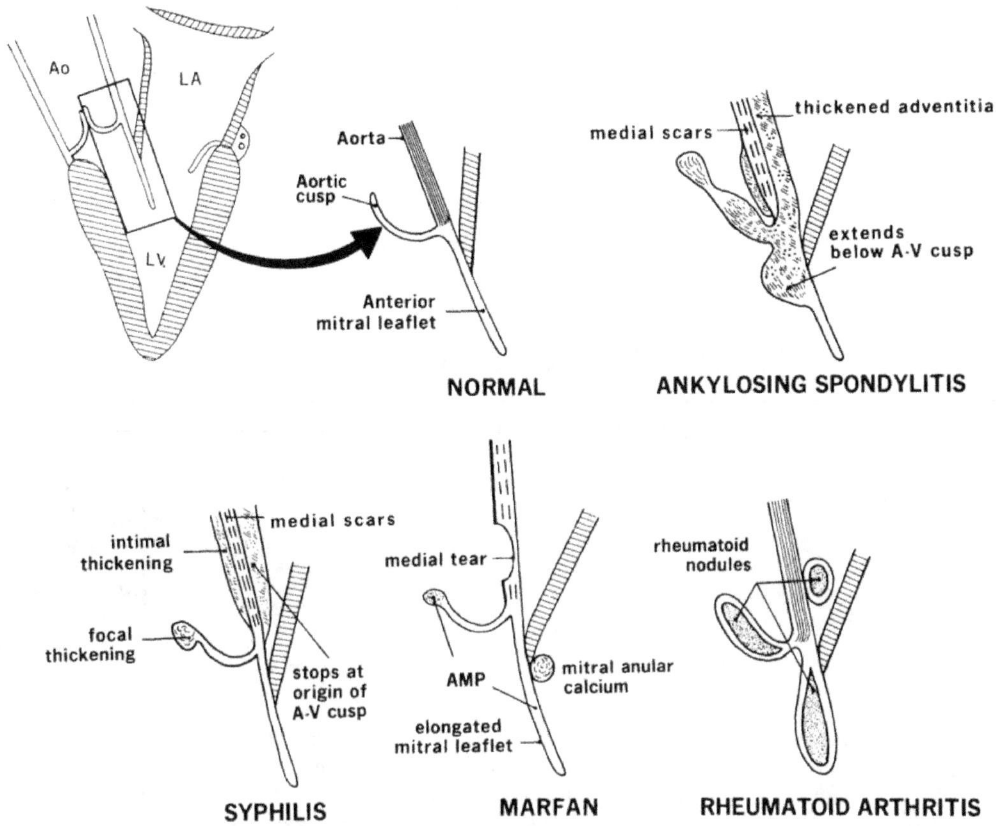

Figure 8

Cardiovascular lesion of ankylosing spondylitis compared to other conditions associated with aortic regurgitation.

spondylitis for as long as 30 years, but in only about 2% of those with signs of spondylitis for as short as 10 years.[1]

Urethritis, iritis and psoriasis occur in increased frequencies in patients with ankylosing spondylitis.[4, 25] Some patients with Reiter's syndrome (urethritis, iritis and peripheral arthritis) have aortic regurgitation, and when they do spondylitis is nearly always present as well.[25, 26] One of our eight patients had Reiter's syndrome, and all our eight patients had peripheral arthritis. The inflammatory lesion which infiltrates the central joint in ankylosing spondylitis is similar histologically to the lesion observed in the aorta in patients with

---

Figure 7

Morphologic characteristics of cardiac and skeletal involvement in ankylosing spondylitis. The inflamed fibrous tissue which infiltrates the aortic root area is histologically similar to the "pannus" which infiltrates the joints. Shown in **(a)** *is a histologic section through aortic valve* (AV), *anterior mitral leaflet and left atrium* (LA) *from a 35-year-old man (A64-17) with ankylosing spondylitis who died almost two years after aortic valve replacement because of severe regurgitation. The subvalvular area and anterior mitral leaflet are thickened by vascularized and inflamed fibrous tissue* **(c)** *containing a few small bony spicules* **(b)**, *an unusual finding in a valve not heavily calcified. Focal collections of lymphocytes and plasma cells also are present in the same area* **(d)**. *This patient had severe bilateral sacroiliitis* **(e)**. *A histologic section of sacroiliac joint demonstrates infiltration of the joint space with vascularized fibrous tissue* **(f)** *containing focal collections of lymphocytes and plasma cells* **(g)** *causing a "fibrous ankylosis." The latter may progress to a bony ankylosis with total obliteration of joint space.*

Thus, both joint and aortic root area are involved by a similar inflammatory process. The stimulus to this process, however, remains uncertain. (Hematoxylin and eosin stain; ×3½ **(a)**, *×90* **(b)**, *×140* **(c)**, *×560* **(d)**, *×25* **(f)**, *×560* **(g)**.)

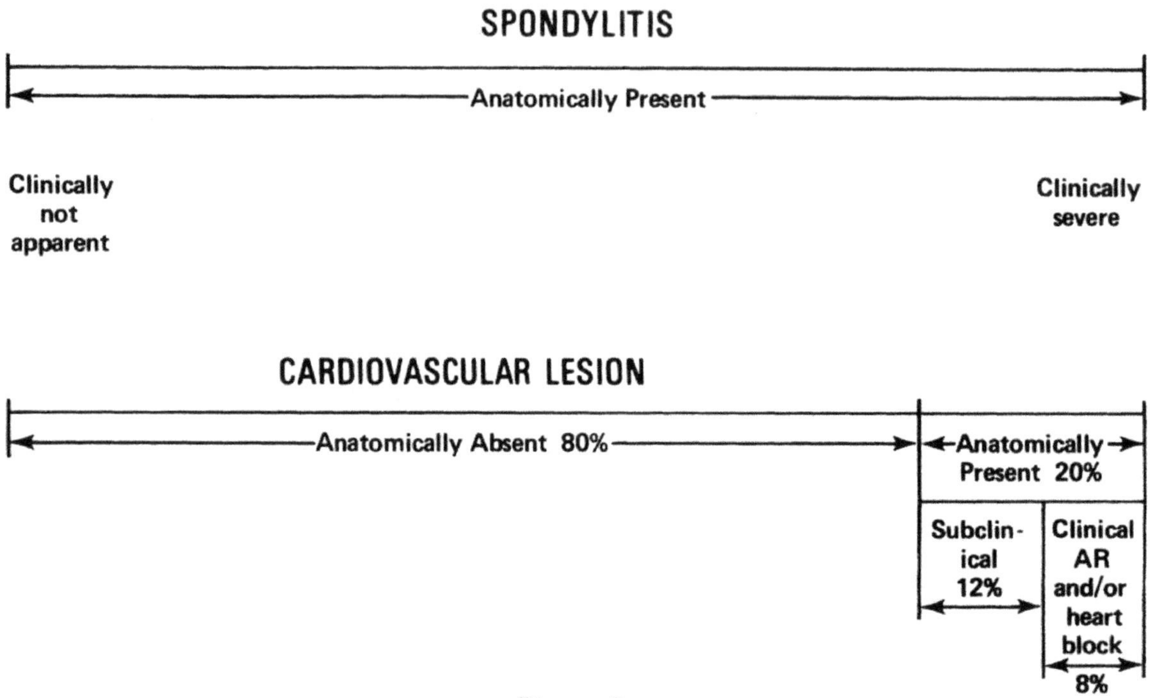

Figure 9

The spectrum of heart disease in patients with ankylosing spondylitis. Cardiovascular disease may be clinically apparent in patients with ankylosing spondylitis of any stage or severity. What proportion of patients with ankylosing spondylitis have anatomic valvular heart disease whether or not it be clinically detectable is unknown. A necropsy study by Davidson et al.,[14] however, suggests that approximately 20% of patients with ankylosing spondylitis have anatomic disease of aortic valve, but less than half of the latter group have clinically detectable valvular dysfunction.

ankylosing spondylitis and aortic regurgitation. Similar inflammatory changes occur in peripheral joints of patients with ankylosing spondylitis.[3, 27] The specificity with which certain target sites in the body are infiltrated by the inflammatory lesion suggest that a common tissue element is involved in ankylosing spondylitis and that the latter might better be termed the "spondylitis syndrome" (table 5).

Table 5

Spondylitis Syndrome

1. Vertebral-sacroiliac joints	Spondylitis sacroiliitis
2. Cardiovascular system	Aortic regurgitation Heart block
3. Eye	Conjunctivitis Iritis
4. Genitourinary system	Urethritis
5. Skin	Psoriasis Keratodermia blennorrhagica
6. Peripheral joints and tendons	Arthritis and tendinitis

Acknowledgment

The gross photographs were taken by Mr. Kensie L. Edwards and the histologic sections were prepared by Ms. Sandra J. Lewis.

References

1. Graham DC, Smythe HA: The carditis and aortitis of ankylosing spondylitis. Bull Rheum Dis **9**: 171, 1958
2. Graham W: Is rheumatoid spondylitis a separate entity? Arthritis Rheum **3**: 88, 1960
3. Cruickshank B: Pathology of ankylosing spondylitis. Bull Rheum Dis **10**: 211, 1960
4. Julkunen H: Rheumatoid spondylitis—clinical and laboratory study of 149 cases compared with 182 cases of rheumatoid arthritis. Acta Rhem Scand Suppl No 4, **172**: 24, 1962
5. Zvaifler NH, Weintraub AM: Aortitis and aortic insufficiency in the chronic rheumatic disorders—A reapraisal. Arthritis Rheum **6**: 241, 1963
6. Mallory TB: Case records of the Massachusetts General Hospital. N Engl J Med **214**: 690, 1936
7. Clark WS, Kulka P, Bauer W: Rheumatoid aortitis with aortic regurgitation. An unusual manifestation of rheumatoid arthritis (including spondylitis). Am J Med **22**: 580, 1957

8. Schilder DP, Harvey WP, Hufnagel CA: Rheumatoid spondylitis and aortic insufficiency. N Engl J Med **255**: 11, 1956
9. Valaitis J, Clifford GP, Montgomery MM: Aortitis with aortic valve insufficiency in rheumatoid arthritis. Arch Pathol **63**: 207, 1956
10. Ansell BM, Bywaters EGL, Doniach I: The aortic lesions of ankylosing spondylitis. Br Heart J **20**: 507, 1958
11. Toone EC, Pierce EL, Hennigar GR: Aortitis and aortic regurgitation associated with rheumatoid spondylitis. Am J Med **26**: 255, 1959
12. Weed CL, Kulander BG, Mazarella JA, Decker JL: Heart block in ankylosing spondylitis. Arch Intern Med **117**: 800, 1966
13. Liu SM, Alexander CS: Complete heart block and aortic insufficiency in rheumatoid spondylitis. Am J Cardiol **23**: 888, 1969
14. Davidson P, Baggenstoss AH, Slocumb CH, Daugherty GW: Cardiac and aortic lesions in rheumatoid spondylitis. Proc Staff Meet Mayo Clinic **38**: 427, 1963
15. Roberts WC, Perloff JK: Mitral valvular disease. A clinicopathologic survey of the conditions causing the mitral valve to function abnormally. Ann Intern Med **77**: 939, 1972
16. Roberts WC, Dangel JC, Bulkley BH: Nonrheumatic valvular cardiac disease: A clinicopathologic survey of 27 different conditions causing valvular dysfunction. Cardiovasc Clin 1973
17. Roberts WC, Kehoe JA, Carpenter DF, Golden A: Cardiovascular lesions in rheumatoid arthritis. Arch Intern Med **122**: 141, 1968
18. Carpenter DF, Golden A, Roberts WC: Quadrivalvular rheumatoid heart disease associated with left bundle branch block. Am J Med **43**: 922, 1967
19. Buchbinder NA, Roberts WC: Left-sided valvular active infective endocarditis. A study of forty-five necropsy patients. Am J Med **53**: 20, 1972
20. Roberts WC: The congenitally bicuspid aortic valve. A study of 85 autopsy cases. Am J Cardiol **26**: 72, 1970
21. Malette WG, Eisman B, Danielson GK, Mazzoleni A, Rams JJ: Rheumatoid spondylitis and aortic insufficiency. J Thorac Cardiovasc Surg **57**: 471, 1969
22. Spangler RD, McCallister BD, McGoon DC: Aortic valve replacement in patients with severe aortic valve incompetence associated with rheumatoid spondylitis. Am J Cardiol **26**: 130, 1970
23. Blumberg B, Ragan C: The natural history of rheumatoid spondylitis. Medicine **35**: 1, 1956
24. Wilkinson M, Bywaters EGL: Clinical features and course of ankylosing spondylitis as seen in follow-up of 222 hospital reference cases. Ann Rheum Dis **17**: 209, 1958
25. Rodman GP, Benedek TG, Shaver JA, Fennell RH: Reiter's syndrome and aortic insufficiency. JAMA **189**: 889, 1964
26. Paulus HE, Pearson CM, Pitts W: Aortic insufficiency in 5 patients with Reiter's syndrome. Am J Med **53**: 464, 1972
27. Cruickshank B: Lesions of cartilaginous joints in ankylosing spondylitis. J Pathol **71**: 73, 1956

Nonrheumatic Valvular Cardiac Disease: A Clinicopathologic Survey of 27 Different Conditions Causing Valvular Dysfunction

William C. Roberts, M.D.,
James C. Dangel, M.D., and
Bernadine H. Bulkley, M.D.

Until relatively recent years most valvular cardiac lesions in adults or older children were believed to be rheumatic in origin. During the past two decades, however, it has become increasingly apparent that rheumatic disease is only one of many causes of valvular dysfunction, and, indeed, not the most common. We have found it helpful to divide functionally significant valvular lesions into two groups: (1) those causing obstruction (with or without regurgitation) and (2) those causing pure regurgitation, i.e., without any element of obstruction (nonobstructive) (Table 1). Rheumatic disease continues to be a major cause of obstructive valve lesions but it plays a far less prominent role as a cause of nonobstructive lesions. Even in the obstructive group, however, the most common lesion is valvular aortic stenosis, which when isolated is rarely rheumatic in origin.[1-4] Mitral stenosis, on the other hand, is usually rheumatic in origin as are most combined valvular lesions.

We also have found it useful to divide the nonobstructive, i.e., purely incompetent, valvular lesions into two groups: (1) those associated with abnormalities of the ascending aorta and (2) those which do not affect the aorta (Table 1). Most lesions affecting the aorta cause aortic regurgitation, and most cases of

Table 1. A classification of nonrheumatic valvular cardiac disease

I. Obstructive lesions
- A. Left-sided
  - 1. Obstruction to left ventricular outflow
    - a. Valvular aortic stenosis
    - b. Subvalvular
      - (1) Discrete
      - (2) Hypertrophic (asymmetric) cardiomyopathy
    - c. Supravalvular
  - 2. Obstruction to left ventricular inflow
- B. Right-sided
  - 1. Obstruction to right ventricular outflow
  - 2. Obstruction to both right ventricular outflow and inflow
    - a. Carcinoid heart disease
- C. Combined left-sided and right-sided

II. Nonobstructive lesions
- A. With involvement of ascending aorta
  - 1. Syphilis
  - 2. Ankylosing spondylitis
  - 3. The Marfan syndrome including forme fruste variety
  - 4. The Hurler syndrome
  - 5. Osteogenesis imperfecta
  - 6. Pseudoxanthoma elasticum
  - 7. Ehlers-Danlos syndrome
  - 8. Takayasu's arteritis
- B. Without involvement of ascending aorta
  - 1. Floppy atrioventricular valve
  - 2. Calcification of atrioventricular valve annuli
  - 3. Papillary muscle necrosis or fibrosis or both
  - 4. Infective endocarditis
  - 5. Congenital malformation
  - 6. Trauma
  - 7. Systemic lupus erythematosus
  - 8. Rheumatoid arthritis
  - 9. Endomyocardial fibrosis with and without eosinophilia
  - 10. Irradiation
  - 11. Idiopathic

pure aortic regurgitation result from abnormalities of the ascending aorta. Because pure aortic regurgitation most frequently results from conditions affecting the aorta rather than the aortic valve cusps, rheumatic disease is not a major cause of isolated aortic regurgitation. Pure mitral regurgitation, in contrast, is the major nonobstructive lesion not involving the aorta.

This report focuses on the nonrheumatic conditions causing valvular dysfunction. Patients with intracardiac or extracardiac shunts with a few exceptions have been excluded. The various entities will be discussed as outlined in Table 1. When possible, concrete data of patients studied at necropsy by the authors will be presented in place of or in addition to information derived from reports of others.

OBSTRUCTIVE LESIONS

Obstruction to Left Ventricular Outflow

Valvular Aortic Stenosis

It is now clear that isolated valvular aortic stenosis (with or without associated aortic regurgitation) is nearly always nonrheumatic in origin, and most commonly represents a congenital malformation of this valve.[1-4] Isolated valvular aortic stenosis is the most common cause of fatal valvular dysfunction in patients over 14 years of age. Of 543 patients with severe (functionally class III or IV [New York Heart Association Classification]) fatal valvular cardiac disease studied at necropsy by us, 182 patients or 34 per cent had isolated valvular aortic stenosis (with or without regurgitation) (Table 2). The second most common valvular

Table 2. Functional classification of valvular heart disease: data in 543 autopsy patients older than age 14 years

Functional Valve Lesion	No. Pts. (%)	Anatomic Classification				
		AV	MV	MV-AV	MV-TV	MV-AV-TV
1. Aortic Stenosis (AS)	182 (34)	158 (87)	0	23 (12.5)	0	1 (.5)
2. Mitral Stenosis (MS)	94 (17)	0	53 (57)	23 (24)	7 (7)	11 (12)
3. AS + MS	66 (12)	0	0	52 (79)	0	14 (21)
4. Aortic Regurgitation (AR)	60 (11)	50 (83)	0	9 (15)	0	1 (2)
5. Mitral Regurgitation (MR)	55 (10)	0	44 (80)	7 (13)	1 (2)	3 (5)
6. MS + AR	34 (6)	0	0	25 (74)	0	9 (26)
7. MR + AR	24 (5)	0	0	20 (83)	0	4 (17)
8. AS + MR	16 (3)	0	0	15 (94)	0	1 (6)
9. Tricuspid Stenosis + MS $\pm$ AS	12 (2)	0	0	0	1 (8)	11 (92)
TOTALS	543	208 (38)	97 (18)	174 (32)	9 (2)	55 (10)

lesion, namely mitral stenosis, is only half as frequent as aortic stenosis (Table 2). When aortic stenosis is the only functional valve lesion the remaining three cardiac valves are usually normal. As shown in Table 2, of the 182 patients with isolated valvular aortic stenosis, the other three cardiac valves were anatomically normal in 87 per cent of them. In contrast, of the 94 patients with isolated mitral stenosis (with or without regurgitation) only 57 per cent had anatomic involvement limited to the mitral valve.

We have found it useful to subdivide patients with valvular aortic stenosis into three groups according to ages[5]: (1) patients less than 15 years old; (2) patients 15 to 65 years old; and (3) patients older than 65 years.[4] Little anatomic data is available in the group less than 15 years of age. The data available tends to indicate that the aortic valves in these young individuals are either unicuspid or bicuspid and only occasionally tricuspid. In the group aged 15 to 65 years, the aortic valve is congenitally malformed in about 60 per cent of them (Table 3). Of the patients older than 65 years of age, the aortic valve is tricuspid in more than 90 per cent and congenitally malformed (biscuspid) in less than 10 per cent (Table 4).

Table 3. Aortic valve structure in clinically isolated aortic stenosis: ages 15–65 years

Valve Structure	No. Pts. (%)	Age Range (Avg.)	No. Males (%)	Hx ARF or chorea	LV-SA PSG (mm. Hg)
1. Unicommissural	18 (12)	16-62 (44)	14 (78)	1	10-158 (78)
2. Bicuspid	72 (46)	16-65 (49)	53 (73)	5	12-165 (91)
3. Tricuspid	57 (37)	21-64 (49)	49 (86)	15	20-155 (82)
MV Normal	36	28-64 (50)	29 (81)	1	20-155 (90)
MV Thickened	21	21-61 (48)	20 (95)	14	20-120 (74)
4. Uncertain	8 (5)	41-58 (52)	7 (87)	0	52-105 (81)
TOTALS	155	16-65 (46)	123 (79)	21 (13%)	10-165 (86)*

* 121 pts.

Table 4. Aortic valve structure in clinically isolated aortic stenosis: ages greater than 65 years

Valve Structure	No. Pts. (%)	Age Range (Avg.)	No. Males (%)	Hx ARF or chorea	LV-SA PSG (mm. Hg)
1. Unicommissural	0				
2. Bicuspid	2 (7)	75 + 79	1 (50)	0	–
3. Tricuspid	25 (93)	66-90 (77)	13 (52)		20-160 (88)
MV Normal	23	66-90 (77)	13 (56)	0	20-160 (92)
MV Thickened	2	74 + 76	0	0	70
4. Uncertain	0				
TOTALS	27	66-90 (78)	14 (52)	0	20-160 (88)

Although valvular aortic stenosis frequently involves a congenitally malformed aortic valve, the stenosis is usually not congenital but acquired, the result of fibrosis and calcification of the malformed cusps. Thus, acquired valvular aortic stenosis is fundamentally of two types: (1) that involving a previously congenitally malformed but initially normally functioning valve and (2) that involving a previously normally formed valve.

Several types of congenitally malformed aortic valves occur. Each type is determined by its number of cusps and commissures. At least two types of *unicuspid* aortic valves exist. In one, the orifice is centrally located and the cusp is devoid of lateral attachments to the wall of the aorta (simple dome or *acommissural* valve). This type valve also is usually the one underlying valvular pulmonic stenosis. Often three remnants of commissures are observed, and the undeveloped commissures have caused it to be confused with tricuspid semilunar valves. A second type of unicuspid valve is the *unicommissural* one.[6] This valve, described by Edwards,[7] is characterized by an eccentrically located orifice with only one lateral attachment to the aortic wall and that at the level of the orifice. From above, this valve has the appearance of an exclamation mark. Remnants of undeveloped commissures also are present in the unicommissural valve.[6] This is the most frequent malformation found in fatal valvular aortic stenosis in children less than one year of age.[8]

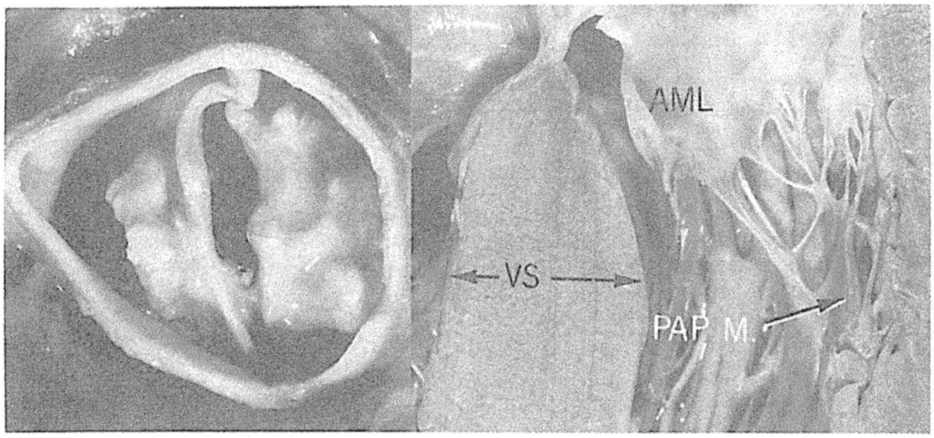

Figure 1. Stenotic congenitally bicuspid aortic valve and atrophied and scarred left ventricular papillary muscle (PAP M.) in a 52-year-old woman (A68–105). She had symptoms of cardiac dysfunction for three years and a murmur of mitral regurgitation as well as a murmur of aortic stenosis. The peak systolic pressure gradient across the aortic valve was 130 mm. Hg. She died of congestive cardiac failure. VS = ventricular septum. AML = anterior mitral leaflet.

The most frequent malformation of the aortic valve is the presence of only two cusps[3] (Fig. 1). The *bicuspid* valve is basically of two types: in one the cusps are located right and left, the commissures anteriorly and posteriorly, a raphe or false commissure, if present, is always in the right cusp, and a coronary artery arises from behind each cusp; in the second type, the cusps are located anteriorly and posteriorly, the commissures right and left, a raphe, if present, is always in the anterior cusp, and both coronary arteries arise in front of the anterior cusp. These two types are divided about equally among patients with congenitally bicuspid aortic valves.

Of 107 patients over 14 years of age with congenitally bicuspid aortic valves studied at necropsy by one of us (W.C.R.), 75 had aortic stenosis, 17 had pure aortic regurgitation, and 15 had functionally normal valves (Table 5). Why one patient with a congenitally bicuspid aortic valve develops stenosis, why another develops infection with subsequent regurgitation, why another (rarely) develops

Table 5. Congenitally bicuspid aortic valve: summary of 107 autopsied patients older than age 14 years

Group	No. Pts.	Age at Death Range (Avg.) Years	Sex M	Sex F	Infective Endocarditis	LV-SA PSG Range (Avg.) mm.Hg	AV Calcium Deposits
AS with or without AR	75	16 – 79 (48)	54	21	6	18 – 165 (94)	73
Pure AR	17	15 – 55 (34)	15	2	14	0 – 0 (0)	5
Functionally normal valve	15	23 – 59 (45)	9	6	0	–	4
TOTALS	107	15 – 79 (46)	78 (72%)	29 (28%)	2 (18%)		82 (77%)

pure regurgitation without infection, and why another never develops any of these complications during an entire lifetime is uncertain. The 15 patients with normally functioning congenitally bicuspid valves (Table 5) were found during routine examination of 1600 hearts at necropsy, none of which had dysfunctioning cardiac valves or shunts. How many patients with bicuspid aortic valves at birth develop complications (stenosis, regurgitation, infection) and how many never develop any of these complications is unknown. The biscuspid condition of the aortic valve appears to be the most common congenital malformation of the heart or great vessels; possibly as many as 2 per cent of births have this anomaly.[3] Stenosis, not infection, is by far the most common complication of the congenitally biscuspid aortic valve.

Occasionally a tricuspid aortic valve is malformed. When this occurs, the cusps are of unequal size. Minor differences in cuspal size are frequent but major differences appear to constitute a congenital malformation. There may be some basis for believing that contact of unequal sized cusps with one another can lead to focal cuspal fibrosis with eventual calcification and stenosis.[2] A quadricuspid aortic valve on rare occasion may be stenotic.[9] Most quadricuspid valves, however, function normally.[9] Although six-cuspid valves may occur (persistent truncus arteriosus), stenosis of these multi-cuspid valves is rare.

Function of the malformed aortic valves at birth is variable. The fewer the number of cusps and commissures the greater the likelihood that the valve is stenotic at birth. The acommissural and unicommissural unicuspid valves are stenotic from birth: the orifices of these valves are small and there is little opportunity for the valvular orifice to alter its size during either phase of the cardiac cycle. Most patients with unicuspid aortic valves have precordial murmurs from birth whereas this is probably not the case in most patients with congenitally bicuspid aortic valves.[6]

Whether or not the bicuspid aortic valve is ever stenotic at birth is unclear. Probably most often this valve becomes stenotic only as it thickens and calcifies. Of 30 patients, mostly children, with congenital valvular aortic stenosis operated upon by Morrow,[10] however, 18 were said to have bicuspid valves, 11 tricuspid, and one a unicommissural unicuspid valve. Unicommissural valves are most frequent in fatal congenital aortic valve stenosis in the first year of life.[8] Tricuspid aortic valves rarely appear to be stenotic at birth. If stenosis is present at birth and the aortic valve is three-cuspid, the stenosis is more usually the result of a very small aortic *annulus* rather than the result of fusion of the cusps. Acquired stenosis of a three-cuspid aortic valve, in contrast, is common. Of 155 patients aged 15 to 65 years with clinically isolated aortic stenosis (with or without regurgitation) studied at necropsy (Table 3), 57 (37 per cent) had tricuspid valves, and among the 27 patients older than age 65 years (Table 4), 25 (93 per cent) had tricuspid valves. In the 15 to 65 year age group, about half of the 57 patients with clinically isolated aortic stenosis had diffuse fibrous thickening of the mitral leaflets as well. The associated diffuse mitral leaflet thickening in them is strong evidence that the etiology of the stenosis in this group is rheumatic.[1] Also, about 70 per cent of this group had positive histories of acute rheumatic fever, whereas only 6 per cent of the other group, i.e., those with anatomically normal mitral valves, with valvular aortic stenosis had positive histories. The etiology of the aortic stenosis in the patients with anatomically normal mitral valves is unsolved. Possibly, as mentioned earlier, minor abnormalities in cuspal size from birth sets the stage for abnormal leaflet contact with resultant fibrosis and finally stenosis.[2]

Stenosis of the aortic valve in patients greater than age 65 years is usually characteristic.[4] The valves are tricuspid, nodular calcific deposits are rather uniformly distributed on the aortic aspects of each cusp, and the commissures are not fused. Obstruction results from the calcific deposits which prevent the cusps from retracting adequately during ventricular systole. Because the commissures are usually not fused, associated aortic regurgitation is infrequent.

Clinically, aortic stenosis in the elderly is characterized by several features which are either absent or more prominent than in younger subjects with this valvular lesion: the systemic arterial pulse pressure may be increased due to systolic hypertension; a harsh right basal systolic murmur may be relatively inconspicuous while a pure musical systolic murmur may be prominent at the apex; a coexisting apical systolic murmur of mitral regurgitation may be related to mitral annular calcification and not to left ventricular failure; and systemic systolic hypertension can result in a comparatively small pressure gradient despite severe left ventricular outflow obstruction.

The cause of the aortic stenosis in elderly patients is uncertain but simple wear-and-tear or degeneration appears to be the most reasonable explanation. The presence in the same hearts of other wear-and-tear lesions such as calcified mitral annuli, calcified coronary arteries, and focal thickening of other valve leaflets supports this contention.

Discrete Left Ventricular Outflow Obstruction (Discrete Subaortic Stenosis [DDS])

Although this congenital malformation does not primarily involve a cardiac valve, it may be confused with valvular aortic stenosis and it may cause secondary damage to the aortic valve cusps (Fig. 2).

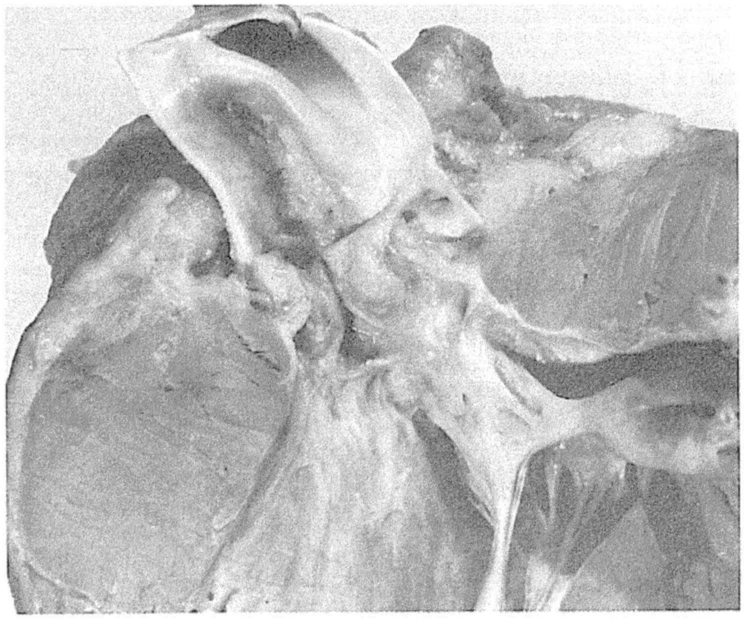

Figure 2. Discrete subaortic stenosis with scarring of the aortic valve. Opened aorta, aortic valve, and left ventricular outflow tract of a 13-year-old boy (A72–115) who died while swimming. Subaortic stenosis had been diagnosed by catheterization at age five. He had two operative procedures (ages five and seven) for removal of the subaortic membrane. Residual gradients of 132 mm. Hg and 60 mm. Hg, respectively, remained after these operations. At necropsy, a tough fibrous membrane was present. The aortic valve cusps were thickened and the aorta was smaller than normal.

We have studied at necropsy seven patients, aged 13 to 47 years (average 24), with DSS (Table 6). Five were male, and two were female. All seven had precordial diastolic murmurs (grade 1–3/6) typical of aortic regurgitation in addition to systolic thrills and loud murmurs (grade 3–5/6) typical of aortic stenosis. The one patient (#6, Table 6) with valvular stenosis also had an ejection click. Left ventricular peak systolic pressure gradients in 6 patients varied from 70 to 170 mm. Hg (avg. 115) and pressure tracings or left ventricular cineangiographic studies in each indicated discrete obstruction in the subvalvular region. The narrowed left ventricular outflow tract area ranged from 0.23 to 0.40 $cm.^2$ (avg. 0.34) in the four patients in whom it was calculated. Two patients, at ages 28 and 41 years respectively, developed infective endocarditis of the aortic valve causing severe regurgitation in each. Five patients underwent operative resection of the subaortic membrane and one also had aortic valve replacement because of aortic regurgitation. Three died within a month of operation and one died suddenly seven years later because of residual obstruction. The patient in whom the aortic valve was replaced died six years postoperatively because of prosthetic dysfunction.

Two of the seven patients with DSS had other congenital cardiovascular malformations—one had a parachute mitral valve (which apparently functioned normally), a small aortic valve "ring," and a small coarctation of the aorta; the second had a large patent ductus arteriosus and mild coarctation of the aorta.

Subaortic "membrane" tissue was present at necropsy in all seven patients.

Table 6. Discrete subaortic stenosis: clinical and necropsy findings

Patient	Age	Sex	Murmurs AS	Murmurs AR	Pressures LV S/D	Pressures SA S/D	Pressures LV-SA PSG	Area of LVOT (cm.^{2})	Operative resection of subvalvular membrane	LV-SA PSG (mm.Hg) postoperative	Anatomic findings: Aortic valve	Anatomic findings: Associated malformations
1. A57–133	18	M	4/6	2/6	156/–	86/55	70	0.4	+	0	Thickened	0
2. A62–305	30	F	5/6	2/6	270/24	100/55	170	0.23	+	10	Thickened	0
3. A64–20	28	M	3/6	2/6	—	—	—	—	0	—	Infected	0
4. 05–23–07	47	F	3/6	3/6	260/55	100/60	160	—	+*	12	Infected	PDA, C of A
5. A60–164	17	M	4/6	1/6	200/8	122/65	78	—	+	—	Thickened	Parachute MV
6. GT71A–215	14	M	4/6	2/6	165/30	85/60	80	0.4	0	—	Bicuspid stenotic	C of A VSD (closed)
7. A72–115	13	M	5/6	1/6	240/9	108/64	132	0.32	+	65	Thickened	0

* Also, aortic valve replacement
AR = aortic regurgitation. AS = aortic stenosis. C of A = coarctation of aorta. LV = left ventricle. LVOT = left ventricular outflow tract. MV = mitral valve. PDA = patent ductus arteriosus. PSG = peak systolic gradient. SA = systemic artery. S/D = systolic/diastolic. VSD = ventricular septal defect.

The discrete membrane (fibrous tissue) was, or had been, located in circumferential fashion on a plane approximately 1 cm. below the base of the aortic cusps corresponding with the ventricular aspect of the basal attachment of the anterior mitral leaflet. The ventricular aspects of the aortic valve cusps in all seven patients were thickened by fibrous tissue. The focal fibrous thickening in each of the six with tricuspid valves caused them to be incompetent. The ascending aorta and aortic root was hypoplastic in two patients (#6 and #7). The ventricular papillary muscles were focally scarred in all patients.

These seven patients emphasize the frequency of acquired lesions of the aortic valve in DSS. The aortic valves may become thickened and incompetent, and resulting jet lesions infected.[11]

Hypertrophic (Asymmetric) Cardiomyopathy with or without Subaortic Stenosis (Idiopathic Hypertrophic Subaortic Stenosis [IHSS])

Like discrete subaortic stenosis, diffuse muscular left ventricular outflow tract obstruction (IHSS) does not primarily involve a cardiac valve but it also may be confused with valvular heart disease and it also secondarily affects a cardiac valve (mitral) to produce varying degrees of regurgitation.

We have studied at necropsy 34 patients with IHSS. Cardiac catheterization had been performed in 28: 17 had systolic pressure gradients (20 to 162 [avg. 93]) at rest between left ventricular body and a systemic artery, and 11 had no pressure gradients at rest. Patients with gradients at rest differed in one respect anatomically from those without gradients at rest: those with gradients had uniformly thickened left ventricular free walls whereas those without gradients at rest had free walls, at least that portion immediately behind posterior mitral leaflet, of normal thickness. The cardiac anatomic features in these 34 patients were: (1) disproportional hypertrophy of the ventricular septae, i.e., the ventricular septae were thicker than the left ventricular free walls (28 patients); (2) small or normal-sized left and right ventricular cavities (31 patients); (3) endocardial mural plaques, left ventricular outflow tract (25 patients); (4) thickened mitral valves (25 patients); (5) dilated left and right atria (32 patients); (6) hypertrophied free walls of all four cardiac chambers (34 patients); (7) normal or nearly normal aortic valve cusps (31 patients); and (8) normal sized aortae (34 patients).

In contrast to discrete subaortic stenosis, the aortic valve is not involved in IHSS. The reason appears to be related to the relatively long distance between the site of left ventricular outflow obstruction and the aortic valve. In IHSS the gradient appears to be located on a plane corresponding to the distal margin of the anterior mitral leaflet. The caudal margin of the endocardial mural plaque in the left ventricular outflow tract also corresponds to the distal margin of the anterior mitral leaflet. The caudal margin of the endocardial mural plaque in the left ventricular outflow tract also corresponds to the distal margin of the anterior mitral leaflet. The caudal extension of this plaque is about 3 to 4 cm. below the base of the aortic valve cusps, and thus any jet produced at the site of obstruction is diffused by the time blood contacts the aortic valve cusps. In discrete subaortic stenosis, in contrast, the obstruction occurs about 1 cm. below the base of the aortic valve cusps, the jet is unable to be diffused before contacting the aortic cusps, and the cusps become thickened and prone to infection.

The cardiac valve which is made abnormal in IHSS is the mitral one. The ventricular aspect of the anterior leaflet is usually thickened by contacting the mural endocardium in the left ventricular outflow tract during ventricular systole. The left ventricular cavity in IHSS is relatively small, and when the left ventricular walls contract, the posterior leaflet is squeezed abnormally so that portions of it contact other portions like an accordian causing focal fibrous thickening. Although it may be impressive in IHSS, the fibrous thickening of the mitral leaflets and chordae tendineae does not appear to be the explanation for mitral regurgitation, which occurs in the majority of patients with IHSS because the mitral regurgitation nearly always disappears following adequate left ventricular myotomy of myectomy.[12] Distortion of the anterior left ventricular papillary muscle during ventricular systole by the massively hypertrophied ventricular septum may better explain the mitral regurgitation in these patients.[13]

Although mitral regurgitation is to be expected in patients with IHSS, the

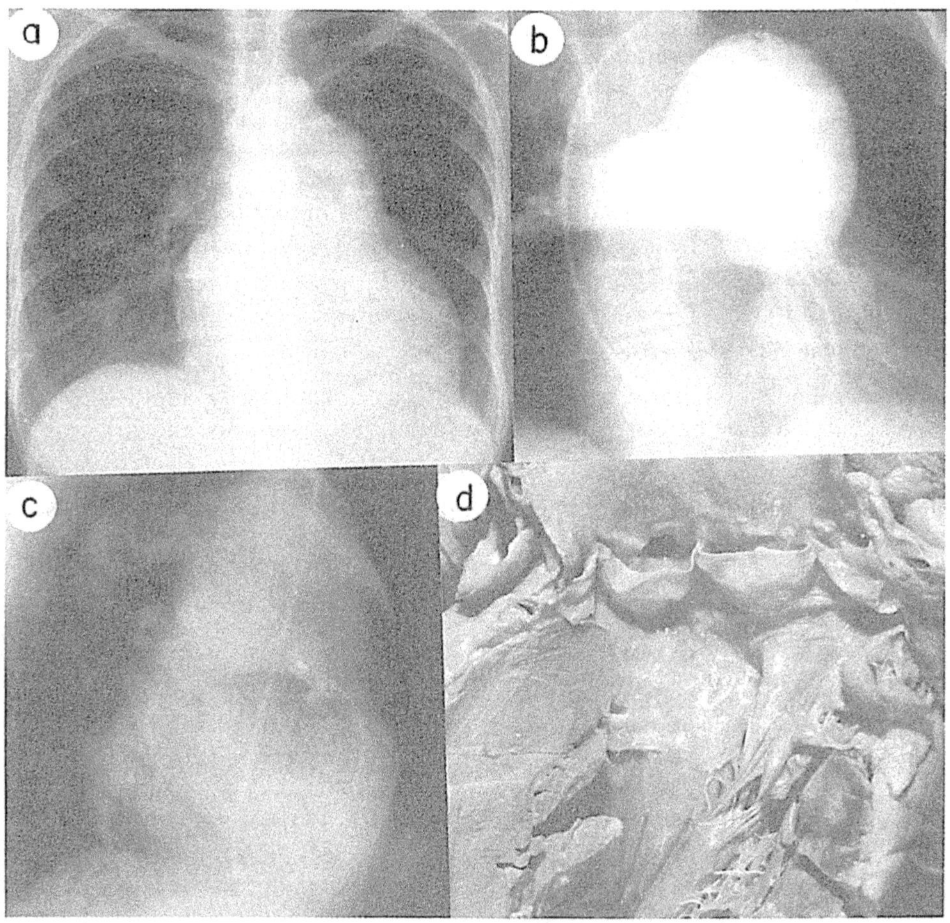

Figure 3. Hypertrophic (asymmetric) cardiomyopathy (idiopathic hypertrophic subaortic stenosis [IHSS]) presenting as pure mitral regurgitation. This 41-year-old woman (A63–77) was found to have a precordial murmur and cardiomegaly on insurance examination at age 33 and overt right-sided

and left-sided congestive cardiac failure, which progressed, appeared at age 38 years. When examined a month before death she was severely ill (functionally class IV). A grade 4/6 blowing pansystolic precordial murmur, loudest along the lower left sternal border, was audible. Electrocardiogram showed atrial fibrillation and a marked clockwise rotation. By x-ray (a, b, c), the heart was enlarged and the pulmonary trunk was aneurysmally dilated. The total serum protein was 5.3 with albumin 1.9 gm. per 100 ml., and 2.2 gm. of protein were measured in the urine in a 24-hour period. The total serum cholesterol was 318 mg. per 100 ml. At catheterization, the pressures (in mm. Hg) were: pulmonary artery, 34/7; right ventricle, 34/5; right atrial mean, 4; pulmonary arterial wedge, mean 11, v14; left ventricle, 112/11; and femoral artery, 122/65. The cardiac output (Fick method) was 1.6 L./min./m.^{2}. Left ventricular cineangiogram disclosed 4 /4 mitral regurgitation. (Retrospective examination of this angiogram was strongly suggestive of hypertrophic cardiomyopathy.) Aortic root injection of contrast material showed no aortic regurgitation. A day before death, cardiotomy was performed to replace the severely incompetent mitral valve. At operation, however, no systolic thrill was palpable over the left atrium which expanded hardly at all during ventricular systole. Examination of the mitral valve after cardiopulmonary bypass was instituted disclosed that the mitral leaflets and chordae were "normal" and that the left ventricular cavity was not dilated. Therefore, valve replacement was not carried out. The patient died the next day because of inadequate cardiac output. At necropsy, a large transmural acute myocardial infarct involved the posterior left ventricular free wall. Histologic study indicated that the infarct was about 14 days old. The mitral leaflets and chordae were focally thickened but the annulus was not dilated and the left ventricular cavity was of normal size. In the outflow tract of the left ventricle, a mural endocardial plaque, in direct apposition to the anterior mitral leaflet, was present (d). Since the aortic valve cusps were normal, it was clear that this endocardial plaque indicated that *hypertrophic cardiomyopathy* was the proper diagnosis. The ventricular septum was nearly twice as thick as was the left ventricular free wall. Thus, this patient demonstrates how IHSS may present as pure mitral regurgitation. The cause of the aneurysmal dilatation of the pulmonary trunk is uncertain. (At operation, a diastolic thrill had been palpated over this artery indicating the presence of pulmonic regurgitation.)

amount of regurgitation is usually minimal or mild. On rare occasions, however, mitral regurgitation is the dominant lesion (Fig. 3) and valve replacement, although hazardous in this condition, has been performed.

Supravalvular Aortic Stenosis (SAS)

Like subaortic stenosis, this condition does not primarily affect a cardiac valve but it too may be confused with valvular aortic stenosis and it also may

Figure 4. Valvular aortic stenosis from arteriosclerosis in homozygous type II hyperlipoproteinemia. a, Opened aortic valve and ascending aorta showing severe atherosclerosis of the aorta and severe fibrous thickening of the aortic valve cusps which are relatively rigid. b, Radiograph of heart at necropsy showing extensive calcific deposits in the ascending aorta and in the coronary arteries. c, Photograph of patient showing xanthomas on elbows, buttocks, and ankles. d, Photomicrograph (hematoxylin-eosin stain X 63) of portion of anterior mitral leaflet showing extensive collections of foam cells. Similar lesions were present in the aortic valve cusps. This 28-year-old man (A70–64), who died suddenly, had xanthomas noted at age two years. He ate low-fat foods most of his life. He was asymptomatic until age 17 years when angina pectoris appeared. At age 23, the first of several episodes of syncope occurred and at age 26 he had an episode of acute pulmonary edema without evidence of acute myocardial infarction. When studied a month later, he had mild exertional dyspnea and angina. He slept flat in bed. Several family members, including both parents, had type II hyperlipoproteinemia. In addition to large widespread tuberotendinous xanthomas, he had a sustained left ventricular lift and a grade 3/6 mid-systolic, ejection-type murmur over the left sternal border with radiation into the neck. He had no signs of congestive cardiac failure. The blood pressure was 115/65 mm. Hg. The heart was of normal size on chest roentgenogram. The initial serum total cholesterol was 588 with beta, alpha, and VLDL fractions 529, 31, and 28 mg. per 100 ml., respectively. The total serum triglyceride was 100 mg. per 100 ml. Protein electrophoresis showed a bifid peak in the beta region with a quantitation of 1.3 gm. per 100 ml. During his last two years he was treated with a low-cholesterol diet and high doses (48 gm. daily) of cholestyramine. The total serum cholesterol fell to 340 mg. per 100 ml., the xanthomas softened slightly and became less yellow. The immediate cause of death was not determined at necropsy.

be associated with fibrous thickening of the aortic valvular cusps. In this condition, the site of obstruction is the ascending aorta, most frequently (66 per cent) on a level corresponding to the most cephalad extension of the aortic valve cusps.[14] Maximal narrowing at this site produces an hourglass type obstruction. The narrowing results both from thickening of the aortic media and from superimposed fibrous intimal proliferation. Less frequently (21 per cent), the supravalvular obstruction results from diffuse hypoplasia of the entire ascending aorta or from a fibrous membrane just above the aortic sinuses associated with a central opening and a more normal-sized aorta (13 per cent).[14] Each of these three anatomic

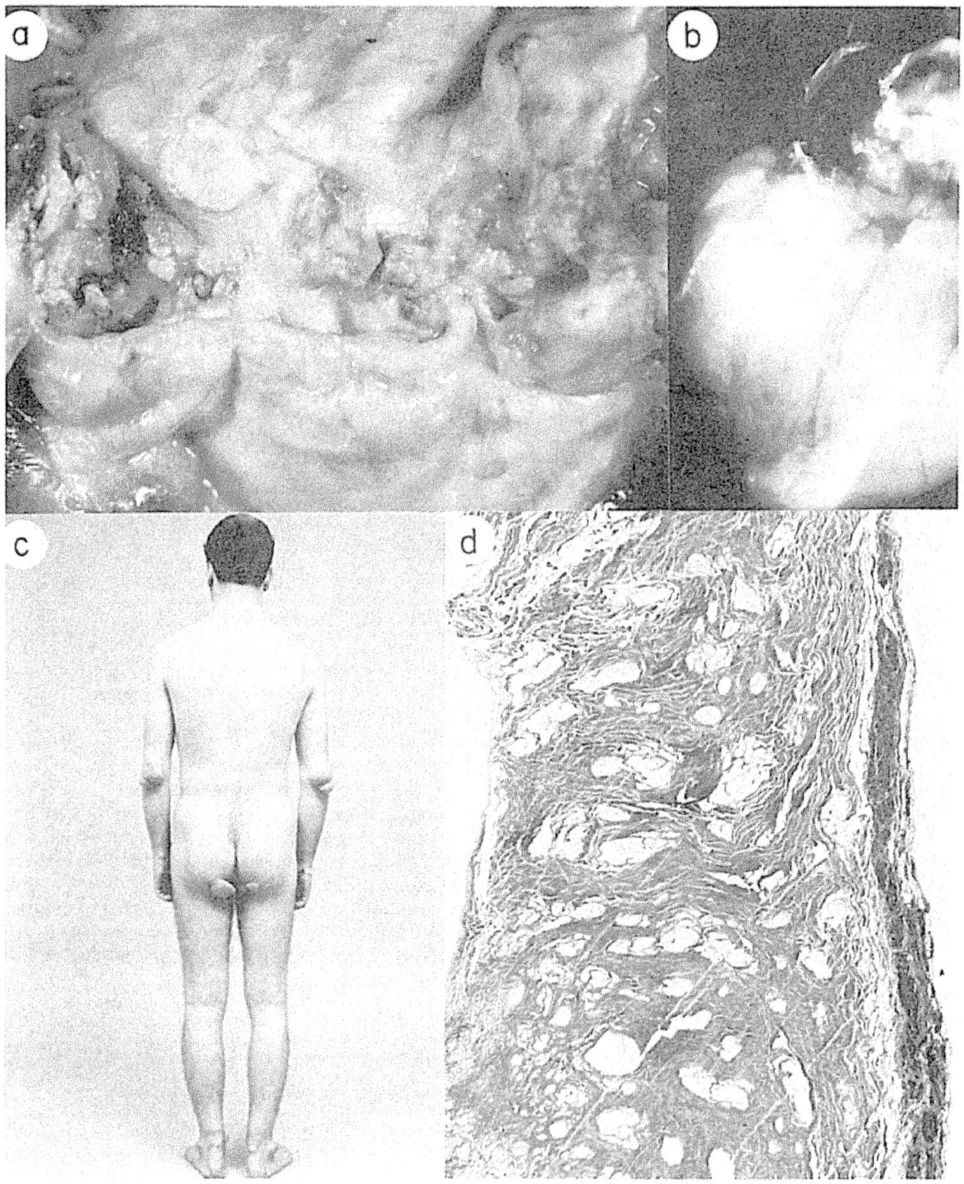

types may be associated with fibrous thickening of the aortic valve cusps, and may produce valvular aortic stenosis. Aortic valve cusps were thickened in 30 per cent of 68 necropsy cases of supravalvular aortic stenosis analyzed from the literature.[14] Occasionally, the margin of one or more cusps may be adherent to the aortic wall at the site of supravalvular obstruction and these deformities may produce aortic regurgitation. We have studied at necropsy two patients with supravalvular aortic stenosis.[15] Both had the hourglass type deformity: in one the aortic valve cusps were normal and in the second the cusps were diffusely thickened and adherent to the area of supravalvular stenosis probably causing valvular dysfunction.

Infection on the intima of the aorta above the aortic valve may complicate supravalvular aortic stenosis and the infection may extend retrogradely to involve the area of narrowing just above the aortic valve and the valve itself.

Although usually congenital in origin, SAS on rare occasion may be acquired. Healing of an aortotomy incision may constrict the aorta in an hourglass-type deformity. Homozygous type II hyperlipoproteinemia may be associated with severe atherosclerosis in the ascending aorta as well as in the aortic valve cusps themselves[16] (Fig. 4). Recently, a patient with type II hyperlipoproteinemia was reported as having supravalvular aortic "stenosis."[17]

Obstruction to Left Ventricular Inflow

Congenital Mitral Stenosis

Obstruction to left ventricular inflow at the level of the mitral valve may be congenital in origin or acquired. In the latter, the cause is usually filling defects

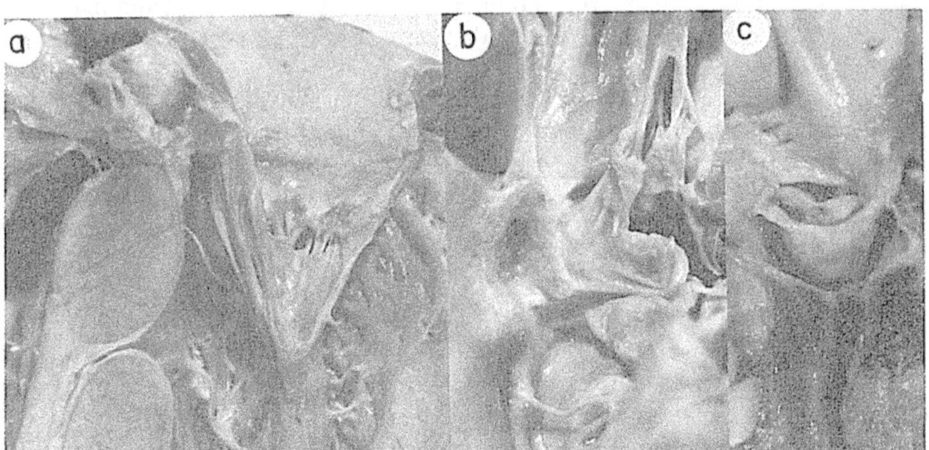

Figure 5. Single left ventricular papillary muscle (a) (Parachute mitral valve), discrete subaortic stenosis (b), and stenotic congenitally bicuspid aortic valve (c) in a 14 year-old boy (GT 71A–215) who had an 80 mm. Hg peak systolic pressure gradient between left ventricle and systemic artery. He had been asymptomatic until one year before death from pulmonary edema. No abnormality of the mitral valve had been appreciated clinically. a, Longitudinal section across mitral and aortic valves and ventricular septum demonstrating the parachute mitral deformity. A defect in the muscular portion of the ventricular septum had closed spontaneously by fibrous-tissue proliferation. b, View of discrete subaortic stenosis from left ventricle. c, View of bicuspid, stenotic aortic valve from above.

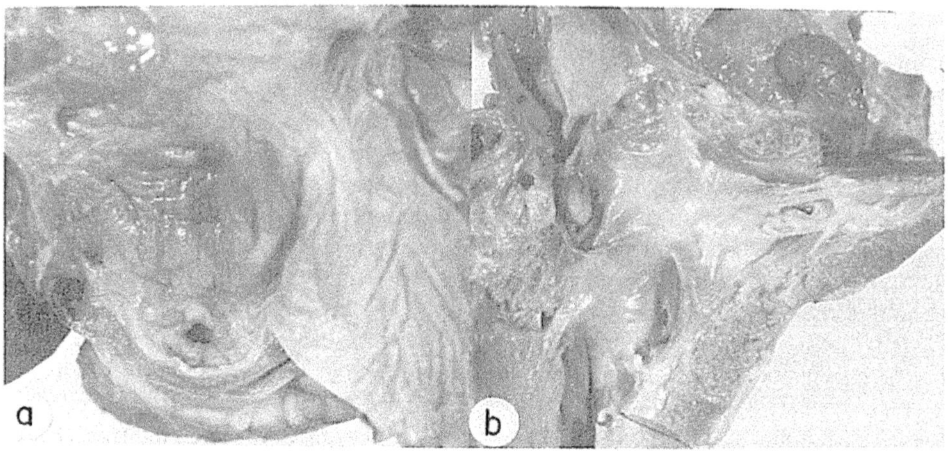

Figure 6. Congenital mitral stenosis with parachute mitral valve and supravalvular left atrial ring in a young child (A69–264). a, Mitral valve area viewed from left atrium. A fibrous diaphragm with a narrowed central orifice is present at the level of the annulus. The endocardium of the dilated left atrium is severely thickened. b, Opened left ventricle, aortic valve, and aorta. The thickened chordae tendineae insert into a single papillary muscle which is located in an anterolateral position. The valve orifice is stenotic. In addition, this child had a defect in the membranous portion of the ventricular septum (it nearly was closed by septal tricuspid leaflet), a persistent patent ductus arteriosus, and a coarctation of the aorta.

in the left atrium which protrude into the mitral orifice during ventricular diastole. These filling defects include left atrial myxomas,[18] fungal masses[19] and malignant neoplasms.[20] The latter two generally originate in the lung and extend into the left atrium via pulmonary veins.

Nonrheumatic valvular obstruction involving mitral leaflets is virtually limited to congenital anomalies. In one type of congenital mitral stenosis (MS) the leaflets are thickened and fibrosed with rudimentary or fused commissures and short and fused chordae.[21] Anatomically, the valve is funnel-shaped and resembles a rheumatically diseased valve. Another variety is the parachute deformity[22-23] (Figs. 5 and 6), in which the chordae are shortened and converge to insert on a single papillary muscle thus restricting the motion of the leaflets. Left ventricular inflow is limited primarily to openings between chordae. Both anomalies often are complicated by discrete supravalvular fibrous diaphragms arising from the atrial aspect of the valve annuli (Fig. 6). Either the valvular deformity or the annular diaphragm or both may cause obstruction. Parachute mitral valves are usually associated with other developmental anomalies including coarctation of the aorta (often with a bicuspid aortic valve), discrete subvalvular left ventricular outflow obstruction, and supravalvular mitral ring, which may or may not be stenotic. Congenital MS also may result from an arcade type deformity of the valve[24] (Fig. 7).

The hemodymanic consequences of congenital MS are similar to those caused by acquired (rheumatic) MS. Auscultation, however, may differ. Many patients with congenital MS do not have detectable diastolic murmurs, and opening snaps

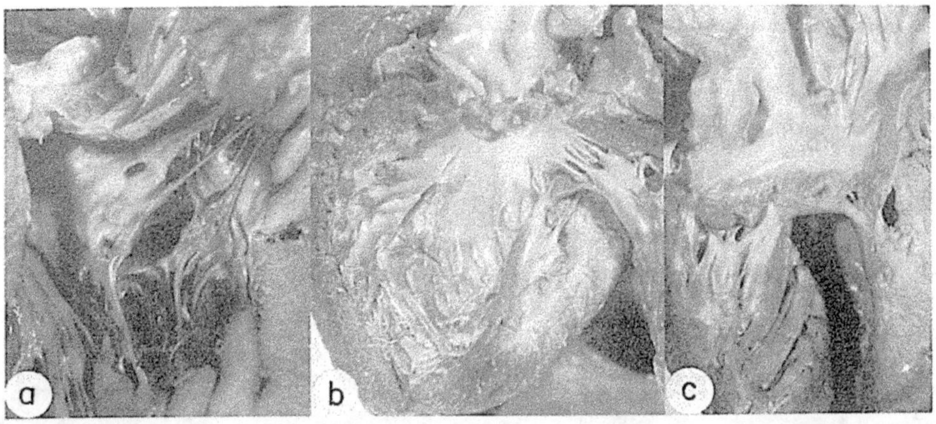

Figure 7. Congenital mitral stenosis due to "arcade" type deformity of the valve. This 3-day-old boy (A67–212), who died during catheterization, was diagnosed clinically as having "hypoplastic left heart." At necropsy, the mitral valve appeared stenotic. a, View of mitral valve from left ventricle. b, Opened left ventricle, aortic valve, and aorta. The endocardium is thickened, and the aortic valve consisted of rudimentary cusps. c, Opened mitral valve showing short chordae tendineae and thickened cuspal margins. The patient also had a large patent ductus arteriosus.

are rare. These auscultatory differences may be explained by their rapid heart rates, by the increased tendency of the right ventricle to occupy the apex and obscure the murmur, and by the severly reduced mobility of the leaflets.[25]

Congenital MS, even when associated with other anomalies, is rare, but when isolated is extremely rare.[26] We have not observed congenital MS as an isolated defect. The heart of a child with a stenotic supravalvular ring and a parachute deformity of the mitral valve is illustrated in Figure 6.

Obstruction to Right Ventricular Outflow

Isolated Valvular Pulmonic Stenosis

Congenital valvular pulmonic stenosis (PS) with intact ventricular septum is the most common form of isolated right ventricular outflow obstruction and comprises about 10 per cent of all major congenital cardiovascular anomalies in patients surviving beyond infancy.[27] The stenotic valve usually has a

Table 7. Isolated congenital pulmonic stenosis: clinical and necropsy findings

Patient	*Age (yrs.)*	*Sex*	*Duration (yrs.) symptoms*	*Cyanosis*	*Right-sided CHF*	*RV-PA PSG (mm. Hg)*	*Heart weight (gm.)*	*Pulmonic valve*	*VC-PFO*
1. A55–59	4	F	2	+	+	124	270*	Dome	+
2. A64–135	43	F	35	+	+	161	400	Dome	+
3. NNMC# A71–24	38	F	—	0	+	88	450	Bicuspid	0

* Expected weight = 75 gm.
CHF = congestive heart failure. PA = pulmonary artery. PSG = peak systolic gradient. RV= right ventricle. VC-PFO = valvular competent patent foramen ovale.

domed shape or funnel shape with a small (less than 5 mm.) opening at the apex. Three raphes extend from the valve to the pulmonary trunk and these probably represent vestigial commissures. Rarely, three separate cusps are identifiable but when this occurs additional developmental defects usually are present.[28] The mean age of death in unoperated patients with isolated PS is 25 years.[29] Older patients with this malformation may develop calcific deposits in the valve.[30,31]

We have studied at necropsy three patients with isolated congenital valvular PS (Table 7, Figs. 8–11). All three died within two months of pulmonic val-

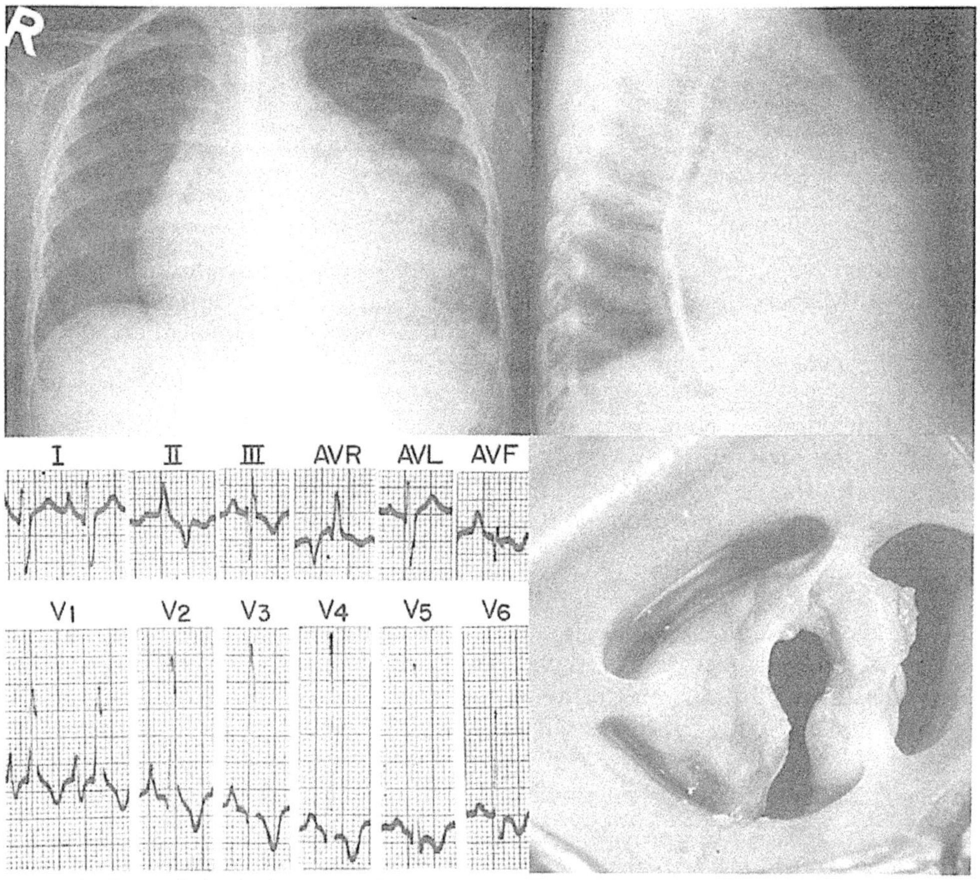

Figure 8. Congenital valvular pulmonic stenosis. Posteroanterior and lateral chest roentgenograms, electrocardiogram, and pulmonary valve from a four-year-old girl (A55–59) who died just after pulmonic valvulotomy. A precordial murmur had been heard at six months of age and by two years cyanosis was present. By age three she was in right-sided cardiac failure and had episodes of precordial pain. Chest roentgenogram reveals severe cardiomegaly with marked right ventricular enlargement and decreased pulmonary vascular markings. Electrocardiogram shows right atrial enlargement and right ventricular hypertrophy. The cardiac size and monophasic R waves in V_1 through V_6 contrast sharply with those of the adult patient in Figure 9. A single incision had been made in the valve at operation but the domed structure, small central orifice, and fused commissures with raphes attached to the wall of the pulmonary trunk are well preserved.

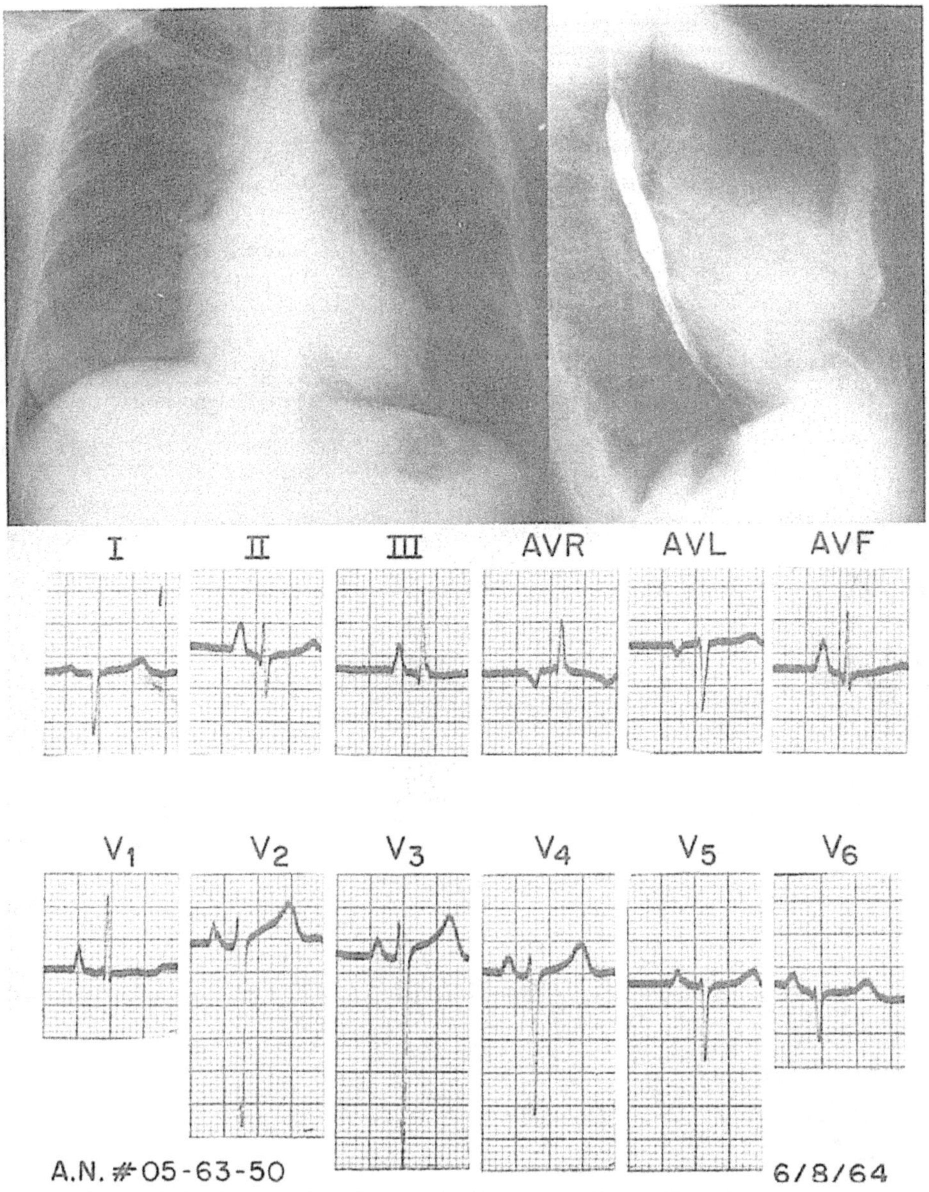

Figure 9. Congenital valvular pulmonic stenosis. Posteroanterior and lateral chest roentgenograms and electrocardiogram of a 43-year-old woman (A64–135) who died during pulmonic valvulotomy. She had symptoms of cardiac dysfunction since age five years. For several years before death she had episodes of severe precordial pressure and dyspnea associated with mild exertion. Despite these symptoms she underwent two normal pregnancies and worked on a factory assembly line until hospitalization. On examination, she was cyanotic with clubbed fingers and toes. Chest roentgenogram revealed right atrial and right ventricular enlargement, a prominent pulmonary segment, normal to decreased pulmonary vascular markings, and pectus carinatum. Electrocardiogram showed right axis deviation (120 degrees) and right atrial and right ventricular hypertrophy.

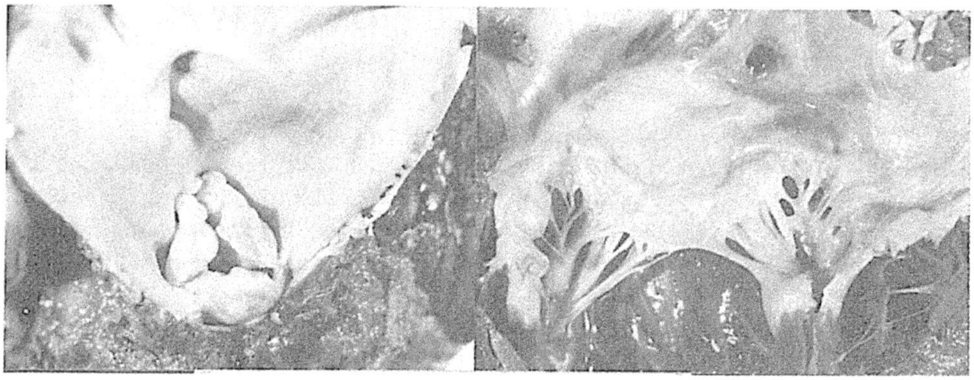

Figure 10. Congenital valvular pulmonic stenosis. Anatomic findings from woman whose electrocardiogram and roentgenogram are depicted in Figure 9. *Left,* Opened pulmonary trunk showing stenotic three-cuspid pulmonic valve after commissurotomy. *Right,* Although there was no clinical evidence of mitral valve dysfunction, the mitral leaflets and chordae were thickened.

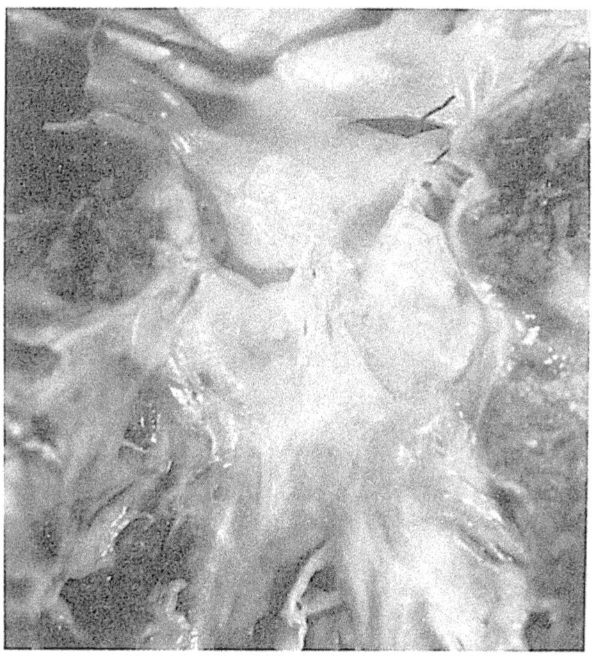

Figure 11. Pulmonic valve stenosis with bicuspid valve. Opened pulmonic valve and pulmonary trunk of a 34-year-old woman (NNMC# A71-24) who died of sepsis from an infected hematoma several months after pulmonic valvulotomy. The cusps are thickened and stiff.

vulotomy. Two had dome-shaped valves and one had a congenitally bicuspid valve. The valves in each were thickened, scarred, and stiff.

Congenitally bucuspid pulmonic valves are rare in comparison with the frequency of congenitally bicuspid aortic valves. Although they are commonly associated with other congenital cardiovascular malformations, particularly tetralogy of Fallot, congenitally bicuspid pulmonic valves appear to be extremely rare in patients with isolated pulmonic stenosis.[32] Indeed, we have found no reports describing isolated pulmonic stenosis complicating the congenitally bicuspid valve.

Obstruction to Both Right Ventricular Outflow and Inflow

The Carcinoid Syndrome

First recognized as a distinct entity in 1954,[33] this syndrome is caused by a metastasizing carcinoid tumor located usually in the small intestine, occasionally in the bronchus[34] or stomach,[35] and rarely elsewhere. The tumor produces several biologically active substances, including serotonin (5-hydroxytryptamine), histamine, and kinin peptides (bradykinin).[36] Diagnosis is established on the basis of increased urinary excretion of 5-hydroxyindole acetic acid (HIAA), a breakdown product of serotonin.[37] Dermal flushing and diarrhea occur in almost all patients with the syndrome; wheezing occurs in approximately a third, and a peculiar but specific cardiac disease is present in over one half.[38,39] Of 32 necropsy patients with the carcinoid syndrome studied by us, 18 had carcinoid heart disease and 14 did not (Table 8).

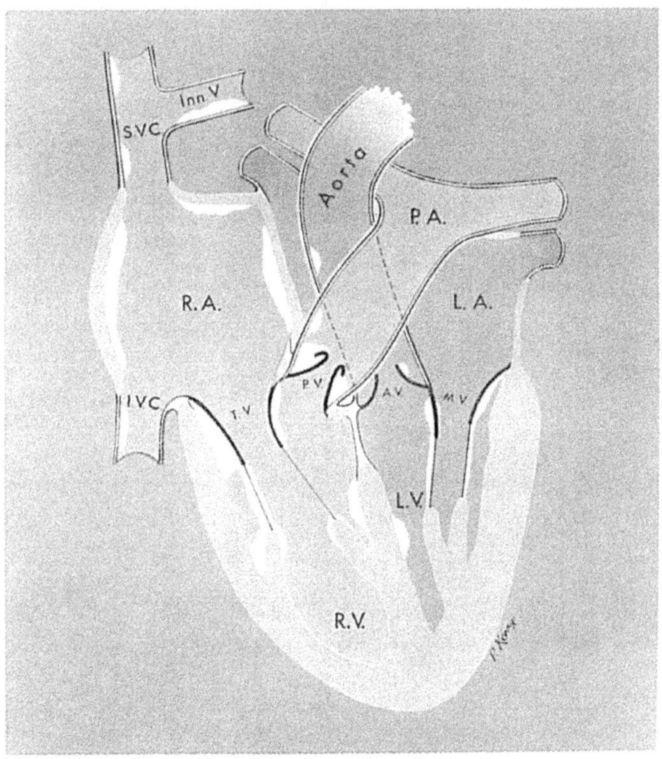

Figure 12. Carcinoid heart disease. Summary diagram demonstrating (in white) the sites where fibrous plaques occur in patients with the carcinoid syndrome. In patients with abdominal carcinoid tumors the lesions are always more numerous and more extensive on the right side of the heart. The white plaques often are extensive in right atrium (R.A.) and tricuspid (T.V.) and pulmonic (P.V.) valves. The lesions have not been observed in the pulmonary arteries (P.A.) except in the immediate vicinity of the valve or in the left atrium (L.A.). Inn. V. = innominate vein. S.V.C. = superior vena cava. I.V.C. = inferior vena cava. R.V. = right ventricle. M.V. = mitral valve. L.V. = left ventricle. A.V. = aortic valve.

Table 8. The carcinoid syndrome: clinical and necropsy data

	No. pts.	Ages range (avg.) (years)	F	M	Length of illness (mo.) (avg.)	Diarrhea	Flushing	Asthma	Precordial murmur	Urinary 5-HIAA excretion (mg./24 hrs.)	Small intestinal primary	Hepatic metastases	Organ weights (gm.) Liver	Heart	Spleen
With heart disease	18*	32–69 (53)	8	10	10–156 (58)	18	17	8	18	120–1270 (418)	18	18	1600–7400 (2723)	200–475 (283)	40–475 (159)
Without heart disease	14†	28–75 (56)	4	10	12–108 (45)	13	14	4	8‡	14–900 (284)	10 ¶	13	500–6100 (3015)	150–450 (284)	30–730 (247)
TOTALS	32	28–75 (55)	12	20	10–156 (53)	31	31	12	26	14-1270 § (357)§	28 ¶	31	1600–7400 (2847)	150–475# (285)	30–730** (200)

* 3 black; 15 white
† All white
‡ One had a large atrial septal defect; another had a large left atrial myxoma; another had severe valvular aortic stenosis.
§ The range and average are of the highest values for each patient.
¶ Bronchus in three; stomach in one.
\# Only four (two from each group) of 32 hearts weighed more than 400 gm. and each patient had a history of systemic hypertension.
** Weight more than 300 gm. in five patients, two with and three without carcinoid heart disease.

The cardiovascular lesions associated with the carcinoid syndrome are pathognomonic and bear little resemblance to those in other cardiac diseases.[38] The involvement consists of focal or diffuse collections of a peculiar type of fibrous tissue which is deposited on the endocardium of the valvular cusps and cardiac chambers and on the intima of the great veins, coronary sinus, and occasionally great arteries (Figs. 12–14). The valvular cusps per se and mural endocardium are normal, and are clearly separated from the fibrosing process by the endocardial elastic membrane. The deposits, which are often referred to as fibrous, white, or carcinoid plaques, are most frequent and extensive in the right side of the

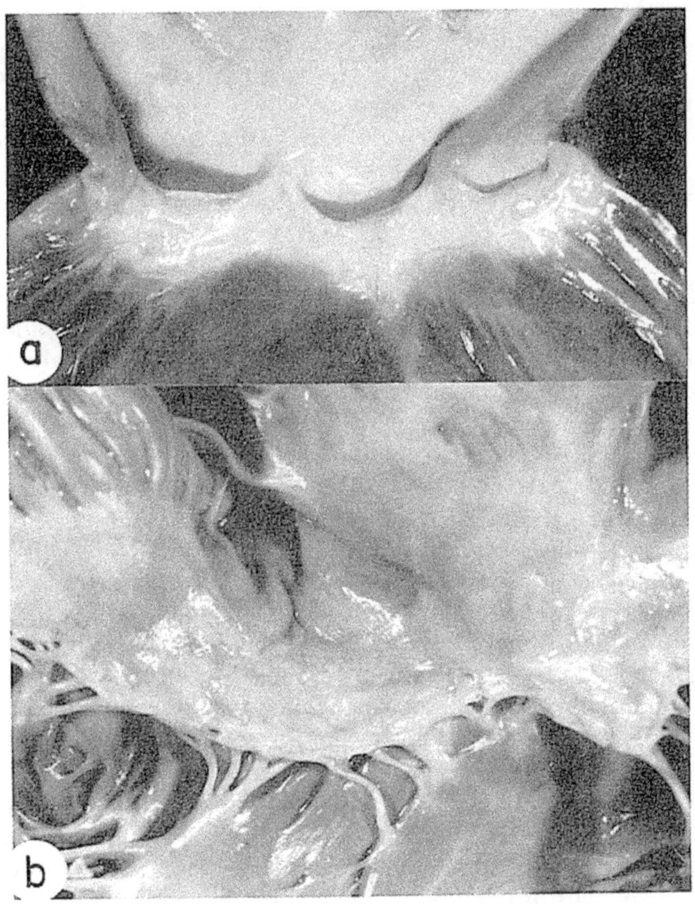

Figure 13. Carcinoid heart disease. Opened pulmonic (a) and tricuspid (b) valves in a 61-year-old woman (A72–96) who had had diarrhea and dermal flushing for 12 months. She had evidence clinically of tricuspid regurgitation and pulmonic stenosis. She developed severe ascites and subcutaneous edema and died of massive gastrointestinal hemorrhage. A carcinoid tumor was present in the ileum and carcinoid metastases were present in abdominal lymph nodes and in liver. The heart was small (240 gm.) but she was cachectic. Carcinoid plaques were present on tricuspid and pulmonic valves, right atrial endocardium, and coronary sinus. The pulmonic valve ring was constricted and the cusps were retracted (a). The tricuspid valve cusps and chordae also were thickened and contracted (b).

heart. Of our 18 patients with carcinoid heart disease, plaques were present on the tricuspid and pulmonic valves in all: on right atrium in 17, right ventricle in 11, vena cava in 7, coronary sinus and veins in 8, and pulmonary trunk in 4. In every patient the tricuspid and pulmonic valves were contracted, relatively rigid, and both stenotic and incompetent. The predominant hemodynamic lesion of the tricuspid valve, however, was regurgitation, and that of the pulmonic valve, stenosis. The diffuse deposition of fibrous tissue on the endocardium of the right atrium causes its wall to be relatively noncompliant.[39] The deposits on the right ventricle, in contrast, are always small and functionally insignificant.

Left-sided cardiac lesions in the carcinoid syndrome are more common than initially believed and occurred in seven patients: mitral valve lesion in all seven, left ventricle in three, aortic valve in one, and ascending aorta in one. Although two patients had diffuse mitral valvular deposits, the valvular orifices did not appear stenotic or incompetent. The aortic valve carcinoid plaque occurred in only one of the three cusps and caused no valvular dysfunction. No patients with left-sided lesions had intracardiac or extracardiac shunts nor carcinoid tumor in the lungs. The right-sided cardiac lesions in these seven patients were always more extensive than the left-sided ones. Carcinoid plaquing limited entirely to the left side of the heart, however, has been reported with bronchial carcinoid.[40]

With the exception of the anterior tricuspid and anterior mitral leaflets, the fibrous plaques were located on the ventricular surfaces of the atrioventricular cusps. The deposits on the posterior and septal tricuspid leaflets adhered these cusps to the underlying right ventricular wall, and the semilunar valvular deposits were located entirely within the sinuses.

The right ventricle and right atrium were mildly hypertrophied and dilated in each of the 18 patients with carcinoid heart disease, but, overall, the hearts of the 18 patients with carcinoid heart disease were identical in weight to those of the 14 patients without cardiac involvement (Table 8). Four patients had hearts weighing more than 400 gm. and each had histories of systemic hypertension. Interstitial and replacement myocardial fibrosis is not part of carcinoid heart disease and if present can be attributed to another condition.

Carcinoid plaques are composed of layers of collagen and acid mucopolysaccharide; the cellular elements are narrow, elongated, arranged parallel to the surface of the plaque, and stain intensely with phosphotungstic acid hematoxylin. The distinctive histologic feature of carcinoid plaques, however, is the absence of elastic tissue. The underlying internal elastic lamina of the endocardium is intact. Electron-microscopic examination shows that the carcinoid plaque consists of smooth muscle cells, fibrils of young and developing collagen, layered material similar to that of basement membranes of smooth muscle cells, and small spicules of unknown composition.[41]

The most useful clinical finding for distinguishing patients with carcinoid heart disease from those without is the presence of a precordial murmur suggestive of tricuspid regurgitation or pulmonic stenosis. The most frequent murmur in the 18 patients with cardiac involvement was fairly harsh in quality, grade 1 to 3/6 in intensity, systolic in time, and located along the upper left sternal border. Less frequently, a systolic blowing murmur which increased with inspira-

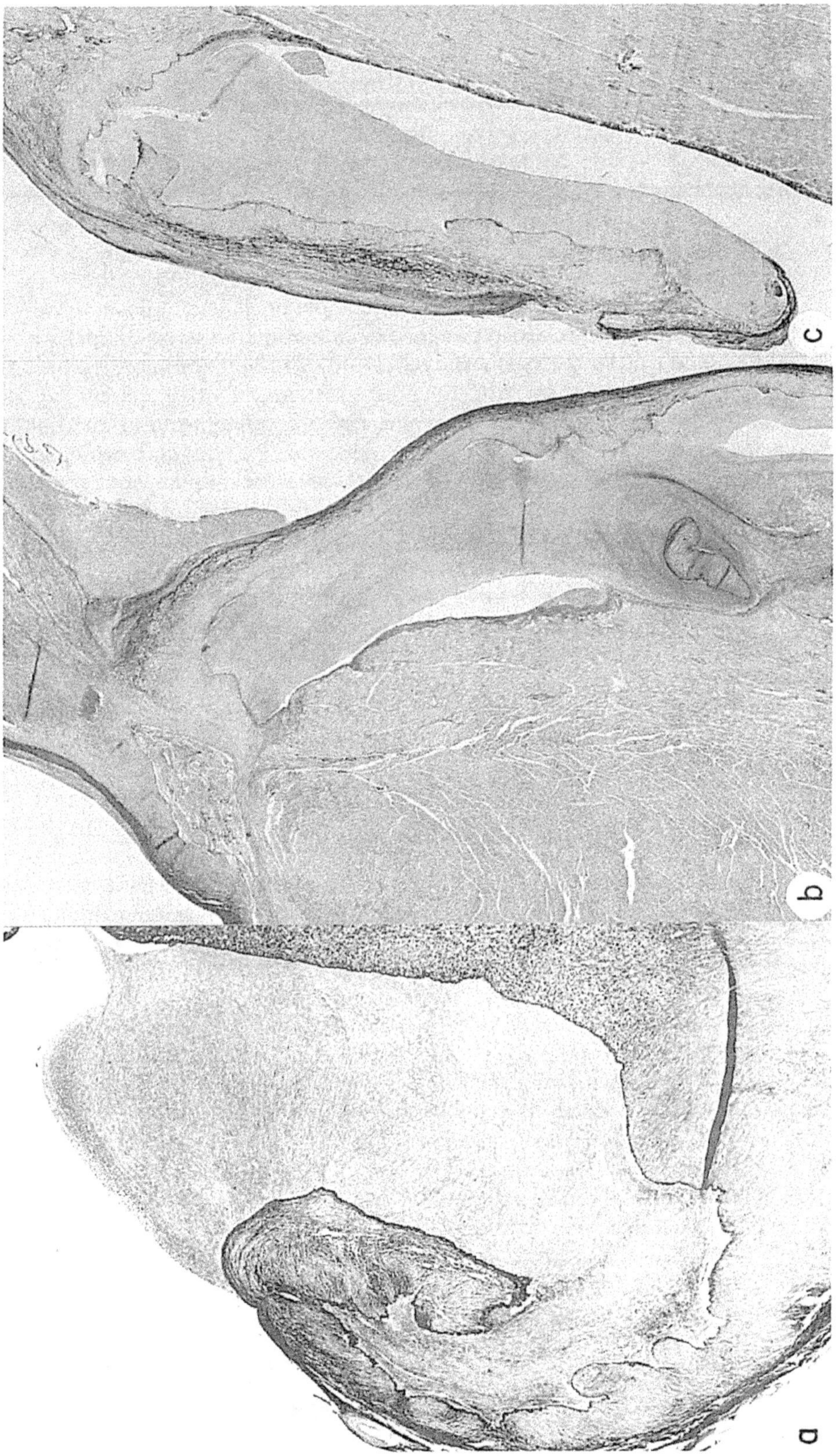

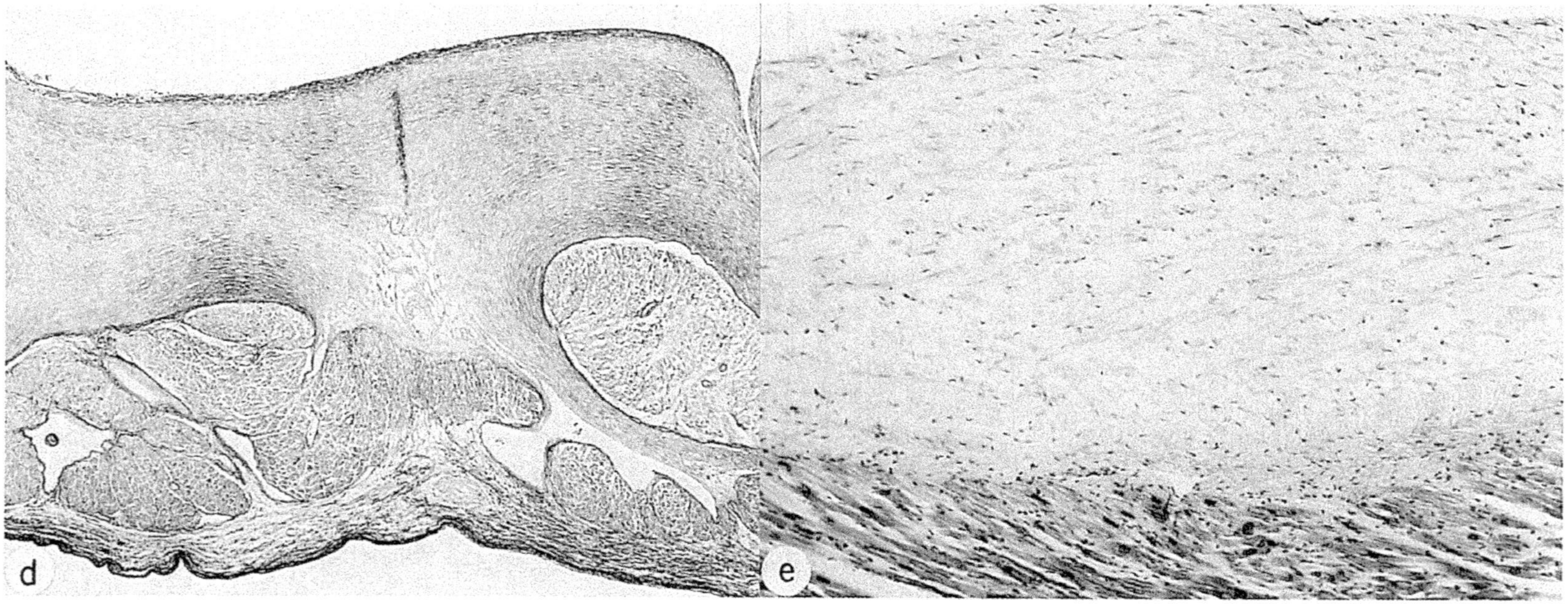

Figure 14. Carcinoid heart disease. Photomicrographs of carcinoid plaques in pulmonic valve (a), tricuspid valve (b), mitral valve (c), and right atrium (d and e). a, The carcinoid plaque which consists of an unusual type of elastic fiber, is located entirely on the sinus side of the cusp, i.e., the side which does not have the initial contact with the blood stream. The normal valve cusp is clearly separated from the superimposed fibrous tissue by a black staining elastic membrane (A61–68). b, Tricuspid valve showing extensive carcinoid plaquing on the ventricular aspect of the cusp. The plaque adheres the valve leaflet to the underlying mural endocardium. The penetrating portion of the atrioventricular bundle also is visible on this section (A61–193). c, Posterior mitral leaflet. The carcinoid plaque is on the undersurface of the cusp, which remains normal (A61–193). d, Right atrial wall showing a large carcinoid plaque superimposed on normal right atrial endocardium (A59–223). e, Close-up of carcinoid atrial plaque showing that it consists of strap cells, arranged parallel to its surface, separated by an amorphous ground substance (A61–193). a-d, Elastic van Gieson stains. e, Hematoxylin-eosin stain. [Reduced 15 per cent from × 39(a), × 14(b), × 18(c), × 40(d), and × 108 (e).]

tion was heard along the lower left sternal border. In none of the seven patients with mitral carcinoid disease was the diagnosis apparent clinically. Prominent v waves often were detectable in the superficial jugular veins; a waves were occasionally prominent also. The liver was sometimes pulsatile.

The chest roentgenogram and electrocardiogram are of little value in determining the presence or absence of carcinoid heart disease. Although the lateral chest roentgenogram sometimes discloses enlargement of the right ventricle, the overall size of the heart on posteroanterior projection is usually normal. Low voltage, the most frequent electrocardiographic abnormality in patients with this syndrome, occurred in 9 of 18 patients with carcinoid heart disease and in 3 of the 14 patients without it. Electrocardiographic evidence of right ventricular hypertrophy occurred in only 2 patients, and evidence of right atrial enlargement (peaked P waves) occurred in 4 of 18 patients with carcinoid heart disease.

Cardiac catheterization in patients with carcinoid heart disease has disclosed tricuspid regurgitation and pulmonic stenosis to be the most frequent valvular lesions. The right atrial pressures are commonly very elevated, and probably higher than would be expected with rheumatic tricuspid regurgitation of similar severity.[39] Although the cardiac output has been reported to be elevated in patients with the carcinoid syndrome without carcinoid heart disease, it is generally normal or low in patients who have carcinoid heart disease.

One of the best means of producing severe right-sided failure in animals is by making the pulmonary trunk stenotic and the tricuspid valve incompetent. These are the two principal valvular lesions which occur in patients with carcinoid heart disease. This cardiac disease, however, does not appear to decrease longevity. The length of illness from onset of symptoms to death in the 18 patients with carcinoid heart disease averaged 58 months, and in the 14 without it, 45 months. Peripheral edema and ascites appear to be worse in patients with carcinoid cardiac disease, but these signs appear to result more commonly from associated hepatic dysfunction (due to metastases) and hypoalbuminemia.

The pathogenesis of the carcinoid plaque is uncertain. An intriguing feature of the carcinoid plaque is the lack of varying stages of development. No "early" lesions have been observed. All plaques are similar whether on valvular or mural endocardium. Initially, serotonin was believed to cause the endocardial fibrosis, but there is no evidence to substantiate this belief. It has not been possible to produce the cardiac lesions in animals by giving serotonin or other substances, and urinary levels of the breakdown product of serotonin (5-hydroxyindole acetic acid) and blood serotonin levels have been similar in patients with the carcinoid syndrome with and without cardiac involvement.[42] Serotonin initially also was believed to be responsible for the dermal flush in this syndrome, but this hypothesis has been discounted.[43] A kinin peptide, such as bradykinin, appears the more likely cause of the flush,[43] and it may also cause the carcinoid endocardial lesions, but this has not been demonstrated. Our identification of the cells in carcinoid plaques as smooth muscle cells is of interest in this respect since the clinical features of the carcinoid syndrome, i.e., flushing, wheezing, and diarrhea, are mediated through effects on smooth muscle. The same circulating factor responsible for the aforementioned clinical manifestations may stimulate smooth muscle cells in endocardium to proliferate and to synthesize collagen and basement membrane-like material. The importance of other unknown factors in the formation of carcinoid endocardial plaques is shown by the selective localization of the plaques and by their lack of elastic tissue.

Combined Stenosis of Right and Left-Sided Cardiac Valves

Stenosis of multiple valves usually indicates rheumatic heart disease. Rarely, however, one valve on both right and left sides of the heart may be stenotic when the etiology is congenital rather than rheumatic. The usual combination is congenital pulmonic and aortic stenosis,[44-45] and rarely tricuspid stenosis with aortic or mitral stenosis or both.[46] The occurrence of combined congenital pulmonic and mitral stenosis also is rare,[47] but we have studied two such patients at necropsy. Mitral stenosis was diagnosed only at catheterization in one, and never clinically in the second.[48] The latter patient underwent pulmonic valvulotomy, and died shortly thereafter of pulmonary edema, the consequence of the undiagnosed and untreated mitral stenosis.[48] Both patients had dome-shaped pulmonic valves. The mitral valve leaflets and chordae in one were thickened, stiff, and shortened; the other had a parachute mitral valve.

Stenotic right-sided lesions regardless of etiology protect to varying degrees against pulmonary vascular congestion resulting from associated mitral stenosis. When both right and left-sided stenotic lesions are present the left-sided stenosis should be relieved first. Unfortunately, the same conditions which delay the onset of incapacitating symptoms may obscure the clinical diagnosis of mitral stenosis as was true in both our patients.

NONOBSTRUCTIVE LESIONS

With Involvement of Ascending Aorta

Syphilis

Syphilis remains an important cause of severe aortic regurgitation. We have studied at necropsy nine patients with aortic regurgitation secondary to syphilitic aortitis (Table 9). Six were men, three were women, and their ages ranged from 19 to 80 years. Serological tests for syphilis were positive in six of the eight patients in whom the tests were performed. No patient had received penicillin at the time of the primary infection. In seven of nine patients, symptoms of congestive cardiac failure developed within three years of detection of a precordial murmur. In each, aortic regurgitation was severe, caused congestive failure, and was responsible for death in all but one. The latter patient died of a stroke.

At necropsy, the hearts weighed 600 to 850 gm. (avg. 695), and in each the left ventricular cavities were dilated and their walls, hypertrophied. The ascending aorta was diffusely dilated in all patients. In seven, the entire ascending aorta was involved by the luetic process and in the other two, the process was limited to that portion behind the sinuses of Valsalva (Figs. 15–17). The luetic process caused the aortic wall to be up to four times thicker than normal. The thickening

Table 9. Aortic regurgitation secondary to syphilis: clinical and necropsy observations

Patient	Age	Sex	STS	Age (yrs.) onset		Conduction disturbances by ECG	Pressures (mm./Hg)		Heart weight (gm.)	Saccular AA aneurysm
				Murmur	CHF		LV	SA		
1. A58–280	19	M	+	17	17	0	105/33	148/33	800	0
2. A61–192	37	M	0	34	32	0	160/20	170/50	600	+
3. A4344	44	M		43	43	1°HB	175/5	175/85	850	+
4. 70A–369	50	M	+	50	50	0	—	160/50	720	+
5. A65–31	53	M	+	53	48	0	143/18	152/40	600	+
6. A64–223	56	F	0	52	55	0	106/25	108/27	800	0
7. A67–43	69	M	+	63	63	1°HB	—	170/50*	640	0
8. A69–226	69	F	+	56	54	0	—	200/90*	650	+
9. A72–137	80	F	+	44	60	0	—	210/70*	600	0

AA = ascending aorta. CHF = congestive heart failure. LV = left ventricle. SA = systemic artery. STS = serologic test for syphilis. 1°HB = prolonged P–R interval (P–R greater than 0.20 sec.).
* Arm cuff pressure.

was due to both intimal proliferation and to dense adventitial scarring (Fig. 16). The aortic media, in contrast, was not thickened, and many of its elastic fibers had been replaced by scar tissue. The walls of the vasa vasorum were thickened and their lumens were narrowed. Collections of lymphocytes and plasma cells surrounded many vasa vasorum. Arteriosclerotic plaques were superimposed on the diseased aorta in all patients, including the 19-year-old. No spirochetes were found on special stains of aorta. The aortic "annuli" were dilated in all nine patients, preventing coaptation of the aortic valve cusps. The distal margins of the cusps were thickened in all patients, but the valves remained mobile and

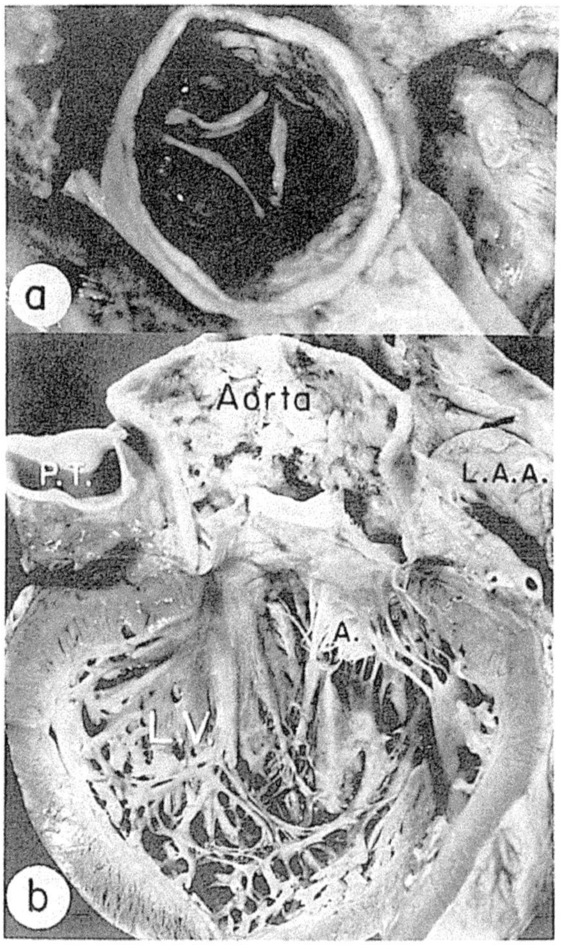

Figure 15. Cardiovascular syphilis with severe aortic regurgitation. Shown here is the aortic valve from above (a) and the opened aorta, aortic valve, and left ventricle (b) in a 69-year-old man (A67–43) who died of congestive cardiac failure. His blood pressure was 170/50 mm. Hg. The regurgitation resulted from inability of the cusps to coapt during ventricular diastole (a). Dilatation of the aortic root stretched the cusps between any two commissures but no one commissure was widened. The wall of the entire ascending aorta is involved by the syphilitic process. The left ventricle (L.V.) is very dilated. P.T. = pulmonary trunk. A. = anterior mitral leaflet. L.A.A. = left atrial appendage.

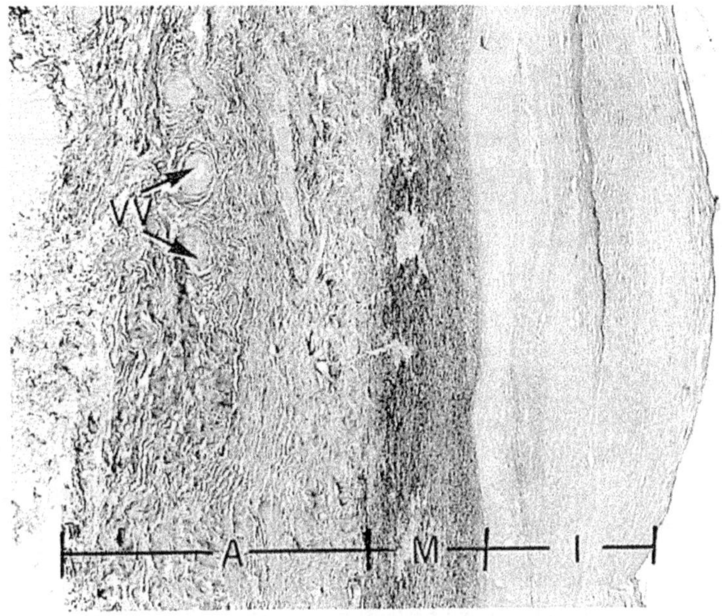

Figure 16. Syphilis of the aorta. Photomicrograph of a cross section of aortic wall from a 55-year-old man (DCGH #72A–115) with luetic aortitis. The intima (I) is thickened by fibrous tissue. The media (M) is thinned due to elastic fiber degeneration. The stellate scars resulted from focal disruption of the darkly staining elastic fibers. The adventitia (A) also is thickened by a dense scarring process and the vasa vasorum (VV) are severely thickened by the obliterative endocarditis. Infiltrate of lymphocytes, not evident at this magnification, are present in the adventitia. Elastic tissue stain; × 21.

otherwise grossly and histologically normal. In only two patients were the commissures widened.

Aortic regurgitation occurs in about 30 per cent[49-51] of patients with cardiovascular syphilis. The regurgitation is due primarily to aortic root dilatation, the result of destructive aortitis. Stretched across a dilated aortic annulus, the cusps are unable to meet in diastole and a central regurgitant stream results. The fibrosis of the rolled free margins of the aortic valve cusps appears to be secondary to regurgitation and not due to a valvulitis per se. The sparing of the valvular cusps might result from their being relatively avascular.

Syphilitic aortitis is a focal disease of the ascending aorta with skip areas that are grossly and histologically normal. The site of disease in the aorta is the major determinant of valvular dysfunction. All our patients with aortic regurgitation had severe aortic root involvement and variable involvement of other portions of ascending aorta. Extensive destruction of ascending aorta, even with formation of aneurysms, may occur in the absence of aortic regurgitation if the aortic wall immediately behind the sinuses is spared (Fig. 17). Thus, the aortic root is the important determinant of aortic valve function and alteration in its structure may prevent normal valve closure.

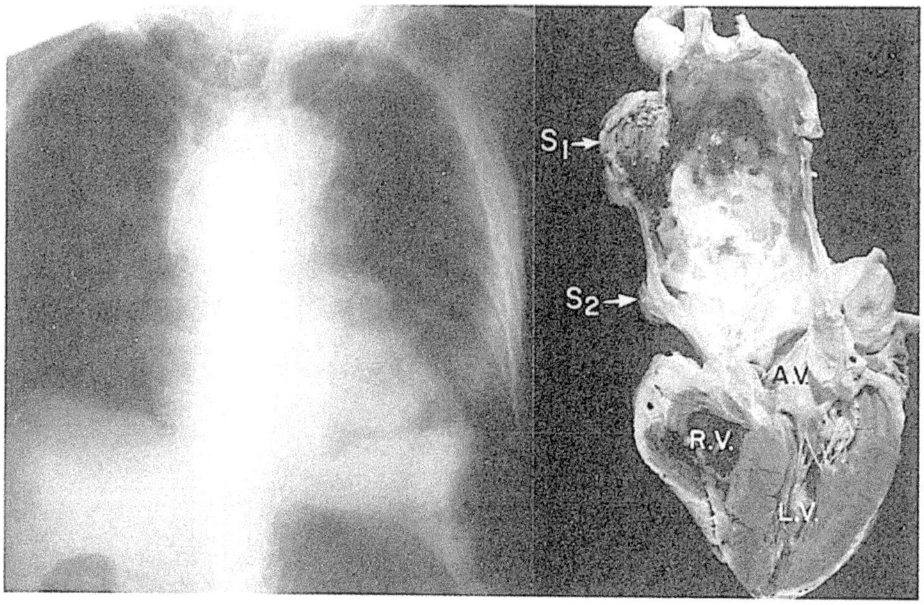

Figure 17. Cardiovascular syphilis without aortic regurgitation. Incidental finding in an 81-year-old man (A67–177) who died of pneumonia but never had evidence of cardiac dysfunction. Syphilitic aortitis led to severe destruction and aneurysmal dilatation of aorta, and formation of two smaller saccular aneurysms (S and S_2). Chest roentgenogram demonstrates a diffusely dilated aorta with a calcified wall. In contrast to the patient illustrated in Figure 15, aortic regurgitation did not occur in this patient since the walls of the sinuses of Valsalva were not involved by the syphilitic process. Neither aortic root nor left ventricle (L.V.) was dilated. R.V. = right ventricle. A.V. = aortic valve.

Ankylosing Spondylitis

We have studied eight patients with combined ankylosing spondylitis and aortic regurgitation (Table 10). All were men, aged 34 to 57 years. All had severe (functionally class III or IV) congestive cardiac failure and signs and symptoms of joint involvement consistent with ankylosing spondylitis. In all eight patients, the joint symptoms antedated those of congestive cardiac failure, in seven of them by 10 to 20 years. In five of the eight patients, however, precordial murmurs of aortic regurgitation were noted at the same time, or within one year of onset of joint symptoms. Serologic test (VDRL) for syphilis was negative in all patients. Conduction disturbances were present in six of eight patients: five had prolonged (greater than 0.20 sec.) P–R intervals, one associated with right bundle branch block and another with left bundle branch block; and one had complete heart block. At catheterization, the left ventricular and systemic arterial diastolic pressures were equal in five of seven patients studied. Aortic valve replacement was carried out in five patients. Death in seven patients was directly related to the aortic valvular disease and occurred at an average of six years from the onset of congestive cardiac failure; the eighth patient died of lung carcinoma.

At necropsy, the hearts weighed 520 to 1100 gm. (avg. 756). The aortic valve cusps were shortened and thickened, particularly at their attachments. Focal calcific deposits were present along the bases of the cusps in four patients, and in one the deposit extended to the anterior mitral leaflet and membranous septum. The ascending aorta was diffusely dilated. The thickening was limited to the

Table 10. Ankylosing spondylitis: clinical and necropsy observations

Patient	Age (years) at death	Sex	Age (years) onset arthritis	Age (years) onset cardiac disease: Murmur	CHF	Duration (years) of arthritis	Duration (years) of cardiac disease: Murmur	CHP	Conduction disturbances by ECG	Pressures (mm. Hg) LV	SA	AR	Heart weight (gm.)	AV cusps thick	short	Sub AV ridge	Thickening of aorta of sinuses
1. A61–99	52	M	24	37	43	28	15	9	1°HB RBBB	160/18	168/30	+	850	+	+	+	+
2. A61–262	55	M	45	45	53	15	15	2	1°HB	114/40	124/40	+	680	+	+	+	+
3. A61–274	34	M	18	31	31	16	3	3	1°HB	100/22	120/25	+	700	+	+	+	+
4. A64–17	35	M	6	6	29	29	29	6	0	170/12	170/50	+	840	+	+	+	+
5. A66–127	57	M	42	41	55	16	17	2	0	—	180/40	+	520	+	+	+	+
6. A68–142	38	M	13	14	32	25	24	6	1°HB	170/16	190/20	+	1100	+	+	+	+
7. A68–300	54	M	40	40	48	14	14	6	CHB	170/52	170/50	+	750	+	+	+	+
8. A68–350	46	M	18	38	38	28	8	8	LBBB	128/32	128/32	+	610	+	+	+	+
Averages	46		26	32	41	21	16	6									

AR = aortic regurgitation. AV = aortic valve. CHB = complete heart block. CHF = congestive cardiac failure. 1°HB = first degree heart block (P–R interval greater than 0.20 sec.). LBBB = left bundle branch block. LV = left ventricle. RBBB = right bundle branch block. SA = systemic artery.

most proximal 3 to 4 cm. of ascending aorta, and the wall behind the sinuses of Valsalva was always involved. The thickening resulted from dense connective tissue in the adventitia of the aorta. The adventitial scarring continued downward in the groove between the anterior mitral leaflet and the aortic valve cusps, producing a fibrous ridge between the base of the aortic valve cusps and the anterior mitral leaflet (Fig. 18). In four patients the fibrous tissue involved the membranous ventricular septum as well. A few mononuclear cells were present in the adventitia of the aorta, and the lumens of the vasa vasorum were narrowed by extensive intimal fibrous proliferation and medial hypertrophy. The media of the aorta behind the sinuses showed evidence of severe degeneration, and the overlying intima was thickened by proliferated fibrous tissue.

Although aortic regurgitation has been described previously in ankylosing spondylitis,[52-57] the distinctive morphologic features of the cardiovascular lesion have not been clearly defined. The aortic valve cusps, particularly near their aortic attachments, are shortened and diffusely thickened by fibrous tissue. The extension of the dense adventitial fibrosis below the attachments of the aortic valve cusps to anterior mitral leaflet and membranous ventricular septum distinguished these patients morphologically from those with aortic regurgitation of other etiologies. The extension of the scarring process below the aortic valve also explains the frequency of conduction disturbances in ankylosing spondylitis.

Although the aortic valve cusps are abnormal in as high as 20 per cent,[56] aortic regurgitation is said to occur clinically in only about 3 per cent of patients with ankylosing spondylitis.[56,58,59] Symptoms of arthritis usually antedate the cardiac disease by 10 to 20 years. In five of our patients and in patients described by others,[54,59-62] precordial murmurs were noted within two years of the onset of joint symptoms. Symptoms of cardiac dysfunction, however, developed much later. This observation suggests that the joints and the aortic root area may be attacked at the same time, but that it takes many years for the sclerosing process to produce aortic regurgitation.

Ankylosing spondylitis has been described as a benign disease.[62-64] Seven of our eight patients, however, died of consequences of aortic regurgitation at a mean age of 46 years with death occurring within six years of the first symptoms of heart disease. The age at death in the 16 patients with ankylosing spondylitis and aortic regurgitation reported by Clark et al.[54] was 45 years, and the interval from the onset of symptomatic heart disease to death was six years. In contrast, the overall mortality of patients with ankylosing spondylitis has been reported to be similar to that of the general population.[64] Thus, the presence of aortic regurgitation appears to be a prime determinant of whether or not ankylosing spondylitis shortens life.

The Marfan Syndrome

This heritable disorder involves the bones, joints, eye, heart, and blood vessels.[65] The extremities are long and thin (dolichostenomelia), the ligaments and joint capsules are redundant, the lenses are dislocated (ectopia lentis), the ascending aorta is dilated, and one or both left-sided cardiac valves usually are incompetent.

We have studied at necropsy 11 patients with the classic features of the

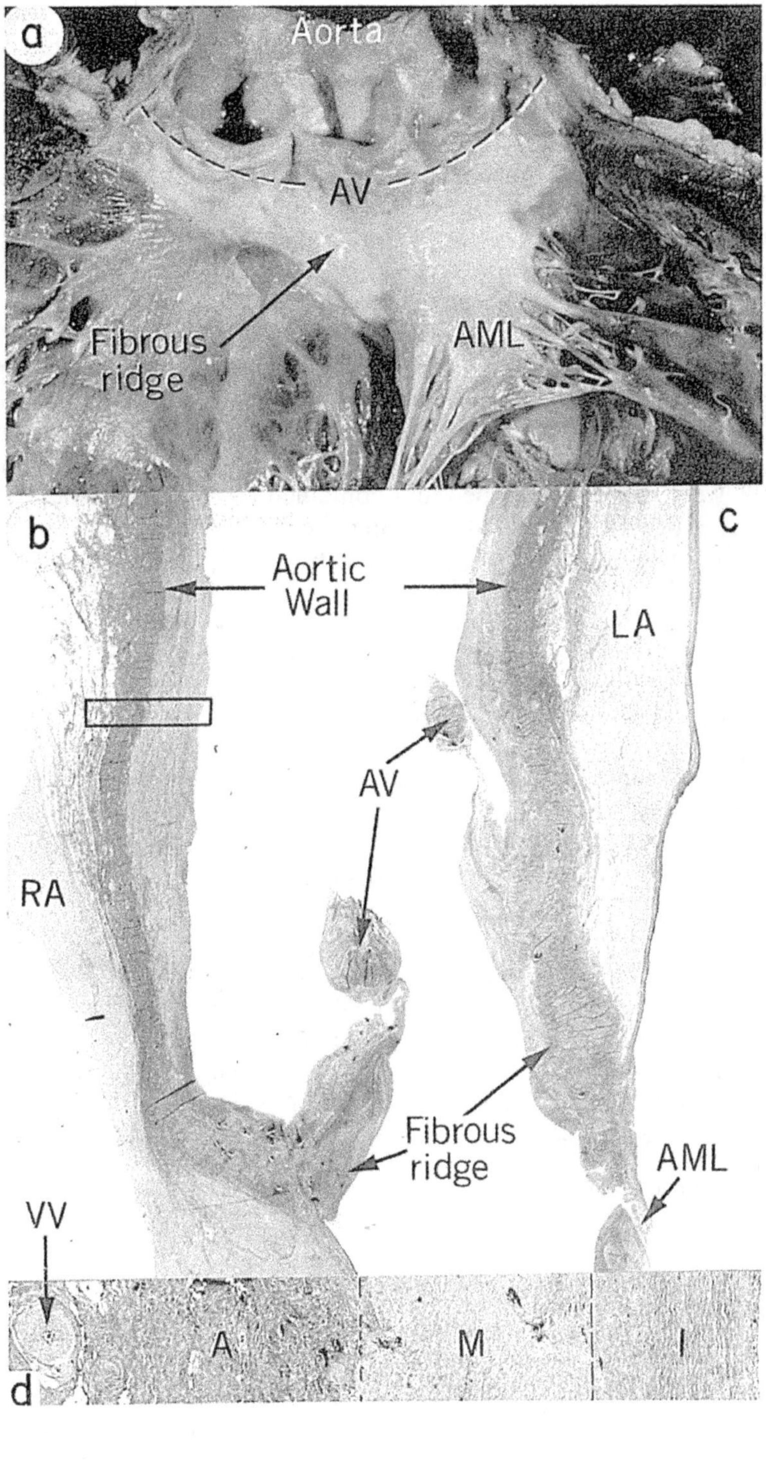
a
Aorta
AV
Fibrous ridge
AML
b
c
Aortic Wall
LA
AV
RA
Fibrous ridge
AML
VV
A
M
I
d

Marfan syndrome and four other patients without the bone, joint, or eye features of the syndrome but with similar lesions in the ascending aorta (Table 11) (Figs. 19–22). The youngest died of congestive cardiac failure from mitral regurgitation at two days of age and the oldest, at age 59 years of congestive failure from aortic regurgitation. Thirteen were males, two were females; 12 were white and three, black. Fourteen had congestive cardiac failure, and the fifteenth died suddenly of rupture of the ascending aorta before congestive failure had appeared. All 15 had precordial murmurs consistent with mitral regurgitation, and 12 had murmurs of aortic regurgitation. Operations to alleviate valvular regurgitation were performed in eight patients, and in another, an aortic coarctation was resected.

At necropsy (or operation), the ascending aorta was dilated in 13 patients, all but one of whom had had clear evidence of aortic regurgitation. The sinuses of Valsalva were especially dilated and their walls, thinner than normal. In addition, focal outpouching was present in the ascending aorta in these 13 patients. Their walls were markedly thinned and contained few if any elastic fibers. The intima of these thinned areas had an orange-peel appearance whereas the other areas of intima usually were grossly normal. Elastic fibers in the grossly normal portions of aorta, however, also were severly decreased in number and the amount of acid mucopolysaccharide material, focally increased. Few medial scars were present in any portion of ascending aorta. Neither adventitia nor intima was thickened and the vasa vasorum were not narrowed.

Other than mild focal thickening of their margins, the aortic valve cusps were grossly normal (Fig. 22). On histologic study, however, the aortic cusps, as well as the mitral ones, contained increased quantities of acid mucopolysaccharide material. The mitral valve leaflets and chordae were elongated, both transversely and longitudinally, in most patients, and in several the leaflets and chordae were focally thickened. In four patients calcific deposits were present in the mitral annuli behind the posterior mitral leaflets. All four valve annuli in all 15 patients were dilated.

The two major functional valve lesions in the Marfan and Marfan-like (forme fruste) syndromes are mitral regurgitation[65-71] and aortic regurgitation.[65,71] All 15 of our patients had clinical evidence of mitral regurgitation and 13 of them had aortic regurgitation. The aortic regurgitation appears to result from dilatation of the aortic root, the result of massive degeneration of elastic fibers (and probably

Figure 18. Ankylosing spondylitis associated with aortic regurgitation and complete heart block. This 54-year-old man (A68–300) had crippling ankylosing spondylitis which progressed over a 14-year period. Coincident with his initial skeletal symptoms was the development of a murmur of aortic regurgitation. He subsequently developed congestive cardic failure and complete heart block. a, The aortic valve cusps are shortened and thickened and a dense fibrous band or ridge extends along the base of the cusps to the anterior mitral leaflet. b, Photomicrograph of longitudinal section through right coronary cusp, right atrium (RA), and adjacent aortic wall. The latter is thickened by intimal proliferation and by dense adventitial scar which extends below the base of the valve forming the fibrous ridge. c, Photomicrograph of a longitudinal section through left coronary cusp, left atrium (LA), and anterior mitral leaflet (AML). Dense scar extends from adventitia of aorta below the aortic valve to the AML. d, Close-up of full thickness of aortic wall showing dense fibrosis of adventitia (A) with narrowing of lumen of vasa vasorum (VV), degeneration of medial (M) elastic tissue, and thickening of intima (I) by fibrous tissue proliferation. These changes are virtually indistinguishable from the changes seen in syphilitic aortitis. b and c, Elastic tissue stains. d, Hematoxylin-eosin stain. [× 3.5 (b), × 2.5 (c), and × 24 (d).]

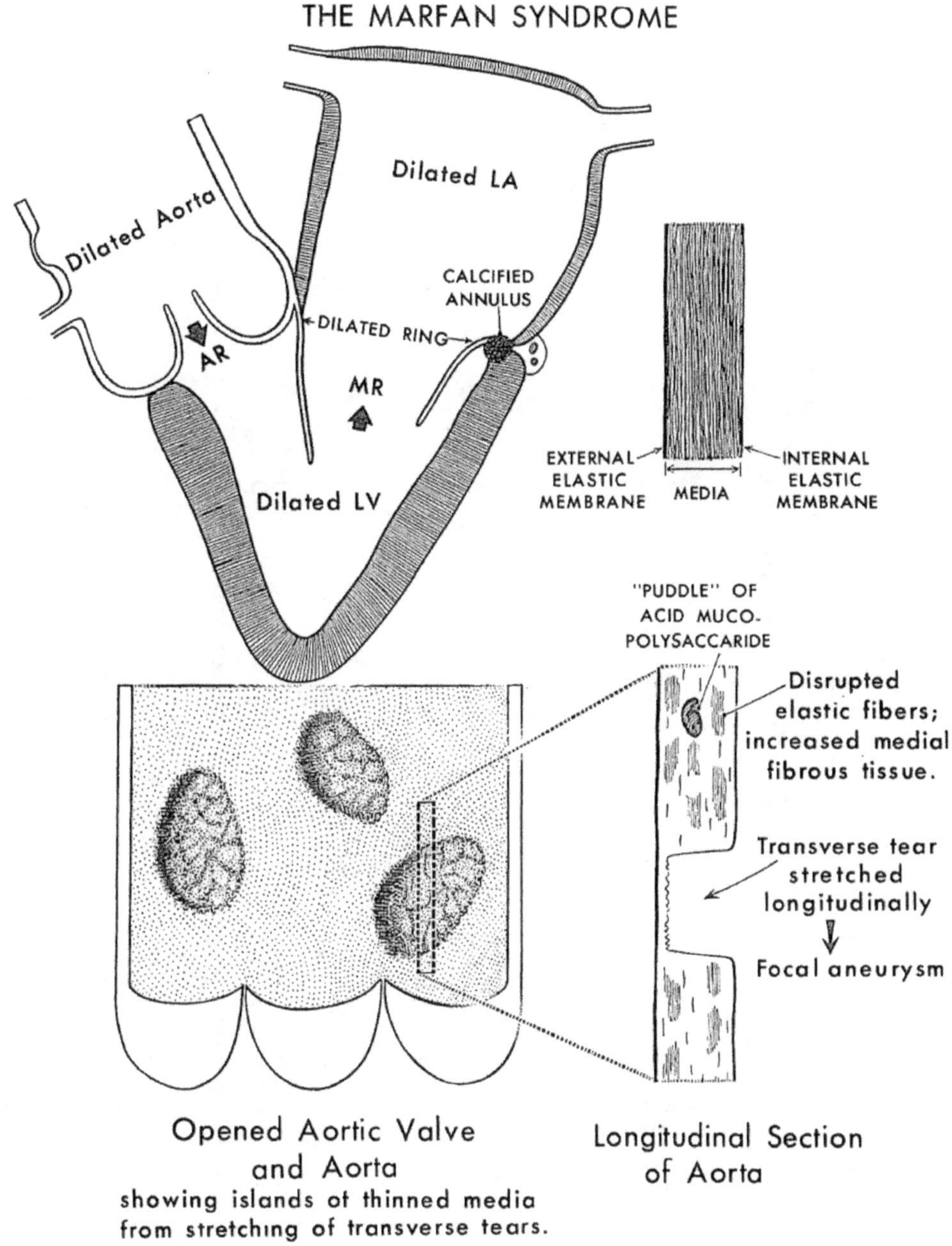

Figure 19. Diagram demonstrating the various cardiovascular abnormalities found in the Marfan syndrome. The aortic regurgitation appears to be related primarily to dilatation of the aorta. The mitral regurgitation probably results from a combination of factors: dilatation of the left ventricular cavity altering the papillary muscle–mitral leaflet angle; dilatation of the mitral annulus; calcification of the mitral annulus; and elongation of the mitral leaflets and chordae allowing prolapse of the leaflets into left atrium during ventricular systole. Shown on top right is a longitudinal section of normal aorta. At bottom right is a longitudinal section in a patient with the Marfan syndrome. There is severe loss of elastic fibers, deposition of abnormal amounts of acid mucopolysaccharide material, and tears in the wall. These tears expand to cause islands of thinning noted in the view of the opened aortic valve and aorta.

Table 11. The Marfan syndrome and its forme fruste variety

Patient	Age (yrs.)	Sex	CHF	Murmurs AR	Murmurs MR	SA press. (mm. Hg)	Operation AVR	Operation AAR	Ascending aorta: Medial degen.	Ascending aorta: Diffuse aneurysm	Ascending aorta: Complete rupture	Heart weight (gm.)	Ca^{++} MV annulus	Other lesions
The Marfan syndrome														
1. A56-132	31	M	+	2/6	4/6	135/40¶	O*	O	+	+	O	700	+	Hx IE
2. A58-150	15	M	+	3/6	3/6	150/0	O	O	+	+	O	750	O	Hx IE
3. A58-206	36	F	+	4/6	2/6	—	O	O	+	+	O	750	O	O
4. A59-134	20	M	+	3/6	3/6	160/60¶	O	O†	O	+	O	850	+	C of A† bicuspid AV
5. A63-25	28	M	+	0	5/6	130/80¶	O	O	O	O	O	850	+	O
6. A64-224	21	M	+	4/6	2/6	158/62¶	+‡	+	+	+	O	700	+	O
7. A65-64	41	M	+	5/6	1/6	105/35¶	+	+	+	+	O	750	O	An., desc. thoracic aorta
8. A67-120	21	M	O	O§	2/6	130/80§	O	O	+	+	+	460	O	O
9. A69-278	48	F	+	4/6	2/6	150/40¶	+	+	+	+	O	520	O	O
10. A67-236	2 days	M	+	O	4/6	—	O	O	+	O	O	—	O	O
11. 37468	47	M	+	4/6	2/6	108/39¶	+	+	+	+	O	—	O	O
The forme fruste variety														
12. A68-197	52	M	+	3/6	2/6	160/60¶	+	+	+	+	O	850	O	O
13. A70-102	32	M	+	4/6	2/6	110/45¶	+	+	+	+	O	650	O	C of A bicuspid AV
14. A59-169	59	M	+	3/6	2/6	190/80¶	O	O	+	+	O	820	O	O
15. 37429	48	M	+	3/6	2/6	135/54¶	+	+	+	+	O	900	O	Bicuspid AV

* This patient underwent insertion of a Hufnagel ball-value prosthesis in his descending thoracic aorta in 1956 and died from rupture of the proximal aortic suture line a month later.

† This patient died in the operating room from bleeding after insertion of a conduit proximal and distal to the coarctation of the aorta.

‡ Replacement of the ascending aorta and aortic valve was performed nine months before death and mitral valve replacement (for mitral regurgitation) was carried out 15 days before death.

§ This recording was at age 12 (nine years before sudden death). Since his ascending aorta was quite dilated at necropsy, it is highly likely that aortic regurgitation was present and the systemic arterial diastolic pressure was low for some time before death.

¶ Direct pressure recording during catheterization.

AAR = ascending aorta replacement. An. = aneurysm. AR = aortic regurgitation. AV = aortic valve. AVR = aortic valve replacement. Ca^{++} = calcium. CHF = congestive cardiac failure. C of A = coarctation of aorta. degen. = degeneration. desc. = descending. Hx = history of. IE = infective endocarditis. MR = mitral regurgitation. MV = mitral valve. SA systemic artery.

also of some smooth muscle cells) of the media. The especially severe dilatation of the sinuses of Valsalva appears to cause peripheral migration of the aortic valve cusps which tilt or prolapse toward left ventricle. The focal thickening of the cuspal margins appears to be secondary to the aortic regurgitation and not a factor in causing it.

At least four factors are important in causing mitral regurgitation in this syndrome: (1) Papillary muscle dysfunction resulting from the tremendous left ventricular dilatation.[72,73] The dilatation appears to alter the angle of pull of these structures making it more difficult for the leaflets to coapt during ventricular systole. (2) Dilatation of the mitral annulus. This annulus is probably more dilatated in patients with the Marfan or Marfan-like syndromes than in any other condition. (3) Calcification of the mitral annulus.[74] It is well known that calcific deposits in the annulus of the posterior leaflet can inhibit the sphincter-like action of this ring, an action which occurs normally during ventricular systole. (4) Floppiness of the mitral leaflets. Not only are the leaflets stretched transversely as the annulus dilates, but they also are stretched longitudinally by the dilating left ventricular cavity. It is possible that the increased quantities of acid-mucopolysaccharide material in the mitral leaflets allow this abnormal stretching. The chordae tendineae also are stretched and this in turn allows abnormal prolapsing of the leaflets toward left atrium during ventricular systole. Possibly none of the four factors alone could account for severe regurgitation, but in combination severe regurgitation may result. Tricuspid regurgitation and floppy tricuspid valve leaflets and chordae tendineae also may occur in this condition as illustrated by our patient #11 and as described by others.[68]

Although floppiness of the atrioventricular valves is a prominent feature of the Marfan and Marfan-like syndromes, the major cause of cardiovascular dysfunction results from involvement of ascending aorta. The major lesion here appears to be degeneration of elastic fibers and not the presence of increased quantities of acid-mucopolysaccharide material. In our view, the latter deposits have been too strongly emphasized and therefore the name *medial cystic necrosis* is probably not the most appropriate one. Dissection of the aorta did not occur in any of our 15 patients. What has been called "dissection" may represent tears beginning in the intima and extending for varying distances into the media or through the media to be enclosed by adventitia.

The occurrence of congenitally bicuspid aortic valves in three of our 15 patients is a frequency too high to be attributed to chance alone. Bicuspid aortic valves were present in one of the 11 patients with the Marfan syndrome and in two of the four without the syndrome but with similar lesions in the ascending aorta. Two of the three also had aortic coarctation. It is possible that the ascending aorta is structurally congenitally weak in patients with congenitally malformed aortic valves. If this postulate is correct, it might be reasoned that congenitally weak elastic fibers in the ascending aorta are more likely to degenerate than are structurally normal elastic fibers. If coarctation also is present the increased pressure in the ascending aorta might accelerate the elastic-fiber-degeneration process. When aortic elastic fibers degenerate, the spaces may be filled with acid-mucopolysaccharide material to produce a lesion which is typical of that

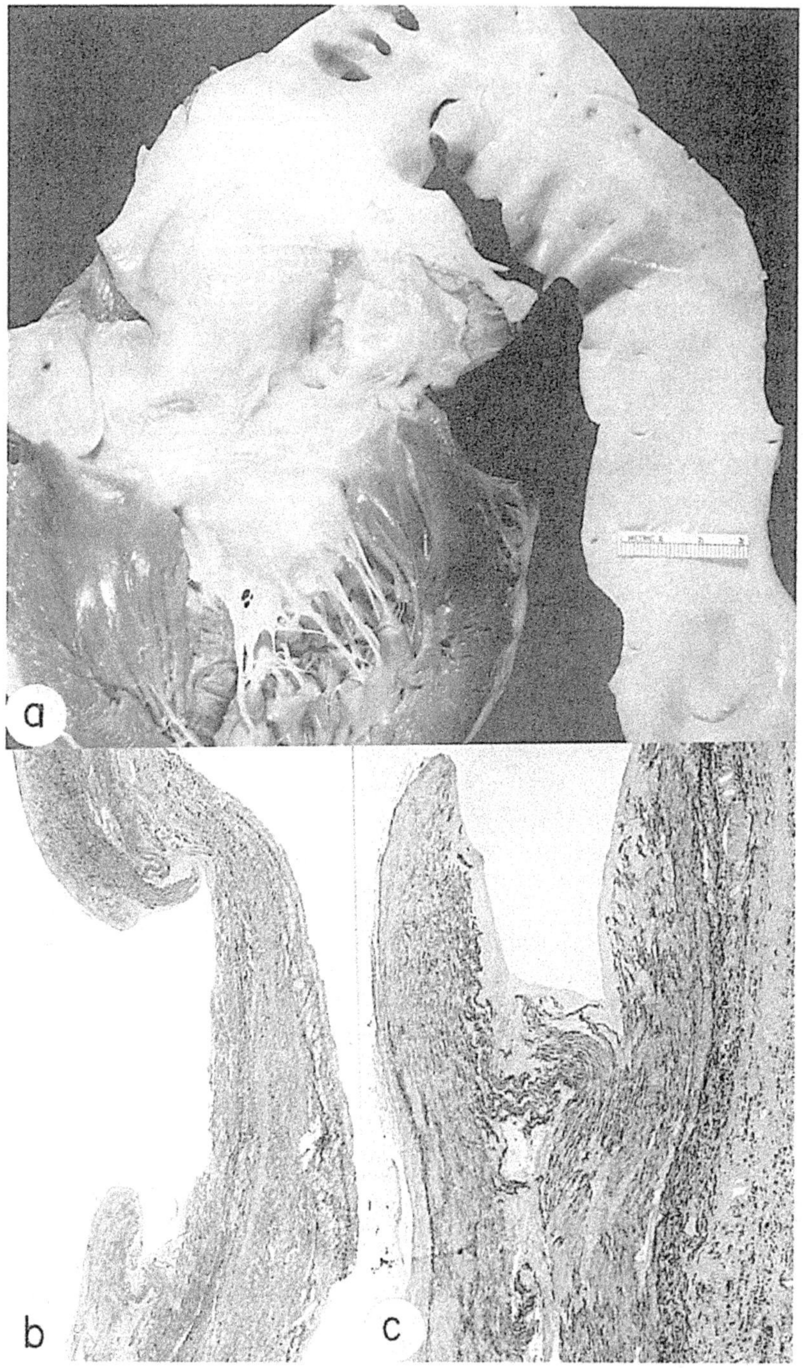

Figure 20. The Marfan syndrome. This 21-year-old man (A67–120) with typical skeletal and optic features of this syndrome had always been asymptomatic. He was found dead in his parked car after playing in a band during the several previous hours. At necropsy, the precordial sac was filled with blood. A through-and-through rupture had occurred in the ascending aorta (a) just above the aortic valve. In addition, several partial ruptures or tears also were present in ascending aorta. A histologic section of one tear is shown in b. A close-up of an adjacent section of b is shown in c. There is severe degeneration of elastic fibers of the media. b and c, Elastic tissue stains. [× 7 (b) and × 18 (c).]

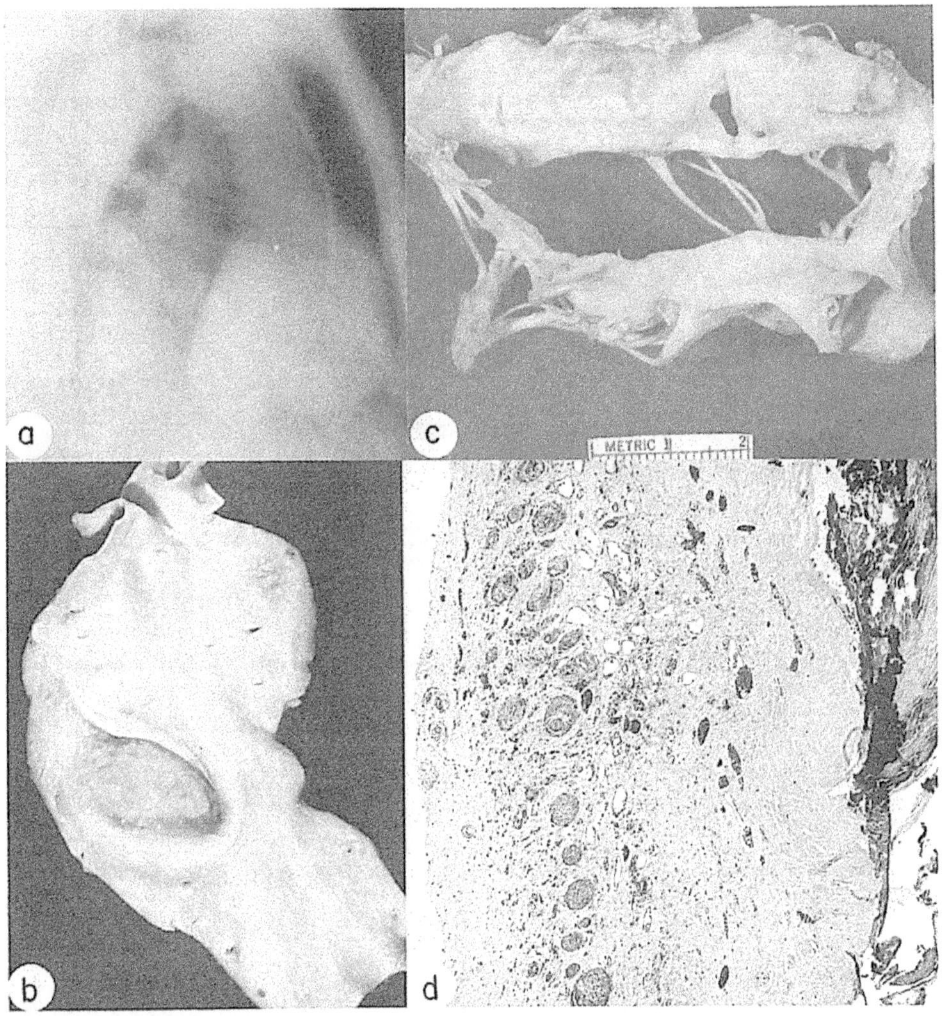

Figure 21. The Marfan syndrome with both aortic and mitral regurgitation in a 21-year-old man (A64–224). This patient had a precordial murmur at birth. Four siblings also had the Marfan syndrome. He was asymptomatic until about one year before death when episodes of rapid atrial fibrillation appeared. He had one episode of sudden heavy retrosternal chest pain 10 months before death. He died after replacement of both aortic and mitral valves with prostheses. The ascending aorta had been resected at operation. a, Lateral aortogram showing dilatation of the aortic sinuses, a typical cardiovascular feature of the Marfan syndrome. b, Excised ascending aorta showing two punched out aortic tears or splits. The nontorn portion of aorta grossly appears normal but histologically the aorta showed extensive loss of elastic fibers and focal collections of acid mucopolysaccharide material. c, Excised mitral valve. The leaflets are thickened, the annulus is dilated, and focal deposits of calcium are present at the line of excision (annulus). d, Histologic section of portion of mitral leaflet, which is thickened by vascularized fibrous tissue. Vascularization of valvular leaflet at one time was considered typical of rheumatic heart disease but this is not so as demonstrated here. Also, a deposit of calcium (near the annulus) is present. Hematoxylin-eosin stain. (Reduced 25 per cent from × 56.)

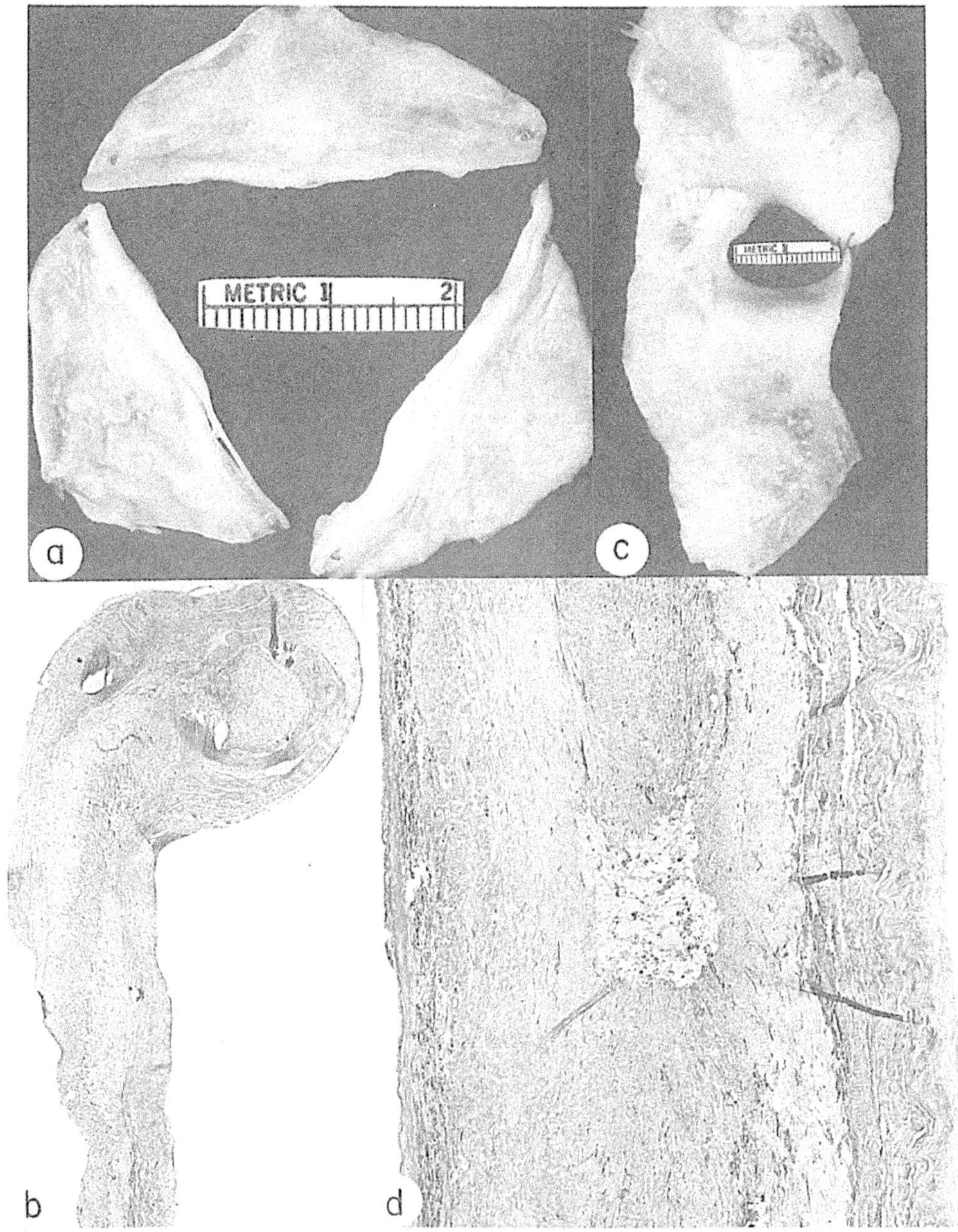

Figure 22. The Marfan syndrome with severe aortic regurgitation in a 41-year-old man (A65–64). This patient underwent replacement of his aortic valve and ascending aorta two months before death from complications of the nephrotic syndrome. At necropsy, he was found to have a large aneurysm filled with organized thrombus in the descending thoracic aorta. a, Excised aortic valve showing mild thickening of the margins of each of the three cusps. Otherwise, the aortic valve grossly appears normal. This is the typical appearance of the aortic valve in a patient with the Marfan syndrome. b, Photomicrograph of portion of one aortic valve cusp showing increased spongiosa and therefore increased acid-mucopolysaccharide material. c, Excised ascending aorta. d, Photomicrograph of portion of ascending aorta showing virtual total disappearance of elastic fibers and a puddle of acid-mucopolysaccharide material. b, Hematoxylin-eosin stain. d, Elastic van Gieson stain. [Reduced 15 per cent from × 24 (b) and × 58 (d).]

Table 12. The Hurler syndrome: data in three necropsy patients

Patient	Age-race-sex	Cardiac symptoms	Murmur	CE by x-ray	ECG	Cardiac involvement: Heart weight (gm.)	All four valves	Mural endocardium of four chambers	Cor. art.	Myocardium	MV annulus Ca^{++}
1. A65-89	6 WF	0	+	Slight	Normal*	95(101)†	+	+	+	+	0
2. A66-199	9 WM	0	0	0	LAE	110(138)†	+	+	+	+	+
3. A70-236	12 WM	0	+	Slight	RAE, RAD, VPCs	150(169)†	+	+	+	+	+

* Recorded eight years before death.
† Expected weight for age and sex.

Ca^{++} = calcium. CE = cardiac enlargement. Cor. art. = coronary artery. LAE = left atrial enlargement. MV = mitral valve. RAD = right axis deviation. VPCs = ventricular premature contractions. RAE = right atrial enlargement.

which occurs in the Marfan syndrome in subjects with three-cuspid aortic valves. Furthermore, aortic medial degeneration with cystic necrosis also has been observed in patients with valvular aortic stenosis.[75,76] The stenosis in most of the latter patients probably is superimposed on a congenitally malformed aortic valve.

The Hurler Syndrome (Mucopolysaccharidosis I)

Virtually all patients with this syndrome have anatomically abnormal cardiac valves. Three children (one girl, two brothers) with typical clinical, chemical, and morphologic features of this syndrome were studied (Table 12). Each had moderate dwarfism, grotesque facial appearances, protuberant abdomens, joint contractures, and mental retardation. Acid mucopolysaccharides, mainly chondroitin sulfate B and heparitin sulfate, in increased amounts were found in the urine of each patient. Although none had symptoms of cardiac dysfunction, two had precordial systolic murmurs (grade 2/6 intensity), loudest at the apices, two had slight cardiomegaly by chest roentgenograms, and two had abnormal electrocardiograms.

At necropsy, each heart was smaller than normal, the ventricular walls were

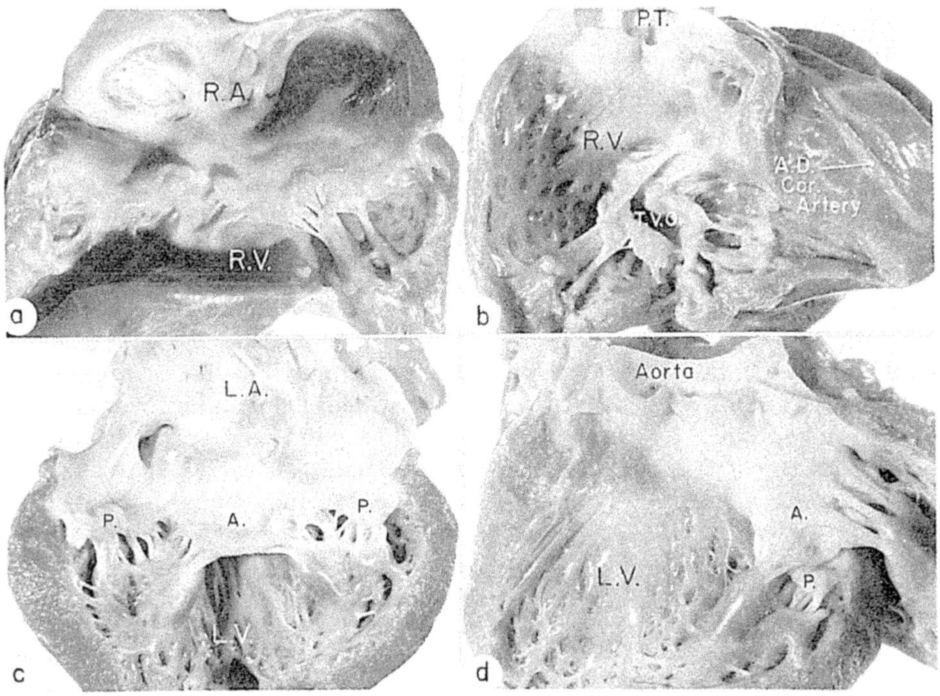

Figure 23. The Hurler syndrome. Opened right (a and b) and left (c and d) sides of the heart in a six-year-old girl (A65–89) with typical features of the Hurler syndrome. She had a precordial murmur but no evidence of cardiac dysfunction. All four cardiac valves and the mural endocardium of all four chambers were thickened. a, Opened right atrium (R.A.), tricuspid valve, and right ventricle (R.V.). b, Opened pulmonary trunk (P.T.) and right ventricle (R.V.) showing the thickened valves and the tricuspid valve orifice (T.V.O.). The anterior descending (A.D.) coronary (Cor.) artery is thickened. c, Opened left atrium (L.A.), mitral valve, and left ventricle (L.V.). A. = anterior mitral leaflet. P. = posterior mitral leaflet. d, Opened left ventricle (L.V.) and aorta showing thickening of both valves and the mural endocardium.

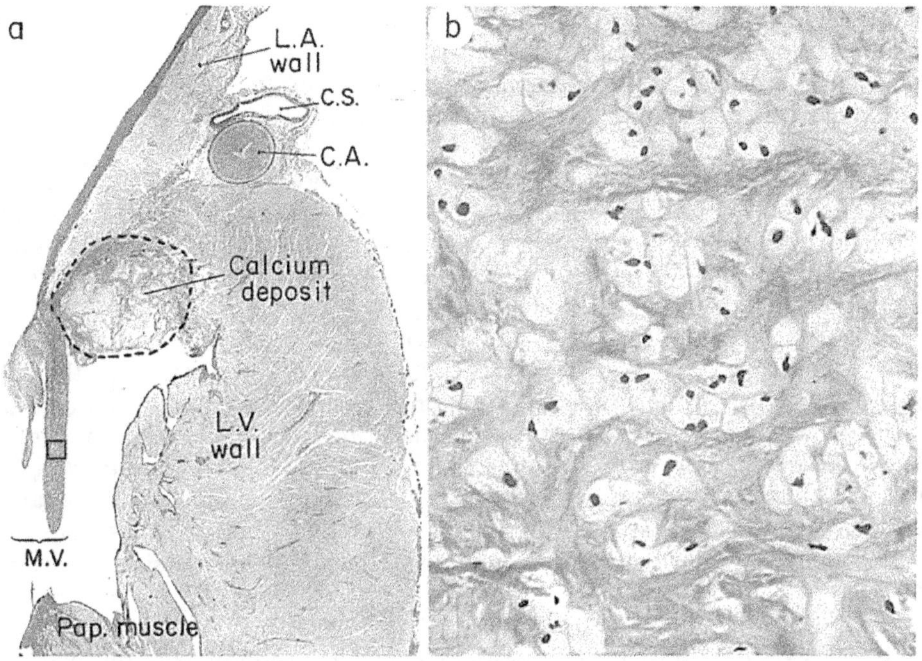

Figure 24. The Hurler syndrome. a, Photomicrograph of section of left atrium (L.A.), posterior mitral valve (M.V.) leaflet, and left ventricular (L.V.) wall showing a heavy deposit of calcium in the mitral annular region and an extremely narrowed coronary artery (C.A.). A close-up of calcium deposit area seen in (a) from a portion of a chorda tendinea is shown in (b). These are typical Hurler cells with vacouloted cytoplasm. These cells were present in valve leaflets, mural endocardium, and in coronary arteries. This patient was a 9-year-old boy (A65–89) without evidence of cardiac dysfunction. a, Elastic tissue stain. b, Hematoxylin-eosin stain. [Reduced 25 per cent from × 4.5 (a) and × 290 (b).]

firmer than normal in consistency, and the mural endocardium of all four chambers of all three patients was diffusely thickened, more on the left than right. The leaflets of all four cardiac valves and many chordae tendineae of all three patients were diffusely thickened (Fig. 23). The mitral and aortic valves were thickened the most, followed by the tricuspid and pulmonic valves. In two patients, calcific deposits were present in mitral annuli (Fig. 24), and smaller calcific deposits were present on the anterior mitral leaflets and on the aortic aspects of one or more aortic valvular cusps. In no patient did the anatomic abnormalities appear to produce clinically significant valvular dysfunction. The lumens of the major coronary arteries were narrowed at some sites more than 75 per cent. Despite the narrowing, however, no myocardial necrosis was observed and fibrosis was limited to the left ventricular papillary muscles (in the two brothers only). Many yellow and fibrous atherosclerotic plaques were present in the aorta of each patient.

Histologic studies disclosed that the valvular thickening and the coronary luminal narrowing were due mainly to the presence of large cells with clear cytoplasm (gargoyle, Hurler, clear or balloon cells) and to bundles of fibrous tissue between the cells. The membranous ventricular septa and atrioventricular valve annuli were thickened by similar clear cells and by collagenous and calcific deposits. The thickening of the mural endocardium resulted primarily from proliferation of elastic fibrils (endocardial fibroelastosis), but a few clear cells also were observed.

Electron microscopic study[77,78] of valvular endocardium and of proliferated tissue within the lumens of the coronary arteries disclosed large clear vacuolated cells and lipid deposits. Although they appeared normal by light microscopic examination, the cardiac muscle cells were found to contain organized lipid and amorphous material by electron microscopy.

Virtually all patients with the Hurler syndrome have been found at necropsy to have anatomically abnormal hearts. Furthermore, all portions of the heart have been shown to be involved, including valvular and mural endocardium, coronary arteries, myocardial fibers, cardiac fibrous skelton, and epicardium. The involvement consists of proliferation of fibrous tissue within which is enmeshed varying numbers of gargoyle cells and ground substance containing acid-mucopolysaccharide material. The result of this involvement is thickening of the valvular leaflets and chordae tendineae, thickening of mural endocardium, and narrowing of the lumens of the coronary arteries.

Of the four cardiac valves, the one most frequently involved in the Hurler syndrome is the mitral. Of 40 necropsy patients with the Hurler syndrome gathered from the literature by Okada et al.,[79] the mitral was involved in 90 per cent, the pulmonic in 20 per cent, and the aortic and tricuspid, each in about 40 per cent. In each of our three patients all four cardiac valves were thickened and contained numerous gargoyle cells.

Another valvular abnormality in this syndrome, one rarely commented on in previous publications, is the occurrence of mitral annular calcification. The Hurler syndrome is probably the most common cause of annular calcification in childhood. Small calcific deposits also may occur on the ventricular aspect of the anterior mitral leaflet and on the aortic aspects of the aortic valvular cusps.

Although there may be no functional consequence of the valvular involvement in the Hurler syndrome, valvular regurgitation of some degree probably occurs eventually in most patients. Because leaflet and chordal thickening is more severe on the left than on the right side of the heart, the mitral valve is the one involved by annular calcification, and the left-sided pressures are higher, regurgitation is usually limited to the mitral or aortic valve or both. Although precordial murmurs have been described in many patients with the Hurler-Hunter syndrome, including one of Hunter's original two patients,[80] hemodynamic and angiographic observations were not reported until 1965 when Krovetz et al.[81] demonstrated mitral regurgitation in six and aortic regurgitation in one of 15 children. Only one of the seven had auscultatory evidence of valvular dysfunction. Although regurgitation is the usual valvular lesion of the Hurler syndrome, mitral stenosis was described at necropsy in a five-year-old child with atypical gargoylism.[82]

Although it is a striking anatomic finding, valvular involvement does not explain the sudden cardiovascular collapse or progressive congestive cardiac failure which causes about 50 per cent of the deaths in this syndrome. Systemic hypertension, coronary arterial luminal narrowing, and lipid deposits in myocardial fibers are probably more important factors.

Other Heritable Disorders of Connective Tissues Associated with Cardiac Valvular Regurgitation

Occurrence of cardiac valvular lesions in pseudoxanthoma elasticum (PXE) and in the Ehlers-Danlos (E-D) syndrome is not well known. About 10 patients with either PXE or E-D and valvular lesions have been described.[65,83-90] Elongated mitral and tricuspid valve leaflets and chordae (floppy valves) have been observed in both conditions, and aortic regurgitation, the result of severe degeneration of elastic fibers of the aorta with or without dissecting aneurysm, has been seen in the E-D syndrome. Dilated aortic roots with severe aortic regurgitation were observed in three men with *osteogenesis imperfecta* (OI) studied by Criscitiello et al.[91] One had had probable infective endocarditis as well. Other patients with aortic and mitral valvular incompetence associated with OI also have been reported.[92] Although not proved, it appears reasonable to believe that the valvular lesions accompanying OI, PXE and E-D syndrome are the result of an underlying disorder of connective tissue.

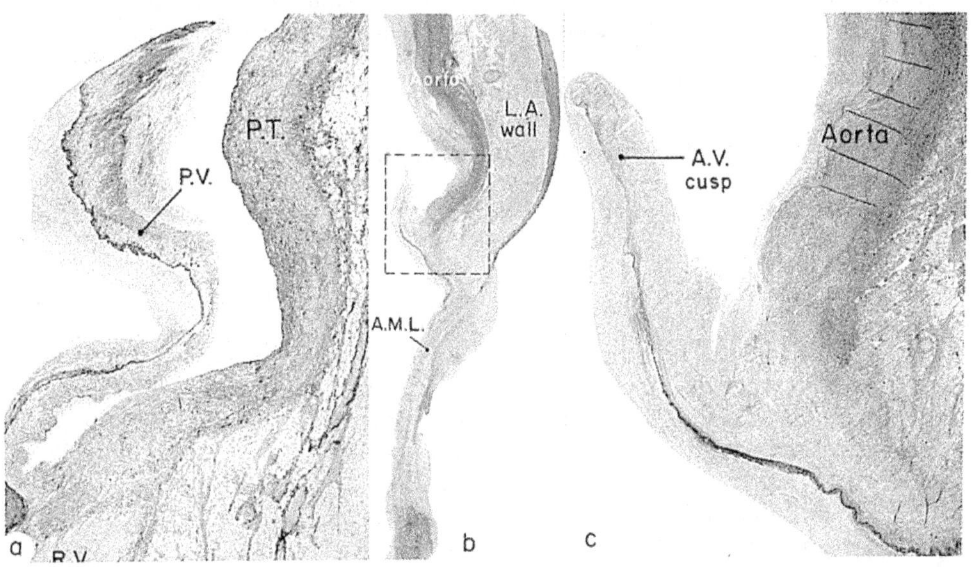

Figure 25. Valvular lesions in Takayasu's arteritis. This 46-year-old woman (A66–237) had panarteritis involving aorta and all vessels arising from it. She presented with fever of unknown origin and changing precordial murmurs. All four cardiac valves were thickened and both atrioventricular valves were mildly incompetent. Histologic sections of three cardiac valves are shown here. a, Pulmonic valve (P.V.) cusp is delineated by the black-staining elastic membrane. Superimposed on this membrane is fibrous tissue which contains few elastic fibers. P.T. = pulmonary trunk. R.V. = right ventricle. b, Section includes anterior mitral leaflet (A.M.L), aortic valve cusp, and walls of the aorta and left atrium (L.A.). Both mitral and aortic leaflets are diffusely thickened as is the wall of the aorta. c, Close-up of aortic valve (A.V.) shown in b. The cusp per se is normal but fibrous tissue, devoid of elastic fibers, is superimposed on it. a-c, Elastic tissue stains. [Reduced 40 per cent from × 15 (a), × 3 (b), and × 11 (c).]

Takayasu's Arteritis

Takayasu's disease is a panarteritis of the aorta and its major branches leading to progressive vascular occlusion. This rare syndrome occurs predominantly in women and is characterized by fever, elevation of erythrocyte sedimentation rate, and diminished or absent peripheral pulses. Vascular compromise most frequently causes neurologic dysfunction. Since any branch of aorta may be affected, however, its clinical manifestations are protean and may include angina pectoris, myocardial infarction, and sudden death.[93-97]

Although considered a disease of arteries, Takayasu's syndrome may cause valvular dysfunction before or after peripheral pulses disappear.[98] One such patient studied by us at necropsy had both tricuspid and mitral regurgitation.[98] The aorta and all four cardiac valves were involved by an unusual fibrosing process (Fig. 25) which may be unique for this condition. The fibrous tissue contained mononuclear cells, mainly lymphocytes, and vascular channels and no elastic fibers. The fibrous tissue was superimposed on both surfaces of the valvular leaflets, which appeared intact. The mural endocardium was focally involved by a similar process. Although aortic, mitral, and tricuspid regurgitation have been described clinically in at least 20 patients with Takayasu's arteritis, few gross and no other histologic descriptions of these valves have appeared. The cause of the diffuse valvular and focal endocardial fibrosis in these patients is uncertain, but it is reasonable to believe that its etiology is the same as that causing the panarteritis and aortitis.

NONOBSTRUCTIVE LESIONS

Without Involvement of Ascending Aorta

The Floppy Valve

The floppy valve as a cause of mitral valvular dysfunction is a relatively new concept. The innocence of apical systolic clicks and late systolic murmurs was refuted by Barlow[99] in 1963 when he demonstrated by left ventricular cineangiocardiography mild mitral regurgitation in these patients. He also suggested that the mid-late systolic clicks were not extracardiac in origin, but resulted from "snapping of fibrosed chordae." Subsequent reports confirmed his observations, and demonstrated prolapse of the posterior mitral leaflet into left atrium coincident with the regurgitant murmur.[101-103] Using intracardiac phonocardiograms, Criley et al.[100] showed that the systolic click coincided with maximum prolapse of the valve leaflet into left atrium. Hence, a syndrome of "mid-late systolic click and late systolic murmur" became synonymous with the "billowing or ballooning mitral leaflet syndrome" or "floppy valve syndrome." Although by cineangiocardiography the valve lesions appeared similar, the clinical syndrome was described in many conditions, including the Marfan syndrome, trauma, atrial septal defect, hypertrophic (asymmetric) cardiomyopathy, and even ischemic and rheumatic heart disease.[66, 104-110] The syndrome was described in all ages, newborn to elderly. In most patients valve dysfunction was asymptomatic. Electrocardiographic abnormalities, namely T wave and ST segment changes suggestive of posterior

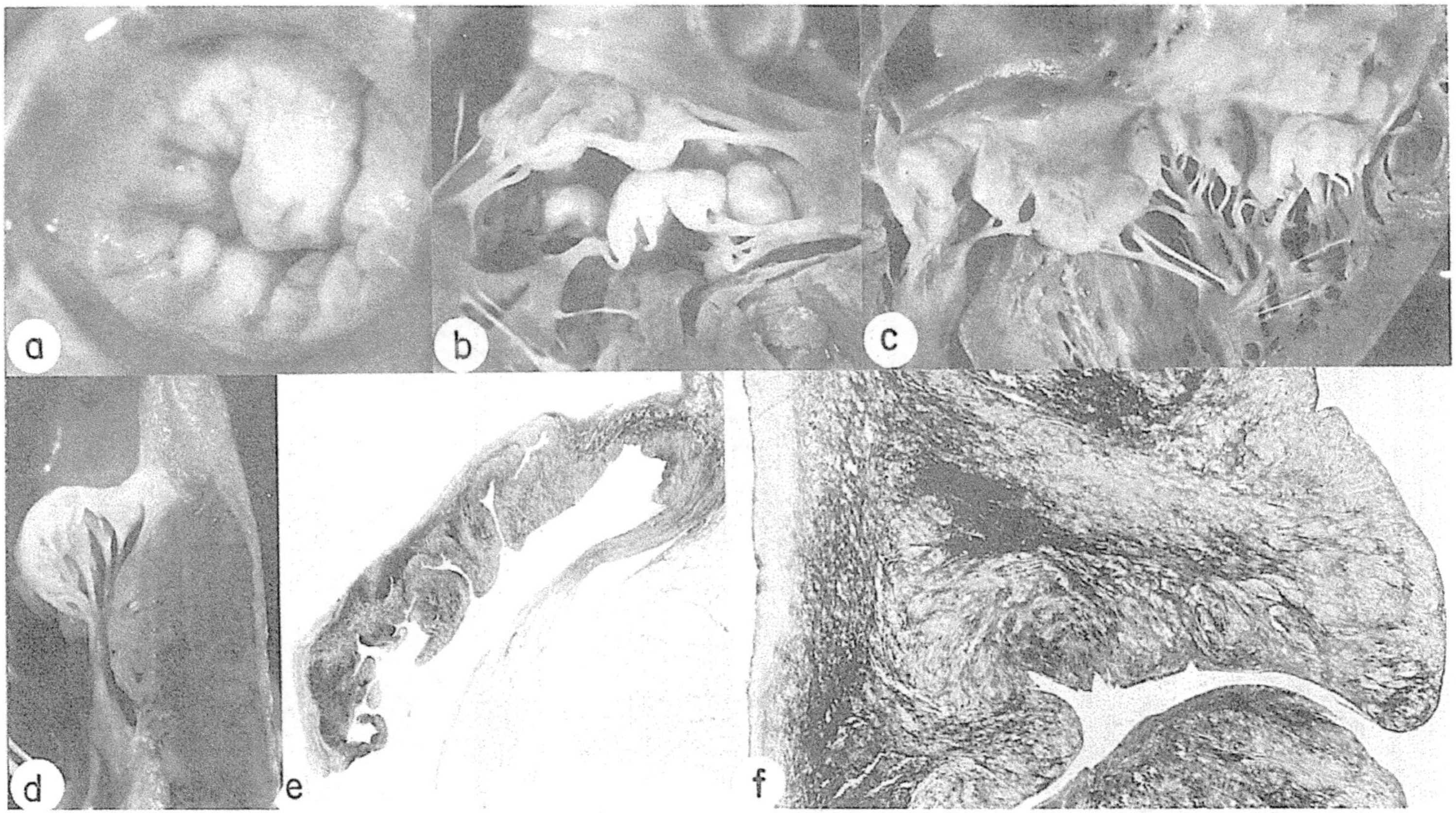

Figure 26. Floppy mitral valve, an incidental necropsy finding. This 18-year-old girl (A71–172), who died of Ewing's sarcoma, never had symptoms of cardiac dysfunction despite an active life. She had a mid-systolic click and a grade 3/6 ejection type systolic murmur over the precordium, left axilla, and back, loudest over the apex. At necropsy, she had an Ebstein's malformation of the tricuspid valve in addition to the floppy mitral valve. The mitral valve leaflets are elongated, but in contrast to those seen in Figure 27 the chordae are not elongated. a, Prolapsed mitral valve leaflets as viewed from left atrium. b, View of floppy leaflets from left ventricle. c, Opened mitral valve showing elongated and focally thickened anterior and posterior leaflets. d, Longitudinal section through left atrium, posterior mitral leaflet, and left ventricle showing the billowed posterior leaflet. e, Photomicrograph of the leaflet demonstrates focal thickening and increased acid-mucopolysaccharide (AMP) deposits. f, Higher power magnification showing AMP deposits (dark-staining). e and f, Acid-mucopolysaccharide stains (Rinehart). [Reduced 10 per cent from × 5(e) and × 36 (f).]

wall ischemia, were frequent, prompting still another name, "the auscultatory-electrocardiographic syndrome."

Necropsy observations[109-113] (Figs. 26–29) on patients with clear-cut clinical evidence of the floppy mitral valve syndrome have been sparse. A major reason for the sparcity of morphologic data is the good prognosis of most patients with this clinical complex. The term "floppy valve syndrome," however, also has been used to describe patients with morphologic evidence of a floppy leaflet whether or not clinically detectable valvular dysfunction is present and therefore includes a wide spectrum of patients. Floppy valve has become synonymous with *myxomatous degeneration,* a histologic description which needs further clarification.

In most valvular heart diseases, the spongiosa component of leaflets is either partially or completely replaced by the fibrous component. In the condition under consideration, the spongiosa is the component which proliferates. Because the spongiosa is the portion of the valve which contains acid-mucopolysaccharide

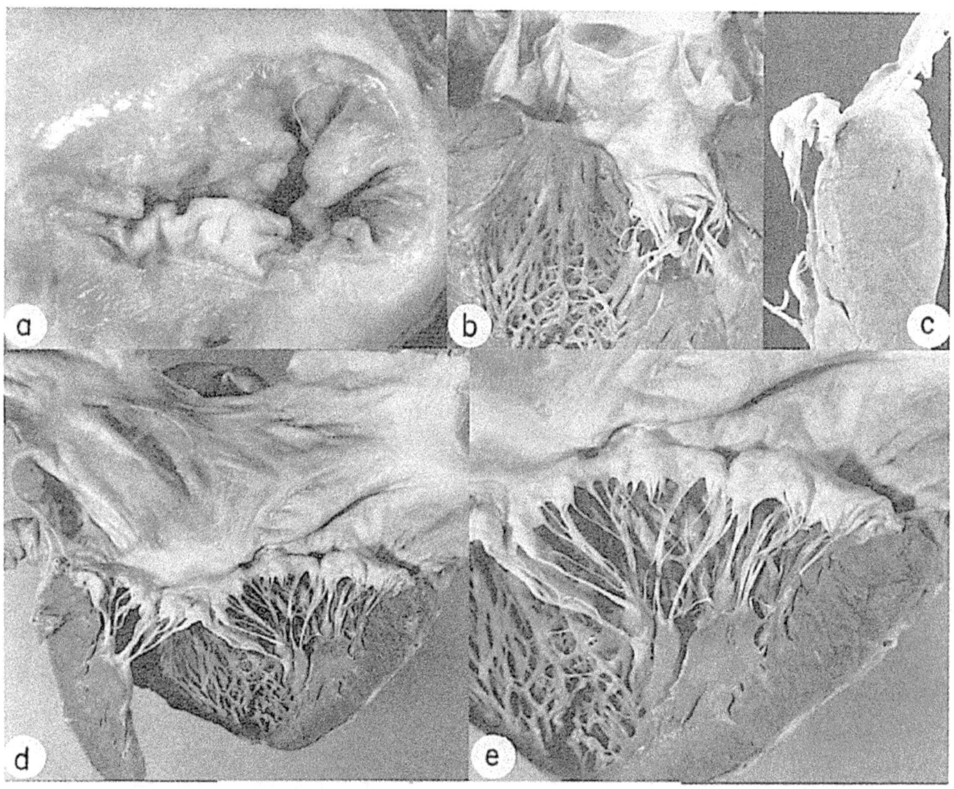

Figure 27. Floppy mitral valve. This 70-year-old man (A71–152), who died of gastric carcinoma, had had a grade 3/6 pansystolic blowing murmur. He never had symptoms of cardiac dysfunction. a, Mitral valve as viewed from left atrium. The leaflets protrude toward the atrium because the chordae tendineae are too long. Photographs of opened mitral valve and left ventricle (b, d, e) show elongated chordae and voluminous anterior and posterior mitral leaflets. A longitudinal section (c) through the left atrium, posterior mitral leaflet, and left ventricle shows the billowed leaflet and small calcific deposits in the annulus.

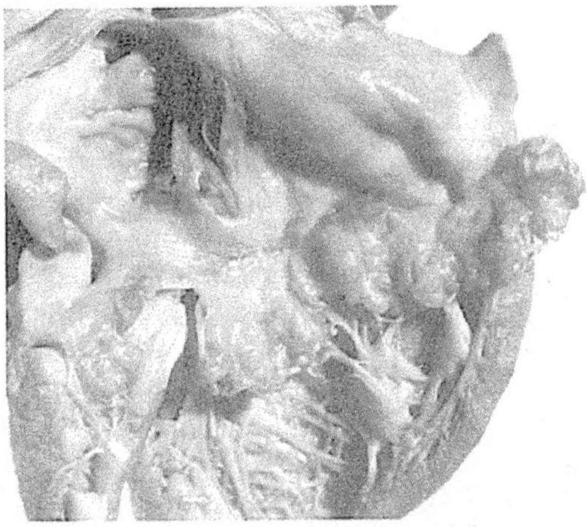

Figure 28. Floppy mitral valve. This two-day-old boy (A67–236), with long toes and fingers and a high-arched palate, had a grade 3/6 precordial systolic murmur typical of mitral regurgitation. Shown here is the opened left atrium, mitral valve, and left ventricle. The mitral leaflets are considerably elongated in both longitudinal and transverse dimensions. The left atrium is dilated. This case is important because it shows that the floppy valve may be present from birth.

(AMP) material, there is an increased amount of AMP in floppy leaflets. In the floppy valve the spongiosa has been described as being disorganized, giving rise to what has been called mucoid or myxomatous degeneration, but little information regarding normal organization of the spongiosa is available for comparison.

Because spongiosa (and therefore AMP material) is part of the normal valve, it is not surprising that it also is part of the diseased valve. Most cardiac valves, excised for either stenosis or incompetency or both, contain myxoid stroma.[110] Stenotic valves, however, appear to contain a much smaller percentage of myxoid material than do purely incompetent valves.

A wide spectrum of leaflet abnormalities may be associated with an isolated increase in valvular myxoid stroma. In some patients the change is evident only by histologic examination, and grossly the leaflet appears normal. We have called this change grade 1 on a scale of 1 to 4. When myxoid stroma is increased enough to cause valve leaflet to be grossly abnormal, the leaflet may prolapse without causing valvular incompetence (grade 2), the valve may prolapse and be mildly incompetent (grade 3), or the valve may be moderately to severely incompetent with or without congestive cardiac failure (grade 4). Similar myxomatous changes also have been described in tricuspid, aortic, and pulmonic valves, most frequently in the Marfan and Marfan-like syndromes, and they also may be incompetent.[68,114,115]

The common denominator of the floppy valve syndrome is an abnormal prolapse of one or both mitral valve leaflets toward left atrium during ventricular systole. Whether or not mitral regurgitation (MR) is a consequence of leaflet prolapse is determined by the extent of the prolapse. Abnormal prolapse without MR generally results in a systolic click without an accompanying murmur (stage I) (Table 13). Additional prolapse generally produces mild MR as manifested by a late systolic murmur with retention of the systolic click (stage II) (Barlow syndrome). Severe prolapse produces moderate to severe MR as manifested by prolongation of the murmur throughout systole (pansystolic) and disappearance of the systolic click (stage III). Thus, MR represents a consequence of the prolapsing (floppy) mitral valve. Other complications, namely infective endocarditis,

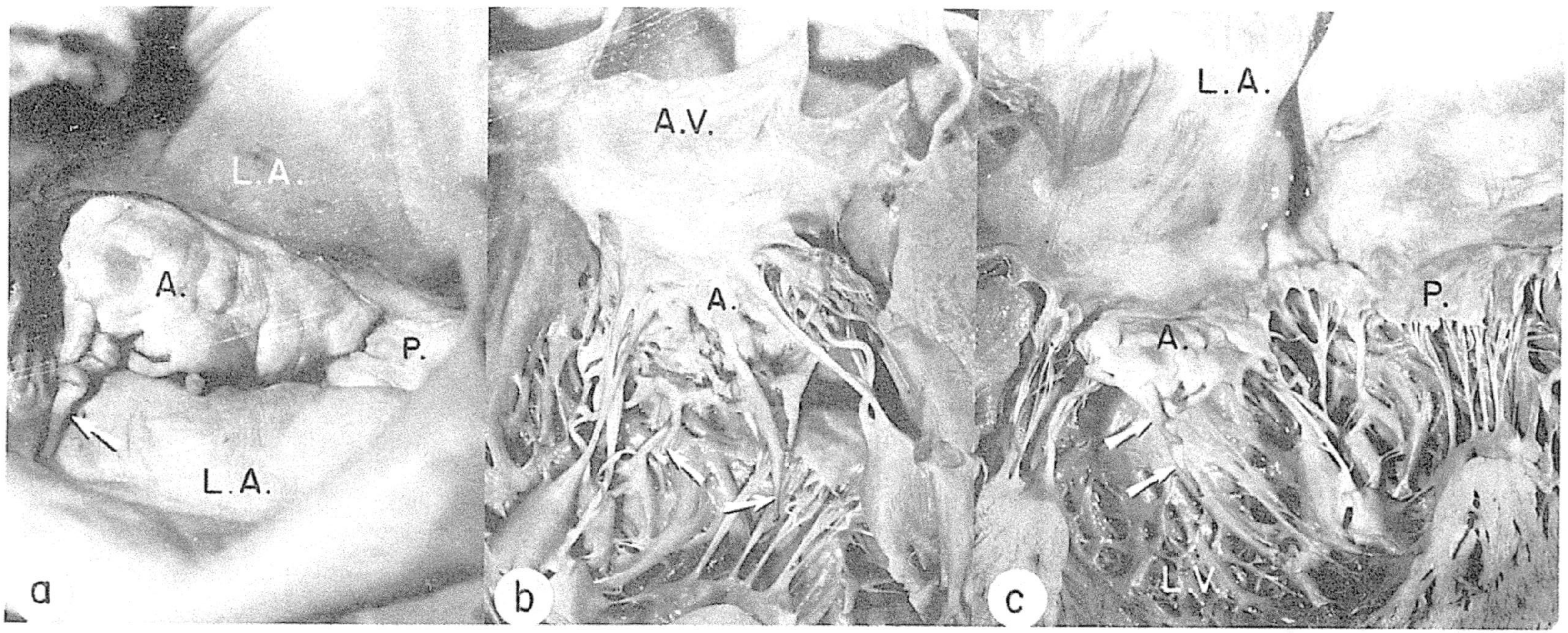

Figure 29. Prolapsed anterior mitral leaflet with chordae, probably involving an initially focally floppy valve. This 71-year-old man (A67–66) had a precordial murmur first noted at age 20 and it suddenly increased from grade 2/6 to 4/6 two years before death when heart failure appeared. At necropsy, the mitral regurgitation was explained by rupture of the chordae attached to the anterior mitral leaflet. There was no clinical or necropsy evidence of active endocarditis or of myocardial infarction. a, Left atrial (L.A.) view showing prolapsed anterior (A.) mitral leaflet. P. = posterior mitral leaflet. b, Opened aortic valve (A.V.) and left ventricle showing aortic aspect of anterior mitral leaflet (A.). The leaflet is thickened and two chordae are ruptured (arrows). c, Opened left atrium, mitral valve and left ventricle (L.V.). Arrows point to a ruptured chorda. The posterior mitral leaflet (P.) is normal. The case may represent spontaneous rupture of chordae tendineae in association with floppy mitral valve.

Table 13.

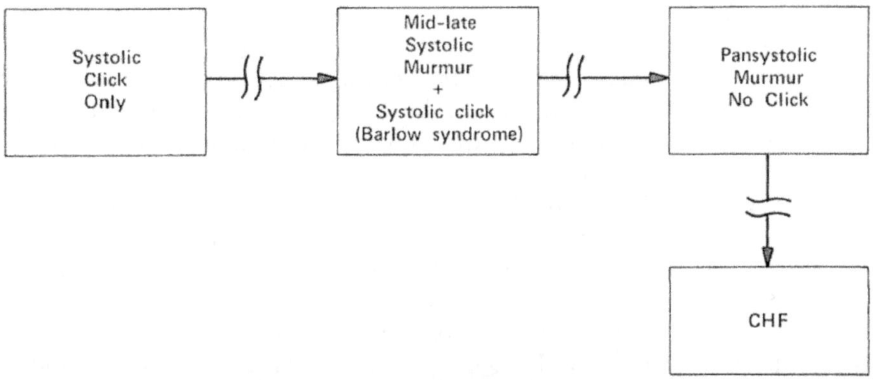

rupture of chordae tendineae without infection, rupture of valvular leaflet, calcification of the mitral annulus, arrhythmias, chest pain, and sudden death may occur at any of the three stages. Although probably most patients enter the scene at stage I, initial entrance may be at stage II or III. Although little information is available regarding progression from stage I to stage III, it appears reasonable to believe that progression is in this order even though one may remain only briefly at one stage or skip stage II entirely.

The actual frequency with which mitral regurgitation complicates myxomatous degeneration of the mitral valve is uncertain. A recent necropsy study of 35 patients with these valves disclosed that less than 25 per cent had mitral regurgitation and more than 50 per cent had symptoms of cardiac dysfunction.[111] It is well established that floppy mitral valves have a predisposition to develop infective endocarditis, and therefore antibiotics before operative procedures are warranted. It is less well appreciated that spontaneous rupture of chordae tendineae may be a complication of floppiness,[111] and even less well recognized that myxomatous degeneration may result in aneurysmal dilatation and rupture of a mitral leaflet. Whether or not calcification of the mitral annulus is a complica-

Table 14. Cause of prolapse (overshooting) of mitral valve leaflet(s) into left atrium during ventricular systole

I. Abnormal leaflets only
   A. Elongation
      1. Focal
      2. Diffuse
II. Abnormal chordae tendineae only
   A. Elongation
   B. Rupture
III. Abnormal leaflets and chordae
IV. Normal leaflets and chordae
   A. Shortened left ventricular cavity (old age)
   B. Necrosis, fibrosis, or ischemia of papillary muscle(s)
   C. Rupture of papillary muscle
      1. Whole trunk
      2. One or more heads

tion of floppiness is uncertain. It is frequently seen in the elderly, and appears to be accelerated by conditions which elevate left ventricular pressure and cause increased wear and tear on the valve. The snapping back of the mitral leaflet in systole may cause added stress on the mitral annulus and also accelerate or increase the likelihood of calcification of the annulus. Calcification of the annulus in the Marfan syndrome may be an expression of this complication of floppiness.

The causes of abnormal prolapse of mitral valve leaflets into left atrium during ventricular systole may be divided anatomically into four categories (Table 14). The mitral leaflets themselves may be enlarged (redundant) leading to billowing of the valve. This had been described most frequently in association with histologic changes of myxomatous degeneration of leaflet and marked increase in acid-mucopolysaccharide material. These histologic changes may not be unique to this syndrome, however, since the aging process may lead to anatomic and functional floppy mitral valves which show little or no evidence of mucoid degeneration microscopically.[116-118] Chordae tendineae which are ruptured or elongated may cause the leaflets to prolapse. The resulting laxity of the valve may lead secondarily to stretching and elongation of the leaflets. In the Marfan syndrome, abnormality in both mitral chordae and leaflets may result in billowing of the valve. An inborn defect of connective tissue of leaflet and chorda appears responsible. Intrinsically normal valves may become floppy because of left ventricular wall abnormalities. The shrunken left ventricular cavity of old age may cause the mitral valve to be redundant. A dysfunctioning or ruptured left ventricular papillary muscle may lead to slackening of the mitral valve in systole with prolapse into left atrium. A left ventricular contraction ridge has been seen by cineangiocardiography in some patients with the billowing mitral leaflet syndrome. This ridge may represent an abnormality of papillary muscle or of adjacent left ventricular wall, that is either cause or consequence of the valvular lesion.[104,119]

Thus, floppiness of the mitral valve is an anatomic and functional abnormality of diverse etiology and it is an important cause of nonrheumatic valvular regurgitation.

Calcification of the Mitral Annulus

Calcification of the mitral annulus is one of the most frequent abnormalities of the heart. Mitral annular calcification is generally considered to be a disease of elderly women. Indeed, of 14 patients with massive mitral annular calcification reported by Korn et al.[120] in 1962, all were women and all were over 65 years of age. It is incorrect, however, to believe that this entity is reserved entirely for a particular sex at a particular time in life. During the past four years one of us (W.C.R.) has examined at necropsy the hearts of 95 patients in whom varying amounts of calcium involved the mitral annulus. Of the 95 patients, 46 were male and 49 were female. Sixty-five patients (27 male, 38 female) were greater than 65 years of age and 30 patients (19 male, 11 female) were less than 66 years of age. Of the latter 30 patients, 8 were less than 40 years of age: three of them had the Marfan syndrome; two had the Hurler syndrome; and three had metabolic disturbances with hypercalcemia.

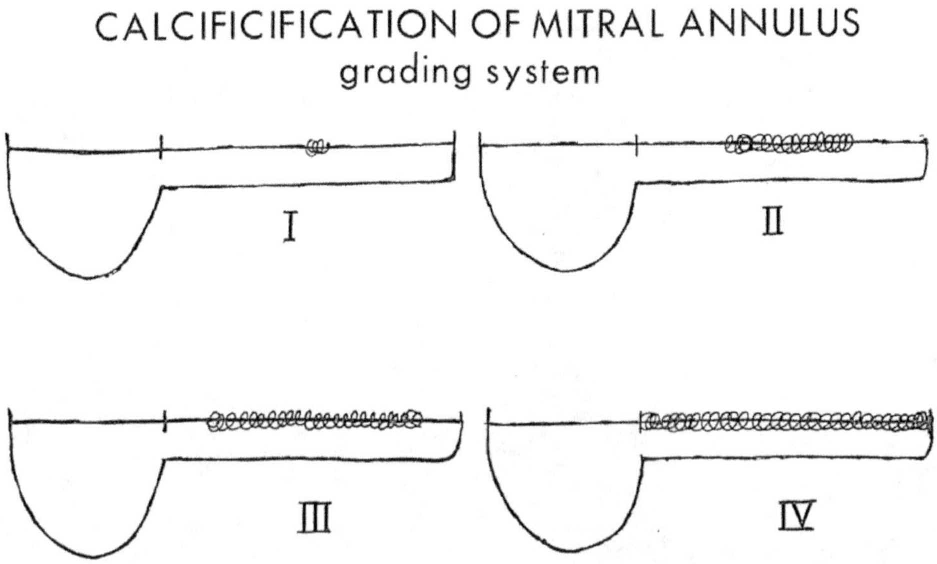

Figure 30. Method of grading mitral annular calcification. Grade I indicates only a single small deposit, grade II a large single or more than one small deposit. Grades III and IV represent extensive deposits. The entire annulus behind the posterior leaflet is involved in grade IV and, on rare occasion, calcific deposits also may extend across the anterior leaflet.

The extent of mitral annular calcification was graded 1+ to 4+ (Fig. 30): 49 patients (30 male, 19 female) had 1+ or 2+ deposits, and 46 (16 male, 30 female) had 3+ or 4+ deposits. Thus, this condition is as frequent in both sexes, but the larger deposits (those likely to be seen on chest roentgenogram) are more frequent in women. The smaller deposits (grade 1+ and 2+) have no functional importance. The larger deposits (grade 3+ and 4+) (Fig. 31), in contrast, may produce mitral regurgitation. Although stenosis has been mentioned as a possible complication of massive mitral annular calcification, obstruction has never been confirmed hemodynamically. Wide-open severe mitral regurgitation, likewise, is probably never due to mitral annular calcification.

Among patients with calcific deposits in the mitral annulus, similar calcific deposits often also are observed in the aortic valve cusps and in the extramural or epicardial coronary arteries. Of the 95 patients with mitral annular calcification,

Figure 31. Calcification of the mitral valve annulus. This 71-year-old woman (PH# A72–68) had had second degree heart block with ventricular rates as low as 40 beats per minute for two years. Bundle of His studies by Dr. Ross Fletcher had showed normal conduction through the atrioventricular node with block distal to the atrioventricular bundle. A pacemaker had been inserted 23 months before death. She died suddenly after climbing a flight of stairs at home. Necropsy disclosed acute myocardial infarction with rupture of the left ventricular apex and a blood-filled tense pericardial sac. Necropsy disclosed a large calcific deposit in the area behind the posterior mitral leaflet (a, b, c). Calcium had extended from this area into the ventricular septum in the area of the atrioventricular bundle. a, Radiograph at necropsy of the heart with pacing catheter in the right ventricle. Electrocardiogram at necropsy disclosed that the pacemaker was functioning normally, firing at 70 beats per minute. Calcific deposits also are present in the walls of the coronary arteries and aorta. b, Longitudinal section showing calcific deposit beneath the posterior mitral leaflet. c, Radiograph of heart specimen from above showing circumferential extent of the mitral annular calcific deposits.

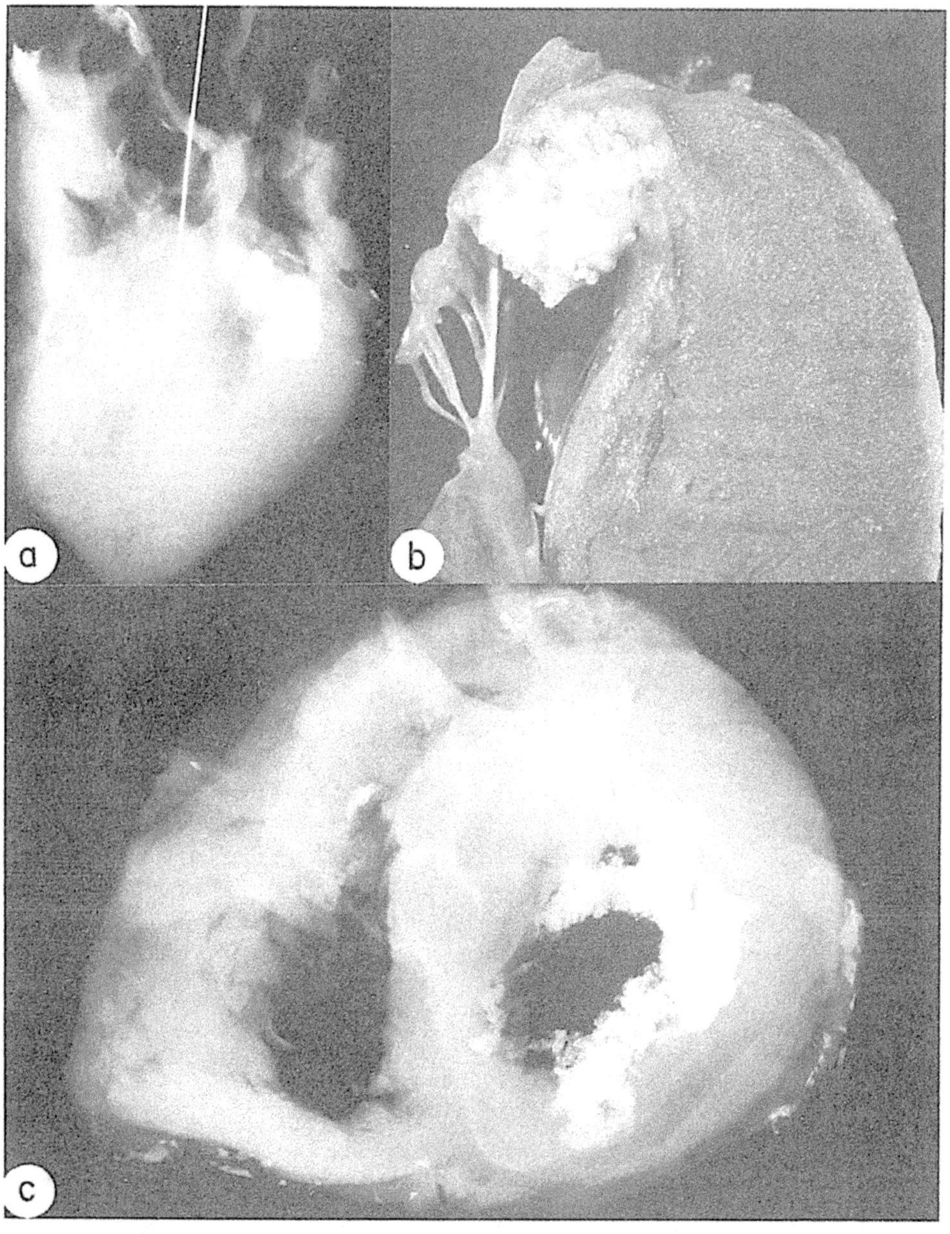
a
b
c

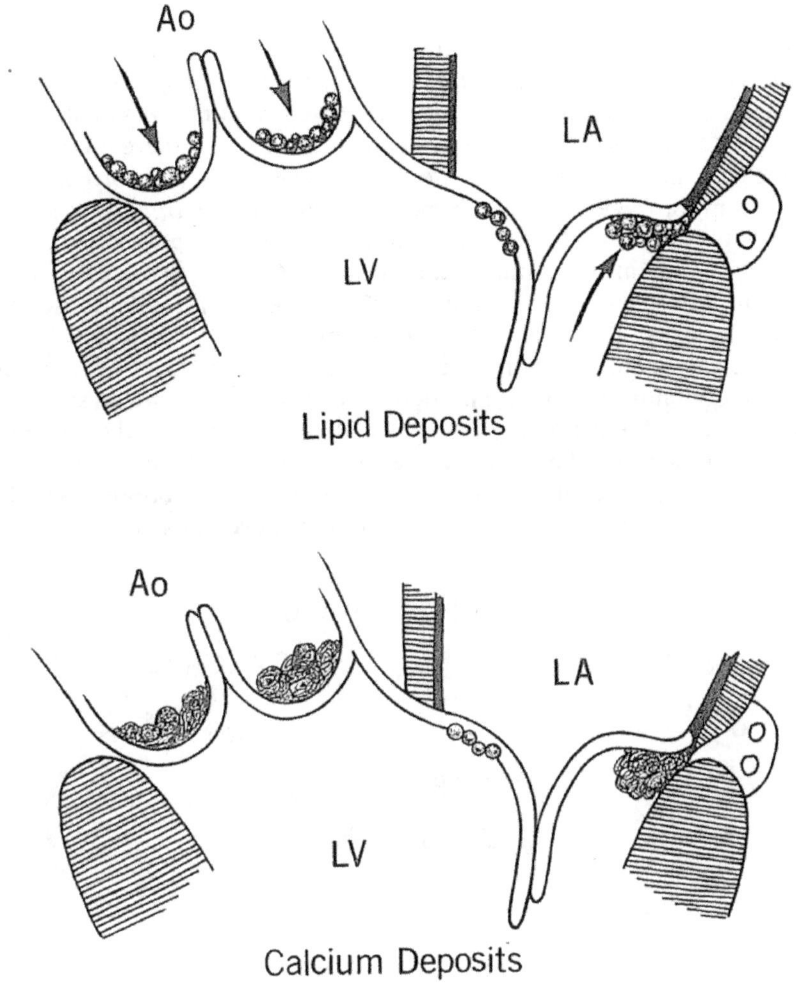

Figure 32. The cause of calcification of the mitral annulus is uncertain. Since most patients with mitral annular calcific deposits also have calcific deposits in the aortic valve cusps and coronary arteries, it seems reasonable to believe that the cause of the calcification in each of these sites is similar. In young adults, yellow deposits are nearly always seen on the ventricular surface of both mitral leaflets and on the aortic surfaces of the aortic valve cusps. The lipid may be both intracellular and extracellular. Degeneration of the lipid probably leads to the calcification. The latter occurs behind the posterior mitral leaflet and on the aortic aspects of the cusps because these are the sites of high pressure and there is nowhere else for the blood to go, so, in effect, it is pushed into the valve leaflets. In contrast, the high pressure on the anterior leaflet is reflected off into the aorta. In other words, the impact of pressure contacts the posterior mitral leaflet and aortic valve cusps at right angles to the cusps, whereas the angle of contact with the anterior leaflet approaches a 180 degree angle.

68 (72 per cent) also had calcific deposits in the aortic valve and in 35 of them the deposits were so extensive that the aortic valve orifice appeared stenotic. Large peak systolic pressure gradients were recorded across the aortic valve in several.[4] The aortic valve in this situation usually contains calcific deposits only on its aortic surfaces, the commissures are not fused, and there is no associated incompetence.[4] Calcific deposits were observed grossly in the coronary arteries in 83 (87 per cent) of the 95 patients. Nine of 12 patients *without* coronary arterial calcific deposits were less than 53 years of age. Of the 65 patients greater than 65 years of age with mitral annular calcification, 62 (95 per cent) had calcific deposits in the coronary arteries and 51 (78 per cent) had calcific deposits in the aortic valve cusps. Thus, deposits of calcium in these three locations—mitral annulus, aortic valve, and coronary artery—are seen most frequently in the elderly and suggest a common etiology. The deposits occur on the undersurface, i.e., ventricular surface of the posterior mitral leaflet at or below the annulus and on the aortic surfaces of the aortic valve cusps. Foam (lipid-containing) cells are common in these locations in younger adults. Probably, breakdown of these lipid deposits is responsible for the calcification at these sites (Fig. 32).

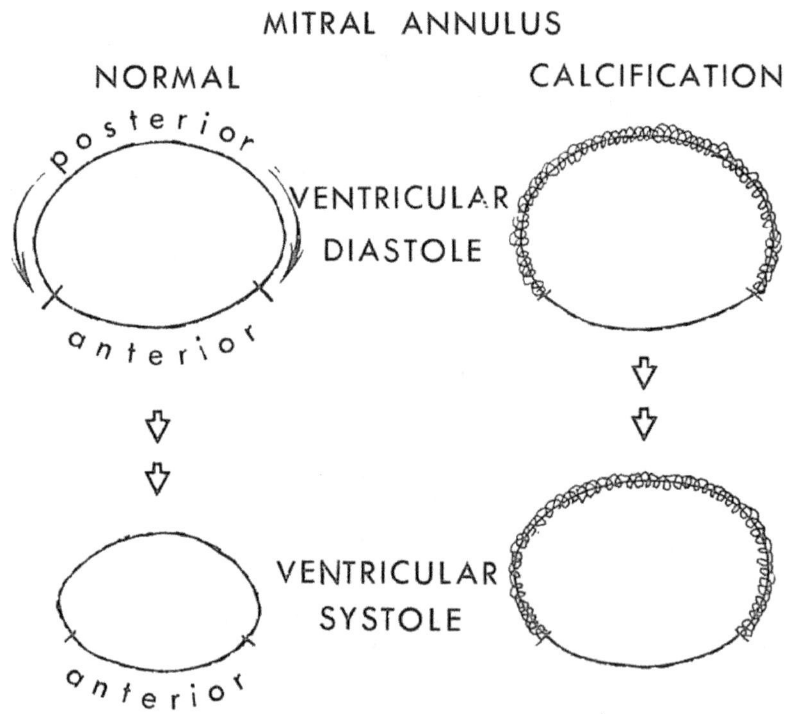

Figure 33. The mechanism of mitral regurgitation in patients with calcification of the mitral annulus is depicted here. During ventricular systole the base of the left ventricle contracts like a sphincter. Included in the base of the left ventricle is the annulus behind the posterior mitral leaflet. Thus, this circumference decreases during systole. If, however, the annulus behind the posterior mitral leaflet is calcified, the sphincter-like contraction of the left ventricular base no longer takes place. Thus, the area of the mitral orifice is not decreased and mild degrees of mitral regurgitation may be the result.

Calcification in the mitral annular area appears to be accelerated by conditions which elevate left ventricular pressure, namely systemic hypertension, aortic valvular stenosis, and hypertrophic cardiomyopathy,[121] and by conditions which accelerate atherosclerosis, for example, diabetes mellitus. The former conditions increase the mitral closing pressure and the latter appear to increase the supply of lipids. An intrinsic defect of the fibrous skeleton of the heart appears to be the explanation for early mitral annular calcification in the Marfan and Hurler syndromes. The mechanism by which mitral regurgitation is produced in patients with calcified mitral annuli is discussed in Figure 33.

In contrast to calcification of the mitral annulus, calcification of the tricuspid valve annulus is rare and the deposits are always focal and usually small. Tricuspid annular calcification may occur in two circumstances: (1) In patients with heritable connective tissue defects. We have observed tricuspid annular calcification in a patient with the Marfan syndrome and in another with the Hurler syndrome. (2) In patients with right ventricular hypertension from any cause. This is by far the most common underlying abnormality in these patients. We have observed tricuspid annular calcific deposits in patients with so-called pure pulmonic stenosis, primary pulmonary hypertension, and tetralogy of Fallot. Others have made similar observations.[122-124]

Papillary Muscle Dysfunction

A significant advance in clinical cardiology during the decade of the 1960s was the appreciation of the important contribution of the left ventricular papillary muscles to maintenance of mitral valve competence during ventricular systole. It is now well recognized that hypoxia, necrosis, or fibrosis of the left ventricular papillary muscles may be associated with varying degrees of mitral regurgitation. Discrepancies exist, however, in correlating papillary muscle structure with function. Although it most commonly results from coronary atherosclerosis, papillary muscle necrosis or fibrosis may occur when the coronary arteries are normal. Patients without clinical evidence of mitral valve dysfunction at necropsy have had severe necrosis or fibrosis or both, of one or both left ventricular papillary muscles; severe mitral regurgitation during or after acute myocardial infarction has been found at necropsy to be associated with normal papillary muscles, normal mitral leaflets and chordae tendineae, and normal-sized mitral annuli. This section seeks to clarify these discrepancies. Types and causes of papillary muscle damage are outlined in Table 15.[72]

Transient ischemia of papillary muscles is believed to be common and probably results in varying degrees of mitral regurgitation.[73] A murmur of mitral regurgitation may occur during an attack of angina pectoris and be absent during pain-free periods. Transient systolic murmurs during and after myocardial infarction probably result from papillary muscle ischemia. Arterial perfusion of the left ventricular papillary muscles even may be influenced by body position.[125] Possibly, transient ischemia of papillary muscles occurs during emotional stress in individuals with normal or nearly normal coronary arteries in a manner similar to that which leads to constriction of the peripheral vascular beds during anxiety or during cigarette smoking.

Table 15. Spectrum of left ventricular papillary muscle disease

I. Anatomically normal papillary muscles but papillary muscle dysfunction
   A. Transient ischemia
   B. Left ventricular dilatation from any cause
      1. Generalized
      2. Localized
   C. Necrosis or fibrosis in adjacent left ventricular free wall
      1. With coronary arterial narrowing
      2. Without coronary arterial narrowing
   D. "Small" left ventricular cavity (hypertrophic cardiomyopathy)

II. Necrosis or fibrosis of papillary muscle(s) without rupture
   A. With coronary arterial narrowing
      1. Acute myocardial infarction
      2. Healed myocardial infarction
   B. Without coronary arterial narrowing
      1. Acute
         a. Shock
         b. Acute valvular regurgitation (infective endocarditis)
      2. Chronic
         a. Anemia
         b. Left ventricular outflow obstruction
            (1) Valvular aortic stenosis
            (2) Discrete and diffuse subaortic stenosis
            (3) Supravalvular aortic stenosis
         c. Systemic hypertension
         d. Origin of left coronary artery or of both coronary arteries from pulmonary trunk
         e. Primary endocardial fibroelastosis of left ventricle
         f. Endomyocardial disease and eosinophilia
            (1) Löffler's fibroplastic parietal endocarditis
            (2) Endomyocardial fibrosis of Davies
         g. Idiopathic cardiomegaly (primary or diffuse myocardial disease)
         h. Focal myocardial disease
            (1) Idiopathic
            (2) "Neurogenic" heart disease
               (a) Progressive muscular dystrophy
               (b) Friedreich's ataxia
               (c) Myotonic muscular dystrophy

III. Necrosis or fibrosis of papillary muscle(s) with rupture
   A. Acute myocardial infarction from coronary heart disease
   B. Trauma
   C. Miscellaneous

IV. Infiltrative diseases of papillary muscles
   A. Pyogenic abscess
   B. Granulomas
      1. Aschoff bodies
      2. Sarcoid
   C. Amyloid
   D. Neoplasm
   E. Calcium
   F. Iron
   G. Other

V. Congenital malformations of papillary muscle(s)
   A. Single papillary muscle (parachute mitral valve syndrome)
   B. Accessory papillary muscle
   C. Abnormally large and malpositioned papillary muscles
   D. Abnormally small and malpositioned papillary muscle
   E. Insertion of papillary muscle directly into mitral leaflet

VI. Miscellaneous afflictions of papillary muscle(s)
   A. Excision, partial or complete, during mitral valve replacement
      1. Atrophy of nonexcised portion of papillary muscle after valve replacement
      2. Left ventricular aneurysm at site of papillary muscle excision
   B. Disuse atrophy after excision of mitral leaflets and chordae without excision of papillary muscle(s)

Left ventricular dilatation is a frequent cause of papillary muscle dysfunction.[126] Although the papillary muscles may contract normally under such circumstances, the spatial relationships between them, chordae tendineae, and orifices are altered by the caudal and lateral migration of the left ventricular walls away from the mitral annuli. The valve leaflets thus are pulled downward toward the left ventricle and consequently the mitral orifice becomes incompetent.

Although it may accompany left ventricular dilatation, mitral annular dilatation is probably an infrequent cause of mitral regurgitation, and most cases of mitral regurgitation attributed to annular dilatation probably result from papillary muscle dysfunction. Mitral annular dilatation must be massive to cause regurgitation for at least two reasons: (1) normally the surface area of the mitral leaflets is about two times the area of the mitral orifice and (2) the mitral ring has a sphincter-like action which causes the annulus to contract during ventricular systole.[127] Furthermore, a fibrous skeleton at the base of the heart inhibits mitral annular dilatation. Indeed, in the dilated heart the widest diameter occurs not at the left ventricular base, the area which includes the mitral annulus, but in the midportion of the chamber between apex and base.

It is now well appreciated that dilated left ventricles, per se, with or without fibrosis or necrosis of ventricular walls, may be associated with mitral regurgitation. It is less well recognized that mitral regurgitation may be associated with necrosis or fibrosis of the left ventricular free wall without accompanying left ventricular dilatation or papillary muscle or mitral valve lesions. Necrotic or scarred myocardium adjacent to papillary muscles, which fail to move or move paradoxically during ventricular systole, and the abnormal ventricular contraction may lead to abnormal papillary-muscle anchoring with resulting mitral regurgitation. Anatomic left ventricular aneurysms unassociated with papillary muscle necrosis or fibrosis also may cause mitral regurgitation by a similar mechanism. In hypertrophic cardiomyopathy the septal hypertrophy bends or distorts the papillary muscles causing mitral regurgitation.[72,73]

Necrosis or fibrosis of one or both left ventricular papillary muscles is extremely common. It may be focal or diffuse, involve only one papillary muscle or both, and auscultatory mitral regurgitation may or may not be present. Experimental studies show[128] that mitral regurgitation is not a consequence of fibrosis of papillary muscles alone. The free wall beneath the papillary muscle must also be fibrotic for mitral regurgitation to occur. We have observed at necropsy many patients who had no audible precordial murmurs in life but had extensive fibrosis or necrosis of one or both left ventricular papillary muscles. Papillary muscle fibrosis or necrosis causing mitral regurgitation, however, does not necessarily assure the appearance of a precordial murmur. Several patients without a regurgitant murmur have been shown to have mitral regurgitation by cineangiocardiography, and at necropsy to have extensive necrosis or fibrosis of papillary muscle and of left ventricular free wall.[129] Silent mitral regurgitation during acute myocardial infarction has been attributed to a diminished flow velocity across the mitral valve secondary to diminished myocardial contractility.

The most common cause of papillary muscle necrosis or fibrosis is narrowing of the coronary arterial lumen by atherosclerosis. The posteromedial papillary

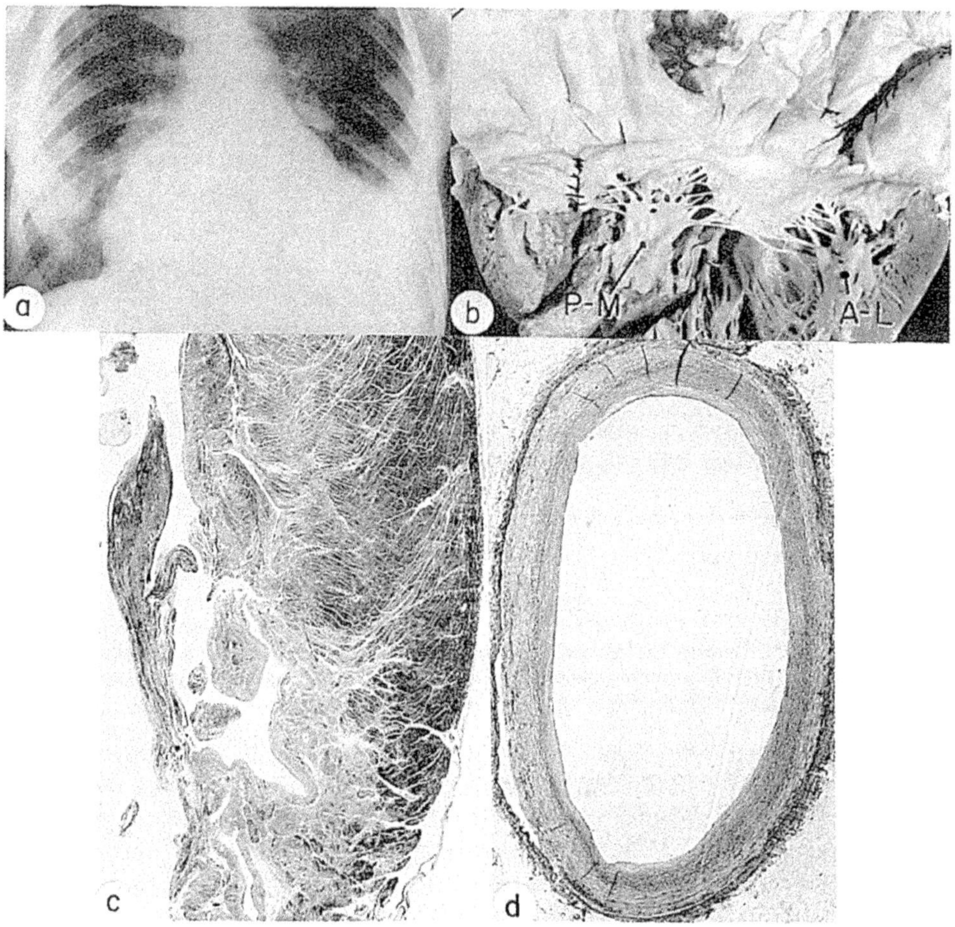

Figure 34. Possible focal myocarditis with subsequent fibrosis causing severe mitral regurgitation in an 84-year-old man (A66–213). A precordial murmur had been known to be present for 44 years. During his last 20 years he had periodic overt congestive cardiac failure and a grade 4/6 pansystolic blowing murmur typical of mitral regurgitation. He never had chest pain, systemic hypertension, rheumatic fever, or infective endocarditis. The heart was enlarged (a). The mitral leaflets and chordae tendineae were virtually normal. The posteromedial (P-M) papillary muscle was diffusely fibrotic as was the adjacent left ventricular free wall beneath it (b). No other myocardial scars were present and the coronary arteries were wide open. c, Longitudinal section of posteromedial papillary muscle and adjacent left ventricular free wall. Both are severely scarred and thinned. d, Section of right coronary artery which is wide open. All his coronary arteries were widely patent. c, Masson stain. d, Elastic van Gieson stain. [Reduced 30 per cent from × 4 (c) and × 21 (d).]

muscle is usually involved in posterior wall infarction, but in anterior wall infarction the anterolateral papillary muscle may be spared. Necrosis or fibrosis of one or both left ventricular papillary muscles may be unassociated with luminal narrowing of the extramural coronary arteries (Fig. 34). Inadequate oxygenation of the papillary muscles may occur if the amount of oxygen in the blood is low (i.e., anemia) or if the cardiac output for any reason is below a critical level. To perfuse the apices of the papillary muscles the coronary arteries must extend

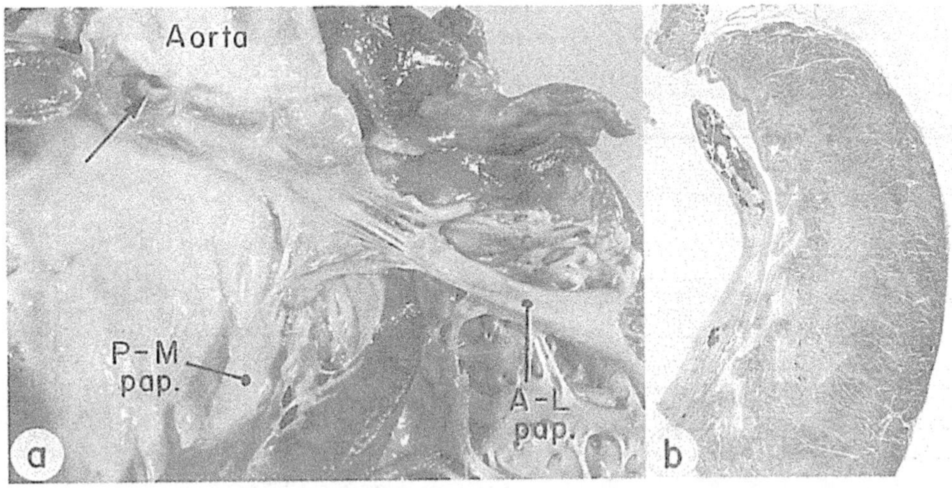

Figure 35. Mitral regurgitation due to origin of left coronary artery from the pulmonary trunk. Severe fibrosis and calcification in the anterolateral left ventricular papillary muscle in a nine-month-old girl (A56–14) in whom the left coronary artery arose from the pulmonary trunk. She had had evidence of congestive cardiac failure since age three weeks. Examination at age eight months disclosed a grade 3/6 systolic precordial murmur consistent with mitral regurgitation. The heart was huge, and electrocardiogram showed evidence of left ventricular hypertrophy and ischemia. She died during cardiac operation. At necropsy, the left ventricle was considerably dilated and its endocardium showed diffuse fibroelastosis (a). The anterolateral papillary muscle was severely thinned, scarred and calcified (b). b, Hematoxylin-eosin stain. [Reduced 15 percent from × 4 (b).]

through the entire thicknesses of the myocardial free walls, turn up hill, and ascend distances of at least one and often two thicknesses of the free wall. Hence, the papillary muscles (particularly the posteromedial one) are the most sensitive markers of inadequate myocardial oxygenation. Foci of necrosis also are common in patients with fatal severe valvular regurgitation of recent onset. Among 47 patients dying of active valvular infective endocarditis, 34 (72 per cent) had necrotic lesions in one or both left ventricular papillary muscles and none had significant narrowing of the extramural coronary arteries.[130-132] Severely diminished cardiac output with resultant poor myocardial perfusion appeared to cause the papillary muscle necrosis in them.

Fibrosis with atrophy of the papillary muscles is seen in patients with primary

Figure 36. Diagrammatic representation of the types of, and possible consequences of, papillary muscle rupture during acute myocardial infarction. It is likely that rupture of the entire trunk (*left*) is incompatible with survival in any patient since a major portion of the support to both valve leaflets is destroyed. With rupture of an apical head (*right*), survival would appear to depend on the extent to which the function of the left ventricle has been impaired by the infarct. With severely impaired ventricular function, the additional burden of even modest mitral regurgitation may be intolerable, and death will ensue. If the left ventricle is less severely compromised, survival is possible for weeks or months, but congestive cardiac failure will almost invariably develop. *Lower*, Rupture of a portion of one papillary muscle during acute myocardial infarction in a 51-year-old man (S67–813) who underwent mitral valve replacement three months after the onset of infarction. Preoperatively, the pulmonary arterial pressure was 60/28 (mean 40); pulmonary arterial wedge pressure, mean 28, v42; left ventricular pressure 74/17; and cardiac index, 1.7 L./min./m^2. Shown here is the excised mitral valve (by Dr. Andrew G. Morrow). The leaflets are normal but the posteromedial papillary muscle is necrotic and fibrotic and a portion of it is entwined in chordae tendineae at the margin of the anterior mitral leaflet. This is a view of the ventricular aspects of the leaflets.

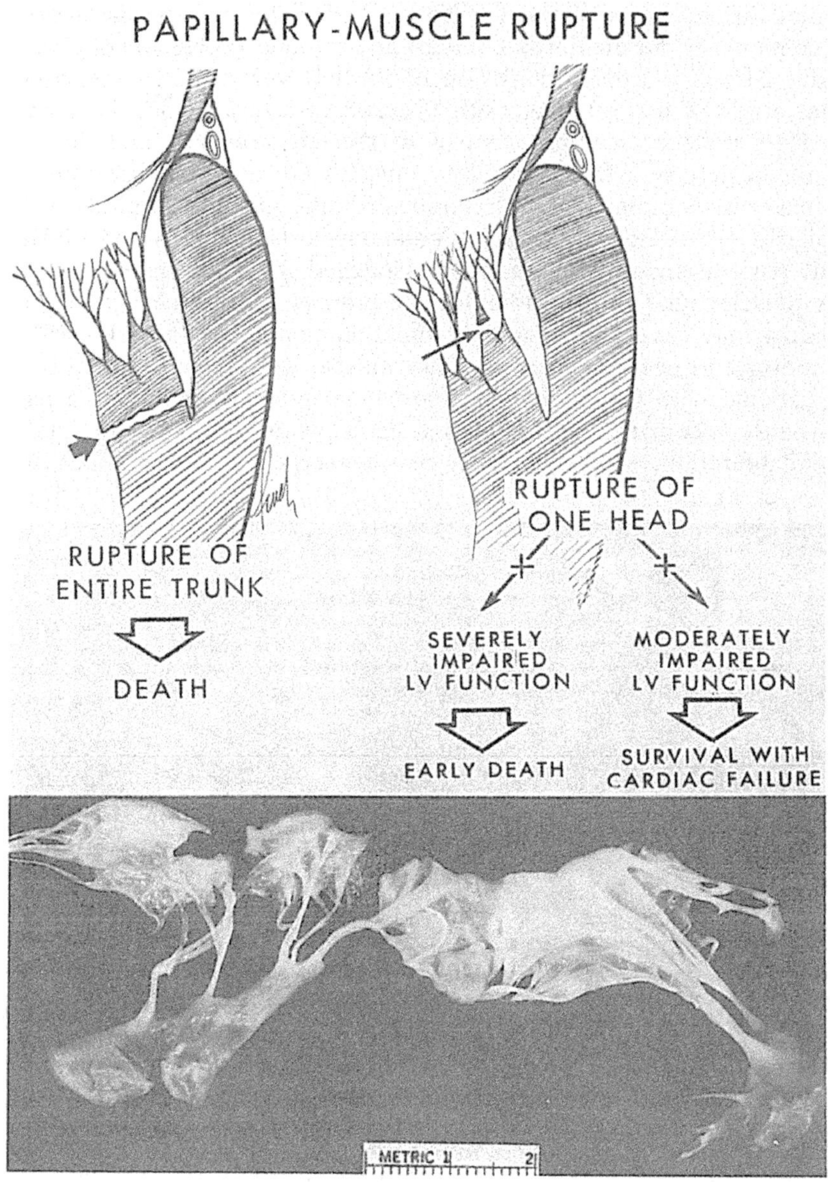
PAPILLARY-MUSCLE RUPTURE
RUPTURE OF ENTIRE TRUNK
DEATH
RUPTURE OF ONE HEAD
SEVERELY IMPAIRED LV FUNCTION
EARLY DEATH
MODERATELY IMPAIRED LV FUNCTION
SURVIVAL WITH CARDIAC FAILURE
METRIC 1 2

endocardial fibroelastosis of the left ventricle.[133] The endocardial scarring as well as the papillary muscle fibrosis may be an anatomic expression of chronically inadequate coronary arterial perfusion of the left ventricle. In the congenital condition, origin of the left[134] or both[135] coronary arteries from the pulmonary trunk, diffuse endocardial fibroelastosis of the left ventricle, and fibrosis and atrophy of the left ventricular papillary muscles are associated lesions. These patients may present clinically with features of pure mitral regurgitation[136] (Fig. 35). Similarly, the African conditions, endomyocardial fibrosis and Löffler's fibroplastic parietal endocarditis may be associated with scarring of one or both papillary muscles, and rarely, patients with primary or secondary forms of cardiomyopathy may have scarred and dysfunctioning papillary muscles.[137-140]

In contrast to necrosis of a papillary muscle which occurs in over 50 per cent of patients with fatal acute myocardial infarction, rupture of a papillary muscle is rare, occurring in less than 1 per cent of patients with fatal acute myocardial infarction. The rupture may be of two types (Fig. 36).[141] One involves

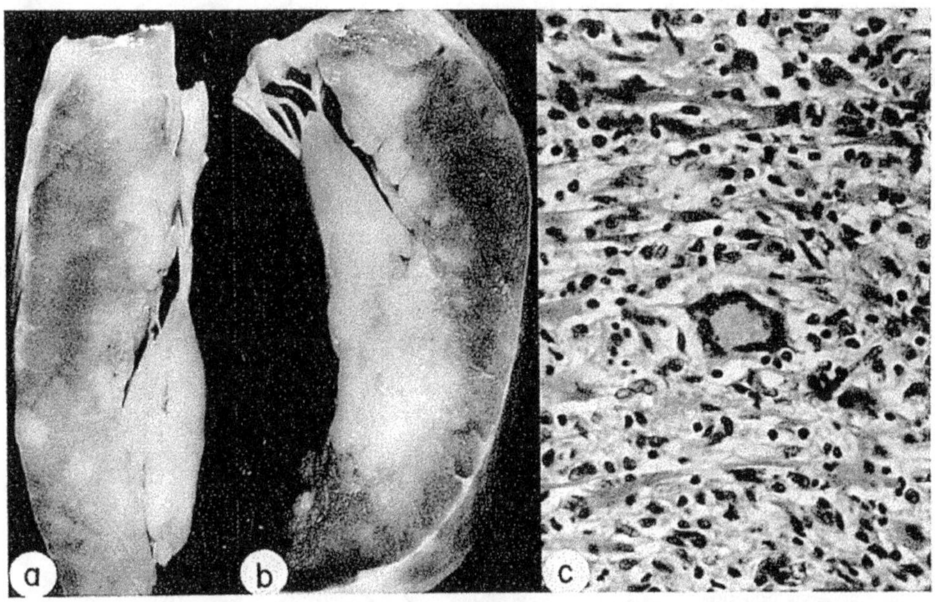

Figure 37. Sarcoidosis of papillary muscles causing mitral regurgitation. Anterolateral (a) and posteromedial (b) left ventricular papillary muscles in a 26-year-old woman (PGGH A-70-541) who was asymptomatic until 10 days before death when dyspnea appeared. The dyspnea rapidly worsened, and when hospitalized on the day of death she was in acute pulmonary edema. The blood pressure was 80/70 mm. Hg, heart rate 160 beats/minute, and a grade 3–4/6 pansystolic blowing apical murmur, which radiated into the axilla, was audible. Chest roentgenogram showed congested lungs, cardiomegaly, and prominent hilar adenopathy. Electrocardiogram showed nonspecific ST–T wave changes and atrial hypertrophy. Several hours after admission ventricular fibrillation occurred; she was resuscitated, but complete heart block appeared. A transvenous pacemaker was inserted, but asystole occurred shortly thereafter. At necropsy, large firm white deposits were present in the walls of all four cardiac chambers and completely replaced both left ventricular papillary muscles (a and b). On histologic section, the firm white areas represented hard granulomas typical of sarcoidosis (c). Similar hard granulomas were present in lymph nodes, liver, spleen, and lung. Stains for acid-fast organisms, other bacteria, and fungi were negative. (Specimen was kindly provided by Dr. James Hutchinson.) c, Hematoxylin-eosin stain. [Reduced 25 per cent from × 400 (c).]

the entire central muscle belly of the papillary muscle, and this type rupture is incompatible with survival since half the support of each valve leaflet is destroyed and mitral regurgitation of overwhelming severity results. The second type of rupture involves only one or two apical heads of a papillary muscle. The resulting mitral regurgitation is of lesser magnitude and immediate survival is then dependent upon the degree to which the function of the left ventricle has been impaired by the infarct. In patients who survive after papillary muscle rupture, the functional capacity of the left ventricle also governs the extent of clinical and hemodynamic improvement after mitral valve replacement.

The papillary muscles are subject to various infiltrative processes just like any other portion of myocardium.[72,142] Pyogenic abscesses, Aschoff bodies, granulomas,[142] neoplasms,[143-145] amyloid,[146] and iron[147] have all been observed in these structures. Congestive heart failure from severe mitral regurgitation may be the initial symptom of sarcoidosis[72] (Fig. 37).

Infective Endocarditis

Infective endocarditis (IE) continues to be a major cause of fatal valvular heart disease. Clinical and necropsy observations in 57 necropsy patients with IE have recently been reported[130,131] from this laboratory and major findings from these studies are summarized in Table 16. Although IE may involve both right-sided and left-sided cardiac valves, or mural endocardium only,[148] it is useful to separate cases with right-sided vegetations (with or without associated left-sided vegetations) from those with isolated left-sided vegetations (Table 16).

The frequency with which infection attacks previously normal as opposed to previously abnormal valves is somewhat uncertain. It has long been stated

Table 16. Infective endocarditis: data in 57 necropsy patients

	Isolated Left-sided Vegetations	Isolated Right-sided Vegetations	Right and Left-sided Vegetations	Totals
Patients	45	6	6	57
Ages (years): Range (avg)	17-70(38)	25-65(40)	1-62(40)	1-70(39)
Males	32(71%)	3	5	40(70%)
Females	13(29%)	3	1	17(30%)
Alcoholics	7(15%)	1	4	12(21%)
Heroin addicts	6(13%)	4	0	10(18%)
Acute meningitis	6(13%)	2	3	11(19%)
Acute pneumonia	4(9%)	5	5	14(25%)
Antemortum diagnosis	36(80%)	3	2	41(72%)
Previous symptomatic H.D.	12(27%)	0	1	13(23%)
Rheumatic H.D.	10(22%)	0	0	10(18%)
Congenital H.D.	8(18%)	0	1	9(16%)
Anatomically normal valve	24(53%)	6	5	35(61%)
Anatomically abnormal valve	21(47%)	0	1	22(39%)
Functionally normal	10(22%)	–	1	11(19%)
Functionally abnormal	11(24%)	–	0	11(19%)
Stenosis	7(15%)	–	0	7(12%)
Incompetent	4(9%)	–	0	4(7%)
Staphylococcus	12(27%)	5	1	18(32%)
Streptococcus	9(20%)	0	1	10(18%)
Pneumococcus	4(9%)	1	3	8(14%)
Acute myocarditis	23(51%)	1	2	26(46%)
Papillary muscle necrosis	22/39(56%)	0	3	25/50(50%)

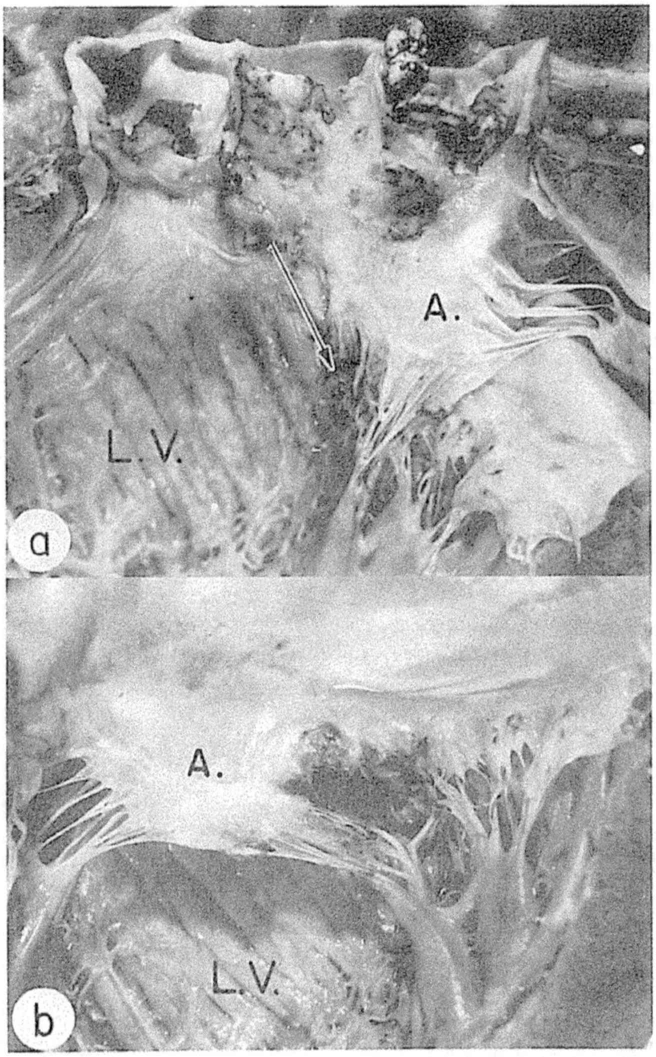

Figure 38. Streptococcus faecalis endocarditis involving both aortic and mitral valves in a 61-year-old man (DCGH# 71A-120). Symptoms and signs of active infective endocarditis appeared three weeks after catheterization of his urinary bladder. Both valves probably were normal before they became sites of infection. a, Opened left ventricle (L.V.) and aortic valve. The vegetations have partially destroyed each cusp causing severe aortic regurgitation. Vegetation on the left ventricular outflow endocardium, mitral leaflet, and chordae tendineae almost certainly resulted from retrograde spread of the aortic vegetations by the aortic regurgitant stream (arrow). A. = anterior mitral leaflet. b, Opened mitral valve showing vegetations at the posteromedial commissure area. Many chordae have ruptured.

that IE tends to affect persons with known valvular heart disease, but that the cardiac condition is compensated, i.e., the patient is usually asymptomatic before infection appears. This view indicates, therefore, that infection tends to involve valves which are anatomically abnormal but functionally normal. From a necropsy standpoint, however, fatal active IE more frequently involves previously anatomically normal valves (Figs. 38–41). Of our 45 necropsy patients with left-sided IE, the affected valve was previously anatomically normal in 24 (53 per cent), and of the 21 (47 per cent) affecting previously anatomically abnormal valves, only 11 of them had been functionally abnormal (valve stenosis in seven, pure incompetency in four). Of our 12 patients with right-sided vegetations, the involved valve had been anatomically normal before IE in 11, and functionally normal in all 12. Because infection of previously anatomically normal valves is nearly always by virulent organisms, and because the infective process can more easily destroy a thin, delicate (normal) valve as opposed to a thick, tough (abnormal) valve, the frequency of involvement by IE of previously anatomically normal

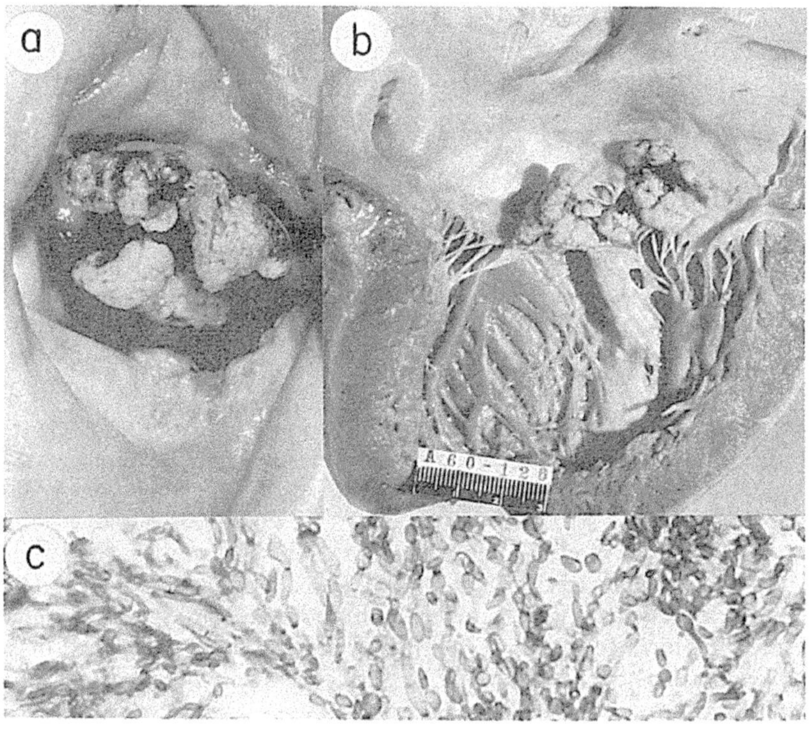

Figure 39. Candida parapsilosis endocarditis on a previously normal mitral valve of a 68-year-old man (A60–126) with chronic lung disease and coronary heart disease. Five months before death he had fever, and 45 days later he was hospitalized. A grade 2/6 apical systolic murmur was present. Despite amphotericin B therapy, blood cultures remained positive, and he died of congestive heart failure. A large embolus to the left common iliac artery occurred during hospitalization. a, Mitral valve viewed from left atrium showing huge vegetations on both leaflets. b, Opened left heart showing large vegetations on both mitral leaflets. Although they were large, the vegetations did not destroy the valvular leaflets or rupture chordae tendineae. c, Photomicrograph of portion of vegetation showing spores and pseudomycelia of Candida species. Methenamine silver stain × 500.

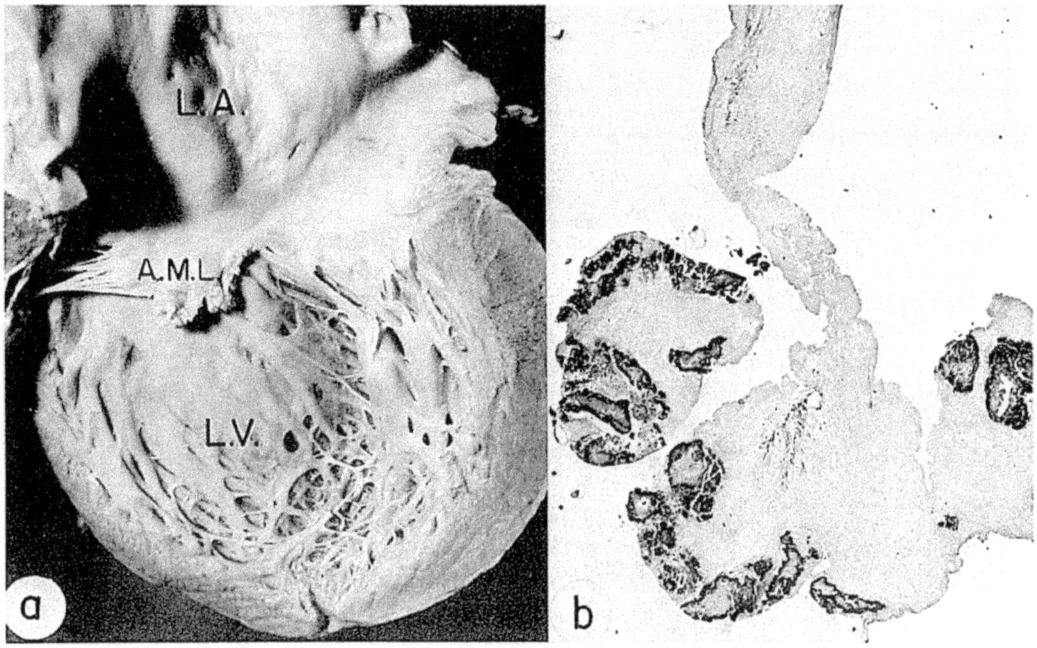

Figure 40. Acute mitral regurgitation from rupture of chordae tendineae secondary to Streptococcus faecalis endocarditis in a 24-year-old woman (A62–19) who had been well until five months earlier when symptoms of infective endocarditis appeared shortly after an abortion. Despite antibiotic therapy, severe congestive cardiac failure and pulmonary hypertension developed. The vegetation healed but she died of results of rupture of many mitral chordae tendineae. a, Opened left atrium (L.A.), mitral valve, and left ventricle (L.V.) showing severence of all chordae on the posterior half of the anterior mitral leaflet (A.M.L.). The valve before infection was normal. b, Histologic section of portion of anterior mitral leaflet showing calcific deposits, almost certainly a consequence of healing of the vegetation. Hematoxylin-eosin stain × 16.

valves in a necropsy study might be abnormally high. The incidence of IE, however, is clearly greater among persons with underlying valvular heart disease as opposed to the incidence of IE among persons with previously normal hearts. But, because there are many more persons with four normal valves compared to persons with one or more abnormal ones, this numerical difference alone may explain the greater frequency with which normal valves are involved by IE. The frequency of certain predisposing factors (malignancy, heroin addiction, alcoholism, long-term intravenous catheters, etc.) allowing entrance of virulent or unusual organisms or alterations in host defense mechanisms also is important in explaining the frequency of IE on normal valves.

Valvular dysfunction is by no means an inevitable consequence of active IE. It was unequivocally a consequence of IE in 59 per cent, and possibly as high as 74 per cent, of our 45 patients with left-sided IE but in none of our six patients with isolated right-sided vegetations. Congestive cardiac failure is common in fatal IE. It occurred in 74 per cent of our patients with left-sided IE, and in each was the result of valvular dysfunction, not the result of associated myocardial lesions. Although the latter occurred in 87 per cent of the patients

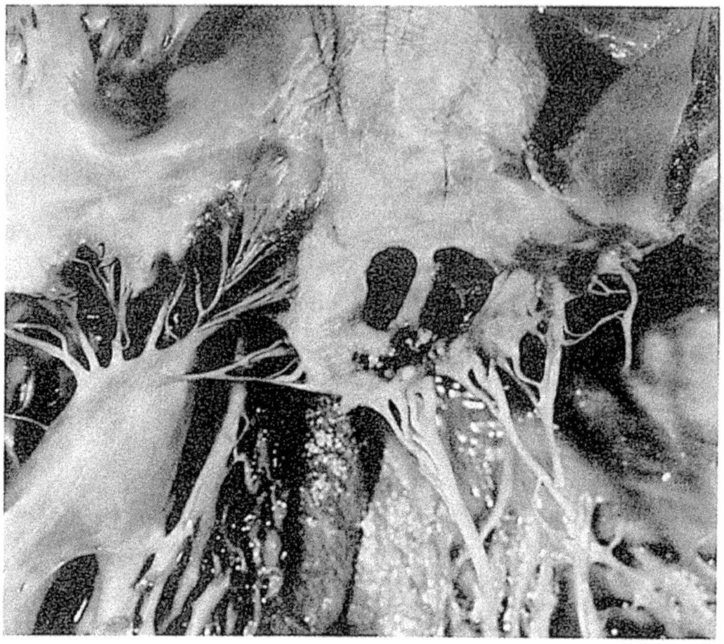

Figure 41. Infective endocarditis with perforation of mitral leaflet and severe regurgitation. This young woman (A69–154) had been well until the appearance of infective endocarditis about one year before death. The infection was "cured" by antibiotics but mitral regurgitation was a consequence. She died of progressive congestive cardiac failure from mitral regurgitation. Perforation of a mitral valve cusp by infection, as shown here, is infrequent. Mitral regurgitation in infective endocarditis far more commonly results from rupture of chordae tendineae. It appears that the valve shown here was anatomically normal before infection appeared.

with isolated left-sided vegetations, in none did they appear large or diffuse enough to account by themselves for congestive cardiac failure. Papillary muscle necrosis was present in 58 per cent, but in none did it appear to cause mitral regurgitation. Valve ring abscesses occurred in 12 or 31 per cent of patients with aortic valve vegetations and in none of 26 with mitral valve vegetations. Ring abscesses indicate severe destruction of valvular cusps and severe valvular dysfunction, and they also usually indicate that the infection is the result of a highly virulent organism. Aortic regurgitation, when it occurred, was the result of destruction (tears or perforations) of the cusps by the infective process. Mitral regurgitation resulted from rupture of chordae tendineae by the infective process, and only 2 of 26 patients with mitral vegetations had cuspal perforations.

Of the 12 patients with right-sided cardiac valvular vegetations, six also had vegetations on left-sided cardiac valves (Table 16). In only one of the latter, however, was the IE definitely primary on the left side of the heart. The tricuspid valve was the site of IE in 11 patients and the pulmonic valve in one. The organisms responsible for the IE were Staphylococcus aureus in six patients, Diplococcus pneumoniae in four, Alpha streptococcus in one and Aspergillus flavus in one.

Five patients were alcoholics, four were heroin addicts, two had blood dyscrasias, and one had congenital cardiac disease (ventricular septal defect). The IE in each of the nine patients with alcoholism or heroin addiction and in the one with congenital heart disease was primary in the heart; in the remaining two patients, it was secondary to generalized infection affecting many body organs. Acute pneumonia was a dominant clinical feature in 10 of the 12 patients and appeared to be secondary to dislodgment of material from the right-sided cardiac vegetations. Six patients also had acute meningitis. Although the vegetations caused considerable damage to the right-sided cardiac valves, evidence of cardiac dysfunction was either absent or attributable to acute *cor pulmonale* secondary to the acute pneumonia. The tetrad of chronic alcoholism, acute pneumonia, acute meningitis, and infective endocarditis is common.[149] In 9 of the 12 patients the right-sided vegetations did not extend to involve the basal attachments of the leaflets to the annuli. Thus, in these nine patients total excision of the valve leaflets would have eradicated their valvular endocarditis.

The two major causes of acute valvular regurgitation are acute myocardial infarction and IE. Among 55 patients with fatal pure mitral regurgitation studied by one of us (W.C.R.), rupture of mitral chordae tendineae was the second most frequent etiology and IE was the most common cause of rupture.[150] Since infection most commonly involves previously normal valves, valvular destruction may be rapid and lead to severe regurgitation and decompensation. Rupture of previously normal mitral chordae leads to sudden severe elevation of left atrial pressures and the left atrial v waves may be similar in magnitude to the left ventricular systolic pressure (ventricularization of left atrial pressure) (Fig. 42). This circumstance occurs because the left atrium does not dilate initially, and as a consequence the high left atrial pressure is reflected to the pulmonary circuit with resulting severe pulmonary and right ventricular hypertension. When the left atrium finally dilates in pure mitral regurgitation from this mechanism, its pressure, along with that in the pulmonary vessels and right ventricle, also decreases.[150]

Although many reports have appeared on active IE, few reports have appeared on the morphologic aspects of *healed* IE. Recently, a study from this laboratory[151] examined cardiac valves in 59 patients with positive histories of IE searching for anatomic evidence of healed IE. Of the 59 patients, healed cuspal perforations were present in 16, healed ruptured chordae tendineae in 15, and healed ring abscesses in 5. A total of 30 of the 59 patients had one or more of these anatomic findings. Thus, about half of the patients with positive histories of IE had clear-cut anatomic evidences of IE. The relationship of healed valvular perforations and

Figure 42. Diagram depicting the two extremes of the spectrum of pure mitral regurgitation. When severe mitral regurgitation appears suddenly in individuals with previously normal or near-normal hearts, the left atrium (LA) is relatively small and the high pressure within it is reflected back into the pulmonary vessels and right ventricle (RV). The anatomic indicator of this latter physiologic event is severe hypertrophy of the left atrial and right ventricular walls and marked intimal proliferation and medial hypertrophy of the pulmonary arteries (PA), arterioles, and veins (PV). In the other extreme, the left atrial cavity is of giant size and its wall is thin. It is thus able to "absorb" the left ventricular (LV) pressure without reflecting it back into the pulmonary vessels or right ventricle. As a consequence, the pulmonary vessels remain normal and the right ventricular wall does not thicken. PT = pulmonary trunk. RA = right atrium.

THE SYNDROME OF MITRAL REGURGITATION

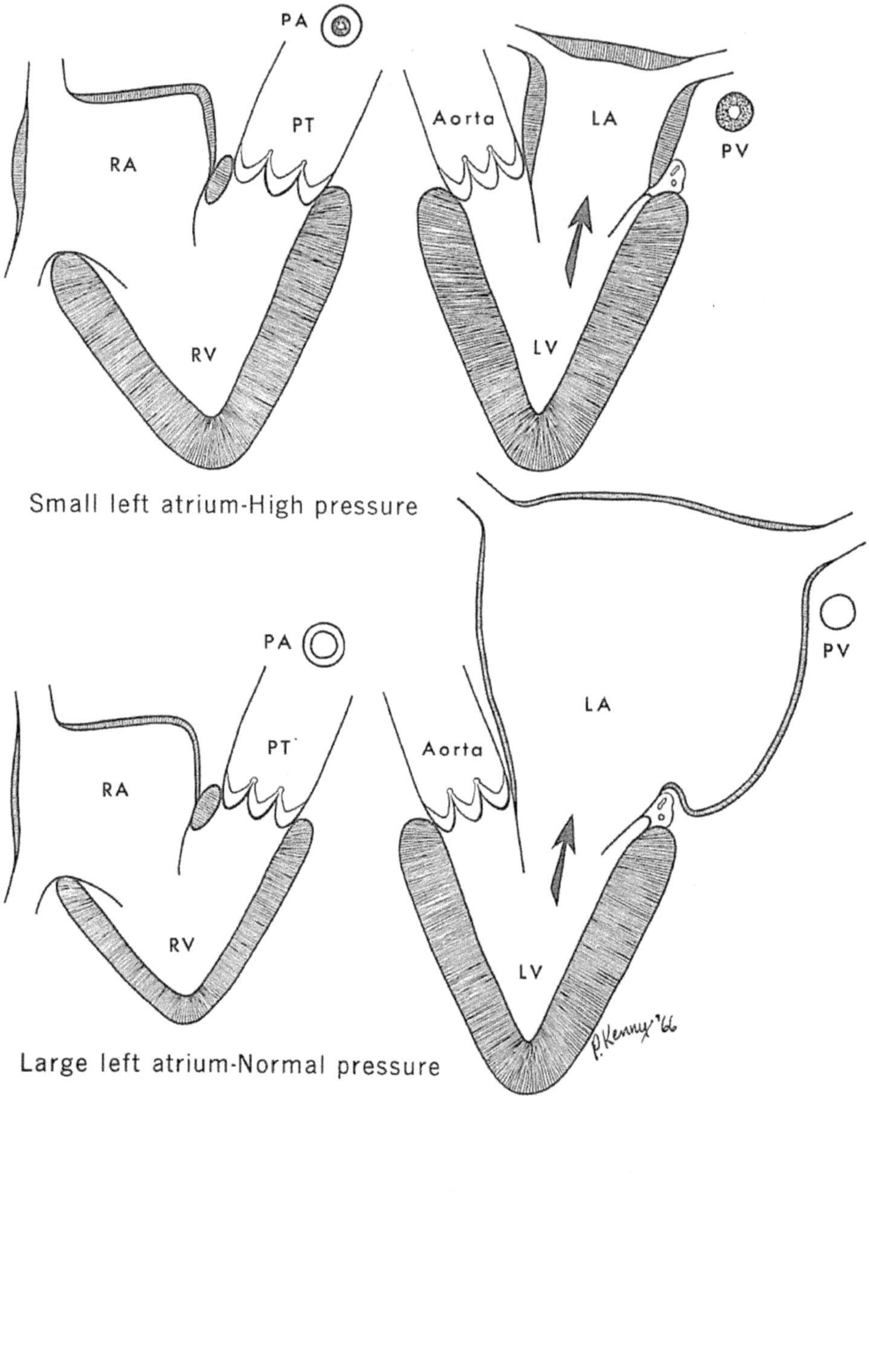

Table 17. Ebstein's anomaly: clinical and necropsy fiindings

Patient	Age	Sex	Age (yrs.) onset of symptoms	Cyanosis	Precordial murmurs: Systolic	Precordial murmurs: Diastolic	CE by x-ray	Electrocardiogram: SVA	Electrocardiogram: P Pulmonale	Electrocardiogram: RBBB	Cause of death	Necropsy findings: DDDTV (0-4+)	Necropsy findings: Associated lesions
1. A57-55	20	M	14	+	+	0	+	+	+	+	Operation*	4+	VI-PFO
2. A58-122	31	F	8	+	+	0	0	0	+	+	Operation†	3+	ASD, anomalous left SVC
3. A66-217	26	M	24‡	0	+‡	0	0	+	0	+	Sudden§	2+	Stenotic bicuspid AV
4. A68-2	18	F	15	0	+	0	0	+	0	0¶	SVA, VA	1+	0
5. A71-172	18	F	—#	0	+	0	0	0	0	0	Ewing's sarcoma	4+	Floppy MV
6. NNMC A72-97	37	F	33	+	+	0	+	+	0**	+	CHF heart block	4+	ASD

* Closure of valvular incompetent patent foramen ovale (VI-PFO) shortly before death.
† Closure of fossa ovale type atrial septal defect shortly before death.
‡ Symptoms and murmur consistent with aortic stenosis.
§ Ventricular fibrillation 18 days after aortic valve repair.
¶ Wolff-Parkinson-White pattern.
\# Asymptomatic.
** Atrial fibrillation.

ASD = atrial septal defect, fossa ovale type. AV = aortic valve. CE = cardiac enlargement. CHF = congestive heart failure. DDDTV = degree of downward displacement of tricuspid valve. MV = mitral valve. RBBB = right bundle branch block. SVA = supraventricular arrhythmias. SVC = superior vena cava. VA = ventricular arrhythmias.

ruptured chordae tendineae to antecedent positive histories of active IE also was examined. Of 18 patients with valve perforations, all 18 had had positive histories of active IE. Of 43 patients with healed ruptured chordae tendineae, only 15 (35 per cent) had had positive histories of active IE.

Congenital Tricuspid Regurgitation

Congenital tricuspid regurgitation most commonly is the result of displacement of the basal attachment of one or more tricuspid valve leaflets into right ventricle. This downward displacement is the characteristic feature of the malformation first described in 1866 by Ebstein.[152] Now over 300 patients have been reported with *Ebstein's anomaly* including one series of 108 patients.[153]

We have studied at necropsy six patients, aged 18 to 37 years, with Ebstein's anomaly (Table 17) (Figs. 43–46). Four were women. Three had been cyanotic, and they were the only ones with atrial septal defects. All six had systolic murmurs, but in two (#2 and #4) they appeared to be caused by associated mitral and aortic lesions and not by tricuspid regurgitation. None had diastolic murmurs. Four had ventricular diastolic gallops. Four had supraventricular arrhythmias. Roentgenograms revealed globular-shaped hearts (Fig. 43) in only two. The degree of caudal displacement of the tricuspid valve leaflets varied. Two (#1 and #5) of the three patients with the most marked downward displacement (Figs. 43–45) had classic clinical features of the anomaly and both had severe congestive failure

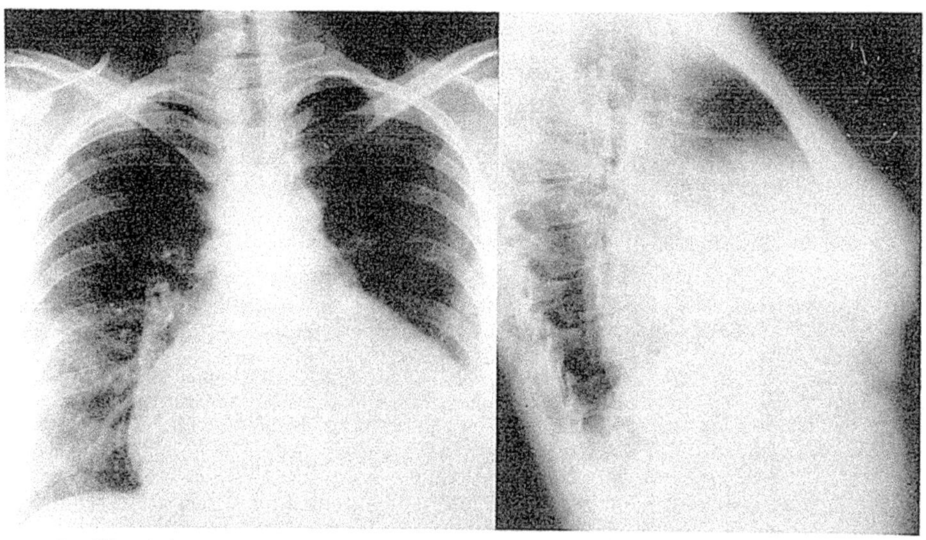

Figure 43. Ebstein's anomaly. Posteroanterior and lateral chest roentgenograms of a 37-year-old woman (NNMC A72–97) who died of severe cardiac failure and heart block. She had had profound cyanosis, chest pain, and episodes of syncope. At necropsy, severe downward displacement of the septal and posterior leaflets of the tricuspid valve and parchment-like thinning of the atrialized portion of right ventricle were found. In addition, a fossa-ovale type atrial septal defect was present. The radiograph reveals globular-shaped cardiomegaly in contrast to the patient in Figures 44 and 45 whose anatomic findings were similar in type and severity.

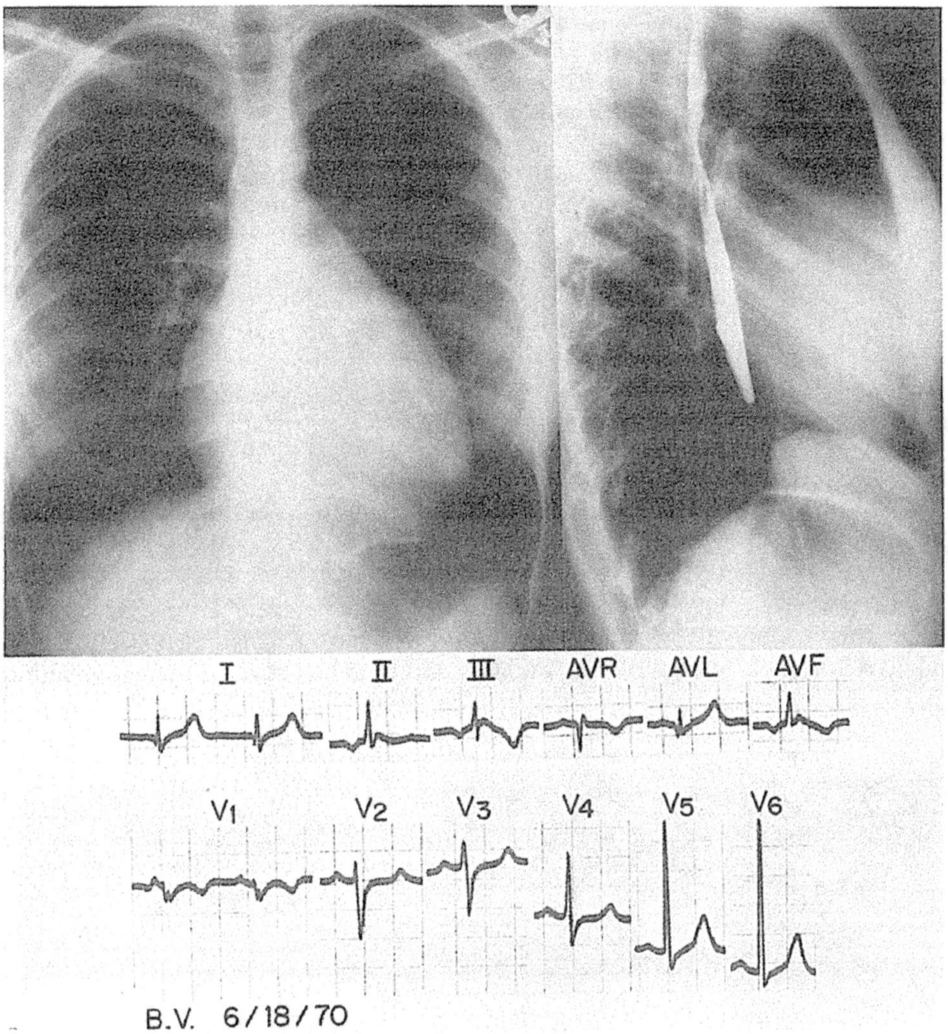

Figure 44. Severe Ebstein's anomaly of tricuspid valve, an incidental necropsy finding. Posteroanterior and lateral chest roentgenogram and electrocardiogram from the patient (A71–172) whose anatomic findings are demonstrated in Figure 45. The roentgenogram suggests right atrial enlargement and borderline cardiomegaly. The anteroposterior thoracic width, however, is narrow. The electrocardiogram reveals an atrioventricular junctional rhythm without tachycardia and an abnormally superior T wave vector. The P amplitude is normal and there are no clearcut defects in atrioventricular or intraventricular conduction.

before death or operation. In contrast, the patients with less caudal displacement did not die of congestive cardiac failure (Fig. 46). The displacement involved primarily the septal and posterior tricuspid valve leaflets, the basal attachments of these leaflets were displaced caudally from 2 to 8 cm. below the normal tricuspid valve annuli. In two patients (#5 and #6) functioning right ventricle was limited to outflow tract. In all patients one or more leaflets adhered to the ventricular walls by short chordae. An accessory tricuspid valve orifice was present in two patients. The tricuspid valve "annuli" were dilated in five patients. Right atrial and right ventricular dilatation was present in all and varied from mild to severe. In two patients the atrialized portion of the right ventricle was parchment-like.

The tricuspid valve in Ebstein's malformation is usually incompetent. Decompensation in these patients, however, appears to result primarily from inadequate pumping of the right ventricle and not from tricuspid regurgitation.[154,155] The portion of right ventricle cephalad to the displaced tricuspid leaflets is atrialized, i.e., the muscle is thin and contracts poorly, if at all. The functioning mass of right ventricular muscle may be reduced to outflow portion. As a result, pulmonary blood flow may decrease and the right atrial and systemic venous pressures may rise. Prognosis in patients with Ebstein's anomaly depends, in general, on the degree of caudal displacement of the tricuspid leaflets and the magnitude of associated valvular incompetency.[156] The average life expectancy is 37 years.[27,157] In its most severe form Ebstein's anomaly has been the presumed cause of intrauterine and perinatal death,[158,159] but survival into the seventh and eight

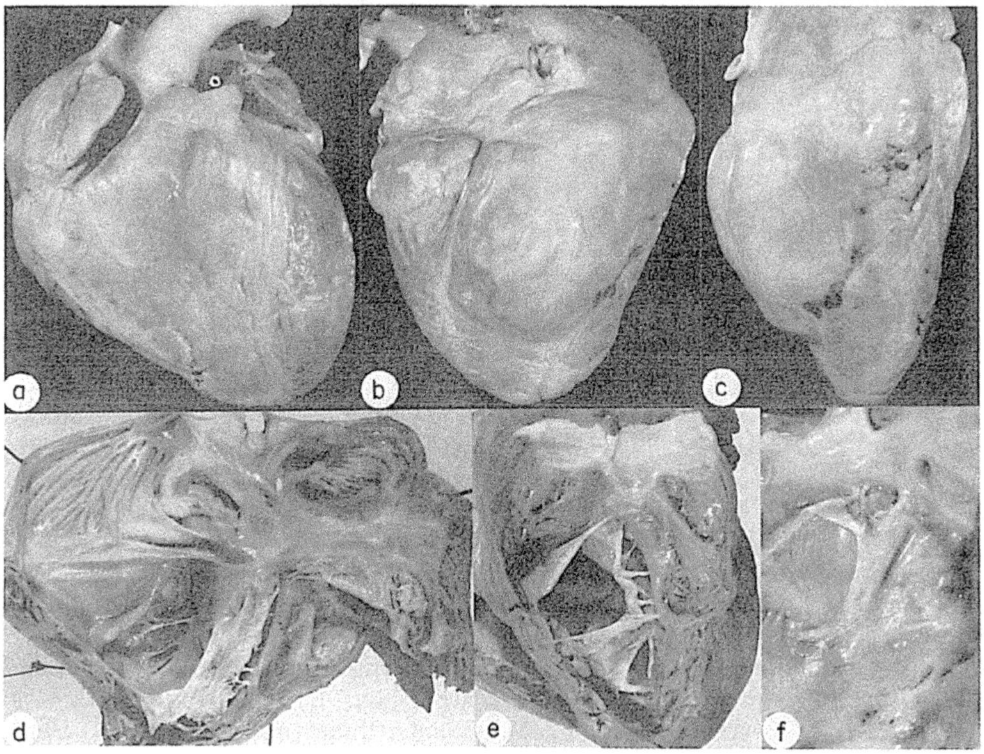

Figure 45. Severe Ebstein's anomaly of the tricuspid valve, an incidental necropsy finding. This 18-year-old girl (A71–172), who died of Ewing's sarcoma, had no symptoms of cardiac dysfunction despite an active life. a, b, and c, Anterior, posterior, and lateral views, respectively, of the external aspect of the heart demonstrating a thinned, parchment-like (atrialized) right ventricular wall bulging posteriorly above the attachment of the tricuspid leaflets. d, Opened right atrium and ventricle showing marked downward displacement of the posterior and septal tricuspid leaflets. The atrialized portion of right ventricle behind the posterior leaflet is the part that bulges (b and c). e, Tricuspid valve from above displaced deep into right ventricular cavity. Two valvular orifices are present. f, Intact atrial septum from left atrium with valvular-competent foramen ovale. The patient was never cyanotic.

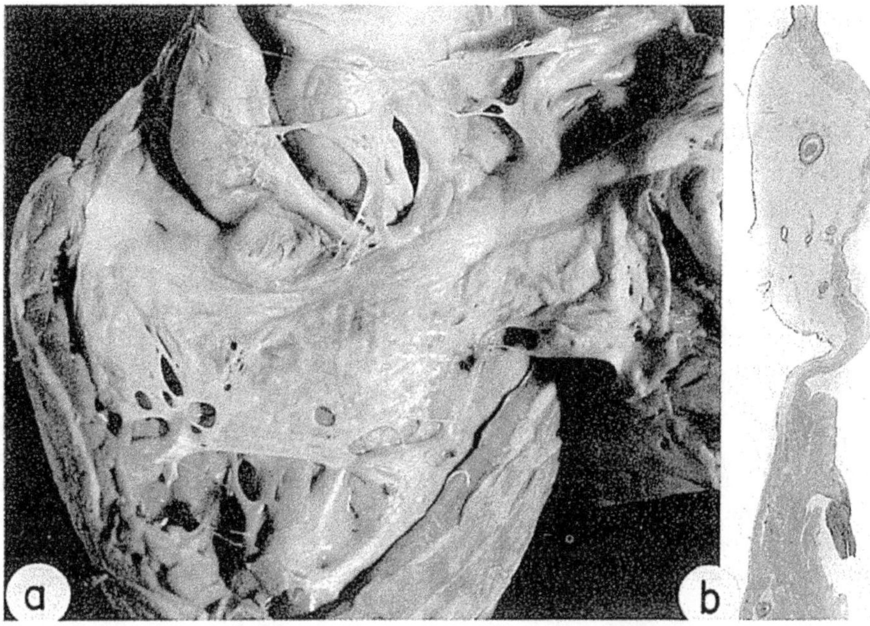

Figure 46. Mild Ebstein's anomaly in two patients. a, Opened tricuspid valve of a 25-year-old man (A66–217) who died 20 days after operation for severe valvular aortic stenosis. Tricuspid valvular dysfunction was not suspected clinically. At necropsy, it was seen that the tricuspid leaflets inserted into the right ventricular wall just below the annulus fibrosis. The tricuspid leaflets were bound down to the ventricular endocardium. b, Photomicrograph of a longitudinal section through right atrioventricular sulcus including a portion of right atrium and right ventricle. The basal attachment of the leaflet of the tricuspid valve is to the ventricular wall 1.8 cm. below the annulus. Hematoxylin-eosin stain × 2. This 18-year-old girl (A68–2) had a systolic precordial murmur of unknown cause and type B Wolff-Parkinson-White syndrome. She died of ventricular tachycardia and fibrillation during treatment of one of many episodes of supraventricular tachycardia. At necropsy, the right atrium, right ventricle, and tricuspid annulus were dilated.

decades may occur.[27,157,158,160,161] Death most frequently (about 40 per cent) results from congestive cardiac failure, another 20 per cent from supraventricular arrhythmias, and the remainder from miscellaneous causes.[158] About 75 per cent of these patients have an atrial septal defect with some right-to-left shunting. Most defects are valvular-incompetent patent foramina ovale.[153,160]

The clinical features of Ebstein's anomaly were first well described in 1950 by Engle et al.[162] The typical patient is fatigued, dyspneic, often cyanotic, and has a large, "quiet" globular heart, gallop rhythm, systolic and scratchy diastolic murmurs, right bundle branch block, and occasionally atrioventricular conduction delay (Wolff-Parkinson-White [type B] in 10 per cent). Diagnosis of this anomaly, however, may be difficult. Of our six patients, three (#2, #3, and #4) were not diagnosed correctly despite repeated clinical examinations. Some patients may be acyanotic, asymptomatic, and devoid of diagnostically useful physical findings.[163] In this situation, the electrocardiogram may be helpful.[164] Diagnosis in patients surviving past the fourth decade may be confused with more common forms of acquired heart disease, as was true of our patient #5 in whom the initial diagnosis was coronary heart disease. Unless strongly suspected, diagnosis of Ebstein's anomaly may be easily missed at catheterization.[165]

Pure Congenital Pulmonic Regurgitation

Isolated pure congenital pulmonary regurgitation (PR) is rare. It may complicate idiopathic dilatation of the pulmonary trunk,[166] hypoplasia or aplasia[167-170] of the pulmonic cusps, congenitally bicuspid[171,172] or quadricuspid[9] valves or malformed tricuspid valves. The congenitally aplastic or bicuspid pulmonic valve is usually associated with other congenital cardiac malformation, notably tetralogy of Fallot.[173] Of 158 patients reported with congenitally quadricuspid pulmonic valves, only four appeared incompetent.[9]

The natural history of congenital PR is unclear. When secondary to an aplastic valve, severe congestive heart failure and death have occurred in infancy.[167,168] Death in adults with pure congenital PR may be sudden[171] or after periods of progressive right-heart failure.[172] Evidence of right ventricular dysfunction without symptoms of congestive cardiac failure also may occur in adults.[174] Most reported patients, however, are young and asymptomatic. Although they may have abnormal right ventricular and pulmonary arterial pulsations and enlarged pulmonary trunks, the right ventricular and pulmonary arterial pressures are usually normal. The presumed benign nature of congenital PR is derived from reports of older adults with little or no evidence of cardiac decompensation.[170,175,176]

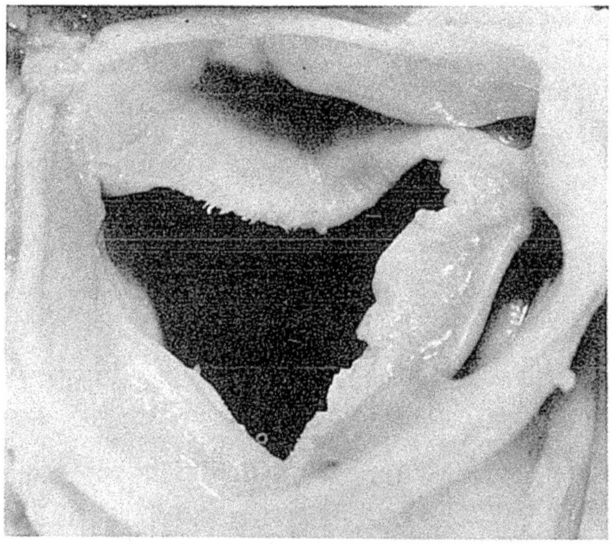

Figure 47. Congenital pulmonic valvular regurgitation in a 67-year-old man (36451) who died suddenly of a myocardial infarction. He had been told that he had "heart disease" at age 35, and cardiomegaly was known to be present at age 40. At age 49 he was found to be in congestive cardiac failure with cardiomegaly and a prominent pulmonary arterial segment on roentgenogram. Systolic and diastolic precordial murmurs were present and the electrocardiogram disclosed complete right bundle branch block. The clinical diagnosis at this time was valvular aortic stenosis and regurgitation. At age 58, pulmonic stenosis and regurgitation were diagnosed after catheterization. Right ventricular systolic pressure was 44 mm. Hg and a 10 mm. Hg peak systolic pressure gradient between right ventricle and pulmonary trunk was recorded on pullback. At necropsy all three pulmonic valve cusps were hypoplastic, thickened, and retracted. The valve did not appear stenotic. The right ventricle was severely dilated.

We have studied a 67-year-old man with isolated congenital PR who died of consequences of systemic atherosclerosis. Cardiac disease had been diagnosed when he was about 35 years of age and his heart was enlarged by age 40. At necropsy, the pulmonic valve was tricuspid but congenitally malformed and severely incompetent (Fig. 47).

Congenital Mitral Regurgitation

Congenital abnormalities of the mitral valve resulting in regurgitation are most often associated with other congenital cardiovascular anomalies. We have studied at necropsy, however, nine patients with fatal congenital mitral regurgitation (MR) presenting with this valve lesion (Table 18). Six were females, three were males, and they ranged in age from 9 months to 44 years. The MR in four patients was associated with and possibly caused by *diffuse endocardial fibroelastosis* of the left ventricle.[133,177,178] Two patients had *congeni-*

Table 18. Congenital mitral regurgitation: clinical and necropsy data

Autopsy number	*Age (yrs.)*	*Sex*	*Age (yrs.) murmur first heard*	*ECG*	*Pressures (mm. Hg)* PA (s/d)	LA (V/mean)	LV (s/d)	SA (s/d)	*LV angio (MR = 1-4+)*
Diffuse endocardial fibroelastosis									
1. A61-133	9	F	7	AF LAH, LVH	30/12	14/8	—	—	—
2. A62-120	8	M	3	AF LVH, RVH	66/36	32/21	102/12	116/72	—
3. A63-33	14	F	7	↑PR LAE, LVH RVH	65/26	23/19	120/20	120/70	+++
4. A66-54	14	F	5	LAE, RVH	58/5*	19/11	95/10	111/63	++++
Corrected transposition of the great arteries									
5. A63-142	44	F	26	$S_{1,2,3}$ QSV_1	98/41	50/34	139/24	—	—
6. UKMC A158-71	22	F	Birth	—	—	—	—	—	—
Partial atrioventricular canal									
7. A59-253	13	M	6	AF LAD, LVH	55/15	27/15	—	—	++++
Origin of left coronary artery from pulmonary trunk									
8. A56-14	9 mo.	F	8 mo.	ALMI	50/—	—	—	—	—
Parachute mitral valve									
9. A66-189	22	M	19	LBBB, LAE	54/28	30/30	96/29	96/67	++++

* Right ventricular pressure. Pulmonary artery not entered.

AF = atrial fibrillation. ALMI = anterolateral myocardial infarction. ECG = electrocardiogram. LA = left atrium. LAD = left axis deviation. LAE = left atrial enlargement. LBBB = left bundle branch block. LV = left ventricle. LVH = left ventricular hypertrophy. MR = mitral regurgitation. PA = pulmonary artery. ↑PR = interval >0.20 sec. QSV_1 = Q and S wave in lead V_1. RVH = right ventricular hypertrophy. $S_{1,2,3}$ = S wave standard leads 1, 2, and 3. SA = systemic artery. s/d = systolic/diastolic.

tally corrected transposition (CCT).[179] During life, one was believed to have rheumatic MR[180] and the second underwent mitral valve replacement shortly before death. Anamalies of the left-sided or systemic atrioventricular valves (anatomic tricuspid valve) in CCT are extremely common (about 80 per cent).[179,181] Although the usual cause of MR in these patients is an Ebstein-type malformation of the so-called mitral valve, neither of our patients with CCT had this anomaly. The mitral leaflets and chordae, however, in each were malformed. Another patient also was considered before cardiac catherization to have severe rheumatic MR, but at operation the severe MR was found to be the result of a complete cleft in the anterior mitral leaflet. Thus, this patient's condition is an example of *partial persistent atrioventricular canal* presenting as MR.[182-184] A small defect (1 cm. size) was found in the lowermost portion of the atrial septum in this patient but the amount of shunting through the defect was small. *Parachute mitral valve* (single papillary muscle) may cause massive MR (patient #8).[185,186] This anomaly most commonly, however, produces stenosis.[187] *Origin of the left coronary artery from the pulmonary trunk* may cause severe fibrosis and atrophy of one or both left ventricular papillary muscles with resulting MR. Indeed, MR may be the presenting or major clinical feature of this condition.[134,136] Another cause of congenital MR is the *arcade type deformity of the mitral valve*.[188] We have studied at necropsy one patient with this anomaly. The patient also had a patent ductus arteriosus and therefore is not included herein. Arcade mitral valve may occur, however, without associated shunts.[188,189] It is well to keep in mind that severe anatomic malformations of the mitral valve may occur without any functional consequence. An example is the double orifice mitral valve.[190]

Isolated Congenital Pure Aortic Regurgitation

Aortic regurgitation (AR) commonly occurs in patients with congenitally malformed aortic valves, particularly the bicuspid one.[3] The degree of AR, however, is usually mild unless the valve has previously been the site of infection. Of 17 necropsy patients with fatal pure AR complicating a congenitally bicuspid aortic valve, infective endocarditis was the cause of the fatal AR in 15 of them.[3,15] The congenitally unicuspid aortic valve appears never to be a cause of pure AR.[6] A quadricuspid aortic valve, an extremely rare malformation, on occasion may lead to pure AR. At least four patients with quadricuspid aortic valves and pure AR have been reported.[9] Although a unicuspid, bicuspid or quadricuspid aortic valve represents a congenital malformation, the aortic valve may be tricuspid and still congenitally malformed. In this situation, one cusp is probably smaller than the other two (see below). Usually, however, pure AR complicating a tricuspid aortic valve represents an acquired lesion.

We have studied at necropsy four patinets with fatal pure AR unassociated with infective endocarditis or shunts (Table 19). The murmur of AR was recognized in all before the age of 18 years and none had clinical or necropsy evidence of acute rheumatic fever. Two patients had bicuspid aortic valves: in one (#1), a fibrous band, extending from the margin of one cusp to the wall of ascending

Table 19. Congenital aortic regurgitation: clinical and necropsy findings

Patient	Age	Sex	Age (yrs.) murmur first heard	Murmurs "AS"	Murmurs AR	Murmurs AF	ECG	Pressures (mm. Hg) BA (s/d)	Pressures (mm. Hg) LV (s/d)	Valve replacement	No. AV cusps	AV calcium	Heart weight (gm.)
1. A66-6	27	M	17	2/6	3/6	2/6	↑PR, LVH, LAD	126/54	125/25	+	2	0	800
2. A66-233	18	M	5	3/6	3/6	2/6	LVH, LVS, LAD	122/40†	—	+*	3	0	570
3. A66-234	23	M	8	5/6	4/6	3/6	LVH	120/45	120/11	+	2	0	600
4. A68-325	51	F	17	3/6	3/6	3/6	↑PR LVH	210/80†	—	+	4	0	520

* Replacement of right coronary cusp only.
† Indirect.

AF = Austin Flint. AR = aortic regurgitation. AS = "aortic stenosis." AV = aortic valve. BA = brachial artery. ECG = electrocardiogram. LV = left ventricular. LVH = left ventricular hypertrophy. LVS = left ventricular strain. ↑PR = interval >0.20 sec. LAD = left axis deviation. s/d = systolic/diastolic.

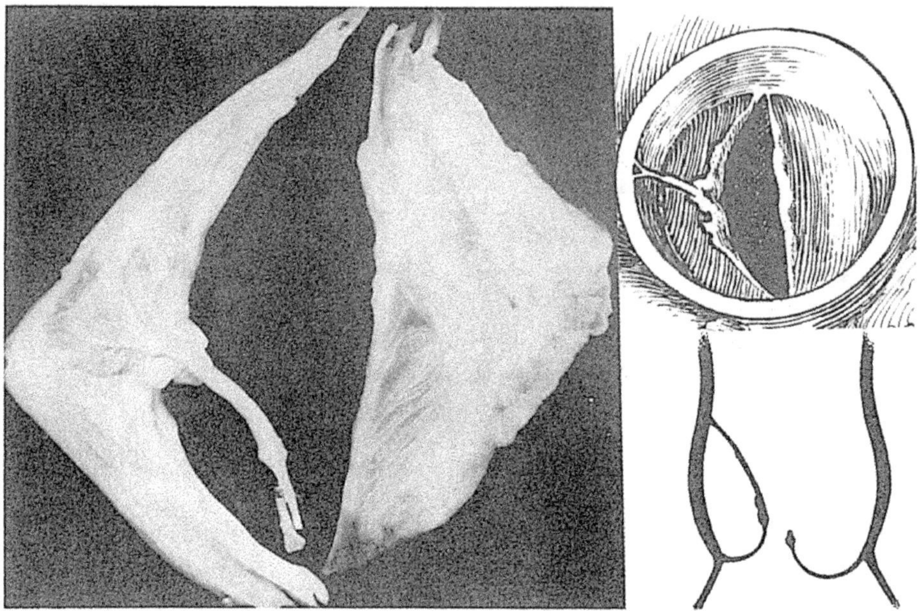

Figure 48. Congenital aortic regurgitation with bicuspid aortic valve. Surgical specimen and diagrams of the aortic valve in situ of a 27-year-old man (A66–6) who was found to have aortic regurgitation at age 17. At age 25 years, evaluation confirmed free aortic regurgitation and he underwent successful prosthetic aortic valve replacement by Dr. Andrew G. Morrow. Thirteen months postoperatively he died suddenly while playing football. Attached to the free margin in the mid-portion of one cusp is a fibrous band which inserts onto the wall of the aorta. This structure prevented closure of the valve during ventricular diastole with resultant severe aortic regurgitation.

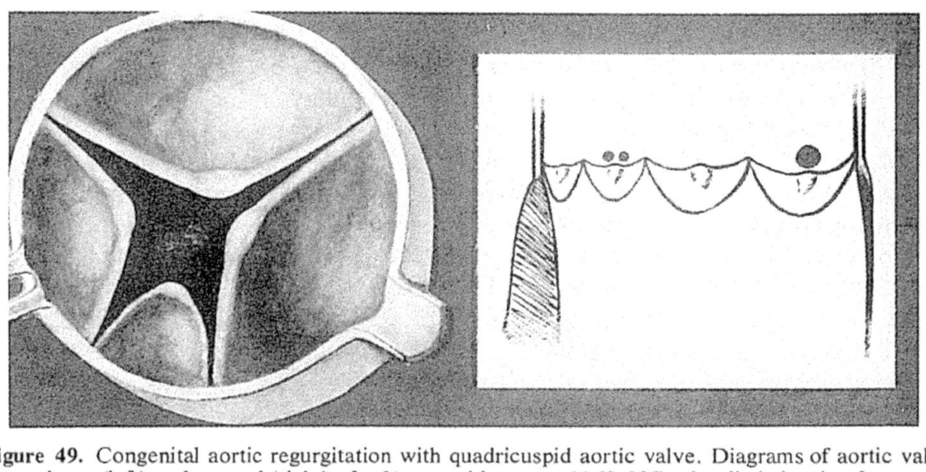

Figure 49. Congenital aortic regurgitation with quadricuspid aortic valve. Diagrams of aortic valve from above (left) and opened (right) of a 51-year-old woman (A68–325) who died shortly after aortic valve replacement. A precordial murmur had been heard at age 17 years. At age 45, she developed congestive cardiac failure and signs of free aortic regurgitation. The aortic valve had four cusps, two hypoplastic ones and two normal ones.

aorta, pulled the cusp cephalad preventing coaptation during ventricular diastole (Fig. 48); in the second (#3), the mechanism of AR is uncertain. Likewise, the mechanism of AR in the patient with a tricuspid aortic valve is uncertain. A murmur of AR had been heard in him at age five years, and a valvular operation was carried out when he was 13 years old. The patient with a quadricuspid aortic valve had two hypoplastic cusps which prevented cuspal coaptation during ventricular diastole[9] (Fig. 49).

Trauma

The heart and vessels may be injured by either blunt or penetrating trauma, and both may lead to valvular regurgitation.

Penetrating trauma results from the passage of projectiles into or through the cardiovascular structures. The speed of entry, the type of projectile, and the structures penetrated determine the kind of injury which results and the length of survival. Laceration or avulsion or both of myocardium or great vessel usually leads to rapid death from hemorrhage into the pericardial sac (cardiac tamponade) or elsewhere. Damage to the cardiac valves from penetrating trauma is rare. Of 456 fatalities from penetrating wounds of the heart and aorta compiled in 1958,[191] the valves were damaged in only a few patients and none survived longer than several days. During the past 14 years, other studies of penetrating cardiac trauma have revealed isolated patients with valvular damage and most of them died quickly.[192-195] Significant valvular regurgitation from penetrating trauma to the aortic,[196-201] mitral,[202,203] or tricuspid[203] valves has been described and recognized clinically in about 10 patients. Valve replacement or repair is necessary.

Blunt or compressive trauma, in contrast to the penetrating variety, is a more common cause of clinically apparent valvular dysfunction (Fig. 50). Since injury to the intracardiac structures may occur without damage to the myocardium or vessels, the patient is more likely to survive until signs of valvular dysfunction appear. Excessive physical effort or strain, a form of blunt trauma, commonly damages only valvular or supporting structures. Like other forms of blunt trauma, the diagnosis of valvular damage may be masked initially by cardiac contusion, pericardial effusion, or myocardial rupture.

Aortic regurgitation (AR) is the most common clinically recognized valvular lesion resulting from blunt trauma.[204] Nevertheless, it is an infrequent consequence and limited almost exclusively to men. Only two of 64 reported patients with AR from nonpenetrating trauma were women.[205,206] The AR may result from muscular strain or from some type of thoracic compression. Of 44 necropsy patients reviewed by Howard in 1928,[205] 30 had AR secondary to muscular strain. Since his review, however, only two additional patients have been described in the English literature as having AR from this mechanism.[207,208] Compressive thoracic trauma, mainly from automotive steering wheel injuries, today is by far the most common cause of valvular regurgitation from nonpenetrating trauma.[206] Although it appears to be an immediate consequence of blunt chest trauma, AR is not always clinically evident or diagnosed in the early post-trauma period, apparently because it is masked by other consequences of the trauma

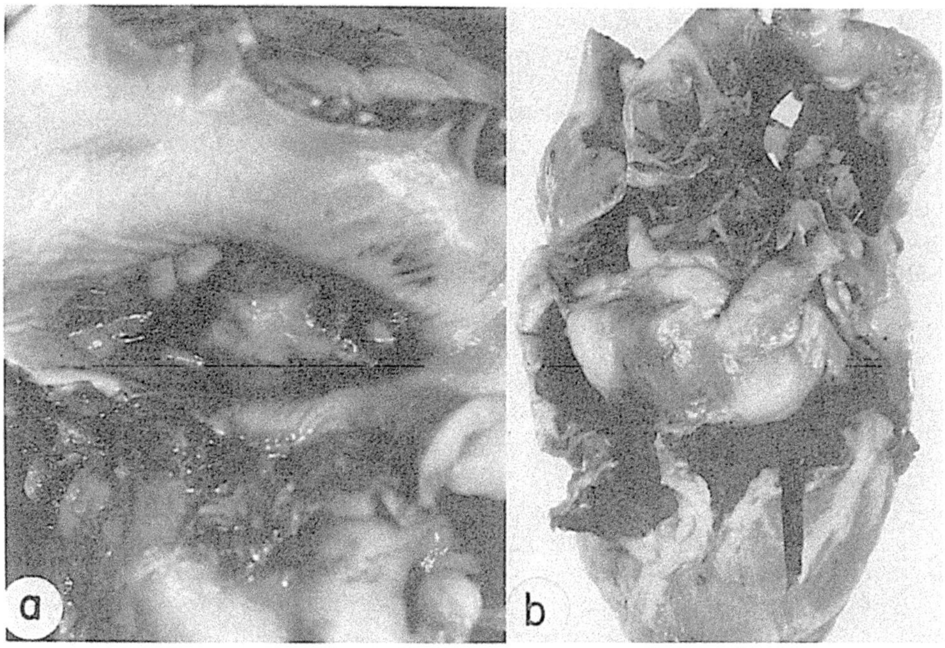

Figure 50. Mitral regurgitation from blunt trauma in a 23-year-old man (NNMC #A71–72) who died instantaneously in an airplane crash. a, Mitral valve viewed from left atrium. The anterior leaflet is flail due to rupture of papillary muscles. b, External aspect of the heart viewed anteriorly. In most cases when blunt trauma results in severe mitral regurgitation, extensive injury to myocardium and great vessels also occurs. This patient sustained an 80 per cent circumferential transmural laceration of both ventricles as well as a large tear in the ascending aorta. Thus, the prolapse of the mitral leaflet was of no consequence.

or because medical attention has not been sought. The murmur of AR may not be detected until weeks or months after the event when symptoms of cardiac dysfunction appear.[209] It has been described as cooing, whistling, buzzing, humming, or whining in character. The AR results from detachment of one or more cusps with prolapse or from tearing or fenestration of one or more cusps without detachment, or from both. Cuspal detachment, similar to that produced by trauma, however, may occur without a clear history of trauma (Fig. 51). The left anterior cusp appears to be the one most commonly involved. Valvular reconstruction or replacement is frequently required for survival.[206]

Atrioventricular valvular regurgitation from blunt trauma is even less common than AR. Of 546 patients described by Parmley et al.,[204] 39 had anatomic evidence of mitral (MR) or tricuspid regurgitation and all but one of them had associated myocardial rupture with rapid death (Fig. 50). By 1964, 18 patients with mitral valve damage due to blunt trauma had been reported in the English literature.[210] Leaflet damage appears to be the least common cause of MR and was responsible in only one patient, described by McLaughlin et al.,[210] and in one patient described subsequently.[211] Rupture of chordae tendineae due to trauma or exertion has long been implicated as a couse of MR, but it too appears to be an infrequent cause of the hemodynamic lesion. Rupture of a papillary muscle by trauma is rare. Sanders et al. in 1957 collected six cases[212] and at least two more have

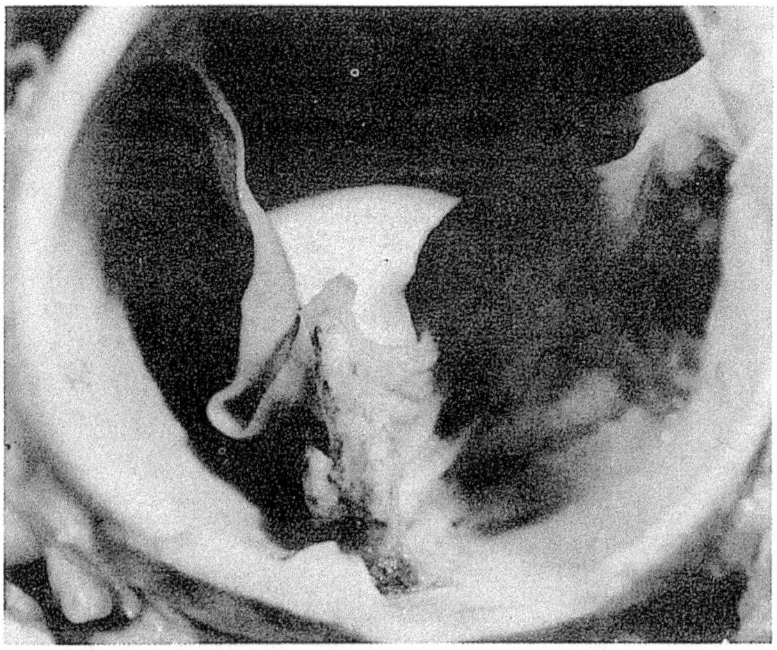

Figure 51. Possible traumatic aortic regurgitation without history of trauma in a 47-year-old man (37266) with no symptoms of cardiac dysfunction until two weeks before death when he suddenly developed fulminant congestive heart failure. Clinical signs of free aortic regurgitation were present and he was treated for infective endocarditis (despite no supporting clinical features and negative blood cultures). At necropsy, the commissure between two of the aortic cusps was torn loose from the aorta causing prolapse of these cusps into left ventricle. The tricuspid aortic valve and aorta were otherwise normal. There was no evidence of infective endocarditis.

been described subsequently.[213,214] All patients had severely compressed thoraces with fulminant pulmonary edema, shock, and rapid death.

Tricuspid regurgitation due to blunt trauma is less common than MR but better tolerated. Several patients have survived over 20 years.[215-218] Parmley et al.[204] described a five-month survivor among their 39 patients with traumatic atrioventricular valve incompetence, and he had a ruptured right ventricular papillary muscle. Associated myocardial rupture is infrequent in trauma-indiced tricus-

Table 20. Systemic lupus erythematosus (SLE): clinical and necropsy data in 26 patients

	No. pts.	*Ages (years) Range (avg.)*	*F*	*M*	*Age onset symptoms SLE range (avg.) (years)*	*Duration (yrs.) of symptoms range (avg.)*	*CHF*	*Renal failure*	*HT*
1. With L-E endocarditis	12	17-61 (30)	11	1	14-61 (26)	1-9 (4)	6	8	10
2. Without L-E endocarditis	14	8-55 (31)	13	1	7-55 (29)	0.5-7 (2)	2	10	9
TOTALS	26	8-61 (31)	24	2	7-61 (28)	0.5-9 (3)	8	18	19

* Purulent in one and granulomatous in one.
AV = aortic valve. CHF = congestive heart failure. HT = hypertension. L-E = lupus-erythematosus. MV = mitral valve.

pid regurgitation and was present in only one of 26 patients previously reported.[219] Symptoms often appeared within days of violent chest trauma but were usually mild. When evaluated weeks to years later because of progressive clinical decompensation, signs of florid tricuspid regurgitation were invariably present. The proper clinical diagnosis was occasionally confused by associated lesions such as traumatic ventricular septal defect, traumatic constrictive pericarditis (secondary to longstanding hemopericardium), and congenital atrial septal defect.[219,220] One patient was followed clinically for many years with the diagnosis of Ebstein's anomaly.[216] The incompetence in 21 patients in whom anatomic data was available resulted primarily from ruptured chordae tendineae and papillary muscles, but six of them also sustained a laceration or avulsion of one or more valve leaflets. Of the 26 patients, 15 underwent tricuspid valvular repair or replacement.[215-221]

Systemic Lupus Erythematosus

Congestive heart failure and systemic hypertension (usually of renal origin) are the predominant cardiovascular consequences of systemic lupus erythematosus (SLE). Valvular lesions also are frequent and often unique but rarely of functional significance.

We have studied at necropsy 26 patients with SLE, and 12 (46 per cent) had valvular lesions consistent with atypical verrucous endocarditis (Table 20). There were no significant differences in age, sex, duration of illness, presence of precordial murmurs, or presence of systemic hypertension between patients with and without SLE endocarditis. All but two had received steroid therapy. Seven of 12 Libman-Sacks (L-S) endocarditis had diffuse fibrinous pericarditis, and only two of 14 without L-S endocarditis had pericarditis and in them it was due to infection. Mitral valvular lesions were present in 12 patients (Figs. 52, 53), one of whom also had aortic valvular verrucae. Only one of the 12 patients had clinical evidence of valvular dysfunction. The pulmonic and tricuspid valves were normal in all 12 patients. The involved leaflets were thickened to some degree by vascularized fibrous tissue in all 12 patients. The mural endocardium beneath the involved leaflets was similarly involved in most patients. In addition, seven patients had valvular lesions variously described in the past as "raised or flat, dry or wet, granular or smooth, single or conglomerate, yellow or gray, tawny or pink, pinhead to 4 mm. in size, shaped like beads or pyramids,

Table 20. (Continued)

Precordial murmur	*Steroid therapy*	*Heart weight (gm.) range (avg.)*	*Valvular involvement MV*	*AV*	*Diffuse pericarditis*	*Hematoxylin bodies in heart*	*Valve leaflet fibrin and/or necrosis*	*Leaflet or mural endocardial fibrous thickening*
6	11	270-600 (385)	12	1	7	7	10	12
7	13	180-400 (306)	0	0	2*	0	0	0
13	24	180-600 (343)	12	1	9	7	10	12

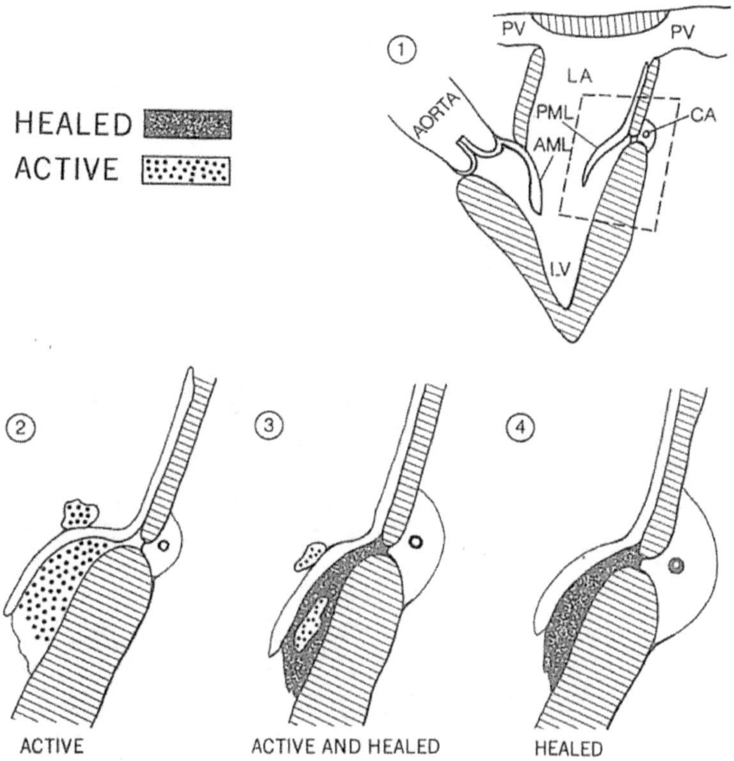

Figure 52. Lupus erythematosus (LE) endocarditis. 2, Active lesions of LE endocarditis, or verrucae, are accumulations of fibrin and cellular debris and project from either surface of the valve leaflet. When located on the atrial surface they usually appear like polyps or vegetations, but when located on the under surface of the leaflet they become adherent to leaflet and mural endocardium and may go unnoticed. 3, As the process heals fibrous tissue appears and it may lead to shortening and thickening of leaflet and chordae. 4, Healed LE endocarditis with fibrous scarring of valve and no evidence of the earlier active process. This complete healing may be a consequence of steroid therapy. The amount of adipose tissue in the atrioventricular sulcus progressively increases, and the lumens of the coronary arteries may become narrowed by atherosclerosis. PV = pulmonic veins. LA = left atrium. LV = left ventricle. CA = coronary artery. AML = anterior mitral leaflet. PML = posterior mitral leaflet.

arranged in mulberry-like clusters or in trails."[222-224] These lesions considered active and represent the verrucae of classic L-S endocarditis. They may be located on either side of a valvular cusp but most frequently are found on the under or ventricular surface of the posterior mitral leaflet or in the valve ring and they infrequently involve the anterior mitral leaflet.

Histologically, the verrucae consist of fibrin partially surrounded by varying quantities of cellular and vascularized fibrous tissue. In seven patients, hematoxylin bodies were present. The fibrin usually appeared to be organizing into fibrous tissue which was continuous with the involved leaflet and usually with the mural endocardium. As the process "heals," fibrous scarring of the undersurface of the posterior mitral leaflet and of the chordae may shorten and thicken these

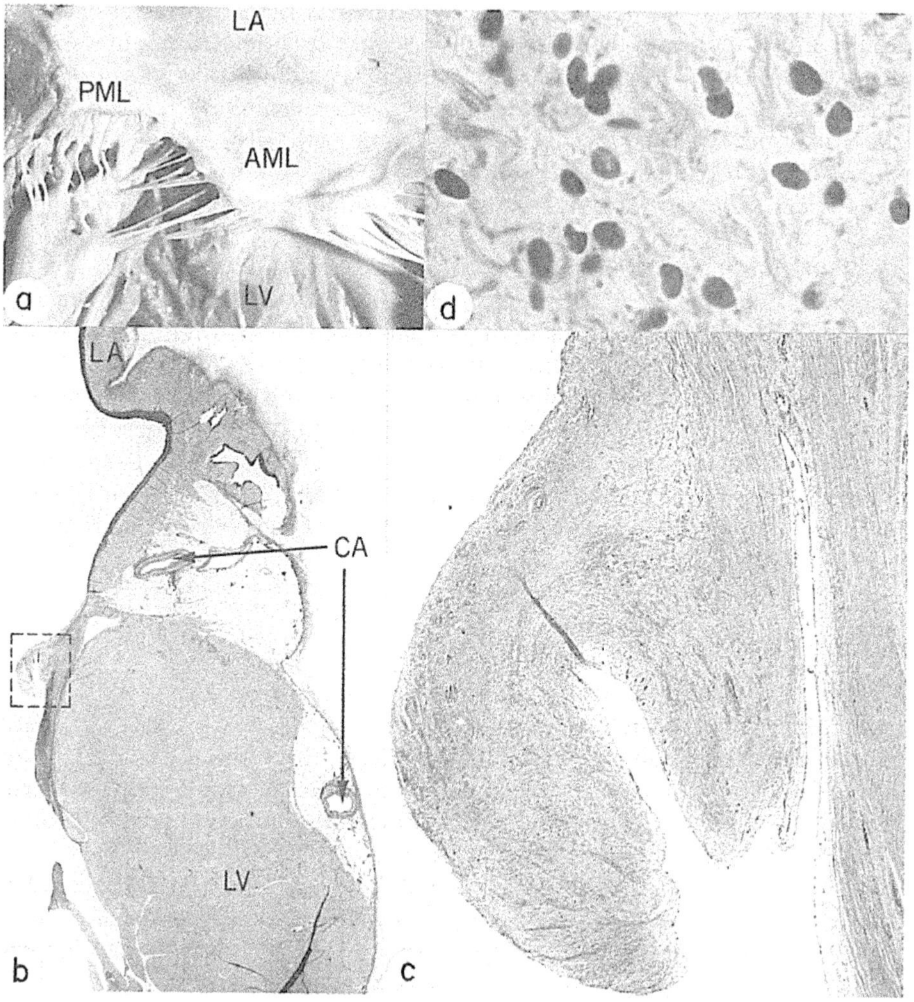

Figure 53. Active and healed lupus erythematosus (LE) endocarditis. This 22-year-old woman (A61–294), who had systemic LE for four years, died of renal failure. She had received steroids for three years. At necropsy, she had a diffuse fibrous pericarditis. a, Her mitral valve was thickened and the under surface of the posterior mitral leaflet (PML) was adherent to left ventricular (LV) mural endocardium. AML = anterior mitral leaflet. LA = left atrium. b, Longitudinal section through left atrium (LA), posterior mitral leaflet, and left ventricle (LV) demonstrating a thickened, contracted leaflet and thickening of the mural endocardium beneath it. c, Photomicrograph of the posterior mitral leaflet shown (----) in b. There is proliferation of vascularized fibrous tissue. Here "active" inflammatory changes are present in the leaflet. d, Numerous hematoxylin bodies were present within the loose posterior mitral leaflet. These bodies are pathognomonic of SLE. b, Elastic tissue stain. c and d, Hematoxylin-eosin stains. [Reduced 25 per cent from × 3.2 (b), × 37 (c), and × 690 (d).]

structures and in one patient this process was severe enough to cause clinically apparent mitral regurgitation. In addition, this same patient had active lesions, including verrucae on two valves and extensive necrosis of the base of the posterior mitral leaflet.

Although Libman-Sacks (L-S) endocarditis, probably better termed lupus erythematosus (LE) endocarditis, is a frequent anatomic finding in SLE, clinically detectable valvular dysfunction in these patients is rare. Moreover, precordial murmurs are detected as frequently (50 per cent) in patients without as in those with endocarditis.[225-227] Steroid therapy may be altering the morphology and location and possibly the frequency of LE endocarditis. Early reports described endocarditis in 33 to 65 per cent of patients with SLE.[228,229] More recent studies[230,231] involving steroid-treated lupus patients reported endocarditis in 13 to 50 per cent; 46 per cent of our 26 patients had endocarditis and only two had not received steroids. An equal frequency of involvement of valves on both sides of the heart in patients with SLE was stressed in early writings.[222-224] In contrast, none of our patients had right-sided valvular lesions and of the 12 with valvular lesions, the mitral valve was involved in each. Others have found a similar preponderance of mitral involvement by LE endocarditis.[230-232] The valvular lesions of SLE also appear to be smaller and fewer in number in the steroid-treated compared to nonsteroid-treated patients. Gross[223] described extensive multivalvular involvement and frequent necrosis of valvular tissue in many of his 23 necropsy patients. In contrast to his findings, the endocarditis in our patients was more limited, and healed lesions were more frequent than active ones.

Rheumatoid Arthritis

Rheumatoid arthritis (RS) is associated with a unique form of valvular heart disease. We have studied at necropsy three patients with RA and cardiac rheumatoid nodules (Table 21). Each had had symptoms of RA for over 15 years. Each had had pansystolic precordial murmurs and one, a diastolic blowing murmur. One patient had left a bundle branch block and another, a prolonged P–R interval. Only one patient had congestive heart failure, and it was mild.

At necropsy, their hearts weighed 260, 350, and 550 gm. respectively. In each, the pericardial space was diffusely obliterated by fibrous adhesions. In two patients, numerous rheumatoid nodules were present in all four cardiac valves (Fig. 54), in membranous ventricular septum, in myocardium of both ventricles, in endocardium of both atria, and in pericardium. In the third patient, rheumatoid nodules were present only in mitral valve and in left ventricular myocardium immediately beneath the posterior leaflet (Fig. 55). The rheumatoid nodules were histologically similar to those classically seen in subcutaneous tissue.

In all three patients the mitral valves were thickened, and the normal cuspal tissue was replaced by rheumatoid nodules. With one exception, the rheumatoid nodules were located *within* the valve leaflets and were enclosed by a border of fibrous tissue. In one patient, however, the nodule had erupted with extrusion of its central necrotic material. The involved aortic valves (two patients) were

Table 21. Rheumatoid arthritis: clinical and necropsy findings

	Age (yrs.)	Sex	Age (yrs.) at onset of arthritis	Duration (yrs.) of arthritis	CHF	Precordial murmur		Heart weight (gm.)	Location, rheumatoid nodules		
						Systolic	Diastolic		Pericardium	Myocardium	Valves
1. A66-100	65	F	50	15	+	+	+	550	+	+	MV, AV, TV, PV
2. A67-1	72	M	36	36	0	+	0	350	+	+	MV, AV TV, PV
3. A69-19	67	F	27	40	0	+	0	260	0	+	MV

AV = aortic valve. CHF = congestive heart failure. MV = mitral valve. PV = pulmonic valve. TV = tricuspid valve.

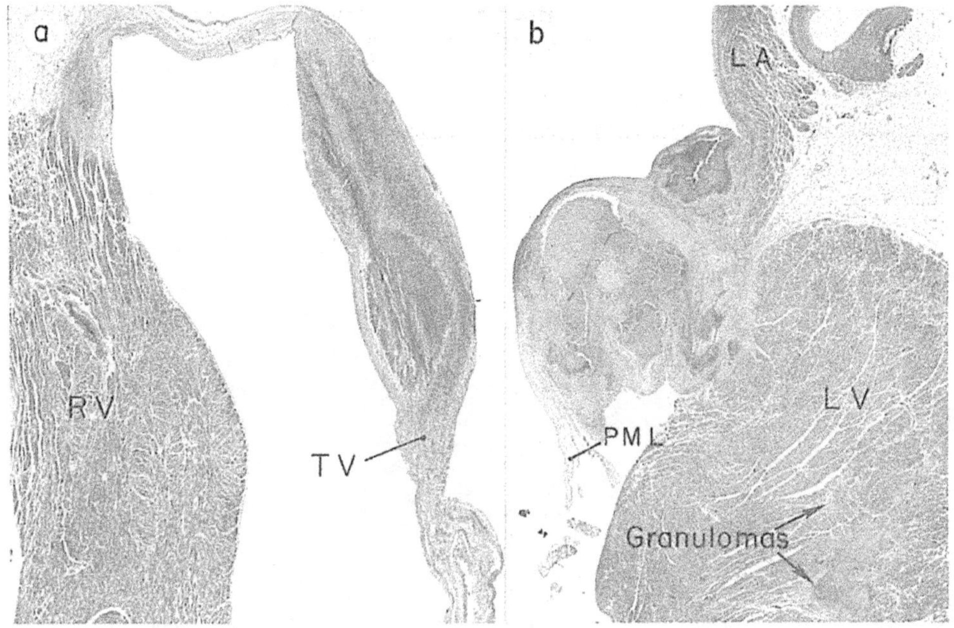

Figure 54. Valvular lesions of rheumatoid arthritis. This 72-year-old man (A67–1) had rheumatoid arthritis for 36 years. He had a grade 1/6 systolic precordial murmur for several years but no signs of cardiac dysfunction, despite extensive involvement of pericardium, myocardium, and endocardium by rheumatoid nodules. a, Tricuspid valve (TV) leaflet showing a typical rheumatoid granuloma within the substance of the leaflet. RV = right ventricle. b, A large rheumatoid granuloma within posterior mitral leaflet (PML). A smaller nodule involves endocardium of left atrium (LA) as well. Arrows indicate rheumatoid granulomas within left ventricular (LV) wall. a and b, Hematoxylin-eosin stain. [Reduced 30 per cent from × 12 (a) and × 6.5 (b).]

similarly thickened by numerous rheumatoid nodules. In the two patients with right-sided valvular lesions, the nodules were localized to the basal attachments of tricuspid and pulmonic valve cusps with little disruption of the normal valve structure.

Although nonspecific forms of pericarditis, myocarditis, and coronary arthritis have been observed at necropsy in patients with rheumatoid arthritis (RA),[233-236] rheumatoid nodules (granulomas) similar to subcutaneous nodules are pathognomonic and occur in the heart in 1 to 3 per cent of necropsied patients with this condition.[237] At least 24 patients with rheumatoid granulomas involving cardiac valves or valvular rings have been reported[235] (Table 22). Nine of the 24 patients had auscultatory evidence of mitral or aortic regurgitation or both, and 11 had hearts weighing more than 300 gm. Most frequently, the valvular lesions were focal. In two of our three patients the mitral and aortic valvular lesions were diffuse and the valves incompetent. Although coronary arterial narrowing is frequent, cardiac dysfunction in RA often can be explained on the basis of valvular cardiac disease.

Although rheumatoid nodules in hearts of patients with RA have been well described, little attention has been given to the exact location of these lesions

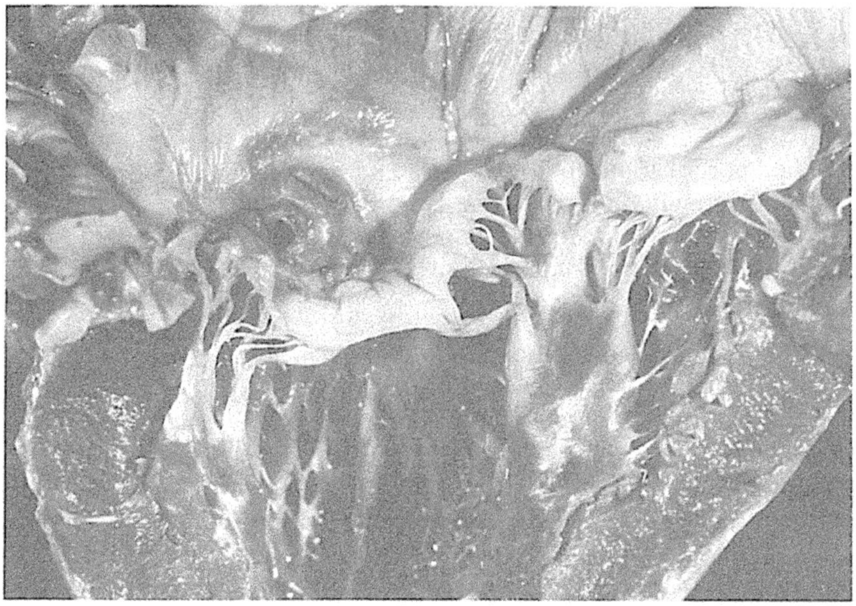

Figure 55. Erupted rheumatoid nodule of mitral valve. This 67-year-old woman (A69–19) had rheumatoid arthritis for 47 years. She had a grade 2/6 systolic murmur but no symptoms of cardiac dysfunction. Shown here is the opened mitral valve. A large rheumatoid nodule, which has erupted, is present in the anterior leaflet. The valve is probably mildly incompetent.

Table 22. Rheumatoid nodules in cardiac valves

Mitral	19	
Aortic	11	
Tricuspid	5	
Pulmonic	4	
	39	of possible 96 valves involved in 24 necropsy patients

in the valve leaflets and rings. The location and size of the cardiac rheumatoid nodules were similar in two of our three patients. The lesions grossly were yellow, firm, smooth, and focal or diffuse. On the tricuspid valve the lesions were focal and located at the basal attachment of the septal and anterior leaflets. The posterior tricuspid leaflets were uninvolved. A single nodule was present at the basal attachment of a pulmonic valvular cusp in both patients with extensive lesions. These right-sided cardiac lesions did not interfere with valvular function because most of the valvular tissue was uninvolved. In contrast to the right-sided lesions in the two patients, those on left-sided cardiac valves were diffuse; nearly all areas of both mitral and aortic leaflets were thickened.

Histologically, the lesions were located within the valve leaflets leaving a border of fibrous tissue to enclose the necrotic material. This fibrous capsule probably represents the original and uninvolved valve tissue. Thus, the process appears to begin as a reaction within the core or central portion of the valve leaflet preserving peripheral portions. The valvular involvement in rheumatoid heart disease is in direct contrast to that of carcinoid heart disease, in which the valve itself remains normal and atypical fibrous tissue is deposited on the surface of the valvular cusp. Also, it differs from rheumatic valvular disease in which the entire leaflet, both its central and peripheral portions, is involved, often leaving no residual normal or near-normal valvular tissue. Cardiovascular differences between rheumatoid arthritis, syphilis, ankylosing spondylitis, and the Marfan syndrome are summarized in Table 23.

Table 23. Cardiovascular manifestations of conditions causing aortic regurgitation

	Syphilis	*Ankylosing Spondylitis*	*Rheumatoid arthritis*	*Marfan*
Avg. age	50	45	70	30
Sex	Men	Men	Women	Men
Aortic regurgitation	++++	++++	+	++++
Mitral regurgitation	0	++	+	+++
Conduction disturbances	+	++++	++	+
Serology (STS)	+	0	0	0
Morphology of aorta				
Thickened adventitia	++++	++++	+	+
Degenerated media	+++	+++	0	++++
Intimal proliferation	+++	+++	0	+
Vasa vasora abnormal	++++	++++	0	0
Calcium	++	+	0	0
Aneurysms	+++	0	0	+++
Rupture	+	0	0	+
Dissection	0	0	0	+
Limited to sinuses	0	+	0	0
Morphology of aortic valve				
Cuspal thickening				
Diffuse	0	+	0	0
Focal	+	0	+	+
Cuspal calcification	0	0	0	0
↑AMP	0	0	0	+
Shortening	0	+	0	0
Commissural abnormality	+	+	0	0

The reason the cardiac valves are involved at all in RA is unclear. If vasculitis is considered to be an intrinsic part of the development of the subcutaneous nodules, as proposed by Sokoloff et al.,[238] then involvement of valvular blood vessels must occur. The cardiac valves, however, contain few blood vessels. Certainly, if vasculitis predisposes to the development of rheumatoid granulomas, these lesions might be expected to be much more frequent in the myocardium than in the endocardium (valves), although this is not the situation.

Endomyocardial Disease with and without Eosinophilia

In 1936 Löffler described two patients with "fibroplastic parietal endocarditis with blood eosinophilia."[239] Since then about 100 patients with this condition have been reported, some under the heading "eosinophilic leukemia."[139,140,142] These conditions are characterized by endocardial fibrosis of one or both ventricles, blood eosinophilia, and usually mitral regurgitation. Death characteristically results from congestive cardiac failure.

The endocardial thickening is located primarily in the inflow tracts of the ventricles. It appears to begin in the apices and progresses retrogradely to involve the endocardium beneath the posterior mitral leaflet and occasionally to involve that behind the posterior or septal tricuspid valve leaflet. Superimposed on the fibrotic mural endocardium is fibrin thrombus. The posterior mitral leaflet may adhere to the underlying mural endocardium and lead to mitral regurgitation. A similar process may cause tricuspid regurgitation. The left ventricular cavity may be prevented from expanding adequately during ventricular diastole by the thickened mural endocardium and the cavity may be considerably decreased in size by thrombus.

We have studied at necropsy six patients, all men, aged 25 to 52 years, with endomyocardial disease and eosinophilia.[139,140,142] Each had symptoms from 11 to 42 months (avg. 24). The highest leukocyte counts ranged from 79,000

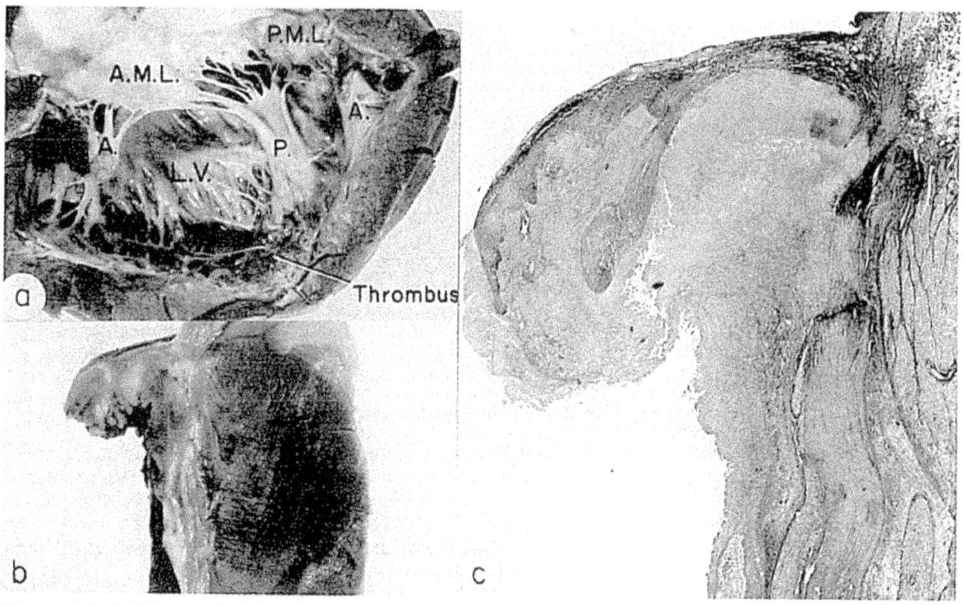

Figure 56. Löffler's fibroplastic parietal endocarditis with thickening of the mitral valve and papillary muscle fibrosis. This 35-year-old man (A65–211) had been well until 12 months before death when recurring headaches, weakness, weight loss, and anorexia appeared and he sought his physician. He was found to have leukocytosis with 70 per cent eosinophils on differential smear. Precordial examination showed no murmur. He died of congestive cardiac failure with chronic eosinophilia and hepatosplenomegaly. At necropsy, the heart weighed 430 gm. and the coronary arteries were clean. Both left ventricular papillary muscles were extensively scarred and mural thrombi were present at the apices of both ventricles. a, Opened left ventricle (L.V.) and mitral valve. Both posteromedial (P.) and anterolateral (A.) papillary muscles are severely scarred and the endocardium covering them is thckened. Much organizing fibrous tissue is present behind the posterior mitral leaflet (P.M.L.). A.M.L. = anterior mitral leaflet. b, Longitudinal section including posterior mitral leaflet and left ventricular well. c, Photomicrograph of posterior mitral leaflet seen in b. The thickening is due to vascularized fibrous tissue located entirely on the ventricular aspect of the cusp and on the mural endocardium. The leaflet is made immobile by its adherence to the underlying mural endocardium.

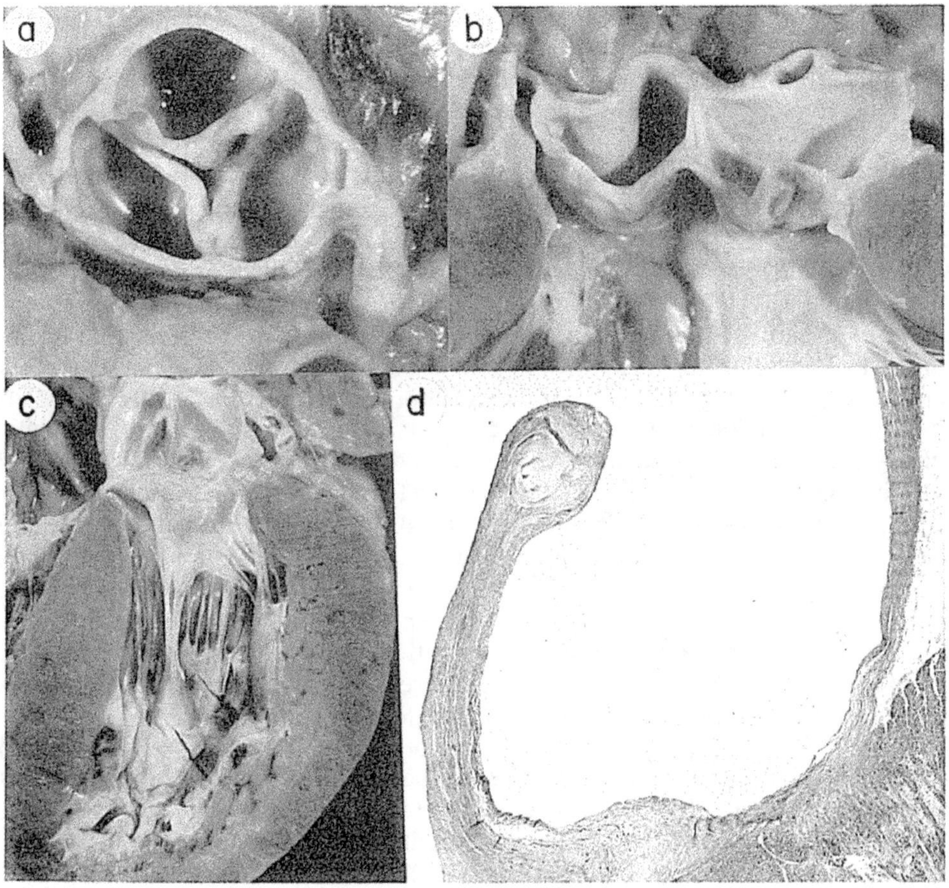

Figure 57. Löffler's fibroplastic parietal endocarditis (LFPE) associated with valvular aortic stenosis. It is well known that patients with LFPE may have mitral regurgitation secondary to extensive thickening of mural endocardium with superimposed thrombosis in the left ventricular inflow tract. That aortic valvular disease can be a part of LFPE is uncertain but highly suggestive from the case shown here. This 46-year-old man (A71–250) had been well until 42 months before death when fatigue and headache were noted and he was found to have eosinophilia (70 per cent). During the next 40 months his white count ranged from 40,000 to 60,000 per cu. mm. and the per cent of eosinophils from 70 to 90. When examined initially no precordial murmur was audible but when examined 22 months before death a grade 2/6 systolic ejection murmur and a grade 1/6 diastolic blowing murmur were audible over the cardiac base and along the left sternal border. Electrocardiogram showed left ventricular hypertrophy and strain and left atrial abnormality. By seven months before death, the precordial systolic murmur had increased to grade 4/6 intensity and the diastolic murmur, to grade 3/6 intensity. He died of progressive congestive cardiac failure. At necropsy, the heart weighed 520 gm. Each of the three valve cusps were thickened and two of the commissures were fused. a, Aortic valve from above. b, Opened aortic valve showing one fused commissure. The adherence of the commissures was produced by thrombus formation on the ventricular aspects of the cusps adjacent to the commissures. d, Photomicrograph of a portion of one aortic valve cusp. The cuspal thickening resulted from fibrous proliferation. Close-up disclosed that the underlying cusp was normal and that the thickening resulted from superimposition of vascularized fibrous tissue on the ventricular aspects of the cusps. c, Left ventricle and aortic valve showing severe endocardial thickening in apical one third of the chamber. The mitral valve is normal. d, Hematoxylin-eosin stain. [Reduced 15 per cent from × 7 (d).]

to 108,000 per cu. mm. and the highest percentage of eosinophils on differential smear of peripheral blood, from 35 to 90 per cent. Although greatly increased in number, the eosinophils appeared structurally normal in each patient. All six patients had overt right-sided and left-sided congestive cardiac failure, which was the dominant clinical feature in each patient, and the major cause of death. Four had precordial murmurs; in three they were consistent with mitral regurgitation and in one, murmurs of aortic stenosis and regurgitation were present. At necropsy, the hearts weighed 420 to 530 gm. (avg. 472). All four cardiac chambers were mildly dilated and the walls of all four chambers were mildly thickened. In each patient, the endocardium in left ventricular inflow tract and apex was thickened by dense fibrous tissue, devoid of elastic fibrils, and overlain by fibrin-platelet-leukocyte-erythrocyte thrombi. Right ventricular apical endocardial scars were present in every patient, with superimposed mural thrombi in two. Left ventricular subendocardial scarring occurred in all six patients. Eosinophilic leukocytes, usually few in number, were found in sections of heart. The mitral regurgitation in three patients appeared to result from the adherence of the posterior mitral leaflets to the underlying mural endocardium (Fig. 56). The aortic valve cusps in the patient with clinical evidence of aortic stenosis and regurgitation were thickened by vascularized fibrous tissue which was superimposed on the ventricular aspects of each of the three cusps (Fig. 57) in a manner directly opposite that causing leaflet thickening in patients with carcinoid heart disease. In addition, two of the three commissures were fused by a fibrin-platelet process similar to that of the mural thrombosis in the left ventricular cavity.

Endomycardial fibrosis (EMF) without eosinophilia (less than 15 per cent) has been observed in the African and their hearts are similar in many respects to those observed in Löffler's fibroplastic parietal endocarditis. One of us (W.C.R.) has examined the hearts of 16 patients with fatal EMF and cardiac dysfunction. Their ages ranged from 3 to 50 years (avg. 27); 11 were males and 5 females. Cardiac symptoms were present from 2 weeks to 24 months (avg. 7 months).

At necropsy, the hearts weighed 370 to 500 gm. Endocardial fibrous tissue devoid of elastic fibers was present in the left ventricle in all patients, and in 14 it was severe. Right ventricular endocardial fibrosis was present in 13. The endocardial fibrosis was located almost exclusively in the ventricular inflow tracts, and frequently beneath the posterior mitral or posterior and septal tricuspid valve leaflets. When the endocardial scars were small, they were usually limited to the ventricular apices. The configuration of the heart, i.e., the size of the various cardiac chambers and of the pulmonary trunk, depend primarily on which ventricle contained the largest deposits of endocardial scar tissue or superimposed thrombi or both. When the amount of endocardial plaquing was severe in the left ventricle and absent, mild, or moderate in the right ventricle, the heart usually had the appearance of a mitral stenotic heart, i.e., the left atrium, pulmonary trunk, right ventricle, and right atrium were dilated; the left ventricular cavity was small, being constricted by the extensive endocardial scarring. The left ventricle in this situation appears to be noncompliant and acts to some extent as an impediment to flow. The mitral lesion in this circumstance, however, is not stenotic unless another disease, i.e., rheumatic, coexists, but the mitral orifice in EMF is frequently made incompetent by the mural endocardial fibrosis which adheres to the undersurface of the posterior mitral leaflet causing the latter to be immobile. When the right ventricular endocardial scarring is more severe than that in the left ventricle, the right ventricle acts as an impediment to flow. The right atrium dilates, at times even to giant proportions (as it did in one of the 16 patients), the right ventricle is usually constricted, and the left atrium and left ventricle remain more or less normal in size. This type of heart may be viewed as the tricuspid incompetent one. When the amount of endocardial plaquing is similar in both ventricles, each atrium becomes quite dilated and the ventricular cavities usually remain small or at least not dilated.

Although it is usually confined to the inflow tract, the ventricular endocardial fibrosis in EMF on rare occasion may extend into the left ventricular outflow tract as it did in one of the 16 patients, and it also may be present in the atria. Also, in one patient both atria contained large endocardial plaques. Infective endocarditis may complicate EMF; three of the 16 patients had superimposed bacterial endocarditis of the mitral valve causing rupture of several chordae tendineae in each patient.

Radiation

Irradiation may produce several morphologic changes in the heart; the most frequent is thickening of parietal and visceral paricardia with or without development of pericardial effusion or tamponade. The second most frequent change reported has been interstital and perivascular myocardial fibrosis of varying degrees. Although mural endocardial thickening has been described from irradiation, cardiac valvular lesions produced by this means have not been described. We have studied 11 necropsy patients who received large doses of radiation to the chest and at necropsy each had lesions involving one or more cardiac valves. All 11 had lymphomas. Only two had clinical evidence of cardiac dysfunction and each had constrictive pericarditis.[145] No patient had evidence of cardiac dysfunction from valvular lesions. Precordial murmurs were recorded in five patients; one had right ventricular outflow tract obstruction secondary to tumor;[145] in the other four patients the cause of the precordial murmurs (grade 1/6 to 2/6) is uncertain. Four had pericardial friction rubs. The number of rads received to mediastinum in the 11 patients ranged from 3,000 to 6,000 (average 4,400). The time interval from completion of irradiation to death ranged from one to eight years (avg. three).

Abnormally large collections of serous fluid were present in the body cavities of all patients. Five had pericardial effusions (100 to 375 ml.) and four had obliterated pericardial sacs from fibrous adhesions. Seven patients had focal or diffuse fibrinous or fibrofibrinous pericarditis. The hearts in the 11 patients weighed 170 to 290 gm. (avg. 220). The right ventricular mural endocardium was focally thickened in all 11 patients. The tricuspid and mitral valve leaflets and chordae tendineae were focally thickened in all 11 patients, the aortic valve in eight, and the pulmonic valve in one (Fig. 58). The extramural coronary arteries in all 11 patients were normal.

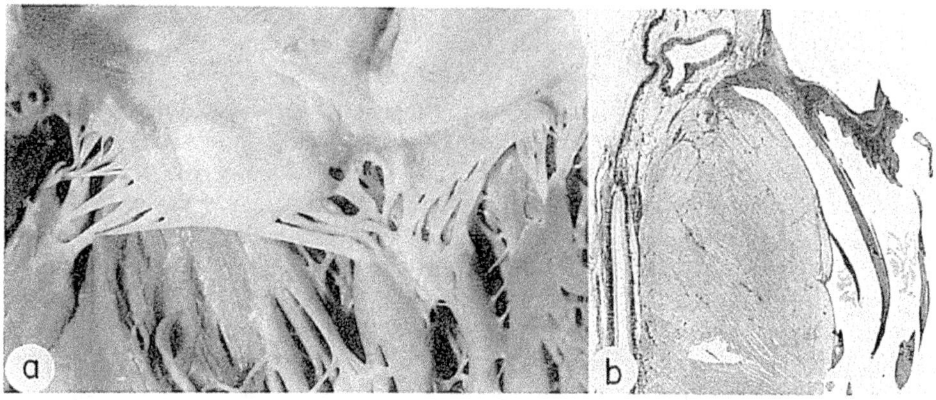

Figure 58. Radiation-induced valvular heart disease. This 29-year-old woman (A71–141) with Hodgkin's disease for four years received total body irradiation including 5335 rads to the anterior chest. A grade 1/6 systolic precordial murmur consistent with mitral regurgitation was audible. At necropsy, the pericardial sac was obliterated by fibrous adhesions. The tricuspid, mitral, and aortic valvular cusps were focally scarred and the mural endocardium of both ventricles was thickened. The myocardium appeared normal. a, Opened mitral valve showing fibrous thickening of the anterior leaflet and of its attached chordae. b, Longitudinal section of thickened posterior mitral leaflet with adjacent left atrial and left ventricular walls. b, Elastic van Gieson stain. [Reduced 20 per cent from × 3.5 (b).]

The valvular lesions in the 11 patients described almost certainly were the consequence of irradiation. All patients were relatively young, none had histories of acute rheumatic fever or infective endocarditis or other types of known valvular disease. The distribution of the lesions also was peculiar in that they involved mainly the tricuspid and mitral valves and the lesions were about as severe on the tricuspid as on the mitral valve. The valvular thickenings were focal: the anterior tricuspid leaflet and anterior mitral leaflet always were more involved than the posteriorly-located leaflets. In no patient were the valvular lesions extensive enough to cause dysfunction of the valve.

Idiopathic

Although a reasonable explanation for valvular dysfunction can usually be provided by necropsy examination of the heart and great arteries, the latter examination on occasion may fail to be enlightening in patients known to have varying degrees of valvular dysfunction during life. Such was the case in the patient described in Figure 59.[240] Mild degrees of aortic regurgitation in the elderly occasionally may be difficult at times to attribute to aortic root dilatation alone. Patients with systemic hypertension may have whiffs of aortic regurgitation, and at necropsy the aortic valve and aorta may be normal. An anatomic explanation of tricuspid regurgitation is often lacking.

SUMMARY

This review has focused on nonrheumatic causes of valvular cardiac disease. A quick survey of the structural alterations observed in a few of these conditions is shown in Figure 60. It appears clear that there are relatively few causes of

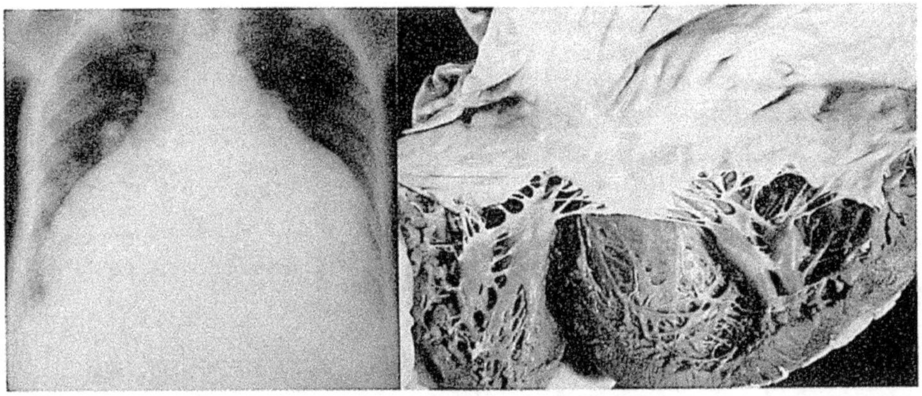

Figure 59. Mitral regurgitation of unknown etiology. This 60-year-old woman (A66–95) had been known to have congestive cardiac failure since age 34. She never had an illness consistent with or diagnostic of acute rheumatic fever or of infective endocarditis. A precordial murmur consistent with mitral regurgitation was heard when she was 43 years old, and her heart was shown enlarged by chest roentgenogram at this time. Thyrotoxicosis was diagnosed and treated at age 50. Although elevated blood pressures (180/105 mm. Hg) had been recorded during her 40s, the pressures were normal during her 50s. The congestive heart failure became severe during her last five years and the pansystolic murmur increased in intensity (to grade 4/6) and a murmur of tricuspid regurgitation also appeared. She was in atrial fibrillation for 26 years. The chest roentgenogram shown here was taken when she was 60 years old. At necropsy, the cause of the mitral regurgitation was not determined. The opened mitral valve (right) shows very pliable, only minimally thickened leaflets and the chordae are not thickened. The left atrium was enormously dilated. The papillary muscles and free wall myocardium are free of foci of fibrosis or necrosis. The mitral annulus is dilated but this in itself does not appear adequate to explain the severe mitral regurgitation. Thus, mitral regurgitation may be present clinically for years and necropsy may fail to provide an explanation for the valvular dysfunction.

valvular stenosis. When a rheumatic etiology is eliminated, most valvular stenotic lesions are congenital in origin, or, in the case of the aortic valve, the result of wear and tear of aging. In contrast to the relatively few causes of valvular stenosis, there are numerous causes and conditions associated with pure valvular regurgitation. Therefore, it is useful to separate valve dysfunction not into predominately stenotic or predominately incompetent lesions, but into purely incompetent lesions and those with elements of stenosis. Purely incompetent valvular lesions may be further divided into those which affect the ascending aorta and into those in which the aorta is normal. The latter primarily are the conditions causing pure mitral regurgitation and the former, the conditions causing aortic regurgitation.

The puzzle of valvular heart disease is beginning to be put together from a morphologic standpoint, but the end of the road is a long way from the beginning and there are many roadblocks and detours along the way.

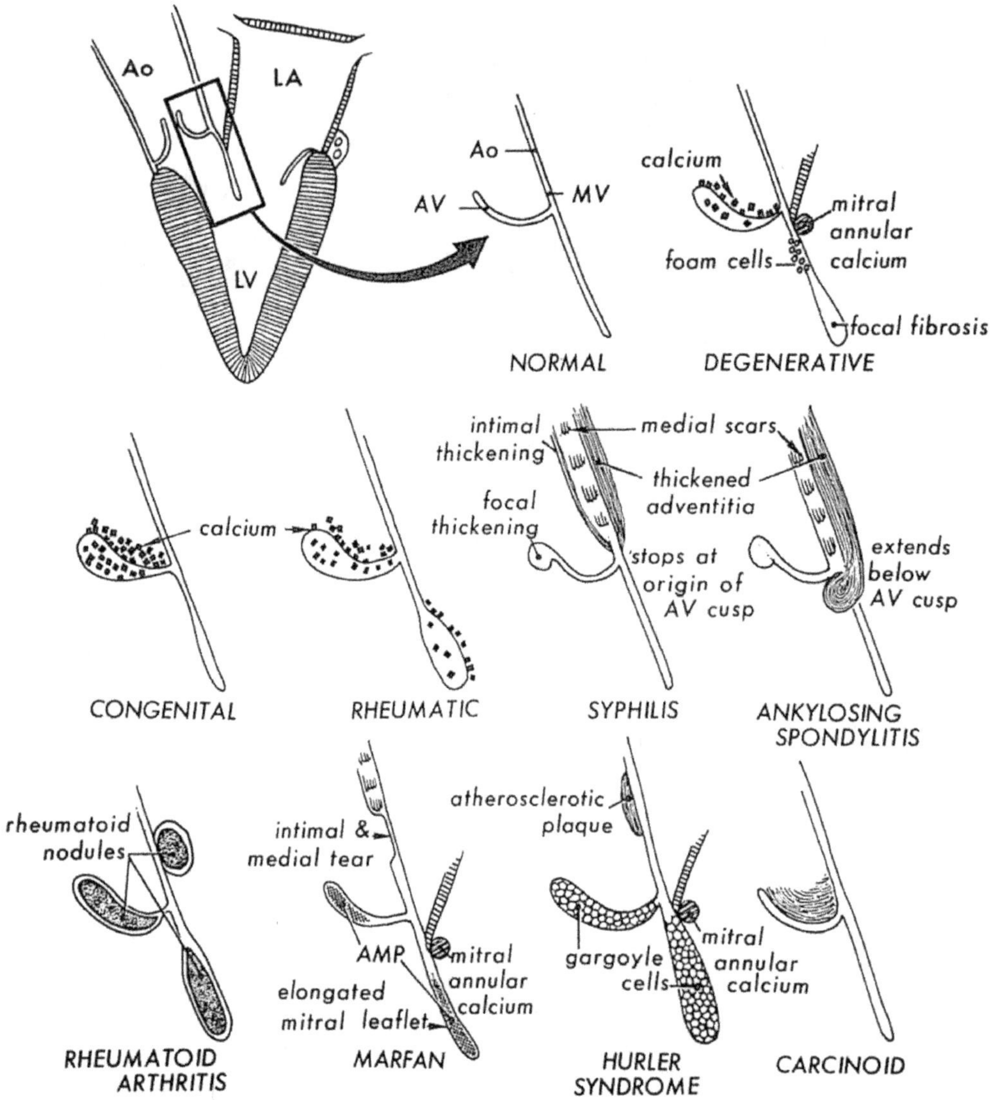

Figure 60. Diagrammatic portrayal of some of the conditions affecting the mitral and aortic valve leaflets. Degenerative, congenital, and rheumatic conditions frequently are associated with some degree of valvular stenosis. Syphilis never affects the mitral leaflets but ankylosing spondylitis extends below the aortic valve and may even lead to some mitral regurgitation. Rheumatoid arthritis, floppy valves with or without the Marfan syndrome, and the Hurler syndrome produce purely incompetent lesions. Carcinoid usually affects, or more severely affects, the right-sided cardiac valves but carcinoid plaques also have been observed on the mitral and aortic leaflets. Ao = aorta. LV = left ventricle. LA = left atrium. AV = aortic valve. MV = mitral valve. AMP = acid-mucopolysaccharide material.

REFERENCES

1. Roberts, W. C.: *Anatomically isolated aortic valvular disease. The case against its being of rheumatic origin.* Am. J. Med. 49:151, 1970.

2. Roberts, W. C.: *The structure of the aortic valve in clinically isolated aortic stenosis. An autopsy study of 162 patients over 15 years of age.* Circulation 42:91, 1970.

3. Roberts, W. C.: *The congenitally bicuspid aortic valve. A study of 85 autopsy cases.* Am. J. Cardiol. 26:72, 1970.

4. Roberts, W. C., Perloff, J. K., and Constantino, T.: *Severe valvular aortic stenosis in patients over 65 years of age. A clinicopathologic study.* Am. J. Cardiol. 27:497, 1971.

5. Roberts, W. C.: *Valvular, subvalvular and supravalvular aortic stenosis. Morphologic features.* Cardiovasc. Clin. 5 (1):97, 1973.

6. Falcone, M. W., Roberts, W. C., Morrow, A. G., and Perloff, J. K.: *Congenital aortic stenosis resulting from a unicommissural valve. Clinical and anatomic features in twenty-one adult patients.* Circulation 44:272, 1971.

7. Edwards, J. E.: *Pathologic aspects of cardiac valvular insufficiencies.* Arch. Surg. 77:634, 1958.

8. Moller, J. H., Nakib, A., Eliot, R. S., and Edwards, J. E.: *Symptomatic congenital aortic stenosis in the first year of life.* J. Pediatr. 67:728, 1966.

9. Hurwitz, L. E., and Roberts, W. C.: *The quadricuspid semilunar valve.* Am. J. Cardiol. (in press).

10. Morrow, A. G., Goldblatt, A., and Braunwald, E.: *Congenital aortic stenosis. II. Surgical treatment and the results of operation.* Circulation 27:426, 1963

11. Morrow, A. G., Fort, L., III, Roberts, W. C., and Braunwald, E.: *Discrete subaortic stenosis complicated by aortic valvular regurgitation. Clinical, hemodynamic, and pathologic studies and the results of operative treatment.* Circulation 20:1003, 1959.

12. Morrow, A. G.: *Hypertrophic subaortic stenosis. Some physiologic concepts and the role of operative treatment.* Arch. Surg. 99:677, 1969.

13. Adelman, A. G., McLoughlin, M. J., Marquis, Y., Auger, P., and Wigle, E. D.: *Left ventricular cineangiographic observations in muscular subaortic stenosis.* Am. J. Cardiol. 24:689, 1969.

14. Peterson, T. A., Todd, D. B., and Edwards, J. E.: *Supravalvular aortic stenosis.* J. Thorac. Cardiovasc. Surg. 50:734, 1965.

15. Roberts, W. C.: *Pathologic aspects of valvular and subvalvular (discrete and diffuse) aortic stenosis, in* Kidd, B. S. L., and Keith, I. D. (eds.): *The Natural History and Progress in Treatment of Congenital Heart Defects. An International Symposium Sponsored by the Ontario Heart Foundation in Co-operation with the Hospital for Sick Children and the University of Toronto.* Charles C Thomas, Springfield, 1971, p. 221.

16. Roberts, W. C., Ferrans, V. J., Levy, R. I., and Fredrickson, D. S.: *Cardiovascular pathology in hyperlipoproteinemia. Anatomic observa-*

tions in 41 necropsy patients with normal or abnormal serum lipoprotein patterns. Am. J. Cardiol. (in press).

17. Wennevold, A., and Jacobsen, J. G.: *Acquired supravalvular aortic stenosis in familial hypercholesterolemia. A hemodynamic and angiographic study*. Am. J. Med. 50:823, 1971.

18. Ferrans, V. J., and Roberts, W. C.: *Structural features of cardiac myxomas. Histology, histochemistry and electron microscopy*. Hum. Pathol. 4:111, 1973.

19. Buchbinder, N. A., and Roberts, W. C.: *Active infective endocarditis confined to mural endocardium. A study of six necropsy patients*. Arch. Pathol. 93:435, 1972.

20. MacLowery, J. D., and Roberts, W. C.: *Metastatic choriocarcinoma of the lung. Invasion of pulmonary veins with extension into left atrium and mitral orifice*. Am. J. Cardiol. 18:938, 1966.

21. Ferencz, C., Johnson, A. L., and Wiglesworth, F. W.: *Congenital mitral stenosis*. Circulation 9:161, 1954.

22. Shone, J. D., Sellers, R. D., Anderson, R. C., Adams, P., Jr., Lillehei, C. W., and Edwards, J. E.: *The developmental complex of "parachute mitral valve," supravalvular ring of left atrium, subaortic stenosis, and coarctation of aorta*. Am. J. Cardiol. 11:714, 1963.

23. Glancy, D. L., Chang, M. Y., Dorney, E. R., and Roberts, W. C.: *Parachute mitral valve. Further observations and associated lesions*. Am. J. Cardiol. 27:309, 1971.

24. Castaneda, A. R., Anderson, R. C., and Ewards, J. E.: *Congenital mitral stenosis resulting from anomalous arcade and obstructing papillary muscles. Report of correction by use of ball valve prosthesis*. Am. J. Cardiol. 24:237, 1969.

25. Van Den Horst, R. L., and Hastreiter, A. R.: *Congenital mitral stenosis*. Am. J. Cardiol. 20:773, 1967.

26. Shem-Tov, A., Yahini, J. H., Deutsch, V., Katznelson, D., and Neufeld, H. N.: *Congenital mitral stenosis*. Cardiologica 54:65, 1969.

27. Fontana, R. S., and Edwards, J. E.: *Congenital Cardiac Disease: A Review of 357 Cases Studied Pathologically*. W. B. Saunders Co., Philadelphia, 1962.

28. Koretzky, B. S., Moller, J. H., Korns, M. E., Schwartz, C. J., and Edwards, J. E.: *Congenital pulmonary stenosis resulting from dysplasia of the valve*. Circulation 40:43, 1969.

29. Campbell, M.: *Natural history of congenital pulmonary stenosis*. Br. Heart J. 31:394, 1969.

30. Roberts, W. C., Mason, D. T., Morrow, A. G., and Braunwald, E.: *Calcific pulmonic stenosis*. Circulation 37:973, 1968.

31. Rodriguez, G. R., Bennette, K. R., and Lehan, P. H.: *Calcification of the pulmonic valve*. Chest 59:160, 1971.

32. Hudson, R. E. B.: *Cardiovascular Pathology*. Edward Arnold Ltd., London, 1965, p. 1953.

33. THÖRSON, A., BIÖRCK, G., BJÖRKMAN, G., AND WALDENSTRÖM, J.: *Malignant carcinoid of the small intestine with metastases to the liver, valvular disease of the heart (pulmonic stenosis and tricuspid regurgitation without septal defects), peripheral vasomotor symptoms, bronchoconstriction, and an unusual type of cyanosis. A clinical and pathologic syndrome.* Am. Heart J. 47:795, 1954.

34. MELMON, K. L., SJOERDSMA, A., AND MASON, D. T.: *Distinctive clinical and therapeutic aspects of the syndrome associated with bronchial carcinoid tumors.* Am. J. Med. 39:568, 1965.

35. OATES, J. A., AND SJOERDSMA, A.: *A unique syndrome associated with secretion of 5-hydroxytryptophan by metastatic gastric carcinoids.* Am. J. Med. 32:333, 1962.

36. OATES, J. A., MELMON, K., SJOERDSMA, A., GILLESPIE, L., AND MASON, D. T.: *Release of kinin peptide in the carcinoid syndrome.* Lancet 1:514, 1964.

37. SJOERDSMA, A., WEISSBACH, H., AND UDENFRIEND, S.: *A clinical, physiologic and biochemical study of patients with malignant carcinoid (argentaffinoma).* Am. J. Med. 20:520, 1956.

38. ROBERTS, W. C., AND SJOERDSMA, A.: *The cardiac disease associated with the carcinoid syndrome (carcinoid heart disease).* Am. J. Med. 36:5, 1964.

39. ROBERTS, W. C., MASON, D. T., AND WRIGHT, L. D., JR.: *The nondistensible right atrium of carcinoid disease of the heart.* Am. J. Clin. Pathol. 44:627, 1965.

40. VON BERNHEIMER, H., EHRINGER, H., HEISTRACHER, P., KRAUPP, O., LACHNIT, V., OBIDITSCH-MAYER, I., AND WENZL, M.: *Biologisch aktives, nicht metastasierendes Bronchuscarcinoid mit Linksherz-syndrom.* Wien. Klin. Wochenschr. 72:867, 1960.

41. FERRANS, V. F., AND ROBERTS, W. C.: *Ultrastructural features of the carcinoid cardiac plaque.* (In preparation).

42. SJOERDSMA, A., WEISSBACH, H., TERRY, L. L., AND UDENFRIEND, S.: *Further observations on patients with malignant carcinoid.* Am. J. Med. 23:5, 1957.

43. LEVINE, R. J., AND SJOERDSMA, A.: *Pressor amines and the carcinoid flush.* Ann. Intern. Med. 58:818, 1963.

44. BROCK, R.: *The surgical treatment of pulmonary stenosis.* Br. Heart J. 23:337, 1961.

45. HORLICK, L., AND MERRIMAN, J. E.: *Congenital valvular stenosis of pulmonary and aortic valves with atrial septal defect.* Am. Heart J. 54:615, 1957.

46. SALAZAR, E., BENAVIDES, P., CONTRERAS, R., AND ESPINO-VELA, J.: *Congenital mitral and tricuspid stenosis.* Am. J. Cardiol. 16:358, 1965.

47. VAN DEN HORST, R. L., AND HASTREITER, A. R.: *Congenital mitral stenosis.* Am. J. Cardiol. 20:773, 1967.

48. ROBERTS, W. C., GOLDBLATT, A., MASON, D. T., AND MORROW, A. G.: *Combined congenital pulmonic and mitral stenosis.* N. Engl. J. Med. 267:1298, 1962.

49. MARTLAND, H. S.: *Syphilis of the aorta and heart.* Am. Heart J. 6:1, 1930.

50. Carr, J. G.: *The gross pathology of the heart in cardiovascular syphilis.* Am. Heart J. 6:30, 1930.

51. Heggtveit, H. A.: *Syphilitic aortitis. A clinicopathologic autopsy study of 100 cases.* Circulation 29:346, 1964.

52. Clark, W. S., and Bauer, W.: *Cardiac changes in rheumatoid arthritis.* Ann. Rheum. Dis. 7:39, 1948.

53. Schilder, D. P., Harvey, W. P., and Hufnagel, C. A.: *Rheumatoid spondylitis and aortic insufficiency.* N. Engl. J. Med. 255:11, 1956.

54. Clark, W. S., Kulka, J. P., and Bauer, W.: *Rheumatoid aortitis with aortic regurgitation.* Am. J. Med. 22:580, 1957.

55. Graham, D. C., and Smythe, H. A.: *The carditis and aortitis of ankylosing spondylitis.* Bull. Rheum. Dis. 9:171, 1958.

56. Davidson, P., Baggenstross, A. H., Slocumb, C. H., and Daugherty, G. W.: *Cardiac and aortic lesions in rheumatoid spondylitis.* Proc. Mayo Clin. 36:427, 1963.

57. Liu, S. M., and Alexander, C. S.: *Complete heart block and aortic insufficiency in rheumatoid spondylitis.* Am. J. Cardiol. 23:888, 1969.

58. Bernstein, L.: *Cardiac complications in spondyl-arthritis ankylopoietica.* Rheumatism 7:18, 1951.

59. Toone, E. C., Pierce, E. L., and Hennigar, G. R.: *Aortitis and aortic regurgitation associated with rheumatoid spondylitis.* Am. J. Med. 26:255, 1959.

60. Valaitis, J., Pilz, C. G., and Montgomery, M. M.: *Aortitis with aortic valve insufficiency in rheumatoid arthritis.* Arch. Pathol. 63:207, 1957.

61. Malette, W. G., Eisman, B., Danielson, G. K., Mazzoleni, A., and Rams, J. J.: *Rheumatoid spondylitis and aortic insufficiency.* J. Thorac. Cardiovasc. Surg. 57:471, 1969.

62. Gleckler, W. J.: *Rheumatoid spondylitis with carditis.* Am. J. Med. 16:284, 1954.

63. Bernstein, C., and Broch, O. J.: *Cardiac complications in spondyl-arthritis ankylopoietica.* Acta Med. Scand. 135:185, 1949.

64. Blumberg, B., and Ragan, C.: *Natural history of rheumatoid spondylitis.* Medicine 35:1, 1956.

65. McKusick, V. A.: *Heritable Disorders of Connective Tissue,* ed. 3. C. V. Mosby Co., St. Louis, 1966.

66. Read, R. C., Thal, A. P., and Wendt, V. E.: *Symptomatic valvular myxomatous transformation (the floppy valve syndrome). A possible forme fruste of the Marfan syndrome.* Circulation 32:897, 1965.

67. Ragib, G., Jue, K. L., Anderson, R. C., and Edwards, J. E.: *Marfan's syndrome with mitral insufficiency.* Am. J. Cardiol. 16:127, 1965.

68. Shankar, K. R., Hultgren, M. K., Laver, R. M., and Diehl, A. M.: *Lethal tricuspid and mitral regurgitation in Marfan's syndrome.* Am. J. Cardiol. 20:122, 1967.

69. DIETZMAN, R. H., PETER, E. T., WANG, Y., AND LILLEHEI, R. C.: *Mitral insufficiency in Marfan's syndrome. A case report of surgical correction.* Dis. Chest 51:650, 1967.

70. CROCKER, D. W.: *Marfan's syndrome confined to the mitral valve region: two cases in siblings.* Am. Heart J. 76:538, 1968.

71. JORTNER, R., SHAHIN, W., ESHKOL, D., GUERON, M., AND LEVY, M. J.: *Cardiovascular manifestations and surgery for Marfan's syndrome.* Dis. Chest 56:24, 1969.

72. ROBERTS, W. C., AND COHEN, L. S.: *Left ventricular papillary muscles. Description of the normal and a survey of conditions causing them to be abnormal.* Circulation 46:138, 1972.

73. PERLOFF, J. K., AND ROBERTS, W. C.: *The mitral apparatus. Functional anatomy of mitral regurgitation.* Circulation 46:227, 1972.

74. GROSSMAN, M., KNOTT, A. P., JR., AND JACOBY, W. J., JR.: *Calcified annulus fibrosis with mitral insufficiency with Marfan's syndrome.* Arch. Intern. Med. 121:561, 1968.

75. MCKUSICK, V. A., LOGUE, R. B., AND BAHNSON, H. T.: *Association of aortic valvular disease and cystic medial necrosis of the ascending aorta. Report of four instances.* Circulation 16:188, 1957.

76. HEATH, D., EDWARDS, J. E., AND SMITH, L. A.: *The rheologic significance of medial necrosis and dissecting aneurysm of the ascending aorta in association with calcific aortic stenosis.* Proc. Mayo Clin. 33:228, 1958.

77. LAGUNOFF, D., ROSS, R., AND BENDITT, E. P.: *Histochemical and electron microscopic study of a case of Hurler's disease.* Am. J. Pathol. 41:273, 1962.

78. FERRANS, V. F., AND ROBERTS, W. C.: *Ultrastructural features of cardiac lesions of the Hurler syndrome.* In preparation.

79. OKADA, R., ROSENTHAL, I. M., SCARAVELLI, G., AND LEV, M.: *A histopathologic study of the heart in gargoylism.* Arch. Pathol. 84:20, 1967.

80. HUNTER, C.: *A rare disease in two brothers.* Proc. R. Soc. Med. 10:104, 1917.

81. KROVETZ, L. J., LORINCZ, A. E., AND SCHIEBLER, G. L.: *Cardiovascular manifestations of the Hurler syndrome. Hemodynamic and angiographic observations in 15 patients.* Circulation 31:132, 1965.

82. VANACE, P. W., FRIEDMAN, S., AND WAGNER, B. M.: *Mitral stenosis in an atypical case of gargoylism: a case report with pathologic and histochemical studies of the cardiac tissues.* Circulation 21:80, 1960.

83. FRIEDEN, J., HURWITT, E. S., AND LEADER, E.: *Ruptured aortic cusp with an heritable disorder of connective tissue.* Am. J. Med. 33:615, 1962.

84. TUCKER, D. H., MILLER, D. E., AND JACOBY, W. J.: *Ehlers-Danlos syndrome with a sinus of Valsalva aneurysm and aortic insufficiency simulating rheumatic heart disease.* Am. J. Med. 35:715, 1963.

85. MADISON, W. R., JR., BRADLEY, E. J., AND CASTILLO, A. J.: *Ehlers-Danlos syndrome with cardiac involvement.* Am. J. Cardiol. 11:689, 1963.

86. BROWELL, J. M., JR., AND DREKE, E. H.: *Aortic valve lesions associated with osteogenesis imperfecta.* Henry Ford Hosp. Med. Bull. 14:245, 1966.

87. GREEN, G. J., SCHUMAN, B., AND BARRON, J.: *Ehlers-Danlos syndrome complicated by acute hemorrhagic diverticulitis with an unusual mitral valve abnormality*. Am. J. Med. 41:622, 1966.

88. HUANG, S., GANRAJ, K., STEELE, H., AND PARK, J. O.: *Cardiac involvement in pseudoxanthoma elasticum*. Am. Heart J. 74:680, 1967.

89. HECKMAN, B. A., AND STEINBERG, I.: *Congenital heart disease (mitral regurgitation) in osteogenesis imperfecta*. Am. J. Roentgenol. Radium Ther. Nucl. Med. 103:601, 1968.

90. GOODMAN, R. W., BABA, M., AND WOOLEY, C. F.: *Observations on the heart in a case of combined Ehlers-Danlos and Marfan syndromes*. Am. J. Cardiol. 24:134, 1969.

91. CRISCITIELLO, M. G., RONAN, J. A., BESTERMAN, E. M. M., AND SCHOENWETTER, W.: *Cardiovascular abnormalities in osteogenesis imperfecta*. Circulation 31:255, 1965.

92. JORRIOD, J., ROTHLIN, M., AND UEHLINGER, E.: *Anomalies cardiovasculaires de la Maladie de Lobstein*. Schweiz. Med. Wochenschr. 98:795, 1968.

93. ALLEN, E. V.: *Primary arteritis of the aortic arch*. Circulation 11:486, 1955.

94. KALMANSOHN, R. B., AND KALMANSOHN, R. W.: *Thrombotic obliteration of the branches of the aortic arch*. Circulation 15:237, 1957.

95. NASU, T.: *Pathology of pulseless disease*. Angiology 14:225, 1963.

96. STRACHAN, R. W.: *The natural history of Takayasu's arteriopathy*. J. Med. 33:57, 1964.

97. ROBERTS, W. C., AND WIBIN, E. A.: *Idiopathic panaortitis, supraaortic arteritis, granulomatous myocarditis and pericarditis*. Am. J. Med. 41:453, 1966.

98. ROBERTS, W. C., MACGREGOR, R. R., DEBLANC, H. J., BEISER, G. B., AND WOLFF, S. M.: *The prepulseless phase of pulseless disease, or pulseless disease with pulses. A newly recognized cause of cardiac disease, monoclonal gammopathy and fever of unknown origin*. Am. J. Med. 46:313, 1969.

99. BARLOW, J. B., POCOCK, W. A., MARCHAND, P., AND DENNY, M.: *The significance of late systolic murmurs*. Am. Heart J. 66:443, 1963.

100. CRILEY, J. M., LEWIS, K. B., HUMPHRIES, J. O., AND ROSS, R. S.: *Prolapse of the mitral valve: Clinical and cine-angiocardiographic findings*. Br. Heart J. 28:488, 1966.

101. STANNARD, M., SLOMAN, J. G., HARE, W. S., AND GOBLE, A. J.: *Prolapse of the posterior leaflet of the mitral valve. A clinical, familial and cineangiographic study*. Br. Med. J. 3:71, 1967.

102. BARLOW, J. B., BOSMAN, C. K., POCOCK, W. A., AND MARCHAND, P.: *Late systolic murmurs and non-ejection ('mid-late') systolic clicks; An analysis of 90 patients*. Br. Heart J. 30:203, 1968.

103. JERESATY, R. M.: *Ballooning of the mitral valve leaflets. Angiographic study of 24 patients*. Radiology 100:45, 1971.

104. EHLERS, K. H., ENGLE, M. A., LEVIN, A. R., GROSSMAN, H., AND FLEMING, R. J.: *Left ventricular abnormality with late mitral insufficiency and abnormal electrocardiogram*. Am. J. Cardiol. 26:333, 1970.

105. Edynak, G. M., and Rawson, A. J.: *Ruptured aneurysm of the mitral valve in a Marfan-like syndrome*. Am. J. Cardiol. 11:674, 1963.

106. Pocock, W. A., and Barlow, J. B.: *Etiology and electrocardiographic features of the billowing posterior mitral leaflet syndrome*. Am. J. Med. 51:731, 1971.

107. McDonald, A., Harris, H., Jefferson, K., Marshall, J., and McDonald, L.: *Association of prolapse of posterior cusp of mitral valve and atrial septal defect*. Br. Heart J. 33:383, 1971.

108. Pocock, W. A., and Barlow, J. B.: *An association between billowing posterior mitral leaflet syndrome and congenital heart disease, particularly atrial septal defect*. Am. Heart J. 81:720, 1971.

109. Davis, R. H., Schuster, B., Knoebel, S. B., and Fisch, C.: *Myxomatous degeneration of the mitral valve*. Am. J. Cardiol. 28:449, 1971.

110. Kern, W. H., and Tucker, B. L.: *Myxoid changes in cardiac valves: pathologic, clinical and ultrastructural studies*. Am. Heart J. 84:294, 1972.

111. Pomerance, A.: *Ballooning deformity (mucoid degeneration) of atrioventricular valves*. Br. Heart J. 31:343, 1969.

112. Sherman, E. B., Char, F., Dungan, W. T., and Campbell, G. S.: *Myxomatous transformation of the mitral valve producing mitral insufficiency. Floppy valve syndrome*. Am. J. Dis. Child. 119:171, 1970.

113. Edwards, J. E.: *Mitral insufficiency resulting from 'overshooting' of leaflets*. Circulation 43:606, 1971.

114. Bowers, D.: *An electrocardiographic pattern associated with mitral valve deformity in Marfan's syndrome*. Circulation 23:30, 1961.

115. Frable, W. J.: *Mucinous degeneration of the cardiac valves: the floppy valve syndrome*. J. Thorac. Cardiovasc. Surg. 58:62, 1969.

116. Pomerance, A.: *Cardiac pathology and systolic murmurs in the elderly*. Br. Heart J. 30:687, 1968.

117. Pomerance, A.: *Ageing changes in human heart valves*. Br. Heart J. 29:222, 1967.

118. Sell, S., and Scully, R. E.: *Aging changes in the aortic and mitral valves*. Am. J. Pathol. 46:345, 1965.

119. Kittredge, R. D., Shimomura, S., Cameron, A., and Bell, A. L.: *Prolapsing mitral valve leaflets; cineangiographic demonstrations*. Am. J. Roentgenol. Radium Ther. Nucl. Med. 109:84, 1970.

120. Korn, D., De Sanctis, R. W., and Sell, S.: *Massive calcification of the mitral annulus*. N. Engl. J. Med. 267:900, 1962.

121. Ewy, G. A., Marcus, F. I., Bohajalian, O., Burke, H. L., and Roberts, W. C.: *Muscular subaortic stenosis. Clinical and pathologic observations in an elderly patient*. Am. J. Cardiol. 22:126, 1968.

122. Rogers, J. B., Chandler, N. W., and Franch, R. H.: *Calcification of the tricuspid annulus.* Am. J. Roentgenol. Radium Ther. Nucl. Med. 106:550, 1969.

123. Cooksey, J. D., Parker, B. M., and Weldon, C. S.: *Atrial septal defect and calcification of the tricuspid valve.* Br. Heart J. 32:409, 1970.

124. Arnold, J. R., Ghahramani, A. R., Hernandez, F. A., and Sommer, L. S.: *Calcification of annulus of tricuspid valve (observation in two patients with congenital pulmonary stenosis).* Chest 60:229, 1971.

125. Brody, W., and Criley, J. M.: *Intermittent severe mitral regurgitation: hemodynamic studies in a patient with recurrent acute left-sided heart failure.* N. Engl. J. Med. 283:673, 1970.

126. Burch, G. E., De Pasquale, N. P., and Phillips, J. H.: *The syndrome of papillary muscle dysfunction.* Am. Heart J. 75:399, 1968.

127. Brock, R. C.: *The surgical and pathological anatomy of the mitral valve.* Br. Heart J. 14:489, 1952.

128. Mittal, A. K., Langston, M., Jr., Cohn, K. E., Selzer, A., and Kerth, W. J.: *Combined papillary muscle and left ventricular wall dysfunction as a cause of mitral regurgitation: An experimental study.* Circulation 44:174, 1971.

129. Falcone, M. W., Ronan, J. A., Jr., and Roberts, W. C.: *Silent mitral regurgitation complicating silent myocardial infarction: hemodynamic and morphologic decumentation.* Chest 62:226, 1972.

130. Roberts, W. C., and Buchbinder, N. A.: *Right-sided valvular infective endocarditis. A clinicopathologic study of twelve necropsy patients.* Am. J. Med. 53:7, 1972.

131. Buchbinder, N. A., and Roberts, W. C.: *Left-sided valvular active infective endocarditis. A study of forty-five necropsy patients.* Am. J. Med. 53:20, 1972.

132. Roberts, W. C., and Buchbinder, N. A.: *Papillary muscle necrosis in active valvular infective endocarditis.* Am. J. Cardiol. 29:287, 1972.

133. Moller, J. H., Lucas, R. B., Jr., Adams, P., Jr., Anderson, R. C., Jorgens, J., and Edwards, J. E.: *Endocardial fibroelastosis. A clinical and anatomic study of 47 patients with emphasis on its relationship to mitral insufficiency.* Circulation 30:759, 1964.

134. Noren, G. R., Raghib, G., Moller, J. H., Amplantz, K., Adams, P., Jr., and Edwards, J. E.: *Anomalous origin of the left coronary artery from the pulmonary trunk with special reference to the occurrence of mitral insufficiency.* Circulation 30:171, 1964.

135. Roberts, W. C.: *Anomalous origin of both coronary arteries from the pulmonary artery.* Am. J. Cardiol. 10:595, 1962.

136. Burchell, H. B., and Brown, A. L., Jr.: *Anomalous origin of coronary artery from pulmonary artery masquerading as mitral insufficiency.* Am. Heart J. 63:388, 1962.

137. Marcus, F. I., Gomez, L., Glancy, D. L., Ewy, G. A., and Roberts, W. C.: *Papillary muscle fibrosis in primary myocardial disease.* Am. Heart J. 77:681, 1969.

138. Perloff, J. K., Roberts, W. C., de Leon, A. C., and O'Doherty, D.: *The distinctive electrocardiogram of Duchenne's progressive muscular dystrophy. An electrocardiographic-pathologic correlative study.* Am. J. Med. 42:179, 1967.

139. Roberts, W. C., Buja, L. M., and Ferrans, V. J.: *Löffler's fibroplastic parietal endocarditis, eosinophilic leukemia, and Davis' endomyocardial fibrosis: The same disease at different stages?* Pathol. Microbiol. 35:90, 1970.

140. Roberts, W. C., Liegler, D. G., and Carbone, P. P.: *Endomycardial disease and eosinophilia: A clinical and pathologic spectrum.* Am. J. Med. 46:28, 1969.

141. Morrow, A. G., Cohen, L. S., Roberts, W. C., Braunwald, N. S., and Braunwald, E.: *Severe mitral regurgitation following acute myocardial infarction and ruptured papillary muscle: Hemodynamic findings and results of operative treatment in four patients.* Circulation 38 (Suppl.): II-124, 1968.

142. Roberts, W. C., and Ferrans, V. J.: *Morphologic observations in the cardiomyopathies, in* Fowler, N. O. (ed.): *The Cardiomyopathies.* Grune & Stratton, New York, 1973, (in press).

143. Roberts, W. C., Bodey, G. P., and Wertlake, P. T.: *The heart in acute leukemia. A study of 420 autopsy cases.* Am. J. Cardiol. 21:388, 1968.

144. Glancy, D. L., and Roberts, W. C.: *The heart in malignant malanoma. A study of 70 autopsy cases.* Am. J. Cardiol. 21:555, 1968.

145. Roberts, W. C., Glancy, D. L., and DeVita, V. T., Jr.: *Heart in malignant lymphoma (Hodgkin's disease, lymphosarcoma, reticulum cell sarcoma and mycosis fungoides). A study of 196 autopsy cases.* Am. J. Cardiol. 22:85, 1968.

146. Buja, L. M., Khoi, N. B., and Roberts, W. C.: *Clinically significant cardiac amyloidosis. Clinicopathologic findings in 15 patients.* Am. J. Cardiol. 26:394, 1970.

147. Buja, L. M., and Roberts, W. C.: *Iron in the heart. Etiology and clinical significance.*. Am. J. Med. 51:209, 1971.

148. Buchbinder, N. A., and Roberts, W. C.: *Active infective endocarditis confined to mural endocardium. A study of six necropsy patients.* Arch. Pathol. 93:435, 1972.

149. Buchbinder, N. A., and Roberts, W. C.: *Alcoholism—An important but unemphasized factor predisposing to infective endocarditis with reemphasis on the syndrome of pneumococcal endocarditis, meningitis and pneumonitis in alcholics.* Arch. Intern. Med. (in press).

150. Roberts, W. C., and Perloff, J. K.: *Mitral valvular disease. A combined clinical and pathologic survey of the conditions causing the mitral valve to function abnormally.* Ann. Intern. Med. 77:939, 1972.

151. Roberts, W. C., Buchbinder, N. A., and Morrow, A. G.: *Healed infective endocarditis: An anatomic study of patients with histories of active*

infective endocarditis and a clinical analysis of anatomically confirmed cases of healed rupture of mitral chordae tendineae or of perforation of mitral or aortic valve cusps. (in preparation).

152. SCHIEBLER, G. L., GRAVENSTEIN, J. S., AND VAN MIEROP, L. H. S.: *Ebstein's anomaly of the tricuspid valve. Translation of the original description with comments.* Am. J. Cardiol. 22:867, 1968.

153. VACCA, J. B., BUSSMANN, D. W., AND MUDD, J. G.: *Ebstein's anomaly, complete review of 108 cases.* Am. J. Cardiol. 2:210, 1958.

154. KEZDI, P., AND WENNEMARK, J.: *Ebstein's malformation: Clinical findings and hemodynamic alterations.* Am. J. Cardiol. 2:200, 1958.

155. SPENCER, F. C.: *Surgery of the tricuspid valve.* Cardiovasc. Clin. 3(2):301, 1971.

156. BECKER, A. E., BECKER, M. J., AND EDWARDS, J. E.: *Pathologic spectrum of dysplasia of the tricuspid valve. Features in common with Ebstein's malformation.* Arch. Pathol. 91:169, 1971.

157. MARKOUS, N., AND VANDER VEER, J. B.: *Ebstein's anamaly and life expectancy. Report of a survival to over age 79.* Am. J. Cardiol. 18:100, 1966.

158. GENTON , E., AND BLOUNT, S. G.: *The spectrum of Ebstein's anomaly.* Am. Heart J. 73:395, 1967.

159. NEWFELD, E. A., COLE, R. B., AND PAUL, M. H.: *Ebstein's malformation of the tricuspid valve in the neonate. Functional and anatomic pulmonary outflow tract obstruction.* Am. J. Cardiol. 19:727, 1967.

160. MAYER, F. E., NADAS, A. S., AND ONGLEY, P. A.: *Ebstein's anomaly. Presentation of 10 cases.* Circulation 16:1057, 1957.

161. HARRIS, R. H. D.: *Ebstein's anomaly: Discovered in a 75 year old subject in the dissecting laboratory.* Canad. Med. Assoc. J. 83:653, 1960.

162. ENGLE, M. A., PAYNE, T. P. B., BRUINS, C., AND TAUSSIG, H. B.: *Ebstein's anomaly of the tricuspid valve. Report of three cases and analysis of the clinical syndrome.* Circulation 1:1246, 1950.

163. POCOCK, W. A., TUCKER, R. B. K., AND BARLOW, J. B.: *Mild Ebstein's anomaly.* Br. Heart J. 31:327, 1969.

164. LOWE, K. G., AND EMSLIE-SMITH, D.: *Scalar, vector and intracardiac electrocardiograms in Ebstein's anomaly.* Br. Heart J. 30:617, 1968.

165. MOLES, S. S., JACOBY, W. J., JR., AND MCINTOSH, H. D.: *Ebstein's malformation. Discordant intracavitary electrocardiographic and pressure relationship.* Am. J. Cardiol. 14:720, 1964.

166. BRAYSHAW, J. R., AND PERLOFF, J. K.: *Congenital pulmonary insufficiency complicating idiopathic dilatation of the pulmonary artery.* Am. J. Cardiol. 10:282, 1962.

167. SMITH, R. D., DUSHANE, J. W., AND EDWARDS, J. A.: *Congenital insufficiency of the pulmonary valve. Including a case of fetal cardiac failure.* Circulation 20:554, 1959.

168. ITO, T., ENGLE, M. A., AND HOLSWADE, G. R.: *Congenital insufficiency of the pulmonic valve. A rare cause of neonatal heart failure.* Pediatrics 28:712, 1961.

169. D'Cruz, I. A., Leudrum, B. L., and Novak, G.: *Congenital absence of the pulmonary valve.* Am. Heart J. 68:728, 1964.

170. Pouget, J. M., Kelly, C. E., and Pilz, C. G.: *Congenital absence of the pulmonic valve. Report of case in a 73 year old man.* Am. J. Cardiol. 19:732, 1967.

171. Ford, A. B., Hellerstein, H. K., Wood, C., and Kelley, H. B.: *Isolated congenital bicuspid pulmonary valve: Clinical and pathologic study.* Am. J. Med. 20:474, 1956.

172. Dickens, J., Raber, G. T., and Goldberg, H.: *Dynamic pulmonary regurgitation associated with a bicuspid valve.* Ann. Intern. Med. 48:851, 1958.

173. Miller, R. A., Leu, M., and Paul, M. H.: *Congenital absence of the pulmonary valve. The clinical syndrome of tetralogy of Fallot with pulmonary regurgitation.* Circulation 26:266, 1962.

174. Nemickas, R., Roberts, J., Gunnar, R., and Tobin, J. R., Jr.: *Isolated congenital pulmonic insufficiency.* Am. J. Cardiol. 14:456, 1964.

175. Holmes, J. C., Fowler, N. O., and Kaplan, S.: *Pulmonary valvular insufficiency.* Am. J. Med. 44:851, 1968.

176. Rokseth, R.: *Isolated pulmonic valvular regurgitation.* Acta Med. Scand. 185:489, 1969.

177. Carney, E. K., Braunwald, E., Roberts, W. C., Aygen, M., and Morrow, A. G.: *Congenital mitral regurgitation. Clinical, hemodynamic and angiographic findings in nine patients.* Am. J. Med. 33:223, 1962.

178. Ainger, L. E.: *Mitral and aortic valve incompetence in endocardial fibroelastosis. Diagnostic and hemodynamic significance.* Am. J. Cardiol. 28:309, 1971.

179. Berry, W. B., Roberts, W. C., Morrow, A. G., and Braunwald, E.: *Corrected transposition of the aorta and pulmonary trunk. Clinical, hemocynamic and pathologic findings.* Am. J. Med. 36:35, 1964.

180. Roberts, W. C., Ross, R. S., and Davis, F. W., Jr.: *Congenital corrected transportation of the great vessels in adulthood simulating rheumatic valvular disease.* Bul. Johns Hopkins Hosp. 144:157, 1964.

181. Schiebler, G. L., Edwards, J. C., Burchell, H. B., Dushane, J. W., Ongley, P. A., and Wood, E. H.: *Congenital corrected transposition of the great vessels. A study of 33 cases.* Pediatrics 27:851, 1961.

182. Braunwald, E., Ross, R. S., Morrow, A. G., and Roberts, W. C.: *Differential diagnosis of mitral regurgitation in childhood: clinical pathological conference at the National Institutes of Health.* Ann. Intern. Med. 54:1223, 1961.

183. Brockenbrough, E. C., Braunwald, E., Roberts, W. C., and Morrow, A. G.: *Partial persistent atrioventricular canal simulating pure mitral regurgitation.* Am. Heart J. 63:9, 1962.

184. MacLeod, C. A.: *Endocardial cushion defects with severe mitral insufficiency and small atrial septal defect.* Circulation 26:755, 1962.

185. Glancy, D. L., Chang, M. Y., Dorney, E. R., and Roberts, W. C.: *Parachute mitral valve. Further observations and associated lesions.* Am. J. Cardiol. 27:309, 1971.

186. Scheiken, R. M., Freidman, S., Waldhausen, J., and Johnson, J.: *Isolated congenital mitral insufficiency: Pathologic and surgical variations in five children.* J. Pediatr. Surg. 6:49, 1971.

187. Shone, J. D., Sellers, R. D., Anderson, R. C., Adams, P., Jr., Lillehei, C. W., and Edwards, J. E.: *The developmental complex of "parachute mitral valve," supravalvular ring of left atrium, subaortic stenosis and coarctation of the aorta.* Am. J. Cardiol. 11:714, 1963.

188. Layman, T. E., Edwards, J. E.: *Anomalous mitral arcade. A type of congenital mitral insufficiency.* Circulation 35:389, 1967.

189. Davachi, F., Moller, J. H., and Edwards, J. E.: *Diseases of the mitral valve in infancy. An anatomic review of 55 cases.* Circulation 43:565, 1971.

190. Rosenberg, J., and Roberts, W. C.: *Double orifice mitral valve. Study of the anomaly in two calves and a summary of the literature in humans.* Arch. Pathol. 86:77, 1968.

191. Parmley, L. F., Mattingly, T. W., and Manion, W. C.: *Penetrating wounds of the heart and aorta.* Circulation 17:953, 1958.

192. Yao, S. T., Vanecko, R. M., Printen, K, and Shoemaker, W. C.: *Penetrating wounds of the heart. A review of 80 cases.* Ann. Surg. 168:67, 1968.

193. Jones, E. W., and Helmsworth, J.: *Penetrating wounds of the heart: Thirty years' experience.* Arch. Surg. 96:671, 1968.

194. Sugg, W. L., Rea, W. J., Ecker, R. R., Webb, W. R., Rose, E. F., and Shaw, R. R.: *Penetrating wounds of the heart: An analysis of 459 cases.* J. Thorac. Cardiovasc. Surg. 56:531, 1968.

195. Wilson, R. F., and Bassett, J. S.: *Penetrating wounds of the pericardium and its contents.* J.A.M.A. 195:513, 1966.

196. Mulder, D. G.: *Stab wound of the heart.* Ann. Surg. 160:287, 1964.

197. Bland, E. F., and Beebe, G. W.: *Missiles in the heart. A twenty year follow-up report of World War II cases.* N. Engl. J. Med. 274:1039, 1965.

198. Riemer, R.: Indiscussion of paper by Sugg, W. L., et al.: *Penetrating wounds of the heart.* J. Thorac. Cardiovasc. Surg. 56:545, 1968.

199. Berger, R. L., Gibson, H., Reimer, R. W., and Ramaswamy, K.: *Traumatic aortic regurgitation, ventricular septal defect and fistula of the sinus of Valsalva.* N. Engl. J. Med. 281:887, 1969.

200. Hutchinson, J. E., Beach, P. M., Kaplan, S., and Garvey, J. W.: *Management of penetrating cardiac trauma.* N. Y. State J. Med. 71:1932, 1971.

201. Cleveland, R. J., Kemp, E. V., and Lower, R. R.: *Acute aortic valve insufficiency as a result of a bullet wound. Report of a case of successful treatment.* J. Thorac. Cardiovasc. Surg. 55:123, 1968.

202. Hardy, J. O., and Timmis, H. H.: *Repair of intracardiac gunshot wounds. Report of three cases.* Ann. Surg. 169:906, 1969.

203. Pate, J. W., and Richardson, R. L.: *Penetrating wounds of the cardiac valves.* J.A.M.A. 207:309, 1969.

204. Parmley, L. F., Manion, W. C., and Mattingly, T. W.: *Nonpenetrating traumatic injury of the heart.* Circulation 18:371, 1958.

205. Howard, C. P.: *Aortic insufficiency due to rupture by strain of a normal aortic valve.* Can. Med. Assoc. J. 19:12, 1928.

206. Loop, F. D., Hofmeir, G., and Groves, L. K.: *Traumatic disruption of the aortic valve.* Cleve. Clin. Q. 38:187, 1971.

207. Najafi, H., Dye, W. S., Javid, H., Hunter, J. A., and Julian, O. C.: *Rupture of an otherwise normal aortic valve: Report of two cases and review of the literature.* J. Thorac. Cardiovasc. Surg. 56:57, 1968.

208. Spurny, O. M., and Hara, M.: *Rupture of the aortic valve due to strain.* Am. J. Cardiol. 8:125, 1961.

209. Levine, R. J., Roberts, W. C., and Morrow, A. G.: *Traumatic aortic regurgitation.* Am. J. Cardiol. 10:1962.

210. McLaughlin, J. S., Cowely, R. A., Smith, G., and Matheson, M. A.: *Mitral valve disease from blunt trauma.* J. Thorac. Cardiovasc. Surg. 48:261, 1964.

211. Goggin, M. J., Thompson, F. D., and Jackson, J. W.: *Deceleration trauma to the heart and great vessels after road traffic accidents.* Br. J. Med. 2:767, 1970.

212. Sanders, R. J., Neubuerger, K. T., and Ravin, A.: *Rupture of papillary muscles: Occurrence of rupture of the posterior muscle in posterior myocardial infarction.* Dis. Chest 31:316, 1957.

213. Gomez, A. R., and Jackson, H. A.: *Traumatic rupture of a papillary muscle in a child.* Am. Heart J. 7:522, 1966.

214. Fry, W. A., and Basinger, C. E.: *Traumatic rupture of a papillary muscle of the heart.* Dis. Chest 51:100, 1967.

215. Brandenburg, R. O., McGoon, D. C., Campeau, L., and Guilliani, E.: *Traumatic rupture of the chordae tendineae of the tricuspid valve. Successful repair 24 years later.* Am. J. Cardiol. 18:911, 1966.

216. Tachovsky, T. H., Giuliani, E. R., and Ellis, F. H.: *Prosthetic valve replacement for traumatic tricuspid insufficiency. Report of a case originally diagnosed as Ebstein's malformation.* Am. J. Cardiol. 26:200, 1970.

217. Morgan, J. R., and Forker, A. D.: *Isolated tricuspid regurgitation.* Circulation 43:559, 1971.

218. Croxson, M. S., O'Brien, K. P., and Lowe, J. B.: *Traumatic tricuspid regurgitation. Long term survival.* Br. Heart J. 33:750, 1971.

219. Kremer, R., Chalant, C. H., Hekster, C., Timmermans, A., Gielan, A., and Lavenne, F.: *Insuffisance Tricuspidienne it communication Interventriculaire dues a un Traumatisme Ferme du Thorax, Correction Surgicale.* Acta Cardiol. (Brux.) 22:381, 1967.

220. Shabetai, R., Vadakepat, A., Danielson, G., and Bryant, L.: *Traumatic hemopericardium with tricuspid incompetence.* J. Thorac. Cardiovasc. Surg. 57:294, 1969.

221. Yamada, J, Nagaoka, H., Kondo, N., Taniguchi, K., and Shintomi, Y.: *Surgical treatment of teaumatic tricuspid insufficiency.* Bull. Tokyo Med. Dent. Univ. 17:319, 1970.

222. Libman, E., and Sacks, B.: *A hitherto undescribed form of valvular and mural endocarditis*. Arch. Intern. Med. 33:701, 1924.

223. Gross, L.: *The cardiac lesions in Libman-Sacks disease; with a consideration of its relationship to acute diffuse lupus erythematosus*. Am. J. Pathol. 16:375, 1940.

224. Klemperer, P., Pollack, A. D., and Baehr, G.: *Pathology of disseminated lupus erythematosus*. Arch. Pathol. 32:569, 1941.

225. Griffith, G. C., and Vural, I. L.: *Acute and subacute disseminated lupus erythematosus: A correlation of clinical and post mortem findings in eighteen cases*. Circulation 3:492, 1951.

226. Bennet, J. C., Claybrook, J., Kinsey, H., and Holley, H. L.: *The clinical manifestations of systemic lupus erythematosus*. J. Chronic Dis. 13:411, 1961.

227. Kong, T. Q., Kellum, R. E., and Haserick, J. R.: *Clinical diagnosis of cardiac involvement in systemic lupus erythematosus*. Circulation 26:7, 1962.

228. Baehr, G., Klemperer, P., and Schifrin, A.: *A diffuse disease of the peripheral circulation (usually associated with lupus erythematosus and endocarditis)*. Trans. Assoc. Am. Physicians 50:139, 1935.

229. Humpries, E. M.: *The cardiac lesions of acute disseminated lupus erythematosus*. Ann. Intern. Med. 28:12, 1948.

230. Shearn, M. A.: *The heart in systemic lupus erythematosus*. Am. Heart J. 58:452, 1959.

231. Hejtmancik, M. R., Wright, J. C., Quint, R., and Jennings, I. L.: *The cardiovascular manifestations of systemic lupus erythematosus*. Am. Heart J. 68:119, 1964.

232. Harvey, A. M., Schulman, L. E., Tumulty, P. A., Conley, C. L., and Schoenrich, E. H.: *Systemic lupus erythematosus: Review of the literature and clinical analysis of 138 cases*. Medicine 33:291, 1954.

233. Baggenstoss, A. H., and Rosenberg, E. F.: *Cardiac lesions associated with chronic fectious arthritis*. Arch. Intern. Med. 67:241–258, 1941.

234. Liebowitz, W. B.: *The heart in rheumatoid arthritis (rheumatoid disease)*. Ann. Intern. Med. 58:102, 1963.

235. Roberts, W. C., Kehoe, J. A., Carpenter, D. F., and Golden, A.: *Cardiac valvular lesions in rheumatoid arthritis*. Arch. Intern. Med. 122: 141, 1968.

236. Carpenter, D. F., Golden, A., and Roberts, W. C.: *Quadrivalvular rheumatoid heart disease associated with left bundle branch block*. Am. J. Med. 43:922, 1967.

237. Sokoloff, L.: *The heart in rheumatoid arthritis*. Am. Heart J. 45:635, 1953.

238. Sokoloff, L., McCluskey, R. T., and Bunim, J. J.: *Vascularity of the early subcutaneous nodule of rheumatoid arthritis*. Arch. Pathol. 55:475, 1953.

239. Löffler, W.: *Endocarditis parietalis fibroplastica mit Bluteosinophilie*. Schweiz. Med. Wochenschr. 66:817, 1936.

240. Roberts, W. C., Ross, R. S., Eggleston, J. C., and Massumi, R. A.: *Chronic mitral regurgitation of unresolved etiology in the elderly. A clinicopathologic study of two patients*. Johns Hopkins Med. J. 122:26, 1968.

The Hypertensive Diseases

Evidence that Systemic Hypertension is a Greater Risk Factor to the Development of Other Cardiovascular Diseases than Previously Suspected

"Here, in twentieth-century America, millions of people are sitting or walking around quite unaware that their bodies carry hidden time bombs ticking toward the moment of detonation."

The Honorable Elliot L. Richardson

WILLIAM C. ROBERTS, M.D.
Bethesda, Maryland

This report summarizes the clinical frequencies of systemic hypertension and necropsy evidence of cardiomegaly in various cardiovascular conditions (Table I), termed "the hypertensive diseases" because of their frequent association with systemic hypertension. Although long recognized as a major risk factor, systemic hypertension appears to be an even greater risk factor to the development of various cardiovascular conditions than previously appreciated. Hypertension by itself appears to be the sole underlying factor in most cases of nontraumatic cerebral arterial or aortic (dissection = partial rupture) rupture. In association with hyperlipidemia, hypertension clearly accelerates atherosclerosis and its devastating consequences.

Other than age and sex, systemic hypertension, hyperlipidemia and cigarette smoking are the three major factors that increase the risk of having symptomatic cardiovascular disease. Of the three, two are correctable, smoking by abstinence and hypertension by certain drugs. As yet, it is uncertain whether the reduction of serum lipid levels will decrease the frequency of symptomatic cardiovascular disease. Among patients with symptomatic cardiovascular disease, however, hypertension is more common than hyperlipidemia, and reducing the blood pressure level clearly decreases the frequency of complications of hypertension [1–4]. This report examines several cardiovascular disorders, termed "the hypertensive diseases," as consequences, in whole or in part, of systemic hypertension* (Table I). If cardiomegaly (heart weight greater than

* At what level of blood pressure normotension becomes hypertension is debatable. Certain studies [5] have emphasized that the frequency of complications increase with increasing increments of blood pressure. Although both levels might be considered normal, the person with a systolic pressure of 130 mm Hg is at greater risk of fatal or nonfatal complications than is the person with a systolic pressure of 110 mm Hg. The World Health Organization has defined systemic hypertension as systolic pressure greater than 160 mm Hg or diastolic pressure greater than 95 mm Hg or both. This study defines hypertension as systolic pressure greater than 140 mm Hg or diastolic pressure greater than 90 mm Hg or both. Because the pressure tends to increase with age, persons more than 65 years old are excluded from this analysis.

From the Section of Pathology, National Heart and Lung Institute, National Institutes of Health, Bethesda, Maryland 20014. Requests for reprints should be addressed to Dr. William C. Roberts, Bldg 10A, Rm 3E30, National Institutes of Health, Bethesda, Maryland 20014. Manuscript accepted February 28, 1975.

TABLE I The Frequencies of Systemic Hypertension and Cardiomegaly in Various Cardiovascular Conditions (The Hypertensive Diseases)

Condition	% with Hypertension*	% with Cardiomegaly at Necropsy†
Sudden death	50	70
Angina pectoris	50	75
Acute myocardial infarction‡	50	75
Complications of acute myocardial infarction		
A. Rupture of left ventricular free wall	70	85
B. Rupture of ventricular septum	70	85
C. Rupture of papillary muscle	70	85
D. Left ventricular aneurysm (healed)	70	80
Aneurysm of aorta		
A. Fusiform, sacular or cylindric	60	80
B. Dissecting	80	95
Atherothrombotic obstruction of abdominal aorta or of its branches	70	?
Cerebrovascular accident (stroke)		
A. Atherothrombotic cerebral infarction	50	70
B. Intracerebral hemorrhage	>90	>90
C. Lacunar softenings	>90	>95
D. Charcot-Bouchard aneurysm	>90	>95
Renal failure	>90	>90
Miscellaneous		
A. Calcific aortic valve disease of the elderly	50	70
B. Calcification of the mitral anulus	40	60

* Blood pressure = systolic >140 or diastolic >90 mm Hg. Limited to persons less than 66 years of age.
† Heart weight = women >350 and men >400 g.
‡ Transmural type. Nearly all patients with fatal subendocardial necrosis have cardiomegaly.

400 g in men; greater than 350 g in women) is utilized as an indicator of hypertension, in addition to or in place of the blood pressure measurement, then hypertension is probably an even more common precursor of symptomatic vascular disease than previously realized. Therefore, cardiomegaly at necropsy is recorded (Table I) when this information is available. (To be sure, ischemic heart disease, particularly when associated with congestive cardiac failure, appears capable of enlarging myocardial fibers and, in some patients undoubtedly does so, it appears more reasonable in most cases to attribute the cardiomegaly to hypertension.)

SUDDEN CORONARY DEATH

About 50 per cent of the deaths from ischemic heart disease are sudden (ventricular fibrillation [6], and sudden death is the initial coronary event in about 25 per cent of patients with fatal ischemic heart disease [7–16]). Of the 526 sudden coronary deaths (greater than 24 hours from onset of chest pain) reported by Kuller and associates [16], 38 per cent of those who died had histories of hypertension and 40 per cent had hearts weighing more than 500 g. Thus, probably well over 50 per cent of them had hearts weighing more than 400 g. Among the blacks, the hearts in 55 per cent weighed more than 600 g. Among 24 patients studied personally who had a sudden coronary death (less than 6 hours from onset of chest pain) at least 55 per cent had a positive history of hypertension and 65 per cent had cardiomegaly at necropsy [17].

ANGINA PECTORIS

Most investigators have found that angina pectoris is more frequently found in hypertensive than in normotensive persons [18–27], and this association increases continuously as blood pressure levels rise [27]. Hypertension is present in about 50 per cent of men with angina; this percentage is much higher in women [18]. Indeed, Eppinger and Levine [18] in 1934 considered "the rarity of normal blood pressure in women with angina pectoris helpful in diagnosis of the presence of angina." The percentage of patients with fatal angina (without previously clinically diagnosed myocardial infarction) who have cardiomegaly at necropsy is uncertain, but it is probably about 75 per cent. The major reason for this uncertainty is that most patients with angina pectoris usually either die suddenly and are therefore placed in the "sudden coronary death" category, or they die after an acute myocardial infarction and are then included in the "myocardial infarction" category. Of 72 patients with angina preceding the first diagnosed acute myocardial infarction reported by Francis et al. [22], about 50 per cent had a history of hypertension; at necropsy about 70 per cent had cardiomegaly.

ACUTE MYOCARDIAL INFARCTION

Over-all, about 60 per cent of the patients with fatal acute transmural myocardial infarction have a positive history of hypertension, and about 80 per cent have cardiomegaly at necropsy [28–38]. Not only does hypertension increase the risk of having an acute myocardial infarction, but it also increases the immediate and long-term mortality after an infarction [39–44]. The reason hypertension worsens the prognosis from an acute myocardial infarct is uncertain, but it is probably because hypertension increases the frequency of major complications. Although hypertension is a common precursor of myocardial infarction, the latter is the most common natural cure of hypertension. (Other natural cures include constrictive pericarditis and extensive cardiac amyloidosis [45].)

CARDIAC COMPLICATIONS OF ACUTE MYOCARDIAL INFARCTION

Rupture of the heart during acute myocardial infarction, be it of the left ventricular free wall, ventricular septum (acquired ventricular septal defect) or papillary muscle, is rare in the absence of left ventricular hypertrophy, and its most common cause is systemic hypertension [46]. When rupture occurs, it is nearly always during the first acute myocardial infarction and in patients without previous congestive cardiac failure [46]. Therefore, myocardial scars are rare in patients who die shortly after rupture of a papillary muscle or after perforation of the ventricular septum or left ventricular free wall [46]. Of 42 patients with rupture of the ventricular septum (19 patients) or left ventricular free wall (23 patients) studied personally at necropsy [46], at least 35 (80 per cent) had a positive history of hypertension, none had previous evidence of congestive cardiac failure, and none had clinical evidence of a previous acute myocardial infarction. At necropsy, all had hypertrophied left ventricular free walls, and in 40 (95 per cent) the hearts were increased in weight. Only four had left ventricular scars, and each was small and subendocardial in location. Thirteen of the 42 patients had dilated left ventricular cavities, but in each the dilatation almost certainly was absent before they had the fatal acute myocardial infarct. Rupture may occur more frequently in patients in whom hypertension persists during the acute myocardial infarction, but its presence immediately preceding the rupture is not necessary. The recent study by Snell and Sobel [47] indicates that lowering the blood pressure during an acute myocardial infarction in the hypertensive patient improves the prognosis.

It is also likely that left ventricular aneurysm is found more frequently after an acute myocardial infarction in patients with previous hypertension than in those with previous normotension. A healed anatomic left ventricular aneurysm, for example, is virtually never observed at necropsy except in quite large hearts. The left ventricle may be viewed as being capable of accommodating a systolic pressure of less than 140 mm Hg; when the pressure is higher and acute myocardial infarction occurs, the chances of aneurysmal formation are greater.

ANEURYSM OF AORTA

Just as left ventricular aneurysm from acute myocardial infarction appears to be more frequent in hypertensive than in normotensive patients, abdominal aortic aneurysm (etiology atherosclerosis) [48–53] and dissecting aortic aneurysm [54–70] (other than the type associated with the Marfan and Marfan-like syndromes) are far more frequent in the hypertensive subject. Indeed, both types of aneurysm are infrequent in patients whose hearts are of normal weight. The association of hypertension with aortic dissecting aneurysm has been appreciated for years, but the high frequency of hypertension in patients with abdominal fusiform aneurysms is not commonly appreciated. Burchell [65] stated 20 years ago that "if Marfan's syndrome and pregnancy are excluded . . . aortic dissection is always associated with hypertension . . ." Dissection of the ascending and transverse aorta also is far more frequent in patients with untreated coarctation of the aorta than in those without aortic coarctation [71]. The higher the blood pressure, the greater the likelihood of aortic dissection [65]. Thus, the frequency of aortic dissection in patients with accelerated or malignant hypertension is higher than in patients with "benign" (one of medicine's worse terms) hypertension [65].

It is also likely that generalized aortic dilatation ("senile ectasia") occurs more frequently in the hypertensive than in the normotensive subject. The numbers of elastic fibers in the aorta normally decrease with age, with resultant weakening of its wall [72]. Consequently, the higher the intraluminal pressure, the more the aortic expansion. Precordial diastolic, basal, blowing murmurs in the elderly person may result from this aortic dilatation, and these murmurs are more frequent in the hypertensive than in the normotensive person [73].

ATHEROTHROMBOTIC OBSTRUCTION OF THE ABDOMINAL AORTA OR OF ITS BRANCHES

The syndrome of thrombotic obliteration of the aortic bifurcation, described by Leriche in 1940 [74], is often associated with hypertension [75–79]. Hypertension was present in each of the four patients he described in 1948 [77], in seven of 11 patients described by Kekwick et al. [78], and in nine of 13 patients described by Gunning and associates [79]. Atherosclerotic obstruction of arteries in the legs (arteriosclerosis obliterans) with intermittent claudication also occurs more frequently in the hypertensive than in the normotensive person [80–85]. Information regarding the weight of the heart in a large series of patients with obstructed abdominal aortas or more peripheral arteries is unavailable, but it is highly likely that most patients with this condition also have cardiomegaly at necropsy.

CEREBROVASCULAR ACCIDENTS

Atherothrombotic (nonembolic) Cerebral Infarction. After age, hypertension is the most common and potent precursor of atherothrombotic cerebral infarction (ACI), which accounts for 60 to 80 per cent of all strokes [86–101]. Its contribution is direct [93]. In patients with asymptomatic, casual hypertension the risk of ACI is about four times that of normotensive subjects [93]. The frequency of hypertension in patients with ACI has been reported to be from 50 to 75 per cent [86,87,89,91–94]. Heart weight is increased in the majority of patients with fatal ACI, and evidence of left ventricular hypertrophy on the electrocardiogram increases the risk of cerebral infarction ninefold (only a threefold increase, however, after adjustment for coexisting hypertension) [95]. Of patients with hypertensive heart disease, one-half will have one or more cerebral infarcts at necropsy [89,101]. As with acute myocardial infarction, the presence of hypertension increases the mortality rate at the time of the ACI [87,92,93,95]. Furthermore, although a person who survives a cerebral infarction for more than a month is more likely to die of cardiac disease than of a subsequent stroke [96,100], the frequency of a new ACI after recovery from the first one is greater in the hypertensive than in the normotensive person [92]. Treatment of hypertension clearly diminishes the frequency of ACI [1–4]. The frequency of hypertension and of electrocardiographic evidence of left ventricular hypertrophy in patients with transient ischemic attacks,* a frequent percursor of ACI, is probably similar to that of patients with ACI alone [95,102–104].

Primary Intracerebral Hemorrhage (Significant hemorrhage into the brain parenchyma, unassociated with trauma, arterial aneurysms, inflammatory vascular lesions, arteriovenous or angiomatous formations, neoplasms or blood dyscrasias). Primary intracerebral hemorrhage almost always is preceded by hypertension [93], and some investigators define primary intracerebral hemorrhage as a disease exclusively of hypertensive persons. Millikan et al. [105] include the presence of systemic hypertension as one of their four criteria for the clinical diagnosis of nontraumatic intracerebral hemorrhage. The hearts of patients with primary intracerebral hemorrhage are nearly always increased in weight. Of 347 patients (193 males, 154 females) with primary intracerebral hemorrhage, 89 per cent had left ventricular hypertrophy at necropsy: the hearts in 87 per cent of the women weighed more than 400 g and the hearts in 91 per cent of the men weighed more than 420 g [106].

Lacunar Softenings. Lacunar strokes or infarcts are small infarcts, usually multiple and cystic, of the basal ganglia or pons resulting from occlusion of penetrating branches chiefly from the middle or posterior cerebral or basal arteries [107,108]. At their peak they cause a relatively minor neurologic deficit, which, although it appears submaximal, actually represents the total maximal stroke and not the initial stage of a devastating paralysis. Prognosis is good. Four lacunar strokes have been identified [109]: (1) pure motor hemiplegia and hemiparesis; (2) pure sensory stroke; (3) a syndrome in which cerebellar ataxia is combined with weakness of the corresponding leg; and (4) dysarthria and clumsiness of one hand. Systemic hypertension nearly always is a precursor of the lacunar softening, the most common cause of stroke in persons over 60 years of age [107–109].

Charcot-Bouchard Aneurysm. Miliary aneurysms of very small cerebral arteries were described in 1868 by Charcot and Bouchard in 60 elderly patients who died of cerebral hemorrhage [110]. These aneurysms occur on small perforating arteries of less than 1 mm diameter, especially in basal ganglia and subcortical regions. The media disappears at the neck of the aneurysm whose walls consist of intima and adventitia. Cole and Yates [111] found these intracerebral microaneurysms at necropsy in 46 per cent of 100 hypertensive patients and in only 7 per cent of 100 normotensive patients matched for age and sex. Massive intracerebral hemorrhage occurred in 20 of the 100 hypertensive patients, 18 of whom had microaneurysms. In contrast, massive intracere-

* Transient (10 to 30 minutes) disturbances of neurologic function of 24 hours' duration occurring in the territory of supply of the carotid or vertebrobasilar arteries and believed on clinical grounds to be associated with atherosclerotic disease in those arteries or in their branches [102].

bral hemorrhage occurred in only 1 of the 100 normotensive patients, and no microaneurysm was found in that patient. The microaneurysms are age dependent: they occurred in 71 per cent of the hypertensive patients aged 65 to 69 years and in only 10 per cent of the hypertensive patients less than 50 years of age. All 18 patients with microaneurysms and normotension were more than 65 years of age.

It is likely that these microaneurysms are responsible for most primary intracerebral hemorrhages in patients over 40 years of age with hypertension [110–112]. These aneurysms clearly are unrelated to atherosclerosis, and they provide the explanation for the much closer relationship between cerebral hemorrhage and hypertension than that between cerebral infarction and hypertension. The latter obviously is the result of atherosclerosis and more analogous to myocardial infarction. Cerebral hemorrhage involves small cerebral arteries, the medial weakening leading to aneurysm and rupture, and therefore more analogous to dissecting aortic aneurysm.

RENAL FAILURE

Renal disease is both a cause and an effect of hypertension. Hypertension can be produced by parenchymal renal diseases (glomerulonephritis, pyelonephritis, tumor, cysts) and by renal arterial and renal ostial disease, the most common being atherosclerosis. Although the pathologic features of the parenchymal renal diseases are often distinctive, their separation from nephrosclerosis, the most common renal consequence of hypertension, is often not easy. Thus, determining whether renal disease is the cause or the consequence of hypertension may be difficult. Classically, in nephrosclerosis the kidneys are involved uniformly, the weights are usually normal, their surfaces are diffusely finely "granular," fibrotic and the lumens of the vascular channels, particularly the arterioles, are narrowed [113]. There appears to be some relationship between the severity of the hypertension, especially the diastolic pressure, and the arterial and arteriolar damage. Of patients with "benign" essential (primary) hypertension, about 10 per cent have renal failure and then relatively late. In the accelerated or malignant phase of hypertension, the renal arteriolar changes appear soon after the striking elevation of pressure, and the resulting damage to the kidneys is usually severe. The vascular lesions are accompanied by severe parenchymal damage including hemorrhagic infarction of glomeruli, tubular degeneration and cellular infiltration of the interstitium. In contrast to patients with mild essential hypertension, those with accelerated hypertension frequently present initially with azotemia, and, if untreated, usually die within a year with evidence of advanced renal failure.

It is difficult to arrive at a precise figure regarding the percentage of patients with parenchymal renal disease who have hypertension. If the disease is one primarily of glomeruli (glomerulonephritis) the figure is high. If it is one involving primarily the tubules and interstitium (pyelonephritis), the figure is low. If both kidneys are involved uniformly, this percentage tends to be lower than when only one kidney is involved but that one severely. It is clear, however, that nearly all patients who die in chronic renal failure have hypertension and left ventricular hypertrophy.

MISCELLANEOUS CONSEQUENCES OF HYPERTENSION

Calcific deposits in the **aortic valve** and **mitral anulus** are extremely common in elderly patients and in them have been attributed to the consequences of wear and tear [114,115]. Their frequency is higher in patients with hypertension than in those with normotension [115]. Furthermore, these calcific deposits tend to occur at younger ages in persons with hypertension than in normotensive persons [115]. Hypertension greatly increases the closing pressures on both mitral and aortic valves, and thus, the amount of resulting wear and tear. The calcific deposits are located on the aortic aspects of the aortic valve cusps and, if extensive enough, may produce stenosis from the immobility imparted to the cusps by the heavy calcific deposits [114]. Similar calcific deposits are located on the undersurface of the posterior mitral leaflet and, if extensive enough, can cause the mitral valve to be incompetent [115] and rarely, stenotic [116].

Not only does hypertension increase or accelerate the development of calcific deposits in the aortic valve and mitral anulus, it also is associated with a marked increased frequency of **calcific deposits in the coronary arteries.** Nearly 90 per cent of patients with hypertension studied by Frink and associates [117] had calcific deposits in their coronary arteries by roentgenographic examination of the heart at necropsy, whereas less than 50 per cent of those with normal pressures had coronary calcific deposits.

Although usually asymptomatic (indeed, some physicians believe that hypertensive persons may feel better than normotensive persons— "supernormal"), headaches, pounding precordia and arterial pulses, local bleeding (nosebleeds), increased risk from operations and other trauma (because of more rapid blood loss), increased rubor of skin (a cosmetic irritant), etc., may be consequences of elevated blood pressure levels. Because of their tendency to raise the blood pressure level immediately, certain types of exercises, calisthenics (push-ups) or weight lifting, and sexual intercourse may be more dangerous in the hypertensive person. A recent study suggests a higher incidence of **cancer,** primarily of the lung and colon, in hypertensive persons than in normotensive persons [118].

COMMENTS

Systemic hypertension acts as a major risk factor in the development of cardiovascular disease in two ways: (1) by increasing the deposition of atherosclerotic plaques (intimal lesions) in major arteries most commonly causing luminal **narrowing** with resulting organ ischemia or infarction or both, and (2) by weakening the media of certain arteries causing **aneurysms** which may or may not rupture. Its affect on the arterial media is direct whereas its effect on the arterial intima is indirect. Hypertension is the only known major underlying factor in two conditions: intracerebral microaneurysm (with or without rupture) and dissecting aortic aneurysm (excluding patients with the Marfan and Marfan-like syndrome [110]), both of which are associated with medial weakening or disruption. Reduction in blood pressure clearly leads to a reduction in the incidence of nontraumatic intracerebral hemorrhage and of dissecting aortic aneurysm [2–4]. Thus, both of these conditions are virtually preventable simply by maintaining a normal blood pressure.

The more common consequence of hypertension, however, is its ability to increase the amount of atherosclerotic plaquing in various arteries. This effect, however, is not direct because hypertension in population groups with normal (less than 200 mg/100 ml) serum cholesterol levels do not have more or larger atherosclerotic plaques than do the normotensive persons in those populations. Hypertension, for example, is by far the most common cardiovascular disease in the black African [119]. Yet, complicated atherosclerotic plaques (as opposed to fatty and fibrous plaques), the only ones capable of producing significant luminal narrowing [17,120], have not been reported in either the hypertensive or the normotensive black African. Experimentally, however, lipid-induced atherosclerosis clearly is accelerated by hypertension [121–123]. Furthermore, certain complications of atherosclerosis, angina pectoris, myocardial infarction, sudden coronary death, atherothrombotic cerebral infarction, intermittent claudication, are clearly more frequent in hypertensive persons in the affluent or developed countries than in normotensive persons residing in the same countries [14–16,18,82,93,95]. Thus, hypertension accelerates or increases atherosclerosis only in hypercholesterolemic (serum cholesterol greater than 200 mg/100 ml) population groups and not in those with normal serum cholesterol levels.

Other examples in human subjects of hypertension's increasing atherosclerosis are provided by patients with coarctation of the aorta and by those with pulmonary hypertension. Among patients with aortic isthmic coarctation, atherosclerotic plaques are always more frequent and more extensive proximal to the narrowing than distal to it. Pulmonary atherosclerotic plaques develop in young persons with severely elevated pulmonary arterial pressures whereas plaques in these arteries are virtually never observed in young persons with normal pulmonary arterial pressures. Indeed, pulmonary hypertension may accelerate the development of atherosclerosis in the pulmonary circulation to a greater extent than may systemic hypertension accelerate the development of atherosclerosis in the systemic circulation. Among patients with balanced pulmonary and systemic systolic pressures, for example, the amount of atherosclerosis is usually considerably more extensive in the pulmonary circuit than in the systemic circuit.

Although hypercholesterolemia (serum cholesterol greater than 200 mg/100 ml) may be necessary for hypertension to accelerate atherosclerosis, a certain level of blood pressure is required for atherosclerosis to develop no matter what the level of serum cholesterol. The serum cholesterol level is similar in both venous and arterial blood in the same person. Yet, atherosclerotic plaques do not develop in veins under normal pressure no matter what the serum cholesterol level. However, in veins subjected to increased pressure, such as occurs in arteriovenous fistulas or in veins used for arterial bypass [124], arteriosclerotic plaques do develop. This phenomenon also is seen in the portal and mesenteric vasculature of patients with portal hypertension [125].

The mechanism by which hypertension accelerates atherosclerosis is uncertain. Possibly, the higher pressure increases intimal damage, which provides a nidus for thrombus or lipid deposition with subsequent plaque formation. Likewise, the mechanism by which hypertension causes medial weakening is uncertain. Although the media of aorta normally contain acid mucopolysaccharide (AMP) material, the amount of AMP (and "cystic medial necrosis") in the aortic media is increased in persons with systemic hypertension compared to that in normotensive subjects of similar age [126]. This small quantitative increase in AMP, however, does not provide, in my view, an adequate explanation for the occurrence of dissecting aortic aneurysm. Indeed, the amount of AMP is not increased at sites of aortic rupture compared to nonruptured sites. The mechanism of cerebral aneurysm formation is not understood either. Possibly, focal thinning of the media is a common occurrence at birth, and the thinned media thereafter progressively bulges simply as a response to the increased intra-arterial pressure. Certainly there is no increased amount of AMP in the cerebral arteries which are purely muscular arteries. The presence of aortic medial dissection and of cerebral microaneurysm is unrelated to the occurrence of atherosclerosis. Indeed, the greater the amount of atherosclerosis, the less the likelihood of aortic dissection or of cerebral aneurysm rupture.

Although recognized for some time as a major risk factor to the development of ischemic heart disease, systemic hypertension is the only risk factor (other than advanced age) which increases mortality during an acute myocardial infarction and during the first six years after recovery from an acute myocardial infarction [127–130]. The explanation for the increased mortality during acute myocardial infarction is uncertain, but it probably is the increased frequency of rupture of the left ventricular free wall, ventricular septum or papillary muscle, or the increased propensity to the development of left ventricular aneurysm or both in the hypertensive subject compared to the normotensive person. The explanation for the poorer long-term prognosis after recovery from an acute myocardial infarction in the hypertensive person is less certain. It is likely that in hypertensive persons larger areas of myocardial necrosis develop at the time of acute myocardial infarction than in normotensive persons and thus larger myocardial scars remain. The greater the amount of scarring, the greater the likelihood of persistent left ventricular failure, and congestive heart failure is considerably more frequent in the hypertensive than in the normotensive patient [131]. Kannel and associates [131] considered hypertension a causative factor in 75 per cent of their patients with congestive cardiac failure. The incidence of congestive cardiac failure increased in both their female and male patients at all ages with increasing systolic or diastolic pressure. Even in the absence of overt congestive cardiac failure, the function of the hypertrophied, hypertensive left ventricle often is impaired with a decreased ejection rate and prolonged tension-time index [132].

Despite its being such a devastating risk factor to the development of cardiovascular disease and despite its being the most responsive of the cardiovascular diseases to medical therapy, systemic hypertension is the most neglected, by both physician and patient, of all major cardiovascular diseases. It has been found, from community studies, that just under one half of the adults in the U.S.A. who have hypertension are aware that they have it (Figure 1) [133].

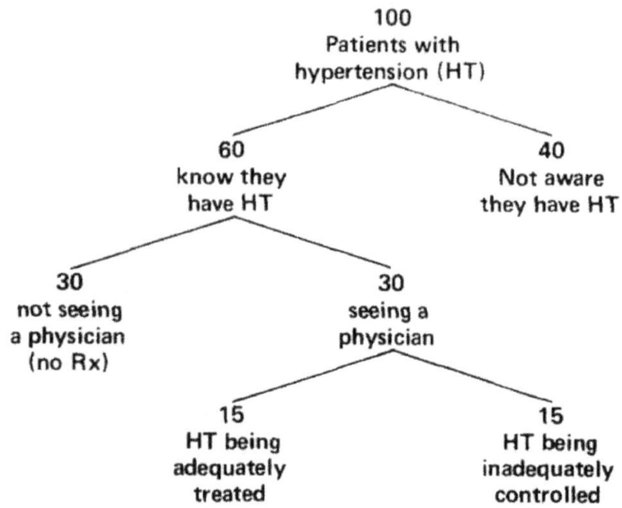

Figure 1. *Incidence of hypertension based on data collected by Wilber and Barrow [133].*

Furthermore, only half of those who are aware of their hypertension are receiving therapy, and of them, only half are receiving proper therapy. Another study, which entailed reviewing charts of patients discharged from four hospitals, disclosed that the blood pressure had been recorded on admission in only 75 of every 100 patients, and of them 30 had hypertension (Figure 2) [134]. A diagnosis of hypertension, however, appeared as part of the discharge diagnosis in only 2 of these 30 patients. Obviously, the only way to prevent the development of complications of hypertension is first, to recognize the occurrence of an elevated systemic arterial pressure and second, to lower it.

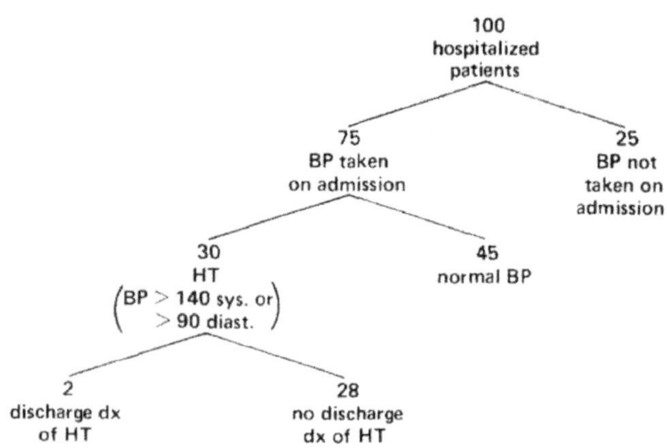

Figure 2. *Blood pressure recorded in patients on their admission to the hospital based on data collected by Frohlich et al. [134]. BP = blood pressure; diast. = diastolic; dx = diagnosis; HT = hypertension; and sys. = systolic.*

REFERENCES

1. Hamilton M, Thompson EN, Wisniewski TKM: Role of blood pressure control in preventing complications of hypertension. Lancet 1: 235, 1964.
2. Veterans Administration Cooperative Study Group on anti-hypertensive agents. Effects of treatment on morbidity in hypertension. Results in patients with diastolic blood pressures averaging 115 through 129 mm. Hg. JAMA 202: 1028, 1967.
3. Veterans Administration Cooperative Study Group on Anti-hypertensive agents. Effects of treatment on morbidity in hypertension. II. Results in patients with diastolic blood pressure, averaging 90 through 114 mm. Hg. JAMA 213: 1143, 1970.
4. Freis ED: Effectiveness of drug therapy in hypertension: present status. A review. Circ Res 28 and 29 (suppl): II-70, 1971.
5. Kannel WB, Gordon T, Schwartz MJ: Systolic versus diastolic blood pressure and risk of coronary heart disease. The Framingham Study. Am J Cardiol 27: 335, 1971.
6. Lown B, Kosowsky BD, Klein MD: Pathogenesis, prevention, and treatment of arrhythmias in myocardial infarction. Circulation 39 and 40 (suppl): IV-261, 1969.
7. Moritz AR, Zamcheck N: Sudden and unexpected deaths in young soldiers: diseases responsible for such deaths during World War II. Arch Pathol 42: 459, 1946.
8. Spain DM, Bradess VA, Mohr C: Coronary atherosclerosis as a cause of unexpected and unexplained death. JAMA 174: 384, 1960.
9. Kuller L: Sudden and unexpected non-traumatic deaths in adults: a review of epidemiological and clinical studies. J Chronic Dis 19: 1165, 1966.
10. Kuller L, Lilienfeld, A, Fisher R: Epidemiological study of sudden and unexpected deaths due to arteriosclerotic heart disease. Circulation 34: 1056, 1966.
11. Kuller L, Lilienfeld A, Fisher R: An epidemiological study of sudden and unexpected deaths in adults. Medicine 46: 341, 1967.
12. Shapiro S, Weinblatt E, Frank CW, Sager RV: Incidence of coronary heart disease in a population insured for medical care (HIP). Myocardial infarction, angina pectoris, and possible myocardial infarction. Am J Public Health 59: 1 (Part II), 1969.
13. Fulton M, Julian DG, Oliver MF: Sudden death and myocardial infarction. Circulation 39 and 40 (suppl): IV-182, 1969.
14. Chiang BN, Perlman LV, Fulton M, Ostrander LD Jr, Epstein FH: Predisposing factors in sudden cardiac deaths in Tecumseh, Michigan. Circulation 41: 31, 1970.
15. Gordon T, Kannel WB: Premature mortality from coronary heart disease. The Framingham study. JAMA 215: 1617, 1971.
16. Kuller LH, Cooper M, Perper J, Fisher R: Myocardial infarction and sudden death in an urban community. Bull NY Acad Med (2nd Series) 49: 532, 1973.
17. Roberts WC, Buja LM: The frequency and significance of coronary arterial thrombi and other observations in fatal acute myocardial infarction. A study of 107 necropsy patients. Am J Med 52: 425, 1972.
18. Eppinger EC, Levine SA: Angina pectoris. Some clinical considerations, with special reference to prognosis. Arch Intern Med 53: 120, 1934.
19. Block WJ Jr, Crumpacher EL, Dry TJ: Prognosis of angina pectoris, observations in 6,882 cases. JAMA 150: 259, 1952.
20. Richards DW, Bland EF, White PD: Completed 25 year follow-up study of 456 patients with angina pectoris. J Chronic Dis 4: 423, 1956.
21. Seim S: Angina pectoris: a prognostic study. Acta Med Scand 166: 255, 1960.
22. Francis RL, Achor RWP, Brown AL, Jr: Angina pectoris preceding initial myocardial infarction. A clinicopathologic study. Arch Intern Med 112: 226, 1963.
23. Shurtleff D: The Framingham Study. An Epidemiological Investigation of Cardiovascular Disease, Sect 26. (Kannel WB, Gordon T, eds), U.S. Government Printing Office, Washington, D.C. 1970.
24. Roseman RH, Friedman M, Straus R, Jenkins CD, Zyzanski SJ, Wurm M: Coronary heart disease in the Western collaborative group study. J Chronic Dis 23: 173, 1970.
25. Chapman JM, Coulson , Clark VA, Borun ER: The differential effect of serum cholesterol, blood pressure and weight on the incidence of myocardial infarction and angina pectoris. J Chronic Dis 23: 631, 1971.
26. Kannel WB, Feinleib M: Natural history of angina pectoris in the Framingham study. Prognosis and survival. Am J Cardiol 29: 154, 1972.
27. Medalie JH, Snyder M, Groen JJ, Neufeld HN, Goldbourt U, Riss E: Angina pectoris among 10,000 men. 5 year incidence and univariate analysis. Am J Med 55: 583, 1973.
28. Nathanson, MH: Disease of the coronary arteries. Clinical and pathologic features. Am J Med Sci 170: 240, 1925.
29. Parkinson J, Bedford DE: Cardiac infarction and coronary thrombosis. Lancet 1: 4, 1928.
30. Levine SA: Coronary thrombosis. Its various clinical features. Medicine 8: 245, 1929.
31. Bartels, EC, Smith HL: Gross cardiac hypertrophy in myocardial infarction. Am J Med Sci 184: 452, 1932.
32. Master AM, Jaffe HL, Dack S: The treatment and the immediate prognosis of coronary artery thrombosis (267 attacks). Am Heart J 12: 549, 1936.
33. Levy H, Boas EP: Coronary artery disease in women. JAMA 107: 97, 1936.
34. Rosenbaum FF, Levine SA: Prognostic value of various clinical and electrocardiographic features of acute myocardial infarction. I. Immediate prognosis. Arch Intern Med 68: 913, 1941.
35. Levine SA, Rosenbaum FF: Prognostic value of various clinical and electrocardiographic features of acute myocardial infarction. II. Ultimate prognosis. Arch Intern Med 68: 1215, 1941.
36. Billings FT, Kalstone BM, Spencer JL, Ball OT, Meneely GR: Prognosis of acute myocardial infarction. Am J Med 7: 356, 1949.
37. Zinn WJ, Crosby RS: Myocardial infarction. I. Statistical analysis of 679 autopsy-proved cases. Am J Med 8: 169, 1950.
38. Mulcahy R, Hickey N, Maurer B: Coronary heart disease in women. Study of risk factors in 100 patients less than 60 years of age. Circulation 36: 577, 1967.
39. Bland EF, White PD: Coronary thrombosis (with myocardial infarction) ten years later. JAMA 117: 1171, 1941.
40. Cole DR, Singian EB, Katz LN: The long term prognosis following myocardial infarction, and some factors which affect it. Circulation 9: 321, 1954.
41. Biörck G, Sievers J, Blomqvist G: Studies on myocardial infarction in Malmö 1935–1954. III. Follow-up studies from a hospital material. Acta Med Scand 162: 81, 1958.
42. Beard OW, Hipp HR, Robins M, Taylor JS, Ebert RV, Beran LG: Initial myocardial infarction among 503 veterans. Five-year survival. Am J Med 28: 871, 1960.
43. Pell S, D'Alonzo CA: Immediate mortality and five-year survival of employed men with a first myocardial infarction. N Engl J Med 270: 915, 1964.

44. Kannel WB, Gordon T, Castelli WP, Margolis JR: Electrocardiographic left ventricular hypertrophy and risk of coronary heart disease. The Framingham study. Ann Intern Med 72: 813, 1970.
45. Buja LM, Khoi NB, Roberts WC: Clinically significant cardiac amyloidosis. Clinicopathologic findings in 15 patients. Am J Cardiol 26: 394, 1970.
46. Roberts WC, Ronan JA Jr, Harvey WP: Rupture of the left ventricular free wall (LVFW) or ventricular septum (VS) secondary to acute myocardial infarction (AMI): an occurrence virtually limited to the first transmural AMI in a hypertensive individual. Am J Cardiol 35: 166, 1975.
47. Shell WE, Sobel BE: Protection of jeopardized ischemic myocardium by reduction of ventricular afterload. N Engl J Med 291: 481, 1974.
48. Estes JE Jr: Abdominal aortic aneurysm: A study of one hundred and two cases. Circulation 2: 258, 1950.
49. Crane C: Arteriosclerotic aneurysm of the abdominal aorta. Some pathological and clinical correlations. N Engl J Med 253: 954, 1955.
50. Wheelock F, Shaw RS: Aneurysm of the abdominal aorta and iliac arteries. N Engl J Med 255: 72, 1956.
51. Brindley P, Stembridge VA: Aneurysms of the aorta. A clinicopathologic study of 369 necropsy cases. Am J Pathol 32: 67, 1956.
52. Sommerville RL, Allen EV, Edwards JE: Bland and infected arteriosclerotic abdominal aortic aneurysms: a clinicopathologic study. Medicine 38: 207, 1959.
53. Halpert B, Willms RK: Aneurysms of the aorta. An analysis of 249 necropsies. Arch Pathol 74: 163, 1962.
54. MacCallum WG: Dissecting aneurysm. Bull Johns Hopkins Hosp 20: 9, 1909.
55. Tyson MD: Dissecting aneurysms. Am J Pathol 7: 581, 1931.
56. Shennan T: Dissecting aneurysms. Medical Research Council. Special Report Series, No. 193, London. His Majesty's Stationary Office, 1934.
57. Weiss S: The clinical course of spontaneous dissecting aneurysm of the aorta. Med Clin North Am 18: 1117, 1935.
58. McGeachy TE, Paullin JE: Dissecting aneurysm of the aorta. JAMA 108: 1690, 1937.
59. Glendy RE, Castleman B, White PD: Dissecting aneurysm of aorta: clinical and anatomic analysis of 19 cases (13 acute) with notes on differential diagnosis. Am Heart J 13: 129, 1937.
60. David P, McPeak EM, Vivas-Salas E, White PD: Dissecting aneurysm of the aorta: a review of 17 autopsied cases of acute dissecting aneurysm of the aorta encountered at the Massachesetts General Hospital from 1937 to 1946 inclusive, eight of which were correctly diagnosed ante mortem. Ann Intern Med 27: 405, 1947.
61. Levinson DC, Edmeades DT, Griffith GC: Dissecting aneurysm of the aorta. Its clinical, electrocardiographic and laboratory features. Report of fifty-eight autopsied cases. Circulation 1: 360, 1950.
62. Gore I, Seiwert VJ: Dissecting aneurysm of the aorta. Pathologic aspects; an analysis of eighty-five fatal cases. Arch Pathol 53: 121, 1952.
63. Gore I: Pathogenesis of dissecting aneurysm of the aorta. Arch Pathol 53: 142, 1952.
64. Gore I: Dissecting aneurysms of the aorta in persons under forty years of age. Arch Pathol 55: 1, 1953.
65. Burchell HB: Aortic dissection (dissecting hematoma; dissecting aneurysm of the aorta). Circulation 12: 1068, 1955.
66. Halpert B, Brown CA: Dissecting aneurysms of the aorta. Study of 12 cases. Arch Pathol 60: 378, 1955.
67. Hirst AE Jr, Jones VJ Jr, Kime SW Jr: Dissecting aneurysm of aorta: A review of 505 cases. Medicine 37: 217, 1958.
68. De Bakey ME, Henly WS, Cooley DA, Crawford ES, Morris GC Jr: Surgical treatment of dissecting aneurysm of the aorta. Analysis of seventy-two cases. Circulation 24: 290, 1961.
69. Lindsay J Jr, Hurst JW: Clinical features and prognosis in dissecting aneurysm of the aorta. A re-appraisal. Circulation 35: 880, 1967.
70. Gore I, Hirst AE Jr: Dissecting aneurysm of the aorta. Cardiovasc Clin 5: 239, 1973.
71. Reifenstein GH, Levine SA, Gross RE: Coarctation of the aorta: review of 104 autopsied cases of "adult type" two years of age or older. Am Heart J 33: 146, 1947.
72. Ashworth CT, Haynes DM: Lesions in elastic arteries associated with hypertension. Am J Pathol 24: 195, 1948.
73. Puchner TC, Huston JH, Hellmuth GA: Aortic valve insufficiency in arterial hypertension. Am J Cardiol 5: 758, 1960.
74. Leriche R: De la rèsection du carrefour aortoiliaque avec double sympathectomie lombaire pour thrombose artèritique de l'aorte: Le syndrome de l'oblitèration terminoaortique par artèrite. Presse mėd 48: 601, 1940.
75. Gross H, Philips B: Complete occlusion of the abdominal aorta: a review of seven cases. Am J Med Sci 200: 203, 1940.
76. Lueth HC: Thrombosis of the abdominal aorta: a report of four cases showing the variability of symptoms. Ann Intern Med 13: 1167, 1940.
77. Leriche R, Morel A: The syndrome of thrombotic obliteration of the aortic bifurcation. Ann Surg 127: 193, 1948.
78. Kekwick A, McDonald L, Semple R: Obliterative disease of the abdominal aorta and iliac arteries with intermittent claudication. Q J Med 21: 185, 1952.
79. Gunning AJ, Hackett MEJ, MacKenzie JR, Oliver DO, Pickering GW, Tibbs DJ: A clinicopathological study of aorto-iliac thrombosis (the Leriche syndrome). Q J Med 35 (N.S.): 475, 1966.
80. Juergens JL, Barker NW, Hines EA Jr: Arteriosclerosis obliterans: review of 520 cases with special reference to pathogenic and prognostic factors. Circulation 21: 118, 1960.
81. Tillgren C: Obliterative arterial disease of the lower limbs. II. A study of the cause of disease. Acta Med Scand 178: 103, 1965.
82. Kannel WB, Skinner JJ Jr, Schwartz MJ, Shurtleff D: Intermittent claudication. Incidence in the Framingham study. Circulation 41: 875, 1970.
83. Kannel WB, Shurtleff D: The natural history of arteriosclerosis obliterans. Cardiovasc Clin 3: 37, 1971.
84. Schenk EA: Pathology of occlusive disease of the lower extremities. Cardiovasc Clin 5: 287, 1973.
85. Lippmann HI: Peripheral vascular disease today. Bull NY Acad Med 49: 674, 1973.
86. Hicks SP, Warren S: Infarction of the brain without thrombosis. An analysis of one-hundred cases with autopsy. Arch Pathol 52: 403, 1951.
87. David NJ, Heyman A: Factors influencing the prognosis of cerebral thrombosis and infarction due to atherosclerosis. J Chronic Dis 11: 394, 1960.
88. Low-Beer T, Phear D: Cerebral infarction and hypertension. Lancet 1: 1303, 1961.
89. Vost A, Wolochow DA, Howell DA: Incidence of infarcts of the brain in heart disease. J Pathol Bact 88: 463, 1964.
90. Prineas J, Marshall J: Hypertension and cerebral infarction. Br Med J 1: 14, 1966.
91. Louis S, McDowell F: Stroke in young adults. Ann Intern Med 66: 932, 1967.
92. Baker RN, Schwartz WS, Ramseyer JC: Prognosis among survivors of ischemic stroke. Neurology 18: 933, 1968.
93. Kannel WB, Wolf PA, Verter J, McNamara PM: Epidemiologic assessment of the role of blood pressure in

stroke. The Framingham Study. JAMA 214: 301, 1970.

94. Heyden S, Heyman A, Goree JA: Nonembolic occlusion of the middle cerebral and carotid arteries—a comparison of predisposing factors. Stroke 1: 363, 1970.

95. Kannel WB: Current status of the epidemiology of brain infarction associated with occlusive arterial disease. Stroke 2: 295, 1971.

96. Whisnant JP, Fitzgibbons JP, Kurland LT, Sayre GP: Natural history of stroke in Rochester, Minnesota, 1945 through 1954. Stroke 2: 11, 1971.

97. Kannel WB, Gordon T, Wolf PA, McNamara P: Hemoglobin and the risk of cerebral infarction: The Framingham Study. Stroke 3: 409, 1972.

98. Wolf PA, Kannel WB, McNamara PM, Gordon T: The role of impaired cardiac function in atherothrombotic brain infarction: The Framingham Study. Am J Public Health 63: 52, 1973.

99. Siekert RG, Reagan TJ: Clinical and pathologic correlations in ischemic cerebrovascular disease. Cardiovasc Clin 5: 311, 1973.

100. Matsumoto N, Whisnant JP, Kurland LT, Okazaki H: Natural history of stroke in Rochester, Minnesota, 1955 through 1969: an extension of a previous study, 1945 through 1954. Stroke 4: 20, 1973.

101. Hudson AJ, Hyland HH: Hypertensive cerebrovascular disease: a clinical and pathologic review of 100 cases. Ann Intern Med 49: 1049, 1958.

102. Marshall J: The natural history of transient ischaemic cerebro-vascular attacks. Q J Med 33: 309, 1964.

103. Acheson J, Hutchinson EC: Observations on the natural history of transient cerebral ischaemia. Lancet 2: 871, 1964.

104. Whisnant JP, Matsumoto N, Elveback LR: Transient cerebral ischemic attacks in a community: Rochester, Minnesota, 1955 through 1969. Mayo Clin Proc 48: 194, 1973.

105. Millikan CH, Siekert RG, Whisnant JP: The clinical pattern in certain types of occlusive cerebrovascular disease. Circulation 22: 1002, 1960.

106. Stehbens WE: Pathology of the Cerebral Blood Vessels. Saint Louis, C.V. Mosby Co., 1972, p 284.

107. Fisher CM: Lacunes: small deep cerebral infarcts. Neurology 15: 774, 1965.

108. Fisher CM: The arterial lesions underlying lacunes. Acta Neuropath 12: 1, 1969.

109. Fisher CM: A lacunar stroke. The dysarthria-clumsy hand syndrome. Neurology 17: 614, 1967.

110. Pickering G: Hypertension. Definitions, natural histories and consequences. Am J Med 52: 570, 1972.

111. Cole FM, Yates PO: The occurrence and significance of intracerebral micro-aneurysms. J Pathol Bact 93: 393, 1967.

112. Fisher CM: Cerebral miliary aneurysms in hypertension. Am J Pathol 66: 313, 1972.

113. Bell ET, Clawson BJ: Primary (essential) hypertension. A study of four hundred and twenty cases. Arch Pathol 5: 939, 1928.

114. Roberts WC, Perloff JK, Costantino T: Severe valvular aortic stenosis in patients over 65 years of age. A clinicopathologic study. Am J Cardiol 27: 497, 1971.

115. Roberts WC, Perloff JK: Mitral valvular disease. A clinicopathologic survey of the conditions causing the mitral valve to function abnormally. Ann Intern Med 77: 939, 1972.

116. deLeon AC, Hammer WJ, Roberts WC: Mitral stenosis resulting from calcification of the mitral anulus. (In preparation).

117. Frink RJ, Achor RWP, Brown AL Jr, Kincaid OW, Brandenburg RO: Significance of calcification of the coronary arteries. Am J Cardiol 26: 241, 1970.

118. Dyer AR: High blood pressure: A risk factor for cancer mortality? Circulation 49 and 50: III-100, 1974.

119. Hutt MSR: Pathology of African cardiomyopathies. Pathol Microbiol 35: 37, 1970.

120. Roberts WC: Coronary thrombosis and fatal myocardial ischemia. Circulation 49: 1, 1974.

121. Bronte-Stewart B, Heptinstall RH: The relationship between experimental hypertension and cholesterol. Induced atheroma in rabbits. J Pathol Bact 68: 407, 1954.

122. Moses C: Development of atherosclerosis in dogs with hypercholesterolemia and chronic hypertension. Circulation Res 2: 243, 1954.

123. Wakerlin GE, Moss WG, Kiely JP: Effect of experimental renal hypertension on experimental thiouracil-cholesterol atherosclerosis in dogs. Circulation Res 5: 426, 1957.

124. Vlodaver Z, Edwards JE: Pathologic analysis in fatal cases following saphenous vein coronary arterial bypass. Chest 64: 555, 1973.

125. Moyer JH, Flynn J: The role of arterial hypertension in coronary atherosclerosis, Coronary Heart Disease (Russek HI, Zohman BL, eds), Philadelphia, J.B. Lippincott, 1971, p 137.

126. Carlson RG, Lillehei CW, Edwards JE: Cystic medial necrosis of the ascending aorta in relation to age and hypertension. Am J Cardiol 25: 411, 1970.

127. Norris RM, Bensley KE, Caughey DE, Scott PJ: Hospital mortality in acute myocardial infarction. Br Med J 3: 143, 1968.

128. Norris RM, Brandt PWT, Caughey DE, Lee AJ, Scott PJ: A new coronary prognostic index. Lancet 1: 274, 1969.

129. Norris RM, Caughey DE, Deeming LW, Mercer CJ, Scott PJ: Coronary prognostic index for predicting survival after recovery from acute myocardial infarction. Lancet 2: 485, 1970.

130. Norris RM, Caughey DE, Mercer CJ, Scott PJ: Prognosis after myocardial infarction. Six-year follow-up. Br Heart J 36: 786, 1974.

131. Kannel WB, Castelli WP, McNamara PM: Role of blood pressure in the development of congestive heart failure. N Engl J Med 287: 781, 1972.

132. Frohlich ED, Tarazi RC, Dustan HP: Clinical-physiological correlations in the development of hypertensive heart disease. Circulation 44: 446, 1971.

133. Wilber JA, Barrow JG: Reducing elevated blood pressure. Experience found in a community. Minn Med 52: 1303, 1969.

134. Frohlich ED, Emmott C, Hammarsten JE, Linehan WM, Pollack D, Horsley AW: Evaluation of the initial care of hypertensive patients. JAMA 218: 1036, 1971.

Choosing a Substitute Cardiac Valve: Type, Size, Surgeon

WILLIAM C. ROBERTS, MD, FACC

Bethesda, Maryland

Certain ideal characteristics of substitute cardiac valves are analyzed for each of the four basic types of available substitute cardiac valves. Of the four, the caged disc prosthesis is the least desirable: It obstructs, it clots and it degenerates. Each of the other three types of substitute cardiac valves has more favorable characteristics. Ideally, the caged ball prosthesis might be limited to patients with predominantly regurgitant lesions because of the problem of prosthetic disproportion. The tilting disc has favorable hemodynamic and wear characteristics, but long-term anticoagulant therapy is essential, as with the caged ball and caged disc types of prosthesis. The porcine xenograft appears to be desirable, but patients with sufficient implantation time (more than 5 years) for proper evaluation are just beginning to be studied and, therefore, final judgment must be reserved. Assuming that valve replacement is to be carried out in a large medical center by a surgical team experienced in this procedure, the results of this operation today are dependent more on the type and size of substitute valve inserted than on the surgeon who inserts the valve. It is therefore important for the cardiologist to become more informed about the various types of prosthetic cardiac valves and to become a member of the team deciding which type and size of cardiac valve are most suitable for his (or her) patient.

In the annals of cardiology the decade of the 1960's will probably be remembered most as the decade during which cardiac valve replacement became a successful reality. This tremendous accomplishment has brought new life to several hundred thousand persons since the first successful (survival more than 3 months) cardiac valve replacement in September 1960. Despite this success, the ideal cardiac valve is still not available or, if available, not adequately tested. This review will examine the various advantages and disadvantages of available substitute cardiac valves and, in addition, will examine the determinants of the results of cardiac valve replacement.

Available Prosthetic Valves

Of the nearly 50 different substitute cardiac valves introduced during the past 2 decades, many have been discarded and, of those remaining, usually several modifications have been made. At present, four basic types of substitute cardiac valves are in use: (1) caged ball, (2) caged disc, (3) tilting disc, and (4) tissue valve. The caged ball was the first prosthesis used successfully for the treatment of cardiac valve disease; it was placed in the descending thoracic aorta by Hufnagel in 1953 for treatment of severe aortic regurgitation.[1,2] Although utilized unsuccessfully for aortic valve replacement (subcoronary insertion) in 1960 by Harken et al.,[3,4] the caged ball was first used successfully for mitral valve replacement in the same year by Starr and Edwards.[5] Although first utilized in the descending thoracic aorta as treatment for aortic regurgitation in 1956,[6–8] the aortic valve homograft was introduced for aortic valve replacement

From the Pathology Branch, National Heart, Lung, and Blood Institute, National Institutes of Health, Bethesda, Md. 20014. Manuscript received March 17, 1976; accepted March 31, 1976.

Address for reprints: William C. Roberts, MD, National Institutes of Health, Bldg 10A, Rm. 3E 30, Bethesda, Md. 20014.

in 1962[9–12] (later[13] for mitral valve replacement), and the heterograft aortic valve was first used for aortic valve replacement in 1967.[14–16] The caged disc appeared in 1965[17,18] and the tilting disc in 1967.[19–22] Flow through the caged ball and caged disc is peripheral, through the tilting disc semicentral, and through the tissue valve central.

Characteristics of Prosthetic Valves

There are at least six ideal characteristics of a good prosthetic cardiac valve (Table I): (1) It has good hemodynamic characteristics, that is, it is *nonobstructive* or nearly so, and completely *competent* or nearly so; (2) it is *nonthrombogenic;* (3) it *does not degenerate,* wear out or vary; (4) it *does not significantly alter blood components;* (5) *it can be inserted without undue difficulty* (that is, exquisite technical skill is not required

TABLE I

Substitute Cardiac Valves: General Characteristics

Type	Year Intro-duced	Ob-struc-tive	In-com-petent	Throm-botic	Hemo-lytic	De-gener-ates
Caged ball	1960	+	0	+	+	+
Caged disc	1965	+	0	+	+	+
Tilting disc	1967	+	0	+	0	0
Tissue valve						
Homograft	1962	0	+	0	0	+
Xenograft	1965	+	0	0	0	?

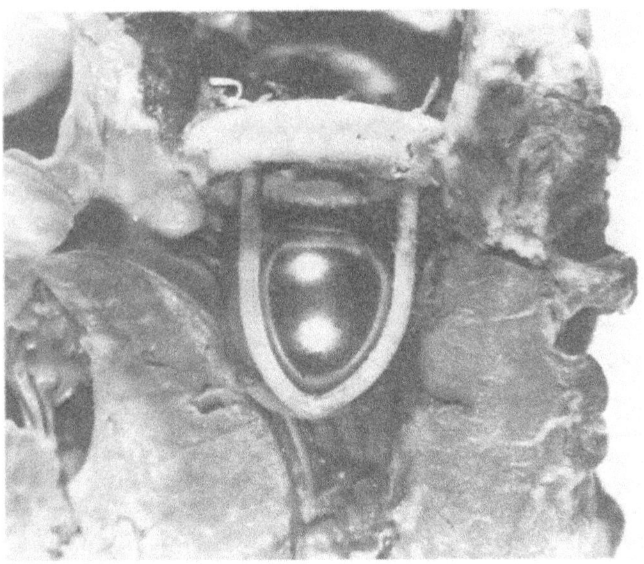

FIGURE 1. Prosthetic mitral stenosis after replacement with a ball valve prosthesis. Shown is longitudinal section of the heart of a woman with severe isolated mitral stenosis. The valve was replaced in July 1974 with a size 3M Starr-Edwards prosthesis. The prosthesis is too large for the normal-sized left ventricular cavity, and both struts and poppet contact the endocardium of the left ventricle causing obstruction to left ventricular inflow. The patient could not be separated from cardiopulmonary bypass.

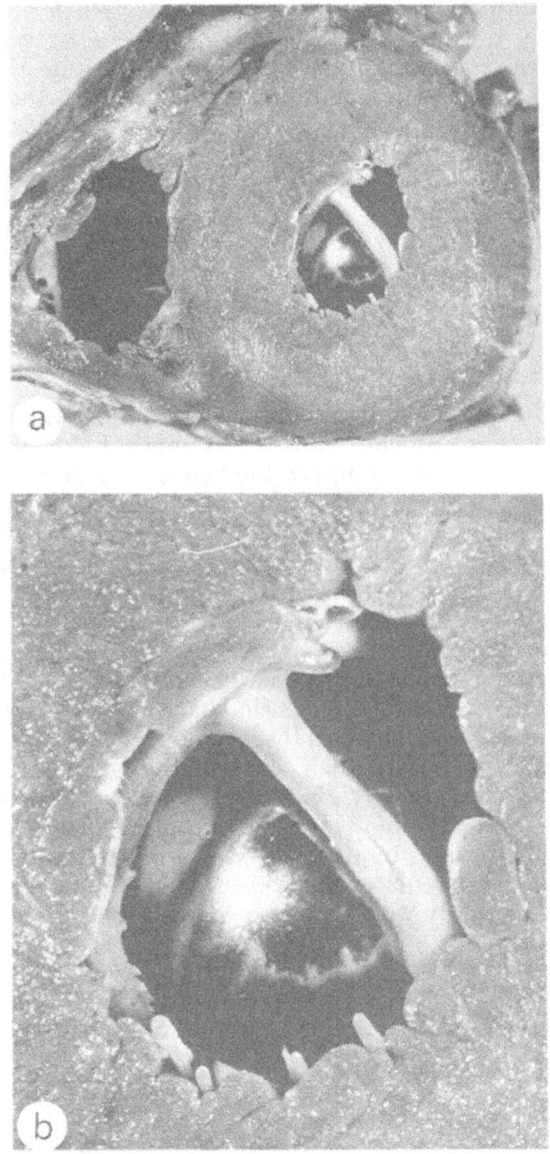

FIGURE 2. Prosthetic mitral stenosis after replacement of a stenotic mitral valve (7 mm Hg mean diastolic gradient between left ventricle and pulmonary capillary wedge position) with a size 4M model 6320 Starr-Edwards prosthesis. This 58 year old man also had his stenotic aortic valve (103 mm Hg peak systolic pressure gradient between left ventricle and brachial artery) replaced with a size 9A model 2320 Starr-Edwards prosthesis. The immediate postoperative period was complicated by the low cardiac output syndrome. Late postoperatively, however, the patient became asymptomatic. At cardiac catheterization 6 1/2 months postoperatively, the mean diastolic gradient across the mitral prosthesis was 11 mm Hg and no systolic gradient was present across the aortic prosthesis. The mitral valve area preoperatively was 2.0 and, postoperatively, 1.6 cm^2. The patient died suddenly 5 days after the postoperative catheterization. *At necropsy,* as shown in the above photographs, the mitral prosthesis is too large for the normal-sized left ventricular cavity (shown here as it appears during ventricular systole). Thus, not only did the mitral prosthesis appear obstructive at necropsy but the pressure gradient was considerably greater postoperatively than preoperatively. Although this patient had been asymptomatic postoperatively, he had considerable prosthetic mitral stenosis. **a,** transverse section of the cardiac ventricles. Each of the cloth-covered struts contacts endocardium of the left ventricle and the metal poppet occupies too much space in the left ventricular cavity, as seen in the closer view **(b).**

for its insertion); and (6) it *does not disturb the patient.*

Analysis of each of the four types of substitute cardiac valves for the first four of these ideal characteristics should separate the good ones from the bad ones. The degree of difficulty or ease in inserting each of the four basic types of currently employed substitute valves is similar because all have rigid or semirigid frames and cloth-covered sewing rings. Furthermore, with the possible exception of the recent metal track Starr-Edwards prosthesis, none of the substitute valves now used make noise audible to the patient.

Caged Ball Valve

The caged ball prosthesis (Harken, Starr-Edwards, Magovern, Smeloff-Cutter, Braunwald-Cutter, De Bakey) clearly belongs in the "good" category. More information on it is available than on any of the other prostheses because it has been the one used most widely and for the longest time; however, it is not necessarily the best prothesis. It has had a number of modifications (a word not always synonymous with "improvements") during the past 16 years, and generally has adequate but not the best hemodynamic characteristics.[23–35] Although the introduction of cloth covering on the struts and base has diminished the incidence of clinical events compatible with emboli, this prosthesis continues to have a tendency to form thrombus, and anticoagulant agents are required.[35] It hemolyzes erythrocytes, more frequently and more severely after aortic than after mitral valve replacement and also more frequently and more severely with the cloth-covered than with non-cloth-covered models.[36–43] Hemolysis, however, is rarely a major clinical problem with any prosthesis because the bone marrow is capable of replacing the destroyed erythrocytes without development of anemia or thrombocytopenia.

Degeneration of the silicone rubber poppet was common in the caged ball prostheses inserted before 1967,[44–62] but no degeneration or variance has been reported in the metallic (stellite 21) hollow poppet introduced at that time. The silicone rubber poppet models continue to be employed in some major centers and it is likely that poppet degeneration eventually will occur in them. Such was the case with the Braunwald-Cutter aortic valve prosthesis, which has been withdrawn from the market.[63] Wear of cloth covering on both struts and orifice occurred in some of the completely cloth-covered caged ball prostheses, but strut cloth wear has not been observed since introduction of the metal track in the latest Starr-Edwards models.

Obstructive complications: A problem with the caged ball prosthesis is that it may occupy too much space within either the ventricle or aortic root, and, because flow is entirely peripheral, there may not be adequate space between the surface of the poppet and the endocardium of the ventricle or the intima of the ascending aorta to accommodate blood flow adequately[64–78] (Fig. 1 to 3). This situation occurs most frequently when mitral valve replacement is performed in a patient, usually a woman, with pure mitral stenosis and a normal aortic valve. In this circumstance the left ventricle may not be of adequate size to accommodate the mitral prosthesis, and one or more struts of the

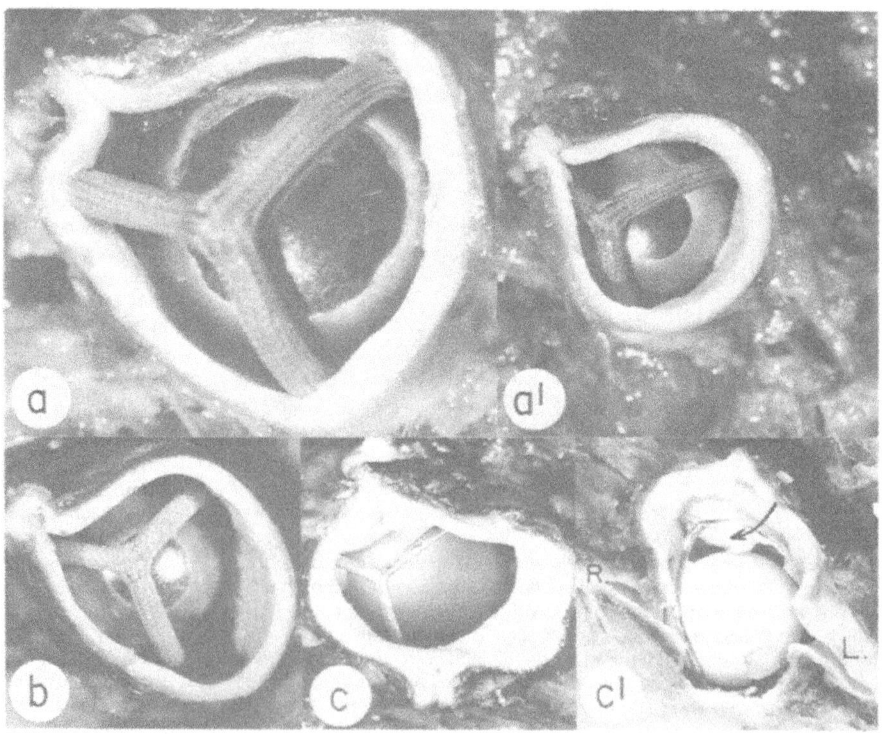

FIGURE 3. Prosthetic aortic stenosis secondary to disproportion between the size of the caged ball prosthesis and the size of the ascending aorta. The aortic prostheses, even though small (8A, Starr-Edwards), are too large for the aortas into which they had been placed. The struts of the cages contact the aortic walls, which protrude between the struts to contact the poppets and restrict their movement. **a, a**[1], from a 45 year old woman who had had mitral stenosis (11 mm Hg mean diastolic gradient between the left atrium and left ventricle) and pure aortic regurgitation (2+/4+). She died several hours after operation. **b,** from a 55 year old woman who also had severe mitral stenosis (17 mm Hg mean diastolic gradient between the left atrium and left ventricle) and pure aortic regurgitation (4+/4+). She died in the operating room. **c, c**[1], from a 25 year old man also with severe mitral stenosis (18 mm Hg mean diastolic gradient between the left atrium and left ventricle) and pure aortic regurgitation (2+/4+). The patient also died on the day of operation several hours after entering the recovery room.

prosthesis may burrow into the myocardial wall preventing adequate descent of the poppet, with resulting obstruction to left atrial emptying.[64] This occurrence is obviously most likely when a large prosthesis is utilized, but it may occur when even the smallest caged ball prosthesis is used to replace a purely stenotic mitral valve. Fatal obstruction to left ventricular outflow occurs most commonly in the patient with combined mitral and aortic valve disease. In most such patients, whether the aortic valve lesion is stenosis or pure regurgitation, the aortic root is usually not dilated and consequently the space available in the aortic root to accommodate the caged ball may be limited. A particularly dangerous circumstance is combined mitral and aortic stenosis. In this circumstance, the left ventricular wall is hypertrophied but its cavity is not dilated. Insertion of a mitral caged ball into a hypertrophied nondilated left ventricle may obstruct left ventricular inflow or outflow. Because ventricular inflow obstruction is probably even more common after tricuspid than after mitral valve replacement with a caged ball prosthesis, utilization of this prosthesis in the tricuspid position may be unwise.[74–78]

Real and potential prosthetic disproportion (prosthesis too large or ventricular cavity or aorta too small) occur most frequently with the caged ball prosthesis although none of the various types of substitute cardiac valves are completely immune from it (Fig. 4 to 7). Therefore, it may be most wise to limit the use of this type of prosthesis to patients with purely incompetent or at least predominantly incompetent valve lesions, that is, to patients in whom volume overload has produced a large left ventricular cavity or ascending aorta. Use of the caged ball prosthesis in patients with purely stenotic or predominantly stenotic valve lesions appears unnecessary because of the availability of other excellent substitute cardiac valves.

Caged Disc Valve

The caged disc prosthesis (Kay-Shiley, Cross-Jones, Hufnagel, Kay-Suzuki, Beall, Harken, Cooley-Bloodwell-Cutter, Cooley-Cutter) is in my view the least desirable prosthetic cardiac valve now in use. Because of its "low profile" configuration, this prosthesis was introduced as an alternative to the caged ball prosthesis and was initially believed to be particularly useful in the patient with the "small left ventricle," (pure mitral stenosis). This device, however, has proved to be highly thrombogenic[79–85] and the most obstructive of all the prosthetic valves now in use.[86–99] In a recent study, although the pulmonary arterial pressures had decreased and the cardiac indexes had increased, the mean diastolic pressure gradient across the mitral prosthesis (Beall type) was not significantly different from preoperative values.[99] In addition, the nonmetallic discs have shown evidence of degeneration,[87,97,100–113] and strut fracture of uncertain cause with dislodgment of the disc occluder has been reported.[96,107] Hemolysis with this prosthesis is universal.[97,114] This device was

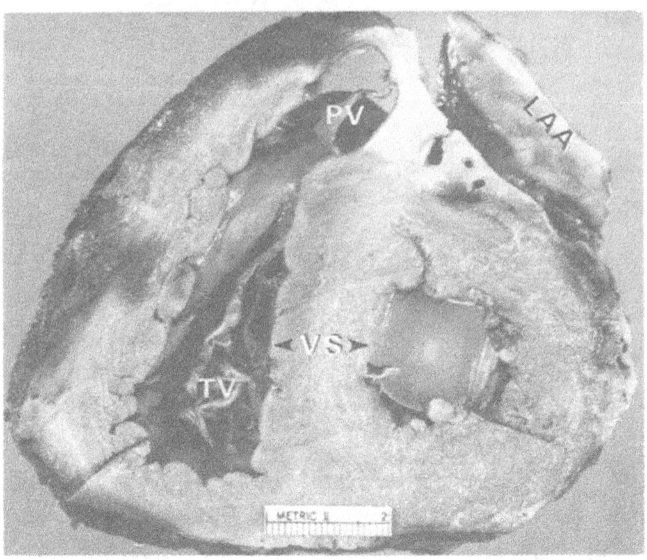

FIGURE 4. Prosthetic stenosis after replacement of the mitral valve with a caged disc prosthesis. Shown is a transverse section of the cardiac ventricles in a 57 year old woman who died in the operating room after replacement of a severely stenotic mitral valve with a no. 19 Hufnagel discoid prosthesis. The margins of the disc contact the left ventricular endocardium at several sites and movement of the disc is impeded. In addition to mitral stenosis and severe pulmonary hypertension (95/45 mm Hg), the aortic valve was mildly stenotic (peak systolic pressure gradient 34 mm Hg). LAA = left atrial appendage; PV = pulmonary valve; TV = tricuspid valve; VS = ventricular septum.

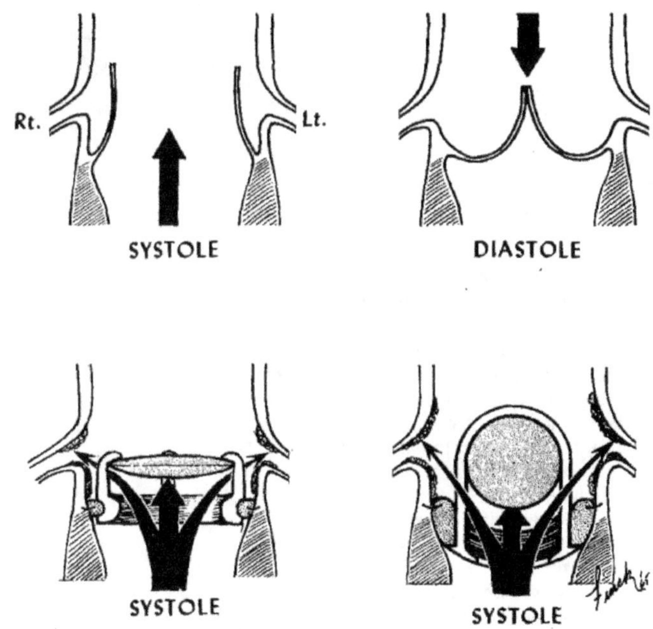

FIGURE 5. Diagram delineating flow across the normal aortic valve (**upper**) and across a caged disc and caged ball prosthesis (**lower**). Normally, flow across the aortic valve is central and nearly laminar. Flow across the prostheses is entirely peripheral and therefore turbulent. Intimal proliferation in the proximal ascending aorta is an expected consequence of this peripheral flow.[45,46] On rare occasion, this intimal proliferation may extend into one or both coronary arteries. It is likely that this intimal proliferation will progressively increase with time. Flow across a tissue valve is certainly more laminar than across either the caged disc or caged ball. Lt. = left; Rt. = right.

utilized briefly in the aortic position[89,90,97] but its use in this location was abandoned because of its obstructive, thrombogenic and wear characteristics.

More recently, a new type of caged disc, the Cooley-Cutter biconical disc, has been introduced for use in both atrioventricular and semilunar valve positions.[115–117] This newer prosthesis, which has a semidiamond-shaped occluder rather than a flat one (like all other caged discs) also has entirely peripheral flow characteristics and is therefore unlikely to have ideal hemodynamic features. Furthermore, intimal proliferation in the aortic root (where the coronary ostia are located) remains a potential problem with the peripheral flow type of prosthesis and is probably most severe with use of the caged disc[97] (Fig. 5). Also very worrisome is disc cocking, a potential problem with all caged discs[80,82,83,102,110–113,118,119] including the newly introduced one, and its frequency of occurrence is entirely unknown (Fig. 8). Possibly, nonfatal transient cocking is common, and fatal cocking of the caged disc may occur and be totally unrecognized at necropsy.

Tilting Disc Valve

The tilting disc prosthesis (Wada-Cutter, Lillehei-Kastor, Björk-Shiley) of the latter two types (the first type has been discontinued[120]) has proved to be a good prosthesis for replacement of tricuspid, mitral and aortic valves. Its semicentral flow usually allows minimal gradients,[121–127] its effect on red blood cell survival is minimal[128,129] and there has been no evidence of disc wear (variance) since the introduction of the carbon pyrolyte disc. This prosthesis, however, has a tendency to clot, and anticoagulant agents are required.[129–135] Because movement of the disc is in close proximity to the sewing ring, the chances of interference to it by contact with adjacent mural endocardium or aortic intima is small, but, as with all prostheses, a potential problem if a large model is utilized in a small ventricle or aorta[129] (Fig. 6 and 7).

Tissue Valves

Tissue valves, in the form of aortic homografts, were first utilized for aortic valve replacement in 1962.[9–12]

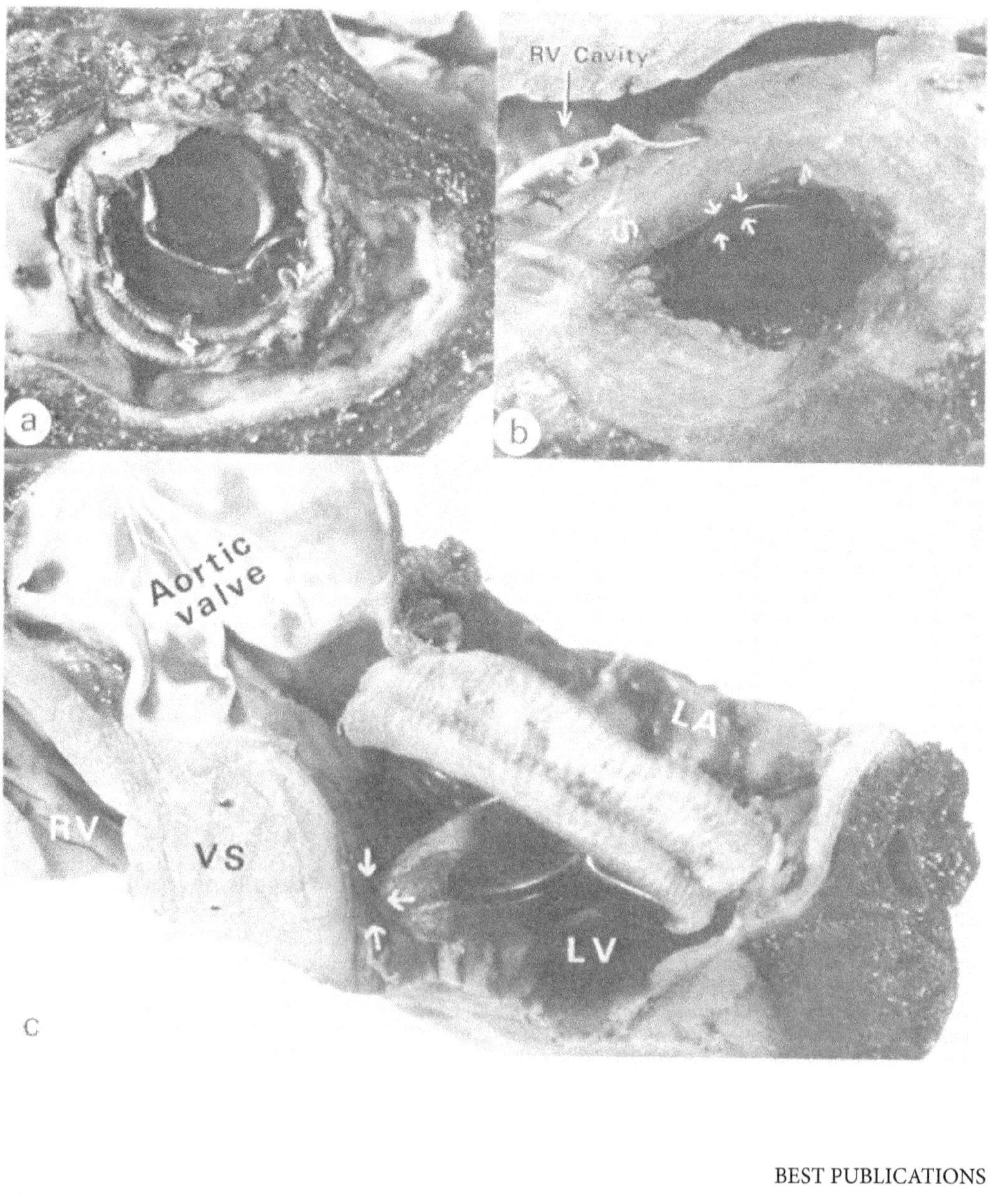

FIGURE 6. Prosthetic malfunction after replacement of a severely stenotic mitral valve with the largest-sized (31 mm) Björk-Shiley prosthesis in a 54 year old man. Although the prosthesis appears to have opened well, the occluder (disc) was prevented from seating by the ventricular septum, which "moved inward" during ventricular systole. The patient could not be separated from cardiopulmonary bypass. **a,** prosthesis as it *should appear* when viewed from left atrium during simulated ventricular systole. It fills most of the "floor" of this chamber. **b,** view of mitral prosthesis from below as it *did appear* during ventricular systole. The margin (**arrows**) of the disc contracted the ventricular septum (VS), preventing seating of the disc. RV = right ventricular. **c,** longitudinal cut of the heart again showing the disc as it appeared during ventricular systole. The margins (**arrows**) of the disc contact the ventricular septum. LA = left atrium; LV = left ventricle.

The initial results were gratifying: The valve lesions were usually ameliorated, and anticoagulant therapy was not required. The problem proved to be accelerated wear and tear with development of incompetency.[136–140] Other tissue valves followed—namely, fascia lata, dura mater, parietal pericardium—but all proved to be poor valve substitutes because they became stiff and relatively immobile.[141–145] The fresh antibiotic-sterilized homograft remains in use, but now the most commonly employed tissue valve is the porcine xenograft attached to a semiflexible stent[146] and preserved by a glutaraldehyde process.[146–153] (The graft failed when preserved in formalin.[141,154])

Porcine xenograft: Enthusiasm for this substitute valve is increasing. Although relatively few late postoperative hemodynamic studies have been reported, a pressure gradient across the porcine bioprosthesis has been recorded in all three valve positions despite its central flow. Among 56 patients studied late postoperatively after mitral valve replacement, the mean diastolic gradient averaged 6 mm Hg,[148,151,152] but of 37 patients studied at the National Heart, Lung, and Blood Institute, no gradient was recorded across the mitral porcine valve in 16 patients. Of 11 patients studied late postoperatively after tricuspid valve replacement with a porcine xenograft, the mean diastolic gradient averaged 4 mm Hg.[152] Hemodynamic data after aortic valve replacement with the porcine xenograft are virtually nonexistent: Among five patients studied late postoperatively at the National Heart, Lung, and Blood Institute, the peak systolic pressure gradients ranged from 10 to 35 mm Hg (average 18).[146] Other data are not available, to my knowledge.

Clinical episodes compatible with emboli are rare after valve replacement with the porcine xenograft and, therefore, its use rarely requires anticoagulant therapy. The porcine xenograft does not damage blood elements. The major concern is its wear characteristics. The en-

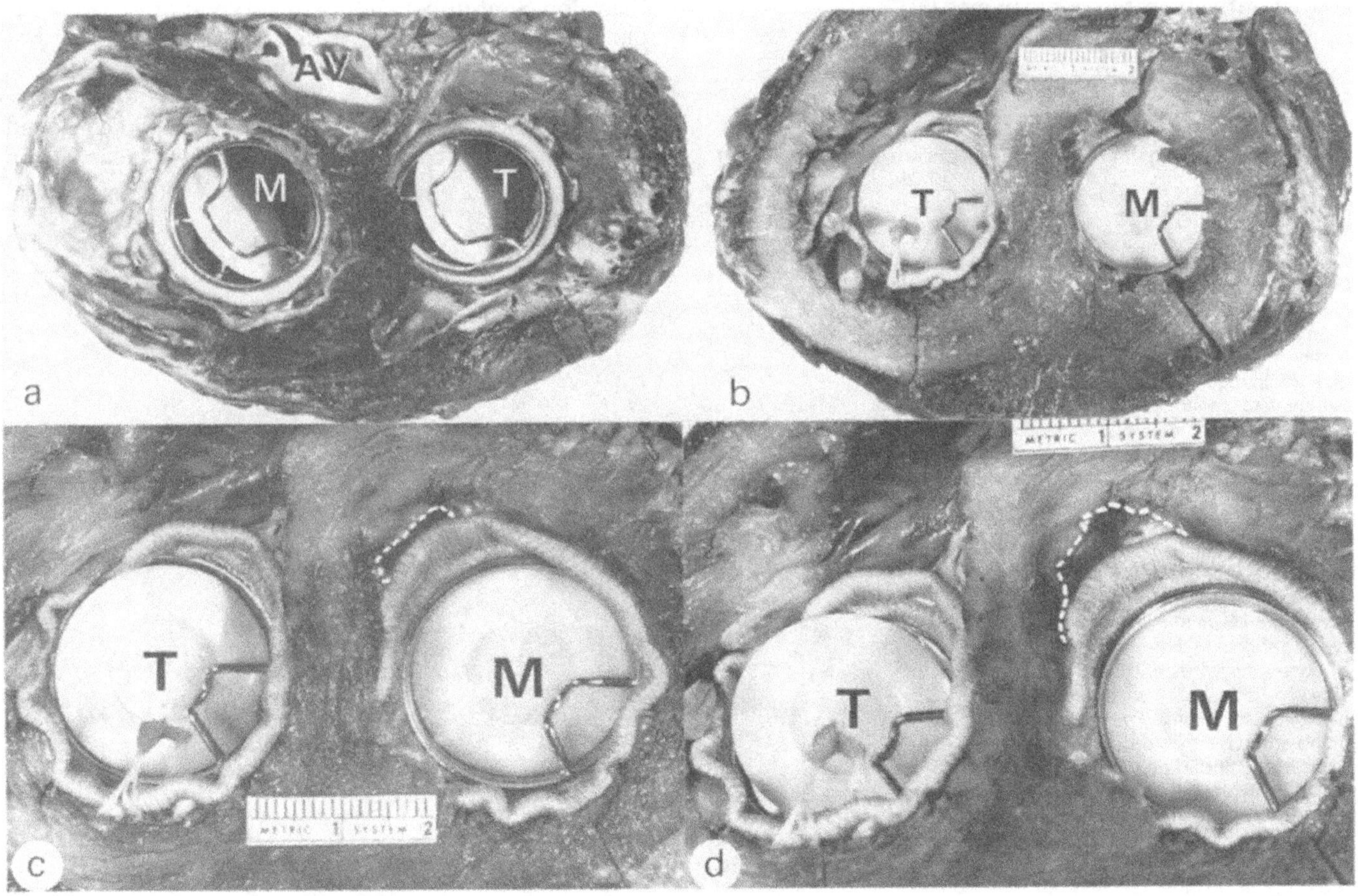

FIGURE 7. Prosthetic-ventricular chamber disproportion after replacement of both mitral and tricuspid valves with tilting-disc (Björk-Shiley) prostheses in a 64 year old woman with severe mitral stenosis, severe pulmonary hypertension and functional tricuspid regurgitation. At operation in April 1975, both mitral and tricuspid anuli readily accepted a 31 mm Björk sizer and, consequently, size 31 mm Björk-Shiley prostheses were inserted in both positions. The patient died in the operating room. At necropsy, the major problem appeared to be obstruction to left ventricular emptying (**b, c, d**) and, of lesser importance, failure of the tricuspid valve occluder to seat completely (**b, c, d**). **a,** heart during simulated ventricular diastole from the atrial aspect after most of the atrial walls have been excised. Both prostheses occupy most of the "floor" of each atrium. AV = aortic valve; M = mitral valve prosthesis; T = tricuspid valve prosthesis. **b,** view of both prostheses from below. The left ventricular outflow tract is nearly completely obliterated in this view by the mitral prosthesis. The tricuspid valve disc is prevented from seating completely. **c** and **d,** close-up views of both prostheses from the ventricular aspects showing interference to closure of the tricuspid occluder and severe obstruction to left ventricular outflow by the mitral prosthesis. The retained fragment of right ventricular papillary muscle and chordae tendineae potentially could have interfered with movement of the tricuspid valve occluder. The aortic valve was normal and the left ventricular cavity was of normal size.

couraging feature at this time is that there have been extremely few "valve failures"[146–153] and, indeed, no other substitute valve has had so few problems in its first 5 years. Nevertheless, relatively few patients (estimated to be about 500) have had this substitute valve in place for longer than 5 years, and signs of cusp degeneration, should they occur, are likely to occur after this period.

It is likely that the cusps of the porcine valve will be subject to changes that affect all natural left-sided cardiac valves, namely, lipid deposition and calcification.[155–157] These changes occur on the native valves, on the aortic aspects of the aortic valve cusps and on the ventricular aspects of the mitral valve cusps. Such changes will probably occur more rapidly in this substitute valve than in the natural valve, but, at least by 5 years, calcific deposits in the substitute valve cusps have been infrequent and minimal.[158] Small thrombi have been observed on the sinus aspects of the porcine cusps and possibly it is the organization of these minute thrombi that has led to the calcific deposits, at this point almost entirely microscopic in size.[141]

Factors Determining Outcome of Valve Replacement

At least six major factors appear to determine the result of valve replacement in a particular patient: (1) the type of the substitute valve inserted; (2) the size of the substitute valve inserted; (3) the experience and technical skill of the surgeon; (4) the adequacy of the "pump team," anesthesiologists and surgeons, physicians and nurses providing postoperative care; (5) the presence of associated (diagnosed or undiagnosed) or uncorrected cardiac disease or previous pericardiotomy; and (6) the preoperative status of the patient. The relative effect of each of these factors on the outcome of valve replacement will be examined next.

Assuming that the cardiac operation will take place in a large medical center where several cardiac operations are performed weekly by a surgeon or group of surgeons experienced in cardiac valve replacement, the most important factor determining the long-term outcome of valve replacement is the type of substitute valve inserted. At a conference on prosthetic valves for cardiac surgery held in Chicago[159] on September 9 and 10, 1960, it was observed that there were no living survivors of total cardiac valve replacement. After Starr's successful replacement of the mitral valve with a caged ball prosthesis on September 21, 1960, survival after valve replacement using the caged ball prosthesis rapidly became commonplace. The caged ball was the first prosthesis used for cardiac valve replacement by many surgeons whose previous valve operations had consisted entirely of mitral commissurotomy and yet, nearly from

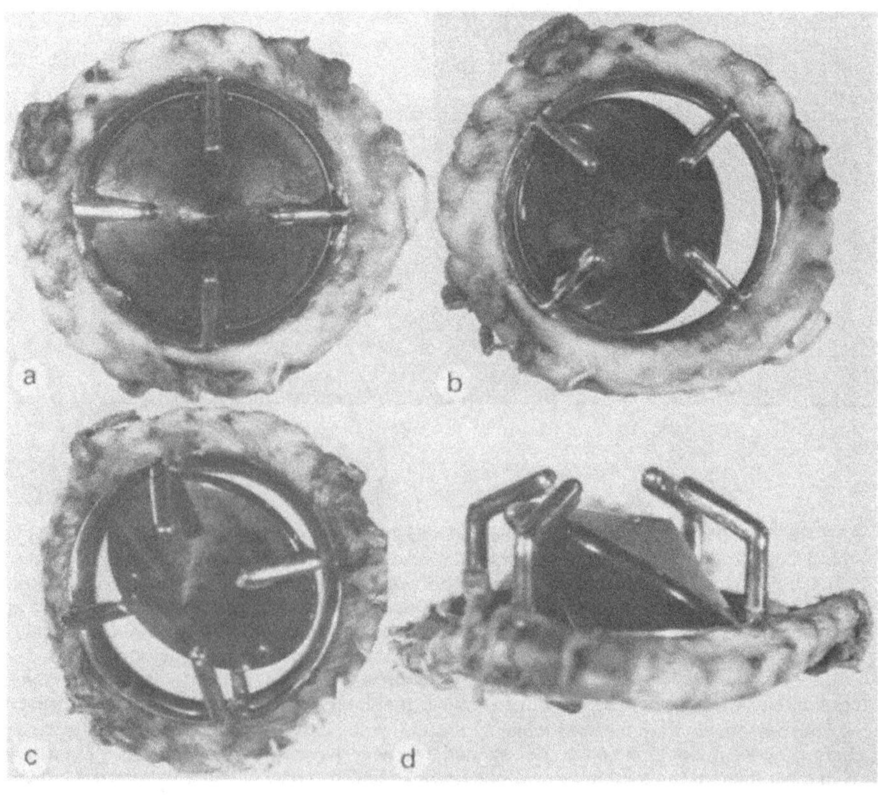

FIGURE 8. Various views of the Cooley-Cutter biconical caged disc prosthesis that had been inserted in the aortic valve position 4 months earlier in a 30 year old man because of severe pure aortic regurgitation. Late postoperatively the patient had severe aortic regurgitation (blood pressure 170/20 mm Hg) and fatal pulmonary edema. At necropsy, half of the circumference of the prosthesis had detached from the anulus, and there was no evidence of active infective endocarditis. The cause of the detachment, therefore, is uncertain, but at operation, continuous sutures had been utilized except for four interrupted sutures (one in each of the four quadrants). These four views of this prosthesis show potential types of cocking that are possible with any type of caged disc prostheses. A photograph of the closed prosthesis as it should appear in ventricular diastole is shown in **a**. For the occluder to ascend in the aortic position properly, pressure must be exerted on all portions of the occluder more or less equally. If pressure is exerted unequally for any reason, cocking may occur (**b, c, d**). One of the good features of the caged ball prosthesis is that the poppet ascends, in the aortic position, irrespective of the angle at which the blood is ejected from the left ventricle. Not so with the caged disc. If the prosthesis is inserted at a nonright angle to the aortic "anulus," the force of ejection may not be applied equally to all portions of the disc occluder. The result may be asymmetric opening of the prosthesis, and systolic cocking may be a precursor to diastolic cocking. In other words, the range of error for insertion of a caged disc in the aortic position is probably not as great as that inherent to the other three types of substitute cardiac valves discussed.

the beginning, rapid success was achieved using this device.

Choice of Valve Prosthesis

Choice of type of prosthesis: Because the decision regarding the type of substitute valve to be chosen for a particular patient is crucial, consideration might be given to the following questions: (1) Who *does* choose the type of prosthesis to be inserted? and (2) Who *should* choose the type of prosthesis to be inserted? From the beginning, that is, 1960, the surgeon has determined the type of prosthesis to be inserted in a particular patient. What are factors that determine a surgeon's preference for a prosthesis? The major one is previous experience, including personal experience and that of colleagues. The choice of prosthesis by a particularly prominent surgeon or by the trainer of a new cardiovascular surgeon may be especially influencing. Some surgeons who started with the caged ball, for example, and had satisfactory results are reluctant to change. One is simply more comfortable with the device one has used before. Change of prosthesis or model when it proves not to be ideal is admirable, and best exemplified by Cooley's experience with 34 different types or models of prosthetic cardiac valves.[116]

The choice of prosthesis by some surgeons has been influenced by personal involvement in the development of a particular prosthesis. Admitting that a prosthesis of someone else's design is better than one of one's own design is, at best, difficult. There may be inherent conflict when the same surgeon participates in the design of, and in the insertion of, a particular prosthesis. There have been many examples of this potential conflict during the past 16 years.

Again, assuming that valve replacement is to be performed in a large medical center with an experienced cardiovascular surgical team, long-term survival is more dependent on the type of prosthesis inserted than on the surgeon who inserts the prosthesis. Thus, if I personally were to undergo valve replacement, I would first choose the type of prosthesis and, second, the surgeon whose results with this particular prosthesis were excellent. In my view, the referring cardiologist is not fulfilling his responsibility by simply referring his patient to a surgeon irrespective of the type of prosthesis the surgeon most frequently utilizes. To use a caged disc, at least one of those with a flat occluder, is unwise in my view and, to date, few hemodynamic or other data are available to allow proper evaluation of the biconical type of caged disc. Although some surgeons periodically employ all four types of available substitute cardiac valves, most generally use only one or two types. If the patient has mitral stenosis or combined mitral and aortic valve disease (and in this circumstance the aortic "root" is usually small) or if the patient is small, referral to a surgeon who only, or nearly always, uses the caged ball prosthesis would not appear ideal. The fewest problems with valve replacement now appear to be with the porcine xenograft, but this too may change. Patients requiring valve replacement who have real or potential bleeding tendencies should have a porcine xenograft because anticoagulant therapy is required with use of any of the other three substitute valves.

Cardiologists in large medical centers usually refer their patients requiring valve replacement to the surgeons in the same medical center even though they may not necessarily be pleased with or involved in the choice of the substitute valve to be used. Ideally this choice would be made by both the cardiologist and the surgeon in light of all the data known about a particular patient. Greater participation by cardiologists in valve selection would require their acquisition of greater knowledge of such valves than they now generally have. Obviously, who chooses the type of substitute valve for a particular patient is not important so long as the choice is the right one, but surgeons do not necessarily have a monopoly on that right choice. The point is that the era of the "one-valve surgeon" may be over: ". . . Selection of the most favorable valve substitute for implantation should be individualized to each patient's specific anatomical, hemodynamic, and hematological needs".[160] It no longer appears proper for a surgeon to use only one type of substitute valve for all patients.

Determination of the size of prosthesis to insert: This determination, to my knowledge, has always been made in the operating room with the patient on cardiopulmonary bypass and after the insertion of various sizers placed through the valve orifice after excision of the native valve. But does this method best determine the size of a prosthesis to be inserted? My view is no. With the patient on cardiopulmonary bypass and with various retractors pulling on the heart, the surgeon may be able to insert large sizing devices and, therefore be led to insert a large prosthesis when, in actuality, with the patient off cardiopulmonary bypass and all retractors withdrawn, the valve orifice is much smaller (Fig. 6 and 7). Therefore, the size of the valve to be inserted might best be determined, not exclusively on the basis of sizing devices at operation, but at least in part on the basis of the hemodynamic valve lesion or lesions before operation with consideration of the lean weight of the patient. A small woman with pure mitral stenosis and a normally functioning aortic valve should have a relatively small prosthesis. Recently (1975), I saw the hearts at necropsy of two patients with severe isolated mitral stenosis who each had the largest tilting disc prosthesis (Björk-Shiley 31 mm). At operation in each, the sizing devices had apparently indicated that the valve orifice was capable of accommodating this large prosthesis. Yet fatal malfunction of the prosthesis because of its large size and each patient's "small" left ventricle occurred by mechanisms delineated in Figures 6 and 7. If the largest prosthesis is used in a small woman with pure mitral stenosis, what size of device should be used in a large man with pure mitral regurgitation? Thus, the decision regarding the size of prosthesis to insert might roughly be determined at the preoperative conference or consultation and based on the hemodynamic valve lesion and body weight and not entirely on the dimensions measured in the operating room.

Surgical Skill and Experience

Although I have thus far placed greatest emphasis on the type and size of the prosthetic valve inserted, the technical skill and experience of the surgeon are obviously extremely important and experience is probably more important than technical skill. (One of the finest examples of technical skill in the field of cardiac valve surgery is the placing of a porcine xenograft on a semi-flexible cloth-covered stent. This procedure is performed by women before the tissue valve is shipped to surgeons.) There is no question that results of valve replacement are better among experienced than among nonexperienced surgeons, although the technical skills of the latter might be greater. The "occasional open heart surgeon," as emphasized by Eiseman and Spencer,[161] no matter how great his technical skill, is not the ideal cardiac surgeon. Certain technical factors, however, might be taken into consideration by the referring physician. Should prosthetic valves be inserted with continuous or interrupted sutures? It appears most reasonable that interrupted sutures would be less likely to be associated with "massive" prosthetic regurgitation (prosthetic disruption), and yet continuous or nearly continuous sutures are commonly employed by some surgeons.[162] If the world's "best" surgeon uses the world's worst prosthesis or inserts it by noninterrupted suture, the result may not be ideal.

Other Determinants of Results

The three other determinants of the results of cardiac valve replacement are self-evident. Obviously, the entire surgical team must be a good one. The patients with associated heart disease—for example, coronary heart disease or previous thoracotomy—do not do as well as patients without these complications.[61,62] The less sick the patient before operation the greater are his (or her) chances of survival after operation, but the sicker the patient before operation, usually the more dramatic is the change after operation.

Acknowledgment

I thank Dr. Johanna M. van der Bel-Kahn, Associate Professor of Pathology, University of Cincinnati, Cincinnati, Ohio, for allowing me to study with her two patients with a bioconical disc prosthesis in the aortic valve position.

Addendum

Recently, some hemodynamic data have been reported concerning patients with a porcine (Hancock) xenograft valve in the aortic position. Cohn et al.[163] studied seven patients postoperatively and found they had a peak systolic pressure gradient at rest of 5 to 32 mm Hg (average 16 mm Hg). Morris[164] studied 23 patients postoperatively whose peak systolic pressure gradient at rest ranged from 6 to 58 mm Hg (mean 23 mm Hg). The higher pressure gradients tended to occur in the patients who had the smaller bioprostheses.

References

1. **Hufnagel CA, Harvey WP:** The surgical correction of aortic regurgitation. Preliminary report. Bull Georgetown Univ Med Center 6:60–61, 1953
2. **Hufnagel CA, Harvey WP, Rabil PJ, et al:** Surgical correction of aortic insufficiency. Surgery 35:673–683, 1954
3. **Harken DE, Soroff HS, Taylor WJ, et al:** Partial and complete prostheses in aortic insufficiency. J. Thorac Cardiovasc Surg 40:744–762, 1960
4. **Harken DE, Taylor WJ, Lefemine AA, et al:** Aortic valve replacement with a caged ball valve. Am J Cardiol 9:292–299, 1962
5. **Starr A, Edwards ML:** Mitral replacement: clinical experience with a ball-valve prosthesis. Ann Surg 154:726–740, 1961
6. **Murray G:** Homologous aortic-valve-segment transplants as surgical treatment for aortic and mitral insufficiency. Angiology 7:446–471, 1956
7. **Kerwin AJ, Lenkei SC, Wilson DR:** Aortic-valve homograft in the treatment of aortic insufficiency. Report of nine cases, with one followed for six years. N Engl J Med 266:852–857, 1962
8. **Beall AC, Morris GC, Cooley DA, et al:** Homotransplantation of aortic valve. J Thorac Cardiovasc Surg 42:497–506, 1961
9. **Ross DN:** Homograft replacement of the aortic valve. Lancet 2:487, 1962
10. **Duran CG, Gunning AJ:** A method for placing a total homologous aortic valve in the subcoronary position. Lancet 2:488–489, 1962
11. **Barratt-Boyes BG:** Homograft aortic valve replacement in aortic incompetence and stenosis. Thorax 19:131–150, 1964
12. **Barratt-Boyes BG, Lowe JB, Cole DS, et al:** Homograft valve replacement for aortic valve disease. Thorax 20:495–504, 1965
13. **Angell WW, Wuerflein RD, Shumway NE:** Mitral valve replacement with the fresh aortic valve homograft: experimental results and clinical application. Surgery 62:807–813, 1967
14. **Binet JP, Duran CG, Carpentier A, et al:** Heterologous aortic valve transplantation. Lancet 2:1275, 1965
15. **Ionescu MI, Wooler GH, Smith DR, et al:** Mitral valve replacement with aortic heterografts in humans. Thorax 22:305–313, 1967
16. **Carpentier A, Blondeau Ph, Laurens B, et al:** Mitral valve replacement with frame-mounted aortic heterografts. J Thorac Cardiovasc Surg 56:388–394, 1968
17. **Hufnagel CA, Conrad PW:** Comparative study of some prosthetic valves for aortic and mitral replacement. Surgery 57:205–210, 1965
18. **Kay EB, Suzuki A, Demaney M, et al:** Comparison of ball and disc valves for mitral valve replacement. Am J Cardiol 18:504–514, 1966
19. **Wada J:** Knotless suture method and Wada hingeless valve. Jpn J Thorac Surg 15:88–94, 1967
20. **Wada J, Komatsu S, Kamata K:** Cardiac valve replacement with Wada-Cutter prosthesis. Ann Thorac Surg 14:38–46, 1972
21. **Kaster RL, Lillehei CW:** A new cageless free-floating pivoting disc prosthetic heart valve: design, development and evaluation. In, Digest of the 7th International Conference on Medical and Biological Engineering. Stockholm, 1967, p 387
22. **Björk VO:** A new tilting disc valve prosthesis. Scand J Thorac Cardiovasc Surg 3:1–10, 1969
23. **Mason DT, Ross J Jr, Gault JH, et al:** Combined prosthetic replacement of the mitral and aortic valves. Preoperative and postoperative hemodynamic studies at rest and the left ventricular response to muscular exercise. Circulation 35, 36:Suppl I:I-15–I-23, 1967

24. **McHenry MM, Smeloff EA, Davey TB, et al:** Hemodynamic results with full-flow orifice prosthetic valves. Circulation 35, 36:Suppl I:I-24–I-33, 1967
25. **Glancy DL, O'Brien KP, Reis RL, et al:** Hemodynamic studies in patients with 2M and 3M Starr-Edwards prostheses: evidence of obstruction to left atrial emptying. Circulation 39, 40:Suppl I:I-113–I-118, 1969
26. **Reis RL, Glancy DL, O'Brien K, et al:** Clinical and hemodynamic assessments of fabric-covered Starr-Edwards prosthetic valves. J Thorac Cardiovasc Surg 59:84–91, 104–108, 1970
27. **Rodriguez L:** Haemodynamic and angiographic findings in patients with isolated aortic valvular disease before and after insertion of a Starr-Edwards aortic ball-valve prosthesis. Scand J Thorac Cardiovasc Surg [Suppl] 5:1–39, 1970
28. **Winter TQ, Reis RL, Glancy DL, et al:** Current status of the Starr-Edwards cloth-covered prosthetic cardiac valves. Circulation 45, 46:Suppl I:I-14–I-24, 1972
29. **Björk VO, Olin C, Rodriguez L:** Comparative results of aortic valve replacement with different prosthetic heart valves. J Cardiovasc Surg 13:268–271, 1972
30. **Levine FH, Copeland JG, Morrow AG:** Prosthetic replacement of the mitral valve. Continuing assessments of the 100 patients operated upon during 1961–1965. Circulation 47:518–526, 1973
31. **O'Rourke RA, Peterson KL, Braunwald NS:** Postoperative hemodynamic evaluation of a new fabric-covered ball-valve prosthesis. Circulation 47, 48:Suppl III:III-74–III-79, 1973
32. **Bonchek LI, Anderson RP, Starr A:** Mitral valve replacement with cloth-covered composite-seat prostheses. The case for early operation. J Thorac Cardiovasc Surg 67:93–109, 1974
33. **Bonchek LI, Starr A:** Ball valve prostheses: current appraisal of late results. Am J Cardiol 35:843–854, 1975
34. **Brawley RK, Donahoo JS, Gott VL:** Current status of the Beall, Björk-Shiley, Braunwald-Cutter, Lillehei-Kaster and Smeloff-Cutter cardiac valve prostheses. Am J Cardiol 35:855–865, 1975
35. **Smithwick W III, Kouchoukos NT, Karp RB, et al:** Late stenosis of Starr-Edwards cloth-covered prostheses. Ann Thorac Surg 20:249–255, 1975
36. **DeCesare W, Rath C, Hufnagel C:** Hemolytic anemia of mechanical origin with aortic-valve prosthesis. N Engl J Med 272: 1045–1050, 1965
37. **Walsch JR, Starr A, Ritzmann LW:** Intravascular hemolysis in patients with prosthetic valves and valvular heart disease. Circulation 39, 40:Suppl I:I-135–I-140, 1969
38. **Wallace HW, Kenepp DL, Blakemore WS:** Quantitation of red blood cell destruction associated with valvular disease and prosthetic valves. J Thorac Cardiovasc Surg 60:842–852, 1970
39. **Roberts WC, Morrow AG:** Renal hemosiderosis in patients with prosthetic aortic valves. Circulation 36:390–398, 1966
40. **Roberts WC, Morrow AG:** Causes of death and other anatomic observations after cardiac valve replacement. Adv Cardiol 7: 226–247, 1972
41. **Weily HS, Genton E:** Altered platelet function in patients with prosthetic mitral valves. Effects of sulfinpyrazone therapy. Circulation 42:967–972, 1970
42. **Steele PP, Weily HS, Davies H, et al:** Platelet survival time following aortic valve replacement. Circulation 51:358–362, 1975
43. **Ahmad R, Manohitharajah SM, Deverall PB, et al:** Chronic hemolysis following mitral valve replacement. A comparative study of the Björk-Shiley, composite-seat Starr-Edwards, and frame-mounted aortic homograft valves. J Thorac Cardiovasc Surg 71:212–217, 1976
44. **Starr A, Pierie WR, Raible DA, et al:** Cardiac valve replacement. Experience with the durability of silicone rubber. Circulation 33, 34:Suppl I:I-115–I-123, 1966
45. **Roberts WC, Morrow AG:** Late postoperative pathological findings after cardiac valve replacement. Circulation 35, 36:Suppl I:I-48–I-62, 1967
46. **Roberts WC, Morrow AG:** Anatomic studies of hearts containing caged-ball prosthetic valves. Johns Hopkins Med J 121:271–295, 1967
47. **Laforet EG:** Death due to swelling of ball component of aortic ball-valve prosthesis. N Engl J Med 276:1025–1027, 1967
48. **Roberts WC, Morrow AG:** Fatal degeneration of the silicone rubber ball of the Starr-Edwards prosthetic aortic valve. Am J Cardiol 22:614–620, 1968
49. **Sanderson RG, Hall AD, Thomas AN:** The clinical diagnosis of ball variance in a mitral valve prosthesis. Ann Thorac Surg 6: 473–475, 1968
50. **Collins JJ Jr, Berg EJ, Harken DE:** Silicone ball variance. A clinical and pulse duplicator study. Ann Thorac Surg 6:546–551, 1968
51. **Bonnabeau R, Lillehei W:** Mechanical "ball failure" in Starr-Edwards prosthetic valves. A report of three cases. J Thorac Cardiovasc Surg 56:258–264, 1968
52. **Leatherman LL, Leachman RD, McConn RG, et al:** Malfunction of mitral ball-valve prostheses due to a swollen poppet. J Thorac Cardiovasc Surg 57:160–163, 1969
53. **Roberts WC, Morrow AG:** Late postoperative pathologic findings following cardiac valve replacement with Starr-Edwards prostheses. In, Proceedings of Second National Conference on Prosthetic Heart Valves. Springfield, Ill, Charles C Thomas, 1969, p 365–393
54. **Hylen JC, Kloster FE, Starr A, et al:** Aortic ball variance: diagnosis and treatment. Ann Intern Med 72:1–8, 1970
55. **Roberts WC, Levinson GE, Morrow AG:** Lethal ball variance in the Starr-Edwards prosthetic mitral valve. Arch Intern Med 126:517–521, 1970
56. **Connolly DC, Harrison CE, Ellis FH Jr:** Ball variance in a Starr-Edwards prosthetic mitral valve causing acute pulmonary edema (diagnosis by auscultation before onset of symptoms). Mayo Clin Proc 45:20–24, 1970
57. **Metzger CC, Magovern GJ, Leonard JJ:** Ball variance in a sutureless mitral valve prosthesis. A report of two cases and a clue to early diagnosis. J Thorac Cardiovasc Surg 61:699–704, 1971
58. **Schluger J, Mannix EP Jr, Wolf RE:** Auscultatory and phonocardiographic sign of ball variance in a mitral prosthetic valve. Am Heart J 81:809–816, 1971
59. **Hylen JC, Hodam RP, Kloster FE:** Changes in the durability of silicone rubber in ball-valve prostheses. Ann Thorac Surg 13: 324–329, 1972
60. **Roberts WC, Bulkley BH, Morrow AG:** Pathologic anatomy of cardiac valve replacement: a study of 224 necropsy patients. Prog Cardiovasc Dis 15:539–587, 1973
61. **Barnhorst DA, Oxman HA, Connolly DC, et al:** Isolated replacement of the mitral valve with the Starr-Edwards prosthesis. An eleven-year review. J Thorac Cardiovasc Surg 71:230–237, 1976
62. **Barnhorst DA, Oxman HA, Connolly DC, et al:** Long-term follow-up of isolated replacement of the aortic or mitral valve with the Starr-Edwards prosthesis. Am J Cardiol 35:228–233, 1975
63. **Pluth JR, Broadbent JC, Barnhorst DA, et al:** Aortic and mitral valve replacement with cloth-covered Braunwald-Cutter prosthesis. A three-year follow up. Ann Thorac Surg 20:239–248, 1975
64. **Roberts WC, Morrow AG:** Mechanisms of acute left atrial thrombosis after mitral valve replacement. Pathologic findings indicating obstruction to left atrial emptying. Am J Cardiol 18: 497–503, 1966
65. **Roberts WC, Lambird PA, Gott VL, et al:** Fatal aortic regurgitation following replacement of the mitral and aortic valves. A mechanical complication of double valve replacement. J Thorac Cardiovasc Surg 52:189–192, 1966
66. **Roberts WC, Morrow AG:** Causes of early postoperative death following cardiac valve replacement. Clinico-pathologic correlations in 64 patients studied at necropsy. J Thorac Cardiovasc Surg 54:422–437, 1967
67. **Robicsek F, Sanger PW, Daugherty HK, et al:** Fatal arrhythmias caused by the pressure of the ball-valve prosthesis upon the left ventricular myocardium. Dis Chest 52:813–816, 1967
68. **Quattlebaum FW, Kalke B, Edwards JE, et al:** Obstruction of the aorta by prosthetic aortic valve. J Thorac Cardiovasc Surg 55: 231–237, 1968
69. **Kalke B, Korns ME, Goott B, et al:** Engagement of ventricular myocardium by open-cage atrioventricular valvular prosthesis. J Thorac Cardiovasc Surg 58:92–94, 1969
70. **Najafi H, Ostermiller WE Jr, Javid H, et al:** Narrow aortic root

complicating aortic valve replacement. Arch Surg 99:690–694, 1969

71. **Ibarra-Pérez C, Rodriguez-Trujillo F, Perez-Redondo H:** Engagement of ventricular myocardium by struts of mitral prosthesis. Fatal complications of use of open-cage cardiac valves. J Thorac Cardiovasc Surg 61:403–404, 1971
72. **Shepherd RL, Glancy DL, Stinson EB, et al:** Hemodynamic confirmation of obstruction to left ventricular inflow by a caged-ball prosthetic mitral valve. J Thorac cardiovasc Surg 65:252–254, 1973
73. **Seningen RP, Bulkley BH, Roberts WC:** Prosthetic aortic stenosis. A method to prevent its occurrence by measurement of aortic size from preoperative aortogram. Circulation 49:921–924, 1974
74. **Vander Veer JB Jr, Rhyneer GS, Hodam RP, et al:** Obstruction of tricuspid ball-valve prostheses. Circulation 43, 44:Suppl I:I-62–I-67, 1971
75. **Bache RJ, From AHL, Castaneda AR, et al:** Late thrombotic obstruction of Starr-Edwards tricuspid valve prosthesis. Chest 61:613–616, 1972
76. **Assad-Morrell JL, Tajik AJ, Anderson MW, et al:** Malfunctioning tricuspid valve prosthesis. Clinical, phonocardiographic, echocardiographic and surgical findings. Mayo Clinic Proc 49:443–447, 1974
77. **Baxter RH, Bain WH, Rankin RJ, et al:** Tricuspid valve replacement: a five-year appraisal. Thorax 30:158–161, 1975
78. **Malcolm AD, Ahuja SP, Chamberlain MJ:** Malfunction of tricuspid valve prosthesis shown by isotope angiocardiography. J Thorac Cardiovasc Surg 71:134–136, 1976
79. **Paton BC:** Reoperation for fibrinous stenosis of disc mitral valve prosthesis. J Thorac Cardiovasc Surg 57:726–731, 1969
80. **Horsley HT, Rappoport WJ, Vigoda PS, et al:** Fatal malfunction of Edwards low-profile mitral valves. Circulation 41, 42:Suppl I:II-39–II-42, 1970
81. **Mullen DC, Shull WH, Daugherty HK, et al:** Emergency thrombectomy of the prosthetic mitral valve. Vasc Surg 4:137–141, 1970
82. **Demany MA, Zimmerman HA:** Thrombosis of a mitral disc-valve prosthesis: diagnostic importance of the absent opening click. Am Heart J 80:816–819, 1970
83. **Gunstensen J:** Acute dysfunction of Starr-Edwards mitral prostheses. Thorax 26:163–166, 1971
84. **Stross JK, Willis PW, Kahn DR:** Diagnostic features of malfunction of disc mitral valve prostheses. JAMA 217:305–308, 1971
85. **Balkoura-Christopoulos MH, Resnekov L, Kittle CF:** Malfunction of a disc mitral valve prosthesis: detection by phonocardiography. Chest 63:624–626, 1973
86. **Linhart JW, Barold SS, Hildner FJ, et al:** Clinical and hemodynamic findings following replacement of the mitral valve with a Beall valve prosthesis (Dacron velour-covered Teflon-disc valve). Circulation 39, 40:Suppl I:I-127–I-134, 1969
87. **Vogel JHK, Paton BC, Overy HR, et al:** Abnormal hemodynamic function after disc mitral valve replacement. Circulation 39, 40:Suppl I:I-141–I-147, 1969
88. **Björk VO, Olin C, Aström H:** Results of aortic valve replacement with the Kay-Shiley disc valve. Scand J Thorac Cardiovasc Surg 3:93–106, 1969
89. **Kay EB, Suzuki A, Tambi A, et al:** Comparative analysis of the Starr-Edwards ball valve, the Kay-Suzuki disc valve and transplant valves in the surgical correction of aortic valve disease. Am J Cardiol 25:535–545, 1970
90. **Olin C:** Evaluation of the Kay-Shiley disc valve prosthesis in the aortic position. Clinical and haemodynamic results, and experimental comparison with other prosthetic aortic valves. Scand J Thorac Cardiovasc Surg [Suppl] 7:1–37, 1970
91. **Ramsey HW, Williams JC Jr, Vernon CR, et al:** Hemodynamic findings following replacement of the mitral valve with the Beall valve prosthesis. J Thorac Cardiovasc Surg 62:624–630, 1971
92. **Rogers AK, Morgan JR, Forker AD, et al:** Supravalvular stenosis after disc mitral valve replacement. J Thorac Cardiovasc Surg 62:810–812, 1971
93. **Reid JA, Stevens TW, Sigwart U, et al:** Hemodynamic evaluation of the Beall mitral valve prosthesis. Circulation 45, 46:Suppl I: I-1–I-7, 1972
94. **Shepherd RL, Glancy DL, Reis RL, et al:** Hemodynamic function of the Kay-Shiley prosthetic cardiac valve. Observations after mitral or tricuspid valve replacement. Chest 63:323–326, 1973
95. **Hawe A, Frye RL, Ellis FH Jr:** Late hemodynamic studies after mitral valve surgery. J Thorac Cardiovasc Surg 65:351–358, 1973
96. **Beall AC Jr, Morris GC Jr, Howell JF Jr, et al:** Clinical experience with an improved mitral valve prosthesis. Ann Thorac Surg 15: 601–606, 1973
97. **Roberts WC, Fishbein MC, Golden A:** Cardiac pathology after valve replacement by disc prosthesis. A study of 61 necropsy patients. Am J Cardiol 35:740–760, 1975
98. **Wellons HA Jr, Strauch RS, Nolan SP, et al:** Isolated mitral valve replacement with the Kay-Shiley disc valve. Actuarial analysis of the long-term results. J Thorac Cardiovasc Surg 70:862–868, 1975
99. **Fernandez J, Morse D, Spagna P, et al:** Results of mitral valve replacement with the Beall prosthesis in 209 patients. J Thorac Cardiovasc Surg 71:218–225, 1976
100. **Behrendt DM, Austen WG:** Current status of prosthetics for heart valve replacement. Prog Cardiovasc Dis 15:369–401, 1973
101. **Carey JS, Hughes RK:** A complication of mitral-valve replacement with caged-lens prosthesis. Ann Thorac Surg 6:77–81, 1968
102. **Vasko JS, Leighton RF:** Acute massive mitral regurgitation resulting from disc-valve malfunction. Ann Thorac Surg 6:564–569, 1968
103. **Robinson JJ, Hildner FJ, Greenberg JJ:** Disc variance of Beall mitral valve. Ann Thorac Surg 11:11–17, 1971
104. **Detmer DE, McIntosh CL, Boretos JW, et al:** Polypropylene poppets for low-profile prosthetic heart valves. Ann Thorac Surg 13:122–127, 1972
105. **Berroya RB, Escana FB Jr:** Mitral disc-valve variance. Thorax 27:87–89, 1972
106. **Hildner FJ, Robinson MJ:** Complications of Beall valve prosthesis. Am J Cardiol 30:922, 1972
107. **Nathan MJ:** Strut fracture. A late complication of Beall mitral valve replacement. Ann Thorac Surg 16:610–613, 1973
108. **Shaw TRD, Turner RWD:** Sudden mechanical malfunction of Hammersmith mitral valve prostheses due to wear of polypropylene. J Thorac Cardiovasc Surg 67:579–583, 1974
109. **Hughes DA, Leatherman LL, Norman JC, et al:** Late embolization of prosthetic mitral valve occluder with survival following reoperation. Ann Thorac Surg 19:212–215, 1975
110. **Low HBC, Lefemine AA:** Acute mitral insufficiency due to jamming of a disc-valve prosthesis. Ann Thorac Surg 4:71–73, 1967
111. **Hopeman AR, Treasure RL, Hall RJ:** Mechanical dysfunction in caged-lens prostheses. J Thorac Cardiovasc Surg 60:51–59, 1970
112. **Oliva PB, Johnson ML, Pomerantz M, et al:** Dysfunction of the Beall mitral prosthesis and its detection by cinefluoroscopy and echocardiography. Am J Cardiol 31:393–396, 1973
113. **Hammer WJ, Hearne MJ, Roberts WC:** Cocking of a poppet disc prosthesis in the aortic position. A cause of intermittent aortic regurgitation. J Thorac Cardiovasc Surg 71:259–261, 1976
114. **Williams JC Jr, Vernon CR, Daicoff GR, et al:** Hemolysis following mitral valve replacement with the Beall valve prosthesis. J Thorac Cardiovasc Surg 61:393–396, 1971
115. **Cooley DA, Okies JE, Wukasch DC, et al:** Ten-year experience with cardiac valve replacement: results with a new mitral prosthesis. Ann Surg 177:818–826, 1973
116. **Wukasch DC, Sandiford FM, Reul GJ Jr, et al:** Complications of cloth-covered prosthetic valves: results with a new mitral prosthesis. J Thorac Cardiovasc Surg 69:107–116, 1975
117. **Cooley DA, Sandiford FM, Wukasch DC, et al:** Mitral valve replacement with a new prosthesis. Experience with 366 patients. J Cardiovasc Surg (Torino): special no:378–383, 1975
118. **Edgett JW, Nelson WP, Hall RJ, et al:** A complication of valve replacement by a caged-lens prosthesis. Circulation 36:422–426, 1967
119. **Hammermeister KE, Dillard DH, Kennedy JW:** Severe, intermittent, mitral regurgitation in a Cross-Jones valve. Report of a case with angiocardiographic and hemodynamic observations. J Thorac Cardiovasc Surg 58:575–580, 1969

120. **Roe BB, Fishman NH, Hutchinson JC, et al:** Occluder disruption of Wada-Cutter valve prosthesis. Ann Thorac Surg 20:256–264, 1975
121. **Björk VO, Holmgren A, Olin C, et al:** Clinical and hemodynamic results of aortic valve replacement with the Björk-Shiley tilting disc valve prosthesis. Scand J Thorac Cardiovasc Surg 5: 177–191, 1971
122. **Lepley D, Reuben CF, Flemma RJ, et al:** Experience with the Björk-Shiley prosthetic valve. Circulation 47, 48:Suppl III:III-51–III-55, 1973
123. **Böök K:** Mitral valve replacement with the Björk-Shiley tilting disc valve. A clinical and haemodynamic study in patients with isolated mitral valve lesions. Scand J Thorac Cardiovasc Surg [Suppl] 12:1–28, 1974
124. **Lillehei CW, Kaster RL, Coleman M, et al:** Heart-valve replacement with Lillehei-Kaster pivoting disk prosthesis. NY State J Med 8:1426–1438, 1974
125. **Björk VO, Henze A, Holmgren A:** Five years' experience with the Björk-Shiley tilting-disc valve in isolated aortic valvular disease. J Thorac Cardiovasc Surg 68:393–404, 1974
126. **Björk VO, Henze A, Holmgren A:** Long-term results with the Björk-Shiley tilting disc valve in aortic valvular disease. Isr J Med Sci 11:161–172, 1975
127. **Starek PJK, Wilcox BR, Murray GF:** Hemodynamic evaluation of the Lillehei-Kaster pivoting disc valve in patients. J Thorac Cardiovasc Surg 71:123–128, 1976
128. **Slater SD, Sallam IA, Bain WH, et al:** Haemolysis with Björk-Shiley and Starr-Edwards prosthetic heart valves: a comparative study. Thorax 29:624–631, 1974
129. **Roberts WC, Hammer WJ:** Cardiac pathology after valve replacement with a tilting disc prosthesis (Björk-Shiley type): a study of 46 necropsy patients and 49 Björk-Shiley prostheses. Am J Cardiol 37:1024–1033, 1976
130. **Messmer BJ, Okies JE, Hallman GL, et al:** Mitral valve replacement with the Björk-Shiley tilting-disc prosthesis. J Thorac Cardiovasc Surg 62:938–946, 1971
131. **Messmer BJ, Okies JE, Hallman GL, et al:** Early and late thromboembolic complications after mitral valve replacement. A comparative study of various prostheses. J Cardiovasc Surg 13:281–289, 1972
132. **Messmer BJ, Okies JE, Hallman GL, et al:** Aortic valve replacement: two years' experience with the Björk-Shiley tilting-disc prosthesis. Surgery 72:772–779, 1972
133. **Henze A, Carlsson S, Björk VO:** Mortality and pathology following aortic valve replacement with the Björk-Shiley tilting disc valve. Scand J Thorac Cardiovasc Surg 7:7–16, 1973
134. **Ben-Zvi J, Hildner FJ, Chandraratna PA, et al:** Thrombosis on Björk-Shiley aortic valve prosthesis. Clinical, arteriographic, echocardiographic and therapeutic observations in seven cases. Am J Cardiol 34:538–544, 1974
135. **Byrd CL, Yahr WZ, Greenberg JJ:** Long-term results of "simple" thrombectomy for thrombosed Björk-Shiley aortic valve prostheses. Ann Thorac Surg 20:265–273, 1975
136. **Ross D:** Biologic valves. Their performance and prospects. Circulation 45:1259–1272, 1972
137. **Angell WW, Shumway NE, Kosek JC:** A five-year study of viable aortic valve homografts. J Thorac Cardiovasc Surg 64:329–339, 1972
138. **Wallace RB, Londe SP, Titus JL:** Aortic valve replacement with preserved aortic valve homografts. J Thorac Cardiovasc Surg 67:44–52, 1974
139. **Wallace RB:** Tissue valves. Am J Cardiol 35:866–871, 1975
140. **Moore CH, Martelli V, Al-Janabi N, et al:** Analysis of homograft valve failure in 311 patients followed up to 10 years. Ann Thorac Surg 20:274–281, 1975
141. **Yarbrough JW, Roberts WC, Reis RL:** Structural alterations in tissue cardiac valves implanted in patients and in calves. J Thorac Cardiovasc Surg 65:364–375, 1973
142. **Ionescu MI, Pakrashi BC, Mary DAS, et al:** Replacement of heart valves with frame-mounted tissue grafts. Thorax 29:56–67, 1974
143. **Nuno-Conceicão A, Puig LB, Verginelli G, et al:** Homologous dura mater cardiac valves. Structural aspects of eight implanted valves. J Thorac Cardiovasc Surg 70:499–508, 1975
144. **Mary DAS, Pakrashi BC, Catchpole RW, et al:** Tissue valves in the mitral position. Five years' experience. Br Heart J 37: 1123–1132, 1975
145. **Olsen EGJ, Al-Janabi N, Salamão CS, et al:** Fascia lata valves: a clinicopathological study. Thorax 30:528–534, 1975
146. **Reis RL, Hancock WD, Yarbrough JW, et al:** The flexible stent. A new concept in the fabrication of tissue heart valve prostheses. J Thorac Cardiovasc Surg 62:683–695, 1971
147. **Stinson EB, Griepp RB, Shumway NE:** Clinical experience with a porcine aortic valve xenograft for mitral valve replacement. Ann Thorac Surg 18:391–401, 1974
148. **Horowitz MS, Goodman DJ, Fogarty TJ, et al:** Mitral valve replacement with the glutaraldehyde-preserved porcine heterograft. Clinical, hemodynamic, and pathological correlations. J Thorac Cardiovasc Surg 67:885–895, 1974
149. **Carpentier A, Deloche A, Relland J, et al:** Six-year follow-up of glutaraldehyde-preserved heterografts. With particular reference to the treatment of congenital valve malformations. J Thorac Cardiovasc Surg 68:771–782, 1974
150. **Brown JW, Myerowitz PD, Cann MS, et al:** Clinical and hemodynamic comparisons of Kay-Shiley, Starr-Edwards no. 6520, and Reis-Hancock porcine xenograft mitral valves. Surgery 76:983–991, 1974
151. **Johnson AD, Daily PO, Peterson KL, et al:** Functional evaluation of the porcine heterograft in the mitral position. Circulation 50, 51:Suppl I:I-40–I-48, 1975
152. **McIntosh CL, Michaelis LL, Morrow AG, et al:** Atrioventricular valve replacement with the Hancock porcine xenograft: a five year clinical experience. Surgery 78:768–775, 1975
153. **Pipkin RD, Buch WS, Fogarty TJ:** Evaluation of aortic valve replacement with a porcine xenograft without long-term anticoagulation. J Thorac Cardiovasc Surg 71:179–186, 1976
154. **Zudhi N, Hawley W, Voehl V, et al:** Porcine aortic valves as replacement for human heart valves. Ann Thorac Surg 17:479–491, 1974
155. **Roberts WC, Perloff JK, Constantino T:** Severe valvular aortic stenosis in patients over 65 years of age. A clinicopathologic study. Am J Cardiol 27:497–506, 1971
156. **Roberts WC, Perloff JK:** Mitral valvular disease. A clinicopathologic survey of the conditions causing the mitral valve to function abnormally. Ann Intern Med 77:939–975, 1972
157. **Roberts WC, Dangel JC, Bulkley BH:** Nonrheumatic valvular cardiac disease: a clinicopathologic survey of 27 different conditions causing valvular dysfunction. Cardiovasc Clin 5:333–446, 1973
158. **Hancock WD:** Personal communication, November 1975
159. **Merendino KA, Morrow AG, Lillehei CW, et al:** Prosthetic Valves for Cardiac Surgery. Springfield, Ill, Charles C Thomas, 1961, p 86
160. **Braunwald NS:** The fabric-covered prosthetic heart valve. Present status and future development. Ann Thorac Surg 20:360–363, 1975
161. **Eiseman B, Spencer FC:** The occasional open-heart surgeon. Circulation 31:161–162, 1965
162. **Fernandez J:** Insertion of Björk-Shiley aortic prosthesis by continuous suture technique. Ann Thorac Surg 17:587–590, 1974
163. **Cohn LH, Sanders JH Jr, Collins JJ Jr:** Aortic valve replacement with the Hancock porcine xenograft. Presented at the Society of Thoracic Surgeons, Washington, DC, January, 1976
164. **Morris DC:** Hemodynamic evaluation of porcine xenograft valve. Presented at the Annual Scientific Sessions of the American College of Cardiology, New Orleans, February, 1976

Sarcoidosis of the Heart

A Clinicopathologic Study of 35 Necropsy Patients (Group I) and Review of 78 Previously Described Necropsy Patients (Group II)

WILLIAM C. ROBERTS, M.D.
Bethesda, Maryland

HUGH A. McALLISTER, Jr., M.D.
Washington, D.C.

VICTOR J. FERRANS, M.D., Ph.D.
Bethesda, Maryland

Certain clinical and morphologic observations are described in 35 necropsy patients with cardiac sarcoidosis (group IA and IB), and similar observations are summarized in 78 previously described necropsy patients with cardiac sarcoidosis (group IIA and IIB). All patients had non-necrotic ("hard") granulomas in lymph nodes and either sarcoid granulomas in the heart (108 patients) or transmural myocardial scarring (five patients) unassociated with coronary arterial narrowing, i.e., healed granulomas. The 113 patients (groups I and II) whose data are analyzed also were divided into those in whom cardiac dysfunction clearly was the result of sarcoid granulomatous infiltration of the heart (89 patients) (groups IA and IIA), and those in whom cardiac dysfunction, if present, was clearly not the result of sarcoid involvement of the heart (24 patients) (groups IB and IIB).

Analysis of the 89 patients in groups IA and IIA disclosed that death was *sudden* (arrhythmia) in 60 (67 per cent), secondary to progressive *congestive cardiac failure* in 20 (23 per cent), from *recurring pericardial effusion* in three (3 per cent) and from other or unknown causes in six (7 per cent). Sudden death was the initial manifestation of sarcoidosis in 10 (17 per cent) of the 60 patients who died suddenly. Other than premature ventricular beats, *ventricular tachycardia* was the most common arrhythmia (17 patients), and *complete heart block* was the most common conduction disturbance (25 patients). *Complete bundle branch block* occurred in 21 patients. *Ventricular aneurysm* (eight patients) and *papillary muscle dysfunction* (possibly 16 patients) were other cardiac disturbances observed.

Although *corticosteroid therapy* tends to cause fibrous replacement of myocardial sarcoid granulomas, a possible consequence of this medication is the development of ventricular aneurysm.

Most patients with cardiac sarcoidosis causing dysfunction (groups IA and IIA) presented initially with manifestations related to the heart. Furthermore, most patients with cardiac sarcoidosis have little or no clinical evidence of dysfunction of an organ system other than the heart. Usually the course in patients with extensive cardiac sarcoidosis is not prolonged.

From the Pathology Branch, National Heart, Lung and Blood Institute, National Insitutes of Health, Bethesda, Maryland; and the Cardiovascular Department, Armed Forces Institute of Pathology, Washington, D.C. Requests for reprints should be addressed to Dr. William C. Roberts, Building 10A, Room 3E-30, National Institutes of Health, Bethesda, Maryland 20014.

Manuscript accepted October 6, 1976.

Sarcoidosis, a systemic granulomatous disease of undetermined etiology and pathogenesis, most often involves lymph nodes, lungs, liver, spleen, skin, eyes, phalangeal bones and parotid glands, but other organs and tissues also may be affected. Cardiac involvement in patients with sarcoidosis has been reported on many occasions, but most reports are isolated case studies. The present study is a clinicopathologic analysis of a relatively large number of necropsy patients with cardiac sarcoidosis. It focuses on the varying types of functional and morphologic cardiac alterations in patients with cardiac sarcoidosis and, in addition, summarizes previous reports of this condition.

METHODS

The data on all the necropsy patients having cardiac sarcoidosis studied in the Pathology Branch, National Heart, Lung and Blood Institute, and in the Cardiovascular Registry of the Armed Forces Institute of Pathology are included in this analysis. A total of 35 patients was available for study (groups IA and IB). Prerequisites for inclusion in this study included (1) the presence of sarcoid-type, i.e., "hard" (non-necrotic) granulomas in lymph nodes, and (2) either the presence of sarcoid-type granulomas in the heart or the presence of transmural myocardial scarring unassociated with significant luminal narrowing of the extramural coronary arteries. The clinical and necropsy records, and the histologic sections from all body organs were reviewed. Excluding the one patient in whom the atrioventricular node and bundle were serially sectioned (sections cut a thickness of 6 μ and every fifth section was stained by hematoxylin and eosin), a total of 230 histologic sections of heart were examined, an average of six per patient (range one to 20). At least one histologic section of left ventricle was examined in every patient. Sections of other portions of the heart were available for reexamination in 31 patients: these included the ventricular septum (27 patients), the right ventricular free wall (25 patients), the right atrial wall (16 patients) and the left atrial wall (14 patients). The autopsy protocols also were examined for information regarding the presence or absence of granulomas in the various portions of the heart. Information was obtained regarding the presence or absence of sarcoid-type granulomas in lymph nodes (all patients) and lung, liver, and spleen (32 patients). Weights of the heart were available in 30 patients, and of the spleen, liver and both lungs in each of 20 patients. The available clinical information was examined in all 35 patients. Similar information was obtained on previously described cases of cardiac sarcoidosis. The classification used to group the 35 personally studied patients and the 78 previously described cases of cardiac sarcoidosis is outlined in Table I.

RESULTS

Certain clinical and morphologic observations in the 35 personally studied patients (groups IA and IB) are summarized in Tables II and III. For analysis of the cardiac disturbances, the 35 patients were subdivided into those in whom cardiac dysfunction clearly was the result of sarcoid granulomatous infiltration of the heart (26 patients, group IA, Table II), and those in whom cardiac dysfunction, if present, was clearly not the result of sarcoid granulomatous infiltration of the heart (nine patients, group IB, Table III).

At necropsy, 25 of these 26 patients (group IA) had grossly visible, usually large, granulomas in their hearts; the remaining patient had transmural myocardial scars unassociated with significant coronary arterial luminal narrowing. The other nine patients (group IB) were subdivided according to their predominant clinical features as shown in Table III. All nine of these patients had sarcoid granulomas in their hearts, but these granulomas were small; in eight patients they were visible only by histologic examination. This report focuses primarily on the 26 patients with cardiac dysfunction clearly secondary to sarcoid infiltration of the heart (group IA).

Observations in the Patients with Cardiac Dysfunction Secondary to Cardiac Sarcoidosis (Group IA). Cardiac dysfunction in the 26 patients in whom it was caused by cardiac sarcoidosis was variously manifested by arrhythmias and conduction disturbances, congestive cardiac failure and recurring pericardial effusions (Table II). These cardiac disturbances accounted for death in 25 of the 26 patients.

Arrhythmias or **conduction disturbances**, or both, were documented in 16 of these patients; electrocar-

TABLE I Cardiac Sarcoidosis: Necropsy Patients Analyzed

		Causing Cardiac Dysfunction (Subgroup A)		Not Causing Cardiac Dysfunction (Subgroup B)	
	Totals	No.	%	No.	%
Personally studied patients (group I)	35	26	74	9	26
Previously described patients (group II)	78	63	81	15	19
Totals	113	89	79	24	21

diograms were never recorded in six of the remaining 10 patients. Episodes of **ventricular tachycardia** were documented by electrocardiogram in five patients; 12 patients had ventricular premature beats. Four patients, two of whom also had episodes of ventricular tachycardia, had **atrial arrhythmias:** atrial fibrillation in two, atrial tachycardia in one and frequent atrial premature beats in one.

Heart block was confirmed by electrocardiogram in seven patients: prolongation of the P-R interval in one patient and complete heart block in six. In five of them the third degree heart block was present from two to six months; in the sixth patient it appeared about 2 hours before death. Three of the five patients with long-term complete heart block had syncope, which was the initial manifestation of sarcoidosis in each of them. Among the five patients with long-term complete heart block, the conduction disturbance, once it appeared, was persistent thereafter in four and periodic in one. In the latter patient, fibrous scarring associated with lymphocytic-cell infiltration was present at necropsy in the most cephalad portion of the muscular ventricular septum, whereas in the four patients with permanent complete heart block, large granulomas were still

TABLE II Cardiac Sarcoidosis Causing Cardiac Dysfunction: Clinical and Morphologic Observations in 26 Personally Studied Patients (Group IA)

	Mode of Death				
	Sudden	Congestive Heart Failure	Pericardial Effusion	Noncardiac	Totals
Patients (no.)	17	6	2	1	26
Age (yr)					
Range	21–74	26–73	35–47	34	21–74
Average	36	51	41	34	40
Race					
Black	9	3	2	0	14 (54)
White	7	2	0	1	10 (38)
Unknown or other	1	1	0	0	2 (8)
Sex					
Male	10	2	1	1	14 (54)
Female	7	4	1	0	12 (46)
Duration of symptoms (mo)					
Range	0–53	1–18	16, 18	48	0–53
Average	9*	7	17	48	11
Atrial arrhythmia	3	1	0	0	4 (15)
Ventricular premature beats	9	2	1	0	12 (46)
Ventricular tachycardia	5	0	1	0	6 (23)
Complete heart block	4	1	0	1	6 (23)
Syncope	3	0	0	0	3 (12)
Left bundle branch block	0	1	0	0	1 (12)
Right bundle branch block	1	1	0	0	2
Congestive heart failure	2	6	0	0	8 (31)
Diagnosis of sarcoid in life	5	0	2	1	8 (31)
Corticosteroid therapy	2	0	0	1	3 (12)
Heart weight (g)					
Range	300–550	300–660	350, 570	310	300–660
Average	430	536	460	310	428
Cardiac granulomas					
Left ventricle	17	6	2	0	25 (96)
Ventricular septum	15	4	0	0	19 (73)
Right ventricle	10	2	0	0	12 (46)
Papillary muscle	11	5	1	0	17 (65)
Atria	2	1	0	0	3 (12)
None	0	0	0	1	1 (4)
Ventricular aneurysm	2	0	0	0	2 (8)
Cardiac mural thrombi	0	0	0	1	1 (4)
Noncardiac granulomas					
Lymph node	17	6	2	1	26 (100)
Lung	15	4	1	0	20 (77)
Liver	11	4	2	1	18 (69)
Spleen	11	4	2	1	18 (69)
Other	6	2	2	1	11 (42)

NOTE: Figures in parentheses are per cents.

* This average includes six patients whose initial manifestation of sarcoidosis was sudden death.

present at necropsy in the most cephalad portion of the muscular ventricular septum. In addition to the six patients with complete heart block, three others had **complete bundle branch block** (right in two; left in one); one of these patients also had episodes of ventricular tachycardia, and another had atrial fibrillation.

It is presumed that an arrhythmia or a conduction disturbance was the cause of **sudden death,** which was the mode of death in 17 (65 per cent) of the 26 patients. Sudden death was the initial manifestation of sarcoidosis in six (35 per cent) of the 17 patients who died suddenly, and in each, death occurred during exertion. In none of these six patients was an electrocardiogram ever recorded. Of the remaining 11 patients who died suddenly, five had recurring episodes of ventricular tachycardia, and four others had complete heart block, three of whom had episodes of syncope (Stokes-Adams attacks). Of the remaining two patients who died suddenly, one was known to have ventricular premature beats, but he had always been asymptomatic and without any recognized features of sarcoidosis; the second patient, a 26 year old woman, began to lose weight about three years before her death, had a persistent cough, a right Horner's syndrome, and pulmonary lesions and hilar lymphadenopathy. Fatal rapid atrial fibrillation developed shortly after the patient underwent an open biopsy of lung.

Congestive cardiac failure occurred in eight of the

TABLE III Cardiac Sarcoidosis Not Causing Cardiac Dysfunction: Clinical and Morphologic Observations in Nine Personally Studied Patients (Group IB) and in 15 Previously Described Patients (Group IIB)

	Group IB (9 patients)			Group IIB (15 patients)			
Data	Respiratory Failure	Nonsarcoid Cardiac Dysfunction	Noncardiac and Non-pulmonary	Respiratory Failure	Nonsarcoid Cardiac Dysfunction	Noncardiac and Non-pulmonary	Totals
Patients	4	3	2	10	3	2	24*
References	. . .	. . .	. . .	[51–59, 61]	[22, 63, 64]	[60, 62]	[22, 51–64]
Ages (yr)							
Range	30–59	28–50	38–43	28–58	40–68	72, 83	28–83
Average	40	39	40	45	52	77	45
Race							
Black	3	2	1	3	0	0	9 (37)
White	1	1	1	4	2	1	10 (42)
Unknown	0	0	0	3	1	1	5 (21)
Sex							
Male	2	2	0	8	2	2	16 (67)
Female	2	1	2	2	1	0	8 (33)
Duration of symptoms (mo)							
Range	24–96	10–168	0–12	5–84	36–54	. . .	0–96
Average	72	71	6	36	45		46
Atrial arrhythmia	0	0	0	1	0	0	1 (4)
Ventricular premature beats	0	0	0	0	1	0	1 (4)
Bundle branch block	0	0	0	0	1	1	2 (8)
Congestive heart failure	. . .	3	0	. . .	3	0	6 (25)
Diagnosis of sarcoid during life	4	1	0	8	2	0	10 (42)
Corticosteroid therapy	2	0	0	0	1	0	3 (12)
Heart weight (g)							
Range	300–400	370–950	280–460	250–420	520–870	340	250–950
Average	345	623	370	336	670	340	440
Cardiac granulomas							
Left ventricle	4	3	2	3/3	. . .	2	14/14 (100)
Ventricular septum	1	1	0	2/3	. . .	1	5/14 (36)
Right ventricle	2	2	1	3/3	. . .	2	10/14 (71)
Papillary muscle	. . .	1	. . .	0/3	. . .	. . .	1/6 (17)
Atria	0	0	0	0/3	. . .	. . .	0
Noncardiac granulomas							
Lymph node	4	3	2	9/9	3	2	23/23 (100)
Lung	4	2	2	9/9	1	2	20/23 (87)
Liver	4	3	2	6/9	1	2	18/23 (78)
Spleen	4	2	2	7/9	1	2	18/23 (78)
Other	3	2	1	5/9	1	0	12/23 (52)

NOTE: Figures in parentheses are per cents.

* None of these 24 patients had ventricular tachycardia, complete heart block, syncope, cardiac aneurysm, intracardiac thrombi, or completely healed myocardial granulomas.

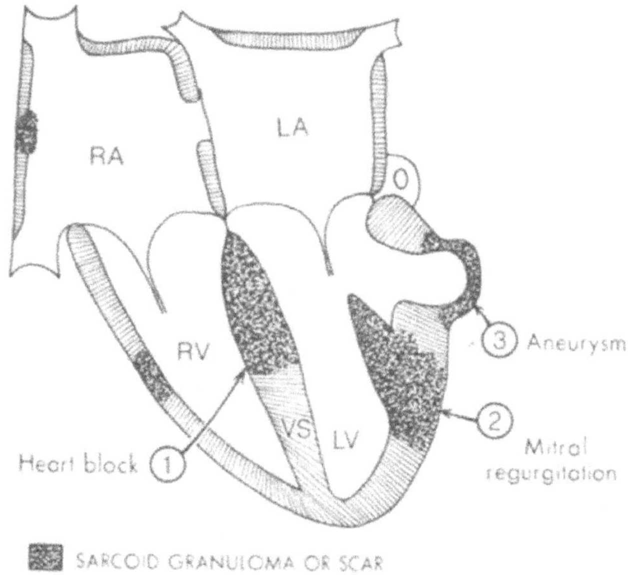

Figure 1. *Diagram showing the most common sites of sarcoid granulomas or scars in the heart and the most frequent functional consequences of these lesions.*

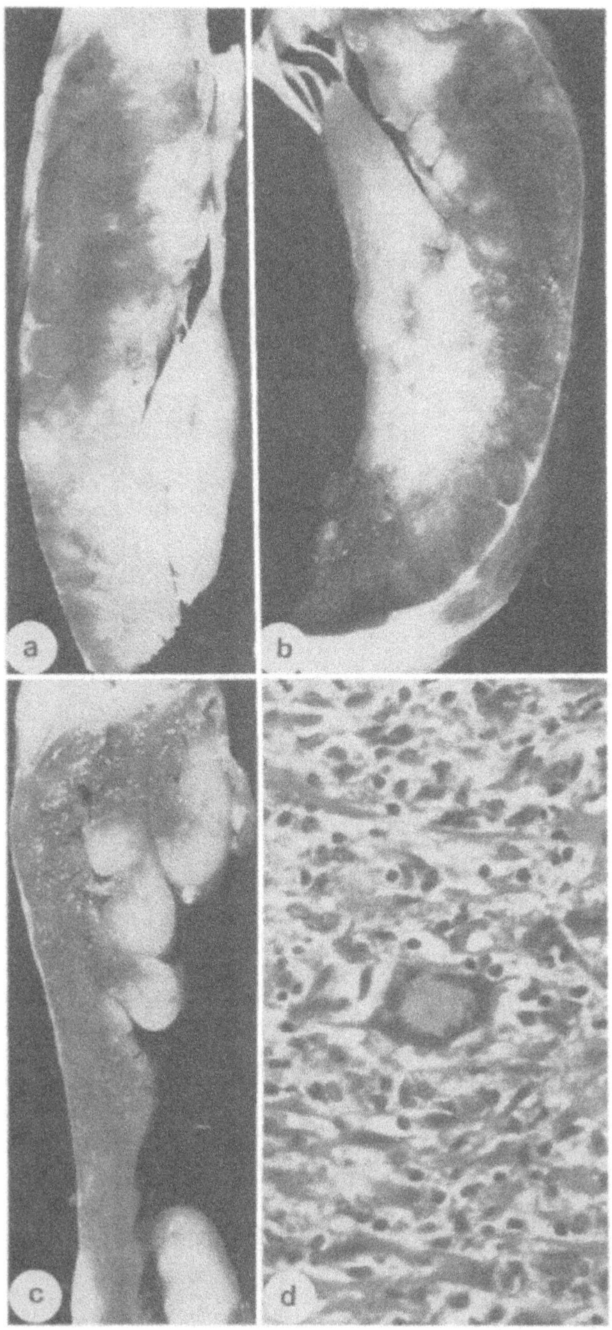

Figure 2. *The heart in a 26 year old black woman (A-70-541) who had been asymptomatic until 10 days before her death when dyspnea appeared. The dyspnea rapidly worsened, and when the patient was hospitalized on the day of death, she was in acute pulmonary edema. The blood pressure was 80/70 mm Hg, heart rate 160 beats/min and a grade 3-4/6 pansystolic blowing murmur, which radiated to the axilla, was audible. A chest roentgenogram showed congested lungs, cardiomegaly and prominent hilar adenopathy. Electrocardiogram showed nonspecific S-T segment and T-wave changes and atrial hypertrophy. Complete heart block developed and the patient died shortly thereafter.* ***a*** *and* ***b****, longitudinal sections of left ventricular free wall at sites of the papillary muscles. The latter are totally replaced by firm, white deposits, several of which also infiltrate the free wall.* ***c****, longitudinal section of right atrial wall showing similar white deposits.* ***d****, histologic section of a portion of a white deposit in the heart showing typical sarcoid granulomas. Similar hard granulomas were present in lymph nodes, liver, spleen and lung. Hematoxylin and eosin stain; original magnification X 400 (****d****), reduced by 12 per cent.*

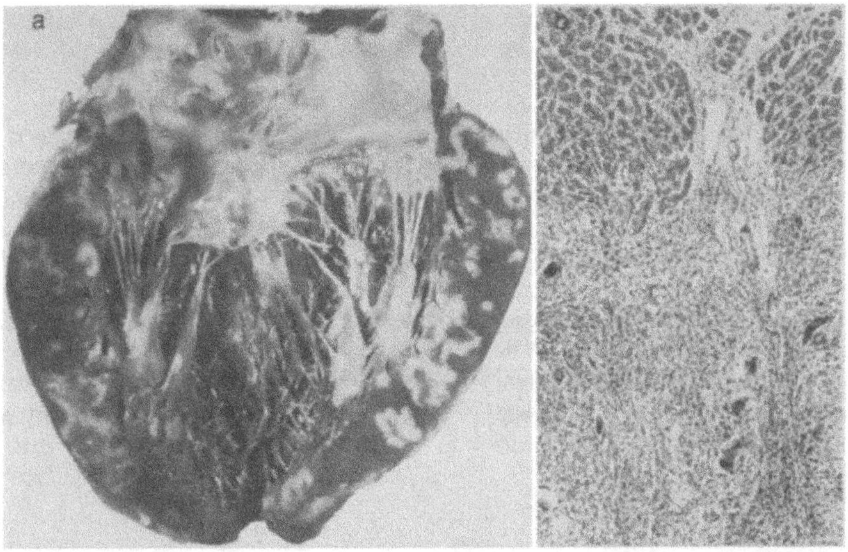

Figure 3. *Opened left atrium, mitral valve and left ventricle (**a**) and photomicrograph of a portion of the left ventricular wall (**b**) in a 28 year old black man (A-70-55) who died suddenly on his job as a construction worker. He had been well until two days earlier when he complained of "pain in his neck," but this had not prevented him from performing his usual activities. He had never sought medical care. At necropsy, sarcoid granulomas were found in the mediastinal lymph nodes, lung and heart. The heart weighed 420 g. Numerous sarcoid granulomas are present in the left ventricular free wall and in both papillary muscles. The posteromedial one is virtually replaced by the granulomas. Hematoxylin and eosin stain (**b**); original magnification × 100, reduced by 26 per cent.*

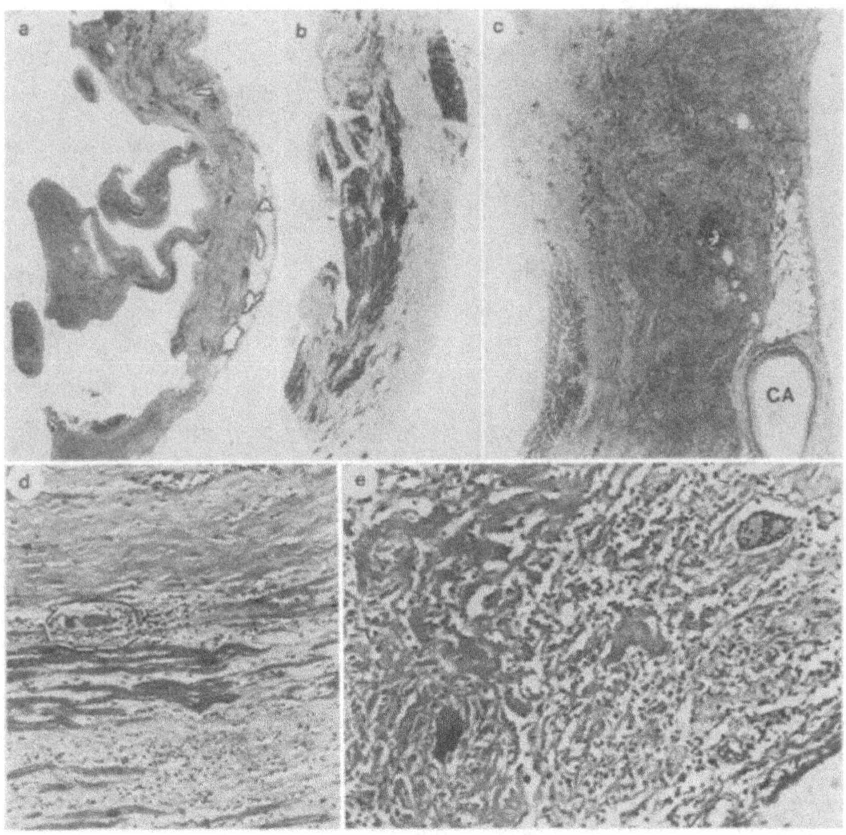

Figure 4. *Photomicrographs of the posterior left ventricular free wall in a 44 year old, extremely obese (260 pounds), white woman (A73-128) in whom evidence of congestive cardiac failure developed months before her death. A chest roentgenogram showed mild cardiomegaly and "pulmonary congestion." Several days before death, ventricular tachycardia developed suddenly. Episodes of this arrhythmia occurred until her death. Diagnosis of sarcoid was not suspected during life. **a, b, c,** longitudinal sections of left ventricular posterior wall at three different sites. In **a** and **c** there is complete transmural replacement of the wall primarily by fibrous tissue which contains occasional granuloma. The posteromedial papillary muscle is also completely replaced by sarcoid (**a**). Mainly the epicardial half of the portion shown in **b** is replaced. The coronary arteries (CA), one of which is shown in **c,** were wide open. In **d** only one granuloma (dashed circle) is present but the amount of fibrous tissue is extensive. In **e** more granulomas are seen. Far more granulomas were present in the lymph nodes than in the heart. Some also were found in the liver, spleen and lungs. Masson trichrome stain (**a** and **b**), hematoxylin and eosin stain (**c**, **d** and **e**); original magnification × 3 (**a** and **b**), × 15 (**c**), × 140 (**d**) and × 200 (**e**), reduced by 40 per cent.*

26 patients. Two of the eight patients had mild failure and died suddenly; the other six had progressive and eventually fatal failure. The left ventricular walls were extensively infiltrated by sarcoid granulomas in all eight patients with congestive cardiac failure. Of the six patients with severe, fatal heart failure, two had loud (grade 3–4/6) precordial, apical, systolic murmurs consistent with mitral regurgitation. At necropsy, both patients had extensive infiltration of their left ventricular papillary muscles by sarcoid granulomas; thus each had papillary muscle dysfunction as a result of myocardial sarcoidosis. Two patients had changes on the electrocardiogram that suggested recent myocardial infarction; one patient presented with acute failure, was symptomatic for only about one month and, during life, was considered to have the failure on the basis of acute myocardial infarction. Two patients, each of whom had had chronic failure for at least six months, had an acute exacerbation of the failure several days before death; at necropsy, each had large pulmonary emboli.

Recurring pericardial effusion was the cause of cardiac dysfunction in two of the 26 patients. The

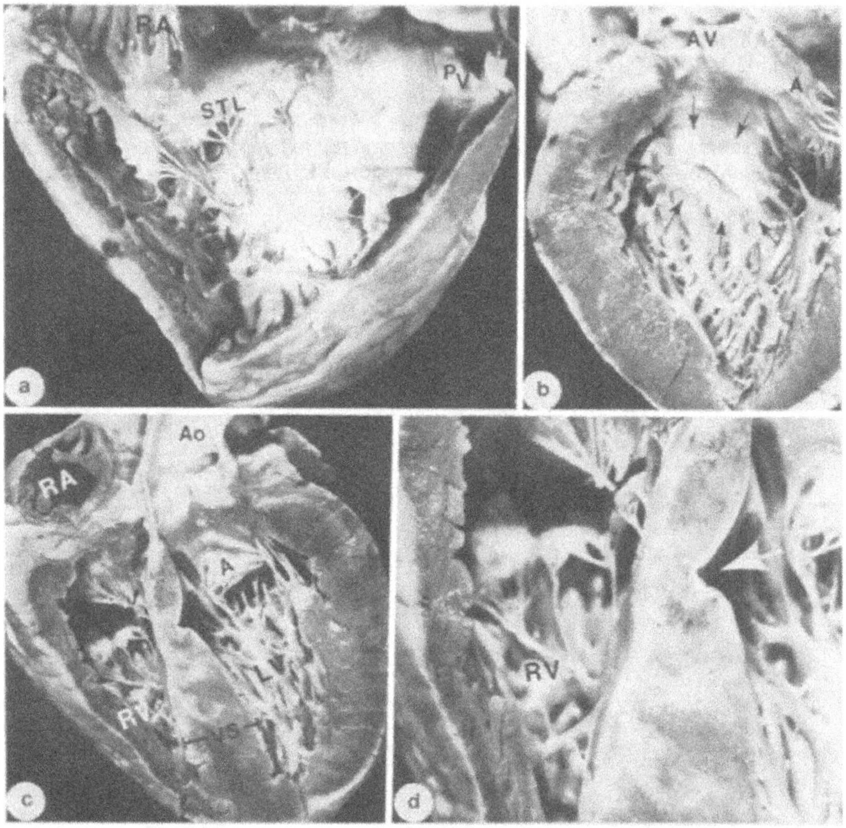

Figure 5. *Heart in a 30 year old black man (73-12-1146) who, three years before his death, was found to have bilateral pulmonary infiltrates. Open biopsy at that time disclosed sarcoidosis. He was asymptomatic until about 12 months before death when he noted occasional palpitations. Seven months before death he had the sudden onset of dyspnea, severe weakness and sweating, and he was found to have supraventricular tachycardia with a ventricular rate of 260 beats/min. Cardioversion restored his rhythm to sinus mechanism. An electrocardiogram shortly thereafter showed complete right bundle branch block, left ventricular hypertrophy and changes suggesting anteroseptal myocardial infarction of indeterminate age. A chest roentgenogram showed bilateral pulmonary infiltrates. Other electrocardiograms during this hospitalization showed atrial, nodal and ventricular premature beats, and periodic nodal tachycardia. Prednisone therapy was started at this time, initially 40 mg daily, and three months before death, 25 mg daily. The supraventricular tachycardia recurred thereafter about once a month until death despite prednisone, procainamide, diphenylhydantoin, and transiently, transvenous pacemaker, therapy. He was found dead in a hotel room while on a trip. At necropsy, the heart weighed 450 g. A small focus of fibrous pericardial adhesions was present posteriorly. The walls of both cardiac ventricles were hypertrophied. The endocardium of the right ventricular aspect of the ventricular septum was white and thick (**a**). RA = right atrium; PV = pulmonic valve; STL = septal tricuspid leaflet. A small indentation surrounded by white thick endocardium (**arrows**) was present on the left ventricular aspect of the ventricular septum (**b**). On longitudinal section (**c**) the cephalad portion of the ventricular septum (VS) was thinned and extensively infiltrated by firm white tissue which histologically was typical of sarcoid. LV = left ventricle; RV = right ventricle; A = anterior mitral leaflet; Ao = aorta. A close-up view of the sarcoid-infiltrated ventricular septum is shown in **d.** The indentation (**arrow**) of the ventricular septum is well shown.*

effusions had recurred over periods of 16 and 18 months, respectively, and both patients had huge cardiac silhouettes on chest roentgenogram. The diagnosis of sarcoidosis was established in each by biopsy of parietal pericardium one and two days, respectively, before death. At open biopsy, each patient had approximately 800 ml of serous pericardial effusion; at necropsy, each had sarcoid granulomas in the parietal pericardium, and both had left ventricular myocardial granulomas. Granulomas in one patient were small and in the second patient, huge.

Morphologic Observations. The weight of the heart in the 26 patients ranged from 310 to 700 g (average 461 g). The average weight among the 17 patients who died suddenly was less than that in the six patients with fatal congestive cardiac failure. Cardiac granulomas were observed grossly in 25 of the 26 hearts, and in the remaining one transmural myocardial scars were present. Sarcoid granulomas were present in the left ventricular free wall of all 25 patients, in the ventricular septum in at least 19 patients, in the right ventricular wall in 12 patients, in the right atrial wall in three patients and in the left atrial wall in two. The granulomas were most extensive in the left ventricular free wall and usually transmural (involving more than half of the thickness of the wall) (Figures 1 through 4). The deposits in the atrial wall were small (<1 cm) in all but one patient (Figure 2), in whom they were extensive in the right

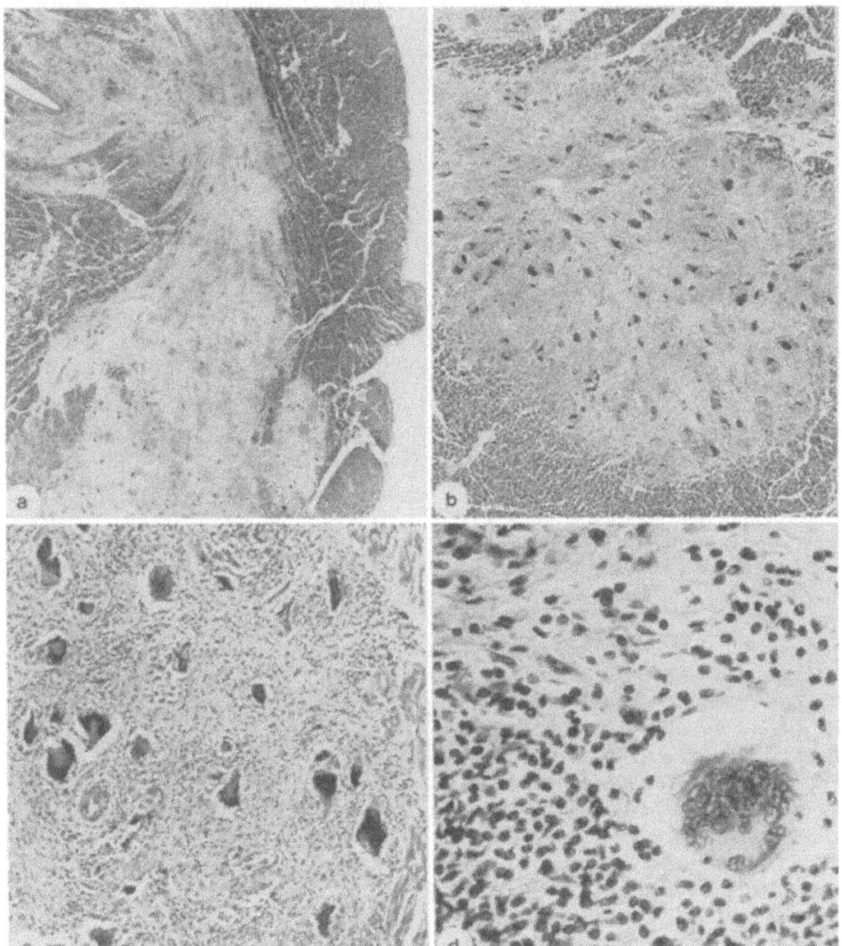

Figure 6. *Extensive, myocardial sarcoid in a 49 year old extremely obese (220 pounds) Indian woman (A-5559) who had been asymptomatic until two months before death when she fainted, and an electrocardiogram showed complete heart block with a ventricular rate of 32 beats/min. A chest roentgenogram disclosed mild cardiomegaly. Thereafter, she became quite dyspneic with only mild exertion. She collapsed while in the bathroom, and resuscitation was unsuccessful. Diagnosis of sarcoidosis was never suspected during life. At necropsy, the heart weighed 430 g. The entire cephalad portion of the ventricular septum, the entire anterolateral papillary muscle and several portions of left ventricular free wall were replaced by sarcoid granulomas.* ***a,*** *low power view of the ventricular septum showing extensive replacement of myocardium by sarcoid.* ***b, c*** *and* ***d,*** *progressive higher power views showing numerous giant cells, mononuclear cells and fibrous tissue. Hematoxylin and eosin stains; original magnification × 11 (****a****), × 35 (****b****), × 130 (****c****) and × 185 (****d****), reduced by 40 per cent.*

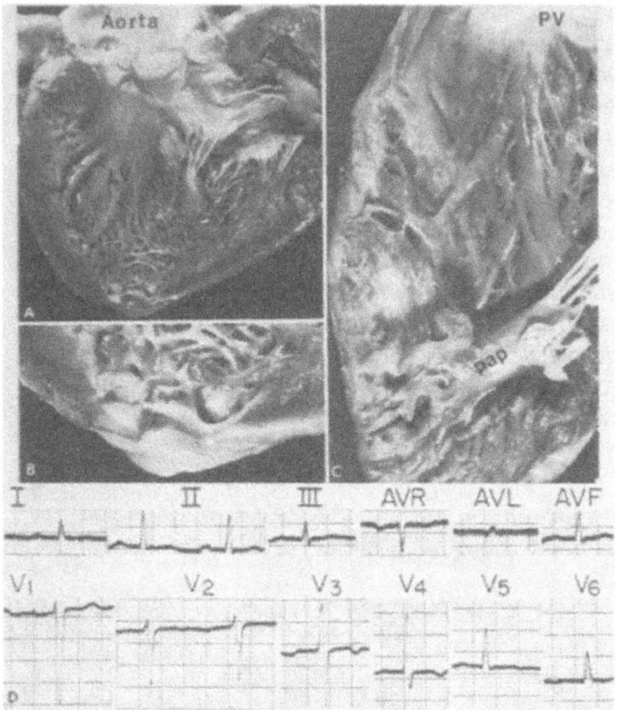

***Figure 7.** Heart and electrocardiogram in a 34 year old man (A68-10) who noted swelling in his neck at age 29. Biopsy of the excised lump at age 30 disclosed that it consisted of lymph nodes infiltrated by hard granulomas. A diagnosis of sarcoidosis therefore was made. The liver was within normal limits on biopsy at age 31. A chest roentgenogram showed prominent bilateral hilar adenopathy, and prednisone therapy (10 to 20 mg daily) was begun and continued thereafter until his death. Five months later cryptococcal meningitis developed, but it was eradicated by amphotericin therapy. One year before death marked hypercalcemia developed. About one month before death a high degree of atrioventricular block developed, which at times progressed to complete heart block. The patient died of complications of peptic ulcer perforation. At necropsy the heart weighed 320 g. Both ventricular cavities were mildly dilated. Mural thrombi were present at the apices of both ventricles. The apical left ventricular wall beneath the thrombi was fibrotic; a small area of scarring was present in the basal anterior left ventricular wall, and the anterior right ventricular wall was focally scarred. Histologic study of the scarred areas disclosed some mononuclear cells but no giant cells. The area of the atrioventricular node and bundle was serially sectioned: considerable scarring with some mononuclear cells was present in the conduction tissue, but the node and bundle and proximal bundle branches were not interrupted at any point. Although no granulomas were observed in this patient's heart, it is nevertheless highly likely that the myocardial scars were the result of "healed" sarcoid granulomas. The myocardial scarring, for example, was similar to that observed in the lymph nodes, and the coronary arteries were normal. The healing appears to have been the result of steroid therapy given for three years. **A,** opened left ventricle (LV). At the apex is a thrombus, better seen in **B.** The myocardium beneath the thrombus is scarred. **C,** right ventricular wall shows severe focal scarring. Pap = papillary muscle. **D,** electrocardiograms recorded three days before death.*

atrium. The granulomas grossly were white and firm. In addition to the left ventricular free wall, granulomas often were observed in the left ventricular papillary muscles (at least 17 patients) (Figures 1, 2 and 3) and in the ventricular septum (at least 19 patients), primarily its cephalad portion (Figures 5 and 6). Of the six patients with complete heart block, five had granulomas in the most cephalad portion of the muscular ventricular septum (Figures 5 and 6), and one had scar tissue in this area (Figure 7). In the one patient in whom serial sections were studied (Figure 5), the atrioventricular bundle and the proximal portions of the right and left bundle branches were partially destroyed by granulomas. In a number of patients, large portions of the left ventricular free wall and ventricular septum were completely replaced by sarcoid granulomas (Figures 2 through 6). The white granulomas usually were visible on the endocardial surface of the left ventricle and, in several patients, they were grossly visible on the epicardial surface. Electron microscopic examination of a sarcoid granuloma in the myocardium was performed in one patient; ultrastructurally, the granulomas were similar to those present in the lungs (Figure 8). In several patients without grossly visible epicardial granulomas, histologic examination of the atrioventricular sulci and epicardium disclosed sarcoid granulomas. In each of the two patients with recurring pericardial effusions, sarcoid granulomas were present in both visceral and parietal pericardia (Figure 9).

Left ventricular aneurysm was present at necropsy in two patients, each of whom had myocardial granulomas. Sudden death was the initial manifestation of sarcoidosis in both patients.

In addition to occurring in the lymph nodes, granulomas consistent with sarcoidosis were present in the lung in 20 patients; in the liver in 18; in the spleen in 18 and in other organs or tissues in 11. The average weight of the liver and spleen was only slightly increased despite the presence of granulomas in these organs. The liver ranged in weight from 1,250 to 2,300 g (average 1,755 g) and the spleen, from 120 to 350 g (average 244 g). The weights of the lungs (together) were usually increased: they ranged from 800 to 1,600 g (average 1,132 g).

Observations in the Patients in Whom Cardiac Dysfunction, if Present, was Not Secondary to Cardiac Sarcoidosis (Group IB). In contrast to the 26 patients described, each of these nine patients had small (microscopic-sized in eight) myocardial sarcoid granulomas (Table III). Four had extensive pulmonary sarcoidosis resulting in cor pulmonale. Three had cardiac dysfunction on the basis of nonsarcoid cardiac conditions: valvular heart disease in two causing pure aortic regurgitation of uncertain etiology in one, and combined mitral and aortic regurgitation in one, presumably rheumatic in origin (this patient underwent mitral valve replacement three months before a fatal cerebral embolus); the third patient, a 50 year old man, had severe coronary atherosclerosis with a documented acute myocardial infarction nine years before his death and congestive cardiac failure probably on that basis. The myocardial granulomas in each of these three patients were minute and visible only by histologic examination. None of these nine patients had arrhythmias or conduction disturbances. None of the five patients without respiratory insufficiency had symptoms or signs definitely attributable to sarcoidosis. The diagnosis of

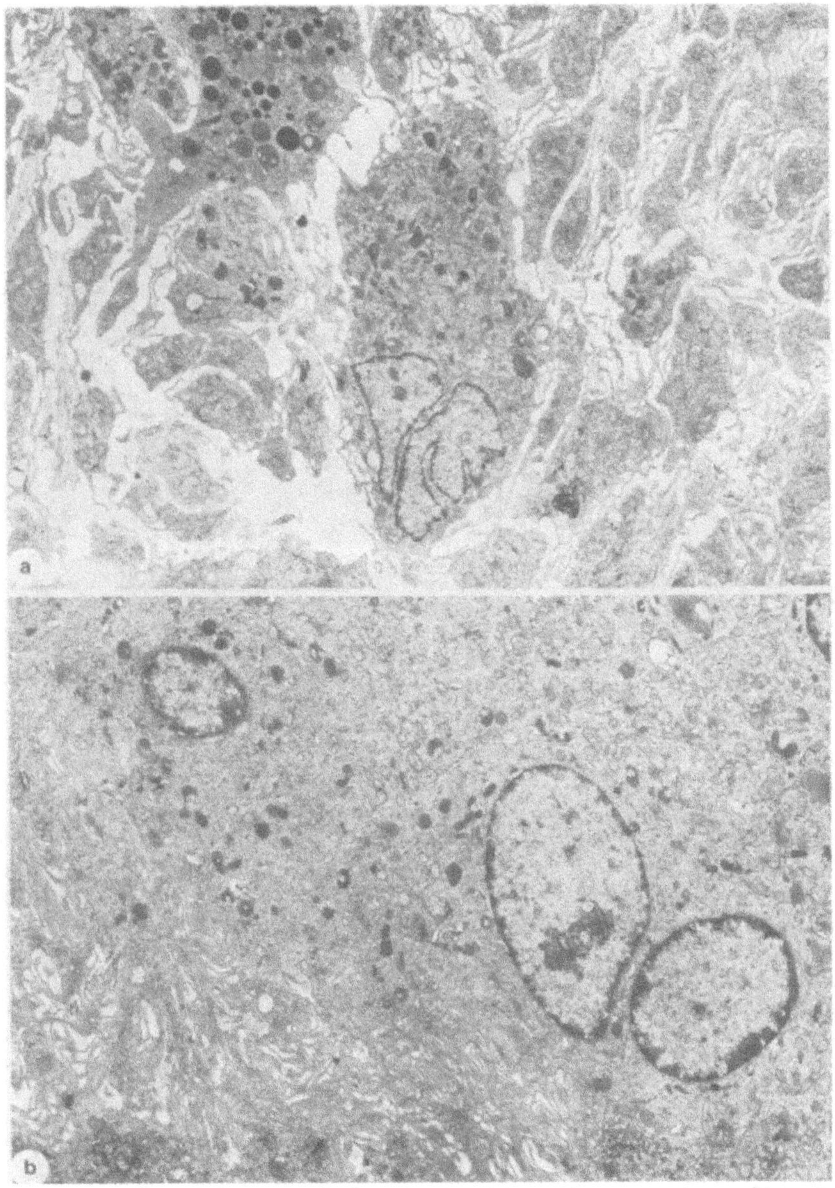

Figure 8. *Electron micrographs of portions of sarcoid granuloma from a biopsy specimen of lung tissue from a 24 year old white man. Similar granulomas were observed ultrastructurally in the myocardium in the one patient examined in the present study, but preservation of the myocardial tissue was not nearly as good as that of the lung biopsy specimen.* ***a,*** *in this electron micrograph an epithelioid cell is present in the central area; it has a multilobulated nucleus and numerous cytoplasmic dense bodies. The surface of this cell is highly irregular, with many flap- and pocket-like projections. Similar projections are present on the surfaces of adjacent cells. A macrophage-like cell is present at the upper left; it contains many large dense bodies.* ***b,*** *portion of multinucleated giant cell (same tissue as in* ***a****) showing parts of 4 nuclei and moderate numbers of dense bodies, mitochondria and cisterns of endoplasmic reticulum. The surface of this cell (lower left) is highly convoluted with complex, interdigitating folds. Original magnification × 6,000 (****a****) and × 7,500 (****b****), reduced by 38 per cent.*

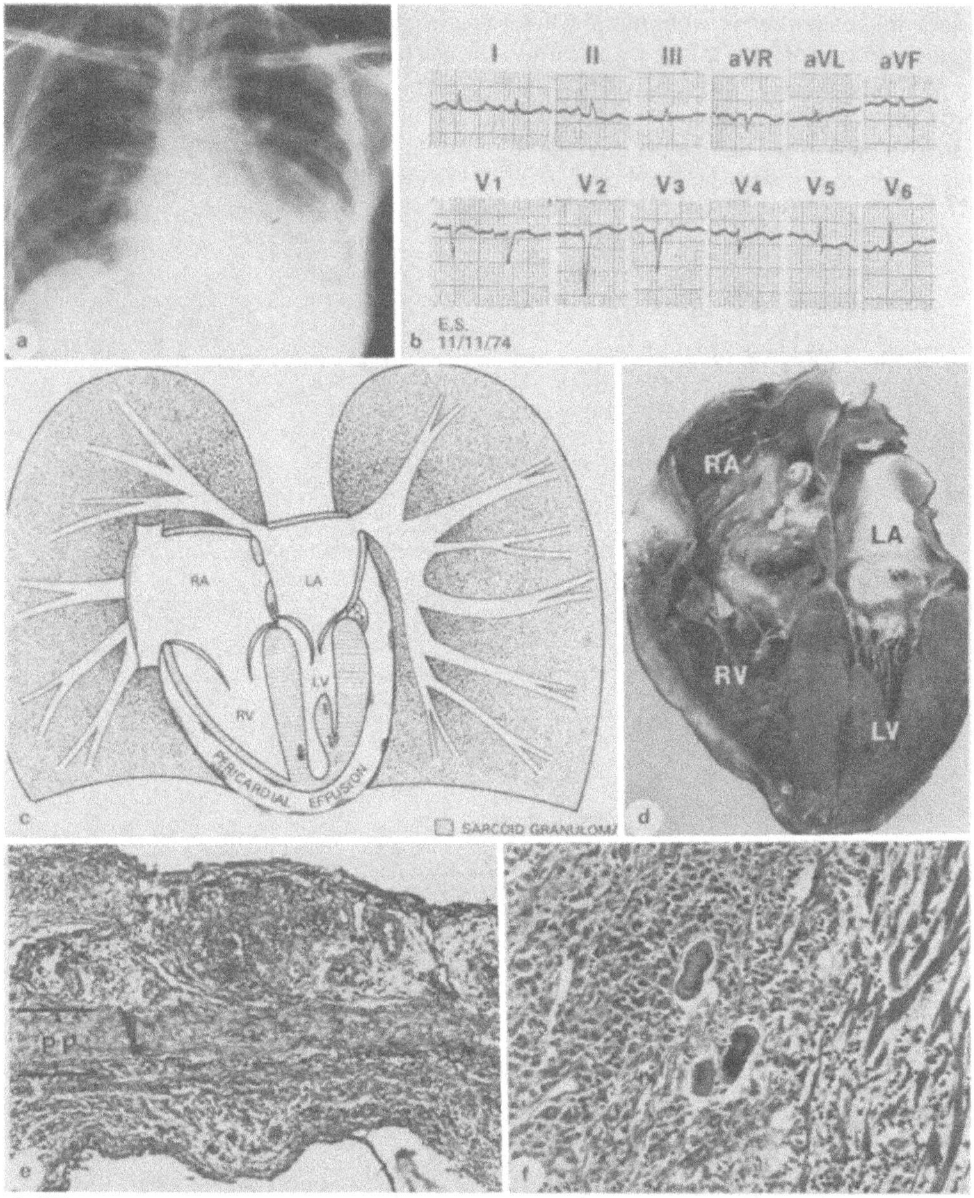

Figure 9. *Chest roentgenogram, electrocardiogram, diagram of heart and lungs, longitudinal cut of heart, and photomicrographs of parietal pericardium and left ventricular papillary muscle in a 47 year old black woman (74-A-223) who was well until 15 months before death when she noted exertional dyspnea, cough and retrosternal chest pain. Hospitalization a month later disclosed distended neck veins, a pericardial friction rub and bilateral pulmonary rales. A chest roentgenogram showed pulmonary "congestion" and mild cardiomegaly. A right-sided cardiac angiogram disclosed a large pericardial effusion. During her four month period in the hospital, infiltrates appeared in the lower lobes of both lungs, but a definite diagnosis was not made. During the next 10 months, she had only dyspnea on severe exertion and an occasional nonproductive cough. A week before death, she had the sudden appearance of severe dyspnea. Physical examination disclosed pulsus paradoxicus (12 mm Hg), distended neck veins and hepatosplenomegaly; roentgenography (**a**) disclosed bilateral pleural effusions, a large cardiac silhouette and interstitial pulmonary infiltrates. An electrocardiogram (**b**) showed low voltage and sinus tachycardia. An echocardiogram showed an echo-free space behind the posterior left ventricular wall. The pulmonary arterial pressure was 30/10 (mean 15) mm Hg. At open thoracotomy (for diagnostic purposes), 800 ml of straw-colored fluid was found in the pericardial sac (protein content = 2.5 g/100 ml; glucose = 105 mg/100 ml). The patient died three days later from progressive "respiratory insufficiency." At necropsy, many sarcoid granulomas were found in both lungs (**c**), hilar lymph nodes, liver and spleen. The parietal pericardium was thickened and contained many sarcoid granulomas (**e**). No lesions were noted on gross examination of the myocardium (**d**), but histologic study did disclose several sarcoid granulomas in the left ventricular free wall and papillary muscles. Granulomas also were present in the epicardium (**c**). The thickness of the normal parietal pericardium (PP) is shown in (**e**). Hematoxylin and eosin stains; original magnification × 85 (**e**) and × 220 (**f**), reduced by 38 per cent.*

noncardiac sarcoidosis was established by biopsy during life in five of the nine patients, and cardiac sarcoidosis was not diagnosed during life in any.

Granulomas were found at necropsy in the left ventricular myocardium in nine patients, in the ventricular septum in two, in the right ventricle in five, and in the atrium in none. In addition to their being present in lymph nodes in all nine patients, granulomas also were present in the lungs in eight, the liver in nine, the spleen in eight and in other organs or tissues in six. The weights of the liver ranged from 830 to 2,600 g (average 1,907 g); the spleen, from 70 to 400 g (average 211 g); and the lungs together, from 760 to 2,800 g (average 1,336 g).

Review of Data on Previously Described Patients with Cardiac Sarcoidosis (Group II). At least 78 necropsy patients have been described with sarcoid granulomas

TABLE IV Cardiac Sarcoidosis Causing Cardiac Dysfunction: Clinical and Morphologic Observations in 63 Previously Described Patients (Group IIA)

	Mode of Death					
Data	Sudden	Congestive Heart Failure	Pericardial Effusion	Non-cardiac	Uncertain	Totals
Patients (no.)	43	14	1	1	4	63
References	[1–34]	[10, 33, 35–44]	[47]	[2]	[48–54]	[1–51]
Age (yr)						
Range	18–76	24–67	27	42	18–38	18–76
Average	43	33	27	42	27	40
Race						
Black	13	10	1	1	2	27 (43)
White	14	2	0	0	1	17 (27)
Unknown or other	16	2	0	0	1	19 (30)
Sex						
Male	18*	9	0	1	2	30/62 (48)
Female	24*	5	1	0	2	32/62 (52)
Duration of symptoms (mo)						
Range	0–180	25–72	60	108	2–12	0–180
Average	27†	29§	60	108	7	28
Atrial arrhythmia	5	4	0	...	2	11 (17)
Ventricular premature beats	12	5	1	...	3	21 (33)
Ventricular tachycardia	8	4	0	...	1	13 (21)
Complete heart block	16	0	0	1	2	19 (30)
Syncope	14	1	0	1	1	17 (27)
Left bundle branch block	2	1	0	...	1	4 }
Right bundle branch block	8	2	0	...	1	11 } (32)
Indeterminate bundle block	3	1	0	...	1	5 }
Congestive heart failure	10	14	1	...	2	27 (43)
Diagnosis of sarcoid in life	10	5	0	...	1	16 (25)
Corticosteroid therapy	8	3	0	0	1	12 (19)
Heart weight (g)						
Range	225–640	320–660	745	...	300–450	225–745
Average	439‡	549§	745	...	385¶	476
Cardiac granulomas						
Left ventricle	28/30	9/9	1	0	2/2	40/41 (98)
Ventricular septum	27/30	4/9	1	0	1/2	33/41 (80)
Right ventricle	10/30	5/9	1	0	0/2	16/41 (39)
Papillary muscle	10/30	2/9	...	0	0/2	12/41 (29)
Atria	9/30	2/9	1	0	0/2	12/41 (29)
None	2	1	0	1	0	4 (6)
Ventricular aneurysm	4	2	0	0	0	6 (15)
Cardiac mural thrombi	0	4	0	0	0	4 (10)
Noncardiac granulomas						
Lymph node	41/41	12/12	1	1	4	59/59 (100)
Lung	35/41	9/12	1	0	4	49/59 (83)
Liver	22/41	8/12	1	0	4	35/59 (59)
Spleen	20/41	7/12	0	0	3	30/59 (51)
Other	9/41	6/12	1	0	1	17/59 (29)

* Sex not stated in one patient.
† Information from 30 patients; average includes four patients whose initial manifestation of sarcoidosis was sudden death. The average in the 26 patients with symptoms was 32 months.
‡ Eighteen patients.
§ Ten patients.
¶ Two patients.

(75 patients) or nonischemic myocardial scars, i.e., healed granulomas (three patients), in their hearts and sarcoid granulomas in at least one other body organ (Tables III and IV). The 78 patients were subdivided into two groups: (1) 63 patients with cardiac dysfunction resulting from extensive cardiac sarcoidosis (group IIA) [1–51] (Table IV) and (2) 15 patients with minute cardiac granulomas and either no (12 patients) cardiac dysfunction [51–62] or cardiac dysfunction (three patients) [22,63,64] not on the basis of cardiac sarcoidosis (group IIB) (Table III). Observations in these two groups of previously described cases are added to those in the personally studied patients and summarized in Table V.

Analysis of these 63 patients (group IIA, Table III) indicates that 43 died suddenly [1–34], 14 from progressive congestive cardiac failure [10,33,35–46], one from recurring pericardial effusion [47], one from noncardiac (suicide) [2] and four from unknown causes [48–51]. Sudden death was the initial manifestation of sarcoidosis in four of the 43 patients who died suddenly [4,6,12,27]; in the other 39 patients, symptoms were present from five days to 180 months (average 27 months). Electrocardiograms, obtained in 53 of the 63 patients, disclosed atrial **arrhythmias** in 11 [5,25–27,31,33,36,42,46,48,51], **ventricular premature beats** in 19 [7,12,16–18,20,27,28,31,34,35,37,40,45,46,49–51], **ventricular tachycardia** in 12 [10,17,27–29,32–35,37,39,40], **complete heart block** in 19 [2,7,11,13–16,20–24,30,31,49,50], second degree heart block in four [14,24,25,47], prolonged (>0.20 sec) P-R interval in five [18,27,36,40,46] and **complete bundle branch block** in 18 (left = three, right = 11, indeterminate = four) [5,7,11,14,16,18–20,25,26,31,33,36,41,46,51]. None of the 19 patients with complete heart block had ventricular tachycardia. Clinical evidence of **congestive cardiac failure** was present in 26 (50 per cent) [7,10,17,19,23,25–27,29,32,33,35–46,48,51] of the 52 patients in whom it was mentioned. The diagnosis of sarcoidosis was established during life in only 16 (25 per cent) of the 63 patients [3,10,14–16,22,27,29,31,34,37,38,40,44,46,51]. Twelve of the 63 patients received corticosteroid therapy at some time [15,19,20,22,27–29,34,44–46,51].

At necropsy, the **cardiac weight,** available in 31 of the 63 patients, ranged from 225 to 745 g (average 476 g). Although granulomas were present in "the heart" or "myocardium" of 60 patients, the **specific chambers involved** were mentioned in 44 patients: the left ventricle in 40 (91 per cent), the ventricular septum in 33 (75 per cent), the right ventricle in 16 (36 per cent) and

TABLE V Cardiac Sarcoidosis: Summary of Personally Studied and Previously Described Patients

Data	Causing Cardiac Dysfunction (Groups IA and IIA)	Not Causing Cardiac Dysfunction (Groups 1B and IIB)
Patients (no.)	89	24
Age (yr)		
Range	18–76	28–83
Average	40	45
Race		
Black	41	9
White	27	10
Unknown	0	3
Sex		
Male	45	16
Female	44	5
Unknown	0	3
Symptoms (mo)		
Range	0–180	0–96
Average	22	46
Syncope	20 (22)	0
Congestive heart failure	35 (39)	6 (25)
Atrial arrhythmia	15 (17)	1 (4)
Ventricular premature beats	33 (37)	1 (4)
Ventricular tachycardia	19 (21)	0
Complete heart block	25 (28)	0
Complete bundle branch block	23 (26)	2 (8)
Diagnosis of sarcoid in life	24 (27)	15 (62)
Corticosteroid treatment	15 (17)	3 (12)
Ventricular aneurysm	8 (9)	0
Intracardiac thrombi	5 (6)	0

NOTE: Figures in parentheses are per cents.

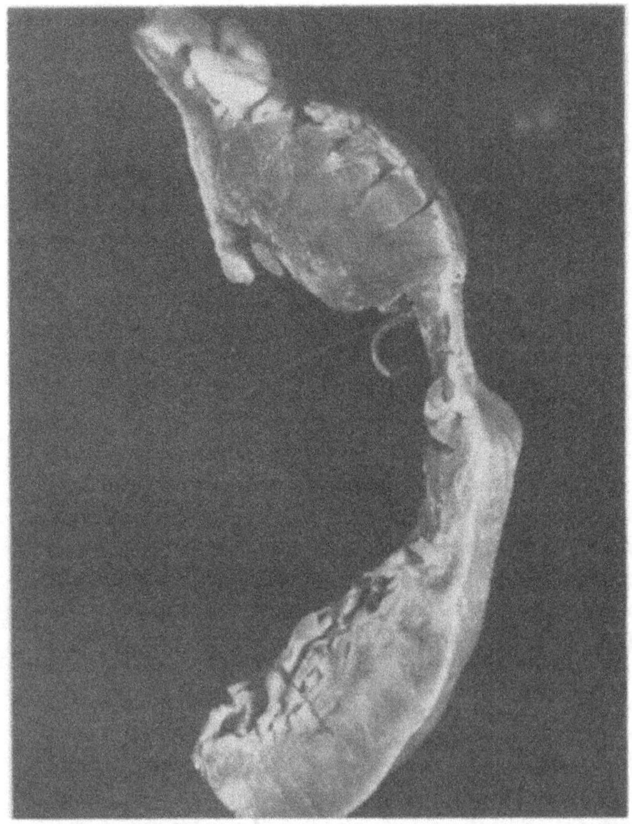

Figure 10. *Longitudinal section of left ventricular free wall showing an area of thinning which during life resulted in an aneurysm. This 49 year old black woman (A72-144), reported earlier by Chun and associates [34] and also examined by one of us (WCR), had 20 episodes of ventricular tachycardia during a 38-month period. She was treated with prednisone most of that time. She died suddenly. At necropsy, the wall of the left ventricular aneurysm consisted entirely of fibrous tissue and the coronary arteries were normal. No sarcoid granulomas were present in the heart but they were present in lymph nodes, spleen, liver and bone marrow. The heart weighed 470 g. It is believed that sarcoid granulomas were present in the heart at one time but that the prednisone therapy caused their healing with development of the above illustrated aneurysm.*

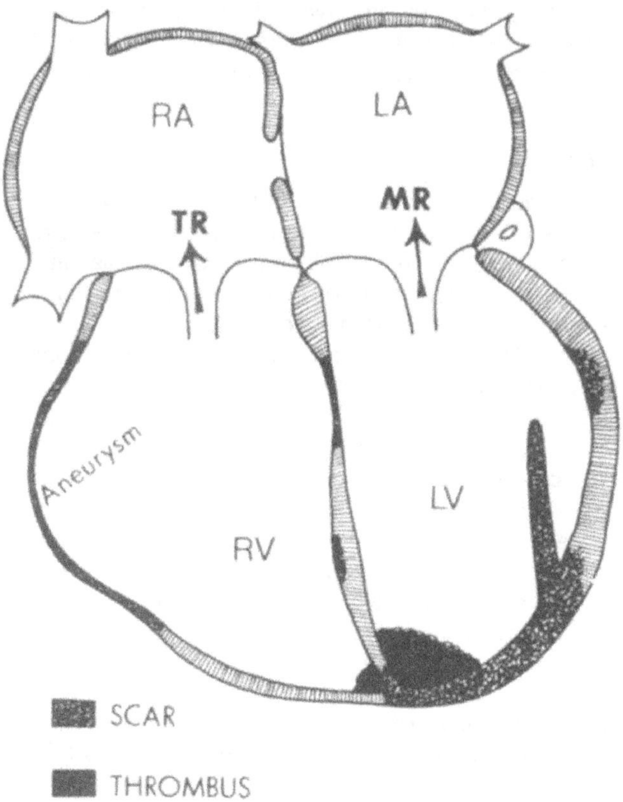

Figure 11. *Diagram of heart in a 37 year old white man (BIH A74-275) who was described in a New England Journal of Medicine CPC by Harthorne and Freiman [46]. (The heart was examined by one of us [WCR] through the courtesy of Walter H. Abelmann and David G. Freiman.) This case is of particular importance because the patient's course was eight years. During this period he had multiple arrhythmias, bilateral bundle branch block with prolongation of the P-R interval, systemic emboli, and progressive cardiomegaly, so that by necropsy both ventricles were enormously dilated and the right ventricular wall, so thinned that it was aneurysmal. Scars also were present in the left ventricular free wall and ventricular septum but no granulomas were present in the heart. Indeed, although sarcoid granulomas had been present in lymph nodes in an earlier biopsy, at necropsy no sarcoid granulomas were present in any organ. It is believed that corticosteroid therapy (two years) contributed to the disappearance of the granulomas. His heart at necropsy was very similar to the typical heart of idiopathic cardiomyopathy of the ventricular dilated type except for the presence of the healed granulomas (scars).*

the atrium in 12 (right atrium in eight, left atrium in seven and unspecified in one) (27 per cent). In at least 12 patients [1,3–6,10,12,14,18,32,40,43] sarcoid granulomas were stated to be present in one or more papillary muscles. The cardiac granulomas were visible grossly in all patients. One or more **ventricular aneurysms** were present in six patients [19,29,33,34,44,46] (Figures 10 and 11), and intracardiac thrombi in four patients [10,35,42,46] (Figure 11), all of whom had congestive cardiac failure. The specific location of sarcoid granulomas in organs other than the heart was described in 59 patients: lymph nodes in 59 (100 per cent); lung in 49 (83 per cent); liver in 35 (59 per cent); spleen in 31 (53 per cent) and other organs in 17 (29 per cent).

Observations in the previously described 15 patients in whom cardiac dysfunction, if present, was not secondary to cardiac sarcoidosis (group IIB) are summarized in Table II [22,51–64]. In contrast to the patients in group IIA, men were more numerous than women (12:3), the duration of symptoms was longer (average 38 months), arrhythmias and conduction defects were infrequent, the diagnosis of sarcoidosis was made in life in 10 of the 15 patients, and one patient died suddenly. The heart weights, available in 10 patients, were normal in seven and increased in the three patients with cardiac dysfunction from valvular disease of nonsarcoid origin. The cardiac sarcoid granulomas were minute in all 15 patients and usually visible only by histologic examination. Other body organs involved by sarcoid included the lymph nodes in all 15 patients, the lung in 12, the liver in nine, the spleen in 10 and other body organs or tissues in six.

COMMENTS

Study of our 35 patients (group I) and the 78 previously described necropsy patients (group II) allows certain general conclusions regarding cardiac sarcoidosis, and these items will be discussed in the following order: (1) the portions of the heart involved anatomically by sarcoid granulomas; (2) the determinants of whether or not cardiac sarcoidosis causes cardiac dysfunction; (3) the clinical types of cardiac dysfunction and their probable anatomic explanations; (4) the determinants of whether or not cardiac dysfunction from cardiac sarcoidosis is diagnosed clincally; (5) the modes of death and length of illness; (6) the effect of corticosteroid therapy on cardiac sarcoid granulomas and (7) the differences between cardiac sarcoidosis and idiopathic granulomatous (giant cell) myocarditis.

No portion of the heart is immune to infiltration by sarcoid granulomas. The granulomas may involve the pericardium, myocardium and endocardium, but of the three, the myocardium is, by far, the one most frequently involved. The portion of myocardium most frequently involved by sarcoid granulomas is the left ventricular free wall, followed by the ventricular septum, the right ventricle and, lastly, the atrial wall. Why the left ventricular free wall is the one most frequently involved and the atrial wall the one least frequently involved is uncertain, but the explanation may simply be that the largest fraction of the total myocardial mass is in the left ventricle, including the ventricular septum, and the smallest fraction is in the atrium. (Interestingly, the left ventricular wall also is the most frequent portion of myocardium invaded by secondary neoplasms of the heart [65–67].) Sarcoid granulomas within the left ventricle appear to be most common in the papillary muscles and in the free walls immediately beneath them. The cephalad half of the ventricular septum is more often involved than the caudal half. It is probable that the left ventricular papillary muscles and the cephalad portion of the ventricular septum are the preferential locations in the heart for sarcoid granulomas, but since these sites often are not incised at necropsy small granulomas in these locations may be missed. Thus, it is possible that the frequency of cardiac involvement by granulomas in patients with sarcoidosis may be higher than generally appreciated because of inadequate examination of these two structures.

Involvement of the epicardium (visceral pericardium) and mural endocardium by granulomas usually represents an extension of the myocardial involvement into these layers of the heart. None of our patients or those previously described had epicardial or mural endocardial involvement without concomitant myocardial sarcoid granulomas. The occurrence of sarcoid granulomas in the adipose tissue adjacent to the coronary arteries, particularly the atrioventricular sulci, however, is unusual, whereas this portion of the heart is the area most frequently invaded by metastatic neoplasm [65–67]. Although their occurrence on the mediastinal aspect of the parietal pericardium is common, the occurrence of sarcoid granulomas on the cardiac (serous) aspect of the parietal pericardium is unusual. Such an occurrence, however, was observed in each of our two patients with recurring pericardial effusions. Rarely, valvular endocardium may contain sarcoid granulomas: in one of our 35 patients these granulomas were present on the pulmonic valve cusps, but they were not of sufficient size to cause valvular malfunction. Sarcoid involvement of the tricuspid valve has also been reported [39].

Whether or not cardiac dysfunction occurs as a consequence of cardiac sarcoidosis is dependent on at least three factors: (1) the number of sarcoid granulomas in the heart, i.e., the amount of ventricular myocardium replaced by granulomas versus the amount of uninvolved ventricular myocardium; (2) the amount of ventricular wall scarring, i.e., the amount of ventricular myocardium replaced by scar versus the amount of uninvolved ventricular myocardium, and (3) the location of the granulomas or scars within the heart. Of our 26 patients in whom cardiac dysfunction resulted from cardiac sarcoid (Table I), 23 had large, granulomas or scars on the left ventricular wall: two had recurring pericardial effusions and sarcoid granulomas in the pericardium, and one had a scar in the most cephalad portion of ventricular septum resulting in complete heart block. The amount of myocardium replaced by sarcoid granulomas was minute in each of our nine patients who had cardiac sarcoidosis and no cardiac dysfunction as a result of the cardiac granulomas (Table II). Indeed, in eight of these nine patients the cardiac granulomas were observed only by histologic examination. This also was the situation in the 15 patients described by others as having cardiac sarcoidosis but no cardiac dysfunction as a result of that infiltration (Table II).

The types of cardiac dysfunction produced by cardiac sarcoidosis include: (1) arrhythmias, primarily ventricular ones; (2) high degrees of atrioventricular block and complete bundle branch block; (3) sudden death; (4) congestive cardiac failure; (5) papillary muscle dysfunction; (6) "acute myocardial infarction"; (7) ventricular aneurysm and (8) recurring pericardial effusion.

Other than premature ventricular beats, ventricular tachycardia was the most frequent major arrhythmia, occurring in at least six (23 per cent) of our 26 patients (group IA) and in at least 12 (19 per cent) of 63 previously described patients with cardiac dysfunction resulting from cardiac sarcoidosis (group IIA). The occurrence of ventricular tachycardia in these patients usually indicates extensive sarcoid granulomatous involvement of the heart or extensive scarring as a result of healing of the granulomas. Atrial arrhythmias, present in four (15 per cent) patients in group IA and in 11 (17 per cent) of the 63 patients in group IIA did not appear to be direct consequences of cardiac sarcoidosis because only two of the 15 patients with atrial arrhythmias had sarcoid granulomas in the atrial walls at necropsy. The atrial arrhythmias more likely were consequences of atrial dilatation arising as a result of the ventricular malfunction.

Severe conduction disturbances also were common. Complete heart block was documented in six (23 per cent) patients in group IA and in 19 (30 per cent) of the 63 patients in group IIA. Of the 25 patients with complete heart block, 17 (68 per cent) also had episodes of syncope (Stokes-Adams attacks). In each of our five patients and in most if not all of the 19 previously described patients with complete heart block, the cephalad portion of the muscular ventricular septum, and especially that portion in the vicinity of the atrioventricular bundle, was extensively infiltrated by sarcoid granulomas or, in one patient, by scar tissue. In our one patient with complete heart block in whom serial histologic sections of the atrioventricular node and bundle were examined, partial destruction of the atrioventricular bundle and complete disruption of the bundle branches from their origin were observed. Similar observations have been made by Morales and associates [33]. Thus, complete heart block in these patients appears to result from interruption of the conduction pathways by either sarcoid granuloma or scar or both.

Complete bundle branch block also was common. It occurred in three (12 per cent) of our patients (group IA) and in 20 (32 per cent) of the patients in group IIA. The bundle branch block was right in 13, left in five and indeterminate in five. The patients with bundle branch block also had either granulomas or scars in the cephalad portion of the ventricular septum, but the amount of granulomatous or scar tissue appeared to be less extensive than that in patients with complete heart block.

Sudden death is the most common cardiac manifestation of clinically significant cardiac sarcoidosis. It occurred in 17 (65 per cent) of the patients in group IA and in 43 (68 per cent) of the patients in group IIA. That the sudden death in these 60 patients was of cardiac origin cannot be unequivocally proved, but many had had preceding arrhythmias or complete heart block, and ventricular fibrillation was confirmed terminally in several of them. Thus, sarcoidosis is an important but neglected cause of sudden cardiac death. Sudden death may be the initial manifestation of sarcoidosis. This was the case in six (35 per cent) of our 17 patients who died suddenly and in four (9 per cent) of the 43 previously described patients who died suddenly. Among these 10 patients (age range, 18 to 53 years [average 31]), death occurred during exertion in eight, and, although none had had symptoms, one had had ventricular premature beats documented by electrocardiogram. Of the remaining 50 patients who died suddenly, complete heart block had been present in 20 (40 per cent), ventricular tachycardia in 12 (24 per cent), ventricular premature beats in 11 (22 per cent) and atrial arrhythmias in seven (14 per cent). Of the 50 patients who died suddenly (excluding the 10 in whom sudden death was the initial manifestation of sarcoidosis), either complete heart block or a ventricular arrhythmia had been documented by electrocardiogram in 38 (76 per cent); of the remaining 12 patients, four had atrial arrhythmias, one had complete right bundle branch block, and seven never had an electrocardiogram recorded. Thus, ventricular arrhythmias and complete heart block are bad omens in patients with sarcoidosis.

Congestive cardiac failure is another common form of cardiac dysfunction in patients with extensive cardiac

TABLE VI Cardiac Sarcoidosis: Cardiac Aneurysm

Case No.	Reference	Age (yr)	Sex	Precordial Murmur	CHF	CHB	VT	SD	Length of Illness (mo)	CS Rx	Length of CS Rx (mo)	Site of Aneurysm RV	Site of Aneurysm LV	Myocardial Granuloma	Myocardial Transmural Scarring	Heart Weight (g)
1	Hines, Sancetta [19]	44	F	+	+	0	0	+	17	+	3	+	+	0	+	465
2	Duvernoy, Garcia [29]	30	F	+	+	0	+	+	30	+	—	0	+	+	—	—
3	Morales et al. [33]	41	M	—	—	0	0	+	—	—	—	0	+	+	—	—
4	Chun et al. [34]	49	F	+	—	0	+	+	38	+	30	0	+	0	+	470
5	Clark, Blount [44]	28	M	+	+	0	0	0	12	+	—	+	0	+	+	650
6	Freiman [46]	37	M	+	+	0	0	0	96	+	24	+	0	0	+	700
7	Present study	21	M	—	0	—	—	+	0	0	—	0	+	+	0	400
8	Present study	41	F	—	0	—	—	+	0	0	—	0	+	+	0	300

NOTE: 0 = absent; + = present; — = no information available; CHB = complete heart block; CHF = congestive heart failure; CS Rx = corticosteroid treatment; LV = left ventricle; RV = right ventricle; SD = sudden death; VT = ventricular tachycardia.

sarcoidosis. It occurred in eight (31 per cent) (fatal in six) of the patients in group IA and in 27 (43 per cent) (fatal in 14) of the patients in group IIA. With rare exception these 35 patients with congestive cardiac failure had extensive granulomas or scars in the left ventricular free wall, with or without similar involvement of the ventricular septum. The patients with congestive failure, however, had varying clinical features. In some, consequences of complete heart block or ventricular tachycardia dominated the clinical course and the failure was episodic. Most patients, however, had chronic failure.

Precordial systolic murmurs may be consequences of cardiac sarcoidosis. They were noted in four (15 per cent) of the patients in group IA and in 12 (19 per cent) [10,16,17,19,29,32,34,37,43,46,50] of the patients in group IIA. The murmurs usually were apical in location and varied from grade 1 to 5 (on a scale of 6) in intensity. Cardiac catheterization was performed in five patients [19,29,34,43,46] with precordial murmurs; in each of the four patients [19,29,43,46] in whom pulmonary arterial pressures were recorded, mild to moderate pulmonary hypertension was present and in one [43] the pulmonary arterial wedge pressure was greatly increased (v waves to 66 mm Hg). The cause of the murmurs in most of the 16 patients is unclear, but papillary muscle dysfunction is the most likely explanation. Although sarcoid granulomas in papillary muscle were described at necropsy in 29 (33 per cent) of the 89 patients in group IIA (no mention of papillary muscle in at least 27 patients) with cardiac dysfunction from cardiac sarcoidosis, precordial murmurs had been recorded in only six of them. Conversely, of the 16 patients with precordial murmurs, in only six (38 per cent) were sarcoid granulomas noted in their left ventricular papillary muscles at necropsy. Thus, although sarcoid infiltration into one or both left ventricular papillary muscles and into the free walls beneath them may produce papillary muscle dysfunction with mitral regurgitation, more often, the presence of a precordial murmur in these patients is not indicative of sarcoid in these structures. More often, the murmurs appear to result from altered papillary muscle dynamics due to dilatation of the left ventricle.

Ventricular aneurysm may be a consequence of cardiac sarcoidosis. A ventricular aneurysm occurred in two (8 per cent) of the patients in group IA and in six (10 per cent) of the patients in group IIA (Table VI). The aneurysm may involve either or both ventricular walls; it may be discrete and relatively small in the left ventricle, as illustrated by the patient described by Chun and associates [34] (Figure 10), or it may be diffuse and involve a large portion of the right ventricular wall, as occurred in the patient described by Freiman [46] (Figure 11) and in the patient described by Clark and

Blount [44]. Scarring or thinning of the ventricular septum may be associated with protrusion of the septum toward the right ventricle, producing, in effect, an internal cardiac aneurysm. Such was the probable case in the patient described by Hines and Sancetta [19]. The aneurysmal wall may or may not contain sarcoid granulomas: of the eight patients with ventricular aneurysms from cardiac sarcoidosis whose data are summarized in Table III, five had residual granulomas in the heart and three had none. In each of the latter three patients, the aneurysmal wall consisted entirely of fibrous tissue. The dominant component of the aneurysmal wall, however, in the other five patients also appears to have been fibrous tissue. The myocardial scarring and aneurysmal formation in these patients may have been related in part to the administration of corticosteroids. Of the 89 patients in groups IA and IIA, only nine (seven previously described [15,19,22,27,29,34,46]) had received corticosteroid therapy for longer than one month, and five of these nine patients were among the eight with ventricular aneurysms. The eight patients with ventricular aneurysms were young (range 21 to 49 years [average 36 years]). In only one [29] was the presence of a ventricular aneurysm recognized during life (by left ventricular angiography). Six of the eight patients died suddenly, and in two sudden death was the initial manifestation of sarcoidosis; the other two patients died of progressive congestive cardiac failure, and it is likely that their ventricular aneurysms contributed to, or were responsible for, the congestive failure. None of the eight patients had significant coronary arterial luminal narrowing. The occurrence of either right or left ventricular aneurysm in the absence of significant coronary arterial luminal narrowing is quite suggestive of cardiac sarcoidosis (which may or may not have "healed").

Excision of a left ventricular aneurysm of sarcoid origin at times may be beneficial. Lull and associates [68] described such an aneurysm, "the size of a tennis ball," which was resected in a 22 year old man with evidence of sarcoidosis for five months. Preoperatively, the patient had had episodes of ventricular tachycardia unresponsive to therapy with corticosteroids or antiarrhythmic agents. After aneurysmectomy, the ventricular arrhythmia, at the time of the report, was "no longer a problem." Although histologic examination of the wall of the resected aneurysm disclosed mainly fibrous tissue, a few sarcoid-type granulomas were present.

Although an effusion into a body cavity is an unusual feature of sarcoidosis, recurring pericardial effusion on occasion may be a prominent clinical manifestation of cardiac sarcoidosis. Such was the case in two (8 per cent) of the patients in group IA and in one (2 per cent) [47] patient in group IIA. A living patient with recurrent pericardial effusion secondary to pericardial sarcoidosis also was described by Shiff and associates [69]. This patient, a 31 year old woman, had a 1,000 ml serous effusion and multiple sarcoid granulomas on the epicardium. A possibly similar patient was described by Bailey [70]. The three necropsy patients were 27, 35 and 47 years of age, respectively, and two were women. Each had huge cardiac silhouettes typical of pericardial effusion. Two underwent thoracotomy shortly before death because of cardiac tamponade from large (800 ml each) pericardial effusions. At necropsy two of the three patients also had severe pulmonary sarcoidosis with considerable right ventricular hypertrophy, but the third had no sarcoid granulomas in the lung. Pericardial adhesions were present in one patient. All three had epicardial sarcoid granulomas; in addition, two had large and one had minute myocardial granulomas. Marked dilatation of both ventricles secondary to active or healed myocardial sarcoidosis may produce a "water-bottle" configuration of the cardiac silhouette on chest roentgenogram and mimic a large pericardial effusion. This situation occurred in the patient described by Clark and Blount [44]. Their patient proved to have only a small pericardial effusion but aneurysmal dilatation of both cardiac ventricles.

Because of its ability to cause arrhythmias, conduction disturbances, precordial murmurs, huge cardiac silhouettes, ventricular aneurysm and electrocardiographic evidence of "myocardial damage," cardiac sarcoidosis may mimic other cardiac conditions. In at least eight (31 per cent) of the patients in group IA and in five (8 per cent) [9,18,19,25,36] of the patients in group IIA, the initial clinical diagnosis was "acute myocardial infarction." The myocardial damage evident on the electrocardiogram may be the consequence of a sudden arrhythmia or complete heart block, or it may result entirely from the replacement of myocardium by sarcoid granulomas. Chest pain simulating acute myocardial infarction also was described in a patient described by Stephen [9] and in another described by Forbes and Usher [18]. Electrocardiograms were not diagnostic of, but compatible with, acute myocardial infarction in both patients; if necropsy had not been performed, coronary heart disease would have remained their diagnosis. Papillary muscle dysfunction in cardiac sarcoidosis may mimic valvular heart disease. The presentation of features of congestive cardiac failure associated with a large cardiac silhouette obviously may mimic idiopathic dilated cardiomyopathy [71] as well as pericardial effusion. The occurrence of very dilated ventricular cavities, particularly when associated with intracardiac thrombi, may even suggest this diagnosis at necropsy. Five of the 89 analyzed patients with cardiac dysfunction from cardiac sarcoidosis (groups IA and IIA) had intracardiac thrombi at

TABLE VII Cardiac Sarcoidosis: Effect of Corticosteroid Therapy on the Cardiac Granulomas

Case No.	Reference	Age (yr)	Sex	VT	CHB	CHF	Length of Illness (mo)	Length of CS Rx (mo)	SD	Cardiac Granulomas				Heart Weight (g)	No. of Cardiac Granulomas	Cardiac Aneurysm	
										LV	VS	RV	Atria			RV	LV
1	Porter [15]	19	M	0	+	0	24	7	+	+	+	+	—	—	—	0	0
2	Hines, Sancetta [19]	44	F	0	0	+	17	3	+	0	0	0	0	465	Few	0	+
3	Johansen [22]	43	M	0	+	0	108	108	+	0	+*	0	0	500	Few	0	0
4	Bashour et al. [27]	48	F	+	0	+	10	9	+	+	+	—	—	500	Few	0	0
5	Duvernoy, Garcia [29]	30	F	+	0	+	31	7	+	+	—	—	—	—	Few	0	+
6	Chun et al. [34]	49	F	+	0	—	38	30	+	0	0	0	0	470	0	0	+
7	Freiman [46]	37	M	0	0	+	96	24	0	0	0	0	0	700	0	+	0
8	Present study	30	M	+	0	0	53	7	+	+	+	+	0	450	Few	0	0
9	Present study	34	M	0	+	0	48	36	0	0	0	0	0	310	0	0	0

NOTE: 0 = absent; + = present; — = no information available; * = microscopic-sized; CHB = complete heart block; CHF = congestive heart failure; CS Rx = corticosteroid treatment; LV = left ventricle; RV = right ventricle; SD = sudden death; VS = ventricular septum; VT = ventricular tachycardia.

necropsy; four of the five had had severe congestive cardiac failure.

Another type of cardiac involvement in some patients with sarcoidosis is calcification of the mitral anulus. Although ectopic and metastatic calcification is a well recognized occurrence in patients with sarcoidosis [72,73,83], calcification of the mitral anulus has not been described previously in this condition. Nevertheless, one of the conditions which predisposes to mitral anular calcification is hypercalcemia, irrespective of its cause [74,75]. Because hypercalcemia is a recognized manifestation of sarcoidosis, it therefore is reasonable to believe that mitral anular calcification should occur with increased frequency in this condition. We found minimal deposits of calcium in the mitral anulus in one of our 35 patients with cardiac sarcoidosis (group I). This man was only 34 years of age, but he had severe hypercalcemia [76]. We found heavy mitral anular calcific deposits in another patient (not included in this study) who also had severe hypercalcemia from sarcoidosis but no cardiac sarcoid granulomas or myocardial scars (Figure 12). Both of these patients also received corticosteroid therapy for several years, and this medication possibly might also predispose to mitral anular calcification.

The effect of corticosteroid therapy on patients with cardiac sarcoid granulomas has received little attention. Analysis of the data on our and previously described necropsy patients with cardiac sarcoidosis strongly suggests that this medication promotes healing of the cardiac granulomas. Only three of the patients in group IA and only 12 of the patients in group IIA received corticosteroid therapy at some time; only nine of these 15 patients received this medication for longer than one month. Certain clinical and morphologic observations in them are summarized in Table VII. Of these nine patients, four had no sarcoid granulomas in the heart—only myocardial scars at sites preferentially involved by sarcoid—and each of the remaining five patients had mainly myocardial scars with relatively few residual granulomas. The four patients without any cardiac granulomas were the only ones among the entire group of 113 patients (Tables II through IV) who had no cardiac granulomas, and three of the four also had one or more cardiac aneurysms at sites of myocardial scarring. Only one of the eight patients with a cardiac aneurysm had not received corticosteroid therapy. Thus, the evidence is substantial that corticosteroid therapy can cause healing of cardiac granulomas but that a possible consequence of this healing is the development of a cardiac aneurysm (Figure 13). The administration of corticosteroids over a period of several weeks during acute myocardial infarction resulting from severe coronary atherosclerosis also can lead rapidly to the development of a cardiac aneurysm [77].

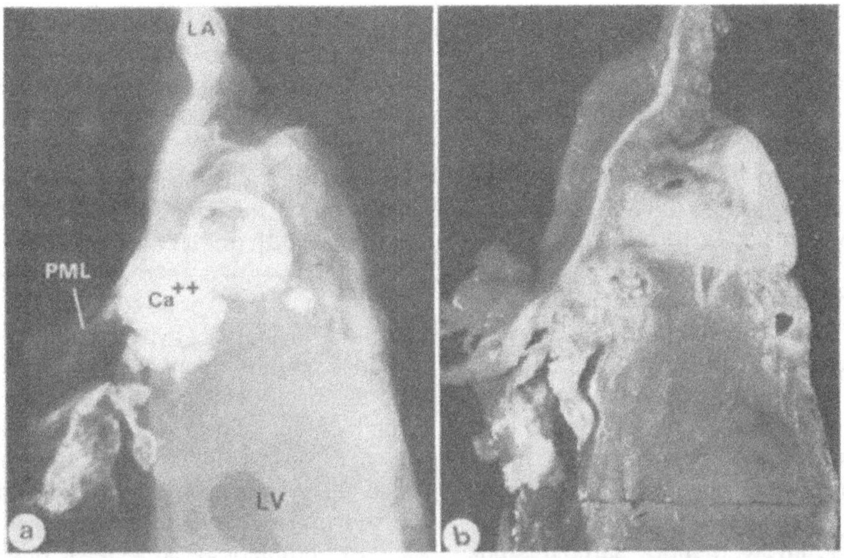

Figure 12. *Longitudinal cut of left atrium (LA), posterior mitral leaflet (PML) and left ventricle (LV) in a 44 year old black woman (A75-12) who had had evidence of noncardiac sarcoidosis for 18 years. Hypercalcemia developed and she died from rupture of a peptic ulcer, apparently a consequence of corticosteroid therapy. A surprise finding at necropsy was the presence of large calcific deposits (Ca++) in the mitral anular region as shown here. A tongue of calcium also protruded from the anular area into the space just behind the posterior mitral leaflet. Hypercalcemia, and possibly also prolonged corticosteroid therapy, are precursors to mitral anular calcification.* ***a,*** *roentgenogram.* ***b,*** *specimen itself.*

Indirect evidence that corticosteroid therapy causes "shrinkage" of the cardiac sarcoid granulomas is demonstrated by the reported diminution in the frequency of arrhythmias, conduction disturbances and electrocardiographic evidence of myocardial damage after initiation of this medication [78–81].

Sarcoid granulomas in the heart may be more responsive to corticosteroid therapy than are sarcoid granulomas located in other body organs. Of the four patients with no residual cardiac sarcoid granulomas, only one [46] had no residual granulomas in other body organs at necropsy. (Lymph node biopsy in the patient before he was given corticosteroid therapy had disclosed many sarcoid granulomas.) Of the other five patients with few cardiac sarcoid granulomas, all appeared to have relatively larger numbers of granulomas in other body organs. Obviously, a possible explanation for this observation is that the area for sarcoid granulomatous infiltration is larger in the liver or lung than in the heart; in other words, the area for granulomatous

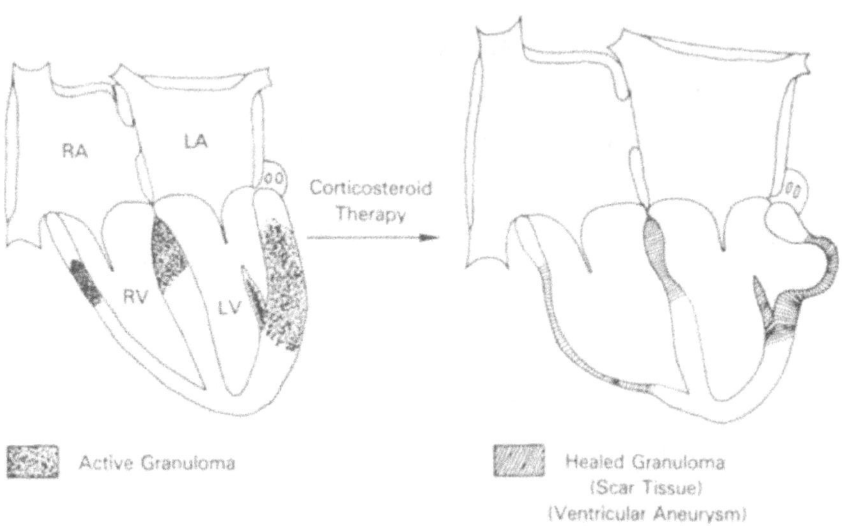

Figure 13. *Diagram showing the good and bad effects of corticosteroid therapy in patients with cardiac sarcoidosis.*

infiltration in the heart is smaller than that of some other body organs.

The majority of patients, in whom cardiac sarcoidosis causes cardiac dysfunction, present initially with manifestations related to the heart rather than to involvement of other body organs or systems. The initial manifestation of sarcoidosis in 23 (88 per cent) of the patients in group IA was related to the heart. Among the previously described 63 patients (group IIA), information regarding the initial manifestation was available in 38: in 28 (74 per cent) of them the initial manifestation was related to signs or symptoms of cardiac dysfunction. Furthermore, in the majority of these 89 patients (26 plus 63) there was never any clinical evidence of dysfunction of an organ system other than the heart. Indeed, the occurrence of symptomatic involvement of another body system by sarcoid generally indicates that symptom-producing cardiac involvement by sarcoid is unlikely to occur. Fleming [80], in search of patients with cardiac sarcoid, surveyed the chest, eye and skin clinics in his hospital in which patients with other forms of sarcoidosis were being followed and found this search unprofitable in revealing patients with cardiac sarcoid. Thus, cardiac sarcoidosis severe enough to cause cardiac dysfunction tends to be an all or none process: if it causes cardiac dysfunction, it tends not to cause dysfunction of another organ system; conversely, if it causes dysfunction of a noncardiac organ system, it infrequently causes cardiac dysfunction.

Although signs or symptoms of cardiac dysfunction from cardiac sarcoidosis may be present for many years, more often the course is not prolonged. The duration of symptoms of cardiac dysfunction from cardiac sarcoidosis was 12 months or less in 19 (73 per cent) of the patients in group IA and in 26 (58 per cent) of the 45 previously described patients (information not available in 18) in group IIA.

Although it appears to be the major cause of giant cell myocarditis, sarcoidosis is not the only condition in which giant cells unassociated with stainable organisms occur in the heart. Giant cells also have been observed in the hearts of patients with infective endocarditis [82], rheumatoid arthritis [83], Takayasu's arteritis [84], Wegener's granulomatosis [85] and, rarely, in patients with coronary heart disease with or without systemic hypertension [71]. "Idiopathic" granulomatous (giant cell) myocarditis has been reported by a number of investigators [86–94], but in many such reports the condition described may not have been "isolated" and, therefore, almost surely [86–90] or probably [91–94] was **cardiac sarcoidosis.** If the latter condition is defined as the presence of "hard" granulomas in at least one other body organ (always lymph node) in addition to the heart, then many patients described as having "isolated" giant cell or granulomatous myocarditis in actuality had cardiac sarcoidosis. It is probable that many patients reported to have isolated granulomatous (giant cell) myocarditis also had giant cells in lymph nodes but that these structures were not examined histologically. In several described patients and in a few of our patients with cardiac sarcoidosis, the lymph nodes were not enlarged grossly; if the nodes had not been studied histologically, sarcoidosis would not have been diagnosed. Thus, a diagnosis of "isolated granulomatous (giant cell) myocarditis" is justified only after thorough exclusion of extracardiac sarcoidosis. In contrast to Davies et al. [90], we believe that "idiopathic giant cell myocarditis" and "cardiac sarcoidosis" cannot be distinguished by histologic examination of the heart alone.

REFERENCES

1. Brosig W: Zur tuberkulösen Erkrankung des Herzmuskels. Zentralbl Allg Pathol 72: 161, 1939.
2. Longcope WT, Fisher AM: The effect of Schaumann's disease upon the heart and its mechanism. Acta Med Scand 108: 529, 1941.
3. Bates GS, Walsh JM: Boeck's sarcoid: observations on seven patients, one autopsy. Ann Intern Med 29: 306, 1948.
4. Scotti TM, McKeown CE: Sarcoidosis involving the heart. Report of case with sudden death. Arch Pathol 46: 289, 1948.
5. Vogt H: Morbus Besnier-Boeck-Schaumann. Klinische und pathologische-anatomie Studie. Helv Med Acta 16 (suppl 25): 1, 1949.
6. Kulka WE: Sarcoidosis of the heart. A cause of sudden and unexpected death. Circulation 1: 772, 1950.
7. Simkins S: Boeck's sarcoid with complete heart block mimicking carotid sinus syncope. Report of a case. JAMA 146: 794, 1951.
8. Oille WA, Ritchie RC, Barrie HJ: The age of lesions in a case of myocardial sarcoidosis. Can Med Assoc J 68: 277, 1953.
9. Stephen JD: Fatal myocardial sarcoidosis. A case of sudden death. Circulation 9: 886, 1954.
10. Powell LW Jr: Sarcoidosis of the myocardium. NC Med J 15: 28, 1954.
11. Gottfarb AG, Wahlgren F: Adams-Stokes syndrom framkallat av morbus Besnier-Boeck-Schaumann (sarcoidosis). Nord Med 52: 985, 1954.
12. Clinicopathologic conference. Cardiac arrhythmia. US Armed Forces Med J 8: 855, 1957.
13. Peacock RA, Lippschutz EJ, Lukas A: Myocardial sarcoidosis. Circulation 16: 67, 1957.
14. Poon TP, Forbus WD: Sudden death due to myocardial sarcoidosis, with a comment on the etiology of sarcoid. Arch Intern Med 104: 771, 1959.
15. Porter GH: Sarcoid heart disease. N Engl J Med 263: 1350, 1960.
16. Phinney AO Jr: Sarcoid of the myocardial septum with complete heart block. Report of two cases. Am Heart J 62: 270, 1961.
17. Chamovitz DL, Culley AW, Carlson KE: Cardiac sarcoidosis. Report of a case with paroxysmal ventricular tachycardia.

JAMA 182: 574, 1962.
18. Forbes G, Usher A: Fatal myocardial sarcoidosis. Br Med J 2: 771, 1962.
19. Hines JD, Sancetta SM: Myocardial sarcoidosis simulating healed myocardial infarction. Ohio State Med J 59: 689, 1963.
20. Smith WP: Primary sarcoid heart disease. Report of a case. J Fla Med Assoc 51: 652, 1964.
21. Chomette G, Auriol M, Daddi G, et al.: Localisations cardiaques massives d'une sarcoïdose de Besnier-Boeck-Schaumann. Ann Anat Pathol (Paris) 10: 177, 1965.
22. Johansen A: Isolated myocarditis versus myocardial sarcoidosis. A contribution to the discussion regarding points of resemblance between these and a report of three illustrative cases. Acta Pathol Microbiol Scand 67: 15, 1966.
23. Shimada N, Ishihara Y, Kojima A, et al.: Three cases of granulomatous myocarditis with giant cells. Acta Pathol Jap 17: 503, 1967.
24. Miyaji T, Ohara M, Funaki M, et al.: [A case of myocardial sarcoidosis with Adams-Stokes syndrome]. J Jap Soc Intern Med 56: 260, 1967.
25. Contreras R, Sánchez Torres G, Durán Rodríquez P: Sarcoidosis cardiaca. Arch Inst Cardiol Mex 37: 20, 1967.
26. Hishimoto Y, Takano Y, Tagaki M: Case of fatal myocardial sarcoidosis preceded by cardiac symptoms. Jap J Clin Med 26: 1244, 1968.
27. Bashour FA, McConnell T, Skinner W, et al.: Myocardial sarcoidosis. Dis Chest 53: 413, 1968.
28. Rajasenan V, Cooper ES: Myocardial sarcoidosis, bouts of ventricular tachycardia, psychiatric manifestations and sudden death. A case report. J Natl Med Assoc 61: 306, 1969.
29. Duvernoy WFC, Garcia R: Sarcoidosis of the heart presenting with ventricular tachycardia and atrioventricular block. Am J Cardiol 28: 348, 1971.
30. Rossi L: Sarcoid heart disease. Br Med J 1: 546, 1973.
31. Ghosh P, Fleming HA, Gresham GA, et al.: Myocardial sarcoidosis. Br Heart J 34: 769, 1972.
32. Zoneraich S, Gupta MP, Mehta J, et al.: Myocardial sarcoidosis presenting as acute mitral insufficiency. Chest 66: 452, 1974.
33. Morales AR, Levy S, Davis J, et al.: Sarcoidosis and the heart. Pathology Annual 1974 (Sommers SC, ed), New York, Appleton-Century-Crofts, 1974, p 139.
34. Chun SK, Andy JJ, Jilly P, et al.: Ventricular aneurysm in sarcoidosis. Chest 68: 392, 1975.
35. Johnson JB, Jason RS: Sarcoidosis of the heart. Report of a case and review of the literature. Am Heart J 27: 246, 1944.
36. Yesner R, Silver M: Fatal myocardial sarcoidosis. Am Heart J 41: 777, 1951.
37. Adickes GC, Zimmerman SL, Cardwell ES: Sarcoidosis with fatal cardiac involvement. Ann Intern Med 35: 898, 1951.
38. Arkless HA, Gokcebay TM, Mendell TH: Sarcoidosis of the heart. Am J Cardiol 1: 648, 1958.
39. Stein MH, Gross JM, Shulman H: A case of cardiac sarcoidosis manifested by uncontrollable ventricular tachycardia. Review of cardiac manifestations in sixteen cases of sarcoidosis. Am J Cardiol 10: 864, 1962.
40. Ferrans VJ, Hibbs RG, Black WC, et al.: Myocardial degeneration in cardiac sarcoidosis. Histochemical and electron microscopic studies. Am Heart J 68: 159, 1965.
41. Carvalhal S dos S, Rocha JC: Un caso de sarcoidose com comprometimento de coraçao. Rev Assoc Med Brasil 11: 89, 1965.
42. Deneberg M: Sarcoidosis of the myocardium and aorta. A case report. Am J Clin Pathol 43: 445, 1965.
43. Raftery EB, Oakley CM, Goodwin JF: Acute subvalvular mitral incompetence. Lancet 2: 360, 1966.
44. Clark EJ, Blount AW: A fatal case of myocardial sarcoidosis. Lancet 86: 568, 1966.
45. Bruno MS, Ober WB: Clinico-pathologic conference. Intractable heart failure with long-standing granulomatous disease. NY State J Med 68: 2790, 1968.
46. Case Records of the Massachusetts General Hospital. Case 46–1975. Harthorne JW, Freiman DG. N Engl J Med 293: 1138, 1975.
47. Gozo EG Jr, Cosnow I, Cohen HC, et al.: The heart in sarcoidosis. Chest 60: 379, 1971.
48. Cotter EF: Boeck's sarcoid. Autopsy in a case with visceral lesions. Arch Intern Med 64: 286, 1939.
49. Hirayama J: Ein Fall von diffuser spezifischer Myocarditis mit zahlreichen Riesenzellen. Trans Soc Pathol Jap 29: 261, 1939.
50. Botti RE, Young FE: Myocardial sarcoid, complete heart block and aortic stenosis. Ann Intern Med 51: 811, 1959.
51. Nissen AW, Berte JB: Cardiac arrhythmias in sarcoidosis. Arch Intern Med 113: 275, 1964.
52. Bernstein M, Konzlemann FW, Sidlick DM: Boeck's sarcoid. Report of a case with visceral involvement. Arch Intern Med 44: 721, 1929.
53. Nickerson DA: Boeck's sarcoid. Report of six cases in which autopsies were made. Arch Pathol 24: 19, 1937.
54. Spencer J, Warren S: Boeck's sarcoid. Report of a case, with clinical diagnosis confirmed at autopsy. Arch Intern Med 62: 285, 1938.
55. Granström KO, Gripwall E, Kristofferson CE, et al.: A case of uveoparotid fever (Heerfordt) with autopsy findings. Acta Med Scand 126: 307, 1946.
56. Skavlem JH, Ritterhoff RJ: Coexistent pulmonary asbestosis and sarcoidosis. Am J Pathol 22: 493, 1946.
57. Gendel BR, Young JM, Greiner DJ: Sarcoidosis. A review with twenty-four additional cases. Am J Med 12: 205, 1952.
58. Gilg I: Sarcoidosis involving the heart. Acta Derm Venereol 33: 318, 1953.
59. Brun J, Turiaf J, Perrin LF, et al.: Coeur et sarcoidose de Besnier-Boeck-Schaumann. Presse Med 63: 284, 1955.
60. Pascoe HR: Myocardial sarcoidosis. Report of a case with unexpected death. Arch Pathol 77: 299, 1964.
61. Peison B: Sarcoidosis of the heart associated with myocarditis: report of case. Ill Med J 130: 317, 1966.
62. Smith LH Jr: Case Records of the Massachusetts General Hospital. Weekly Clinicopathological Exercises. Case 8–1974. N Engl J Med 290: 504, 1974.
63. Laroche C, de Gennes J-L, Hazard J, et al.: Maladie de Besnier-Boeck-Schaumann avec manifestations polyarticulaires et localisations endo-myo-péricardiques mortelles. Bull Mém Soc Med Hôp Paris 71: 908, 1955.
64. Thorbjarnarson B, Glenn F: Sarcoidosis associated with sudden death during mitral valvulotomy. Arch Surg 73: 862, 1956.
65. Roberts WC, Bodey GP, Wertlake PT: The heart in acute leukemia. A study of 420 autopsy cases. Am J Cardiol 21: 388, 1968.
66. Glancy DL, Roberts WC: The heart in malignant melanoma. A study of 70 autopsy cases. Am J Cardiol 21: 555, 1968.
67. Roberts WC, Glancy DL, DeVita VT Jr: Heart in malignant lymphoma (Hodgkin's disease, lymphosarcoma, reticulum cell sarcoma and mycosis fungoides). A study of 196 autopsy cases. Am J Cardiol 22: 85, 1968.
68. Lull RJ, Dunn BE, Gregoratos G, et al.: Ventricular aneurysm due to cardiac sarcoidosis with surgical cure of refractory ventricular tachycardia. Am J Cardiol 30: 282, 1972.
69. Shiff AD, Blatt CJ, Colp C: Recurrent pericardial effusion secondary to sarcoidosis of the pericardium. A biopsy-proven case. N Engl J Med 281: 141, 1969.
70. Bailey RR: Systemic sarcoidosis with pericarditis and pericardial effusion. N Z Med J 65: 704, 1966.
71. Roberts WC, Ferrans VJ: Pathologic anatomy of the cardiomyopathies. Idiopathic dilated and hypertrophic types,

infiltrative types, and endomyocardial disease with and without eosinophilia. Hum Pathol 6: 287, 1975.

72. Lathan SR, Block RA, McLean RL: Sarcoidosis with metastatic calcification. Am J Med 44: 1000, 1968.
73. Fujita N, Torres A, Sharma OP: Ectopic calcification in sarcoidosis. JAMA 227: 556, 1974.
74. Roberts WC: Calcification of the mitral anulus: a study of 87 necropsy patients (abstract). Circulation 45 & 46 (Suppl II): 107, 1972.
75. Roberts WC, Perloff JK: Mitral valvular disease. A clinicopathologic survey of the conditions causing the mitral valve to function abnormally. Ann Intern Med 77: 939, 1972.
76. Bell NH, Bartter FC: Studies of ^{47}Ca metabolism in sarcoidosis: evidence for increased sensitivity of bone to vitamin D. Acta Endocrinol (Kbh) 54: 173, 1967.
77. Bulkley BH, Roberts WC: Steroid therapy during acute myocardial infarction. A cause of delayed healing and of ventricular aneurysm. Am J Med 56: 244, 1974.
78. Gold J, Cantor P: Sarcoid heart disease. A case with unusual electrocardiogram. Arch Intern Med 104: 101, 1959.
79. Unsigned Editorial. Myocardial sarcoidosis. Lancet 2: 1351, 1972.
80. Fleming HA: Sarcoid heart disease. Br Med J 1: 174, 1973.
81. Strauss GS, Lawton BR, Wenzel FJ, et al.: Detection of covert myocardial sarcoidosis by scalene node biopsy. Chest 69: 790, 1976.
82. Buchbinder NA, Roberts WC: Left-sided valvular active infective endocarditis. A study of forty-five necropsy patients. Am J Med 53: 20, 1972.
83. Roberts WC, Kehoe JA, Carpenter DF, et al.: Cardiac valvular lesions in rheumatoid arthritis. Arch Intern Med 122: 141, 1968.
84. Roberts WC, Wibin EA: Idiopathic panaortitis, supra-aortic arteritis, granulomatous myocarditis and pericarditis. A cause of pulseless disease and possibly left ventricular aneurysm in the African. Am J Med 41: 453, 1966.
85. Walton EW: Giant-cell granuloma of the respiratory tract (Wegener's granulomatosis). Br Med J 2: 265, 1958.
86. Jonas AF Jr: Granulomatous myocarditis. Bull Johns Hopkins Hosp 64: 45, 1939.
87. Kean BH, Koekenga MT: Giant cell myocarditis. Am J Pathol 28: 1095, 1952.
88. Tesluk H: Giant cell versus granulomatous myocarditis. Am J Clin Pathol 26: 1326, 1956.
89. Long WH: Granulomatous (Fiedler's) myocarditis with extracardiac involvement. A case report with sudden death. JAMA 177: 184, 1961.
90. Davies MJ, Pomerance A, Teare RD: Idiopathic giant cell myocarditis—a distinctive clinico-pathological entity. Br Heart J 37: 192, 1975.
91. Manger D: A case of fatal subacute myocarditis of unknown etiology. Am J Med Sci 198: 246, 1939.
92. Saphir O: Isolated myocarditis. Am Heart J 24: 167, 1942.
93. Dilling NV: Giant-cell myocarditis. J Pathol Bacteriol 71: 295, 1956.
94. Rab SM, Choudhury GM, Choudhury AR: Giant-cell myocarditis. Lancet 2: 172, 1963.

THE AUTOPSY: ITS DECLINE AND A SUGGESTION FOR ITS REVIVAL

William C. Roberts, M.D.

Abstract The hospital autopsy rate in the United States dropped from 41 per cent in 1964 to 22 per cent in 1975. This reduction is attributable to a declining interest for many reasons by clinicians, surgeons, pathologists, families of the deceased and hospital administrators and hospital accreditors. Various advances in medicine and surgery in recent years have not replaced the value of the autopsy; indeed they have increased the potential information to be gained from it. For interest in autopsies to be revived among physicians and surgeons, pathologists must provide more expert information from the autopsy. To provide the type of information sought from autopsies by physicians and surgeons, the training of pathologists must be altered so that there can be more specialization in anatomic pathology and more subspecialization in the various organ systems, as in internal medicine. In addition, the means of communication between anatomic pathologists and clinicians needs altering so that important clinical questions are recognized by pathologists, and the answers sought and promptly, understandably and diplomatically communicated to physicians and surgeons. Moreover, the large body of information obtained in recent years from autopsies alone needs to be better recognized by clinicians so that they may better understand the value of these examinations. (N Engl J Med 299:332-338, 1978)

THE hospital autopsy rate (number of autopsies performed in a hospital divided by the number of hospital deaths) in the United States and in other Western countries continues to decline.[1-4] This fall is due both to a decrease in the absolute number of autopsies performed and to an increase in the number of deaths in hospitals. Shortly after World War II, the hospital autopsy rate in the United States was nearly 50 per cent. By 1964, the mean autopsy rate in all United States hospitals was 41 per cent; by 1970 it was 29 per cent, by 1973, 22.2 per cent, and by 1975, 21.7 per cent.[1,4] Breakdown of the hospitals analyzed in 1975 disclosed lower average rates in the smaller nonteaching (those without any residency program) hospitals than in the larger nonteaching hospitals, and lower rates in the smaller teaching (at least one approved residency training program) hospitals than in the larger or major teaching (an approved residency training program in at least three specialties) hospitals.[4] This rate is also lower in older patients, in women and in certain fatal conditions (cerebrovascular disease, for example, as compared to cardiovascular disease, respiratory disease and cancer).[3]

In recent years many papers, editorials and letters to the editor have attested to the value and importance of the autopsy,[5-63] including four symposia on the subject.[12-17,20-25,35,45-61] Most of these publications were written by pathologists. The present report summarizes some of these reported observations, including reasons for the decline in the autopsy rate, and suggests ways by which interest in the autopsy might be revived. But a review of the purposes of the autopsy is appropriate:

The autopsy is a check on the accuracy of the clinical diagnoses, historical data and "instruments of precision" used for diagnostic purposes. The autopsy nearly always provides additional diagnoses, and occasionally (in about 25 per cent of cases[64-66]) it alters completely the previous-

From the Pathology Branch, National Heart, Lung, and Blood Institute, Bldg. 10A, Room 3E-30, National Institutes of Health, Bethesda, MD 20014, where reprint requests should be addressed to Dr. Roberts.

ly prevailing major clinical diagnoses. Thus, it clearly improves the accuracy of medical records and statistics.

The autopsy is a check on the appropriateness of medical and surgical therapy, including indications and effect, as well as complications. The autopsy should prevent the burying of diagnostic and therapeutic mistakes with the dead.[32]

The autopsy provides data on both new and old diseases, drugs and surgical procedures. This information may come initially from study of the single case and later from compilation of autopsy findings from many cases. Study of multiple autopsies of the same condition brings together the different stages of a given disease and provides information on the entire range of any disorder.[22] The autopsy allows study not only of the effects of a natural disease on the various organs but also of the effects of a medication or operative procedure on that disease. It improves enormously the accuracy of certain epidemiologic data and is a resource for study of the effects of environmental hazards on health and the effectiveness of certain sanitary conditions. Death certificates without autopsy verification provide inaccurate figures on the incidence of various diseases.[67] Finally, autopsies of patients with one disease or condition may serve as controls for studies of patients with other conditions. Thus, the autopsy serves as a large research resource to study natural disease, the incidences of particular diseases in particular geographic areas and during various periods, the effects of medicine and surgery on natural diseases and another basis for evaluation of a drug or an operative procedure.

The autopsy provides information beneficial to the deceased's family.[47] It may remove guilt on the part of the immediate family members because of a belief that they may have contributed to death. It provides a sense of comfort and understanding by giving the more precise cause of death. It obviously may be useful for determining insurance benefits. It may provide knowledge of the presence or absence of a contagious or hereditary disease, and may provide the experience of charity that comes from the general gift of medical knowledge to society or the specific gift of an organ to another in need.

The autopsy is a provider of organs (kidney, heart, liver, bone marrow and vascular conduit), *tissues* (cornea, cartilage, fascia and skin) *and extracts* (such as blood and growth hormone) *for the benefit of the living.*

And, finally, *the autopsy clarifies real or potential medicolegal deaths.* The post-mortem examination is essential if the guilty are to be brought to justice and convicted, and if the innocent are to be set free.[10]

All six of the reasons given above contribute, or should contribute, to *patient care*. Five of the six (all but the provider of organs) contribute to the *education* of professionals and society as a whole. Five of the six (all but the information for the family) contribute or may contribute to *research,* and four (the first three and the last) contribute to what has been called "quality control" of medical care. Just as "surgical pathology" serves as a quality control for operative procedures, the autopsy serves the same function for both accuracy of clinical diagnosis and appropriateness of therapy.

If these purposes of autopsies are appropriate, why has the hospital autopsy rate dropped so sharply in recent years? The reasons for the decline are many and complex but may be summarized simply by a declining interest by physicians and surgeons, by pathologists themselves, by families of the deceased, and by hospital administrators and hospital accreditors.

The declining interest in autopsies by physicians and surgeons is the result of at least eight factors. First of all, they believe that the autopsy will provide today little or no information not already available during life from various clinical tests or learned at operation. Secondly, the findings at autopsy are not communicated by the pathologist to the physician or surgeon adequately, understandably, promptly or diplomatically; important clinical questions are ignored or the answers to them are unreasonable, inconsequential findings of little or no clinical relevance too often receive the major focus, and the long written autopsy reports filled with pathology jargon are difficult to decipher, much less to correlate with the clinical findings. Thirdly, lack of knowledge by the pathologist of the patient's fatal condition may prevent proper interpretation of the autopsy findings. Fourthly, the physician or surgeon may fear that the autopsy will uncover a finding that shows error in diagnosis or treatment and thus increase the chance of a malpractice suit. The fifth factor is a desire not to upset the bereaved family further by requesting an autopsy, and inadequate time to plow through the red tape necessary to obtain permission for autopsy, including the finding of the pathologist after 5 p.m. or on weekends to perform the post-mortem study. The sixth is inadequate time or desire to witness the autopsy being performed or to attend the conference that might discuss the findings in his patient. The seventh is an attitude that death represents physician failure, and a desire to forget that failure as quickly as possible and go on to the next case. And the eighth is lack of appreciation that new knowledge is frequently derived from autopsies, particularly from study of a number of patients with the same condition.

The declining interest in autopsies by pathologists themselves also has several explanations. For one thing, this disagreeable task is too often thankless. Clinicians and surgeons often show little enthusiasm for autopsies on their patients, infrequently attend the autopsy or the conference discussing its findings, and too often make the pathologist feel servile, defensive or inferior.

Also, there is a far greater interest in other activities (namely, clinical pathology, surgical pathology, and "research"), and the autopsy is too often viewed as an interruption of these other endeavors. Autopsies are considered the least important activity of most pathology departments, and this attitude is readily visible. The autopsy is the only form of free medical service remaining in all medicine.[23] Because no party pays directly for the autopsy, it is difficult in most medical centers for pathologists to make a living just doing autopsies. The least experienced (intern or resident) physician or the pathologist-in-training performs the autopsies. Staff pathologists, at least at teaching hospitals, have only secondary or advisory roles in "the autopsy service." The youngest staff pathologist too often is appointed chief of the autopsy service. The autopsy reports are typed last by the secretaries, the paraffin blocks on autopsies are cut last by the technicians, and the staff pathologists delay "the signing out" of autopsies to the last because of other more important duties.

Moreover, there is a belief that no meaningful medical information will come from study of autopsies. In the university centers this attitude translates to "academia is outside the morgue." Academic advancement comes from publication of the results of research supported by grants, and no grants support autopsies.

Finally, there is the belief that all autopsies must be "complete," including extensive histologic examination of all organs.

The declining interest in autopsies by families of the deceased is also understandable. The families of the deceased have sensed a lack of interest in autopsies on the part of many physicians and surgeons. Too often today no request for an autopsy is even made to the families of the deceased, or physicians and surgeons tell them that an autopsy will not be necessary because the underlying disease or cause of death is "obvious." Secondly, morticians have discouraged families of the deceased from giving permission for autopsy, which delays the embalming procedure and causes it to take more time. Thirdly, families who have had experience with autopsies are often dissuaded from permitting another autopsy on a family member because of the previous failure of the attending physician to inform the family promptly or at all of the findings at autopsy. Obviously, no family will benefit from an autopsy without knowledge of its findings. Fourthly, stories of lack of adherence to the autopsy permit by the pathologist may be a minor factor — permits restricting the autopsy examination to the chest, for example, must not have one or more abdominal organs examined or excised through the diaphragm. Fifthly, some families fear that the autopsy might mutilate the body of their loved ones. Sixthly, religious objections to autopsies still persist in some areas. Seventhly, belief that the deceased "has suffered enough" is still highly prevalent. And, finally, red tape involved in permission for autopsy occasionally discourages families of the deceased as well as the professionals.

The declining interest in autopsies by hospital administrators and hospital accreditors plays some part. In the late 1960's the Board of Commissioners of the Joint Commission on Accreditation of Hospitals (composed of 16 physicians and four nonphysicians) rewrote the hospital-accreditation standards; the report was published in 1971 (*Accreditation Manual for Hospitals*). They eliminated the previously held minimum autopsy-rate requirement of 20 per cent for hospital accreditation. Although the elimination of this fixed quota rate has been widely interpreted as a lowering of the importance of the autopsy, the intent of the board apparently was not to de-emphasize the autopsy's importance but to place emphasis on the quality and interpretation of autopsies performed rather than on the number performed.[35] Hospital administrators may applaud the declining hospital rate because this decrease is saving money.

If autopsies are important, and clearly most anatomic pathologists believe that they are, what can be done to revive interest in them, to upgrade the standards of their performance, to increase the amount of information derived from them and to increase the number done? At least six factors appear important to accomplish these goals. The first and most important is that more expert information must be provided from the autopsy and communicated to clinicians and surgeons. Secondly, direct monetary support for the autopsy must be made available. Thirdly, the method by which permission for the autopsy is granted must be changed. Fourthly, the concept that all autopsies must be "complete" must be discarded. Fifthly, a campaign to educate the medical profession and society as a whole might be made to make both more aware of discoveries gained from the autopsy in the past and its importance as a contributor to medical knowledge now. And, finally, the findings at autopsy must be better communicated to the families of the deceased.

To provide more information to clinicians and surgeons from the autopsy, the pathologist must have greater expertise in certain subspecialties of medicine, particularly in cardiovascular disease. The most frequent cause of death in the United States is cardiovascular disease (54 per cent of deaths[68]), and yet the number of pathologists who are expert in this subspecialty is minuscule. As a consequence, the majority of autopsies are performed by nonspecialists in the condition responsible for the patients' death. I have never met anyone who entered pathology because he or she was interested in cardiovascular disease, and, indeed, few enter pathology because they wish to study the remains of victims of disease. Not only is cardiovascular disease, usually in the form of coronary heart disease, the most common cause of death among adults in the United States but heart disease in the form of congenital malformations is the most common cause of hospital death of patients in the pediatric age group in the United States. For an autopsy to be performed on a patient with fatal cardiovascular disease by a non-cardiovascular expert, supervised by another pathologist who has little or no interest in the "autopsy service," much less expertise in cardiovascular disease, provides minimal information and engenders little excitement or respect on the part of the cardiologist or cardiac surgeon. It is analogous to a precordial examination in a patient with valvular heart disease by a urologist as contrasted to one by a cardiologist.

How can this greater expertise on the part of pathologists be achieved? First of all, and most importantly, the training of anatomic pathologists needs to be altered. Training in pathology today is almost entirely of a generalist type, consisting typically of two years in anatomic pathology and two years in clinical pathology (clinical chemistry, hematology and microbiology). At the end of four years the board-qualified pathologist is an expert in nothing and too often only superficially informed on a broad spectrum of subjects. Anatomic pathology and clinical pathology have virtually nothing in common: in anatomic pathology various tissues and organs are studied for structural changes; in clinical pathology various fluids (such as blood, urine, and effusions) are studied for the presence or absence of — or the amount of — certain substances. Historically, "pathology" meant anatomic pathology, but gradually microbiology, hematology and finally chemistry were outgrowths so that, today, most "pathologists" spend most of their time in clinical pathology and comparatively little in anatomic pathology. Expertise in the latter has consequently suffered. Thus, for a first step to revitalize anatomic pathology, clinical pathology should be entirely separate, and training should be focused on one or the other. To emphasize this separation, the word "pathology" might be reserved for anatomic pathology, and what had been called "clinical pathology" might best be called "laboratory medicine."

After separation from clinical pathology, anatomic pathology might be subdivided into two divisions (namely, surgical pathology and medical [autopsy] pathology) with both, however, remaining under the umbrella of "anatomic pathology." Surgical pathology focuses primarily on histologic examination of tissues, organs or smears obtained at operation, and medical pathology focuses primarily on gross examination of organs and tissues removed at autopsy. Obviously, there is a good bit of overlap between surgical and medical pathology so constituted, but there may be considerable expertise in one and little in the other. I have seen some excellent surgical pathologists who were poor medical (autopsy) pathologists and vice versa because one is primarily a microscopical expertise, and the other primarily a gross expertise. Cancer is the major subspecialty of the surgical pathologist, and cardiovascular disease, the major subspecialty of the medical pathologist.

To become an excellent surgical pathologist, the pathologist might ideally complete a surgical internship, one year in surgical pathology, one year in medical (autopsy) pathology, and one year in diagnostic radiology. The ideal training for the medical pathologist might include a medical internship, one year in autopsy pathology, six months in surgical pathology, six months in diagnostic radiology and one year in a chosen medical subspecialty — for example, cardiovascular or gastrointestinal disease.

Diagnostic radiology should be extremely important to the anatomic pathologist, particularly the medical pathologist and the surgical bone pathologist. Radiography concerns gross pathology, presenting it in two-dimensional rather than in three-dimensional fashion. There is no better way to study a chest radiograph than to view it adjacent to a longitudinal view of a sectioned, fixed lung at autopsy. Thus, diagnostic radiology and medical (autopsy) pathology are dealing with the same subject matter and there needs to be considerably more overlap between the two for the benefit of both. There is far more rationale, in my view, for placing anatomic pathology and diagnostic radiology under the same umbrella than for putting anatomic pathology and clinical pathology together in the same department.

For the anatomic medical pathologist intent on practicing in a large teaching hospital, specialization in a particular organ system or region of the body is essential for a meaningful contribution to medical care, medical education or the fund of medical knowledge. Possibly, subdivision initially into only four medical pathology specialties — namely, chest, abdominal, hematologic and neurologic diseases — might be a useful beginning. It is worth noting that there has never been any question about separating neuropathology from the rest of anatomic pathology, just as neurology for years has been separated from the remainder of the department of medicine.

The purpose of this new approach to training in surgical pathology and medical pathology, particularly the latter, is to narrow the communication gap between pathologists and clinicians and surgeons. The medical pathologist subspecializing in cardiovascular disease, for example, must be a member of the clinical team, participating in the medical and surgical cardiovascular conferences and even ward rounds, so that the pathologist understands the clinicians' and surgeons' questions and speaks their language. This type of relation is ideal for all subspecialties of medical pathology in academic or large training centers. At the same time, this association could make the clinicians and surgeons more aware of the type of information that can be derived from autopsy or other morphologic studies. Specialization for the medical pathologist must be full time, or nearly so, in the large teaching hospitals if pathologists are to have meaningful influence.

Not only must more expert information be obtained from the autopsy but this information must be communicated back to the physicians and surgeons promptly, understandably and diplomatically. Before the autopsy is started, the clinician or surgeon should be called by the pathologist to touch base on important clinical problems and questions to be answered. The autopsy, at least in large medical centers, must be vigorously supervised, if not performed, by a senior pathologist experienced and vitally interested in the condition or primary organ system affected by the patient to be studied. After completion of the autopsy, a second call to the physician or surgeon is useful to describe the findings. The final written autopsy report should contain simple, understandable diagrams, a minimum of inconsequential descriptive detail, explanations of the cause (or causes) of the major clinical problems and a description of the unusual features or new information provided by the clinicopathological analysis. Conferences on autopsy patients should not be held in autopsy rooms but in well ventilated, comfortable conference rooms where learning is a pleasurable rather than a disagreeable experience. Various graphics obtained during life, such as radiographs, electrocardiograms, echocardiograms and angiograms, should be brought to the review conference and re-examined in light of the autopsy findings. There is no better way to study an echocardiogram than to examine it beside the heart itself. Organs must be demonstrated and photographed in ways that are understandable to clinicians and surgeons.[69] Organs must be retained at least for a while and made available for clinicians and surgeons to examine at their convenience. Becoming intimately familiar with the major morphologic aspects of disease enormously improves one's clinical acumen. The pathologist must bring to his clinical colleagues the excitement and enthusiasm that new knowledge inspires in him. He cannot be hesitant in pointing out errors in diagnosis or management, but tact and diplomacy are essential and an air of friendship and professional respect and goodwill must be created and maintained.

A second factor necessary to revive interest in the hospital autopsy is direct monetary support for this service.[23] There is no provision in existing health or life-insurance policies or Medicare–Medicaid policies to pay directly for the autopsy, estimated to cost today about $1,000.[55] Medicare does not recognize the autopsy as being a direct medical service to a patient.[56] (A cadaver is not considered a patient.) Likewise, research grants provide no support for the autopsy.[9] Hospitals recover the expenses of the autopsy by building its cost back into their overall rate structure by either a loading of the daily service charge or ancillary service charges. Thus, indirectly third-party carriers and private-pay patients provide funds for the autopsy. With the push to "cost accounting" in all areas of medicine, the autopsy cost will come under additional scrutiny, but it should be viewed as a medical professional service and financed accordingly. For medical (autopsy) pathology to survive and contribute in a meaningful way to medical care, education and knowledge, specialization in this area is essential. At present, specialization in a non-income-producing field of pathology is at best difficult.

A third means to revive interest in the autopsy is to alter the method by which permission for it is granted. At present in the United States, most autopsies are done only when the patient's physician requests it, the patient's relatives give consent for it, and the pathologist agrees to perform it. Thus, the patient's physician and the next of kin of the deceased usually must get together shortly after the patient's death. Too often, however, contact at this time is not possible. The patient may have died during the night, so that neither physician nor next of kin was at the hospital, or the address and telephone number of the nearest relative are not known to the deceased's physician.[48] At other times, cumbersome and outmoded state laws are factors limiting consent for autopsy. As pointed out by Prutting,[20] "in New York State, for example, when a surviving spouse dies, permission for autopsy must be obtained from all living children. It doesn't matter whether one of them is sheepherding in Australia or canoeing on an isolated lake in Canada." The system regarding autopsies in some Scandinavian countries appears ideal. It is understood, when a patient enters a hospital in those countries, that if death ensues, there will be an autopsy unless the family signs a form within 12 hours of death specifying that one is not desired.

Another factor that might help to revive interest in autopsies — at least among anatomic pathologists — is to eliminate the concept that all autopsies must be complete. A "complete" autopsy means extensive gross and histologic examination of all body organs. It is certainly ideal to examine all body organs grossly in all autopsies, but it is not necessary to prepare histologic sections from all body organs in every autopsy. As mentioned above, over 50 per cent of autopsies in the United States are on patients with fatal cardiovascular disease. Histologic examination of these patients can often be limited to the heart and lungs. The non-thoracic organs can be examined rapidly in these patients, so that emphasis can be placed on the heart or other portions of the vascular system. Too often, in a patient with fatal cardiac disease, there will be one histologic section prepared of heart and 29 others of other body organs that are normal except for "congestion." The diagnoses at autopsy can in most cases be completed from the gross examination alone. Histologic descriptions in autopsy protocols are unnecessary, and any diagnoses provided by histologic study that were not apparent grossly can be added as a supplementary report. In this way, autopsy reports to clinicians and surgeons are not delayed, and the shorter this interval between autopsy and submission of the report to the deceased's physician or surgeon, the greater the desire of the latter to obtain autopsies.

It is more important to vary the extent of the examination than to decrease the numbers of autopsies. The ideal hospital autopsy rate is 100 per cent. This rate should be the goal of large teaching hospitals. Many small (<200 beds) hospitals do not have full-time pathologists, and purposes of the autopsy at community hospitals may be somewhat different from those at large teaching medical centers. The higher the autopsy rate at a hospital, the less the selectivity factor and, therefore, the greater the value of the findings. For example, if one were studying the causes of death, determined at autopsy, in patients dying early after cardiac-valve replacement, the causes observed might be quite different in a hospital where the autopsy rate was 20 per cent from those observed in a hospital where the rate was 95 per cent. When the hospital autopsy rate is low, it is likely that the percentage of "technical errors" as a cause of death would be considerably less than in the hospital where the autopsy rate is quite high.

There has been much discussion in recent years concerning the ideal autopsy rate. Reinstatement of a required specific hospital rate for accreditation has been advocated, but I am not convinced that this move would be useful. Another view is that some statistically determined sample of all patients dying in a hospital should have an autopsy, and in this way the sampling error produced by autopsy requests only on the most interesting patient could be eliminated. An autopsy rate might be established for each hospital service (such as medicine, general surgery or neurosurgery). Still another view is that every physician and surgeon should have a specified autopsy rate to be given hospital privileges. Another view is that the hospital autopsy rate should be determined by the number of house officers (interns, residents and fellows) on the hospital staff.

A fifth means of reviving interest in the autopsy is to make physicians more aware of more recent contributions of the autopsy to medical knowledge. Its contributions to knowledge on cardiovascular disease alone in the past 30 years have been enormous. It is amazing how one can be aware of the increase in structural knowledge in recent years and not recognize the importance of the autopsy. Both Angrist[23] and Gall[22] prepared long lists of diseases in which initial or highly important descriptions of them were the result of careful autopsy studies.

And, finally, more interest in autopsies by nonprofessionals might arise if they obtained more information on their autopsied relatives. The pathologist, in collaboration with the patient's physician or surgeon, should provide to the family of the deceased a carefully interpreted report of the autopsy, oral or written, soon after its performance. As emphasized by Goodale,[60] the public deserves to be better educated about health and disease, about medical procedures in general and about autopsies in particular. What better way to educate them than by explaining the findings of autopsies to family members?

References

1. Walsh CJ: Autopsy rates in U.S. hospitals. PAS Rep 12(6):1-4, 1974
2. Waldron HA, Vickerstaff L: Necropsy rates in the United Birmingham Hospitals. Br Med J 2:326-328, 1975
3. Cameron HM, McGoogan E, Clarke J, et al: Trends in hospital necropsy rates: Scotland 1961-74. Br Med J 1:1577-1580, 1977
4. Lowe JA, Davis CJ: Need we revive falling autopsy rates?: time trends in PAS hospitals in the United States. PAS Rep 15(12):1-7, 1977
5. Klemperer P: The autopsy. JAMA 161:175-176, 1956
6. Karsner HT: The autopsy. JAMA 161:176, 1956
7. Angrist AA: Effective use of the autopsy in medical education: its role in correlation and integration. JAMA 161:303-309, 1956
8. Cannon PR: Clinical lessons learned in the morgue. JAMA 161:730-732, 1956
9. Angrist A: A plea for grant support of the autopsy. Arch Pathol 63:318-321, 1957
10. *Idem:* The role of the forensic pathologist: Sherlock Holmes or medical and social scientist. JAMA 182:929-931, 1962
11. Prutting J: Final contribution. N Engl J Med 272:51-52, 1965
12. Hazard JB: The autopsy. JAMA 193:805-806, 1965
13. Angrist A: What remedies for the ailing autopsy? JAMA 193:806-808, 1965
14. McManus JFA: The autopsy as research. JAMA 193:808-810, 1965
15. Bohrod MG: Uses of the autopsy. JAMA 193:810-812, 1965
16. Madden SC: How many autopsies? JAMA 193:812-813, 1965
17. Davidson CS: The autopsy in the age of molecular biology. JAMA 193:813-814, 1965
18. Wilson RR: In defense of the autopsy. JAMA 196:1011-1012, 1966
19. Prutting J: Lack of correlation between antemortem and postmorten diagnoses. NY State J Med 67:2081-2084, 1967
20. *Idem:* Symposium on medical progress and the postmortem: introduction. Bull NY Acad Med 44:793-798, 1968
21. McManus JFA: Types of research and the postmortem. Bull NY Acad Med 44:799-807, 1968
22. Gall EA: The necropsy as a tool in medical progress. Bull NY Acad Med 44:808-829, 1968
23. Angrist A: Breaking the postmortem barrier. Bull NY Acad Med 44:830-842, 1968
24. Teare RD: The Scotland Yard autopsy. Bull NY Acad Med 44:843-853, 1968
25. Helpern M: Comments on the value of the autopsy. Bull NY Acad Med 44:854-861, 1968
26. Mottet NK, Kohnen P: Should your hospital have a multipurpose autopsy service? Hosp Pract 5(8):77-89, 1970
27. Spiro RK: A backward glance at the study of postmortem anatomy. Int Surg 56:27-40, 101-112, 1971
28. Prutting J: Abolition of percentage requirement for accreditation of hospitals: et tu Brute. NY State J Med 72:2507-2509, 1972
29. Hasson J: The autopsy — the key to quality control in medical care. NY State J Med 72:2509-2510, 1972
30. Hernandez JA: Autopsies. JAMA 223:1157-1158, 1973
31. Wheelock MC: Autopsies. JAMA 223:1157, 1973
32. Prutting J: The autopsy. JAMA 224:1295-1296, 1973
33. King LS, Meehan MC: A history of the autopsy: a review. Am J Pathol 73:514-544, 1973
34. Hasson J, Gross H: The autopsy and quality assessment of medical care. Am J Med 56:137-140, 1974
35. Ebert RV, Porterfield JD, Trump BF, et al: A debate on the autopsy: its quality control function in medicine. Hum Pathol 5:605-618, 1974
36. Castleman B, Chase RA, Ranchod M: Role of the autopsy in the teaching of gross anatomy. N Engl J Med 291:1413-1414, 1974
37. Munan L, Kelly A: The postmortem examination. JAMA 233:418, 1975
38. Burrows S: The postmortem examination: scientific necessity or folly? JAMA 233:441-443, 1975
39. Swank RL: Postmortem examination. JAMA 235:21, 1976
40. Szanto PB: The value of the autopsy. Int Surg 61:326-327, 1976
41. DeRoy AK: The autopsy as a teaching-learning tool for medical undergraduates. J Med Educ 51:1016-1018, 1976
42. Sampson CC: Declining necropsy rates: a peril to quality medical practice. J Natl Med Assoc 69:617, 1977
43. Reviving the hospital necropsy. Br Med J 1:1560, 1977
44. Gambino SR: The autopsy — an essential component of clinical pathology. Med Lab Observ 9:115-116, 1977
45. Williams MJ, Peery TM: The autopsy, a beginning, not an end. Am J Clin Pathol 69:215-216, 1978
46. Dorsey DB: A perspective on the autopsy. Am J Clin Pathol 69:217-219, 1978

47. Reynolds RC: Autopsies — benefits to the family. Am J Clin Pathol 69:220-222, 1978
48. Prutting J: Autopsies — benefits for clinicians. Am J Clin Pathol 69:223-225, 1978
49. Derman H: The contribution of the autopsy to hospitals. Am J Clin Pathol 69:226-227, 1978
50. Hartmann WH: Contributions of the autopsy to medical education. Am J Clin Pathol 69:228-229, 1978
51. Trump BF, Mergner WJ, Jones RT, et al: The use and application of autopsy in research. Am J Clin Pathol 69:230-234, 1978
52. Gantner GE: The autopsy and the law. Am J Clin Pathol 69:235-238, 1978
53. Anderson RE: The autopsy — benefits to society. Am J Clin Pathol 69:239-241, 1978
54. Yesner R: Medical center hospital costs. Am J Clin Pathol 69:242-244, 1978
55. Pontius EE: Financing mechanisms for autopsy. Am J Clin Pathol 69:245-247, 1978
56. Orsini LA: Health insurance and the autopsy. Am J Clin Pathol 69:248-249, 1978
57. Penner DW: Cost effectiveness of the autopsy in maintaining and improving the standard of patient care. Am J Clin Pathol 69:250-252, 1978
58. Saladino AJ, Dailey ML: The problem-oriented postmortem examination. Am J Clin Pathol 69:253-257, 1978
59. Peery TM: The autopsy data bank: a proposal for pathologists to contribute to the health care of the nation. Am J Clin Pathol 69:258-259, 1978
60. Goodale F: The future of the autopsy. Am J Clin Pathol 69:260-262, 1978
61. Lind CJ Jr: Caveat prosector: the pathologist and autopsy law. Am J Clin Pathol 69:263-265, 1978
62. Wissler RW: The pathos of pathology and a possible cure. Am J Clin Pathol 69:267-275, 1978
63. Kaplan RA: The autopsy — to be or not to be. Hum Pathol 9:127-129, 1978
64. Bauer FW, Robbins SL: An autopsy study of cancer patients. I. Accuracy of the clinical diagnoses (1955 to 1965) Boston City Hospital. JAMA 221:1471-1474, 1972
65. Britton M: Diagnostic errors discovered at autopsy. Acta Med Scand 196:203-210, 1974
66. *Idem:* Clinical diagnostics: experience from 383 autopsied cases. Acta Med Scand 196:211-219, 1974
67. Accuracy of mortality statistics. Br Med J 2:445-446, 1967
68. United States National Center for Health Statistics. Vital and Health Statistics. Vital Statistics of the United States 1973, Vol. 2. Mortality. (DHEW Publication No. [HRA] 77-1101). Washington, DC, Government Printing Office, 1977, pp 184, 214
69. Roberts WC: Examining the heart at necropsy, Cardiac Radiology. Edited by E Carlsson. St Louis, CV Mosby (in press)

Right Ventricular Infarction Complicating Left Ventricular Infarction Secondary to Coronary Heart Disease

Frequency, Location, Associated Findings and Significance From Analysis of 236 Necropsy Patients With Acute or Healed Myocardial Infarction

JEFFREY M. ISNER, MD, FACC
WILLIAM C. ROBERTS, MD, FACC

Bethesda, Maryland

Right ventricular infarction associated with left ventricular infarction was identified by gross examination at necropsy in 33 (14 percent) of 236 patients with transmural myocardial infarction. Right ventricular infarction occurred exclusively as a complication of posterior left ventricular infarction. Associated right ventricular infarction occurred in none of the 97 patients with isolated anterior wall infarction of the left ventricle, but in 33 (24 percent) of the 139 patients with posterior left ventricular infarction. Transmural infarction of the posterior ventricular septum was an additional prerequisite for right ventricular infarction. Of the 139 patients with infarction of the posterior left ventricular wall, 74 had no transmural infarction of the ventricular septum and none of these 74 had associated right ventricular infarction. In contrast, of the 65 patients with infarction of the posterior left ventricular wall and transmural infarction of the ventricular septum, 33 (50 percent) had associated right ventricular infarction.

Among the 33 patients with right ventricular infarction, the infarct was limited to the posterior right ventricular free wall in 27 (82 percent); in the other 6 patients (18 percent) it extended to involve the anterolateral right ventricular free wall. Among patients with a posterior left ventricular infarct, those with a right ventricular infarct had right ventricular dilatation nearly three times ($P < 0.05$) more frequently than the patients without a right ventricular infarct. Comparison of the same two groups disclosed no differences in the patients' age, sex, extent of coronary arterial luminal narrowing, right ventricular hypertrophy, right ventricular thrombi or duration of symptoms of myocardial ischemia.

Hemodynamic data in four patients with a right ventricular infarct disclosed previously reported characteristic hemodynamics of right ventricular infarction in only one patient. Recognition of right ventricular infarction is important because it implies specific therapy, namely, aggressive volume administration. Clinical evidence of *posterior left ventricular infarction* and *right ventricular dilatation* should arouse strong suspicion of associated right ventricular infarction.

From the Pathology Branch, National Heart, Lung, and Blood Institute, National Institutes of Health, Bethesda, Maryland. Manuscript received May 15, 1978; revised manuscript received July 11, 1978, accepted July 12, 1978.
Address for reprints: William C. Roberts, MD, Building 10A, Room 3E-30, National Institutes of Health, Bethesda, Maryland 20014.

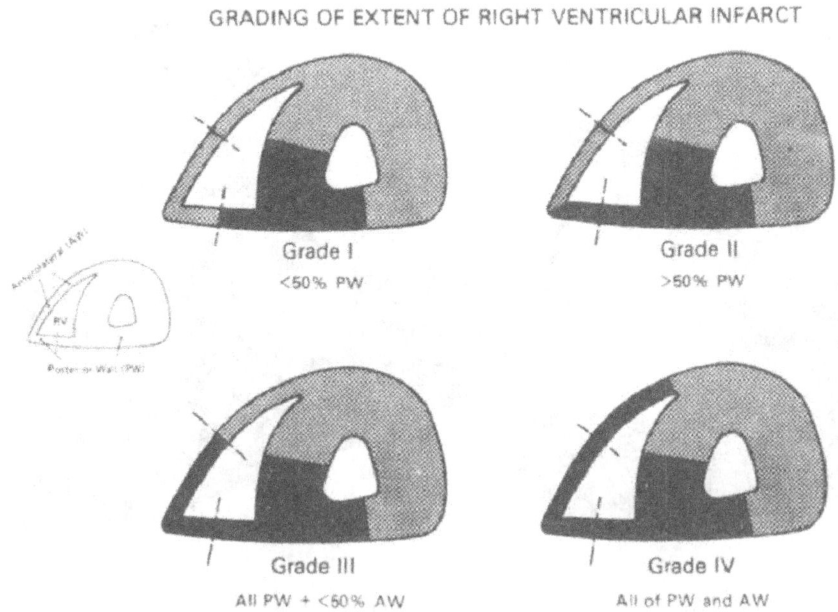

FIGURE 1. Diagram of transverse slices of cardiac ventricles illustrating the scheme used to grade the extent of the right ventricular (RV) infarct. The right ventricular infarct was classified as grade I when it involved less than 50 percent of the posterior wall (PW) of the right ventricle; grade II when it was limited to the posterior wall but involved more than 50 percent of it; grade III when it involved all of the posterior wall and some, but less than 50 percent, of its anterolateral wall (AW); and grade IV when it involved all of the right ventricular posterior wall and more than 50 percent of the anterolateral wall.

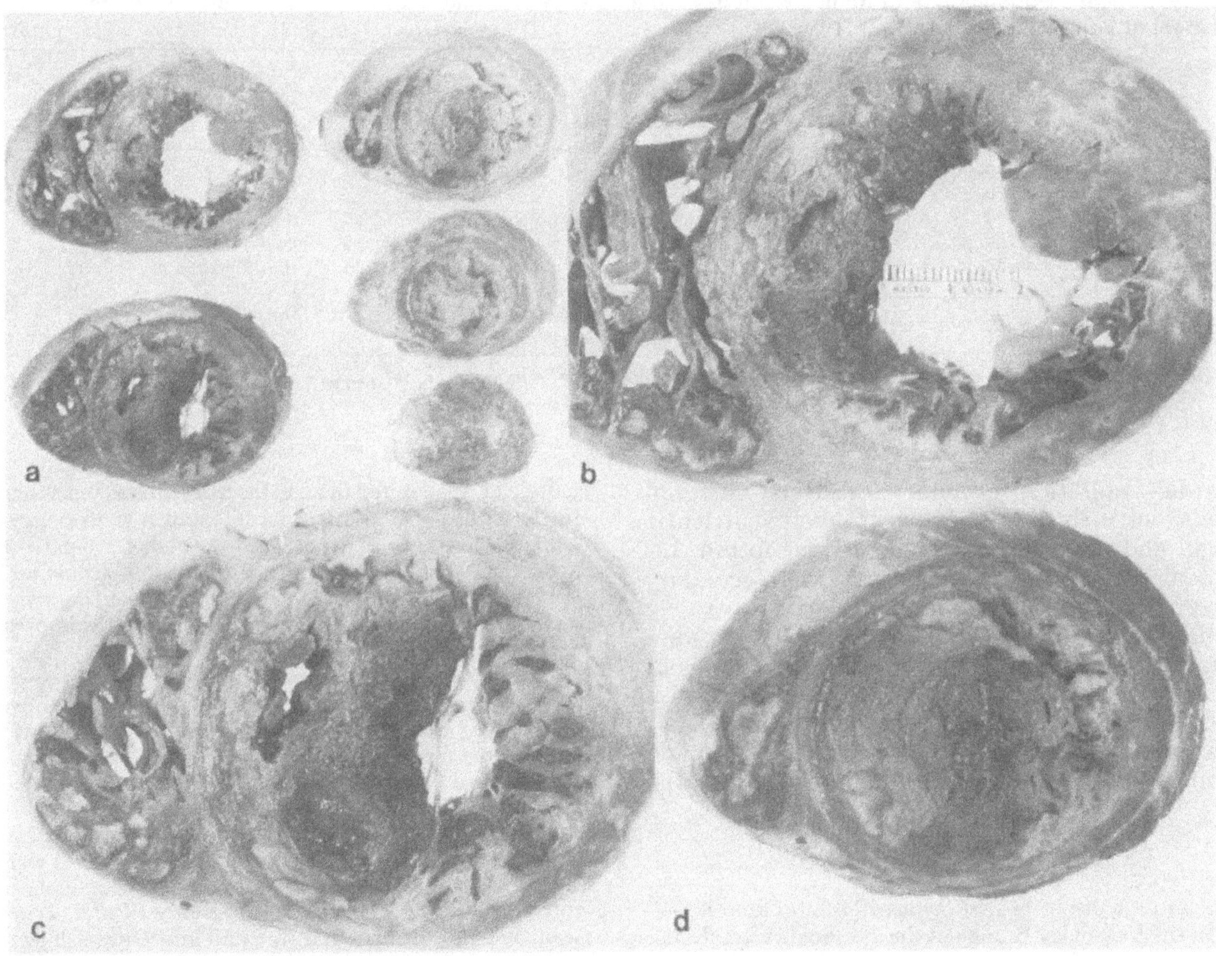

FIGURE 2. Transverse slices of cardiac ventricles illustrating acute myocardial infarction of the right ventricular wall associated with infarction of the ventricular septum and the posterior and anterior walls of the left ventricle in a 66 year old man. The patient had the onset of typical clinical features of acute myocardial infarction beginning 25 days before death. The electrocardiogram showed changes consistent with an acute inferior wall myocardial infarct. Death occurred suddenly. **a,** transverse sections of the cardiac ventricles. **b,** close-up view of the upper left slice in **a,** showing thrombus in both ventricular cavities and necrosis of most of the septum. **c,** close-up view of the bottom left slice in **a,** showing necrosis of the entire septum and all of the posterior right and left ventricular free walls. **d,** close-up view of the upper right slice in **a.** In this slice the infarct is circumferential.

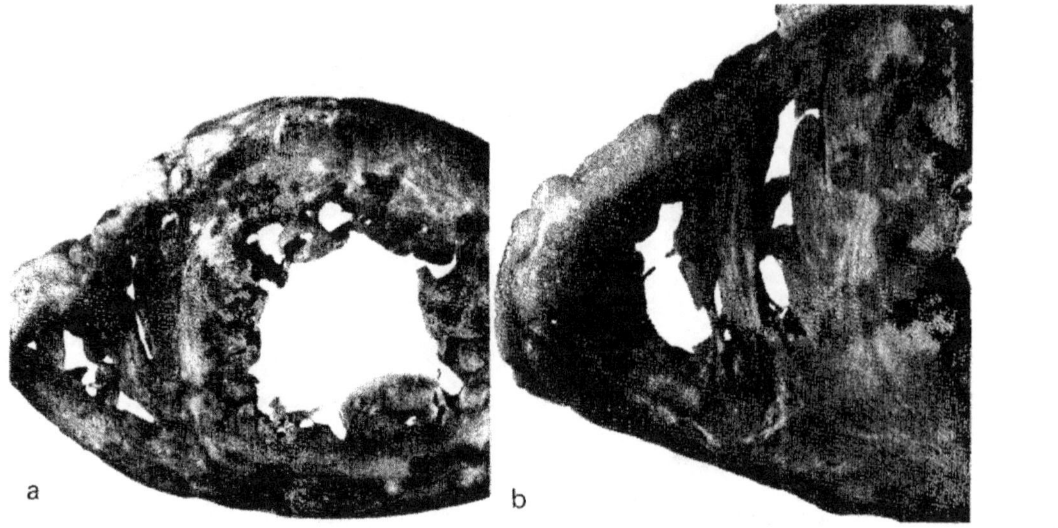

FIGURE 3. Patient 1 (Table IV). Acute right ventricular infarction associated with extensive necrosis of left ventricle in a 57 year old man who died 3 days after the onset of severe chest pain. The electrocardiogram showed changes of acute inferior myocardial infarction. The hemodynamic findings did not suggest associated right ventricular infarction. **a** and **b**, close-up views of two transverse slices of cardiac ventricles showing necrosis of the right ventricle that is limited to but involves more than 50 percent of the posterior wall (grade II). There is associated transmural necrosis of the ventricular septum.

TABLE I

Frequency of Right Ventricular Infarct Among Necropsy Patients With Transmural Left Ventricular Infarction and Relation to Involvement of Ventricular Septum

	Patients								
		Age (yr)		Sex					
LV Infarct	no.	Range	Average	M	F	Transmural VS MI	RV MI	No Transmural VS MI	RV MI
Anterior	97	26–90	69	67	30	68	0	29	0
Acute	60	26–90	74	36	24	43	0	17	0
Healed	37	31–80	60	31	6	25	0	12	0
Posterior	139	26–93	62	99	40	65	33 (51%)	64	0
Acute	56	38–93	64	37	19	32	16 (29%)	24	0
Healed	83	26–93	61	62	21	33	17 (20%)	50	0
Totals	236	26	65	166 (70%)	70 (30%)	133	33 (25%)	103	0

LV = left ventricular; MI = myocardial infarct; RV = right ventricular; VS = ventricular septal.

Myocardial infarction secondary to coronary arterial narrowing virtually always involves the left ventricular free wall and often also the ventricular septum. Involvement of the right ventricular free wall secondary to coronary luminal narrowing has until recently rarely been diagnosed clinically, and few morphologic studies have focused on its frequency or extent. The present study examines the frequency of right ventricular infarction in patients with associated transmural left ventricular infarction and determines its extent and relation to the site of the infarction of the left ventricle.

Patients Studied and Methods

All cases of acute or healed myocardial infarction accessioned in the Pathology Branch of the National Heart, Lung, and Blood Institute from January 1969 to February 1978 were reviewed. Patients with acute or healed myocardial infarction who had associated primary valvular heart disease, infiltrative myocardial disease or hypertrophic cardiomyopathy or who had cardiac surgery at any time were excluded. In addition, patients whose myocardial infarct involved only papillary muscle or was limited in all areas to less than 50 percent of the thickness of the left ventricular free wall or ventricular septum (subendocardium) were excluded. A total of 236 patients were accepted for study. By *gross* inspection, transmural (involvement of greater than the inner half of the myocardial wall) infarction of the left ventricular wall was present in each.

On the basis of reexamination of the hearts, the patients were classified into two major groups: (1) those with transmural myocardial necrosis (acute infarct), and (2) those with transmural myocardial fibrosis (healed infarct). When both fibrosis and necrosis were visible grossly in the same heart (34 patients), the group in which the patient was placed was determined by which feature was dominant by visual examination of the heart specimens. The hearts were then further subdivided by location of the left ventricular infarct into two additional groups: (1) anterior wall, and (2) posterior wall. The right ventricular free wall infarcts are shown by the diagrammatic scheme in Figure 1.

The hearts were weighed and the maximal thickness of the free wall of the right ventricle was measured. The size of both ventricular cavities was judged normal or dilated by visual inspection. The presence or absence of ventricular thrombi was recorded.

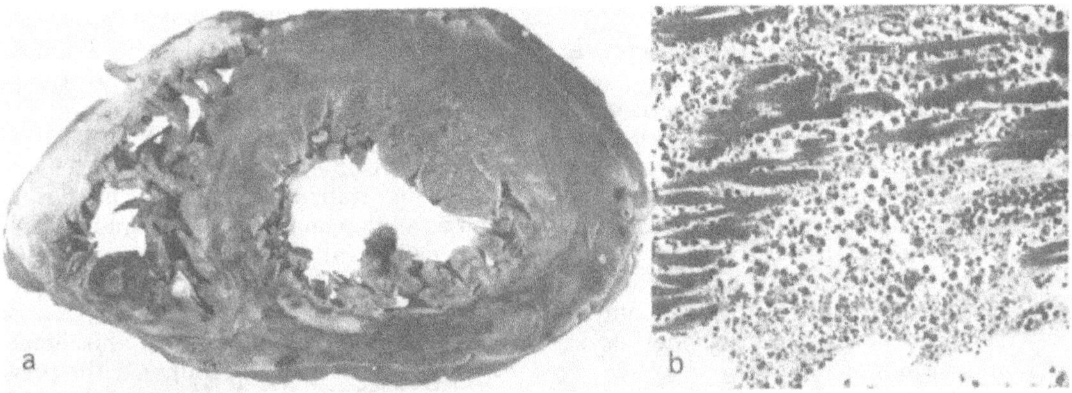

FIGURE 4. Acute right ventricular infarction. **a,** transverse slice of cardiac ventricles illustrating acute infarction of the right ventricle associated with infarction of the posterior wall of the left ventricle in an 82 year old woman who had the onset of typical clinical features of acute infarction 23 days before death. Her last 5 days were complicated by multiple arrhythmias, congestive heart failure and shock. The electrocardiogram was typical of acute myocardial infarction, posterior ("inferior") wall. **b,** photomicrograph of right ventricular wall necrosis from a 68 year old man with acute myocardial infarction involving the right ventricle (grade II), septum and posterior wall of left ventricle. Acute infarction in this patient was complicated by rupture of the ventricular septum 1 day before death. (Phosphotungstic acid hematoxylin stain X212, reduced by 18 percent.)

The coronary arteries were excised intact and sectioned with a method described elsewhere.[1] Briefly, the excised arteries were cut at 5 mm intervals at right angles to the longitudinal axis of the vessels, and each 5 mm long segment was labeled consecutively, processed in alcohols and xylene, embedded in paraffin and cut. A single Movat-stained histologic section was examined from each 5 mm segment.

The clinical records of each of the 236 patients were reviewed. Hemodynamic data were available in 21 patients.

Results

Incidence and relation to anterior, posterior and septal infarction: Of the 236 patients, 116 had an acute and 120 had a healed left ventricular myocardial infarct. The findings in these patients are summarized in Table I and various, mainly morphologic, cardiac findings in several patients are illustrated in Figures 1 to 7. The myocardial infarcts in 236 patients involved the anterior wall in 97 patients and the posterior wall in the other 139. The age and sex of patients with anterior and posterior left ventricular myocardial infarcts were similar. Of the 97 patients with an *anterior* left ventricular infarct (acute in 60 [62 percent] and healed in 37 [38 percent]), none had an associated right ventricular infarct; of the 139 patients with a *posterior* left ventricular infarct (acute in 56 [40 percent] and healed in 83 [60 percent]), 33 (24 percent) had an associated

TABLE II

Right Ventricular Infarction: Morphologic Features

RVMI	Patients no.	Patients Age (yr)	RV Features D	RV Features H	RV Features T	Grade of RV MI I	Grade of RV MI II	Grade of RV MI III	Grade of RV MI IV
Acute	16	46–86 (m 65)	2	1	3	6	9	0	1
Healed	17	26–80 (m 56)	10	0	0	3	8	5	1
Totals	33	26–86 (m 62)	12	1	3	9	17	5	2

D = dilatation; H = hypertrophy; M = mean; MI = myocardial infarct; RV = right ventricular; T = thrombus.

TABLE III

Status of Right Ventricle and Coronary Arteries in Patients With Posterior Wall Left Ventricular Myocardial Infarct (MI) With and Without Associated Right Ventricular (RV) Infarct

					Patients With Histologic Study of Coronary Arteries (no. [%])			
						With >75% Narrowing* of		
LVMI	Cases (no.)	D (no. [%])	H (no. [%])	T (no. [%])	Total (no. [%])	RCA	LAD	LCx
With RV MI	33	12[36]	1[3]	3[9]	28[85]	26[93]	20[74]	20[74]
Without RV MI	106	10[9]	5[5]	4[4]	59[56]	50[85]	46[78]	45[76]

* More than 75 percent narrowing of cross-sectional area by plaque. D = dilatation; H = hypertrophy; LAD = left anterior descending coronary artery; LCx = left circumflex coronary artery; RCA = right coronary artery.

right ventricular infarct. Of the total of 236 patients, 133 had transmural infarction of the ventricular septum (Table I), 68 with anterior and 65 with posterior left ventricular infarction. All 33 patients with right ventricular infarction were among the 65 with posterior left ventricular infarction associated with transmural infarction of the ventricular septum. Of the 74 patients with posterior left ventricular infarction without associated transmural infarction of the ventricular septum, none had a right ventricular infarct. None of the patients with an isolated anterior left ventricular infarct had an associated right ventricular infarct whether or not the ventricular septum was involved.

Clinical and morphologic features: Certain clinical and morphologic features of the patients with right ventricular myocardial infarction are summarized in Tables II and III. Only 1 of the 33 patients had hypertrophy of the right ventricular wall (more than 5 mm thick), whereas 12 had right ventricular dilatation. Antemortem thrombus was found in the right ventricle of three patients. The infarct of the right ventricle was limited to its posterior wall (types I and II) (Fig. 2 to 4, 6 and 7) in 36 patients and to both the posterior and anterolateral right ventricular free walls (types III and IV) in the other 7 (Fig. 5 and 9 to 11).

Comparison of the 33 patients with a posterior left ventricular wall infarct and associated right ventricular wall infarction and the 106 patients with a posterior left ventricular wall infarct *without* associated right ventricular wall infarction disclosed no significant differences in the patients' age, sex, length of survival after onset of symptoms of myocardial ischemia (range 1 to 23 days [mean 8] in all groups) or the presence of right ventricular hypertrophy or thrombus (Tables II and III). Right ventricular dilatation, however, was significantly ($P < 0.05$) more frequent among the group with a posterior left ventricular infarct and associated right ventricular wall infarction.

Coronary arterial findings: The three major (right, left anterior descending and left circumflex) coronary

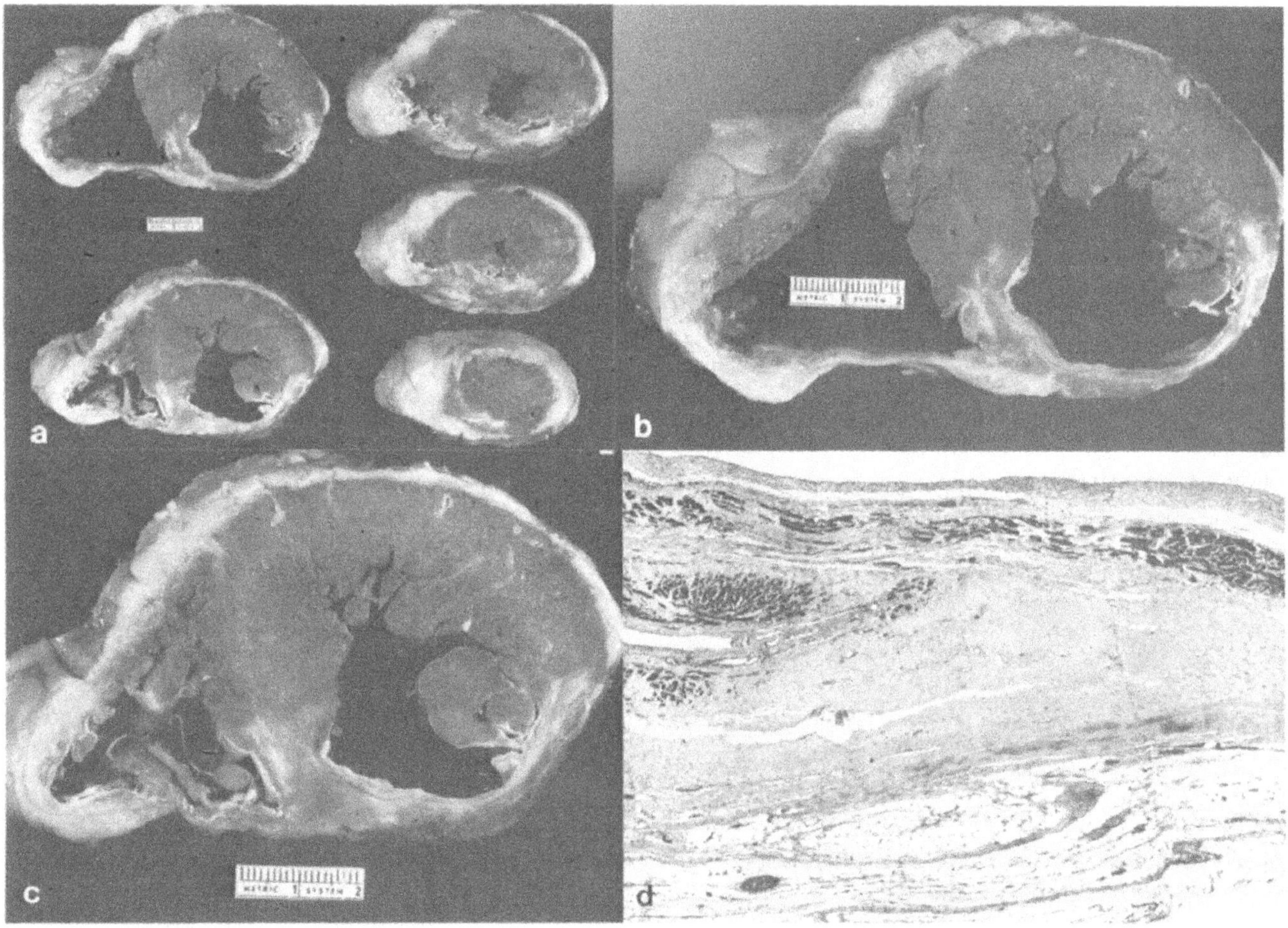

FIGURE 5. Transverse slices of cardiac ventricles **(a, b, c)** and photomicrograph of healed right ventricular infarct **(d)** from a 73 year old man who had had an "inferior" wall myocardial infarct at age 68. The patient was subsequently treated with digoxin and diuretic agents for "mild" congestive heart failure. He died 5 years later from complicatons of eye surgery. **a,** transverse cardiac ventricular slices. **b,** close-up view of slice at upper left in **a**. There are healed posterior right and left ventricular infarcts with thinning of the right (grade II) and left ventricular free walls and the posterior portion of ventricular septum. Both ventricular cavities are dilated. **c,** close-up view of slice at bottom left in **a,** showing additional scarring of the anterolateral wall of the right ventricle. **d,** photomicrograph showing transmural scarring of the right ventricular free wall. (Movat stain ×27, reduced by 25 percent.)

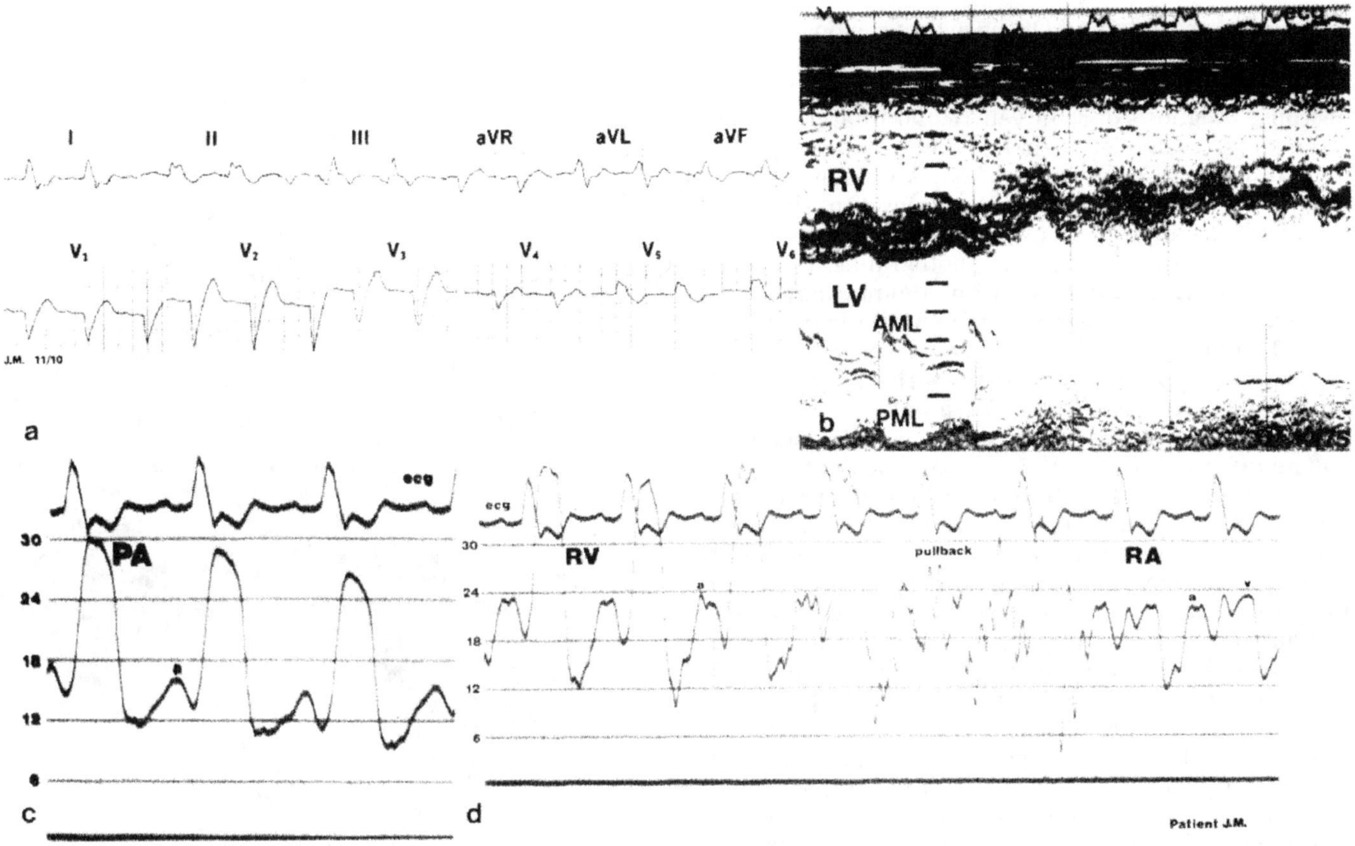

FIGURE 6. Clinical findings recorded in a 48 year old man with healed right ventricular myocardial infarction. The infarction had occurred 7 years before the recordings presented here, and the patient died of progressive congestive heart failure 2 years after the recordings. **a,** electrocardiogram showing S-T segment elevation in lead III, complete left bundle branch block and absent or small R waves in leads V_1 to V_4. **b,** echocardiogram showing biventricular dilatation and abnormal septal motion. AML = anterior mitral leaflet; LV = left ventricle; PML = posterior mitral leaflet; RV = right ventricle. **c,** pulmonary arterial (PA) pressure recording showing a prominent *a* wave. **d,** pullback tracing from the right ventricle (RV) to the right atrium (RA), demonstrating an elevated (18 mm Hg) end-diastolic pressure and prominent *a* waves in the right ventricular pressure tracing.

arteries were examined in detail in 87 (63 percent) of the 139 patients with a left ventricular posterior wall infarct (Table III). Twenty-eight of the 87 had an associated right ventricular infarct and 59 did not. No significant differences were observed among the patients with posterior left ventricular infarcts in the percent of those with and without right ventricular infarction who had more than 75 percent cross-sectional area luminal narrowing by old atherosclerotic plaques in one or more of the three major coronary arteries. The degree of narrowing of the right coronary artery was similar in the patients with and without right ventricular infarction. The percent of patients whose right coronary artery was narrowed more than 75 percent in cross-sectional area by old atherosclerotic plaque was significantly ($P < 0.05$) greater than that of patients whose left anterior descending coronary artery was narrowed to this degree, whether or not infarction involved the right ventricular wall.

TABLE IV

Right Ventricular Infarction: Hemodynamic Features

Case no.	State of MI	Grade of RV MI	Pressures (mm Hg) RA Mean	RV(s/d)	PA (s/d)	PAW Mean
1	Acute	II	5	47/10	41/25	24
2	Healed	II	5	35/5	35/15	15
3	Healed	III	7	30/5	28/12	8
4	Healed	III	23	32/23	34/20	20

MI = myocardial infarction; PA = pulmonary arterial; PAW = pulmonary arterial wedge; RA = right atrial; RV = right ventricular; s/d = systolic/diastolic.

Hemodynamic data: Of the 21 patients who had undergone cardiac catheterization, 4 had an associated right ventricular wall infarct (Table IV). In one of the four, the right atrial mean pressure was higher than the mean pulmonary arterial wedge pressure, and both the right ventricular and pulmonary arterial pressure tracings were deformed by a prominent atrial *a* wave (Fig. 6). Hemodynamic data in the other three patients with a right ventricular infarct were consistent with an isolated left ventricular wall infarct with or without left ventricular decompensation.

Comments

Although right ventricular wall infarction secondary to coronary arterial narrowing has recently received attention from the hemodynamic[2-6] and radioisotopic[7,8] standpoints, it has received little attention from a morphologic standpoint. Of the eight previous reports mentioning infarction of the right ventricular free wall at necropsy,[2,3,7,9–13] only two[10,11] actually focused on the necropsy diagnosis of right ventricular infarction and, when an associated left ventricular infarct was present, most did not describe its location. Although four reports[7,11–13] showed photographs of infarcts of the right ventricular wall, the extent of the infarcts was rarely described or discernible in the photographs.

Right ventricular infarction: a complication of transmural posteroseptal left ventricular infarction: The present study is based on reexamination of the hearts in 236 necropsy patients with transmural left ventricular myocardial infarction secondary to coronary luminal narrowing. Of the 236 patients, 33 (14 percent) had an infarct involving the right ventricular free wall and all of them had a posteriorly located left ventricular infarct. None of the 97 patients with isolated anterior wall left ventricular infarction had associated right ventricular infarction. Thus, among patients with fatal myocardial infarction secondary to severe coronary arterial luminal narrowing, right ventricular infarction occurred only when the left ventricular infarct involved its posterior wall. Of our 139 patients with a posterior left ventricular infarct, 33 (24 percent) had an associated right ventricular infarct. Even among the patients with a posteriorly located left ventricular infarct, however, transmural infarction of the ventricular septum was a prerequisite for development of right ventricular infarction. Of the 139 patients with a posterior left ventricular infarct, 74 did not have transmural infarction of the ventricular septum and none of the 74 had an associated right ventricular infarct. In contrast, of the 65 with transmural infarction of the ventricular septum, 33 (50 percent) had an associated right ventricular infarct. Thus, *right ventricular infarction among our patients was a complication exclusively of transmural posteroseptal left ventricular infarction.*

The extent of the right ventricular necrosis or fibrosis ranged from less than one half of the posterior right ventricular free wall adjacent to the ventricular septum (nine patients) to involvement of the entire right ventricular free wall (two patients). Among the 33 patients with right ventricular infarction, the infarct was limited to the posterior right ventricular free wall in 26 (79 percent); in the remaining 7 (21 percent), both the posterior and anterolateral walls of the right ventricle were involved.

Role of right ventricular hypertrophy and dilatation: Previous investigators have proposed that right ventricular hypertrophy was either an important predisposing factor[10,14] or an absolute prerequisite[15] for the development of right ventricular myocardial infarction. The results of our study do not confirm this speculation. Right ventricular hypertrophy, in fact, was more frequent among our patients without associated right ventricular infarct. It was observed at necropsy in only 1 (3 percent) of our 33 patients *with* a right ventricular infarct, and in 12 (6 percent) of 203 patients with a left ventricular myocardial infarct unassociated with a right ventricular infarct. Furthermore, although one patient had a history of clinically diagnosed "chronic obstructive pulmonary disease," none had necropsy evidence of cor pulmonale. Although extensive right ventricular scarring has been described in various entities associated with right ventricular hypertrophy (including chronic pulmonary emboli[16] and hypertrophic cardiomyopathy[17] in the absence of significant coronary arterial luminal narrowing), such cases were excluded from the present study unless they were associated with left ventricular scarring *and* significant coronary arterial luminal narrowing.

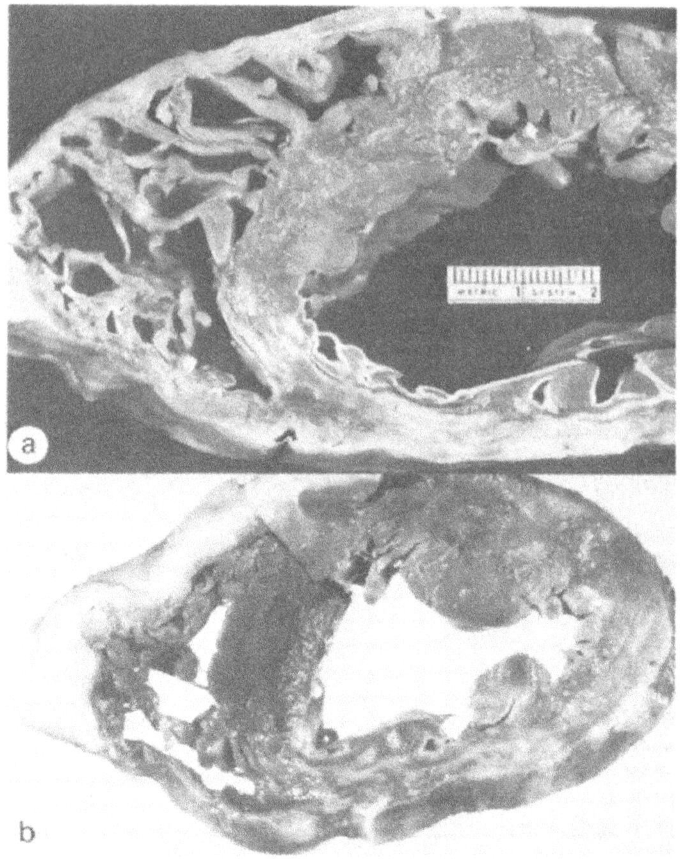

FIGURE 7. Transverse slices of cardiac ventricles showing healed right ventricular infarcts in two patients. **a,** the clinical findings in the patient whose grade III right ventricular wall infarct is shown here are shown in Figure 6. **b,** the posterior right ventricular wall is thinned as is the posterior portion of ventricular septum and posterior portion of left ventricular wall in this 56 year old woman who had an acute myocardial infarct 5 months before death.

Right ventricular dilatation was the single anatomic feature distinguishing our patients from those without right ventricular myocardial infarction. Among the 139 patients with a posterior wall left ventricular infarct, the right ventricular cavity was dilated in 12 (36 percent) of the 33 patients with and in 10 (9 percent) of 106 patients without an associated right ventricular infarct (Table III). This difference (36 versus 9 percent) is significant ($P < 0.05$). Also, for comparison, right ventricular dilatation occurred in only 16 (16 percent) of the 97 patients with an anterior wall left ventricular infarct, a significantly ($P < 0.05$) lower percent than in our patients with a right ventricular infarct.

Right ventricular mural thrombus: This is another necropsy finding reported to be more frequent among patients with associated right ventricular wall infarction than among patients with an isolated left ventricular wall infarct.[10] However, in our 237 patients with a left ventricular wall infarct, right ventricular thrombus occurred with similar frequency in those with and in those without an associated infarct of the right ventricular wall. Of our 139 patients with a posterior wall left ventricular infarct, right ventricular thrombus occurred in 3 (9 percent) of the 33 patients with and in 4 (4 percent) of the 106 patients without an associated right ventricular infarct; of our 97 patients with an anterior wall left ventricular infarct, right ventricular thrombus occurred in 8 patients (8 percent).

Role of severe right versus left coronary arterial narrowing: Several previous investigators have noted a particularly high frequency of severe luminal narrowing by atherosclerotic plaques of the right coronary artery in patients with a right ventricular infarct associated with a left ventricular infarct. These previous studies, however, did not compare the frequency of severe narrowing of this artery among patients with a right ventricular infarct and those with an isolated left ventricular infarct. Furthermore, the previous studies did not compare the frequency of severe narrowing of the right coronary artery by atherosclerotic plaques with the frequency of severe narrowing of either the left anterior descending or left circumflex coronary artery. Among our patients with posterior wall left ventricular infarction, the percent with greater than 75 percent cross-sectional area luminal narrowing by atherosclerotic plaques of the right coronary artery was similar (about 90 percent) in the patients with and without right ventricular infarction. All our patients with right ventricular infarction had severe (greater than 75 percent cross-sectional area) luminal narrowing of the coronary artery responsible (dominant) for perfusing the posterior ventricular wall (that is, either the right or the left circumflex artery).

Clinical diagnosis: Diagnosis during life of right ventricular infarction in patients with left ventricular infarction secondary to severe coronary arterial luminal narrowing is at best difficult. If the left ventricular infarct is limited to the anterior wall, the chance of an associated right ventricular infarct is minimal. Thus, a *posterior location* of the left ventricular infarction is a prerequisite for right ventricular infarction. Nearly a quarter of all our patients with posterior wall infarction of the left ventricle had associated right ventricular infarction. Thus, if the left ventricular infarct is posterior and transmural, there is a 1 in 4 chance that there will be an associated right ventricular infarct. If, however, the ventricular septum is transmurally infarcted in association with a posterior left ventricular free wall infarction, the chance of an associated right ventricular infarction becomes 1 in 2. But the electrocardiogram is not helpful in distinguishing infarction limited to the posterior left ventricular wall from that involving both posterior and septal walls. The echocardiogram might show diminished motion of the ventricular septum in this circumstance, but the reliability of this technique to determine transmural septal infarction is unproved. One finding suggestive of right ventricular infarction is right ventricular dilatation, an occurrence nearly 3 times more frequent in our patients with than in those without right ventricular infarction. Right ventricular hypertrophy is rare in patients with right ventricular infarction secondary to coronary narrowing and is therefore not helpful from a diagnostic standpoint.

Hemodynamic findings: role in clinical diagnosis: Before the introduction of newer, noninvasive techniques, the clinical diagnosis of right ventricular myocardial infarction had been limited to cardiac catheterization. The finding of elevated right atrial (or right ventricular end-diastolic) pressure out of proportion to left atrial (or left ventricular end-diastolic) pressure has been suggested as the characteristic hemodynamic profile of right ventricular infarction.[2] Such hemodynamic abnormalities have been confirmed in at least five patients by necropsy.[2,3,7,13] No previous reports, however, have described hemodynamic findings in patients in whom the diagnosis of right ventricular myocardial infarct was first established at necropsy. Three of our four patients with necropsy-confirmed right ventricular myocardial infarction had a hemodynamic profile that was *not* suggestive of associated right ventricular infarction (Table IV). The nondiagnostic hemodynamics in at least one of these three patients were not simply a function of the temporal relation of the catheterization to the infarction because the right-sided cardiac catheterization was performed during the period of acute myocardial infarction. An alternative explanation for the nondiagnostic hemodynamic findings in one or all three of these patients is that they were obscured by relative hypovolemia. Rigo et al.[7] described two patients with cardiogenic shock and a low left ventricular filling pressure in whom the characteristic hemodynamic profile of right ventricular infarction complicating left ventricular infarction was unmasked by volume administration. Thus, it is possible that had our three patients with right ventricular infarction and "nondiagnostic" hemodynamics been stressed with volume or exercise, diagnostic hemodynamic findings might have developed.

Nevertheless, it appears that the hemodynamic profile previously considered characteristic of right ventricular infarction is less diagnostically sensitive than thought and that right ventricular infarction may occur in the presence of normal or near normal intracardiac pressures. Conversely, in the absence of pericardial or valvular heart disease, the hemodynamics described for right ventricular infarction appear to be relatively specific. Hemodynamic findings in 17 other necropsy patients with left ventricular infarction without associated right ventricular infarction disclosed no intracardiac pressure recordings typical of those observed in patients with right ventricular infarction, that is, no false positives.

Simulation of hemodynamics of constrictive pericarditis: The intracardiac pressures characteristic of right ventricular infarction may persist for years after anatomic healing of the infarct, and these pressure tracings may simulate those observed in patients with pericardial heart disease. Our Patient 4 (Table IV) at cardiac catheterization performed 2 years after healing of the acute myocardial infarct still had hemodynamics characteristic of those observed during the period of acute infarction (Fig. 6). Furthermore, the pressure tracings in this patient disclosed prominent *a* waves in both the right ventricle and major pulmonary arteries, findings identical to those described in patients with constrictive pericarditis. Raabe and Chester[13] and Lorell et al.[3] recently pointed out that among patients with acute left ventricular infarction associated with right ventricular infarction the intracardiac hemodynamics could simulate those in patients with pericardial constriction. As in patients with combined acute right and left ventricular wall myocardial infarcts, the characteristic hemodynamic abnormalities in patients with pericardial constriction may not be manifest until the patients are stressed with volume loading or with exercise.[18]

Clinical recognition and determinants of right ventricular dysfunction: Cumulative clinical experience with right ventricular myocardial infarction complicating left ventricular myocardial infarction has clearly established the existence of a specific hemodynamic syndrome of right ventricular dysfunction characterized by underfilling of the left ventricle as a result of impaired right ventricle contractility.[2-8,13] In such patients, right ventricular dilatation is the sole compensatory mechanism by which right ventricular contractility may be augmented. Under such circumstances, volume administration may be critical to maintain a maximal right ventricular filling pressure. Indeed, supplemental volume administration in patients with *elevated* right-sided pressures and a *normal* or near-normal left ventricular filling pressure (that is, patients with right ventricular infarction) has produced marked hemodynamic improvement. Thus, it becomes important to recognize clues to the often occult syndrome of right ventricular dysfunction or right ventricular infarction. Our study suggests that evidence of an "inferior" myocardial infarct combined with evidence of right ventricular dilatation should make one particularly suspicious of the presence of right ventricular infarction.

The amount of hemodynamic data available in patients with proved right ventricular infarction is inadequate to permit conclusions regarding the relation between the extent of the right ventricular infarct and the degree of hemodynamic decompensation. It is likely that the ability of the right ventricle to contribute adequately to left ventricular filling is more a function of the integrity of the ventricular septum than of the integrity of the right ventricular free wall. Starr et al.[19] and others[20,21] have demonstrated in dogs that experimental destruction of the right ventricular free wall does not produce adverse hemodynamic consequences. The contribution of the contracting ventricular septum is apparently great enough to compensate for the loss of participation of the right ventricular free wall. It might be expected that an infarct limited to the juxtaseptal portion of the right ventricular free wall (grade I) or even limited to the entire posterior wall (grade II) would be too small to affect right ventricular function. Yet of our 12 patients with right ventricular dilatation in association with right ventricular infarction, 11 had right ventricular infarction limited to the posterior wall (grade I in 3 and grade II in 8). If right ventricular dilatation constitutes a sign of right ventricular dysfunction, then the latter was not simply a function of the anatomic extent of the right ventricular infarct. It is more likely that the extent of septal involvement (present to a greater degree in all our patients with a right ventricular infarct) was the principal determinant of right ventricular decompensation. In addition, acute myocardial ischemia can in itself lead to acute reduction in ventricular contractility.

Newer, noninvasive methods of diagnosis: Recent reports of echocardiographic and radioisotopic findings in patients with acute myocardial infarction suggest that it may be possible to establish the diagnosis of right ventricular myocardial infarction reliably by noninvasive means. Sharpe et al.[8] demonstrated right ventricular dilatation with M mode echocardiography in five of six patients with acute right ventricular myocardial infarction. Similar results were demonstrated with gated scintigraphy.[7] The frequency of right ventricular dilatation among our patients with right ventricular infarction supports the validity of these noninvasive findings in patients with right ventricular infarction. Additional abnormalities demonstrated on radioisotopic studies in patients with right ventricular infarction include segmental or generalized right ventricular contraction abnormalities and increased right ventricular uptake of technetium pyrophosphate. Of the five patients described by Sharpe et al.[8] with increased uptake of this radionuclide in the right ventricular free wall each had increased uptake in the ventricular septum and posterior left ventricle. This observation is consistent with our finding of consistent involvement of the septum and posterior wall of the left ventricle in patients with right ventricular myocardial infarction.

Role of coronary blood supply to right ventricle: The basis for the apparently exclusive association of right ventricular infarct with infarction of the posterior wall of the left ventricle may be the specific anatomy of the coronary blood supply to the right ventricle. The bulk of the right ventricular myocardium is consistently supplied by numerous branches of the coronary artery supplying the posterior wall of the left ventricle (usually [90 percent[22]] the right coronary artery); with a left dominant system, the circumflex coronary artery supplies both right ventricular and posterior left ventricular branches. Thus, infarction of the right ventricle can result only when the vascular supply to the posterior wall of the left ventricle is compromised as well. In contrast, the anteriormost portion of the right ventricle, including the anterior paraseptal region, has a *dual* blood supply that consists of right ventricular branches from the left anterior descending coronary artery and, most importantly, the conus branch of the right coronary artery. The latter is insurance for the right ventricle in cases of anterior left ventricular infarction; conversely, atherosclerotic narrowing of the right coronary artery proximal to or involving the conus branch probably accounts for most cases of circumferential (type IV) right ventricular myocardial infarction.

References

1. **Roberts WC, Buja LM:** The frequency and significance of coronary arterial thrombi and other observations in fatal acute myocardial infarction. A study of 107 necropsy patients. Am J Med 52:425–443, 1972
2. **Cohn JN, Guiha NH, Broder MI, Limas CJ:** Right ventricular infarction. Clinical and hemodynamic features. Am J Cardiol 33: 209–214, 1974
3. **Lorell B, Gold HK, Pohost GM, Dinsmore RE, Leinbach RC, Hutter AM, De Sanctis RW:** Right ventricular infarction: Clinical features, emphasizing its resemblance to cardiac tamponade (abstr). Am J Cardiol 41:409, 1978
4. **Rackley CE, Russell RO:** Right ventricular function in acute myocardial infarction. Am J Cardiol 33:927–929, 1974
5. **Wells DE, Befeler B:** Dysfunction of the right ventricle in coronary artery disease. Chest 66:230–235, 1974
6. **Zone DD, Botti RE:** Right ventricular infarction with tricuspid insufficiency and chronic right heart failure. Am J Cardiol 37: 445–448, 1976
7. **Rigo P, Murray M, Taylor DR, Weisfeldt ML, Kelly DT, Strauss HW, Pitt B:** Right ventricular dysfunction detected by gated scintiphotography in patients with acute inferior myocardial infarction. Circulation 57:483–490, 1978
8. **Sharpe DN, Botvinick EH, Shames DM, Schiller NB, Massie BM, Chatterjee K, Parmley WW:** The non-invasive diagnosis of right ventricular infarction. Circulation 57:483–490, 1978
9. **Wartman WB, Hellerstein HK:** The incidence of heart disease in 2,000 consecutive autopsies. Ann Intern Med 28:41–65, 1948
10. **Wade WG:** The pathogenesis of infarction of the right ventricle. Br Heart J 21:545–554, 1959
11. **Laurie W, Woods JD:** Infarction (ischemic fibrosis) in the right ventricle of the heart. Acta Cardiol 18:399–411, 1963
12. **Erhardt LR:** Clinical and pathological observations in different types of acute myocardial infarction. A study of 84 patients deceased after treatment in a coronary care unit. Acta Med Scand [Suppl] 560:7–78, 1974
13. **Raabe DS, Chester AC:** Right ventricular infarction. Chest 73: 96–99, 1978
14. **Peter RH, Ramo BW, Ratliff N, Morris JJ:** Collateral vessel development after right ventricular infarction in the pig. Am J Cardiol 29:56–60, 1972
15. **James TN:** The coronary circulation and conduction system in acute myocardial infarction. Prog Cardiovasc Dis 10:410–449, 1968
16. Case Records of the Massachusetts General Hospital (Case 42-1963). New Engl J Med 268:1403–1410, 1963
17. **Roberts WC, Ferrans VJ:** Pathologic anatomy of the cardiomyopathies. Idiopathic dilated and hypertrophic types, infiltrative types, and endomyocardial disease with and without eosinophilia. Hum Pathol 6:287–342, 1975
18. **Bush CA, Stang JM, Wooley CF, Kilman JW:** Occult constrictive pericardial disease. Diagnosis by rapid volume expansion and correction by pericardiectomy. Circulation 56:924–930, 1977
19. **Starr I, Jeffers WA, Mead RH:** The absence of conspicuous increments in venous pressure after severe damage to the right ventricle of the dog and a discussion of the relation between clinical congestive failure and heart disease. Am Heart J 26:291–301, 1943
20. **Bakos ACP:** The question of the function of the right ventricular myocardium: an experimental study. Circulation 1:724–732, 1950
21. **Kagan A:** Dynamic responses of the right ventricle following extensive damage by cauterization. Circulation 5:816–823, 1952
22. **James T:** Anatomy of the Coronary Arteries. New York, Paul B Hoeber, 1961, p 51–60

Congenital Cardiovascular Abnormalities Usually "Silent" until Adulthood: Morphologic Features of the Floppy Mitral Valve, Valvular Aortic Stenosis, Discrete Subvalvular Aortic Stenosis, Hypertrophic Cardiomyopathy, Sinus of Valsalva Aneurysm, and the Marfan Syndrome

William C. Roberts, M.D.

Congenital heart disease most commonly consists of *defects* (absent tissue) in cardiac septa causing shunts, *obstructions* (excess tissue) at or near valvular levels, *anomalous connections* between arteries and veins or between arteries or veins and cardiac chambers, and *combinations* of these three malformations. Less commonly, a congenital cardiovascular malformation consists of an improperly formed tissue which functions normally or almost normally at birth and during the early decades of life, but later causes cardiac dysfunction. This chapter describes certain morphologic features in six of these conditions.

FLOPPY ATRIOVENTRICULAR VALVE

Delineation of the click-late systolic murmur syndrome was a major addition to cardiologic knowledge in the 1960s.[1-5] It is now apparent that the click-late systolic murmur is common, probably occurring in 5 percent or more of persons older than 15 years.[6,7] Although generally not considered as such, the click-systolic murmur syndrome, probably in the majority of persons, is a form of congenital heart disease and, therefore, is the most common congenital heart disease. The auscultatory manifestations, however, are usually not manifest until adulthood.

The click-murmur syndrome may be viewed from both auscultatory and morphologic standpoints as manifesting three stages (Fig. 1): (1) systolic click(s) only, (2) click(s) plus a mid-to-late systolic murmur, and (3) pansystolic murmur only. Although progression from stage one to stage three has been documented in relatively few patients, it appears likely that this is the natural sequence of events in some patients. In others, there may be no progression from stage 1; patients in stage 2 may revert to stage 1; patients in stage 1 may lose their click(s) altogether; and patients appearing in stage 3 (pansystolic murmur) may have had no documentation of stages 1 and 2. This condition in stages 1 and 2 is usually unassociated with symptomatic evidence of cardiac dysfunction; the rare exceptions are patients with arrhythmias and/or chest pain. Patients in stage 3 may have congestive heart failure because of the associated severe mitral regurgitation. The stage 3 floppy mitral valve appears to be a major cause, possibly the most common, of severe *pure* mitral regurgitation requiring valve replacement. As a consequence, there is considerable anatomic information available on the floppy mitral valve which produces a pansystolic murmur (stage 3) and causes severe mitral regurgitation.[8-18] In contrast, there is relatively little anatomic information available in patients with systolic click(s) only (stage 1) or those with both click(s) and late systolic murmur (stage 2).

THE SPECTRUM OF MITRAL VALVE PROLAPSE

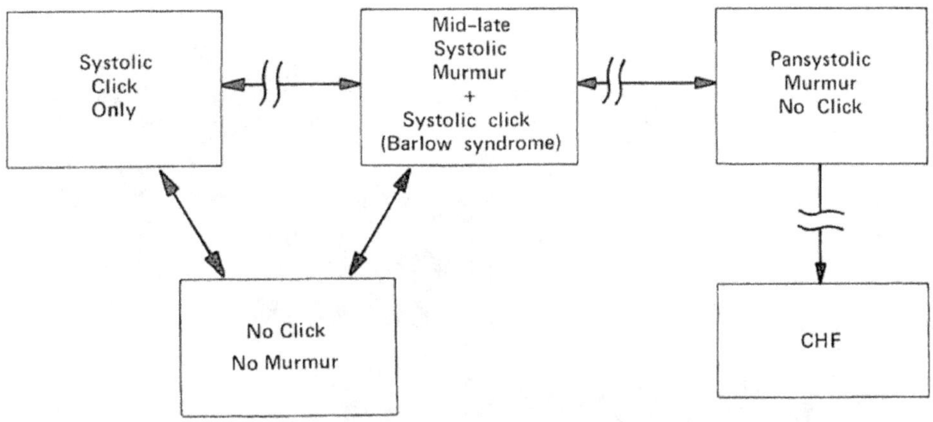

Figure 1. Diagram showing likely auscultatory progression in the prolapsing mitral valve syndrome. CHF = congestive heart failure.

Several names applied to this syndrome describe to some extent what the valve looks like anatomically; "prolapsing posterior mitral leaflet," "prolapsing mitral valve," "billowing or ballooning mitral leaflet syndrome," "overshooting or hooded mitral valve," "floppy mitral valve," and "myxomatous" or "mucinous degeneration of the mitral valve." The common anatomic denominator of the floppy mitral valve is either *excessive leaflet tissue* or *excessive length of chordae tendineae,* or both. Of these, the most common is excessive leaflet tissue. The excess most commonly results from an increase in the transverse or commissure-to-commissure dimension of the leaflet (width). This excess may be focal, involving only a portion of one or both leaflets, or it may be diffuse, involving both leaflets but not necessarily uniformly. The increase in transverse dimension causes the circumferences of the leaflets, measured on a line corresponding to the distal margin of the posterior leaflet, to be much larger than the circumference of the mitral valve anulus; in the normal valve the two are equal. The result is analogous to an accordian not fully extended, or better, a skirt gathered at the waist. The leaflets or the opened normal mitral valve are flat or smooth (like the mucosa of the ileum) whereas those of the opened floppy mitral valve are undulating (like the mucosa of the duodenum or jejunum).

Excessive leaflet tissue also results when there is an increase in the longitudinal or base-to-distal margin dimension of the leaflet (length). Again, this increase may be focal, involving portions of one or both leaflets, or diffuse when both leaflets are involved throughout, though not necessarily uniformly. In some patients there may be an increase in both the transverse and longitudinal dimensions of the leaflets.

Excessive length of chordae tendineae may be an additional cause of mitral valve prolapse. Again, all chordae may be elongated (diffuse) or just a few of them (focal). Elongation of chordae by itself is probably the least frequent mechanism of prolapse. In some patients there appears to be both excessive leaflet tissue and excessive length of chordae tendineae.

Opportunities for structural study of a mitral valve associated with click(s) only have been extremely rare. Figure 2 depicts such a valve. This child was examined while alive by Dr. John Barlow of Johannesburg, South Africa, who by auscultation heard three systolic clicks and no precordial murmur. The child had no symptoms of cardiac dysfunction and died of leukemia; necropsy revealed a perfectly competent mitral valve but three distinct foci where leaflet overlapped adjacent leaflet. The leaflets otherwise were

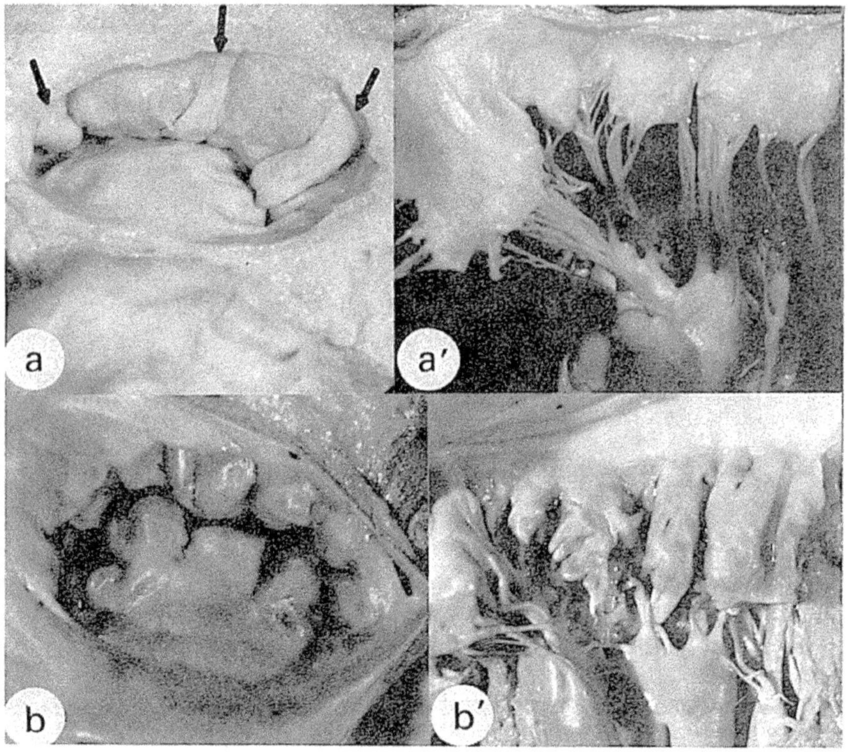

Figure 2. Mitral valves of two children, aged 9 and 13, who died of leukemia. Neither had symptoms of cardiac dysfunction. *a* and *a′*, Mitral valve as viewed from left atrium (a) and after opening (a′). Three areas of leaflet overlap (arrows) are present with the valve intact and the orifice is competent. The leaflets are devoid of scallops and relatively smooth (a′). This child had three systolic clicks during life but no precordial murmur. *b* and *b′*, Mitral valve as viewed from left atrium (b) and after opening (b′). Both leaflets of this valve, in contrast to the valve above, are highly scalloped causing the orifice to be incompetent. This child had a systolic click and a late systolic murmur. (The children whose valves are shown here were examined by Dr. John Barlow in Johannesburg, South Africa, and the auscultatory findings described above were those of Dr. Barlow. I am indebted to him for allowing me to photograph each of these hearts.)

smooth and notably devoid of so-called scallops. There are no reported anatomic descriptions, to my knowledge, of mitral valves producing one or more systolic clicks without an associated precordial systolic murmur. I recently learned, however, of a young woman in her 20s who had, on different occasions, one or more systolic clicks without murmur, associated with recurring arrhythmias. She died during an arrhythmia and a competent pathologist described the mitral valve at necropsy as "entirely normal."

The opportunity to examine the mitral valves (at necropsy) of patients who had systolic click(s) plus a mid-to-late systolic murmur (Barlow syndrome) also is infrequent since this stage is usually asymptomatic. Death in stage 2—as in stage 1—is usually from a noncardiac cause. The mitral valves of three such patients are illustrated in Figures 2 to 4. In this stage the most characteristic feature is leaflet scalloping, which represents excessive leaflet due to an increase in the transverse or commissure-to-commissure dimension of the leaflet. The mitral anulus, as in stage 1, is not dilated. The chordae tendineae may or may not be elongated and they may even be shorter than normal.

The major anatomic characteristic of stage 3 "floppiness" is dilatation of the mitral anulus.[19] Normally, the mitral anulus in adults measures about 9 cm. in circumference.

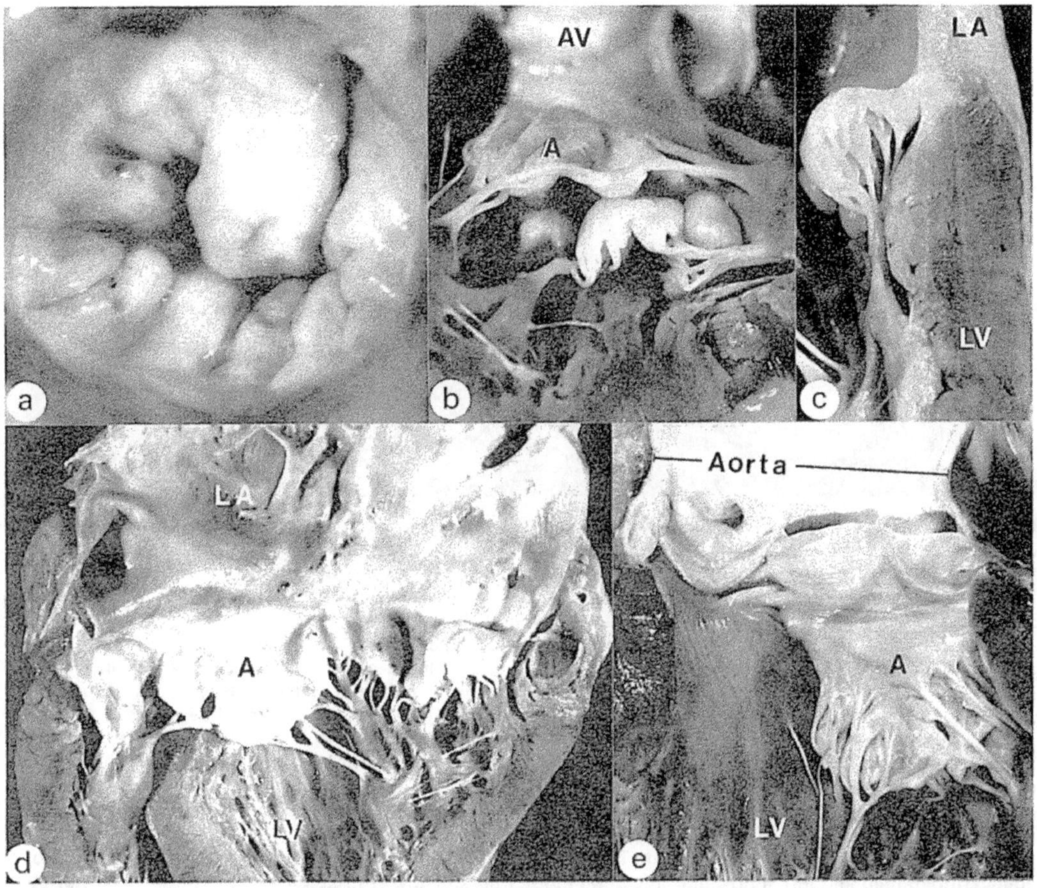

Figure 3. *Floppy mitral valve* in an 18-year-old girl who died of Ewing's sarcoma. She never had symptoms of cardiac dysfunction despite an active life. She had a mid-systolic click and a grade 3/6, ejection-type systolic murmur over the precordium, loudest over the apex. Necropsy revealed Ebstein's anomaly of the tricuspid valve. The mitral valve leaflets shown are elongated transversely, but the chordae are not elongated. *a*, Mitral valve as viewed from left atrium showing marked scalloping. *b*, Same valve as viewed from left ventricle. (A = anterior mitral leaflet; AV = aortic valve) *c*, Longitudinal section of left atrium (LA), billowing posterior mitral leaflet and left ventricle (LV). *d*, Opened mitral valve. *e*, View of anterior mitral leaflet (A) from the left ventricular (LV) aspect. The mitral leaflets and chordae tendineae contained excessive amounts of acid mucopolysaccharide material.

In patients with left ventricular dilatation from any cause with or without mitral regurgitation, the circumference of the mitral anulus usually dilates slightly, to about 11 cm. or less than 25 percent.[19] Among patients with floppy mitral valves associated with severe mitral regurgitation, the circumference of the mitral anulus generally increases by well over 50 percent of normal dimensions (15 to 18 cm.).[19] When the anulus dilates to this extent, the leaflets may "stretch" or flatten transversely, and this stretching diminishes the amount of scalloping. In addition, the left ventricular dilatation may cause longitudinal stretching of the leaflets. The amount of scalloping in the stage 3 valves, therefore, appears to be less than that observed in the stage 2 valves.

Microscopically, the floppy mitral valve leaflets contain an excessive amount of acid mucopolysaccharide material. Both the normal and the floppy mitral leaflet consists of two elements, the fibrosa and the spongiosa. The fibrosa consists of fibrous tissue (collagen), and the spongiosa, of mucoid or myxomatous material high in acid

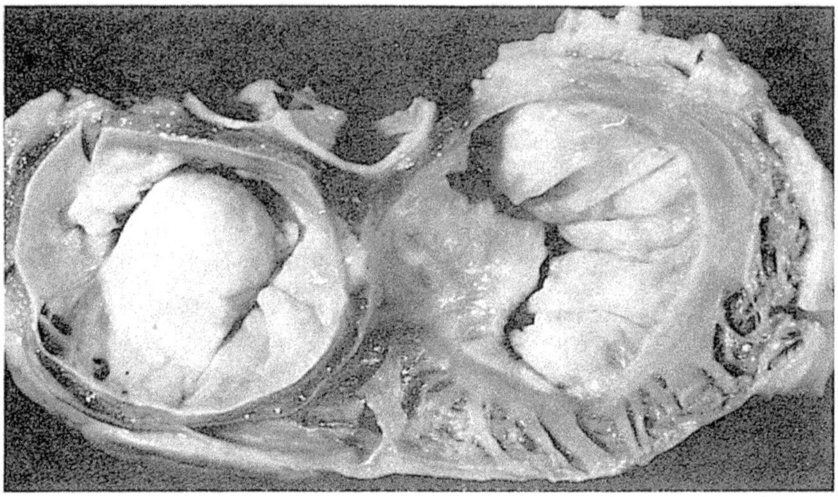

Figure 4. *Floppy mitral valve* (left) and *floppy tricuspid valve* (right) in a 51-year-old man who died suddenly at a dance. Although always asymptomatic, he was found to have a precordial systolic murmur when he was 36 years old. When evaluated about one year before death, he had a systolic murmur; echocardiogram disclosed the classic "hammocking" of the mitral leaflets during ventricular systole, and left ventricular angiography also showed "classic" mitral leaflet prolapse during ventricular systole.

At necropsy, at least one third of the posterior mitral leaflet had prolapsed toward left atrium; several chordae tendineae to this prolapsed segment were thickened and a few were absent, indicating that rupture had occurred. The anterior mitral leaflet appeared normal from the left ventricular aspect, but from the left atrial aspect it was thickened as a result of abnormal contact by the large prolapsed segment of posterior leaflet. All chordae tendineae from the anterior leaflet were elongated, whereas those from the posterior leaflet were thickened. The tricuspid-valve leaflets also were elongated but only mildly thickened compared to the mitral leaflets. There was no clinical evidence of dysfunction of the tricuspid valve. Both atria were mildly dilated. The coronary arteries were normal in course and size and free of significant luminal narrowing. The myocardial walls were free of foci of necrosis or fibrosis.

This case is an example of sudden death in a previously asymptomatic patient with classical auscultatory, echocardiographic and left ventricular angiographic features of the systolic click–late systolic murmur syndrome.

mucopolysaccharide material. In most valve diseases the fibrosa element proliferates and may entirely replace the spongiosa element. In the floppy mitral valve the spongiosa element comprises the more central portion of the leaflet, and appears to proliferate with a far less proportional increase in the fibrosa element. The resulting proliferated myxoid or myxomatous stroma, however, does not appear abnormal, i.e., degenerated, simply increased in amount. Thus, the term myxoid or myxomatous "degeneration" for this condition is not appropriate. The fibrosa element makes up the periphery of the leaflet, and is also increased focally in this condition. The fibrosa element may be subdivided into two components, the *auricularis,* which normally is a thin layer forming the atrial or contact aspect of the leaflet, and the *ventricularis,* which normally is a relatively thick layer which covers the ventricular aspect of the leaflet. The atrial aspect of the floppy mitral leaflet often is focally thickened. This change is considered secondary to abnormal friction from contact between the prolapsed segment of the leaflet and its "opposite number," i.e., the other leaflet, or between two prolapsed segments of the same leaflet.[17,18] The changes on the ventricular surface of the leaflet consist of connective tissue "pads" forming primarily in the interchordal segments. This proliferation of fibrous tissue may extend into adjacent chordae tendineae and onto ventricular endocardium behind the posterior mitral leaflet.[18] The interchordal collections of fibrous tissue are considered responses to the tension and stretching that occurs at the undersurface of prolapsed leaflet or segment of leaflet.[18] This increase in fibrous tissue,

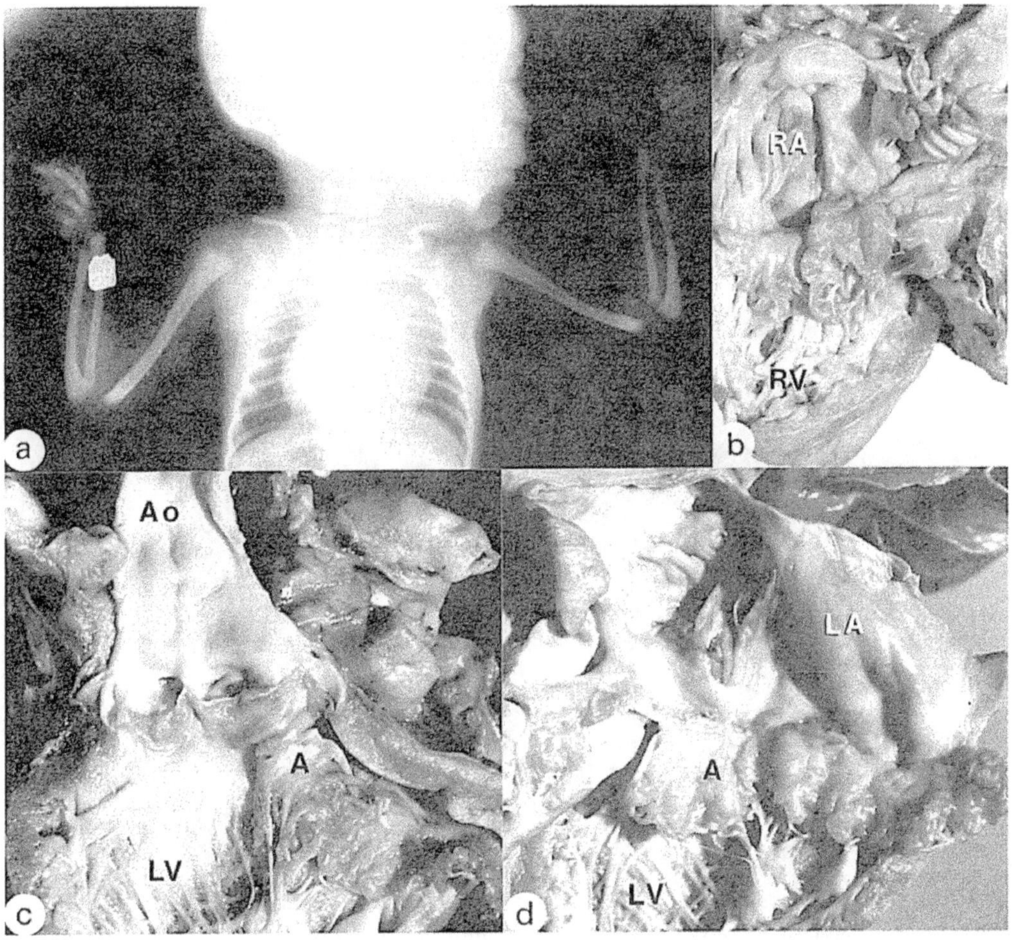

Figure 5. Congenital *floppy mitral valve* and *floppy tricuspid valve* in a 2-day-old boy who had long toes and fingers, a high-arched palate, and a grade 3/6 precordial systolic murmur typical of mitral regurgitation. The heart was enlarged *(a)* and he died of congestive cardiac failure. At necropsy, the intima of the ascending aorta (Ao) was wrinkled *(c)* suggesting that the underlying media was abnormal at this early stage. Shown here is the opened aorta, aortic valve, and left ventricle (LV) (A = anterior mitral leaflet). *(d)* Opened left atrium (LA), mitral valve, and left ventricle (LV). The mitral leaflets are considerably elongated in both longitudinal and transverse dimensions. The left atrium (LA) is dilated. *b*, The tricuspid valve leaflets also are elongated in both transverse and longitudinal dimensions (RA = right atrium; RV = right ventricle).

particularly on the ventricular surface of the valve, has, on occasion, caused this type of valve to be considered as rheumatic in origin rather than floppy.[17]

Ultrastructural studies of floppy mitral valves[20] have disclosed alterations of the collagen fibers in the leaflets and in the chordae tendineae. These changes have included fragmentation, splitting, swelling and coarse granularity of the individual collagen fibers, as well as spiraling and twisting of the fibers.[20] Also, some elastic fibers are fragmented and contain cystic spaces. These alterations in the structure of the collagen may be more important than the accumulation of the acid mucopolysaccharide material in that they lead to focal weaknesses in the leaflets. The left ventricular systolic pressure exerted against these weakened areas may lead to prolapse or focal interchordal hooding. Although the actual prolapse of the mitral valve may be acquired and a consequence of the left ventricular systolic (closing) pressure, the focally weak areas of

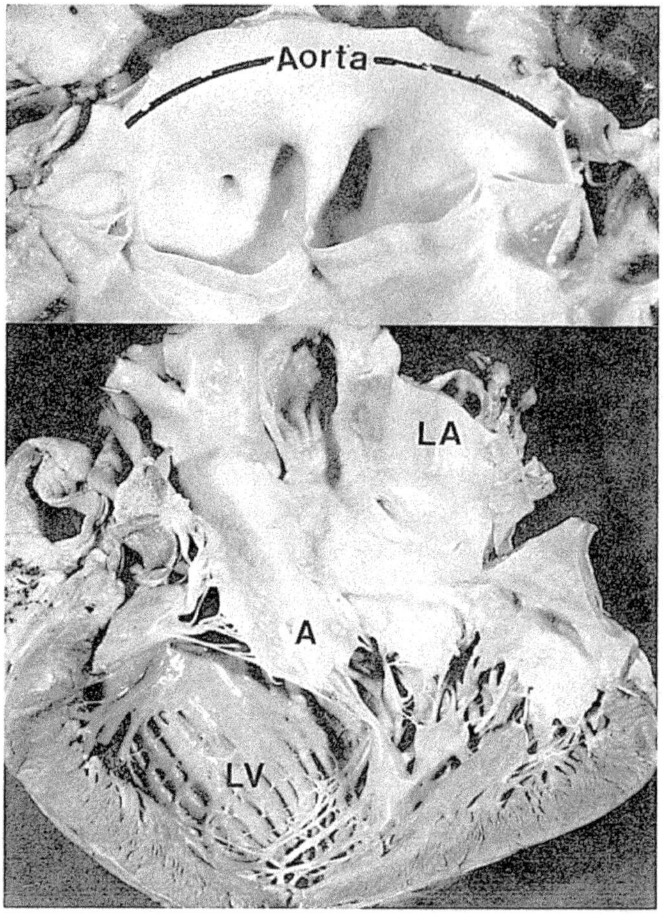

Figure 6. *Floppy mitral valve*—pure mitral regurgitation without aortic disease—in the *Marfan syndrome* in a 28-year-old man who died from severe mitral regurgitation. He had been well until age 24 when he developed exertional dyspnea and hemoptysis and was found to have cardiomegaly. Catheterization was performed at age 25 and the pressures (in mm. Hg) were: pulmonary artery, 19/10; right ventricle, 19/5; right atrial mean, 5; pulmonary arterial wedge mean, 10; and systemic artery 130/80. The cardiac output was 2.3 L./min. He remained functionally class II for the next three years but during his last year of life the congestive heart failure worsened and he became class IV. When examined seven days before his death he was quite ill. A grade 5/6 pansystolic precordial murmur, loudest over the apex, was audible. No diastolic murmur was present. The chest radiograph showed a big heart and severe kyphoscoliosis. Electrocardiogram showed sinus rhythm and left ventricular hypertrophy. He died of progressive heart failure.

At necropsy, the heart was huge (850 gm.). Although the sinuses were dilated, the aorta was entirely normal histologically (top). The mitral leaflets (bottom) were mildly thickened and elongated and the mitral anulus was severely dilated (15 cm.). Calcific deposits were present in the anulus behind the posterior mitral leaflet. The left atrium (LA) was quite dilated as was the left ventricle (LV) (A = anterior mitral leaflet).

the leaflets are probably most often congenital in origin. This focal leaflet weakness may be analogous to the berry aneurysm of the cerebral artery—the weakness in the arterial wall is almost certainly congenital in origin and the later bulging, with or without rupture, is acquired as a consequence of a high intra-arterial pressure. Mitral valve prolapse also may be higher in persons with elevated left ventricular systolic pressures than in persons with normal levels of this pressure. Certainly, calcification of the mitral anulus is more common in hypertensive than in normotensive individuals,[21] and mitral anular calcification is more common in persons with floppy mitral valves

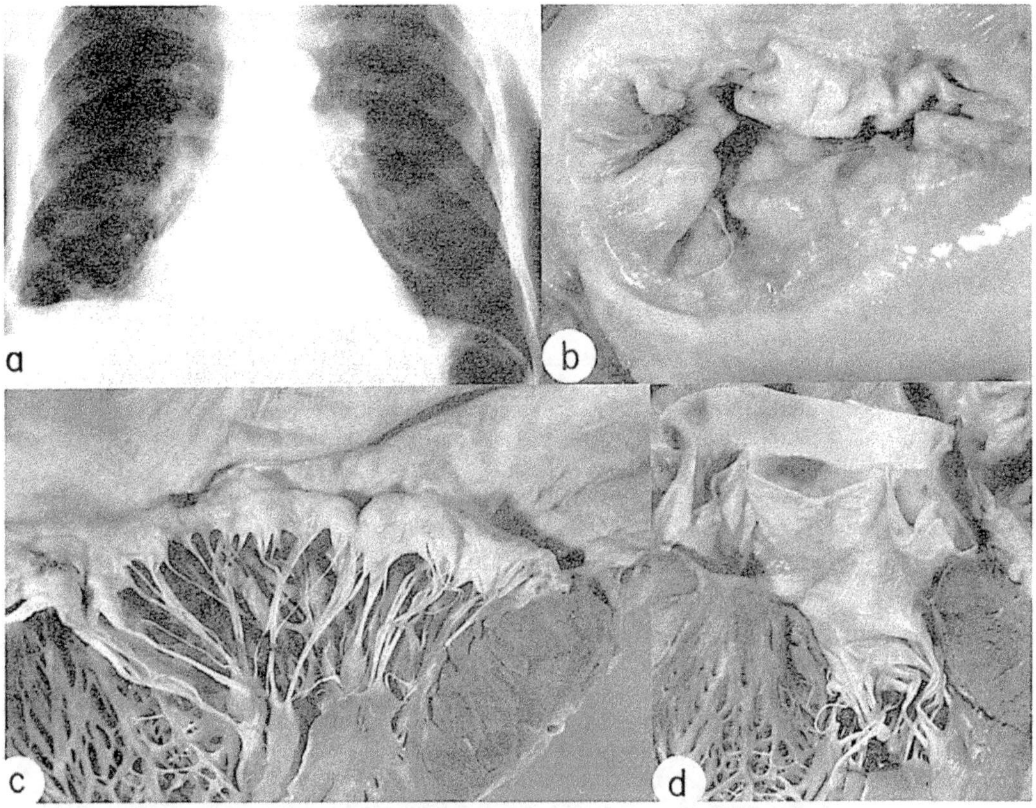

Figure 7. *Floppy mitral valve* in a 70-year-old man who died of gastric carcinoma. During life a grade 3/6 pansystolic blowing murmur was heard, loudest over the apex with radiation to the left axilla. The rhythm was atrial fibrillation. He never had symptoms of cardiac dysfunction. The heart was enlarged by radiograph *(a)*, but at necropsy it weighed only 310 gm. Both atria were quite dilated. The mitral leaflets protruded toward the left atrium *(b)* because the chordae tendineae were too long. A portion of opened mitral valve showing the elongated chordae is shown in *c*. *d*, The opened left ventricle and aortic valve show excessively long chordae. Focal calcific deposits also were present in the mitral anulus.

than it is in individuals of similar age and sex without floppy mitral valves.[21,22] Another factor supporting the concept that the underlying fault of mitral floppiness is congenital is its high frequency in patients with other congenital defects (atrial septal defect)[23–26] or deficiencies (the Marfan syndrome)[14,21,27–34] (Figs. 5–7).

Recognized complications of the floppy mitral valve are listed in Table 1. Because a valve may be floppy or prolapsed without mitral regurgitation, it appears reasonable to consider mitral regurgitation as a complication of floppiness rather than a necessary component of this syndrome. Calcification of the mitral anulus almost surely is the second most frequent complication of mitral floppiness (Fig. 8). Rupture of mitral chordae tendineae may be the consequence of infective endocarditis, or rupture may occur without evidence of infection ("spontaneous" rupture)[35-37] (Figs. 9 and 10). Chordal rupture is probably noninfective more often than infective in origin.[38] Nevertheless, because patients with systolic murmurs are at increased risk to develop infective endocarditis and because infection superimposed on a floppy valve is usually highly destructive, antibiotic prophylaxis against this valvular infection appears warranted.

The cause of the arrhythmias is unclear.[39] There is no anatomic evidence in these patients of "a myocardial factor" or abnormality in course or size of any of the major

Table 1. Complications of prolapsing mitral valve.

1. Mitral regurgitation
2. Calcification, mitral "anulus"
3. Rupture of chordae tendineae
   A. Infective endocarditis
   B. Non-infective ("spontaneous")
4. Infective endocarditis
5. Arrhythmias
6. Chest pain
7. Stroke (transient ischemic attacks)
8. Sudden death

coronary arteries. An attractive but unproven explanation is the considerable friction between chordae tendineae and the underlying left ventricular mural endocardium.[18] The cause of the chest pain which occurs occasionally in these patients is also unknown. Associated coronary arterial disease is clearly not the explanation for the chest pain in the majority of these patients. Acute nonprogressive strokes or transient cereb-

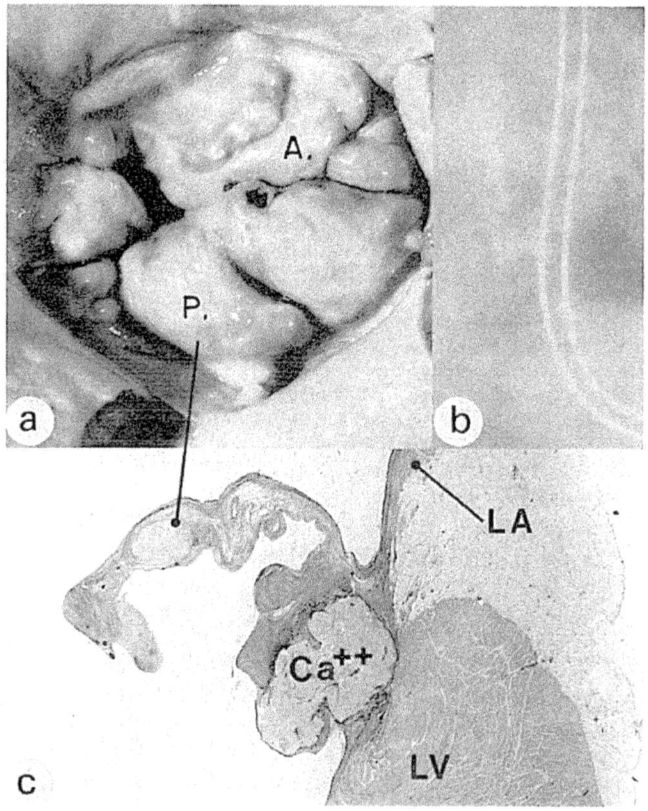

Figure 8. *Floppy mitral valve* and *calcium in the mitral anulus* of a 70-year-old woman who had a grade 3/6 murmur of mitral regurgitation, atrial fibrillation and complete heart block. *a,* Mitral valve from left atrial aspect (A., P. = anterior and posterior mitral leaflets, respectively). *b,* Radiograph taken while the patient was alive shows a C-shaped deposit of calcium in the mitral anular area. Pacing wires also are visible. *c,* Photomicrograph through wall of left atrium (LA), prolapsed posterior leaflet, and left ventricle (LV). The calcium (CA^{++}) in the anular area is apparent.

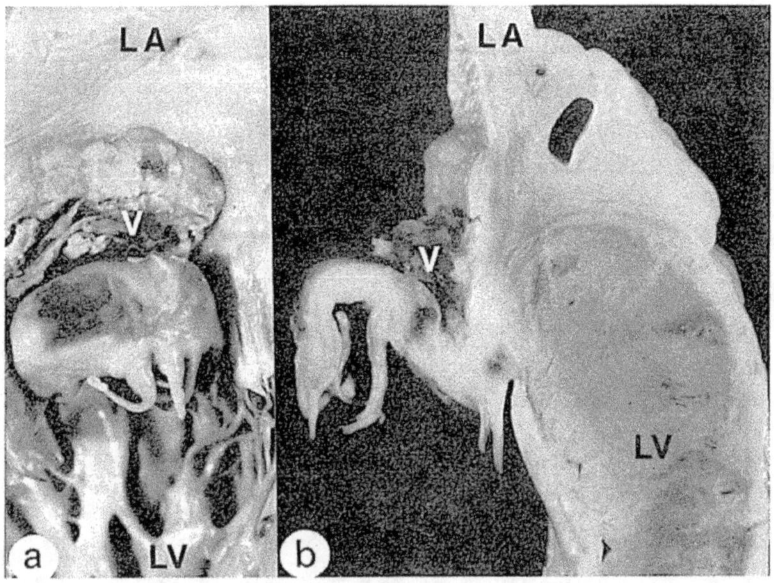

Figure 9. *Floppy mitral valve* with superimposed *Staphylococcus aureus endocarditis* in a 52-year-old man who was known to have a murmur of mitral regurgitation for 10 years. He was asymptomatic, however, until he developed typical clinical features of active infective endocarditis which caused a fatal septic cerebral embolus. Necropsy revealed a portion of posterior mitral leaflet prolapsed toward left atrium (LA) and vegetative (V) material at the acute angle formed by the hooded posterior leaflet and mural endocardium of left atrium. (This junction is a common location of fibrin-platelet deposits in patients with prolapsed posterior mitral leaflets.) *a,* Closeup of hooded segment of posterior leaflet with the superimposed vegetation. *b,* Longitudinal section through left atrium, prolapsed and thickened posterior leaflet and left ventricle (LV).

ral ischemic attacks recently have been noted to occur with increased frequency in these patients.[40] In some patients, small fibrin-platelet thrombi have been observed on the atrial aspects of the prolapsed segments of mitral leaflet at junctions with the left atrial mural endocardium.[18] It has been suggested that dislodgement of these small fibrin-platelet thrombi and their migration to the cerebral arteries is the explanation for the transient cerebral ischemia. It is also possible that these minute thrombi dislodge and embolize to the coronary arteries, triggering an arrhythmia or chest pain or both.[41]

AORTIC VALVE STENOSIS AND THE CONGENITALLY MALFORMED AORTIC VALVE

If papillary muscle dysfunction is excluded, valvular aortic stenosis (AS) is the most common fatal cardiac valve lesion; it was found in 50 percent of patients older than 15 years with valvular heart disease whom I have studied at necropsy.[42-44] Of the patients with AS (with or without aortic regurgitation), the lesion was isolated in 66 percent; in the other 34 percent the mitral valve was stenotic or incompetent or both. The evidence is substantial that the cause of AS, when associated with mitral valve disease, is rheumatic.[44] In contrast, the evidence is substantial that isolated AS (anatomically normal mitral valve) is nonrheumatic in origin.[42-44] This section focuses on patients with isolated AS.[42-50]

In contrast to what was generally believed 30 years ago[51], at least three factors indicate that anatomically isolated aortic valve disease (actually either stenosis or pure regurgitation) is nonrheumatic in origin: (1) the low frequency (about 10 percent) of a positive history of acute rheumatic fever, (2) the absence of Aschoff bodies, and, most

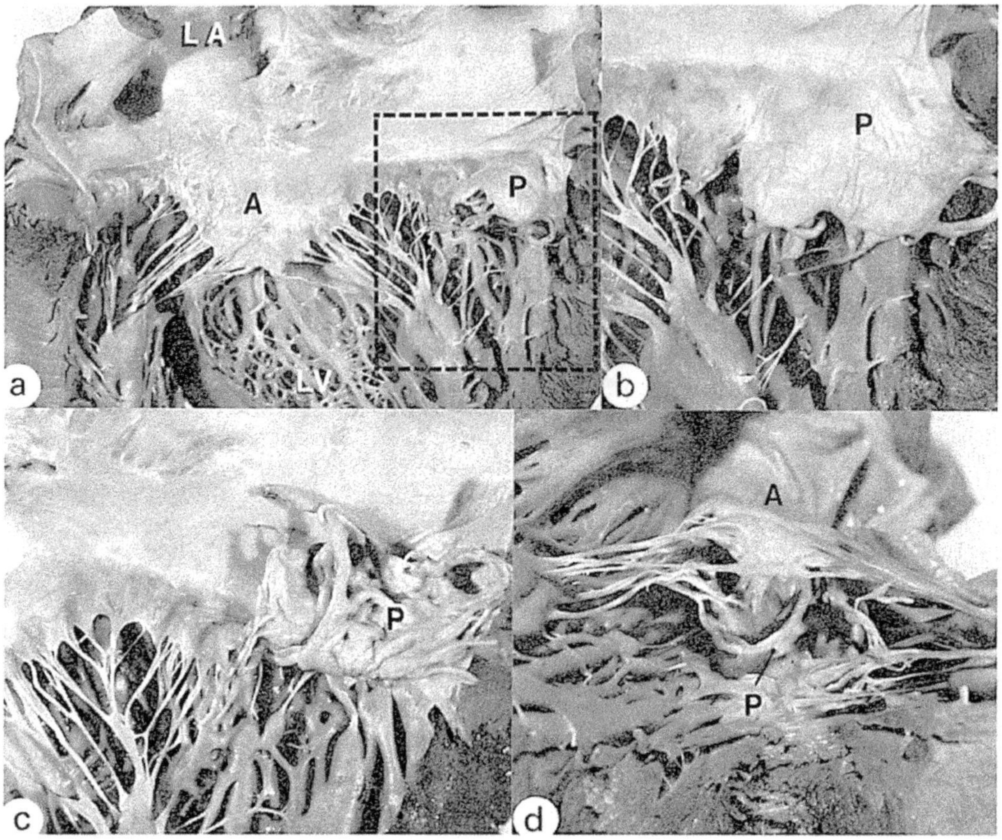

Figure 10. *Floppy mitral valve* in a 38-year-old man who had been well until three years before death, when he experienced a fairly abrupt onset of congestive heart failure. Cardiac catheterization at that time confirmed the presence of pure mitral regurgitation. His blood urea nitrogen at that time was 41 mg./dl. During the next three years he developed severe systemic hypertension (240/140 mm. Hg), severe anemia, severe azotemia (blood urea nitrogen = 230 mg./dl.), and finally, fatal hemorrhagic cardiac tamponade. Necropsy revealed a large segment of posterior mitral leaflet, elongated and prolapsed into the left atrium. Most of the chordae tendineae from this prolapsed segment were ruptured. (The patient never had evidence of infective endocarditis.) The heart weighed 620 gm.

a, Opened left atrium (LA), mitral valve, left ventricle (LV), and prolapsed segment (P). The portion outside the boxed area of mitral leaflets and chordae are normal or near normal (A = anterior mitral leaflet). *b*, Closeup of atrial aspect of the prolapsed segment. *c*, Same view showing the prolapsed segment flipped back into left atrium, exposing its ventricular aspect. *d*, View of mitral valve from left ventricle. In this case mitral prolapse may have been worsened by systemic hypertension; increased closing pressure on the mitral leaflets is created by the elevated systolic pressure.

importantly, (3) the frequency of an underlying congenital malformation of the aortic valve.

The structure of the aortic valve in AS can be correlated to some extent with the age of the patient (Table 2).[43] In patients younger than 15 years, the aortic valve most commonly (60 percent) is congenitally unicuspid and unicommissural;[45,50] in patients 15 to 65 years of age, the valve is most commonly (60 percent) congenitally bicuspid;[46,48] and in patients age older than 65 years, the valve is most commonly (90 percent) tricuspid.[49] The stenosis is either caused by or superimposed on the congenitally malformed aortic valve in virtually all the patients under 15 and in at least 70 percent—possibly as high as 85 percent—of patients between 15 and 65.[43] A congenitally mal-

Table 2. Configuration of aortic valve in isolated aortic stenosis in relation to age

	No. valve cusps	*<age 15 years*	*Age 16-65*	*>age 65 years*
1	1	60%	10%	0
2	2	20%	60%	10%
3	3	15%	25%	90%
4	Uncertain	5%	5%	0

formed (in this case congenitally bicuspid) valve appears to be the underlying condition in only about 10 percent of the patients over 65 with AS.[49]

The unicommissural valve, the only type of unicuspid valve observed in the aortic valve position, was described initially by Edwards in 1958[52] (Figs. 11 and 12). This valve, like all other congenitally malformed aortic valves, tends to become more stenotic with time,[50] in contrast to the congenitally bicuspid aortic valve. But the unicuspid aortic valve is almost certainly stenotic from the time of birth, and the fewer the number of aortic valve cusps and commissures, the greater is the likelihood that the valve is stenotic from birth.[43]

Next to the floppy mitral valve, the congenitally bicuspid aortic valve is the most frequent major congenital malformation of the heart or great vessels (Figs. 13 to 19). It is possible that the frequency of this malformation is as high as 2 percent of all human births.[48] In 1800 hearts studied personally, none of which had cardiac valvular, septal, or great vessel abnormalities causing dysfunction, 17 had normally functioning congenitally bicuspid aortic valves. This frequency of nearly 1 percent is similar to that reported by others who examined hearts for the specific purpose of determining presence or absence of congenitally bicuspid aortic valves. Osler[53] found 10 apparently normally functioning congenitally bicuspid aortic valves in 800 autopsies (750 of which were performed by him), an incidence of 1 percent. Eight additional patients had infective endocarditis involving congenitally bicuspid aortic valves. Thus, 18 of 800 (2 percent) had either normally functioning or infected congenitally bicuspid aortic valves. Grant, Wood, and Jones[54] found apparently normally functioning congenitally bicuspid aortic valves in 12 of 1350 (1 percent) necropsy patients. Osler,[53] Lewis and Grant,[55] and Grant and coworkers[54] appear not to have recognized that the bicuspid condition of this valve may underlie severe stenosis or calcification at this site. Thus, if congenitally bicuspid aortic valves that develop complications (stenosis or incompetency with or without infection) are added to those which function normally during the entire lifetime, the frequency of congenitally bicuspid aortic valves may approach 2 percent of the population.

Among the complications of the bicuspid condition of the aortic valve, stenosis is by far the most frequent; pure regurgitation is next, and the latter lesion is most frequently

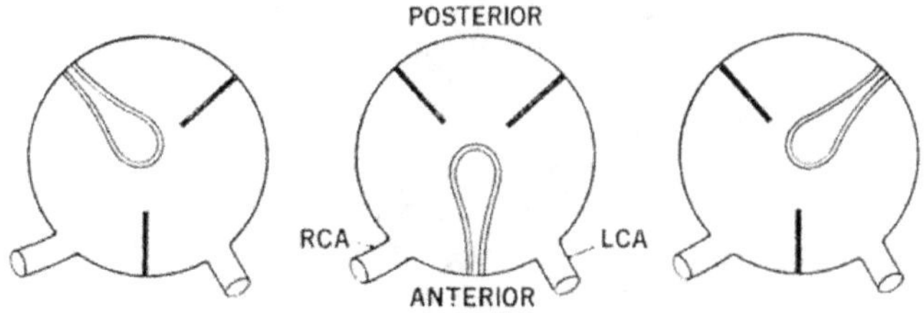

Figure 11. Location of the true commissure in congenitally unicommissural aortic valve stenosis. RCA, LCA = right and left coronary arteries, respectively.

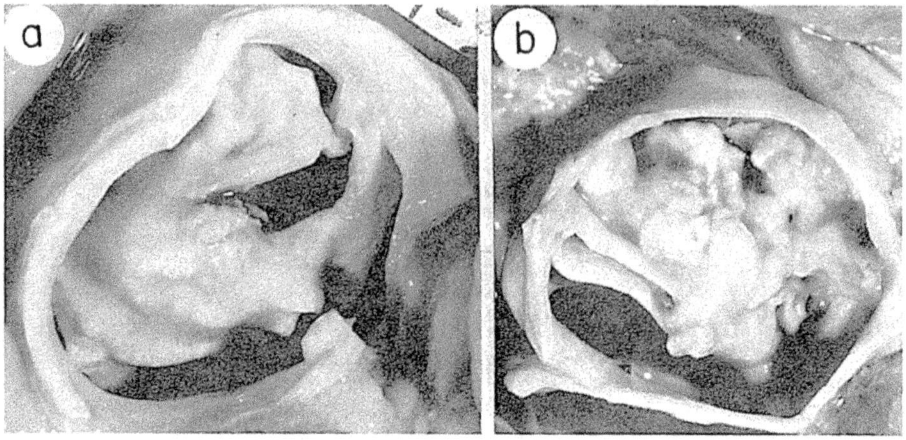

Figure 12. *Congenitally unicommissural stenotic aortic valve* in two men aged 28 *(a)* and 48 years *(b)*.

the result of its being the site of infective endocarditis.[37,38] Why one congenitally bicuspid aortic valve becomes stenotic, another incompetent, and another the site of infective endocarditis is unknown. However, it is clear that stenosis, regurgitation, and infection are complications of the bicuspid condition of the aortic valve and none of them are present at birth. It appears likely that a congenitally bicuspid aortic valve becomes stenotic only as its cusps become fibrotic and calcified; neither cusp of a congenitally bicuspid aortic valve is fibrotic or calcified at the time of birth.

The frequency of development of stenosis or incompetency at the site of a congeni-

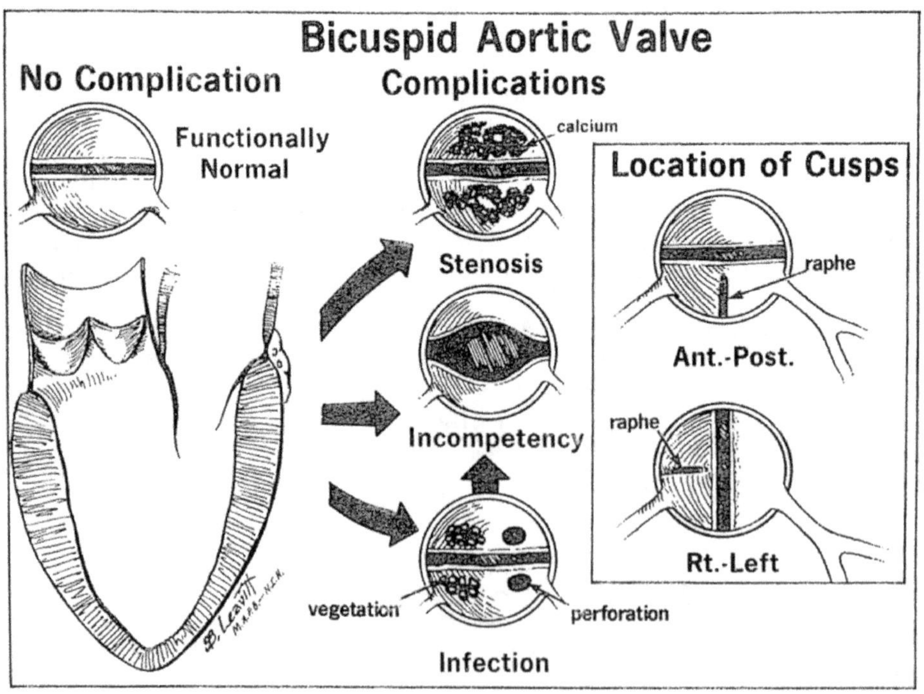

Figure 13. The congenitally bicuspid aortic valve. The location of the cusps and raphes and the acquired complications of the congenital malformation are depicted.

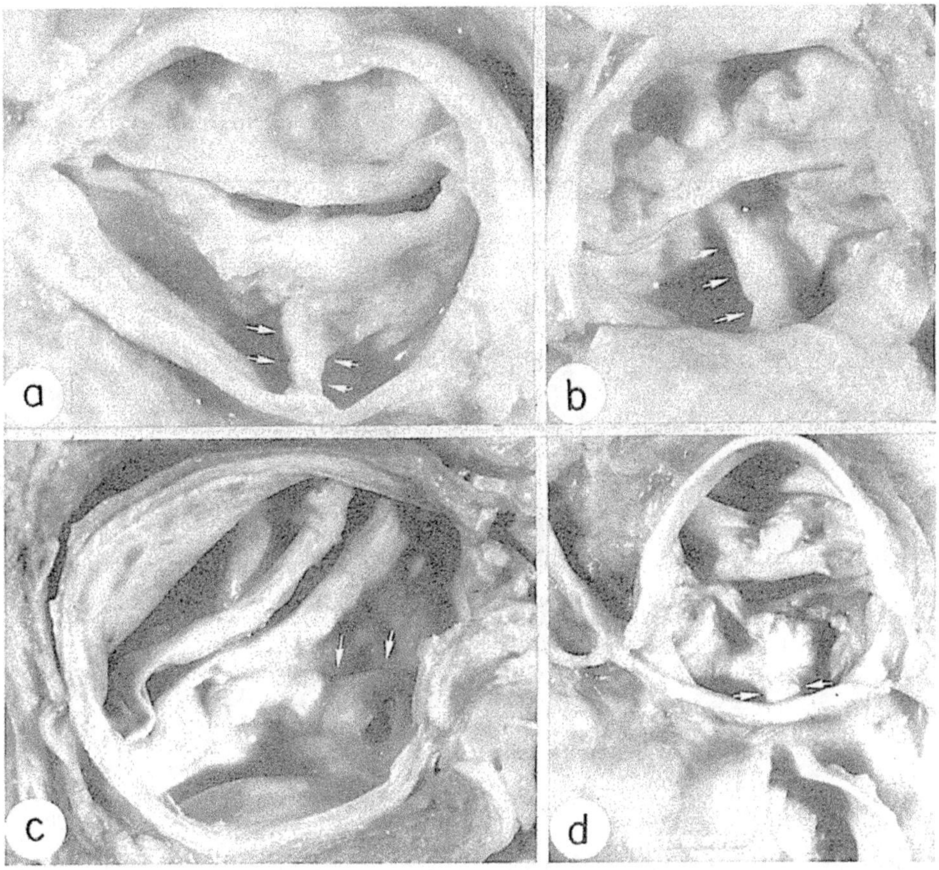

Figure 14. *Calcified, stenotic, congenitally bicuspid aortic valves* in four patients. The cusps are situated anteriorly and posteriorly and the commissures right and left, respectively. Each of the valves has a raphe (white arrows) in the anterior cusp. *a*, Valve of a 61-year-old man. At catheterization two years before his death, the peak systolic gradient (PSG) across the valve was 45 mm. Hg when the cardiac index was 2.6 l./min./m.^{2}. He had complete heart block secondary to destruction of the atrioventricular bundle by calcium. *b*, Valve of a 60-year-old man who suddenly collapsed on the street. Electrocardiogram recorded in the emergency room showed left bundle branch block. His only previous symptom of cardiac dysfunction was mild exertional dyspnea. *c*, Valve of a 75-year-old man who died after resection of an asymptomatic abdominal aortic aneurysm which had been discovered during a routine physical examination. A grade 3/6 murmur consistent with aortic stenosis had been heard, but he had no symptoms of cardiac dysfunction. *d*, Valve of a 51-year-old man. The PSG across this valve was only 18 mm. Hg but it was severely incompetent.

tally bicuspid aortic valve also is unknown. Lewis and Grant[55] concluded that vegetations develop at these sites in about 23 percent of adults (16 of 69) with congenitally bicuspid aortic valves. More information is available regarding the incidence of congenitally bicuspid valves in patients with infective endocarditis involving the aortic valve. Of 31 patients with "subacute infective endocarditis" studied at necropsy by Lewis and Grant,[55] 8 had congenitally bicuspid aortic valves. Such valves were found in 4 of 13 patients with infective endocarditis involving aortic valves studied at necropsy by Starling[56] and in 2 of 22 patients studied at necropsy by Fulton and Levine.[57] These investigators apparently were not aware of the fact that congenitally bicuspid aortic valves could become stenotic.

Of the 157 necropsy patients older than 15 years in whom I found congenitally bicuspid stenotic aortic valves, 99 percent had grossly visible extensive calcific deposits in

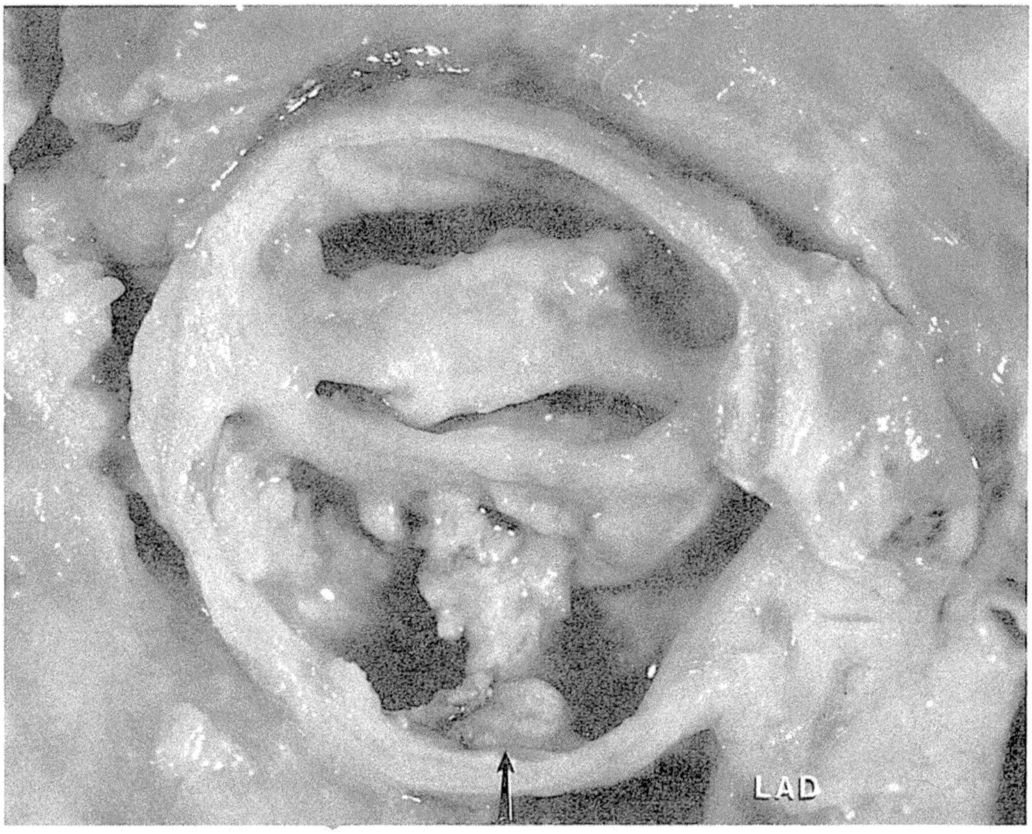

Figure 15. *Congenitally bicuspid, stenotic aortic valve* in an 87-year-old man who developed angina pectoris one year before his sudden death at home. He never had congestive heart failure or syncope. The two cusps are located anteriorly and posteriorly with a raphe (arrow), which is calcified, in the anterior cusp. In addition to the heavy deposits of calcium in the aortic valve, large calcific deposits also were present in the mitral anulus. Aortic stenosis had been diagnosed by physical examination 10 years before he died. LAD = left anterior descending coronary artery.

both cusps. The two patients without calcific deposits were under 30. In contrast, only 5 of the 22 patients with purely incompetent congenitally bicuspid aortic valves had calcific deposits which were focal and small. Calcific deposits are to be expected in adults with stenotic congenitally bicuspid aortic valves. Furthermore, heavy deposits of calcium do not occur in purely incompetent congenitally bicuspid aortic valves; valvular stenosis appears to be a prerequisite for the development of heavy deposits of calcium at this site. Development of infective endocarditis on a heavily calcified valve also is rare.[58] Infective endocarditis was found in only 13 (8 percent) of the 157 patients I studied with stenotic congenitally bicuspid aortic valves; infection was superimposed on a heavily calcified valve in only 4 of them. Of the 22 patients with purely incompetent congenitally bicuspid aortic valves, the valve was the site of vegetative endocarditis in 19 (86 percent), and this infection was the principal cause of incompetency.

The mechanism by which a congenitally bicuspid aortic valve becomes stenotic or incompetent is uncertain. There is no evidence that the valve is stenotic or incompetent at birth. Likewise, there is no evidence that superimposed rheumatic fever or rheumatic heart disease is the cause of the stenosis or incompetency. The explanation advanced by Edwards[59] is attractive. He proposed that it is not mechanically possible for a

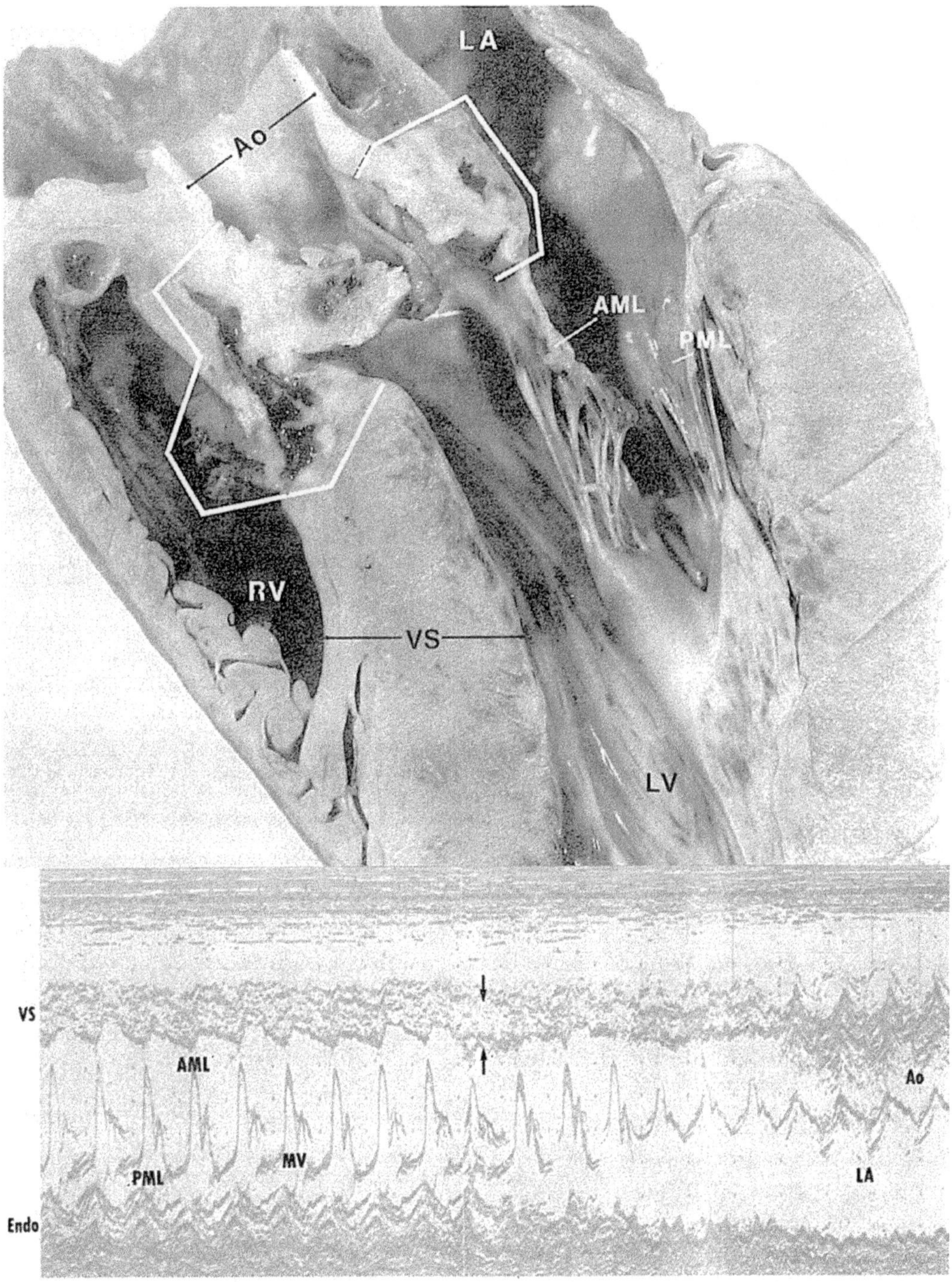

Figure 16. *Congenitally bicuspid aortic valve* with superimposed *Staphylococcus aureus endocarditis* in a 30-year-old man. Before the onset of the infective endocarditis the patient was asymptomatic but before the infection the valve was already mildly stenotic and mildly calcified. Nail biting, to the point of bleeding, apparently was the source of the infection. At necropsy the heart weighed 560 gm. The infection of the aortic valve burrowed into the adjacent soft tissues (brackets) producing large "ring abscesses." Ring abscess caused complete right bundle branch block. There was extensive subendocardial and papillary muscle necrosis of the left ventricle, presumably the result of severely diminished cardiac output. The echocardiogram was recorded several days before death. The arrows in the ventricular septum of the echocardium designate the probable ring abscess. Ao = aorta; LA = left atrium; RV = right ventricle; LV = left ventricle; AML and PML = anterior and posterior mitral leaflets; VS = ventricular septum; MV = mitral valve; Endo = endocardium.

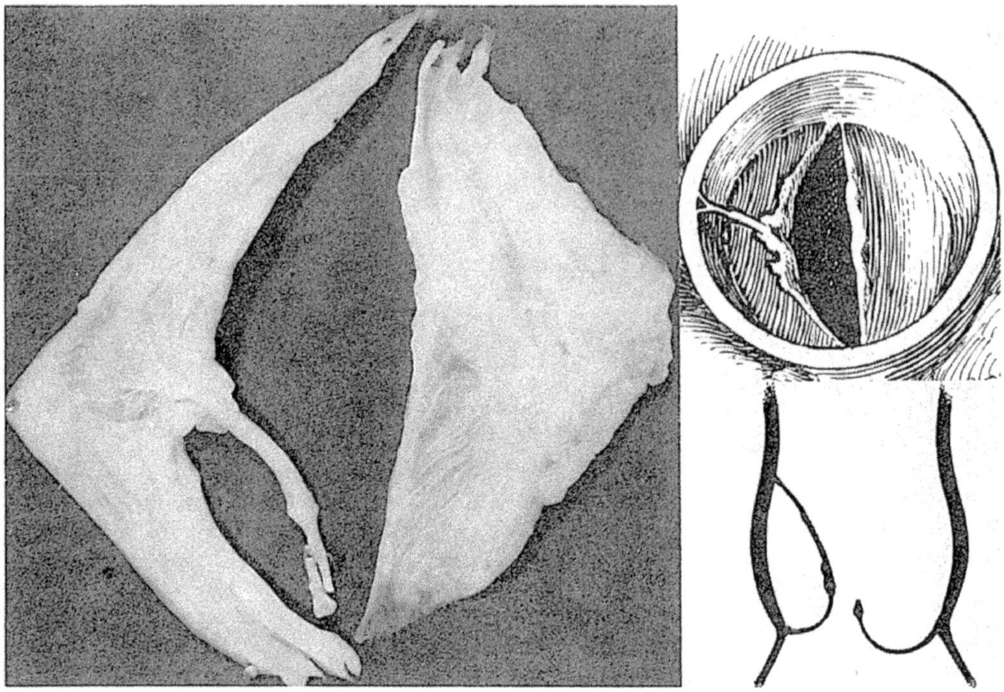

Figure 17. *Purely incompetent congenitally bicuspid aortic valve* in a 27-year-old man who was found to have aortic regurgitation at age 17; he developed exertional dyspnea at age 25. Just before valve replacement, simultaneous left ventricular and brachial arterial pressures were 125/25 and 126/54 mm. Hg, respectively, when the cardiac index was 2.2 l./min./m.². He died suddenly 13 months after valve replacement. The heart weighed 800 gm. Excised aortic valve is pictured at left. The drawing shows the supporting fibrous band that stretched from the margin in the midportion of one cusp to the aortic wall above one sinus of Valsalva (right). This patient is an example of pure severe aortic regurgitation of a congenitally bicuspid valve which was never the site of infective endocarditis.

congenitally bicuspid aortic valve to open and close properly. The distances between lateral attachments of normal aortic valvular cusps along their free margins are curved lines. The extra length allows the cusps to move freely during opening and closing of the valves. In contrast, the distances between lateral attachments of congenitally bicuspid aortic valves along their free margins are almost straight lines. (If the distances were

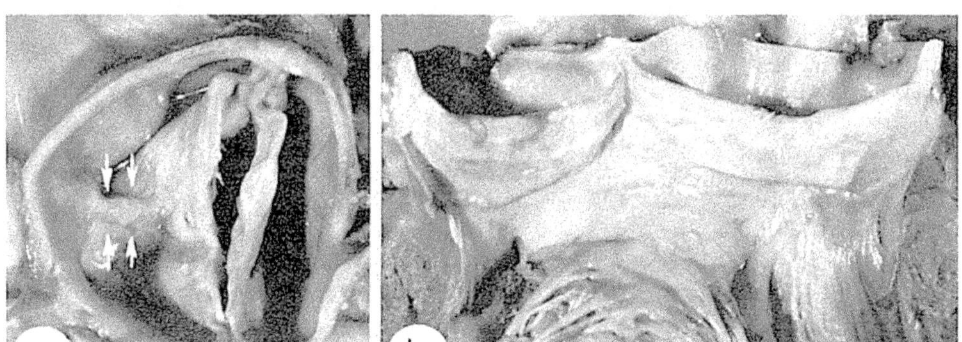

Figure 18. *Functionally normal congenitally bicuspid aortic valve. a,* The right cusp contains the raphe (arrows) and is the larger of the two cusps. *b,* Opened valve.

exactly straight, the valves could not open during ventricular systole.) Consequently, at least one cusp is larger than the other. The excessive length of one or both cusps of a congenitally bicuspid aortic valve produces abnormal contact between the cusps. This abnormal contact, in turn, causes focal fibrous thickening that becomes diffuse with time, eventually causing dystrophic calcification. Thus, stenosis of a congenitally bicuspid aortic valve may be the result of trauma to these cusps produced by their abnormal contact with each other. Although this explanation is appealing, it does not explain why one congenitally bicuspid aortic valve becomes stenotic, another becomes entirely incompetent, and another remains free of complications.

Criteria for differentiating a bicuspid valve of congenital origin from a bicuspid valve of acquired origin have been debated (Fig. 19). There is no controversy over the distinction between a congenitally bicuspid aortic valve devoid of a raphe (false commissure or ridge) and complications (stenosis, incompetency, or infection) and a tricuspid aortic valve devoid of similar complications. There was controversy about the means of differentiating a congenitally bicuspid aortic valve with a raphe from an acquired bicuspid aortic valve resulting from fusion of two cusps at one true commissure.* Osler,[53] from his study of 18 hearts (15 adults), deduced the following characteristics of a congenitally bicuspid aortic valve, all recognizable by gross observation: (1) The raphe is located where the true commissure normally would be, i.e., between the right and left anterior aortic valve cusps; (2) The length of the free margin of the cusp without a raphe is slightly shorter (by an average of 12 percent in his measurements on 7 hearts) than the length of the margin of the cusp containing a raphe, the "conjoint" cusp; (3) The free border of the conjoint cusp is straight or curled and free of nodular thickenings which would indicate bodies of Arantius; (4) The border of attachment of the conjoint cusp, as viewed from the ventricular aspect, presents either the contour of a single semilunar cusp or a shallow groove, indicative of the junction of two cusps; (5) The raphe may be located on the aortic wall alone or may extend onto the cusp for variable distances, but in either case it usually divides the sinus of Valsalva into units of equal size.

In 1923 Lewis and Grant[54] clarified several gross features of "unequivocally" congenital bicuspid aortic valves and presented histologic criteria for differentiating bicuspid valves of "congenital" origin from those of "inflammatory" origin. In contrast to Osler's findings these authors found that fusion could occur not only between right and left anterior cusps but also between right anterior and posterior cusps. A raphe, dividing one of the two cusps, was observed "in about half the cases." The two cusps could be the same size, but usually the conjoined cusp was larger, though less than twice the size of the undivided cusp; or else, "the subdivided cusp is larger than one normal cusp but smaller than two normal cusps." However, Lewis and Grant considered gross distinction between congenital and acquired bicuspid aortic valves unreliable. Elastic tissue stains of transverse sections of congenital raphes showed them to consist mainly of elastic fibers; thus, histologically the raphe was similar to the media of the aorta. In contrast, transverse sections of two fused cusps at a true commissure disclosed that the fused commissure was devoid of elastic fibers and consisted of fibrous valvular tissue. Other investigators[60,61] confirmed these histologic criteria. Koletsky[61] also pointed out that congenital raphes were devoid of vascular channels and inflammatory cells, whereas both were seen in acquired, fused commissures. Since Lewis and Grant de-

*The definition of a *commissure* differs depending on whether a semilunar or an atrioventricular (A-V) cardiac valve is under consideration. The aortic valve commissure is the space between two lateral attachments on the aortic wall. Normally each aortic valve cusp is an independent similar sized unit and adherence of one cusp to another at the narrow space (commissure) between the two cusps is abnormal. In contrast to a semilunar valve, the leaflets of an atrioventricular valve are continuous one with another. Thus, the commissures of the A-V valves are the sites of connection between the unequal sized leaflets, not the spaces between the cusps as in the case of the semilunar valves.

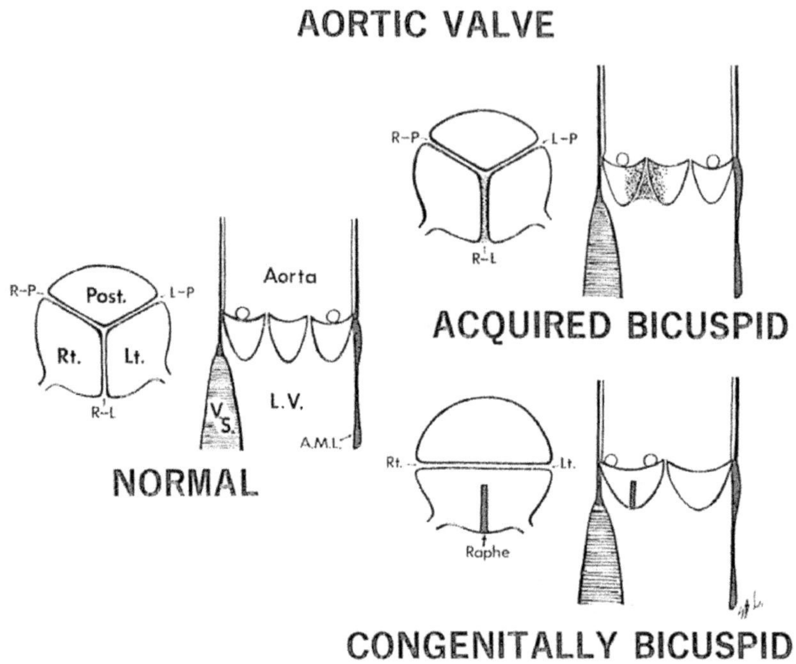

Figure 19. Diagram illustrating differences between *bicuspid aortic valves* of congenital origin as compared to the normal valve. The circumferential distances between each of the three commissures in a normally formed valve are similar. L-P = left-posterior; R-L = right-left, and R-P = right-posterior commissures; Rt., Lt., Post., = right, left, and posterior cusps, respectively; V.S. = ventricular septum; L.V. = left ventricular outflow tract; and A.M.L. = anterior mitral leaflet. In the *acquired bicuspid valve* the circumferential distance between the commissures remains equal, as in a normal valve. The fused commissure is wide, the distal margins of each of the two fused cusps are still usually visible, and the most cephalad margin of the fused commissure is on the same horizontal level as the most cephalad margins of the two nonfused commissures. In the *congenitally bicuspid valve*, the raphe is generally narrow and rarely extends to the free margin of the conjoined cusp or to the cephalad level reached by the two true commissures. The circumferential distances between the two true commissures are greater than this distance between either true commissure and the raphe. The circumferential distance between the true commissures around the conjoined cusp, i.e., the cusp with the raphe, is equal to or slightly greater than the circumferential distance between the true commissures around the cusp devoid of the raphe.

scribed these histologic features, many pathologists have been reluctant to distinguish between congenital and acquired bicuspid aortic valves without microscopic examination of raphes. But however helpful these histologic criteria may be, they are not specific. In some patients certain sections of a raphe show a structure like that of the aortic media, while other sections of the same raphe show only fibrous tissue. Also, the congenital raphe may lose its elastic fibers as the valvular cusps become fibrotic and calcified. The raphe may be the first portion of a congenitally bicuspid aortic valve to calcify, and these deposits destroy existing elastic fibers. Interestingly, Lewis and Grant and others who emphasized the importance of histologic distinction between congenital raphes and fused true commissures were unaware that calcific stenosis was a consequence of a congenitally bicuspid aortic valve. Once the valve is extensively scarred and calcified, histologic examination of the raphe is often fruitless. Furthermore, as Edwards[62] pointed out, in the patient with a bicuspid aortic valve that must be assumed to be congenital—as in infants with aortic coarctation—the raphe may not only be fibrous, but may grossly display features suggesting fusion of two distinguishable, separate cusps.

It appears that tricuspid aortic valves are rarely stenotic at birth. If stenosis is present at birth and the aortic valve has three cusps, the stenosis is usually the result of a very small aortic "anulus" rather than the result of fusion of the cusps; whereas acquired stenosis of a three-cusp aortic valve is common. Of the patients studied personally with clinically isolated AS (with or without regurgitation), aged 16 to 65 years (Table 2), 25 percent had tricuspid valves, and among those over 65, 90 percent had tricuspid valves. In the younger group, about one half of the patients with clinically isolated AS had diffuse fibrous thickening of the mitral leaflets as well. The associated diffuse mitral leaflet thickening is strong evidence that the etiology of AS in this group is rheumatic.[44] Also, nearly 75 percent of this group had positive histories of acute rheumatic fever, whereas 10 percent of the other group, i.e., those with anatomically normal mitral valves and AS, had positive histories.[42,44] The etiology of AS in the patients with anatomically normal mitral valves is unknown. Possibly, as mentioned earlier, minor abnormalities in the sizes of the aortic valve cusps from birth set the stage for abnormal contact of the leaflets with one another, resulting in fibrosis and, finally, stenosis[47] (Fig. 20).

DISCRETE SUBAORTIC STENOSIS

Like valvular AS, discrete subaortic stenosis (DSS), when isolated, usually does not produce symptoms of cardiac dysfunction until adulthood, and it is compatible with a relatively long survival. The average age of death is 35.[63] Unlike valvular AS, however, DSS is rare. In this condition the discrete obstruction is located about 1 cm. caudal to the bases of the aortic valve cusps.[43] The obstruction is on a line corresponding to the site where the atrial septum inserts into the anterior mitral leaflet. The obstruction, at

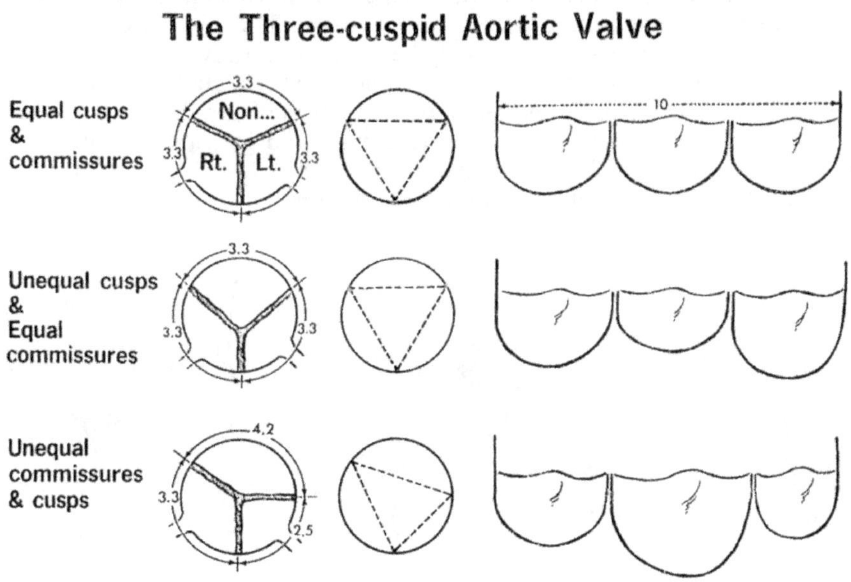

Figure 20. Diagrammatic portrayal of aortic valve cusps equal and unequal in size. *Top row,* The cusps of the aortic valve are equal in size and the circumferential distances between the commissures are equal. The straight-line distances between the commissures (as indicated by the dashed lines in the center circle) also are equal. On the right the aortic valve is opened. *Middle row,* Here the cusps are of unequal size, and they are made unequal by differing cephalocaudal lengths of the individual cusps. The distances between the commissures circumferentially around the aorta and the straight-line distances within the lumen of the aorta are similar to the normal shown in the top panel. *Bottom row,* Here the cephalocaudal lengths of the individual cusps differ and the circumferential distances around the aorta and the straight-line distances within the lumen of the aorta between the commissures (lateral attachments) are different as well.

least in adults, is produced by dense fibrous tissue—not really a "membrane"—which encircles the entire left ventricular outflow tract. The dense fibrous tissue may spread slightly cephalad, approaching the bases of the aortic valve cusps, and caudally for about a centimeter. Because in DSS the obstruction is usually severe and located just below (1 cm.) the aortic valve, the aortic valve cusps are the site of the impact of the blood ejected through the discrete obstruction. As a consequence, the aortic valve cusps become thickened and thus are ideal sites for vegetations. The consequence of cuspal thickening, with or without superimposed infective endocarditis, is development of mild aortic regurgitation. As a result, nearly all adults with DSS have precordial diastolic murmurs of aortic regurgitation in addition to the systolic murmurs of left ventricular outflow obstruction.[64,65] The absence of aortic valve calcific deposits and the absence of dilatation of the ascending aorta in adults, however, helps, before cardiac catheterization, to separate these patients from patients with valvular AS.

Although adequate data is not yet available, it is likely that DSS, on a percentage basis, is the cardiac condition most frequently complicated by infective endocarditis, being more common than that infection's association with congenitally bicuspid or unicuspid aortic valve, prolapsed aortic valve associated with ventricular septal defect, or floppy mitral valve.[58,66] The narrow jet of blood contacting one or more aortic valve cusps under high pressure and velocity provides the ideal circumstance for infective endocarditis to develop. Of five Newfoundland dogs with DSS that were dying naturally, four had active infective endocarditis, which was the cause of death, at necropsy.[66] Among seven patients with DSS whom I studied at necropsy, four had died from active infective endocarditis (Figs. 21 and 22).

Infective endocarditis complicating DSS may be difficult to diagnose clinically, at least before embolic events occur, and early diagnosis in this circumstance is essential to prevent severe damage to the aortic valve cusps. The high pressure jet ejected through the subaortic stenosis damages these cusps naturally, as already mentioned, but when infection is present this damage by the jet is markedly accelerated and the cusps are rapidly destroyed. In patients with destroyed aortic valve cusps and no subaortic stenosis, the consequence is severe aortic regurgitation with progressive left ventricular dilatation and failure. But in patients with destroyed aortic valve cusps associated with DSS, severe aortic regurgitation is prevented by the subaortic obstruc-

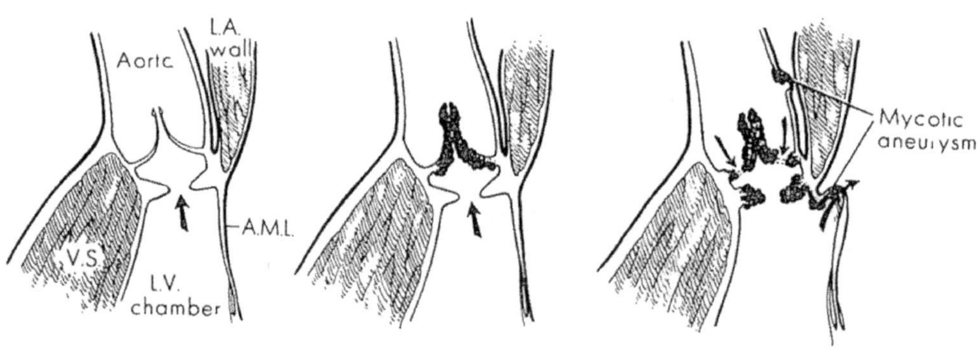

Figure 21. Diagram of aortic-valve region of the patient described in detail in Figure 22. Here the course of the pathologic process suggested by the necropsy findings is illustrated. The left diagram shows the *discrete subvalvular obstruction* before the development of *bacterial endocarditis* when the valve was traumatized by the jet of blood from below. The central diagram depicts the initial formation of bacterial vegetations, exclusively on the aortic valve cusps. As vegetations proliferated, the cusps ruptured (right diagram); the infection then extended to the discrete subvalvular fibrous band and anterior mitral leaflet (A.M.L.) where a mycotic aneurysm formed immediately below the "membrane" where systolic pressure was highest. A second aneurysm in the wall of the ascending aorta resulted from the effects of a systolic jet through the valve. L.A. = left atrium; V.S. = ventricular septum; L.V. = left ventricle.

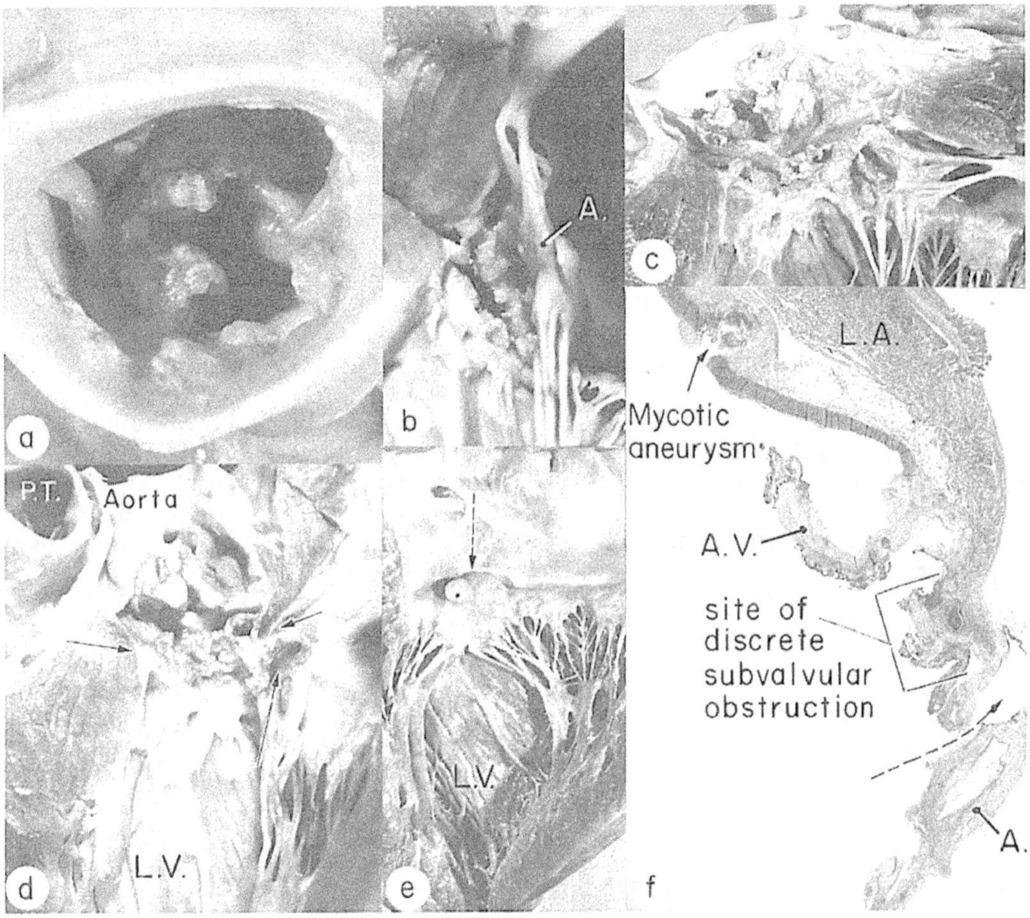

Figure 22. Alpha hemolytic streptococcus endocarditis complicating congenitally *discrete subaortic stenosis* in a 28-year-old man. The infection, which appeared about nine months before death, produced valvular aortic regurgitation. *a*, Aortic valve from above. *b*, Left ventricular outflow tract from below, showing vegetative material on the subvalvular "membrane" and adjacent anterior mitral leaflet (A.). *c*, Opened left ventricular outflow tract showing vegetations on each aortic cusp, on the subvalvular "membrane," and on the ventricular surface of anterior mitral leaflet. *d*, Longitudinal section showing the left ventricular outflow tract. The area of subaortic stenosis is apparent (between the *solid arrows*) and a mycotic aneurysm *(dashed arrow)* is seen in the anterior mitral leaflet. The mitral aneurysm is in the high-pressure portion of the left ventricle (L.V.), i.e., below the discrete subvalvular obstruction. P.T. = pulmonary trunk. *e*, Opened mitral valve showing atrial aspect of the mycotic aneurysm *(dashed arrow)* on the anterior leaflet. *f*, Photomicrograph of section through aorta, left atrium (L.A.), aortic valve (A.V.) cusp, subvalvular "membrane," and anterior mitral leaflet (A.). A mycotic aneurysm is present in the ascending aorta *(solid arrow)* as well as in the anterior mitral leaflet *(dashed arrow)*. Vegetations are present on the aortic valve cusp and on the subvalvular membrane. (Hematoxylin and eosin stain; x 2, reduced 15%)

tion; therefore, the aortic or systemic arterial diastolic pressure does not fall significantly despite an anatomically destroyed aortic valve. As a consequence, the left ventricle does not dilate and congestive cardiac failure may be absent. Because the aortic valve cusps in these patients are previously traumatized by the jet of blood traversing the subaortic stenosis, the infection is superimposed on a previously abnormal valve. In this situation the most common infecting organisms are alpha streptococci, organisms of a relatively low virulence that are compatible with active infective endocarditis over a long period (many months) without antibiotic treatment.[58]

One of the essential reasons for diagnosing DSS before adulthood is to allow operative resection of the "membrane" so that cuspal damage is prevented. When operative treatment is delayed until adulthood, aortic valve replacement is often required in addition to resection of the subaortic "membrane." Then survival becomes dependent on the "survival" of the valvular prosthesis, and anticoagulants usually are required with all of their inherent complications.

A recent anatomic observation in necropsy patients with DSS is severe thickening and luminal narrowing of the intramural coronary arteries located in the ventricular septum.[66] A similar finding has been observed in patients with hypertrophic cardiomyopathy (see next section) and in patients with tunnel subaortic stenosis.[67]

HYPERTROPHIC CARDIOMYOPATHY

In his original description,[68] Teare applied the term *asymmetrical hypertrophy of the heart* to this condition. Subsequently, terms such as *functional subaortic stenosis, diffuse muscular subaortic stenosis, idiopathic hypertrophic subaortic stenosis, hypertrophic obstructive cardiomyopathy,* and *asymmetric septal hypertrophy (ASH)* have been applied. The terms which include the words "stenosis" and "obstruction" appear inappropriate because obstruction is more often absent than present.[69] The terms which emphasize asymmetry of the walls bordering the left ventricular cavity have served a useful purpose in emphasizing a characteristic morphologic feature of this condition,[43] but the ventricular septum may be thicker than the left ventricular free wall in conditions other than hypertrophic cardiomyopathy (HC).[70–77] A few patients (about 5 percent) with HC do not have ASH (i.e., septum thicker than free wall[78,79]) and in rare cases the free wall is not thickened in HC.[78]

Study at necropsy of patients with HC[78] has demonstrated the following morphologic features: (1) greater thickening of the ventricular septum than of the left ventricular free wall (95 percent); (2) small or normal-sized left and right ventricular cavities (95 percent); (3) mural endocardial plaque, left ventricular outflow tract (75 percent, adults only); (4) thickened mitral valve (75 percent, adults only); (5) dilated atria (100 percent, adults only); (6) abnormal intramural coronary arteries (50 percent);[80] and (7) disorganization of myocardial fibers in the ventricular septum (95 percent) (Figs. 23–31; Table 3).

The chief morphologic abnormality in HC resides in the *ventricular septum*. As pointed out by Teare in 1958, the ventricular septum nearly always is thicker than the left ventricular free wall. Among our adult necropsy patients, the maximal thickness of ventricular septum averaged 3.0 cm. and the maximal thickness of left ventricular free wall, 1.8 cm. The thickest portion of the septum is that part located about midway between aortic valve and left ventricular apex. This level corresponds approximately to the apex of right ventricle. Although in all our necropsy patients the ventricular septum was thicker than normal, the left ventricular free wall was usually, though not always, thicker than normal.

Although *ventricular asymmetry* (i.e., a significant difference in maximal thickness of ventricular septum and left ventricular free wall) is a characteristic morphologic feature of HC, about 5 percent of our patients with this condition showed *ventricular symmetry* at necropsy (i.e., equal maximal thickness of the ventricular septum and left ventricular free wall). Thus, although asymmetric septal hypertrophy (ASH) is a highly sensitive marker for HC,[69] it is not specific for this condition. Ventricular septa thicker than left ventricular free walls have been reported in conditions causing thinning of the left ventricular free wall relative to the septum and in conditions causing thickening of the septum relative to the free wall. The most common cause of preferential free wall

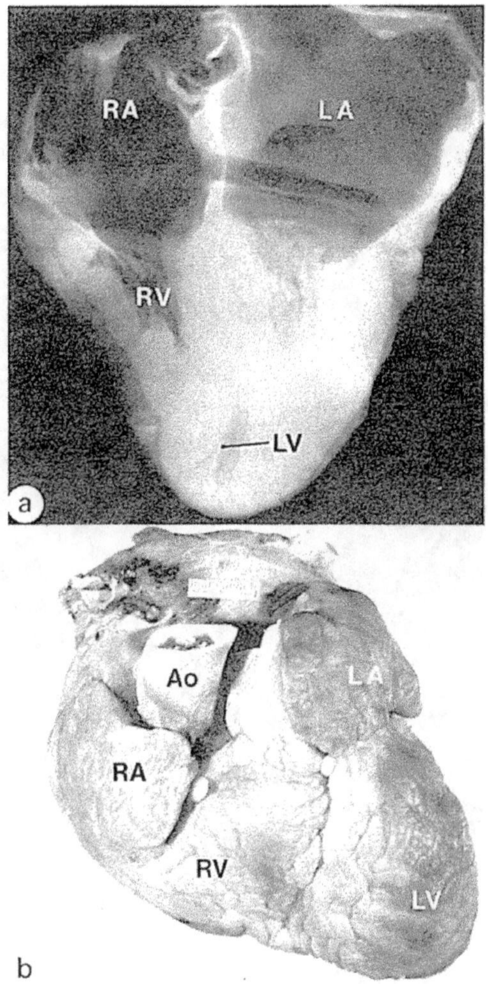

Figure 23. *a*, Radiograph of heart specimen and *b*, the heart itself in a 43-year-old woman with *hypertrophic cardiomyopathy.* Eleven years before she died the peak systolic pressure gradient between left ventricle and aorta was 54 mm. Hg at rest. She had periodic atrial fibrillation, chronic congestive cardiac failure, and an event compatible with cerebral embolus. The radiograph shows very dilated right (RA) and left (LA) atria, small-sized right (RV) and left (LV) ventricular cavities and a ventricular septum thicker than the left ventricular free wall. The exterior view of the specimen also shows very prominent atria. Ao = aorta.

Table 3. Idiopathic dilated (DC) and hypertrophic (HC) cardiomyopathies: morphologic differences

	DC	HC
1. Dilated ventricular cavities	+	0
2. Intracardiac thrombi	+	0
3. Asymmetric septal hypertrophy	0	+
4. Myocardial fiber disorientation	0	+
5. Endocardial plaque, LV outflow tract	0	+
6. Thickened mitral valve	0	+
7. Abnormal intramural coronary arteries	0	+
8. Ventricular scarring (gross)	0 – +	+
9. Thickened ventricular walls	0 – +	+
10. Increased cardiac weight	+	+
11. Dilated atrial cavities	+	+

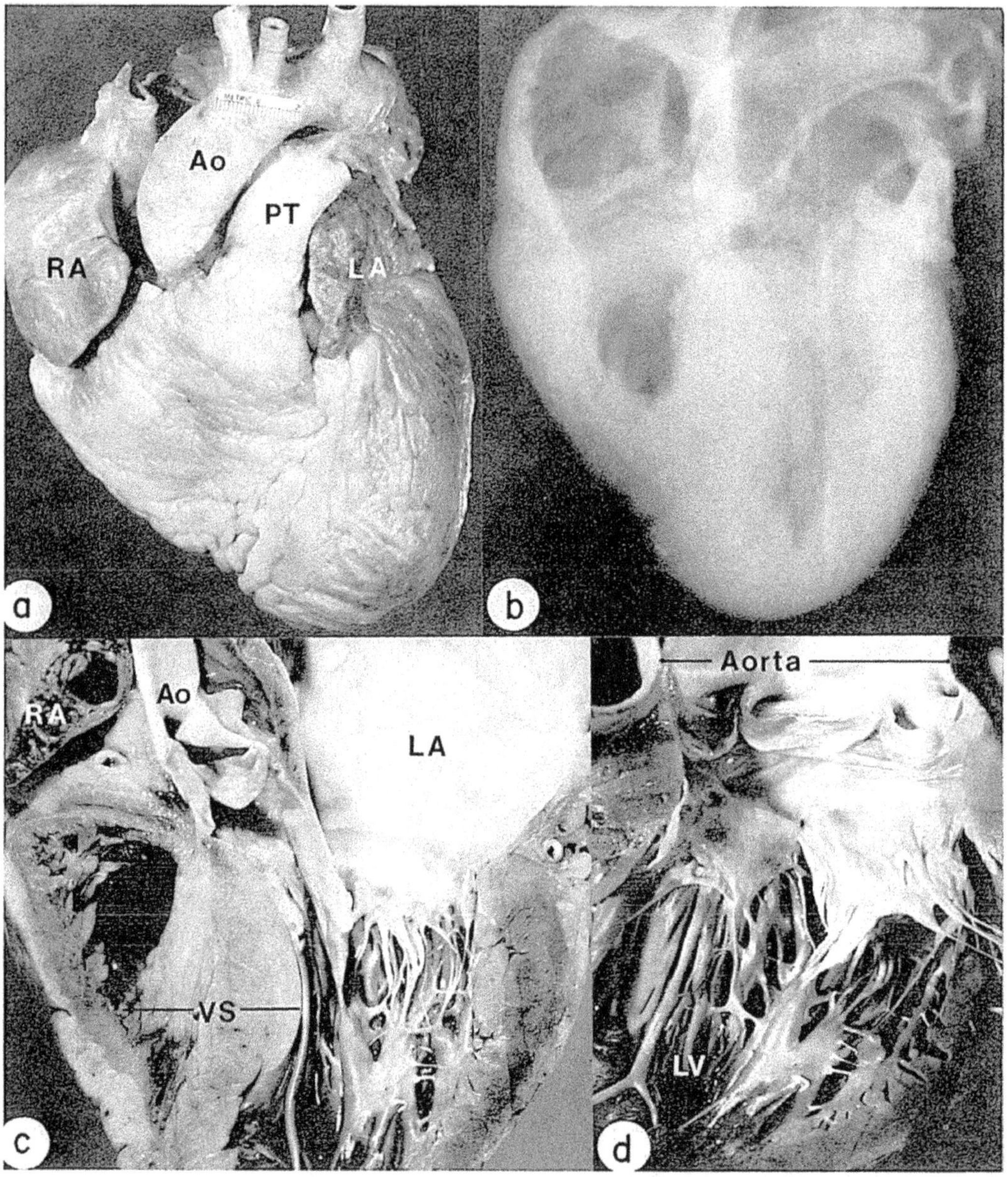

Figure 24. Heart of a 26-year-old man with *hypertrophic cardiomyopathy.* At catheterization three years before his death, a peak systolic pressure gradient of 30 mm. Hg was present between left ventricle and brachial artery and the gradient increased to 85 mm. Hg with provocation (ouabain). The cardiac index was 2.1 l./min./m.^{2}. At another catheterization done only six days before his sudden death, the gradient at rest was zero and it rose to only 33 mm. Hg when provoked (isoproterenol). The cardiac index was 2.0 l./min./m.^{2}. The anatomic features of hypertrophic cardiomyopathy are demonstrated in these photographs. *a,* Exterior view; both right (RA) and left (LA) atria are dilated. Ao = aorta; PT = pulmonary trunk. *b,* Radiograph of specimen showing the ventricular septum to be thicker than left ventricular free wall. *c,* Coronal section; the septum (VS) is clearly thicker than the left ventricular free wall, and an endocardial mural plaque is present in the left ventricular outflow tract in apposition to the anterior mitral leaflet. *d,* A closer view of the plaque and the thickened anterior mitral leaflet.

thinning is myocardial infarction; the most common cause of preferential septal thickening is right ventricular systolic hypertension from any of a variety of conditions.

Among patients with HC, the thickness of the ventricular septum is not dependent on the presence of left ventricular outflow tract obstruction at rest, and, indeed, the thickness of the septum is similar in patients with outflow obstruction at rest and in those without outflow obstruction at rest. Although examination of the septum in patients with HC is not helpful in separating the patients *with* from those *without* left ventricular outflow obstruction at rest, examination of the basal portion of the left ventricular free wall (posterior or posterolateral portion) does permit delineation between these two groups of patients.[81,82] In the patients with the obstructive type of HC, this posterobasal portion of left ventricular free wall represents the thickest portion of free wall, whereas in the patients with the nonobstructive type of HC, this posterobasal portion is thinner than normal and often pointed like a bird's bill (Fig. 25). In the patients with obstruction at rest, the thickest portion of the left ventricular free wall is about midway between the base of posterior mitral leaflet and apex of left ventricle.

Another abnormality in the ventricular septum in patients with HC is focal *myocardial fiber disarray* or disorganization[68,78,81-83] (Fig. 30). This abnormality also was described by Teare in 1958, and occurs in 90 to 100 percent of these patients depending on how "septal disorganization" is defined.[83] Small foci of myocardial fibers not parallel to one another in the ventricular septum are common in normal hearts. When, however, the definition of "septal disorganization" is rigid and quantitation of the amount of disorganization is introduced, about 90 percent of the patients with HC can be clearly delineated from persons with normal hearts or from patients with cardiac conditions other than HC.[83] Studies by Maron and associates[83] have shown that among patients

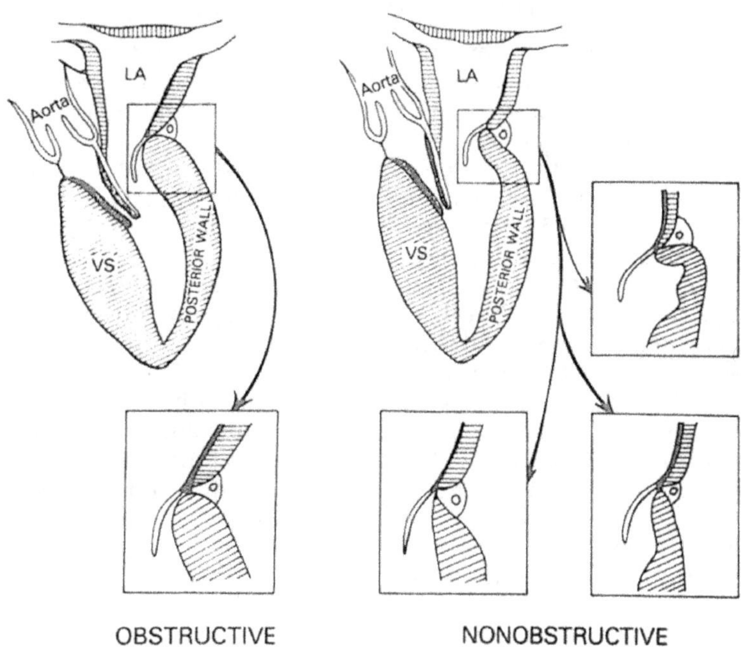

Figure 25. Diagram depicting the configuration and thickness of the posterolateral left ventricular free wall just behind the posterior mitral leaflet in the obstructive and nonobstructive types of *hypertrophic cardiomyopathy*. In the obstructive form, the most basal portion of free wall is rounded and thick. In the nonobstructive form, the most basal portion of left ventricular free wall is pointed and thin. In each type the ventricular septum is much thicker than the left ventricular free wall. The mural endocardium in the left ventricular outflow tract and the anterior mitral leaflet in apposition to it is thickened.

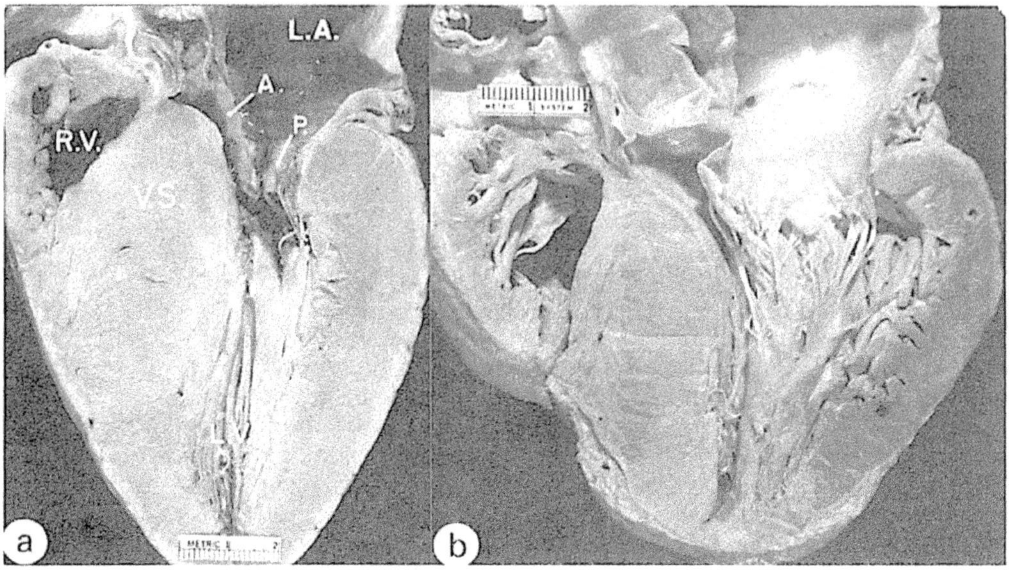

Figure 26. *Hypertrophic cardiomyopathy* in two patients. *a*, Left ventricular outflow obstruction in patient whose gradient at rest was 77 mm. Hg. *b*, Patient with no gradient at rest. The posterobasal portion of left ventricular (L.V.) free wall in the first patient is rounded and thick; this portion of free wall in the second patient is more pointed and thin. The result is a larger left ventricular cavity in the basal portion in *b* than in *a* and, consequently, more room for the mitral valve. The ventricular septum (V.S.) in both patients, however, is severely thickened. A., P. = anterior and posterior mitral leaflets, respectively; R.V. = right ventricle.

with HC nearly 90 percent had 5 percent or more of the area of the ventricular septum showing myocardial fiber disorganization. In contrast, among persons with normal hearts or heart conditions other than HC, less than 5 percent of the area of the ventricular septum showed such disorganization.

Although "septal disorganization" of greater than 5 percent of the area of the ventricular septum occurs in about 90 percent of the patients with HC, about 10 percent of these patients have less than 5 percent of the area of the septum showing disarray and of them a few patients have absolutely no disarray at all.[83] Thus, like ventricular asymmetry, "septal disorganization" of greater than 5 percent of the area of the septum occurs in most patients with HC, but this abnormality may involve a smaller area of the septum, or, rarely, may be entirely absent.

Not only does disorganization of *myocardial fibers* occur; ultrastructural studies have shown disarray of *myofibrils* and *myofilaments* within individual cells.[84] Again, the abnormalities of myofibrils and myofilaments are not absolutely specific for HC, but when disorganization of these subcellular components is found in other cardiac conditions, the abnormal cells are in small numbers. The individual septal myocardial cells in HC also frequently show increased amounts of Z-band material and nonspecific changes of cellular hypertrophy and degeneration.[84]

Myocardial fiber disarray in the left and right ventricular free walls is more difficult to determine by light microscopy than that in the ventricular septum. Ultrastructural examination of the left and right ventricular free walls, however, has disclosed many bizarrely shaped, disorganized cells in the ventricular free walls of patients *without* obstruction whereas the bizarrely shaped and disorganized myocardial fibers are virtually entirely absent from the ventricular free walls in the patients *with* obstruction.[81,82] Thus, the disorientation of groups of myocardial cells and the disarray of myofibrils and myofilaments within individual myocardial cells is not the result of left ventricular outflow obstruction or high intraventricular systolic pressures.

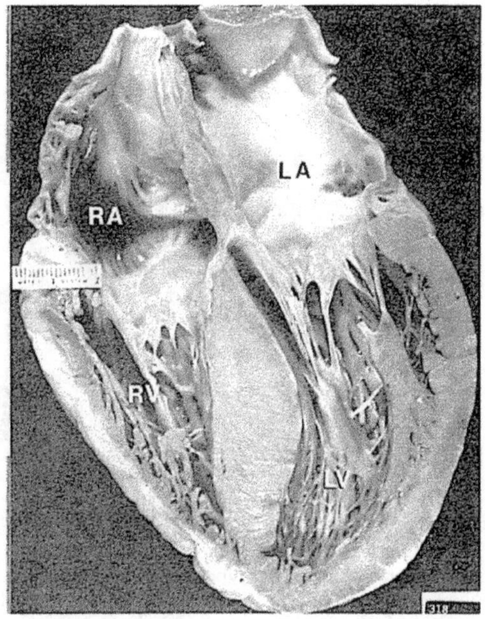

Figure 27. *Hypertrophic cardiomyopathy* (HC) in a 16-year-old girl who was always asymptomatic and died suddenly while jogging. Her mother had HC and three of her four siblings died suddenly. HC had been demonstrated clinically in each of them. The present patient by echocardiograms had systolic anterior motion of the anterior mitral leaflet, an ejection fraction of 87 percent, and no evidence of left ventricular outflow obstruction. She had no precordial murmur. The electrocardiogram had shown narrow Q waves in II, III, and AVF. The heart weighed 310 gm. and the ventricular septum was twice as thick as the left ventricular free wall (19 to 9 mm.). The left ventricular free wall was actually of normal thickness. RA = right atrium; RV = right ventricle; LA = left atrium; LV = left ventricle.

The functional or clinical significance of "septal disorganization" among patients with HC is not entirely clear. Among the patients studied at necropsy by Maron and associates,[83] those with high percentages of disorganization in the septal area were younger, had a higher frequency of premature deaths involving more than one member of the same family,[85,86] and thicker ventricular septa than those with lower percentages. A comparison of the presence or degree of left ventricular outflow obstruction, length of symptoms of cardiac dysfunction, mode of death, arrhythmias, etc., revealed no significant difference between the patients with high percentages and those with low percentages of septal area disorganization.[83]

Another abnormality of ventricular septum with HC is the presence of *abnormal intramural coronary arteries,* found in about one half of the patients[80] (Fig. 31). The abnormalities observed in the intramural coronary arteries in these patients are striking and consist of increased number and size of arteries with thickened walls and narrowed lumens. The thickening results from proliferation of smooth-muscle cells and collagen in both the media and the intima. Also, mucoid deposits (acid mucopolysaccaride material) are more numerous. Like disproportionate septal thickening (causing ventricular asymmetry) and septal disorganization, however, abnormality of the intramural coronary arteries is not specific for HC, though it is certainly more striking in HC than in most other conditions. Similar abnormality of the intramural coronary arteries may be observed in patients and in Newfoundland dogs with discrete subaortic stenosis,[66] in patients with tunnel subaortic stenosis,[67] and in newborns with aortic-valve atresia.[87]

The significance of the changes in the intramural coronary arteries in patients with HC is unknown. Their presence or absence does not correlate with any analyzed clinical parameter including age, sex, presence or degree of left ventricular outflow tract obstruction, presence of cardiac dysfunction including chest pain, or length of symptoms of cardiac dysfunction.

The cause of the striking abnormalities of the intramural coronary arteries also is uncertain. In each of the four conditions in which this degree of abnormality have been observed, namely, HC, discrete and tunnel subaortic stenosis and aortic-valve atresia, the septum is extremely thick and movement of the septum during life as shown by

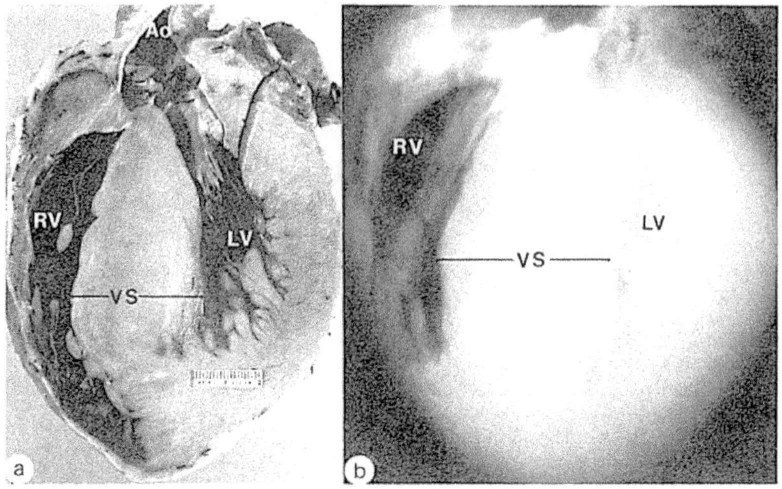

Figure 28. *Hypertrophic asymmetric obstructive* (right-sided) *cardiomyopathy*. This 18-year-old boy described in detail in the text was first studied when he was asymptomatic at age eight; his brother had died suddenly at age nine from idiopathic hypertrophic subaortic stenosis (left-sided obstruction). At catheterization no systolic pressure gradient was observed between the left ventricle and the systemic artery, but a systolic pressure gradient of 35 mm. Hg was recorded between the right ventricle (56/5) and the pulmonary artery (21/9). An electrocardiogram showed right axis deviation, right ventricular hypertrophy, and a right ventricular conduction delay. The child remained asymptomatic until age 12, when he developed chest pain while playing football. Precordial pain recurred frequently thereafter and was precipitated by exertion of decreasing intensity so that he was forced to limit his activities to a sedentary level. When he was restudied at age 13, a grade 1/6 systolic ejection-type precordial murmur was heard which was loudest along the left sternal border. Electrocardiography now showed more severe right ventricular hypertrophy. Cardiac catheterization showed a peak systolic pressure gradient of 118 mm. Hg between the right ventricle (135/7) and pulmonary artery (17/7) and there was no systolic gradient between the left ventricle (108/4) and the brachial artery (108/63 mm. Hg). Resection of the right ventricular outflow myocardium with insertion of a patch at the right ventriculuotomy was performed, and catheterization seven months postoperatively showed virtually no systolic pressure gradient between the right ventricle (30/4 mm. Hg) and the pulmonary artery (28/12). He was asymptomatic. Electrocardiograms now showed a right bundle branch block. This boy apparently remained asymptomatic until the day of death, when he felt faint while driving a car. He pulled over to the side of the road and collapsed. No anatomic explanation for death was revealed at necropsy. His heart weighed 660 gm. The right ventricular (RV) outflow tract was wide open. The ventricular septum (VS) was much thicker than the left ventricular (LV) free wall (1.0 compared to 1.9 cm.), and the right ventricular wall was of normal thickness. The endocardium of the left ventricular outflow tract was not thickened and the mitral valve was normal. Mild interstitial fibrosis involved the ventricular septum. *a*, A longitudinal section of the ventricles shows the disproportionate ventricular septal hypertrophy. The right ventricular cavity is larger than the left. Ao = Aorta. *b*, The radiograph of the heart was taken before it was opened.

echocardiogram is extremely limited. It is possible that the severe septal thickening prevents adequate expansion of these vessels during ventricular diastole and thus reduces flow. The fibrous-smooth muscle cell response, in turn, may serve to obliterate the unused lumen. However, this explanation does not explain the large size of these arteries. It is possible that the proliferation of the smooth-muscle cells in the walls of these arteries represents a response to the same stimulus which is causing severe hypertrophy and abnormal configuration of many striated myocardial cells.

A fourth abnormality of the ventricular septum in adults with HC is the occurrence of a fibrous plaque on the mural endocardium of the outflow portion of the septum[77] (Fig. 24). This fibrous thickening is located in direct apposition to the ventricular aspect of the anterior mitral leaflet and is the result of contact between the valvular and mural endocardium. The mural plaque, in other words, is the anatomic equivalent of the "systolic anterior motion" (SAM) of the anterior mitral leaflet observed on echocar-

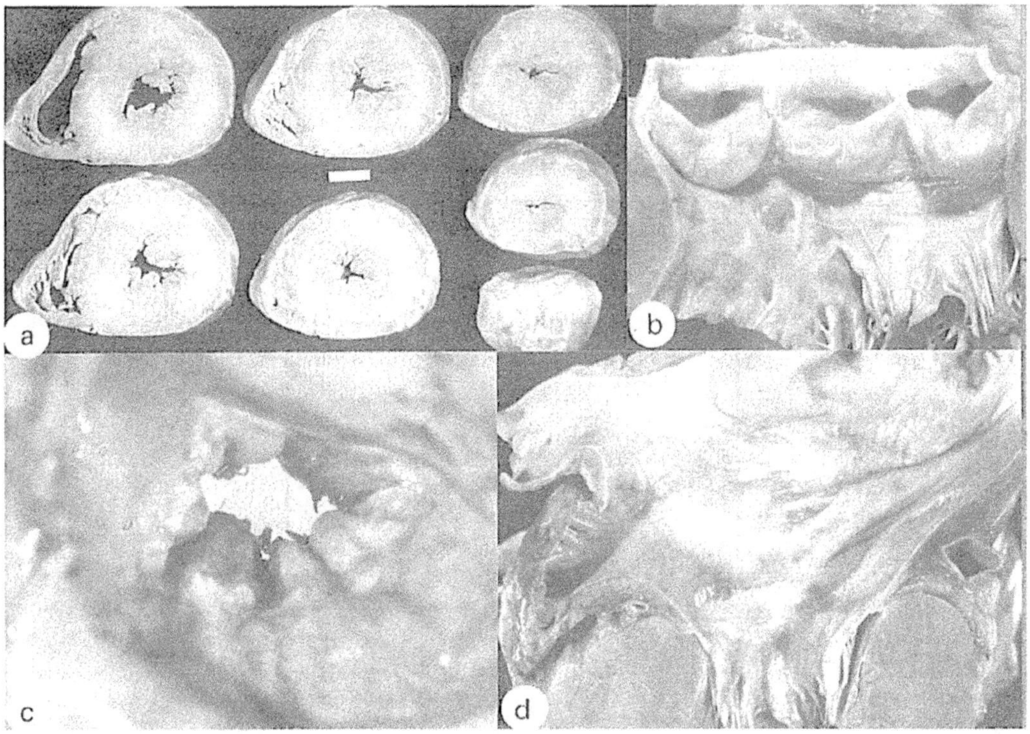

Figure 29. *Hypertrophic cardiomyopathy* in a 53-year-old man who died suddenly at home six weeks after onset of atrial fibrillation. Catheterization when he was asymptomatic (but had cardiomegaly) at age 46 disclosed a left ventricular to systemic arterial peak systolic gradient of 8 mm. Hg at rest, and a gradient of 69 mm. Hg with provocation (isoproteronol). Thereafter, he developed exertional dyspnea, dizziness, and angina. *a*, "Bread loaf" slices of cardiac ventricles. Although the echocardiogram had shown the ventricular septum to be thicker than left ventricular free wall during ventricular diastole, both were of similar thickness at necropsy (25 mm.). *b*, Opened aortic valve showing thickening of the mural endocardium in apposition to the thickened anterior mitral leaflet. *c*, View of mitral valve from left atrium. Thickening of its leaflets is typical of hypertrophic cardiomyopathy. *d*, Opened left atrium and thickened mitral valve. The basal portion of left ventricular wall is rounded and thick.

diogram in patients with HC and occasionally in other conditions.[76] When present in HC, the obstruction almost certainly begins at a level corresponding to the distal margin of the anterior mitral leaflet and with the caudal margin of the septal endocardial plaque. The mural endocardial septal plaque is present more frequently and is thicker in the patients with obstruction at rest compared to those without obstruction at rest.

It appears that HC is primarily a disease of the ventricular septum and that the morphologic abnormalities in it are apparent at the gross, microscopic, and ultrastructural levels. Other portions of the heart, however, are affected in HC but it seems likely that these other abnormalities are secondary to the abnormalities of the ventricular septum. These other abnormalities include *decreased ventricular cavity size* or, at least, lack of ventricular cavity dilatation, *increased atrial cavity size*, varying degrees of interstitial and replacement *myocardial fibrosis* (particularly in the ventricular septum), thickening of the posterior as well as the anterior mitral leaflet and, in elderly patients, calcification of the mitral anulus.[77,88,89]

The cause of the relatively small size of ventricular cavities in HC is unclear. The septum, being on the average about twice normal thickness, surely occupies space normally represented by cavity. The ventricular free walls are, on the average, about a

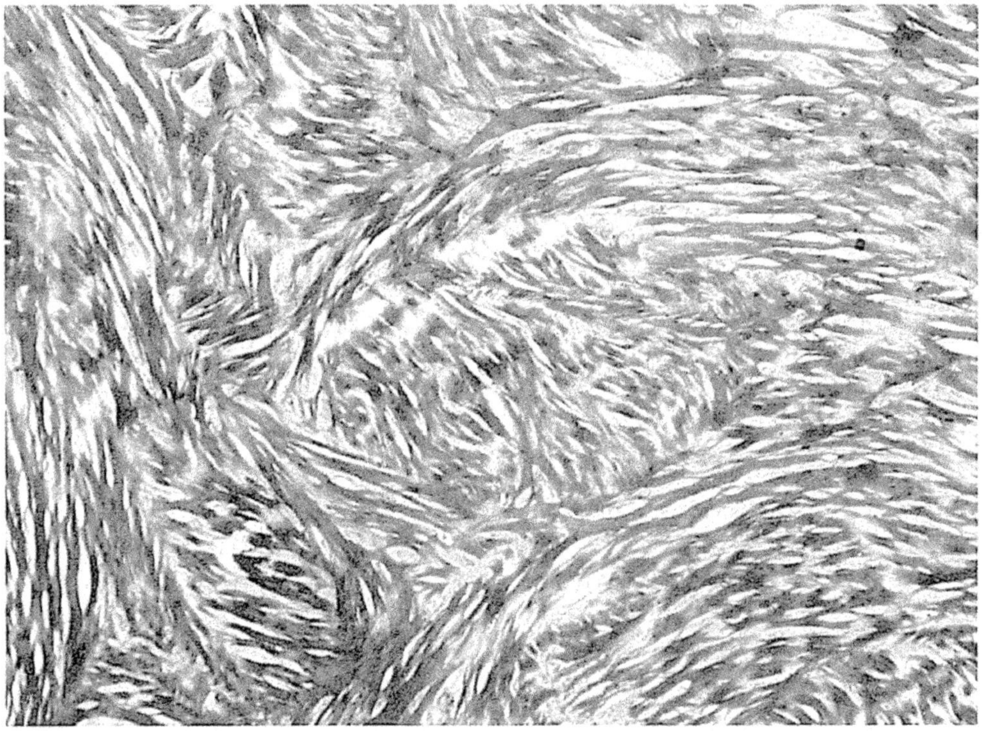

Figure 30. Photomicrograph of portion of ventricular septum in a 19-year-old man with *hypertrophic cardiomyopathy* showing the myocardial fiber disarray typical of this condition. (Masson stain; x 60 magnification)

third thicker than normal; this probably compromises slightly the intracavitary space even further. The greater thickness of the septum makes it relatively noncompliant (as demonstrated by its absent or minimal movement on echocardiogram). Although the left ventricular free wall in HC (by echocardiogram) usually contracts vigorously (in contrast to the septum), it appears to have little capacity to distend outwardly. Whatever the explanation, ventricular cavity size is rarely enlarged in these patients. The patients I have studied with dilated ventricular cavities at necropsy (4 of 65 with HC) have either nonscarred left and/or right ventricular free walls of normal thickness or scarred ventricular free walls of less than normal thickness. Dilatation may occur after operative septotomy-septectomy in HC.[90]

The impression of ventricular cavity size as observed at necropsy in patients with HC may be somewhat misleading because the cavity at necropsy in patients with HC represents the size at the end of ventricular systole.[91] This information was derived by comparing the left ventricular free wall thickness at necropsy to that measured by echocardiogram during life.[91] The thickness at necropsy corresponds to the thickness during ventricular systole, not diastole, which is observed by echocardiogram.

In contrast to the ventricular cavities, the atrial cavities in HC, at least in adults, are always dilated. The dilatation appears to be a response to difficulty in filling the relatively small ventricular caivities.

Not only is the anterior mitral leaflet thickened, but often (more frequently in the patients with obstruction) the posterior mitral leaflet too is thickened. The thickening of both leaflets is probably the consequence of the small left ventricular cavity. It is important to recall that the mitral valve resides in the left ventricle, which because of its

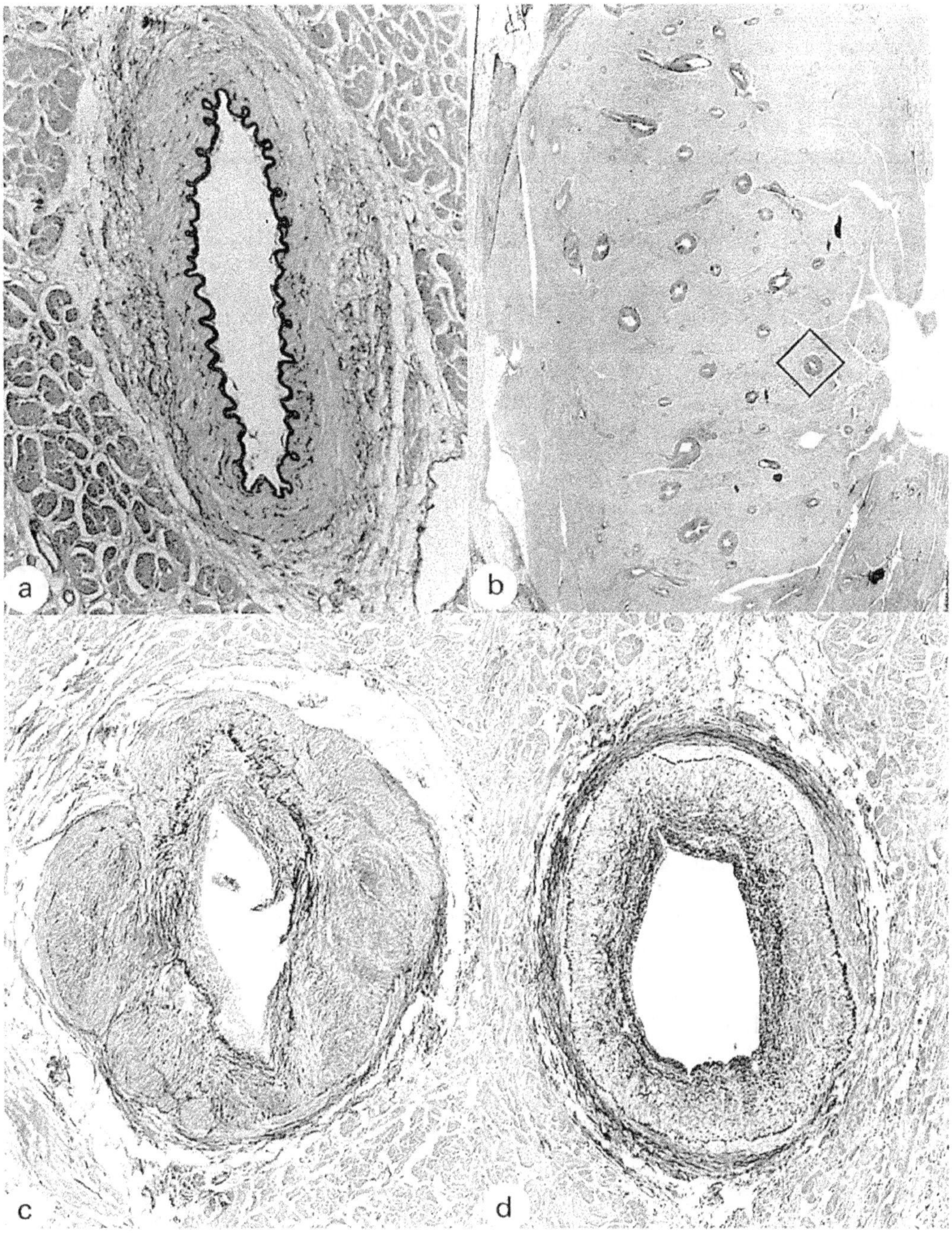

Figure 31. *Intramural coronary arteries in ventricular septum in hypertrophic cardiomyopathy* (HC) in three different patients. *a,* A normal artery (in a patient with HC) x 140. *b,* Low-power (x 4) photomicrograph of portion of ventricular septum showing marked prominence of the intramural coronary arteries in another patient. The arteries appear to be increased in number, size, and wall thickness. *c,* The artery enclosed by the box in *b* is shown here x 90. *d,* This artery, from another patient, has marked intimal thickening by fibroelastic proliferation, in contrast to the artery shown in *c,* which shows no delineation between intima and media. (Elastic van Gieson stains.) (Reduced 18%.)

small size, causes abnormal contact of the leaflets with themselves and also causes the anterior one to contact the septum. In the patients without obstruction, the basal portion of the left ventricular cavity is larger than in the patients with obstruction because of the thinning of the basal portion of free wall posteriorly and laterally. The focal fibrous thickening of the posterior mitral leaflet probably results from abnormal contact during ventricular systole since there is not enough room in the ventricular cavity to easily accommodate the leaflets and chordae. In this respect the ventricle and mitral leaflets mimic the movement of an accordion. The mitral leaflet thickening in HC is somewhat analogous to that which occurs normally as a consequence of aging. With aging, the left ventricular cavity becomes smaller, presumably in response to the lowered cardiac output; the mitral leaflets thicken; the left ventricular muscle becomes less compliant; and the left atrium dilates in response to increased work required to fill the small left ventricle. The same mechanisms appear to be accelerated in HC.

Most patients with HC have some degree of mitral regurgitation. It is not related to anular dilatation because the mitral anulus in this condition is not dilated.[78] Furthermore, the leaflet thickening in and of itself is not extensive enough to cause valvular regurgitation. The most likely explanation appears to be abnormal bending of the papillary muscles, particularly the anterolateral one.[69] These structures may be bent abnormally by the bulging ventricular septum with resulting excessive tension on the chordae tendineae preventing closure of the mitral orifice. Although they are usually present in the papillary muscles in HC, focal scars cannot account for the regurgitation. Although it is usually mild in HC, mitral regurgitation may be the predominant clinical feature of this condition. Despite advocacy by some investigators,[92,93] mitral valve replacement in HC is hazardous and unwarranted for a number of reasons.[94] The small left ventricular cavity is rarely capable of freely accommodating a prosthesis, and the mitral regurgitation in patients with HC nearly always either disappears or is strikingly lessened by adequate partial septectomy-septotomy.

SINUS OF VALSALVA ANEURYSM

Dilatation of each of the three sinuses of Valsalva is a normal consequence of aging and this "senile-type dilatation" appears to be more common in hypertensive than in normotensive persons.[21] In addition to aging, there are at least three other causes of dilatation of each of the three sinuses of Valsalva; these are the Marfan and Marfan-like syndromes,[14] syphilis,[95] and ankylosing spondylitis.[96,97] A congenital type of dilatation of all three aortic sinuses unassociated with other congenital anomalies of the heart or great vessels also has been recorded,[98] but its occurrence, if indeed of congenital origin, must be unique.

In contrast to the common occurrence of dilatation of all three aortic sinuses, aneurysmal dilatation of only one or two of the three sinuses is quite unusual (Figs. 32 to 34). The most common cause is probably infective endocarditis with spread of the infective process into adjacent structures and formation of one or more ring abscesses.[99] Aneurysmal dilatation of only one aortic sinus unassociated with infective endocarditis is extremely rare. In this circumstance the localized aneurysmal dilatation is generally attributed to a congenital absence of media in the wall of the aorta behind the sinus of Valsalva[100] (Fig. 35). The wall of aorta behind the sinus may rupture, and when this occurs, aortic regurgitation into either right ventricle or right atrium is the usual consequence (Fig. 33). Less commonly, the sinus aneurysm may obstruct right ventricular outflow or cause a conduction disturbance.[101]

The basic defect in patients with aneurysms involving only one or two of the three aortic valve sinuses is an absence of a portion or all of the media in the wall of aorta behind the sinus. Just because the media is deficient, however, does not assure the

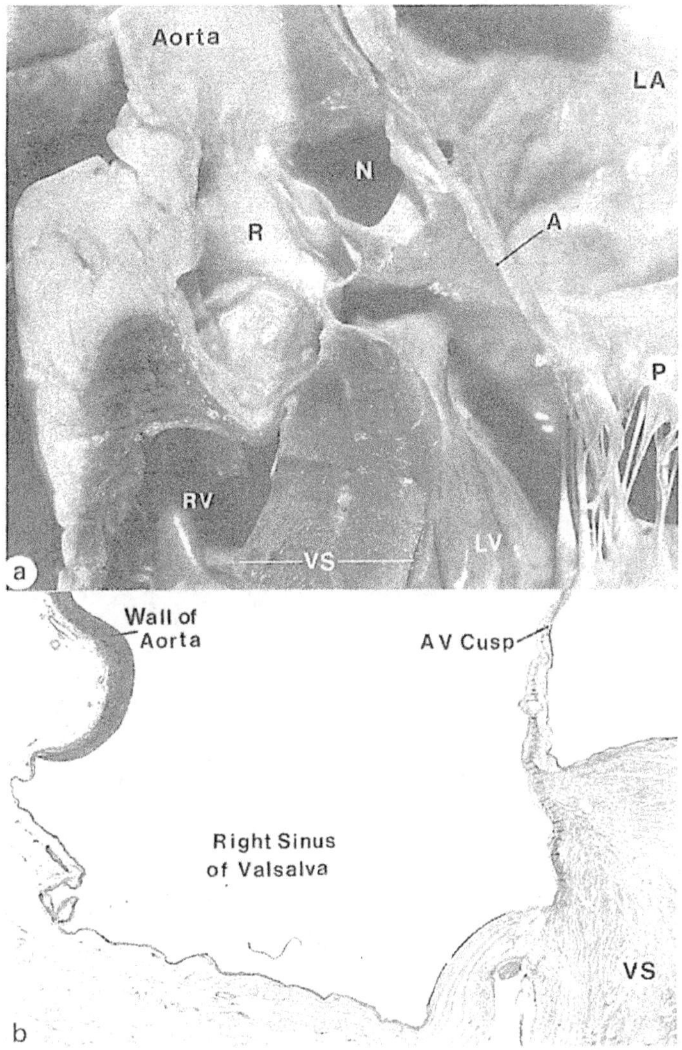

Figure 32. *Unruptured sinus of Valsalva aneurysm* in an 82-year-old man who died of cancer. An unexpected finding at necropsy was aneurysmal dilatation of the right sinus of Valsalva. The right sinus was 2.5 cm. deep and held 15 ml. of fluid, while the left and noncoronary sinuses of Valsalva were only 1.5 cm. deep and held only 5 ml. of fluid.

a, Longitudinal section of heart showing the aneurysmal dilatation of the right (R) sinus of Valsalva. N = noncoronary sinus of Valsalva; A, P = anterior and posterior mitral leaflets, respectively; LA = left atrium; LV = left ventricle; VS = ventricular septum. *b*, Histologic section of wall of right sinus of Valsalva showing the absence of aortic media in the caudal portion of the aneurysm. AV = aortic valve.

appearance of an aortic sinus aneurysm. When a deficiency of aortic media occurs, the wall involved most commonly is that behind the right anterior cusp (about 70 percent of patients); occasionally it is the portion behind the noncoronary (posterior) cusp (about 29 percent); it rarely (< 1%) involves that portion behind the left anterior cusp.[102] The explanation for these differences is uncertain.

Whether or not a sinus of Valsalva aneurysm is ever present from birth is uncertain; most likely the aneurysm is acquired, presumably the result of the aortic pressure. The higher the aortic pressure (for example, in patients with coarctation of the aortic

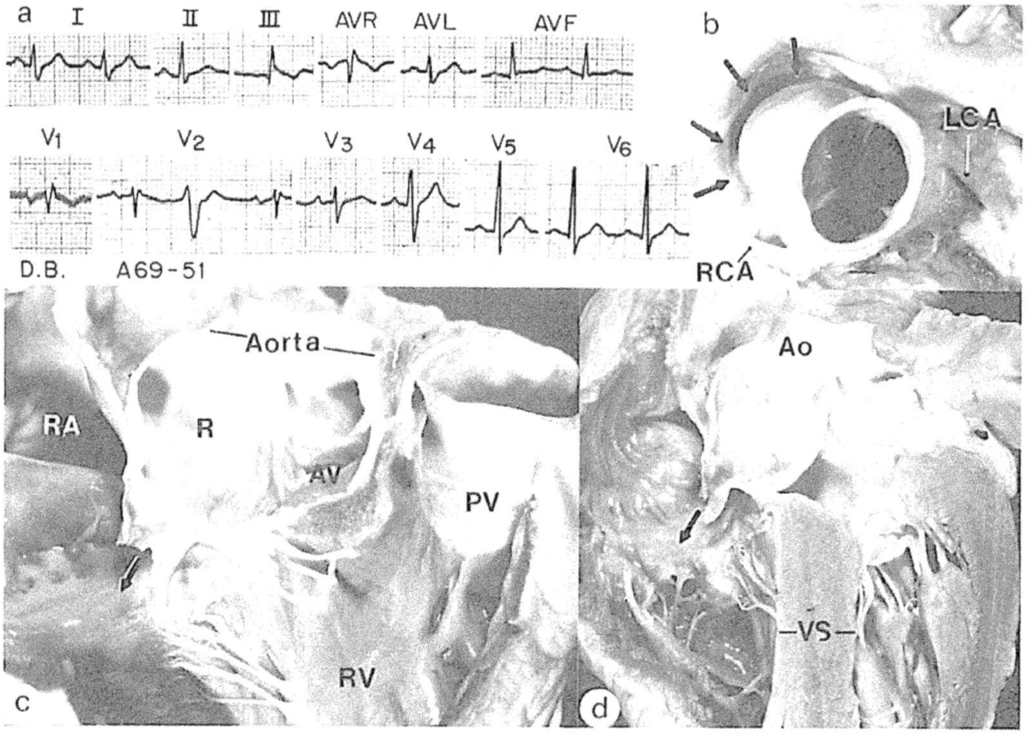

Figure 33. *Rupture of right (R) sinus of Valsalva aneurysm into right ventricle* (RV) in a 31-year-old woman who had been well until about 60 days before death when exertional dyspnea appeared. Eighteen days before death, she developed acute pulmonary edema and a murmur of aortic regurgitation. She died of progressive congestive cardiac failure. *a,* An electrocardiogram taken several days before her death. At necropsy the heart weighed only 300 gm. *b,* An aneurysm of the right sinus of Valsalva was present and bulged to the right (arrows). LCA, RCA = left and right coronary arteries, respectively. *c,* Opened right ventricle (RV) and wall of aorta behind right (R) sinus of Valsalva showing the aneurysm which had ruptured (arrow) into the right atrium (RA) anatomically and into right ventricle functionally. AV = aortic valve; PV = pulmonic valve. *d,* In this view the anterior half of the heart has been removed; the ruptured (arrow) aneurysm's relation to the right side of the heart and to the ventricular septum (VS) is apparent. Ao = aorta.

isthmus), the more likely is the possibility that an aortic sinus aneurysm will develop. The youngest child described with isolated sinus of Valsalva aneurysm was four years old.[103] Although the aneurysm itself may or may not be congenital, the deficiency in aortic media behind the sinus must be congenital.[101]

Both the natural history and the frequency of media-deficient aortic sinus wall are uncertain. The number of persons with a media-deficient aortic sinus wall in whom a sinus aneurysm developed is uncertain, as is the frequency of rupture of a developed sinus aneurysm. Among 78 cases of sinus of Valsalva aneurysm collected from previous publications by Kieffer and Winchell,[104] 59 (76 percent) had ruptured and 19 (24 percent) had not. In some of these cases, however, the aneurysms involved all three sinuses and were therefore probably associated with the Marfan syndrome. Among seven hearts with aneurysm of one aortic sinus studied at necropsy by Edwards and Burchell,[100] four aneurysms had ruptured and three had not. Of six single (one of three sinuses involved) aortic sinus aneurysms which I studied at necropsy, five had ruptured and only one[101] was unruptured. The latter patient was 82 years old; the five patients with ruptured aneurysms ranged in age from 31 to 49 years (average, 38). These figures indicate that among reported cases of aortic sinus aneurysm, rupture is more common than nonrupture. These data are probably considerably biased in favor of ruptured aneurysms;

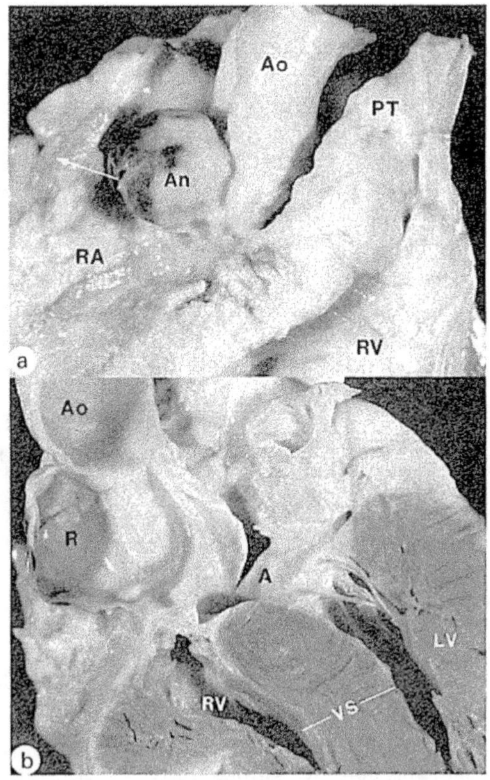

Figure 34. *Rupture of right sinus of Valsalva aneurysm into pericardial sac* in a 33-year-old woman who had been well until she died suddenly while house cleaning. At necropsy the pericardial sac was filled with blood. *a,* The right sinus of Valsalva is exteriorly round and a rupture (arrow) is visible in its right lateral wall. Extravasation was into the pericardial space only and not into a cardiac chamber. An = aneurysm; Ao = aorta; PT = pulmonary trunk; RA = right atrium; RV = right ventricle. *b,* The anterior portion of the heart has been removed again showing the right (R) sinus of Valsalva aneurysm. A = anterior mitral leaflet; LV = left ventricle; VS = ventricular septum.

nonruptured sinus aneurysm may be missed at necropsy, while the nonruptured aneurysm, with few exceptions, produces no evidence of cardiac dysfunction. Therefore, at necropsy there may be no clinical sign or symptom to alert the pathologist to the presence of an aortic sinus aneurysm. Furthermore, incidental necropsy findings, which an aortic sinus aneurysm usually represents, are infrequently reported. Thus, it

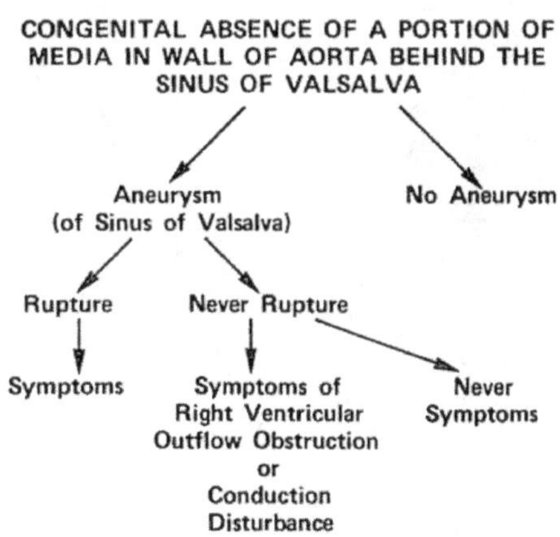

Figure 35. Diagram showing possible outcome in patients with *congenital absence of a portion of media in aortic wall behind sinus of Valsalva.* If no aneurysm occurs, the congenital defect will go unrecognized. If an aneurysm does occur it may or may not rupture. Rupture will virtually always produce clinical symptoms and signs of cardiac dysfunction. If rupture does not occur, symptoms will usually be present only if there is right ventricular outflow obstruction or conduction disturbances.

is likely that the frequency of unruptured aortic sinus aneurysm is considerably greater than has been reported.

On rare occasion an unruptured single aortic sinus aneurysm may produce evidence of cardiac dysfunction. Kerber and associates[105] described clinical and operative findings in a 62-year-old man who had evidence of right ventricular outflow obstruction as the result of an aortic sinus aneurysm's bulging into the crista supraventricularis. Complete heart block has also been described in a patient with unruptured aortic sinus aneurysm.[106] The latter patient, however, also had calcific aortic stenosis, and thus it is not certain that the sinus aneurysm was responsible for the conduction defect.

Rupture of the sinus of Valsalva aneurysm is clearly the most frequent complication of aneurysm involving only one of the three aortic sinuses. Rupture rarely occurs before adulthood. Like all conditions affecting the aorta and the aortic valve, it is more common in males than females (about 4 to 1). Death occurs suddenly if the rupture is into the pericardial space rather than into a cardiac cavity (Fig. 34). Death usually occurs, however, within a year after rupture with regurgitation into a cardiac chamber. Death most commonly is the result of congestive cardiac failure.

THE MARFAN SYNDROME

This inheritable disorder may involve the bones, joints, eyes, heart, and blood vessels. The extremities are long and thin (dolichostenomelia), the ligaments and joint capsules are redundant, the lenses may be dislocated (ectopia lentis), the ascending aorta often is dilated, and one or both left-sided cardiac valves usually are incompetent. Cardiovascular disease is by far the most common cause of death in patients with the Marfan syndrome. Of 18 patients that I studied at necropsy, all fulfilled McKusick's rigid criteria for this syndrome,[107] and all died prematurely from cardiovascular disease (average age, 34; range, 15 to 52). Of 56 decreased patients with this syndrome studied by Murdoch and associates,[108] cardiovascular disease was the cause of death in 52 (93 percent) and the average age at death was 32 years.

A variety of cardiovascular lesions have been observed in the aorta and heart of patients with the Marfan syndrome.[107] The 18 necropsy patients with this syndrome just

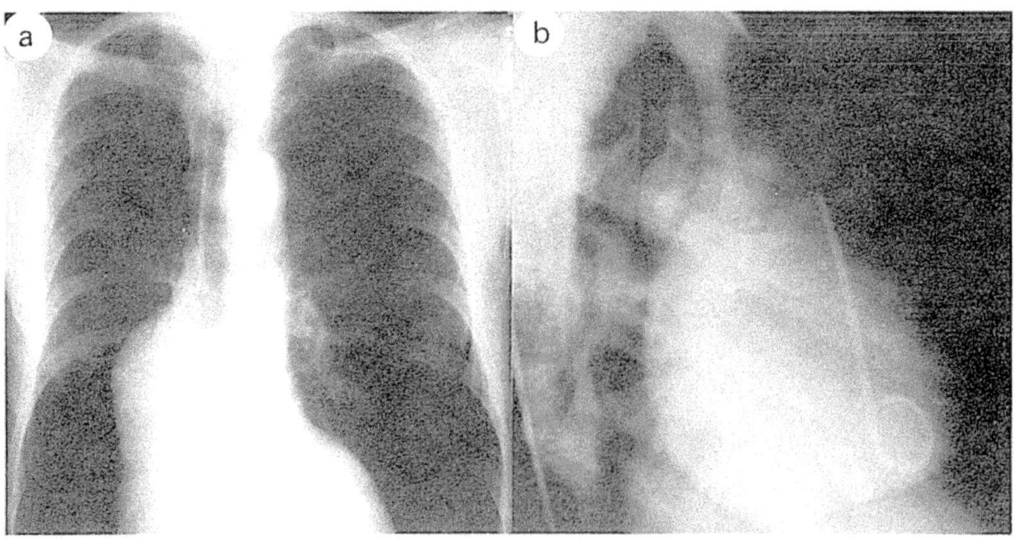

Figure 36. Chest radiograph *(a)* and aortogram *(b)* in a 38-year-old man with *Marfan syndrome*. A large aortic "root" aneurysm is present. (see Figure 37 for additional findings in this patient)

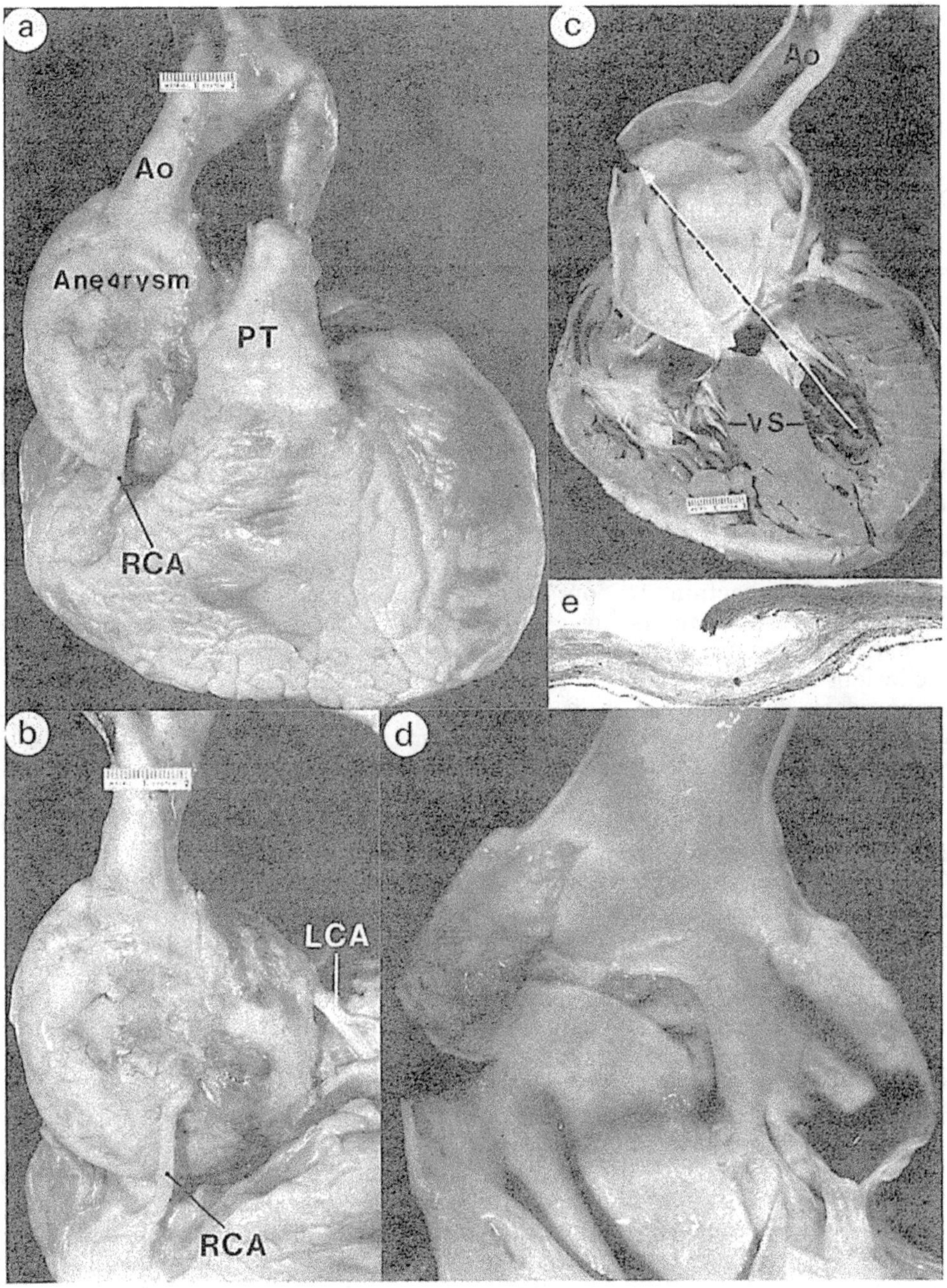

Figure 37. *The Marfan syndrome with rupture of ascending aortic aneurysm* in a 38-year-old black man. The patient was known to have a murmur of aortic regurgitation (aortic pressure 115/55 mm. Hg) but there was no evidence of congestive heart failure. He died suddenly at home and at necropsy the pericardial space was filled with blood and a tear was present in a large aneurysm involving all three sinuses of Valsalva and the proximal tubular portion of ascending aorta. *a*, View of heart shows the size of the aneurysm in comparison to the sizes of other structures. Ao = aorta; PT = pulmonary trunk; RCA = right coronary artery. *b*, A closer view of the large aneurysm with the coronary arteries arising from it. LCA = left coronary artery. *c*, The anterior half of the heart and aorta have now been removed. The dashed line depicts the direction of the blood ejected from the left ventricle. The arrow points to the rupture site in the wall of the aneurysm. The right lateral wall is the site of the rupture. VS = ventricular septum. *d*, Closeup of interior lining of aortic aneurysm at site of rupture. Several healed incomplete tears are present in the wall of the aneurysm and these have been confused with aortic dissections. *e*, Photomicrograph through one of the aortic tears showing massive degeneration of elastic fibers.

mentioned were readily separated into three distinct groups on the basis of their cardiovascular lesions. Group 1 included 12 patients with *saccular aneurysms of ascending aorta* (Figs. 36 to 38). All 12 patients had aortic regurgitation and 6 of them also had associated mitral regurgitation. Their aneurysms involved the sinus portion and the proximal tubular portion of ascending aorta, and two also had saccular aneurysms in the descending thoracic aorta. Histologic study of the wall of the ascending aorta disclosed the typical lesion of this syndrome, i.e., massive degeneration of elastic fibers and increase in mucoid material in the media (Fig. 38).

Group 2 included three patients with *dissection of the entire aorta* (Fig. 39). Before dissection, the aorta was of normal size in all three patients, and histologic study of the aortic wall disclosed that the typical lesion of this syndrome was absent; in fact, except for the dissection itself, the wall of aorta was histologically normal save for some aging changes.[109,110] Only one of the three patients had aortic regurgitation and then only after the dissection; one had mitral regurgitation and two had systemic hypertension before the aortic dissection.

Group 3 included two patients *without aortic saccular aneurysm or aortic disease* but with *pure mitral regurgitation* with floppy mitral leaflets and markedly dilated mitral anuli (Fig. 6). The aorta was of normal size and its wall was histologically normal in both.

Thus, the major lesions in the aorta in patients with this syndrome are saccular root aneurysms and dissection. In contrast to that described clinically by others,[111] our study of 18 necropsy patients suggests that the two rarely go together, since none of these patients had both a saccular aortic aneurysm and aortic dissection. These two aortic lesions may be mutually exclusive. None of the 12 patients with saccular aortic root aneurysms had evidence of dissection, although 9 of the 12 had focal intimal and medial tears in the wall of the saccular aneurysms (Figs. 37 and 38). These aortic tears have been mistakenly called "dissections" in a number of reports. None of the three with aortic dissection had saccular aneurysms of the aorta which was of normal size before the dissection. Histologically, the wall of the aorta varies with the type of lesion. In all 12 patients with aortic root saccular aneurysms, there was massive degeneration of the elastic fibers associated with increased amounts of collagen and mucoid material in the media of the aneurysmal wall. The increased amount of collagen in the aortic wall in these patients may actually prevent longitudinal dissection. In each of the three patients with aortic dissection, the wall of the aorta appeared histologically "normal," i.e., as it does in patients with aortic dissection who do not have the Marfan syndrome,[112] with no changes other than aging. Interestingly, two of the three patients with aortic dissection had evidence of diastolic systemic hypertension, whereas none of the other 16 patients had diastolic hypertension.

The term applied to the characteristic histologic lesion in the aorta in patients with the Marfan syndrome has been "cystic medial necrosis," a term first used by Erdheim in 1929[113] and an outgrowth of the term "medionecrosis" coined by Gsell[114] a year earlier. This term, however, is not ideal because "cysts" as such are infrequent and "necrosis," to my knowledge, has never been observed in the aortic media in this condition. Gsell used the term "medionecrosis" to designate areas in the aortic media with a diminished number of nuclei. Becker[109] recently showed that these areas devoid of nuclei actually consisted of large amounts of fibrous tissue and were a regular feature of the normal, aging aorta. Furthermore, the striking histologic aortic lesion in the Marfan syndrome is *massive degeneration of elastic fibers* in the media and this feature is ignored by the term "cystic medial necrosis." When Erdheim coined this term, stains for elastic fibers were poor or rarely used, and loss or degeneration of elastic fibers are difficult to appreciate on hematoxylin-eosin stained sections. Thus, he apparently could not appreciate this histologic feature of this condition.

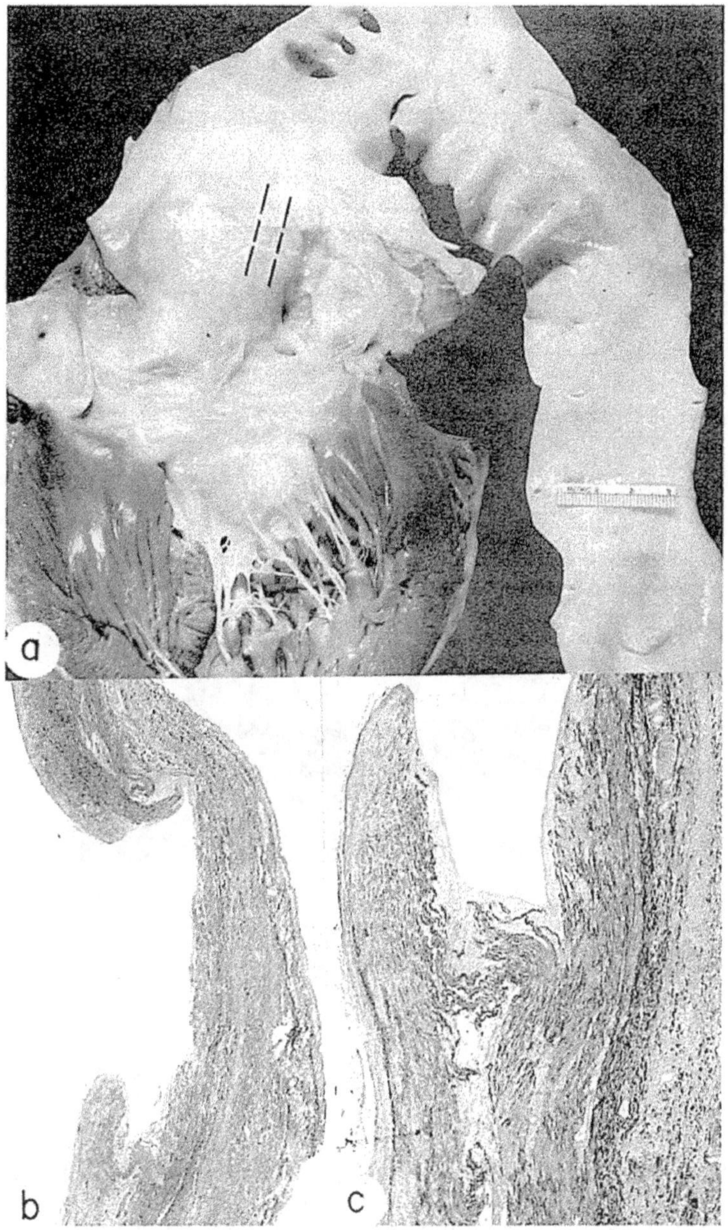

Figure 38. *The Marfan syndrome*. This 21-year-old man had the typical skeletal and optic features of this syndrome but had always been asymptomatic. He was found dead in his parked car after playing in a band for several hours. At necropsy the pericardial sac was filled with blood. *a*, Evidence of a through-and-through rupture is visible in the ascending aorta just above the aortic valve. In addition, several partial ruptures or tears are also present in the ascending aorta. *b*, A histologic section of one tear (shown between dashed lines in *a*). *c*, A closeup of an adjacent section of *b* reveals severe degeneration of elastic fibers of the media. (Elastic tissue stains; *b*, x 7 and *c*, x 18 magnification)

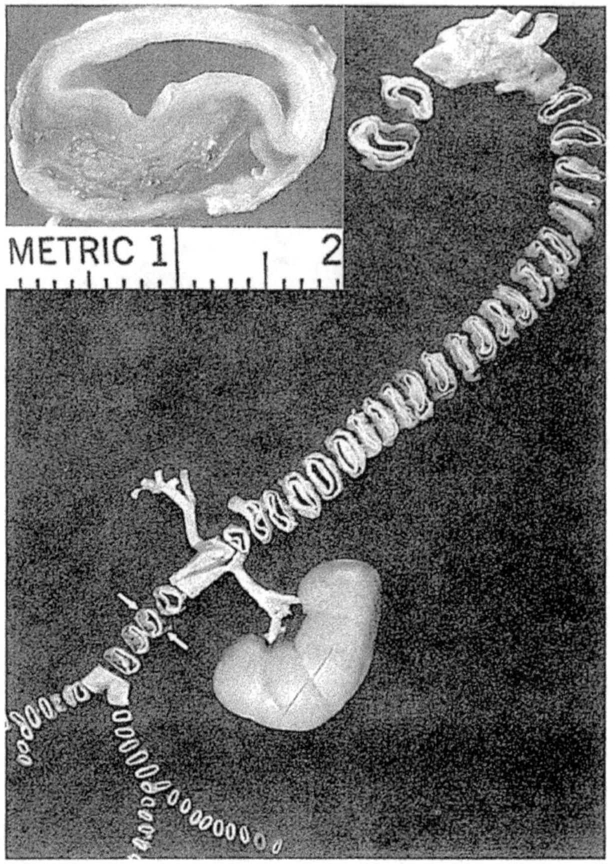

Figure 39. *Aorta* in a 43-year-old man known to have *Marfan syndrome*. He died 15 days after the sudden onset of typical clinical features of *aortic dissection*. Before the aortic dissection there was no precordial murmur. At necropsy, except for the acute dissection, there was no enlargement of the aorta, and except at the site of the entrance into the false channel, there were no tears in the aorta. Shown here is the complete aorta with both true and false channels and a hematoma in the false channel of the abdominal portion. A closeup of the transverse section indicated by the arrows is shown in the upper left. Histologically, there was no evidence of elastic fiber degeneration in the media of aorta. The heart weighed 500 gm. and neither ventricle was dilated. Thus, although this patient had both aortic dissection and Marfan syndrome, the typical histologic aortic medial lesion of this syndrome was absent. Therefore, it is more likely that the systemic hypertension was a more important contributing factor to the aortic dissection.

When elastic fibers disappear from the aortic wall in this condition, the space previously occupied by them appears to be replaced by collagen fibrils and mucoid material. Although the increased acid mucopolysaccharide material has been considered an inherent defect in this condition, it is just as reasonable to believe that this material serves simply as "a filler" for the lost elastic fibers and even smooth muscle cells. It is not clear whether or not the numbers of the elastic lamellae are normal or decreased at the time of birth in patients with the Marfan syndrome; however, aortic root aneurysm, with or without tears, has not been described in newborns with this syndrome. Thus, it appears that although the composition of the aortic media may be defective at birth, the aneurysms form later, presumably as a consequence of intra-aortic pressure on an inherently weak wall. The possible consequences of the inherently or congenitally weakened aortic media is shown diagrammatically in Figure 40.

Aortic regurgitation in patients with the Marfan syndrome is usually the result of

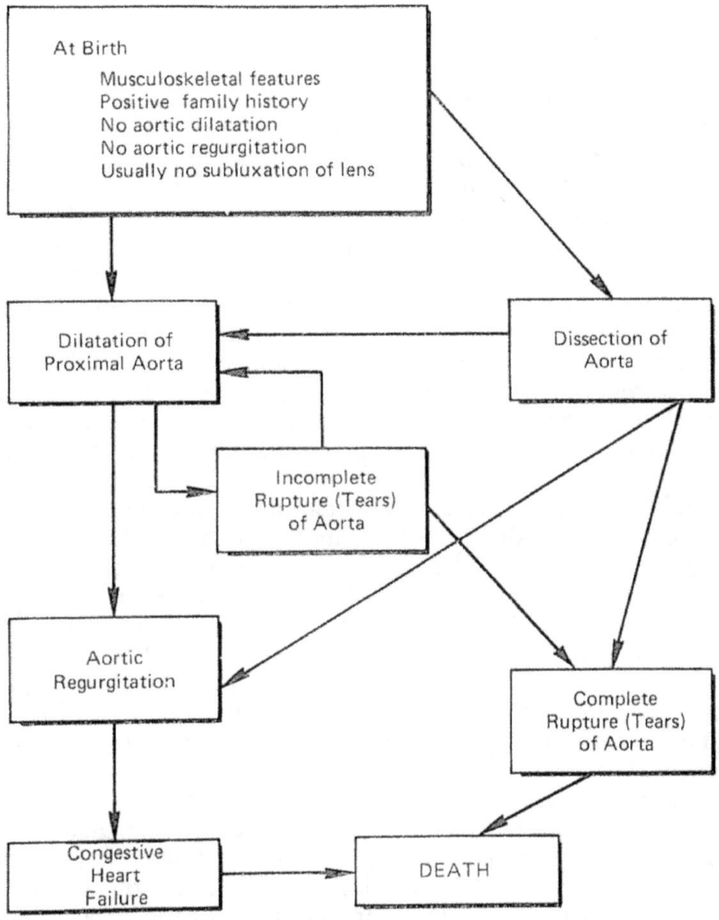

Figure 40. *The Marfan syndrome.* Schema of development of the aortic complications.

severe dilatation of the aortic "root" by the saccular aneurysm. The amount of regurgitation may not, however, correlate directly with the size of the aortic root aneurysm.[111] The aortic regurgitation is the consequence of aortic dissection even less commonly. The aortic valve cusps in patients with the Marfan syndrome appear to have an increased amount of mucoid material (acid mucopolysaccharide), irrespective of the presence of aortic regurgitation.

Mitral regurgitation also is frequent. At least five factors may be important in causing mitral regurgitation in patients with this syndrome. These are (1) floppiness of the mitral leaflets and/or chordae tendineae, (2) dilatation of the mitral anuli, (3) calcification of the mitral anuli, (4) rupture of mitral chordae tendineae, and (5) papillary muscle dysfunction. Of these factors, the first three appear to cause the most severe mitral regurgitation. Of the necropsy patients mentioned, 9 had mitral regurgitation: it was isolated in two and combined with aortic regurgitation in seven. Six of the nine with mitral regurgitation had floppy mitral valves and none of the nine without mitral regurgitation had floppy valves. The "floppiness" involved the posterior mitral leaflet in all six patients. Furthermore, of the nine patients with mitral regurgitation, the circumference of the mitral anulus ranged from 10 to 17 cm. (average, 15 cm.; normal, 9 cm.); of the nine patients without mitral regurgitation this circumference ranged from 9 to 12.5 cm. (average, 11 cm.). In the six patients with floppy mitral valves, the mitral circumference ranged from 14 to 17 cm. (average, 16 cm.). Thus, the average circumference of the mitral anulus in the nine patients with mitral regurgitation (15 cm.) was dilated 67 percent over normal (9 cm.) and in the nine patients without mitral regurgitation it was only 22 percent over normal (12 cm.). It therefore seems reasonable to conclude that both mitral leaflet floppiness and anular dilatation play significant roles in causing mitral regurgitation in these patients. Calcification of the mitral anulus is known to cause or at least be associated with mitral regurgitation.[21] The degree of regurgitation produced by this mechanism alone, however, is nearly always mild or minimal, and the mitral anuli in non-Marfan patients with mitral anular calcification is nearly always of normal or near-normal circumference. Of the 18 patients seen, four had mitral anular calcific deposits with associated mitral regurgitation; three also had floppy mitral leaflets. All four showed a mitral anulus which was quite dilated (range, 13 to 17 cm.; average, 15 cm.). Evidence for rupture of mitral chordae tendineae was found in four of the nine patients with mitral regurgitation. Two of these four patients had histories of infective endocarditis which had healed.[38] All four patients with evidence of mitral chordae rupture had floppy mitral leaflets and dilated mitral anuli (range, 15 to 17 cm.; average, 16 cm.).

The role played by "papillary muscle dysfunction" in causing mitral regurgitation in these patients is less clear.[115] All our 18 patients had dilated left ventricles and all had increased left ventricular masses. The hearts of the 18 patients ranged in weight from 375 to 850 gm. (average, 654 gm.). In 13 of the 18 patients the mitral leaflets were elongated from their basal attachments to their distal margins. This "stretching" probably was the result of the elongation (apex to base) of the left ventricular cavities, resulting primarily from the associated aortic regurgitation. The resulting left ventricular dilatation may have altered the normal angulation between the papillary muscles and the mitral leaflets. Whether or not mitral regurgitation was increased by this mechanism is uncertain.

Although the foregoing discussion concerns only patients with typical features of the Marfan syndrome, the cardiovascular features described in them also occur in patients without the skeletal or ocular manifestations of this syndrome or with histories of this syndrome in other family members. In addition, the characteristic histologic features in the wall of ascending aorta also have been observed in the aorta of patients with congenitally malformed aortic valves, particularly the bicuspid condition, and in patients with aortic stenosis when superimposed on congenitally malformed valves.[116,117] In individuals with the characteristic ascending aortic root aneurysms and histologic evidence of massive elastic-fiber degeneration of aortic media, features of the Marfan syndrome are more often absent than present.

REFERENCES

1. Barlow, J. B., Pocock, W. A., Marchand, P., et al.: *The significance of late systolic murmurs.* Am. Heart J. 66:443,1963.
2. Barlow, J. B., and Bosman, C. K.: *Aneurysmal protrusion of the posterior leaflet of the mitral valve: an auscultatory-electrocardiographic syndrome.* Am. Heart J. 71:166,1965.
3. Criley, J. M., Lewis, K. B., Humphries, J. O., et al.: *Prolapse of the mitral valve: clinical and cine-angiocardiographic findings.* Br. Heart J. 28:488,1966.
4. Stannard, M., Sloman, J. G., Hare, W. S., et al.: *Prolapse of the posterior leaflet of the mitral valve. A clinical, familial and cineangiographic study.* Br. Med. J. 3:71,1967.
5. Barlow, J. B., Bosman, C. K., Pocock, W. A., et al.: *Late systolic murmurs and non-ejection ('mid-late') systolic clicks: An analysis of 90 patients.* Br. Heart J. 30:203,1968.
6. Markiewicz, W., Stoner, J., London, E., et al.: *Mitral valve prolapse in one hundred presumably healthy young females.* Circulation 53:464,1976.
7. Procacci, P. M., Savran, S. V., Schreiter, S. L., et al.: *Prevalence of clinical mitral-valve prolapse in 1169 young women.* N. Engl. J. Med. 294:1086,1976.

8. Promerance, A.: *Ballooning deformity (mucoid degeneration) of atrioventricular valves*. Br. Heart J. 31:343,1969.
9. Sherman, E. B., Char, F., Dungan, W. T., et al.: *Myxomatous transformation of the mitral valve producing mitral insufficiency. Floppy valve syndrome*. Am. J. Dis. Child. 119:171,1970.
10. McCarthy, L. J., and Wolf, P. L.: *Mucoid degeneration of heart valves: Blue valve syndrome*. Am. J. Clin. Pathol. 54:582,1970.
11. Davis, R. H., Schuster, B., Knoebel, S. B., et al.: *Myxomatous degeneration of the mitral valve*. Am. J. Cardiol. 28:449,1971.
12. Edwards, J. E.: *Mitral insufficiency resulting from "overshooting" of leaflets*. Circulation 43:606,1971.
13. Kern, W. H., and Tucker, B. L.: *Myxoid changes in cardiac valves: pathologic, clinical, and ultrastructural studies*. Am. Heart J. 84:294,1972.
14. Roberts, W. C., Dangel, J. C., and Bulkley, B. H.: *Non-rheumatic valvular cardiac disease: a clinicopathologic survey of 27 different conditions causing valvular dysfunction*. Cardiovasc. Clin. 5(2):333,1973.
15. Ranganathan, N., Silver, M. D., Robinson, T. I., et al.: *Angiographic-morphologic correlation in patients with severe mitral regurgitation due to prolapse of the posterior mitral valve leaflet*. Circulation 48:514,1973.
16. Marshall, C. E., and Shappell, S. D.: *Sudden death and the ballooning posterior leaflet syndrome: detailed anatomic and histochemical investigation*. Arch. Pathol. 98:134,1974.
17. Guthrie, R. B., and Edwards, J. E.: *Pathology of the myxomatous mitral valve: nature, secondary changes and complications*. Minn. Med. 59:637,1976.
18. Shrivastava, S., Guthrie, R. B., and Edwards, J. E.: *Prolapse of the mitral valve*. Mod. Concepts Cardiovasc. Dis. 46:57,1977.
19. Bulkley, B. H., and Roberts, W. C.: *Dilatation of the mitral anulus. A rare cause of mitral regurgitation*. Am. J. Med. 59:457,1975.
20. Renteria, V. G., Ferrans, V. J., Jones, M., et al.: *Intracellular collagen fibrils in prolapsed ("floppy") human atrioventricular valves*. Lab. Invest. (in press).
21. Roberts, W. C., and Perloff, J. K.: *Mitral valvular disease. A clinicopathologic survey of the conditions causing the mitral valve to function abnormally*. Ann. Intern. Med. 77:939,1972.
22. Jeresaty, R. M.: *Etiology of the mitral valve prolapse-click syndrome*. Am. J. Cardiol. 36:110,1974.
23. McDonald, A., Harris, A., Jetterson, K., et al.: *Association of prolapse of posterior cusp of mitral valve and atrial septal defect*. Br. Heart J. 33:383,1971.
24. Pocock, W. A., and Barlow, J. B.: *An association between billowing posterior mitral leaflet syndrome and congenital heart disease, particularly atrial septal defect*. Am. Heart J. 81:720,1971.
25. Betriu, A., Wigle, E. D., Felderhof, C. H., et al.: *Prolapse of the posterior leaflet of the mitral valve associated with secundum atrial septal defect*. Am. J. Cardiol. 35:363,1975.
26. Leachman, R. D., Cokkinos, D. V., and Cooley, D. A.: *Association of ostium secundum atrial septal defects with mitral valve prolapse*. Am. J. Cardiol. 38:167,1976.
27. Edynak, G. M., and Rawson, A. J.: *Ruptured aneurysm of the mitral valve in a Marfan-like syndrome*. Am. J. Cardiol. 11:674,1963.
28. Ragib, G., Jue, K. L., Anderson, R. C., et al.: *Marfan's syndrome with mitral insufficiency*. Am. J. Cardiol. 16:127,1965.
29. Read, R. C., Thal, A. P., and Vernon, E. W.: *Symptomatic valvular myxomatous transformation (the floppy valve syndrome); a possible forme fruste of the Marfan syndrome*. Circulation 32:897,1965.
30. Shankar, K. R., Hultgren, M. K., Laver, R. M., et al.: *Lethal tricuspid and mitral regurgitation in Marfan's syndrome*. Am. J. Cardiol. 20:122,1967.
31. Dietzman, R. H., Peter, E. T., Wang, Y., et al.: *Mitral insufficiency in Marfan's syndrome. A case report of surgical correction*. Dis. Chest 51:650,1967.
32. Crocker, D. W.: *Marfan's syndrome confined to the mitral valve region: two cases in siblings*. Am. Heart J. 76:538,1968.
33. Grossman, M., Knott, A. P., Jr., and Jacoby, W. J., Jr.: *Calcified annulus fibrosis with mitral insufficiency with Marfan's syndrome*. Arch. Intern. Med. 121:561,1968.
34. Jortner, R., Shahin, W., Eshkol, D., et al.: *Cardiovascular manifestations and surgery for Marfan's syndrome*. Dis. Chest 56:24,1969.
35. Goodman, D., Kimbiris, D., and Linhart, J. W.: *Chordae tendineae rupture complicating the systolic click-late systolic murmur syndrome*. Am. J. Cardiol. 33:681,1974.
36. Lachman, A. S., Bramwell-Jones, D. M., Lakier, J. B., et al.: *Infective endocarditis in the billowing mitral leaflet syndrome*. Br. Heart J. 37:326,1975.

37. Arnett, E. N., and Roberts, W. C.: *Active infective endocarditis: a clinicopathologic analysis of 137 necropsy patients.* Curr. Probl. Cardiol. 1(7):1,1976.

38. Roberts, W. C., and Buchbinder, N. A.: *Healed left-sided infective endocarditis. A clinicopathologic study of 59 patients.* Am. J. Cardiol. 40:876,1977.

39. DeMaria, A. N., Amsterdam, E. A., Vismara, L. A., et al.: *Arrhythmias in the mitral valve prolapse syndrome. Prevalence, nature and frequency.* Ann. Intern. Med. 84:656,1976.

40. Barnett, H. J., Jones, M. W., Boughner, D. R., et al.: *Cerebral ischemic events associated with prolapsing mitral valve.* Arch. Neurol. 33:777,1976.

41. Roberts, W. C.: *Coronary embolism. A review of causes, consequences and diagnostic considerations.* Cardiovasc. Med. 3:699,1978.

42. Roberts, W. C.: *Anatomically isolated aortic valvular disease. The case against its being of rheumatic etiology.* Am. J. Med. 49:151,1970.

43. Roberts, W. C.: *Valvular, subvalvular, and supravalvular aortic stenosis: morphologic features.* Cardiovasc. Clin. 5(1):97,1973.

44. Roberts, W. C., and Virmani, R.: *Aschoff bodies at necropsy in valvular heart disease. Evidence from an analysis of 543 patients over 14 years of age that rheumatic heart disease, at least anatomically, is a disease of the mitral valve.* Circulation 57:803,1978.

45. Roberts, W. C., and Morrow, A. G.: *Congential aortic stenosis produced by a unicommissural valve.* Br. Heart J. 27:505,1965.

46. Roberts, W. C., and Elliott, L. P.: *Lesions complicating the congenitally bicuspid aortic valve. Anatomic and radiographic features.* Radiol. Clin. North Am. 6:409,1968.

47. Roberts, W. C.: *The structure of the aortic valve in clinically-isolated aortic stenosis. An autopsy study of 162 patients over 15 years of age.* Circulation 42:91,1970.

48. Roberts, W. C.: *The congenitally bicuspid aortic valve. A study of 85 autopsy cases.* Am. J. Cardiol. 26:72,1970.

49. Roberts, W. C., Perloff, J. K., and Costantino, T.: *Severe valvular aortic stenosis in patients over 65 years of age. A clinicopathologic study.* Am. J. Cardiol. 27:497,1971.

50. Falcone, M. W., Roberts, W. C., Morrow, A. G., et al.: *Congenital aortic stenosis resulting from unicommissural valve. Clinical and anatomic features in twenty-one adult patients.* Circulation 44:272,1971.

51. Karsner, H. T., and Koletsky, S.: *Calcific Disease of the Aortic Valve.* J. B. Lippincott, Philadelphia, 1947.

52. Edwards, J. E.: *Pathologic aspects of cardiac valvular insufficiencies.* Arch. Surg. 77:634,1958.

53. Osler, W.: *The bicuspid condition of the aortic valves.* Trans. Assoc. Am. Physicians 2:185,1886.

54. Grant, R. T., Wood, J. E., and Jones, T. D.: *Heart valve irregularities in relation to subacute bacterial endocarditis.* Heart 14:247,1928.

55. Lewis, T., and Grant, R. T.: *Observations relating to subacute infective endocarditis. Part 1. Notes on the normal structure of the aortic valve. Part 2. Bicuspid aortic valves of congenital origin. Part 3. Bicuspid aortic valves in subacute infective endocarditis.* Heart 10:21,1923.

56. Starling, H. J.: *Endocarditis lenta.* Q. J. Med. 16:263,1923.

57. Fulton, M. N., and Levine, S. A.: *Subacute bacterial endocarditis, with special reference to the valvular lesions and previous history.* Am. J. Med. Sci. 183:60,1932.

58. Roberts, W. C.: *Characteristics and consequences of infective endocarditis (active or healed or both) learned from morphologic studies.* In Rahimtoola, S. H. (ed.): *Infective Endocarditis,* Grune & Stratton, New York, 1978, pp. 55–123.

59. Edwards, J. E.: *The congenital bicuspid aortic valve.* Circulation 23:485,1961.

60. Bishop, L. F., Jr., and Trubek, M.: *Bicuspid aortic valve. A differential study between inflammatory and congenital origin.* J. Tech. Meth. 15:111,1936.

61. Koletsky, S.: *Congenital bicuspid aortic valves.* Arch. Intern. Med. 67:129,1941.

62. Edwards, J. E.: *Congenital malformations of the heart and great vessels: C. Malformations of the valves.* In Gould, S. E. (ed.): *Pathology of the Heart and Blood Vessels,* ed. 3. Charles C Thomas, Springfield, Ill., 1968, p. 341.

63. Fontana, R. S., and Edwards, J. E.: *Congenital Cardiac Disease. A Review of 357 Cases Studied Pathologically.* W. B. Saunders, Philadelphia, 1962.

64. Morrow, A. G., Fort, L., III, Roberts, W. C., et al.: *Discrete subaortic stenosis complicated by aortic valvular regurgitation. Clinical, hemodynamic, and pathologic studies and the results of operative treatment.* Circulation 20:1003,1959.

65. Reis, R. L., Peterson, L. M., Mason, D. T., et al.: *Congenital fixed subvalvular aortic stenosis. An anatomical classification and correlations with operative results.* Circulation 43,44(Suppl. I):11,1971.

66. Muna, W. F. T., Ferrans, V. J., Pierce, J. E., et al.: *Discrete subaortic stenosis in Newfoundland dogs: association of infective endocarditis*. Am. J. Cardiol. 41:746,1978.

67. Maron, B. J., Redwood, D. R., Roberts, W. C., et al.: *Tunnel subaortic stenosis. Left ventricular outflow tract obstruction produced by fibromuscular tubular narrowing*. Circulation 54:404,1976.

68. Teare, D.: *Asymmetrical hypertrophy of the heart in young adults*. Br. Heart J. 20:1,1958.

69. Epstein, S. E., Henry, W. L., Clark, C. E., et al.: *Asymmetric septal hypertrophy*. Ann. Intern. Med. 81:650,1974.

70. Maron, B. J., Edwards, J. E., Ferrans, V. J., et al.: *Congenital heart malformations associated with disproportionate ventricular septal thickening*. Circulation 52:926,1975.

71. Maron, B. J., Clark, C. E., Henry, W. L., et al.: *Prevalence and characteristics of disproportionate ventricular septal thickening in patients with acquired or congenital heart disease: echocardiographic and morphologic findings*. Circulation 55:489,1977.

72. Maron, B. J., Savage, D. D., Clark, C. E., et al.: *Prevalence and characteristics of disproportionate ventricular septal thickening in patients with coronary artery disease*. Circulation 57:250,1978.

73. Maron, B. J., Verter, J., and Kapur, S.: *Disproportionate ventricular septal thickening in the developing normal human heart*. Circulation 57:520,1978.

74. Maron, B. J., Edwards, J. E., and Epstein, S. E.: *Disproportionate ventricular septal thickening in patients with systemic hypertension*. Chest 73:466,1978.

75. Spray, T. L., Maron, B. J., Morrow, A. G., et al.: *A discussion on hypertrophic cardiomyopathy*. Am. Heart J. 95:511,1978.

76. Maron, B. J., Gottdiener, J. S., Roberts, W. C., et al.: *Disproportionate ventricular septal thickening (ASH) with systolic anterior motion of the anterior mitral leaflet secondary to valvular heart disease*. Br. Heart J. (in press).

77. Isner, J. M., Falcone, M. W., Virmani, R., et al.: *Cardiac sarcoma causing "ASH" and simulating coronary heart disease*. Am. J. Med. (in press).

78. Roberts, W. C., and Ferrans, V. J.: *Pathologic anatomy of the cardiomyopathies. Idiopathic dilated and hypertrophic types, infiltrative types, and endomyocardial disease with and without eosinophilia*. Hum. Pathol. 6:287,1975.

79. Maron, B. J., Gottdiener, J. S., Roberts, W. C., et al.: *Left ventricular outflow tract obstruction due to systolic anterior motion of the anterior mitral leaflet in patients with concentric left ventricular hypertrophy*. Circulation 57:527,1978.

80. McReynolds, R. A., and Roberts, W. C.: *The intramural coronary arteries in hypertrophic cardiomyopathy*. Am. J. Cardiol. 35:120,1975.

81. Maron, B. J., Ferrans, V. J., Henry, W. L., et al.: *Differences in distribution of myocardial abnormalities in patients with obstructive and nonobstructive asymmetric septal hypertrophy (ASH). Light and electron microscopic findings*. Circulation 50:436,1974.

82. Henry, W. L., Clark, C. E., Roberts, W. C., et al.: *Differences in distribution of myocardial abnormalities in patients with obstructive and non-obstructive asymmetric septal hypertrophy (ASH). Echocardiographic and gross anatomic findings*. Circulation 50:447,1974.

83. Maron, B. J., Epstein, S. E., and Roberts, W. C.: *Cardiac muscle cell disorganization in the ventricular septum: evidence from quantitative histology that it is a highly sensitive marker of hypertrophic cardiomyopathy*. Am. J. Cardiol. 41:435,1978.

84. Ferrans, V. J., Morrow, A. G., and Roberts, W. C.: *Myocardial ultrastructure in idiopathic hypertrophic subaortic stenosis. A study of operatively excised left ventricular outflow tract muscle in 14 patients*. Circulation 45:769,1972.

85. Maron, B. J., Roberts, W. C., Edwards, J. E., et al.: *Sudden death in patients with hypertrophic cardiomyopathy. Characterization of 26 patients without functional limitation*. Am. J. Cardiol. 41:803,1978.

86. Maron, B. J., Lipson, L. C., Roberts, W. C., et al.: *"Malignant" hypertrophic cardiomyopathy. Identification of a subgroup of families with unusually frequent premature deaths*. Am. J. Cardiol. 41:1133,1978.

87. Roberts, W. C., Perry, L. W., Chandra, R. S., et al.: *Aortic valve atresia: a new classification based on necropsy study of 73 cases*. Am. J. Cardiol. 37:753,1976.

88. Ewy, G. A., Marcus, F. I., Bohjalian, O., et al.: *Muscular subaortic stenosis. Clinical and pathologic observations in an elderly patient*. Am. J. Cardiol. 22:126,1968.

89. Roberts, W. C.: *Cardiomyopathy and myocarditis: morphologic features*. Adv. Cardiol. 22:184,1978.

90. Merrill, W. H., Henry, W. L., Maron, B. J., et al.: *Echocardiographic assessment of the left ventricle following myotomy and myectomy for idiopathic hypertrophic subaortic stenosis (IHSS)*. Am. J. Cardiol. 41:435,1978.

91. MARON, B. J., HENRY, W. L., ROBERTS, W. C., ET AL.: *Comparison of echocardiographic and necropsy measurements of ventricular wall thicknesses in patients with and without disproportionate septal thickening.* Circulation 55:341,1977.

92. COOLEY, D. A., LEACHMAN, R. D., AND WUKASCH, D. C.: *Diffuse muscular subaortic stenosis: surgical treatment.* Am. J. Cardiol. 31:1,1973.

93. COOLEY, D. A., GRACE, R. R., WUKASCH, D. C., ET AL.: *Replacement and/or repair of the mitral valve as treatment of idiopathic hypertrophic subaortic stenosis.* Cardiovasc. Dis. Bull. Texas Heart Inst. 3:381,1976.

94. ROBERTS, W. C.: *Operative treatment of hypertrophic obstructive cardiomyopathy. The case against mitral valve replacement.* Am. J. Cardiol. 32:377,1973.

95. ROBERTS, W. C.: *Left ventricular outflow tract obstruction and aortic regurgitations.* In Edwards, J. E., LEV, M., and Abell, M. R. (eds.): *The Heart,* Williams & Wilkins, Baltimore, 1974, pp. 110–175.

96. BULKLEY, B. H., AND ROBERTS, W. C.: *Ankylosing spondylitis and aortic regurgitation. Description of the characteristic cardiovascular lesion from study of eight necropsy patients.* Circulation 48:1014,1973.

97. ROBERTS, W. C., HOLLINGSWORTH, J. F., BULKLEY, B. H., ET AL.: *Combined mitral and aortic regurgitation in ankylosing spondylitis. Angiographic and anatomic features.* Am. J. Med. 56:237,1974.

98. POMERANCE, A., AND DAVIES, M. J.: *Congenital aneurysms of all three sinuses of Valsalva.* J. Pathol. Bacteriol. 89:607,1965.

99. ARNETT, E. N., AND ROBERTS, W. C.: *Valve ring abscess in active infective endocarditis. Frequency, location, and clues to clinical diagnosis from the study of 95 necropsy patients.* Circulation 54:140,1976.

100. EDWARDS, J. E., AND BURCHELL, M. B.: *Specimen exhibiting the essential lesion in aneurysm of the aortic sinus.* Mayo Clin. Proc. 31:407,1956.

101. FISHBEIN, M. C., OBMA, R., AND ROBERTS, W. C.: *Unruptured sinus of Valsalva aneurysm.* Am. J. Cardiol. 35:918,1975.

102. SAKAKIBARA, S., AND KONNO, S.: *Congenital aneurysm of the sinus of Valsalva. Anatomy and classification.* Am. Heart J. 63:405,1962.

103. FOWLER, R. E. L., AND BEVEL, H. H.: *Aneurysms of the sinus of Valsalva.* Pediatrics 8:340,1951.

104. KIEFFER, S. A., AND WINCHELL, P.: *Congenital aneurysms of the aortic sinuses with cardioaortic fistula.* Dis. Chest 38:79,1960.

105. KERBER, R. W., RIDGES, J. D., KRISS, J. P., ET AL.: *Unruptured aneurysm of the sinus of Valsalva producing right ventricular outflow obstruction.* Am. J. Med. 53:775,1972.

106. DURAS, P. F.: *Heart block with aneurysm of the aortic sinus.* Br. Heart J. 6:61,1944.

107. MCKUSICK, V. A.: *Heritable Disorders of Connective Tissue.* C. V. Mosby Co., St. Louis, 1972, pp. 61–223.

108. MURDOCH, J. L., WLAKER, B. A., HALPERN, B. L., ET AL.: *Life expectancy and causes of death in the Marfan syndrome.* N. Engl. J. Med. 286:804,1972.

109. BECKER, A. E.: *Medionecrosis aortae.* Pathol. Microbiol. (Basel) 43:124,1975.

110. SCHLATMANN, T. J. M., AND BECKER, A. E.: *Histologic changes in the normal aging aorta: implications for dissecting aortic aneurysm.* Am. J. Cardiol. 39:13,1977.

111. LEMON, D. K., AND WHITE, C. W.: *Anuloaortic ectasia: angiographic, hemodynamic and clinical comparison with aortic valve insufficiency.* Am. J. Cardiol. 41:482,1978.

112. SCHLATMANN, T. J. M., AND BECKER, A. E.: *Pathogenesis of dissecting aneurysm of aorta. Comparative histopathologic study of significance of medial changes.* Am. J. Cardiol. 39:21,1977.

113. ERDHEIM, J.: *Medionecrosis aortae idiopathica.* Virchows Arch. (Pathol. Anat.) 273:454,1929.

114. GSELL, O.: *Wandnekrosen der Aorta als selbstandige Erkrankung und ihre Beziehung zur Spontanruptur.* Virchows Arch. (path. Anat.) 270:1,1928.

115. ROBERTS, W. C., AND COHEN, L. S.: *Left ventricular papillary muscles. Description of the normal and a survey of conditions causing them to be abnormal.* Circulation 46:138,1972.

116. MCKUSICK, V. A., LOGUE, R. B., AND BAHNSON, H. T.: *Association of aortic valvular disease and cystic medial necrosis of the ascending aorta. Report of four instances.* Circulation 16:188,1957.

117. FUKUDA, T., TADAVARTHY, S. M., AND EDWARDS, J. E.: *Dissecting aneurysm of aorta complicating aortic valvular stenosis.* Circulation 53:169,1976.

The Aorta: Its Acquired Diseases and Their Consequences as Viewed from a Morphologic Perspective

The aorta is the superhighway of the systemic arterial system, and from it arise all major oxygen suppliers of every body organ and tissue. The aorta carries more blood than any other artery in the systemic arterial system, and, therefore, it is the largest systemic artery. It is subjected to aging changes, just like every other tissue and organ in the body, and the major consequence of aging is generalized dilatation. The aorta, obviously, is subject to several diseases, the most important of which are *atherosclerosis* and *dissection,* and although the etiology of neither is known, the means of preventing both is known. In addition to atherosclerosis and dissection, however, the aorta is occasionally the site of *syphilis* and other types of vasculitis, *trauma, congenital anomalies,* and *medial degeneration* with and without the Marfan syndrome. These conditions cause the aorta to *thicken, thin, bulge* (aneurysm), *tear* (partial rupture), *rupture* (through-and-through), *stenose* or *dissect,* or be altered by combinations of these anomalies. This chapter focuses on the morphologic aspects of conditions affecting the aorta, with particular emphasis on atherosclerosis and dissection and their consequences because these are by far the most common aortic diseases.

THE NORMAL AND AGING AORTA

The normal aorta consists of elastic fibers, collagen fibers, smooth muscle cells, and a mucoid ground substance (acid-mucopolysaccharide material). All four of these components change with age.[1] The elastic fibers, which are arranged in parallel layers and which number approximately 56 in the ascending aorta and about 28 in the abdominal aorta,[2] fragment in older persons. The smooth muscle cells appear to decrease in number, and some of those that remain may lose certain organelles, usually the nuclei. The collagen fibers appear to increase with time, probably mainly at the expense of the smooth muscle cells. Also with time, the amount of mucoid ground substance in the wall of the aorta increases. The end result of these changes is weakening of the aorta, so that its lumen enlarges with age. The generalized dilatation of the aorta, which is both a transverse and a longitudinal enlargement, has been given the general name of ''ectasia.''

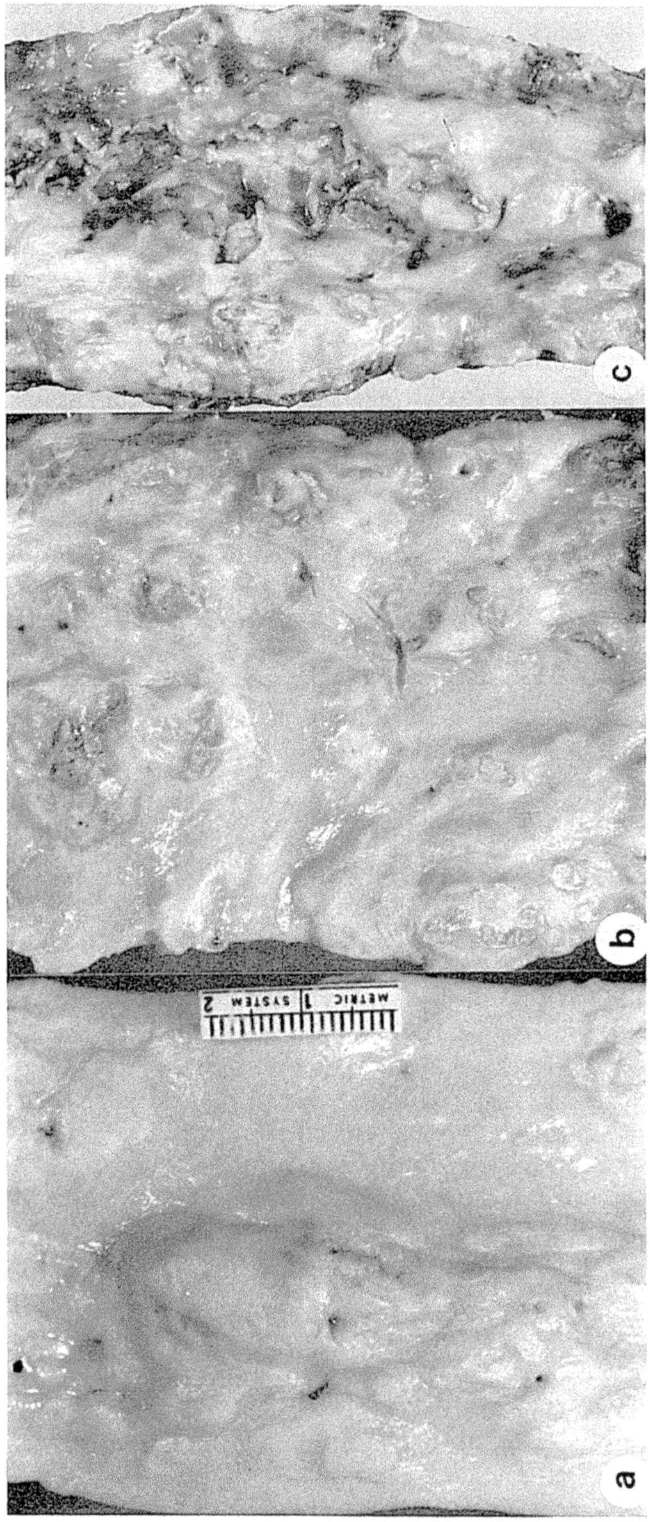
c
b
METRIC 1 SYSTEM 2
a

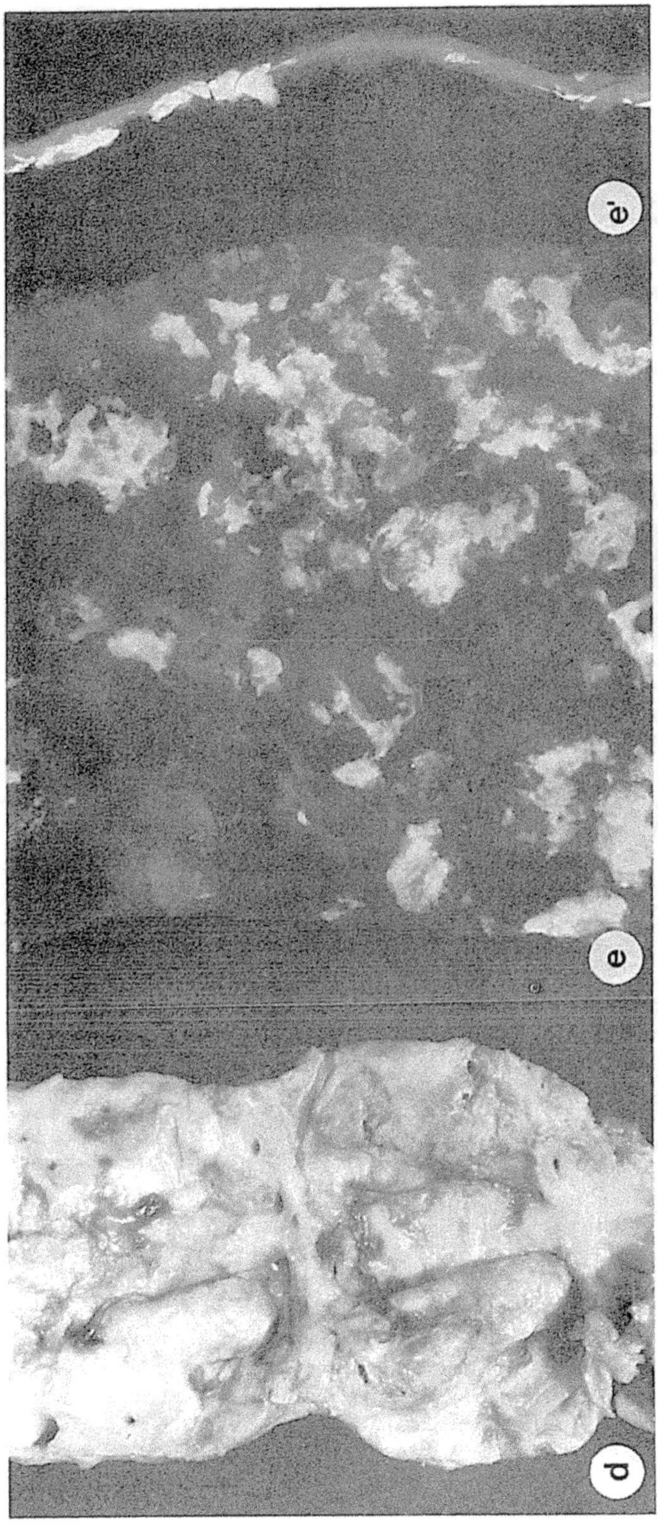

Fig. 1. Opened descending thoracic aortas in 5 different patients showing extensive atherosclerotic plaquing with ulceration and calcification in each (e and e′ are radiographs at necropsy).

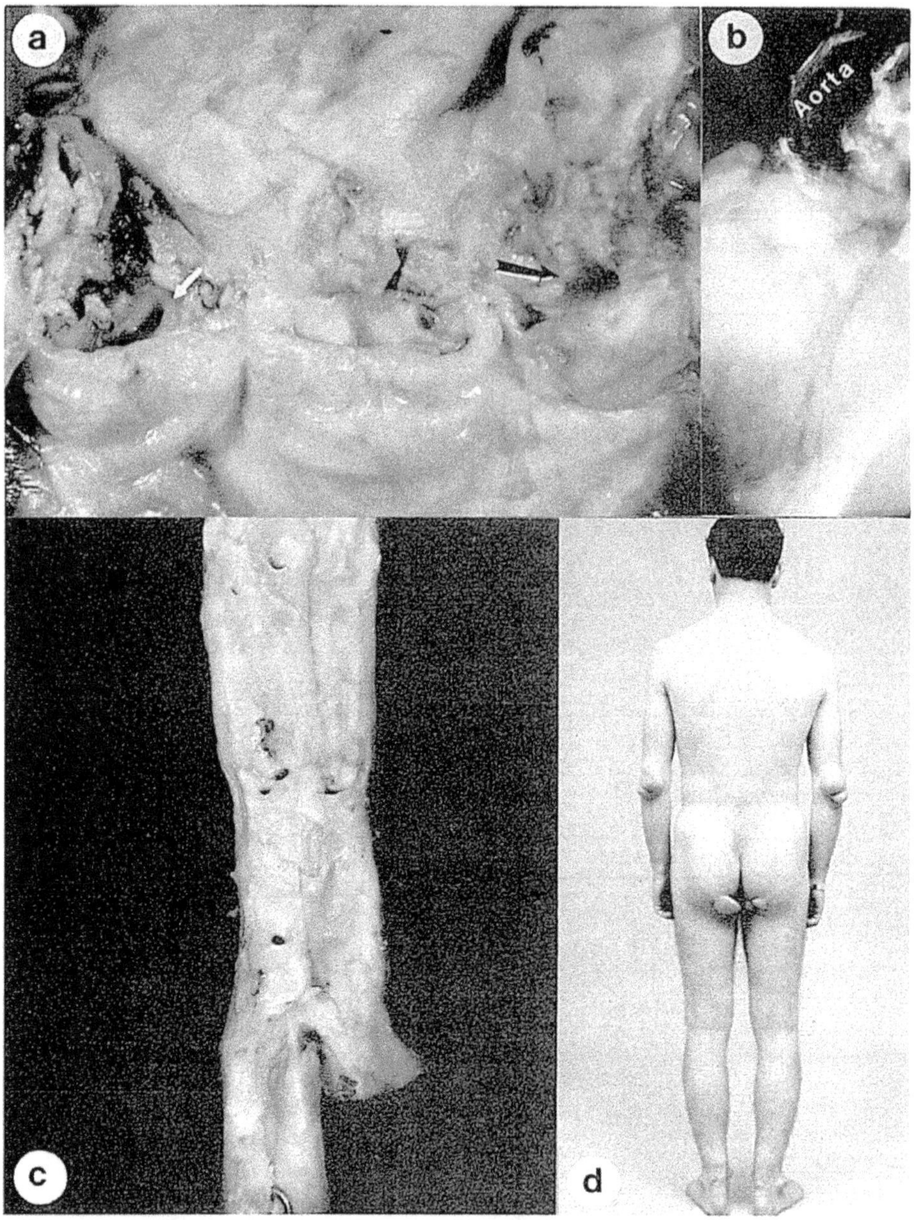

Fig. 2. Severe atherosclerosis in a 28-year-old white man (A70-64) with homozygous type II hyperlipoproteinemia. There is more atherosclerosis in the ascending aorta (*a* and *b*) than in the abdominal aorta (*c*), the reverse of the usual distribution. The atherosclerotic process in the ascending aorta actually invaded the aortic valve cusps, causing them to be rigid and leading to aortic stenosis. In addition, the calcific process (*b*) in the ascending aorta caused severe narrowing of the coronary ostia (arrows). This patient had many xanthomas (*d*). He died suddenly from severe coronary narrowing by atherosclerotic plaques.

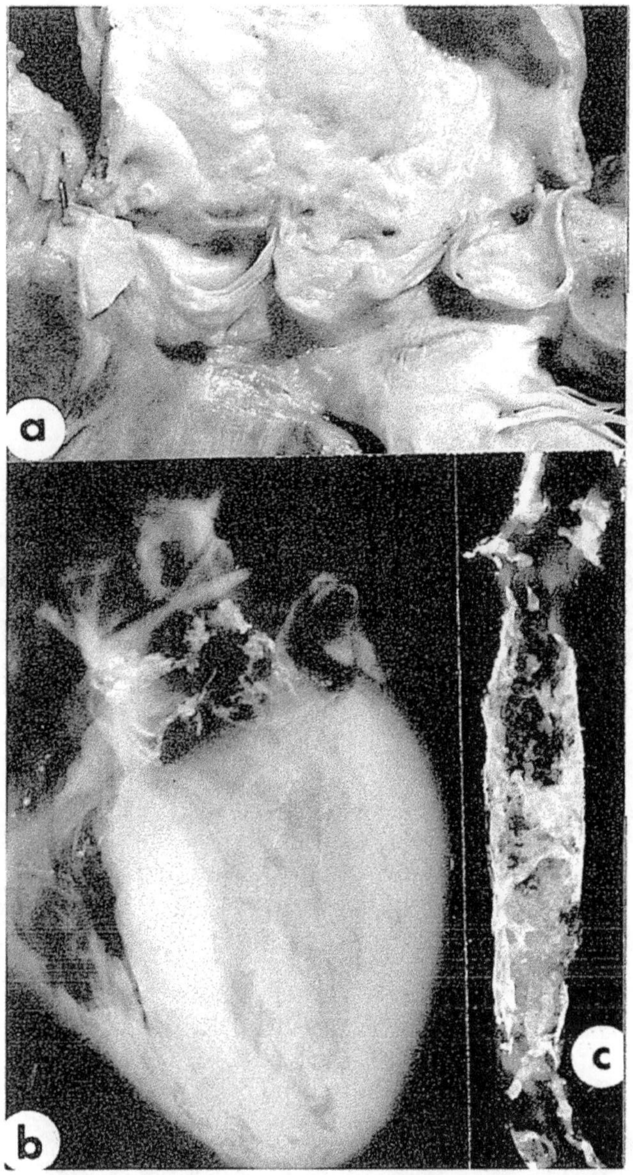

Fig. 3. Heart and aorta in a 51-year-old man (A71-22) with heterozygous type II hyperlipoproteinemia. During life, he had a grade 2/6 systolic ejection murmur interpreted as evidence of "aortic stenosis." At necropsy, small calcific deposits were present on the aortic aspects of each cusp, but the cusps were freely mobile and the valve orifice was not stenotic. (*a*) Opened ascending aorta, aortic valve, and left ventricle. Although extensive atherosclerotic plaquing is present in the ascending aorta, the degree is far less than that observed in the patient with homozygous type II hyperlipoproteinemia (Fig. 2). (*b*) Radiograph of heart disclosing calcific deposits in the aortic valve, root of aorta, and coronary arteries. (*c*) Radiograph of abdominal aorta showing extensive calcific deposits.

By far, the most common disease of the aorta is atherosclerosis (Figs. 1, 2, and 3). This condition, prevalent in all societies where the mean serum total cholesterol level of adults is greater than 200 mg/dl, begins before age 10 years and is manifested by the appearance of yellow dots or streaks in the intima. Although an area not prone to severe atherosclerosis, these yellow dots or streaks are usually first observed in the descending thoracic aorta, most commonly adjacent to the ostia of the intercostal arteries. Interestingly, these yellow dots or streaks do not appear to be related to serum cholesterol in that

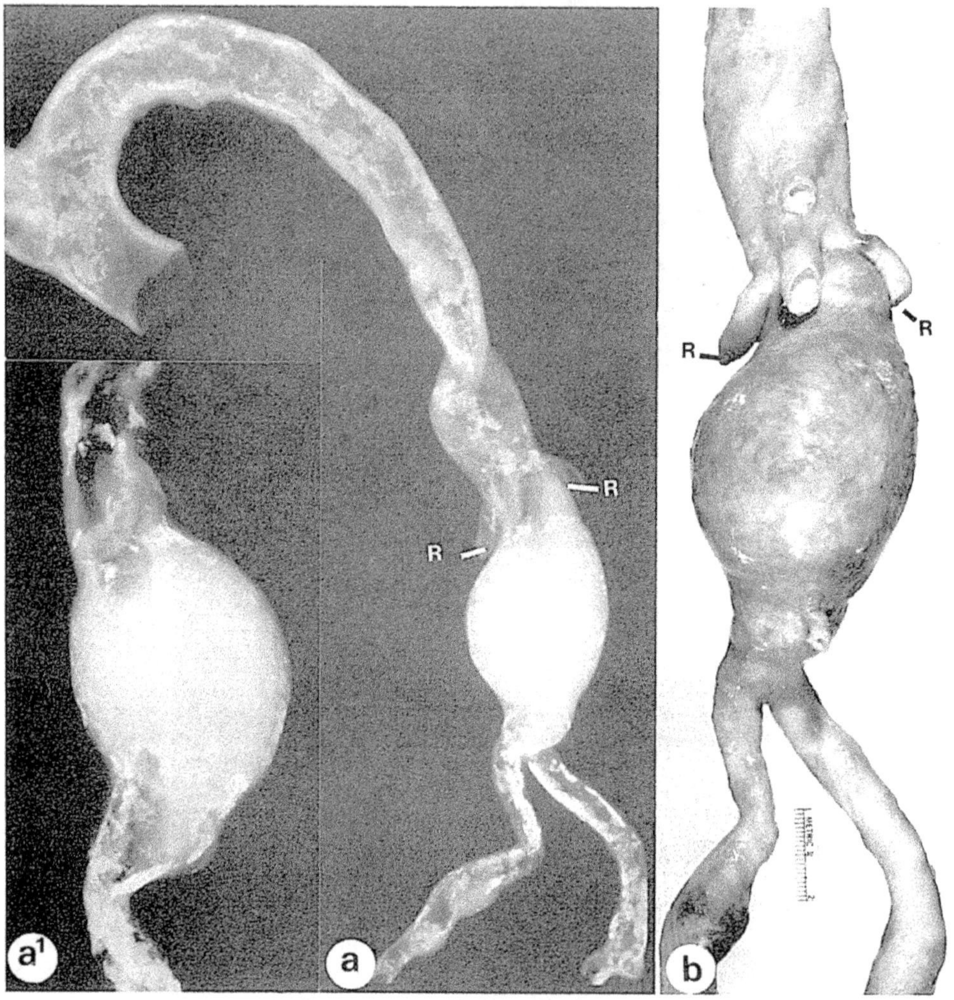

Fig. 4. Asymptomatic abdominal aortic aneurysm in an 89-year-old white woman (A70-164) who died suddenly from coronary heart disease. The aneurysm was never suspected during life. She had no history of systemic hypertension or diabetes mellitus, but the heart weighed 390 gm at necropsy. (*a*) Radiograph of the aorta at autopsy showing extensive calcific deposits. (*a*[1]) Lateral view of the aneurysm showing many calcific deposits in the wall of aorta. (*b*) Exterior view of the aneurysm, which measures nearly 5 cm in maximal transverse width. The aneurysm begins immediately below the renal arteries (R). (*Legend and figure continue on following page.*)

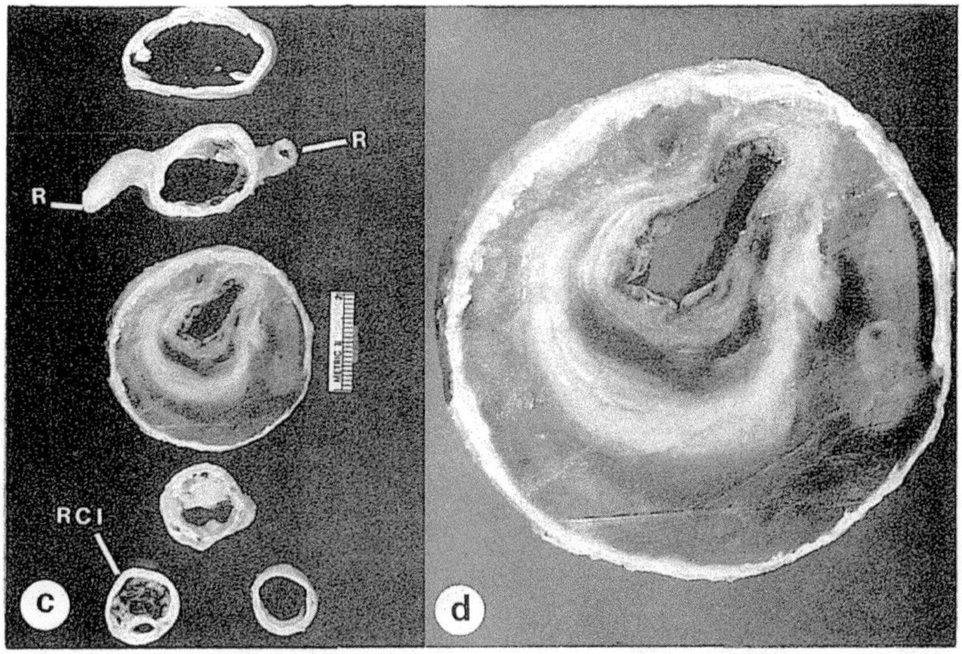

Fig. 4. (*continued*). (*c*) Transverse sections of the abdominal aorta disclosing a large thrombus within the aneurysm. A close-up of the section of the aneurysm is shown in (*d*). Note that the lumen at the site of the aneurysm is much smaller than that above the aneurysm. The lumen of the right common iliac (RCI) artery is >75 percent narrowed in cross-sectional area by thrombus (*c*).

they are just as common in the first two decades of life in persons residing in areas of the world where the average total serum cholesterol levels are under 180 mg/dl as they are in populations where this average level is greater than 200 mg/dl. After age 20, however, fibrosis and complicated atherosclerotic plaques, with few exceptions, are found only in individuals living in areas of the world where the average total serum cholesterol levels are greater than 200 mg/dl.

After age 20 years, atherosclerotic plaques, with rare exceptions, are more extensive in the abdominal portion of aorta than in any other area. As long as the plaques consist entirely of lipid (foam cells), the plaques remain small and, for practical purposes, occur only on the intimal surface of the aorta, that is, on the luminal side of the internal elastic membrane. As the lipid becomes extracellular and is associated with considerable quantities of fibrous tissue and especially calcific deposits, the plaques may cause atrophy of some components of the underlying media. Basically, however, atherosclerosis, whether in the aorta or coronary artery or in any other artery, is an intimal disease, and its effect on the media is purely a secondary phenomenon.

Of all portions of aorta, the area least prone to atherosclerosis—as long as the underlying media is normal—is the ascending aorta. The author has seen a number of patients at necropsy who have had virtually 100 percent intimal surface involvement of the transverse, descending thoracic, and abdominal portions of aorta and, except for a few plaques at the sinotubular junction, virtually no atherosclerotic plaques in the tubular portion of ascending aorta. There are, however, a group of patients that may have more atherosclerosis in the ascending than in the abdominal aorta. These are patients with *type*

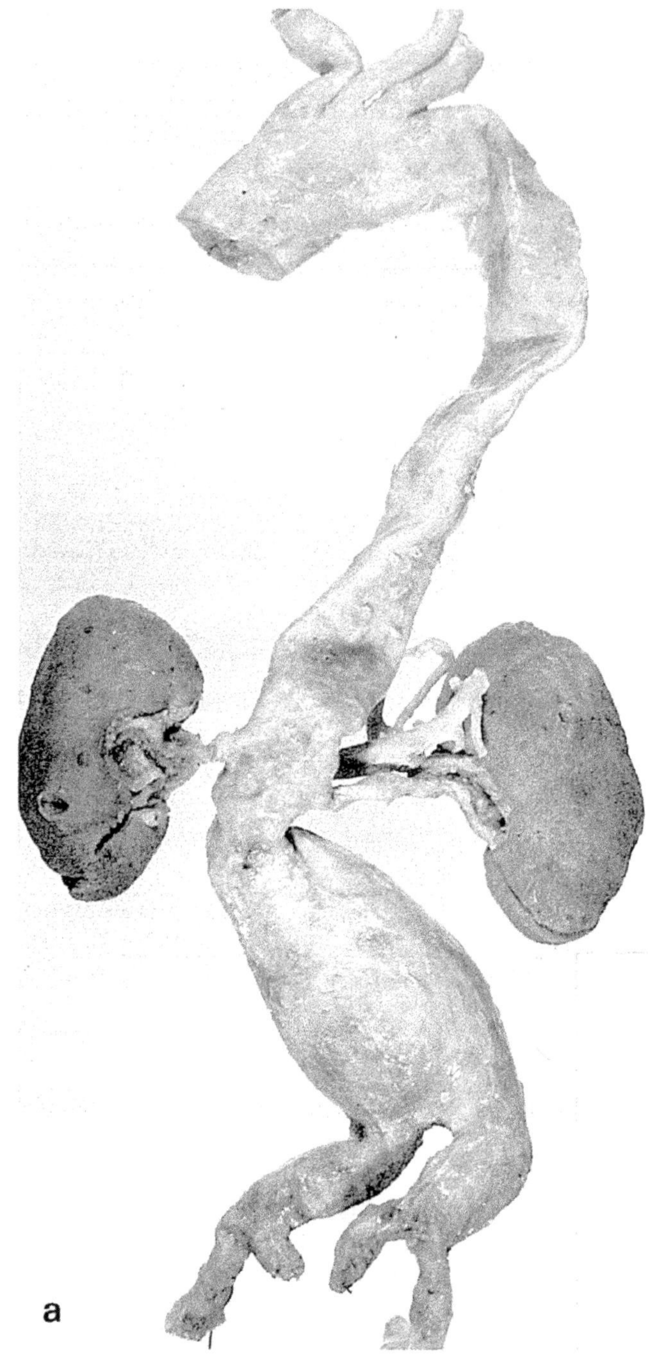

a

Fig. 5. Asymptomatic abdominal aortic aneurysm in a 78-year-old man (DCVAH #78-A-117) who died of bronchogenic carcinoma. He had had both systemic hypertension and diabetes mellitus. At necropsy, the heart weighed 505 gm, and the lumens of both the right and left circumflex coronary arteries were >75 percent narrowed in cross-sectional area by atherosclerotic plaque. (*a*) View of entire aorta showing the fusiform aneurysm of the abdominal portion and of the proximal portions of both common iliac arteries. (*b*) (*facing page*) Radiograph showing extensive calcific deposits in the abdominal aorta and the common iliac arteries. (c, c^{I}, c^{II} and c^{III}) Transverse sections of the entire aorta and the common iliac arteries and their branches showing thrombus occupying

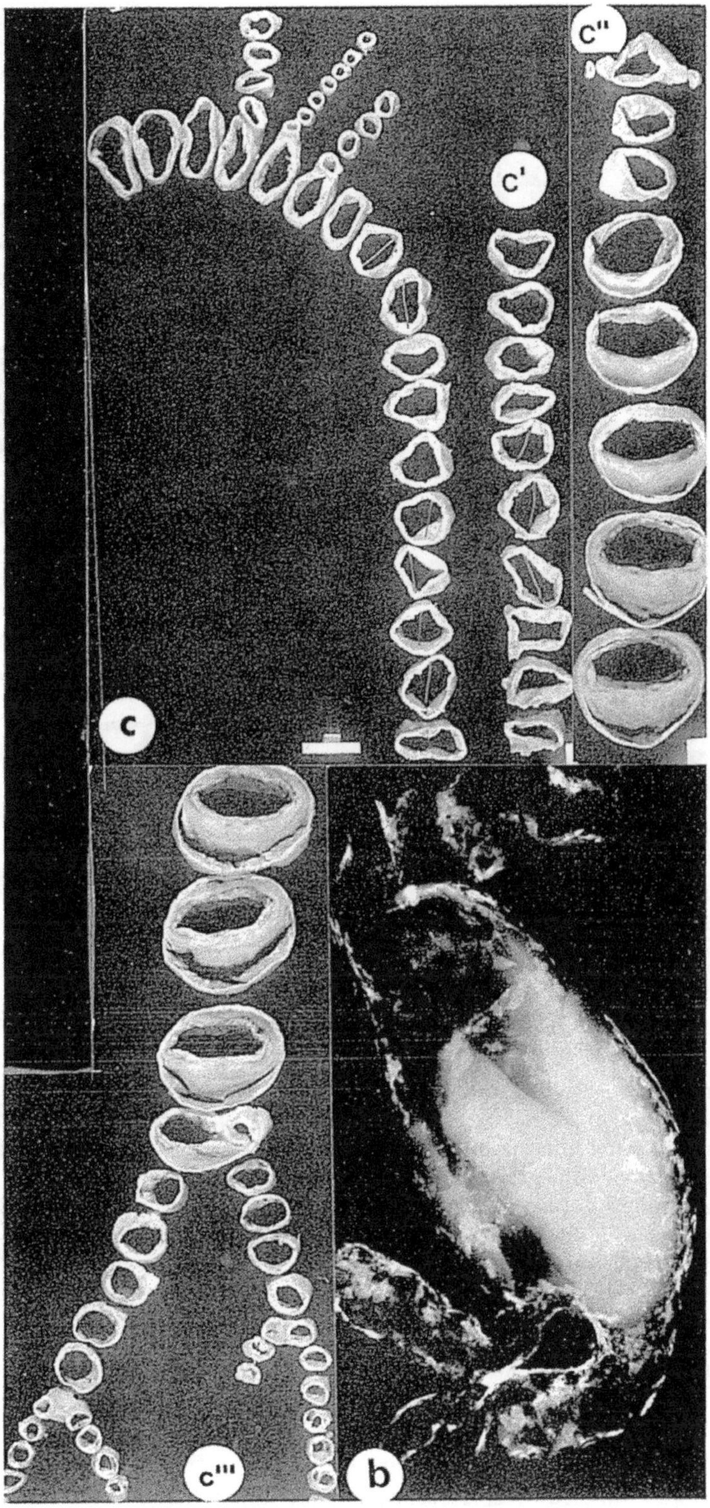

>50 percent of the lumen of the abdominal aortic aneurysm. The lumen of the left femoral artery is severely narrowed.

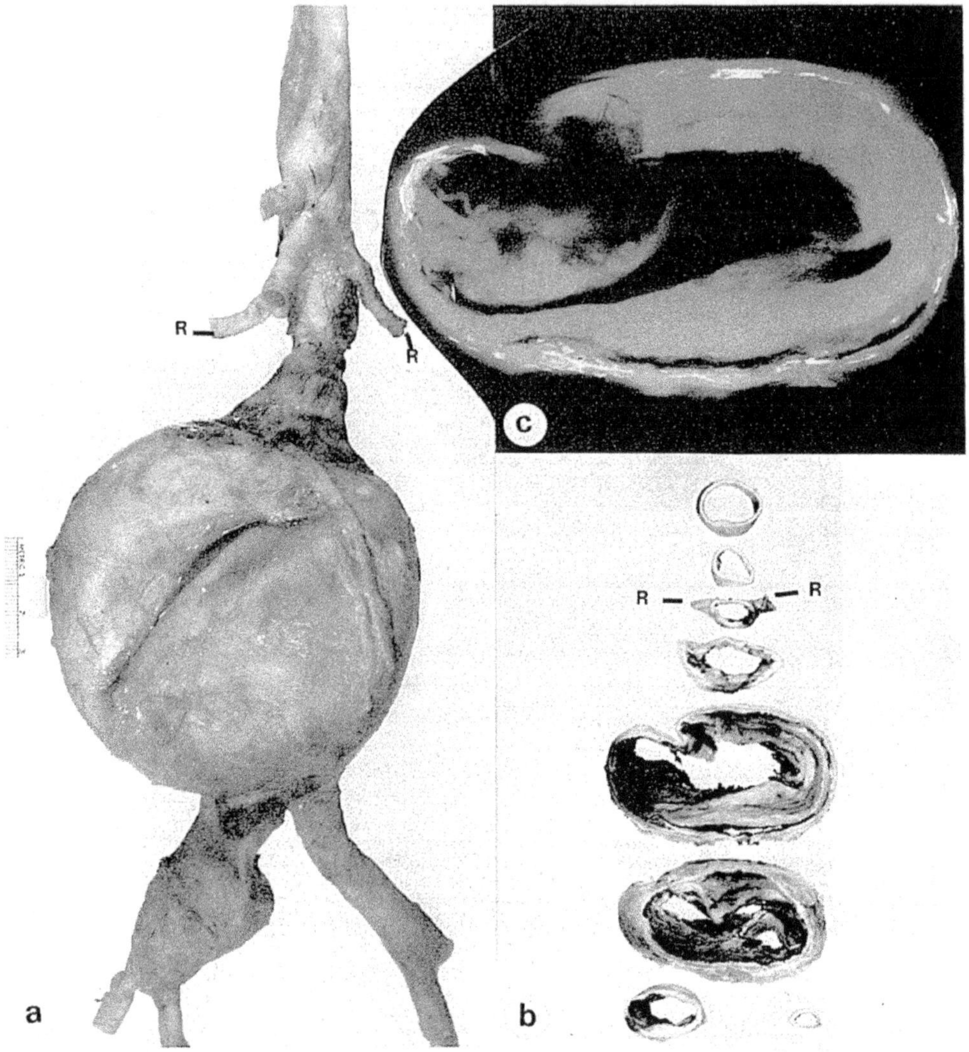

Fig. 6. Asymptomatic abdominal aortic aneurysm in a 57-year-old white man (A71-55) who died of metastatic carcinoma of the tongue. The heart weighed 340 gm. (*a*) Exterior view of abdominal aorta showing the fusiform aneurysm to measure approximately 10 cm in maximal transverse diameter. Another fusiform aneurysm measuring about 3 cm in maximal transverse diameter involves the right common iliac artery. R, renal artery. (*b*) Transverse sections of the abdominal aorta and common iliac arteries showing thrombus within both aneurysms. (*c*) Radiograph of one section of the abdominal aneurysm showing calcific deposits within the arterial wall but none in the thrombus.

II hyperlipoproteinemia, both homozygous and heterozygous, especially for former (Fig. 2).[3] The author has observed massive atherosclerosis with heavy calcific deposits in the ascending aorta in a 28-year-old man with homozygous familial hypercholesterolemia; the plaquing was so extensive that the coronary ostia were severely narrowed and the aortic valve cusps were infiltrated by atherosclerotic material, including foam cells and cholesterol clefts (Fig. 2). Extensive, although lesser degrees of ascending aortic atherosclerosis are observed in patients with heterozygous type II hyperlipoproteinemia (Fig. 3).

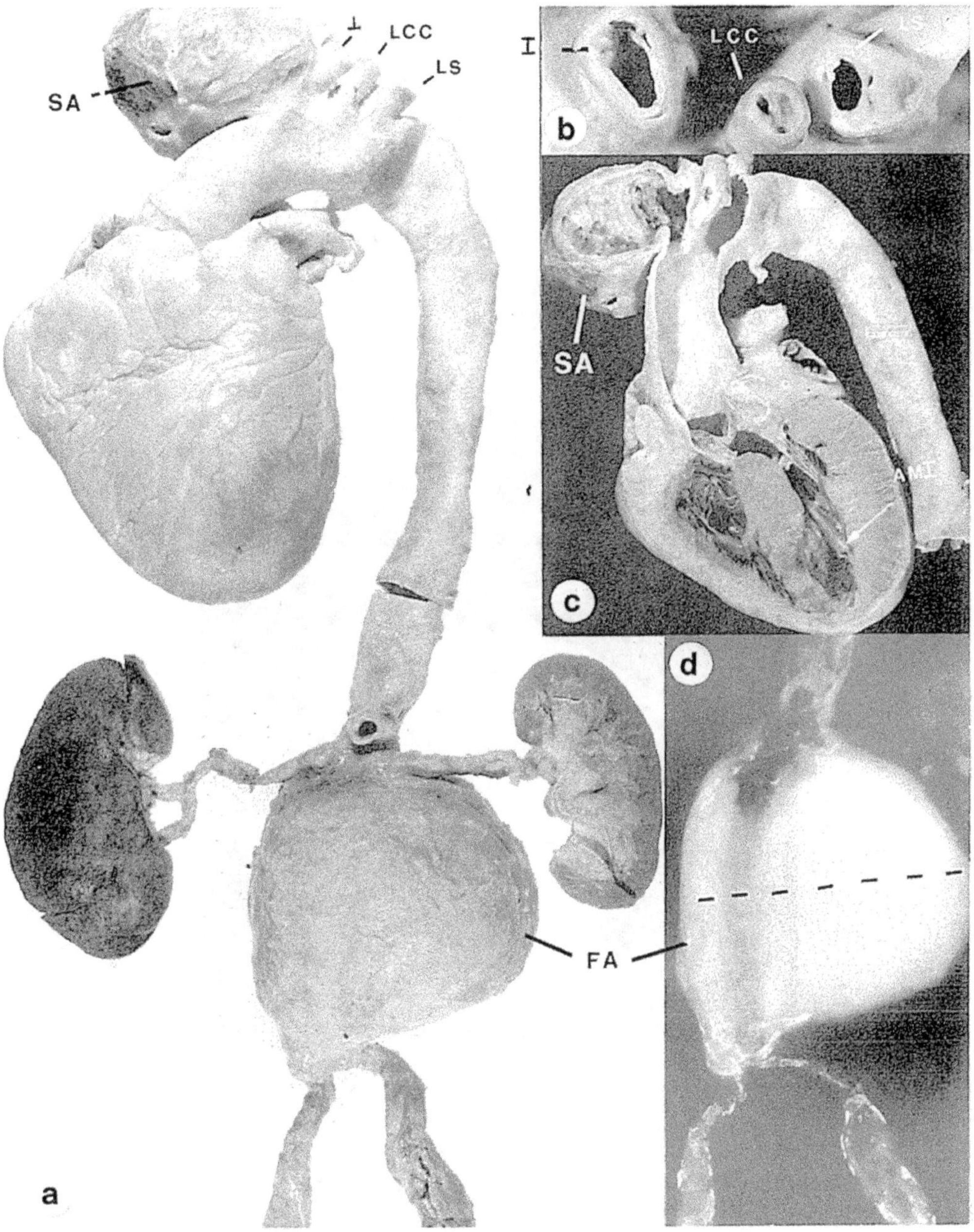

Fig. 7. Saccular ascending aortic aneurysm (SA) and fusiform abdominal aortic (FA) in a 68-year-old white man (GT #76A-33) who died of an acute transmural myocardial infarct. He had had angina pectoris and leg claudication for about 5 years, and an aortic angiogram 4 years before death confirmed a saccular aneurysm arising in the proximal portion of the left innominate artery. He had been known to have systemic hypertension at least since age 50. While recovering from the acute myocardial infarction, he developed anuria, which was attributed to compression of one or both renal arteries by the large abdominal aortic aneurysm, and he died 5 days later.

(*a*) The heart, aorta, common iliac arteries, and kidney showing the saccular aneurysm (SA), which measured up to 8 cm in diameter, arising in the most proximal portion of the innominate (I) artery, and the fusiform abdominal aneurysm (FA), which measured 12 cm in maximal transverse diameter. The abdominal aneurysm pushes both renal arteries cephalad, compressing their lumens. (*b*) Transverse cuts of the innominate, left common carotid (LCC), and left subclavian (LS)

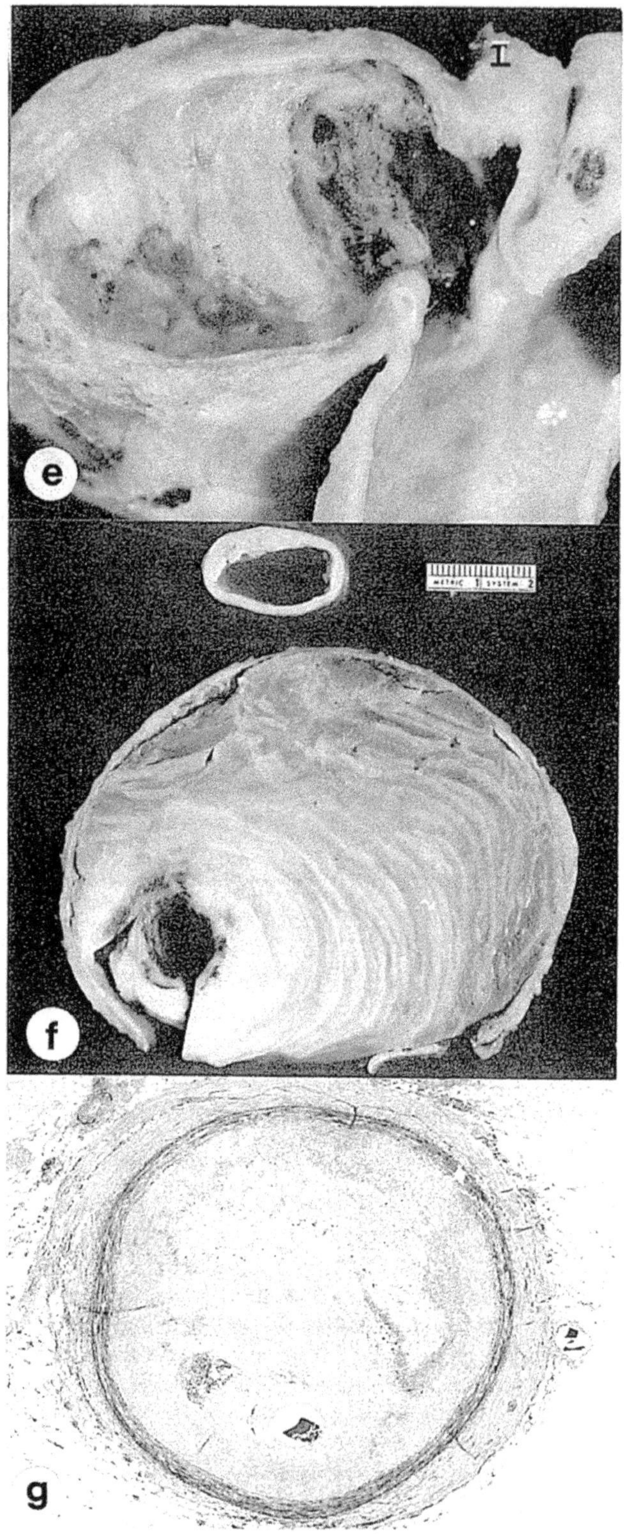

arteries. The lumens of the LCC and LS are narrowed. (*c*) Longitudinal cut of heart and thoracic aorta. The more caudal portion of left ventricle is infarcted (AMI), and a thrombus is present within the left ventricular cavity. The saccular aneurysm, better shown in (*e*), arises from the

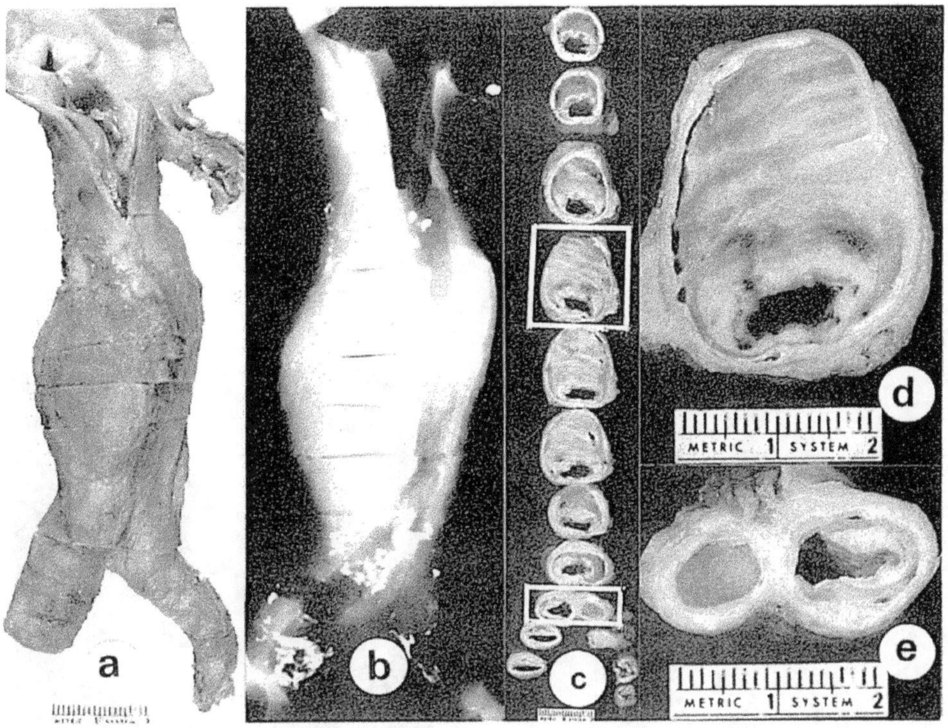

Fig. 8. Symptomatic abdominal aortic aneurysm in a 61-year-old black man (DCVAH #78-A-124) who had a bronchogenic carcinoma but who died from complications of bowel infarction secondary to thrombotic occlusion of the superior mesenteric artery. (*a*) View of abdominal aortic aneurysm. (*b*) Radiograph showing calcific deposits in its wall and severe narrowing of its lumen. (*c*) Transverse sections of the abdominal aortic aneurysm again showing severe narrowing of its lumen by thrombus. (*d*) Close-up of one section in brackets showing laminated thrombus. (*e*) Close-up of the first centimeter of the common iliac arteries (in brackets in *c*) showing complete occlusion of the right one by thrombus.

There are two other conditions in which atherosclerotic plaquing may be extensive in the ascending aorta. One is in patients with *diabetes mellitus,* but the involvement of the ascending portion is not so severe as that in the abdominal portion of aorta. The other condition is *syphilis*. In cardiovascular syphilis, however, the underlying media and adventitia are not normal, so the atherosclerosis in this circumstance appears simply to be one of superimposition on an underlying severely abnormal aorta.

---

innominate (I) artery, and it is virtually completely filled with laminated thrombus. (*d*) Radiograph of the abdominal aneurysm showing the lumen of the aorta within the aneurysm is smaller than the lumen of aorta proximal to the aneurysm. Calcific deposits are present in the walls of both aorta and common iliac arteries. (*f*) Transverse section of abdominal aortic aneurysm (from dashed line in *d*) showing that laminated thrombus occupies most of the area of the aneurysm and that the intraaneurysmal lumen is much smaller than the lumen of aorta just proximal to the aneurysm. A transverse section of aorta just proximal to the origin of the renal arteries is seen to the left of the ruler. (*g*) Photomicrograph (×20, Movat stain) of right coronary artery. The lumens of the left anterior descending and left circumflex coronary arteries also were >75 percent narrowed in cross-sectional area by atherosclerotic plaque.

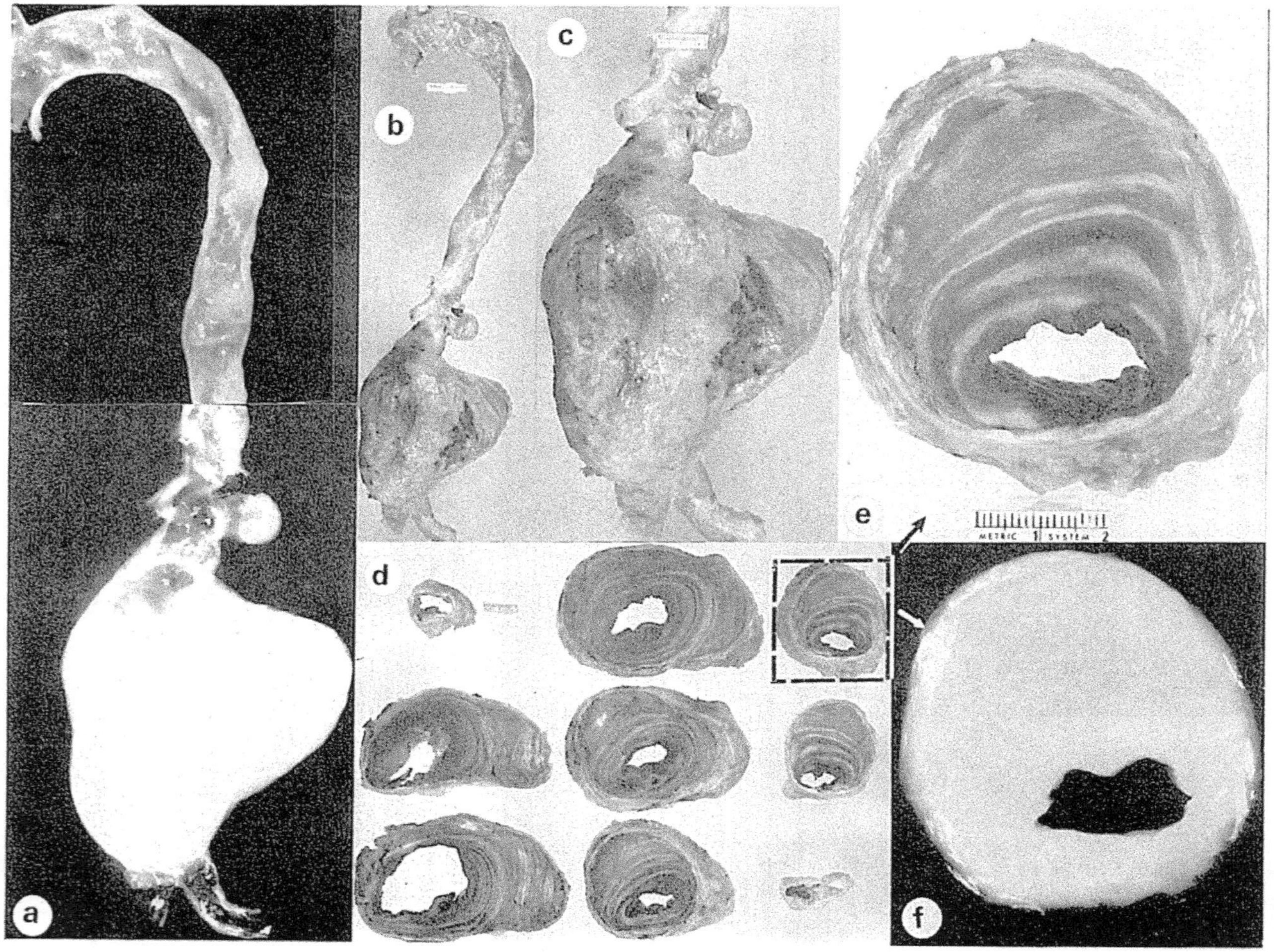

Fig. 9 Rupture of abdominal aortic aneurysm in a 72-year-old white man (DCMEO #78-10-802). He died suddenly shortly after finishing a meal. There apparently was no previous evidence of the presence of an abdominal aneurysm. At necropsy, the heart weighed 590 gm, strongly suggesting that he had had systemic hypertension. A great deal of extravasated blood was present in the retroperitoneal area. (*a*) Radiograph of aorta at necropsy showing a huge abdominal aortic aneurysm measuring approximately 12 cm in maximal transverse diameter. Calcific deposits are present throughout the aorta. In addition to the huge abdominal fusiform aneurysm, six smaller saccular aneurysms are present in the aorta. (*b*) View of entire aorta. (*c*) Close-up of abdominal aneurysm. (*d*) Transverse sections through the abdominal aneurysm showing laminated thrombus with resulting reduction in luminal size. (*e*) Close-up of one section. (*f*) Radiograph of one section showing calcium primarily in the aortic wall and not in the superimposed thrombus.

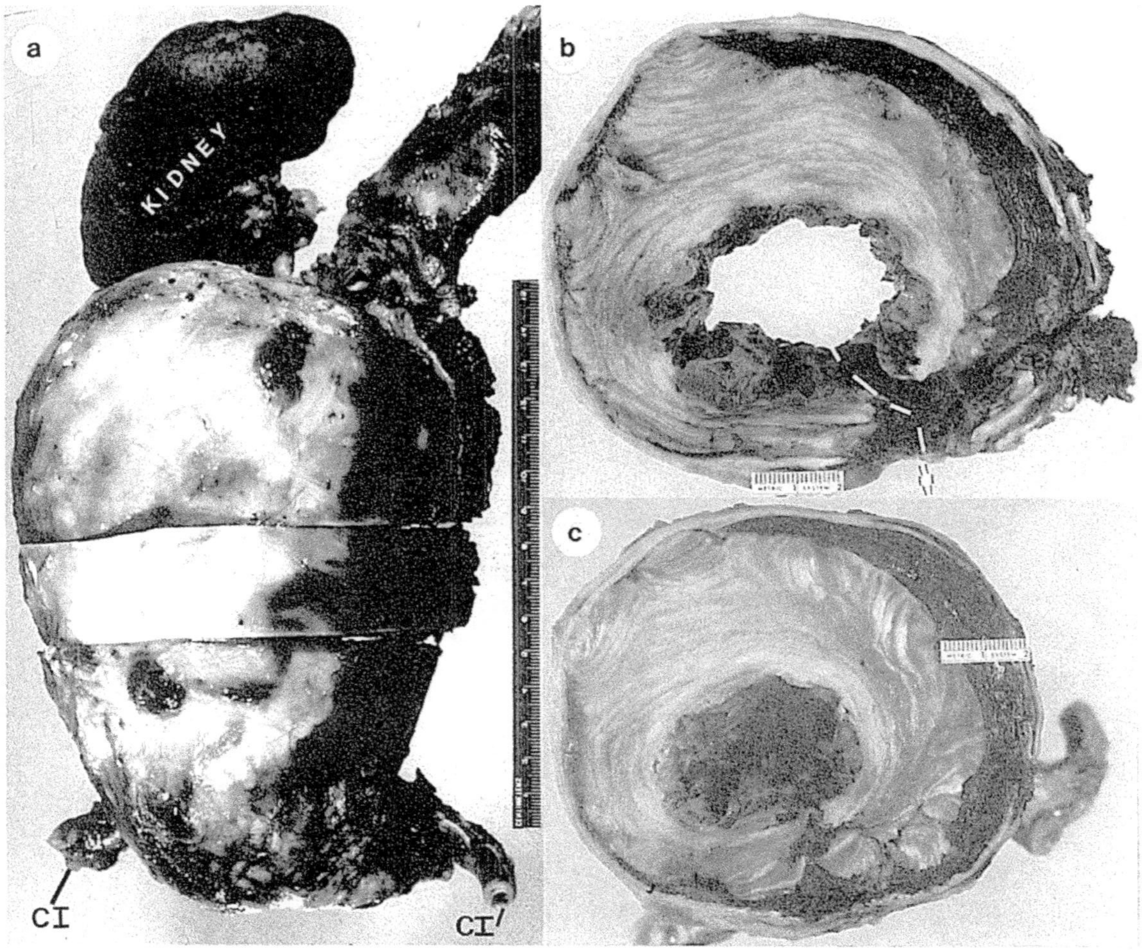

Fig. 10. Ruptured abdominal aortic aneurysm in an 87-year-old white man (NNMC #A73-12) who died 36 hours after operation on an incarcerated inguinal hernia. He had had systemic hypertension for years but never had evidence of cardiac or limb ischemia. The abdominal aortic aneurysm was easily palpated clinically. During the operation for the inguinal hernia, it is likely that the abdominal aortic aneurysm was manipulated, and during his subsequent 36 hours, the blood hematocrit value gradually fell. At necropsy, large quantities of blood were present in the retroperitoneal area. The heart weighed 425 gm. (*a*) Enormous fusiform abdominal aneurysm measuring about 13 cm in maximal transverse diameter and over 18 cm in maximal longitudinal dimension. The abdominal aortic aneurysm with its intra-aneurysmal thrombus weighed 1200 gm. (*b* and *c*) Two transverse sections of the aneurysm showing laminated thrombus and dissection of blood through the thrombus to rupture outside the abdominal aortic wall.

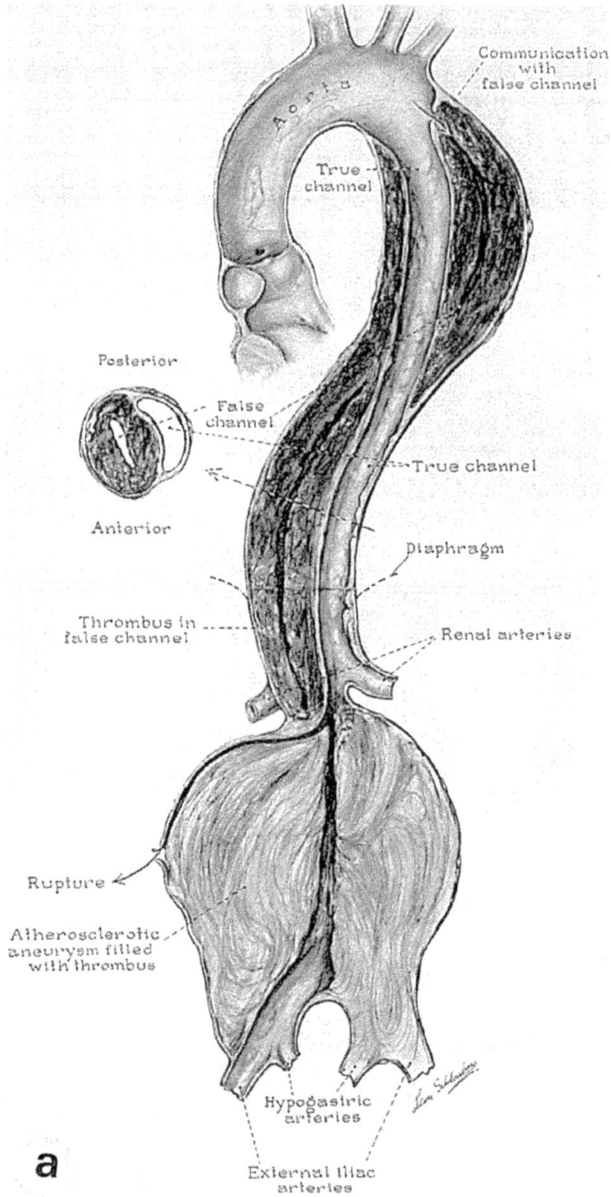

a

Fig. 11. Rupture of a fusiform abdominal aortic aneurysm and healed dissecting aortic aneurysm together in a 67-year-old white man (NNMC #A76-211). He had had systemic hypertension for years and more than one acute myocardial infarct which had healed. Neither fusiform abdominal aortic aneurysm nor aortic dissection had been diagnosed clinically. (*a*) Drawing of the locations of the aortic aneurysms. The dissection stopped at the beginning of the fusiform abdominal aortic aneurysm and began just past the origin of the left subclavian artery. (*Figure and legend continued on following page.*)

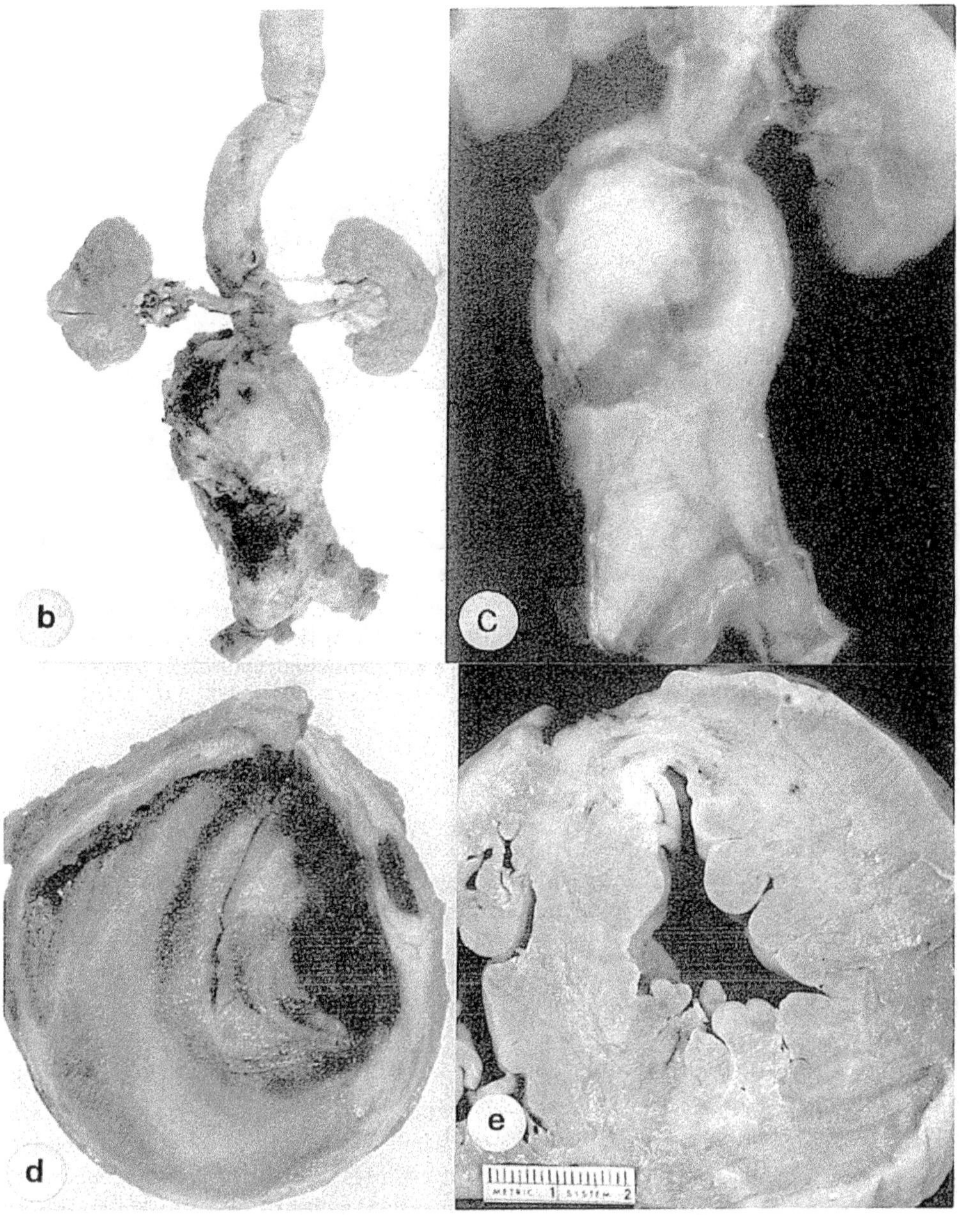

Fig. 11.(*continued*). (*b*) Exterior view of the aorta, kidneys, and fusiform aneurysm. (*c*) Radiograph of fusiform abdominal aneurysm showing a few calcific deposits. (*d*) Transverse section of the abdominal aneurysm showing a severely narrowed lumen. (*e*) Transverse section of left ventricle showing a healed transmural infarct.

The major consequences of severe atherosclerosis of the aorta are luminal *dilatation* (aneurysm) and luminal *obstruction*. Of the two, dilatation is far more common, and aneurysm may affect the transverse, descending thoracic, and abdominal portions of aorta. In contrast, obstruction resulting from atherosclerosis affects only the abdominal portion of aorta, although the lumen of any artery arising from aorta may be made stenotic by atherosclerotic plaques.

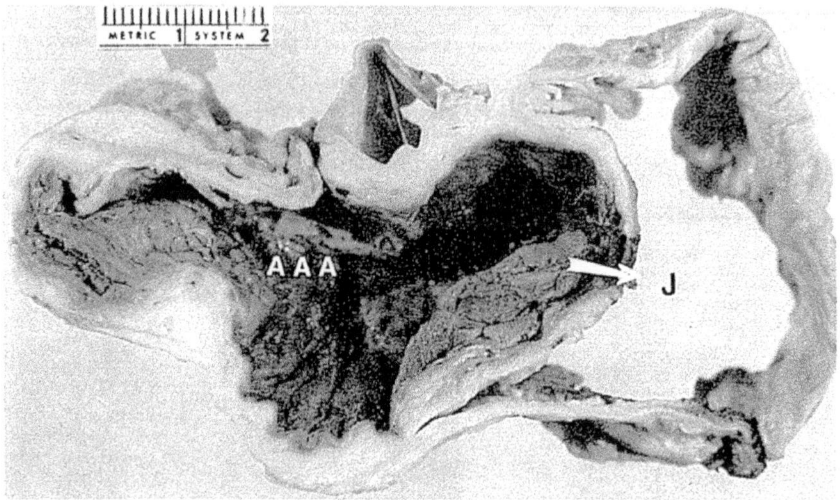

Fig. 12. Rupture of abdominal aortic aneurysm (AAA) into jejunum (J) in a 52-year-old black man (H #A77-136) causing massive bleeding into the bowel. He had been known to have systemic hypertension for at least 5 years, but his heart weighed only 310 gm. The coronary arteries were considerably narrowed, and a small transmural left ventricular scar was present. The rupture into jejunum occurred about 10 cm distal to the duodenojejunal junction. This photograph represents a cross section of the abdominal aortic aneurysm at the site (arrow) of rupture into jejunum.

Aortic Atherosclerotic Aneurysm

Unless there is disease of the underlying media, such as syphilis, the sinus and tubular portions of ascending aorta are not sites of atherosclerotic aneurysmal formation. Furthermore, when the transverse and/or descending thoracic aorta are sites of aneurysm, there usually also is aneurysmal involvement of the abdominal portion of aorta. Most patients with abdominal aortic aneurysms, however, do not have aneurysms in other portions of the aorta. Thus the abdominal portion of aorta is by far the most common site of aneurysm in the aorta.

True aneurysms of the aorta are of two types: fusiform or cylindrical and saccular. In the *fusiform* variety, the entire circumference of the aorta is involved in the wall of the aneurysm (Fig. 4 to 15). This is the most common type of aortic aneurysm, and with extremely rare exception, the abdominal aortic aneurysms are all of the fusiform variety. In the *saccular* variety, only a portion of the aortic wall is incorporated into the wall of the aneurysm (Figs. 7, 9, 15 to 17). This type of aneurysm when of atherosclerotic origin is more common in the transverse and descending thoracic aorta. It also may occur in the abdominal aorta but when it does, it is proximal to the origin of the renal arteries rather than distal to these arteries, which is the characteristic location of the fusiform abdominal aortic aneurysms. The saccular aortic aneurysm usually has a mouth that is smaller than the maximal diameter of the saccular protrusion. In this respect, the saccular aneurysm resembles a false aneurysm, but in the latter circumstance, the wall of the aneurysm was not originally the wall of aorta, whereas in a true saccular aneurysm, the bulging wall was originally the wall of aorta.

In nearly all fusiform and saccular aortic aneurysms, thrombus is located within the aneurysm (Fig. 4 to 17). Although the risk of thrombus is dislodgment of thrombotic

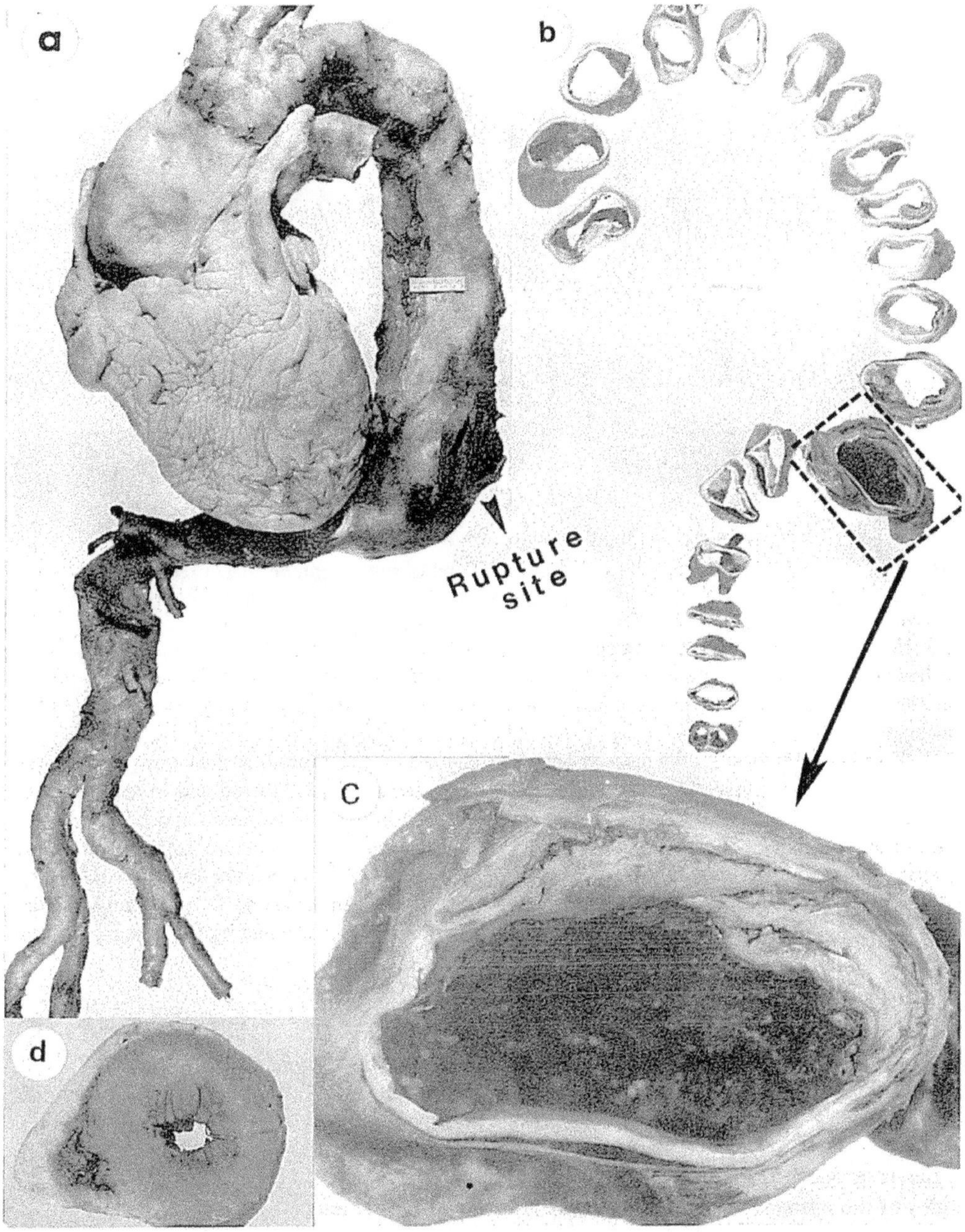

Fig. 13. Ruptured fusiform descending thoracic aortic aneurysm in an 83-year-old white woman (GT #76A-196) who developed left upper quadrant ''abdominal'' pain about 8 hours before death, which was sudden. At necropsy, 1500 ml of blood was found in the left hemithorax. She was known to have had systemic hypertension, angina pectoris, and a large hiatal hernia. (*a*) Heart and aorta and its branches. The aorta is dilated in a fusiform fashion at the level of the diaphragm and the aneurysm ruptured at its site of maximal transverse diameter (5 cm). The aorta is very tortuous. The heart is big. (*b*) Transverse sections of aorta. (*c*) Close-up of a transverse section of the aneurysm. Some intraaneurysmal thrombus is present. (*d*) Transverse section of the cardiac ventricles showing left ventricular hypertrophy.

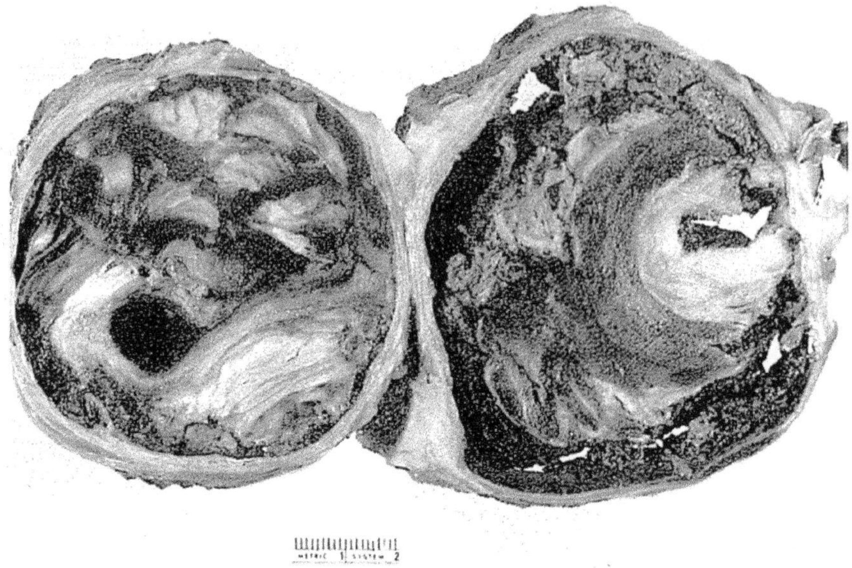

Fig. 14. Fusiform aneurysms of abdominal aorta and of both common iliac arteries (shown here) and healed dissection of the descending thoracic aorta in a 62-year-old black man (DCGH #76A-80). He was known to have had systemic hypertension for many years. When he was 56 years old, he had an illness typical of acute aortic dissection. At age 59, a pulsatile abdominal mass was noted, and it proved to be a fusiform abdominal aortic aneurysm. He died from rupture of the abdominal aneurysm.

At autopsy, the descending thoracic aorta and also the proximal portion of abdominal aorta was the site of a healed dissection. The false channel was aneurysmally dilated and in several areas contained thrombus. A large fusiform aneurysm involved the abdominal aorta and both common iliac arteries, and thrombus was present within the aneurysm. Shown here are both common iliac arteries, which are enormously dilated: each is approximately *8 cm* in maximal transverse diameter, and together the two common iliac aneurysms from aortic bifurcation to femoral canal (groin) weighed 1500 gm! The lumens of both common iliac arteries are narrowed by the intraaneurysmal thrombus.

material with embolism, the intraaneurysmal thrombus serves to protect the aneurysm from rupturing. Rupture of an aortic aneurysm, be it fusiform or saccular, would be far more common were it not for the intraaneurysmal thrombus. The typical saccular aneurysm fills up completely or nearly so with thrombus, which in this circumstance tends not to organize at all. All fusiform aneurysms of significant size (> 4 cm in maximal transverse diameter), for practical purposes, contain laminated thrombus that borders all sides of the intraaneurysmal lumen. The thrombus is so extensive as a rule in the fusiform abdominal aneurysms that the intraaneurysmal lumen is commonly smaller than the lumen of the aorta just proximal to the origin of the aortic aneurysm. The prevention of intraaneurysmal luminal expansion by the thrombus may prevent diagnosis of a fusiform abdominal aneurysm by injection of contrast media proximal to the aneurysm. Likewise, because the lumens of most saccular aortic aneurysms are filled with thrombus, these types of aneurysms are frequently—indeed, probably more frequently than not—missed entirely by aortogram.

Although this complication is prevented or delayed by the intraaneurysmal thrombus, *rupture,* nevertheless, is the most feared and most common fatal or potentially fatal

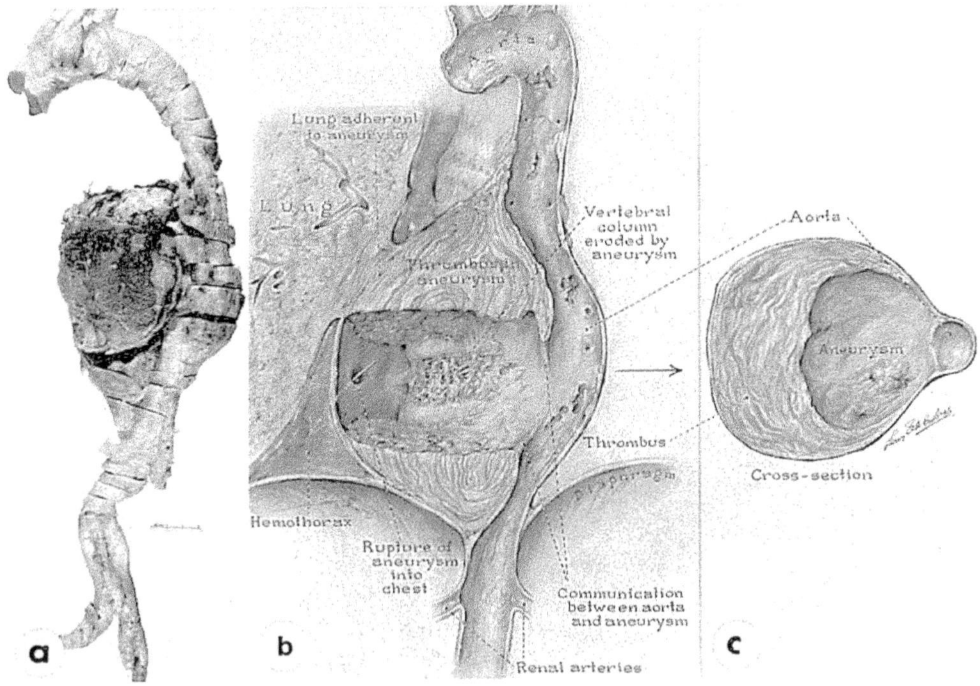

Fig. 15. Saccular descending thoracic aortic aneurysm in a 62-year-old black woman (DCMEO #77-05-440) who began noting intermittent chest pain, unassociated with exertion, about 3 months before death. She refused to seek medical care and was found dead at home. She was known to have had systemic hypertension and severe kyphoscoliosis. At necropsy, 2400 ml of blood was found in one hemithorax. (*a*) Aorta showing a large aortic aneurysm just cephalad to the diaphragm. (*b*) Drawing showing that the aneurysm contained laminated thrombus (*c*) and that the aneurysm burrowed into the vertebral column, causing rupture.

complication of atherosclerotic aortic aneurysm (Figs. 10, 12–15). Compared to the number of aortic aneurysms, however, rupture is relatively infrequent. Although the larger the aneurysm, the greater the likelihood of rupture, most aneurysms, irrespective of size, do not rupture. Fusiform aneurysms less than 5 cm in maximal transverse diameter rarely rupture.[4] Although precise data are not readily available, fusiform aneurysms almost surely have a higher frequency of rupture than do saccular aneurysms. With the saccular aneurysm, most of the intraaneurysmal space is occupied by thrombus, and the communication with the lumen of the aorta is via a small orifice (Figs. 7, 9, 15 to 17). Because the area of communication with the aorta is small, the wall of the aneurysm may not be exposed to the full force of the intraaortic pressure, as is the case with the fusiform aortic aneurysm. In the latter circumstance, the entire wall of the aneurysm is constantly exposed to the full intraaortic pressure.

Why aneurysmal rupture occurs in some patients with aortic aneurysms and not in other similarly aged patients with similarly sized aneurysms is uncertain. Possibly, calcific deposits within the wall of the aorta play a role in rupture. As shown in Figs. 4 to 9 and 11, radiographs of either fusiform or saccular atherosclerotic aortic aneurysms show no calcific deposits within the intraaneurysmal thrombus, which consists essentially of layed fibrin. The calcific deposits when present are located within the wall of aorta, particularly in its more intimal portion. Pressure of the heavy overlying thrombus com-

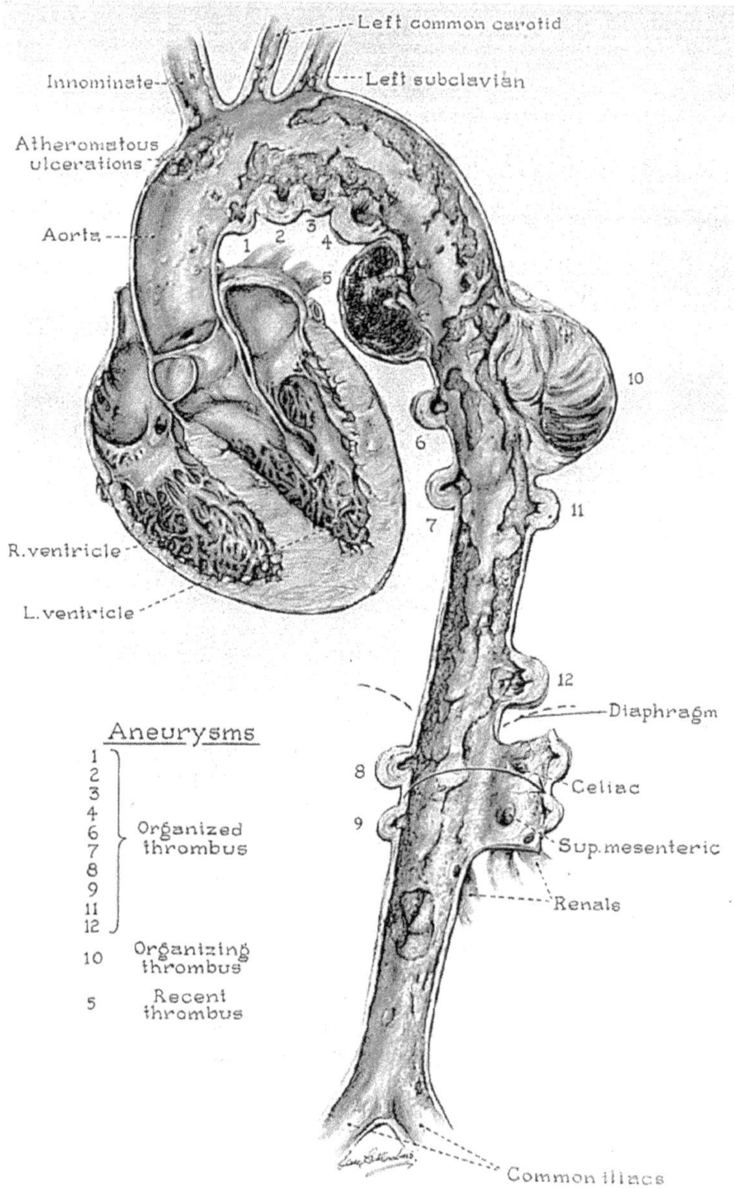

Fig. 16. Multiple asymptomatic saccular aneurysms of aorta in a 66-year-old black woman (H #A76-82) who died from consequences of acute myocardial infarction. She had had systemic hypertension, diabetes mellitus, and angina pectoris. The heart weighed 470 gm.

This drawing shows 12 different saccular aortic aneurysms; all contain thrombus in varying stages of organization. The aorta is severely atherosclerotic. Atherosclerotic type (cholesterol) emboli were found in several small arteries of the kidneys, pancreas, and spleen.

pressing against the calcium-containing aortic wall with the force of the intraabdominal aortic pressure would appear to drive the intimal calcium further into the aortic wall, which becomes thinner as the aneurysm becomes larger.

Another mechanism of aneurysmal rupture is simply compression of the aneurysm against a rigid, nonmovable adjacent structure. The rigid structure adjacent to the aorta, obviously, is the vertebral body. Although descending thoracic aortic aneurysms, particularly, can indent into one or more vertebral bodies (Fig. 15), the aneurysms tend to rupture before the vertebral bodies are damaged very much. Indentation or erosion of vertebral bodies by fusiform abdominal aneurysm is very unusual because the protrusion of the aneurysm is usually only lateral and anterior. A rare cause of aneurysmal rupture is intraaneurysmal infection.[5]

The site of aortic aneurysmal rupture is most dependent on the location of the aneurysm. Abdominal aneurysms most commonly rupture into the *retroperitoneal tissues,* and from there, the extravasated blood may occasionally enter the peritoneal cavity. Descending thoracic aneurysms most commonly rupture into the left *pleurel cavity* because the aorta descends on the left. Rupture of an arch or an isthmic aneurysm may be into other portions of the *respiratory system,* including trachea, left main bronchus, and left lung. Rupture may also be into the *gastrointestinal tract.* The esophagus is the usual site when the ruptured aneurysm is located in the descending thoracic aorta. When the abdominal aorta ruptures into the gastrointestinal tract, it is usually into the duodenum because the third segment of duodenum lies just anterior to the abdominal aorta (Fig. 12).

Aortic Atherosclerotic Obstruction (Figs. 18 and 19)

When severe atherosclerosis affects the coronary, cerebral, and peripheral arteries, the usual consequence is luminal obstruction with or without clinical evidence of organ ischemia. Severe atherosclerosis in the aorta, however, more commonly leads to aneurysmal formation than to luminal obstruction. When aortic obstruction is the consequence of atherosclerosis, the site of obstruction is the abdominal aorta. When abdominal obstruction results from severe atherosclerosis or from its consequences, the lumens of the common iliac arteries are almost always also occluded by the same process. Why the severely atherosclerotic abdominal aorta becomes aneurysmal in some persons and obstructed without aneurysmal formation in others is uncertain. Although the intraaneurysmal lumen may be narrowed in patients with fusiform abdominal aortic aneurysms, most patients with atherosclerotic obstruction of the abdominal aorta have nondilated abdominal aortas. When severe atherosclerosis with superimposed thrombosis causes abdominal aortic obstruction, the wall of the aorta is nearly always severely calcified. Very possibly, it is the heavy deposition of calcium in the wall of the aorta that prevents its expansion. Although the aortic wall in patients with fusiform or saccular aortic aneurysms may also contain some calcific deposits, the extent of the deposits is far less than that observed in the nondilated abdominal aorta obstructed by an atherosclerotic process. It appears that in this circumstance the heavy calcific deposits occur in the wall of aorta before it has had an opportunity to dilate, or in other words, the rigid pipe cannot dilate.

Although slow progressive obstruction of the abdominal aorta by atherosclerosis with superimposed thrombosis may lead to the Leriche syndrome, which includes both buttock claudication and impotency, this process more often results in none of these symptoms and often no evidence of leg ischemia.

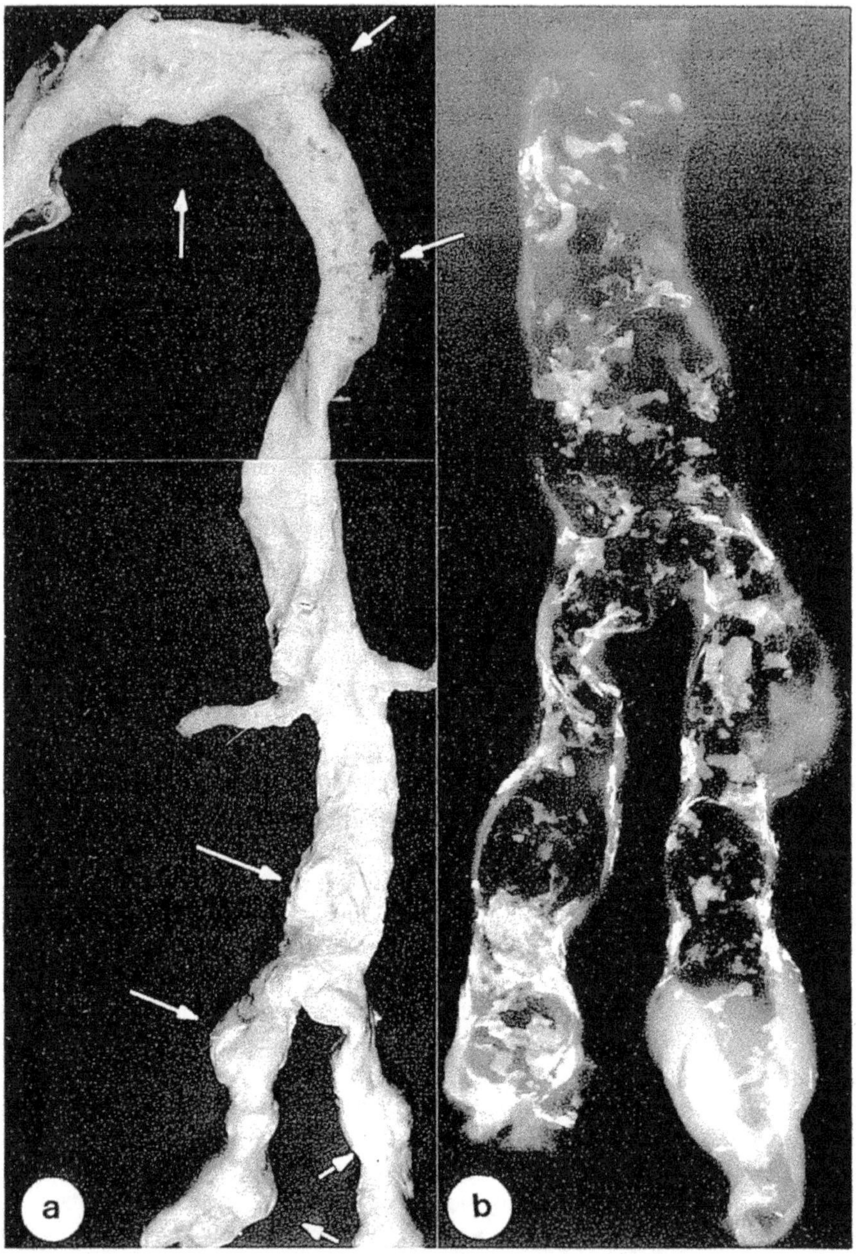

Fig. 17. Multiple asymptomatic saccular aneurysms of aorta in a 78-year-old woman (A71-95) who died of carcinoma of the colon. (*a*) Aorta and common iliac arteries. The arrows designate the aneurysms. (*b*) Radiograph of abdominal aorta and common iliac arteries showing heavy calcific deposits. (*Figure and legend continue on following page.*)

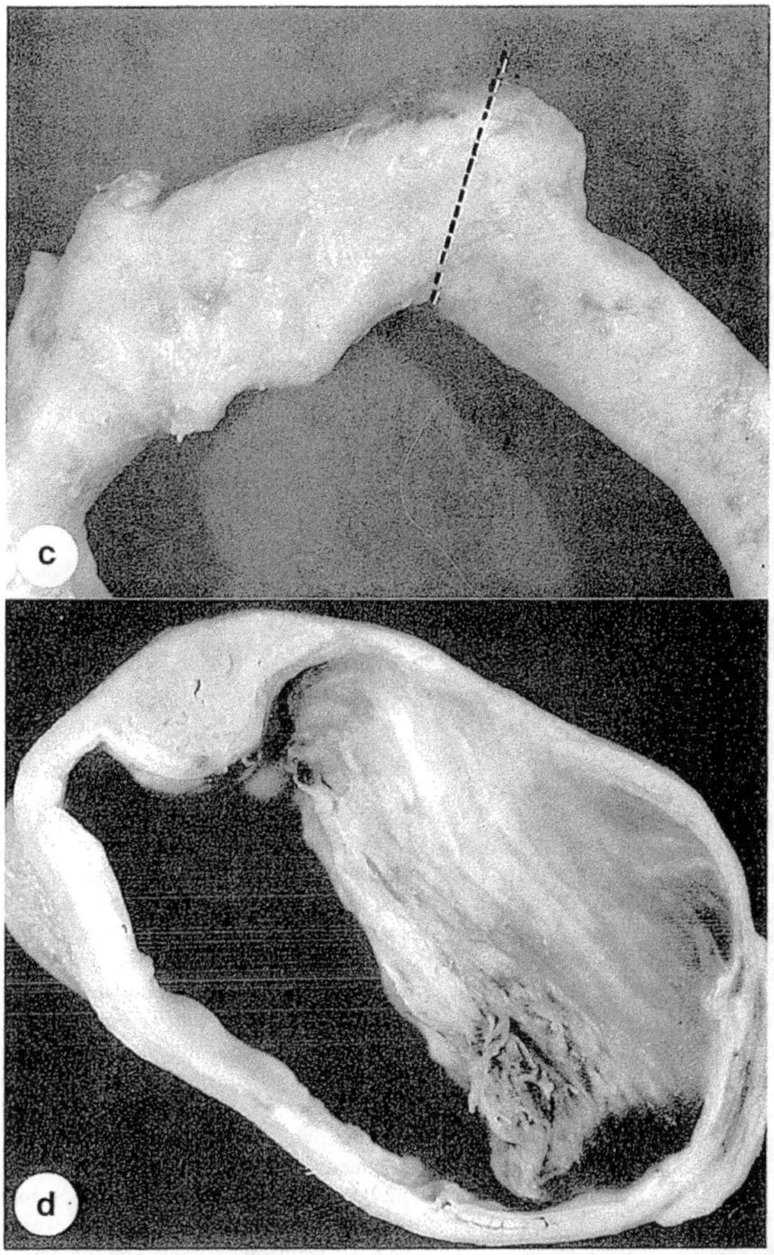

Fig. 17. *(continued).* (*c*) Close-up view of one saccular aneurysm in the descending thoracic aorta. A transverse section (at the site of the dashed line) of this saccular aneurysm is shown in (*d*). The aneurysm contains thrombus.

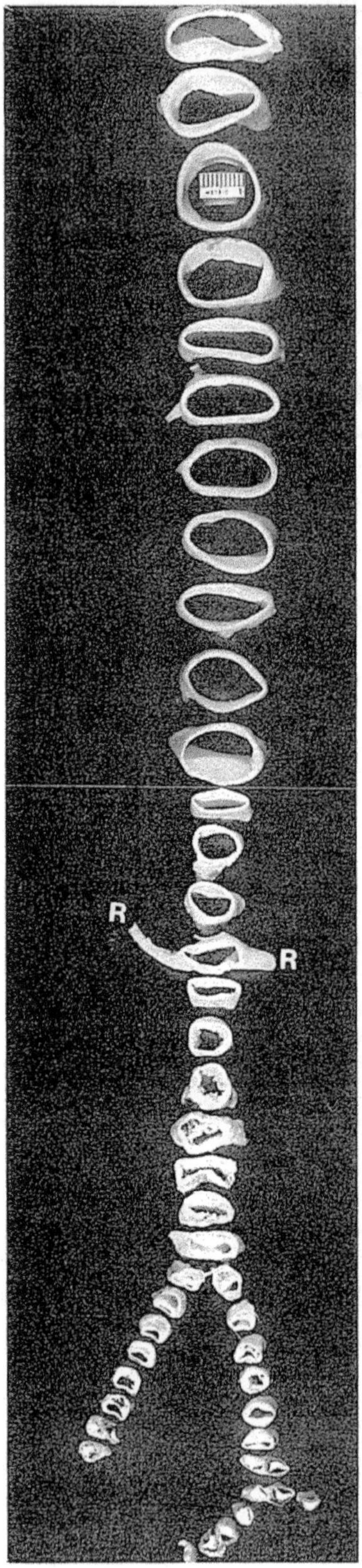

Fig. 18. Occlusive aortoiliac disease in a 52-year-old white man (A78-85) with type II hyperlipoproteinemia. He died suddenly shortly after a meal on the first day of his honeymoon. When he was 21 years old, xanthomas were noted, and when he was 28, he had a well-documented acute myocardial infarction which healed. He had had an endarterectomy on his left femoral artery because of claudication when he was 33 years old. At age 45, angina pectoris appeared, and at age 46, lumbar sympathectomy was performed (without benefit) for right leg claudication. He also had systemic hypertension. At necropsy, the healed myocardial infarct was confirmed. The heart weighed 550 gm. The lumens of the coronary arteries were severely narrowed: the lumens of 39 of 41 5 mm segments of the four major coronary arteries were > 75 percent narrowed in cross-sectional area by atherosclerotic plaque. Shown here are cross sections of aorta and the common iliac arteries. The wall of the aorta down to the origins of the renal (R) arteries, surprisingly, is smooth and nearly free of atherosclerotic plaques. The abdominal portion of aorta and both common iliac arteries are diffusely involved by plaques, and their lumens are narrowed.

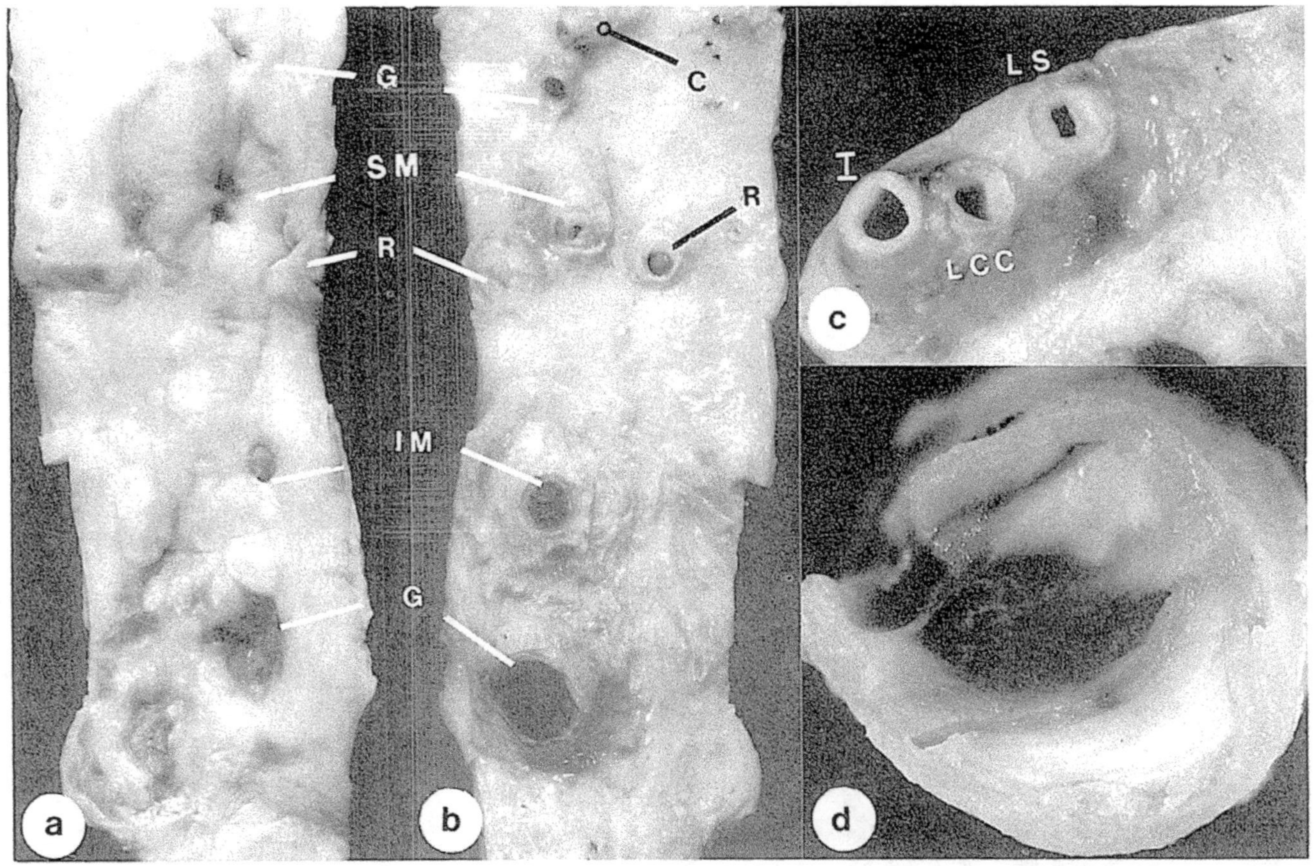

Fig. 19. "Malignant" atherosclerosis of the aorta and its branches in a 34-year-old white man (KMC #76A-171) who developed abdominal angina approximately 19 months before death. An aortogram 13 months before death disclosed complete occlusion of the superior and inferior mesenteric arteries and the right superficial femoral artery and considerable narrowing of both renal arteries. At that time, a portion of gangrenous cecum was resected, and about a month later, a synthetic graft was placed between the aorta and the superior mesenteric artery. Shortly after this

(caption continued on bottom of next page)

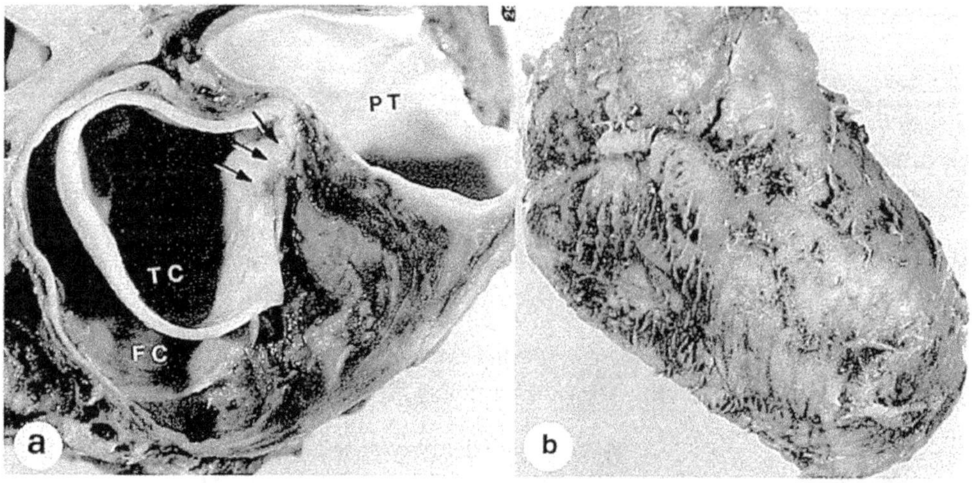

Fig. 20. Acute aortic dissection with rupture into the pericardial sac in a 63-year-old black woman (SH #A78-113). She had been well until 12 days before death, when she developed chest pain and was hospitalized. Electrocardiograms were suggestive of myocardial ischemia. She died suddenly. Aortic dissection had not been suspected during life. At necropsy, the pericardial sac was filled with blood. The dissection involved the entire aorta and the tear or entrance into the false channel was about 2 cm cephalad to the aortic valve. (*a*) Double lumen aorta. TC, true channel; FC, false channel. The arrows designate the site of the aortic tear. (*b*) Hypertrophied heart covered by blood and fibrin.

AORTIC DISSECTION (Figs. 20 to 34)

If systemic hypertension were eliminated, aortic dissection would disappear.[6] Aortic dissection, therefore, represents a therapeutic failure (on the part of the patient or physician or both) in the management of systemic hypertension. The higher the blood pressure, the greater the likelihood of dissection. The only common denominator among patients with aortic dissection is left ventricular hypertrophy, and the most reasonable explanation

---

second operation, he had an acute myocardial infarct. The abdominal angina continued, and 2 months before death, a repeat aortogram disclosed that the conduit between aorta and superior mesenteric artery had become totally occluded and that now both renal arteries were severely narrowed. A third operation was then performed, namely insertion of a conduit between left common iliac artery and left renal artery. He died soon thereafter of infarction of his entire small intestine and of a portion of large intestine. This patient's mother died at age 44 years from an acute myocardial infarct, and his brother died at age 33 from a gangrenous bowel. His father, who is living, has had a stroke. This patient's blood cholesterol, triglyceride, and glucose levels were normal. His blood pressure during his last few months was 210/120 mm Hg, and the elevation was believed to be renal in origin. He smoked about 30 cigarettes daily since age 17 years.

(*a*) Opened interior view and (*b*) exterior view of abdominal aorta showing complete or near complete occlusion of the superior mesenteric (SM), inferior mesenteric (IM), and renal (R) arteries by thrombus superimposed on atherosclerotic plaque and occlusion of both grafts (G) by thrombus. The aorta (a) itself contains many atherosclerotic plaques. (*c*) The three aortic arch arteries. The left subclavian (LS) artery is narrowed. I, innominate; LCC, left common carotid. (*d*) Close-up of a severely narrowed renal artery.

The lumens of the right, left main, left anterior descending, and left circumflex coronary arteries were > 75 percent narrowed in cross-sectional area by atherosclerotic plaque, and a healed transmural left ventricular infarct was present.

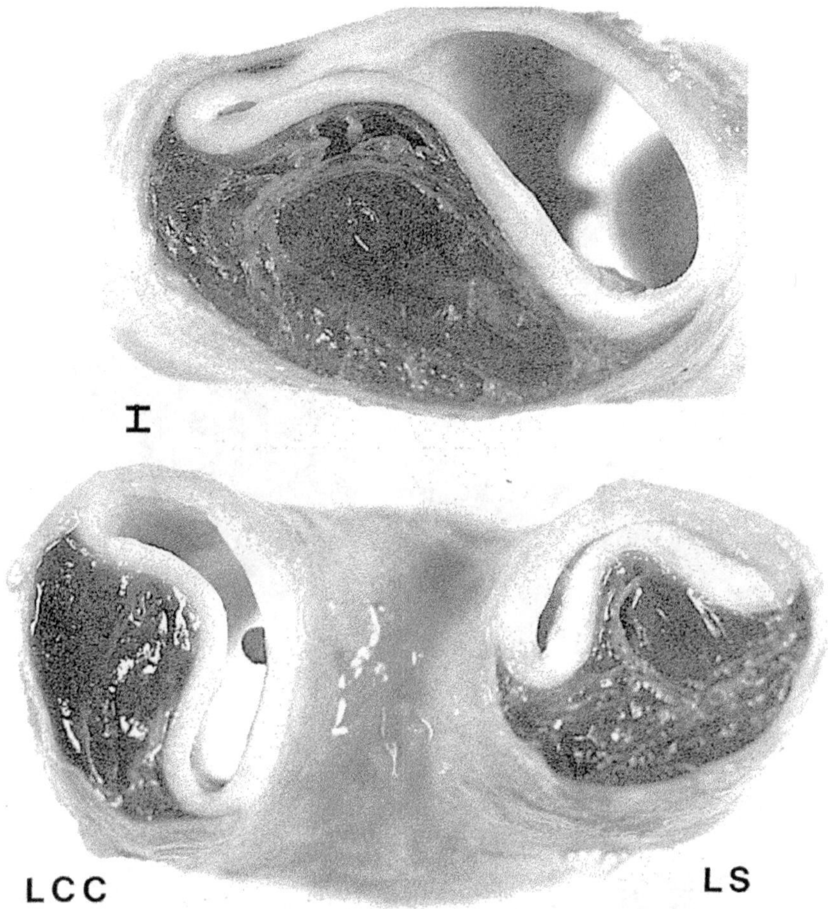

Fig. 21. Acute dissection involving the ascending and transverse portions of aorta with rupture into the pericardial sac in a 71-year-old (HHMC #A-74-81) previously healthy woman. The entrance site was just above the aortic valve, and the exit site was in the transverse aorta. Although both functioned normally, the aortic and pulmonic valves were congenitally bicuspid. The heart weighed 430 gm. The dissection extended into the adventitia of the major pulmonary arteries and into the media of all three arch arteries (shown here), narrowing the lumens of each. I, innominate; LCC, left common carotid, LS, left subclavian artery.

for the hypertrophy, with extremely rare exception is systemic hypertension.[6] Although only about 70 percent of patients with aortic dissection have a history of systemic hypertension, aortic dissection often represents their first serious illness and often the first time that the patient had sought medical care. After dissection, of course, the blood pressure may fall, and by the time of hospitalization, the systemic hypertension may have vanished. Unfortunately, aortic dissection is also one of the more dramatic means of lowering the blood pressure.

Although it is the common denominator in patients with aortic dissection, systemic hypertension cannot by itself be considered the sole cause of aortic dissection. There are estimated to be 25 million Americans with systemic hypertension, and the frequency among them of aortic dissection is quite low. Why one hypertensive patient has aortic dissection and another of similar age and with similarly elevated pressures does not is unclear. The author has studied, by serial sections, the site of the aortic tear at the

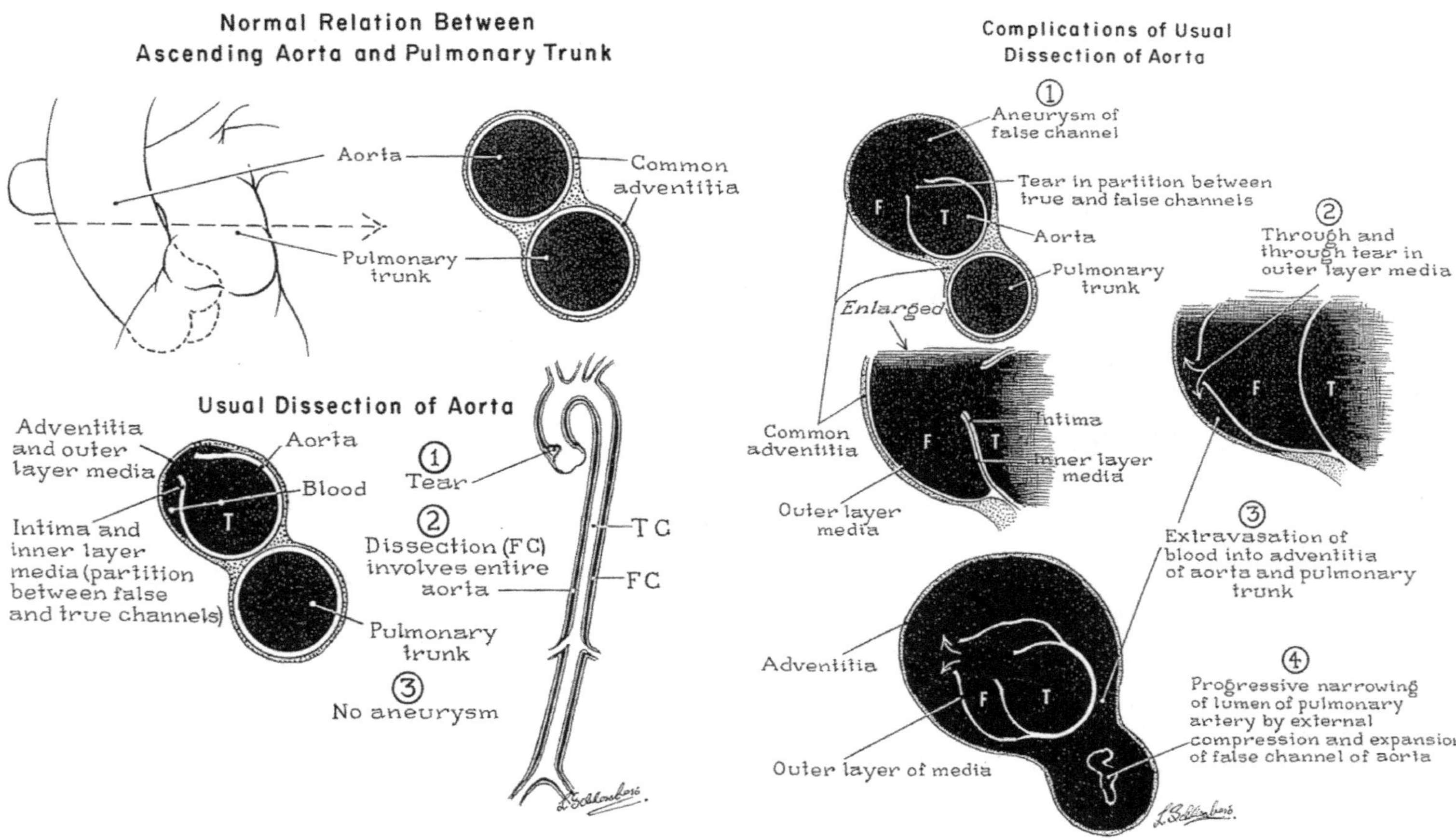

Fig. 22. Diagrams showing the relationship between the adventitia of ascending aorta and pulmonary trunk, the usual aortic dissection, and complications of aortic dissection including adventitial pulmonary dissection with pulmonary arterial luminal narrowing.

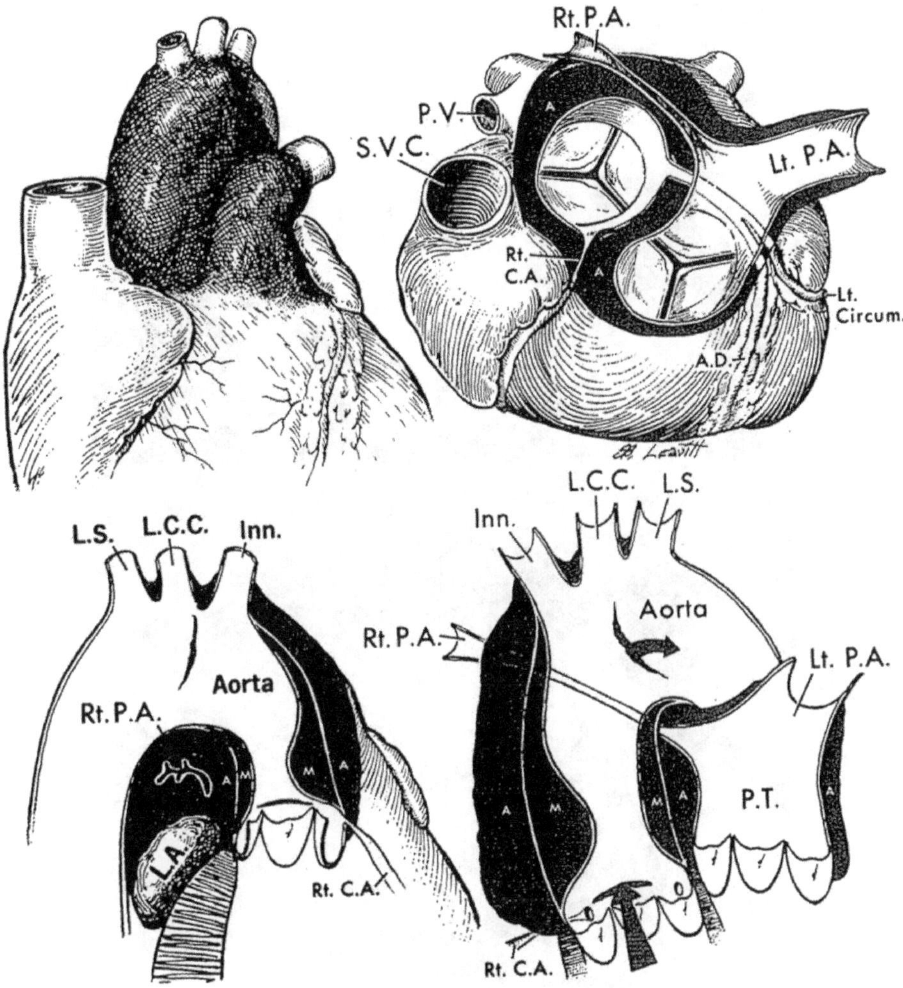

Fig. 23. Dissection of the entire aorta with rupture into the pericardial sac in a 57-year-old man (A69-302) who developed chest pain 17 hours before death. He was known to have had systemic hypertension. (This patient is described in detail elsewhere [Buja LM, Ali N, Fletcher RD, Roberts WC: Stenosis of the right main pulmonary artery. A complication of acute dissecting aneurysm of the ascending aorta. Am Heart J 83:89–92, 1972].)

At necropsy, extravasated blood was present in the adventitia (A) of both ascending aorta and the extrapulmonary pulmonary arteries (PA). Because the ascending aorta and the pulmonary trunk (PT) have a common adventitia, extension of blood into the adventitia of aorta can lead to extension of the blood into the adventitia of pulmonary trunk and into the main right (Rt) and left (Lt) pulmonary arteries. Because the latter has a much lower pressure than the former, the lumen of the major pulmonary arteries can be narrowed by this process.

This drawing shows how aortic adventitial blood may extend into the adventitia of the pulmonary trunk and lead to severe narrowing of the lumen of the right pulmonary artery. The ascending aorta was also narrowed by blood in the false channel as well as in the adventitia. The entrance site of the dissection was just above the aortic valve, and the exit site was in the arch. The lumen of the right coronary artery (Rt CA) was also severely narrowed by the medial (M) and adventitial hematoma. AD, left anterior descending coronary artery; Circum, circumflex coronary artery; LS, left subclavian artery; LCC, left common carotid artery; Inn, innominate artery.

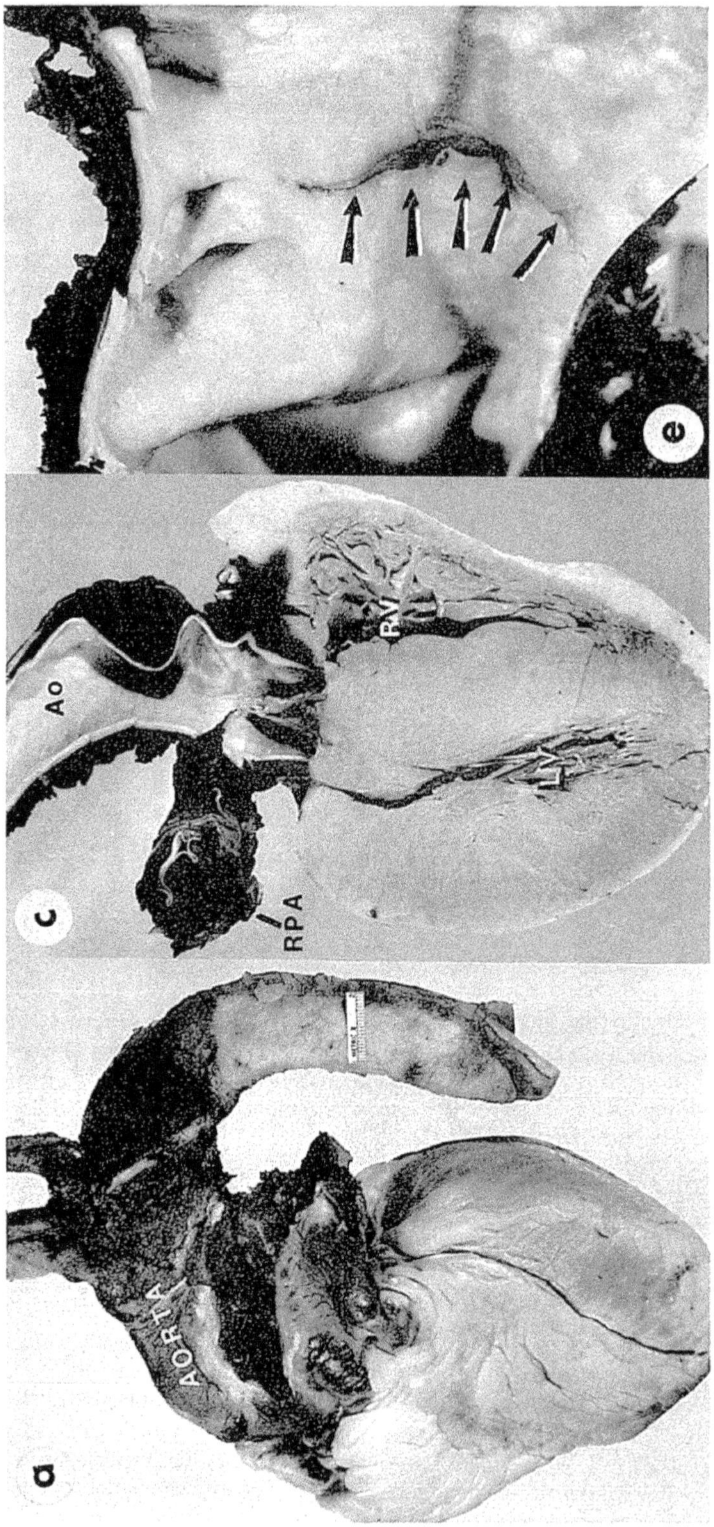
a
AORTA
c
RPA
Ao
RV
LV
e

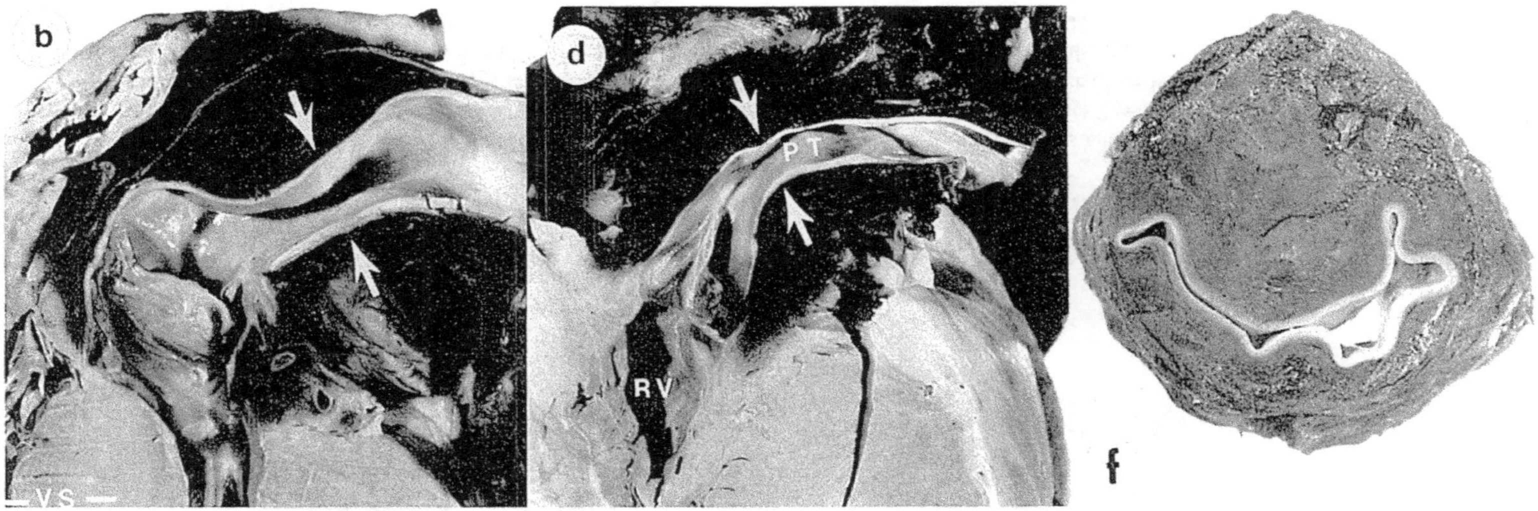

Fig. 24. The heart and major arteries in the patient described in Fig. 23. (*a*) Exterior view showing blood in the adventitia of the aorta and major pulmonary arteries. (*b*) Longitudinal view showing the aortic medial and adventitial hematoma which narrows the aortic lumen (arrows). VS, ventricular septum. (*c*) View of anterior half of heart and great arteries from behind. Ao, aorta; RPA, right pulmonary artery; RV, right ventricle; LV, left ventricle. (*d*) Close-up view of compressed pulmonary trunk (PT) by adventitial hematoma. (*e*) Arrows show exit site of dissection in the transverse aorta. (*f*) Cross section of the right main pulmonary artery, the lumen of which is narrowed by the adventitial hematoma.

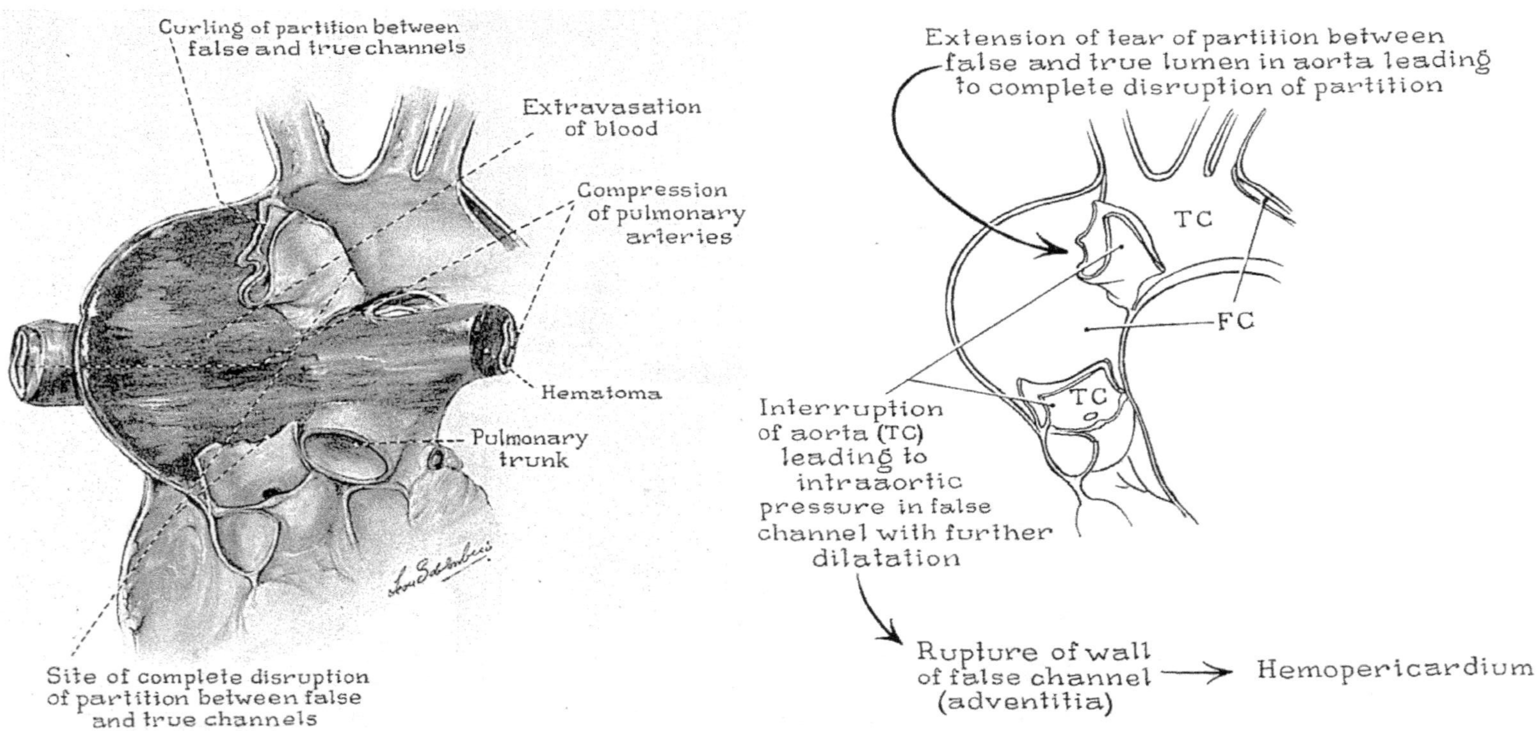

Fig. 25. Dissection of aorta with "intussusception" of partition between true and false channels and rupture into the pericardial sac in a 43-year-old black woman (H #A76-166). Although known to have mild aortic regurgitation for 2 years, she was asymptomatic until about 5 hours before death, when she had the sudden onset of chest and back pain. An hour or so later, her blood pressure was 160/110 mm Hg, and one radial and one femoral arterial pulsation was absent. She died suddenly.

At necropsy, the pericardial sac was filled with blood, and dissection involved the entire aorta. The entrance site of the dissection was in the ascending aorta just above the aortic valve. The tear extended across the entire circumference of the aorta such that the partition between the true and false channels had curled and extended into the transverse aorta, probably causing some obstruction to flow. Blood also extended from the aortic media into the aortic adventitia and from there it dissected into the wall of the pulmonary trunk and then into the adventitia of the main right and left pulmonary arteries, resulting in narrowing of their lumens. TC, true channel; FC, false channel.

beginning of the aortic dissection in many patients and has not observed any intrinsic defect in the wall of the aorta. There is no more acid-mucopolysaccharide material in the aortic media at the site of the aortic tear, or in other parts of the aorta, in the patients with dissection than in age- and sex-matched individuals without aortic dissection.[7]

Although the initiating tear is usually more or less transverse to the direction of flow of blood in the aorta (Figs. 20, 22 to 28, 31), the medial dissection is parallel to the direction of blood flow. Once the blood enters the media via the transverse tear, the time required thereafter to dissect the media of the entire length of the aorta appears to be only a matter of a second or so. Evidence of the rapidity of the longitudinal dissection once it begins is gained from retrograde aortic dissections, which have been observed occasionally during cardiopulmonary bypass. With the arterial cannula in the wall of the femoral artery (rather than within its lumen), the entire length of the aorta has been observed to dissect within a second or so after cardiopulmonary bypass has been initiated. Presumably, the anterograde aortic dissections occur with the same speed and possibly even more rapidly, because in the natural state the aorta is exposed to a pulsatile flow (systolic and diastolic) rather than entirely to a mean pressure.

The location of the dissecting channel (false channel; dissecting hematoma) is nearly always in the outer half of the wall of aorta (Fig. 27). As a consequence, the outer wall of the false channel is very thin, often only a fourth or a fifth as thick as the original wall of aorta. The partition, therefore, between the true and false channels (the inner wall of the false channel) is about three times as thick as the outer wall of the false channel but only about three-fourths as thick as the original wall of aorta. The thinness of the outer wall of the false channel is the anatomic feature that explains the high frequency of rupture of this outer wall and indeed explains why extravasation of blood outside the aorta is more common than rerupture of the inner wall of the false channel into the true channel. If the situation were reversed such that the inner wall of the false channel (partition between the true and false channels) was only a quarter as thick as the outer wall, survival after aortic dissection would be far more common, and rerupture of the separating partition between the two channels would be far more frequent. Of course, the thinner the outer wall of the false channel, the greater the likelihood of fatal rupture, and vice versa.

The dissecting hematoma rarely involves the entire circumference of the aorta. Most commonly, about one-half of the aortic circumference is involved by the longitudinal dissection, and the other half of the aorta remains intact. Although the longitudinal dissection commonly involves about one-half of the aortic circumference, the amount of circumference involved varies somewhat throughout the full length of aorta. The initial transverse tear of aorta infrequently involves as much as one-half of the aortic circumference. More commonly, the transverse tears appear to involve about a third of the aortic circumference. On rare occasion (Fig. 25), however, the aortic tear may involve the entire circumference of aorta.

The portion of aortic circumference involved by the longitudinal dissection is fairly characteristic. With dissections beginning in the ascending portion, the transverse tear is most commonly about 1 to 3 cm above the sinotubular junction of aorta along the right lateral wall. The longitudinal dissection most commonly follows the greater curvature of the ascending, transverse, and descending portions of aorta. Because the arch arteries arise from this greater portion, extension of the dissection into the innominate, left common carotid, and left subclavian arteries is extremely common (Figs. 21 and 27).

Although the initiating transverse tears are most frequently located in the ascending aorta, the ascending portion is not necessarily the most common portion of aorta involved by dissection. The reason is that the more proximal portion of descending thoracic aorta is

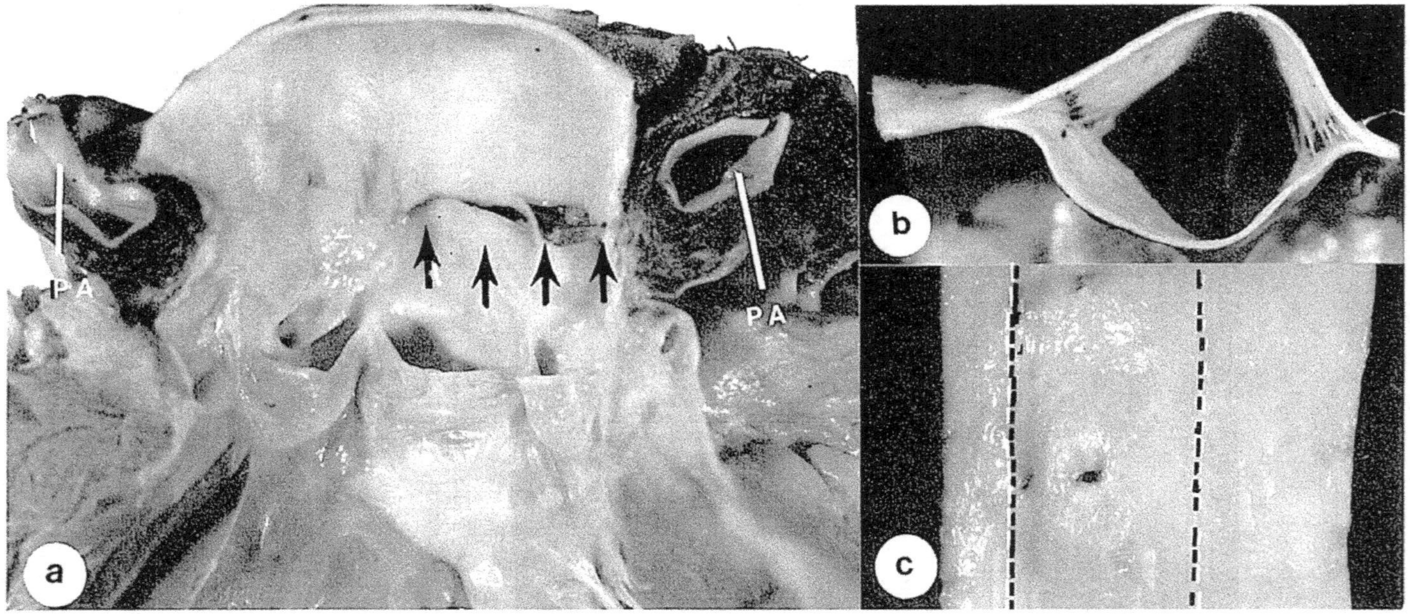

Fig. 26. Dissection involving entire aorta with rupture into pericardial sac in a 41-year-old man (DCMEO #78-08-724) who had the onset of chest pain 1 hour before being found slumped over the steering wheel of his automobile. Because his heart weighed 550 gm, it is reasonable to believe that this patient had had systemic hypertension. (*a*) The aortic tear is located just above the aortic valve. The tear extended into aortic adventitia and from there into the adventitia of the major pulmonary arteries (PA), causing mild narrowing of their lumens. (*b*) The opened area represents the false channel in the media of the descending thoracic aorta. (*c*) This aorta is relatively free of atherosclerotic plaque. The false channel is located beneath the intima between the dashed lines.

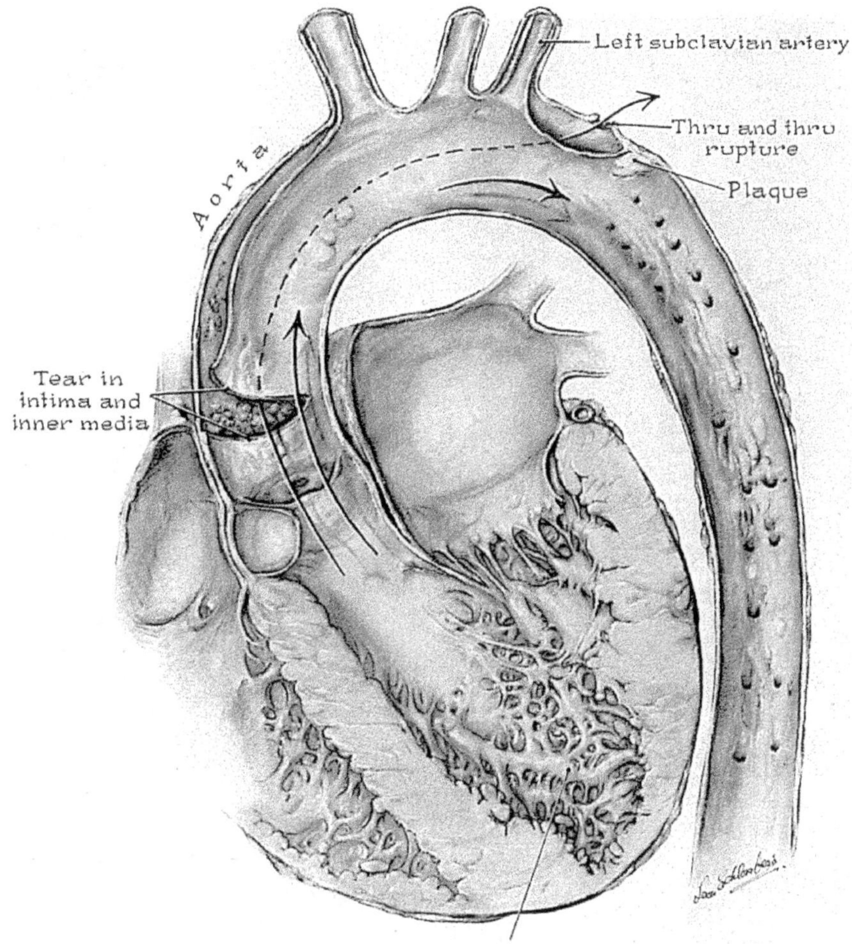

Fig. 27. Acute dissection involving the ascending and transverse portions of aorta with rupture into the left hemithorax in a 25-year-old black woman (DCMEO #78-06-451) who died suddenly at home. She had complained of chest pain about 2 months before death, and her blood pressure at that time was 200/110 mm Hg. She weighed 425 pounds (193 kg). The drawing of the heart and aorta shows the part of the aorta involved by the dissection. The large entrance tear was about 1 cm above the aortic valve. The dissection extended into all three arch arteries. The exit site was just past the aortic isthmus. The aortic dissection appears to have been stopped at this point, because its medial path was interrupted by an overlying intimal atherosclerotic plaque that has burrowed into the underlying media.

the second most common location of the primary tear. As a consequence, because most ascending aortic dissections extend to involve the descending aorta (indeed, usually the entire aorta)and because relatively few primary tears in the descending thoracic aorta extend retrogradely to involve the ascending portion of aorta, the descending thoracic aorta is the most common portion of the aorta to be involved by longitudinal dissection. Dissection limited to the ascending aorta is relatively infrequent (see section on the Marfan syndrome).

The most common sites of reentry or rerupture (secondary rupture) into the true

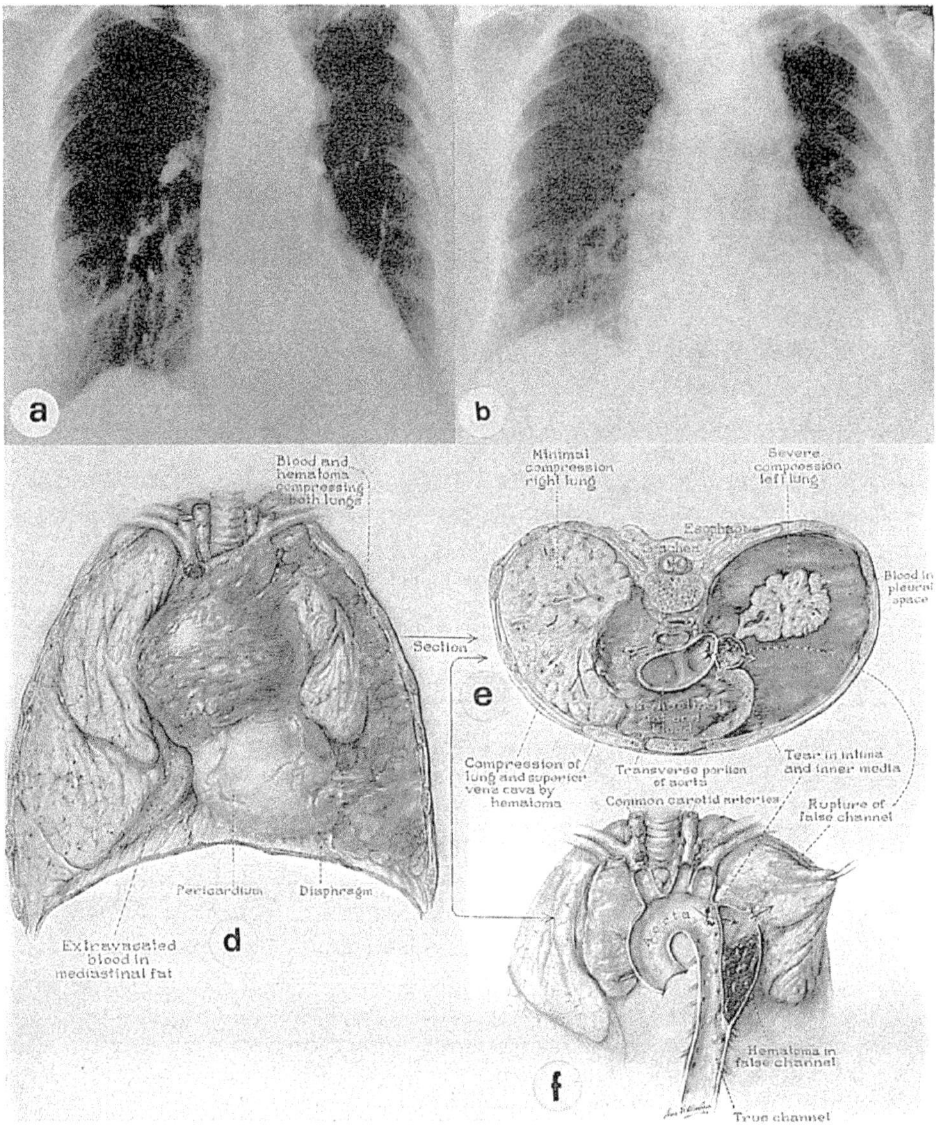

Fig. 28. Acute aortic dissection in a 76-year-old white woman (GT #77A-173). The entrance site is in the descending thoracic aorta with extravasation of blood into anterior mediastinal tissues simulating an ascending aortic dissecting aneurysm. The patient had been well until 14 days before death, when she noted "epigastric" pain and nausea. A chest radiograph (*a*) showed an abnormally shaped thoracic aorta. Electrocardiogram showed left ventricular hypertrophy, and her blood pressure was 200/100 mm Hg. Because of previous esophageal stricture, her chest pain was believed to be related to the esophagus. She felt well thereafter until the day of death, when she suddenly noted dyspnea and profuse sweating; repeat chest radiographs (*b* and *c*) showed further widening of the mediastinum and markedly diminished lung space in the left hemithorax. Her heart stopped shortly thereafter.

At necropsy, the left lung was collapsed, and most of the left hemithorax was filled with blood

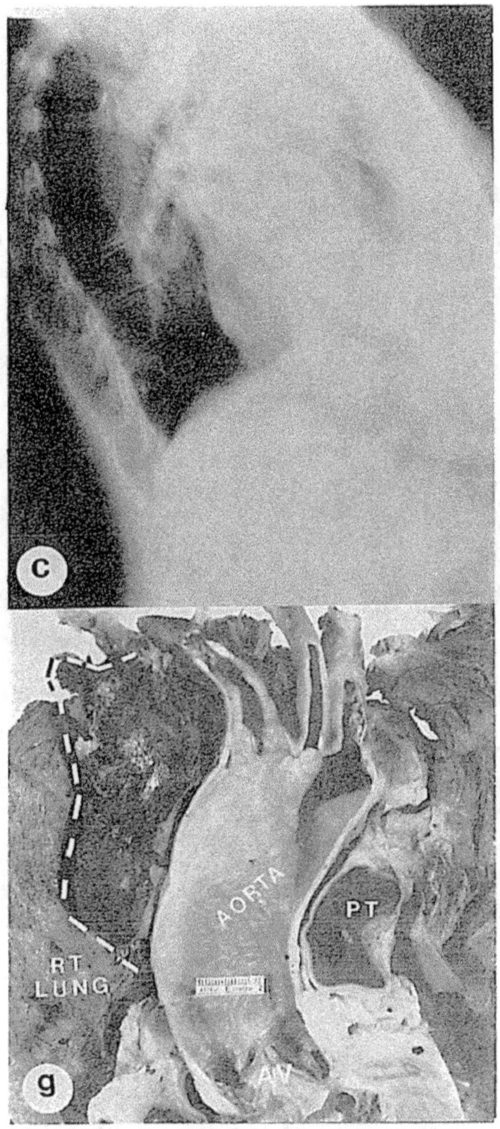

(*d* and *e*). A localized descending thoracic aortic dissection was present (*f*) and the entrance site into the false channel was at the aortic isthmus. The caudal two-thirds of the false channel was filled with thrombus, and the outer wall of the false channel was ruptured. Before the final extravasation of blood into the left hemithorax, blood appears to have dissected more slowly into the mediastinal tissues lying to the right of and anterior to the aorta. Hemorrhage into these mediastinal tissues on chest radiographs simulated dissection of the ascending aorta, which was not the case. (*g*) Close-up view of mediastinal hematoma to the right of the ascending aorta and behind the arch arteries. PT, pulmonary trunk; AV, aortic valve.

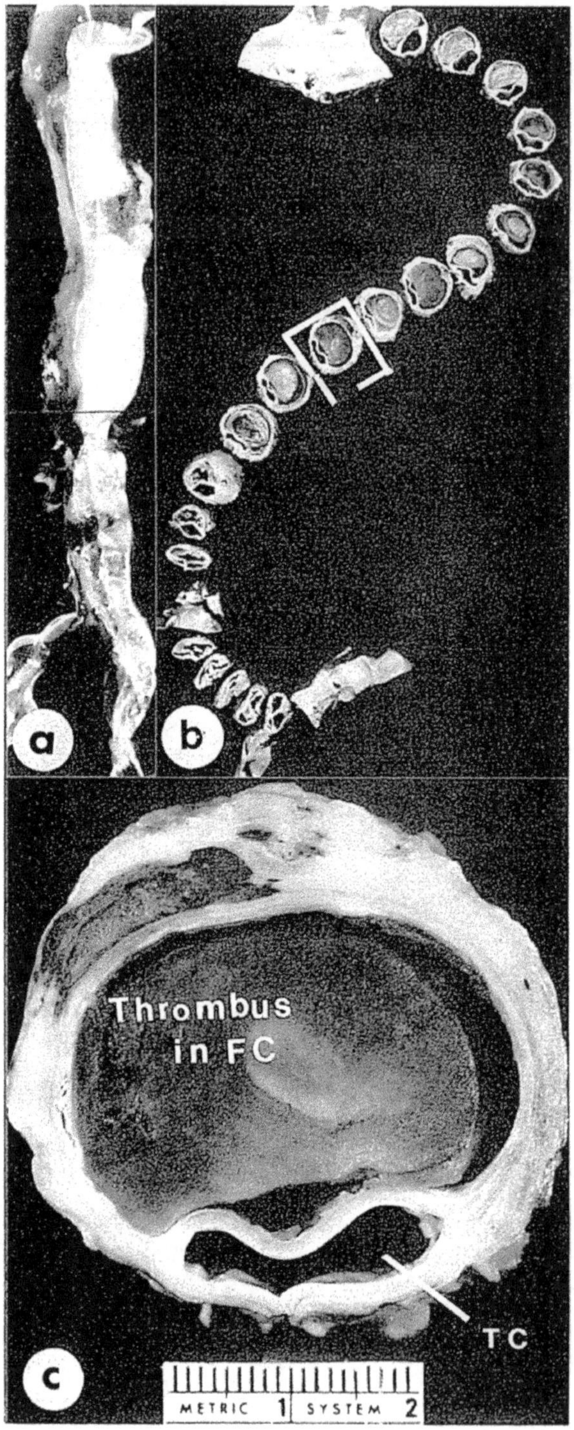

Fig. 29. Clinically silent healed dissection involving the descending thoracic and abdominal aorta in a 58-year-old white man (NNMC #A76-87) who died from complications of habitual alcoholism. He was known to have had systemic hypertension for many years. (*a*) Radiograph of aorta showing a narrowed true channel and thrombus plus heavy calcific depositis in the false channel. The entrance site was just distal to the aortic isthmus, and the exit site was in the left femoral artery.
(Legend continues on bottom of following page.)

lumen from the false lumen are in arteries arising from the aorta rather than in the aorta itself. The transverse, descending thoracic, and abdominal portions of aorta, however, are all sites of rerupture occasionally. At necropsy of patients dying from acute aortic dissection, rupture of the outer wall of the false channel is far more common than rupture of the inner wall of the false channel such that blood reenters the true channel.

Why any longitudinal aortic dissection once begun stops within the aorta has received little attention. Probably, the most common cause of interruption of the longitudinal dissection is extensive atherosclerotic plaquing that has caused underlying medial scarring, which in turn interrupts the longitudinal dissection. A common site of extensive atherosclerotic plaquing is the isthmus of aorta—the vicinity of the ligamentum arteriosum (Fig. 27). Extensive atherosclerosis in the abdominal portion of aorta also may prevent longitudinal dissection in this portion of aorta. Aortic dissection in patients with isthmic coarctation have the longitudinal dissection only in the ascending and transverse aorta. Coarctation is a medial invagination that prevents progression of a longitudinal dissection started upstream. Progression of a longitudinal dissection past a resected aortic coarctation also appears impossible. Fusiform abdominal aortic aneurysms prevent progression of a longitudinal aortic dissection (Fig. 11).

When longitudinal dissection of the aorta commences, it is unlikely that aortic aneurysm is the immediate consequence. In patients with fatal acute aortic dissection who die within minutes after developing signs and symptoms of cardiovascular catastrophe, aortic aneurysm is not often observed at necropsy. In the individuals living several days weeks, or months, however, aneurysm is to be expected. The thin outer wall of the false channel, whether thrombus forms within it or not, protrudes under the force of the intraaortic pressure. The longer the interval, in general, between the onset of aortic disease and death the greater the likelihood that the bulging of the false channel results in a larger aorta than was present before the dissection. In patients surviving the acute dissection, the false channel tends to enlarge progressively thereafter (Figs. 29 to 31, 33, and 34).

Complications of aortic dissection are numerous, and most are well appreciated. The most frequent is rupture of the outer wall of the false channel, and these ruptures are nearly always fatal. When the rupture involves the ascending aorta, the extravasation of blood is nearly always into the pericardial cavity (Figs. 20 to 26). The reason lies in the fact that the parietal pericardium is attached to the ascending aorta at the origin of the innominate artery. As a consequence, virtually all ascending aortic ruptures (the usual site being in the right lateral wall, the site of contact of blood ejected from left ventricle) do so into the pericardial space. When the rupture is relatively slow, blood may extend from the adventitia of aorta into the adventitia of the major pulmonary arteries because the two have a common adventitia (Figs. 20 to 26). Because the intrapulmonary pressure is low and because the extravasated aortic blood is forced into the pulmonary arterial adventitia under systemic arterial pressures, the lumens of the major pulmonary arteries may be narrowed by this mechanism.

Rupture of the descending thoracic aorta is usually into the left hemithorax, and rupture of the abdominal aorta is into the retroperitoneal areas. Rupture generally is in the vicinity of the primary tear, and again, fatal rupture is more common when a secondary tear is not identified.

(*b*) Transverse sections of the aorta again showing that the true channel is narrowed by thrombus in the false channel. (*c*) Close-up view of the section in the brackets in (*b*). TC, true channel; FC, false channel.

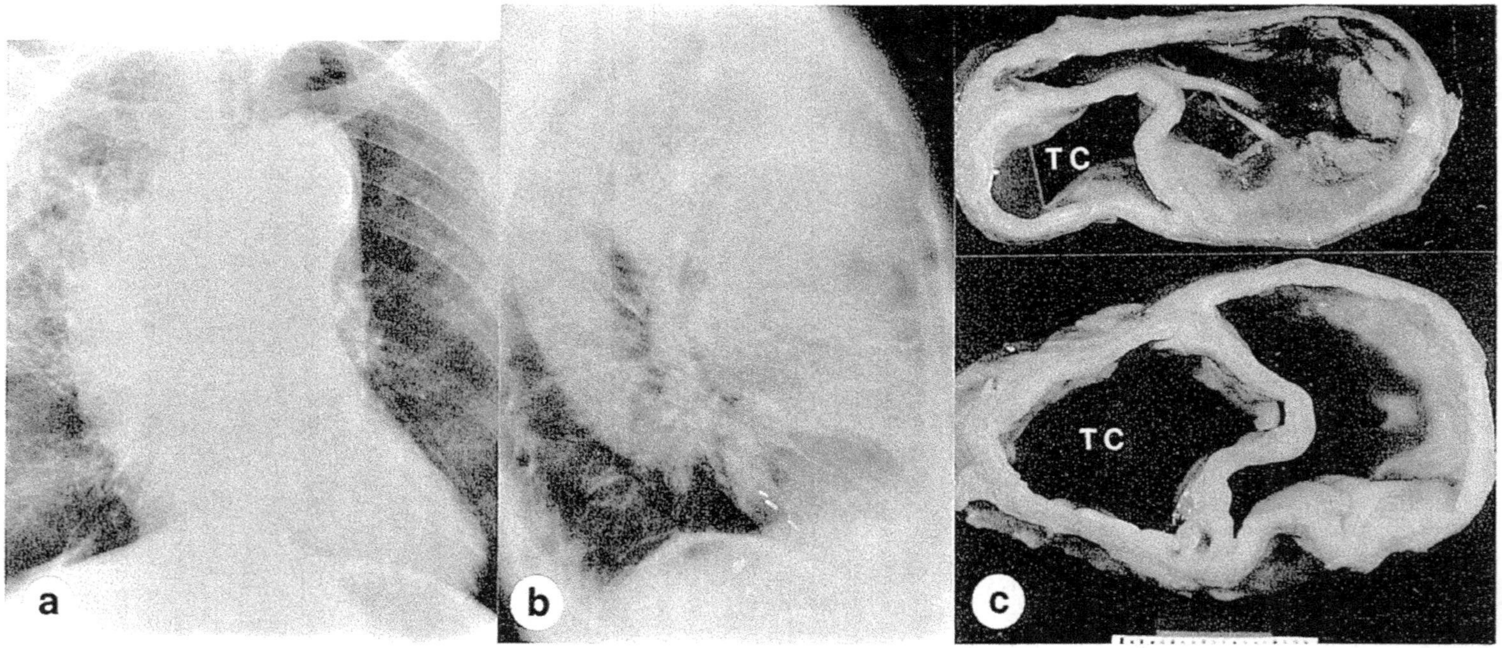

Fig. 30. Clinically silent aortic dissection after resection of an abdominal aortic fusiform aneurysm in a 69-year-old man (DCVAH #-A-178) who died of a bronchogenic carcinoma (*a* and *b*). The abdominal aorta was replaced with a graft about 1 year before death. Dissection of the aorta stopped at the beginning of the graft. There was no history of systemic hypertension, and the heart weighed only 330 gm. (*a* and *b*) Chest radiographs shortly before death. (*d*) Aorta, common iliac arteries, and kidneys. (*e*) Cross sections of aorta to the renal arteries. The dissection began at the aortic isthmus. The false channel is larger than the true channel. Thrombus is present in some portions of the false channel. (*c*) Close-up views of the two bracketed cross sections shown in (*e*). (*f*) Cross sections of the Dacron abdominal aortic graft. Some thrombus is present in its lumen.

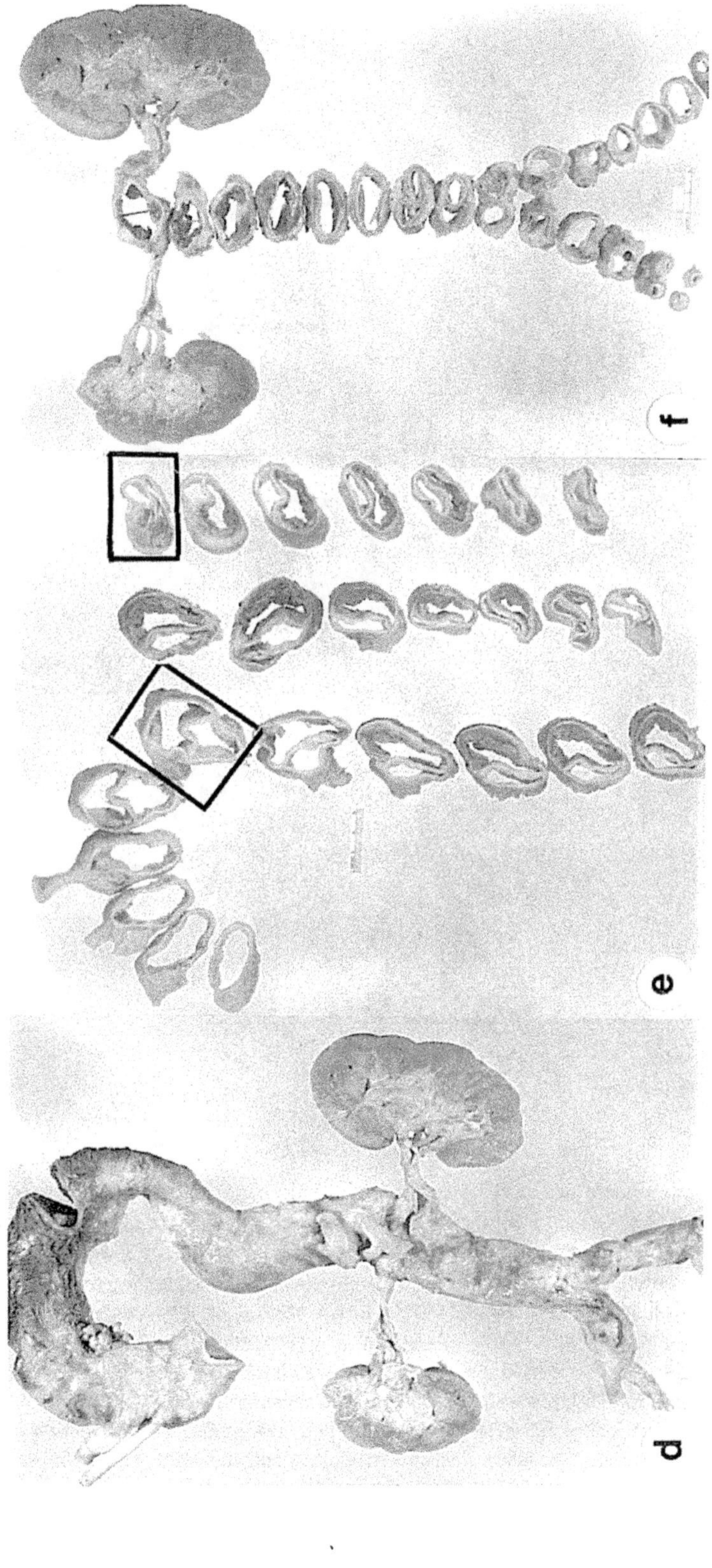
d
e
f

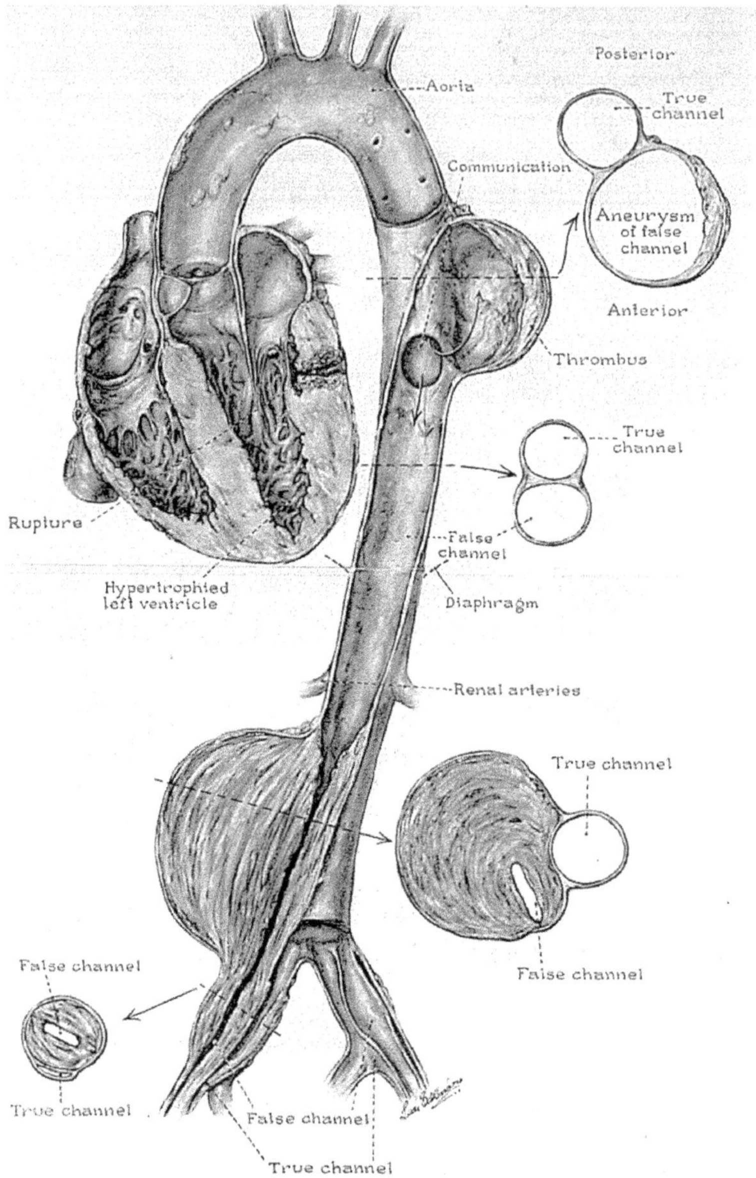

Fig. 31. Asymptomatic healed dissection of the descending thoracic and abdominal aorta in a 63-year-old man (GW #8399) who died of rupture of the left ventricle during acute myocardial infarction. There was no clinical evidence of an aortic dissection. He was known to have had systemic hypertension (blood pressure 180/100 mm Hg). He was asymptomatic until about 12 hours before death, when he had the onset of chest pain of myocardial infarction.

This drawing shows the entrance site into the false channel in the descending thoracic aorta, and the false channel just caudal to this site developed a saccular aneurysm. The false channel in the abdominal aorta also became aneurysmal and filled with thrombus. The dissection extended into both common iliac arteries. The heart was hypertrophied, and the acute transmural left ventricular infarction ruptured, causing massive extravasation of blood into the pericardial sac.

Retrograde longitudinal dissection in the ascending aorta, particularly when it extends into the sinus portion of aorta, may lead to extension of the medial dissection into the media of one or both major coronary arteries, usually the right one. Medial dissection of an artery the size of the coronary artery commonly leads to luminal narrowing, and this in turn may cause fatal myocardial ischemia. A second consequence of dissection in the vicinity of the aortic root is loss of commissural support of one or more aortic valve cusps, and the consequence of this development, of course, is aortic regurgitation.

Extension of the longitudinal dissection into the arteries arising from the aortic arch may lead to arm or cerebral ischemia or both (Fig. 21). Extension into one (usually the left) renal artery may produce signs of renal failure or elevation of the systemic blood pressure; and extension into the celic axis or one or both mesenteric arteries results in signs of abdominal organ insufficiency. Extension into the common iliac arteries or distally may lead to leg ischemia. The dissection may even cause near or complete obstruction of the aorta by a large thrombus of the false channel compressing the lumen of the true channel (Fig. 29).

Although most aortic dissections are fairly rapidly fatal, some certainly are not, and the latter go on to "heal." When "healing" occurs, a reentry opening reconnecting the false channel with the true channel is usually identified. The "healed" false channel usually progressively dilates. Its interior lining is covered initially by a fibrin layer, and sizable focal thrombi usually develop in the false channel (Figs. 29 to 34). Occasionally, the lumen of the false channel is entirely obliterated by thrombus. The latter situation is the most favorable type of development, for the thrombus tends to protect against rupture. The interior lining of the false channel eventually is covered by fibrous tissue (collagen) over which other thrombi develop, and between the thrombi and the underlying fibrous layer, lipid deposition occurs. With time, the wall of the false channel is made thicker than that of the true channel by the overgrowth of fibrous tissue (Fig. 34). On rare occasion, the wall of the false channel may become calcified (Fig. 29). Examination of the interior lining of the false channel provides a bit of evidence for the thrombogenic origin of atherosclerotic plaques. At times, the false channel will become enormously dilated (aneurysmal), sometimes in a rather uniform manner and at other times with large focal outpouchings suggesting saccular aneurysmal formation (Fig. 31).

THE MARFAN SYNDROME

The Marfan syndrome, an inheritable disorder, may involve the bones, joints, eyes, heart, and blood vessels (Figs. 35 to 37). The extremities are long and thin (dolichostenomelia), the ligaments and joint capsules are redundant, the lenses may be dislocated (ectopia lentis), the ascending aorta is often dilated, and one or both left-sided cardiac valves usually are incompetent. Cardiovascular disease is by far the most common cause of death in patients with the Marfan syndrome. Of 18 personally studied necropsy patients fulfilling McKusick's rigid criteria for this syndrome,[8] all died from cardiovascular disease, and in each case, death was premature (average age, 34 years; range, 15 to 52). Of 56 deceased patients with this syndrome studied by Murdoch and associates,[9] cardiovascular disease was the cause of death in 52 (93 percent), and the average age at death was 32 years.

A variety of cardiovascular lesions have been observed in the aorta and heart of patients with the Marfan syndrome.[8] The 18 personally studied necropsy patients with this

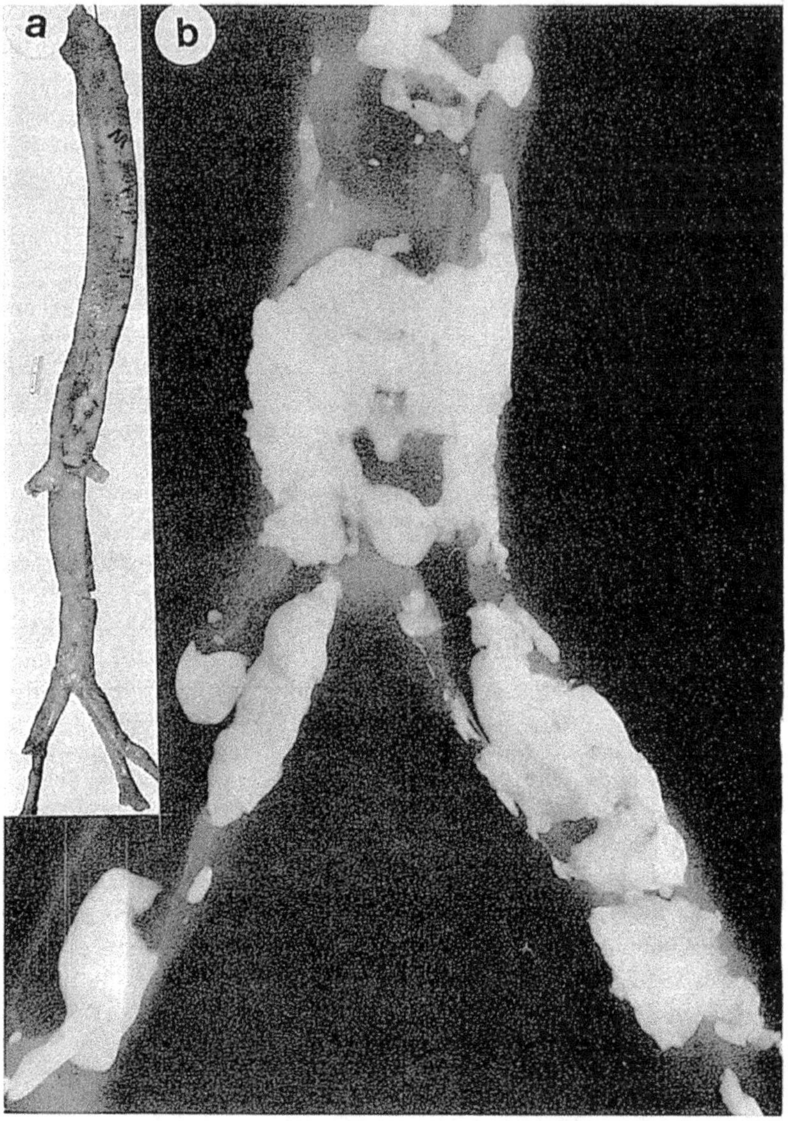

Fig. 32. Acute dissection of the entire aorta during left femoral arterial cannulation for cardiopulmonary bypass for mitral and aortic valve replacement in a 56-year-old white woman (A74-130). At the time of operation, the aortic dissection was apparent immediately after institution of cardiopulmonary bypass. It was believed that the cannula in the left femoral artery had pierced a plaque, and perfusion created a false channel in the media. The patient lived 20 days after the double valve replacement.

At necropsy, the aorta was only mildly dilated if at all (*a*). The abdominal portion of aorta and both common iliac arteries contained heavy calcific deposits (*b*) and the lumens of both were considerably narrowed. (Preoperatively, the patient had not complained of leg claudication.) *Figure and legend continue on following page.*

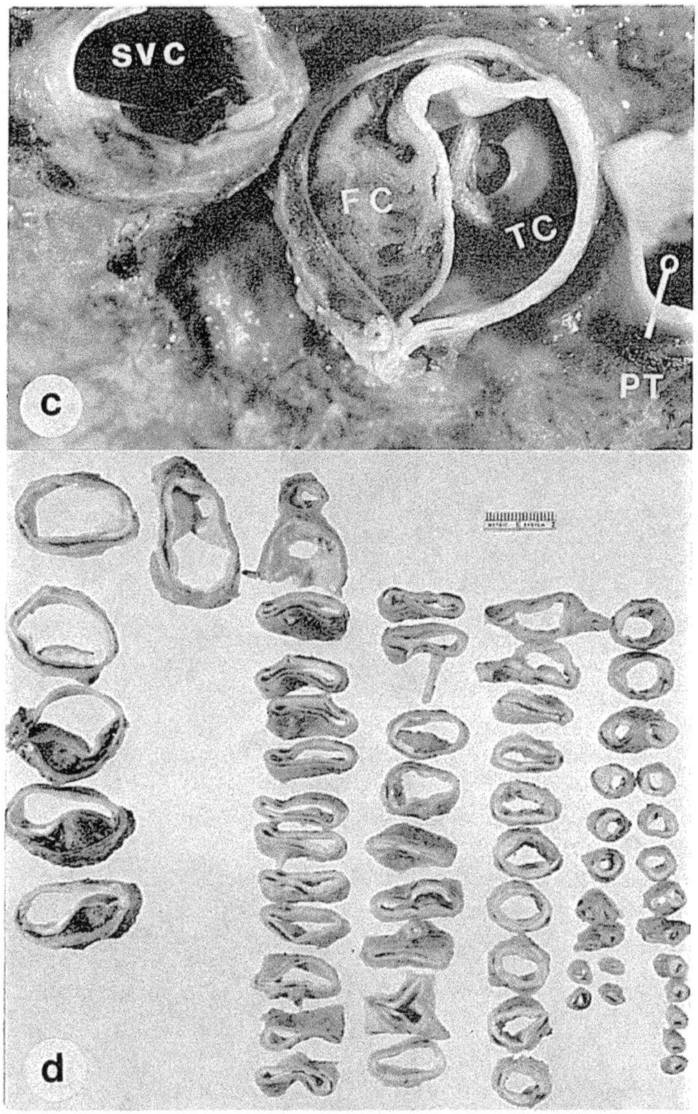

Fig. 32.(*continued*). (*c*) View of ascending aorta with a thombus in the false channel (FC). A caged-ball prosthesis (Starr-Edwards type) is visible in the true channel (TC). PT, pulmonary trunk; SVC, superior vena cava. (*d*) Cross-sections of aorta beginning (lower left) just above the aortic valve and ending (lower right) with the common iliac arteries.

syndrome were readily separated into three distinct groups on the basis of their cardiovascular lesions. Group 1 included 12 patients with *fusiform aneurysms of ascending aorta* (Figs. 35 and 36). All 12 patients had aortic regurgitation, and 6 also had associated mitral regurgitation. In each, the aneurysm involved the sinus portion and the proximal tubular portion of ascending aorta. Two patients also had fusiform aneurysms in the descending thoracic aorta. Histologic study of the wall of the ascending aorta disclosed the typical lesion of this syndrome, that is, massive degeneration of elastic fibers and increase in mucoid material in the media (Fig. 35).

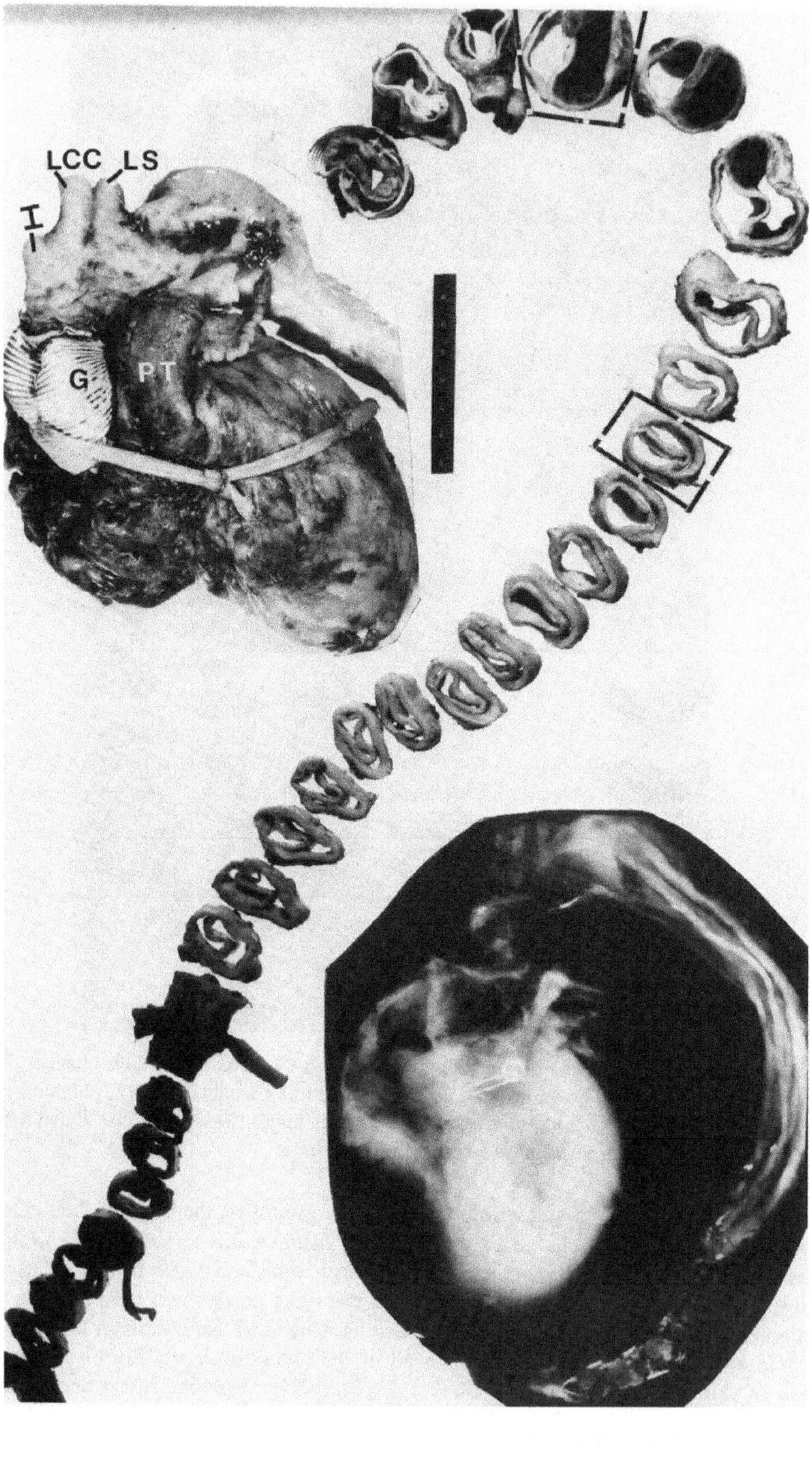
LCC
LS
I
G
PT

Group 2 included 3 patients with *dissection of the entire aorta*. Before dissection, the aorta was of normal size in each of these 3 patients, and histologic study of the aortic wall disclosed that the typical lesion of this syndrome was absent, and indeed, except for the dissection itself, the wall of aorta was histologically normal save for some aging changes.[1] Only 1 of the 3 patients had aortic regurgitation and that occurred only after the dissection. One had mitral regurgitation. Two of the 3 patients had systemic hypertension before the aortic dissection.

Group 3 included 2 patients *without aortic fusiform aneurysm or aortic disease* but with *pure mitral regurgitation* with floppy mitral leaflets and markedly dilated mitral anuli. The aorta was of normal size, and histologically, its wall was normal in each patient.

Thus, the major lesions in the aorta in patients with this syndrome are fusiform root aneurysms and dissection. In contrast to that described clinically by others,[10] from study of the 18 necropsy patients described above, it appears that the two lesions rarely occur together; at least, none of the 18 patients studied personally had both a fusiform aortic aneurysm and an aortic dissection. These two aortic lesions may be mutually exclusive. None of the 12 patients with fusiform aortic root aneurysms had evidence of dissection, although 9 of the 12 had focal intimal and medial tears in the wall of the fusiform aneurysms (Figs. 35 and 36). These aortic tears mistakenly have been called "dissections" in a number of reports. None of the 3 patients with aortic dissection had fusiform aneurysms of the aorta, which was of normal size before the dissection. Histologically, the wall of the aorta appears entirely different. In all 12 patients with aortic root fusiform aneurysms, there was massive degeneration of the elastic fibers associated with increased amounts of collagen and mucoid material in the media of the aneurysmal wall. The increased amount of collagen in the aortic wall in these patients may, in actuality, prevent longitudinal dissection. In each of the 3 patients with aortic dissection, the wall of the aorta histologically appeared "normal," that is, just like that in patients with aortic dissection who do not have the Marfan syndrome—no changes other than aging. Interestingly, 2 of the 3 patients with aortic dissection had evidence of diastolic systemic hypertension, whereas none of the other 16 patients had diastolic hypertension.

The term applied to the characteristic histologic lesion in the aorta in patients with the Marfan syndrome has been "cystic medial necrosis," a term first used by Erdheim in

---

Fig. 33. Healed and healing dissection of the aorta in a 66-year-old white woman (A76-125) who clinically was considered by Victor A. McKusick, M.D., to be a variant of the Ehlers-Danlos syndrome. She had mild valvular aortic stenosis and moderately severe aortic regurgitation (aortic pressure = 150/70 mm Hg; left ventricle = 176/16 mm Hg). For several months, she had complained periodically of back pain. She underwent aortic valve replacement without difficulty, but 3 days postoperatively she had a stroke, and a day later, signs of cardiac tamponade appeared. Reoperation disclosed a dissection beginning near the aortotomy site. A portion of aorta, therefore, was replaced with a graft (*upper left*), and because the left main coronary artery had been severed from the aorta, a conduit (saphenous vein) was inserted between the aortic graft and the left anterior descending and left circumflex coronary arteries. She was unable to be weaned from cardiopulmonary bypass.

At necropsy, the entire aorta was dissected. Most of the dissection had healed or was healing in that the wall of the false channel was thickened by fibrous tissue and the lumen of the false channel in most areas was free of thrombus. Just distal to the aortic isthmus, the aorta was quite dilated, as a result of dilatation of the false channel which in this area contained thrombus. The lower right is a postmortem radiograph that shows a double-channeled aorta.

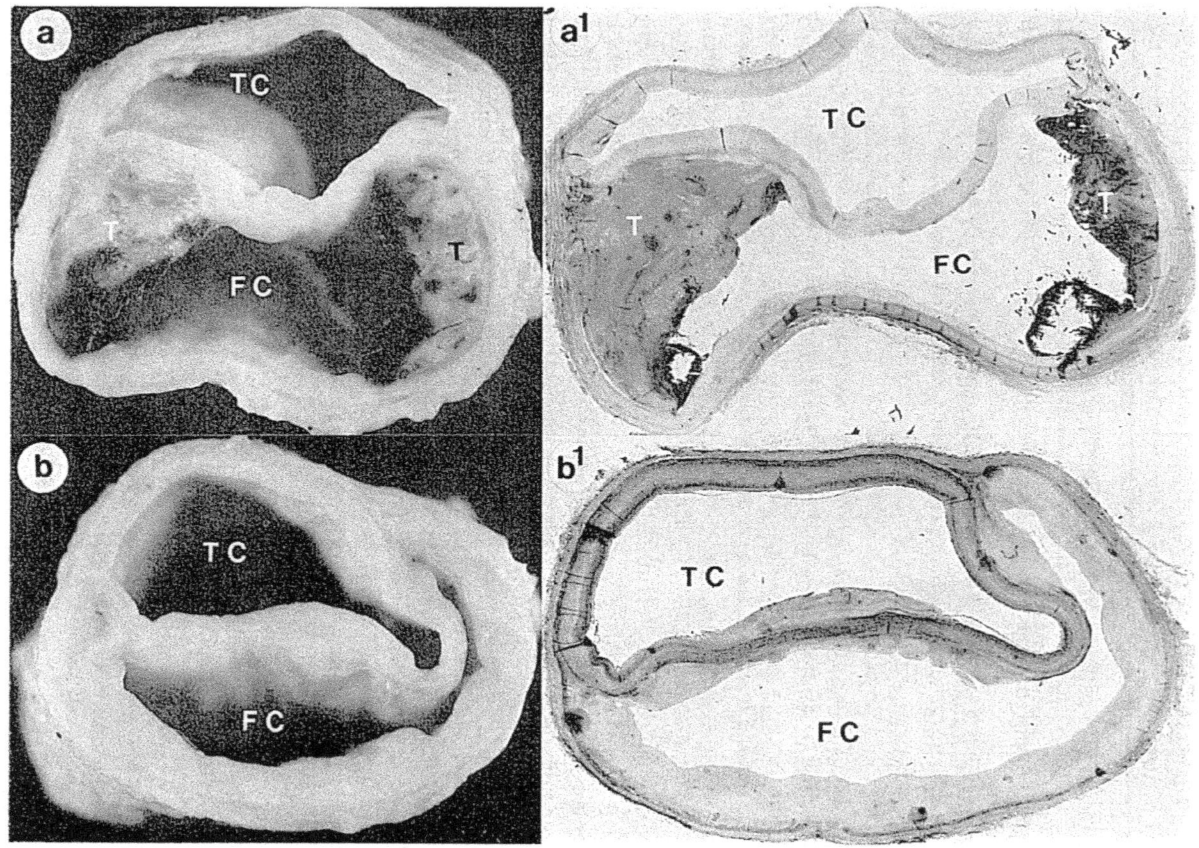

Fig. 34. Transverse sections of aorta from two sites designed in figure (A76-125). The wall of the false channel is thickened by fibrous tissue, which appears to result from organization of thrombus. The media of the aorta is histologically normal. TC, true channel; FC, false channel; T, thrombus. A^1, hematoxylin-eosin stain; b^1, Movat stain.

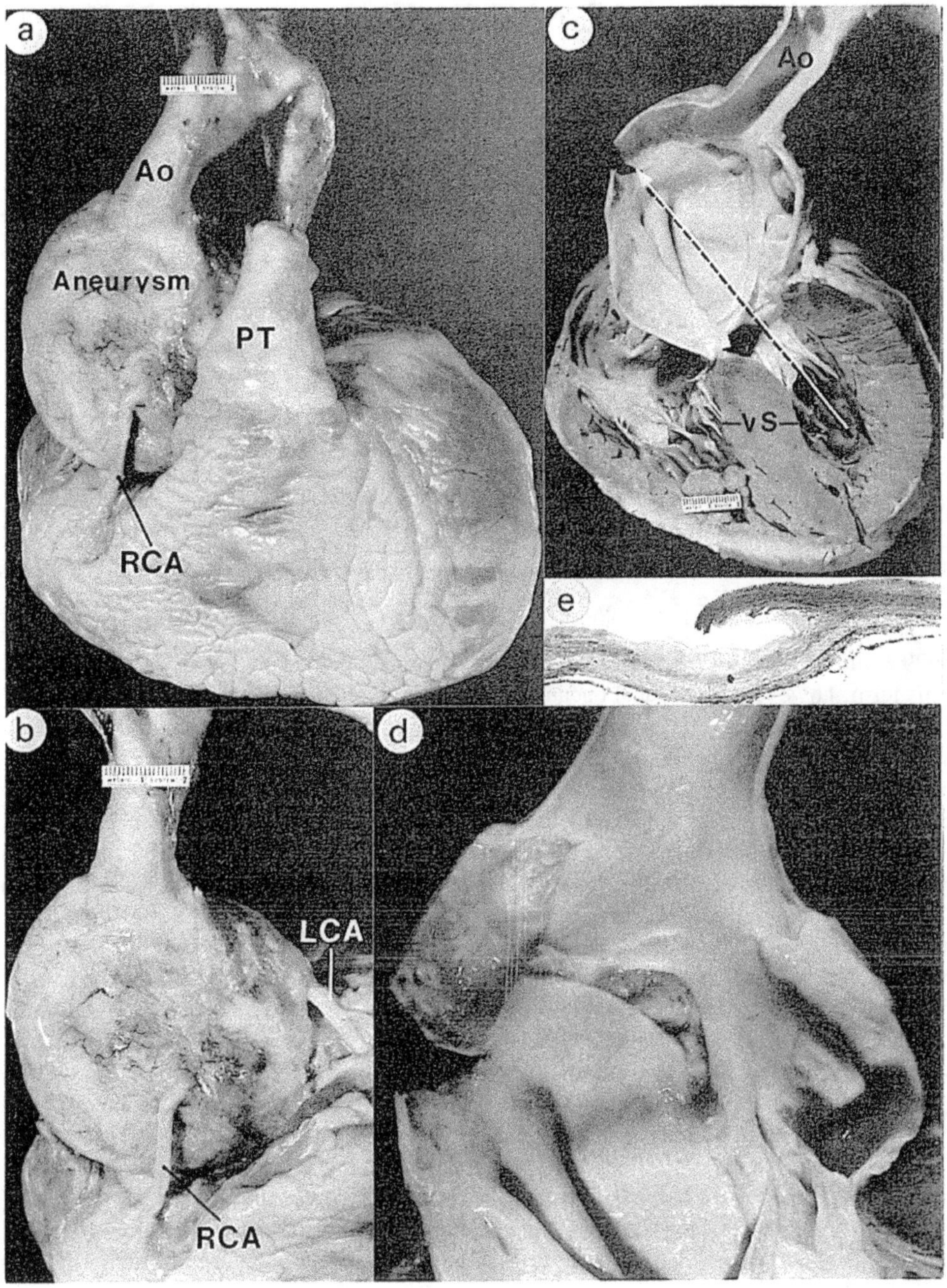

Fig. 35. The Marfan syndrome with rupture of ascending aortic aneurysm in a 38-year-old black man (A73-84). The patient was known to have a murmur of aortic regurgitation (aortic pressure 115/55 mm Hg), but there was no evidence of congestive heart failure. He died suddenly at home, and at necropsy the pericardial space was filled with blood, and a tear was present in a large aneurysm involving all three sinuses of Valsalva and the proximal tubular portion of ascending aorta. (*a*) View of heart shows the size of the aneurysm in comparison to the sizes of other structures. Ao, aorta; PT, pulmonary trunk; RCA, right coronary artery. (*b*) A closer view of the

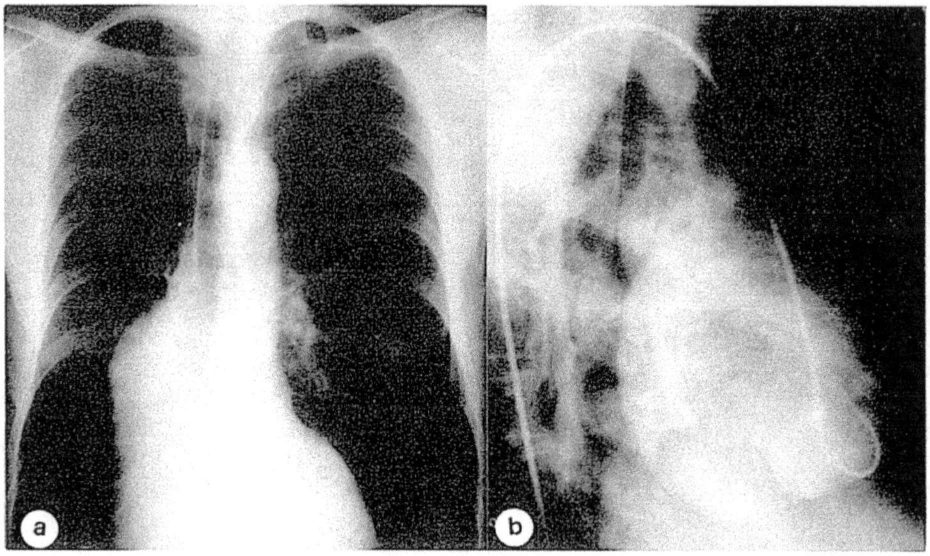

Fig. 36. Posteroanterior chest roentgenogram (*a*) and lateral view aortogram (*b*) in the patient (A73-84) described in Fig. 35.

1929[11] and an outgrowth of the term "medionecrosis" coined by Gsell[12] a year earlier. This term, however, is not ideal because "cysts" as such are infrequent and "necrosis," to my knowledge, has never been observed in the aortic media in this condition. Gsell used the term "medionecrosis" to designate areas in the aortic media with a diminished number of nuclei.[12] Becker recently showed that those areas devoid of nuclei actually consisted of large amounts of fibrous tissue and were a regular feature of the normal aging aorta.[13] Furthermore, the striking histologic aortic lesion in the Marfan syndrome is *massive degeneration of elastic fibers* in the media, and this feature is ignored by the term "cystic medial necrosis." When Erdheim coined this term, stains for elastic fibers were poor or rarely used, and loss or degeneration of elastic fibers is difficult to appreciate on hematoxylin-eosin stained sections. Thus, he apparently did not appreciate this histologic feature of the condition.

When elastic fibers disappear from the aortic wall in this condition, the space previously occupied by them appears to be replaced by collagen fibrils and mucoid material. Although the increased acid-mucopolysaccharide material has been considered an inherent defect in this condition, it is just as reasonable to believe that this material serves simply as "a filler" for the lost elastic fibers and probably also many smooth muscle cells. It is not clear whether or not the number of elastic lamellae is normal or decreased at the time of birth in patients with the Marfan syndrome. Whether normal or decreased, however, aortic-root aneurysm, with or without tears, has not been described in newborns with this

---

large aneurysm with the coronary arteries arising from it. LCA, left coronary artery. (*c*) The anterior half of the heart and aorta have now been removed. The dashed line depicts the direction of the blood ejected from the left ventricle. The arrow points to the rupture site in the wall of the aneurysm. The right lateral wall is the site of the rupture. VS, ventricular septum. (*d*) Close-up of interior lining of aortic aneurysm at site of rupture. Several healed incomplete tears are present in the wall of the aneurysm, and these have been confused with aortic dissection. (*e*) Photomicrograph through one of the aortic tears showing massive degeneration of elastic fibers.

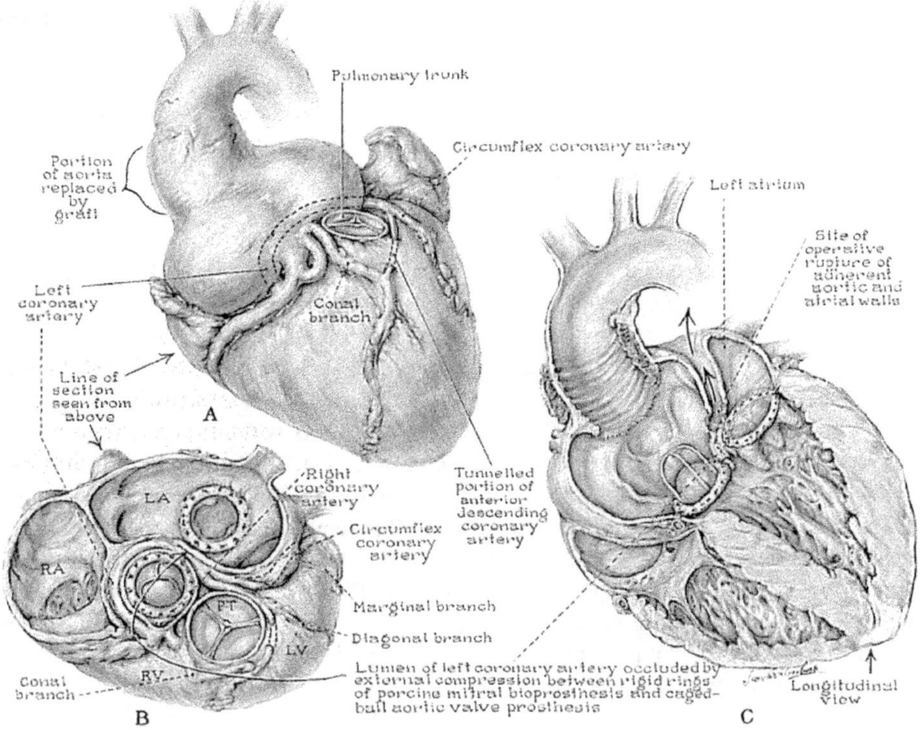

Fig. 37. Drawing of the heart and aorta in a 69-year-old man (A78-155) who had the typical cardiovascular features of the Marfan syndrome but without the skeletal, ocular, or familial features of this syndrome. Although a precordial murmur had been heard when he was 17 years old, he was asymptomatic until age 50, when he had the onset of periodic chest pain believed to be angina pectoris and also some exertional dyspnea. Aortic regurgitation was documented 2 years later, and at age 57, he underwent aortic valve replacement and resection of a portion of the ascending aorta. Histologic study of the excised portion of aorta disclosed massive degeneration of elastic fibers, the typical histologic lesion of the Marfan and forme fruste varieties of this syndrome. Thereafter, he did well for many years but by age 67 he had the reappearance of considerable congestive cardiac failure. At age 69, severe mitral regurgitation was confirmed. He underwent mitral valve replacement but died during the procedure because of massive bleeding caused by tearing of the aorta during mitral replacement.

(*a*) Huge aortic "root" aneurysm. The left main coronary artery arises as the first branch of the right coronary artery. (*b*) In this view, the atria and ascending aorta have been removed to show the caged-ball aortic valve prosthesis and the porcine prosthesis in the mitral position. (*c*) Opened longitudinal view of heart and aorta again showing the massive aortic root aneurysm that was observed at operation 12 years before death.

syndrome. Thus, it appears that although the composition of the aortic media may be defective at birth, the aneurysms form later, presumably as the consequence of the intraaortic pressure's effect on an inherently weak wall.

Aortic regurgitation in patients with the Marfan syndrome is usually the result of severe dilatation of the aortic "root" by the fusiform aneurysm. The amount of regurgitation may not, however, correlate directly with the size of the aortic root aneurysm.[14] Far less commonly, the aortic regurgitation is the consequence of aortic dissection. The aortic valve cusps in patients with the Marfan syndrome appear to have an increased amount of mucoid material (acid mucopolysaccharide), irrespective of whether or not aortic regurgitation is present.

Mitral regurgitation also is frequent. At least five factors may be important in causing mitral regurgitation in patients with this syndrome. These are (1) floppiness of the mitral leaflets and/or chordae tendineae; (2) dilatation of the mitral anuli; (3) calcification of the mitral anuli; (4) rupture of mitral chordae tendineae; and (5) papillary muscle dysfunction. Of these five factors, the first, second, and third appear to be the most important in causing severe degrees of mitral regurgitation. Of the 18 necropsy patients with this syndrome studied personally, 9 had mitral regurgitation, which was isolated in 2 and combined with aortic regurgitation in 7. Of these 9 patients with mitral regurgitation, 6 had floppy mitral valves; of the 9 without mitral regurgitation, none had floppy valves. The "floppiness" involved the posterior mitral leaflet in all 6 patients. Furthermore, of the 9 patients with mitral regurgitation, the circumference of the mitral anulus ranged from 10 to 17 cm (average, 15; normal, 9), and of the 9 patients without mitral regurgitation, this circumference ranged from 9 to 12.5 cm (average, 11). In the 6 patients with floppy mitral valves, the mitral circumference ranged from 14 to 17 cm (average, 16). Thus the average circumference of the mitral anulus in the 9 patients with mitral regurgitation was dilated 67 percent over normal (15 compared to 9), whereas in the 9 patients without mitral regurgitation, the average circumference was only 22 percent over normal (12 compared to 9). It therefore seems most reasonable to conclude that both mitral leaflet floppiness and anular dilatation play significant roles in causing mitral regurgitation in these patients. Calcification of the mitral anulus is known to cause or at least be associated with mitral regurgitation.[15] The degree of regurgitation produced by this mechanism alone, however, is nearly always mild or minimal, and, in addition, the mitral anuli in non-Marfan patients with mitral anular calcification is nearly always of normal or near normal circumference. Of the 18 personally studied necropsy patients, 4 had mitral anular calcific deposits: all 4 had associated mitral regurgitation, but in addition, 3 had floppy mitral leaflets, and in all 4 patients the circumference of the mitral anulus was quite dilated (range, 13 to 17; average, 15). Evidence for rupture of mitral chordae tendineae was found in 4 of the 9 patients without mitral regurgitation. Two of these 4 patients had histories of infective endocarditis that had healed.[16] All 4 patients with evidence of mitral chordae rupture had floppy mitral leaflets and dilated mitral anuli (range, 15 to 17; average, 16).

The role played by "papillary muscle dysfunction" in causing mitral regurgitation in these patients is less clear.[17] Among our 18 patients, the left ventricles were dilated in each, and the left ventricular mass was increased in each. The hearts of the 18 patients ranged in weight from 375 to 850 gm (average, 654). In 13 of the 18 patients, the mitral leaflets from their basal attachments to their distal margins were increased in length. This "stretching" probably was the result of the elongation (apex to base) of left ventricular cavities, resulting primarily from the associated aortic regurgitation. The resulting left ventricular dilatation may have altered the normal angulation between the papillary muscles and the mitral leaflets. Whether or not mitral regurgitation was increased, however, in any patient by this mechanism is uncertain.

Although the above discussion concerned only patients with typical features of the Marfan syndrome, the cardiovascular features described in them also occur in patients without the skeletal or ocular manifestations of this syndrome and without histories of this syndrome in other family members (Fig. 37). In addition, the characteristic histologic features in the wall of the ascending aorta also have been observed in the aorta of patients with congenitally malformed aortic valves, particularly the bicuspid condition, and in patients with aortic stenosis when superimposed on congenitally malformed valves.[18] Of individuals with the characteristic ascending aortic root aneurysms and histologic evidence of massive elastic fiber degeneration of aortic media, more often than not, features of the Marfan syndrome will be absent rather than present.

CARDIOVASCULAR SYPHILIS

Just 60 years after syphilis was first recognized in Europe in the late fifteenth century, anatomists of the day suggested that "the pox" was the cause of aortic aneurysm. It was not until approximately 400 years later, in 1875, however, that irrefutable evidence linking syphilis and aortic aneurysm appeared. By the twentieth century, it was generally accepted that syphilis did involve the aorta in a way grossly and microscopically distinguishable from the effects of atherosclerosis.

Syphilis may involve the cardiovascular system in at least five ways: (1) aortitis, (2) aortic aneurysm, with or without rupture, (3) aortic valvular regurgitation, (4) stenosis of the ostium of one or both coronary arteries, and rarely, (5) gumma formation within the aortic wall or myocardium. Each of the four most common manifestations of cardiovascular syphilis involves the aorta and/or structures closely related to the aortic wall.

Characteristically, *aortitis* resulting from syphilis starts abruptly at the sinotubular junction (superior margin of the sinuses of Valsalva) and extends distally to involve a variable portion of ascending (thoracic) aorta (Figs. 38 to 41). The process occasionally involves the transverse or descending (thoracic) portions of the aorta. Evidence that it can involve the abdominal portion of aorta is unconvincing. The histologic hallmark is infiltration of the adventitia and media of the aortic wall by plasma cells and lymphocytes. The inflammatory cells preferentially cluster around the vasa vasora and the nutrient arteries in the aortic adventitia, and intimal fibrous proliferation may partially or completely occlude the lumens of these small vessels. As a result of inflammation and ischemia, patchy destruction of elastic fibers and smooth muscle cells occurs within the media of the aorta. The focal medial necrosis leads to scarring and contracture of the aortic wall, producing intimal wrinkling, recognized grossly as so-called tree barking. Spirochetes are absent. No one has ever positively observed a spirochete in the wall of aorta. Intimal thickening invariably occurs, even though this layer does not contain inflammatory cells. Atherosclerosis is virtually always superimposed on the medial and adventitial process, causing the ascending aorta to be more plaqued than the abdominal aorta, a reversal of the usual distribution of atherosclerotic lesions. The calcific deposits occur in this superimposed atherosclerotic process.

Aneurysm of the aorta resulting from syphilis occurs because the media is weakened by the interruption of its elastic fibers. Although the aortic wall in syphilis is thicker than normal, it is weaker than normal. The syphilitic aneurysms are usually saccular and always involve the ascending portion with or without involvement of the transverse and descending portions of aorta. Rupture, obviously, is the major complication of syphilitic aneurysm. It may expand into and compress or erode adjacent vital structures, such as superior vena cava, pulmonary artery, sternum, vetebral bodies, trachea, major bronchi, esophagus, recurrent laryngeal nerve, or carotid, innominate, and subclavian arteries. Dissection of the aorta involved by syphilis is extremely rare because the media is interrupted by the more or less transverse scars.

In most patients with cardiovascular syphilis, the process involves only the tubular

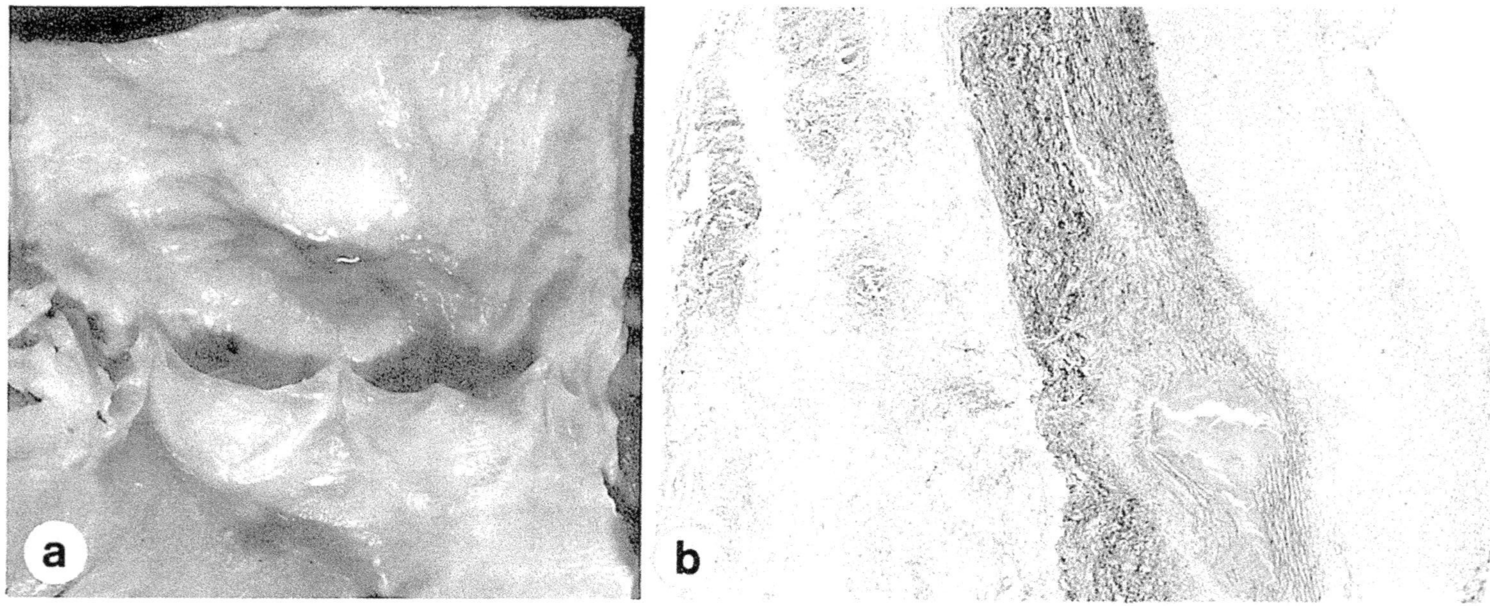

Fig. 38. Cardiovascular syphilis in a 32-year-old woman (DCMEO #76-05-456) who was killed, while walking, by an automobile. She had no symptoms or apparent signs of cardiac dysfunction during life. (*a*) Opened ascending aorta and aortic valve showing much wrinkling of the tubular portion. (*b*) Close-up of portion of tubular ascending aorta showing this portion to be very thick. The media is interrupted at this point (×23). (*c*) Low-power (×4) photomicrograph of aortic-valve (AV) cusp and wall of ascending aorta. The portion of aortic wall below the origin of the coronary artery (CA) is normal, the coronary ostium is narrowed by a fibrous intimal process, and the wall of aorta above the ostium of the coronary artery is markedly thickened by a combination of adventitial and intimal fibrous tissue proliferation. Focal scars are present in the media (Movat stain). (*d*) Vasa vasorum vessel surrounded by mononuclear cells in adventitia of aorta (×380). (*e*) Close-up of the adventitial cells (×1280). This case is of particular interest because the patient was so young. The aorta at this point is only slightly dilated and is free of calcific deposits.

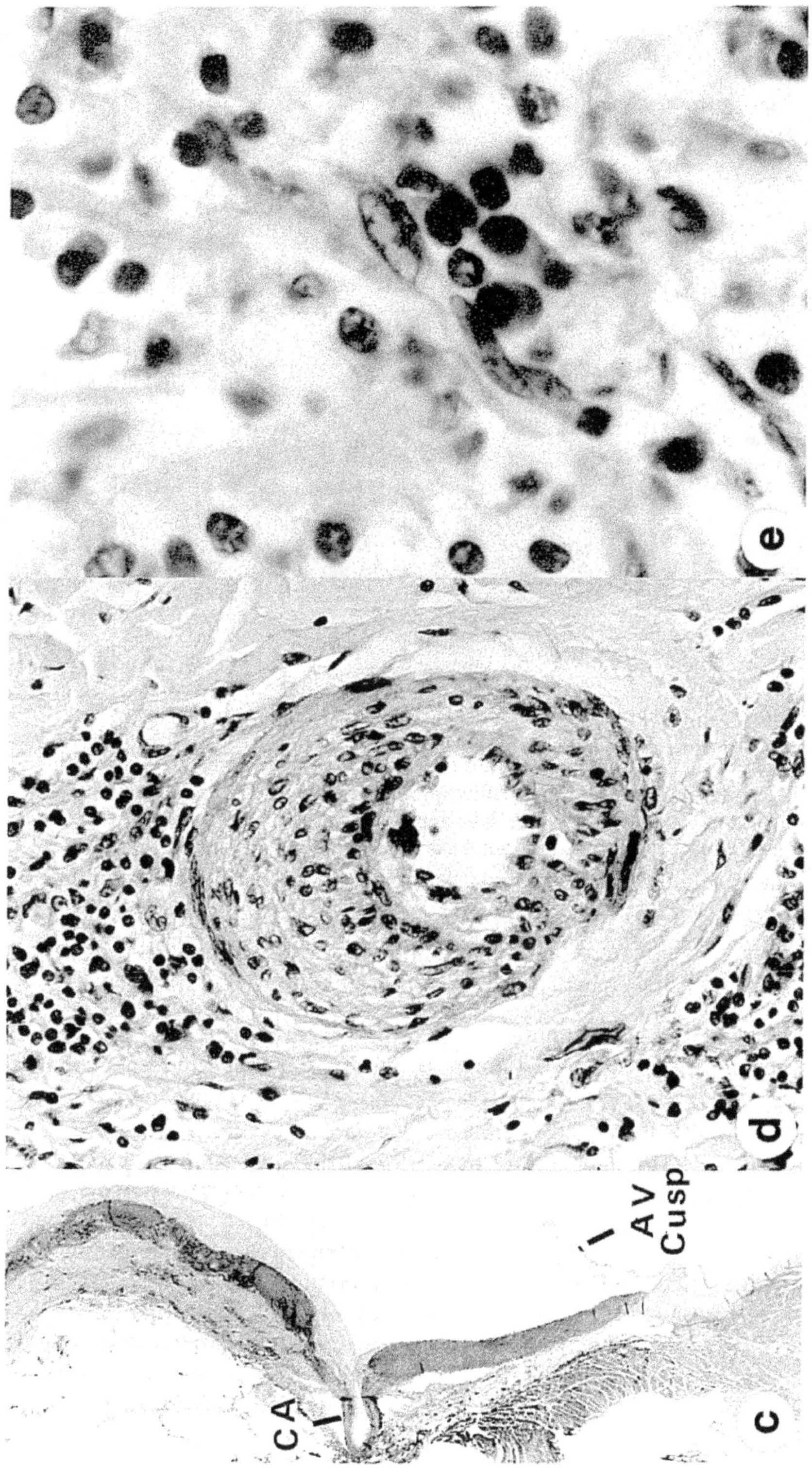
CA
AV
Cusp
c
d
e

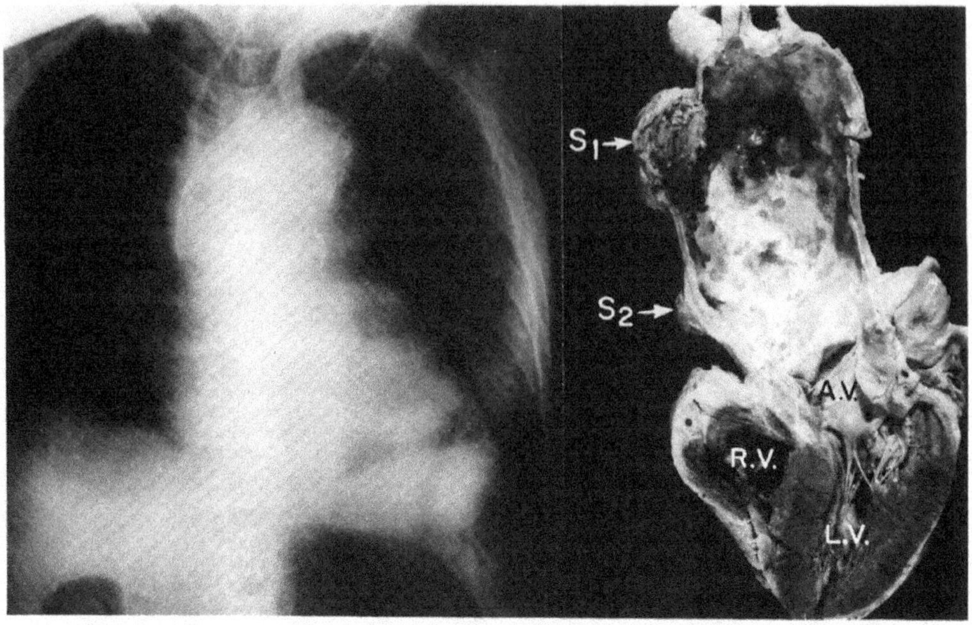

Fig. 39. Cardiovascular syphilis without aortic regurgitation. Incidental finding in an 81-year-old man (A67-177) who died of pneumonia but who had no evidence of cardiac dysfunction. Syphilitic aortitis led to severe destruction and aneurysmal dilatation of aorta and formation of two smaller saccular aneurysm (S and S_2). Chest roentgenogram demonstrates a diffusely dilated aorta with a calcified wall. Aortic regurgitation did not occur in this patient, since the walls of the sinuses of Valsalva were not involved by the syphilitic process. Neither the aortic root nor the left ventricle (LV) was dilated. RV, right ventricle, AV, aortic valve.

portion of ascending aorta. If the tubular portion becomes severely dilated, some degree of *aortic regurgitation* may result, but it is usually not severe. When the process extends into the wall of aorta behind the sinuses of Valsalva, the regurgitation may become severe. The regurgitation, just as in the Marfan-type aorta, is caused by a central leak that results simply from stretching of the margins of the valve cusps between their commissural attachments, the result of dilatation of the aortic "root." The leak is rarely the result of so-called commissural widening. Of approximately 40 necropsy patients with cardiovascular syphilis studied personally, only 1 had commissural widening and that involved only one of the three commissures.

Stenosis of the coronary artery ostium occurs when proliferation of the aortic intima, caused by aortitis, partially or completely obstructs the takeoff of a coronary artery from the aorta (Fig. 38). The narrowing is at the ostium and does not extend into the coronary artery itself. Stenosis, of course, is more likely when coronary ostia are located distal to the sinotubular junction. Generally, they are just proximal to it. Coronary ostial narrowing in syphilis, surprisingly, infrequently produces evidence of myocardial ischemia. On rare occasion, one or both coronary ostia may be dilated (aneurysmal) by the syphilitic process rather than narrowed by it.

With the development of effective chemotherapeutic agents, cardiovascular syphilis has ceased to be a common necropsy finding and cause of death. When antispirochetal therapy is not given or is delayed until the secondary or tertiary stages, however, cardiovascular syphilis may still develop.

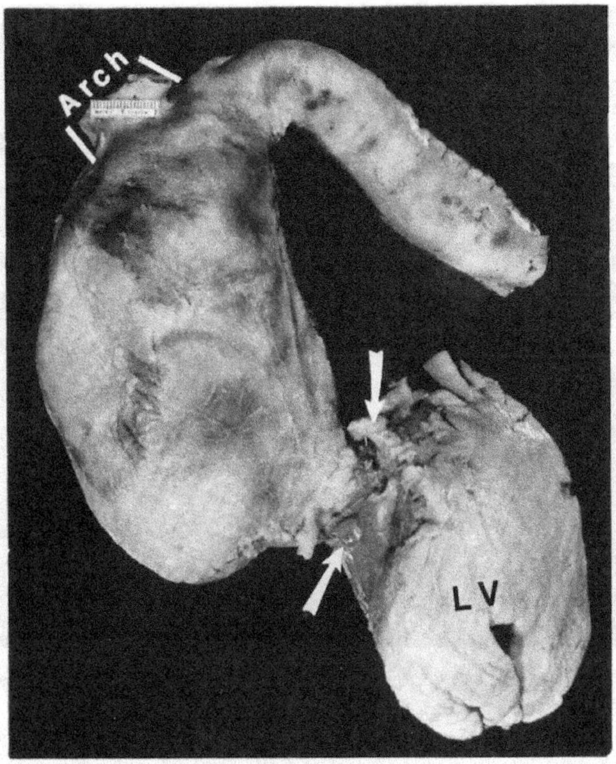

Fig. 40. Syphilitic aortitis with huge ascending aortic fusiform aneurysm in a 79-year-old woman (HH-DB #A75-47). This is the largest syphilitic aortic aneurysm the author has seen. In this fixed state, its maximal transverse diameter is nearly 10 cm and its maximal circumference is 25 cm. In contrast, the circumference of the aortic isthmus was 7 cm. The aneurysm spares the sinus portion of aorta (between the arrows), but it involves the entire transverse aorta as well as the tubular portion of ascending aorta. The entire descending thoracic aorta also was involved by the syphilitic process. All of the heart except the left ventricle has been removed. The aortic aneurysm is larger than the left ventricle. This patient had negative serological findings (both VDRL and FTA-ABS). The cardiovascular syphilis produced no symptoms of cardiac dysfunction. She died of colonic carcinoma. The heart weighed only 330 gm.

ANKYLOSING SPONDYLITIS

Although rheumatoid arthritis and ankylosing spondylitis were recognized as distinct entities just over 20 years ago, only recently has it become appreciated that each produces a distinctive cardiovascular disease.[19–23] Rheumatoid arthritis produces characteristic nodules, but these do not involve the aorta per se.[19,20] Ankylosing spondylitis, however, is a condition that affects the aorta in a manner very similar histologically to syphilis, but its distribution in the aorta is very different from syphilis.[21–23] In contrast to syphilis, an-

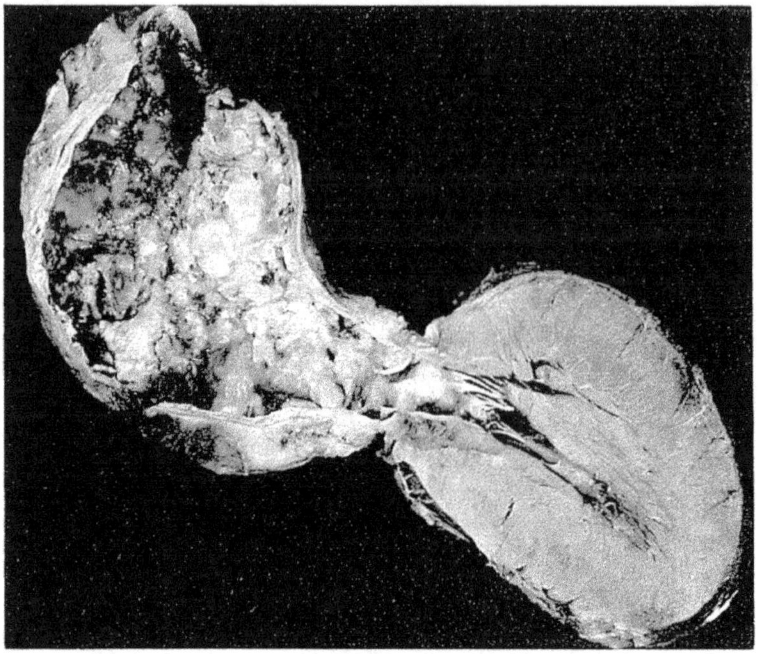

Fig. 41. Ascending aorta and left ventricle in a 67-year-old white woman (GT #77A-2) who died of acute myocardial infarction. Four years before death, serological findings for syphilis were positive (both VDRL and FTA). She had systemic hypertension for about 30 years, and during her last 5 years, she showed intermittent evidence of both cerebral and peripheral ischemia. At necropsy, she had a huge fusiform aneurysm of the ascending aorta, as shown here. The process involved only the tubular portion of ascending aorta and spared the wall of aorta behind the sinuses of Valsalva. As a consequence, the "root" of aorta was not dilated, aortic regurgitation did not occur, and the left ventricular cavity was not dilated. This woman also had a saccular aneurysm of descending thoracic aorta, and this aneurysm also was almost certainly syphilitic in origin. The intima of the entire aorta (except for the sinus portion) was atherosclerotic and tremendously calcified. It appears that atherosclerosis is particularly devastating when superimposed on syphilis, and systemic hypertension is also devastating in this circumstance.

kylosing spondylitis primarily affects the wall of aorta behind the sinuses of Valsalva and extends into the tubular portion of aorta only for a couple of centimeters (Figs. 42 to 45). The area of aorta behind the commissures of the aortic valve appear to be a particularly predisposed site of involvement in ankylosing spondylitis. Also in contrast to syphilis, ankylosing spondylitis extends into the aortic valve cusps, at least to their basal portions, causing them to be thickened, whereas the cusps are spared in syphilis. Also, in ankylosing spondylitis the adventitial process in the aorta extends below the aortic valve into the membraneous and most cephalad portion of muscular ventricular septum and down the anterior mitral leaflet, causing its basal portion to become quite thickened by fibrous tissue. The extension of the aortic adventitial process below the aortic valve occasionally causes conduction disturbances because of the close vicinity of the atrioventricular bundle to the membraneous ventricular septum and causes mitral regurgitation because of the involvement of the anterior mitral leaflet.[23]

Eight necropsy patients with ankylosing spondylitis and aortic regurgitation have been studied personally.[23] All were men aged 34 to 55 years. All had severe congestive

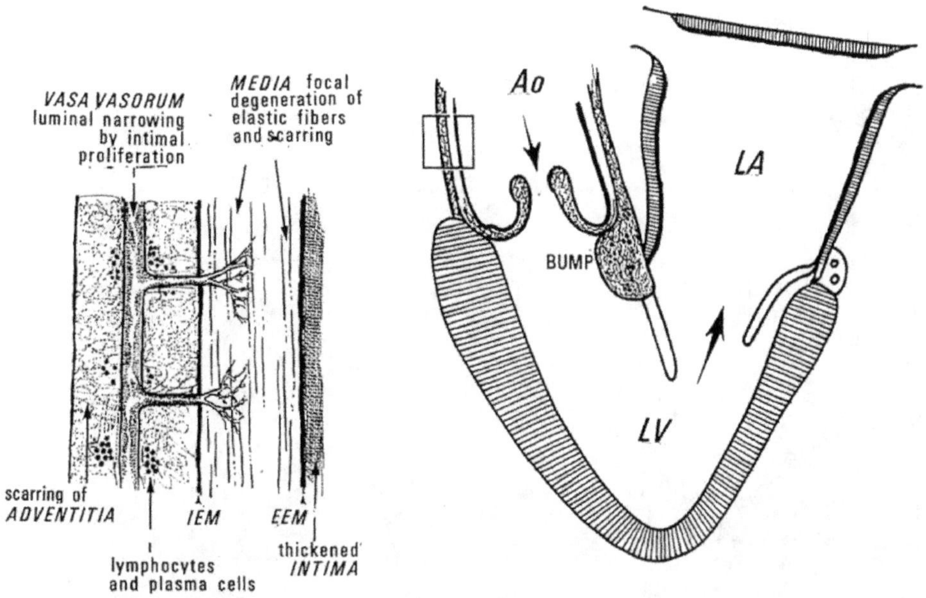

Fig. 42. Diagram depicting the changes observed in the aorta, in aortic valve cusps, and in the area just below the aortic valve in ankylosing spondylitis. The lesion in the aorta is identical to syphilis, but the process is more or less limited to that area behind the sinuses of Valsalva. The fibrosing process extends below the aortic valve to form a ridge or bump at the basal portion of anterior mitral leaflet. The aortic valve cusps are usually thickened diffusely.

cardiac failure and signs and symptoms of joint involvement consistent with ankylosing spondylitis. In all 8 patients, the joint symptoms antedated those of congestive cardiac failure, in 7 of them by 10 to 20 years. In 5 of the 8 patients, however, precordial murmurs of aortic regurgitation were noted at the same time or within 1 year of the onset of joint symptoms. Results of serologic tests for syphilis were negative in all patients. Conduction disturbances were present in 6 patients. At catheterization, the left ventricular and systemic arterial diastolic pressures were equal in 5 of 7 patients studied. Aortic valve replacement was carried out in 5 patients. Death in 7 patients was directly related to the aortic valvular disease and occurred at an average of 6 years from the onset of congestive cardiac failure.

At necropsy, the hearts weighed 520 to 1110 gm (average, 756). The aortic valve cusps were shortened and always thickened at their basal attachments and distal margins and frequently in between. Focal calcific deposits were present along the bases of the cusps in 4 patients, and in 1 they extended to the anterior mitral leaflet and membranous septum. The ascending aorta was diffusely dilated in all 8 patients. The thickening was limited to the most proximal 3 cm of ascending aorta, and the wall behind the sinuses of Valsalva was always involved (Figs. 42 to 45). The thickening resulted from dense connective tissue in the adventitia of the aorta. The adventitial scarring was continuous with similar scarring in the groove between the anterior mitral leaflet and the aortic valve cusps, producing a fibrous ridge between the base of the aortic valve cusps and the anterior mitral leaflet. In 4 patients the fibrous tissue also infiltrated the membranous ventricular septum. A few mononuclear cells were present in the adventitia of the aorta, and the lumens of the vasa vasorum were narrowed by extensive intimal fibrous prolifera-

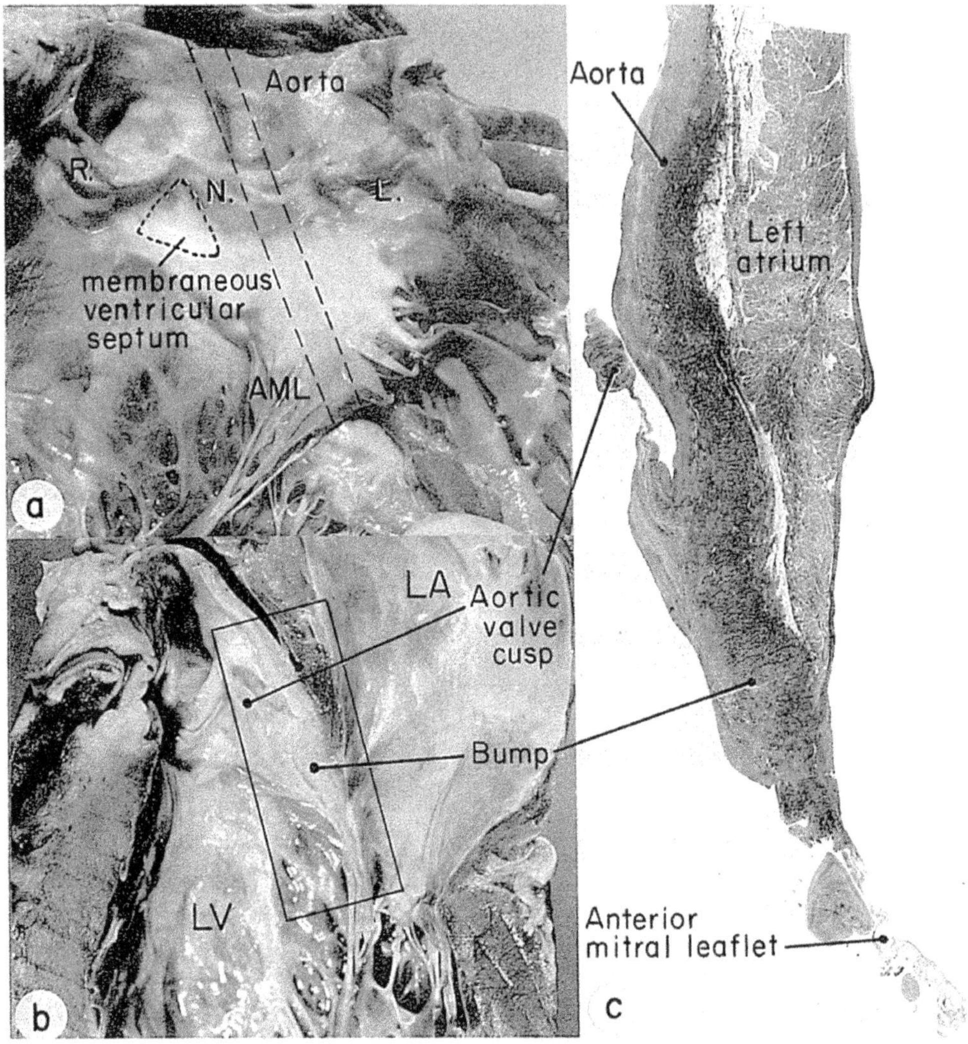

Fig. 43. Part of aorta and heart of a 54-year-old man (A68-300) who presented with aortic regurgitation and left bundle branch block 6 years before death. Four years later, the diagnosis of ankylosing spondylitis was made by retrospective examination of serial "spinal" roentgenograms and by a story of long-standing low back pain. The characteristic features of the cardiovascular lesion are shown. (*a*) Opened left ventricle, aorta, aortic valve, right coronary cusp (R), noncoronary cusp (N), left coronary cusp, and anterior mitral leaflet. The aortic wall thickening is limited to the wall immediately behind and above the sinuses of Valsalva, especially behind the commissures. The basal portion of anterior mitral leaflet (AML) and the membranous septum are thickened by fibrous tissue. The dotted lines indicate the longitudinal cut through noncoronary (N) cusp of aortic valve, left atrium (LA), and ventricle (LV), which is shown in (*b*) and (*c*). The subvalvular fibrous bump beneath aortic valve is best shown in histologic section (*c*). (Phosphotungstic acid-hematoxylin stain; ×3).

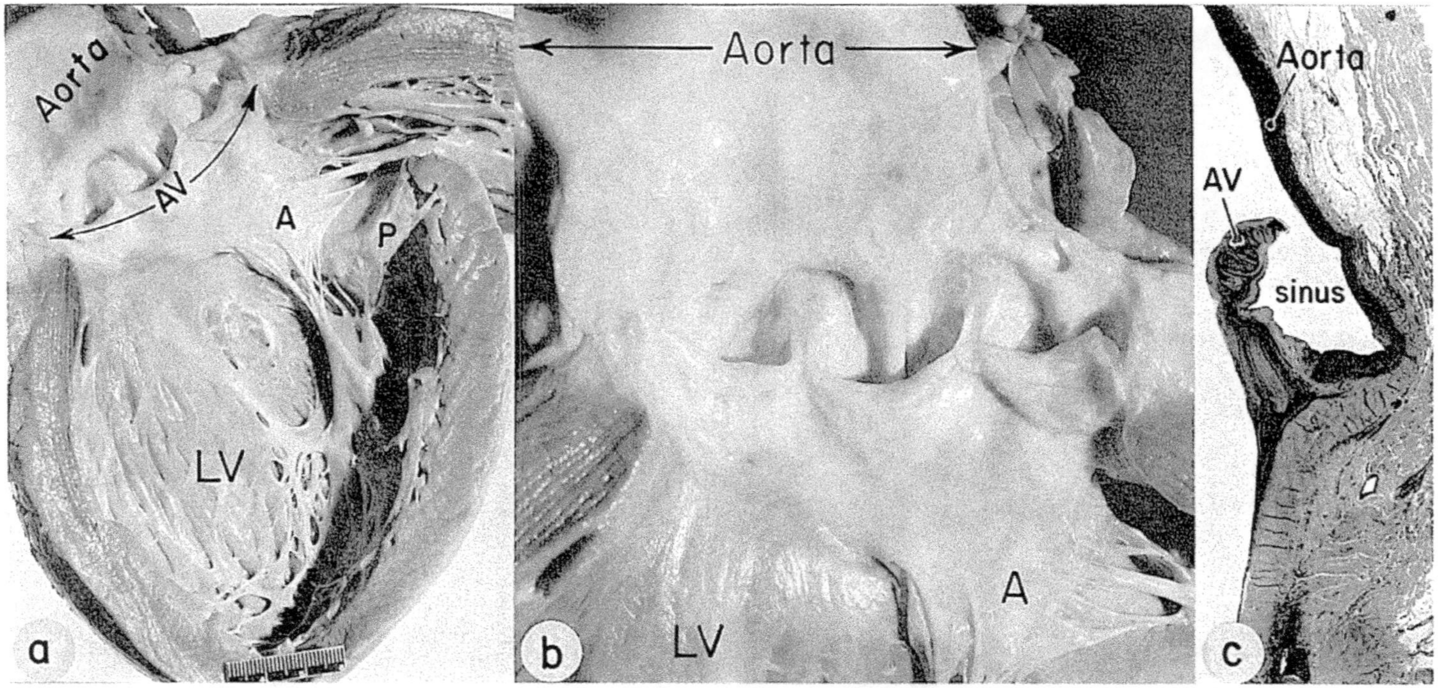

Fig. 44. Aorta and heart in a 55-year-old man (A61-262) with ankylosing spondylitis and intractable congestive cardiac failure from severe aortic regurgitation. (*a*) Opened aorta, aortic valve (AV), and left ventricle (LV). The scarring process of the aortic wall is limited to the region of the sinuses, which are dilated. Fibrous tissue extends below the aortic valve cusps, which are thickened (*b* and *c*). A and P, anterior and posterior mitral leaflets. (*c*: Elastic van Gieson stain; ×3)

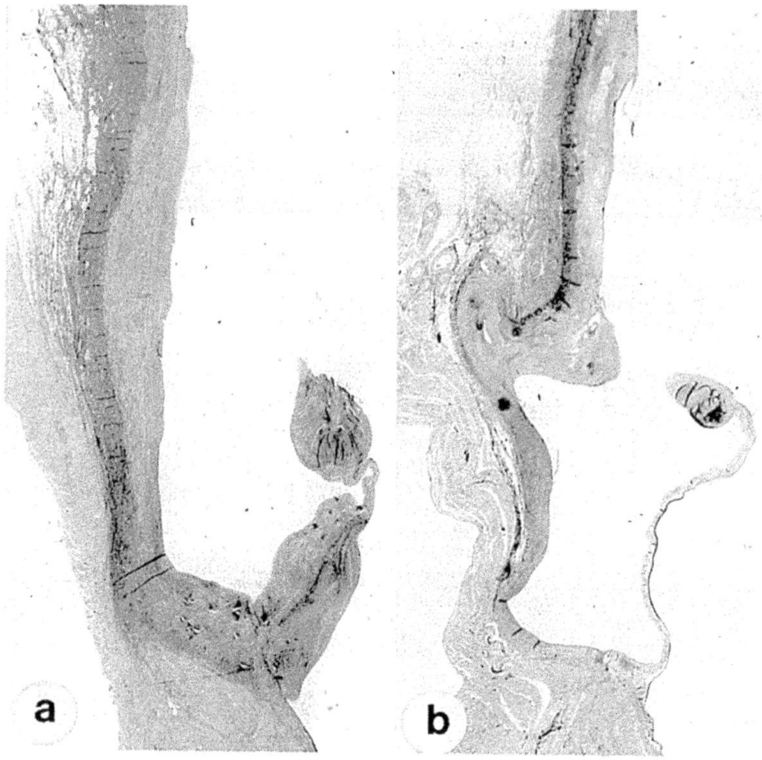

Fig. 45. Longitudinal sections through the wall of the aorta, aortic valve cusps, and ventricular septum from 2 patients: one (*a*) was a 54-year-old man (A68-300) with aortic regurgitation and ankylosing spondylitis, and the other (*b*) was a 69-year-old man (A67-43) with aortic regurgitation and syphilis. In ankylosing spondylitis, the aortic wall behind the sinuses is involved by the scarring process, whereas in syphilis, a similar process frequently begins distal to the sinus of Valsalva. Only the distal margin of the aortic valve is thickened in syphilis, whereas the proximal portions of the cusps are thickened as well in ankylosing spondylitis. (Elastic van Gieson stain; left, ×3.5; right, ×4.)

tion and medial hypertrophy (just as in syphilis). The media of the aorta behind the sinuses showed evidence of severe degeneration, and the overlying intima was thickened by proliferated fibrous tissue.

Although ankylosing spondylitis without cardiovascular involvement has been thought of as a "benign" condition, when complicated by aortic regurgitation the condition is not benign. Seven of the 8 patients studied personally died of consequences of the associated aortic regurgitation at a mean age of 46 years, with death occurring within 6 years of the first symptoms of cardiovascular involvement. The age of death in the 16 patients with ankylosing spondylitis and aortic regurgitation reported by Clark and associates was 45 years, and the interval from the onset of symptomatic heart disease to death also was 6 years.[24] In contrast, the overall mortality of patients with ankylosing spondylitis has been reported to be similar to that of the general population.[25] Thus the presence of aortic regurgitation appears to be a prime determinant of whether or not ankylosing spondylitis shortens life.

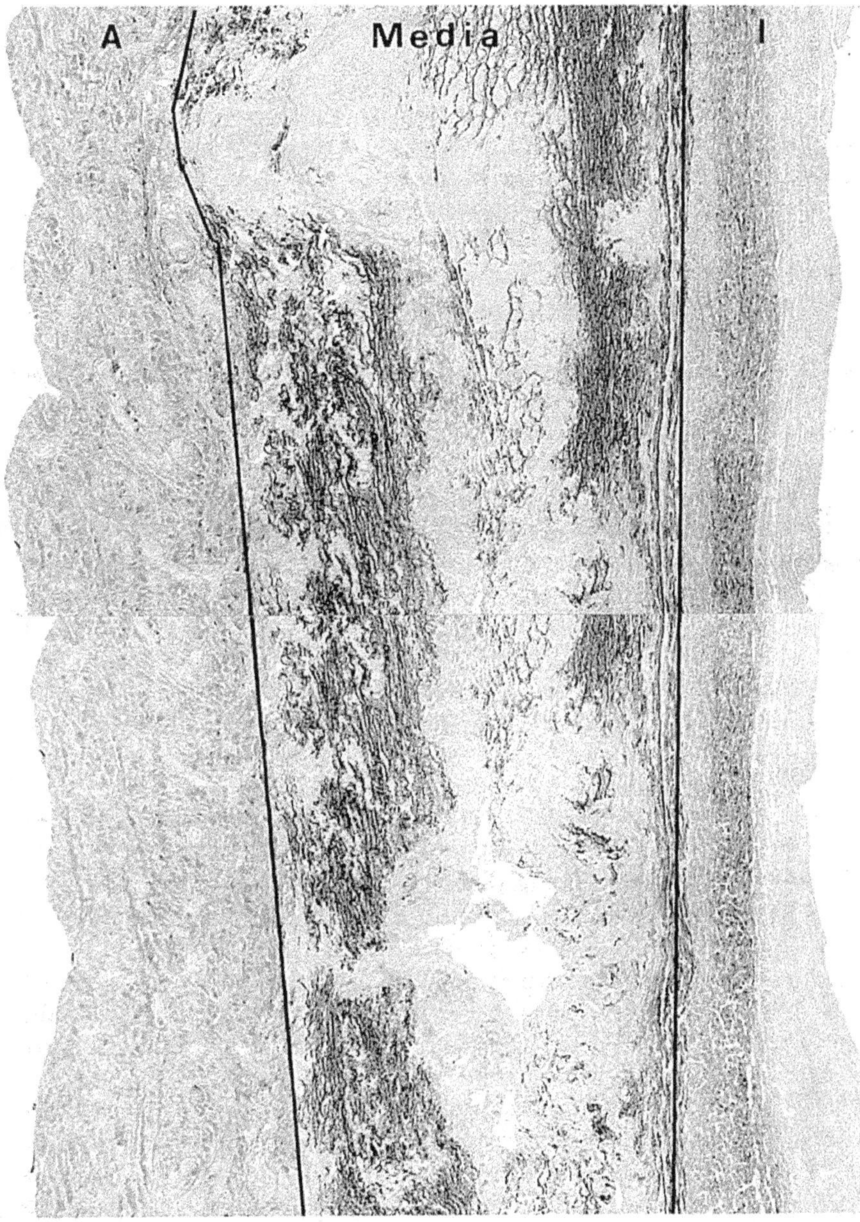

Fig. 46. Aorta involved by idiopathic aortitis in a 43-year-old white woman (GT #75S-6866) who was described in detail elsewhere.[30] She developed complete heart block early in life and evidence of aortic regurgitation (AR) in her early forties. By age 43, the AR was of severe degree, and the aortic valve was replaced. A large biopsy of the aorta showed typical aortitis with involvement of all three layers of the wall. As shown above, there is extensive destruction of the media and thickening by fibrous tissue of the adventitia (A) and intima (I). Granulomatous type inflammation was present in the wall of aorta. (Elastic van Gieson stain, ×45.)

Among patients in whom there is an absence of one or more arterial pulses in the neck or in one or both arms, the name "pulseless disease" or "aortic arch syndrome," among many others, has been applied. Studies during the past 25 years have shown that there is no single etiology for this condition, because severe atherosclerosis, syphilis, dissecting aneurysm, emboli, thrombi, trauma, and congenital anatomic variation all have been shown at times to cause absent or markedly diminished subclavian and carotid arterial pulsations.[26] A large group of patients with pulseless disease, however, do not fit into any of these etiologic categories. This *idiopathic* form of pulseless disease is far more common in the Orient than in the Western world, and it most frequently involves young women ("young female arteritis").

It has become apparent in recent years that idiopathic pulseless disease is simply one clinical variety of a relatively widespread arterial disease. Autopsy and angiographic studies in patients with isolated subclavian and carotid arterial involvement have demonstrated that the disease process nearly always also involves the aorta, sometimes the entire aorta, and any of its branches, including the coronary, intercostal, renal, mesenteric, and common iliac. Histologic study of these involved arteries has shown that all three layers of the wall are involved (panarteritis) but that the actual obstruction of the lumen results mainly from intimal fibrous proliferation [27–30] (Fig. 46). Giant cells may or may not be present in the involved arteries, but when they are, the histologic picture may be identical with that seen in temporal or giant cell arteritis.[27] As in patients with idiopathic pulseless disease, autopsy studies in patients with "temporal arteritis" have shown that the arteritis is widespread and may involve the aorta and many of its branches.

"Idiopathic aortitis" is another condition in which the histology and distribution of the lesions are similar to those seen in idiopathic pulseless disease and temporal arteritis. Despite the anatomic similarities among these three conditions, however, the clinical pictures are different. Patients with *temporal arteritis* are usually men over 65 years of age, and their signs and symptoms are related to the temporal arteries. Patients with *idiopathic pulseless disease* are usually women aged 15 to 40 years, and their clinical manifestations are related to inadequate perfusion of the subclavian and carotid arteries. Patients with idiopathic aortitis are often children (5 to 15 years old), and their symptoms are usually related to systemic hypertension resulting from extension of the arteritis to the renal arteries or ostia. Although patients with temporal arteritis and idiopathic aortitis anatomically may have panarteritis of the subclavian or common carotid arteries, occlusion of the lumens of these vessels in these two conditions is most unusual. Likewise, although aortitis is to be expected in idiopathic pulseless disease and temporal arteritis, aortic aneurysms and coarctations, renal arterial stenoses, and aortic regurgitation are uncommon.

REFERENCES

1. Schlatmann TJM, Becker AE: Histologic changes in the normal aging aorta. Am J Cardiol 39:13, 1977
2. Wolinsky H, Glagov S: A lamellar unit of aortic medial structure and function in mammals. Circ Res 20:99, 1967
3. Roberts WC, Ferrans VJ, Levy RI, et al: Cardiovascular pathology in hyperlipoproteinemia.

Anatomic observations in 42 necropsy patients with normal or abnormal serum lipoprotein patterns. Am J Cardiol 31:557, 1973

4. Darling RC, Messina CR, Brewster DC et al. Autopsy study of unoperated abdominal aortic aneurysms: The case for early resection. Circulation 56 (Suppl 2): 161, 1977
5. Bliss BP, Maini RN, Scott JT: Ruptured abdominal aorta infected with *Salmonella Brandenburg*. Br Med J 4:751, 1968
6. Roberts WC: The hypertensive diseases. Evidence that systemic hypertension is a greater risk factor to the development of other cardiovascular diseases than previously suspected. Am J Med 59:523, 1975
7. Schlatmann TJM, Becker AE: Pathogenesis of dissecting aneurysm of aorta. Am J Cardiol 39:21, 1977
8. Roberts WC: Congenital cardiovascular abnormalities usually "silent" until adulthood: Morphologic features of the floppy mitral valve, valvular aortic stenosis, discrete subvalvular aortic stenosis, hypertrophic cardiomyopathy, sinus of Valsalva aneurysm, and the Marfan syndrome, in Roberts WC (ed): Congenital Heart Disease in Adults. Philadelphia, 1979, p 407 FA Davis Co
9. Murdoch JL, Walker BA, Halpern BL, et al: Life expectancy and causes of death in the Marfan syndrome. N Engl J Med 286:804, 1972
10. McKusick VA: Heritable Disorders of Connective Tissue. St. Louis, CV Mosby Co, 1972, p 61
11. Erdheim J: Medionecrosis aortae idiopathica. Virchows Arch Pathol Anat Physiol 273:454, 1929
12. Gsell O: Wandnekrosen der Aorta als selbstäñdige Erkrankung und ihre Beziehung zur Spontanruptur. Virchows Arch Pathol Anat Physiol 270:1, 1928
13. Becker AE: Medionecrosis aortae. Pathol Microbiol 43:124, 1975
14. Lemon DK, White CW: Anuloaortic ectasia: Angiographic, hemodynamic and clinical comparison with aortic valve insufficiency. Am J Cardiol 41:482, 1978
15. Roberts WC, Perloff JK: Mitral valvular disease. A clinico-pathologic survey of the conditions causing the mitral valve to function abnormally. Ann Intern Med 77:939, 1972
16. Roberts WC, Buchbinder NA: Healed left-sided infective endocarditis. A clinicopathologic study of 59 patients. Am J Cardiol 40:876, 1977
17. Roberts WC, Cohen LS: Left ventricular papillary muscles. Description of the normal and a survey of conditions causing them to be abnormal. Circulation 46:138, 1972
18. McKusick VA, Logue RB, Bahnson HT: Association of aortic valvular disease and cystic medial necrosis of the ascending aorta. Report of four instances. Circulation 16:188, 1957
19. Carpenter DF, Golden A, Roberts WC: Quadrivalvular rheumatoid heart disease associated with left bundle branch block. Am J Med 43:922, 1967
20. Roberts WC, Kehoe JA, Carpenter DF, et al: Cardiac valvular lesions in rheumatoid arthritis. Arch Intern Med 122:141, 1968
21. Roberts WC, Dangel JC, Bulkley BH: Nonrheumatic valvular cardiac disease: A clinicopathologic survey of 27 different conditions causing valvular dysfunction. Cardiovasc Clin 5:333, 1973
22. Bulkley BH, Roberts WC: Ankylosing spondylitis and aortic regurgitation. Description of the characteristic cardiovascular lesion from study of eight necropsy patients. Circulation 48:1014, 1973
23. Roberts WC, Hollingsworth JF, Bulkley BH, et al: Combined mitral and aortic regurgitation in ankylosing spondylitis. Angiographic and anatomic features. Am J Med 56:237, 1974
24. Clark WS, Kulka JP, Bauer W: Rhematoid aortitis with aortic regurgitation. Am J Med 22:580, 1957
25. Blumberg B, Ragan C: Natural history of rheumatoid spondylitis. Medicine 35:1, 1956
26. Ross RS, McKusick VA: Aortic arch syndromes. Diminished or absent pulses in arteries arising from arch of aorta. Arch Intern Med 92:701, 1953
27. Nasu T: Pathology of pulseless disease. A systematic study and critical review of twenty-one autopsy cases reported in Japan. Angiology 14:225, 1963
28. Roberts WC, Wibin EA: Idiopathic panaortitis, supra-aortic arteritis, granulomatous myocarditis and pericarditis. A cause of pulseless disease and possibly left ventricular aneurysm in the African. Am J Med 41:453, 1966
29. Roberts WC, MacGregor RR, DeBlanc HJ Jr, et al: The prepulseless phase of pulseless disease, or pulseless disease with pulses. A newly recognized cause of cardiac disease, monoclonal gammopathy and "fever of unknown origin." Am J Med 46:313, 1969
30. Honig HS, Weintraub AM, Gomes MN, et al: Severe aortic regurgitation secondary to idiopathic aortitis. Am J Med 63:623, 1977

Aortic dissection: Anatomy, consequences, and causes

William C. Roberts, M.D. *Bethesda, Md.*

Despite its recognition at necropsy over 200 years ago and its recognition clinically about 50 years ago, aortic dissection remains a poorly understood condition from several aspects. Because its anatomic features have received relatively little attention in recent years, this report will focus on them and on the major consequences and causes of aortic dissection.

MORPHOLOGIC FEATURES OF AORTIC DISSECTION

All aortic dissections are characterized by separation of their media in a course parallel to that of the flow of blood. In addition to the medial longitudinal dissection, a continuous more or less transverse intimal and medial tear is identified in all but a few (<5%) patients.[1] In nearly 70% of patients (Table I), the tear which marks the beginning of the dissection, is located in the ascending aorta, usually about 2 cm cephalad to the sinotubular junction, which corresponds to the cephalad extension of the aortic valve cusps[1-7] (Figs. 1 to 8). The entrance tear or laceration is in the aortic arch in about 10% of patients, in the descending thoracic aorta (Figs. 9 to 14) (mainly the isthmic portion) in about 20%, and rarely (about 2%) in the abdominal aorta (Fig. 15). The entrance tear, in general, involves about one half the circumference of the aorta, occasionally much less, and rarely, the entire aortic circumference.[8] In contrast to the entrance tear, a reentry tear is identified far less frequently—only in about 10% of the patients collected from previous reports by Hirst et al.[1] (Table II). Its location is the aorta in about half of them (most commonly the abdominal portion, next the descending thoracic portion, and last, the ascending portion), and in the other half a peripheral artery (most commonly one or more iliac arteries).[1] Rarely, a single tear serves as both the entrance to and the exit from the false channel. In this circumstance, flow within the false channel may be both retrograde and anterograde.

Once blood under pressure enters the media via the intimal and medial tear, the time required thereafter to dissect the media of the entire length of the aorta appears to be only one or a few seconds. Evidence of the rapidity of the longitudinal dissection once it begins is gained from retrograde aortic dissection observed during attempted cardiopulmonary bypass, and also by virtual instantaneous death in some victims of spontaneous aortic dissection. Presumably, the anterograde aortic dissections occur with similar speed, possibly even more rapidly because in the natural state the aorta is exposed to a pulsatile flow (systolic and diastolic) rather than entirely to a mean pressure as during cardiopulmonary bypass.

The location of the dissecting channel (false channel, dissecting hematoma) is in the outer half of the aortic media. As a consequence, the outer wall of the false channel is very thin, usually only about a fourth as thick as the original medial wall. The partition, therefore, between the true and false channels (the inner wall of the false channel) is about three times as thick as the outer wall of the false channel and about three fourths as thick as the original medial wall of aorta. The thinness of the outer wall of the false channel is the anatomic feature which explains its high frequency of rupture and also explains why extravasation of blood outside the aorta is more common than rerupture of the inner wall of the false channel into the true channel. If the situation were reversed such that the inner wall of the false channel (partition between the true and false channels) was only a quarter as thick as the outer wall, survival after aortic dissection would surely be far more common and rerupture of the partition between the two channels would be far more frequent. The thinner the outer wall of the false channel, the greater the likelihood of fatal

From the Pathology Branch, National Heart, Lung and Blood Institute, National Institutes of Health.

Received for publication Nov. 14, 1980; accepted Nov. 21, 1980.

Reprint requests: Dr. William C. Roberts, Building 10A, Room 3E30, National Institutes of Health, Bethesda, MD 20205.

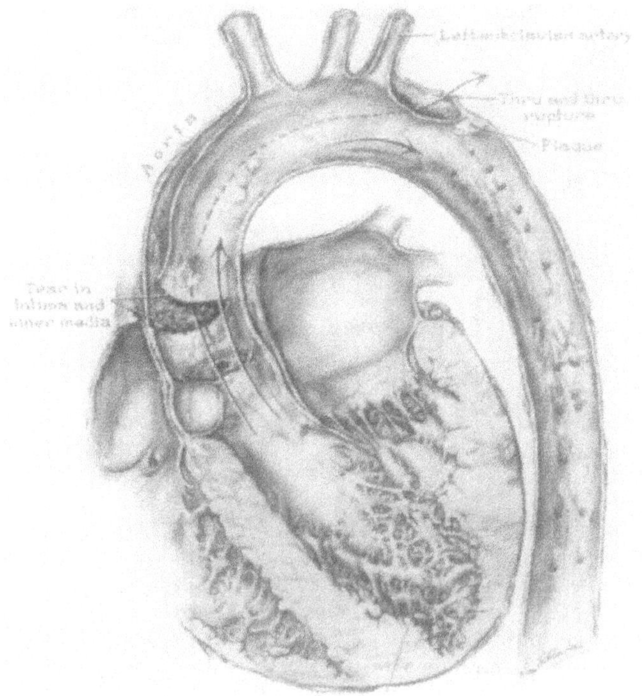

Fig. 1. Acute dissection involving the ascending and transverse portions of the aorta with rupture into the left hemithorax in a 25-year-old black woman (DCMEO No. 78-06-451) who died suddenly at home. She had complained of chest pain about 2 months before death and her blood pressure at that time was 200/110 mm Hg. She weighed 425 pounds (193 kg). Drawing of heart and aorta shows the part of the aorta involved by the dissection. The large entrance tear was about 3 cm above the aortic valve. The dissection extended into all three arch arteries. The exit site was just past the aortic isthmus. The aortic dissection appears to have been stopped at this point because its medial path was interrupted by an overlying intimal atherosclerotic plaque which has burrowed into the underlying media.

rupture, and, conversely, the thicker the outer wall of the false channel, the less the likelihood of fatal rupture. Among patients with aortic dissection surviving as long as 48 hours, necrosis of the dissected aortic wall may occur, and this event further weakens the aortic wall, encouraging its rupture.[9] Aortic wall necrosis was observed histologically in 21 (62%) of 34 necropsy patients with aortic dissection reported by Barsky and Rosen.[9]

Although dissection is a longitudinal separation of media, the percent of aortic circumference involved by the dissection at any particular level of aorta is variable. Most commonly at any level, about one half of the circumference of the aorta is dissected and the wall of the other half of the aorta is intact. The portion of aortic circumference involved by the longitudinal dissection is fairly characteristic. With

Table I. Aortic dissection; sites of primary tear in aorta*

Portion of aorta	*No. (%)*
1. Ascending	244(62)
2. Arch	37(9)
3. Isthmus	62(16)
4. Descending thoracic	41(10)
5. Abdominal aorta	10(3)
Totals	394(100)

*Adapted from Hirst et al., Medicine 37:217, 1958. Produced with permission.

dissections beginning in the ascending portion, the tear usually involves the right lateral aortic wall and thereafter courses downstream along the greater curvature of the ascending, transverse, and descending thoracic portions of aorta,[10] just as peptic ulcer most commonly involves the greater curvature of the stomach. Because the arch arteries arise from this greater curvature portion, extension of the dissection into the innominate, left common carotid, and left subclavian arteries is common (Fig. 8).

Although the initiating tears are most frequently located in the ascending aorta, this portion is not the most common portion of aorta involved by dissection. This is because the more proximal portion of descending thoracic aorta is the second most common location of the primary tear. Consequently, because most ascending aortic dissections extend to involve the descending aorta (indeed, usually the entire aorta) and because relatively few primary tears in the descending thoracic aorta extend retrogradely to involve the ascending portion of the aorta, the descending thoracic aorta is the most common portion of aorta to be involved. Dissection limited to the ascending aorta is infrequent.

Why any aortic dissection, once begun, stops within the aorta with or without rerupture back into the true lumen is a question whose answer has received little attention. The most common cause of interruption of the longitudinal dissection appears to be *extensive atherosclerotic plaquing* which has caused underlying medial scarring or atrophy or both, which in turn interrupts the longitudinal dissection. A common site of extensive atherosclerotic plaquing is the isthmus of aorta—the vicinity of the ligamentum arteriosum (Fig. 1). Extensive atherosclerosis in the abdominal portion of aorta with or without fusiform aneurysm also may prevent longitudinal dissection in this portion (Figs. 9 and 13).

Another cause of interruption of a dissection involving the ascending and/or arch portions of

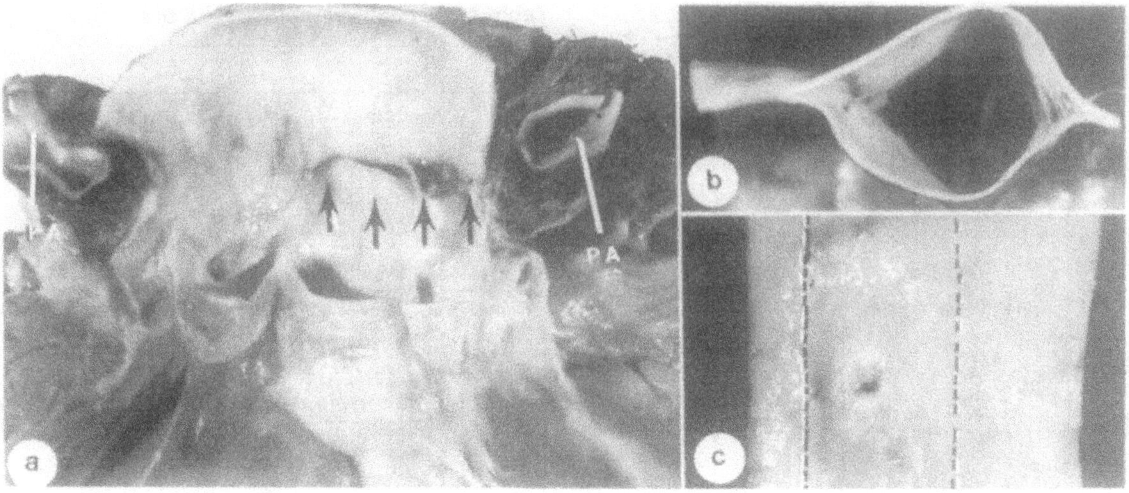

Fig. 2. Dissection involving entire aorta with rupture into pericardial sac in a 41-year-old man (DCMEO No. 78-08-724) who had the onset of chest pain 1 hour before being found slumped over the steering wheel of his automobile. Because his heart weighed 550 gm, it is reasonable to believe that he had had systemic hypertension. **a,** The aortic tear is located just above the aortic valve. The tear extended into aortic adventitia and from there into the adventitia of the major pulmonary arteries (*PA*), causing mild narrowing of their lumens. **b,** The opened area represents the false channel in the media of the descending thoracic aorta. **c,** This aorta is relatively free of atherosclerotic plaque. The false channel is located beneath the intima between the *dashed lines.*

aorta is *aortic isthmic coarctation.* Aortic rupture, usually with dissection, was pointed out by Abbott[11] in 1928 to be a major cause of death in patients with aortic isthmic coarctation. Because aortic isthmic coarctation represents an invagination of media,[12] progression of a longitudinal dissection started upstream cannot pass through a natural coarctation or an aortic coarctation which has been resected and repaired by end-to-end suture anastomosis. Although aortic dissection in patients with aortic isthmic coarctation most commonly involves only the portion of aorta proximal to the coarctation, occasionally the dissection involves only the aorta distal to the coarctation, but never both.[11, 13-15] Of 200 necropsy patients with aortic isthmic coarctation collected from previous reports by Abbot,[11] 38 (19%) had aortic rupture, most because of dissection: in 33, the rupture was proximal and in the other 5 it was distal to the coarctation. Of the 104 necropsy patients with aortic isthmic coarctation reviewed by Reifenstein,[13] 24 (23%) had aortic rupture, nearly all from dissection: in 19, the rupture was proximal and in the other 5 it was distal to the coarctation.

Thus without extensive aortic atherosclerosis or coarctation, the entire aorta distal to the entrance tear usually dissects. Dissection limited to the ascending and transverse portions of aorta when the tear is near the aortic valve therefore generally indicates extensive aortic atherosclerotic plaquing or coarctation at the aortic isthmus. If aortic isthmic coarctation is absent, aortic dissection in patients aged 40 years or less nearly always involves the entire aorta because atherosclerotic plaquing in them is usually mild; aortic dissection in patients past age 65 years has a greater chance of being localized because of the greater probability of heavy atherosclerotic plaquing (at least among persons residing in the Western world), with or without a fusiform aneurysm.

COMPLICATIONS OF ACUTE AORTIC DISSECTION

Various complications and causes of death from acute aortic dissection are listed in Tables III and IV. Death, of course, is the most frequent and it occurs in about 90% of untreated patients with aortic dissection and is more common in the acute cases when a reentry site is absent (or not identified). The most frequent mechanism of death is through-and-through rupture of the aorta.[1] The rupture site is usually near the site of the initial intimal-medial aortic tear. Because the most frequent site of the entrance tear is the ascending aorta, the most frequent site of through-and-through rupture is the ascending aorta and the extravasation of blood in this circumstance is nearly always into the pericardial sac (Fig. 3). Because the parietal pericardium is attached to the ascending aorta just proximal to the origin of the innominate

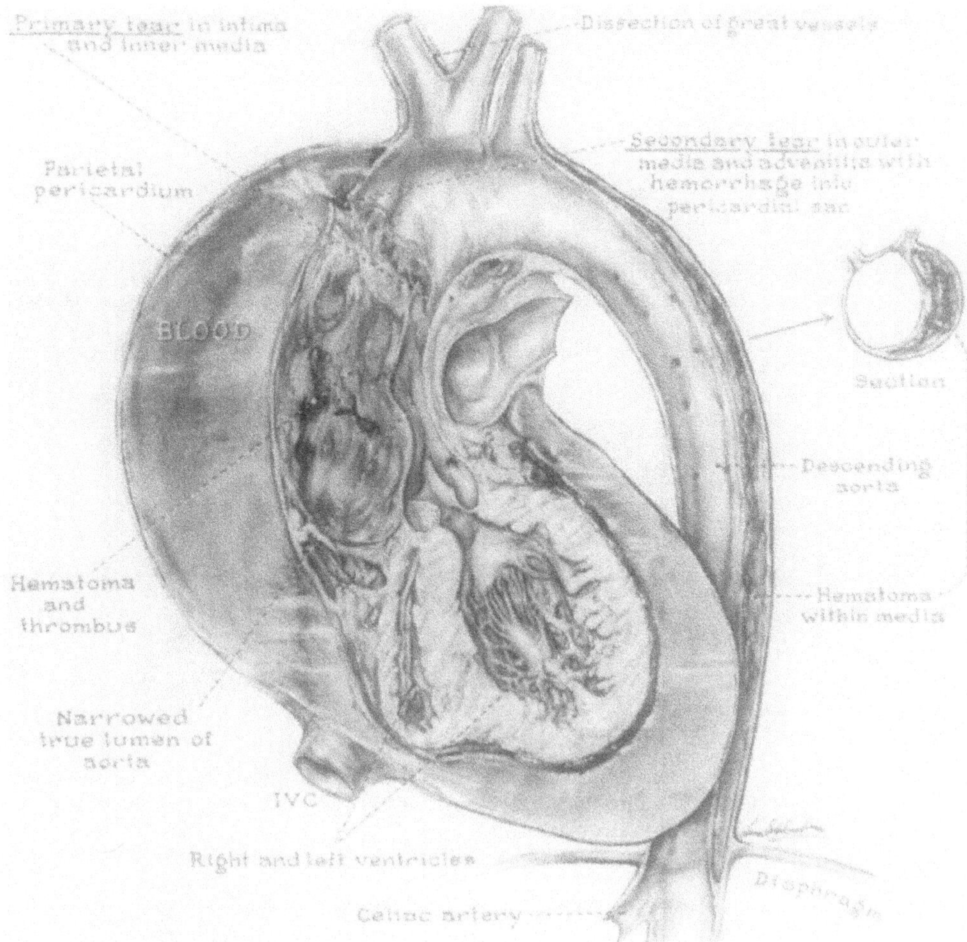

Fig. 3. Dissection with initial tear about 8 cm cephalad to the aortic valve and extending to the diaphragm in a 70-year-old man (H No. A79-153) who died several days after the onset of symptoms resulting from aortic dissection. Thrombus filled the false channel from the tear to the aortic root, causing narrowing of the true channel. The outer wall of the false channel ruptured at the initial tear causing hemopericardium. The weight of the heart was normal.

artery, rupture of any portion of the ascending aorta leads to extravasation into the pericardial sac. The usual site of the through-and-through rupture is the right lateral wall,[10] the site of contact of blood ejected from the left ventricle.

Although rupture of the outer wall of the false channel generally leads to rapid death from hemopericardium, frequently before the final extravasation occurs blood dissects into the adventitia of the wall of the aorta's false channel. Because the ascending aorta and pulmonary trunk have a common adventitia, blood may extend from the adventitia of the aorta into the adventitia of the major pulmonary arteries.[16] Because the intrapulmonary pressure is low and because the extravasated aortic blood is forced into the pulmonary arterial adventitia under systemic arterial pressure, the lumens of the major pulmonary arteries may be narrowed by this dissecting adventitial hematoma, leading to a type of peripheral pulmonary stenosis[16] (Figs. 2, 4 through 7).

Rupture of the aortic arch is most often into the mediastinum, descending thoracic aorta into the left pleural space and abdominal aorta into retroperitoneum.[1]

Extension of the medial dissection or hematoma into an artery arising from the aorta of course may lead to ischemia or necrosis of the organ or tissue normally perfused by that artery. Retrograde longitudinal dissection in the ascending aorta, particularly when it extends into the sinus portion of the aorta, may lead to extension of the medial dissection into the media of a major coronary artery, usually the right coronary artery.[10] Medial dissection of an

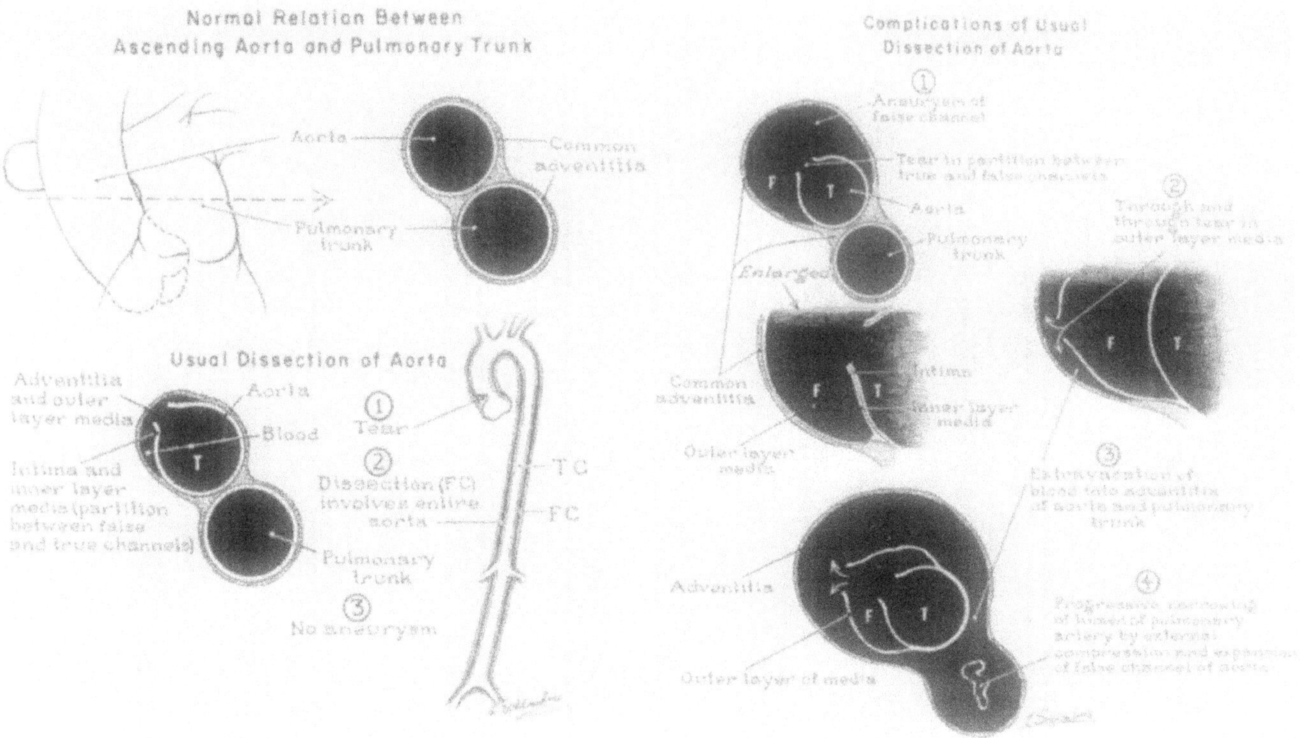

Fig. 4. Diagrams showing the relationship between the adventitia of the ascending aorta and pulmonary trunk, the usual aortic dissection, and complications of aortic dissection including adventitial pulmonary dissection with pulmonary arterial luminal narrowing.

artery the size of a coronary artery commonly leads to luminal narrowing, and this in turn may cause myocardial ischemia which may be fatal. A second consequence of dissection involving the aortic root is loss of commissural support of one or more aortic valve cusps, and the consequence of this development of course is aortic regurgitation.[8] Of 36 necropsy patients with dissection involving the ascending aorta reported by Murray and Edwards,[8] aortic regurgitation occurred in 10 (28%): in eight of 32 with acute dissection, and in two of four with healed dissection. A third complication of retrograde aortic dissection is extension of blood into the free walls and/or septa of the adjacent cardiac atria or ventricles or both, and this may lead to development of an aortico-atrial or aortico-right ventricular fistula or to a high degree of atrioventricular block.[17-21] Of 42 necropsy patients with dissection involving the ascending aorta reported by Thiene et al.,[21] 23 (55%) had extravasation of blood into the wall of the right atrium, eight (19%) into the atrial septum including the "specialized atrioventricular junctional area." Five of these latter patients developed complete atrioventricular dissociation.

Extension of the longitudinal dissection into the arteries arising from the aortic arch may lead to arm or cerebral ischemia, or both (Fig. 8). Extension into one (usually the left[10]) renal artery may produce signs of renal failure, even elevation of the systemic blood pressure, and into the celiac axis or one or both mesenteric arteries signs of abdominal organ insufficiency. Extension into the common iliac arteries or distally may lead to leg and foot ischemia. Dissection of the aorta on occasion may completely shear off or separate one or more arteries arising from the aorta (Fig. 16). When this situation occurs, flow through the branch ceases but extravasation usually is prevented by drainage into the false channel.

True aortic stenosis (as opposed to aortic valve stenosis) may result when a large hematoma or thrombus fills most or all of the false channel with resulting compression of the lumen of the true channel (Figs. 3, 4, and 6). This circumstance is most likely to occur when the dissection occupies a large proportion of the circumference of the aorta. Another unappreciated type of true aortic stenosis occurs when the entrance tear into the medial longitudinal dissection involves the entire circumference of the aorta. In this situation, the partition between the

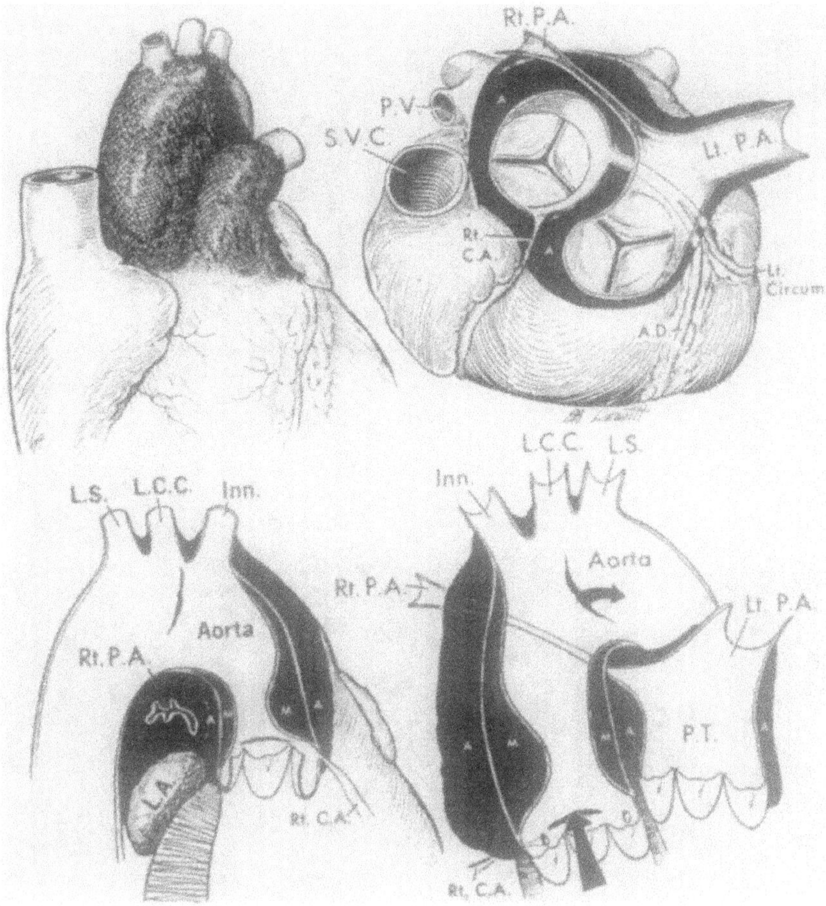

Fig. 5. Dissection of the entire aorta with rupture into the pericardial sac in a 57-year-old man (A69-302) who developed chest pain 17 hours before death. He was known to have had systemic hypertension. (This patient is described in detail elsewhere [Buja LM, Ali N, Fletcher RD, Roberts WC: Stenosis of the right main pulmonary artery. A complication of acute dissecting aneurysm of the ascending aorta. AM HEART J 83:89, 1972].) At necropsy, extravasated blood was present in the adventitia (*A*) of both ascending aorta and the extrapulmonary pulmonary arteries (*PA*). Because the ascending aorta and the pulmonary trunk (*PT*) have a common adventitia, extension of blood into the adventitia of the aorta can lead to extension of the blood into the adventitia of the pulmonary trunk and into the main right (*Rt*) and left (*Lt*) pulmonary arteries. Because the latter has a much lower pressure than the former, the lumen of the major pulmonary arteries can be narrowed by this process. This drawing shows how aortic adventitial blood may extend into the adventitia of the pulmonary trunk and lead to severe narrowing of the lumen of the right pulmonary artery. The ascending aorta also was narrowed by blood in the false channel as well as in the adventitia. The entrance site of the dissection was just above the aortic valve, and the exit site was in the arch. The lumen of the right coronary artery (*Rt CA*) also was severely narrowed by the medial (*M*) and adventitial hematoma. *AD*-left anterior descending coronary artery; *Circum*-circumflex coronary artery; *LS*-left subclavian artery; *LCC*-left common carotid artery; *Inn*-innominate artery.

true and false channels "rolls up" and is propelled into the lumen of the aorta distally, producing in essence an intussusception (Fig. 7).

HEALED AORTIC DISSECTION (double-barrel aorta)

About 10% of all acute aortic dissections heal, and nearly all of them have an identifiable reentry rupture site, usually in the abdominal aorta or iliac artery[1] (Table IV). The entry site most commonly is at or near the aortic isthmus, and therefore obstruction by the dissecting hematoma to the arch branches or coronary arteries is infrequent.

In contrast to its inappropriate use in most patients with acute dissection, the word *aneurysm* is usually appropriate in patients with healed aortic dissection because the false channel usually is quite large (larger than the true channel) and its wall has focal, frequently multiple, saccular aneurysms, most

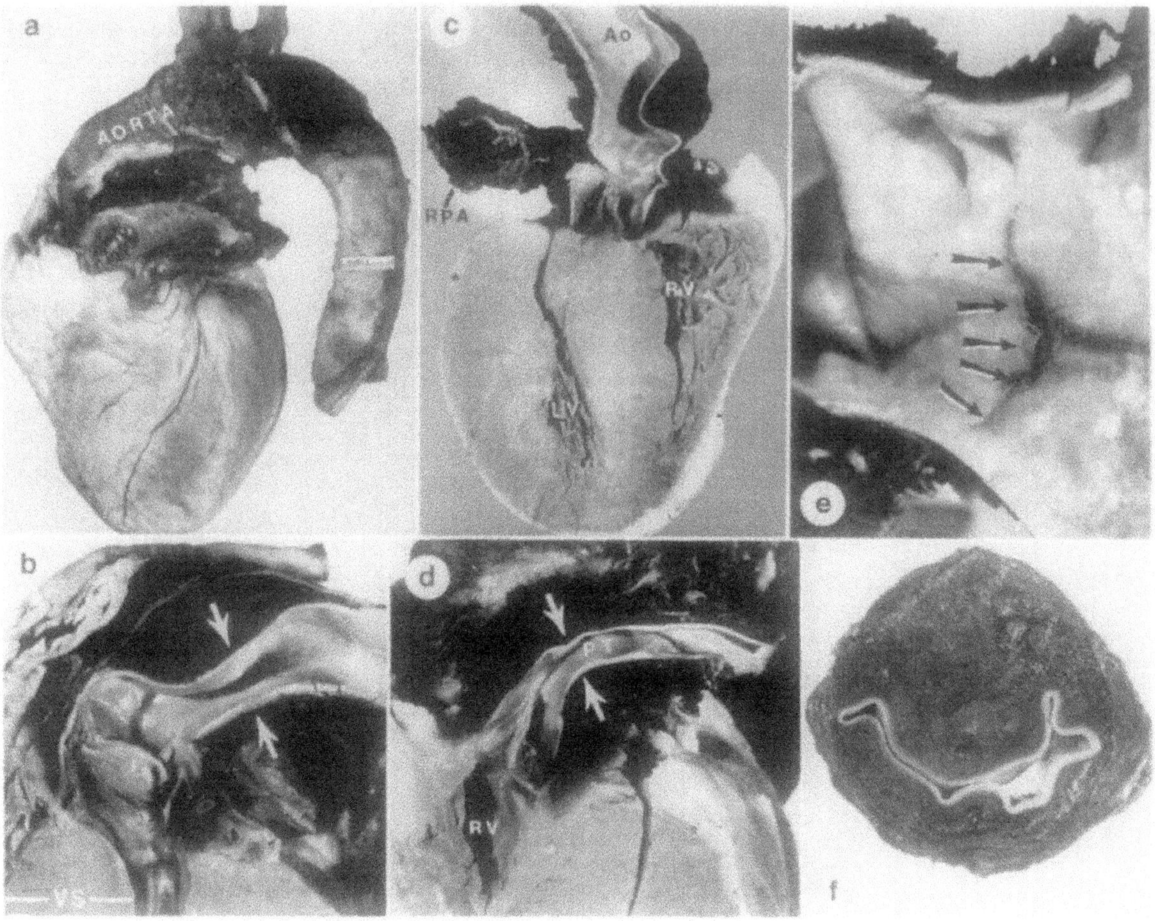

Fig. 6. The heart and major arteries in the patient described in Fig. 5. **a,** Exterior view shows blood in the adventitia of the aorta and major pulmonary arteries. **b,** Longitudinal view showing the aortic medial and adventitial hematoma which narrows the aortic lumen (*arrows*). *VS* = ventricular septum. **c,** View of anterior half of the heart and great arteries from behind. *Ao* = aorta; *RPA* = right pulmonary artery; *RV* = right ventricle; *LV* = left ventricle. **d,** Close-up view of compressed pulmonary trunk (*PT*) by adventitial hematoma. **e,** *Arrows* show exit site of dissection in the transverse aorta. **f,** Cross-section of the right main pulmonary artery. Its lumen is narrowed by the adventitial hematoma.

of which contain thrombi (Figs. 12 to 15). Occasionally, the false channel is filled completely by thrombus (Fig. 9). The lining of the false lumen is usually completely endothelialized and usually yellow atheroma covered by thrombi cover it.

The atheromatous plaques in the false channel provide the rare opportunity of studying plaques known to be present for specified periods of time. If the acute dissection occurred 2 years before death, for example, it can be certain that the atheromatous plaque in the false channel had been present no more than 2 years. Most yellow atheromatous plaques in the false channel are covered by thrombi, an observation suggesting that the underlying plaques are formed by organization of thrombi. At times, healed aortic dissection is found at necropsy and no earlier clinical event compatible with acute dissection had been apparent (clinically silent acute aortic dissection).[22]

In general, survival after dissection and therefore the chance of healing are proportional to the distance of the intimal-medial tear from the aortic valve.[23] Consequently few patients with healed aortic dissection have the initial tear in the ascending aorta. Once healing has occurred, however, the longer the false channel, the longer the survival, in general.

ETIOLOGY

The cause of *spontaneous* (nonoperative-induced) aortic dissection is usually unknown, and intrinsic abnormality in the wall of the aorta is usually not identified. It is known, however, that about 70% of patients with aortic dissection have or have had

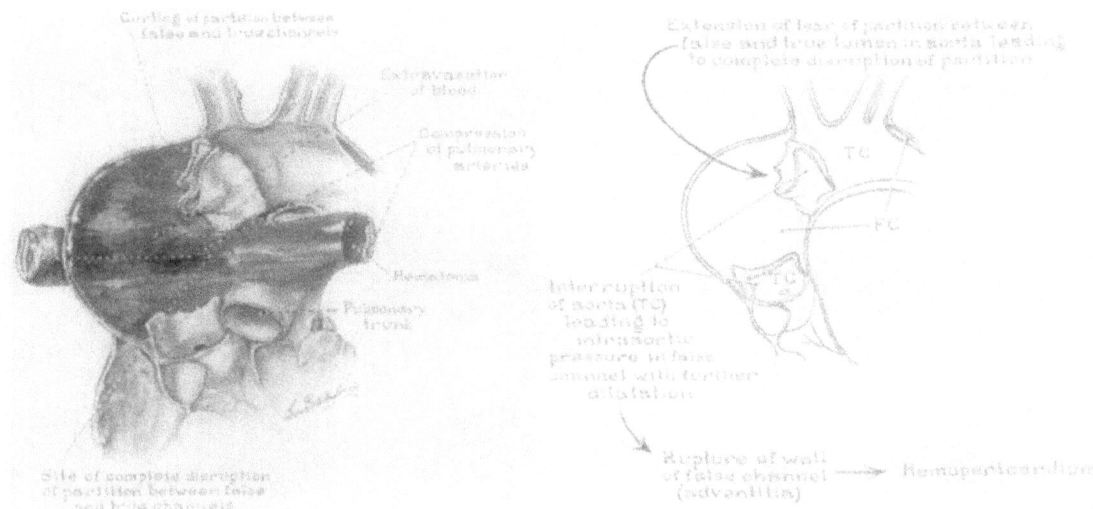

Fig. 7. Dissection of aorta with "intussusception" of partition between true and false channels and rupture into the pericardial sac in a 43-year-old black woman (H No. A76-166). Although she was known to have mild aortic regurgitation for 2 years, she was asymptomatic until about 5 hours before death, when she had the sudden onset of chest and back pain. An hour or so later, the blood pressure was 160/110 mm Hg and one radial and one femoral arterial pulsation was absent. She died suddenly. At necropsy, the pericardial sac was filled with blood and dissection involved the entire aorta. The entrance site of the dissection was in the ascending aorta just above the aortic valve. The tear extended across the entire circumference of the aorta so that the partition between the true and false channels had curled and extended into the transverse aorta, probably causing some obstruction of flow. Blood also extended from the aortic media into the aortic adventitia and from there it dissected into the wall of the pulmonary trunk and from there into the adventitia of the main right and left pulmonary arteries, resulting in narrowing of their lumens. *TC* = true channel; *FC* = false channel.

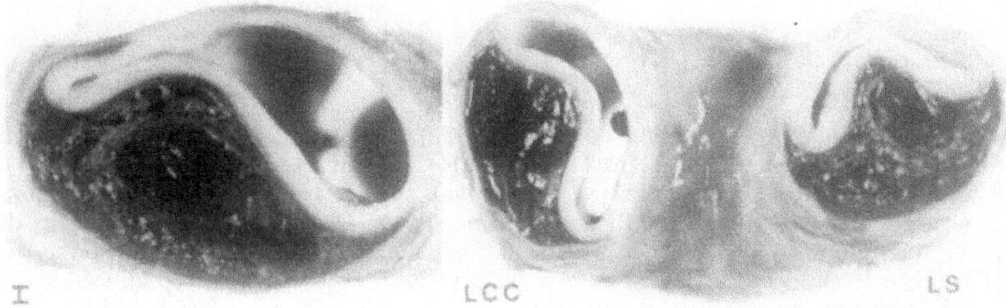

Fig. 8. Acute dissection involving the ascending and transverse portions of aorta with rupture into the pericardial sac in a 71-year-old (HHMC No. A-74-81) previously healthy woman. The entrance site was just above the aortic valve, and the exit site was in the transverse aorta. Although both functioned normally, the aortic and pulmonic valves were congenitally bicuspid. The heart weighed 430 gm. The dissection extended into the adventitia of the major pulmonary arteries and into the media of all three arch arteries (shown here), narrowing the lumens of each. *I*-innominate; *LCC*-left common carotid; *LS*-left subclavian artery.

systemic hypertension by blood pressure measurements, and at necropsy about 90% have left ventricular hypertrophy (heart weight >350 gm in adult women and >400 gm in adult men).[1-3, 6, 7] The most reasonable explanation for the cardiomegaly in most of these patients is systemic hypertension. Often aortic dissection represents the patient's first serious illness and the acute dissection often is the first time that the patient had sought medical care. After the dissection has occurred, of course, the blood pressure usually falls and by the time of hospitalization, the systemic hypertension may have vanished. The dissection in some patients causes death so rapidly that the systemic blood pressure may never be obtained.

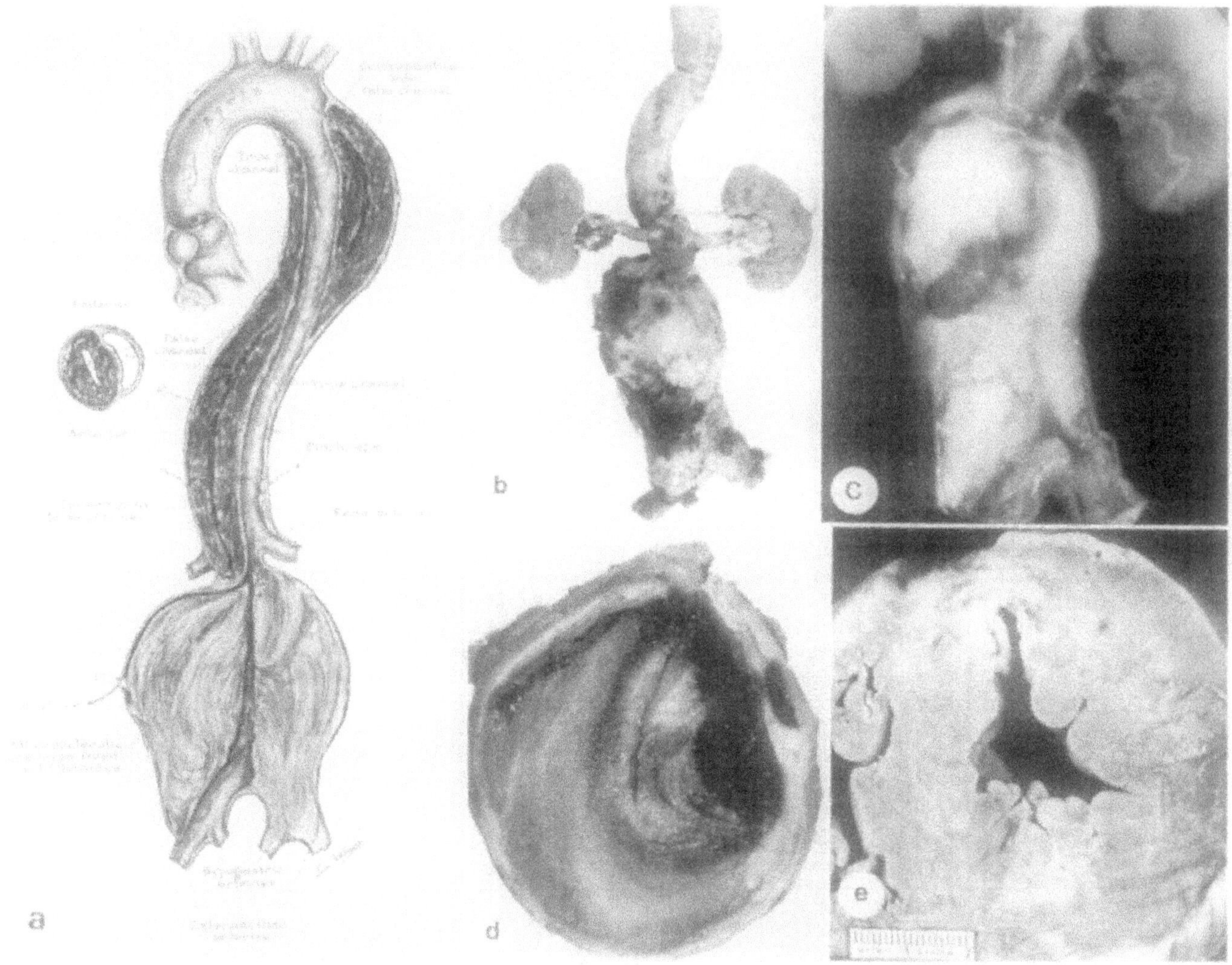

Fig. 9. Atherosclerotic fusiform abdominal aortic aneurysm, which ruptured, and healed dissecting aortic aneurysm in a 67-year-old white man (NNMC No. A76-211). He had had systemic hypertension for years and more than one acute myocardial infarct which had healed. Neither fusiform abdominal aortic aneurysm nor aortic dissection had been diagnosed clinically. **a,** Drawing of the locations of the aortic aneurysms. The dissection stopped at the beginning of the fusiform abdominal aortic aneurysm and began just past the origin of the left subclavian artery. **b,** Exterior view of the aorta, kidneys, and fusiform aneurysm. **c,** Radiograph of fusiform abdominal aneurysm showing a few calcific deposits. **d,** Transverse section of the abdominal aneurysm showing a severely narrowed lumen. **e,** Transverse section of left ventricle showing a healed transmural infarct.

Thus, it is not surprising that the frequency of documentation of systemic hypertension in these patients is no more than 70%.

It is likely that the higher the systemic blood pressure, the greater the likelihood of aortic dissection.[23] Dissection, for example, is much more frequent proximal than distal to an aortic isthmic coarctation.[11, 13, 15] The frequency of aortic dissection appears to be higher in patients with accelerated or malignant hypertension than in those with "benign" systemic hypertension.[23] Aortic dissection occurred in 6 (18%) of 34 patients with malignant hypertension reported by Beaven and Murphy,[24] a percentage much higher than in patients with "benign" hypertension. Additionally, dissection of a major pulmonary artery is a recognized complication of severe pulmonary hypertension, but dissection in the lesser circulation is virtually unheard of in the absence of pulmonary hypertension.[25]

Systemic hypertension appears to act as a major risk factor in the development of cardiovascular disease in two ways[25]: (1) by increasing the deposi-

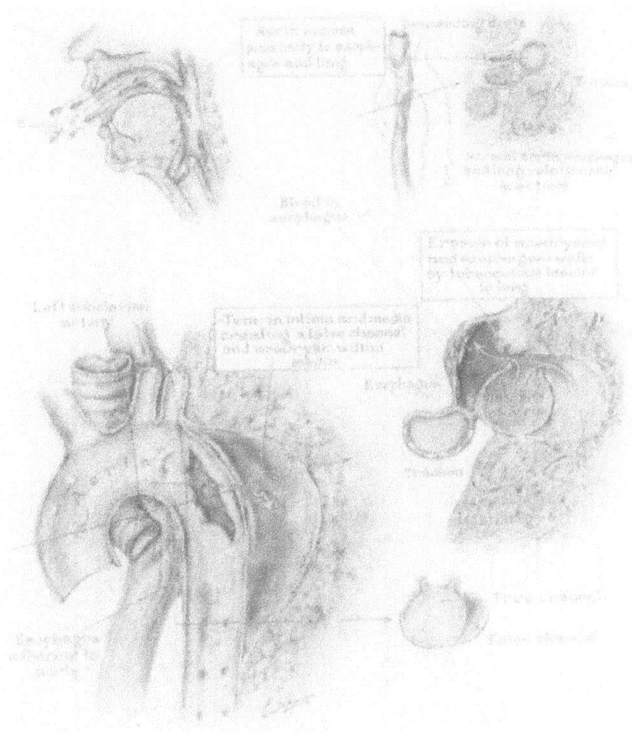

Fig. 10. Drawing of a dissected descending thoracic aorta in a 91-year-old woman (GT No. 80A-126). She collapsed and was found with blood ejecting from her mouth. Necropsy disclosed that the lungs were infected by tuberculous bacilli and that the left lung was adherent to the descending thoracic aorta. The pulmonary infection was the medium which allowed the aorta to rupture into the esophagus, to which it was adherent.

Table II. Aortic dissection; sites of secondary or reentry tear*

Artery	No. (%)
1. Aorta	33(50)
a. Ascending or arch–2	
b. Isthmus and descending thoracic–14	
c. Abdominal–17	
2. Peripheral	33(50)
a. Iliac–22	
b. Carotid–1	
c. Subclavian–1	
d. Not specified–9	
Totals	66(100)

*Adapted from Hirst et al., Medicine 37:217, 1958. Produced with permission.

tion of atherosclerotic plaques (intimal lesions) in major arteries most commonly causing luminal *narrowing* with resulting organ ischemia or infarction or both; and (2) by weakening the media of certain arteries causing *aneurysms* which may or may not rupture or *tears* which may or may not form aneurysms. Its effect on the arterial media is direct, whereas its effect on the arterial intima is indirect. Systemic hypertension is the only known major underlying factor in two conditions: aortic dissection and intracerebral microaneurysm (with or without rupture). Reduction in blood pressure clearly leads to a reduction in the incidence of aortic dissection and of nontraumatic intracerebral hemorrhage.[25]

The more common consequence of systemic hypertension, of course, is its ability to increase the amount of atherosclerotic plaques in various arteries. This effect, however, is not direct because hypertensive persons in population groups with normal (< 180 mg/100 ml) total serum cholesterol levels do not have more or larger atherosclerotic plaques than do normotensive persons in those populations. Hypertension, for example, is by far the

Table III. Aortic dissection: complications

I. Through-and-through rupture of aorta with extravasation of blood into
   - A. Pericardial sac
   - B. Pleural space
   - C. Mediastinum
   - D. Retroperitoneum
   - E. Wall of pulmonary trunk and/or main right and left pulmonary arteries (because of common adventitia with aorta)
     - 1. Peripheral pulmonary stenosis
   - F. Atrial and/or ventricular cardiac septum
     - 1. Atrioventricular conduction defect
   - G. Lung
   - H. Esophagus

II. Partial or complete obstruction by medial hematoma of the lumen of an artery arising from aorta
   - A. Coronary
     - 1. Sudden death
     - 2. Acute myocardial infarction
   - B. Innominate and/or common carotid
     - 1. Syncope, confusion, stroke, coma
   - C. Innominate and/or subclavian
     - 1. Upper limb gangrene, paralysis
   - D. Intercostal and/or lumbar
     - 1. Spinal cord ischemia-paraplegia
   - E. Celiac
   - F. Renal
     - 1. Oliguria
   - G. Mesenteric
     - 1. Bowel ischemia
   - H. Common iliac
     - 1. Lower leg gangrene, paralysis

III. Separation of branch of aorta from aorta

IV. Aortic regurgitation

V. Obstruction of aorta itself (true aortic stenosis)
   - A. By compression of true lumen by medial hematoma
   - B. Intussusception of aorta

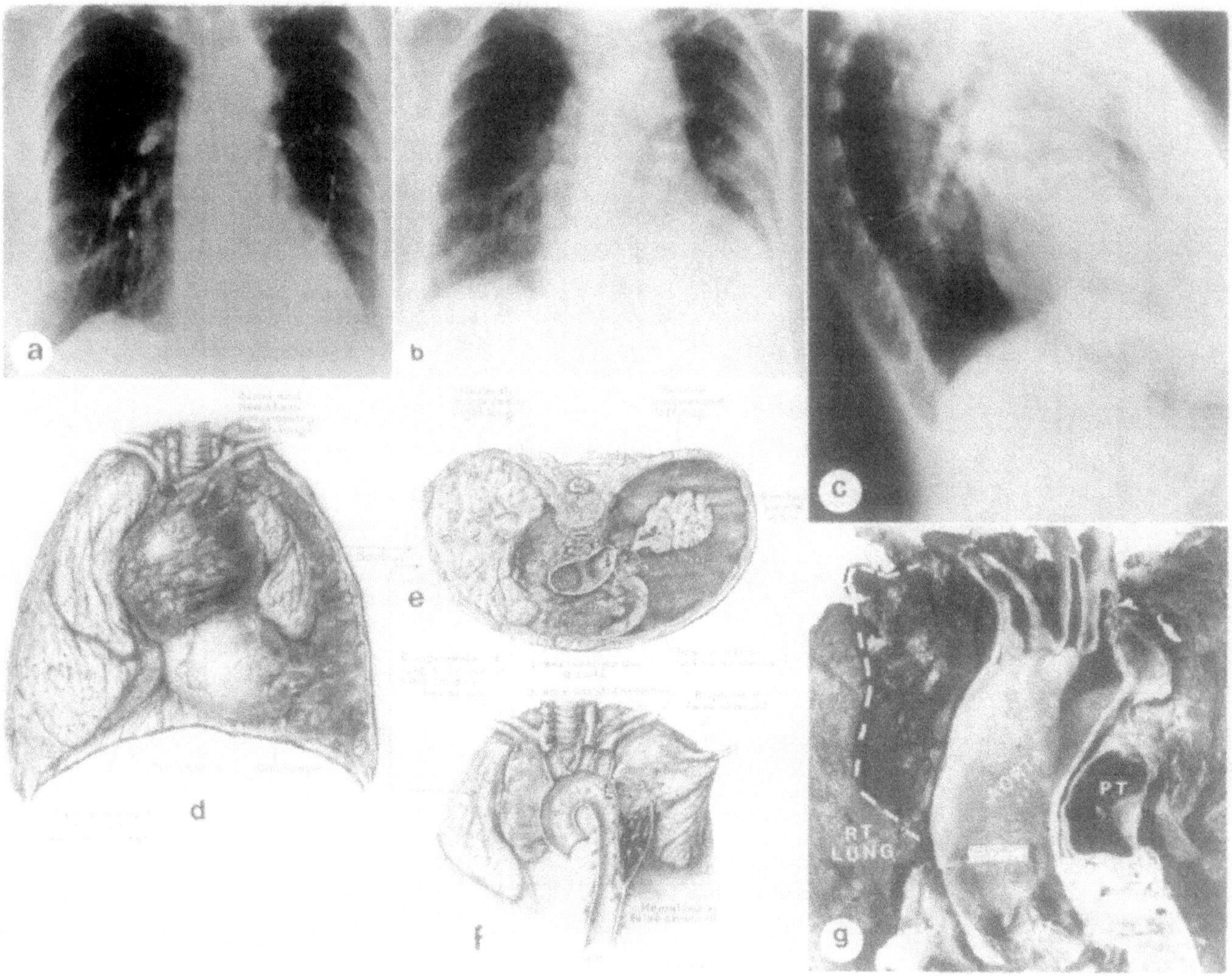

Fig. 11. Acute aortic dissection in a 76-year-old white woman (GT No. 77A-173). The entrance site is in the descending thoracic aorta with extravasation of blood into anterior mediastinal tissues simulating an ascending aortic dissecting aneurysm. The patient had been well until 14 days before death, when she noted "epigastric" pain and nausea. A chest radiograph **(a)** showed an abnormally-shaped thoracic aorta. The ECG showed left ventricular hypertrophy, and her blood pressure was 200/100 mm Hg. Because of previous esophageal stricture, her chest pain was believed to be related to the esophagus. She felt well thereafter until the day of death, when she suddenly noted dyspnea and profuse sweating; repeat chest radiographs (**b** and **c**) showed further widening of the mediastinum and markedly diminished lung space in the left hemithorax. Her heart stopped shortly thereafter. At necropsy, the left lung was collapsed, and most of the left hemithorax was filled with blood (**d** and **e**). A localized descending thoracic aortic dissection was present **(f)** and the entrance site into the false channel was at the aortic isthmus. The caudal two thirds of the false channel was filled with clot, and the outer wall of the false channel was ruptured. Before the final extravasation of blood into the left hemithorax, blood appears to have dissected more slowly into the mediastinal tissues lying to the right of and anterior to the aorta. Hemorrhage into these mediastinal tissues on chest radiographs simulated dissection of the ascending aorta, which was not the case. **g,** Close-up view of mediastinal hematoma to the right of the ascending aorta and behind the arch arteries. *PT*-pulmonary trunk; *AV*-aortic valve.

most common cardiovascular disease in the black African.[26] Yet complicated atherosclerotic plaques (as opposed to fatty and fibrous plaques), the only ones capable of producing significant luminal narrowing, have rarely been reported in either the hypertensive or the normotensive black African. Experimentally, however, lipid-induced atherosclerosis clearly is accelerated by hypertension.[25] Furthermore, certain complications of atherosclerosis (angina pectoris, myocardial infarction, sudden cor-

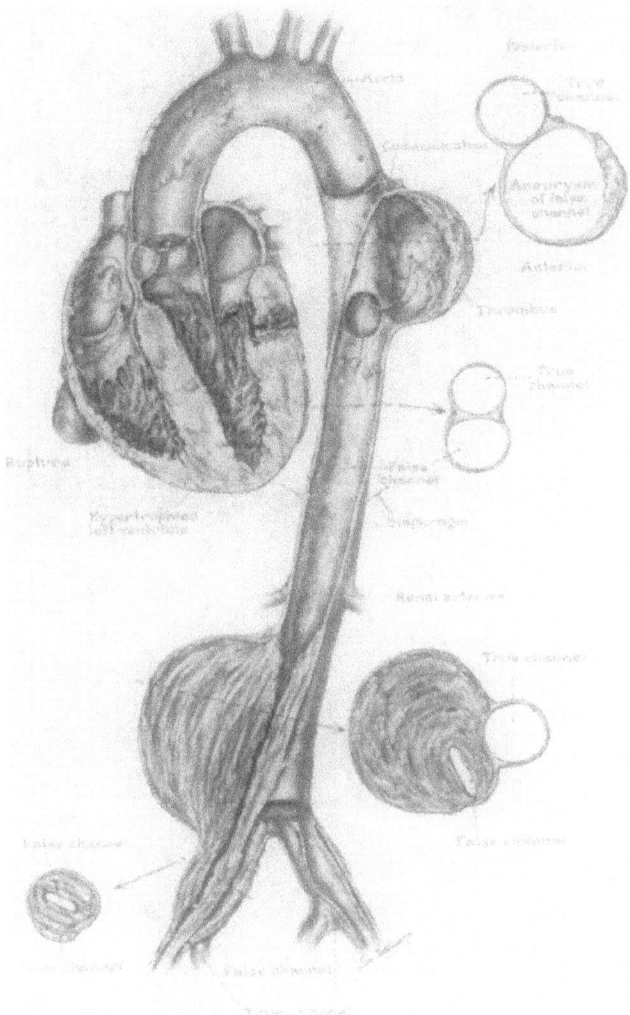

Fig. 12. Asymptomatic healed dissection of the descending thoracic and abdominal aorta in a 63-year-old man (GW No. 8399) who died of rupture of the left ventricle during acute myocardial infarction. There was no clinical evidence of an aortic dissection. He was known to have had systemic hypertension (blood pressure 180/100 mm Hg). He was asymptomatic until about 12 hours before death, when he had the onset of chest pain of acute myocardial infarction. The drawing shows the entrance site into the false channel in the descending thoracic aorta, and the false channel just caudal to this site developed a saccular aneurysm. The false channel in the abdominal aorta also became aneurysmal and filled with thrombus. The dissection extended into both common iliac arteries. The heart was hypertrophied, and the acute transmural left ventricular infarction ruptured, causing massive extravasation of blood into the pericardial sac.

onary death, atherothrombotic cerebral infarction, intermittent claudication) are clearly more frequent in hypertensive persons in the affluent or developed countries than in normotensive persons residing in the same countries.[25] Thus hypertension accelerates

Table IV. Aortic dissection: causes of death

Cause	*Acute dissection (n = 266)*	*Healed dissection (n = 66)*
1. Rupture in	228(86%)	37(56%)
a. Pericardial sac	172	17
b. Pleural space	93	13
c. Mediastinum	32	5
d. Retroperitoneum	16	6
e. Peritoneal space	4	3
f. Bowel	4	1
2. Congestive heart failure	9(3%)	22(33%)
3. Coronary heart disease	5(2%)	0
4. Miscellaneous	24(9%)	9(14%)

*Adapted from Hirst et al., Medicine 37:217, 1958. Produced with permission.

or increases atherosclerosis only in hypercholesterolemic (total seurm cholesterol > 180 mg/100 ml) population groups and not in those with lower total serum cholesterol levels.

Thus, aortic dissection may be viewed as representing a therapeutic failure (on the part of the patient or physician or both) in the management of systemic hypertension. *If systemic hypertension were eliminated, spontaneous aortic dissection would virtually disappear.* Despite its being the common denominator in patients with spontaneous aortic dissection, however, systemic hypertension by itself cannot be viewed as the sole cause of aortic dissection. There are estimated to be 25 million Americans with systemic hypertension, and the frequency of aortic dissection among them is quite low. Furthermore, experimentally the pressure in the aorta can be increased eight times above normal before rupture occurs.[27] Why one hypertensive person has aortic dissection and another of similar age and similarly elevated pressures does not is unclear. There are infrequently any histologic abnormalities present in the wall of the aorta, even at the entrance site into the dissection.[28-30] I have studied by serial sections the site of the proximal aortic tear in many patients and have not observed any intrinsic defect in the aortic wall. There is usually no more acid-mucopolysaccharide material in the aortic media at the site of the aortic tear or in other parts of the aorta in the patients with dissection than in similarly aged individuals of the same sex without aortic dissection.[28-30]

Pregnancy is often listed as one of the "causes" of aortic dissection.[31-34] The actual number of reported patients with aortic dissection occurring during pregnancy, however, is small, and even among them little information on the presence or absence of

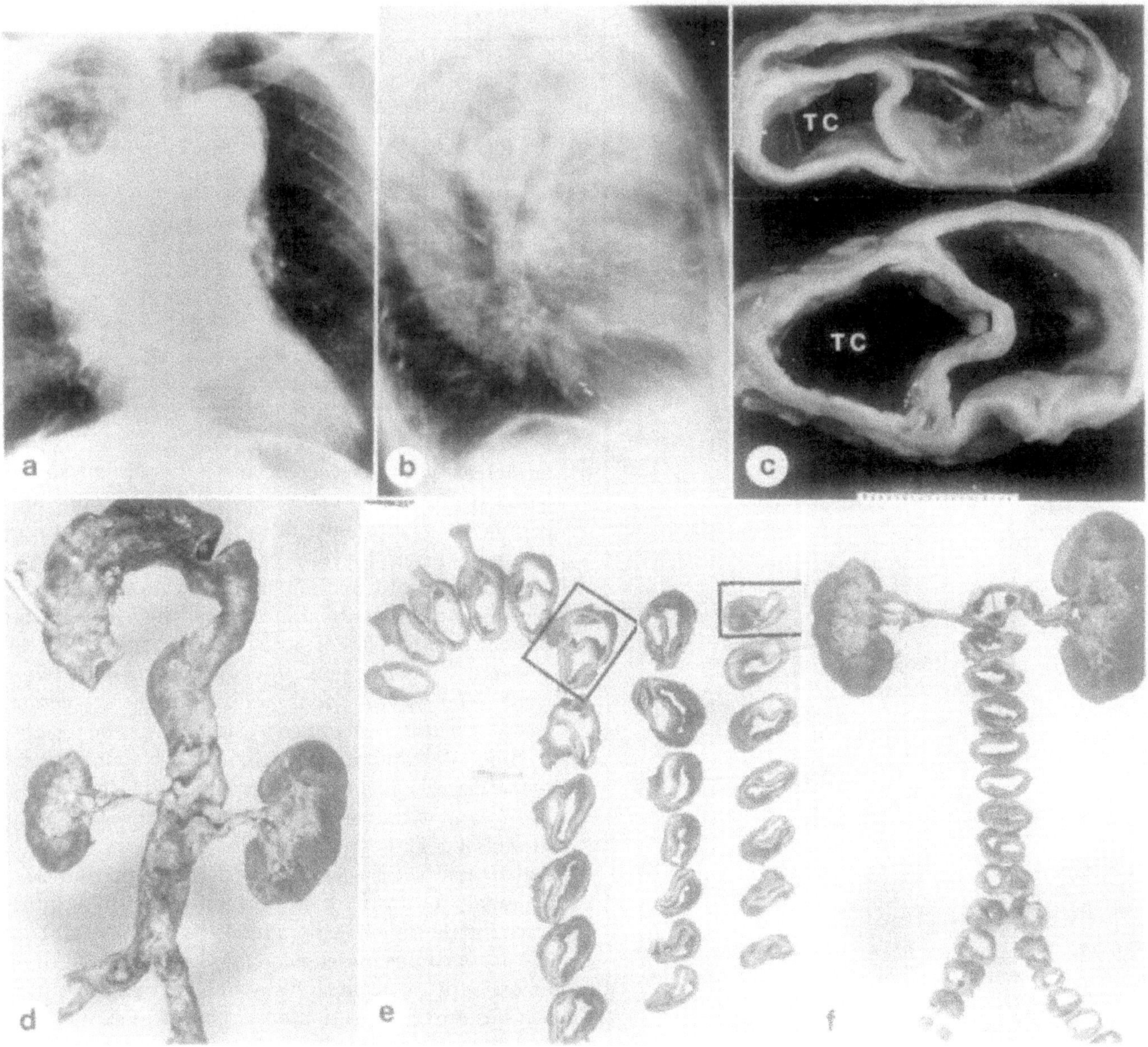

Fig. 13. Clinically silent aortic dissection after resection of an abdominal aortic fusiform aneurysm in a 69-year-old man (DCVAH No. A-178) who died of bronchogenic carcinoma. The abdominal aorta was replaced with a graft about 1 year before death. Dissection of the aorta stopped at the beginning of the graft. There was no history of systemic hypertension, and the heart weighed only 330 gm. Chest radiographs (**a** and **b**) shortly before death. Aorta, common iliac arteries, and kidneys **(d)**. Cross-sections of aorta to the renal arteries **(e)** and below **(f)**, which include the Dacron graft. The dissection began at the aortic isthmus. The false channel is larger than the true channel. Thrombus is present in some portions of the false channel **(c)**. Close-up views of the two bracketed cross-sections are shown in *e*.

hypertension is available. Of 49 women under age 40 years with aortic dissection reported by Schnitker and Bayer,[31] in 24 (49%) the dissection occurred in association with pregnancy: before labor in 20 (usually the third trimester), during labor in two, and shortly after labor in two. Most of the 24 patients were primiparous. The level of the blood pressure was mentioned in only eight of the 24 patients: in two it was elevated. Of 48 patients with aortic dissection associated with pregnancy collected by Pedowitz and Perell,[33] 40 had blood pressures recorded and in 19 (48%) systemic hypertension was present. Systemic hypertension was present in each of the two patients with aortic dissection

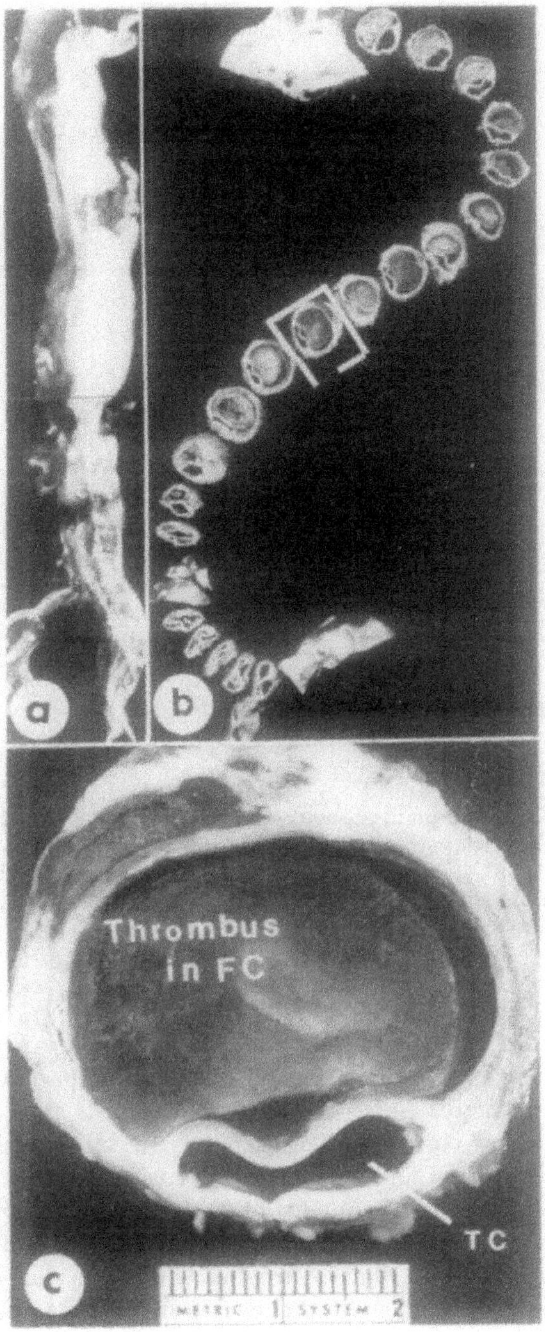

Fig. 14. Clinically silent healed dissection involving the descending thoracic and abdominal aorta in a 58-year-old white man (NNMC No. A76-87) who died from complications of habitual alcoholism. He was known to have had systemic hypertension for many years. **a,** Radiograph of aorta showing a narrowed true channel and thrombus plus heavy calcific deposits in the false channel. The entrance site was just distal to the aortic isthmus, and the exit was in the left femoral artery. **b,** Transverse sections of the aorta again showing that the true channel is narrowed by thrombus in the false channel. **c,** Close-up view of the section in the brackets in *b*. *TC*-true channel; *FC*-false channel.

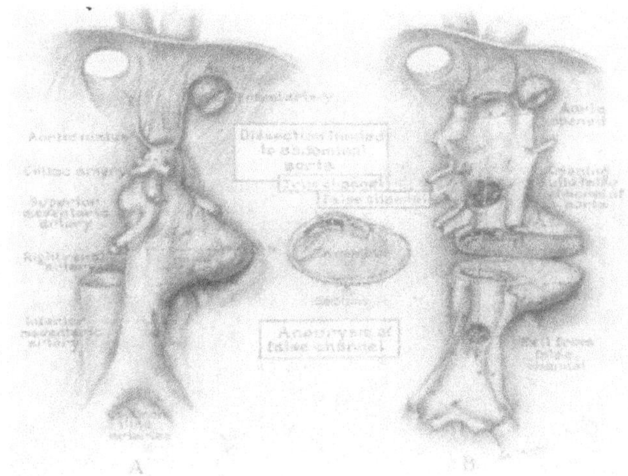

Fig. 15. Healed dissection limited to abdominal aorta in a 78-year-old man (DCMEO No. 80-02-144). The dissection was a surprise finding at necropsy. The patient died from consequences of a subdural hematoma. Most of the false channel is filled by thrombus.

during pregnancy reported by Kitchen[34] and in the one patient reported by Mandel et al.[32] It is well known that the systemic blood pressure and blood volume rise during pregnancy, and therefore it is reasonable to believe that aortic dissection would be more frequent during pregnancy than during non-pregnant periods when similar aged women are compared.

The *Marfan syndrome* and its forme fruste varieties also is listed as a major cause of aortic dissection (Fig. 16). Of 18 necropsy patients with the Marfan syndrome studied personally, three had aortic dissection.[35] Two of the three, however, had systemic hypertension before the aortic dissection occurred, and all three at necropsy had histologically normal aortas and no aortic root aneurysms. Thus, although each of these three patients had both aortic dissection and the Marfan syndrome, the characteristic aortic histologic lesion of the Marfan syndrome was absent, and therefore the aortic dissection in them cannot be attributed to the Marfan-type aorta. In contrast, of 13 other necropsy patients personally studied with the Marfan syndrome having aortic root fusiform aneurysms and the characteristic histologic aortic-medial lesion ("medial cystic necrosis") of this syndrome, none had aortic dissection, although all 13 had intra-aneurysmal tears without dissection.[35] The intimal and medial tears in the wall of the aortic root aneurysms in the Marfan syndrome patients appear to be called "dissections" by many, but infrequently are the

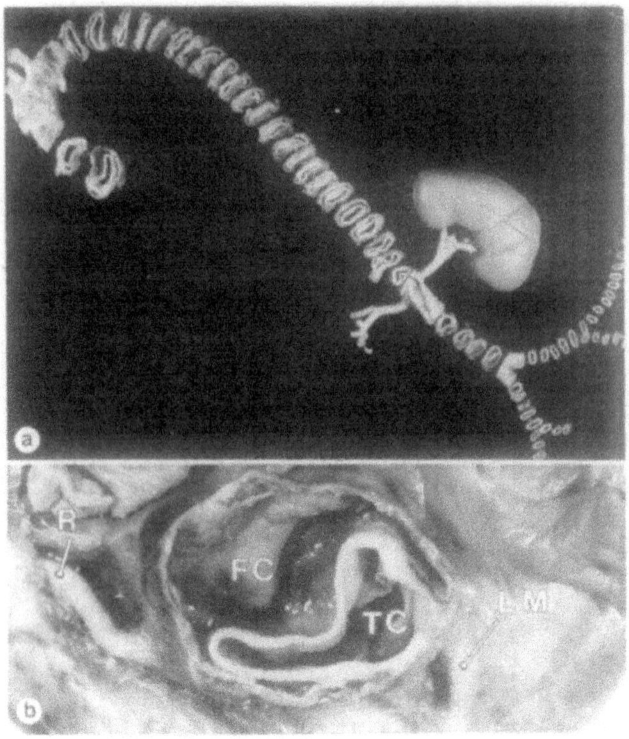

Fig. 16. Aorta **(a)** in a 43-year-old man (GT No. 76A-48) known to have the *Marfan syndrome.* He died 15 days after the sudden onset of typical clinical features of aortic dissection. Before the aortic dissection, there was no precordial murmur. At necropsy, except for the acute dissection, there was no enlargement of the aorta, and except at the site of the entrance into the false channel, there were no tears in the aorta. Shown in **a** is the complete aorta with both true and false channels and a hematoma in the false channel of the abdominal portion. Histologically, the aorta was normal. A close-up view of the aortic root is shown in **b.** *FC* = false and *TC* = true channels; *R* = right and *LM* = left main coronary arteries. The origin of the right coronary artery has been completely separated from the true channel. The heart weighed 500 gm and neither ventricle was dilated. Thus, although this patient had both aortic dissection and the Marfan syndrome, the typical histologic medial lesion of this syndrome was absent. Therefore, it is more likely that the systemic hypertension was a more important contributing factor to the aortic dissection.

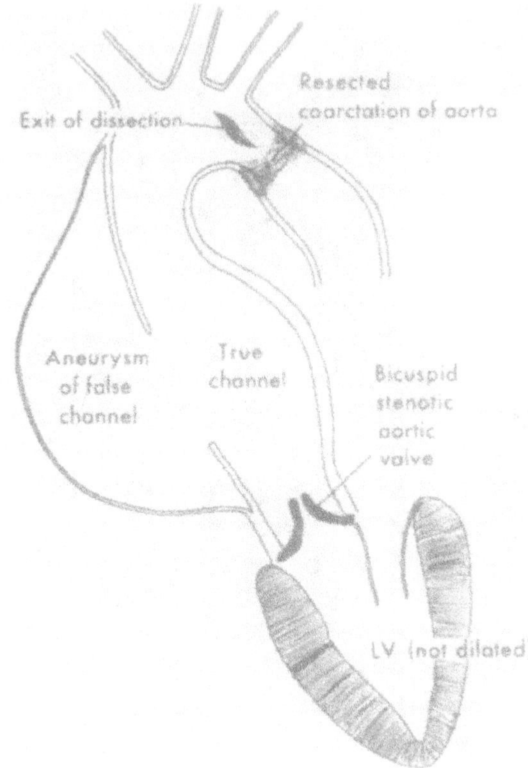

Fig. 17. Diagram in an adult (NNMC No. A73-168) who had an aortic isthmic coarctation resected in childhood and who died of rupture of a dissection involving only the ascending aorta. The aortic valve was congenitally bicuspid and stenotic.

aneurysmal wall tears associated with true longitudinal medial dissection. Indeed, dissection is rare in patients with fusiform aortic root aneurysms.[35]

One type of aortic dissection which may not be associated with systemic hypertension is that occurring in patients with *congenitally bicuspid aortic valves* with or without associated aortic valve stenosis[11, 13, 36-42] (Fig. 8). Of 85 necropsy patients with aortic dissection reported by Gore and Seiwert,[36] 11 (13%) had congenitally bicuspid aortic valves, only one of whom had aortic isthmic coarctation. Of their 11 patients with congenitally bicuspid aortic valves and aortic dissection, nine were less than 40 years of age (range 19 to 39 years).[37] Of 119 necropsy patients with aortic dissection reported by Edwards et al.,[42] 11 (9%) had congenitally bicuspid aortic valves, only three of whom had aortic isthmic coarctation.

Not only is the frequency of congenitally bicuspid aortic valves much higher than expected in patients with aortic dissection, the frequency of aortic dissection is much higher than expected in patients with congenitally bicuspid aortic valves. Of 152 necropsy patients over 20 years of age reported by Fenoglio et al.,[41] eight (5%) had aortic dissection.

Aortic isthmic coarctation clearly is associated with a high frequency of aortic dissection, probably through a double mechanism: (1) by causing systemic hypertension and (2) by having a high frequency of association with the congenitally bicuspid aortic valve (Fig. 17). The latter, particularly in association with aortic isthmic coarctation, appears to be related in some way to a structurally weaker aorta than in patients with three cuspid aortic

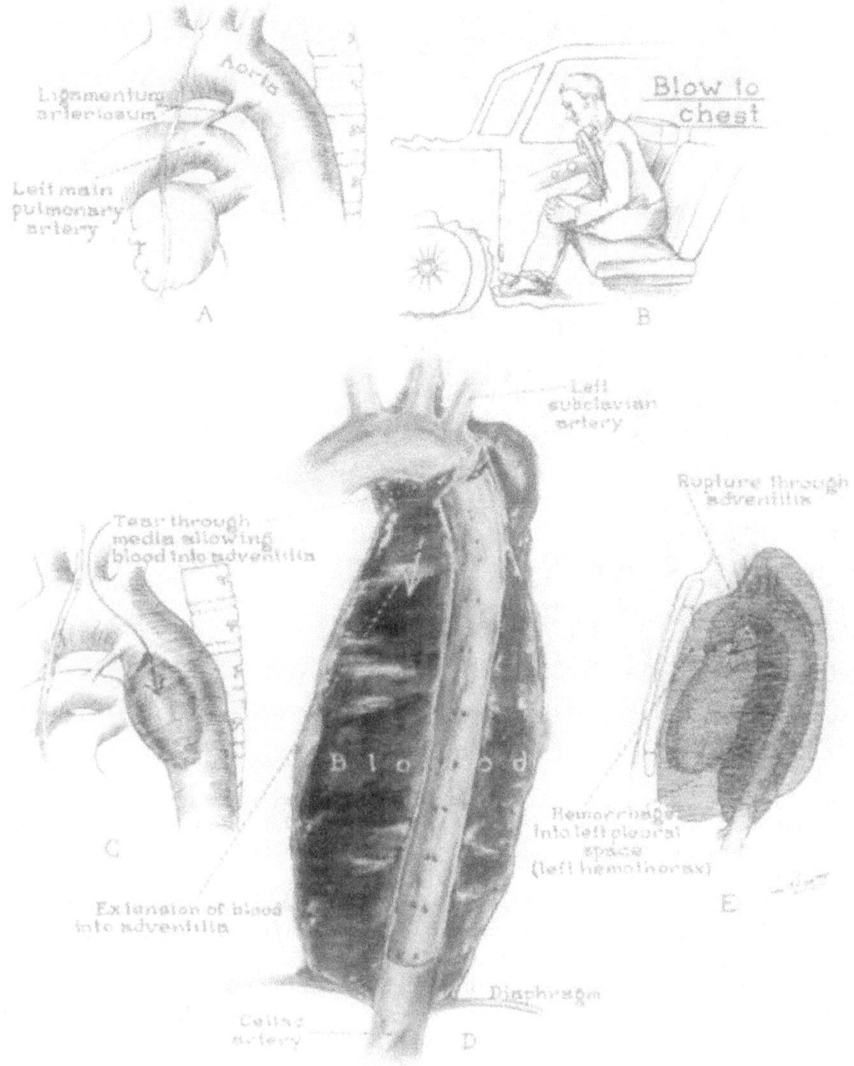

Fig. 18. Drawing of descending thoracic aorta in a 19-year-old man (DCMEO No. 80-01-10) who was in an automobile accident 12 days before death. The aorta was torn **(D)** at the time of the accident but immediate extravasation of blood beyond the media and adventitia did not occur until nearly 2 weeks later. At necropsy, the left pleural space was filled with blood.

valves with or without associated aortic isthmic coarctation. Of 200 necropsy patients with aortic isthmic coarctation reviewed by Abbott,[11] 38 (19%) had aortic rupture usually with dissection, and 17 (45%) of them had congenitally bicuspid aortic valves. All 17 patients were among the 33 in whom the dissection involved only the ascending aorta, thus giving a frequency of fatal proximal aortic dissection in necropsy patients with combined aortic isthmic coarctation and congenitally bicuspid aortic valves of over 50%. Of 104 necropsy patients with aortic isthmic coarctation reviewed by Reifenstein et al.,[13] 24 (23%) had aortic dissection and 10 (42%) of them had congentially bicuspid aortic valves.

Trauma[43] is a well-recognized, although rare, cause of aortic dissection. The truma is usually nonpenetrating and the aortic tear usually occurs in the region of the aortic isthmus (Fig. 18). At this site the aorta is braced by the ligamentum arteriosum.

In recent years, *iatrogenic-induced* traumatic aortic dissections have become more frequent and better recognized[44-56] (Figs. 19 to 21). They are primarily of two types: (1) *canulation*-induced and (2) *aortic-incision*-induced. The former commonly has resulted from insertion of a cardiopulmonary bypass cannula into the femoral artery (Fig. 19) or of an intra-aortic balloon counterpulsation device (Fig. 21). Rather than the tip of the catheter's being

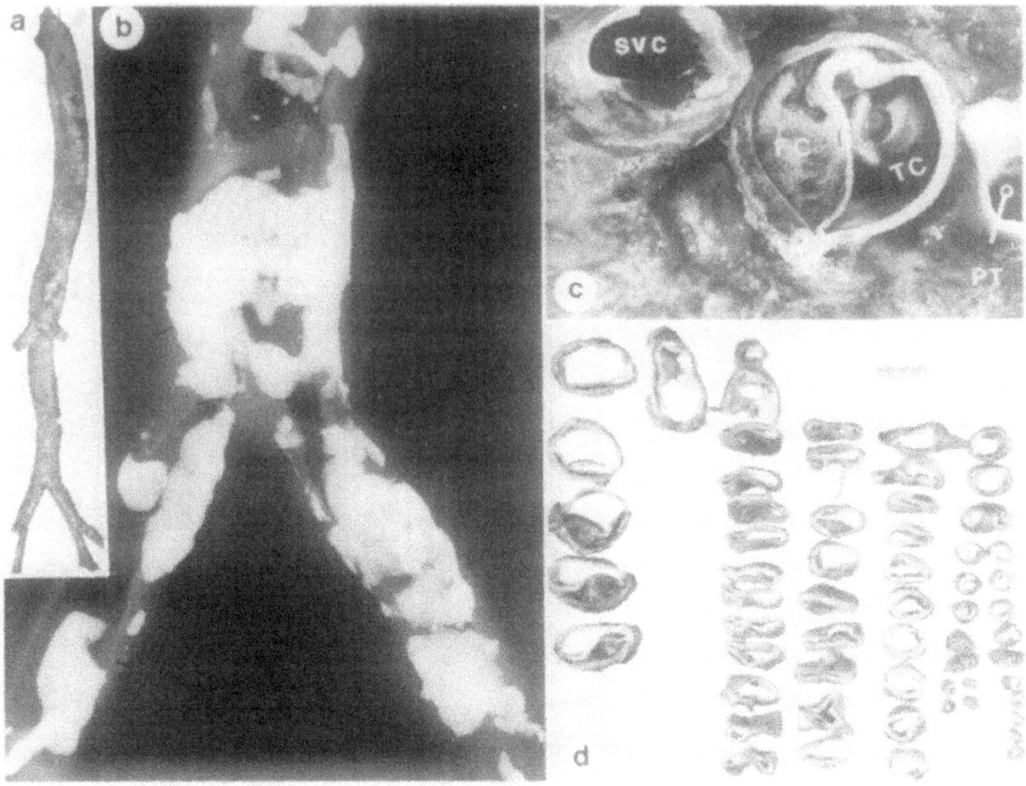

Fig. 19. Acute dissection of the entire aorta during left femoral arterial cannulation for cardiopulmonary bypass for mitral and aortic valve replacement in a 56-year-old white woman (A74-130). At the time of operation, the aortic dissection was apparent immediately after the institution of cardiopulmonary bypass. The cannula in the left femoral artery pierced an atherosclerotic plaque, and perfusion created a false channel in the media. The patient lived 20 days after the double valve replacement. At necropsy, the aorta was only mildly dilated if at all **(a).** The abdominal portion of aorta and both common iliac arteries contained heavy calcific deposits **(b),** and the lumens of both were considerably narrowed. (Preoperatively, the patient had not complained of leg claudication.) **c,** View of ascending aorta with a thrombus in the false channel *(FC).* A caged-ball prosthesis (Starr-Edwards type) is visible in the true channel *(TC). PT* = pulmonary trunk; *SVC* = superior vena cava. **d,** Cross-sections of aorta beginning *(lower left)* just above the aortic valve and ending *(lower right)* with the common iliac arteries.

positioned into the arterial lumen, the tip inadvertently was inserted into the arterial media. When cardiopulmonary bypass was instituted, arterial blood under pressure caused immediate retrograde dissection of the aorta by way of the femoral and iliac artery. Because of these types of accidents, radiographs of the distal aorta and its branches have been recommended before cannulation by this route, particularly in older patients. Cannulation into the proximal aorta has been a safer procedure, but it too has led to aortic dissection, generally not immediate. Incisions into the ascending aorta for insertion of aortocoronary bypass conduits[53, 55] or for replacement of the aortic valve[49, 54] also have been followed, usually late, by aortic dissection originating at the site of aortic incision (Fig. 20).

Atherosclerosis and *syphilis* also have been listed as "causes" of aortic dissection, but both "etiologies" appear highly unlikely. Atherosclerosis is, at least initially, an intimal disease. Later the overlying atherosclerotic plaques may cause atrophy of the underlying media. Dissection, in contrast, is primarily a medial disease, and its course down the aorta may be interrupted by the atrophied media from the overlying atherosclerotic plaques. Furthermore, the entrance tears into dissections most commonly are located in the ascending aorta, and this portion of the aorta tends to be spared or relatively spared by the atherosclerotic process, and rarely are plaques present at the entrance site of the dissection. Additionally, there tends to be an inverse relationship between severe aortic atherosclerosis and aortic dissections. Although there are many exceptions, the greater the extent of aortic atherosclerosis, the less the likelihood of aortic dissection. Syphilis produces transverse medial scars which tend to prevent rather than to predispose to aortic dissection.

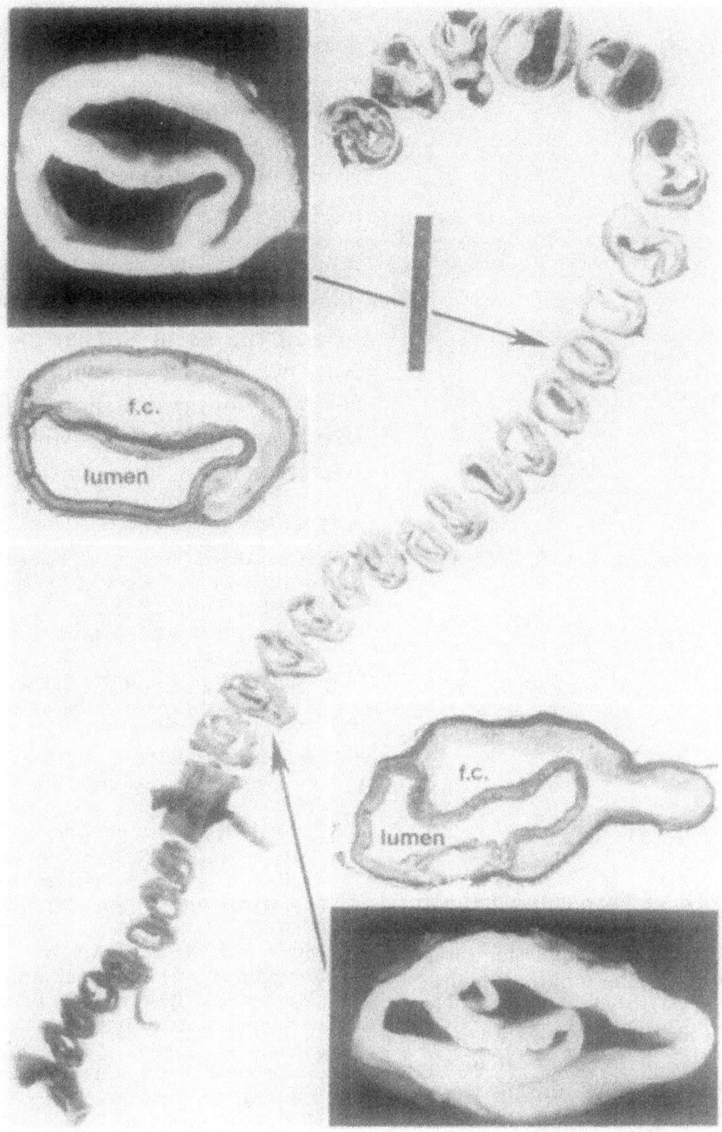

Fig. 20. Healed and healing dissection of the aorta in a 66-year-old white woman (A76-125) who clinically was considered by Victor A. McKusick, M.D. to have a variant of the Ehlers-Danlos syndrome. She had mild valvular aortic stenosis and moderately severe aortic regurgitation (aortic pressure = 150/70 mm Hg; left ventricle = 176/16 mm Hg). For several months, she had complained periodically of back pain. She underwent aortic valve replacement without difficulty, but three days postoperatively she had a stroke, and a day later, signs of cardiac tamponade. Reoperation disclosed a dissection beginning near the aortotomy site. A portion of aorta, therefore, was replaced with a graft, and because the left main coronary artery had been served from the aorta, a conduit (saphenous vein) was inserted between the aortic graft and the left anterior descending and left circumflex coronary arteries. She was unable to be weaned from cardiopulmonary bypass. At necropsy, the entire aorta was dissected. Most of the dissection had healed or was healing in that the wall of the false channel *(f.c.)* was thickened by fibrous tissue and the lumen of the false channel in most areas was free of thrombus. Just distal to the aortic isthmus, the aorta was quite dilated, as a result of dilatation of the false channel which in this area contained thrombus.

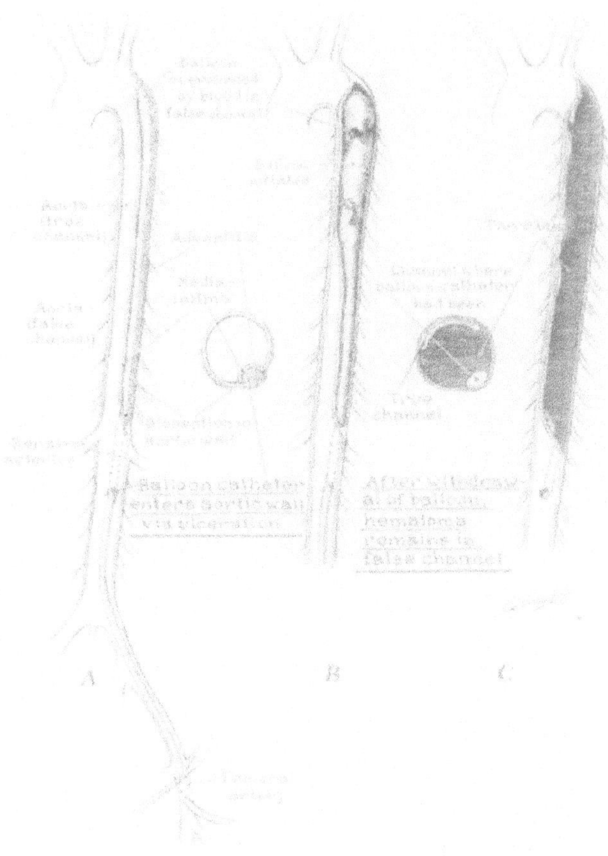

Fig. 21. Drawing of aorta with an intraaortic balloon located in a false channel in a 65-year-old woman (A77-234). The tip of the balloon catheter entered the aortic media at the site of an ulcerated atheromatous plaque located just caudal to the origin of the renal arteries. The balloon functioned successfully for 3 days despite its being located in the false channel **(B)**. After removal of the balloon the patient survived for 28 days, during which time organized thrombus filled the false channel **(C)**.

CONCLUSIONS

Aortic dissection generally is a catastrophic cardiovascular event which in the vast majority of patients is entirely preventable by proper treatment of systemic hypertension. Exactly how systemic hypertension is involved in the pathogenesis of aortic dissection is unclear, but it is clear that aortic dissection would virtually vanish if systemic hypertension disappeared. Patients with congenitally bicuspid aortic valves (with or without associated aortic isthmic coarctation), however, have an increased frequency of aortic dissection compared to individuals with three cuspid aortic valves, irrespective of the presence or absence of systemic hypertension. Most dissections involve the entire aorta. Those which stop within the aorta with or without a reentry site generally do so because of extensive atherosclerotic plaques which may cause atrophy or degeneration of the underlying media, which is where the longitudinal dissection is located. Although there are many exceptions, dissection involving the entire aorta generally indicates relatively mild or absent atherosclerosis. A common and poorly appreciated complication of aortic dissection is stenosis of the lumen of one or more major pulmonary arteries (peripheral pulmonic stenosis) due to extension of blood from the common adventitia of the aorta to that of the pulmonary trunk. Narrowing of the lumen of the true channel of the aorta by compressing hematoma in the false channel (true aortic stenosis) is another unappreciated but not uncommon complication of aortic dissection.

REFERENCES

1. Hirst AE Jr, Johns VJ Jr, Kime SW Jr: Dissecting aneurysm of the aorta: a review of 505 cases. Medicine **37:**217, 1958.
2. Erb BD Tullis IF: Dissecting aneurysm of the aorta. The clinical features of thirty autopsied cases. Circulation **22:**315, 1960.
3. Lindsay J Jr, Hurst JW: Clinical features and prognosis in dissecting aneurysm of the aorta. A re-appraisal. Circulation **35:**880, 1967.
4. Anagnostopoulos CE, Prabhakar MJS, Kittle CF: Aortic dissections and dissecting aneurysms, Am J Cardiol **30:**263, 1972.
5. Gore I, Hirst AE Jr: Dissecting aneurysm of the aorta. Cardiovasc Clin **2:**239, 1973.
6. Talbot S: Clinical features and prognosis of dissecting aneurysms and ruptured saccular aneurysms. Chest **66:**252, 1974.
7. Slater EE, DeSanctis RW: The clinical recognition of dissecting aortic aneurysm. Am J Med **60:**625, 1976.
8. Murray CA, Edwards JE: Spontaneous laceration of the ascending aorta. Circulation **47:**848, 1973.
9. Barsky SH, Rosen S: Aortic infarction following dissecting aortic aneurysm. Circulation **58:**876, 1978.
10. Edwards JE: Manifestations of acquired and congenital diseases of the aorta. Curr Probl Cardiol **3:**1, 1979.
11. Abbott ME: Coarctation of the aorta of the adult type. II. A statistical study and historical retrospect of 200 recorded cases, with autopsy, of stenosis or obliteration of the descending arch in subjects above the age of two years. Am Heart J **3:**392, 574, 1928.
12. Edwards JE, Christensen NA, Clagett OT, McDonald JR: Pathologic considerations in coarctation of the aorta. Proc Staff Meet Mayo Clin **23:**324, 1948.
13. Reifenstein GH, Levine SA, Gross RE: Coarctation of the aorta. A review of 104 autopsied cases of "adult type," 2 years of age or older. Am Heart J **33:**146, 1947.
14. McCombs HL, Crocker DW: Dissecting aneurysm distal to coarctation of the aorta, with long survival. Am Heart J **74:**675, 1967.
15. Edwards JE: Aneurysms of the thoracic aorta complicating coarctation. Circulation **48:**195, 1973.
16. Buja LM, Ali N, Fletcher RD, Roberts WC: Stenosis of the main pulmonary artery: A complication of acute dissecting aneurysm of the ascending aorta. Am Heart J **83:**89, 1972.
17. Perryman RA, Gay WA: Rupture of dissecting thoracic aortic aneurysm into the right ventricle. Am J Cardiol **30:**277, 1972.
18. Yacoub MH, Schottenfeld M, Kittle CF: Hematoma of the

interatrial septum with heart block secondary to dissecting aneurysm of the aorta. A clinicopathologic entity. Circulation **46**:537, 1972.

19. Page AJF, Yacoub MH, Sutton GC: Aorto-right atrial fistula. A rare complication of aortic dissection. Br Heart J **35**:1338, 1973.
20. Spitzer S, Blanco G, Adam A, Spyrou PG, Mason D: Superior vena cava obstruction and dissecting aortic aneurysm. JAMA **233**:164, 1975.
21. Thiene G, Rossi L, Becker AE: The atrioventricular conduction system in dissecting aneurysm of the aorta. AM HEART J **98**:447, 1979.
22. Baer S, Goldburgh HL: The varied clinical syndromes produced by dissecting aneurysm. AM HEART J **35**:198, 1948.
23. Burchell HB: Aortic dissection (dissecting hematoma; dissecting aneurysm of the aorta). Circulation **12**:1068, 1955.
24. Beaven DW, Murphy EA: Dissecting aneurysm during methonium therapy. A report of nine cases treated for hypertension. Br Med J **1**:77, 1956.
25. Roberts WC: The hypertensive diseases. Evidence that systemic hypertension is a greater risk factor to the development of other cardiovascular diseases than previously suspected. Am J Med **59**:523, 1975.
26. Hutt MSR: Pathology of African cardiomyopathies. Pathol Microbiol **35**:37, 1970.
27. Klotz O, Simpson W: Spontaneous rupture of the aorta. Am J Med Sci **184**:455, 1932.
28. Manley G: Histology of the aortic media in dissecting aneurysms. J Clin Pathol **17**:220, 1964.
29. Hirst AE, Gore I: Is cystic medionecrosis the cause of dissecting aortic aneurysm? Circulation **53**:915, 1976.
30. Schlatmann TJM, Becker AE: Pathogenesis of dissecting aneurysm of aorta. Comparative histopathologic study of significance of medial changes. Am J Cardiol **39**:21, 1977.
31. Schnitker MA, Bayer CA: Dissecting aneurysm of the aorta in young individuals, particularly in association with pregnancy. With report of a case. Ann Intern Med **20**:486, 1944.
32. Mandel W, Evans EW, Walford RL: Dissecting aortic aneurysm during pregnancy. N Engl J Med **251**:1059, 1954.
33. Pedowitz P, Perell A: Aneurysms complicated by pregnancy. Part I. Aneurysms of the aorta and its major branches. Am J Obstet Gynecol **73**:720, 1957.
34. Kitchen DH: Dissecting aneurysm of the aorta in pregnancy. J Obstet Gynaecol Br Commonw **81**:410, 1974.
35. Roberts WC: Congenital cardiovascular abnormalities usually "silent" until adulthood: Morphologic features of the floppy mitral valve, valvular aortic stenosis, discrete subvalvular aortic stenosis, hypertrophic cardiomyopathy, sinus of Valsalva aneurysm, and the Marfan syndrome. *In* Roberts WC, editor: Congenital heart disease in adults. Philadelphia, 1979, FA Davis Co, pp 407-453.
36. Gore I, Seiwert VJ: Dissecting aneurysm of the aorta. Pathologic aspects. An analysis of eighty-five fatal cases. Arch Pathol **53**:121, 1952.
37. Gore L: Dissecting aneurysms of the aorta in persons under forty years of age. Arch Pathol **55**:1, 1953.
38. McKusick VA, Logue RB, Bahnson HT: Association of aortic valvular disease and cystic medial necrosis of the ascending aorta. Report of four instances. Circulation **16**:188, 1957.
39. Heath D, Edwards JE, Smith LA: The rheologic significance of medial necrosis and dissecting aneurysm of the ascending aorta in association with calcific aortic stenosis. Proc Mayo Clin **33**:228, 1958.
40. Fukuda T, Tadavarthy SM, Edwards JE: Dissecting aneurysm of aorta complicating aortic valvular stenosis. Circulation **53**:169, 1976.
41. Fenoglio JJ, McAllister HA, DeCastro CM: The congenital bicuspid aortic valve after age 20. Am J Cardiol **39**:164, 1977.
42. Edwards WD, Leaf DS, Edwards JE: Dissecting aortic aneurysm associated with congenital bicuspid aortic valve. Circulation **57**:1022, 1978.
43. Parmley LF, Mattingly TM, Manion WC, Jahnke EJ Jr: Nonpenetrating traumatic injury of aorta. Circulation **17**:1086, 1958.
44. Gaylis H, Laws JW: Dissection of aorta as a complication of translumbar aortography. Br Med J **2**:1141, 1956.
45. Elliott DP, Roe BB: Aortic dissection during cardiopulmonary bypass. J Thorac Cardiovasc Surg **50**:357, 1965.
46. Salama FD, Blesovsky A: Complications of cannulation of the ascending aorta for open heart surgery. Thorax **25**:604, 1970.
47. Cooley DA, Wukasch DC, Hallman GL: Acute dissecting ascending aortic aneurysm resulting from coronary arteriography: Successful surgical treatment. Chest **61**:317, 1972.
48. Wellons HA Jr, Singh R: Acute dissecting aortic aneurysm resulting from retrogarde brachial arterial catheterization. Successful operative intervention. Am J Cardiol **33**:562, 1974.
49. Derkac W, Laks H, Cohn LH, Collins JJ Jr: Dissecting aneurysm after aortic valve replacement. Arch Surg **109**:388, 1974.
50. Benedict JS, Buhl TL, Henney RP: Acute aortic dissection during cardiopulmonary bypass. Successful treatment of three patients. Arch Surg **108**:810, 1974.
51. Williams CD, Suwansirikul S, Engelman RM: Thoracic aortic dissection following cannulation for perfusion. Ann Thorac Surg **18**:300, 1974.
52. Litchford B, Okies JE, Sugimura S, Starr A: Acute aortic dissection from cross-clamp injury. J Thorac Cardiovasc Surg **72**:709, 1976.
53. Lam R, Morton J, Robinson MD, Morales AR: Aortic dissection complicating aorto-coronary saphenous vein bypass. Am J Clin Pathol **68**:729, 1977.
54. Muna WF, Spray TL, Morrow AG, Roberts WC: Aortic dissection after aortic valve replacement in patients with valvular aortic stenosis. J Thorac Cardiovasc Surg **74**:65, 1977.
55. Nicholson WJ, Crawley IS, Logue RB, Dorney ER, Cobbs BW, Hatcher CR Jr: Aortic root dissection complicating coronary bypass surgery. Am J Cardiol **41**:103, 1978.
56. Isner JM, Cohen SR, Virmani R, Lawrinson W, Roberts WC: Complications of the intraaortic balloon counterpulsation device: Clinical and morphologic observations in 45 necropsy patients. Am J Cardiol **45**:260, 1980.

Congenitally Bicuspid Aortic Valve Causing Severe, Pure Aortic Regurgitation Without Superimposed Infective Endocarditis

Analysis of 13 Patients Requiring Aortic Valve Replacement

WILLIAM C. ROBERTS, MD, FACC
ANDREW G. MORROW, MD, FACC
CHARLES L. McINTOSH, MD
MICHAEL JONES, MD
STEPHEN E. EPSTEIN, MD, FACC

Bethesda, Maryland

Although stenosis and infective endocarditis are commonly appreciated complications of the congenitally bicuspid aortic valve, pure *severe* aortic regurgitation complicating this congenital malformation, unassociated with either stenosis or infection, is not well recognized. Among 189 patients who had aortic valve replacement at the National Heart, Lung, and Blood Institute because of isolated pure aortic regurgitation, the congenitally bicuspid aortic valve, never the site of infective endocarditis, was responsible for the aortic regurgitation in 13 (7 percent). This report describes certain clinical and morphologic findings in 13 men, aged 26 to 65 years (mean 43), who required aortic valve replacement because of severe aortic regurgitation secondary to a noninfected, nonstenotic congenitally bicuspid aortic valve. Although not generally recognized, the noninfected congenitally bicuspid aortic valve is an important cause of pure aortic regurgitation severe enough to warrant aortic valve replacement.

The congenitally bicuspid aortic valve frequently becomes stenotic, and because most stenotic valves are also regurgitant, the most frequent circumstance in which aortic regurgitation is found with this congenital anomaly is in association with aortic valve stenosis.[1] In this situation the aortic regurgitation is usually of only mild or moderate degree. Also, the congenitally bicuspid aortic valve is often the site of infective endocarditis.[1] Although it may be superimposed on a stenotic congenitally bicuspid aortic valve, infective endocarditis far more commonly involves the previously normally functioning bicuspid valve or the one previously only slightly regurgitant.[1,2] The usual consequence of the infection in this circumstance is severe pure aortic regurgitation. Mild degrees of pure aortic regurgitation also are commonly observed in patients with a congenitally bicuspid aortic valve and elevated pressure in the ascending aorta from associated aortic isthmic coarctation. However, *severe* aortic regurgitation due to a nonstenotic and noninfected congenitally bicuspid aortic valve is believed to be decidedly infrequent and, indeed, no reports, to our knowledge, have focused specifically on this complication of the bicuspid valve condition. In this report, we describe observations in 13 men who underwent aortic valve replacement because of severe pure aortic regurgitation unassociated with aortic valve stenosis or infective endocarditis.

Clinical Features of Patients

Clinical findings (Table I): At the time of aortic valve replacement, the ages of the 13 men studied ranged from 26 to 65 years (mean 43). Preoperatively, one patient had been in functional class I (New York Heart Association classification[3]), three patients in class II, eight in class III and one in class IV. The one patient who was asymptomatic preop-

From the Pathology, Surgery and Cardiology Branches, National Heart, Lung, and Blood Institute, National Institutes of Health, Bethesda, Maryland. Manuscript received August 4, 1980; revised manuscript received September 16, 1980; accepted September 18, 1980.
Address for reprints: William C. Roberts, MD, Building 10A, Room 3E-30, National Institutes of Health, Bethesda, Maryland 20205.

TABLE I

Clinical and Operative Observations in 13 Men With Aortic Valve Replacement for Pure Severe Aortic Regurgitation and Noninfected Congenitally Bicuspid Aortic Valve

Case	Age (yr) at AVR	Age (yr) M First Heard	Age (yr) Onset of Cardiac Symptoms	Pressures (s/d) (mm Hg) LV	SA	Site of AV Cusps	AV Raphe	AV Ca^{++}	AV Wt (g)
1	26	17	20	125/25	125/54	R-L	+	0	
2	26	13	21	150/24	150/60	A-P	+	0	1.2
3	28	6	27	200/32	235/70	?		0	1.0
4	30	16	29	135/11	160/55	A-P	0	0	0.9
5	30	27	27	118/6	118/52	R-L	+	0	0.7
6	40	11	35	200/32	200/80	A-P	+	+	2.9
7	46	20	44	125/7	130/50	A-P	+	0	?
8	48	13	40	170/12	170/60	?	+	+	2.2
9	49	20	?	118/5	120/58	R-L	0	0	1.5
10	56	27	27	165/17	165/72	A-P	+	0	1.4
11	57	22	44	160/14	170/75	R-L	+	+	1.8
12	63	45	60	155/7	155/55	?	+	+	2.3
13	65	60	65	138/36	160/53	R-L	+	+	1.7

A = anterior; AV = aortic valve; AVR = aortic valve replacement; Ca^{++} = calcium; L = left; LV = left ventricle; M = murmur; P = posterior; R = right; SA = systemic artery; s/d = peak systole/end-diastole; Wt = weight; ? = not known; + = present or positive; 0 = absent or negative.

eratively underwent aortic valve replacement because of severe aortic regurgitation associated with a dilated left ventricular cavity[4] (left ventricular end-systolic cavity dimension on echocardiogram = 56 mm). None of the 13 patients at any time had had clinical evidence of either active infective endocarditis or acute rheumatic fever.

A precordial murmur had been heard for the first time initially as early as age 6 years to as late as age 60 years (mean 23). By auscultation, all 13 patients had grade 3-5/6 murmurs typical of aortic regurgitation, and by aortic root angiograms the degree of aortic regurgitation was graded in each as either 3+/4+ or 4+/4+. The direct aortic diastolic pressures preoperatively ranged from 45 to 80 mm Hg (mean 61). All 13 patients also had basal precordial systolic murmurs, but at catheterization none had a peak systolic pressure gradient between the left ventricle and a major systemic artery or on pullback from the left ventricle to the aorta. Precordial ejection sounds were absent in all 13 patients. Aortic root angiograms were obtained in all patients, but the bicuspid condition of the aortic valve could not be established by this method. Also, the bicuspid nature of the valve was not recognized in any of the seven patients who had echocardiograms.

Three patients (Cases 3, 4 and 6) had aortic isthmic coarctation, with a peak systolic pressure gradient across the coarctation of 70, 50 and 70 mm Hg, respectively. One (Patient 1) had a right aortic arch. No patient had evidence of mitral regurgitation. The father of Patient 2 had had aortic valve replacement because of a stenotic (60 mm Hg peak systolic pressure gradient) congenitally bicuspid aortic valve.

Surgical and morphologic findings: At aortic valve replacement, only two aortic valve cusps were identified in each of the 13 patients (Fig. 1 to 4). In 10 valves, a

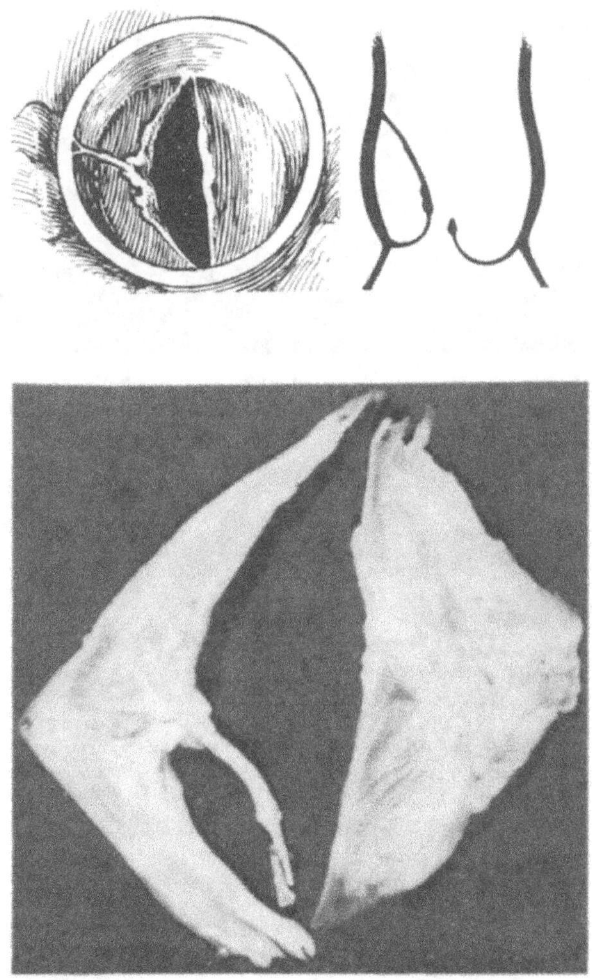

FIGURE 1. Aortic valve in Case 1. The fibrous band on the right cusp (**below**) was attached to the wall of the ascending aorta as shown in the diagram (**above**).

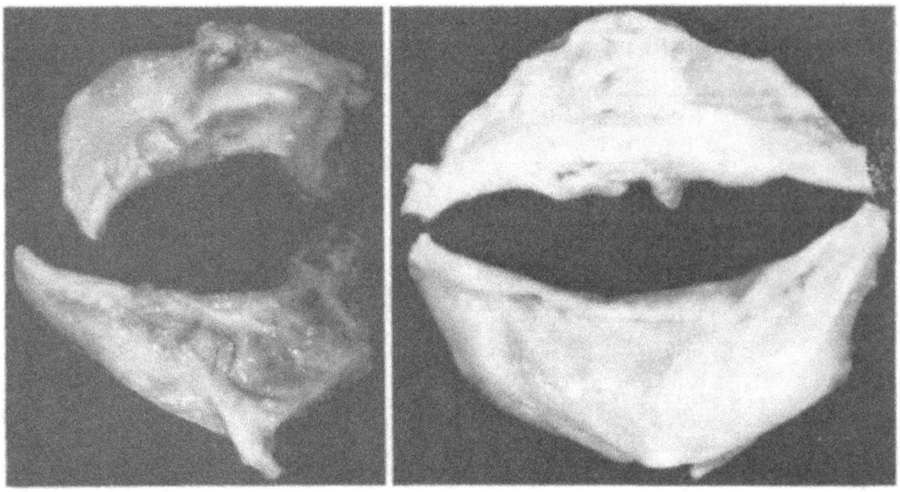

FIGURE 2. Aortic valve in Case 6 (**left**) and Case 7 (**right**). In each valve, the larger cusp is the anterior one. Calcium deposits are present in the valve on the **left**, *but not in the one on the* **right**.

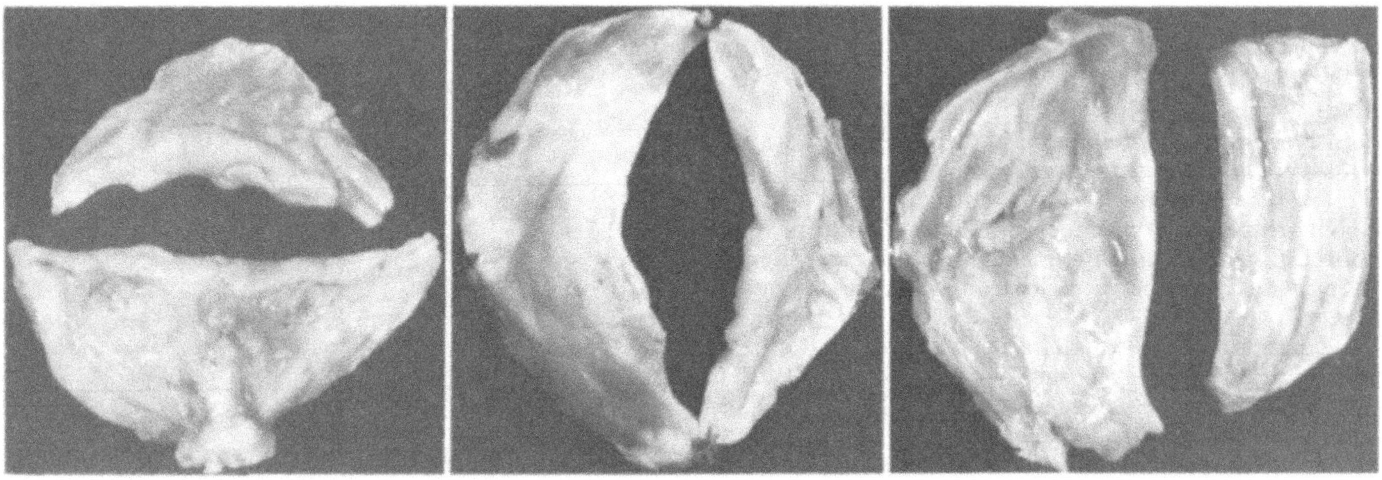

FIGURE 3. Aortic valve in Case 8 (**left**), Case 9 (**middle**) and Case 13 (**right**). The orientation of the cusps is uncertain in Case 8; calcium is present in the raphe in the larger cusp. In both Case 9 and Case 13, the larger cusp is the right one, and the smaller cusp, the left one.

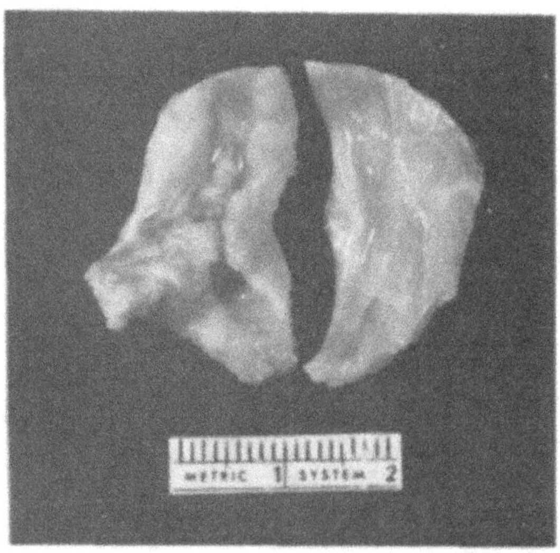

FIGURE 4. Aortic valve in Case 12. The orientation of the two cusps in this patient is not known. The raphe is calcified.

congenital raphe (false commissure) was identified. Each cusp of all 13 aortic valves was thickened by fibrous tissue; no cusp contained vegetations or perforations, indentations, or other evidences of healed infective endocarditis.[5] Calcific deposits, all small, were present in 5 of the 13 excised aortic valves; the deposits in 3 were limited to the raphes.

Comments

Frequency at necropsy of pure regurgitation in bicuspid aortic valve: Each of the 13 patients had aortic regurgitation severe enough to require aortic valve replacement, and at operation each was found to have a congenitally bicuspid aortic valve that neither was stenotic nor had evidence of past infective endocarditis. Furthermore, no patient had had a past clinical illness compatible with active infective endocarditis. Among the complications of a congenitally bicuspid aortic valve, pure severe aortic regurgitation unrelated to infective endocarditis is the least common. Among 200 patients over age 15 years with a congenitally bicuspid aortic valve studied by one of us (W.C.R.) at *necropsy*, only 3 had pure severe aortic regurgitation unassociated with infective endocarditis.[1] Of the 200 necropsy patients, however, 179 had some degree of aortic regurgitation, but it was associated with aortic valve stenosis in 157 and was the result of infective endocarditis in 19; in the remaining 21 patients the bicuspid valve functioned normally. Of 152 necropsy patients with a congenitally bicuspid aortic valve reported on by Fenoglio et al.,[6] 4 apparently had pure aortic regurgitation without evidence of infective endocarditis; however, the severity of the aortic regurgitation in their patients was not stated.

Frequency of congenitally bicuspid valve in pure aortic regurgitation (operative experience): Although the two studies cited provide some information on the frequency of pure aortic regurgitation unassociated with infective endocarditis among *necropsy* patients with a congenitally bicuspid aortic valve, no information is available concerning the frequency of the congenitally bicuspid aortic valve unassociated with infective endocarditis among patients with pure *severe* aortic regurgitation. Accordingly, we reviewed the clinical and operative records and the excised aortic valves in 189 patients aged 18 to 70 years who had aortic valve replacement at the National Heart, Lung, and Blood Institute from 1963 to 1979 because of *isolated* (unassociated with dysfunction of another cardiac valve) *pure* (no element of valve stenosis) aortic regurgitation (Table II). In 13 (7 percent) of the 189 patients the aortic regurgitation was the result of a congenitally bicuspid aortic valve that was not and had not been the site of infective endocarditis. In contrast to the 13 patients that form the basis of this report, only 7 patients (among the 189) had pure aortic regurgitation because of infective endocarditis involving a congenitally bicuspid aortic valve. Thus, the congenitally bicuspid aortic valve unaffected by infective endocarditis is an important cause of pure aortic regurgitation severe enough to warrant aortic valve replacement.

TABLE II

Etiology of Isolated Pure Aortic Regurgitation in 189 Patients Aged 18 to 70 Years Having Aortic Valve Replacement

Cause	Patients n	Patients %
1.* Rheumatic	94	49
2.* Infective endocarditis	41	22
Bicuspid (n = 7)		
Tricuspid (n = 34)		
3. Marfan and Marfan-type	15	8
4.* Congenital (bicuspid valve)	13	7
5.* Prolapse from ventricular septal defect	10	5
6. Syphilis	9	5
7. Aortic dissection	2	7 (items 7–10)
8. Ankylosing spondylitis	2	
9.* With subaortic stenosis	2	4 (items 7–10)
Discrete subaortic stenosis (n = 1)		
Hypertrophic cardiomyopathy (n = 1)		
10. Trauma	1	
Total	189	100

* Aortic regurgitation resulted from abnormality of the aortic valve only and not from abnormality of the aorta.

References

1. **Roberts WC.** The congenitally bicuspid aortic valve. A study of 85 autopsy cases. Am J Cardiol 1960;23:72–83.
2. **Roberts WC.** Characteristics and consequences of infective endocarditis (active or healed or both) learned from morphologic studies. In: Rahimtoola SH, ed. Infective Endocarditis. New York; Grune & Stratton, 1978;55–123.
3. Criteria Committee of the New York Heart Association. Nomenclature and Criteria for Diseases of the Heart and Great Vessels. 8th ed. Boston; Little, Brown, 1979:349.
4. **Henry WL, Bonow RO, Rosing DR, Epstein SE.** Observations on the optimum time for operative intervention for aortic regurgitation. II. Serial echocardiographic evaluation of asymptomatic patients. Circulation 1980;61:484–92.
5. **Roberts WC, Buchbinder NA.** Healed left-sided infective endocarditis: a clinicopathologic study of 59 patients. Am J Cardiol 1977; 40:876–88.
6. **Fenoglio JJ, McAllister HA, DeCastro CM.** The congenital bicuspid aortic valve after age 20. Am J Cardiol 1977;39:164–9.

Effect of Chronic Hypercalcemia on the Heart

An Analysis of 18 Necropsy Patients

WILLIAM C. ROBERTS, M.D.
BRUCE F. WALLER, M.D.
Bethesda, Maryland

Certain clinical and morphologic cardiac observations are described in 18 necropsy patients, aged 33 to 58 years (mean 45 years) (14 women), with chronic hypercalcemia (11.6 to 34.4 mg/dl [19.4]) from one to nine years (mean five years). Primary hyperparathyroidism was present in nine patients and secondary hyperparathyroidism in the other nine (of renal origin in seven). Cardiac valve anular and coronary arterial calcific deposits were present in 10 patients (Group I) including four (mean age 51 years) with considerable narrowing of two or three of the four major epicardial coronary arteries. None of the other eight patients (Group II) had cardiac valve anular or cuspal calcific deposits; only two had coronary calcific deposits, small in each, and none had significant coronary luminal narrowing. Calcium was in the media ("medial calcinosis"), with or without intimal deposition, of the coronary arteries in five patients. Comparison of the patients in Group I to those in Group II disclosed similar mean ages, durations of hypercalcemia and serum calcium levels, but significantly ($p < 0.05$) higher mean total serum cholesterol levels (216 versus 163 mg/dl) and heart weights (426 versus 320 g).

This study demonstrates that chronic hypercalcemia is associated with accelerated deposition of calcium in the cardiac anuli and valvular cusps, in the media and intima of the coronary arteries and in individual myocardial fibers (dystrophic calcification), and that coronary intimal calcification may be associated with or produce luminal narrowing, especially in patients with serum total cholesterol levels over 200 mg/dl. Thus, chronic hypercalcemia may be viewed as a "risk factor" to accelerated coronary atherosclerosis.

During the past 15 years, one (W.C.R.) of us has routinely examined hearts of patients at necropsy before receiving any clinical information about them. On the basis of the cardiac examination at necropsy, the patient's age, sex, clinical diagnosis and clinical features are predicted. Several years ago, a heart was examined in which massive calcific deposits were present in the mitral-valve anulus and coronary arteries, and small calcific deposits were present in the tricuspid-valve anulus and in both pulmonic and aortic-valve cusps. Primarily on the basis of these calcific deposits, it was predicted that the patient had been about 90 years of age. When clinical information was provided, however, it was learned that the patient had been only 44 years old and had died of consequences of primary hyperparathyroidism. Because the cardiac examiner had never missed a patient's age by nearly half a century on the basis of the cardiac examination at necropsy, a search was made of reports describing the heart at necropsy in patients with chronic hypercalcemia. Few focusing on this subject

From the Pathology Branch, National Heart, Lung and Blood Institute, National Institutes of Health, Bethesda, Maryland. Requests for reprints should be addressed to Dr. William C. Roberts, Building 10A, Room 3E30, National Institutes of Health, Bethesda, Maryland 20205. Manuscript accepted March 31, 1981.

TABLE I **Clinical and Necropsy Observations in 10 Necropsy Patients with Hypercalcemia and Calcific Deposits in Cardiac Valves or Anuli**

	Cases										Mean or Subtotal
	1	2	3	4	5	6	7	8	9	10	
Age (yr)	35	39	43	44	45	45	47	52	55	58	46
Race	W	B	B	B	B	W	B	W	B	B	7B, 3W
Sex	M	F	F	F	F	M	F	F	F	M	7F, 3M
Duration (yr) of H	5	1	5	8	6	7	7	7	5	8	5.9
Cause of H = 1°	0	+	+	0	0	+†	0	+	0	0	4
2°	C	0	0	Sar	R†	0	R†	0	R†	R†	6
PA	0	0	0	0	+	+	+	0	+	+	4
SAP (mm Hg)											
Peak systole	130	110	140	170	180	175	200	140	175	180	160
End diastole	70	70	90	100	110	95	110	90	100	110	95
Serum mean values											
Calcium (mg/dl)*	14.2	20.1	17.0	19.2	18.2	16.8	21.6	26.8	21.0	14.6	18.8
Phosphorus (mg/dl)*	4.8	5.2	1.9	5.5	2.9	6.1	6.5	4.1	4.9	9.0	4.2
Albumin (gm/dl)*	3.0	—	2.9	2.5	2.9	2.7	2.4	2.2	2.9	2.7	2.7
TC (mg/dl)	193	—	230	—	180	271	247	164	158	289	216
Mode of death	C	C	HC	Op‡	IE	VA	R	I§	IE	VA	
Heart weight (gm)	330	320	390	440	500	440	600	300	360	580	426
Calcific deposits (0.4+)											
MVA	1+	2+	4+	3+	4+	4+	4+	2+	4+	3+	10
TVA	0	0	2+	0	0	2+	0	0	0	0	2
AV	0	0	2+	0	0	2+	1+	0	0	0	3
PV	0	0	1+	0	0	1+	0	0	0	0	2
CA, intima	2+	0	0	1+	1+	4+	4+	1+	4+	4+	8
CA, media	0	1+	1+	0	1+	1+	0	0	0	0	4
Myocardium	+	+	+	0	+	+	0	+	0	+	7
NV	+	+	+	+	+	+	+	+	+	+	10
LV fibrosis, transmural	0	0	+	0	0	0	+	0	0	+	13
No. 4 CA narrowed >75%	0	0	0	0	0	3	3	0	2	3	11/36

NOTE: AV = aortic valve cusps; C = cancer (bone sarcoma); CA = coronary arteries; F = fibrosis; H = hypercalcemia; HC = hypercalcemia crisis; I = infection; IE = infective endocarditis; MVA = mitral valve anulus; No. = number; NV = nonvascular, e.g. lung, kidney, etc.; Op = operation; PA = pericardial adhesions; PV = pulmonic valve anulus; R = renal disease; SAP = systemic arterial pressure; Sar = sarcoid; TC = total cholesterol; TVA = tricuspid valve anulus; VA = ventricular arrhythmia.

* Based on 10 to 50 values per patient.

† Hemodialysis.

‡ Partial gastrectomy for peptic ulcer.

§ Following bilateral hip fracture.

were found. Accordingly a search of our necropsy files was made for patients with chronic hypercalcemia during life; 18 in whom the serum calcium level was known to have been unequivocally elevated for longer than one year were found. Clinical and necropsy findings in these 18 patients are the focus of this report.

PATIENTS STUDIED AND METHODS

Certain clinical and necropsy observations in the 18 patients are summarized in **Tables I** and **II.** They ranged in age from 33 to 58 years (mean 45 years); 14 were women, four were men; 11 were white and seven were black. Hypercalcemia was known to have been present from one to nine years (mean five years) before death. Its cause was primary hyperparathyroidism (adenoma or hyperplasia) in nine and secondary hyperparathyroidism (renal disease in seven; sarcoidosis in one and osteogenic sarcoma in one) in nine patients. Five patients (Cases 5, 6, 7, 9 and 10) underwent hemodialysis during the last five to eight years of their lives because of chronic renal failure. The serum calcium levels during the period of hypercalcemia ranged from 11.6 to 34.4 mg/dl (mean 19.4 mg/dl), and the serum phosphorus levels, from 1.5 to 16.6 mg/dl (mean 4.9 mg/dl). The serum albumin levels during the period of hypercalcemia ranged from 1.8 to 3.1 g/dl (mean 2.9 g/dl). The total serum cholesterol levels (15 patients) ranged from 119 to 289 mg/dl (mean 192 mg/dl). Only one patient (Case 10, Table I) had clinical evidence of myocardial ischemia, and he had both angina pectoris and acute myocardial infarction which healed. Information regarding a history of cardiac disease in other family members was present in nine of the 18 patients, only one (Case 15) of whom had a parent or sibling with fatal coronary heart disease. The father and two brothers of that patient had histories of acute myocardial infarction. Systemic hypertension (systolic pressure >140 and/or diastolic pressure >90 mm Hg) was present in 14 patients, including all seven patients in whom the hyperparathyroidism was the result of chronic renal disease. Electrocardiograms (**Figures 1** and **2**) in 16 patients disclosed some type of abnormality in 15 (**Table III**); two patients (Cases 3 and 5) did not have electrocardiograms. Ten had shortened QT intervals (corrected for heart rate). Five patients had ventricular arrhythmias (**Table IV**). Roentgenograms (**Figure 3**) disclosed calcific deposits in vascular or

TABLE II **Clinical and Necropsy Observations in Eight Necropsy Patients with Hypercalcemia and Calcific Deposits in Cardiac Valves or Anuli**

	Cases								Mean or Subtotal
	1	2	3	4	5	6	7	8	
Age (yr)	33	35	37	37	43	43	55	58	43
Race	W	W	W	W	W	W	W	W	0B, 8W
Sex	F	F	M	F	F	F	F	F	7F, 1M
Duration (yr) of H	1	6	1.5	1	5	7	1.5	6	3.6
Cause of H = 1°	+	+	0	+	+	+	0	0	5
2°	0	0	R	0	0	0	R	R	3
PA	0	+	+	0	0	0	+	0	3
SAP (mm Hg)									
Peak systole	80	200	145	200	140	160	205	180	164
End diastole	60	100	100	85	95	100	110	90	92
Serum mean values									
Calcium (mg/dl)*	27.4	22.4	15.6	17.4	21.0	24.4	18.6	14.2	19.2
Phosphorus (mg/dl)*	2.9	10.5	1.6	2.9	2.1	4.1	6.3	8.3	4.4
Albumin (gm/dl)*	2.7	2.1	2.8	2.8	2.9	3.3	2.4	2.5	2.7
TC (mg/dl)	187	200	126	170	147	119	—	192	163
Mode of death	P	R	R	Op	Op	Op	R	R	—
Heart weight (gm)	250	370	320	360	200	310	460	380	320
Calcific deposits (0.4+)									
MVA	0	0	0	0	0	0	0	0	0
TVA	0	0	0	0	0	0	0	0	0
AV	0	0	0	0	0	0	0	0	0
PV	0	0	0	0	0	0	0	0	0
CA, intima	0	0	0	1+	0	0	0	0	1
CA, media	0	1+	0	0	0	0	0	0	1
Myocardium	0	0	0	0	0	0	0	0	0
NV	0	1+	0	0	0	0	0	0	1
LV fibrosis, transmural	0	0	0	0	0	0	0	0	0
No. 4 CA narrowed >75%	0	0	0	0	0	0	0	0	0/36

NOTE: AV = aortic valve cusps; C = cancer (bone sarcoma); CA = coronary arteries; F = fibrosis; H = hypercalcemia; HC = hypercalcemia crisis; I = infection; IE = infective endocarditis; MVA = mitral valve anulus; No. = number; NV = nonvascular, e.g. lung, kidney, etc.; Op = operation; P = porphyria; PA = pericardial adhesions; PV = pulmonic valve anulus; R = renal disease; SAP = systemic arterial pressure; TC = total cholesterol; TVA = tricuspid valve anulus; VA = ventricular arrhythmia.

* Based on 10 to 50 values per patient.

nonvascular tissues other than the heart and aorta in at least 10 of the 18 patients. The mode or course of death was as follows: six patients died of chronic renal failure; three during or shortly after operations to excise parathyroid adenomas; two (Cases 2 and 10) of ventricular tachycardia and one (Case 6), of ventricular asystole; two of infection and one each of hypercalcemic crisis, metastatic osteogenic sarcoma, complications of porphyria and shortly after partial gastrectomy for peptic ulcer disease.

RESULTS

Examination of the hearts at necropsy allowed separation of the 18 patients into two distinct groups on the basis of the presence (Group I) (**Figures 4** through **12**) or absence (Group II) (**Figure 13**) of cardiac valvular calcific deposits. All 10 patients in Group I had cardiac deposits in the mitral anulus, and they ranged from massive (4+) to mild (1+) in extent (Figures 4 through 7 and 9 through 11). Calcific deposits involving >75 percent of the anulus beneath the posterior mitral leaflet were classified as 4+; those involving 51 to 75 percent, 3+; 26 to 50 percent, 2+; and 25 percent or less, 1+ [1]. The mitral anular calcific deposits were graded 4+ in five patients, 3+ in two patients, 2+ in two patients and 1+ in one patient. Of the 10 patients with mitral anular calcific deposits, two had similar but less extensive calcific deposits also in the tricuspid valve anular region (Figures 4, 5 and 6) and on the arterial aspects of the pulmonic and aortic valve cusps (Figure 4), and one also had aortic valve calcific deposits without

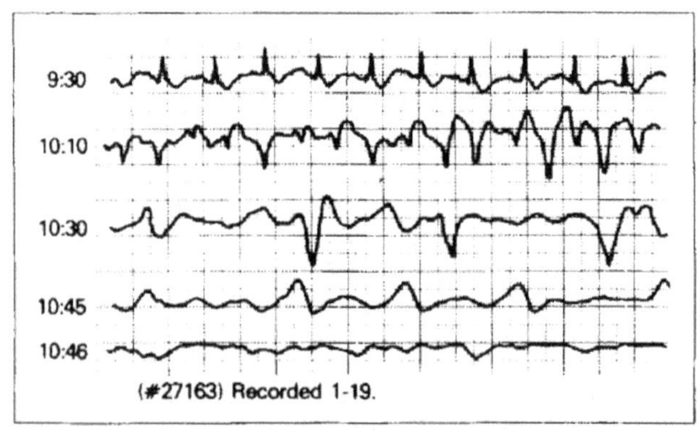

Figure 1. *Case 2 (GT 63A-40). Strips of electrocardiogram recorded during the final 76 minutes of life in a 39 year old woman with hypercalcemia from primary hyperparathyroidism.*

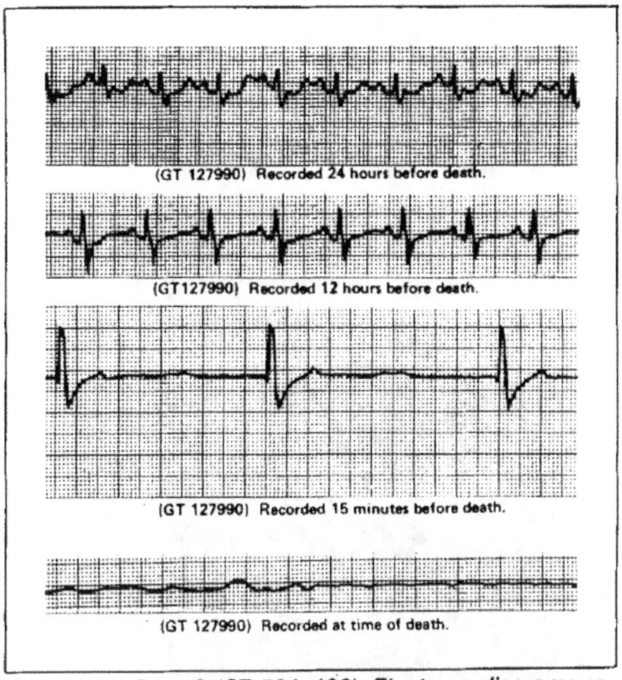

Figure 2. *Case 9 (GT 79A-102). Electrocardiograms recorded 24 hours (upper), 12 hours (upper middle), and 15 minutes before (lower middle) and at time of death (lower).*

TABLE III Electrocardiographic Abnormalities in Chronic Hypercalcemia (In 15 of 16 Patients)

Electrocardiographic Abnormality	Patients (No.)	Group I (8 of 8)	Group II (7 of 8)
T waves flattened	11	3	8
Q-T intervals shortened	10	4	6
Left ventricular hypertrophy	10	4	6
Arrhythmias			
Atrial premature beats	5	3	2
Ventricular premature beats	5	5	0
Ventricular tachycardia	2	2	0
P-R intervals >0.20 sec	3	1	2
Complete heart block	1	1	0
Q wave abnormalities*	1	1	0
	48	24	24

* Characteristic of healed myocardial infarct which was confirmed at autopsy (Case 10)

deposits in the tricuspid valve anulus or pulmonic valve cusps. All 10 patients with mitral anular calcium also had calcific deposits in the coronary arteries: in intimal plaques only in six patients and in both media ("medial calcinosis") and intima in four patients (Figures 7, 9, 11 and 12). In four of the 10 patients with intimal coronary arterial calcific deposits (as part of atherosclerotic plaques), the lumens of two or three of the four major (right, left, main, left anterior descending and left circumflex) coronary arteries were narrowed from 76 to 100 percent in cross-sectional area.

In each of the four patients with 76 to 100 percent cross-sectional area narrowing of the lumen of a major coronary artery and in three additional patients (Cases 1, 11 and 14, Table I), a histologic section of each 5 mm segment of each of the four major coronary arteries was prepared and examined, and the amount of narrowing for each segment was determined for four categories of narrowing (**Table V** and **Figure 14**). In the four patients with severe (>75 percent in cross-sectional area) narrowing of one or more of the four major arteries, 65 (29 percent) of the 224 five millimeter segments of coronary artery were narrowed from 76 to 100 percent in cross-sectional area by atherosclerotic plaque and 74 segments (33 percent) were narrowed 51 to 75 percent; thus, 62 percent of the segments were narrowed >50 percent in cross-sectional area. No 5 mm segment was narrowed >95 percent in cross-sectional area. In the three patients without significant coronary narrowing but with chronic hypercalcemia, none of the 142 five millimeter coronary segments were narrowed 76 to 100 percent in cross-sectional area and only 20 (14 percent) segments were narrowed 51 to 75 percent.

For comparison to the patients with chronic hypercalcemia, 24 necropsy patients (aged 19 to 59 years [mean 39 years]; 11 women, 13 men) were chosen as control subjects and examined in similar fashion. None had evidence of cardiac dysfunction or myocardial ischemia during life; at necropsy, all had normal-sized hearts (range 180 to 380 g [mean 253 g]), and grossly normal myocardial valves and pericardium. All 24 died

TABLE IV Chronic Hypercalcemia and Ventricular Arrhythmias (Five of 16 Necropsy Patients)

Case No.	Age (yr) and Sex	VPB	VT	APB	No. CAs >75 percent	LV F	LV C	V C
1	35, M	+	0	0	0	0	+	+
2	39, F	+	+	0	0	0	+	+
6	45, M	+	0	+	3	0	+	+
8	52, F	+	0	+	0	0	+	+
10	58, F	+	+	0	3	+	+	+

NOTE: C = dystrophic calcium; CA = coronary artery; F = transmural LV fibrosis; LV = left ventricular; V = cardiac valvular; VPB = ventricular premature beats; VT = ventricular tachycardia.

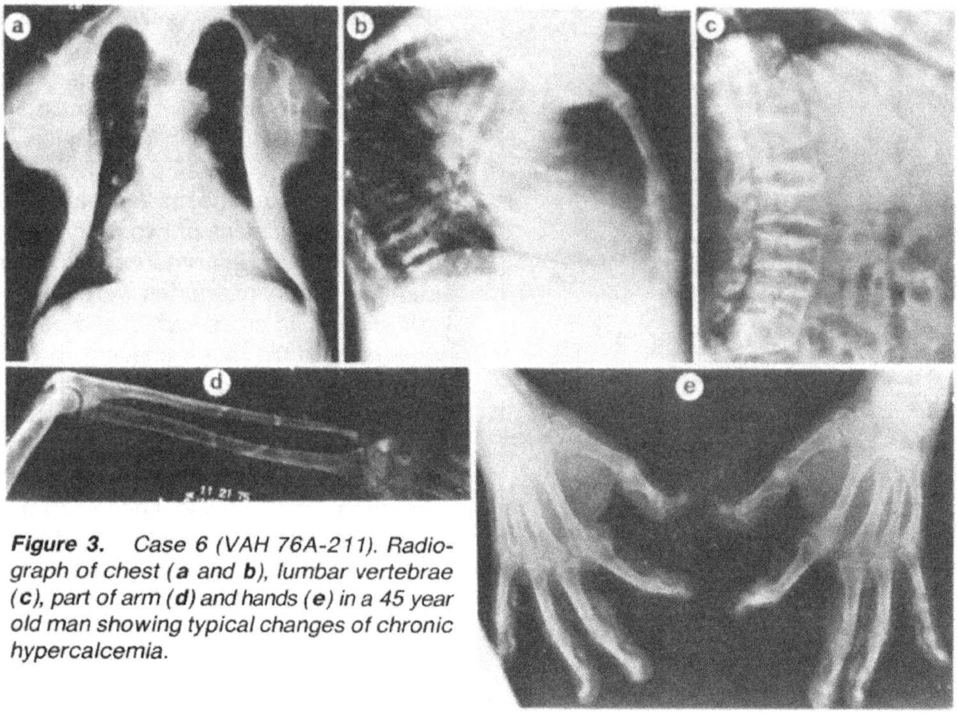

Figure 3. *Case 6 (VAH 76A-211). Radiograph of chest (**a** and **b**), lumbar vertebrae (**c**), part of arm (**d**) and hands (**e**) in a 45 year old man showing typical changes of chronic hypercalcemia.*

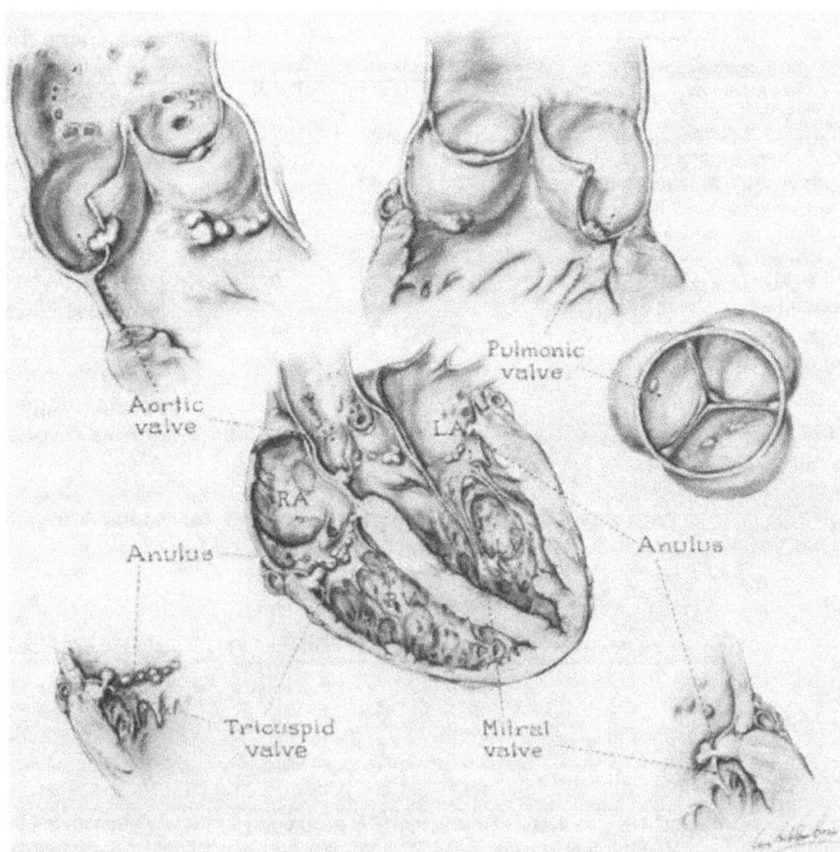

Figure 4. ***Case 3 (H-A-79-73). Drawing of heart showing distribution of calcific deposits in the tricuspid and mitral valve anuli and at the bases of both pulmonic and aortic valve cusps in a 43 year old woman with hypercalcemia secondary to primary hyperparathyroidism.***

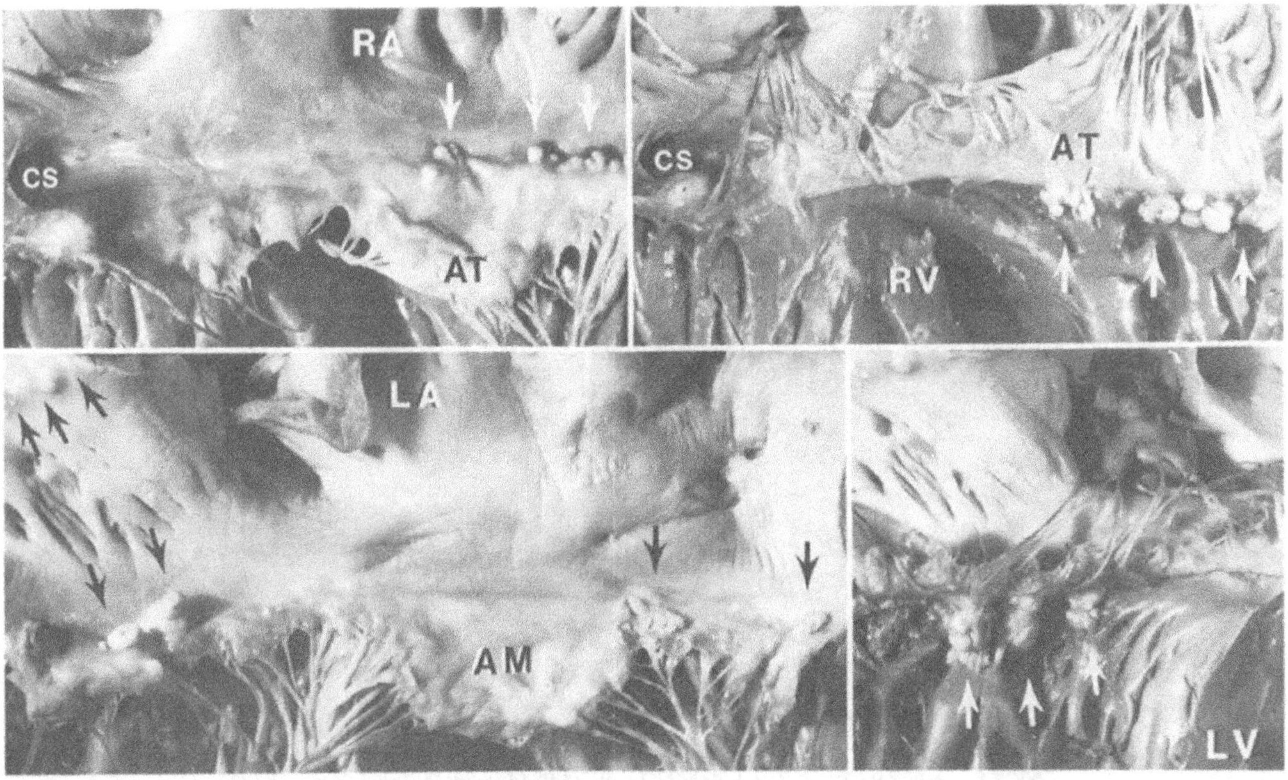

Figure 5. *Case 3 (H-A79-73). Views of the atrioventricular valves in a 43 year old woman with primary hyperparathyroidism.* ***Upper left,*** *opened right atrium (RA) and tricuspid valve. Calcific deposits (arrows) are present on the atrial aspect of the basal attachment of the anterior tricuspid (AT) leaflet. CS = ostium of coronary sinus.* ***Upper right,*** *calcific deposits on the undersurface of the anterior tricuspid leaflet (tricuspid-valve anulus). RV = right ventricle.* ***Lower left,*** *opened left atrium (LA) and mitral valve showing calcific deposits on the mitral valve primarily at its site of attachment and also in the mural endocardium (arrows), AM = anterior mitral leaflet.* ***Lower right,*** *the chordae tendineae have been detached and pulled toward left atrium exposing calcific deposits in the mitral anular region. LV = left ventricle.*

of cancer. Of the 22 in whom the values were known, the serum calcium levels were normal, ranging from 8.0 to 10.4 mg/dl (mean 4.5 mg/dl); of the 22 in whom the value was known, the total serum cholesterol levels ranged from 86 to 208 mg/dl (mean 166 mg/dl) (the value was >180 mg/dl in eight patients). None had calcific deposits in the mitral or tricupsid valve anuli or in the aortic or pulmonic valve cusps. Only one, and that on histologic study only, had calcific deposits in any of the 5 mm segments of the four major coronary arteries and they were in intimal atherosclerotic plaques. Of the 1,027 five millimeter segments of the four major epicardial coronary arteries examined in the 24 control subjects, the lumens of only two 5 mm segments were narrowed 76 to 100 percent in cross-sectional area, and only 53 (5 percent) were narrowed 51 to 75 percent in cross-sectional area by atherosclerotic plaques (Table V).

In addition to the calcific deposits in the intimal (atherosclerotic) plaques of the epicardial coronary arteries (in eight of the 10 patients in Group I), four patients in Group I also had calcific deposits in the media of these arteries (Tables I and II). In each, however, the medial calcific deposits were focal and involved relatively short portions of the total lengths of the major epicardial coronary arteries. Calcific deposits also were observed within individual myocardial fibers (dystrophic calcification) in seven of the 10 patients in Group I. (From three to 13 histologic sections [mean = 7] extending from endocardium to epicardium were examined in each of the 18 patients, including one to eight sections [mean = four] of left ventricular free wall and/or ventricular septum.) Transmural left ventricular scars were present in three of the ten patients in Group I: two of them had narrowing of two or more of the four major coronary arteries >75 percent in cross-sectional area by atherosclerotic plaques, and the third had less coronary arterial narrowing.

None of the eight patients in Group II had calcific deposits in the mitral anulus or in any of the other three cardiac valves or their valvular rings (Tables I and II). Small intimal calcific deposits were present in the walls of one or more epicardial coronary arteries in one patient in Group II and one other patient had calcific deposits in the media (medial calcinosis) (Tables I and II). No patients in Group II had narrowing of any of the four

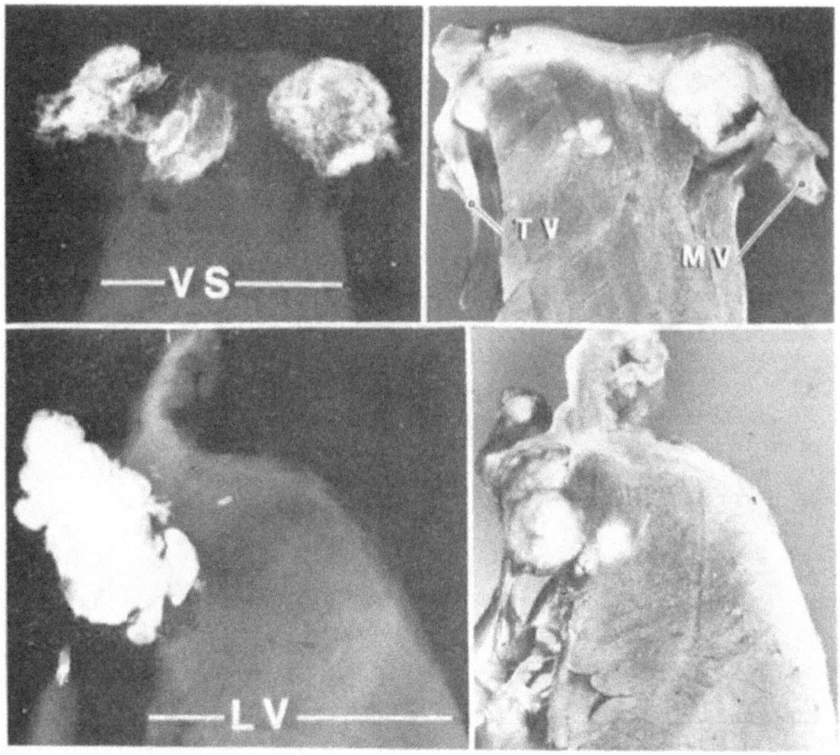

Figure 6. *Case 3 (H-A79-73). Longitudinal sections of basal portions of ventricular septum (VS) (upper) and of left ventricular (LV) free wall (lower) showing calcium in both the tricuspid (TV) and mitral valve (MV) anuli.* ***Left,*** *radiographs.* ***Right,*** *gross photographs of specimen.*

major epicardial coronary arteries >75 percent in cross-sectional area, and examination of each 5 mm long segment of coronary artery in three patients in this group (Group II) disclosed that the lumens in none of the segments were narrowed >50 percent in cross-sectional area (Table V). Calcific deposits were not found in histologic sections of myocardium in any of the eight patients in Group II.

COMMENTS

Analysis of the 18 necropsy patients described herein with chronic hypercalcemia clearly demonstrates an increased frequency of cardiac calcific deposits including an accelerated amount (compared to controls) of coronary arterial atherosclerosis. Of the 18 patients, calcific deposits were present in the mitral valve anuli

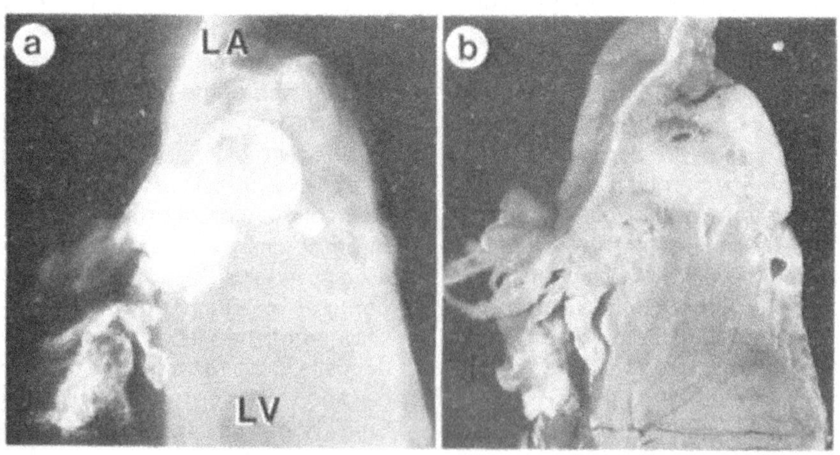

Figure 7. *Case 4 (H-A75-12). Longitudinal section of wall of left atrium (LA) and left ventricle (LV) showing heavy calcific deposits in the mitral anular region and also some deposits in the adjacent coronary artery.* ***a,*** *radiograph.* ***b,*** *gross photograph of same area.*

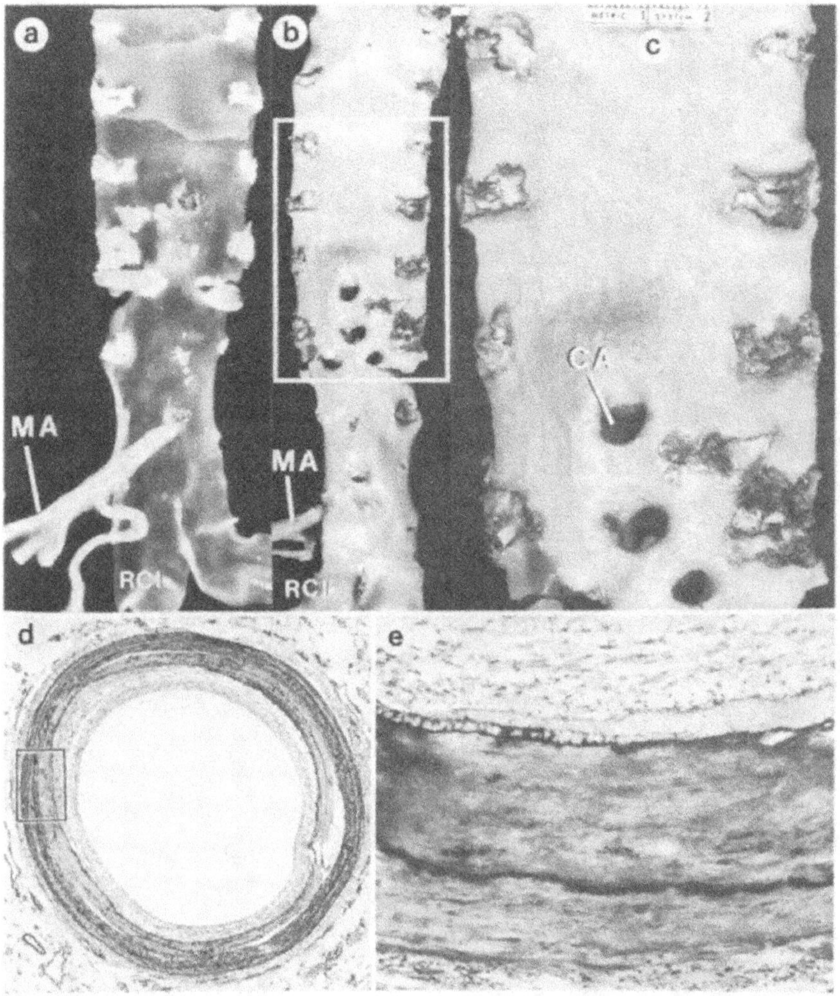

Figure 8. *Case 6 (VAH 76A-211). Abdominal aorta (a,b,c) and photomicrograph of cross-section of mesenteric artery (d and e).* ***a,*** *radiograph of opened aorta showing heavy calcific deposits about each ostium of an intercostal artery and ring-like calcium typical of Monckeberg's medial calcinosis in the mesenteric artery (MA) and its branches. RCI = right common iliac artery.* ***b,*** *opened aorta.* ***c,*** *close-up in area in brackets in b. CA = Celiac axis.* ***d,*** *ring-like calcium in media and* ***e,*** *close-up of area in brackets of d typical of Monckeberg's medial calcinosis. Movat stains, magnification × 28 (b) and × 180 (c).*

in 10, two of whom also had calcific deposits in the tricuspid valve anuli and in both pulmonic and aortic valve cusps. All 10 patients with mitral anular calcific deposits also had calcific deposits in the coronary arteries: in atherosclerotic plaques (intima) in all 10 and in the media ("medial calcinosis") as well in four.

Mitral anular calcific deposits are frequent [1,2], as is well known, in elderly patients residing in the Western World, but they are decidedly infrequent in all areas of the world in persons under 65 years of age (except in patients with connective tissue abnormalities such as the Marfan syndrome [3] and the Hurler syndrome [4]). Our 10 patients with mitral anular calcific deposits, however, were relatively young (mean age 46 years: range 35 to 58 years), and none had either the Marfan or Hurler syndrome.

The occurrence of calcific deposits in the tricuspid-valve anulus, of course, is rare, but two of our 18 patients had such deposits. Of the few patients described with tricuspid-anular calcific deposits, all have had severely increased right ventricular systolic pressure and right ventricular hypertrophy [1]. The latter was absent, and the pulmonic second sound was not described as being of increased intensity in either of our two patients with tricuspid valve anular deposits.

Calcific deposits on the aortic aspects of the aortic-valve cusps also are commonly observed in elderly patients in the Western World, most frequently in as-

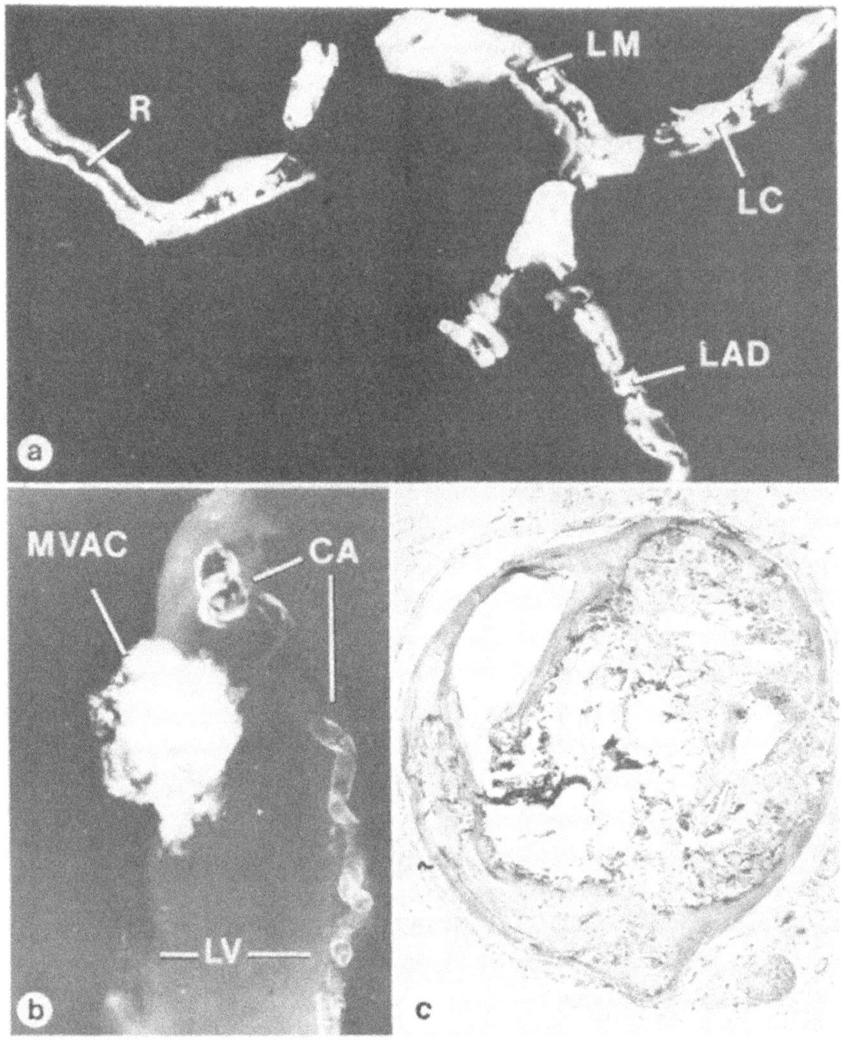

Figure 9. *Case 6 (VAH 76A-211). Major epicardial coronary arteries.* ***a,*** *Radiograph show heavy nonring like calcific deposits in the right (R), left main (LM), left anterior descending (LAD) and left circumflex (LC) coronary arteries of this 45 year old man with hypercalcemia secondary to chronic renal disease.* ***b,*** *radiograph of a longitudinal section of left ventricular (LV) free wall showing heavy mitral valve anular calcium and Monckeberg's ring-like medial calcinosis of one coronary artery (CA).* ***c,*** *photomicrograph of the right coronary artery showing massive intimal, i.e., atherosclerotic, calcific deposits. Movat stain, magnification × 20 (c).*

sociation with mitral anular calcific deposits [5]. Three of our patients, all of whom had much larger mitral anular calcific deposits, had calcific deposits on the aortic-valve cusps without aortic-valve stenosis but each was relatively young (43, 45 and 47 years, respectively).

An extremely rare site of calcific deposits is the pulmonic valve and all patients described with calcific deposits at this site have had pulmonic valve stenosis [6]. Two of our patients had calcific deposits on the arterial aspects of each pulmonic valve cusp, but neither had anatomic nor clinical evidence of pulmonic valve stenosis.

Although calcific deposits in coronary atherosclerotic plaques are common in persons with coronary atherosclerosis, particularly elderly patients and those with diabetes mellitus [7], calcific deposits in the media of one or more epicardial coronary arteries have been reported, to our knowledge, in only one adult patient [8]. Of our 18 patients with chronic hypercalcemia, however, five had medial calcinosis, four of whom also had calcific deposits in superimposed atherosclerotic plaques. Medial calcinosis has been observed frequently, however, in peripheral arteries in hypercalcemic patients [9].

Calcific deposits within individual myocardial fibers

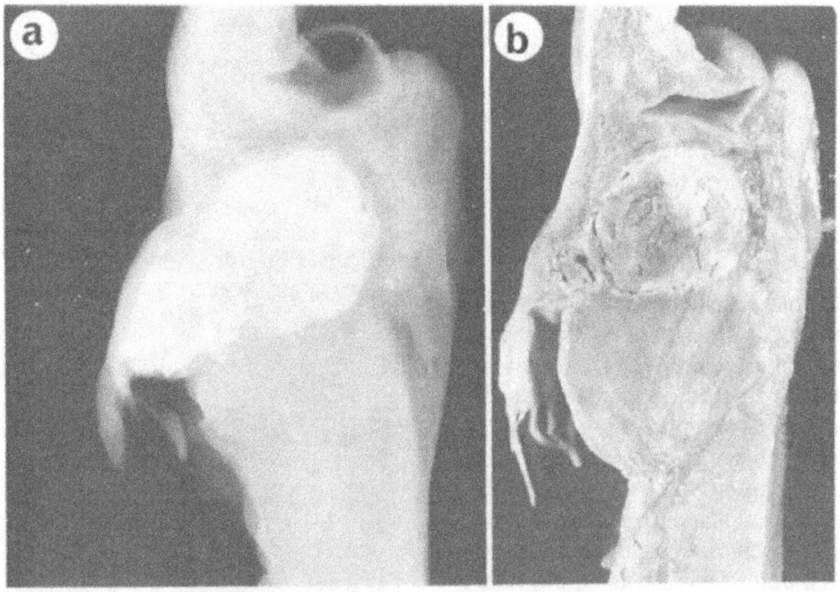

Figure 10. *Case 7 (GW A78-10). Mitral-valve anular calcium in a 47 year old woman with hypercalcemia secondary to renal disease.* ***a,*** *radiograph of longitudinal section of walls of left atrium (LA) and left ventricle (LV) with "massive" calcium beneath the posterior mitral leaflet (PML) with extension into the left ventricular free wall. CS = coronary sinus.* ***b,*** *gross photograph of same area.*

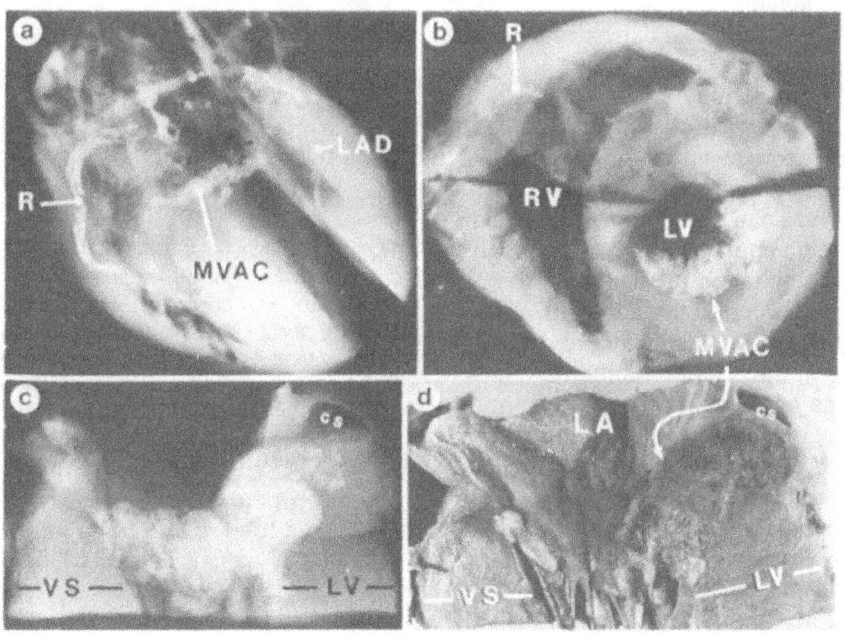

Figure 11. *Case 9 (GT 79A-102). Large calcific deposits in the coronary arteries and mitral anular area in this 55 year old woman with hypercalcemia secondary to chronic renal disease.* ***a,*** *radiograph of heart showing calcium in the right (R) and left anterior descending (LAD) coronary arteries and mitral valve anular area (MVAC).* ***b,*** *radiograph of basal portion of heart better demonstrating the mitral valve anular calcium (MVAC). RV and LV = right and left (LV) ventricular cavities.* ***c,*** *another radiograph of calcium in the mitral anulus from longitudinal view. VS = ventricular septum; CS = coronary sinus.* ***d,*** *gross specimen from which radiograph in c was taken. LA = left atrium.*

(*dystrophic calcification*) [10–12] is observed fairly frequently in patients with chronic renal failure [13–17], hypervitaminosis D [18–24], and in those with prolonged low cardiac output syndromes following cardiac operations [25,26]. Its cause in these latter circumstances is probably related to "global" left ventricular ischemia, because dystrophic myocardial fiber calcification can be produced experimentally by cross-clamping the ascending aorta for prolonged periods [26]. Dystrophic myocardial calcification was observed histologically in seven of our 18 patients with chronic hypercalcemia, all seven of whom had associated cardiac valvular or anular calcific deposits. Because none had clinical evidence of prolonged periods of inadequate cardiac output, this mechanism cannot be implicated in any of these seven patients.

In addition to the cardiac calcific deposits in 12 of our 18 patients, in at least 11 calcific deposits were observed in one or more blood vessels outside the heart and and in one or more other body organs, including kidney, lung and stomach. Thus, the cardiac calcific deposits in our patients were simply part of a systemic calcific process. The renal, pulmonary and gastric calcific deposits were microscopic, however, rather than macroscopic in size, as is usually the case with calcific deposition in previously normal tissues or organs (metastatic calcification).

The cardiac calcific deposits when extensive enough may have functional consequence. The coronary luminal narrowing, of course, may cause myocardial ischemia. One of our patients (Case 10) had clinical evidence of acute myocardial infarction and angina pectoris, and two others had transmural left ventricular scars without clinical evidence of myocardial ischemia. The mitral anular calcific deposits, if severe enough, may produce mitral regurgitation [1] and, on rare occasion, mitral stenosis [27], and the aortic valve deposits, if large enough, can lead to aortic valve stenosis [5]. Calcific deposits in the area of the membranous ventricular septum, as occurred in our Case 1, may extend into the most cephalad portion of muscular ventricular septum and cause varying degrees of heart block [14,28]. Furthermore, the microscopic-sized calcific deposits in alveolar septums can produce restrictive and diffusion ventilatory defects [29,30].

Although its exact mechanism is unclear, chronic hypercalcemia is clearly the common link in our 18 patients; it is, therefore, reasonable to believe that it played the major role in causing the unusual and often extensive cardiovascular calcific deposits [31]. It is also reasonable to believe that the cause of the vascular and nonvascular calcific deposits in our patients was the same.

Although surely playing a major role in producing the vascular cardiac calcific deposits in our patients, chronic hypercalcemia is clearly not the only factor because a third of our 18 patients had no vascular or nonvascular calcific deposits. Comparison of a number of factors between the 10 patients with cardiac valvular and extensive coronary calcific deposits (Group I) and the eight patients without cardiac valvular deposits (two of whom had minimal coronary calcific deposits) (Group II) disclosed no significant differences in ages at death (46 versus 43 years), duration of chronic hypercalcemia (5.9 versus 3.6 years), frequency of systemic hypertension (eight of 10 versus six of eight), cause of the hypercalcemia, or the mean values of the peak serum calcium levels, but significant differences in the mean

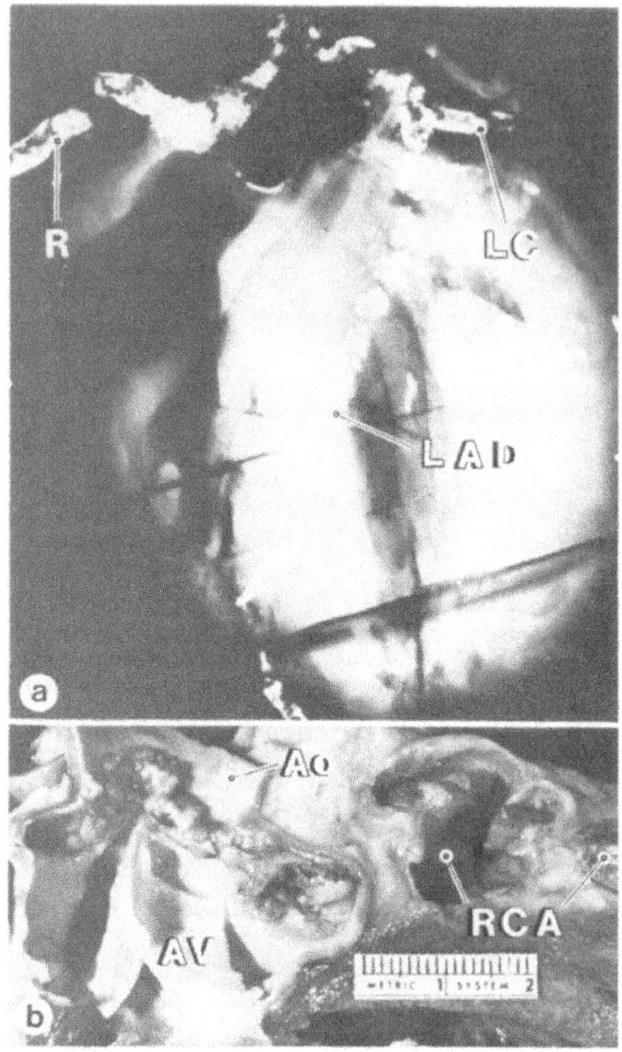

Figure 12. *Case 10 (VAH 77A-190).* ***a,*** *massive calcific deposits in the right (R) left anterior descending (LAD) and left circumflex (LC) coronary arteries and* ***b,*** *in the wall of ascending aorta (Ao) just above the aortic valve (AV) in a 58 year old man with hypercalcemia secondary to chronic renal disease. Portions of the heavily calcified right coronary artery (RCA) are aneurysmally dilated as is shown in b.*

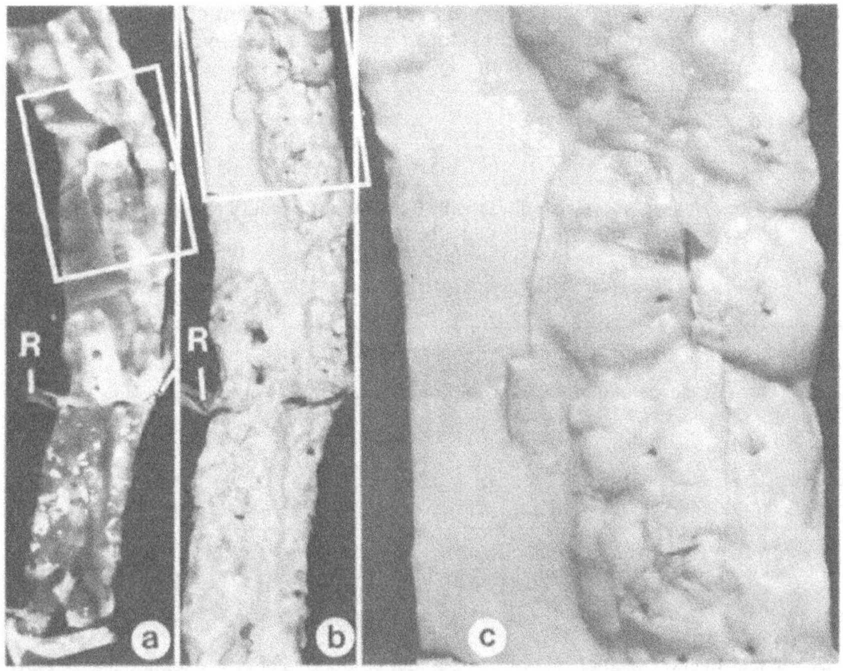

Figure 13. *Case 14 (A79-98). Opened aorta in a 37 year old woman with hypercalcemia secondary to primary hyperparathyroidism.* ***a,*** *radiograph showing calcific deposits in the abdominal portion. R = renal arteries.* ***b,*** *gross photograph of aorta.* ***c,*** *close-up of portion shown in brackets in a and b disclosing large elevated atherosclerotic plaques.*

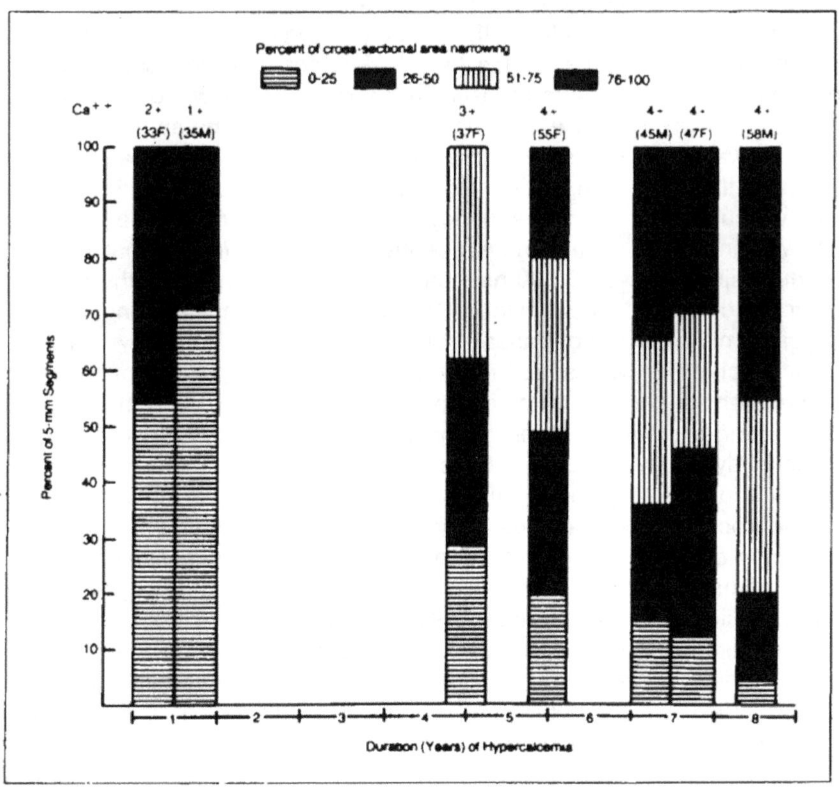

Figure 14. *Bar graphs from seven patients showing relations of duration of hypercalcemia to amount of coronary narrowing in cross-sectional area by atherosclerotic plaques and to amount of calcific deposits in the coronary arteries. The amount of narrowing of the 5 mm segments of the major epicardial coronary arteries (right, left main, left anterior descending, left circumflex) increased as the duration of the hypercalcemia increased. In the 58 year old man who had hypercalcemia for eight years, 45 percent of the 5 mm coronary segments were narrowed from 76 to 100 percent in cross-sectional area, whereas in the 33 year old woman who had known hypercalcemia for only one year, none of the 5 mm coronary segments were narrowed more than 50 percent in cross-sectional area.*

TABLE V **Amount of Cross-sectional Area Narrowing in Each 5 mm Segment of the Right, Left Main, Left Anterior Descending and Left Circumflex Epicardial Coronary Arteries in Seven Patients with Chronic Hypercalcemia and in 17 Control Subjects**

Case No.	Age (yr)	Duration of H (yr)	No. of 5 mm CA Segments Narrowed to Various Degrees 0–25	26–50	51–75	76–100	No. 5 mm CA Segments Examined	Total Coronary Score*	Mean Coronary Score†	Mean % XSA Narrowing Per 5 mm Segment
Four Hypercalcemic Patients with Significant Coronary Narrowing										
6	45	7.0	9(15)	13(21)	18(30)	21(34)	61	173	2.8	61
7	47	7.0	7(13)	17(33)	18(35)	10(19)	52	135	2.6	55
9	55	5.5	12(20)	16(27)	21(35)	11(18)	60	151	2.5	52
10	58	8.0	2(4)	9(18)	17(33)	23(45)	51	164	3.2	71
M or S	51	6.9	30(13)	55(25)	74(33)	65(29)	224	623	2.8	60
Three Hypercalcemic Patients without Significant Coronary Narrowing										
1	35	4.5	15(28)	20(36)	20(36)	0	55	115	2.1	40
11	33	1.0	19(54)	16(46)	0	0	35	51	1.5	22
14	37	1.0	37(71)	15(29)	0	0	52	67	1.3	18
M or S	35	2.2	71(17)	51(36)	20(14)	0	142	233	1.6	27
24 Nonhypercalcemic Controls with Fatal Cancer										
M or S	43	0	791(77)	181(18)	53(5)	2(<1)	1027	1320	1.3	18

NOTE: Figures in parentheses are percents. CA = coronary artery; H = chronic hypercalcemia; M = mean; S = subtotal; XSA = cross-sectional area.

* Sum derived by assigning a number to each segment in each of the four categories of cross-sectional area narrowing as follows: 1 = 0 to 25 percent narrowing; 2 = 26 to 50 percent; 3 = 51 to 75 percent and 4 = 76 to 100 percent.

† Number derived by dividing the total number of 5 mm coronary segments per patient into the total score.

total serum cholesterol levels (216 versus 163 mg/dl [$p < 0.01$]) and the mean *weights of the heart* (426 versus 320 g [$p < 0.05$]). The differences in the mean cholesterol levels, of course, support the thesis that elevation of these levels not only may lead to atherosclerosis but also that its elevation may play a large role in causing calcific deposits in other portions of the heart, particularly the mitral anular region and the aortic valve cusps.

Irrespective of the precise mechanism of the vascular calcific deposits in our patients, it is clear that chronic hypercalcemia is detrimental to the vascular system and that its effect, at least in adults, is worsened by the presence of hypercholesterolemia and possibly also by the presence of systemic hypertension. Additional support, of course, for the role of hypercalcemia, at least in causing vascular and nonvascular calcific deposits, comes from studies of chronic hypervitaminosis D [18–24] in infancy and childhood, and more recently from its association with the congenital syndrome of peculiar elfin faces, mental retardation and supravalvular aortic stenosis [32]. Many necropsy studies, both in human subjects and in nonhuman experimental animals, of patients with hypervitaminosis D have described metastatic and dystrophic calcific deposits in many body organs including the heart, lung, kidney, stomach and walls of blood vessels. The cardiac deposits were located primarily in the media of small coronary arteries (medial calcinosis) and in individual myocardial fibers (dystrophic myocardial calcification). Grossly visible calcific deposits in coronary arteries or valvular cusps or anuli have not been reported previously, to our knowledge, and neither has increased or accelerated coronary atherosclerosis been reported previously in patients with chronic hypercalcemia.

Additionally, this study suggests that chronic hypercalcemia may be a "risk factor" to premature coronary atherosclerosis. Furthermore, although not systematically examined in our 18 patients, the amount of atherosclerotic plaquing present in the aorta was greater than that expected for the age of our patients.

The frequency of chronic hypercalcemia is quite significant. It recently has been estimated that 35,000 to 86,000 new cases of primary hyperparathyroidism appear in the USA yearly [33] and the prolongation of life of patients with chronic renal disease by hemodialysis has yielded an even larger population of patients with chronic hypercalcemia. Comparison of patients with chronic renal disease treated by hemodialysis to those not so treated has demonstrated a higher frequency of metastatic and dystrophic calcification in the group undergoing dialysis [16,17]. Of our 10 patients with valvular or anular calcific deposits, five had long-term hemodialysis varying from three to eight years, and these five patients had the largest and most extensive cardiac calcific deposits. In 1977, Kuzela and associates [17] compared the frequency of metastatic and dystrophic calcification in 56 dialyzed (>6 months) to 18 nondialyzed necropsy patients with fatal chronic renal disease. Although calcific deposits in the kidney, groups, the calcific deposits were clearly larger and involved more body organs in the patients undergoing long-term dialysis than those not dialyzed. Contiguglia and associates [34] demonstrated that the cardiac ease have a calcium:magnesium:phosphorus molar ratio of 5:1:5 and an x-ray diffraction pattern resembling whitlockite, an amorphous microcrystalline compound.

REFERENCES

1. Roberts WC, Perloff JK: Mitral valvular disease. A clinicopathologic survey of the conditions causing the mitral valve to function abnormally. Ann Intern Med 77: 939, 1972.
2. McCarthy JH, Palmer FJ: Incidence and significance of coronary artery calcification. Br Heart J 1974; 36: 499.
3. Roberts WC:Congenital cardiovascular abnormalities usually "silent" until adulthood: morphologic features of the floppy mitral valve, valvular aortic stenosis, hypertrophic cardiomyopathy, sinus of Valsalva aneurysm, and the Marfan syndrome. In: Roberts WC, ed. Congenital heart disease in adults. Philadelphia: F.A. Davis, Co. 1979; 407.
4. Renteria VG, Ferrans VJ, Roberts WC: The heart in the Hurler syndrome. Gross, histologic and ultrastructural observations in five necropsy cases. Am J Cardiol 1976; 38: 487.
5. Roberts WC, Perloff JK, Costantino T: Severe valvular aortic stenosis in patients over 65 years of age. A clinicopathologic study. Am J Cardiol 1971; 27: 497.
6. Roberts WC, Mason DT, Morrow AG, Braunwald E: Calcific pulmonic stenosis. Circulation 1968; 37: 973.
7. Waller BF, Palumbo PJ, Lie JT, Roberts WC: Status of the coronary arteries at necropsy in diabetes mellitus with onset after age 30 years. Analysis of 229 diabetic patients with and without clinical evidence of coronary heart disease and comparison to 183 control subjects. Am J Med 1980; 69: 498.
8. Lachman AS, Spray TI, Kerwin DM, Shugoll GI, Roberts WC: Medial calcinosis of Monckeberg. A review of the problem and a description of a patient with involvement of peripheral, visceral and coronary arteries. Am J Med 1977; 63: 615.
9. Amos RS, Wright V: Monckeberg's arteriosclerosis and metabolic bone disease. Lancet 1980; 2: 248.
10. Gore I, Arons W: Calcification of the myocardium. A pathologic study of thirteen cases. Arch Pathol 1949; 48: 1.
11. Mulligan RM: Metastatic calcification. Arch Path 1947; 43: 177.
12. Fierer JA, Wagner BM, Strebel RF: Metastatic calcification of the myocardium. Am J Cardiol 1970; 26: 423.
13. Herbert FK, Miller HG, Richardson GO: Chronic renal disease, secondary parathyroid hyperplasia, decalcification of bone and metastatic calcification. J Path Bact 1941; 53: 161.
14. Terman DS, Alfrey AC, Hammond WS, et al.: Cardiac calcification in uremia. A clinical, biochemical and pathologic study. Am J Med 1971; 50: 744.
15. Parfitt AM, Massry SG, Winfield AC, DePalma JR, Gordon A: Disordered calcium and phosphorus metabolism during maintenance hemodialysis. Correlation of clinical, roentgenographic and biochemical changes. Am J Med 1971; 51: 319.
16. Meema HE, Oreopoulos DG, deVeber GA: Arterial calcifications in severe chronic renal disease and their relationship to dialysis treatment, renal transplant, and parathyroidectomy. Radiology 1976; 121: 315.
17. Kuzela DC, Huffer WE, Conger JD, Winter SD, Hammond WS: Soft tissue calcification in chronic dialysis patients. Am J Pathol 1977; 86: 403.
18. Vanderveer HL: Hypervitaminosis D and arteriosclerosis. Arch Pathol 1931; 12: 941.
19. Bauer JM, Freyberg RH: Vitamin D intoxication with metastatic calcification. JAMA 1946; 130: 1208.
20. Christensen WR, Liebman C, Sosman MC: Skeletal and periarticular manifestations of hypervitaminosis D. Am J Roentgen 1951; 65: 27.
21. Gillman J, Gilbert C: Calcium, phosphorus and vitamin D as factors regulating integrity of cardiovascular system. Exp Med Surg 1956; 14: 136.
22. Hass GM, Trueheart RE, Taylor CG, Stumpe M: An experimental histologic study of hypervitaminosis D. Am J Pathol 1958; 34: 395.
23. Eisenstein R, Zeruolis L: Vitamin D-induced aortic calcification. An electron microscopic study. Arch Pathol 1964; 77: 27.
24. Friedman WF, Roberts WC: Vitamin D and the supravalvular aortic stenosis syndrome. The transplacental effects of vitamin D on the aorta of the rabbit. Circulation 1966; 34: 77.
25. Roberts WC, Morrow AG: Causes of early postoperative death following cardiac valve replacement. Clinico-pathologic correlations in 64 patients studied at necropsy. J Thorac Cardiovasc Surg 1967; 54: 422.
26. Buja LM, Levitsky S, Ferrans VJ, Souther SG, Roberts WC, Morrow AG: Acute and chronic effects of normothermic anoxia on canine hearts. Light and electronmicroscopic evaluation. Circulation 43 & 44 (suppl): 1971; 144.
27. Hammer WJ, Roberts WC, de Leon AC Jr: "Mitral stenosis" secondary to combined "massive" mitral anular calcific deposits and small, hypertrophied left ventricles. Am J Med 1978; 64: 371.
28. Roberts WC, Wright LD, Morrow AG: Complete heart block and left bundle branch block in valvular heart disease (abstract). Am J Cardiol 1967; 19: 147.
29. Firooznia H, Pudlowski R, Golimbu C, Rafii M, McCauley D: Diffuse interstitial calcification of the lungs in chronic renal failure mimicking pulmonary edema. Am J Roentgen 1977; 129: 1103.
30. Justrabo E, Genin R, Rifle G: Pulmonary metastatic calcification with respiratory insufficiency in patients on maintenance hemodialysis. Thorax 1979; 34: 384.
31. Heuber WC: Metastatic calcification produced by injections of parathyroid extract. Arch Pathol 1927; 3: 14.
32. Garcia RE, Friedman WF, Kaback MM, Rowe RD: Idiopathic hypercalcemia and supravalvular aortic stenosis. Documentation of a new syndrome. N Engl J Med 1964; 271: 117.
33. Heath H III, Hodgson SF, Kennedy MA: Primary hyperparathyroidism. Incidence, morbidity, and potential economic impact in a community. N Engl J Med 1980; 302: 189.
34. Contiguglia SR, Alfrey AC, Miller NL, Runnells DE, LeGeros RZ: Nature of soft tissue calcification in uremia. Kidney Int 1973; 4: 229.

Left ventricular incision midway between the mitral anulus and the stumps of the papillary muscles during mitral valve excision with or without rupture or aneurysmal formation: Analysis of 10 necropsy patients

Certain clinical and morphologic observations are described in 10 patients who had mitral valve replacement (MVR) and *lacerations* of the left ventricular (LV) free wall midway between the anulus of the mitral valve and the stumps of the LV papillary muscles. In five patients the lacerations led to LV free wall *rupture*, with immediate hemopericardium in two and delayed (2 to 4 days) rupture in the other three. Of the other five patients, three developed *aneurysm* of the LV free wall, the mouth of which was located midway between mitral anulus and papillary muscle stumps, the sites of the lacerations observed in the other seven patients. The remaining two patients had midway lacerations which produced neither rupture nor aneurysmal formation. The midway LV lacerations are considered the result of LV incisions made at the time of mitral valve excision, generally in a setting where the left-sided cardiac chambers were only mildly dilated or normal and the tips of the blades of the scissors may have been inadequately visualized during mitral excision. This complication can be prevented by leaving the posterior mitral leaflet and its attached chordae intact or by applying exquisite care during the mitral excision procedure, or both. LV midway rupture may be the most common cause of death early after MVR and operatively induced LV lacerations may lead to LV aneurysm late postoperatively. (Am Heart J 104:1278, 1982.)

William C. Roberts, M.D., Jeffrey M. Isner, M.D., and Renu Virmani, M.D.
Bethesda, Md.

A well-recognized complication of mitral valve replacement (MVR) is left ventricular (LV) or left atrioventricular groove rupture or aneurysmal formation. The most frequently described sites of rupture or aneurysmal formation are the mitral anulus and the LV free wall at the level of the stumps of the papillary muscles.[1-14] The former generally results from inadvertent interruption of the anulus during excision of a heavily calcified mitral valve, or possibly from tearing during insertion of a prosthesis larger than the native mitral ring; and the latter, from excising the papillary muscles with underlying LV free wall because of too vigorous pulling of these structures towards the left atrium before excision. In recent years, a third site of LV rupture or aneurysmal formation after MVR has been described, and that is about midway between the mitral anulus and the stumps of the LV papillary muscles.[15-27] Although the cause of rupture or

From the Pathology Branch, National Heart, Lung and Blood Institute.
Received for publication June 29, 1982; accepted July 8, 1982.
Reprint requests: William C. Roberts, M.D., Pathology Branch, NHLBI-NIH, Bldg. 10A, Room 3E-30, Bethesda, MD 20205.

aneurysm at this site has been discussed, inadvertent incision of the LV wall during mitral valve excision has not been presented as its cause. In this report, certain clinical and morphologic observations are described in 10 necropsy patients who had MVR and lacerations or thinning of the LV free wall midway between the anulus and papillary muscle stumps.

METHODS AND RESULTS

Certain clinical and necropsy observations in the 10 patients are summarized in Table I and illustrated in Figs. 1 to 8. The hearts were submitted to the Pathology Branch, National Heart, Lung and Blood Institute, National Institutes of Health, from seven different medical centers. Lacerations (incisions) or sites of thinning were present in the LV free wall more or less parallel to the mitral anulus and located about midway between the anulus and the stumps of the papillary muscles. The lacerations or thinnings varied from 3.5 to 6 cm in transverse length and involved the posterior and lateral walls in all 10 patients and the anterior wall also in three. In all 10 patients, the two LV papillary muscles were either intact or else only the more apical portions of them had been excised (nine patients) or excised "flush" with the LV endocardium (one patient). No lacerations were present in the LV free wall in the immediate vicinity of either papillary muscle or the mitral anulus. The lacerations were sharp and linear in the five patients dying within 2 days of MVR. In the five patients surviving longer, the LV wall between papillary muscle and anulus was thinned and its interior lining was relatively smooth. Two patients (Nos. 1 and 2, Table I) had lacerations without either LV rupture or aneurysmal formation (Fig. 1). Five patients (Nos. 3 through 7) had through-and-through LV ruptures, two in the operating room at the time of MVR and the other three, 2, 3, and 4 days, respectively, after operation (Figs. 2 to 5). Three patients (Nos. 8 through 10) had LV aneurysms with the mouth of the aneurysm in the LV wall midway between papillary muscle and mitral anulus: one lived 10 days (Fig. 6); one, 3 months (Fig. 7), and one, over 7 years after MVR (Fig. 8).

The type substitute cardiac valve utilized in the 10 patients varied: porcine (Hancock) in five, caged-ball (Starr-Edwards) in four, and tilting disc (Björk-Shiley) in one. Preoperatively, the mitral valve was stenotic in eight patients and purely regurgitant in two. One (No. 3, Table I) of the latter had a prolapsing mitral valve associated with a secundum type atrial septal defect (Fig. 2) and the second (No. 7, Table I) had ruptured chordae tendineae from infective endocarditis involving both mitral and aortic valves (Figs. 4 and 5). Patient No. 7 was the only one having both aortic and mitral valves replaced. In nine patients the MVR was performed via a median sternotomy and an interatrial groove incision; in one (patient No. 3, Table I) the mitral valve was excised and replaced via a large atrial septal defect. Three patients (Nos. 1, 4, and 7) had significant (76% to 100% in cross-sectional area) narrowing by atherosclerotic plaques of one or more of the four major coronary arteries. The ages of the 10 patients ranged from 40 to 68 years (mean 56) and six were women.

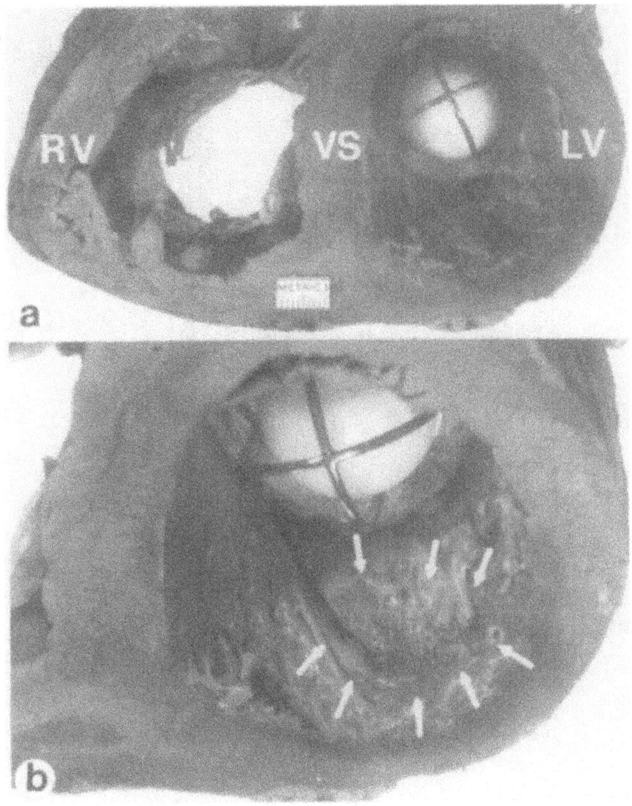

Fig. 1. Patient No. 1 (Table I). **a,** View of both right *(RV)* and left ventricles *(LV)* with Starr-Edwards valve in the mitral position. **b,** Close-up of laceration *(arrows)* in the posterior wall.

DISCUSSION

Summary of presently reported cases. Each of the above 10 patients had linear lacerations extending varying distances through the LV free wall and located more or less transversely about midway between the mitral anulus and the stumps of the LV papillary muscles. Each patient had had MVR with either a mechanical (caged ball or tilting disc) or bioprosthetic cardiac valve. In 5 patients ventricular rupture resulted, either in the operating room (two patients) or up to 4 days later, and 3 patients developed LV aneurysms, the mouths of which were located in the LV wall between the mitral anulus and the stumps of the papillary muscles.

Previously reported patients. Although many reports have described LV rupture or aneurysm formation after MVR, the rupture or aneurysmal

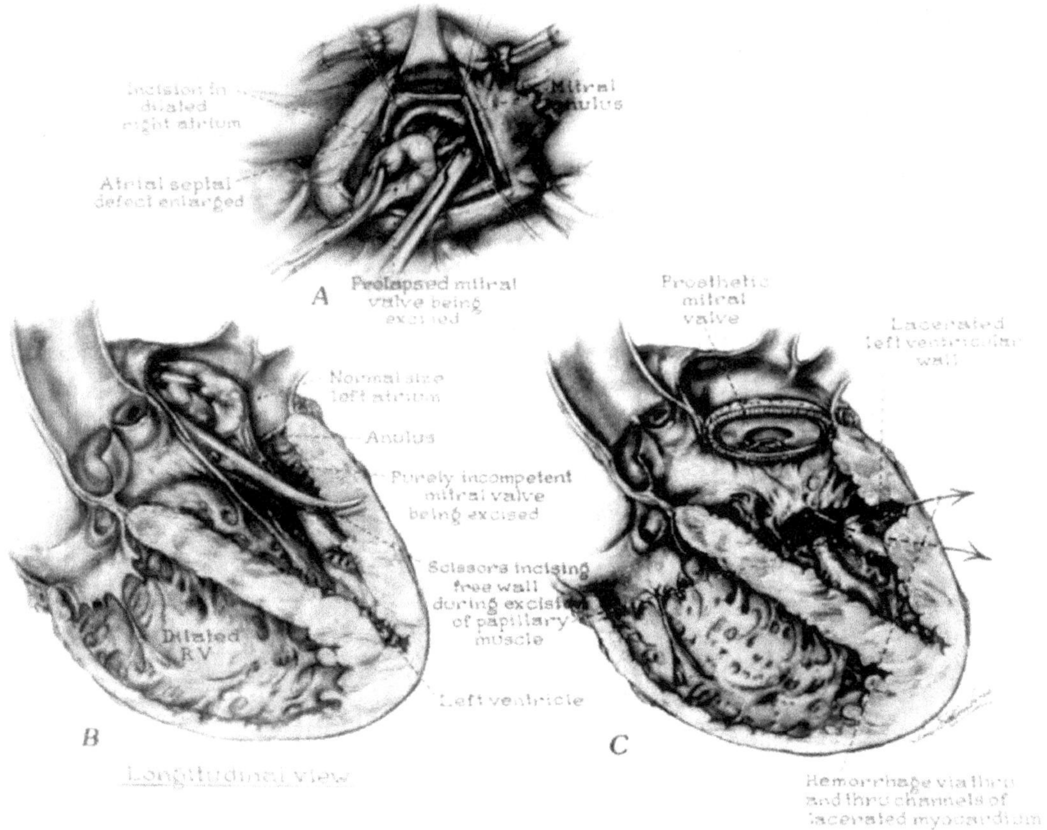

Fig. 2. Patient No. 3. Proposed mechanism of the LV laceration during mitral valve replacement. This patient had an atrial septal defect (ASD) and the mitral valve was excised and replaced via the ASD. Smeloff[5] also described a patient in whom the left ventricle ruptured during MVR via an ASD.

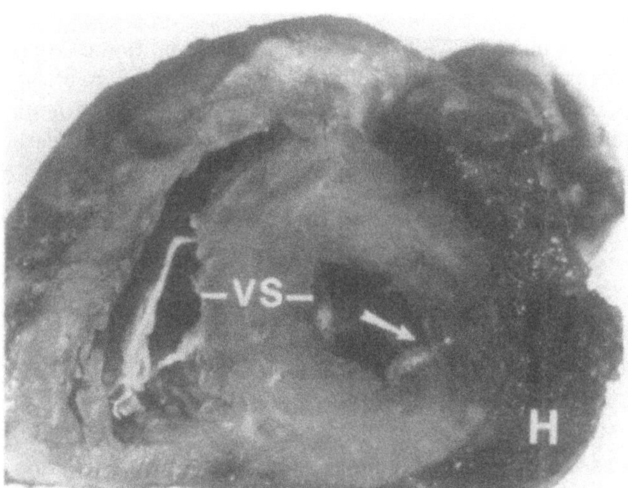

Fig. 3. Patient No. 4. Heart at the level of distal extension of the stumps of the porcine bioprosthesis in the mitral position. Extensive hemorrhage *(H)* is present in the subepicardial adipose tissue surrounding the left ventricle. The *arrow* points to the site of LV rupture. *VS* = ventricular septum.

mouth in most was located at the level of the atrioventricular groove (mitral anulus) or at the stumps of the papillary muscles.[1-14] In several reports, however, it is clear or likely that lacerations, with or without rupture or aneurysm formation, occurred between mitral anulus and the stumps of the papillary muscles.[15-27] Observations in these 36 previously reported patients with this manifestation are summarized in Table II. Of the 36 patients, 27 had died and necropsies were performed in most. The other nine either survived repair of the posterior LV wall rupture (Ref. 16 [cases No. 6 and 8], refs. 19, 22, 25 [case No. 8]) or developed an aneurysm which was later excised.[15,27] Of the 36 patients, LV rupture occurred in 23 (64%), and in 15 it was fatal. Of these 15 patients, fatal rupture occurred in the operating room at the time of MVR or within a few hours after entering the recovery room in 12 patients, and in 2, 4, and 6 days, respectively, after MVR in the other three patients. LV aneurysm developed in six patients, four of whom died: the interval after MVR was 2, 14, 90, and 2112 days,

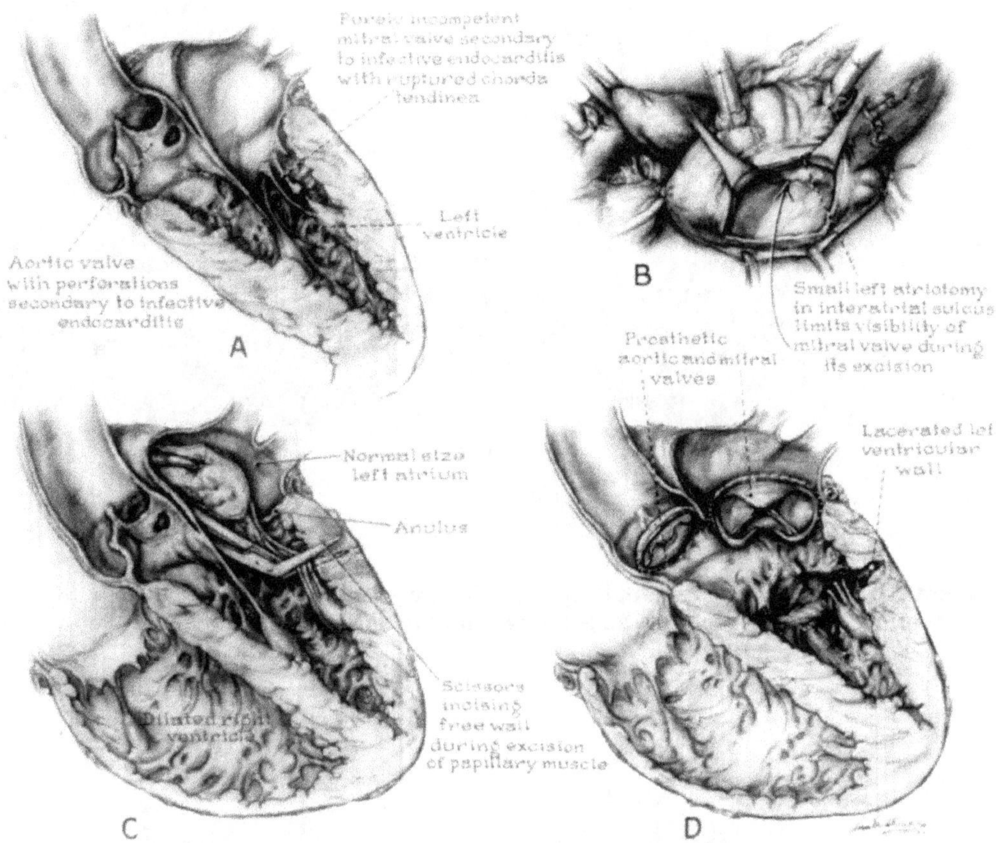

Fig. 4. Patient No. 7. Drawing depicting the mechanism of LV rupture.

Table I. Certain clinical and morphologic observations in the 10 patients with replaced mitral valves and midway left ventricular lacerations or thinnings

Pt	*Age (yr)*	*Sex*	*MS*	*Type mitral prosthesis*	*LVFW*		*Interval (days) MVR to death*	*HW (gm)*	*LV↑ (0-4+)*	*CA↓*
					Rupture	*Aneurysm*				
1	40	M	+	S-E (2M)	0	0	10 hours	490	0	+*
2	55	F	+	Porcine(−)	0	0	2	−	0	0
3	59	F	0	Porcine(−)	+	0	0	−	0	0
4	66	F	+	Porcine(27)	+	0	0	410	0	+*
5	59	F	+	S-E(3M)	+	0	2	400	0	0
6	60	M	+	S-E(3M)	+	0	3	500	0	0
7	44	M	0	Porcine(27)	+	0	4	560	++	+
8	59	M	+	Porcine(33)	0	+	10	475	+	0
9	46	F	+	B-S(−)	0	+	120	−	+	0
10	68	F	+	S-E(3M)	0	+	2464	490	++	0

*Coronary artery bypass grafting.

Abbreviations: CA↓ = one or more of the four major coronary arteries narrowed 76%-100% in cross-sectional area by atherosclerotic plaque; HW = heart weight; LVFW = left ventricular free wall; LV↑ = left ventricular cavity dilated; MS = mitral valve stenosis; MVR = mitral valve replacement; S-E = Starr-Edwards; B-S = Björk-Shiley.

respectively. One patient who had LV rupture repaired at operation at the time of MVR subsequently developed a LV aneurysm at the site of the previous rupture (Ref. 26 [case No. 6]). He died of a cerebral hemorrhage about 65 days after the initial MVR. The remaining six patients had LV lacerations between mitral anulus and papillary muscle stumps and all of them died: four in the operating room or just a few hours thereafter; one, 2 days later, and one, 3 days later.

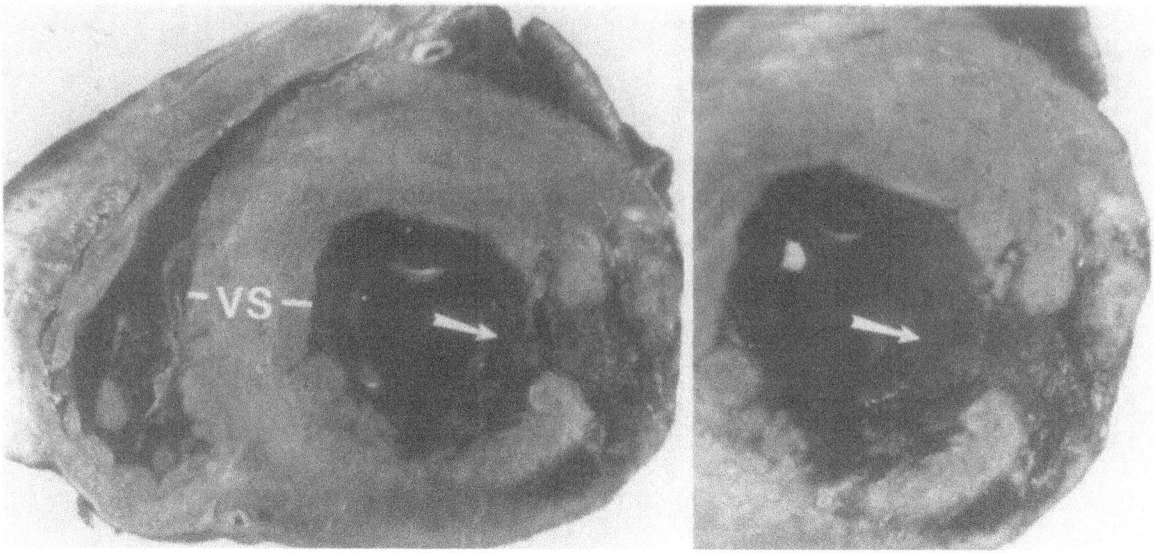

Fig. 5. Patient No. 7. Heart in two views of the patient illustrated in Fig. 4. The *arrows* point to the site of LV free wall rupture. The actual through-and-through rupture did not occur until 4 days postoperatively.

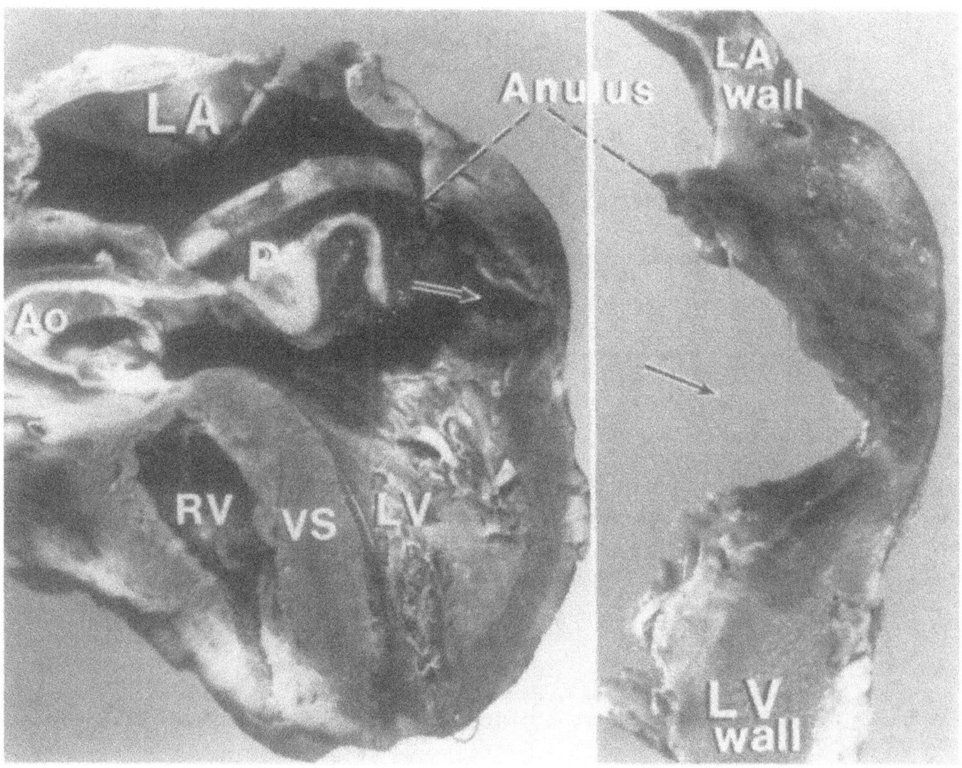

Fig. 6. Patient No. 8. *Left*, Longitudinal view of heart in which an aneurysm developed early postoperatively. *Ao* = aorta; *LA* = left atrial cavity; *LV* = left ventricular cavity; *P* = bioprosthesis; *RV* = right ventricular cavity; *VS* = ventricular septum. *Right*, Longitudinal cut of the LA and LV walls showing the aneurysm *(arrow)* just below the mitral anulus where the porcine bioprosthesis had been attached.

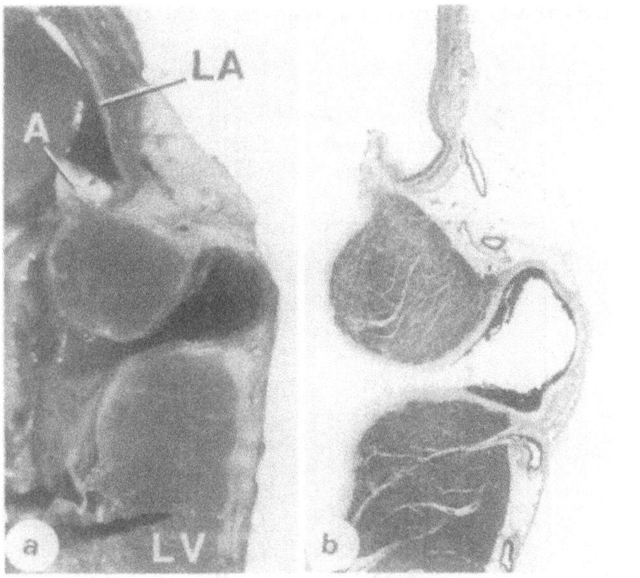

Fig. 7. Patient No. 9. **a,** Left ventricular *(LV)* aneurysm with a small mouth located about midway between the mitral anulus *(A)* and the stumps of the LV papillary muscles. *LA* = left atrial wall. **b,** Photomicrograph of the longitudinal section depicting the aneurysm, the wall of which consists entirely of fibrous tissue. Movat stain.

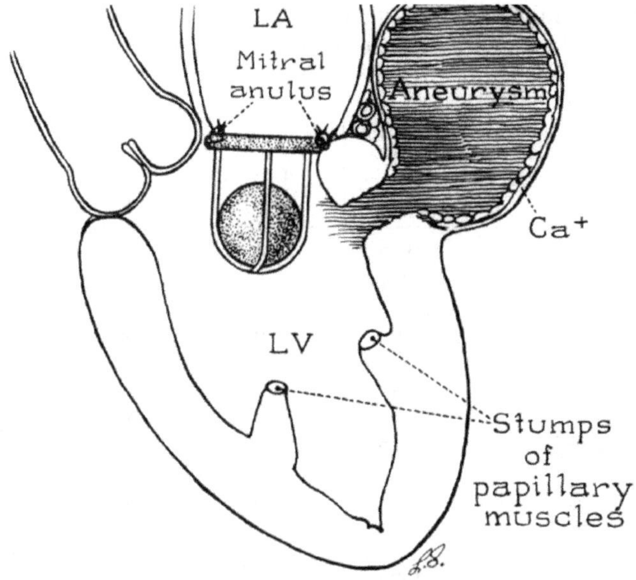

Fig. 8. Patient No. 10. Drawing showing a large submitral aneurysm, the mouth of which is located midway between the mitral anulus and the papillary muscle stumps. The wall of the aneurysm is heavily calcified and this egg-shaped calcific wall was readily visible on chest radiograph during the last few years of life.

The lengths of the LV lacerations were described in 18 patients and ranged from 1 to 6.5 cm. Cobbs et al.[25] described the lengths of the lacerations in six of their seven necropsy patients and they ranged from 4 to 6.5 cm. In the 34 patients in whom the information was provided, the site of the LV rupture or the mouth of the aneurysm or the laceration itself (in those without rupture or aneurysm) involved the LV posterior wall. In five of the seven necropsy patients reported by Cobbs et al.,[25] other or all portions of the LV free wall also were involved by the laceration. In 12[12, 23-25] of the 27 reported necropsy patients, gross photographs illustrated LV lacerations located transversely or obliquely about midway between mitral anulus and papillary muscle stumps. Five additional patients had drawings showing the sites of rupture or the aneurysmal mouth.[15, 19, 22, 27]

Of the 36 previously reported patients, 33 were over 50 years of age and the remaining three were aged 42, 48, and 50 years, respectively. The mean age of 34 patients was 58 years and the two others[20] were aged 70 years or over. Of the 34 in whom the information was provided, 23 (68%) were women and 11 (32%) were men. Preoperatively, 28 (78%) had stenotic mitral valves and eight (22%) had purely regurgitant mitral valves. Of the 28 patients with stenotic mitral valves, five (18%) had had earlier mitral commissurotomies. The type substitute cardiac valves utilized in the 36 patients was as follows: porcine in 14 (Hancock = 13; Carpentier-Edwards = one); caged-ball in 10 (Starr-Edwards = 9; Cutter-Smeloff = one); tilting disc in 10 (all Björk-Shiley); and non-tilting disc in two (Kay-Shiley = one; Beall = one).

Causes of LV lacerations. Although the cause of the ruptures and aneurysms which develop at either the mitral anulus or behind the bases of the papillary muscles during or after MVR are well understood,[1] the cause of the tears, with or without rupture or aneurysm formation, occurring midway between the mitral anulus and LV papillary muscle stumps has not been clearly delineated. Several possibilities have been considered: (1) *Inadvertent removal of calcium within the LV wall.*[16, 22, 26] The calcium in this circumstance represents an extension of calcium from the mitral leaflets and anulus. This possibility seems unlikely as the usual explanation for the *midway* lacerations (i.e., between mitral anulus and papillary muscle stumps), because extension of mitral leaflet calcium, in contrast to mitral anular calcium (an infrequent occurrence in patients with leaflet calcium), into adjacent LV myocardium is a rare occurrence in the setting of mitral stenosis whereas midway LV lacerations (to be discussed

Table II. Summary of previously reported patients with apparent midway left ventricular lacerations at the time of the mitral valve replacement procedure

First author (reference)	*Year*	*Case no.*	*Age (yr)*	*Sex*	*MS*	*Type mitral prosthesis (size)*	*AS*	*AVR*
MacVaugh[15]	1969	1	53	M	+*	S-E(−)	−	+
MacVaugh[16]	1971	6	50	M	+	S-E(3M)	0	0
		8	51	M	+	S-E(2M)	0	0
		9	59	F	+	K-S(No.8)	0	0
		10	53	M	+*	S-E(3M)	+	+
Spellberg[17]	1972	1	42	F	+	S-E(3M)	0	0
		2	57	F	+*	S-E(2M)	0	0
Zacharias[18]	1975	1	53	F	+	S-E(3M)	0	0
		2	69	F	0	S-E(2M)	0	0
		5	56	M	+	C-S(M6)	0	+
Chi[19]	1976	1	54	F	0	Beall(−)	0	0
		2	62	F	+	Hancock(33)	0	0
Stephenson[20]	1978	−	≥70	−	+	S-E(3M)	0	0
		−	≥70	−	+	B-S(29)	0	0
Katske[21]	1979	1	57	F	+	Hancock(31)	0	0
		2	63	F	+	Hancock(29)	0	0
		3	57	F	+*	Hancock(29)	0	0
Engelman[22]	1979	1	53	M	+	B-S(25)	0	0
Miller[23]	1979	1	60	F	+*	B-S(−)	0	0
		2	61	F	+	B-S(−)	+	+
Wild[24]	1980	1	55	M	0	C-E(31)	0	0
Cobbs[25]	1980	1	61	F	+	Hancock(29)	0	0
		2	53	F	+	Hancock(27)	0	+
		3	69	F	0	Hancock(−)	0	0
		4	72	M	0	Hancock(33)	0	0
		5	70	F	+	Hancock(31)	0	0
		6	76	M	0	Hancock(33)	0	0
		7	52	M	0	Hancock(27)	0	0
		8	64	F	+	Hancock(27)	0	0
Gosalbez[26]	1981	1	59	F	+	B-S(31)	−	0
		2	48	F	+	B-S(31)	0	0
		3	58	F	+	B-S(31)	−	0
		4	56	F	+	B-S(31)	−	0
		5	64	F	+	B-S(29)	−	0
		6	56	M	0	B-S(31)	0	0
Sutorius[27]	1981	1	51	F	+	Hancock(30)	0	0

*Previous mitral commissurotomy.

Abbreviations: A = anterior wall of left ventricle; An = aneurysm; AS = aortic valve stenosis; AVR = aortic valve replacement; CA↓ = coronary artery narrowing; C-E = Carpentier-Edwards; C-S = Cutter-Smeloff; K-S = Kay-Shiley; MS = mitral valve stenosis; MVR = mitral valve replacement; P = posterior wall of left ventricle; OR = died in operating room.

below) are common. More importantly, midway lacerations occur in patients having MVR when the operatively excised valve is devoid of calcific deposits. (2) *Stent of a mechanical or bioprosthetic valve's burrowing into the LV wall with or without associated open or closed cardiac massage.* Although this possibly has been considered the likely mechanism by several investigators,[22, 24] this possibility appears highly unlikely, in our view, because of two factors: (a) the stents usually are at a considerable distance from the laceration; and (b) the lacerations have been observed in the hearts of patients with mitral prostheses which are virtually devoid of stents, such as the tilting (Björk-Shiley) and non-tilting (Kay-Shiley) disc prostheses. (3) *Use of cold- and potassium-induced cardioplegia.* Although the cardioplegic myocardium might be more susceptible to stretching than the noncardioplegic myocardium,[25] the lacerations were observed before cold- and potassium-induced cardioplegia was introduced, and the actual technique of mitral excision and/or replacement has changed little since

LV Rupture	LV An	Interval (days) MVR→death	CA↓	LV laceration described	Length (cm) of LV laceration	Location of rupture or aneurysm A	Location of rupture or aneurysm P	Photo of tear	Drawing of tear
0	+	–	–	–	–	–	+	0	+(An)
+	0	–	–	+	2.0	–	+	0	0
+	0	–	–	"Opening"	"Small"	–	+	0	0
+	0	1 hr	–	+	–	–	+	0	0
0	+	90	–	"Orifice"	1.2	–	+	0	0
0	+	2112	–	–	–	–	+	0	0
0	+	2	+	–	2.0	–	+	0	0
+	0	1 hr	–	+	–	–	+	0	0
+	0	<1	0	+	1.5	–	+	0	0
+	0	<1	–	+	2.0	–	+	0	0
+	0	–	–	+	4.0	–	+	0	+
+	0	–	–	+	4.0	–	+	0	+
+	0	<1	–	–	–	–	–	0	0
+	0	6	–	–	–	–	–	0	0
+	0	<1	–	+	–	–	+	+	0
+	0	<1	0	+	0.5	–	+	+	0
+	0	<1	0	+	2.0	–	+	+	0
+	0	–	+	0	2 × 4	–	+	0	+
0	+	14	–	+	–	–	+	+	0
0	0	<1	–	+	4.5	–	+	+	0
0	0	OR	–	+	3.0	–	+	+	0
0	0	3	0	+	4.0	–	+	+	0
+	0	<1	0	+	4.5	+	+	0	0
0	0	OR	0	+	6.5	+	+	+	0
+	0	4	0	+	6.0	+	+	+	0
+	0	2	0	+	5.0	+	+	+	0
0	0	OR	–	+	–	+	+	+	0
0	0	2	+	+	6.0	–	+	+	0
+	0	–	–	0	–	–	+	0	0
+	0	–	–	–	–	–	+	0	0
+	0	OR	–	–	–	–	+	0	0
+	0	<1	–	–	–	–	+	0	0
+	0	OR	–	+	"Large"	–	+	0	0
+	0	OR	–	+	"Large"	–	+	0	0
+	+	65+	–	"Small"	–	–	+	0	0
0	+	–	0	0	–	–	+	0	+

this type of cardioplegia was introduced about 1975. (4) *Older age of the patients.* Although this possibility was suggested by Stephenson et al.,[20] some patients with midway lacerations are not old, and therefore if age is a factor it is clearly not the only one. The older patients may have smaller hearts than younger patients and the latter may be an important contributing factor, as discussed below. (5) *Postoperative elevation of left ventricular systolic pressure.* Although persistence of, or development of, systemic hypertension immediately after MVR has been proposed,[20,21] most patients with midway LV lacerations have normal or low systemic blood pressures. (6) *"Untethered left ventricle" concept.* Cobbs et al.[25] proposed that the interruption of the attachments between mitral anulus and papillary muscle, an occurrence in all patients having MVR at most institutions, transsects "...a major vertical fiberloop—and also removes a longitudinal binder..." and this factor is believed by them to be the likely cause of the midway tears. It seems unlikely to us in view of the fact that midway lacerations, with or without rupture or aneurysmal formation, are relatively uncommon whereas mitral leaflet–papillary muscle continuity is interrupted in nearly all patients having MVR. (7) *Trauma to the LV wall by a canula introduced into the left ventricle at the time of MVR.* This possibility was

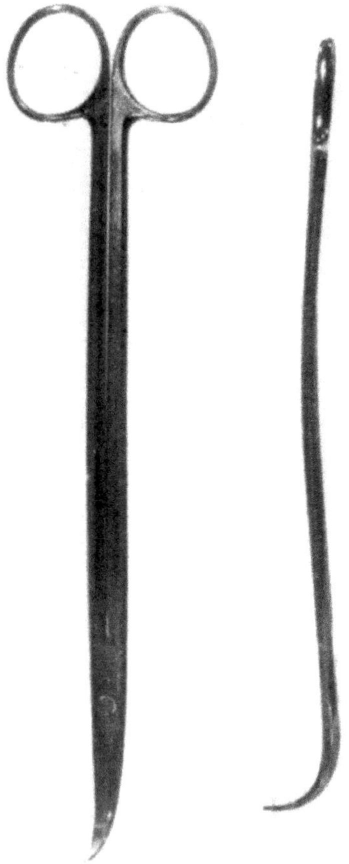

Fig. 9. Two views of nearly 19 cm long scissors with curved blades. They are frequently used for mitral valve excision and are considered the major cause of the midway LV incision.

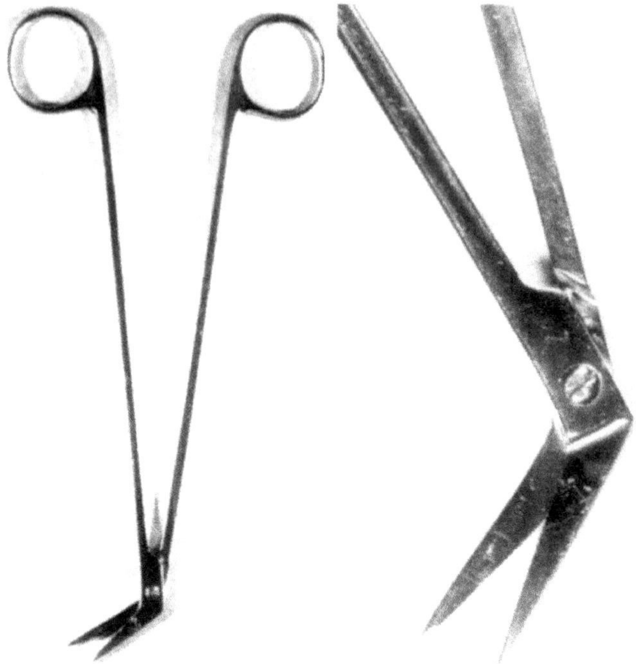

Fig. 10. These scissors are even more dangerous than those shown in Fig. 9 because the tips of the blades are pointed, not rounded. These scissors can lacerate the LV wall readily during either the opening or closing of the blades.

described initially by Björk et al.,[4] but the laceration was not at the midway position. Although in the patient reported by Björk et al. the canula was introduced from the LV apex, we have observed a laceration in the midway position caused by a canula introduced via a right pulmonary vein. (This patient was not included among our 10 patients). Thus, although this possibility appears reasonable in rare circumstances, it clearly is not applicable in most patients because the LV midway laceration has been observed when MVR was carried out without use of a LV drain.

The likely mechanism of the midway LV laceration, in our view, as illustrated by Figs. 2 and 4, is *inadvertent incision of the LV free wall during excision of the mitral valve.* This accident has occurred typically with exposure of the mitral valve via an interatrial groove incision in the setting of a stenotic mitral valve, relatively limited left atrial dilatation, and minimal or no LV dilatation. Thus, exposure of the mitral valve during its excision may be relatively poor. The interatrial groove incision may be only about 5 cm in length, the distance from the interatrial groove incision to the tips of the papillary muscles may be as much as 9 cm, and the relatively small sizes of the left atrium, left ventricle, and mitral anulus prevent adequate visualization of the tips of the scissor blades during mitral valve excision. The scissors themselves are nearly 19 cm long (Fig. 9). Damage to the LV free wall at the level of the chordae tendineae from the posterior mitral leaflet, the midway position, can occur during either the closing or the opening of the scissor blades (Fig. 10).

Evidence that the above described mechanism is the cause of the midway LV laceration is the following: (1) the same type laceration midway between mitral anulus and papillary muscle stump can be produced readily at necropsy by scissors introduced via an interatrial groove incision to incise the chordae tendineae from the posterior mitral leaflet or by opening the scissors within a normal-sized LV cavity. (2) The midway laceration does not occur when the posterior mitral leaflet and its attached chordae tendineae are not removed. Furthermore, the midway laceration is not produced if the chordae from the posterior mitral leaflet are left intact and the valve is removed intact by excising the tips of both papillary muscles and the mitral leaflets circumferentially by an incision a few millimeters toward the orifice from the anulus. Thus, the more intact the excision of the valve, the less likely will the midway laceration occur. (3) The midway laceration is most likely to occur in patients with relatively small left-sided cardiac chambers where visualization of the tips of the scissor blades within the LV cavity is not ideal.

Prevention. Miller et al.[23] proposed that LV rupture (and therefore laceration) can be prevented by not excising the posterior mitral leaflet and by leaving most or all of its chordae tendineae intact. Since doing so, these authors have not observed LV rupture during or after MVR. This advice seems reasonable to us if the mitral valve is replaced with a caged ball prosthesis or a bioprosthesis, but residual mitral leaflet or chordae could potentially interfere with proper closure of the occluders of the more delicate prostheses, namely, the tilting disc (Björk-Shiley, St. Jude Medical Device) or non-tilting disc (Kay-Shiley) prostheses. We suggest simply taking as much care during the mitral valve *excision procedure* as during the *replacement procedure.* If the chordae are left completely intact and only the tips of the papillary muscles are carefully excised, observing at all times the tips of the scissors within the LV cavity, and the leaflets, are incised circumferentially near the anulus, the problem should be prevented.

Frequency. The present subject is of considerable importance because it is a major cause of death early after MVR. Excluding patients in whom rupture occurred at the left atrioventricular junction or at the stumps of the papillary muscles, midway LV rupture occurred in 2 of 14 patients having MVR reported by Stephenson et al.,[20] in 2 of 51 patients having MVR reported by Miller et al.,[23] probably in 11 of 294 patients having MVR reported by Cobbs et al.,[25] and in 4 of 55 patients having isolated MVR reported by Gosalbez et al.[26] Midway LV rupture was the most frequent cause of early death after MVR among the patients reported by both Cobbs et al.[25] and by Gosalbez et al.[26]

REFERENCES

1. Roberts WC, Morrow AG: Causes of early postoperative death following cardiac valve replacement. Clinico-pathologic correlation in 64 patients studied at necropsy. J Thorac Cardiovasc Surg **54**:422, 1967.
2. Treasure RL, Rainer WG, Strevey TE, Sadler TR: Intraoperative left ventricular rupture associated with mitral valve replacement. Chest **66**:511, 1974.
3. Sharratt GP, Ross JK, Monro JL, Johnson AM: Intraoperative left ventricular perforation with false aneurysm formation. Br Heart J **38**:1154, 1976.
4. Björk VO, Henze A, Rodriguez L: Left ventricular rupture as a complication of mitral valve replacement. Surgical experience with eight cases and a review of the literature. J Thorac Cardiovasc Surg **73**:14, 1977.
5. Smeloff EA: Discussion to paper by Björk et al.[4] J Thorac Cardiovasc Surg **73**:21, 1977.
6. Wareham EE: Discussion of paper by Björk VO.[4] J Thorac Cardiovasc Surg **73**:21, 1977.
7. Bloomer WE: Discussion of paper by Björk VO.[4] J Thorac Cardiovasc Surg **73**:21, 1977.
8. Casarotto D, Bortolotti U, Thiene G, Gallucci V, Cevese PG: Rupture of the posterior wall of the left heart at the atrioventricular groove following mitral valve replacement. Acta Chir Belg **76**:297, 1977.
9. Diethrich EB, Koopot R, Kinard SA: Pseudoaneurysm of atrioventricular groove. A late complication of mitral valve replacement. J Thorac Cardiovasc Surg **74**:47, 1977.
10. Wolpowitz A, Barnard MS, Sanchez HE, Barnard CN: Intraoperative posterior left ventricular wall rupture associated with mitral valve replacement. Ann Thorac Surg **25**:551, 1978.
11. Rose AG, Losman JG: Subvalvular left ventricular false aneurysm complicating mitral valve replacement. Arch Pathol Lab Med **102**:285, 1978.
12. Achatzy R, Dittrich H, Jelesijevic V, Knoll D, Lunkenheimer PP, Anyanwu E: Rupture of the ventricle following prosthetic replacement of the mitral valve. Thorac Cardiovasc Surg **27**:48, 1979.
13. Bortolotti U, Thiene G, Casarotto D, Mazzucco A, Gallucci V: Left ventricular rupture following mitral valve replacement with a Hancock bioprosthesis. Chest **77**:235, 1980.
14. Chun PKC, Rajfer SI, Donohue DJ, Bowen TE, Davia JE: Björk-Shiley mitral valvular dehiscence. Documented by radiography, echocardiography, fluoroscopy, and cineangiography. Am Heart J **99**:230, 1980.
15. MacVaugh H III, Joyner CR, Pierce WS, Johnson J: Repair of subvalvular left ventricular aneurysm occurring as a complication of mitral valve replacement. J Thorac Cardiovasc Surg **58**:291, 1969.
16. MacVaugh H III, Joyner CR, Johnson J: Unusual complications during mitral valve replacement in the presence of calcification of the annulus. Ann Thorac Surg **11**:336, 1971.
17. Spellberg RD, O'Reilly RJ: Pseudoaneurysm of left ventricle following mitral valve replacement. Chest **62**:115, 1972.
18. Zacharias A, Groves LK, Cheanvechai C, Loop FD, Effler DB: Rupture of the posterior wall of the left ventricle after mitral valve replacement. J Thorac Cardiovasc Surg **69**:259, 1975.
19. Chi S, Beshore R, Gonzalez-Lavin L: Left ventricular wall rupture after mitral valve replacement: Report of successful repair in 2 patients. Ann Thorac Surg **22**:380, 1976.
20. Stephenson LW, MacVaugh H III, Edmunds LH Jr: Surgery using cardiopulmonary bypass in the elderly. Circulation **58**:250, 1978.
21. Katske G, Golding LR, Tubbs RR, Loop FD: Posterior midventricular rupture after mitral valve replacement. Ann Thorac Surg **27**:130, 1979.
22. Engelman RM, Rousou JH, Wittenberg SA: New technique for repair of posterior left ventricular rupture. J Thorac Cardiovasc Surg **77**:757, 1979.
23. Miller DW Jr, Johnson DD, Ivey TD: Does preservation of the posterior chordae tendineae enhance survival during mitral valve replacement? Ann Thorac Surg **28**:22, 1979.
24. Wild LM, Lajos TZ, Lee AB Jr, Wright J: Left ventricular laceration due to stented prosthesis. Chest **77**:216, 1980.
25. Cobbs BW Jr, Hatcher CR Jr, Craver JM, Jones EL, Sewell CW: Transverse midventricular disruption after mitral valve replacement. Am Heart J **99**:33, 1980.
26. Gosalbez F, de Linera FA, Cofino JL, Naya JL, Rodriguez J, Ortuna A: Isolated mitral valve replacement and ventricular rupture: Presentation of 6 patients. Ann Thorac Surg **31**:105, 1981.
27. Sutorius DJ, Helmsworth JA, Majeski JA, Miller SF: Repair of a subvalvular left ventricular aneurysm following mitral valve replacement. Ann Thorac Surg **32**:92, 1981.

Cardiovascular Disease in the Very Elderly

Analysis of 40 Necropsy Patients Aged 90 Years or Over

BRUCE F. WALLER, MD and WILLIAM C. ROBERTS, MD

Clinical and necropsy observations are described in 40 patients (29 women) aged 90 years and older. The majority (21 patients [57%]) died during the 4 coldest months, and 12 (30%), during the 4 warmest months. At necropsy, 39 had ≥1 major cardiac abnormalities, the most frequent being calcific deposits in the major epicardial coronary arteries in 37 (92%). In 28 patients (70%), 1 or more of the 4 major arteries was narrowed 76 to 100% in cross-sectional area (XSA) by atherosclerotic plaques, an average of 1.9/4.0 per patient: the 12 patients with clinical events compatible with myocardial ischemia (angina pectoris or myocardial infarction) had an average of 2.2/4 and the other 28 patients an average of 1.0/4.0. In 36 patients, a histologic section was examined from each 5 mm long segment from each of the 4 major coronary arteries: of the 1,789 segments, only 6 (<1%) were narrowed 96 to 100% in XSA by plaques; 147 (8%), 76 to 95%; 339 (19%), 51 to 75%; 930 (52%), 26 to 50%, and 367 (21%), 0 to 25%. The average amount of XSA narrowing for the 1,789 segments was about 42%. In 10 patients with clinical evidence of myocardial ischemia, the average amount of narrowing per segment was approximately 55%; in the 26 patients without clinical ischemia, the average was about 38%. Of the 40 patients, 18 (45%) had left ventricular transmural foci of fibrosis or necrosis or both. Of 14 patients with transmural scars, only 1 had a clinical event compatible with acute myocardial infarction; of the 10 with acute myocardial infarction at necropsy, only 4 had typical clinical features of infarction.

Calcific deposits were present in ≥1 aortic valve cusps in 22 patients (55%), causing aortic valve stenosis in 2, and in the mitral anulus in 19 (47%), probably causing mitral valve stenosis in 1.

Amyloid deposits were present in the heart in at least 9 patients; they were grossly visible and caused fatal cardiac dysfunction in 4, and microscopically visible only in 5, causing no cardiac dysfunction. Eight patients (20%) had chronic congestive heart failure; 27 of 39 (69%) had either a history of systemic hypertension or blood pressure >140/90 mm Hg during their final year of life. Precordial murmurs were recorded in 25 (62%) patients—systolic only in 24 and both systolic and diastolic in 1. Data from electrocardiograms were available in 30 patients: 12 (40%) had atrial fibrillation; 12 (40%), abnormal axis; 12, complete bundle branch block; 1, criteria for left ventricular hypertrophy (despite increased cardiac mass in 67%); and 1, low voltage.

All patients had fairly extensive atherosclerosis of the aorta, with aneurysmal formation in 5 with fatal rupture in 3. Five had strokes, which were fatal in 4. At least 5 had leg claudication. Two had massive pulmonary emboli superimposed on chronic obstructive pulmonary disease.

Thus, cardiovascular disease was present at necropsy in 39 of our 40 patients, but frequently it was not diagnosed clinically.

Although the average age at death has increased dramatically during this century, the maximal length of life has not changed.[1] The percentage of individuals surviving for 90 years and beyond, however, is increasing.[2] In 1980, about 1% of the population in the United States was aged 90 years or older.[2] Very few necropsies are performed in patients dying after age 90 years (frequency about 4%)[3] and, therefore, little attention has been focused on the clinical and morphologic frequencies and types of cardiovascular disease observed in these very elderly persons. This report describes the types of cardiovascular disease found at necropsy in 40 patients aged 90 years or over.

From the Pathology Branch, National Heart, Lung, and Blood Institute, National Institutes of Health, Bethesda, Maryland. Manuscript received and accepted September 24, 1982.

Address for reprints: William C. Roberts, MD, Building 10A, Room 3E-30, National Institutes of Health, Bethesda, Maryland 20205.

Patients

General observations: Clinical and morphologic observations in the 40 patients are detailed in Table I. The patients died and underwent necropsy at 12 different hospitals (10 in the Washington, D.C. area [37 patients]); subsequently the heart and frequently the aortas were examined in all 40 patients by 1 of us (WCR). The year of death in 37 patients was between

TABLE I Clinical and Morphologic Observations in 40 Necropsy Patients Aged 90 to 103 Years

											Electrocardiogram						
													BBB		QRS Axis		
Case	Age (yr) & Sex	Race	CP	AP	AMI	AD	CCHF	DM	Hx SH	SAP (mm Hg)	S	AF	R	L	R	L	TC (mg/100 ml)
1	90F	W	+	0	+	0	0	0	+	145/70	0	+	0	+	0	+	—
2	90F	W	+	+	+	0	0	+	0	120/80	0	0	—	—	—	—	—
3	90M	B	+	0	+	+	0	0	+	140/70	0	+	0	+	0	0	236
4	90M	B	0	0	0	+	+	0	0	110/70	0	+	0	+	0	+	250
5	90F	W	+	0	+	+	0	+	+	118/80	0	+	0	+	0	0	—
6	90F	W	0	0	0	0	0	0	0	118/70	0	0	0	0	0	0	—
7	90F	W	0	0	0	0	0	0	+	170/90	0	0	0	0	0	0	223
8	90F	W	0	0	0	0	0	0	+	80/60	0	0	0	0	0	0	—
9	91F	B	0	0	0	0	0	+	+	84/—	0	0	0	0	0	0	—
10	91M	B	0	0	0	0	0	0	+	140/90	0	+	0	0	0	0	—
11	91F	B	0	0	0	0	0	0	+	95/60	0	0	0	0	0	0	—
12	91M	W	0	0	0	0	0	0	+	116/85	+	+	0	0	0	0	—
13	91F	W	+	0	+	+	0	0	+	120/60	0	—	—	—	—	—	283
14	92F	W	+	+	0	+	+	0	0	110/70	0	+	+	0	+	0	—
15	92F	W	0	0	0	0	0	0	+	230/110	0	0	0	0	0	+	—
16	92F	W	+	0	+	0	0	0	0	...	0	—	—	—	—	—	—
17	92F	W	0	0	0	+	+	0	+	100/50	0	+	0	0	0	0	—
18	93F	W	0	0	0	+	0	0	+	...	0	—	—	—	—	—	—
19	93M	W	+	0	+	+	0	0	+	170/60	0	—	—	—	—	—	—
20	93F	B	+	0	+	+	0	+	+	135/60	0	—	—	—	—	—	243
21	93F	W	0	0	0	+	+	0	+	120/70	0	0	0	+	0	+	—
22	93F	W	0	0	+	+	+	0	+	125/80	0	—	—	—	—	—	273
23	95F	W	+	0	+	+	0	0	0	110/70	0	—	—	—	—	—	—
24	95F	W	0	0	0	0	0	0	0	140/60	0	0	0	0	0	0	—
25	95F	W	+	0	0	0	0	+	+	125/100	0	0	0	0	0	+	—
26	95M	B	+	0	0	+	0	0	+	120/115	0	+	+	0	+	+	—
27	96M	W	0	0	0	+	+	0	+	90/70	0	+	+	0	0	+	—
28	95M	W	0	0	0	0	0	0	0	130/70	0	0	0	+	0	+	181
29	95F	W	0	0	0	0	0	0	+	...	0	+	+	0	+	0	235
30	96F	B	0	0	0	+	+†	0	+	140/90	+	—	—	—	—	—	108
31	97F	W	0	0	0	0	0	0	+	118/75	+	+	0	0	0	0	—
32	97F	W	0	0	0	+	0	0	0	140/60	0	0	0	0	0	0	—
33	97F	W	0	0	0	0	0	0	0	...	+	0	0	0	0	0	—
34	97M	W	0	0	0	+	+	0	+	...	0	0	0	0	0	0	—
35	98F	W	0	0	0	0	0	0	0	130/85	0	0	0	0	0	0	—
36	98F	W	0	0	0	0	0	0	0	170/80	0	0	0	+	0	+	165
37	99M	W	+	+	0	0	0	0	+	130/85	+	0	0	0	0	0	—
38	100F	W	0	0	0	0	0	0	0	170/80	0	—	—	—	—	—	—
39	100M	W	0	0	0	0	0	0	0	...	0	0	0	0	0	0	—
40	103F	B	0	0	0	0	0	0	0	110/70	0	0	+	0	0	+	—
Total or mean	(94)		13 (32%)	3 (7%)	10 (25%)	17 (42%)	7 (17%)	5 (12%)	25 (62%)	... ...	4 (10%)	12 (40%)	5 (17%)	7 (23%)	3 (7%)	10 (33%)	220 ...

* Aortic valve stenosis.
† Idiopathic dilated cardiomyopathy.
A = cardiac amyloidosis (++ = massive, grossly visible deposits; + = minute, visible on microscope only); AD = abnormal dyspnea; AF = atrial fibrillation; AMI = acute myocardial infarction clinically; AP = angina pectoris; AV = aortic valve cusp; BBB = bundle branch block; BW = body weight; C = cardiac; CA = coronary artery; CCHF = chronic congestive heart failure; CP = chest pain; DM = diabetes mellitus; F = fibrosis; FAAA = fusiform abdominal aortic aneurysm; HW = heart weight; Hx = history; L = left; LAD = left anterior descending; LC = left circumflex; LV = left ventricular; MCS = mean coronary score; MVA = mitral valve anulus; N = necrosis; O = other; PHD = pericardial heart disease; R = right; S = stroke; SAP = systemic arterial pressure; SH = systemic hypertension; TC = total serum cholesterol; V = vascular.

TABLE I (continued)

Case	Mode of Death			BW (kg)	HW (g)	Calcific Deposits			(%) 5 mm Segments Narrowed to Various Degrees				MCS	Transmural LV			PHD	FAAA
	C	V	O			CA	MVA	AV	0–25	26–50	51–75	76–100		N	F	A		
1	+	0	0	55	550	3+	3+	4 + a	0	17(39)	21(49)	5(12)	2.72	+	0	0	0	0
2	+	0	0	41	340	2+	0	0	...	...	...	...	...	+	0	0	0	0
3	+	0	0	50	450	2+	0	2+	9(18)	16(31)	12(24)	13(27)	2.58	+	+	0	0	0
4	+	0	0	—	520	1+	3+	1+	29(53)	24(44)	2(3)	0	1.51	0	0	++	0	0
5	+	0	0	45	400	2+	2+	1+	16(26)	24(39)	11(18)	10(17)	2.25	+	0	0	0	0
6	0	0	+	45	220	1+	1+	2+	16(37)	13(30)	11(26)	3(7)	1.89	0	0	0	0	0
7	0	0	+	47	270	1+	0	1+	6(16)	25(68)	5(13)	1(3)	2.03	0	0	0	0	0
8	0	+	0	50	505	2+	0	0	0	19(40)	15(32)	12(28)	2.85	0	+	0	0	+
9	0	0	+	60	480	2+	0	0	...	...	...	...	...	0	0	+	0	0
10	0	+	0	—	490	1+	0	1+	33(72)	13(28)	0	0	1.28	0	0	0	0	0
11	0	+	0	46	375	4+	4+	0	9(14)	40(64)	12(19)	2(3)	2.11	0	0	0	0	0
12	+	0	0	65	390	2+	0	1+	16(26)	24(39)	11(18)	10(17)	2.25	0	+	0	0	0
13	+	0	0	—	520	2+	0	0	11(17)	24(37)	16(25)	13(21)	2.48	+	+	0	0	+
14	+	0	0	49	380	1+	1+	1+	10(25)	17(43)	8(20)	5(12)	2.20	0	+	0	+	0
15	0	0	+	50	400	1+	1+	1+	19(33)	39(67)	0	0	1.67	0	0	0	0	0
16	+	0	0	85	280	2+	3+	1+	0	30(70)	8(18)	5(12)	2.42	+	0	0	0	0
17	+	0	0	55	525	2+	4+	4+	3(7)	37(80)	6(13)	0	2.07	0	0	0	0	0
18	0	0	+	—	500	3+	1+	2+	15(23)	46(72)	2(3)	1(2)	1.83	0	+	0	0	0
19	+	0	0	66	470	2+	0	1+	6(14)	14(33)	15(35)	8(18)	2.58	+	+	0	0	0
20	+	0	0	—	510	1+	0	0	0	18(24)	18(42)	18(34)	3.08	+	+	0	0	0
21	+	0	0	—	380	1+	0	0	22(48)	20(43)	4(9)	0	1.61	0	0	++	0	0
22	+	0	0	67	560	3+	3+	2+	7(15)	12(26)	14(31)	12(28)	2.69	+	+	0	0	0
23	+	0	0	—	490	1+	0	0	...	...	...	...	...	+	+	0	0	0
24	0	0	+	58	350	1+	4+	1+	3(6)	31(65)	12(25)	2(4)	2.27	0	0	0	0	0
25	0	+	0	—	460	2+	0	0	18(49)	19(51)	0	0	1.51	0	0	0	0	+
26	0	+	0	47	580	2+	0	0	5(8)	36(59)	19(31)	1(2)	2.26	0	0	0	0	0
27	+	0	0	50	660	3+	2+	2+	9(12)	44(59)	15(20)	7(9)	2.27	0	+	++	0	0
28	0	0	+	—	385	2+	0	1+	12(19)	32(52)	16(26)	2(3)	2.13	0	0	0	0	0
29	0	0	+	52	440	2+	2+	1+	2(3)	48(69)	15(22)	4(6)	2.30	0	+	+	0	0
30	+	0	0	50	630	0	0	0	15(31)	33(69)	0	0	1.69	0	0	0	0	0
31	0	+	0	45	300	2+	4+	1+	11(29)	17(45)	9(24)	1(2)	2.00	0	0	0	0	0
32	0	0	+	55	360	2+	3+	0	19(36)	29(55)	3(5)	2(4)	1.77	0	0	0	0	0
33	0	+	0	41	320	2+	3+	0	8(18)	29(66)	7(16)	0	1.98	0	0	0	0	0
34	+	0	0	68	600	3+	1+	1+	2(5)	24(62)	8(20)	5(13)	2.41	0	0	++	+	+
35	0	0	+	53	360	0	0	0	...	...	...	...	...	0	0	0	0	0
36	0	0	+	52	320	1+	0	0	8(27)	21(70)	1(3)	0	1.77	0	0	0	0	0
37	+	0	0	50	510	2+	0	0	5(11)	22(47)	15(32)	5(10)	2.43	0	+	0	0	0
38	0	+	0	45	280	4+	2+	2+	0	23(58)	12(30)	4(12)	2.51	0	0	+	0	0
39	0	0	+	—	335	2+	0	1+	18(32)	21(37)	16(28)	2(3)	2.04	0	+	+	0	0
40	0	0	+	55	345	0	0	0	5(11)	41(89)	0	0	1.89	0	0	+	0	0
Total (Mean)	19 (47%)	8 (20%)	13 (32%)	(53) ...	431 ...	37 (92%)	19 (47%)	22 (55%)	367 (21%)	930 (52%)	339 (19%)	153 (8%)	2.15 ...	10 (25%)	14 (35%)	4 (10%)	2 (5%)	4 (10%)

1967 and 1982; the other 3 patients had been studied both clinically and at necropsy at the National Institutes of Health in 1954, 1966, and 1967, respectively. The month of death was known in 37 patients: death occurred during 4 cold months (November to February) in 21 (57%); during 4 warm months (June to September) in 11 (30%), and during intermediate weather months in 5 (13%) ($p < 0.05$). (The data throughout this study were analyzed using the t test for paired and unpaired data and linear regression tests to determine correlation coefficients.) The ages of death in the 40 patients ranged from 90 to 103 (mean 94); 29 (72%) were women and 11 (28%) were men; 31 (78%) were white and 9 (22%) were black.

Heart weights and body weights: The weight of the heart was increased (>350 g in women and >400 g in men) in 27 (67%) patients. The hearts in the 29 women ranged from 220 to 630 g (mean 408), and those in the 11 men, from 335 to 660 g (mean 490). The body weights in the 23 women ranged from 41 to 85 kg (mean 52) and the heart weight-body weight ratio, from 0.003 to 0.013 (mean 0.007). Thus, the mean heart weight was 0.7% of the body weight (normal value for younger women is approximately 0.4%[4]). The body weights in 7 men ranged from 47 to 68 kg (mean 50) and the heart weight-body weight ratios, from 0.006 to 0.013 (mean 0.009). Thus, the mean heart weight was 0.6% of the mean body weight (the normal value for younger men is approximately 0.45%[4]).

TABLE II Morphologic Cardiac Observations in 40 Necropsy Patients Aged 90 to 103 Years

	Patients	
	n	%
Coronary arterial disease		
Calcium	37	92
Luminal narrowing 76 to 100% in XSA by atherosclerotic plaques of ≥1 major coronary arteries	28	70
Acute myocardial infarction	10	25
Healed myocardial infarction	14	35
Aortic valve disease		
Calcium	22	55
Stenosis	2	5
Mitral anular disease		
Calcium	19	47
Cardiac amyloidosis (fatal)	4	10
Dilated cardiomyopathy	1	3
Obliterative pericardial disease		
Idiopathic	1	5
Iatrogenic	1	5

Necropsy observations (Table II): *Coronary arterial calcification (Fig. 1 to 6):* Calcific deposits within atherosclerotic plaques were observed grossly in the epicardial coronary arteries in 37 (92%) patients. In 28 patients, radiograms of the heart or of the excised coronary arteries were performed; all patients had calcific deposits in the coronary arteries: 23 (82%), in the left anterior descending, left circumflex, and right coronary arteries, and the other 5 patients, in 2 of these 3 major

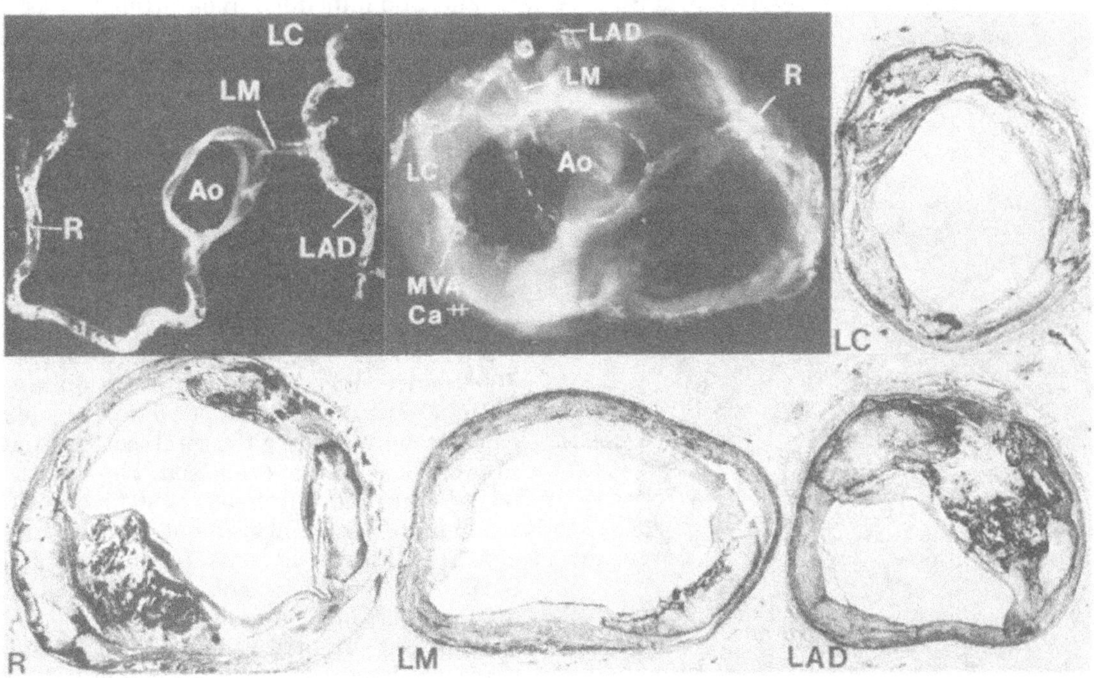

FIGURE 1. Patient 29 (SH #A80-74). Tortuous and heavily calcified coronary arteries in a 95-year-old woman who never had symptoms of cardiac dysfunction and who died from a perforated gastric ulcer. **Top left,** postmortem radiogram of the excised right (R), left main (LM), left anterior descending (LAD), and left circumflex (LC) coronary arteries. **Top center,** radiogram of a portion of the heart after removing the walls of the atria and most of the walls of the ventricles. MVA = mitral valve anulus. **Top right and lower panels,** photomicrographs of coronary arteries at sites of maximal narrowing by calcified atherosclerotic plaques. (Movat stains; magnification ×17, reduced 40%.) This case illustrates extensive calcific deposits in the coronary arteries without significant luminal narrowing.

coronary arteries. In 23 of the 28 patients, the left main coronary artery was studied radiographically: 18 (78%) had calcific deposits. Thus, of 112 major epicardial coronary arteries studied radiographically in 28 patients, 97 (87%) were seen to contain calcific deposits. Of the 37 patients with demonstrated calcific deposits in the epicardial coronary arteries, 26 (70%) also had calcific deposits in either aortic valve cusps or mitral anulus or both. Of the 3 patients without calcium in the coronary arteries, none had calcific deposits in either aortic valve cusps on mital anulus (Fig. 7 and 8).

Coronary arterial atherosclerosis (qualitative studies): At necropsy, 39 of the 40 patients had ≥1 significant cardiac conditions on *gross* examination. One or more of the 4 major (right, left main, left anterior descending, left circumflex) epicardial coronary arteries was narrowed 76 to 100% in XSA by atherosclerotic plaques in 28 (70%) patients; 37 (92%) had grossly palpable calcific deposits in ≥1 major coronary arteries. None of the 28 patients had significant (>75% in XSA) narrowing in the left main coronary artery. Of the other 3 major coronary arteries, 1 was significantly narrowed in 8 patients (29%), 2 were narrowed 76 to 100% by plaques in 15 patients (53%), and 3 arteries were so narrowed in 5 patients (18%). Of the 112 major coronary arteries in these 28 patients, 53 were significantly narrowed, an average of 1.9/4 major coronary arteries per patient. Of the 160 major coronary arteries in the 40 patients, the average number narrowed per patient was 1.3.

Of the 12 patients *with clinical evidence of myocardial ischemia* (angina pectoris or a clinical event diagnosed as or compatible with acute myocardial infarction or both), at least 1 of the 4 major coronary arteries was narrowed 76 to 100% in XSA by plaques: in 10 patients, 2 arteries (right, left anterior descending, or left circumflex) were so narrowed and in the other 2 patients, 3 arteries. Thus, of the 48 major coronary arteries (4 per patient) in these 12 patients, 26 arteries were significantly narrowed, an average of 2.2/4.0 per patient.

Of the 28 patients *without clinical evidence of myocardial ischemia*, at least 1 of the 4 major coronary arteries was narrowed 76 to 100% in XSA by atherosclerotic plaques in 16 patients (57%): in 8 patients, only 1 artery was so narrowed; in 5 patients, 2 arteries; and in 4 patients, 3 arteries. In 12 patients (43%), none of the 4 major coronary arteries was significantly narrowed. Thus, of the 112 major coronary arteries in these 28 patients, 27 (24%) were significantly narrowed, an average of 1.0/4.0 per patient.

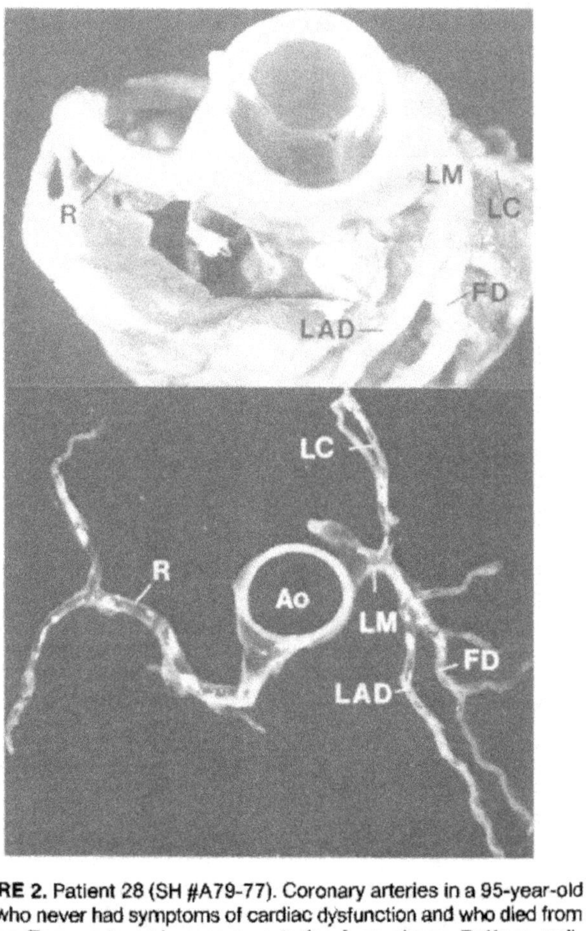

FIGURE 2. Patient 28 (SH #A79-77). Coronary arteries in a 95-year-old man who never had symptoms of cardiac dysfunction and who died from cancer. **Top,** aorta and coronary arteries from above. **Bottom,** radiograms of aortic root (Ao) and excised coronary arteries which contain calcific deposits. FD = first diagonal; LAD = left anterior descending; LC = left circumflex; LM = left main; R = right.

Coronary arterial atherosclerosis (quantitative studies): In 36 patients, including 26 of the 28 in whom 1 or more of the 4 major coronary arteries were significantly narrowed and in 10 of the 12 in whom none of the 4 arteries was significantly narrowed, each of the 4 major coronary arteries was decalcified and cut into 5 mm long segments. Each segment was processed in alcohols and xylene, and imbedded in paraffin. At least 1 histologic section was cut and stained by the Movat method from each segment. Of the 1,789 5 mm segments from the 36 patients (an average of 49 segments per patient [range 30 to 75]), 6 (<1%) were narrowed 96 to 100% in XSA by atherosclerotic plaques; 147 (8%), 76 to 95%; 339 (19%), 51 to 75%; 930 (52%), 26 to 50%; and 367 (21%), 0 to 25%.

A scoring system was utilized to indicate the severity of the coronary narrowing. Every 5 mm long segment was assigned a score of 1 to 4 based on the amount of XSA narrowing by atherosclerotic plaques as follows: 1 = 0 to 25%, 2 = 26 to 50%, 3 = 51 to 75%, and 4 = 76 to 100% narrowing. A total score was obtained for each patient. The mean score per 5 mm segment was then calculated by dividing the total score per patient by the number of segments examined. The total scores for the 36 patients ranged from 53 to 170 (average 107) and the mean score per 5 mm segment, from 1.28 to 3.08 (average 2.15) (Fig. 9). This mean score indicates that each of the 1,789 5 mm segments was narrowed on an average of about 42% in XSA (Fig. 9).

Of the 40 patients, 12 had clinical evidence of myocardial ischemia. Of these 12 patients, the 4 major epicardial coronary arteries were available in their entirety for quantitative studies in 10. Of 467 5 mm coronary segments in these 10 patients, 2 (<1%) were narrowed 96 to 100% in XSA by atherosclerotic plaques; 90 (19%), 76 to 95%; 135 (29%), 51 to 75%; 198 (43%), 26 to 50%;

and 42 (9%), 0 to 25% (Fig. 10). The total score for each of the 10 patients ranged from 88 to 159 (average 120) and the mean score per 5 mm segment of coronary artery, from 2.20 to 3.08 (average 2.59), indicating that each 5 mm segment was narrowed an average of approximately 55% in XSA.

Of the 28 patients without clinical evidence of myocardial ischemia, the 4 major coronary arteries were available for quantitative studies in 26. Of 1,322 5 mm coronary segments examined in these patients, 4 (<1%) were narrowed 96 to 100% in XSA by atherosclerotic plaques; 63 (5%) were narrowed 76 to 95%; 206 (16%), 51 to 75%; 727 (55%), 26 to 50%; and 322 (24%), 0 to 25% (Fig. 10). The total score for each patient ranged from 53 to 170 (average 98) and the mean score per 5 mm segment, from 1.28 to 2.85 (average 2.01) (Fig. 9), indicating that each of the 1,322 5 mm segments was narrowed an average of about 38% in XSA. Of these 26 patients, ≥1 of the 4 major coronary arteries was significantly narrowed in 16. Of the 857 5 mm coronary segments examined in the 26 patients, 4 segments (<1%) had lumens narrowed 96 to 100% in XSA by plaques; 63 (7%), 76 to 95%; 183 (22%), 51 to 75%; 464 (54%), 26 to 50%; and 143 (17%), 0 to 25%. The total score for each of the 16 patients ranged from 56 to 170 (average 111) and the mean score per 5 mm segment, from 1.77 to 2.85 (mean 2.20). Thus, each of the 857 5 mm segments was narrowed an average of approximately 44% in XSA. In

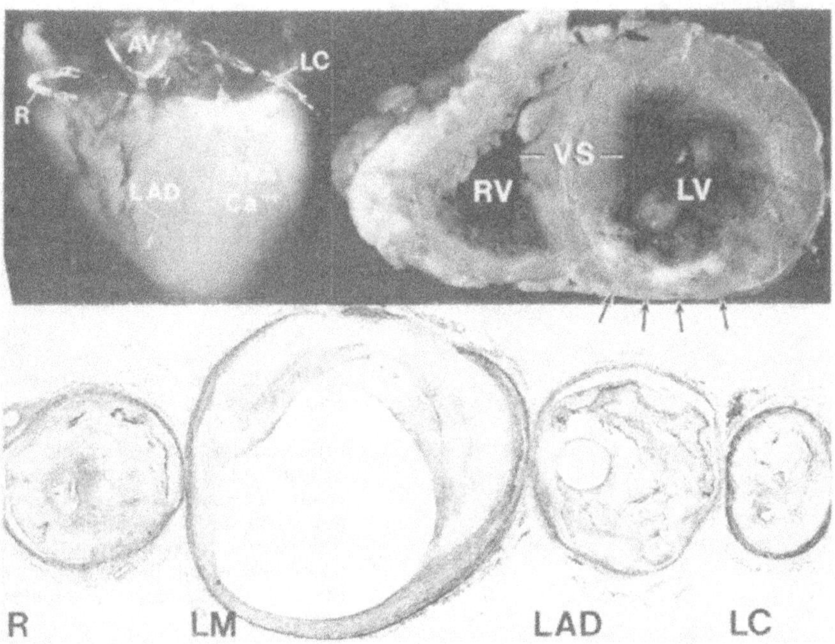

FIGURE 3. Patient 22 (LRC #5). Heart and coronary arteries in a 93-year-old woman who was hospitalized with worsening chronic congestive heart failure. **Top left,** postmortem radiogram showing calcific deposits in the right (R), left anterior descending (LAD), and left circumflex (LC) coronary arteries and in the mitral valve anulus (MVA) and aortic valve. **Top right,** view of right (RV) and left (LV) ventricles and ventricular septum (VS) showing a transmural scar (**arrows**). **Bottom,** coronary arteries at sites of maximal narrowing. LM = left main. (Movat stains; magnification ×17, reduced 40%.)

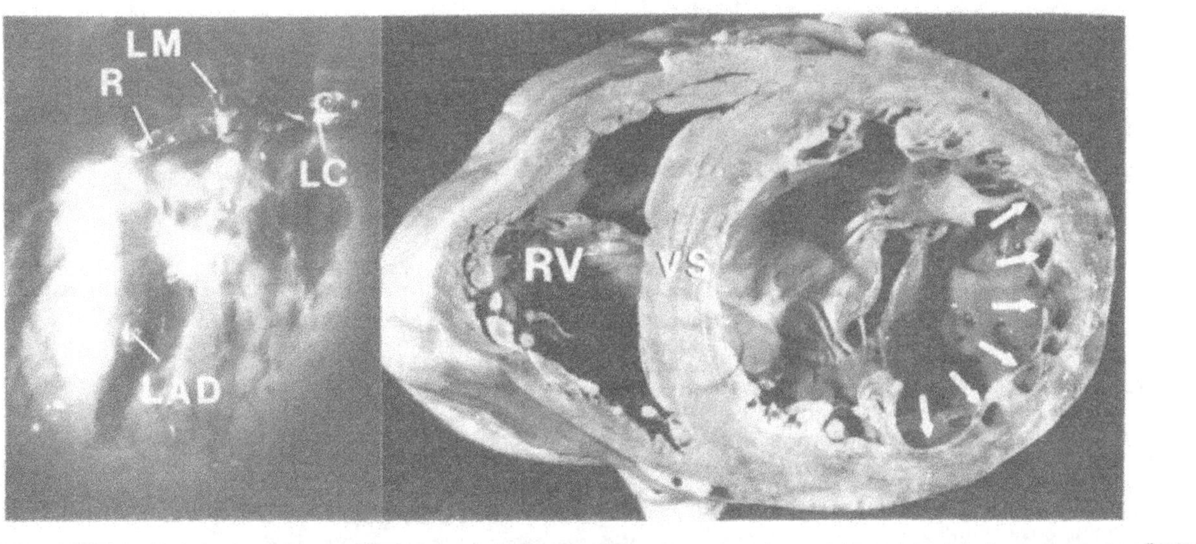

FIGURE 4. Patient 13 (LRC #3). This 91-year-old woman had a "typical" clinical acute myocardial infarct, which was fatal. **Left,** postmortem radiogram showing calcific deposits in the right (R), left main (LM), left anterior descending (LAD), and left circumflex (LC) coronary arteries. **Right,** view of left and right (RV) ventricles showing transmural necrosis and fibrosis (**arrows**) and dilated ventricles. VS = ventricular septum.

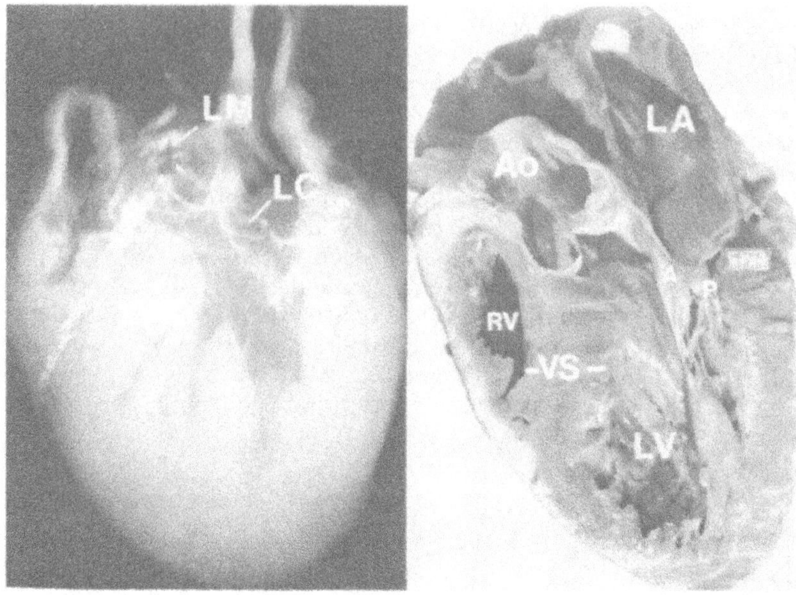

FIGURE 5. Patient 8 (SH #A82-1). This 90-year-old woman had no symptoms of cardiac dysfunction and died from a ruptured fusiform abdominal aortic aneurysm. **Left,** postmortem radiogram of the entire heart showing calcific deposits in the left anterior descending (LAD), left circumflex (LC), and left main (LM) coronary arteries. **Right,** view of heart cut in an anteroposterior fashion (M-mode or long-axis 2-dimensional echocardiographic view) showing a dilated left atrium (LA) and left ventricle (LV). A and P = anterior and posterior mitral valve leaflets; Ao = aorta; RV = right ventricle; VS = ventricular septum.

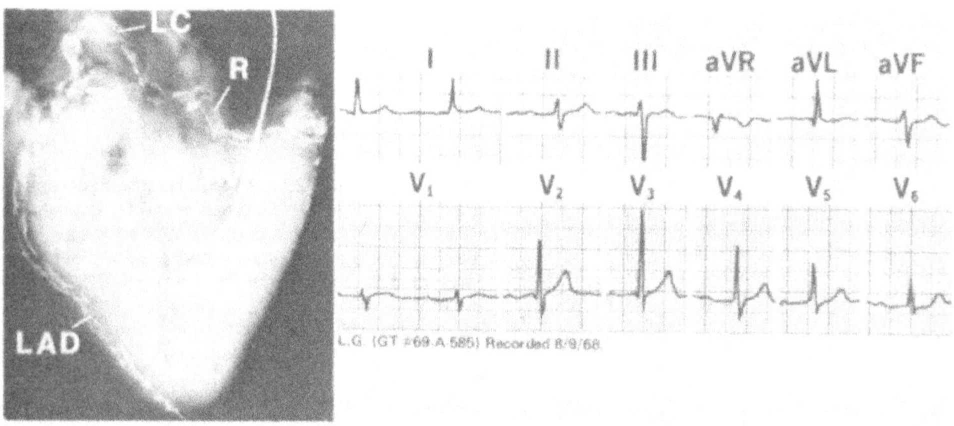

FIGURE 6. Patient 34 (GT #69A-585). This 97-year-old man had complete heart block and had a pacemaker inserted when he was 91 years old. **Left,** radiogram of heart at necropsy showing calcific deposits in the left anterior descending (LAD), left circumflex (LC), and right (R) coronary arteries, and a pacemaker wire in the right ventricle (RV). LV = left ventricle. **Right,** electrocardiogram.

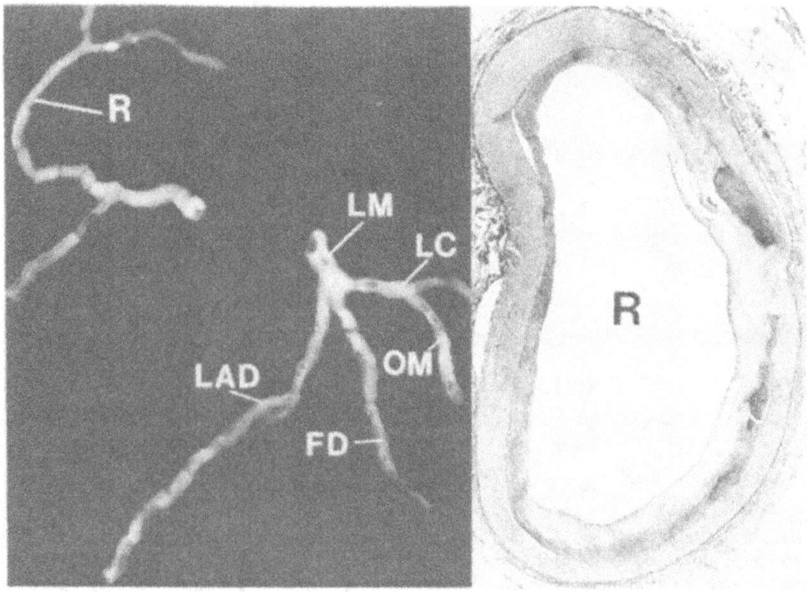

FIGURE 7. Patient 30 (DCGH #68A80). This 96-year-old woman had chronic congestive heart failure from dilated cardiomyopathy. Her total serum cholesterol level was 108 mg/dl. **Left,** postmortem radiogram of the right (R), left main (LM), left anterior descending (LAD), left circumflex (LC), first diagonal (FD), and left obtuse marginal (OM) coronary arteries showing no calcific deposits. **Right,** right coronary artery section devoid of calcium or narrowing. (Movat stain; magnification ×16, reduced 23%.)

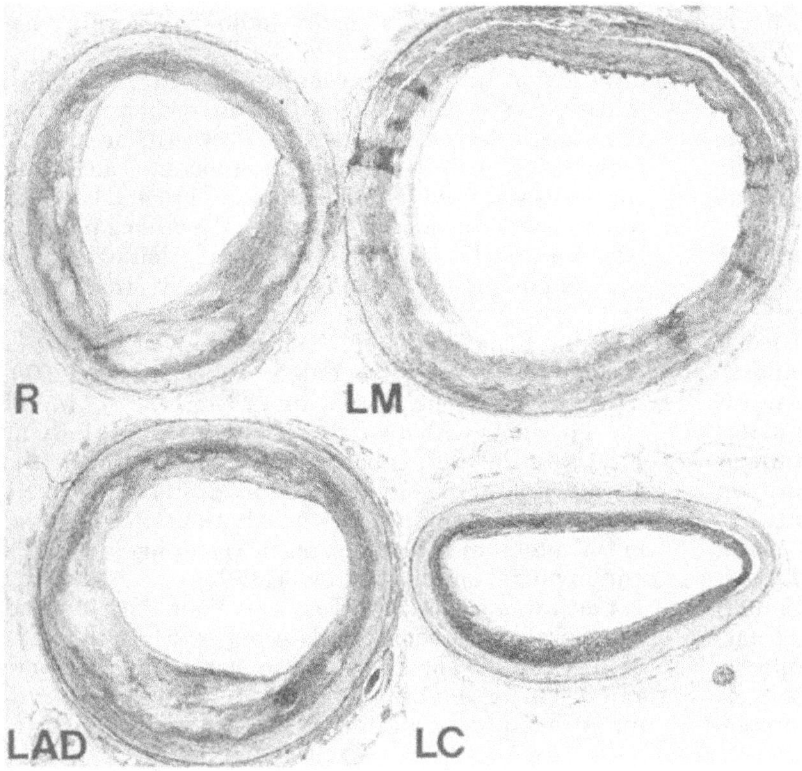

FIGURE 8. Patient 40 (GT #70A301). Right (R), left main (LM), left anterior descending (LAD), and left circumflex (LC) coronary arteries at sites of maximal narrowing in a 103-year-old woman. She never had evidence of cardiac dysfunction and died from complications of a duodenal ulcer. The coronary arteries are devoid of calcium and of significant narrowing. (Elastic van Gieson's stain; magnification ×16, reduced 31%.)

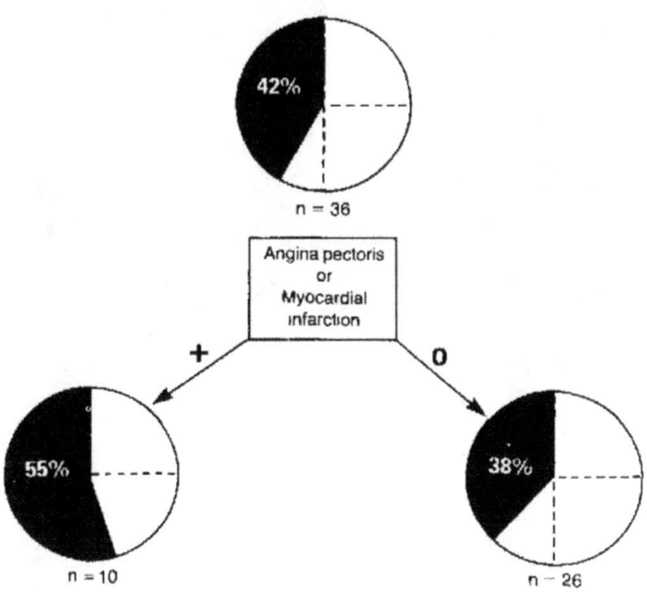

FIGURE 9. Mean percent cross-sectional area narrowing by atherosclerotic plaques in 1,789 5 mm segments of the 4 major epicardial coronary arteries in 36 necropsy patients aged 90 years and older, 10 of whom had angina pectoris or acute myocardial infarction or both and 26 of whom did not. The mean percentage of narrowing for each 5 mm segment differs significantly in the group with clinical evidence of myocardial ischemia (55%) and the group without such evidence (p <0.05).

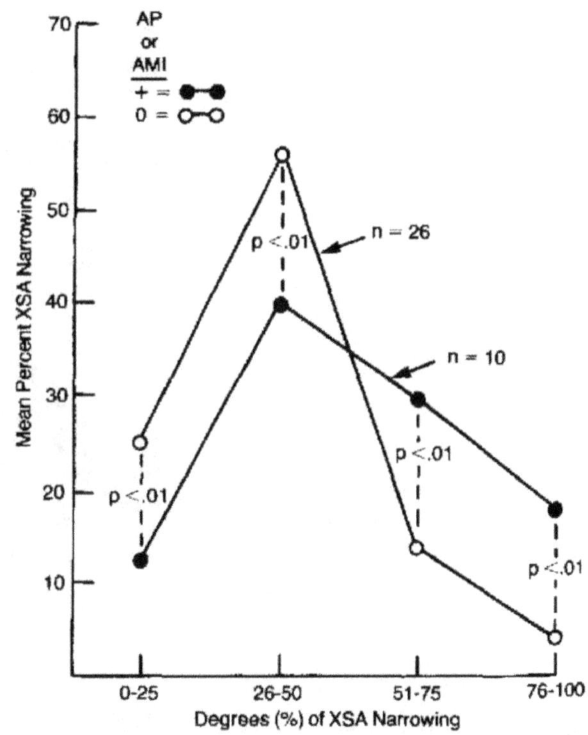

FIGURE 10. Mean percent cross-sectional area (XSA) narrowing by atherosclerotic plaques in the 5 mm segments of the right, left main, left anterior descending, and left circumflex coronary arteries in the 36 patients in whom the 4 major coronary arteries in their entirety were available for examination. The 36 patients were classified into 10 with and 26 without clinical evidence of myocardial ischemia. For each of the 4 categories of narrowing, a highly significant (p <0.01) difference in the amount of narrowing was observed.

the 10 patients without significant narrowing, 465 5 mm segments were examined: 23 (5%) were narrowed 51 to 75% in XSA by plaque; 263 (57%), 26 to 50%; and 179 (38%) ≤25%. The total score for each of these 10 patients ranged from 53 to 138 (average 85) and the mean score per 5 mm segment, from 1.28 to 2.07 (average 1.66). Thus, each of the 465 segments was narrowed an average of approximately 29%.

Left ventricular fibrosis or necrosis or both: Of the 40 patients, 18 (45%) had ≥1 grossly visible foci of transmural (involvement of all the inner one half and a portion of or all of the outer one half of left ventricular wall) sites of necrosis or fibrosis or both (Fig. 3 and 4). Of the 18 patients, 5 had foci of transmural necrosis only, 8 had transmural scars only, 4 had transmural foci of necrosis and fibrosis, and 1 had transmural fibrosis and subendocardial (involvement of less than the inner one half of the left ventricular wall) necrosis. Of the 23 transmural infarcts in 18 patients, 11 (2 acute, 11 healed [10 patients]) were "small"; 9 (7 acute, 2 healed [8 patients]) were "large"; and 2 (both healed [2 patients]) were "intermediate" in size. All 18 patients had narrowing of 76 to 100% in XSA by atherosclerotic plaque of ≥1 of the 4 major epicardial coronary arteries. None of the 10 patients with fatal acute myocardial infarction had a thrombus in a major coronary artery at necropsy.

Valvular and anular calcification (Fig. 11 to 16): Grossly visible calcific deposits were present in ≥1 of the 3 aortic valve cusps (on their aortic surfaces) in 22 patients (55%): in 20 patients, the amount of calcium on the cusps was mild (graded 1+ or 2+/4+) and valvular function was considered normal; in the other 2 patients (Cases 1 and 17) (Fig. 11), the cuspal calcific deposits were extensive (4+/4+) and cuspal mobility was limited, and the orifice in each appeared severely stenotic.[5]

Of the 40 patients, 19 (47%) had grossly visible *mitral anular calcific deposits:* graded 1+ in 5 patients (26%), 2+ in 5 (26%), 3+ in 5 (26%), and 4+ in 4 (22%).[6] In 1 of the 4 patients with 4+ mitral anular calcium (Patient 11), the mitral orifice appeared stenotic (Fig. 13). Of the 40 patients, 26 (65%) had calcific deposits in the aortic valve or mitral anulus or both: in both aortic valve and mitral anulus in 16 (62%), in aortic valve only in 7 (27%), and in mitral anulus only in 3 (11%).

Cardiac amyloidosis (Fig. 17): Four patients had extensive amyloid deposits detected grossly in the walls of all 4 cardiac chambers and in many other body organs.[8] The extent of the deposits in each patient produced symptoms and signs of cardiac dysfunction,

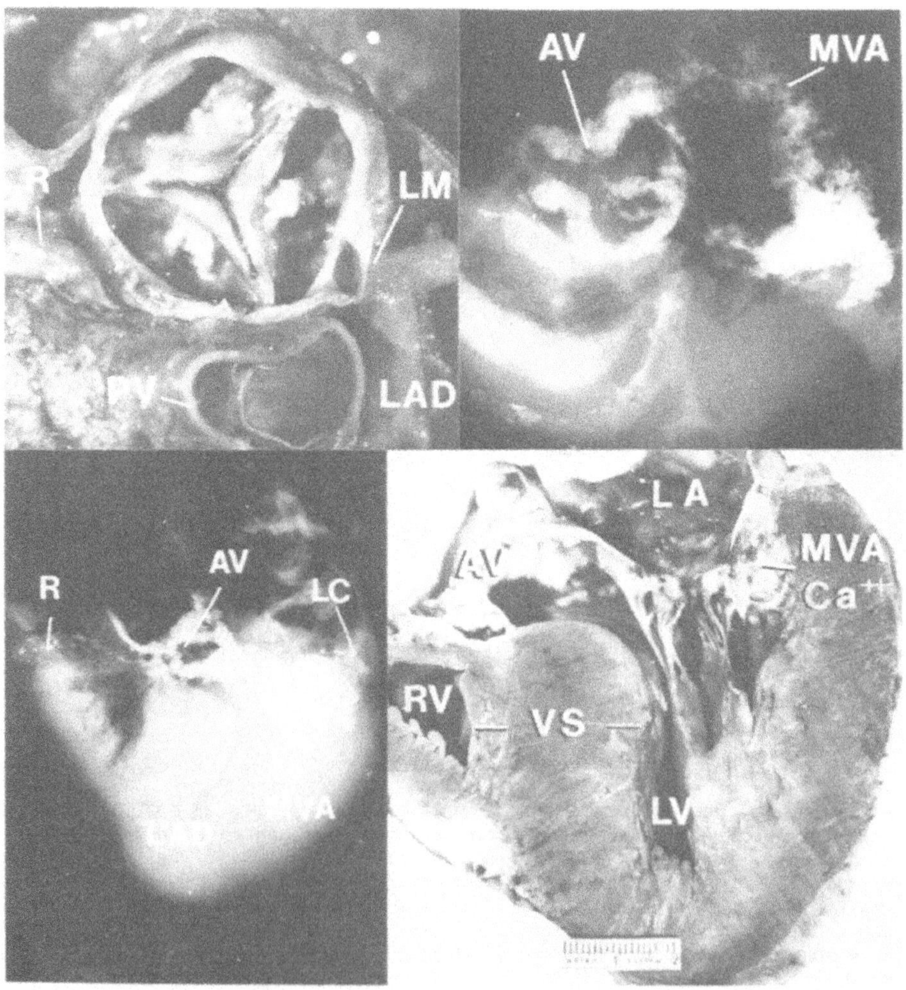

FIGURE 11. Patient 17 (GT #78A58). A 92-year-old woman with clinically recognized and eventually fatal aortic valve stenosis. **Top left,** stenotic aortic valve from above. PV = pulmonic valve; R = right; LM = left main; LAD = left anterior descending coronary arteries. **Top right,** postmortem radiogram showing heavy calcific deposits in the aortic valve (AV) and in mitral valve anular (MVA) region. **Bottom left,** radiogram of the heart at necropsy showing calcific deposits in the coronary arteries, in the aortic valve, and in the mitral anular region. **Bottom right,** long-axis view of heart (M-mode or 2-dimensional long-axis view) showing a small left ventricular (LV) cavity, a thickened and "sigmoid-shaped" ventricular septum (VS), and the stenotic aortic valve just above the right ventricular (RV) outflow tract. LA = left atrium.

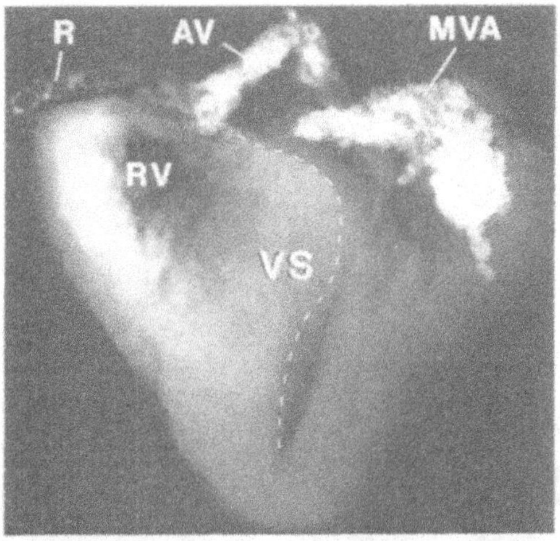

FIGURE 12. Patient 31 (GT #68A-367). Radiogram of the heart showing heavy calcific deposits in the aortic valve (AV), mitral valve anulus (MVA), and right (R) coronary artery. The ventricular septum (VS) has a *S* or sigmoid shape (**dashed line**). RV = right ventricle.

manifested primarily by chronic congestive cardiac failure. The presence of extensive amyloidosis was confirmed by histologic examination. At least 5 other patients also had amyloid deposits. The extent of the cardiac amyloid deposits in these 5 patients, however, was minimal and detectable only by histologic examination. Among the 40 patients, histologic sections (1 to 8 per patient [mean 3]) of left ventricular myocardium extending from endocardium to epicardium were examined in 37: 9 of the 37 patients (24%) had amyloid deposits, which were "massive" in 4 and minimal in 5.

Idiopathic dilated cardiomyopathy: One patient (Case 30) had a large heart (700 g), dilated ventricular cavities without foci of myocardial fibrosis or necrosis, normal valves and pericardia, epicardial coronary arteries virtually free of atherosclerotic plaques, and chronic congestive heart failure. Although a history of systemic hypertension was absent, the blood pressure in the last month of life was recorded as 140/90 mm Hg. The kidneys, however, were near normal. This patient, therefore, fulfills criteria for diagnosis of idiopathic dilated cardiomyopathy. The patient apparently had habitually consumed excessive quantities of alcohol.

Obliterative "pericarditis": Two patients (Cases 14 and 34) had obliterated space between visceral and parietal pericardia by adhesions, some calcified. One (Patient 14) had had talcum powder sprinkled on the epicardium 29 years before death at operation (Beck procedure) for relief of angina pectoris.[9] This patient was the only 1 of the 40 who had undergone a cardiovascular operation. The cause of the obliterative pericardial disease in the other patient was not determined.

Disease of aorta: In 34 of the 40 patients, the status of the aorta was known. In all 34, the aorta was dilated in both its transverse and longitudinal dimensions. The latter produced varying degrees of tortuosity. Some degree of atherosclerotic plaquing was present in the aorta in all 34 patients. The most extensive plaquing involved the abdominal portion. Three patients (Cases 8, 13, and 34) had atherosclerotic fusiform abdominal aortic aneurysms with intraaneurysmal thrombus; death in 1 (Patient 8) was secondary to aneurysmal rupture. One patient (Case 25) had an atherosclerotic fusiform aneurysm of the descending thoracic aorta which ruptured, and 1 patient (Case 11) had a dissection limited to descending thoracic aorta; death was due to rupture of the aneurysm into the esophagus.[10]

Cerebrovascular disease: Extensive cerebral arterial atherosclerosis was described in the necropsy reports in each of the 4 patients (Cases 30, 31, 33, and 38) with clinical strokes.

Pulmonary embolism: Massive pulmonary embolism, that is, thromboembolic material in 1 or both major right and left main pulmonary arteries, was observed at necropsy in 2 patients (Cases 10 and 26). Both had underlying chronic obstructive pulmonary disease.

Clinical observations: *Evidence of coronary heart disease:* Of the 40 patients, 12 (30%) had definite or probable clinical evidence of coronary heart disease as manifested by angina pectoris or acute myocardial infarction or both: 1 patient (Case 14) had angina only, 1

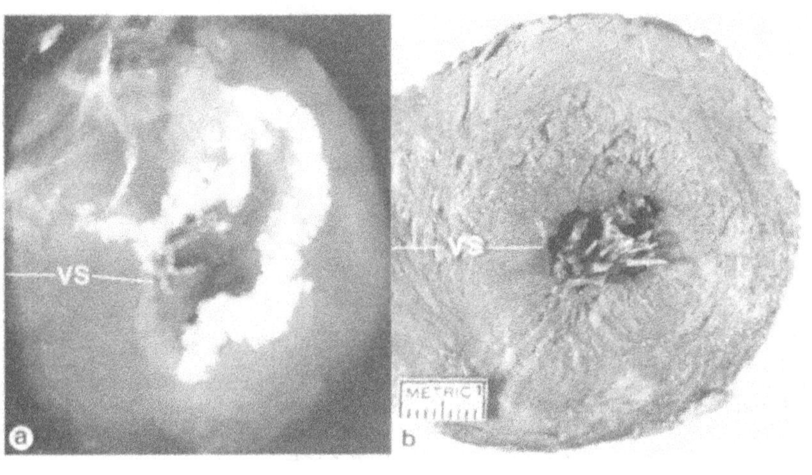

FIGURE 13. Patient 11 (GT #80-A-126). A 90-year-old woman with heavy mitral valve anular calcific deposits which reduced the mitral valve orifice to <1 cm in diameter (**a**). The unusual feature of the mitral calcium in this patient was that it not only was located behind the posterior mitral leaflet (mitral anular region) but it also extended across the anterior mitral leaflet nearly producing a letter *O*, as has been described previously.[7] She died from rupture of a descending thoracic aortic aneurysm. VS = ventricular septum. **b,** view of the left ventricle at the level of the tips of the mitral leaflets showing a very small cavity.

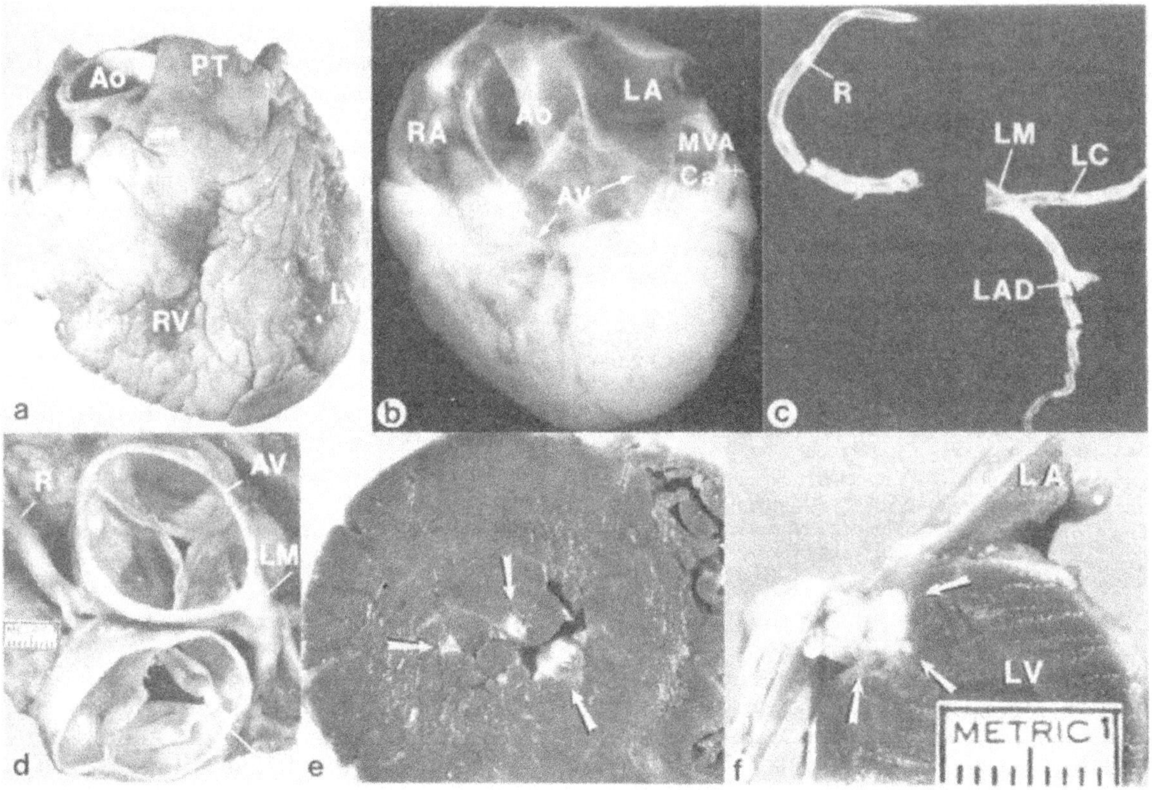

FIGURE 14. Patient 32 (SH #A81-62). A 97-year-old woman who never had clinical evidence of cardiac dysfunction and who died from cancer. **a,** external view of anterior surface of the heart showing an increased amount of subepicardial fat. Ao = aorta; LV = left ventricle; PT = pulmonary trunk; RV = right ventricle. **b,** postmortem radiogram showing calcific deposits in the mitral valve anulus (MVA) and aortic valve (AV). LA = left atrium; RA = right atrium. **c,** radiogram of the excised coronary arteries showing a few calcific deposits. LAD = left anterior descending; LC = left circumflex; LM = left main; R = right. **d,** view of aortic valve (AV) and pulmonic valve (PV) from above. **e,** view of left ventricle showing calcific deposits (**arrows**) in the papillary muscles. **f,** calcific deposits in mitral anular region.

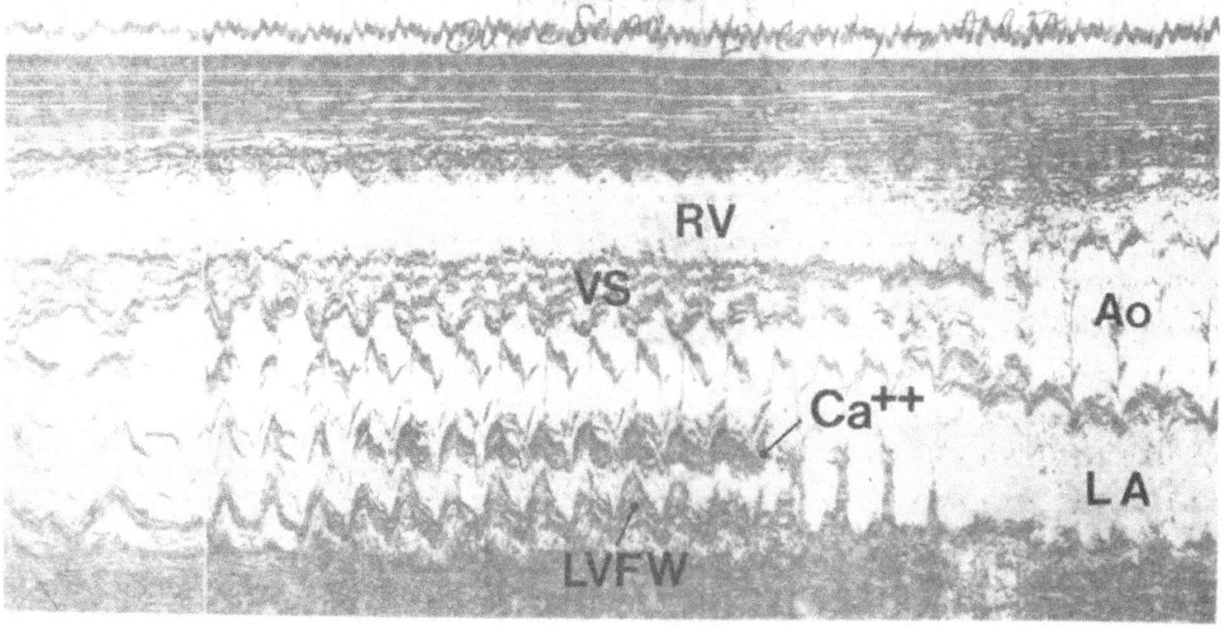

FIGURE 15. Patient 32 (SH #80-18). M-mode echocardiogram obtained 10 months before death from the patient whose heart is shown in Figure 14. The ascending aorta (Ao) has a larger diameter than does the left atrium (LA). The left ventricular (LV) cavity is small. Calcium is present in the mitral anular region. (We thank Dr. Robert Montgomery, Bethesda, Maryland, for allowing us to show this echocardiogram from his patient.)

(Case 37) had angina and a nonfatal acute myocardial infarct 2 years before death. (This patient died 24 hours after onset of increased dyspnea and vague chest pain but at necropsy no myocardial necrosis was visible histologically.) One patient (Case 2) had angina and a fatal acute myocardial infarct, and 9 patients had fatal acute myocardial infarcts which in each was the first one seen clinically. The clinical records regarding anginal attacks in the 3 patients are deficient in details: 2 patients (Cases 2 and 37) were stated to have had angina for "many years" and the third patient (Case 14) had angina for 29 years (since age 63). In none of the 3 patients was there information regarding the frequency of the anginal attacks and only 1 (Patient 37) was known to have taken nitroglycerin tablets.

Ten patients had deaths compatible with acute myocardial infarction. Of these 10 patients, however, only 3 (Cases 13, 16, and 23) had typical "crushing" substernal chest pain associated with typical electrocardiographic changes and enzyme elevations. The remaining 7 patients all were hospitalized because of some acute change in their status; however, acute myocardial infarction was never clearly established in these patients until necropsy. Only 5 of the 7 had chest pain, and it was atypical and not severe. Four had acute worsening of dyspnea. None had typical electrocardiographic features of acute myocardial infarction, but 5 had complete left bundle branch block at admission to the hospital. In 5 of these 7 patients in whom serum enzymes (creatine phosphokinase, lactic dehydrogenase, serum glutamic-oxaloacetic transaminase) were determined, the values were elevated in 4. Of the 14 patients with transmural left ventricular scars, only 1 had a clinical event diagnosed as acute myocardial infarction.

Chronic congestive heart failure was described in 8 patients (20%). In 4 patients (Cases 4, 21, 27, and 34) its cause, as determined initially by necropsy, was diffuse cardiac amyloidosis: in 1 patient (Case 17), its cause was aortic valve stenosis, which was diagnosed clinically; 1 patient (Case 14) had obliterative pericardial disease from the Beck procedure 25 years earlier[9]; 1 patient (Case 30) had cardiomegaly (660 g heart) of uncertain cause clinically (at necropsy the condition was considered idiopathic dilated cardiomyopathy); 1 patient (Case 22) also had congestive heart failure of uncertain cause clinically but at necropsy had a transmural left ventricular scar and severe narrowing of all 3 major epicardial coronary arteries. Of the 8 patients with chronic congestive heart failure, all had cardiomegaly at necropsy and 6 had histories of systemic hypertension during life.

Systemic hypertension: Information regarding "a history of hypertension" or an actual indirect systemic arterial blood pressure recording in the last year of life was available in 39 of the 40 patients: 19 (51%) had "a history" of systemic hypertension; of the 34 patients with actual blood pressure recordings, only 7 had systolic pressures >140 mm Hg or diastolic pressures >90 mm Hg. Of the 39 patients on whom information was available, 27 (69%) had either "a history of hypertension" or a recorded elevated blood pressure in the last year of life. Of the other 12 patients, only 1 (Case 23) had unequivocal cardiomegaly without explanation.

Diabetes mellitus: Five patients, all women, had diabetes mellitus. In 2, its duration was known: 20 years (Patient 5) and 40 years (Patient 20). One patient (Case 5) was treated with insulin; 1 (Case 9) with diet alone; 1 (Case 2) with diet plus tolbutamide; in 2 patients the type therapy received was unknown. Although 3 patients (Cases 2, 5, and 20) had transmural left ventricular scars, none had clinical events compatible with acute myocardial infarction.

Precordial murmurs: Of the 40 patients, 25 (62%) had had precordial murmurs. In all 25, the murmur was

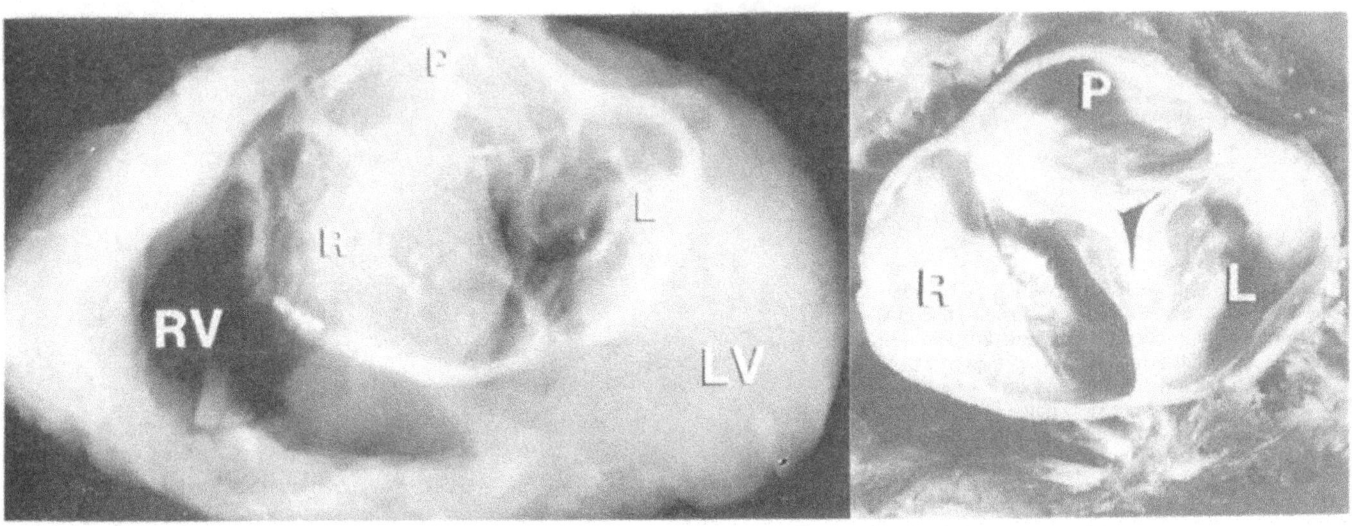

FIGURE 16. Patient 28 (SH #79-77). A 95-year-old man who never had symptoms of cardiac dysfunction and died from sarcoma. The coronary arteries are shown in Figure 2. **Left,** radiogram of heart at necropsy showing considerable enlargement of the aorta in comparison to the ventricles. LV = left ventricle; RV = right ventricle; R = right, L = left, and P = posterior sinuses of Valsalva. **Right,** aortic valve from above. The coronary arteries had been excised before the radiogram and photographs were taken.

described as systolic: apical only in 6; left sternal border only in 8; basal only in 2; all 3 locations in 3; and unspecified in 6. Only 1 (Case 9) of the 25 patients had both diastolic and systolic precordial murmurs. The diastolic murmur appeared to represent mild aortic regurgitation from systemic hypertension. The intensity of the murmur in the 24 patients with purely systolic murmurs was grade 1/6 in 2 patients, grade 2/6 in 5, grade 3/6 in 8, grade 4/6 in 4, and unspecified in 5. The cause of the precordial systolic murmurs was variable and often unclear. Of the 24 patients, 17 (71%) had calcific deposits in either the mitral valve anulus or aortic valve cusps or both: in mitral anulus only in none, in aortic valve only in 4, and in both mitral anulus and aortic valve in 13. In only 4 of the 17 patients, however, was the extent of calcium grade 3 to 4/6. In contrast, of the 15 patients without precordial murmurs recorded, 8 (53%) had calcific deposits in either mitral anulus or aortic valve cusps or both: in 3, the extent of the calcific deposits was either grade 3 or 4/6, but 4 of these 8 patients underwent precordial examination while in severe respiratory distress (3 patients) or in coma (1 patient). The blood hematocrit level ranged from 29 to 46% (mean 39) in the 18 patients with precordial murmurs and known hematocrit values, and from 30 to 57% (mean 38) in the 10 without precordial murmurs but known hematocrit values.

Noncardiac vascular disease: Five patients had strokes, which were fatal in 4 (Cases 12, 31, 33, and 38) and nonfatal in 1 (Case 30). Of the 3 patients with fusiform abdominal aortic aneurysms, only the 1 (Case 8) which ruptured was diagnosed during life. Neither the patient (Case 25) with a ruptured fusiform aneurysm of thoracic aorta nor the patient (Case 11) with rupture of the descending thoracic aorta into the esophagus had the condition diagnosed during life.[10] Five patients (Cases 1, 3, 9, 20, and 25) had leg claudication, requiring amputations in 2 (Cases 3 and 9) for gangrene. In the 2 patients with massive pulmonary embolism, this condition was suspected clinically.

Electrocardiographic data (Fig. 18 and 19) (Tables III and IV): Information on electrocardiograms recorded at age 90 years or later was available in 30 of the 40 patients. In 24 patients, the electrocardiograms were available for reexamination but in the other 6 patients, only the electrocardiographic reports were available. Of the 30 patients, 3 (Cases 1, 3, and 5) had electrocardiograms recorded during the acute illness (recordings 4, 9, and 7 days, respectively, before death). The illnesses, although not diagnosed clinically, were seen at necropsy

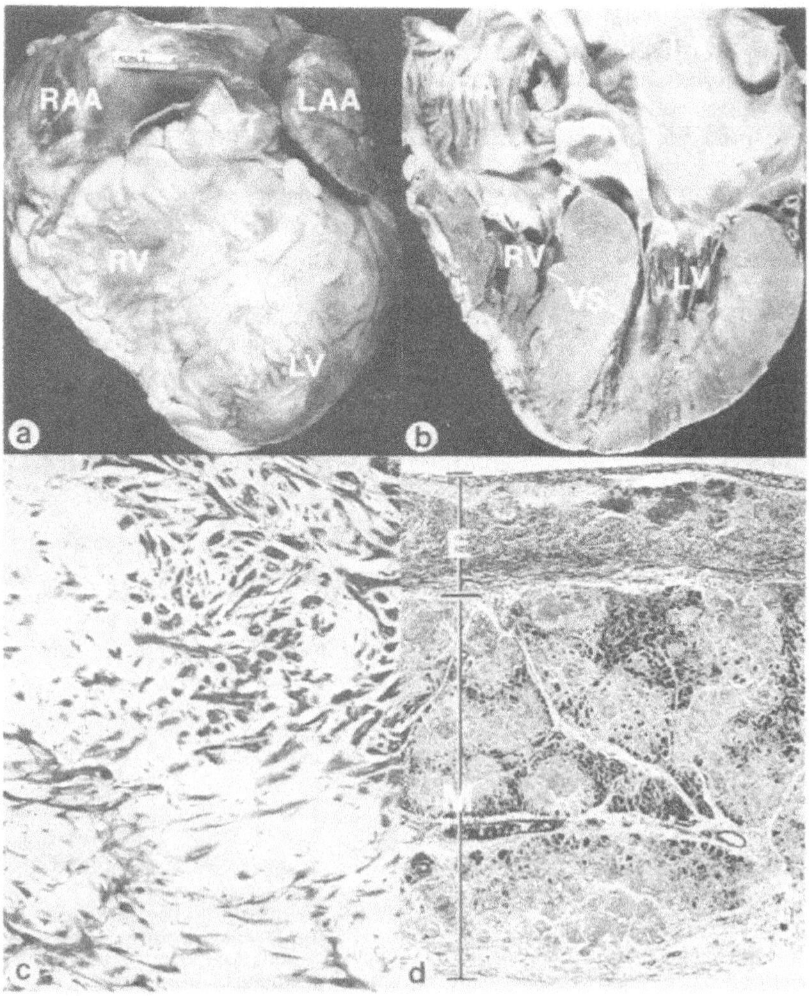

FIGURE 17. Patient 4 (DCGH #69A391), a 90-year-old man with chronic, eventually fatal congestive heart failure from clinically unrecognized cardiac amyloidosis. **a,** external view of the heart showing a prominent left ventricle (LV) and left atrial appendage (LAA). PT = pulmonary trunk; RAA = right atrial appendage; RV = right ventricle. **b,** right-to-left longitudinal cut of the heart (4-chamber, 2-dimensional echocardiographic view) showing thickened ventricular walls and dilated right (RA) and left (LA) atria. VS = ventricular septum. **c,** photomicrograph of a portion of the left ventricle showing extensive amyloid deposits. **d,** photomicrograph of LA wall showing amyloid deposits in endocardium (E) and in myocardium (M). (Hematoxylin-eosin stains; magnification ×100 (**c**) and ×25 (**d**), both reduced 35%.)

to clearly result from acute myocardial infarction. The electrocardiograms in all 3, however, disclosed only atrial fibrillation and complete left bundle branch block and these findings in all 3 patients were known to be present before the fatal acute myocardial infarction. The electrocardiograms in the other 27 patients were not recorded during periods of acute myocardial ischemia. Of the 30 patients on whom electrocardiographic information was available, 8 had clinical evidence of heart disease and 22 did not; the findings are summarized in Table III.

The QRS voltage in all 12 leads in each of 24 patients is summarized in Table IV (Fig. 19). The total 12-lead QRS voltage ranged from 82 to 251 mm (mean 151) (10 mm = 1 mV). In the 19 women, the total voltage ranged from 82 to 251 mm (mean 158), and in the 5 men, from 105 to 154 mm (mean 101) ($p < 0.05$). The total 12-lead QRS voltage did not correlate with either heart ($r = -0.01$) or body weight ($r = -0.2$). The 24 patients in whom the total 12-lead QRS voltage was measured were separated into 2 groups: 8 patients in whom clinical evidence of cardiac dysfunction was present (coronary heart disease in 5, massive cardiac amyloid in 2, aortic valve stenosis in 1) and 16 patients without such evidence. Comparison of the total QRS voltage in the 8 patients with and in the 16 patients without clinical evidence of heart disease disclosed no significant difference (mean 147 mm versus mean 152 mm). Breakdown on the 8 patients with cardiac dysfunction did show some differences: the total 12-lead QRS voltage in the 5 patients with angina pectoris or acute myocardial infarction (Patients 1, 3, 5, 14, and 37) ranged from 123 to 163 mm (mean 143); in the 2 patients with massive cardiac amyloidosis (Patients 21 and 27) it was 102 and 117 mm (mean 109); and in the 1 patient with aortic valve stenosis (Patient 17) it was 238 mm.

Of 29 patients on whom information was available, 18 (62%) received *digitalis* and only 2 appeared to have evidence of digitalis toxicity.

Blood hematocrit levels in the last month of life, known in 29 patients, ranged from 29 to 57% (mean 38).

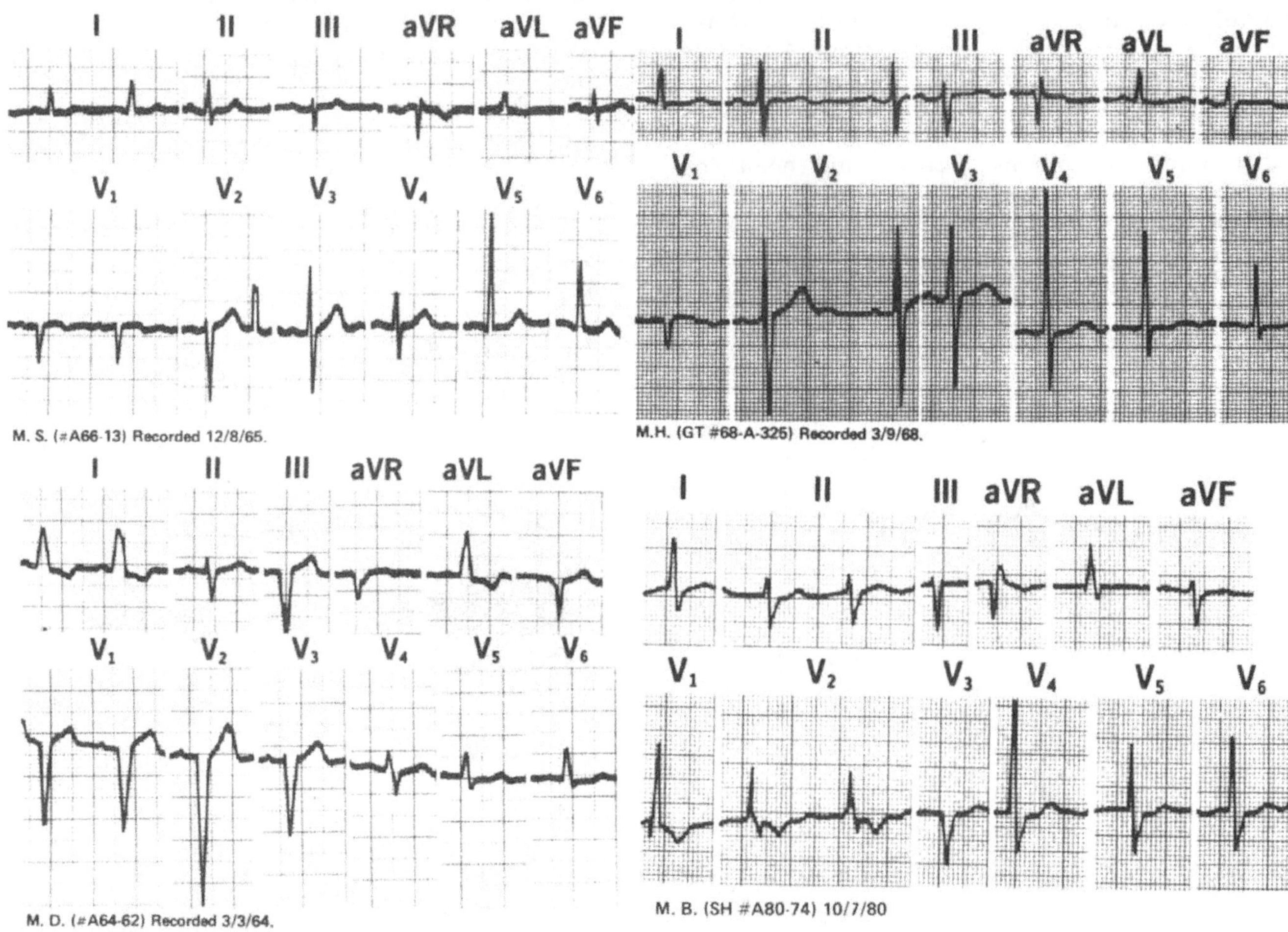

FIGURE 18. Electrocardiograms in 4 patients, each recorded at age 90 years or older. None ever had symptoms of cardiac dysfunction and each died from noncardiac conditions. **Top left,** Patient 7 (A66-13). The electrocardiogram was recorded 43 days before death and it is normal (heart weight 270 g). **Top right,** Patient 15 (GT #68A325). The electrocardiogram was recorded 11 days before death and it shows left QRS axis deviation and a slightly prolonged P-R interval (heart weight 400 g). **Bottom left,** Patient 36 (A64-62). This electrocardiogram was recorded 28 days before death and it shows left-axis deviation and complete left bundle branch block (heart weight 320 g). **Bottom right,** Patient 29 (SH #A80-74). This electrocardiogram was recorded 128 days before death and it shows atrial fibrillation, left-axis deviation, and complete right bundle branch block (heart weight 440 g).

Total serum cholesterol levels recorded at age 90 years or older, available in 10 patients, ranged from 108 to 283 mg/100 ml (mean 220).

Total serum protein values, available in 18 patients, ranged from 5.2 to 8.1 g/100 ml (mean 6.8). Serum albumin values, available in 19 patients, ranged from 2.0 to 4.5 g/100 ml (mean 3.3).

Blood urea nitrogen values, available in 27 patients, ranged from 7 to 70 g/100 ml (mean 33). Most values were obtained during the last month of life and some patients were clearly dehydrated at the time.

Modes of death: Of the 40 patients, 18 (45%) appeared to have died from consequences of cardiac disease, 7 (17%) from noncardiac but vascular problems, and 15 (38%) from noncardiac and nonvascular problems.

Of the 18 patients with cardiac causes of death, 10 had acute transmural myocardial infarcts, 1 (Case 14) had chronic congestive cardiac failure after healing of acute transmural myocardial infarcts, and 1 (Case 37) died in ventricular fibrillation after 24 hours of chest pain and at necropsy was shown to have severe coronary atherosclerosis without myocardial necrosis. Fatal congestive heart failure was due to aortic valve stenosis in 1 (Patient 17), to cardiac amyloidosis in 4 (Patients 4, 21, 27, and 34), and to idiopathic dilated cardiomyopathy in 1 (Patient 30). Of the 7 patients with noncardiac and nonvascular causes of death, 4 (Patients 12, 31, 33, and 38) died from complications of strokes, and the other 3, from rupture of aortic aneurysms (Patients 8, 11, and 25). Of the 15 patients with noncardiac and nonvascular causes of death, 7 (Cases 6, 7, 9, 28, 32, 35, and 36) died from various malignant neoplasms; 3 from nonneoplastic gastrointestional problems (bowel obstruction from adhesions in 1 [Patient 15], perforated gastric ulcer in 1 [Patient 29], and active duodenal ulcer in 1 [Patient 40]); 2 (Patients 24 and 39) from complications of bone fractures after falls; 2 (Patients 10 and 26) from massive pulmonary emboli superimposed on chronic obstructive pulmonary disease; and 1 (Patient 18) from uncertain cause. Of the 7 patients with fatal malignant neoplasms, 3 (Cases 6, 7 and 28) had 2 neoplasms and 4 (Cases 9, 32, 35, and 36) had 1 neoplasm.

Discussion

As in any body organ or tissue, certain changes take place in the cardiovascular system as life progresses. Some of these changes allow easy identification of the very elderly heart when examining cardiac specimens as unknowns. The "normal" elderly heart has relatively small ventricular cavities and relatively large atria and great arteries (Fig. 20). The ascending aorta and left atrium, in comparison with the relatively small left ventricular cavity, appear particularly large. The cor-

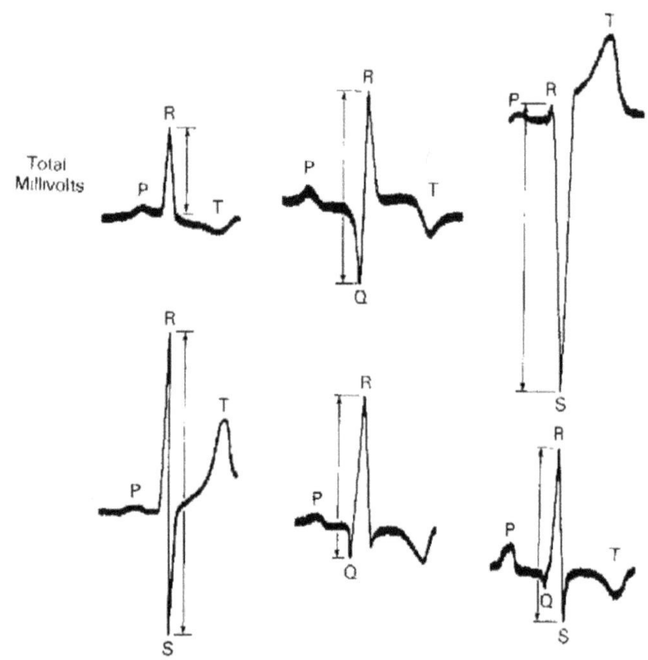

FIGURE 19. Various QRS complexes, and how each was measured. (Reproduced with permission from Siegel RJ, Roberts WC: Electrocardiographic observations in severe aortic valve stenosis: correlative necropsy study to clinical, hemodynamic, and ECG variables demonstrating relation of 12-lead QRS amplitude to peak systolic transaortic pressure gradient. Am Heart J 1982;103:210–221.)

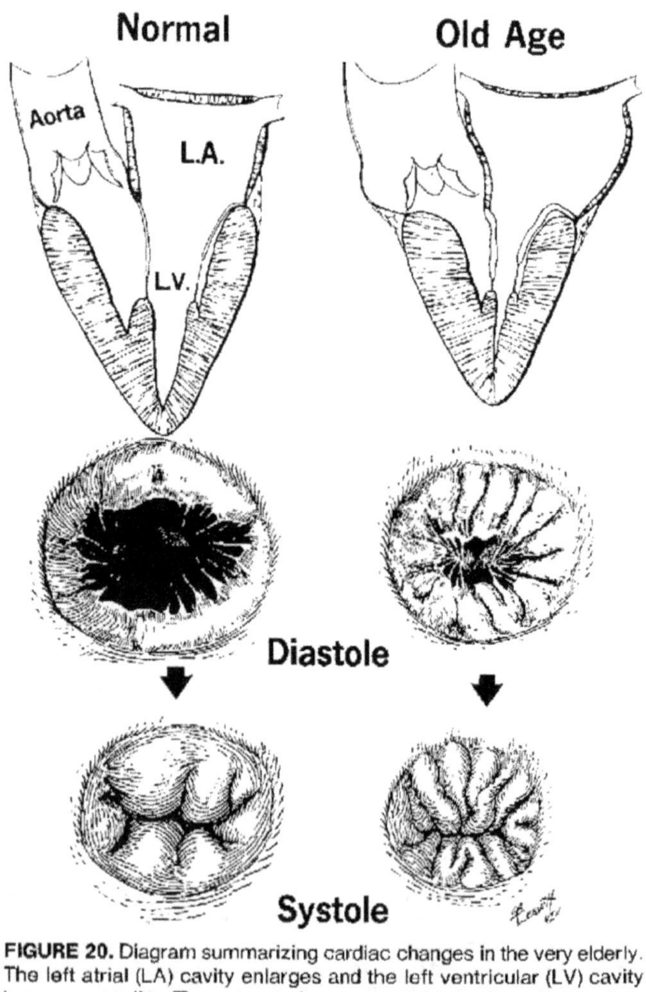

FIGURE 20. Diagram summarizing cardiac changes in the very elderly. The left atrial (LA) cavity enlarges and the left ventricular (LV) cavity becomes smaller. The amount of space available for the mitral leaflets decreases with aging, and consequently the number of scallops in the leaflets appears to increase.

onary arteries increase in both length and width and the former, particularly in association with the decreasing sizes of the cardiac ventricles, results in tortuosity. (The young river is straight and the old one, winding.) The subepicardial adipose tissue increases in amount with aging. The leaflets of each of the 4 cardiac valves thicken with age, particularly the atrioventricular valves, which have a smaller area to occupy in the ventricles because of the diminishing size of the latter. Histologic examination discloses large quantities of lipofuscin pigment in myocardial cells; some contain mucoid deposits ("mucoid degeneration"). These changes appear to affect all population groups of elderly individuals irrespective of where they reside on this earth and irrespective of their level of serum lipids. An elevated systemic arterial pressure appears to both accelerate and amplify these "normal" expected aging cardiac changes.

Both the aorta and its branches and the major pulmonary arteries and their branches enlarge with age. Because the enlargement is in both longitudinal and transverse dimensions, the aorta, like the coronary arteries, tends to become tortuous. This process also is amplified as the vertebral bodies become smaller and the height, somewhat shorter. The major pulmonary arteries appear to be too short and to have too low a pressure to dilate longitudinally.

Although several reports have described cardiovascular finding at necropsy in aged persons, old age was defined as >55,[11] >65,[12] or >75[13] years, and consequently findings in those aged 90 years and over could not be separated from those occurring in the "younger" older persons. The present study appears to be the first to focus entirely on a group of necropsy patients aged 90 years or older. A major finding in our study is the high frequency of calcific deposits in the heart. Of the 40 patients, 37 (92%) had calcific deposits in the epicardial coronary arteries. In most, the deposits were extensive. Although the calcific deposits were located entirely in atherosclerotic plaques, which are located in the intima, the presence of calcific deposits in the coronary arteries in this very elderly population did not necessarily indicate the presence of significant (>75% XSA) luminal narrowing. In contrast, the presence of calcific deposits in epicardial coronary arteries in persons aged <65 years generally indicates the presence of significant luminal narrowing.[14] The calcific deposits tended to occur in each of the 4 major (right, left main, left anterior descending, and left circumflex) epicardial arteries and were always larger in the proximal than in the distal halves of the right, left anterior descending, and left circumflex arteries or, if small, limited to their proximal halves.

Calcific deposits occurred with near equal frequency (55% and 47%) in the aortic valve cusps and in the mitral anular region. The deposits in the aortic valve were located on the aortic aspects of 1 or more of the 3 cusps and usually were unassociated with commissural fusion. The presence or absence of aortic valve stenosis was determined by the quantity of calcium deposited. In 2 patients, the extent of the calcific deposits imparted an immobility to the cusps resulting in aortic valve stenosis. The mitral "anular" calcific deposits, of course, were not limited to the anulus but included the space between the ventricular aspect of the posterior mitral leaflet and the mural endocardium of left ventricular free wall behind posterior mitral leaflet. Often this "anular" calcium extended into the adjacent left ventricular myocardium. Most patients with aortic valve calcium had mitral "anular" calcium and vice versa and all with aortic valvular or mitral "anular" calcium had coronary arterial calcific deposits.

The presence of calcium in the 3 locations in the heart, namely the coronary artery, the aortic valve, and

TABLE III Electrocardiographic Observations in 30 Patients Aged 90 to 103 Years

Abnormality	Clinical Heart Disease: Present* (n = 8)	Clinical Heart Disease: Absent (n = 22)	Total n	Total %
Atrial fibrillation	5	7	12	40
Abnormal QRS axis			12	40
Left (−30 to −90°)	4	6		
Right (+111 to +210°)	1	1		
Complete (QRS ≥0.12 second) BBB			12	40
Left	6	1		
Right	1	4		
Ventricular premature complexes	4	6	10	33
Atrial premature complexes	1	2	3	10
Heart Block			8	27
P-R interval >0.20 second	3	3		
Second degree	0	1		
Third degree (complete)	1†	0		
Q-wave abnormality without BBB			4	13
Q II, III, aV_f	0	1		
Q-S V_1–V_3	0	1		
Both	0	2		
Left ventricular hypertrophy without BBB (R in V_5 or V_6 + S in V_1 ≥35 mm)	1	0	1	3
Low voltage (QRS ≤15 mm in I + II + III)	0	1	1	3

* Coronary heart disease = 3; cardiac amyloidosis = 4; aortic valve stenosis = 1.
† Pacemaker inserted 6 years before death.
BBB = bundle branch block.

TABLE IV Total QRS Voltage in 24 Necropsy Patients Aged ≥90 Years: 8 With (Angina Pectoris [AP] or Acute Myocardial Infarction [AMI] in 5, Amyloid in 2, Aortic Valve Stenosis [AS] in 1) and 16 Without Symptoms of Cardiac Dysfunction

Pt	Age (yr) & Sex	Clinical Heart Disease	Body Wt (Kg)	Heart Wt (g)	QRS (mm) I	II	III	R	L	F	V_1	V_2	V_3	V_4	V_5	V_6	Sum 1 + 11 + 111	Sum R + L + F	Sum 1 − 111 + R − F	Sum $V_1 - V_6$	Total
Patients (n = 8) With Symptoms of Cardiac Dysfunction																					
5	90F	AMI	100	400	8	5	6	6	7	5	11	28	21	12	7	15	19	18	37	94	131
1	90F	AMI + AS	120	540	6	7	8	5	6	6	15	20	14	14	11	11	21	17	38	85	123
3	90M	AMI	110	450	5	8	9	5	6	10	12	24	26	19	11	10	22	21	43	102	145
14	92F	AP	107	380	7	8	9	7	7	8	14	12	20	40	16	15	24	22	46	117	163
17	92F	As	120	525	16	15	14	17	13	12	16	25	34	35	25	16	45	42	87	151	238
21	93F	Amyloid	...	380	10	6	12	5	10	10	9	10	11	14	14	6	28	25	53	64	117
27	96M	Amyloid	126	660	6	5	11	2	8	8	7	18	12	11	9	5	22	18	40	62	102
37	99M	AMI	110	510	7	11	7	8	6	7	22	22	6	18	22	18	25	21	46	108	154
Range (mean)	(93)	...	(137)	(481)	...	...	...	...	...	...	...	...	...	...	...	...	19–45 (26)	17–42 (23)	37–87 (49)	62–151 (98)	102–238 (147)
Patients (n = 16) Without Symptoms of Cardiac Dysfunction																					
6	90F	0	100	220	10	12	8	10	8	8	10	24	27	28	22	14	30	26	56	125	181
7	90F	0	104	270	7	10	6	10	4	7	10	22	30	38	32	17	23	21	44	149	193
8	90F	0	110	505	9	7	13	5	9	9	12	16	13	3	4	7	29	23	52	55	107
11	91F	0	99	375	10	10	6	10	5	6	22	21	25	21	18	14	26	21	47	121	168
15	92F	0	109	400	8	8	9	6	8	8	25	27	33	31	20	13	25	22	47	149	196
24	95F	0	128	350	6	7	4	6	7	5	7	6	5	6	10	13	17	18	35	47	82
29	95F	0	120	440	5	10	10	10	10	8	19	15	33	32	22	20	25	18	43	141	184
25	95F	0	...	460	14	11	12	6	12	10	12	17	18	15	5	4	37	28	65	71	136
28	95M	0	...	385	4	13	10	8	4	11	3	8	11	14	11	8	27	23	50	55	105
31	96F	0	100	300	7	15	10	11	4	11	9	16	17	22	29	28	32	26	58	121	179
32	97F	0	120	360	9	5	3	8	12	5	10	19	16	14	15	10	17	25	42	84	126
33	97F	0	90	320	10	6	10	7	9	6	7	16	15	23	28	23	26	22	48	112	160
35	98F	0	117	360	5	10	8	7	3	8	8	15	14	12	8	5	23	18	41	62	103
36	98F	0	115	320	10	9	15	6	10	10	20	34	18	10	8	9	34	26	60	99	159
39	100M	0	...	335	6	6	1	6	2	3	14	11	2	24	24	12	13	11	24	87	111
40	103F	0	120	345	13	25	37	20	22	13	26	19	16	25	23	12	75	55	130	121	251
Range (mean)	(95)	...	(110)	(359)	...	...	...	...	...	...	...	...	...	...	...	...	13–75 (28)	11–55 (24)	24–130 (52)	47–149 (100)	82–251 (152)

Pt = patient; Wt = weight.

the mitral "anulus," might be termed *the senile cardiac calcification syndrome* and strongly suggests that the etiology of the calcific deposits in each of the 3 locations is similar. It is well appreciated, as already mentioned, that the calcific deposits in the coronary arteries are located in atherosclerotic plaques and, therefore, that the calcific deposits in both aortic valve and mitral anular regions might be viewed as anatomic expressions of the atherosclerotic process. All 3 appear to occur only in populations where the total serum cholesterol level is >150 mg/700 ml. Of our 40 patients, total serum cholesterol levels were available in 10: in only 1 (Patient 30) was the level <150, and in 2 the level was 150 to 200 mg/100 ml. In Patient 30, whose value was 108 mg/100 ml, no calcific deposits were present in any of the 3 sites; in Patient 36 whose level was 165 mg/100 ml, minimal calcific deposits were present only in the coronary arteries; and in Patient 28, whose level was 181 mg/100 ml, small calcific deposits were present in the aortic valve (Fig. 16) and coronary arteries. In contrast, of the 7 patients in whom the total serum cholesterol level was >200 mg/100 ml, calcific deposits were present in either aortic valve or mitral anulus or both in 5 patients and in the coronary arteries in all 7 patients; in each the deposits were larger. Calcific deposits in the coronary artery, aortic valve cusp, and mitral anulus are extremely rare in populations where total serum cholesterol levels are <150 mg/100 ml and, of course, clinical evidence of coronary heart disease in these population groups is extremely rare[15] despite a high prevalence of systemic hypertension.

Of the 40 patients, 28 had narrowing of >75% in XSA of ≥1 of the 4 major epicardial coronary arteries. Of the 28 patients, 17 had transmural foci of left ventricular fibrosis or necrosis (myocardial infarction) and of the 12 with insignificant coronary narrowing, none had grossly visible acute or healed myocardial infarcts. Of the 14 patients with healed myocardial infarcts, only 1 had a clinical event compatible with acute myocardial infarction which healed. Of the 10 patients with acute myocardial infarcts at necropsy, only 3 had typical clinical features of acute myocardial infarction; the other 7 had acute changes in their clinical course and acute myocardial infarction was either suspected or compatible with the acute illness. Angina pectoris was described in 3 patients, 1 of whom was among the 10 with fatal acute myocardial infarcts, and 1 of whom had had a nonfatal acute infarct. Thus, 12 patients had clinical features compatible with coronary heart disease and each was among the 28 with significant narrowing of ≥1 of the major coronary arteries. Conversely, of the 28 patients with significant coronary narrowing at necropsy, 16 (57%) never had either angina pectoris or acute myocardial infarction. Of the total 40 patients, only 12 (30%) had clinical events compatible with coronary heart disease and only in 6 were the clinical events really typical.

In 36 of the 40 patients, each of the 4 major coronary arteries were divided into 5 mm long segments and the degree of XSA narrowing by atherosclerotic plaque was determined for each segment. Of the 1,789 5 mm segments in the 36 patients, the average amount of XSA narrowing by atherosclerotic plaques/segment was 42% (range 19 to 69). Of the 467 5 mm segments in the 10 patients with clinical evidence of coronary heart disease, the average amount of XSA narrowing/segment was 55% (range 43 to 69), and 1,322 segments in the 26 patients without clinical evidence of coronary heart disease, 38% (range 19 to 40) ($p < 0.01$). Among 129 patients aged 22 to 85 years (mean 56), the amount of XSA narrowing by atherosclerotic plaques/segment averaged 67%; in the control subjects, that is, those without symptomatic coronary heart disease, XSA narrowing averaged 32%. The mean percent of 5 mm coronary segments narrowed 76 to 100% in XSA in the 36 patients was 13% (range 2 to 89); of the 10 patients with symptomatic coronary heart disease, the mean was 19% (range 10 to 34); and of the 26 patients without symptomatic coronary heart disease, the mean was 7% (range 2 to 28) ($p < 0.05$). The mean of 19% in patients with symptomatic coronary heart disease aged ≥90 was half that observed in patients aged ≤85 years (mean 56) with fatal coronary heart disease and the mean of 8% was nearly 3 times that observed in the younger patients without fatal coronary heart disease.[16–21]

These detailed morphologic studies of the coronary arteries in these very elderly persons suggest that the degree of severe coronary narrowing necessary to have a fatal or near-fatal coronary event is considerably less than that necessary to have a coronary event in younger patients. Moreover, these studies indicate that these very elderly patients without symptoms of coronary heart disease have distinctly more coronary luminal narrowing by atherosclerotic plaques that do control subjects who are younger, (mean age 52 years).[16–21] The latter observation suggests that coronary heart disease may be underdiagnosed clinically in the very elderly.

Clinical diagnosis of cardiac and other conditions in patients aged 90 years and over appears more difficult than in younger persons. Historic information may be difficult to obtain because of impaired intellect on the part of the patient and an impaired diagnostic pursuit on the part of the physician. Physicians caring for these very elderly persons may focus primarily on the prevention of suffering and only secondarily on accurate diagnosis or longer-term therapy. Patients aged 90 years and over generally have outlived their spouses and private physicians, and often are "inherited" by nursing-home physicians who may have limited access to earlier medical records.

Angina pectoris appears particularly difficult to diagnose in the very elderly because they may not be able to describe this symptom. Acute myocardial infarction also is difficult to diagnose clinically but it is often fatal in the very elderly. Of 11 clinical acute infarcts at or after age 90 years in our patients, 10 were fatal. Only 4 of the 11 acute infarcts were clearly diagnosed clinically; most others were manifest as more dyspnea. Furthermore, the electrocardiogram is not as useful in diagnosis of acute myocardial infarction in the very elderly because left bundle branch block is frequent and it, of course, prevents the appearance of typical changes. Serial recordings of electrocardiograms also appear to be quite infrequent in the very elderly. Only

2 of our 10 patients with fatal acute myocardial infarction had as many as 2 electrocardiograms recorded during the final illness.

Physical examination in the very elderly may be both difficult and misleading. The lack of mobility may prevent proper positioning of the elderly patient for proper examining. Precordial murmurs, although very common (25 of our 40 patients), infrequently indicate significant functional abnormality. Although 22 of our 40 patients had calcific deposits in the aortic valve, only 2 appeared to have actual aortic valve stenosis. Likewise, although 19 of the 40 patients had mitral anular calcific deposits, in only 1 patient did the calcific deposits appear to actually narrow the mitral orifice.

Electrocardiographic abnormalities are common in elderly persons. Of our 30 patients with electrocardiograms available, all had ≥1 abnormalities recorded, the most frequent ones being abnormal axis, atrial fibrillation, and complete bundle branch block. Although 15 of the 30 patients had cardiomegaly (>350 g in women, >400 g in men) at necropsy, only 1 had voltage criteria for left ventricular hypertrophy shown by electrocardiography. Likewise, only 1 had low voltage. Measurement of the QRS amplitude in each of the 12 leads was performed in 24 patients; these measurements have never been recorded previously in elderly individuals. The total QRS voltage was similar in the 8 patients with and in the 16 patients without clinical evidence of cardiac disease (mean 147 mm versus mean 152 mm [10 mm = 1 mV]). Although normal amplitudes of the QRS complexes in all 12 leads in elderly patients are lacking, Simonson[22] provided data on the upper and lower limits of amplitude of the QRS complexes in each of the 12 leads in normal men and women aged 20 to 59 years (means not available). The upper and lower limits of normal for men aged 50 to 59 years was 277 and 36 mm, and for the women 248 and 27 mm, respectively.

Acknowledgment: We thank Filippina Giacometti, Barbara Winterrowd, Margaret Moore, Mary McMahon, Alvado Campbell, and Exa Murray for assistance far beyond the call of duty in the completion of this project.

References

1. **Fries JF.** Aging, natural history, and the compression of morbidity. N Engl J Med 1980;303:130–135.
2. **Siegel JS.** Recent and prospective demographic trends for the elderly population and some implications for health care In: Haynes SG, Feinleib M, eds. Second Conference on the Epidemiology of Aging. U.S. Department of Health and Human Services, Washington DC, NIH Publication No. 80-969, 1980;293.
3. **Kohn RR.** Cause of death in very old people JAMA 1982;247:2793–2797.
4. **Eckner FAD, Brown BW, Davidson DL, Glagov S.** Dimensions of normal hearts after standard fixation by controlled pressure coronary perfusion Arch Pathol Lab Med 1969;88:497–507.
5. **Roberts WC, Perloff JK, Constantino T.** Severe valvular aortic stenosis in patients over 65 years of age. A clinicopathologic study. Am J Cardiol 1971;27:497–506.
6. **Roberts WC, Perloff JK.** Mitral valve disease A clinico-pathologic survey of the conditions causing the mitral valve to function abnormally. Ann Intern Med 1972;77:939–975
7. **Roberts WC, Waller BF.** Mitral valve "anular" calcium forming a complete circle or "O" configuration: clinical and necropsy observations. Am Heart J 1981;101:619–621.
8. **Buja LM, Khoi NB, Roberts WC.** Clinically significant cardiac amyloidosis. Clinicopathologic findings in 15 patients Am J Cardiol 1970;26:394–405.
9. **Beck CS.** Coronary artery disease. A report to William Harvey 300 years later Am J Cardiol 1958;1:38–45
10. **Roberts WC.** Aortic dissection: anatomy, consequences and causes. Am Heart J 1981;101:195–214.
11. **Surgiura M, Hiraoka K, Ohkawa S, Shimada H.** A clinicopathologic study on the heart diseases in the aged. The morphologic classification of 1,000 consecutive autopsy cases. Jpn Heart J 1975;16:526–537.
12. **Pomerance A.** Cardiac pathology in the elderly. In: Noble RJ, Rothbaum DA, eds. Geriatric Cardiology. Philadelphia: FA Davis, 1981: 9–54
13. **Promerance A.** Pathology of the heart with and without cardiac failure in the aged. Br Heart J 1965,27:697–710.
14. **Aldrich RF, Brensike JF, Battaglini JW, Richardson JM, Loh IK, Stone NJ, Passamani ER, Ackerstein H, Seningen R, Borer JS, Levy RI, Epstein SE.** Coronary calcifications in the detection of coronary artery disease and comparison with electrocardiographic exercise testing. Results from the National Heart, Lung, and Blood Institute's Type II Coronary Intervention Study. Circulation 1979;59:1113–1124.
15. **Gelfand M.** Heart disease in the elderly African. Br Heart J 1961;23: 387–392.
16. **Roberts WC, Jones AA.** Quantitation of coronary arterial narrowing at necropsy in sudden coronary death. Analysis of 31 patients and comparison with 25 control subjects. Am J Cardiol 1979;44:39–45
17. **Roberts WC, Virmani R.** Quantification of coronary arterial narrowing on clinically-isolated unstable angina pectoris. An analysis of 22 necropsy patients. Am J Med 1979;67:792–799.
18. **Roberts WC, Jones AA.** Quantification of coronary arterial narrowing at necropsy in acute transmural myocardial infarction: analysis and comparison of findings in 27 patients and 22 controls. Circulation 1980;61:786–790.
19. **Virmani R, Roberts WC.** Quantification of coronary arterial narrowing and of left ventricular myocardial scarring in healed myocardial infarction with chronic, eventually fatal, congestive heart failure Am J Med 1980;68: 831–838.
20. **Cabin HS, Roberts WC.** True left ventricular aneurysm and healed myocardial infarction. Clinical and necropsy observations including quantification of degrees of coronary arterial narrowing. Am J Cardiol 1980;46:754–763
21. **Virmani R, Roberts WC.** Non-fatal healed transmural myocardial infarction and fatal non-cardiac disease. Qualification and quantification of coronary arterial narrowing. Br Heart J 1981;45:434–441.
22. **Simonson F.** Differentiation Between Normal and Abnormal in Electrocardiography. St Louis: CV Mosby, 1961:328.

Morphologic Features of the Normal and Abnormal Mitral Valve

WILLIAM C. ROBERTS, MD

Anatomic and functional features of the normal and abnormal mitral valve are reviewed. Of 1,010 personally studied necropsy patients with severe (functional class III or IV, New York Heart Association) cardiac dysfunction from primary valvular heart disease, 434 (43%) had mitral stenosis (MS) with or without mitral regurgitation (MR): unassociated with aortic valve stenosis or regurgitation or with tricuspid valve stenosis in 189 (44%) patients, and associated with aortic stenosis in 152 (35%), with pure (no element of stenosis) aortic regurgitation in 65 (15%) patients, and with tricuspid valve stenosis with or without aortic valve stenosis in 28 (6%) patients. The origin of MS was rheumatic in all 434 patients. Of the 1,010 necropsy patients, 165 (16%) had pure MR (papillary muscle dysfunction excluded): unassociated with aortic valve stenosis or regurgitation or with tricuspid valve stenosis in 97 (59%) patients, and associated with pure aortic regurgitation in 45 (27%) and with aortic valve stenosis in 23 (14%) patients. When associated with dysfunction of the aortic valve, pure MR was usually rheumatic in origin, but when unassociated with aortic valve dysfunction it was usually nonrheumatic in origin. Review of operatively excised mitral valves in patients with pure MR unassociated with aortic valve dysfunction disclosed mitral valve prolapse (most likely an inherent congenital defect) as the most common cause of MR. Excluding the patients with MR from coronary heart disease (papillary muscle dysfunction), mitral prolapse was the cause of MR in 60 (88%) of the other 68 patients, and a rheumatic origin was responsible in only 3 of the 68 patients, all 68 of whom were >30 years of age.

Mitral anular calcification in persons aged >65 years is usually associated with calcific deposits in the aortic valve cusps and in the coronary arteries. Because calcium in each of these 3 sites is common in older individuals residing in the Western World, it is most reasonable to view mitral anular calcification in older individuals as a manifestation of atherosclerosis. Mitral anular calcium appears to be extremely uncommon in persons with total serum cholesterol levels <150 mg/dl. Mitral anular calcium may produce mild MR and, if the deposits are heavy enough, MS.

This report reviews anatomic findings in both the normally and abnormally functioning mitral valve. Major attention is directed to anatomic observations which have clinical usefulness. This review focuses primarily on studies carried out in my laboratory during the past 20 years.

From the Pathology Branch, National Heart, Lung, and Blood Institute, National Institutes of Health, Bethesda, Maryland. Manuscript received and accepted December 3, 1982.

Address for reprints: William C. Roberts, MD, Building 10A, Room 3E30, National Institutes of Health, Bethesda, Maryland 20205.

Normal Mitral Valve (Fig. 1)

The mitral valve, in comparison with the semilunar valves, is a complex structure consisting of 4 major components: leaflets, chordae tendineae, papillary muscles, and anulus.[1,2] Unlike the other 3 cardiac valves, each of which has 3 cusps, the mitral valve consists of only 2 *leaflets*. The anterior one has a much longer basal-to-margin length than does the posterior leaflet, but the length of the anular attachment of the posterior leaflet (about 6 cm) is about twice that of the anterior leaflet (about 3 cm) (Fig. 1). Although the basal-to-margin lengths and the lengths of the basal attachments

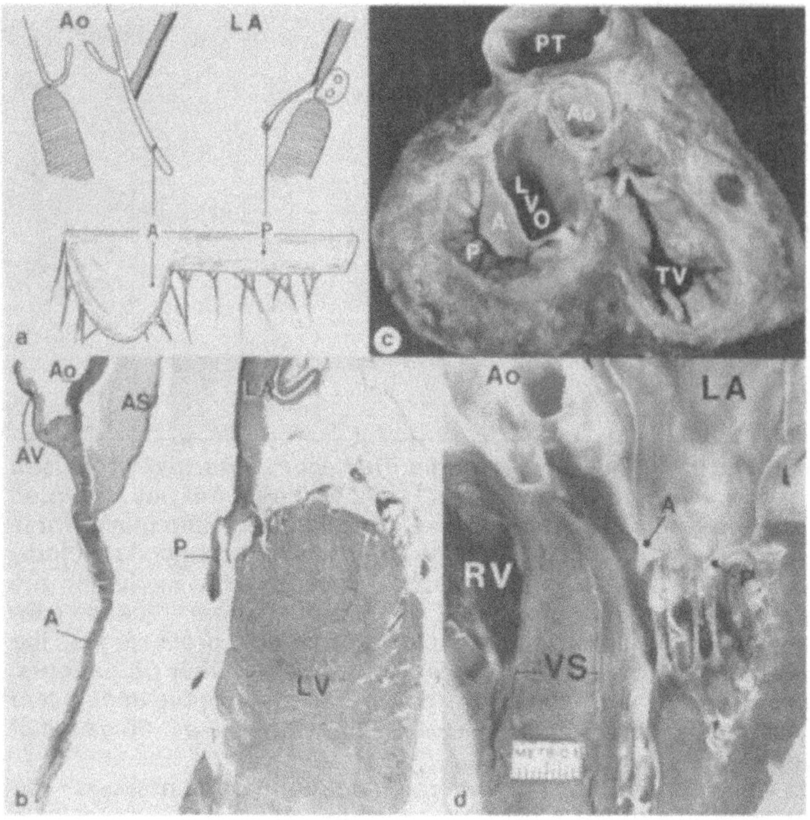

FIGURE 1. Normal mitral valve. **a,** diagram showing relation of anterior (A) and posterior (P) mitral leaflets to one another and to left atrium (LA), aortic valve (AV), and aorta (Ao). The inflow and outflow tracts of the left ventricle are divided by the anterior leaflet. The basal attachment of the posterior leaflet is twice as long as that of the anterior leaflet, although the basal-to-margin length of the anterior leaflet is twice that of the posterior leaflet. **b,** histologic sections of the mitral valve confirming the observations depicted in **a.** One section includes the anterior (A) mitral leaflet, the aortic valve cusp (AV), the wall of the aorta (Ao), and the atrial septal (AS) wall, and the other includes the left atrial and left ventricular free walls with intervening posterior mitral leaflet. (Elastic van Gieson stains; magnification ×4.5 and ×3, reduced 45%). **c,** view of the heart from above after excision of the atria. The anterior (A) mitral leaflet separates the left ventricular inflow from outflow (LVO). PT = pulmonary trunk; TV = tricuspid valve. **d,** longitudinal cut of the left ventricle, mitral valve, aorta, and left atrium, as would be seen by M-mode echocardiogram.

of each mitral leaflet are quite different, the surface area of each leaflet is virtually identical. The posterior leaflet has a true bundle of fibrous tissue (the anulus) separating the myocardium of left atrium from the myocardium of left ventricle. The posterior leaflet, in a large sense, is simply an extension of mural endocardium from the free walls of the left atrium. In contrast to the posterior mitral leaflet, the anterior leaflet does not have a true anulus but is continuous with the wall of the ascending aorta, aortic valve, membraneous ventricular septum, and atrial septum. The area of the leaflets is about 2.5 times that of the area of the mitral orifice at the level of the mitral anulus. In contrast to the semilunar cusps, which are independent or discontinuous of each other, the 2 mitral leaflets are continuous with each other, being connected at the commissures.

Chordae tendineae from both mitral leaflets insert into both papillary muscles. About 5 times as many

TABLE I Functional and Anatomic Classification of Valvular Heart Disease in 1,010 Necropsy Patients Aged ≥15 Years*

Functional Class	Patients (n [%])	Anatomic Class (n [%]) AV	MV	MV-AV	TV-MV	TV-MV-AV
1. Aortic stenosis (AS)	292 (29)	256 (87.5)	0	35 (12.1)	0	1 (0.3)
2. Mitral stenosis (MS)	189 (19)	0	117 (62)	40 (21)	13 (7)	19 (10)
3. MS + AS	152 (15)	0	0	120 (79)	0	32 (21)
4. Aortic regurgitation (AR)	119 (12)	107† (90)	0	10 (8)	0	2 (2)
5. Mitral regurgitation (MR)	97 (10)	0	85 (88)	8 (8)	1 (1)	3 (3)
6. MS + AR	65 (6)	0	52 (80)	0	0	13 (20)
7. MR + AR	45 (4)	0	0	39 (87)	0	6 (13)
8. AS + MR	23 (2)	0	0	21 (91)	0	2 (9)
9. Tricuspid stenosis + MS ± AS	28 (3)	0	0	0	4 (14)	24 (86)
Totals	1,010 (100)‡	363 (36)	254 (25)	273 (27)	18 (2)	102 (10)

AV = aortic valve; MV = mitral valve; TV = tricuspid valve.

* Excludes patients with mitral regurgitation secondary to coronary heart disease (papillary muscle dysfunction), carcinoid heart disease, and hypertrophic cardiomyopathy and those with infective endocarditis limited to 1 or both right-sided cardiac valves. Tricuspid valve regurgitation was present in many patients in most of the 9 functional groups. All patients were in functional class III or IV (New York Heart Association), and more than half had 1 or more cardiac operations.

† In many patients, the aortic valve cusps actually were normal and the regurgitation was the result of disease of the aorta (Marfan and Marfan-like syndromes, syphilis, systemic hypertension, healed aortic dissection).

‡ The hearts in all 1,010 patients were examined and classified by WCR.

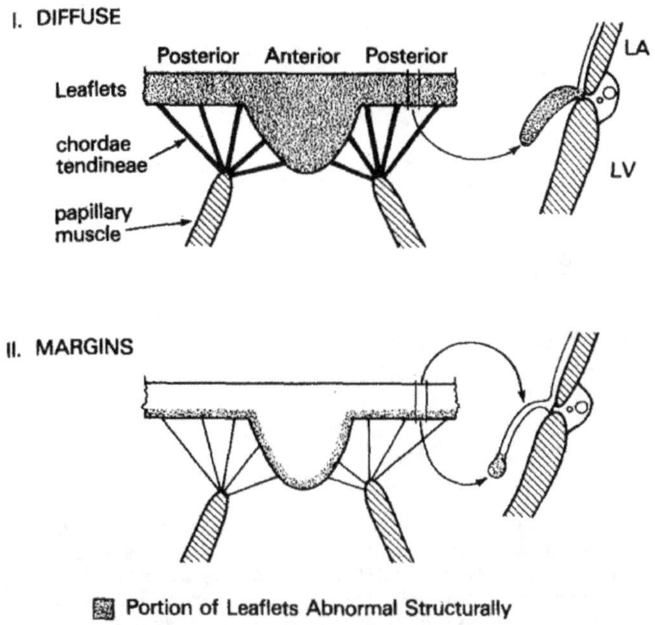

FIGURE 2. Diagram showing the 2 types of anatomic involvement of the mitral valve in rheumatic heart disease. Thickening of chordae are not required for diagnosis, only thickening of the leaflets, either diffusely or on all margins. LA = left atrium; LV = left ventricle. (Reprinted, by permission, from Roberts and Virmani.[11])

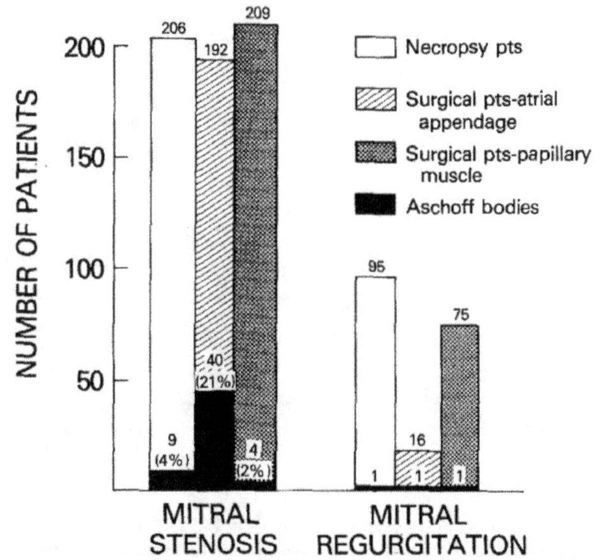

FIGURE 3. Bar graph demonstrating number and percentage of patients (pts) undergoing operations for either mitral stenosis (with or without mitral regurgitation) and pure mitral regurgitation in whom Aschoff bodies were found in either the left atrial appendage or left ventricular papillary muscle.

chordae are attached to leaflets as to papillary muscles. On an average, 24 chordae tendineae are attached to the papillary muscles (12 to each), and 120 chordae are attached to the leaflets.[3] The chordae insert onto the undersurfaces—that is, the ventricular surfaces—of both leaflets. The chordae subdivide as they progress from papillary muscle to leaflet. The subdivisions may be viewed as primary (first order), secondary (second order), and tertiary (third order) chordae. The spaces between the chordae serve as secondary orifices between left atrium and left ventricle. Obviously, the major orifice is the area between the leaflets, but much blood passes between the interchordal spaces. Therefore, fusion of chordae tendineae may narrow the mitral inlet.

The 2 *left ventricular papillary muscles* are preferably designated anterolateral and posteromedial.[3] There is considerable variation in the appearances of these 2 structures in the same person, and comparison of corresponding structures in different persons discloses considerable variation. The anterolateral papillary muscle is generally the more uniform of the 2. It usually consists of a single trunk that protrudes more into the cavity than does the posteromedial one. The posteromedial papillary muscle is generally smaller than the anterolateral structure and often consists of 2 or 3 smaller pillars rather than a single pillar. The posteromedial muscle usually has several connections to the left ventricular wall in addition to the base of the major trunk. Both papillary muscles are attached to the left ventricular free wall roughly at the junction of the caudal third and middle thirds.

With aging, the mitral valve, like other tissues, changes; this change consists mainly of focal fibrous thickening of both leaflets and chordae. The left ventricular cavity becomes smaller (presumably because the cardiac output decreases) as we grow older,[2,4] and consequently less area becomes available in the left ventricle to accommodate the mitral leaflets and chordae. The leaflets then contact one another abnormally during ventricular systole and focal fibrous thickening results. Since the left ventricular cavity diminishes with age, the mitral *anulus* does also. The latter change further increases the abnormal contact of the mitral leaflets with one other and furthers the leaflet scarring. This scarring from aging, however, is not enough to cause mitral dysfunction.

Abnormal Mitral Valve

Mitral Stenosis

The essential hemodynamic fault caused by mitral stenosis (MS) is the inability of the left atrium to empty normally.[2] In sinus rhythm, left atrial contraction serves to augment its emptying, but atrial contraction is lost in atrial fibrillation. The obstruction, represented by a pressure gradient across the valve, results in pulmonary venous obstruction which may be apparent on chest roentgenography.

Of the 9 single or combined cardiac valve lesions severe enough to be fatal, MS, in my experience, ranks second[5,6] (Table I). Of 1,010 patients >14 years of age with functionally severe (class III or IV, New York Heart Association) valvular cardiac disease whom I had studied at necropsy up to 1980, 434 (44%) had MS.[2] Only aortic valve stenosis was more common.[7-9] Mitral

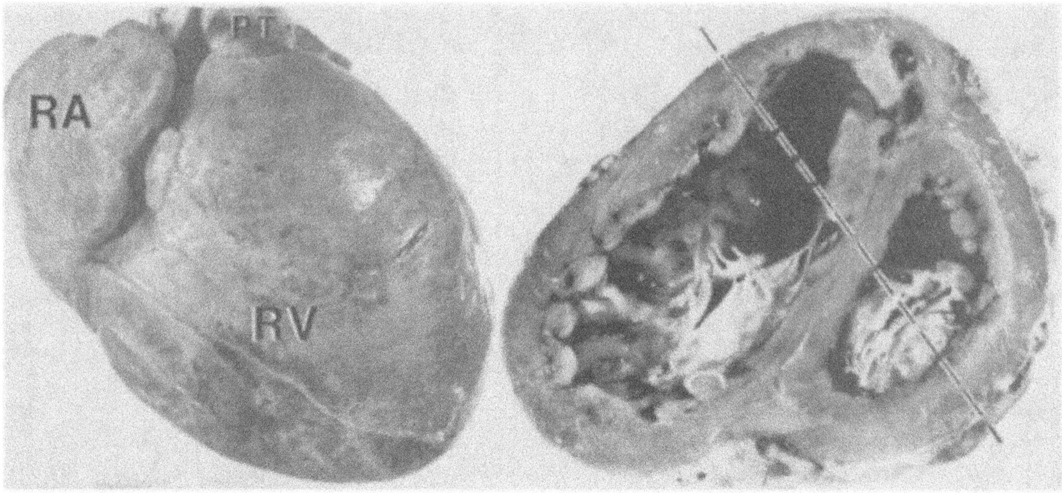

FIGURE 4. Heart in a 16-year-old boy (NIH #A77-232) who had acute rheumatic fever at age 6 years and chronic congestive heart failure beginning at age 10 years. By examination, the patient had evidence of severe mitral stenosis and tricuspid regurgitation. At cardiac catheterization 10 hours before death, the right ventricular pressure was 100/20 and the left ventricular pressure, 100/10 mm Hg. Neither pulmonary arterial wedge or left atrial pressures were obtained. Left ventriculogram disclosed no mitral regurgitation and a normal-sized left ventricular cavity. The patient had acute pulmonary edema after catheterization and underwent closed mitral commissurotomy as a terminal procedure on the ward. At necropsy, the heart weighed 450 g (the patient weighed 43 kg). The right atrium (RA) and ventricle (RV) were huge, and the thickness of the free walls of both ventricles were similar. Both mitral and tricuspid valve leaflets were diffusely thickened but free of calcific deposits. No Aschoff bodies were present. The **dashed straight line** is the line of the M-mode beam. PT = pulmonary trunk.

stenosis occurred alone in 189 (44%) patients and in combination with other functional valvular lesions in the other 245 (56%) patients. Mitral stenosis was rheumatic in origin in all 434 patients.[10,11]

Although a functional classification of valvular heart disease is most useful from physiologic and therapeutic standpoints, an anatomic classification is helpful from an etiologic standpoint. Five anatomic categories have proved useful: isolated mitral, isolated aortic, combined mitral and aortic, combined tricuspid and mitral with

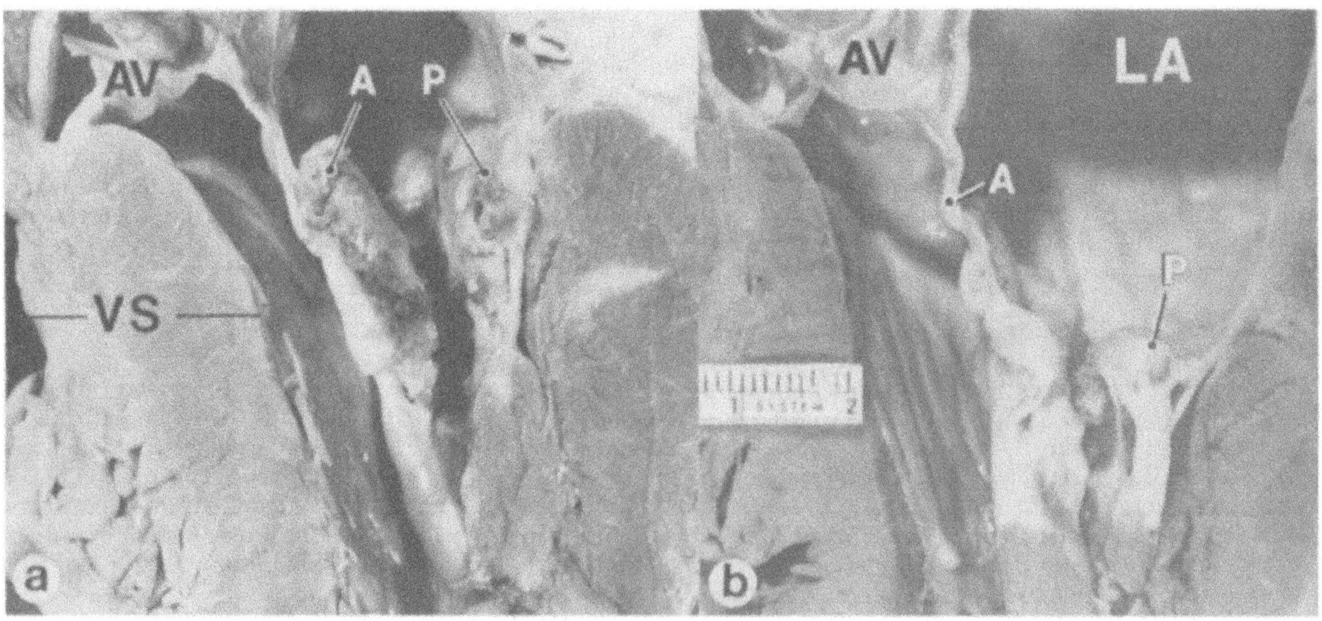

FIGURE 5. Longitudinal views, as would be seen by M-mode echocardiogram, of 2 hearts of patients with severe mitral stenosis. **a,** in a 55-year-old man (GT #74A-69) with equal peak systolic pressures in the right and left ventricles and no associated mitral regurgitation. The patient died from massive bleeding during cannulation of the aorta for planned mitral valve replacement. Both anterior (A) and posterior (P) mitral leaflets are heavily calcified. AV = aortic valve; VS = ventricular septum. **b,** in a 64-year-old woman (GT #78A-129) with right and left ventricular peak systolic pressures of 100 and 135 mm Hg, respectively, and an 18 mm Hg mean diastolic gradient between pulmonary arterial wedge position and left ventricle just before closed mitral commissurotomy 3 years before death. This patient died of progressive congestive cardiac failure. The heart weighed 410 g. The amount of calcium in the thickened mitral leaflets is relatively mild. LA = left atrium.

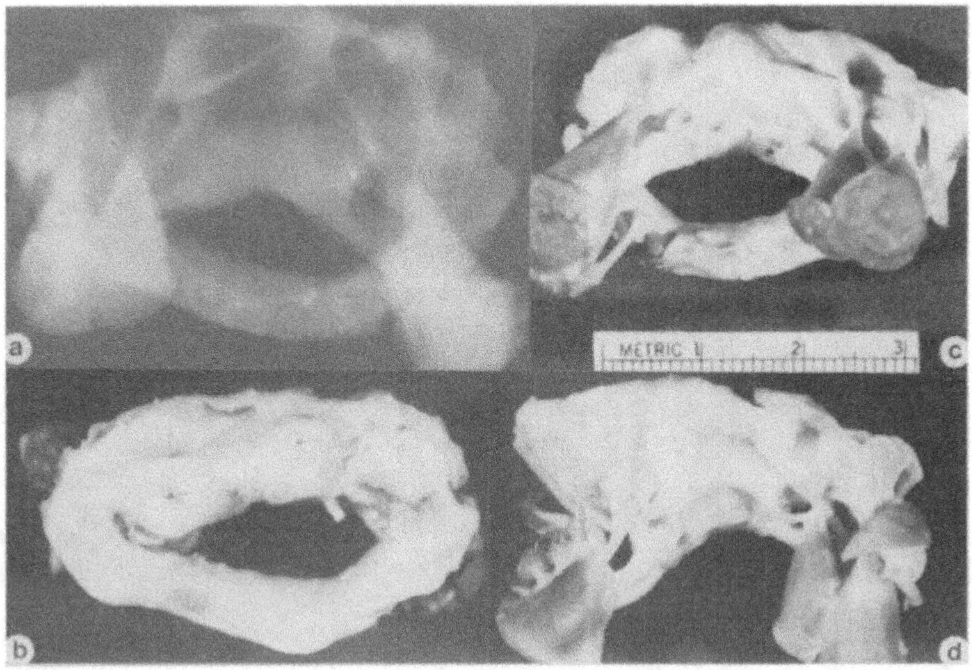

FIGURE 6. Operatively excised stenotic mitral valve in a 40-year-old woman with only a minute calcific deposit in the anterior leaflet. The mean diastolic gradient between the pulmonary arterial wedge position and the left ventricle was 13 mm Hg, the peak pulmonary arterial systolic pressure was 50 mm Hg, and 3+/4+ mitral regurgitation was present by left ventriculogram. **a,** radiogram of operatively excised valve. **b,** view from left atrial aspect. **c,** view from left ventricular aspect. **d,** view of anterior leaflet and papillary muscles. (Reprinted, by permission, from Lachman and Roberts.[18])

or without aortic, and both tricuspid and mitral (Table I). Anatomically isolated aortic valve disease is never rheumatic in origin.[5] Isolated mitral disease causing MS is, with rare exception, rheumatic in origin, but isolated mitral disease causing pure regurgitation is usually nonrheumatic in origin.[12] Anatomic valve disease involving more than 1 cardiac valve is usually rheumatic in origin. Isolated anatomic disease of the tricuspid or pulmonic valves, or both, is usually congenital or infectious in origin or is associated with the carcinoid syndrome.[13–17]

A valve may function normally and yet be anatomically abnormal. Only 62% of the 189 patients with isolated MS (with or without mitral regurgitation [MR]) had anatomic involvement limited to the mitral valve[6] (Table I). In contrast, 88% of the 292 patients with clinically isolated aortic valve stenosis (with or without regurgitation) had anatomic disease limited to the aortic valve only.

Rheumatic heart disease may be viewed as a disease of the mitral valve; other valves also may be involved both anatomically and functionally, but anatomically the mitral valve is always involved[11] (Fig. 2). To my knowledge, *Aschoff bodies* have never been found in hearts without anatomic disease of the mitral valve.[11] Of the first 543 patients with severe valvular heart disease whom I studied at necropsy, 11 (27%) had Aschoff bodies, and all had anatomic mitral valve disease. The ages of the 11 patients with Aschoff bodies ranged from 18 to 68 years (mean 38) and 9 had a history of acute rheumatic fever earlier in life. Clinical study revealed that 9 of the 11 patients had MS with or without dysfunction of 1 or more other cardiac valves, 1 had isolated pure aortic regurgitation, and 1 had both mitral and aortic regurgitation. All 11 patients had diffuse fibrous thickening of the mitral valve leaflets and all but 1 had diffuse anatomic lesions of at least 2 other cardiac valves. No patient with anatomic lesions limited to the aortic valve had Aschoff bodies. Thus, among patients with chronic valvular heart disease, Aschoff bodies, the only anatomic lesion pathognomonic of rheumatic heart disease, usually indicate diffuse anatomic lesions of 1 or more other cardiac valves. The functional mitral lesion is usually stenosis.

Although they are rare at necropsy in patients with fatal chronic valvular heart disease, Aschoff bodies are fairly common in the heart in patients having mitral valve commissurotomy for MS.[10] Among 481 patients undergoing various mitral valve operations, Aschoff bodies were found in 40 (21%) of 191 operatively excised left atrial appendages, in 4 (2%) of 273 operatively excised left ventricular papillary muscles (1 per patient), and in 1 (6%) of 17 patients with both left atrial appendage and papillary muscle operatively excised (Fig. 3). Of the 45 patients with Aschoff bodies, 44 had MS preoperatively, and only 1, a 10-year-old boy, had pure MR. Sinus rhythm was present in 38 (84%), and atrial fibrillation in 7 (16%). Perioperatively, only 1 of the 45 patients with Aschoff bodies had clinical or laboratory stigmata compatible with acute rheumatic fever, and 58% had an illness compatible with acute rheumatic fever at any time.

Rheumatic heart disease not only is a disorder of the cardiac valves; it also affects mural endocardium, pericardium, and myocardium. On histologic study, the atrial walls virtually always have increased amounts of fibrous tissue in both myocardial interstitium and in the mural endocardium, atrophy of some and hypertrophy of other myocardial cells, and hypertrophy of smooth muscle cells of the mural endocardium. In all patients with rheumatic MS, the leaflets are diffusely thickened, either by fibrous tissue or calcific deposits or both; the

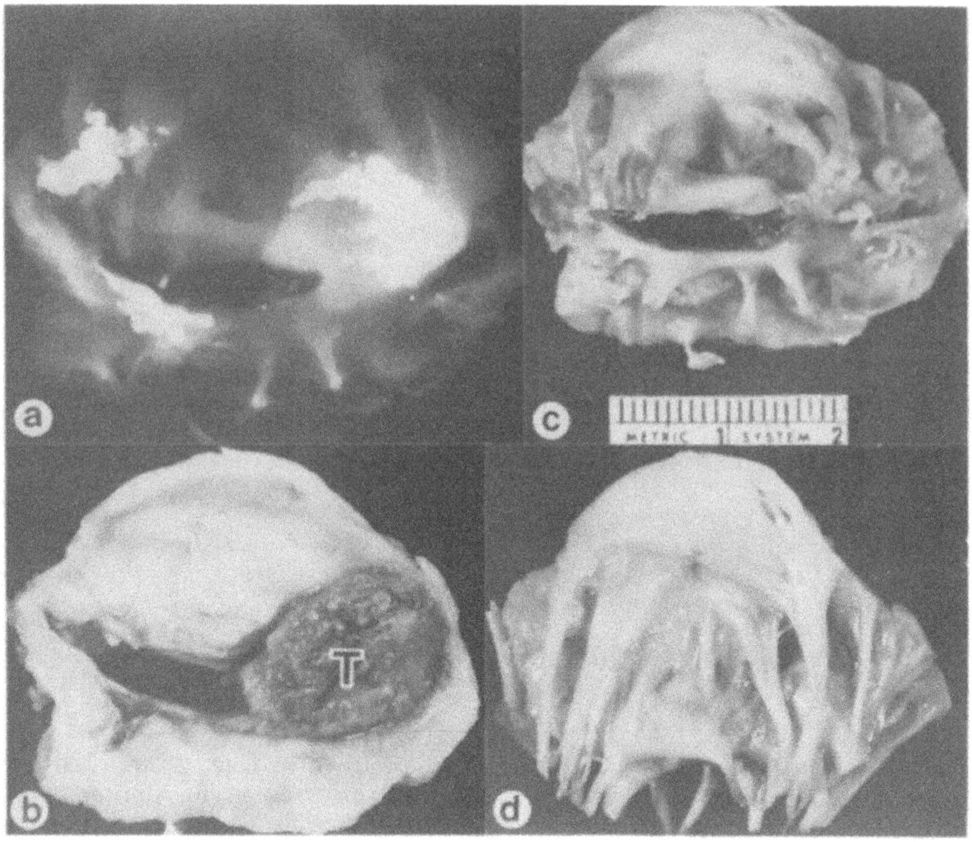

FIGURE 7. Operatively excised stenotic mitral valve in a 72-year-old woman (S76-76) who had had an embolus to a femoral artery 5 years earlier. **a,** radiogram of the operatively excised valve showing focal calcific deposits. **b,** view of the valve from the left atrial aspect showing an oval thrombus (T) over half of the orifice. No thrombus was present in the left atrial cavity. **c,** view of the valve from the left ventricular aspect. The orifice is eccentric. **d,** view of the anterior leaflet.

commissures are usually fused, and the chordae tendineae are shortened and usually fused to some degree (Fig. 4 to 8). The great obstruction to this funnel-shaped valve occurs at its apex, which is within the left ventricular cavity. The primary orifice, located at the level of the anulus, is far less narrowed. Fusion may involve 1 or both commissures. When only 1 is fused or 1 is fused more than the other, the stenotic orifice is eccentrically located. A centrally located orifice indicates symmetrical commissural fusion. In rheumatic MS, the chordae tendineae are occasionally so retracted that the leaflets appear to insert directly into the papillary muscles. When this occurs, the MS is always severe because the interchordal spaces are almost entirely obliterated. Sometimes chordae inserting into 1 papillary muscle are well preserved, whereas those inserting into the other papillary muscle are partially or completely fused. Mitral commissurotomy on a valve in which the leaflets insert almost directly into the papillary muscle(s) usually must include a splitting of the papillary muscle(s) as well as the commissure(s). If there are normally about 120 third-order chordae and about 24 first-order chordae, in MS these numbers are usually halved and, on occasion, even reduced to just 1.

The amount of *calcium* in the leaflets of stenotic mitral valves varies considerably[18] (Figs. 6 to 8). Generally, calcium is more frequent and in larger quantity in men than in women, in older than in younger patients, and in patients with higher compared with those with lower pressure gradients between left atrium and left ventricle[18] (Fig. 9). The rapidity with which calcium develops also varies considerably; it is present at a younger age in men than in women.[18] Lachman and I[18] determined the presence or absence and the extent of calcific deposits in operatively excised stenotic mitral valves by radiography of the excised valve in 164 patients aged 26 to 72 years. The extent of the mitral calcific deposits was determined by the percentage of the valvular circumference containing the deposits: grade 0 (14 patients); grade I = 1 to 25% (43 patients); grade II = 26 to 50% (34 patients); grade III = 51 to 75% (39 patients); and grade IV = 76 to 100% (34 patients). The amount of calcific deposits in the stenotic mitral valves correlated with *sex* and with the *mean diastolic pressure gradient across the mitral valve* ($p < 0.05$) (Fig. 9), but it did not correlate with the patient's age (after age 25 years), cardiac rhythm, pulmonary arterial or pulmonary arterial wedge pressure, previous mitral commissurotomy, presence of thrombus in the body of left atrium, or the presence of disease of 1 or more other cardiac valves.

Among the 164 patients with MS having mitral valve replacement and roentgenography of the excised mitral valve, 14 had no mitral calcium and 43 had only trace or minimal mitral calcific deposits. Thus, we[19] wondered why these 57 patients had mitral replacement rather than mitral commissurotomy. Of the 57 patients, 37 had moderate to severe MR and, therefore, clearly deserved mitral valve replacement. The remaining 20 had absent or minimal calcific deposits, but, nevertheless, they too

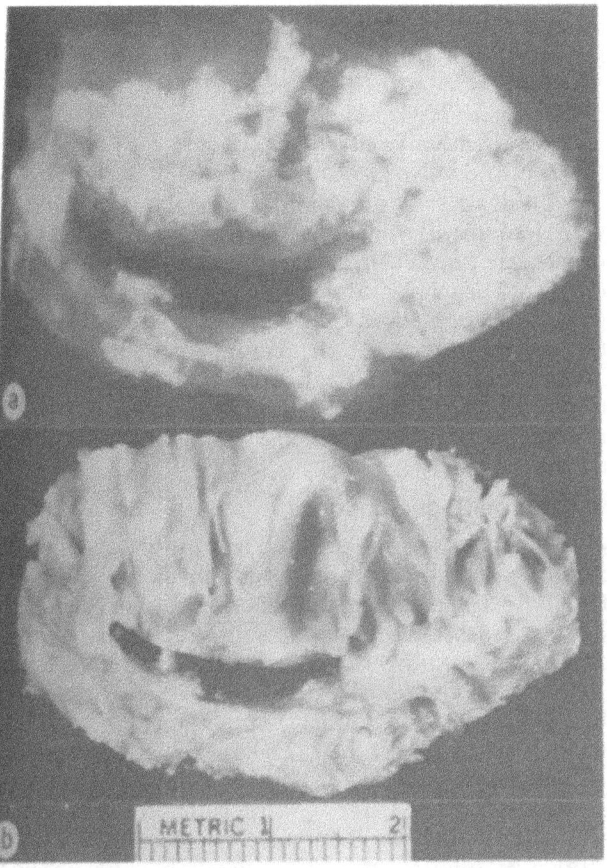

FIGURE 8. Operatively excised stenotic heavily calcified mitral valve in a 53-year-old woman (S67-867) in whom the mean diastolic gradient between the pulmonary arterial wedge position and the left ventricle was 26 mm Hg. She also had 1+/4+ mitral regurgitation by left ventriculogram; a thrombus was present in the body of left atrium. **a**, radiogram of the operatively excised valve. **b**, view of the valve from the left ventricle after excision of the papillary muscle. The orifice is eccentric. (Reprinted, by permission, from Lachman and Roberts.[18])

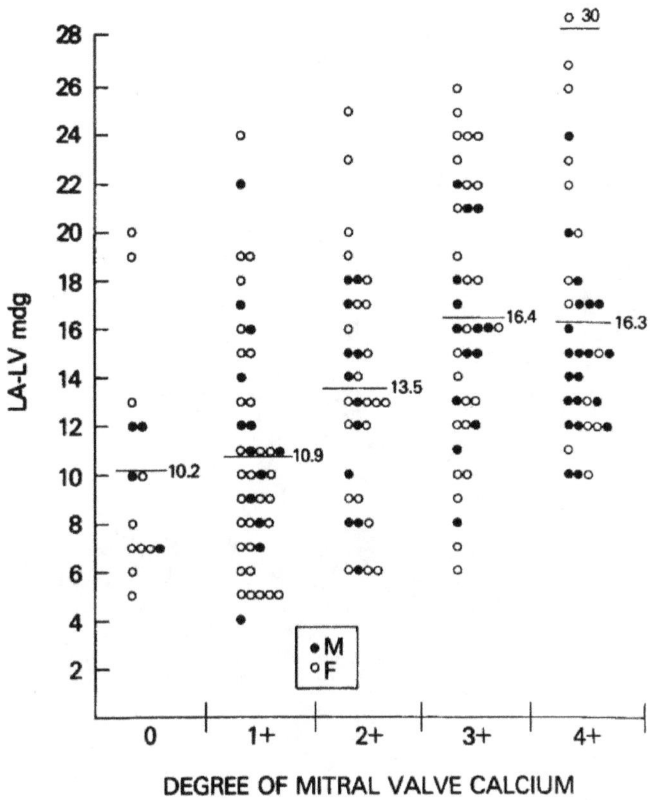

FIGURE 9. Relation between the left atrial (LA) left ventricular (LV) mean diastolic gradient (mdg) and degree of mitral valve calcium. (Reprinted, by permission, from Lachman and Roberts.[18])

had mitral valve replacement. Although in the prevalve replacement era all 20 patients almost surely would have been considered good or ideal candidates for mitral commissurotomy, other factors swung the surgeon to valve replacement rather than commissurotomy. These factors included the need to replace 1 or more other cardiac valves (13 patients), the utilization of cardiopulmonary bypass allowing visual inspection rather than simple palpation of the diseased mitral valve (all 20 patients), relatively little experience with mitral commissurotomy in 4 of the 5 surgeons (17 patients), displeasure with attempted commissurotomy (3 patients), previous mitral commissurotomy (11 patients), and incorrect identification of mitral calcific deposits (2 patients). Even though mitral commissurotomy has been in use for 30 years, the mere alternative of valve replacement may have altered the definition of the stenotic mitral valve previously considered ideal for mitral commissurotomy.

A major complication of MS is *thrombus formation in the left atrial cavity*. The thrombus may be limited to atrial appendage (most common) or be located in both left atrial appendage and body (Fig. 10). The latter group hereafter will be referred to as "left atrial body thrombus." Left atrial body thrombus was observed in 5% of 1,010 personally studied necropsy patients with fatal valvular heart disease; all had severe MS (Table I). Left atrial body thrombus was not observed in any of the 165 patients with pure MR with or without aortic valve dysfunction. All patients with left atrial body thrombi had atrial fibrillation. Comparison of these necropsy patients with 46 patients with MS operated upon at the National Heart, Lung, and Blood Institute and in whom thrombus was found at operation in the left atrial body disclosed that 42 (91%) patients had atrial fibrillation. In contrast, of 40 living patients undergoing mitral valve replacement for pure MR and operated upon at the National Heart, Lung, and Blood Institute, none had thrombus in the body of the left atrium, although 75% had atrial fibrillation. *Thrombus appears to occur in the body of the left atrium only in patients with MS, and atrial fibrillation without MS is incapable of forming a thrombus in the left atrial body.*

Calcific deposits on the mural endocardium of the left atrium are indicative of previous organization with calcification of left atrial thrombi. Histologically, the "calcific thrombi" also contain cholesterol clefts and are identical to atherosclerotic plaques. The observation that left atrial thrombi can organize into lesions iden-

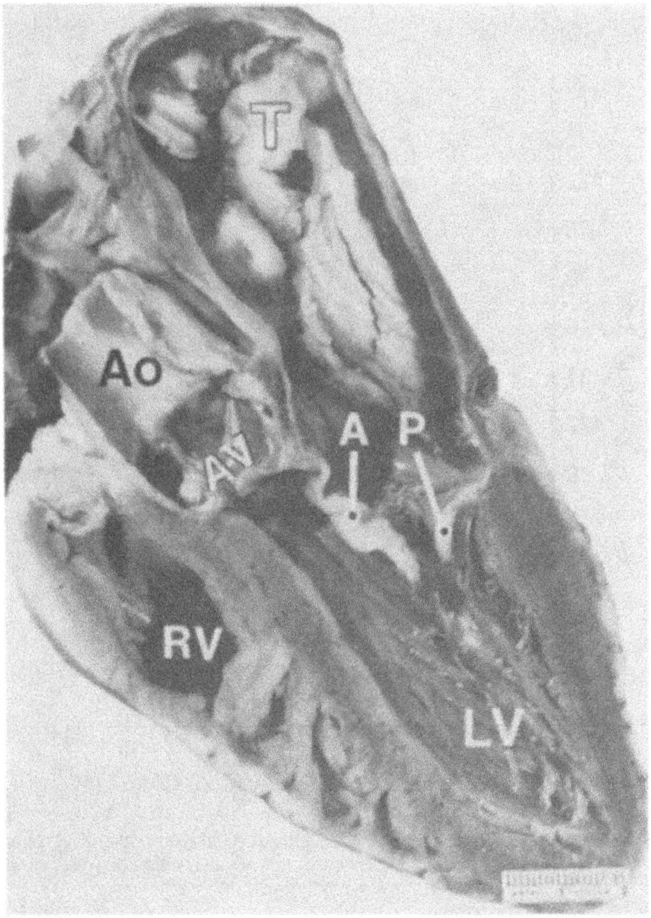

FIGURE 10. Long-axis view of the heart in a 53-year-old woman (GT#77A-190) in whom a huge thrombus (T) was found in the body of the left atrium at necropsy. The mitral valve is quite stenotic. The aortic valve (AV) is normal. A = anterior and P = posterior mitral leaflet; Ao = aorta; LV = left ventricle; RV = right ventricle. Mitral valve commissurotomy had been recommended when the patient was 40 years of age, but she declined. Her last 2 years were characterized by chronic progressive congestive cardiac failure complicated by anemia from multiple myeloma. The patient had chronic atrial fibrillation, but never had cardiac catheterization, a cardiac operation, or evidence of systemic emboli.

tical to atherosclerotic plaques supports the view that atherosclerotic plaques may be the result of organization of thrombi. If calcific deposits form on left atrial body endocardium before the left atrial cavity has had time to dilate, this cavity may be prevented thereafter from dilating. The elevated left atrial pressure may lead more rapidly to pulmonary venous, pulmonary arterial, and right ventricular dilatation with subsequent tricuspsid regurgitation and development of huge right atrial dilatation.[20]

Nonrheumatic causes of MS include *congenital anomalies*[21] (Fig. 11); *neoplasms* (Fig. 12) (particularly myxoma[22]) protruding through the mitral orifice from the left atrium (but malignant neoplasms primary or secondary in the lung may grow into the mitral orifice by way of the pulmonary veins[23]); *large vegetations from active infective endocarditis*[24,25]; and *massive mitral anular calcific deposits*, particularly when associated with small-sized left ventricular cavities and left ventricular outflow tract obstruction[26] (Fig. 13). A relatively new, acquired cause of MS is a *mechanical prosthetic or bioprosthetic cardiac valve.*[27–29] Since the native mitral valve is within the left ventricle, a prosthetic mitral valve also is located within this cavity. The prosthesis must be small enough for the contracting left ventricular wall not to interfere with movement of the prosthetic poppet or disk. When the prosthesis is too large for the cavity into which it was inserted, the poppet may be prevented from moving adequately and may therefore obstruct left atrial emptying. The latter state is far more common than obstruction to left ventricular emptying by the prosthesis. Thrombus formation on a mitral prosthesis also may obstruct left atrial emptying.

Pure Mitral Regurgitation

In contrast to MS, which has mainly 1 cause (rheumatic), pure MR has numerous causes.[2,3,12,16,17,23,30–60] Of the 1,010 patients with functionally severe valvular heart disease, excluding papillary muscle dysfunction, studied personally at necropsy, 165 (16%) had pure (no element of stenosis) MR[5] (Table I); the MR was isolated in 97 of these patients (59%) and associated with aortic valve dysfunction in 68 (41%) (aortic regurgitation in 45 and aortic stenosis in 23). In the 68 patients with associated aortic valve dysfunction, the origin of the valvular disease was rheumatic. Of the 97 patients with clinically isolated pure MR, the aortic valve or the tricuspid valve or both was anatomically abnormal (mild diffuse scarring) in 12 and therefore the cause of the mitral valve dysfunction in these patients was also rheumatic in origin (Table I). Of the remaining 85 patients, the origin of the pure MR was usually nonrheumatic, most commonly ruptured chordae tendineae from infection on a previously normal valve or spontaneous rupture with underlying prolapsing (or floppy) mitral leaflet(s).

Why the mitral valve affected by acute rheumatic fever becomes stenotic in some patients and purely regurgitant in others (mainly children) is unknown. Although the cause may be similar (rheumatic), the structural alterations in the purely regurgitant mitral valve are quite different from those in the stenotic valve. The purely regurgitant rheumatic valve infrequently contains calcific deposits, its commissures are virtually never fused, and its chordae tendineae are only mildly thickened, if at all; chordal fusion is infrequent (Fig. 14). It is often difficult to explain adequately the mechanism of MR in a valve made purely regurgitant by consequences of rheumatic fever. The mitral anuli in children with rheumatic MR usually are dilated but this mechanism is most often not applicable in adults with rheumatic MR.

Rheumatic disease is never limited to endocardium. Inflammatory cells are nearly always found in atrial walls of patients dying with acute rheumatic fever.[61] The inflammation appears to weaken the walls, and superimposed MR tends to dilate the chamber out of proportion to the dilation that would occur with similar degrees of MR into a left atrium with previously normal

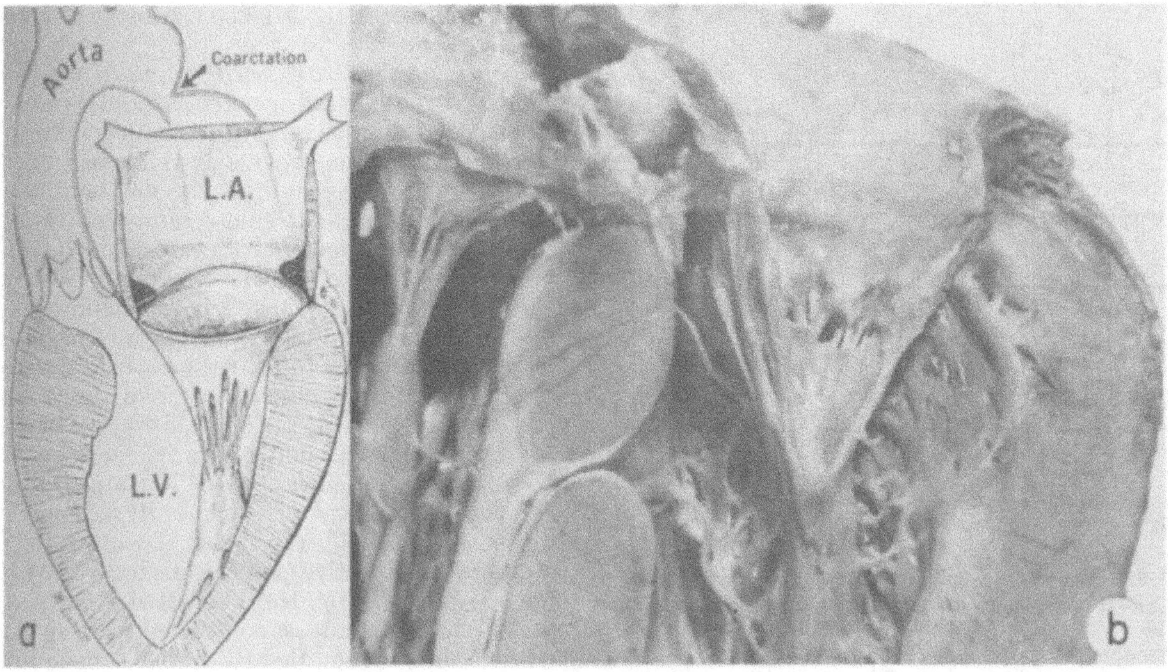

FIGURE 11. Parachute mitral valve causing mitral stenosis in a 14-year-old boy (GT #71A-215) who presented clinically with signs of left ventricular outflow obstruction. The peak systolic gradient between the left ventricle (L.V.) and a systemic artery was 80 mm Hg. Obstruction was caused by a small aortic "anulus" with a bicuspid aortic valve and by discrete obstruction just below the aortic valve. At necropsy, the mitral valve showed a parachute configuration, and all of its chordae inserted into a single left ventricular papillary muscle. Preoperatively, the left atrial mean pressure was 30 mm Hg, and the pulmonary arterial systolic pressure was 50 mm Hg. It was not realized while the patient was alive, however, that the mitral valve was stenotic. In addition, a functionally insignificant coarctation of the aorta was present. A ventricular septal defect had closed spontaneously. L.A. = left atrium. (Reprinted, by permission, from Roberts and Cohen.[3])

walls.[41] What causes the left atrium to dilate enormously in some patients with rheumatic MR is uncertain. Possibly, the patients with so-called giant atria have had more frequent or more severe attacks of acute rheumatic fever, with particularly severe destruction of atrial myocardial fibers. When the left atrium in pure MR is giant in size (Fig. 15), intimal proliferation is rarely found in the pulmonary veins or arteries, and the right ventricular walls are not hypertrophied.[41,47] The larger the left atrial cavity in pure MR, the lower its intracavity pressure. Since the right ventricular walls in these patients are usually not hypertrophied (because the right ventricular systolic pressures are normal or near normal), tricuspid regurgitation is infrequent. In contrast, patients with large left atria from MS or from combined MS and MR have elevated left atrial, pulmonary venous, pulmonary arterial, and right ventricular pressures; the right ventricular walls therefore are

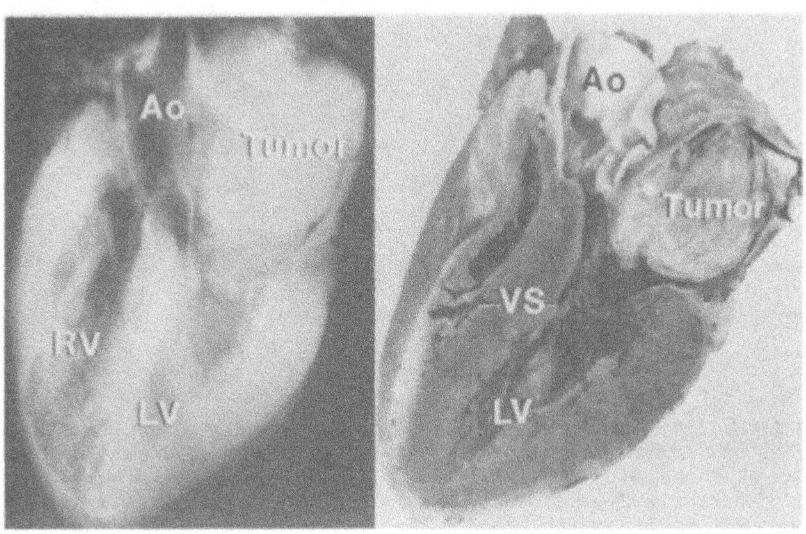

FIGURE 12. Metastatic ovarian carcinoma to the lung with extension into the pulmonary veins and from there into the left atrial body to partly obstruct the mitral orifice in a 44-year-old woman (NNMC #A76-150) who had been asymptomatic until 6 weeks before death, when evidence of congestive heart failure appeared. A precordial murmur was not recorded. **a,** radiogram of heart at necropsy showing a mass in the left atrium and **b,** a long-axis view of heart. Ao = aorta; LV = left ventricle; RV = right ventricle; VS = ventricular septum.

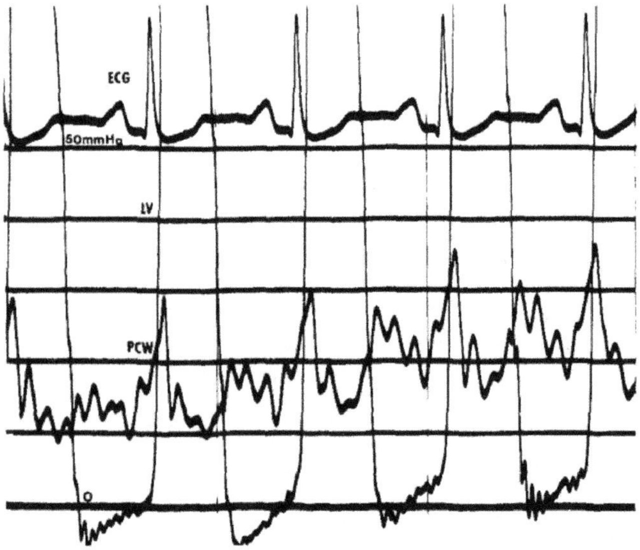

FIGURE 13. Simultaneous, equisensitive recording of pulmonary arterial wedge (PCW) and left ventricular (LV) pressures in a 70-year-old woman (GT #74A-287) with severe (153 mm Hg peak systolic gradient) aortic valve stenosis and massive (4+/4+) mitral anular calcium producing a 15 mm Hg mean diastolic pressure gradient at the level of the otherwise anatomically normal mitral valve. Thus, heavy mitral anular calcific deposits in the setting of left ventricular outflow obstruction can produce "mitral stenosis." ECG = electrocardiogram. (Reprinted, by permission, from Hammer et al.[26])

hypertrophied. Thus, tricuspid regurgitation is a common consequence.

Rupture of mitral chordae tendineae is another common cause of fatal or potentially fatal pure MR.[41,42] The normal chordae tendineae are the ones most likely to rupture, not the previously thickened ones. Thus, rupture of 1 or several thick chordae tendineae in patients with MS is extremely rare. The cause of the rupture varies. Infective endocarditis is the most common cause of acute rupture[41] (Fig. 16). Of 42 patients with healed ruptured mitral chordae tendineae studied by Buchbinder and me, however, only 14 had had infective endocarditis. Infective endocarditis causes acute severe MR by chordal rupture and rarely by leaflet perforation[16] (Fig. 17). The syndrome of acute severe MR associated with normal- or near-normal–sized left atria and severe elevations of left atrial, pulmonary venous, pulmonary arterial, and right ventricular pressures is usually the result of rupture of chordae tendineae by infective endocarditis involving previously normal valves[41] (Fig. 18). The left atrial myocardial fibers in these patients, as contrasted to those in patients with chronic rheumatic MR, have not been previously damaged by rheumatic fever, and, therefore, the left atrial wall is capable of responding to the sudden elevation of left atrial pressure by vigorous contractions, leading to myofiber hypertrophy. The ventricular sys-

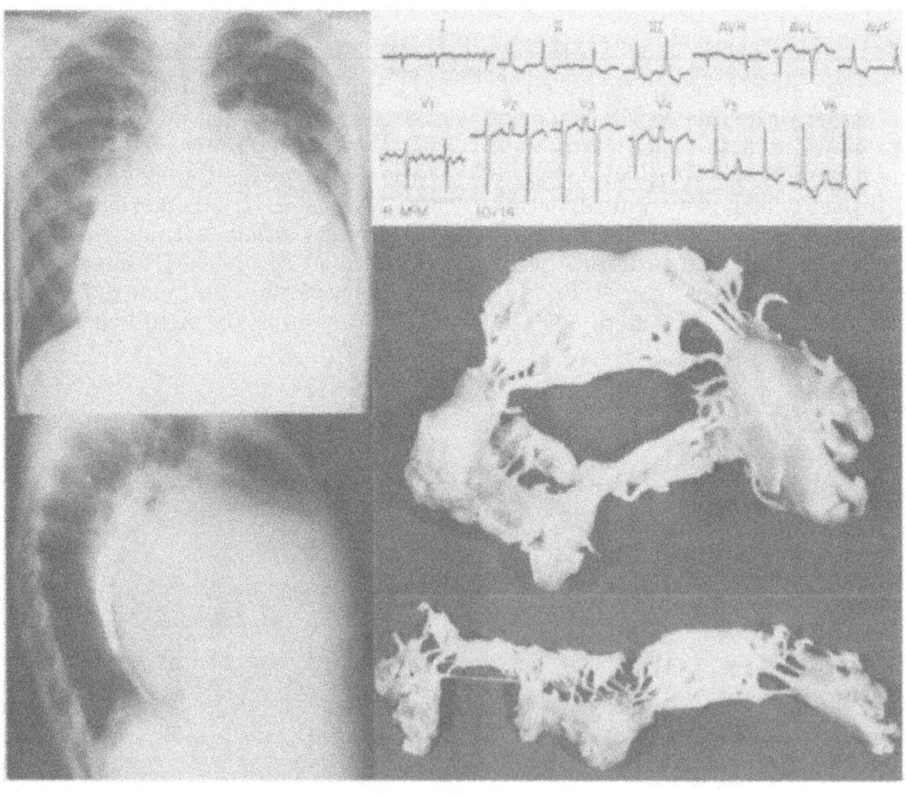

FIGURE 14. Pure mitral and tricuspid valve regurgitation of rheumatic origin in a 15-year-old girl (A63-230) who died 2 days after mitral valve replacement. Shown are posteroanterior and lateral radiograms and an electrocardiogram immediately preoperatively and the intact and opened operatively excised mitral valve. The patient had acute rheumatic fever at ages 6 and 8 years and a prominent "malar flush." The right ventricular and femoral arterial peak systolic pressures were 70 and 110 mm Hg, respectively, preoperatively. The mitral leaflets are diffusely thickened but only mildly so. No Aschoff bodies were present.

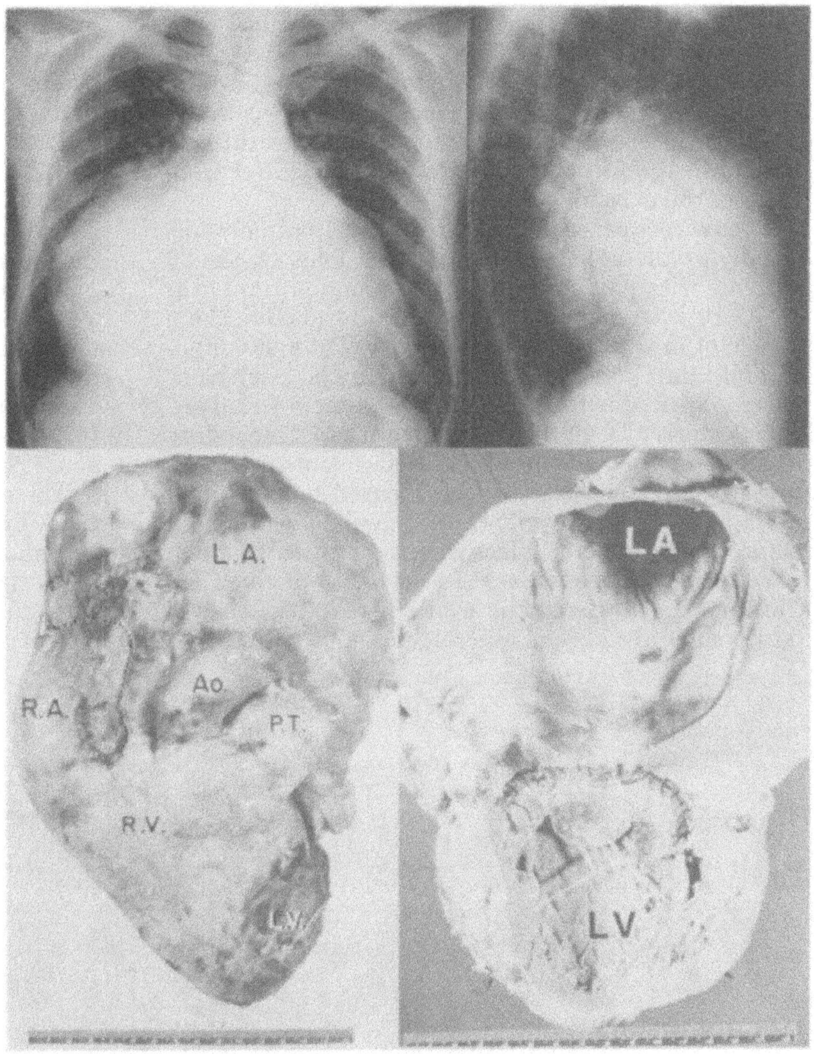

FIGURE 15. Giant-sized left atrium (LA) in a 49-year-old man (A61-84) with severe mitral regurgitation combined with mitral stenosis of rheumatic origin. The right and left ventricular peak systolic pressures were 30 and 100 mm Hg, respectively. The left atrium was entered by a needle inserted into the right mid-axillary line. The patient died 6 hours after mitral replacement. **Lower left,** the giant-sized left atrium is apparent. The **dotted line** outlines the right atrium (RA). Ao = aorta; LV = left ventricle; PT = pulmonary trunk; RV = right ventricle. **Lower right,** opened left atrium, mitral valve, and left ventricle (LV). The ruler units are in centimeters.

tolic pressures in these patients are reflected quickly into the vasculature of the lungs, and severe medial and intimal thickening of the pulmonary arteries and veins progress rapidly. The already diseased left atrium, in contrast, appears to respond to volume load by dilating, not by contracting. Thus, the smaller the left atrial cavity in pure MR, the thicker the right ventricular wall, and, conversely, the larger the left atrial cavity, the thinner the right ventricular wall[41] (Fig. 18).

A relatively new cause of acquired pure MR is *fistulas around the bases of prosthetic and bioprosthetic valves.*[29] Small peribasilar leaks around mitral prostheses are difficult to diagnose clinically without injecting contrast material into the left ventricle.

Although for years rheumatic heart disease has been considered the major cause of significant MR, most patients with rheumatic heart disease and MR also have some degree of MS as well. Of patients with *isolated* (aortic valve function normal), *pure* (no element of stenosis) MR severe enough to warrant mitral valve replacement, *mitral valve prolapse* is now recognized as the most common etiology (Fig. 19 to 22). My associates and I[12] recently reviewed the records and operatively excised mitral valves of 97 patients aged 32 to 78 years (mean 54) (57 men), who underwent mitral valve replacement because of $3^+/4^+$ or $4^+/4^+$ MR as determined by left ventricular angiography. Of the 97 patients, the cause of the MR was leaflet prolapse in 60 (62%), papillary muscle dysfunction from coronary heart disease in 29 (30%), infective endocarditis involving apparently previously normal mitral valve in 5 patients, and rheumatic heart disease in 3 patients (Fig. 23). Of the 60 patients with mitral prolapse, 13 had ruptured chordae tendineae and all 5 patients with infective endocarditis had ruptured chordae.

The circumference of the mitral anuli in the patients with prolapsed valves without ruptured chordae was significantly larger than those in the patients in other groups and in 18 control subjects, both of which were normal (Fig. 24 and 25). Likewise, the areas of the excised leaflets in the prolapsed valves were much larger than in the other groups and in the control subjects, both of which were normal (Fig. 26). The product of the circumference (in centimeters) multiplied by the area (in centimeters squared) calculated for the normal valves ranged from 45 to 140 cm^3 (average 91). The average product was 150 cm^3 in the prolapsed valves with ruptured chordae, and 273 cm^3 in the prolapsed valves with intact chordae. The products were 87, 93, and 106 cm^3, respectively, in the valves regurgitant because of papillary muscle dysfunction, infective endocarditis, or rheumatic disease; these products did not differ from those of the normal valves.

The correct cause of the MR in the 97 patients was usually predictable from the history alone. Of the 29 patients with papillary muscle dysfunction from atherosclerotic coronary heart disease, all had clinical evidence of myocardial ischemia: history of acute myocardial infarction which had healed in 24, a left ventricular aneurysm from a silent infarction in 1, and angina pectoris in 4. Of the 5 patients with MR secondary to infective endocarditis, 4 had well-documented episodes of infection that had been cured by antibiotic therapy; none had evidence of valvular dysfunction before the episode of infective endocarditis. Of the 3 patients with MR secondary to a rheumatic origin, 2 had a history of acute rheumatic fever, whereas this item was positive in only 5 of the other 94 patients. Clinical diagnosis of mitral valve prolapse was by a process of exclusion. Only 2 (3%) of the 60 patients had historical evidence of previous acute myocardial infarction; 5 (8%) had a history of acute rheumatic fever and 4 (7%) had a history of active infective endocarditis. Compared with the 5 patients classified as having ruptured chordae tendineae on previously normal valves (4 of whom had a history of infective endocarditis), the 4 patients with healed infective endocarditis and mitral prolapse were older (mean age 61 years versus 42 years), had previous systolic murmurs of MR before the episode of infective endocarditis (4 of 4 versus 0 of 5), and had a longer mean duration of congestive heart failure (11 months versus 4 months). Thus, of the 60 patients with prolapse, 51 (85%) had no historical evidence of myocardial ischemia, acute rheumatic fever, or infective endocarditis.

The origin of the MR also was suggested preoperatively by more objective means. All 29 patients with MR secondary to coronary disease had abnormal Q waves by electrocardiogram, whereas abnormal Q waves were present in only 4 of the 60 patients with mitral prolapse and in none of the 8 patients with MR from either in-

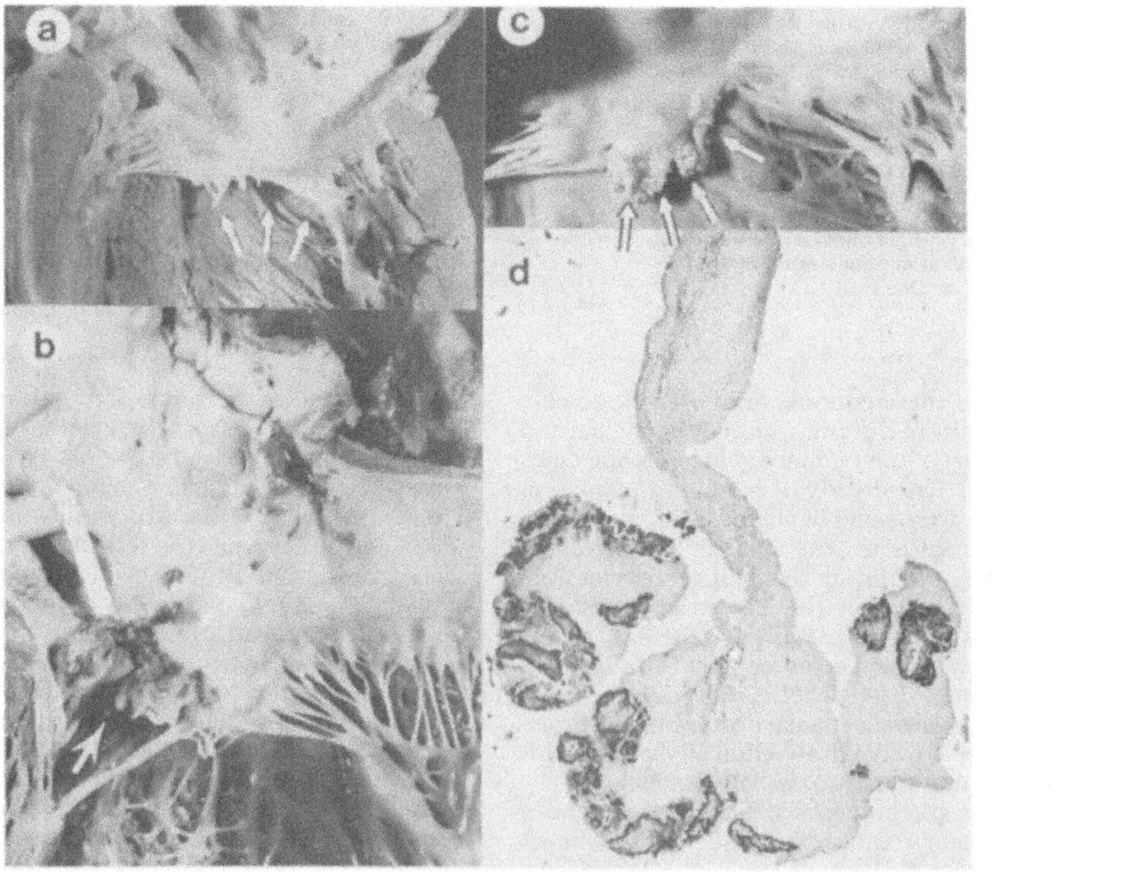

FIGURE 16. Ruptured mitral chordae tendineae (**short arrows**) in 3 patients: **a,** in a 29-year-old woman (A63-97) who had had Staphylococcus epidermidis endocarditis 5 years earlier on what appears to have been a previously anatomically normal valve. The peak systolic pulmonary arterial pressure was 105 mm Hg and the left atrial V wave, 35 mm Hg. **b,** in a 19-year-old girl (A61-221) who had had Streptococcus group D endocarditis 16 months earlier. The peak systolic pulmonary arterial pressure was 70 mm Hg and the left atrial V wave, 36 mm Hg. **c** and **d,** in a 24-year-old woman (A62-19) who had had enterococcus endocarditis 5 months earlier. The peak systolic pulmonary arterial pressure was 72 mm Hg and the left atrial V wave, 66 mm Hg. **d,** histologic section of mitral leaflet at site of chordal rupture showing calcific deposits. Hematoxylin and eosin stain. (Reprinted, by permission, from Roberts et al.[41])

fective endocarditis or rheumatic disease. Atrial fibrillation was significantly ($p < 0.05$) more common in the patients in whom the MR resulted from coronary disease: in 7 (24%) of these 29 patients, in only 4 (7%) of the 60 patients with mitral prolapse, and in 2 of the 8 patients with either infective endocarditis or a rheumatic origin. Of the 60 patients with prolapse, 43 had M-mode echocardiograms; in 32 (74%) prolapse was demonstrated. Of the 29 patients with coronary heart disease, M-mode echocardiograms were done in 22; only 2 (9%) demonstrated prolapse. Of the 8 patients with MR from infective endocarditis or rheumatic etiologies, 7 had

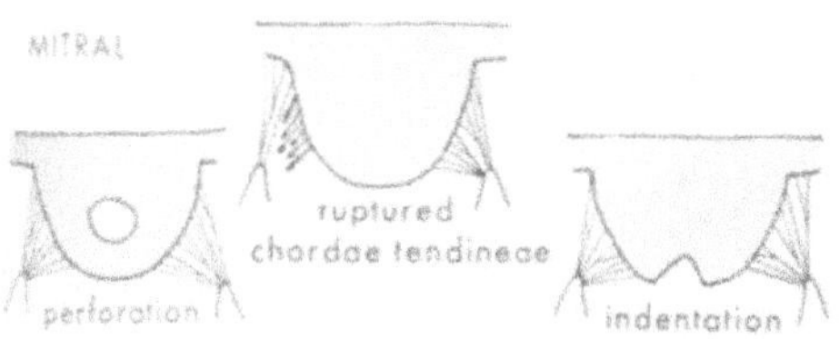

FIGURE 17. Types of mitral valve damage resulting from infective endocarditis.

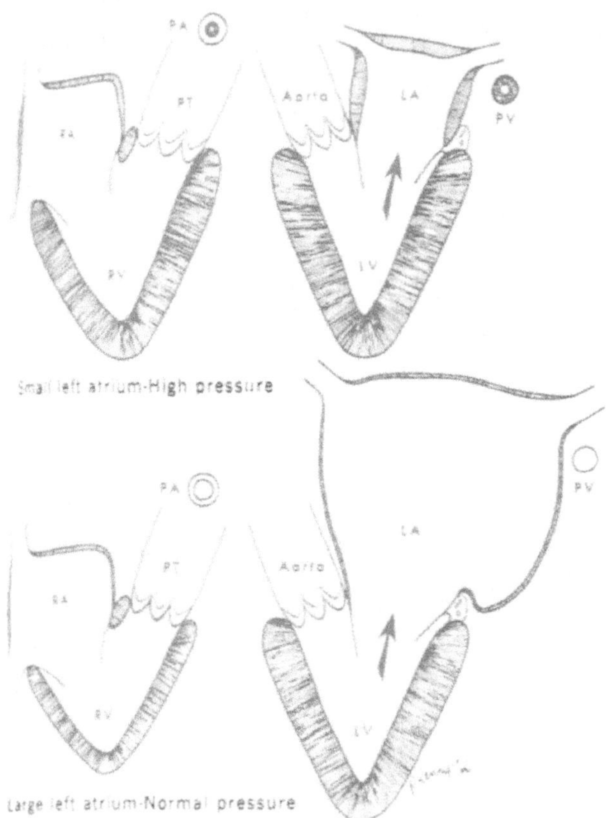

FIGURE 18. Diagram depicting the 2 extremes of the spectrum of pure mitral regurgitation. When severe mitral regurgitation appears suddenly in individuals with previously normal or near-normal hearts, the left atrium (LA) is relatively small and the high pressure within it is reflected back into the pulmonary vessels and right ventricle (RV). The anatomic indicator of this latter physiologic event is severe hypertrophy of the left atrial and right ventricular walls and marked intimal and medial thickening of the pulmonary arteries (PA), arterioles, and veins (PV). In the other extreme, the left atrial cavity is of giant size and its wall is thin. It is thus able to "absorb" the left ventricular (LV) pressure without reflecting it back into the pulmonary vessels or right ventricle. As a consequence, the pulmonary vessels remain normal and the right ventricular wall does not thicken. PT = pulmonary trunk; RA = right atrium. (Reprinted, by permission, from Roberts et al.[47])

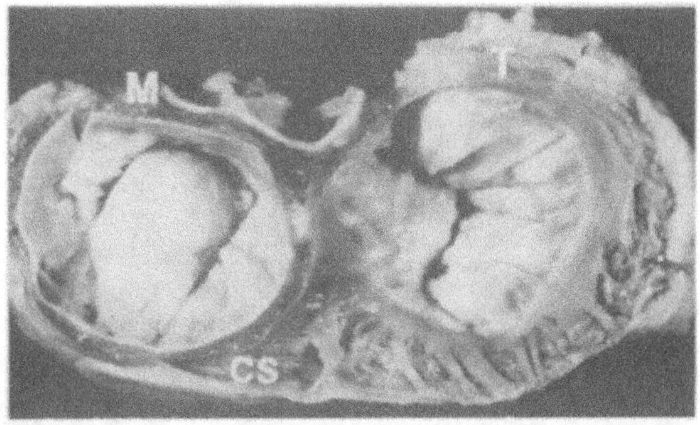

FIGURE 19. Prolapsing mitral (M) and tricuspid (T) valves from the atrial sides in a 55-year-old man (DCMEO #77-05-359) who died suddenly and unexpectedly while at a dance. The patient was known to have had a precordial systolic click and a late systolic murmur since age 36 years but had always been asymptomatic. The M-mode echocardiogram was typical of mitral prolapse. At necropsy, a huge prolapsing "scallop" of the posterior mitral leaflet was present and at least 1 chorda tendinea to this leaflet had ruptured. The leaflet area of the tricuspid valve also was considerably increased. CS = coronary sinus.

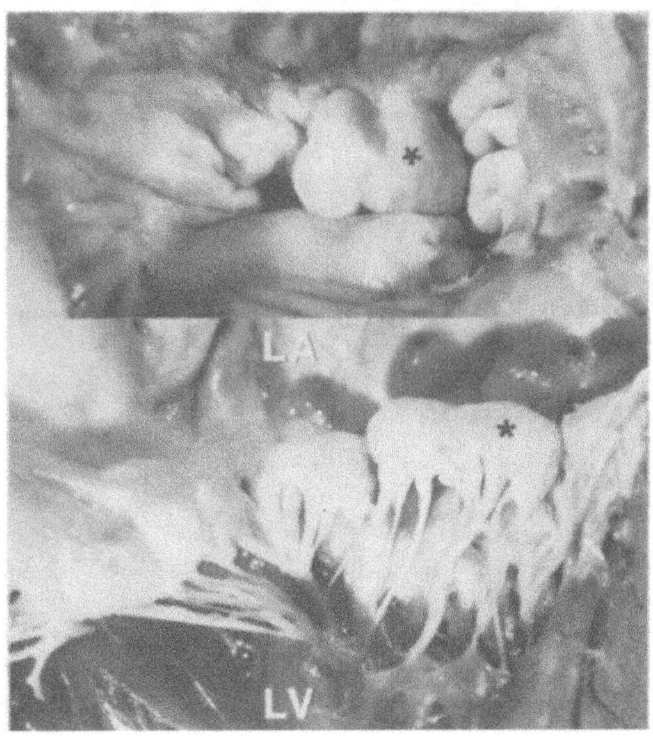

FIGURE 20. Prolapsed mitral valve from above (**top**) and after opening (**bottom**) in an 88-year-old woman who died when hit by an automobile. The patient had had no symptoms of cardiac dysfunction. The **asterisk** indicates the most prolapsed portion of posterior mitral leaflet. The mural endocarium beneath the posterior leaflet is thickened by fibrous tissue. LA = left atrium; LV = left ventricle.

echocardiograms; none demonstrated prolapse. Left ventriculograms, performed in all 97 patients, indicated prolapse in only 16 (27%) of the 60 prolapse patients and in none of the other 37 patients with other causes. Selective coronary angiograms were performed in 53 (55%) of the 97 patients. All 29 with MR secondary to coronary heart disease had significant (>50% diameter reduction) coronary narrowing demonstrated angiographically in at least 2 of the 3 major coronary arteries. Of the 60 patients with mitral prolapse, coronary angiograms were

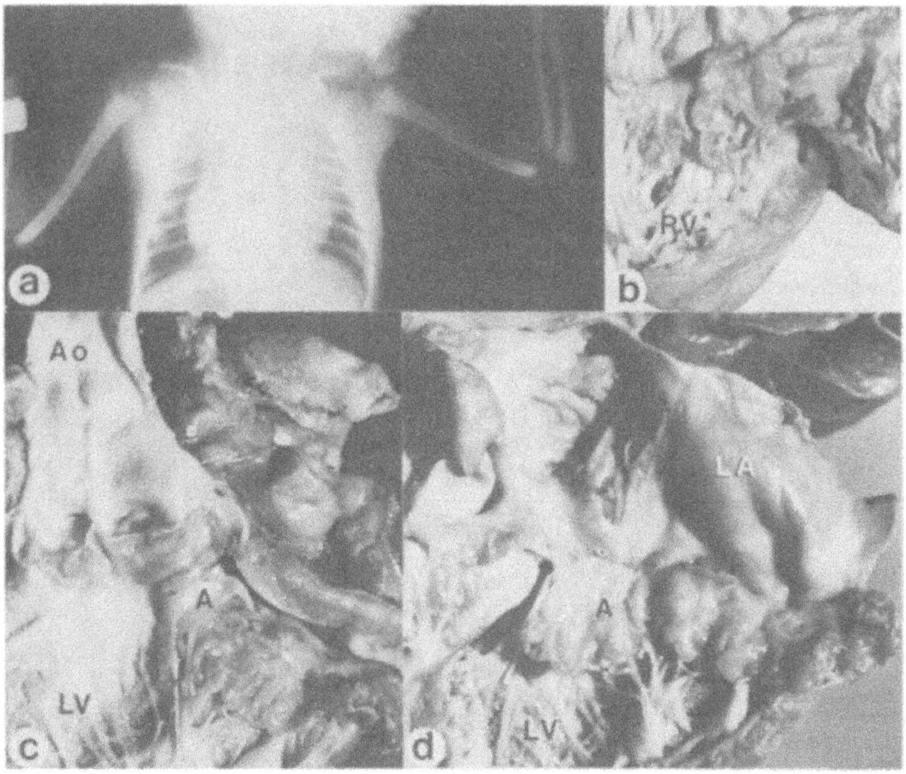

FIGURE 21. Congenital floppy mitral valve and floppy tricuspid valve in a 2-day-old boy (A67-236) who had long toes and fingers, a high-arched palate, and a grade 3/6 precordial systolic murmur typical of mitral regurgitation when examined. The heart was enlarged (**a**) and the infant died of congestive cardiac failure. At necropsy, the intima of the ascending aorta (Ao) was wrinkled (**c**), suggesting that the underlying media was abnormal at this early stage. Shown here are the opened aorta, aortic valve, and left ventricle (LV). A = anterior mitral leaflet. **d,** opened left atrium (LA), mitral valve, and left ventricle (LV). The mitral leaflets are considerably elongated in both longitudinal and transverse dimensions. The left atrium is dilated. **b,** the tricuspid valve leaflets also are elongated in both transverse and longitudinal dimensions. RA = right atrium; RV = right ventricle. (Reprinted, by permission, from Roberts and Honig.[40])

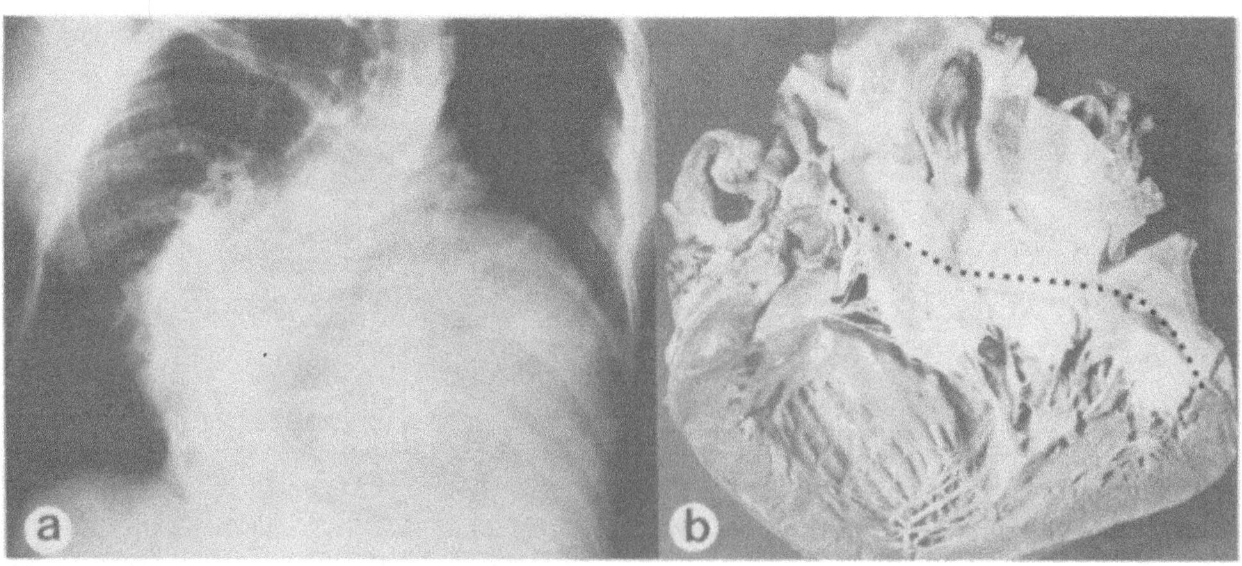

FIGURE 22. Posteroanterior chest roentgenogram (**left**) and opened left atrium, mitral valve, and left ventricle (**right**) in a 28-year-old man (A63-25) who had the onset of exertional dyspnea 4 years before death and evidence of overt congestive heart failure for 1 year before death. He never had a murmur of aortic regurgitation. At necropsy, the aorta was normal both grossly and histologically. The mitral valve anulus (**dotted line**) is greatly dilated (17 cm) and the length of the cusps from basal attachment to distal margin is elongated without elongation of the chordae tendineae. The vertebral column is greatly deformed (**left**). (Reprinted, by permission, from Roberts and Honig.[40])

performed in 23; only 3 (13%) had significant coronary narrowing, limited in each to 1 (right) coronary artery. Auscultation and hemodynamic data at cardiac catheterization were not helpful in delineating the origin of the MR. None of the 97 patients—including the 60 classified as having prolapse—had systolic clicks and the systolic precordial murmurs in all 97 patients were holosystolic. The average pulmonary arterial, left atrial (or pulmonary arterial wedge), and left ventricular pressures were similar in the 97 patients irrespective of the origin of the MR. The systolic systemic arterial pressures, however, were significantly higher in the patients with mitral prolapse and ruptured chordae tendineae than in those with mitral prolapse and intact chordae tendineae.

Surprisingly, few reports are available describing the various causes of MR in large numbers of patients. Furthermore, we[12] were unable to find any reports concerning the causes of pure MR in groups of patients in whom any associated MS or aortic valve dysfunction had been excluded by appropriate hemodynamic and angiographic studies. The most frequently cited report describing patients with MR appears to be that by Selzer and Katayama,[62] who summarized findings in

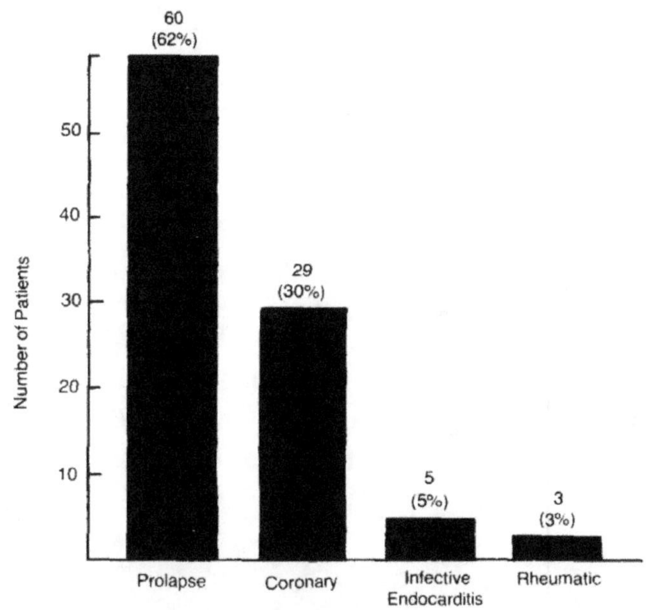

FIGURE 23. Bar graph showing the 4 conditions causing chronic, isolated, pure mitral regurgitation in 97 patients with operatively excised valves. (Reprinted, by permission, from Waller et al.[12])

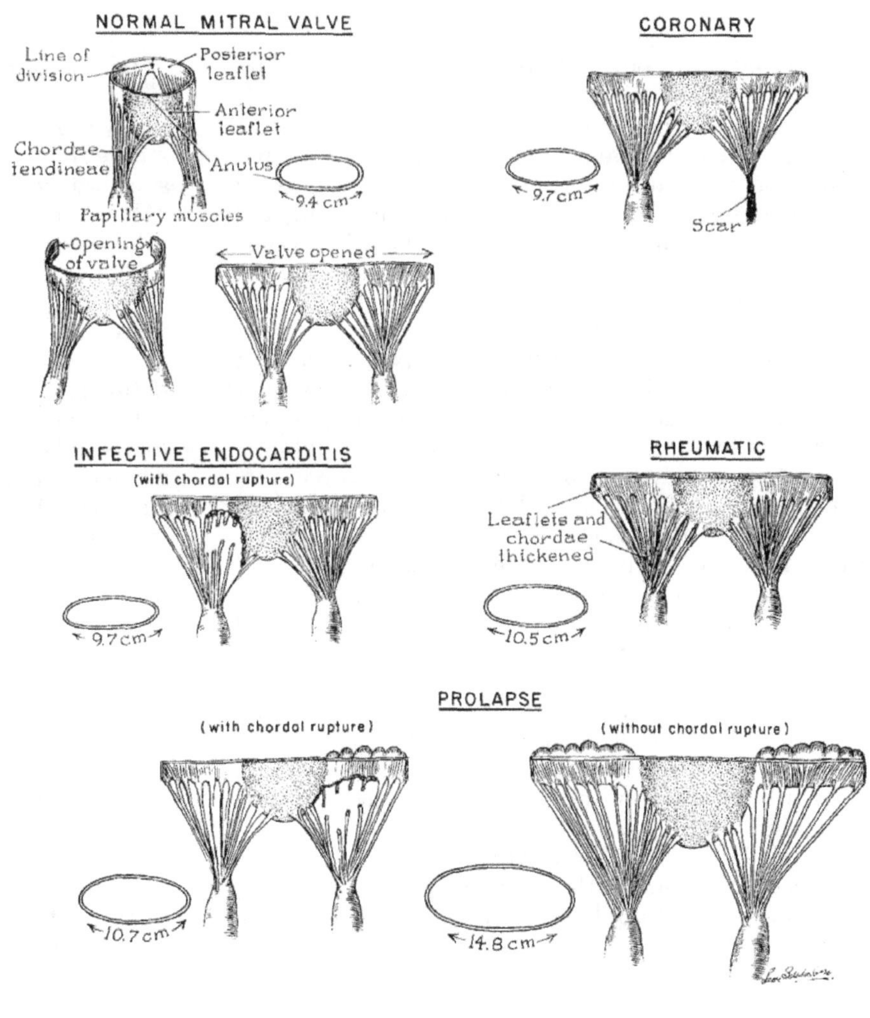

FIGURE 24. Diagram showing morphologic variations in mitral valve "anular" circumference and leaflet area in 4 conditions causing isolated, pure mitral regurgitation. (Reprinted, by permission, from Waller et al.[12])

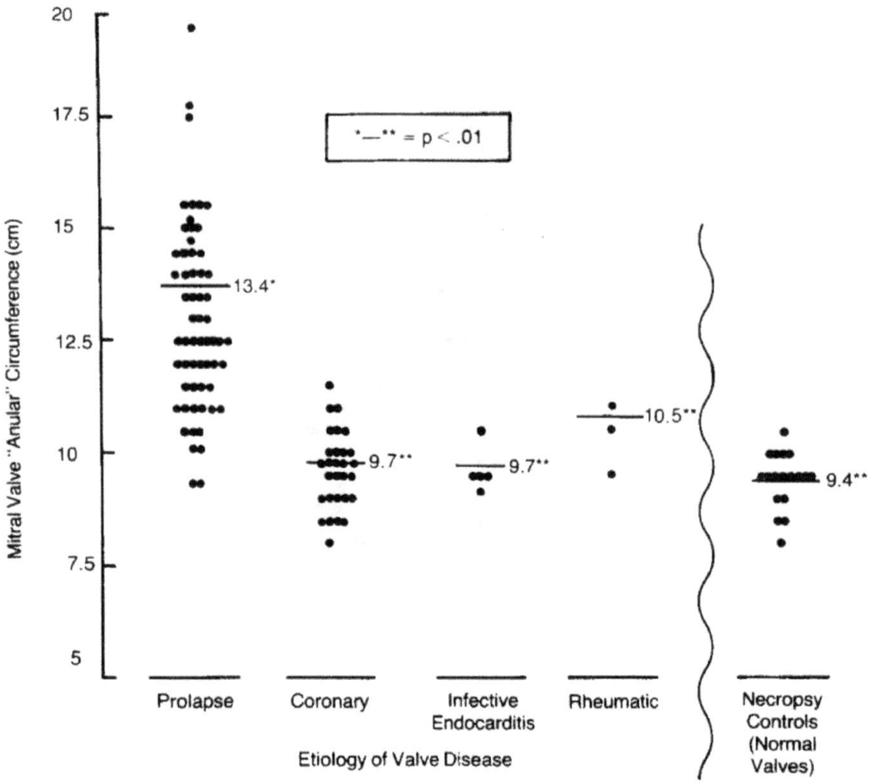

FIGURE 25. Graph showing mitral valve "anular" circumference (in centimeters) in each of the 97 patients with operatively excised mitral valves in the 4 conditions causing chronic, isolated, pure mitral regurgitation, and in 18 necropsy control valves. (Reprinted, by permission, from Waller et al.[12])

230 patients. Although 212 of their 230 patients had pure MR defined as the "absence of a late diastolic gradient across the valve . . . except in tachycardia" at the time of cardiac catheterization, some of their patients had MS at other times. Of their 230 patients, 88 were classified as having MR of rheumatic origin, and I suspect that nearly half (42 patients) had MS at some time in their course: 5 had had mitral commissurotomies for MS and severe MR developed subsequently; 8 of their rheumatic patients had MR only after the development of infective endocarditis, and it is probable that 1 or more previously had had MS; and 33 (38%) of their 88 rheumatic patients had sizeable calcific deposits in their mitral valves, a finding quite unusual in patients without some degree of MS. (Only 4 of our 97 patients had grossly visible calcific deposits in their excised mitral valves.) It is also difficult to compare the observations in our patients with those reported by Selzer and Katayama because of differences in patient selection. We[12] studied only patients who were in functional classes III and IV (New York Heart Association) because of congestive heart failure; all underwent mitral valve replacement and all had their valves examined by the same observer. Seventy (30%) of the 230 patients reported by Selzer and Katayama were in functional classes I or II, and mitral valve operations were performed in just over half of the 230 patients. Additionally, they included children, which we did not. Finally, we excluded patients with any aortic valve dysfunction, which may or may not have been the case in the study by Selzer and Katayama.

In the past, rheumatic heart disease has been considered the most common cause of severe MR, but it is likely that most or many patients so classified in older studies had some degree of MS. Because there has been such a strong tendency in the past to believe that severe MR was usually the result of rheumatic heart disease, other causes commonly have not been sought and definitions of "rheumatic" MR have not been precisely stated. Before 1963, most prolapsing or floppy mitral valves almost certainly were called "rheumatic" in origin at necropsy or operation. Our report[12] morphologically defined a prolapsed mitral valve which can cause severe MR; its anular circumference and leaflet area are clearly increased over that of other valves causing MR, except when the chordae tendineae of the prolapsing valve are ruptured. It is hoped that this definition will prevent indiscriminate labeling of mitral disease in the future as rheumatic when other evidences of previous rheumatic carditis are lacking.

Congenital MR is usually associated with other anomalities.[2,6,30–40] "*Isolated*" congenital MR is usually accompanied by *endocardial fibroelastosis of the left ventricle*. It is sometimes difficult, however, to determine what causes the mitral valve to be regurgitant in this circumstance. Neither is it always clear why the mitral valve is frequently regurgitant in patients with *partial atrioventricular canal* (endocardial cushion defect).[30,31,37] Nearly all patients with partial atrioventricular canal have a cleft, either partial or complete, in the anterior mitral leaflet. It would be easy to attribute the MR to the cleft, but the MR usually disap-

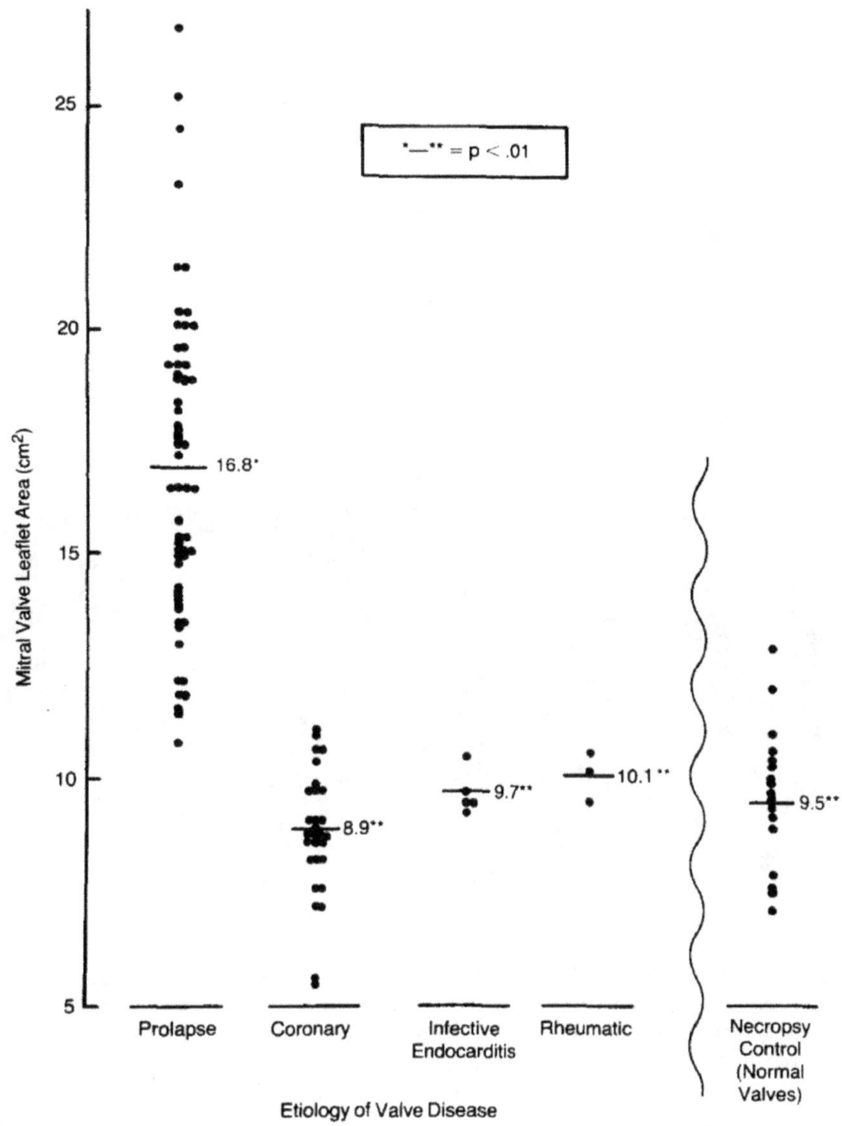

FIGURE 26. Graph showing mitral valve leaflet area (in centimeters squared) in each of the 97 patients with operatively excised mitral valves in the 4 conditions causing chronic, isolated, pure mitral regurgitation and in 18 necropsy control valves. (Reprinted, by permission, from Waller et al.[12])

pears after operative closure of the associated defect in the lowermost portion of the atrial septum (ostium primum defect), irrespective of whether the cleft in the anterior mitral leaflet is closed by suture. For the same reason, it is unlikely that the anomalous chordae tendineae that insert onto the crest of the ventricular septum play a significant role in the production of MR. It is helpful to think of partial atrioventricular canal as a syndrome consisting of 5 components: (1) defect in the lowermost portion of atrial septum; (2) cleft in the anterior mitral leaflet; (3) absence of tissue, either partial or complete, in the septal tricuspid valve leaflet; (4) anomalous chordae tendineae from the anterior mitral leaflet to the crest of ventricular septum; and (5) ventricular septal defect. The syndrome may include all 5 components or may have as few as 2; most commonly, the first 4 components are present. A cleft in the anterior mitral leaflet may occur, however, in the absence of a defect in the lowermost portion of the atrial septum.[63] These individuals usually present with evidence of isolated MR or with features of isolated ventricular septal defect. Of 21 necropsy patients with a cleft in the anterior mitral leaflet unassociated with a defect in the lowermost portion of the atrial septum reported by Segni and Edwards,[63] 11 had no defect in any portion of the atrial or ventricular septa and the other 9 had associated defects, usually ventricular septal defect or a fossa ovale type atrial septal defect or both. Occasionally, the ostium primum defect may be so small that the shunt through it is missed or is only trivial; these patients also may present with essentially pure MR.[30,31]

Corrected transposition is an entity that has produced much confusion. Corrected transposition and complete transposition are quite different; the only thing they have in common is the word "transposition." Complete transposition is essentially 1 defect: the great arteries are transposed, so that the aorta arises from the right ventricle and the pulmonary trunk from the left ventricle. In corrected transposition, the great arteries

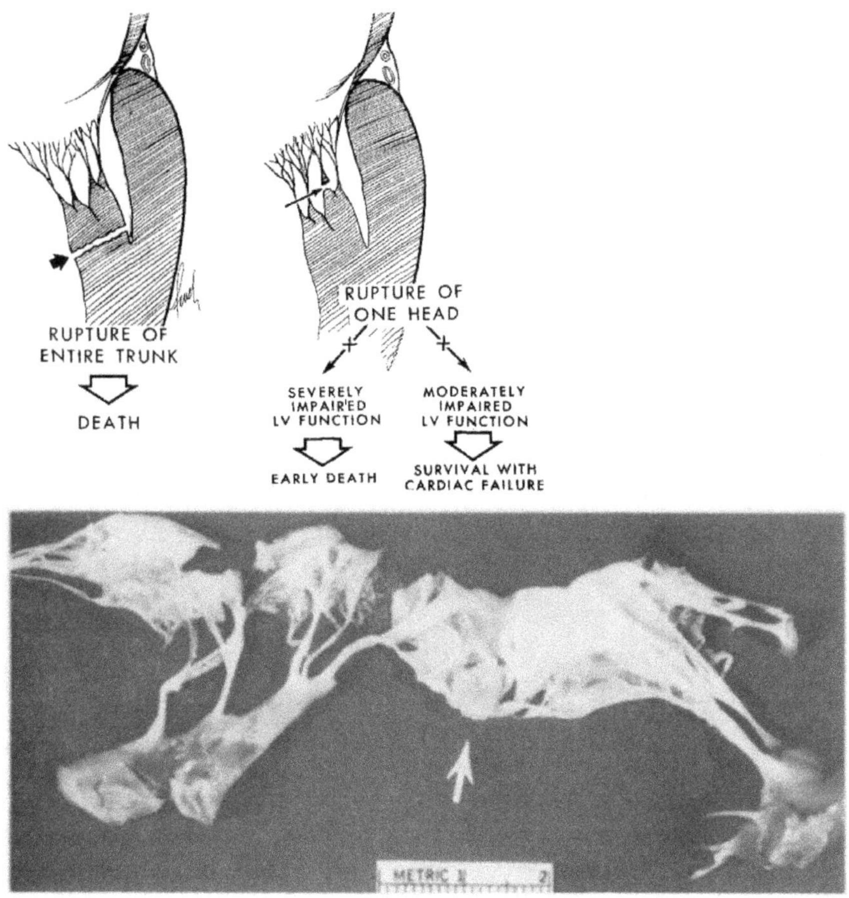

FIGURE 27. Top, diagram of the types of, and possible consequences of, papillary muscle rupture during acute myocardial infarction. It is likely that rupture of the entire trunk (**left**) is incompatible with survival in any patient since a major portion of the support to both valve leaflets is destroyed. With rupture of an apical head (**right**), survival would appear to depend on the extent to which the function of the left ventricle has been impaired by the infarct. With severely impaired ventricular function, the additional burden of even modest mitral regurgitation may be intolerable, and death will ensue. If the left ventricle is less severely compromised, survival is possible for weeks or months, but congestive cardiac failure will almost invariably develop. **Bottom,** rupture of a portion of 1 papillary muscle during acute myocardial infarction in a 51-year-old man (S67-813) who underwent mitral valve replacement 3 months after the onset of the infarction. Preoperatively, the pulmonary arterial pressure was 60/28 mm Hg; pulmonary arterial wedge pressure, mean 28, v42; left ventricular pressure 74/17 mm Hg; and cardiac index, 1.7 liters/min/m^2. The leaflets are normal but the posteromedial papillary muscle is necrotic and fibrotic and a portion of it (**arrow**) is entwined in chordae tendineae at the margin of the anterior mitral leaflet. This is a view of the ventricular aspects of the leaflets. LV = left ventricular. (Reprinted, by permission, from Roberts and Perloff.[2])

also are transposed, but, in addition, the ventricles, atrioventricular valves, coronary arteries, and conduction system are inverted. Patients with complete transposition die because they have inadequate communications between the 2 circuits. Patients with corrected transposition theoretically should be able to live a full lifespan, but usually this is not the case because associated defects—namely, ventricular septal defect or regurgitation of the left-sided atrioventricular valve, or both—cause the heart to function abnormally. Abnormalities of the left-sided atrioventricular valve, a systemic valve but anatomically a tricuspid valve, are the most common associated anomalies in corrected transposition.[64] Of the anomalies, the most frequent is the Ebstein-type malformation. These valves are intrinsically regurgitant because the chordae are short and the leaflets are closely adherent to the ventricular endocardium.

A mitral valve may be abnormal anatomically and yet function entirely normally. A congenital malformation illustrating this point is the *double-orifice mitral valve*, which looks like a double-barreled shotgun.[65] Generally, both orifices are totally competent and the patient should be asymptomatic.

Papillary Muscle Dysfunction

Rupture of a portion of a papillary muscle was not appreciated until 15 years ago.[48] The original concept of papillary muscle rupture was rupture of its entire trunk, caused either by myocardial infarction from coronary narrowing or by trauma (Fig. 27). Complete transsection of a left ventricular papillary muscle is incompatible with life because about 60 chordae tendineae are thus disrupted. More frequent is rupture of a portion of a papillary muscle. In this situation, the largest amount of MR is probably caused by the rupture, but all these patients have severe necrosis of the remaining portion of the papillary muscle and the latter probably contributes to the regurgitation. When 1 head of a papillary muscle is ruptured, about 10 third-order chordae tendineae are disrupted.

Necrosis or fibrosis of a papillary muscle without rupture is far more common than rupture. Table II lists conditions frequently associated with papillary muscle dysfunction, particularly necrosis or fibrosis.[3] Although coronary arterial luminal narrowing is the most frequent cause of papillary muscle necrosis or fibrosis, many other conditions may be accompanied by papillary muscle lesions. The papillary muscles are fibrotic or necrotic in so many conditions because they are the last structures in the heart to be perfused by arterial blood. Of the 2 left ventricular papillary muscles, the posteromedial one has the poorer blood supply, and, consequently, lesions are more frequent in it than in the anterolateral muscle. The posteromedial muscle receives its oxygen mainly from blood passing through the right coronary artery. The mouth of this artery may be >15 cm from the apex of the posteromedial muscle. To perfuse it, blood must pass through the entire thickness of left ventricular wall, turn uphill (so to speak), and ascend a distance equivalent to 2 more full thicknesses of left ventricular wall. Thus, the apices of the papillary muscles are the sites farthest from the coronary ostia, and they receive oxygen only after the other myocardium has had an opportunity to extract its oxygen needs. Although the surfaces of the papillary muscles are entirely bathed by intracavitary ventricular blood, only a small amount of oxygen diffuses into these structures from the intracavitary blood.

The most common cause of papillary muscle necrosis or fibrosis is *narrowing of the coronary arterial lumen by atherosclerotic plaques.* The posteromedial papillary muscle is usually involved in acute posterior myocardial infarction. In anterior wall infarction, however, the anterolateral papillary muscle may be spared, presumably because its blood supply is better than that of the posteromedial muscle. Since infarction limited to the ventricular septum or to the lateral portion of the left ventricular free wall (that is, the portions of the left ventricular wall unassociated with papillary muscles) is rare, the papillary muscles are usually involved when myocardial infarction occurs. It is, therefore, surprising that papillary muscle dysfunction is not more frequent during or after acute myocardial infarction.

In patients with *left ventricular outflow obstruction*, lesions often occur in the papillary muscles. Valvular aortic stenosis, whether in infants or in adults, when superimposed on a congenitally malformed valve, either unicuspid or bicuspid, is nearly always associated with fibrosis and atrophy of at least the posteromedial papillary muscle. Rheumatic valvular aortic stenosis combined with organic MS or MR, however, infrequently is associated with papillary muscle fibrosis or atrophy. Nearly all adult patients with discrete subaortic stenosis or hypertrophic cardiomyopathy with or without diffuse subaortic stenosis have small fibrous scars in both left ventricular papillary muscles, but atrophy of 1 or both muscles is uncommon.[39]

Foci of necrosis also are common in patients with fatal *severe valvular regurgitation of recent onset.* Among 47 patients dying of active valvular infective endocarditis and examined personally, 34 (72%) had necrotic lesions in 1 or both left ventricular papillary muscles; none had significant narrowing of the extramural coronary arteries. Most patients had pure aortic regurgitation, but some had pure MR secondary to the active infective endocarditis. Severely diminished cardiac output resulting in poor myocardial perfusion was believed the cause of the papillary muscle necrosis in these patients.

Small fibrous scars in the papillary muscles are common in patients with *systemic hypertension*, but atrophy of these muscles is infrequent in this condition, unless coronary heart disease also is present. In left ventricular hypertrophy of any cause, the hypertrophy of the papillary muscles should probably be proportional to that of the left ventricular free wall or ventricular septum. This proportional hypertrophy usually exists in patients with systemic hypertension but is infrequent in patients with left ventricular outflow obstruction.

Fibrosis with atrophy of the papillary muscles is to be expected in patients with primary *endocardial fibroelastosis* of the left ventricle. Histologically, the thickened endocardium in this condition is similar to the media of the aorta, being characterized by elastic fibrils running parallel to one another and to the surface. Primary left ventricular endocardial fibroelastosis may be an anatomic expression of chronically inadequate coronary arterial perfusion of the left ventricle; since the posteromedial papillary muscle is the least well-perfused portion of the heart, this structure is affected the most. In the congenital anomaly, origin of the left or both coronary arteries from the pulmonary trunk, diffuse endocardial fibroelastosis of the left ventricle is nearly always an associated lesion.[33] Fibrosis and atrophy of the left ventricular papillary muscles are to be expected in this anomaly, and these patients may present clinically with features of pure MR.

Foci of fibrosis or necrosis in the left ventricular papillary muscles are infrequent in patients with dilated cardiomyopathy.[54,66] Rarely, *myocarditis* may be localized to papillary muscle and adjacent left ventricular free wall.[67] Patients with the *neurogenic heart diseases* (Friedreich's ataxia, progressive muscular dystrophy, and myotonic muscular dystrophy) generally have scarred left ventricular papillary muscles, especially the posteromedial ones.[68] The African cardiomyopathy, *endomyocardial fibrosis*, may be associated with extensive scarring of the papillary muscles.[54] In this condition the posteromedial muscle is usually covered by a thrombus or by dense fibrous tissue that probably represents organized thrombus. Likewise, *Löffler's fibroplastic parietal endocarditis*, which may be 1 stage of endomyocardial fibrosis,[53] is usually associated with extensive scarring of 1 or both papillary muscles.

The papillary muscles are subject to various infiltrative processes, just like any other portion of myo-

TABLE II Spectrum of Left Ventricular Papillary Muscle Dysfunction

I. Rupture of papillary muscle
  A. Total ("belly" or trunk)
    1. Rapid death
    2. Survival—not described
  B. Partial ("head")
    1. Rapid death
    2. Survival but chronic congestive cardiac failure
II. Fibrosis or necrosis of papillary muscle without rupture
  A. With coronary arterial narrowing
    1. Acute myocardial infarct
    2. Healed myocardial infarct
  B. Without coronary arterial narrowing
    1. Acute
    2. Chronic
      a. Valvular, subvalvular (discrete and diffuse) and supravalvular aortic stenosis
      b. Systemic hypertension
      c. Origin of left coronary artery from pulmonary trunk
      d. Primary endocardial fibroelastosis
      e. Endomyocardial fibrosis
      f. *Löffler's fibroplastic parietal endocarditis*
      g. Diffuse (primary) myocardial disease
      h. Focal myocardial disease
        1. Idiopathic
        2. "Neurogenic" heart disease
        3. Infectious
III. Normal or near-normal papillary muscles but severe fibrosis or necrosis in adjacent left ventricular free wall with and without coronary arterial narrowing

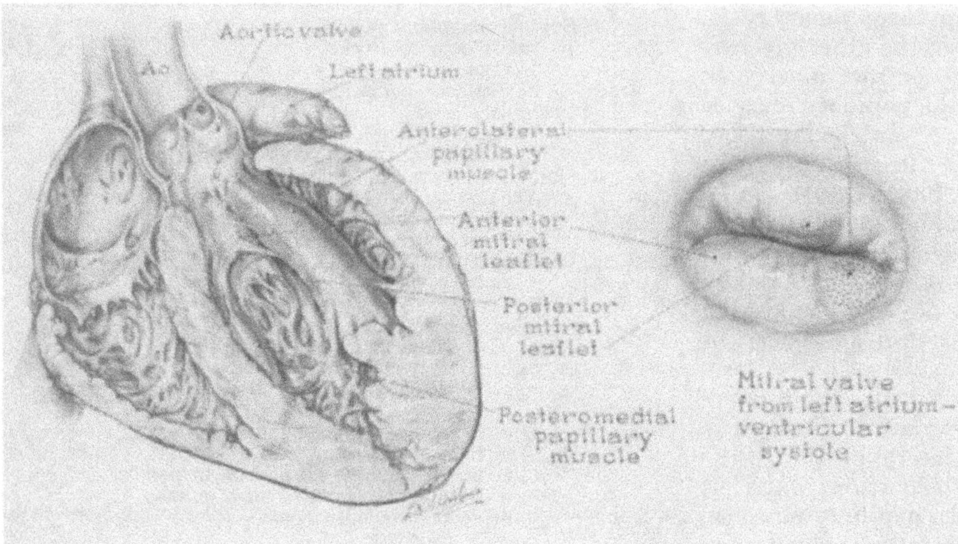

FIGURE 28. Drawing of heart in a 23-year-old man (DCMEO #80-02-134) who died from idiopathic dilated cardiomyopathy. An incidental finding at necropsy was the insertion of the anterolateral papillary muscle directly onto the anterior mitral leaflet. This congenital anomaly has been observed personally in about 5 cases at necropsy. It appears to have no functional significance. Ao = aorta.

cardium. *Pyogenic abscesses, Aschoff bodies, granulomas,*[67] *neoplasms,*[69–71] *amyloid,*[72] *iron,*[73] *and air*[74] have all been observed in these structures. Congestive heart failure from severe MR may be the initial symptom of cardiac *sarcoidosis.*[67]

The most frequent congenital malformation of papillary muscles is the occurrence of only 1 such muscle in the left ventricle. In this condition, described as the *parachute mitral valve*, all mitral chordae tendineae are attached to the 1 left ventricular papillary muscle (Fig. 11). The resulting mitral valve is usually stenotic, but it may be purely regurgitant or it may function normally.[35] The single papillary muscle is usually associated with other malformations, including a supramitral valve ring, diffuse subaortic stenosis, and coarctation of the aorta. Other malformations, including valvular aortic stenosis, ventricular septal defect, and valvular pulmonic stenosis, also may occur.

There may be not only 1 too few papillary muscles but also 1 too many. An *accessory papillary muscle* is usually of no functional significance, but it has been seen in association with congenital MR. When 2 papillary muscles are present, 1 or both may still be congenitally malformed. One or both papillary muscles may be abnormally large and malpositioned with attachment onto the anterior mitral leaflet, creating the potential at least for valvular stenosis or regurgitation (Fig. 28). Both papillary muscles also may be poorly developed and small. This finding is particularly characteristic with origin of the left coronary artery or both coronary arteries from the pulmonary trunk. In this situation, the papillary muscles arise more cephalad than normal from the left ventricular free wall.

Both left ventricular papillary muscles usually are excised either completely or incompletely at operations to replace the mitral valve. The myocardium of the free wall at the sites of excision of these muscles is always infiltrated by inflammatory cells when this area is examined in the early postoperative period. With time, these areas are covered by dense fibroelastic tissue simulating the composition of the media of the aorta. If the papillary muscles are not excised when the mitral leaflets and chordae tendineae are excised during mitral valve replacement, the papillary muscles atrophy and are focally replaced by fibrous tissue; the myocardial cells become disorganized.[75] When the papillary muscles are excised at operation, each is grasped by a clamp extending through the mitral orifice from the left atrium. If the papillary muscles are pulled too vigorously by the clamp during their excision, portions of left ventricular free wall also may be excised. The result may be perforation or severe thinning of the left ventricular wall. The latter may lead to the formation of a functioning or anatomic aneurysm or both.[76,77]

Mitral Anulus

Although it may accompany left ventricular dilation, mitral anular dilation, except in patients with prolapsing or floppy mitral valves,[12] is a rare cause of MR[59]; in the past, most patients with MR that was believed the result of mitral anular dilation probably had papillary muscle dysfunction. Mitral anular dilation to a degree capable of causing MR probably does not occur except in association with mitral valve prolapse because the surface area of the mitral leaflets is more than twice the area of the mitral orifice, and the anulus contracts during ventricular systole.[2] The mitral ring has a sphincter-like action because the mitral orifice is smaller during ventricular systole than during diastole. In patients with dilated left ventricles, the widest diameter does not occur at the left ventricular base, the area that includes the mitral anulus, but in the midportion of the chamber between apex and base (Fig. 29). In fact, the base of the left ventricle is prevented from dilating freely because the "fibrous skeleton" is attached to it, whereas the midportion of the left ventricle is not so restricted. Indeed, severe left ventricular dilation may occur without any dilation of the mitral anulus.

Although it is now well known that MR may occur in patients with dilated left ventricles from any cause

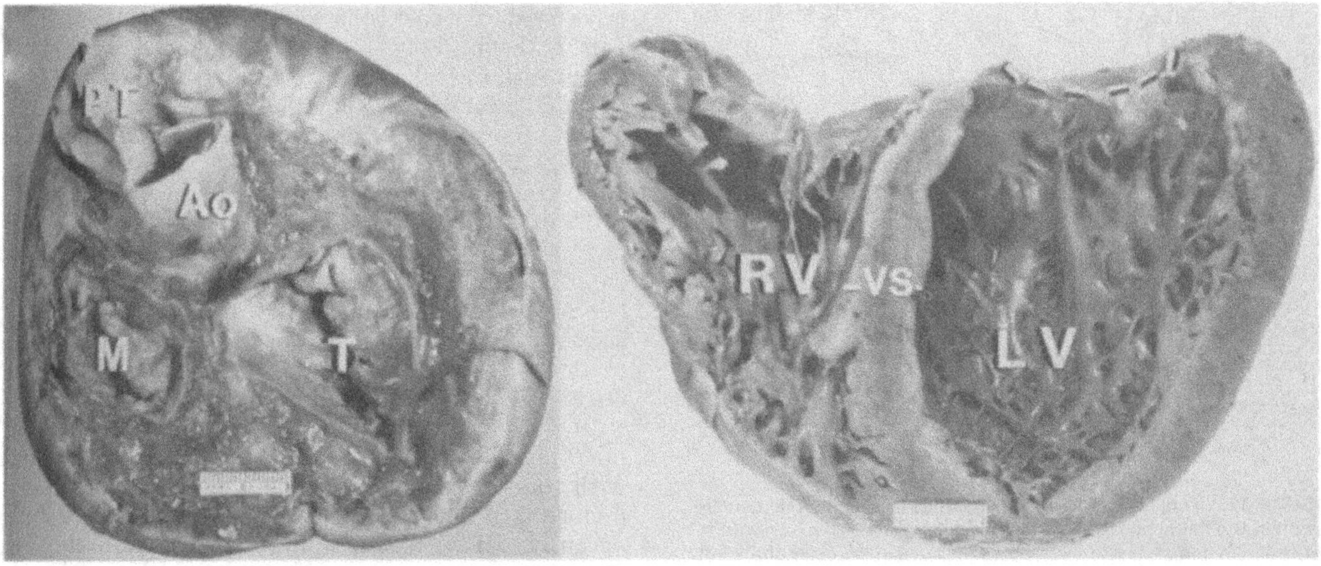

FIGURE 29. The heart of a 34-year-old man (DCGH #74A-65) with idiopathic dilated cardiomyopathy and clinical evidence of both tricuspid and mitral regurgitation of severe degree. Both ventricles are considerably dilated. The greatest increase in dimension of the right (RV) is in the area of the tricuspid valve anulus. The tricuspid valve orifice (T) admitted 4 fingers readily, indicating its proximal diameter to be about 8 cm. In contrast, the maximal diameter of the left ventricle (LV) was about midway between the apex and the mitral anulus. The mitral orifice (M) only admitted 2 fingers, indicating that its maximal diameter was about 4 cm. The mitral regurgitation resulted, therefore, not from anular dilatation, which was mild, but probably from altered angulation of the left ventricular papillary muscles. Ao = aorta.

without associated left ventricular necrosis or fibrosis, it is less well recognized that necrosis or fibrosis of the left ventricular free wall, unassociated with left ventricular dilation or papillary muscle or mitral tissue lesions, also may be associated with MR. Generally, the scarring or necrosis of the myocardium adjacent to the papillary muscles fails to move or moves paradoxically during ventricular systole, and the abnormal ventricular contraction may lead to abnormal papillary muscle anchoring, resulting in MR. Anatomic left ventricular aneurysms unassociated with papillary muscle necrosis or fibrosis may cause MR by the same mechanism.

Abnormal pulling on the papillary muscles unassociated with left ventricular necrosis or fibrosis or cavity

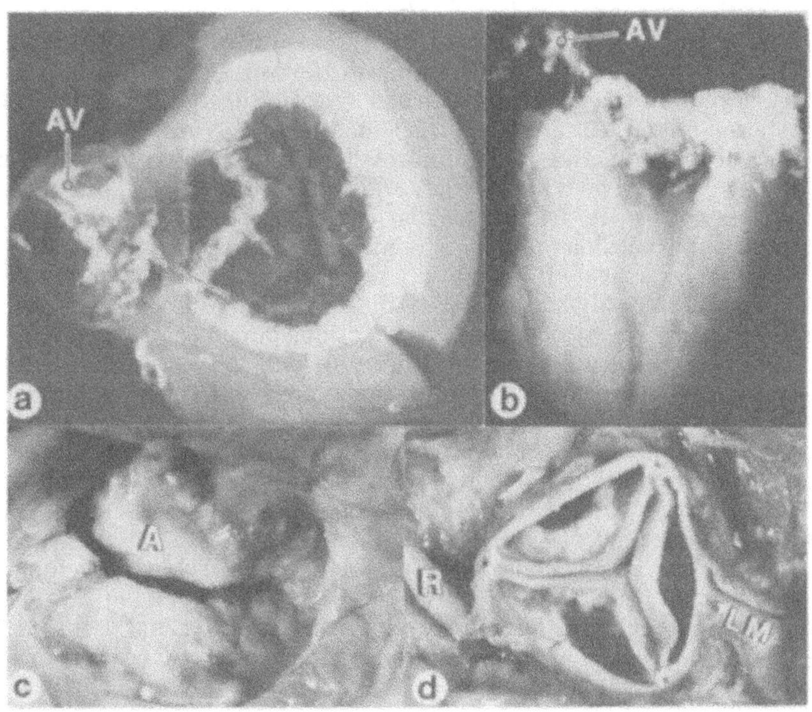

FIGURE 30. Massive calcific deposits in the mitral anulus (**a, b,** and **c**), aortic valve (AV) (**a, b,** and **d**), and coronary arteries (**a** and **b**) in an 82-year-old man (NNMC #A70-200) who had Paget's disease of bone. The short bar of calcium between the lines in **a** is that extending across the anterior (A) mitral leaflet. The radiogram in **a** is a cephalad-caudal orientation, and that in **b**, a lateral view. The mitral valve as observed from the left atrium is shown in **c,** and the aortic valve from the aorta in **d.** LM and R = left main and right coronary arteries. (Reprinted, by permission, from Roberts and Waller.[79])

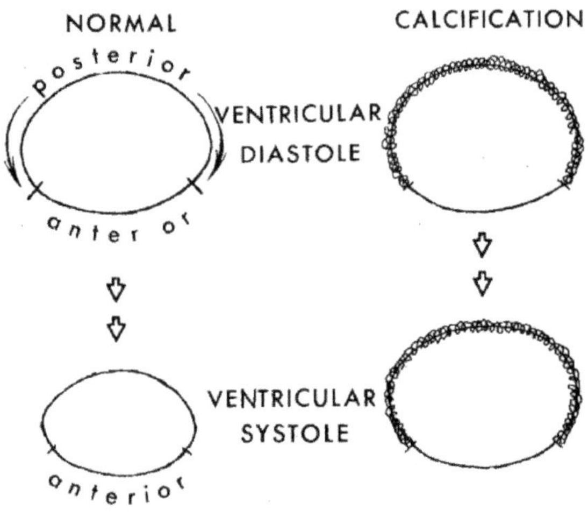

FIGURE 31. Mechanism of mitral regurgitation in patients with calcification of the mitral anulus. During ventricular systole, the base of the left ventricle contracts like a sphincter. Included in the base of the left ventricle is the anulus behind the posterior mitral leaflet. Thus, this circumference decreases during systole. If, however, the anulus behind the posterior mitral leaflet is calcified, the sphincter-like contraction of the left ventricular base may be prevented from occurring. The area of the mitral orifice thus is not decreased, and mild degrees of mitral regurgitation may result. (Reprinted, by permission, from Roberts and Perloff.[2])

dilation may occur in patients with *hypertrophic cardiomyopathy*; this mechanism may account for their MR.[51,54] The huge thickening of the ventricular septum may distort or bend the anterolateral papillary muscle and prevent proper contraction of this structure during ventricular systole. In addition to actual bending of the anterolateral left ventricular papillary muscle, however, the mitral leaflets in adults with hypertrophic cardiomyopathy are always thickened. The thickening of the anterior mitral leaflet appears to be the result of its contact with the mural endocardium in the left ventricular outflow tract during ventricular systole. But the posterior mitral leaflet also is thickened, probably a result of its contacting itself abnormally during ventricular systole. The mitral leaflets and chordae tendineae are within the left ventricular cavity, which in hypertrophic cardiomyopathy is relatively small; as a consequence, space within the left ventricle may be inadequate to easily accommodate the mitral leaflets and chordae, and with vigorous contractions portions of the posterior leaflet contact other portions of the same leaflet abnormally. Fibrous thickening is the consequence. The MR in hypertrophic cardiomyopathy usually disappears after operative excision or incision of myocardium in the left ventricular outflow tract.[51]

Calcification of the mitral anulus is one of the more frequent abnormalities of the heart. Mitral anular calcification is generally considered to be a disease of elderly women. Indeed, of 14 patients with "massive" mitral anular calcification reported by Korn et al[78] 21 years ago, all were women and all were over 65 years of age. It is incorrect, however, to believe that this entity is reserved for a particular sex at a particular time in life. During the past 14 years I have examined over 300 patients with mitral anular calcium at necropsy. Of the first 200 analyzed systematically, 47% were men and 53% were women. Of the 200 patients, 141 (70%) were over age 65 years and 17 (8%) were aged 45 years or less. The extent of the mitral anular calcium was graded 1^+ to 4^+: in 110 patients (55%) the deposits were graded 1^+ or 2^+ and in 90 patients (45%) grade 3^+ or 4^+. The calcium in 198 patients was limited to the anular region behind posterior mitral leaflet, usually forming a C-shaped configuration; in 2 patients, the calcium extended across the anterior mitral leaflet to form an O-shaped configuration[79] (Fig. 30). Of the 38 patients with 4^+ deposits, 76% were women. Thus, although mitral anular calcium of any degree appears to occur with similar frequency in men and women, the larger deposits (those likely to be seen on the chest roentgenogram) are more frequent in women. Calcium deposits also were present on the aortic aspects of the aortic valve cusps in 138 (69%) of the 200 patients (64 [32%] of whom had aortic valve stenosis) and in the coronary arteries in 168 (84%) patients.

Factors predisposing to mitral anular calcium were found in 80% of the 200 patients. These included elevation (>140 mm Hg) of left ventricular systolic pressure (142 patients), diabetes mellitus (39 patients), chronic hypercalcemia (9 patients),[80] prolapsing mitral valve (6 patients), the Marfan syndrome (5 patients),[40] left-to-right shunt (secundum type atrial septal defect) (3 patients), and the Hurler syndrome (2 patients).[46] Mitral anular calcium also may form late at sites of attachment of prosthetic mitral valves.[81]

The association of mitral anular calcium with calcific deposits in the coronary arteries and aortic valve cusps, the lack of mitral anular deposits in persons living in environments where the total serum cholesterol is ≤150 mg/dl, and the frequent occurrence of factors predisposing to atherosclerosis in patients with mitral anular calcium supports a common etiologic basis for both mitral anular calcium and atherosclerosis.

The functional consequences of mitral anular calcium are 2, namely MR or MS, and rarely, if ever, both. The presence of either MR or MS is a function of the amount of anular calcium present and also probably the size of the left ventricular cavity. The most common functional consequence, of course, is MR, which is nearly always of only mild degree and never of severe degree except in a patient with associated mitral anular dilatation in the setting of mitral valve prolapse.[12] The frequency of a murmur typical of MR is nearly always present in patients with $4^+/4^+$ anular deposits and is rarely the consequence of anular deposits if the extent of the latter is only $1^+/4^+$. The mechanism of MR in patients with mitral anular calcium is depicted graphically in Figure 31. Mitral stenosis as a consequence of mitral anular calcium has been observed only in the presence of huge ($4^+/4^+$) mitral anular deposits associated with severe left ventricular hypertrophy without dilatation, usually the consequence of associated left ventricular outflow obstruction.[25]

References

1. **Perloff JK, Roberts WC.** The mitral apparatus. Functional anatomy of mitral regurgitation. Circulation 1972;46:227–239.
2. **Roberts WC, Perloff JK.** Mitral valvular disease. A clinicopathologic survey of the conditions causing the mitral valve to function abnormally. Ann Intern Med 1972;77:939–975.
3. **Roberts WC, Cohen LS.** Left ventricular papillary muscles. Description of the normal and a survey of conditions causing them to be abnormal. Circulation 1972;46:138–154.
4. **Waller BF, Roberts WC.** Cardiovascular disease in the very elderly. An analysis of 40 necropsy patients aged 90 years or over. Am J Cardiol 1983;51:403–421.
5. **Roberts WC.** Anatomically isolated aortic valvular disease. The case against its being of rheumatic etiology. Am J Med 1970;49:151–159.
6. **Roberts WC, Dangel JC, Bulkley BH.** Non-rheumatic valvular cardiac disease: a clinicopathologic survery of 27 different conditions causing valvular dysfunction. Cardiovasc Clin 1973;5:333–446.
7. **Roberts WC.** The structure of the aortic valve in clinically-isolated aortic stenosis. An autopsy study of 162 patients over 15 years of age. Circulation 1970;42:91–97.
8. **Roberts WC.** The congenitally bicuspid aortic valve. A study of 85 autopsy cases. Am J Cardiol 1970;26:72–83.
9. **Roberts WC, Perloff JK, Costantino T.** Severe valvular aortic stenosis in patients over 65 years of age. A clinicopathologic study. Am J Cardiol 1971;27:497–506.
10. **Virmani R, Roberts WC.** Aschoff bodies in operatively excised atrial appendages and in papillary muscles. Frequency and clinical significance. Circulation 1977;55:559–563.
11. **Roberts WC, Virmani R.** Aschoff bodies at necropsy in valvular heart disease. Evidence from an analysis of 543 patients over 14 years of age that rheumatic heart disease, at least anatomically, is a disease of the mitral valve. Circulation 1978;57:803–807.
12. **Waller BF, Morrow AG, Maron BJ, Del Negro AA, Kent KM, McGrath FJ, Wallace RB, McIntosh CL, Roberts WC.** Etiology of clinically isolated, severe, chronic, pure mitral regurgitation: analysis of 97 patients over 30 years of age having mitral valve replacement. Am Heart J 1982;104: 276–288.
13. **Roberts WC, Sjoerdsma A.** The cardiac disease associated with the carcinoid syndrome (carcinoid heart disease). Am J Med 1964;36:5–34.
14. **Glancy DL, Marcus FI, Cuadra M, Ewy GA, Roberts WC.** Isolated organic tricuspid valvular regurgitation. Causes and consequences. Am J Med 1969;46:989–996.
15. **Andy JJ, Sheikh MU, Ali N, Barnes BO, Fox LM, Curry CL, Roberts WC.** Echocardiographic observations in opiate addicts with active infective endocarditis. Frequency of involvement of the various valves and comparison of echocardiographic features of right- and left-sided cardiac valve endocarditis. Am J Cardiol 1977;40:17–23.
16. **Arnett EN, Roberts WC.** Active infective endocarditis: a clinicopathologic analysis of 137 necropsy patients. Curr Probl Cardiol 1976;1:1–76.
17. **Roberts WC.** Characteristics and consequences of infective endocarditis (active or healed or both) learned from morphologic studies. In: Rahimtoola SH, ed. Infective Endocarditis. New York: Grune & Stratton, 1978:55–123.
18. **Lachman AS, Roberts WC.** Calcific deposits in stenotic mitral valves. Extent and relation to age, sex, degree of stenosis, cardiac rhythm, previous commissurotomy and left atrial body thrombus from study of 164 operatively-excised valves. Circulation 1978;57:808–815.
19. **Roberts WC, Lachman AS.** Mitral valve commissurotomy versus replacement. Considerations based on examination of operatively excised stenotic mitral valves. Am Heart J 1979;98:56–62.
20. **Roberts WC, Humphries JO, Morrow AG.** Giant right atrium in rheumatic mitral stenosis. Atrial enlargement restricted by mural calcification. Am Heart J 1970;79:28–35.
21. **Glancy DL, Roberts WC.** Congenital obstructive lesions involving the major pulmonary veins, left atrium, or mitral valve: a clinical, laboratory, and morphologic survey. Cathet Cardiovasc Diagn 1976;2:215–252.
22. **Ferrans VJ, Roberts WC.** Structural features of cardiac myxomas. Histology, histochemistry, and electron microscopy. Hum Pathol 1973;4:111–146.
23. **MacLowry JD, Roberts WC.** Metastatic choriocarcinoma of the lung. Invasion of pulmonary veins with extension into the left atrium and mitral orifice. Am J Cardiol 1966;18:939–941.
24. **Roberts WC, Ewy GA, Glancy DL, Marcus FI.** Valvular stenosis produced by active infective endocarditis. Circulation 1967;36:449–451.
25. **Waller BF, McManus BM, Roberts WC.** Mitral valve stenosis produced by or worsened by active bacterial endocarditis. Chest 1982;82:498–500.
26. **Hammer WJ, Roberts WC, de Leon AC Jr.** "Mitral stenosis" secondary to combined "massive" mitral anular calcific deposits and small, hypertrophied left ventricles. Am J Med 1978;64:371–376.
27. **Shepherd RL, Glancy DL, Stinson EB, Roberts WC.** Hemodynamic confirmation of obstruction to left ventricular inflow by a caged-ball prosthetic mitral valve. Case report. J Thorac Cardiovasc Surg 1973;65:252–254.
28. **Jones AA, Otis JB, Fletcher GF, Roberts WC.** A hitherto undescribed cause of prosthetic mitral valve obstruction. J Thorac Cardiovasc Surg 1977; 74:116–117.
29. **Roberts WC.** Complications of cardiac valve replacement: characteristic abnormalities of prostheses pertaining to any or specific site. Am Heart J 1982;103:113–122.
30. **Braunwald E, Ross RS, Morrow AG, Roberts WC.** Differential diagnosis of mitral regurgitation in childhood: clinical pathological conference at the National Institutes of Health. Ann Intern Med 1961;54:1223–1242.
31. **Brockenbrough EC, Braunwald E, Roberts WC, Morrow AG.** Partial persistent atrioventricular canal simulating pure mitral regurgitation. Am Heart J 1962;63:9–17.
32. **Carney EK, Braunwald E, Roberts WC, Aygen M, Morrow AG.** Congenital mitral regurgitation. Clinical, hemodynamic, and angiocardiographic findings in nine patients. Am J Med 1962;33:223–235.
33. **Roberts WC.** Anomalous origin of both coronary arteries from the pulmonary artery. Am J Cardiol 1962;10:595–600.
34. **Roberts WC, Ross RS, Davis FW Jr.** Congenital corrected transposition of the great vessels in adulthood simulating rheumatic valvular disease. Bull Johns Hopkins Hosp 1964;114:157–172.
35. **Glancy DL, Chang MY, Dorney ER, Roberts WC.** Parachute mitral valve. Further observations and associated lesions. Am J Cardiol 1971;27: 309–313.
36. **Roberts WC, Glancy DL, Seningen RP, Maron BJ, Epstein SE.** Prolapse of the mitral valve (floppy valve) associated with Ebstein's anomaly of the tricuspid valve. Am J Cardiol 1976;38:377–382.
37. **Waller BF, Sheikh MU, Roberts WC.** Prolapsing atrioventricular valve in partial atrioventricular defect. Am Heart J 1981;101:108–110.
38. **Cabin HS, Roberts WC.** Epstein's anomaly of the tricuspid valve and prolapse of the mitral valve. Am Heart J 1981;101:177–180.
39. **Roberts WC.** Congenital cardiovascular abnormalities usually "silent" until adulthood: morphologic features of the floppy mitral valve, valvular aortic stenosis, hypertrophic cardiomyopathy, sinus of Valsalva aneurysm, and the Marfan syndrome. In: Roberts WC, ed. Congenital Heart Disease in Adults. Philadelphia: FA Davis, 1979:407–453.
40. **Roberts WC, Honig HS.** The spectrum of cardiovascular disease in the Marfan syndrome: a clinico-morphologic study of 18 necropsy patients and comparison to 151 previously reported necropsy patients. Am Heart J 1982;104:115–135.
41. **Roberts WC, Braunwald E, Morrow AG.** Acute severe mitral regurgitation secondary to ruptured chordae tendineae. Clinical, hemodynamic, and pathologic considerations. Circulation 1966;33:58–70.
42. **Roberts WC, Buchbinder NA.** Healed left-sided infective endocarditis: a clinicopathologic study of 59 patients. Am J Cardiol 1977;40:876–888.
43. **Carpenter DF, Golden A, Roberts WC.** Quadrivalvular rheumatoid heart disease associated with left bundle branch block. Am J Med 1967;43: 922–929.
44. **Roberts WC, Kehoe JA, Carpenter DF, Golden A.** Cardiac valvular lesions in rheumatoid arthritis. Arch Intern Med 1968;122:141–146.
45. **Roberts WC, Hollingsworth JF, Bulkley BH, Jaffe RB, Epstein SE, Stinson EB.** Combined mitral and aortic regurgitation in ankylosing spondylitis. Angiographic and anatomic features. Am J Med 1974;56:237–243.
46. **Renteria VG, Ferrans VJ, Roberts WC.** The heart in the Hurler syndrome. Gross, histologic and ultrastructural observations in five necropsy cases. Am J Cardiol 1976;38:487–501.
47. **Roberts WC, Ross RS, Eggleston JC, Massumi RA.** Chronic mitral regurgitation of unresolved etiology in the elderly. A clinicopatholigic study of two patients. Johns Hopkins Med J 1968;122:26–36.
48. **Morrow AG, Cohen LS, Roberts WC, Braunwald NS, Braunwald E.** Severe mitral regurgitation following acute myocardial infarction and ruptured papillary muscle. Hemodynamic findings and results of operative treatment in four patients. Circulation 1968;37,38:Suppl II:II-124–II-132.
49. **Falcone MW, Ronan JA Jr, Roberts WC.** Silent mitral regurgitation complicating silent myocardial infarction: hemodynamic and morphologic documentation. Chest 1972;62:226–228.
50. **Glancy DL, Stinson EB, Shepherd RL, Itscoitz SB, Roberts WC, Epstein SE, Morrow AG.** Results of valve replacement for severe mitral regurgitation due to papillary muscle rupture or fibrosis. Am J Cardiol 1973;32:313–321.
51. **Roberts WC.** Operative treatment of hypertrophic obstructive cardiomyopathy. The case against mitral valve replacement. Am J Cardiol 1973; 32:377–381.
52. **Roberts WC, Liegler DG, Carbone PP.** Endomyocardial disease and eosinophilia. A clinical and pathologic spectrum. Am J Med 1969;46:28–42.
53. **Roberts WC, Buja LM, Ferrans VJ.** Löffler's fibroplastic parietal endocarditis, eosinophilic leukemia, and Davies' endomyocardial fibrosis: the same disease at different stages? Pathol Microbiol 1970;35:90–96.
54. **Roberts WC, Ferrans VJ.** Pathologic anatomy of the cardiomyopathies. Idiopathic dilated and hypertrophic types, infiltrative types, and endomyocardial disease with and without eosinophilia. Hum Pathol 1975;6:287–342.
55. **Harley JB, McIntosh CL, Kirklin JJW, Maron BJ, Gottdiener J, Roberts WC, Fauci AS.** Atrioventricular valve replacement in the idiopathic hypereosinophilic syndrome. Am J Med 1982;73:77–81.
56. **Fauci AS, Harley JB, Roberts WC, Ferrans VJ, Gralnick HR, Bjornson BH.** The idiopathic hypereosinophilic syndrome. Clinical, pathophysiologic, and therapeutic considerations. Ann Intern Med 1982;97:78–92.
57. **Bulkley BH, Roberts WC.** Systemic lupus erythematosus as a cause of severe mitral regurgitation. New problem in an old disease. Am J Cardiol 1975;35:305–308.
58. **Bulkley BH, Roberts WC.** The heart in systemic lupus erythematosus and the changes induced in it by corticosteroid therapy. A study of 36 necropsy patients. Am J Med 1975;58:243–264.
59. **Bulkley BH, Roberts WC.** Dilatation of the mitral anulus. A rare cause of mitral regurgitation. Am J Med 1975;59:457–463.
60. **Brosius FC III, Waller BF, Roberts WC,** Radiation heart disease. Analysis of 16 young (aged 15 to 33 years) necropsy patients who received over 3,500 rads to the heart. Am J Med 1981;70:519–530.
61. **Glancy DL, Massumi RA, Roberts WC.** Fatal acute rheumatic fever in childhood despite corticosteroid therapy. A note on the spectrum of childhood rheumatic fever. Am Heart J 1969;77:534–537.
62. **Selzer A, Katayama F.** Mitral regurgitation: clinical patterns, pathophysiology, natural history. Medicine 1972;51:337–350.
63. **di Segni E, Edwards JE.** Cleft anterior leaflet of mitral valve with intact septa. A study of 20 cases. Am J Cardiol 1983;51:919–926.
64. **Berry WB, Roberts WC, Morrow AG, Braunwald E.** Corrected transposition of the aorta and pulmonary trunk. Clinical, hemodynamic and pathologic

findings. Am J Med 1964;36:35–53.
65. **Rosenberg J, Roberts WC.** Double orifice mitral valve. Study of the anomaly in two calves and a summary of the literature in humans. Arch Pathol 1968;86:77–80.
66. **Marcus FI, Gomez L, Glancy DL, Ewy GA, Roberts WC.** Papillary muscle fibrosis in primary myocardial disease. Am Heart J 1969;77;681–685.
67. **Roberts WC, McAllister HA Jr, Ferrans VJ.** Sarcoidosis of the heart. A clinicopathologic study of 35 necropsy patients (group I) and review of 78 previously described necropsy patients (group II). Am J Med 1977;63: 86–108.
68. **Perloff JK, Roberts WC, deLeon AC Jr, O'Doherty D.** The distinctive electrocardiogram of Duchenne's progressive muscular dystrophy. An electrocardiographic-pathologic correlative study. Am J Med 1967;42: 179–188.
69. **Roberts WC, Bodey GP, Wertlake PT.** The heart in acute leukemia. A study of 420 autopsy cases. Am J Cardiol 1968;21:388–412.
70. **Glancy DL, Roberts WC.** The heart in malignant melanoma. A study of 70 autopsy cases. Am J Cardiol 1968;21:555–571.
71. **Roberts WC, Glancy DL, DeVita VT Jr.** Heart in malignant lymphoma (Hodgkin's disease, lymphosarcoma, reticulum cell sarcoma and mycosis fungoides). A study of 196 autopsy cases. Am J Cardiol 1968;22:85–107.
72. **Buja LM, Khoi NB, Roberts WC.** Clinically significant cardiac amyloidosis. Clinicopathologic findings in 15 patients. Am J Cardiol 1970;26:394–405.
73. **Buja LM, Roberts WC.** Iron in the heart. Etiology and clinical significance. Am J Med 1971;51:209–221.
74. **Roberts WC, Berard CW.** Gas gangrene of the heart in clostridial septicemia. Am Heart J 1967;74:482–488.
75. **Pirolo JS, Hutchins GM, Moore GW, Weisfeldt ML.** Myocyte disarray develops in papillary muscles released from normal tension after mitral valve replacement. Circulation 1982;66:841–846.
76. **Roberts WC, Bulkley BH, Morrow AG.** Pathologic anatomy of cardiac valve replacement: a study of 224 necropsy patients. Progr Cardiovasc Dis 1973;15:539–587.
77. **Roberts WC, Isner JM, Virmani R.** Left ventricular incision midway between the mitral anulus and the stumps of the papillary muscles during mitral valve excision with or without rupture or aneurysmal formation. Analysis of 10 necropsy patients. Am Heart J 1982;104:1278–1287.
78. **Korn D, DeSanctis RW, Sell S.** Massive calcification of the mitral annulus. A clinicopathological study of fourteen cases. N Engl J Med 1962;267: 900–909.
79. **Roberts WC, Waller BF.** Mitral valve "anular" calcium forming a complete circle or "O" configuration: clinical and necropsy observations. Am Heart J 1981;101:619–621.
80. **Roberts WC, Waller BF.** Effect of chronic hypercalcemia on the heart. An analysis of 18 necropsy patients. Am J Med 1981;71:371–384.
81. **Bulkley BH, Morrow AG, Roberts WC.** Calcification of prosthetic valve anuli: a late complication of cardiac valve replacement. Am Heart J 1974;87: 129–133.

Cardiac Amyloidosis Causing Cardiac Dysfunction: Analysis of 54 Necropsy Patients

WILLIAM C. ROBERTS, MD and BRUCE F. WALLER, MD

Clinical and morphologic findings are described in 54 necropsy patients (32 men [59%]) aged 21 to 97 years (mean 64) with cardiac amyloid deposits extensive enough to cause fatal cardiac dysfunction. Chronic congestive heart failure (CHF) was present in 46 (85%). The duration of CHF, known in 39 patients, ranged from 1 to 108 months (mean 18) and lasted ≤12 months in 25 patients (64%). All 8 patients without CHF died suddenly and unexpectedly. Systemic arterial pressures were recorded in the last 3 months of life in 43 patients: the peak indirect systolic pressure was ≤130 mm Hg and the diastolic pressure <90 mm Hg in all. Electrocardiograms, recorded in the last 6 months of life in 40 patients, were abnormal in each: low voltage in 35 (63%); "myocardial infarction pattern" in 33 (83%); abnormal QRS axis in 29 (73%); arrhythmias in 29 (73%); first, second, or third degree heart block in 28 (45%); and complete bundle branch block in 7 (18%). In 30 patients, the QRS amplitude in all 12 leads was measured: in the 15 men it ranged from 60 to 197 mm (mean 99) (10 mm = 1 mV) and in the 15 women from 58 to 199 mm (mean 109). Diagnosis of amyloidosis was established by biopsy of noncardiac organs or tissues during life in only 18 (33%) patients. During life the condition simulated hypertrophic cardiomyopathy in 5 patients, constrictive pericardial disease in 3, and coronary heart disease (because of angina pectoris) in 4.

At necropsy, the hearts ranged in weight from 300 to 900 g (mean 554), and all but 1 had a "rubbery," noncompliant consistency. In addition to their presence in myocardial interstitium (53 patients) and in intramural coronary arteries (54 patients), amyloid deposits were present grossly in mural endocardium in all 54 patients and in valvular endocardium in 46 (85%). The cardiac ventricles were not dilated in 43 patients (80%), but both atria were dilated in all 54 patients. Intracardiac thrombi were present in 14 patients (26%). Cardiac amyloidosis must be considered in any elderly patient with chronic CHF unassociated with chest pain when blood pressure is normal and the electrocardiogram discloses low voltage and a pattern of "healed myocardial infarction."

In 1970, clinical and necropsy findings in 15 patients with cardiac dysfunction secondary to cardiac amyloidosis were reported from this laboratory.[1] During the past 13 years we have studied at necropsy an additional 39 patients with fatal cardiac amyloidosis. This report summarizes clinical and morphologic findings in these 54 patients with cardiac amyloid deposits extensive enough to cause cardiac dysfunction, with particular emphasis on electrocardiographic observations.

Patients Studied and Findings

Clinical findings: The 54 patients ranged in age at death from 21 to 97 years (mean 64). The 32 men (59%) ranged in age from 32 to 97 years (mean 65) and the 22 women (41%) from 21 to 93 years (mean 62) (Fig. 1). Thirty-eight (70%) were white and 16 (30%) were black. Of the 54 patients, 46 (85%) had clinical evidence of congestive heart failure (CHF) at some time. The duration of CHF was discernible in 39 of the 46 patients and ranged from 1 to 108 months (mean 18): for ≤12 months in 25 patients (64%), from >12 to 24 months in 6 patients (15%), from >24 to 36 months in 3 patients (8%), and from 60 to 108 months (mean 82) in 5 patients (13%). The duration of CHF in 18 women ranged from 1 to 72 months (mean 18) and in 25 men from 2 to 108 months (mean 22). Each of the 8 patients (15%) without clinical evidence of CHF died suddenly and unexpectedly: in 3 sudden death was the first evidence of amyloidosis, 2 had familial amyloidosis, 2 had multiple myeloma, and 1 clinically had presumed alcoholic cirrhosis (which at necropsy actually was massive hepatic amyloid infiltration). The 8 patients dying suddenly without ever having clinical evidence of CHF ranged in age from 21 to 88 years (mean 56) and the 46 patients with CHF from 32 to 97 years (mean 65). Chest pain was present at some time during amyloid illness in 8 patients (15%), 4 of whom were considered to have angina pectoris.[2,3] Of the 4 patients (aged

From the Pathology Branch, National Heart, Lung, and Blood Institute, National Institutes of Health, Bethesda, Maryland. Manuscript received and accepted April 12, 1983.

Address for reprints: William C. Roberts, MD, Building 10A, Room 3E30, National Institutes of Health, Bethesda, Maryland 20205.

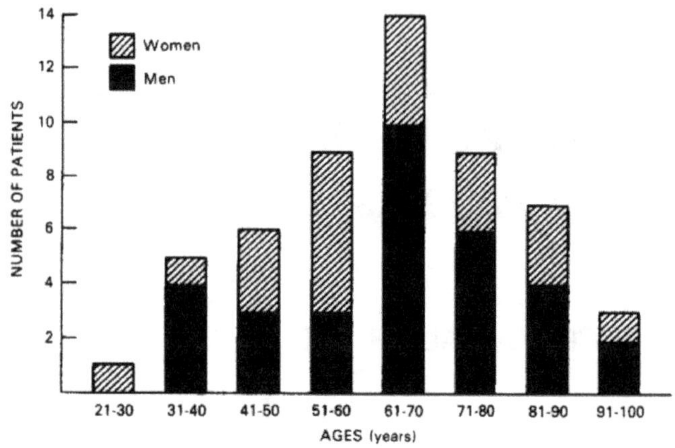

FIGURE 1. Age and sex distribution in the 54 necropsy patients with cardiac amyloidosis extensive enough to cause cardiac dysfunction.

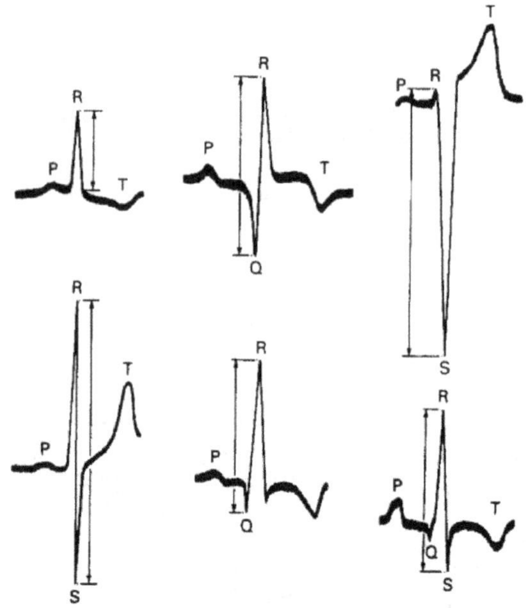

FIGURE 2. Various QRS complexes showing how each was measured.

67 to 89 years [mean 80]) with angina, 2 at necropsy had 1 or more of the 4 major (right, left main, left anterior descending, and left circumflex) epicardial coronary arteries narrowed 76 to 100% in cross-sectional area by atherosclerotic plaques.

Seven patients (13%) had histories of illnesses considered compatible with acute myocardial infarction that healed, but electrocardiographic and enzymatic documentation of myocardial necrosis at the time was unavailable. Grossly visible left ventricular scars, however, were absent at necropsy in all 7 patients, indicating that the histories of acute myocardial infarction in them were fallacious.

Four patients (7%) had 1 or more episodes of syncope. One patient was among the 4 with familial amyloidosis with peripheral neuropathy and postural hypotension. The mechanism of the syncope in the other 3 patients was not determined.

Systemic arterial pressure recordings during the last 3 months of life were available in 43 (80%) of the 54 patients. Although 24 (44%) of the 54 patients had a history of "hypertension," in none of the 43 patients (including the 24) with indirect blood pressure recordings available during the last 3 months of life was the systolic pressure >130 mm Hg or the diastolic pressure >90 mm Hg. The range of systolic arterial pressures during the last 3 months of life was 80 to 130 mm Hg (average 102) and of diastolic pressures 40 to 90 mm Hg (average 66).

The cardiac silhouette was enlarged on chest roentgenogram during the last few months of life in 39 (72%) of 54 patients. In several patients, however, earlier radiographs had shown the cardiac silhouette to be of normal size.

Adequate information on precordial examinations during the last few months of life was available in 44 of the 54 patients, 36 (82%) of whom had precordial murmurs. They were of a blowing type and consistent with mitral or tricuspid regurgitation, or both, in 35 (97%): grade 1 to 2/6 in 26, grade 3/6 in 7, and grade 4/6 in 2 patients. In addition, 1 patient had a murmur typical of valvular aortic stenosis (grade 3/6), which was confirmed to be present and was the type typically observed in the elderly.[4] At least 22 patients had third heart sounds (S_3) and at least 8 patients had fourth heart sounds (S_4).

Reports of 1 or more electrocardiograms recorded in the last 6 months of life were available in 40 patients, and all were abnormal (Table I). Of the 40 patients, electrocardiograms, recorded 0 to 160 days (mean 41) before death, were available for reexamination in 30 (Table II). In each of these 30 patients (15 women and 15 men), the QRS amplitude in all 12 leads was measured (Fig. 2). The total 12-lead QRS amplitude in the 15 men (mean age 52 years) ranged from 60 to 197 mm (mean 99) (10 mm = 1 mV) and in the 15 women (mean age 65 years) from 58 to 199 mm (mean 109). The heart weights in the 15 men ranged from 410 to 750 g (mean 570), and in the 15 women from 370 to 900 g (mean (494) (p <0.01). Some electrocardiograms are illustrated in Figures 3 to 6.

Information regarding digitalis therapy was available in 40 patients, and 31 of them received this drug. At least 12 (39%) of the 31 patients developed physical or electrical signs, or both, considered typical of digitalis toxicity.

M-mode echocardiograms were performed in the last few months of life in 11 patients. The findings are summarized in Table III and illustrated in Figures 6 and 7.

Cardiac catheterization was performed in the last few months of life in 10 patients (19%), and the findings are summarized in Table IV.

TABLE I Cardiac Amyloid Causing Cardiac Dysfunction: Electrocardiographic Observations in 40 Patients*

Abnormality [No. (%)]	No. of Patients (%)
1. Low voltage (QRS ≤15 mm in I + II + III)	25 (63)
2. Myocardial infarct pattern	33 (83)
Anterior = 26 (79)	
Posterior = 2 (6)	
Both = 5 (15)	
3. Abnormal QRS axis	29 (73)
Right (+111 to +210°) = 6 (21)	
Left (−30 to −90°) = 23 (79)	
4. Arrhythmias	29 (73)
Atrial fibrillation = 9 (31)	
Atrial or junctional tachycardia = 10 (34)	
Ventricular premature complexes = 21 (72)	
5. Heart block	18 (45)
P-R interval >0.20 = 9 (50)	
2° AV block = 4 (22)	
3° AV block = 5 (28)	
6. Complete bundle branch block (QRS ≥0.12)	7 (18)
Right = 5	
Left = 2	

AV = atrioventricular.
* Numbers in parentheses represent percentages.

Of the 54 patients, the amyloidosis was primary in 42 (78%), associated with multiple myeloma in 7 (13%), and familial in 5 (9%). None of the 54 patients had "secondary" amyloidosis.

Diagnosis of amyloidosis was established by biopsy of noncardiac organs or tissues during life in 18 patients (33%), including 5 of the 8 patients without and in 13 (28%) of the 46 patients with chronic CHF. Of the 21 patients having undergone biopsy of noncardiac organs or tissues, findings in 18 were positive for amyloid: rectum, 6 of 6; gingiva, 3 of 4; liver, 3 of 3; tongue, 2 of 3; kidney, 1 of 2; and each of prostate gland, thyroid gland, and lymph node, 1 of 1. In addition, endomyocardial biopsy of the right ventricular aspect of the ventricular septum was performed in 1 patient, but amyloid was not observed on histologic examination.

Of the 46 patients with chronic CHF, biopsy of a noncardiac organ or tissue was performed in 10 and all findings were positive for amyloid. In addition to these 10 patients, amyloidosis was considered the most likely cause of chronic CHF in 9 other patients. The cause of chronic CHF was never established during life in the remaining 27 patients (59%). Of the 11 patients having undergone M-mode echocardiography, the maximal thickness of the ventricular septum was greater than that of the left ventricular free wall in 5, and as a consequence hypertrophic cardiomyopathy was the suspected diagnosis clinically in each of them (Fig. 8 and 9). One of these 5 patients also had undergone cardiac catheterization, and hypertrophic cardiomyopathy continued to be the most likely clinical cardiac diagnosis after that procedure. Inability to differentiate clinically between constrictive pericardial disease and restrictive cardiomyopathy led to thoracotomy in 3 patients. At operation, all 3 had normal visceral and parietal pericardia and normal amounts of pericardial fluid. Each of these 3 patients died within 5 days of thoracotomy.

Eight patients had transient episodes of chest pain. In 4 the pain was consistent with angina pectoris, and a diagnosis of coronary heart disease was made in each. At necropsy, however, only 2 of the 4 patients had significant narrowing of an epicardial coronary artery by atherosclerotic plaque. Of the 4 patients with chest pain not consistent with myocardial ischemia, 1 had significant narrowing of 1 or more epicardial coronary arteries by atherosclerotic plaques. One of the latter 4 patients was 1 of the 3 with clinical pericardial constriction syndrome. The cause of chest pain in the other 2 was unclear. All 8 patients with chest pain had chronic CHF, and 2 had a history of acute myocardial infarction in the remote past. All 8 patients had luminal narrowing of many intramural coronary arteries by amyloid deposits.

Morphologic findings: The hearts in all 54 patients were examined initially by 1 of us (WCR), and 40 were reexamined together by both of us. Heart weights, available in 50 of the 54 patients, ranged from 300 to 900 g (mean 554). Of the 22 women, heart weights, available in 19, ranged from 300 to 900 g (mean 484) and 17 (89%) of the 19 weighed >350 g (a weight considered the upper limit of normal in adult women). Of the 32 men, heart weights (available in 31) ranged from 410 to 900 g (mean 596) and all 31 weighed >400 g (a weight considered the upper limit of normal in men).

TABLE II Electrocardiographic QRS Voltage (mm) in Each of 12 Leads in 15 Men and 15 Women With Cardiac Amyloidosis Causing Fatal Cardiac Dysfunction

Case	Necropsy Number	Age (yr) at Death	Interval (Days) ECG to Death	Leads I	II	III	R	L	F	V_1	V_2	V_3	V_4	V_5	V_6	Total QRS 12-Lead	Heart Weight (g)
Men																	
1	A63-125	32	88	6	10	6	8	4	7	11	23	16	14	11	9	125	700
2	Vt. MCV A75-174	35	56	4	4	3	4	3	4	5	9	9	11	13	8	77	750
3	A65-159	38	10	2	4	6	2	5	6	5	19	11	6	9	7	82	410
4	A70-254	38	2	2	2	5	1	3	3	4	18	16	16	9	5	84	600
5	A79-25	45	2	5	4	8	2	6	6	12	27	21	22	30	15	158	780
6	A81-6	46	13	5	5	5	4	4	3	2	10	17	19	19	13	106	545
7	NNMC 80A-15	49	107	6	3	4	3	6	3	14	20	15	12	9	4	99	850
8	A60-19	54	0	4	4	1	4	3	3	10	10	3	10	8	5	65	550
9	A56-81	55	23	2	3	2	2	1	3	5	9	11	11	7	4	60	480
10	A61-190	55	2	2	4	5	3	4	5	3	15	14	12	12	6	85	535
11	GT 74A-259	62	9	2	3	3	2	2	3	1	6	23	21	11	2	79	470
12	A65-232	65	103	7	20	12	11	3	15	8	15	24	32	27	23	197	560
13	A69-187	68	5	5	5	7	3	6	6	13	16	11	9	8	6	95	550
14	A67-241	68	35	9	5	6	7	7	3	11	7	13	15	12	6	101	420
15	A66-151	69	59	4	3	5	3	5	4	7	10	11	8	5	4	69	450
Mean		52	34	4.3	5.3	5.2	3.9	4.1	4.9	7.4	14.3	14.3	14.5	12.7	7.8	99	570
Women																	
1	A65-25	21	58	5	5	5	5	5	3	11	28	30	16	10	12	135	530
2	A68-23	48	50	4	3	3	3	3	3	5	7	9	8	9	8	65	450
3	GT 80A-262	50	91	4	3	3	2	3	3	11	24	20	18	11	14	116	460
4	A68-277	53	15	3	2	3	1	3	3	6	10	10	10	4	3	58	370
5	HU A77-19	54	51	5	2	8	2	7	6	7	15	15	4	7	6	84	420
6	Wil., D. WMC A79-24	55	8	1	8	9	4	5	9	14	21	17	9	9	5	110	430
7	SH A81-47	61	0	2	6	6	5	3	6	6	19	21	16	9	8	107	385
8	GT 71A-67	67	76	8	8	8	7	6	7	7	19	18	17	14	8	127	650
9	GT 81A-90	70	42	3	4	2	3	1	3	3	11	14	9	8	7	68	485
10	GT 71A-435	72	70	5	14	12	9	6	12	3	4	12	24	12	8	121	480
11	SH A79-76	75	30	7	10	7	6	12	5	16	18	17	17	15	15	145	510
12	GT 79A-127	78	49	3	5	4	4	2	3	4	9	16	17	21	9	97	520
13	WHC A82-120	82	6	5	8	12	4	7	10	8	18	34	41	25	27	199	900
14	GT 79A-195	89	160	3	5	1	4	2	3	3	9	14	18	20	9	91	440
15	Sibley A80-99	93	3	10	6	12	5	10	10	9	10	11	14	14	6	117	380
Mean		65	47	4.5	5.9	6.3	4.3	5.0	5.7	7.5	14.8	17.2	15.8	12.5	9.7	109	494
Total (mean)		58	41	4.4	5.6	5.8	4.1	4.6	5.3	7.5	14.5	15.8	15.2	12.6	8.7	104	532

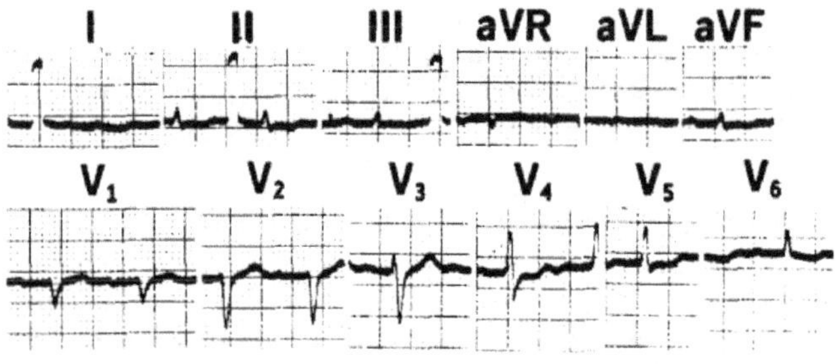

FIGURE 3. Electrocardiogram in a 55-year-old man (A56-81) recorded 23 days before death. The patient never had congestive heart failure. The heart weighed 480 g. The total 12-lead QRS voltage is only 60 mm. R waves are absent in leads V_1 and V_2 and small in V_3.

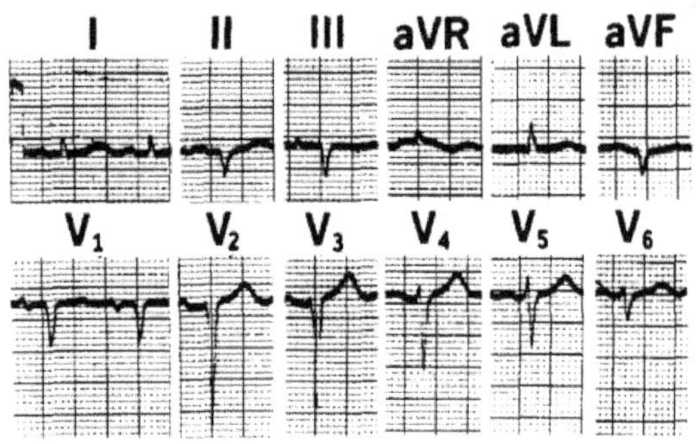

FIGURE 4. Electrocardiogram in a 55-year-old man (A61-190) recorded 2 days before death. The heart weighed 535 g and the total 12-lead QRS voltage is 85 mm. The voltage is decreased. The axis is leftward, Q waves are present in leads II, III, and aVF, and R waves are absent or small in the precordial leads.

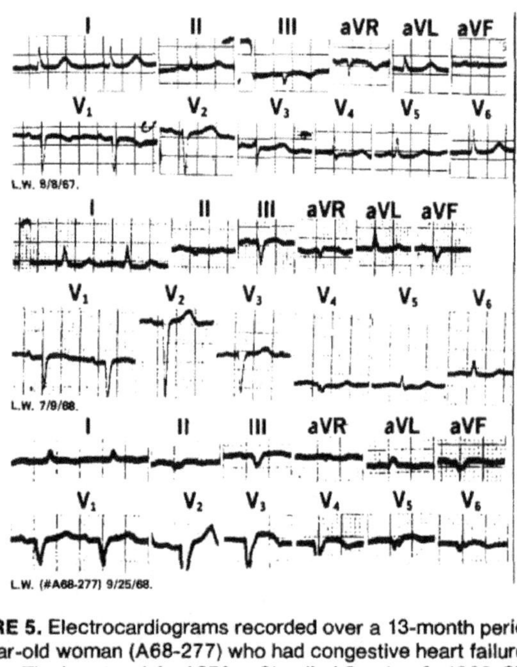

FIGURE 5. Electrocardiograms recorded over a 13-month period in a 53-year-old woman (A68-277) who had congestive heart failure for 5 months. The heart weighed 370 g. She died October 9, 1968. She had low voltage, left axis deviation, and absent R waves in the precordium. On the final electrocardiogram, the total 12-lead QRS voltage is 58 mm.

The hearts in 53 of the 54 patients were firm and rubbery, and this noncompliant consistency of the walls of all 4 cardiac chambers usually allowed the diagnosis of cardiac amyloidosis to be made immediately at necropsy without knowledge of clinical findings (Fig. 7 to 10). Both atria in all 54 patients on gross inspection were dilated, usually to a moderate degree. In contrast, the cardiac ventricles on gross inspection were of normal size in 43 patients (80%) and dilated in 11 (20%). The patients with dilated ventricles usually had other conditions that probably caused the dilatation: coronary heart disease

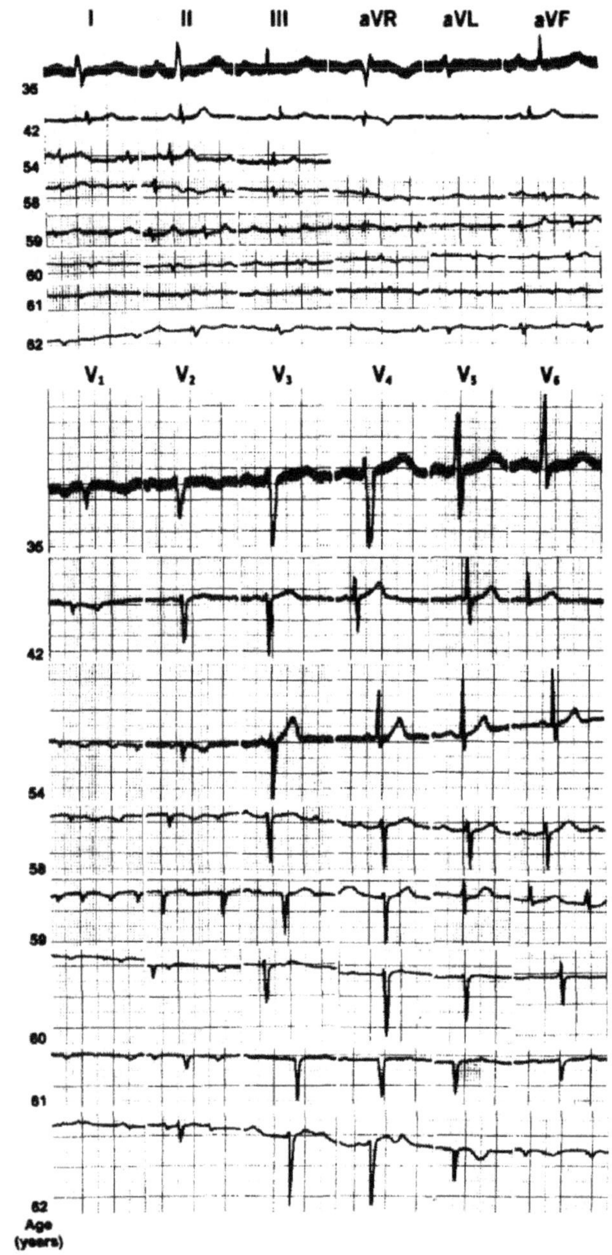

FIGURE 6. Electrocardiograms over a 27-year period in a 62-year-old man (GT 74A-259) who had congestive heart failure for 96 months and, at necropsy, a heart weighing 470 g. The QRS voltage progressively diminished, the axis changed, and R waves disappeared from the precordial leads. While taking digitalis, he developed atrial tachycardia with 2:1 block. The total 12-lead QRS voltage on the final electrocardiogram recorded 9 days before death was 79 mm.

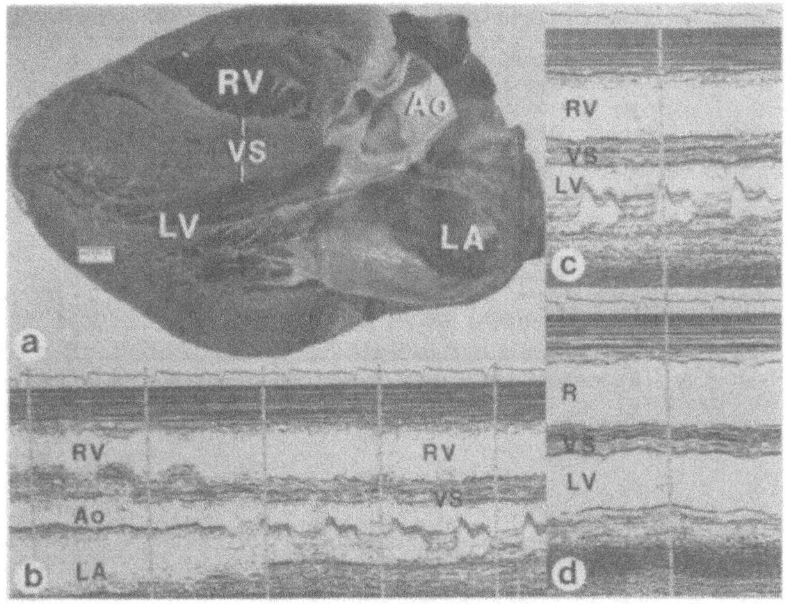

FIGURE 7. Cardiac amyloid with anasarca and pulmonary emboli. Longitudinal view of heart, weighing 545 g, in a 46-year-old man (A81-6) who had been well until 25 months before death, when parathesias and shoulder pain were noted. During his last 3 months he had severe congestive heart failure. When hospitalized 8 days before death, he had anasarca and third and fourth cardiac sounds. Electrocardiography showed a left atrial abnormality, right axis deviation, and poor R-wave progression over the precordium. Echocardiograms (**b, c, and d**) disclosed the ventricular septum (VS) and left ventricular (LV) free walls to be of similar thickness and each moved hardly at all. Both the left atrium (LA) and right ventricle (RV) were dilated. The pressures in mm Hg were: mean pulmonary artery wedge pressure, 27; pulmonary artery, 60/30; RV, 60/16; left ventricle, 90/26; and brachial artery, 90/60. He died from ventricular tachyarrhythmias. The heart in a longitudinal axis view is shown in **a.** The myocardium had the typical firm, rubbery appearance of extensive amyloidosis. Several pulmonary emboli may be the explanation of the right ventricular dilatation. Ao = aorta.

with left ventricular transmural scarring or chronic lung disease. The maximal thickness of the ventricular septum was identical or nearly so to the maximal thickness of the left ventricular free wall in 50 patients (93%); in the other 4 (7%) the septum was >1.3 times thicker than the free wall.

By gross examination, amyloid deposits (focal, tan, and waxy-appearing) were observed (and confirmed histologically) in the mural endocardium of 1 or both atria in all 54 patients and in valvular endocardium of 1 or more cardiac valves in 46 patients (85%) (Fig. 11): in the leaflets of the tricuspid valve in 45 patients (83%), the mitral valve in 43 patients (80%), the pulmonic valve in 29 patients (54%), and the aortic valve in 29 patients (54%). In 27 patients (50%), amyloid deposits were observed grossly in the leaflets of all 4 cardiac valves.

Focal transmural left ventricular lesions were observed grossly in 9 patients (17%) (Fig. 8); on histologic examination the lesions consisted entirely of fibrous tissue in 7 patients (13%) and of amyloid deposits in 2 (4%).

At least 3 histologic sections of heart were examined in each patient. In every patient, at least 1 section of left ventricular wall and at least 1 section of atrial wall were examined. Amyloid deposits, readily identified on hematoxylin-eosin stains, were confirmed by either congo red or crystal violet stains or both. In the chamber walls, the amyloid deposits were located in (1) interstitium, that is, between myocardial fibers, not within them in all but 1 patient,[4] (2) endocardium, often of all 4 chambers but always of 1 or both atria in all patients, and (3) within the walls of several intramural coronary arteries in all patients (Fig. 12). Additionally, amyloid deposits often were found in the lumina of some intramural coronary arteries, causing severe (>75% in cross-sectional area) narrowing of some lumina. Despite numerous sections of the major epicardial coronary arteries, no amyloid deposits were observed. At least 1 and usually multiple cardiac valves contained amyloid deposits, but none were judged to have deposits of sufficient quantity to cause valvular dysfunction. In several patients in whom histologic sections included coronary sinus, amyloid deposits were visible histologically in the wall of this structure.

In all 54 patients, amyloid deposits were observed in 1 or more other body organs. No patient had amyloid limited to the heart.

TABLE III **M-Mode Echocardiographic Observations in 11 Necropsy Patients With Fatal Cardiac Amyloidosis***

Case	Age (yr) & Sex	Interval (Days) Cath to Death	VS		LV Wall		VS/LV Ratio		LV Cavity		LA Cavity		Ascending Aorta	
			ES	ED	ES	ED	ES	ED	ES	ED	ES	ED	ES	ED
1	21F	90	14	12	21	14	0.7	0.9	20	36	28	22	24	20
2	40M	...	...	20	...	20	...	1.0	...	...	...	36	...	41
3	45M	15	28	24	18	15	1.6	1.6	24	32	...	58	...	...
4	46M	62	14	14	18	14	0.7	1.0	36	40	36	40	34	30
5	54F	...	...	20	...	20	...	1.0	...	...	...	36	...	41
6	55F	334	30	26	18	15	1.7	1.7	26	36	...	30	...	27
7	55F	150	25	24	26	20	0.9	1.2	29	33	35	30	40	38
8	62M	300	19	19	22	18	0.9	1.1	38	42	20	18	38	30
9	63M	15	35	25	25	16	1.4	1.6	...	...	...	...	...	...
10	78F	169	12	9	13	8	0.9	1.1	36	48	45	40	35	31
11	89F	13	20	19	18	10	1.1	1.9	55	65	45	42	35	32

* All measurements in millimeters.
Cath = catheterization; ED = end-diastole; ES = end-systole; LV = left ventricular; VS = ventricular septum.

TABLE IV Hemodynamic Data in 9 Necropsy Patients With Fatal Cardiac Amyloidosis

Case	Age (yr) & Sex	Interval (Days) Cath to Death	Right Atrium*			PAW*			RV* (s/d)	PA* (s/d)	LV* (s/d)	SA* (s/d)	CI (liters/min/m²)
			a	v	m	a	v	m					
1	35M	90	...	...	11	...	...	25	52/16	48/28	100/24	100/70	...
2	38M	4	24	22	21	...	...	34	56/18	61/34	110/12	110/65	1.3
3	45M	14	12	13	11	28	38	30	60/11	65/33	100/28	100/64	1.7
4	46F	180	10	8	7	...	42	28	50/9	65/33	98/28	98/70	1.6
5	46M	360	...	...	20	...	...	27	60/16	60/30	90/26	90/65	...
6	47F	90	15	14	12	21	28	20	36/12	36/17	110/20	110/80	2.2
7	70M	7	...	...	...	...	...	30	50/	50/30	...	110/60	...
8	78F	150	14	11	10	...	30	26	70/2	70/30	100/20	100/60	2.3
9	96M	7	...	...	17	...	...	34	60/18	60/30	...	90/70	...

a = peak of a wave averaged for several beats; Cath = cardiac catheterization procedure; CI = cardiac index; LV = left ventricle; m = mean; PA = pulmonary artery; PAW = pulmonary arterial wedge; RV = right ventricle; SA = systemic artery; s/d = systolic/diastolic; v = peak of v wave averaged for several beats.

* Measurements in mm Hg.

Thrombi were observed grossly in 1 or more of the 4 cardiac chambers in 14 (26%) of the 54 patients: in 1 chamber only in 8 patients, in 2 chambers in 3 patients, in 3 chambers in 1 patient, and in all 4 chambers in 1 patient. Of the 22 cardiac chambers that contained thrombi (mainly fibrin in all) in the 14 patients, the right atrial appendage contained thrombi in 10 patients (isolated in 5); the left atrial appendage contained thrombi in 7 patients (isolated in 2); the right ventricle con-

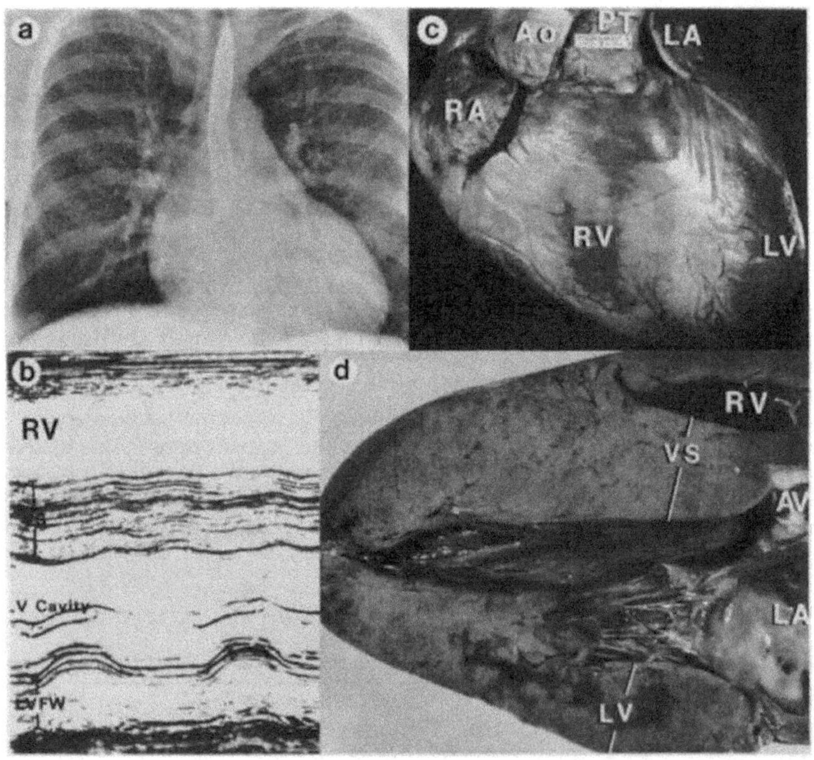

FIGURE 8. Cardiac amyloidosis simulating hypertrophic cardiomyopathy. Chest radiograph (a), M-mode echocardiogram just caudal to the tips of the mitral leaflets (b), exterior view of heart (c), and longitudinal axis view of heart (d) in a 46-year-old man (A79-25) who noted dyspnea while walking 24 months before death. M-mode echocardiography 1 month later disclosed the ventricular septum (VS) to be 1.7 times thicker than the left ventricular free wall (LVFW). The anterior mitral leaflet moved anteriorly during ventricular systole. The left atrial cavity was 30 mm in diameter. The pressures in mm Hg were: mean pulmonary arterial wedge, 5; pulmonary artery, 17/6; right ventricle (RV), 17/3; left ventricle (LV), 130/11; and aorta (Ao), 115/70. Clinically, the patient at that time was considered to have hypertrophic cardiomyopathy. Nine months before death, he had transient sudden left-sided weakness with slurred speech, worsened dyspnea, transient chest pain, and the carpal-tunnel syndrome was noted. Now the mean pulmonary arterial wedge pressure was 23; right ventricular pressure, 47/7; LV, 95/25; and Ao, 95/65 mm Hg. Echocardiogram now showed the ventricular septum to be 2.0 cm and the LVFW 1.5 cm; SAM now was absent. The left atrium (LA) now was 55 mm in diameter. A third catheterization performed 10 days before death showed the mean pulmonary wedge pressure to be 32 and that in the RV 65/11 mm Hg. The cardiac index was 1.4 liters/min/m². The heart was enlarged (a). M-mode echocardiogram (b) now showed the VS to be 2.6 cm and the LVFW 1.5 cm thick. Cardiac amyloidosis was never diagnosed clinically. At necropsy, the heart weighed 780 g. In addition to the usual interstitial myocardial amyloid, large deposits of amyloid were visible grossly on the LVFW (d). The VS is thicker than the free wall. The epicardial coronary arteries were virtually free of atherosclerotic plaques. AV = aortic valve; PT = pulmonary trunk; RA = right atrium; SAM = systolic anterior motion of the anterior mitral leaflet.

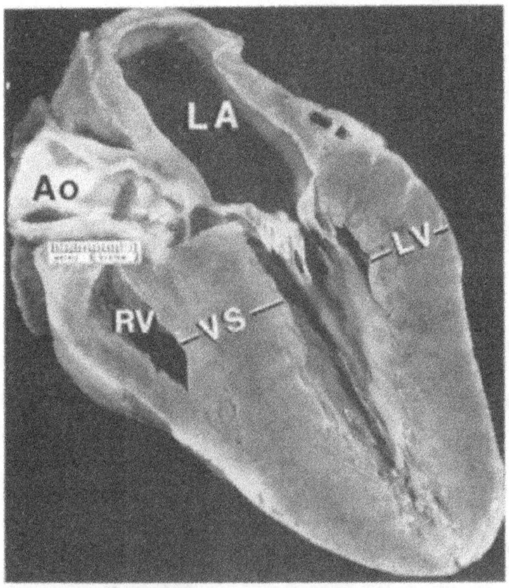

FIGURE 9. Cardiac amyloidosis simulating hypertrophic cardiomyopathy. Long-axis view of heart in a 55-year-old woman (WMC#A79-24) who had been well until 6 months before death when she developed periorbital purpura, pedal edema, and right-arm pain. When syncope occurred a month later, she was hospitalized and found to have multiple myeloma. Electrocardiography disclosed both atrial and ventricular arrhythmias and electrophysiologic studies disclosed distal H-V block. She never had congestive heart failure. On the day of death at home she fainted and soon thereafter had fatal cardiac arrest. The heart weighed 430 g and it had the typical amyloid consistency. A long-axis view is shown. The ventricular septum (VS) is thicker than the left ventricular (LV) free wall. The left atrium (LA) is dilated. Ao = aorta; RV = right ventricular cavity.

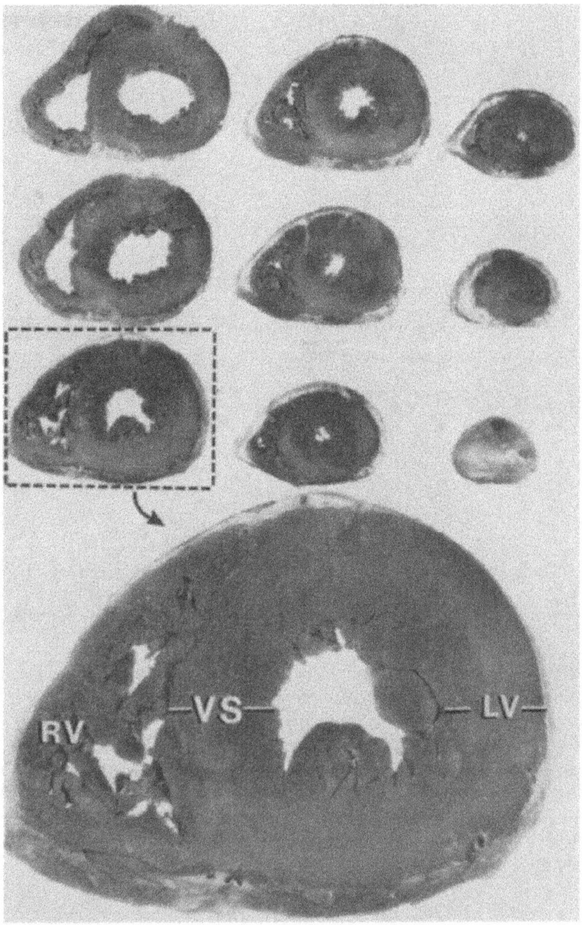

FIGURE 10. Massive ventricular amyloid deposits. Transverse cuts of the ventricles in the 49-year-old man (NNMC#A80-15), described in detail in Figure 3. This uniform appearance of the ventricular walls is the most common finding in extensive cardiac amyloidosis. LV = left ventricle; RV = right ventricle; VS = ventricular septum.

tained thrombi in 2 patients (none isolated), and the left ventricle contained thrombi in 3 patients (isolated in 2). Thus, of the 22 chambers with thrombi, 17 were atrial appendages and 5 were ventricles. None of the 5 ventricles containing thrombi appeared dilated by gross inspection. Of the 14 patients with intracardiac thrombi, 13 had clinical evidence of CHF and 1 died suddenly without evidence at any time of CHF: 2 (of 13) had chronic atrial fibrillation; 2 had clinical evidence of either pulmonary or systemic emboli, and 5 had severe narrowing of 1 or more epicardial cardiac arteries by either atherosclerotic plaque (4 patients) or fibrin-platelet embolus (1 patient). The latter patient was reported on previously.[2]

In addition to the extensive cardiac amyloid deposits, 8 patients (15%) had narrowing >75% in cross-sectional area by atherosclerotic plaques of 1 or more of the 4 major (right, left main, left anterior descending, and left circumflex) epicardial coronary arteries: in 5 patients, 3 of the 4 major arteries were so narrowed; in 1 patient 2 arteries, and in 2 patients 1 artery. The ages of these 8 patients ranged from 65 to 96 years (mean 78); 6 were men and 2 were women. Four had had periodic chest pain, considered angina pectoris in 2. One patient died suddenly and unexpectedly. At necropsy none had foci of myocardial necrosis, but 4 had healed transmural left ventricular infarcts, all of which had been clinically silent.

Calcific deposits were present in the mitral anulus in 7 patients (13%) and in 1 or more aortic valve cusps in 9 patients (17%). In 6 patients, the calcific deposits were present in both mitral anulus and in aortic valve cusps, in 3 patients they were limited to aortic valve cusps, and in 1 patient they were limited to mitral anulus. In 2 of the 9 patients with aortic valve calcium, the deposits appeared extensive enough to cause narrowing of the aortic valve orifice. In none of the 7 patients with mitral anulus calcium did the calcific deposits appear to cause clinically significant mitral dysfunction. All 10 patients (19%) with either mitral anular or aortic valve cuspal calcific deposits, or both, had calcific deposits in 1 or more of the 4 major epicardial coronary arteries, and in each patient they were within atherosclerotic plaques.

Discussion

Patients with cardiac amyloid deposits may readily be separated into 2 major groups: (1) those with amyloid deposits too small to produce cardiac dysfunction, and (2) those with amyloid deposits large enough to produce cardiac dysfunction which eventually is fatal. The finding of minute cardiac amyloid deposits in the heart in elderly persons at necropsy is common,[5–13] but patients with minute cardiac deposits, whether they be young or old, are not included in the present analysis. Each of our 54 patients had heavy cardiac amyloid deposits that caused fatal cardiac dysfunction. All but 1 had firm, rubbery ventricular and usually atrial walls with amyloid deposits in the interstitium (between myocardial cells) of the walls of all 4 chambers, in mural and usually in valvular endocardium, and in the in-

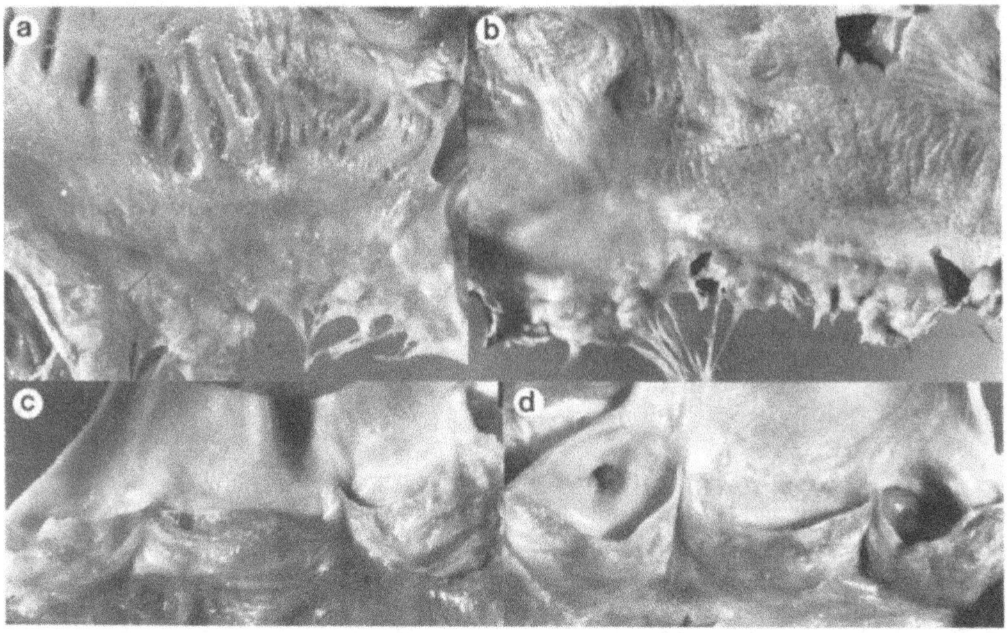

FIGURE 11. Endocardial amyloidosis. Opened right atrium and tricuspid valve (**a**), opened left atrium and mitral valve (**b**), opened pulmonic valve and pulmonary trunk (**c**), and opened aortic valve and aorta (**d**). The mural endocardium of each chamber and the cusps of all 4 cardiac valves contain amyloid deposits. The ventricular myocardium (shown in Figure 4) also contained massive quantities of amyloid, as did the pulmonary trunk. This 49-year-old man (NNMC#A80-15) had been well, but an automobile accident prompted an examination 10 months before death. Both pedal edema and hepatomegaly were found, the blood pressure was elevated (160/100 mm Hg), the heart was enlarged (cardiothoracic ratio 0.55), and electrocardiogram disclosed no R waves in leads V_1–V_3, nonspecific ST-T wave abnormalities, and low voltage. Echocardiogram was normal. Hepatic biopsy yielded amyloid. He remained asymptomatic until 4 months before death, when extensive subcutaneous edema appeared and pericardial effusion (700 ml) was found. The systemic blood pressure was then 120/80 mm Hg. His condition progressively worsened thereafter. He became acutely dyspneic at home and died.

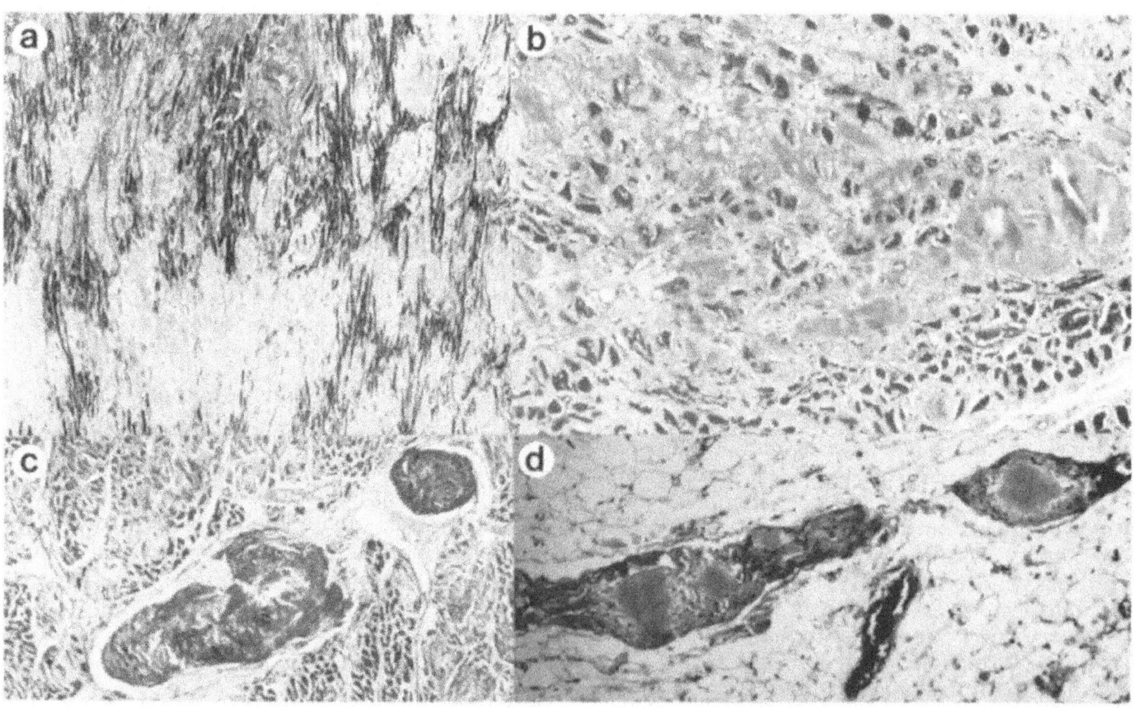

FIGURE 12. Location of amyloid in myocardium (**a** and **b**), intramural coronary artery (**c**) and epicardial nerve (**d**). **a,** massive interstitial myocardial amyloid observed in a longitudinal section in an 89-year-old man (A69-259) with chronic congestive heart failure (CHF) and a heart weighing 520 g. In this section, more amyloid than myocardial fibers are present. **b,** massive interstitial myocardial amyloid observed in cross section in a 68-year-old man (H-A76-143) who had CHF for 36 months. **c,** amyloid occluding the lumens of intramural coronary arteries in a 67-year-old man (A69-187) with chronic CHF and a heart weighing 550 g. **d,** amyloid in epicardial nerves in a 74-year-old man (A58-190) who died suddenly from familial amyloidosis and had a heart weighing 700 g. (Hematoxylin-eosin stain [**a**] ×25 and [**d**] ×100; Movat stain [**b**] ×100; Masson stain [**c**] ×39, all reduced 25%.)

tramural coronary arteries. The 1 patient without interstitial myocardial amyloid had amyloid filling the lumina of most intramural coronary arteries.[3] Additionally, several patients had amyloid in the epicardium but never in the walls or lumina of the major epicardial coronary arteries. All our 54 patients with cardiac amyloid had amyloid deposits in 1 or more noncardiac body organs. We suspect that cardiac amyloid severe enough to cause clinical evidence of cardiac dysfunction is never limited exclusively to the heart.

Although a diagnosis of cardiac amyloidosis was established clinically in less than half of our 54 patients, most were studied clinically before echocardiography and radionuclide angiography became commonly performed procedures. Echocardiography is now often one of the first clues to the diagnosis of cardiac amyloidosis,[14–19] and myocardial technetium-99m pyrophosphate scintigraphy may be diagnostic of this condition.[20–23] Thus, cardiac amyloidosis severe enough to cause cardiac dysfunction almost surely will be suspected hereafter in a majority rather than in a minority of patients. Clinically, diagnosis of cardiac amyloidosis should be suspected in an older patient with evidence of CHF, poorly responsive and/or particularly sensitive to digitalis, unassociated with chest pain or systemic hypertension, and in the presence of cardiomegaly by chest radiograph but low voltage by electrocardiogram. The echocardiogram, rather than showing dilatation of the left ventricle, shows this chamber to be of normal or near-normal size and the ventricular walls to move poorly, and these findings can be confirmed by hemodynamic and angiographic studies.[24–27] Biopsy of either noncardiac or cardiac[28] tissue is required for absolute diagnosis.

Severe cardiac amyloidosis is 1 of the causes of spontaneous cure of systemic hypertension. Although nearly half of our 54 patients had had either a history of systemic hypertension or recordings of elevated systemic arterial pressures, or both, all had systolic systemic pressures $\leq$130 mm Hg and diastolic systemic pressures $\leq$90 mm Hg in the last 3 months of life. The average recorded peak systolic arterial pressure in the last 3 months of life in our patients was 102 mm Hg and the diastolic pressure was 70 mm Hg. Thus, if the systemic arterial pressure is elevated in a patient with CHF, the chance that the CHF is the result of cardiac amyloidosis is minimal. Additionally, none of our patients had evidence of left ventricular hypertrophy by electrocardiogram in their final 3 months, although several had had left ventricular hypertrophy by electrocardiogram >1 year earlier.

The length of time necessary to develop cardiac amyloid deposits extensive enough to cause cardiac dysfunction is uncertain. One clue to the amount of time required can be gained by study of the systemic arterial pressures over several years. We have now observed several patients with systolic systemic pressures in the vicinity of 180 mm Hg; during a period of 4 to 5 years this pressure gradually decreased to about 100 mm Hg without use of antihypertensive agents. Thus, a gradual but spontaneous decrease in systemic arterial pressure also might be a clue to the development of cardiac amyloidosis.

Cardiac amyloidosis needs to be added to the list of great cardiac masqueraders. Initially, it was cardiovascular syphilis that was stated to frequently simulate other cardiac conditions. In recent years, hypertrophic cardiomyopathy has become the most prominent masquerader. The QRS and T-wave changes on the electrocardiogram in cardiac amyloidosis are similar to those produced by healed myocardial infarction secondary to coronary atherosclerosis. The presence of a nondilated left ventricle and the presence of a ventricular septum thicker than the left ventricular free wall by echocardiogram has suggested the presence of hypertrophic cardiomyopathy. Five of our 11 patients with echocardiograms were suspected of having hypertrophic cardiomyopathy because of the combination of these findings. Simulation of cardiac amyloidosis clinically to pericardial constriction has long been recognized.[1,24–27] Three of our 54 patients underwent thoracotomy because of suspected pericardial constriction. Cardiac amyloidosis may present as pericardial tamponade.[29] Its delayed left ventricular filling may simulate mitral stenosis on rare occasions.[30]

Although amyloid deposits are always more extensive in "working" than in "conducting" myocardium,[1,31,32] arrhythmias and conduction disturbances are common (Table I). Some of these disturbances, however, may be the result of aging rather than the result of extensive cardiac amyloidosis.[13,33] In our patients, left-axis deviation (58%), atrial fibrillation (23%), and bundle branch block (18%) were common, but these also are relatively common in elderly patients without cardiac amyloidosis.[13,33] The frequency of low voltage (63%) and a healed myocardial infarction pattern (83%), however, was striking in our patients, and each of these should raise the possibility of cardiac amyloidosis in a patient with CHF of unclear cause.

This report provides for the first time measurements of QRS voltages in each of the 12 leads of an electrocardiogram in patients with cardiac amyloidosis. Simonson[34] provided data on the upper and lower limits of amplitude of the QRS complexes in each of the 12 leads in normal men and women aged 20 to 59 years. (The mean for normal subjects is not available.) The upper and lower limits of normal for men aged 50 to 59 years were 277 and 36 mm and for women 248 and 27 mm, respectively. The upper and lower limits of amplitude in all leads in 30 of our 54 patients (Table II) were 199 and 58 mm, respectively, and averaged 104 mm. For our 15 women from whom the data were available, the total 12-lead QRS voltage ranged from 58 to 199 mm (mean 109) and for our 15 men from 60 to 197 mm (mean 99).

In comparison, Siegel and Roberts[35] determined the total 12-lead QRS voltage in 50 patients (aged 16 to 65 years) with severe and fatal isolated aortic valve stenosis. The upper and lower limits of amplitude in all 12 leads in their 50 patients were 417 and 144 mm, respectively, and averaged 260 mm. In their 14 women with aortic stenosis, the total 12-lead QRS voltage averaged 277 mm and in their 36 men, 249 mm. The average heart weight of their 14 women with aortic stenosis was 521 g, and the heart weight in our 15 women with severe cardiac amyloidosis and available total 12-lead

QRS voltage was 494 g. The difference, however, in average total 12-lead QRS voltage (277 mm versus 109 mm) was a factor of 2.5 times. The mean heart weight of the 36 men with aortic stenosis studied by Siegel and Roberts[35] was 639 g and that of our 15 men with fatal cardiac amyloidosis and available total 12-lead QRS voltage was 570 g. The average total 12-lead QRS voltage in the 36 men with aortic stenosis, however, was 249 mm compared with only 99 mm in our 15 men with fatal cardiac amyloid, again a 2.5-fold difference. Thus, although the sum of the QRS voltage in leads I, II, and III may not fulfill criteria of "low voltage," that is, ≤15 mm, the total QRS voltage in all 12 leads in severe cardiac amyloidosis is usually considerably lower than normal, and particularly small in proportion to the weight of the heart.

References

1. **Buja LM, Khoi NB, Roberts WC.** Clinically significant cardiac amyloidosis. Clinicopathologic findings in 15 patients. Am J Cardiol 1970;26:394–405.
2. **Barth RF, Willerson JT, Buja LM, Decker JL, Roberts WC.** Amyloid coronary artery disease, primary systemic amyloidosis and paraproteinemia. Arch Intern Med 1970;127:627–630.
3. **Saffitz JE, Sazama K, Roberts WC.** Amyloidosis limited to small arteries causing angina pectoris and sudden death. Am J Cardiol 1983;51:1234–1235.
4. **Roberts WC, Perloff JK, Costantino T.** Severe valvular aortic stenosis in patients over 65 years of age. A clinicopathologic study. Am J Cardiol 1971;27:497–506.
5. **Brandt K, Cathcart ES, Cohen AS.** A clinical analysis of the course and prognosis of forty-two patients with amyloidosis. Am J Med 1968;44: 955–959.
6. **Schwartz P.** Amyloidosis. Cause and manifestation of senile deterioration. Springfield, IL: Charles C Thomas, 1970:395.
7. **Kyle RA, Bayrd ED.** Amyloidosis: review of 236 cases. Medicine 1975; 54:271–300.
8. **Hodkinson HM, Pomerance A.** The clinical significance of senile cardiac amyloidosis: a prospective clinico-pathological study. Quart J Med 1977; 46:381–387.
9. **Smith RRL, Hutchins GM, Moore GW, Humphrey RL.** Type and distribution of pulmonary parenchymal and vascular amyloid. Correlation with cardiac amyloid. Am J Med 1979;66:96–104.
10. **Westermark P, Johansson B, Natvig JB.** Senile cardiac amyloidosis: evidence of two different amyloid substances in the aging heart. Scand J Immunol 1979;10:303–308.
11. **Cornwell GG III, Westermark P.** Senile amyloidosis: a protean manifestation of the aging process. J Clin Pathol 1980;33:1146–1152.
12. **Wright JR, Calkins E.** Clinical-pathological differentiation of common amyloid syndromes. Medicine 1981;60:429–448.
13. **Waller BF, Roberts WC.** Cardiovascular disease in the very elderly. Analysis of 40 necropsy patients aged 90 years or older. Am J Cardiol 1983;51: 403–421.
14. **Child JS, Levisman JA, Abbasi AS, MacAlpin RN.** Echocardiographic manifestations of infiltrative cardiomyopathy. A report of seven cases due to amyloid. Chest 1976;70:726–731.
15. **Borer JS, Henry WL, Epstein SE.** Echocardiographic observations in patients with systemic infiltrative disease involving the heart. Am J Cardiol 1977;39:184–188.
16. **Child JS, Krivokapich J, Abbasi AS.** Increased right ventricular wall thickness on echocardiography in amyloid infiltrative cardiomyopathy. Am J Cardiol 1979;44:1391–1395.
17. **Siqueira-Filho AG, Cunha CLP, Tajik AJ, Seward JB, Schattenberg TT, Giuliani ER.** M-mode and two-dimensional echocardiographic features in cardiac amyloidosis. Circulation 1981;63:188–196.
18. **St John Sutton MG, Reichek N, Kastor JA, Giuliani ER.** Computerized M-mode echocardiographic analysis of left ventricular dysfunction in cardiac amyloid. Circulation 1982;66:790–799.
19. **Bhandari AK, Nanda NC.** Myocardial texture characterization by two-dimensional echocardiography. Am J Cardiol 1983;51:817–825.
20. **Wizenberg TA, Muz J, Sohn YH, Samlowski W, Weissler AM.** Value of positive myocardial technetium-99m-pyrophosphate scintigraphy in the noninvasive diagnosis of cardiac amyloidosis. Am Heart J 1982;103: 468–473.
21. **Schiff S, Bateman T, Moffatt R, Davidson R, Berman D.** Diagnostic considerations in cardiomyopathy: unique scintigraphic pattern of diffuse biventricular technetium-99m-pyrophosphate uptake in amyloid heart disease. Am Heart J 1982;130:562–563.
22. **Sobol SM, Brown JM, Bunker SR, Patel J, Lull RJ.** Noninvasive diagnosis of cardiac amyloidosis by technetium-99m-pyrophosphate myocardial scintigraphy. Am Heart J 1982;103:563–566.
23. **Falk RH, Lee VW, Rubinow A, Hood WB Jr, Cohen AS.** Sensitivity of Technetium-99m-pyrophosphate scintigraphy in diagnosing cardiac amyloidosis. Am J Cardiol 1983;51:826–830.
24. **Chew C, Ziady GM, Raphael MJ, Oakley CM.** The functional defect in amyloid heart disese. The "stiff heart" syndrome. Am J Cardiol 1975;36: 438–444.
25. **Meaney E, Shabetai R, Bhargava V, Shearer M, Weidner C, Mangiardi, LM, Smalling R, Peterson K.** Cardiac amyloidosis, constrictive pericarditis and restrictive cardiomyopathy. Am J Cardiol 1976;38:547–556.
26. **Swanton RH, Brooksby IAB, Davies MJ, Coltart DJ, Jenkins BS, Webb-Peploe MM.** Systolic and diastolic ventricular function in cardiac amyloidosis. Studies in six cases diagnosed with endomyocardial biopsy. Am J Cardiol 1977;39:658–664.
27. **Tyberg TI, Goodyer AVN, Hurst VW III, Alexander J, Langou RA.** Left ventricular filling in differentiating restrictive amyloid cardiomyopathy and constrictive pericarditis. Am J Cardiol 1981;47:791–796.
28. **Schroeder JS, Billingham ME, Rider AK.** Cardiac amyloidosis. Diagnosis by transvenous endomyocardial biopsy. Am J Med 1975;59:269–273.
29. **Brodarick S, Paine R, Higa E, Carmichael KA.** Pericardial tamponade, a new complication of amyloid heart disease. Am J Med 1982;73:133–135.
30. **Shenoy UA, Peric-Golia L.** Primary cardiovascular amyloidosis manifesting as mitral stenosis. Hum Pathol 1982;13:768–770.
31. **Ridolfi RL, Bulkley BH, Hutchins GM.** The conduction system in cardiac amyloidosis. Clinical and pathologic features of 23 patients. Am J Med 1977;62:677–686.
32. **Bharati S, Lev M, Denes P, Modlinger J, Wyndham C, Bauernfeind R, Greenblatt M, Rosen KM.** Infiltrative cardiomyopathy with conduction disease and ventricular arrhythmia: electrophysiologic and pathologic correlations. Am J Cardiol 1980;45:163–173.
33. **Fisch C.** Electrocardiogram in the aged: an independent marker of heart disease? Am J Med 1981;70:4–6.
34. **Simonson F.** Differentiation between normal and abnormal in electrocardiography. St. Louis: CV Mosby, 1961:328.
35. **Siegel RJ, Roberts WC.** Electrocardiographic observations in severe aortic valve stenosis: correlative necropsy study to clinical, hemodynamic, and ECG variables demonstrating relation of 12-lead QRS amplitude to peak systolic transaortic pressure gradient. Am Heart J 1982;103:210–221.

Hypertrophic cardiomyopathy: a common cause of sudden death in the young competitive athlete

B. J. MARON, S. E. EPSTEIN AND W. C. ROBERTS

Cardiology and Pathology Branches, National Heart, Lung and Blood Institute, National Institutes of Health, Bethesda, Maryland, USA

KEY WORDS: Sudden death, hypertrophic cardiomyopathy, athletes.

The causes of sudden, unexpected death in highly-conditioned competitive athletes are summarized. In the vast majority of young athletes (less than 35 years of age) sudden death is due to underlying structural cardiovascular disease. Hypertrophic cardiomyopathy appears to be the most common cause of such deaths and may account for about one-half of the sudden deaths in a youthful athletic population. Cardiovascular abnormalities that appear to be less frequent important causes of sudden death include anomalous origin of the left coronary artery from the anterior sinus of Valsalva, ruptured aorta (due to cystic medial necrosis), idiopathic concentric left ventricular hypertrophy and coronary artery atherosclerosis. Other diseases which are probably particularly uncommon causes of sudden death in the young athlete include mitral valve prolapse, aortic valvular stenosis, acute myocarditis, QT interval prolongation syndromes, hypoplasia of the coronary arteries or sarcoidosis. Cardiovascular disease in young athletes is usually unsuspected during life. In only about 25% of those competitive athletes who die suddenly is underlying disease identified prior to participation and rarely is the correct clinical diagnosis made. In contrast, when sudden death occurs in older competitive or recreational athletes (over 35 years of age) it is usually due to coronary artery disease.

Introduction

Highly conditioned competitive athletes epitomize the most healthy segment of our society. For this reason, the occurrence of sudden death in an athlete is particularly shocking and tragic (Fig. 1). For many years our ignorance of the causes of such catastrophes was clothed in esoteric sounding phrases, such as 'sudden death syndrome', which merely masked the fact that the precise causes were unknown. Recently, careful morphologic studies performed after death have revealed that a variety of congenital or acquired structural malformations of the heart and great vessels are responsible for the vast majority of sudden deaths that occur in athletes[1-5].

Sudden death in young competitive athletes

Considering the large numbers of participants in competitive and recreational athletic programs, sudden death must be considered an uncommon event. Nonetheless, an occasional young athlete, apparently in excellent health, will die suddenly and unexpectedly. Such individuals participate in a variety of sports and most commonly are high school athletes at the time of death[1]; however, some young athletes reach the collegiate or even professional level[6] of competition before dying suddenly. Usually such catastrophes occur during or just following exertion on the athletic field and death is thereby often attributed to intense physical activity. However, while extreme effort may be the precipitating cause of death in some instances, the underlying cause of death in the vast majority of young athletes (less than 35 years of age) is a congenital cardiovascular malformation[1]. Despite the fact that these malformations are present at birth, individuals so afflicted can compete for many years without either being aware of their cardiovascular disease or experiencing significant symptoms.

In our series of 29 young competitive athletes who died suddenly, 28 had a structural cardiovascular disease identified at necropsy that represented an unequivocal or probable cause of death[1] (Fig. 2).

Address correspondence to: Dr Barry J. Maron, Senior Investigator, National Heart, Lung, and Blood Institute, Building 10, Room 7B-15, Bethesda, Maryland 20205, USA.

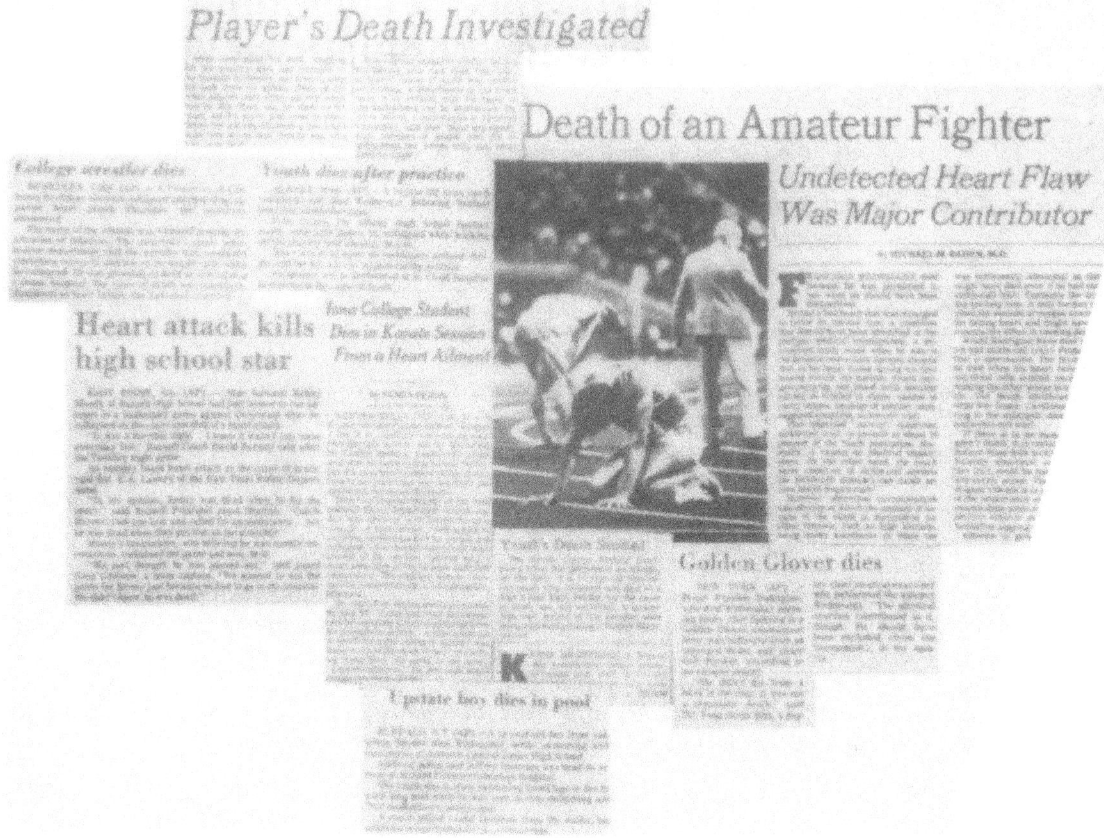

Player's Death Investigated

Death of an Amateur Fighter

Undetected Heart Flaw Was Major Contributor

College wrestler dies

Youth dies after practice

Heart attack kills high school star

Iona College Student Dies in Karate Season From a Heart Ailment

Golden Glover dies

Upstate boy dies in pool

Figure 1 Media reports of sudden unexpected deaths in young athletes.

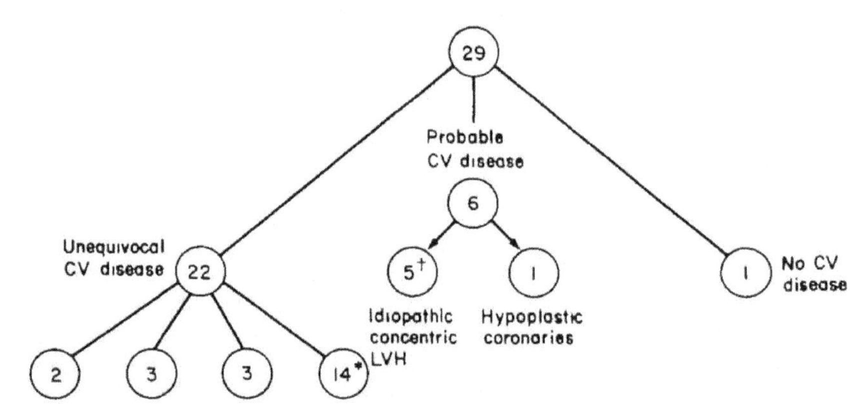

Figure 2 Diagram summarizing the cause of death in 29 competitive athletes. CV = cardiovascular; LVH = left ventricular hypertrophy. The asterisk indicates that this group includes one patient who also had anomalous origin of the left coronary artery from the anterior sinus of Valsalva. The daggar indicates that this group includes one patient who had gross and histologic findings at necropsy consistent with mitral valve prolapse, as well as a family history of that condition.

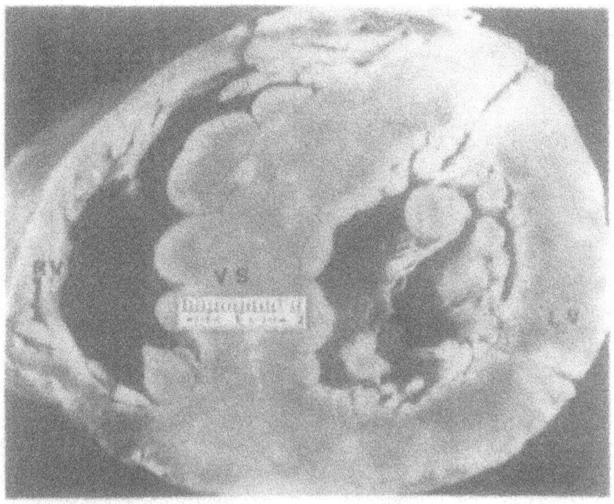

Figure 3 Heart of a 13 year old male (gridiron) football player showing disproportionate thickening of the ventricular septum (VS) with respect to the posterior left ventricular free wall (LV). RV = right ventricular wall.

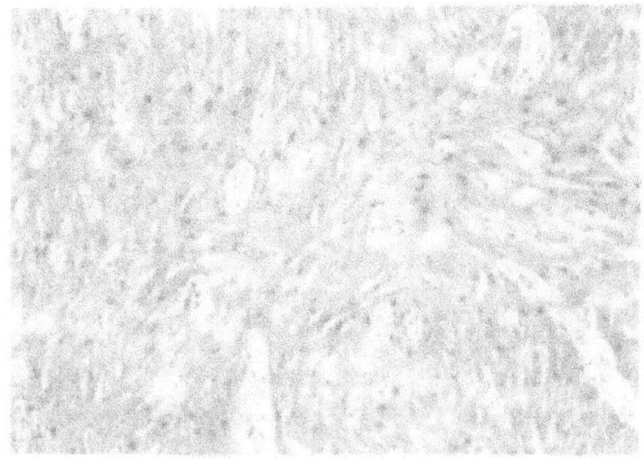

Figure 4 Histologic section of ventricular septal myocardium from a 14 year old competitive athlete, showing marked cellular disorganization in which adjacent cardiac muscle cells are oriented at oblique and perpendicular angles to each other.

HYPERTROPHIC CARDIOMYOPATHY

The most common cause of such deaths appears to be ***hypertrophic cardiomyopathy***, which occurred in almost one-half (i.e. 14) of the athletes. Each of these individuals had a hypertrophied, nondilated left ventricle in the absence of another cardiac or systemic disease that could produce left ventricular hypertrophy (such as valvular, hypertensive or coronary heart disease or infiltrative cardiomyopathy)[7]. The heart weights in these 14 patients were all increased over normal[8] and ranged from 360 to 630 g (mean 475 g). None of the 12 patients with blood pressure recordings during life had systemic hypertension. Mild to moderate right ventricular dilatation also was present in five patients.

For the diagnosis of hypertrophic cardiomyopathy to be made, each of these patients also had to have at least one of the following characteristic features of the disease: (1) asymmetric septal hypertrophy (ventricular septal-to-left ventricular free wall thickness ratio $\geqslant 1 \cdot 3$; range $1 \cdot 3$ to $2 \cdot 2$)[9–11] Fig. 3); (2) marked disorganization of cardiac muscle cells in the ventricular septum[12] involving at least 5% of the relevant areas of the tissue section[13] (Fig. 4); (3) clinical or echocardiographic evidence of hypertrophic cardiomyopathy in one or more closely related family members[14]. Seven of the 14 athletes with hypertrophic cardiomyopathy had both asymmetric septal hypertrophy and marked ventricular septal cellular disorganization and three had asymmetric septal hypertrophy without disorganization. The other four athletes had concentric (symmetric) left ventricular hypertrophy (septal – free wall ratio $<1 \cdot 3$), including two with marked septal disorganization and two without disorganization; each of these four athletes had at least one first degree relative with echocardiographic evidence of hypertrophic cardiomyopathy.

Abnormal intramural coronary arteries (two or more per tissue section) were identified in the ventricular septal myocardium of four athletes with hypertrophic cardiomyopathy. The abnormal arteries had thickened walls (due to intimal proliferation or medial hypertrophy or both) and narrowed lumens. One other athlete with hypertrophic cardiomyopathy showed marked narrowing (due to fibromuscular hyperplasia) of only the arteries to the sinoatrial and atrioventricular nodes. The conduction system was otherwise normal, as were the other intramural coronary arteries.

In athletes with hypertrophic cardiomyopathy the scalar electrocardiogram may show a wide variety of alterations (Figs 5 and 6). It should also be emphasized that electrocardiographic abnormalities in patients with hypertrophic cardiomyopathy may be similar to those in some athletes *without* underlying heart disease. However, in such athletes without cardiac disease the inversion of T waves may normalize with exercise or isoproterenol infusions[15] or spontaneously after deconditioning (Fig. 7).

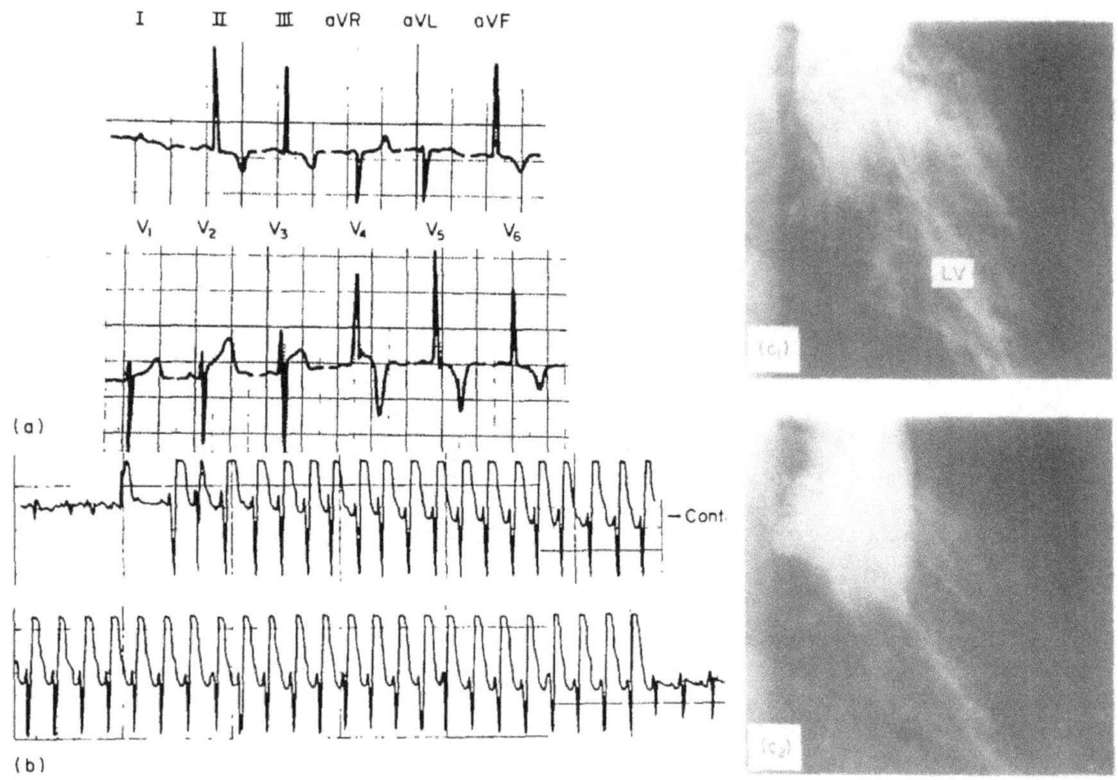

Figure 5 Electrocardiographic and angiographic findings in a 23 year old collegiate basketball player in whom the diagnosis of hypertrophic cardiomyopathy was made at necropsy. (a) Standard 12-lead ECG obtained under basal conditions showing marked symmetric T-wave inversion (as much as 15 mm in depth), as well as left ventricular hypertrophy. (b) Four-second period of ventricular tachycardia that occurred in the second minute of recovery and terminated spontaneously, after a routine treadmill exercise test. (c) Left ventricular angiocardiogram in diastole (c_1) and end-systole (c_2) showing marked cavity obliteration (ejection fraction of 95%). LV = left ventricular cavity. Electrocardiograms have been retraced for clarity.

IDIOPATHIC CONCENTRIC LEFT VENTRICULAR HYPERTROPHY

Five other athletes had a hypertrophied, nondilated left ventricle unassociated with a cardiac lesion that could produce left ventricular hypertrophy; heart weights were increased[8] and ranged from 420 to 530 g. However, each of these five hearts differed from the other hearts in this study considered to represent hypertrophic cardiomyopathy by virtue of *the absence of* (1) asymmetric septal hypertrophy (septal–free wall thickness ratios ranged from 1·0 to 1·2). (2) disorganization of cardiac muscle cells in the ventricular septum; and (3) clinical or echocardiographic evidence of hypertrophic cardiomyopathy in closely related family members.

The five patients with idiopathic concentric left ventricular hypertrophy ranged in age from 16 to 28 years. Two were normotensive, but blood pressure recordings had not been obtained during life in the other three. In three of these five patients the degree of left ventricular wall thickening was particularly marked (i.e. 20 to 23 mm) (Fig. 8); in the other two patients, left ventricular wall thickening was only moderate (thicknesses of 16 and 18 mm). The magnitude of ventricular wall thickening that these athletes with idiopathic concentric left ventricular hypertrophy exhibited at necropsy greatly exceeded that which could be considered to be 'physiologic' ventricular hypertrophy produced by athletic conditioning[16,17].

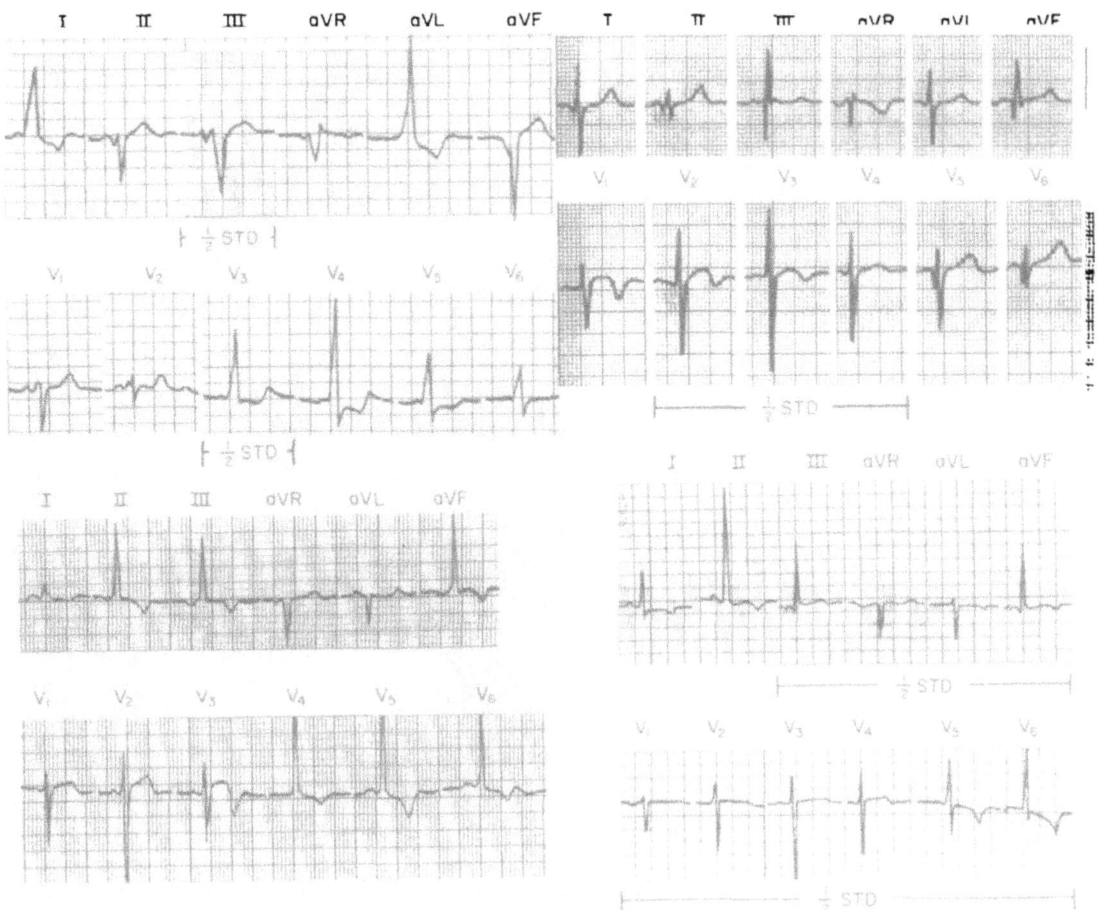

Figure 6 Electocardiograms showing the spectrum of abnormalities in four athletes with hypertrophic cardiomyopathy. Although cardiovascular disease was suspected in each athlete during life, a clinical diagnosis other than hypertrophic cardiomyopathy had been made in each. *Top left:* From a 14 year old wrestler showing Wolff–Parkinson–White pattern, left axis deviation, diffuse T-wave inversion in leads I, AVL and V_4 to V_6 and probable left ventricular hypertrophy. *Top right:* From a 17 year old (gridiron) football player showing deep Q waves in leads III, AVF, V_5 and V_6 and probable left ventricular hypertrophy. *Bottom left:* From a 20 year old basketball player showing deep symmetric T-wave inversion in leads II, III, AVF and V_5 to V_6 and left ventricular hypertrophy. Compare with a similar ECG from another athlete shown in Fig 5(a). *Bottom right:* From a 30 year old tennis player showing left ventricular hypertrophy with 'strain' and diffuse T-wave flattening and inversion. Electrocardiograms have been retraced for clarity.

Two of the five athletes with idiopathic concentric left ventricular hypertrophy had an associated cardiac malformation. In one, a 17 year old football (soccer) player with a 530 g heart, the anterior and posterior mitral leflets had an appearance consistent with relatively mild mitral valve prolapse; the leaflets were thickened, gelatinous and mildly scalloped with excessive mucoid material observed histologically. This patient's mother and two siblings had clinical or echocardiographic evidence of mitral valve prolapse.

In addition, this athlete (and one other with concentric ventricular wall thickening) had an anatomic alteration of the artery to the atrioventricular node, consisting of severe fibromuscular hyperplasia of the vessel wall and marked narrowing of the lumen (Fig. 9). One additional athlete with concentric ventricular wall thickening had a similar alteration in the artery to the atrioventricular node.

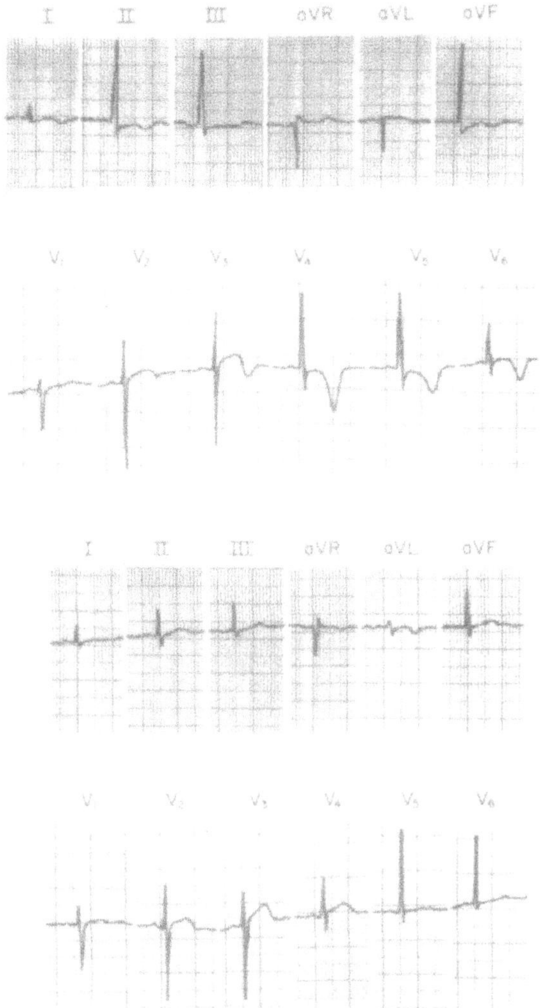

Figure 7 Serial 12-lead ECGs obtained under basal conditions from a professional basketball player *without* underlying structural cardiac disease. *Top:* Recorded during a period of time when the athlete was highly conditioned and competing actively in his sport, showing diffuse T-wave inversion that is particularly deep and symmetric in leads V_4 to V_6. *Bottom:* Three years later at a time when the athlete was no longer training and was deconditioned; the deep T-wave inversions have virtually normalized, although T-waves in V_5 and V_6 still appear flattened.

The conducting tissue was otherwise normal in these latter two athletes. None of the athletes who had idiopathic concentric left ventricular hypertrophy, with or without alterations in the artery to the atrioventricular node, had abnormal intramural

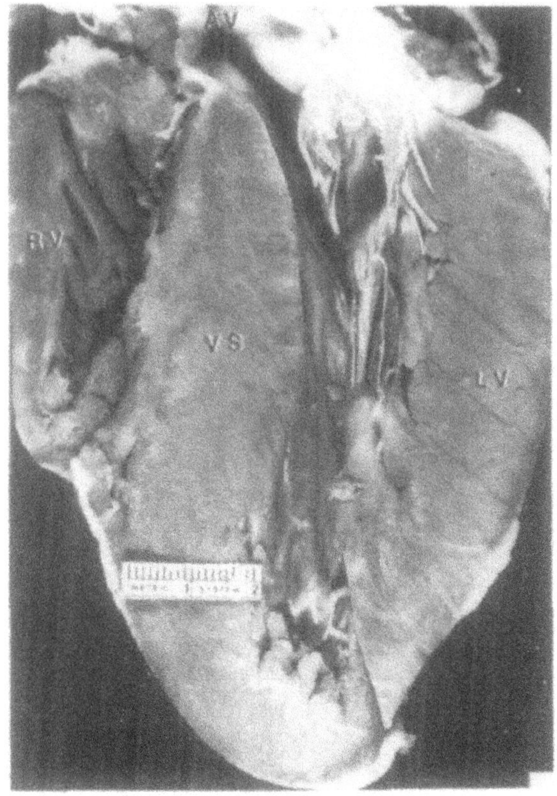

Figure 8 Heart of a 17 year old soccer player showing marked idiopathic concentric (symmetric) thickening of the ventricular septum (VS) and left ventricular free wall (LV). RV = right ventricular wall; AV = aortic valve.

coronary arteries in other areas of ventricular myocardium.

CONGENITAL CORONARY ARTERY ANOMALY

In addition to hypertrophic cardiomyopathy and idiopathic concentric left ventricular hypertrophy, a number of other malformations of the heart and blood vessels may be responsible for sudden death in young athletes. In three of our 29 patients, the left main coronary artery had an anomalous origin from the right (anterior) sinus of Valsalva and followed a course through the narrow area between aorta and main pulmonary artery[18]. Because the left coronary artery followed this unusual course, it necessarily assumed a very acute angle at its origin from the aorta (Fig. 10). It is believed that this acute bend is potentially hazardous. During severe exertion (when the great vessels expand), the left main coronary artery probably becomes severely kinked and

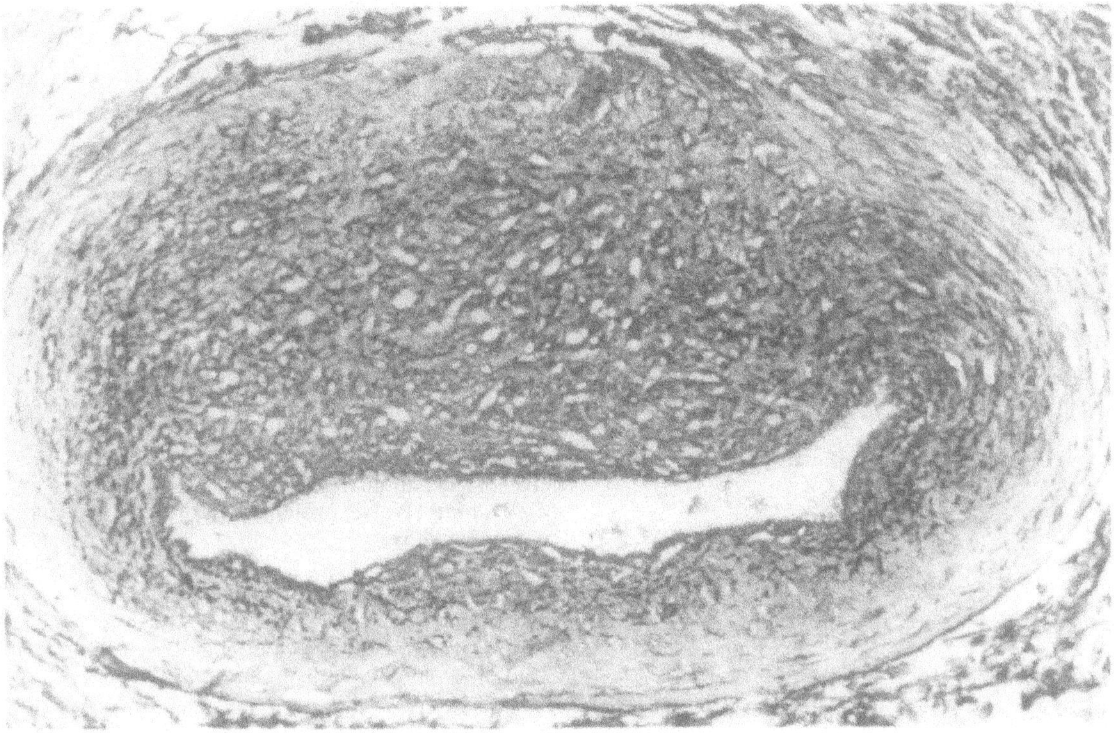

Figure 9 Small artery to atrioventricular node of a 17 year old basketball player with idiopathic concentric left ventricular hypertrophy. The lumen is markedly narrowed due to extreme thickening of the arterial wall.

narrowed, thereby critically diminishing the myocardial oxygen supply.

AORTIC RUPTURE

Two athletes died suddenly from rupture of the aorta. These individuals showed decreased numbers of elastic fibers in their aortic media that produced intrinsic weakening of the wall ('cystic medial necrosis'). Eventually, when such a malformed aorta is unable to maintain the normal blood pressure to which it is exposed, aortic rupture occurs. It is of interest that individuals with cystic medial necrosis may successfully participate in competitive athletics for many years without experiencing a catastrophic event. Many such individuals also have the systemic manifestations of the Marfan syndrome, potentially facilitating their clinical recognition (such as one of our two patients).

CORONARY HEART DISEASE

Three athletes had acquired abnormalities of the coronary arteries. These patients were 24, 26 and 28 years of age. Two of the three athletes showed severe atherosclerosis in each of the three major extramural coronary arteries (>75% cross-sectional area luminal narrowing by atherosclerotic plaque), including one with total occlusion of the right coronary artery by an antemortem thrombus and hemorrhage into atherosclerotic plaque. This athlete, a 28 year old professional (gridiron) football player had a large myocardial infarct that was about 2 months old in the posterior left ventricular wall at necropsy[6]. The remaining patient had 50% cross-sectional area luminal narrowing of the left anterior descending coronary artery by atherosclerotic plaque and no, or only minimal, atherosclerosis in each of the other two major extramural coronary arteries. However, the left anterior descending artery was completely occluded by an antemortem thrombus 2 cm from the bifurcation of the left main coronary artery.

OTHER CAUSES OF SUDDEN DEATH

Certain other cardiovascular diseases such as isolated mitral valve prolapse, QT interval prolongation syndromes, acute myocarditis and

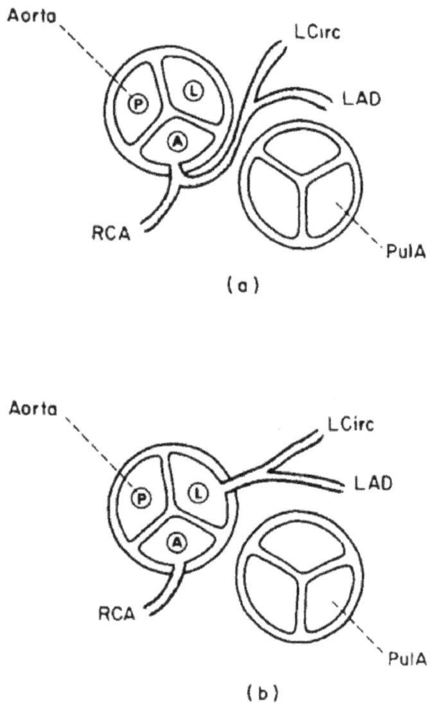

Figure 10 (a) A diagrammatic representation of anomalous origin of the left coronary artery from the right (anterior) sinus of Valsalva. Note the acute leftward and posterior course of the left coronary artery between the aorta and pulmonary artery. (b) Normal origins of the left coronary artery from the left sinus of Valsalva and of the right coronary artery from the right sinus of Valsalva are shown for comparison. A = anterior (right) coronary sinus; L = left coronary sinus; P = posterior (noncoronary) sinus; LAD = left anterior descending coronary artery; LCirc = left circumflex coronary artery; PulA = pulmonary artery; RCA = right coronary artery.

sarcoidosis did not appear in our study group and are probably less common causes of sudden death in athletes. Also, lesions such as aortic valvular stenosis would likely have been identified early in life because of a loud heart murmur or some other obvious physical finding, thereby leading to eventual disqualification from competitive athletics. Infrequently, sudden death may occur in young athletes who have no demonstrable organic heart disease. In such individuals (one of the 29 athletes in our series) death was probably due to a primary arrhythmia that arose independently of any structural abnormality of the heart that could be demonstrated at autopsy.

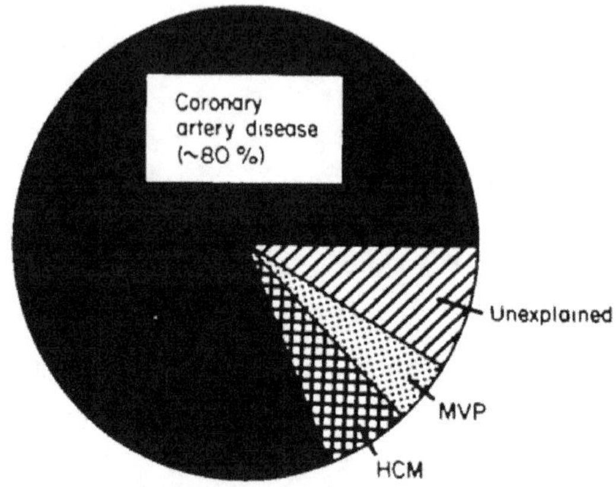

Figure 11 Causes of sudden death in older athletes (>35 years of age). Approximate prevalence figures have been summarized from the literature[2-4]. MVP = mitral valve prolapse; HCM = hypertrophic cardiomyopathy.

CLINICAL FEATURES

Cardiovascular disease had been suspected by an examining physician during life in only seven of our 29 athletes (two with transient symptoms and five who were asymptomatic). In the latter five asymptomatic athletes, the suspicion of cardiovascular disease initially arose because of a heart murmur in two, a family history of heart disease in one, identification of ventricular tachycardia on an exercise electrocardiogram (Fig. 5(b)) performed as a routine part of a preparticipation athletic examination in one, and during evaluation for the Marfan syndrome in one.

In six of the seven athletes in whom cardiovascular disease was suspected during life, hypertrophic cardiomyopathy was confirmed at necropsy. However, in only one of those six athletes was the correct diagnosis of hypertrophic cardiomyopathy made clinically. In the other five athletes, the diagnosis during life was 'normal athletic heart' in three, ventricular septal defect in one and Wolff–Parkinson–White syndrome in one. Each of these five athletes with hypertrophic cardiomyopathy had a distinctly abnormal electrocardiogram, and one also had an abnormal left ventricular angiocardiogram (Fig. 5(c)).

SUDDEN DEATH IN OLDER ATHLETES

Increasing numbers of middle-aged or older individuals (over the age of 35) are now participating in competitive and recreational sports, as well as in physical conditioning programs (such as jogging and swimming). Superior physical fitness at any age, however, does not assure protection against exercise-related death. Similar to young competitive athletes, older athletes may harbor occult cardiovascular disease and die suddenly and unexpectedy while participating in athletic activities. However, unlike the more youthful athletes previously discussed, the cause of death in older athletes is usually not a congenital malformation of the heart. Rather, in the vast majority of instances (about 80%) the cause of sudden death in older athletes is coronary heart disease[2-4] (Fig. 11). The remaining 20% of such deaths are due to other diseases such as mitral valve prolapse or hypertrophic cardiomyopathy[19] or, in some instances, no cause of death is established at necropsy.

References

(1) Maron BJ, Roberts WC, McAllister HA, Rosing DR, Epstein SE. Sudden death in young athletes. Circulation 1980; 62: 218–29.

(2) Thompson PD, Stern MP, Williams P, Duncan K, Haskell WL, Wood PD. Death during jogging or running. A study of 18 cases. JAMA 1979: 242: 1265–7.

(3) Waller BF, Roberts WC. Sudden death while running in conditioned runners aged 40 years or over. Am J Cardiol 1980; 45: 1292–300.

(4) Virmani R, Rabinowitz M, McAllister HA. Nontraumatic death in joggers: a series of 30 autopsy patients. Am J Med 1982: 72: 874–82.

(5) James TN, Froggatt P, Marshall TK. Sudden death in young athletes. Ann Int Med 1967: 67: 1013–21.

(6) Roberts WC, Maron BJ. Sudden death while playing professional football. Am Heart J 1981: 102: 1061–3.

(7) Maron BJ, Epstein SE. Hypertrophic cardiomyopathy: a discussion of nomenclature. Am J Cardiol 1979: 43: 1242–4.

(8) Gould SE. Pathology of the heart and blood vessels, 3rd edn. Springfield, Illinois: Charles C. Thomas, 1968: 1139.

(9) Henry WL, Clark CE, Epstein SE. Asymmetric septal hypertrophy (ASH): echocardiographic identification of the pathognomonic anatomic abnormality of IHSS. Circulation 1973: 47: 225–33.

(10) Menges H, Brandenburg RO, Brown AL. The clinical, hemodynamic, and pathologic diagnosis of muscular subvalvular aortic stenosis. Circulation 1961: 24: 1126–36.

(11) Roberts WC. Valvular, subvalvular and supravalvular aortic stenosis: Morphologic features. Cardiovasc Clin 1973: 5: 104–26.

(12) Teare D. Asymmetrical hypertrophy of the heart in young patients. Br Heart J 1958: 20: 1–8.

(13) Maron BJ, Roberts WC. Quantitative analysis of cardiac muscle cell disorganization in the ventricular septum of patients with hypertrophic cardiomyopathy. Circulation 1979; 59: 689–706.

(14) Maron BJ, Nichols PF, Pickle LW, Muvihill JJ. Patterns of inheritance in hypertrophic cardiomyopathy. Circulation (submitted for publication).

(15) Zeppilli P, Pirrami MM, Sassara M, Fenici R. T wave abnormalities in top-ranking athletes: effects of isoproterenol, atropine and physical exercise. Am Heart J 1980: 100: 213–22.

(16) Morganroth J, Maron BJ, Henry WL, Epstein SE. Comparative left ventricular dimensions in trained athletes. Ann Int Med 1975: 82: 521–4.

(17) Roeske WR, O'Rourke RA, Klein A, Leopold G, Karliner JS. Noninvasive evaluation of ventricular hypertrophy in professional athletes. Circulation 1976: 53: 286–292.

(18) Cheitlin MD, De Castro CM, McAllister HA. Sudden death as a complication of anomalous left coronary origin from the anterior sinus of Valsalva. A not-so-minor congenital anomaly. Circulation 1974: 50: 780–7.

(19) Noakes TD, Rose AG, Opie LH. Hypertrophic cardiomyopathy associated with sudden death during marathon racing. Br Heart J 1979: 41: 624–7.

Loogen If I understood you correctly, you say this giant T inversion is sometimes found in men or in athletes without any other signs of heart disease. What is your policy in such cases? Do you allow them to go on in sports or do you recommend thorough investigation – that means invasive methods, determination of lactate production, and all the other steps that are necessary to exclude a cardiac disease?

Maron I think, certainly, an ECG like that demands a careful non-evasive workup to exclude particularly hypertrophic cardiomyopathy and mitral valve prolapse. But having not found those conditions, I think that I would construe the ECG to be innocent, even though it is dramatic in appearance. This is particularly true since we know that such ECGs may be dynamic, in the sense that they may revert to normal (often with deconditioning). I have been to Italy to speak to a group of sport medicine physicians who had followed athletes in Italy for the 20 years or so since the last Olympiad was in Rome. They have accumulated, over the years, hundreds of ECGs in athletes. These ECGs looked just like the one I showed and they are not indicative of organic heart disease. For the most part such athletes continue to compete and lead active lives.

Kuhn We have observed four people who were not champions, but very active athletes. In three of them we found pronounced asymmetric septal hypertrophy with giant negatives T-waves. In three athletes left ventricular angiography was performed. There was the complete picture of hypertrophic non-obstructive cardiomyopathy. We are not quite sure how to interpret this. I should like to speculate that there is a latent hypertrophic process in these patients and that physical activity during sports would lead to the manifestation of the disease.

Secondly, I should like to comment on the case you showed with an abnormally thickened septum of more than 20 mm. There is an echocardiographic study performed by Dr Ross of Cologne. He found that septal thickness of more than 15 mm hardly ever occurs in athletes. So from this evidence I would suggest that this is really a hypertrophy in the sense of hypertrophic cardiomyopathy. I have now tried to review the literature on autopsy findings in athletes, mainly in Germany, and what I found several times was a diagnosis of myocarditis or chronic myocarditis. However, at autopsy the hearts were described as having a weight of more than 700 or even 800 g, and a septal thickness of more than 20 mm. So I have no doubt that these patients did not have myocarditis, because there were only a few or no inflammatory cells present.

Maron Certainly, in the United States, medical examiners who are responsible for providing a diagnosis after death have a tendency to over-diagnose myocarditis. The awareness of a condition such as hypertrophic cardiomyopathy has not been great, and a few round cells in the myocardium has often been enough to ensure the diagnosis of myocarditis. Myocarditis certainly can be a cause of sudden death in young people, but I think that much of the older literature is a little misleading.

Das I think Dr Maron has addressed the question I had in mind, particularly concerning the four patients, for whom no ideology was discerned. I wonder whether detailed investigation for active myocarditis was carried out in the four patients that you mentioned.

Maron You mean the four patients with idiopathic left ventricular hypertrophy? Certainly, these are not instances of myocarditis. The amount of hypertrophy seen in those four patients would have to be considered pathologic from what we know about a living population of athletes studied echocardiographically. It's pathologic because the athlete is dead and because it represents an obvious increase in left ventricular mass.

Frank Mine is more of a comment rather than a question. I'd like to congratulate Dr Maron on his restraint with the four patients with symmetrical hypertrophy. I remember discussing this with him at an evening meeting and we came to the conclusion that the only way we're going to understand hypertrophic cardiomyopathy as an entity – if indeed it is an entity – was by exclusion of cases that missed one more of the important characteristics of the condition. So, in the absence of myocardial fibre disarray and in the absence of first-degree relatives demonstrating a positive echo, I think that it is quite proper that we continue to call this group idiopathic left ventricular hypertrophy.

Harmjanz In rather young patients having giant T-waves and left ventricular hypertrophy we observed, on a number of occasions, a slowly arising delay in left ventricular exitation up to left ventricular bundle branch block while the patient underwent cardiac catheterization; this declined in a stepwise manner within about 10 beats. I want to ask whether you had the same experience in your cases?

Maron We don't really have much experience catheterizing this type of patient. This is a retrospective study and most of the limited catheterization data is from other institutions. I really couldn't give you an answer to that.

The Floating Heart or the Heart too Fat to Sink: Analysis of 55 Necropsy Patients

WILLIAM C. ROBERTS, MD, and JOHN D. ROBERTS*

Certain clinical and morphologic findings are described in 55 patients whose hearts at necropsy contained so much fat that they floated in water. The patients were 47 to 89 years old (mean 67). Symptomatic coronary heart disease was present in 28 (51%) and valvular heart disease (mitral stenosis) in 3 (5%). The heart at necropsy was enlarged (>350 g for women and >400 g for men) in 45 patients (82%). The mean heart weight for the 31 women was 470 g and for the 24 men, 515 g. In addition to the severe increase in fat in the atrioventricular sulci and over both ventricles, the amount of fat in the atrial septum was increased in all patients. In 14 patients (25%), the thickness of the atrial septum cephaled to the fossa ovale was ≥2 cm. Excessive fat in this location is called "lipomatous hypertrophy of the atrial septum." Of the 16 patients (29%) with fatal acute myocardial infarction, 7 (44%) had rupture of either the left ventricular free wall or ventricular septum. The high frequency of cardiac rupture in these patients supports the contention that rupture during acute myocardial infarction is more common in the fatty than in the non-fatty heart.

(Am J Cardiol 1983;52:1286–1289)

It is well appreciated that very obese people tend to float in water more easily than non-obese people. It is also well appreciated that fat tends to accumulate in the subepicardial area of the heart in adults and that the amount tends to increase with age and with increase in adipose tissue in other parts of the body. For years we have classified hearts at necropsy as having increased, decreased or normal amounts of subepicardial fat. Quantitation of the subepicardial fat, however, has been difficult without considerable destruction of the heart itself. About 2.5 years ago we began placing hearts with obviously increased amounts of subepicardial fat into large containers of water and made note of those that floated and those that did not. This report analyzes certain clinical and morphologic findings in 55 patients whose heart at necropsy floated in water.

Patients and Findings

The 55 patients ranged in age from 47 to 89 years (mean 67); 36 (65%) were ≥65 years of age and 3 (5%) were ≤50 years. Of the 55 patients, 31 (56%) were women and 24 (44%) were men. Although body weight and height are lacking in most of the 55 patients, most were described as obese. One patient lost >50 pounds during her last few months of life from cancer. She was described as "cachetic," but nevertheless, the heart contained massive quantities of fat. Symptoms of cardiac dysfunction occurred during life in 32 patients (58%): from coronary heart disease in 28 (51%) and from valvular heart disease (mitral stenosis) in 3 (5%). Of the 28 patients with sympto-

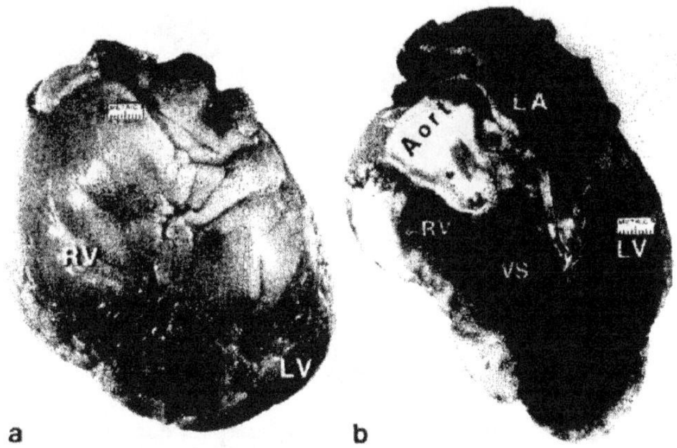

FIGURE 1. Exterior of heart (**a**) and long-axis view of heart (**b**) from a 72-year-old woman (SH #A81-36) who died of consequences of chronic obstructive pulmonary disease. At necropsy, the heart weighed 350 g; the entire anterior surface of the heart was covered by deposits of fat (**a**) and the right ventricular myocardium was infiltrated by fat cells (**b**). LA = left atrial cavity; LV = left ventricle; RV = right ventricle; VS = ventricular septum.

* Student volunteer, Christchurch School, Christchurch, Virginia.

From the Pathology Branch, National Heart, Lung, and Blood Institute, National Institutes of Health, Bethesda, Maryland. Manuscript received and accepted August 22, 1983.

Address for reprints: William C. Roberts, MD, Building 10A, Room 3E-30, National Institutes of Health, Bethesda, Maryland 20205

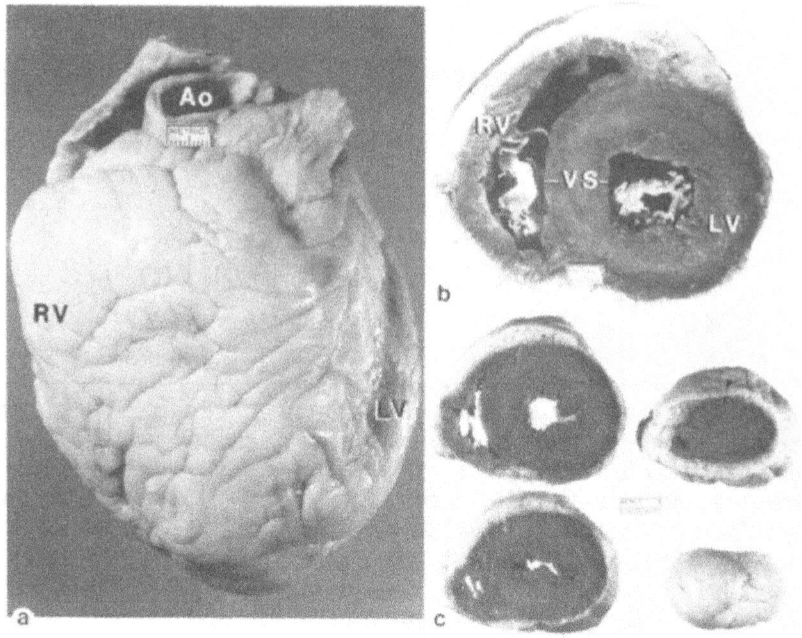

FIGURE 2. Heart from a 67-year-old man (SH#A82-11) who died of rupture of an abdominal aortic aneurysm. His heart weighed 470 g and he had had systemic hypertension during life. **a**, the right ventricle (RV) is completely covered by fat. Ao = aorta; LV = left ventricle. **b**, transverse section of the cardiac base exposing both atrioventricular valves and fat covering the entire right ventricle. VS = ventricular septum. **c**, remainder of transverse sections of the cardiac ventricles.

matic coronary heart disease, 16 had isolated acute myocardial infarction, 4 had isolated angina pectoris, 1 had a fatal acute myocardial infarct preceded by angina, 4 had sudden death attributed to coronary narrowing from atherosclerosis, and 3 had angina for several months before sudden coronary death. Of the 55 patients, at least 21 (38%) had a history of elevated blood pressure and 6 (11%) were habitual alcoholics. Three patients took prednisone chronically.

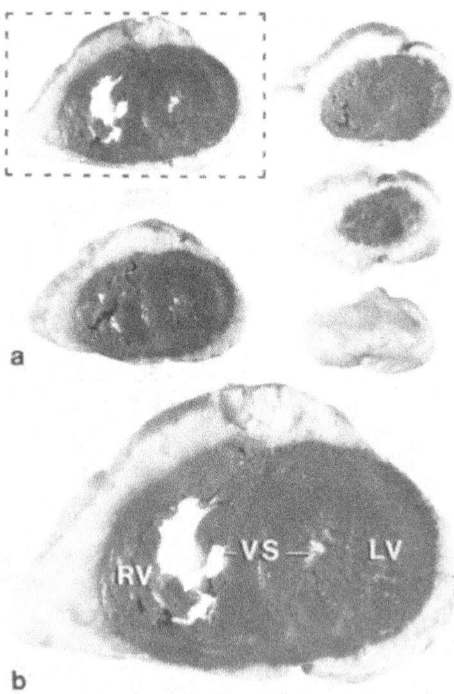

FIGURE 3. Cardiac ventricles from a 67-year-old man (DCVAH #82A-100) who died of consequences of chronic obstructive pulmonary disease. At necropsy, the heart weighed 570 g and huge deposits of fat surrounded most of the right (RV) and left (LV) ventricles. **a**, five 1-cm-thick transverse cuts of the cardiac ventricles. **b**, a close-up of 1 portion (the one in brackets in **a**).

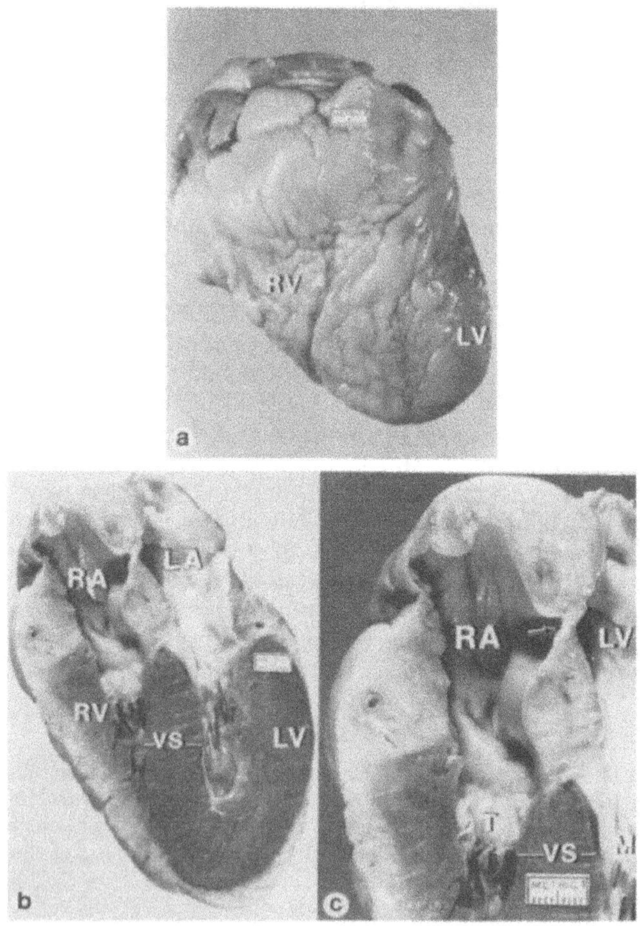

FIGURE 4. Heart from a 53-year-old cachetic woman (SH#A82-19) who died of metastatic breast carcinoma. She never received corticosteroid therapy. At necropsy, the heart weighed 300 g. **a**, exterior anterior view. LV = left ventricle; RV = right ventricle. **b**, 4-chamber view showing huge deposits of fat in the right atrioventricular sulcus, over the entire right ventricle, apical portion of left ventricle and in the atrial septum. LA = left atrium; RA = right atrium; VS = ventricular septum. **c**, close-up of atrial septum showing large deposits of fat (lipomatous hypertrophy) in the atrial septum cephalad and caudal to the fossa ovale region (**arrow**). The maximal thickness of the atrial septum was 1.7 cm. M = mitral leaflet; T = tricuspid leaflet.

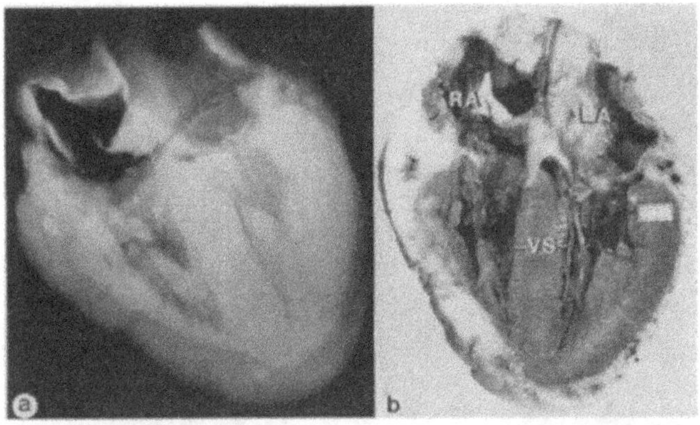

FIGURE 5. Heart from a 67-year-old woman (GT#82A-116) who died of metastatic carcinoma. She received prednisone daily during her last 7 months of life. She had periodic atrial fibrillation and premature atrial contractions during her last 7 years of life. At necropsy, the heart weighed 315 g and all epicardial surfaces of both ventricles were covered with fat. **a**, radiograph of the heart at necropsy showing the less radiodense epicardial fat overlying the ventricular walls. **b**, 4-chamber view. Fat also infiltrates the right ventricular wall. LA = left atrium; RA = right atrium; VS = ventricular septum. The atrial septum is up to 2.3 cm thick (lipomatous hypertrophy) due to fatty infiltration.

The cause of death in the 55 patients was as follows: coronary heart disease in 26 (47%) (sudden in 7, acute myocardial infarction in 16, and death during cardiac catheterization in 1 and shortly after aortocoronary bypass operation in 2); mitral stenosis in 3; rupture of aortic aneurysm in 3; stroke in 2; consequences of alcoholism in 2; cancer in 11; and miscellaneous causes in 8. Of the 16 patients (29%) with fatal acute myocardial infarction, 7 (44%) had rupture of either left ventricular free wall (5 patients) or ventricular septum (2 patients).

At necropsy, each heart floated in water (Fig. 1 to 7). The weight range of the hearts in the 31 women was 265 to 880 g (mean 470) and that of the 24 men was 330 to 710 g (mean 515). Of 31 women, the hearts weighed >350 g in 24 (77%), and of 24 men, the hearts weighed >400 g in 21 (88%).

Of the 4 major (right, left main, left anterior descending and left circumflex) epicardial coronary arteries, ≥1 was narrowed >75% in cross-sectional area by atherosclerotic plaques in 30 of the 55 patients (55%): only 1 artery in 4 patients; 2 arteries in 6 patients; 3 arteries in 18 patients and all 4 arteries in 2 patients. In 25 patients (45%), ≥1 foci of fibrosis or necrosis or both were present in the left ventricular wall; scar only was present in 9, necrosis only in 10, and both were present in 6.

In all 55 patients, more fat than normal was present in the atrial septum. In 14 of the 55 patients (25%), the thickness of the atrial septum cephalad to the fossa ovale region was ≥2.0 cm.

Calcific deposits were present in the mitral valve anulus in 10 patients (18%) and on the aortic aspect of ≥1 aortic valve cusp in 7 (13%). In neither location were the calcific deposits large enough to cause valve stenosis.

Discussion

In the last century and the first decade of this century, *the fatty heart* received considerable attention. Sudden death was often attributed to the fatty heart at the turn of the century. Other than a historic article appearing in the *British Heart Journal* in 1972,[1] little attention has been paid to the fatty heart in recent years. The present study points out that the heart can acquire enough adipose tissue on its walls to allow it to

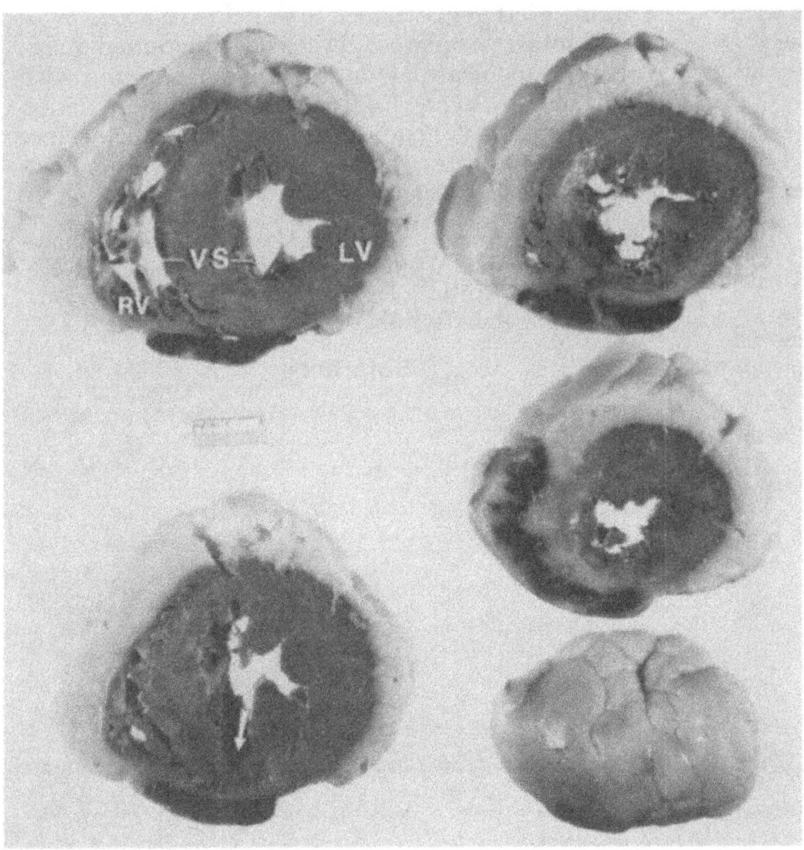

FIGURE 6. Transverse slices of the cardiac ventricles in an 81-year-old man (FSH#4207) who died of rupture of the left ventricular free wall 6 days after the onset of acute myocardial infarction. The slice in the **upper left** is at a level just below the atrioventricular valves and the slice in the **lower right** is at the apex. The site of the rupture is shown by the **arrow** in the **lower left** slice. Blood has focally infiltrated the subepicardial fat. Fat is present on the endocardium of right ventricle (RV) (**upper left**) and on left ventricular (LV) endocardium (**lower left**). VS = ventricular septum.

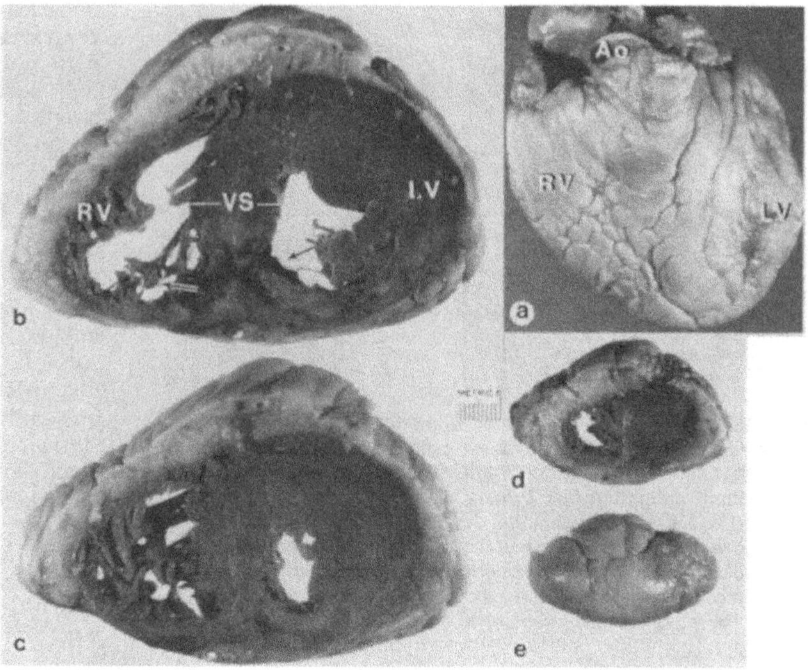

FIGURE 7. Exterior of heart (**a**) and transverse slices of the cardiac ventricles (**b** to **e**) in a 70-year-old man (SH#A81-54) who died of consequences of rupture of the ventricular septum (VS) 3 days after onset of acute myocardial infarction. Fat covers the entire right ventricle (RV) and most of the left ventricle (LV) (**a**). Ao = ascending aorta. **b**, slice showing the site (**arrows**) of rupture in the septum. The ruler is applicable only to the slices shown in **b** and **c**. The slices shown in **d** and **e** are at or near the apex and have been less enlarged than the slices shown in **b** and **c**.

float in water. In almost all 55 hearts examined, the entire surface of the right ventricular wall was covered by fat, which also extended into its myocardial wall. The surface of the left ventricle was rarely completely covered by fat, but in a few cases, nearly so. In a few cases, fat deposits were present on the mural endocardium focally of the right ventricle and, less often, of the left ventricle. The largest deposits of fat in all 55 cases were in the atrioventricular sulci, which are, of course, the locations of the right and left circumflex coronary arteries.

In all 55 patients, more fat than normal was present in the atrial septum. In 14 of the 55 patients (25%), the atrial septum cephalad to the fossa ovale region was ≥2.0 cm thick. Deposition of excessive fat in this area is called "lipomatous hypertrophy of the atrial septum," an acquired abnormality that may be associated with an increased frequency of atrial arrhythmias.

Our 55 cases of the floating heart were observed during a recent 29-month period, during which time one of us (WCR) examined at necropsy 1,135 hearts of patients >40 years old at death. Of these cases, the hearts were free of significant cardiac disease in 58 (5%). Thus, our 55 cases of floating heart represent 5% of hearts of patients >40 years old examined at necropsy. Our youngest patient with a floating heart was 47 years old.

One of us (WCR) has noted through the years that persons who die of rupture of either the ventricular septum or left ventricular free wall during acute myocardial infarction almost always have increased quantities of subepicardial fat. Of our 55 patients with floating hearts, 16 had fatal acute myocardial infarction and of them 7 (44%) had cardiac rupture, a much higher percentage of rupture among patients with acute myocardial infarction than expected.

Acknowledgment: We thank M. M. M. Moore (photographs), Barbara E. Winterrowd (photograph labeling), Filippina Giacometti (histology), Alvado Campbell (specimen organization) and Mary McMahon (typing).

Reference

1. **Bedford E.** The story of fatty heart. *A disease of Victorian times.* Br Heart J 1972;34:23–28.

Major anomalies of coronary arterial origin seen in adulthood

William C. Roberts, M.D. *Bethesda, Md.*

Both coronary arteries normally arise, of course, from ostia located in the sinus of Valsalva portions of the aorta. The right coronary artery (RCA) arises from the right aortic sinus, usually but not always in its central portion, and the left main (LM) coronary artery arises from the left aortic sinus, nearly always from its central portion. If the aorta contains only two cusps or one cusp rather than its usual three, the location of the coronary ostia are usually as they would be were the valve tricuspid rather than bicuspid or unicuspid. A deviation of origin of a coronary artery from the normal falls under the category of "anomaly of coronary arterial origin," and these anomalies will be reviewed in this article. Anomalies of origin are particularly common in hearts in which other major congenital cardiovascular malformations are present. This review, however, will be limited to those anomalies of origin observed in hearts without other major malformations of the heart or great vessels (Table I).

ORIGIN OF 1 OR MORE CORONARY ARTERIES FROM THE PULMONARY TRUNK *AND* ORIGIN OF 1 OR MORE CORONARY ARTERIES FROM THE AORTA

When both right and LM coronary arteries arise from the pulmonary trunk (PT) or when only one coronary artery is present and it arises from the PT, survival past 1 year of life is impossible unless an associated anomaly is present which allows persistence of pulmonary hypertension after birth (Fig. 1). In these two circumstances, no coronary artery arises directly from the aorta.

When one coronary artery, however, arises from the PT and one or more coronary arteries arise from the aorta, survival past 15 years of age may occur. The most common anomaly in this category is origin of the LM coronary artery from the PT and origin of the RCA from the aorta (Fig. 1). Far less common is origin of the right or left anterior descending coronary artery (LAD) from the PT, and these anomalies are usually associated with survival into adulthood (Fig. 1).

Left main from the pulmonary trunk

Historic background. This anomaly was described first by Maude Abbott in 1908.[1] Her patient was a woman who lived for 60 years, and this is the longest survival reported with this anomaly. Abriskossoff[2] in 1911 first described findings in an infant with this anomaly. In 1933, Bland et al.[3] described clinical and necropsy findings in a 3-month-old boy with this anomaly, and subsequently this anomaly in infants has often been referred to as the"Bland-White-Garland Syndrome." The infant described by Bland et al. was the son of a physician who observed "... the paroxysmal attacks of acute discomfort precipitated by the exertion of nursing." These attacks, which also included inspiratory and expiratory grunts followed by marked pallor and cold sweats, were interpreted by Bland et al. as evidence of angina pectoris. The ECG (three limb leads only) disclosed marked T wave inversions and the chest radiograph showed marked enlargement of the cardiac silhouette. The clinical diagnosis in the infant was "congenital idiopathic hypertrophy of the heart." The coronary anomaly was discovered at necropsy.

Frequency. This anomaly was observed only once among 357 patients with congenital heart disease studied at necropsy by Fontana and Edwards[4] from January, 1920, through June 30, 1954, dates which precede cardiopulmonary bypass operations. Fontana and Edwards[4] also found published reports describing 58 necropsy patients with origin of the LM from the PT. More than half of the 58 patients died between ages 3 and 6 months; 46 patients (79%) were dead by 13 months of age; the remaining 12 patients (21%) lived longer than 15 years. The major cause of death during the first year of life was congestive heart failure; 8 of the 12 adults died suddenly and unexpectedly. Fontana and Edwards[4]

From the Pathology Branch, National Heart, Lung, and Blood Institute, National Institutes of Health.

Received for publication Oct. 7, 1985; accepted Nov. 8, 1985.

Reprint requests: William C. Roberts, M.D., Bldg. 10A, Room 3E-30, NIH, Bethesda, MD 20892.

Table I. Anomalies of coronary arterial origin

I. *Origin of 1 or more coronary arteries from the pulmonary trunk (PT) and 1 or more coronary arteries from the aorta*
  - A. Left main (LM) from PT
  - B. Right (R) from PT
  - C. Left anterior descending (LAD) from PT
  - D. Left circumflex (LC) from PT
  - E. Accessory coronary artery from PT

II. Origin of 1 or 2 coronary arteries from the pulmonary trunk without origin of a coronary artery from the aorta
  - A. R and LM from PT
  - B. "Single coronary artery" from PT

III. *Anomalous origin of 1 or more coronary arteries from the aorta*
  - A. LM and R from right aortic sinus
  - B. LM and R from left aortic sinus
  - C. LM and R from the posterior aortic sinus
  - D. R and LC from right aortic sinus (or LC from R) and LAD from left sinus
  - E. R and LAD from right aortic sinus (or LAD from R) and LC from left sinus
  - F. R from posterior aortic sinus and LM from left sinus
  - G. LM from posterior aortic sinus and R from right sinus
  - H. LAD and LC from a separate ostium in the left aortic sinus and R from right aortic sinus

IV. *Origin of only 1 coronary artery from the aorta without origin of a coronary artery from the PT (single coronary ostium)*
  - A. From the right aortic sinus
    - 1. R crosses crux and continues as the LC which continues as the LAD
    - 2. LM from R
      - a. Coursing of LM posterior to aorta before dividing into LAD and LC
      - b. Coursing of LM between aorta and PT before branching into LAD and LC
      - c. Coursing of LM anterior to PT
      - d. Coursing of LM in ventricular septum beneath right ventricular infundibulum
    - 3. LAD and LC from R with coursing of LC posterior to aorta and LAD anterior to right ventricle (RV)
    - 4. LAD from R with coursing anterior to RV with R crossing crux to form LC
    - 5. LAD from R with coursing between aorta and PT with R crossing crux to continue as LC
    - 6. LAD from R with coursing between aorta and PT and LC from R with retroaortic course
    - 7. LAD from R coursing anterior to RV, LC from R coursing between aorta and PT
    - 8. LAD from R coursing retroaortic with R crossing crux to continue as LC
    - 9. LAD from R with coursing to left side in ventricular septum beneath right ventricular outflow tract and LC from R with retroaortic course to left atrioventricular sulcus
  - B. From left aortic sinus
    - 1. LAD and LC from single coronary artery with LC crossing crux to continue as R
    - 2. R, LAD, and LC from single coronary artery
      - a. R posterior to aorta
      - b. R between aorta and PT
      - c. R anterior to RV
    - 3. R and LC from single coronary artery and LAD from R
      - a. R between aorta and PT
      - b. R posterior to aorta
    - 4. R and LAD from single coronary artery and of LC from LAD
      - a. R between aorta and PT
      - b. R posterior to PT
  - C. From posterior aortic sinus
    - 1. Single coronary artery between aorta and PT with trifurcation into R, LAD, and LC
    - 2. Single coronary artery to left of PT with trifurcation into R, LAD, and LC
    - 3. Single coronary artery to right and when anterior to aorta giving rise to R and LM which subdivides into LAD and LC

found no reports of death in patients with this anomaly from age 13 months to 16 years. Thus, if a patient with this anomaly is able to survive the first year of life, the chances are good that the child will survive until adulthood. Origin of the LM from the PT occurs about equally often in both sexes. I have studied at necropsy 11 patients (seven females) in whom the LM arose from the PT: nine were aged 1 to 18 months (means seven); 1 was 3.5 years old, and one died suddenly at age 41 years. The latter patient was known to have a continuous precordial murmur but never had symptoms of cardiac dysfunction. Her sudden death was clearly the result of the coronary anomaly.

The frequency of this anomaly among adults having coronary arterial angiograms for suspected ischemic heart disease is of course quite low. Among 1750 adults having coronary angiograms reported by Thomas et al.[5] two had origin of the LM from the PT: one was a 45-year-old woman and the other was a 40-year-old woman. Among 9152 patients having coronary angiograms reported by Donaldson et al.,[6] six had origin of the LM from the PT.

Flow in the anomalous artery. Why some patients with anomalous origin of the LM coronary artery from the PT die during the first year of life or soon thereafter and why others survive into adulthood (without operative intervention) is related to the development of collaterals between the coronary artery attached to the ascending aorta (the right

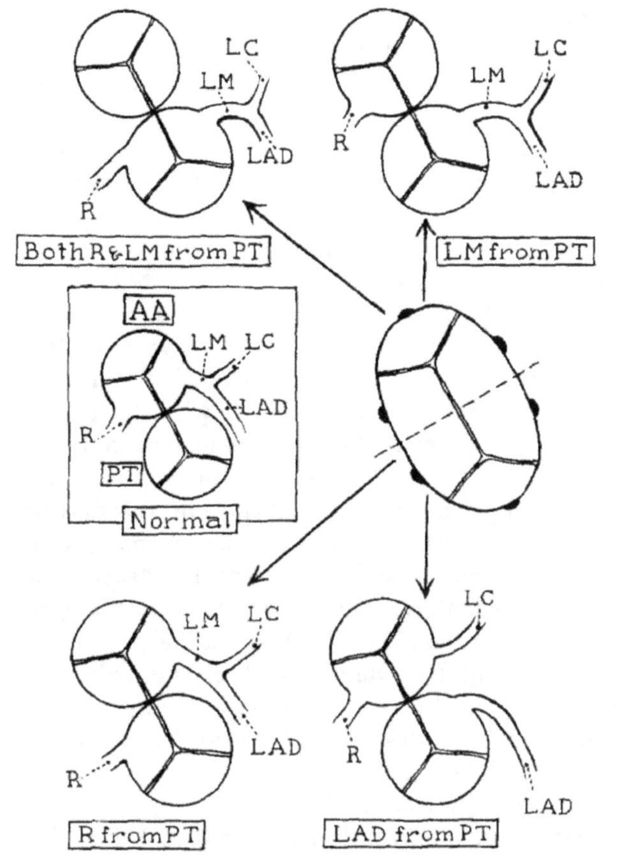

Fig. 1. Diagram illustrating the common arterial trunk arising from the heart in its early development with six potential coronary arterial ostia and the possible coronary anomalies resulting when inappropriate ostia do not regress. *AA* = ascending aorta; *LAD* = left anterior descending coronary artery; *LC* = left circumflex coronary artery; *LM* = left main coronary artery; *PT* = pulmonary trunk; *R* = right coronary artery.

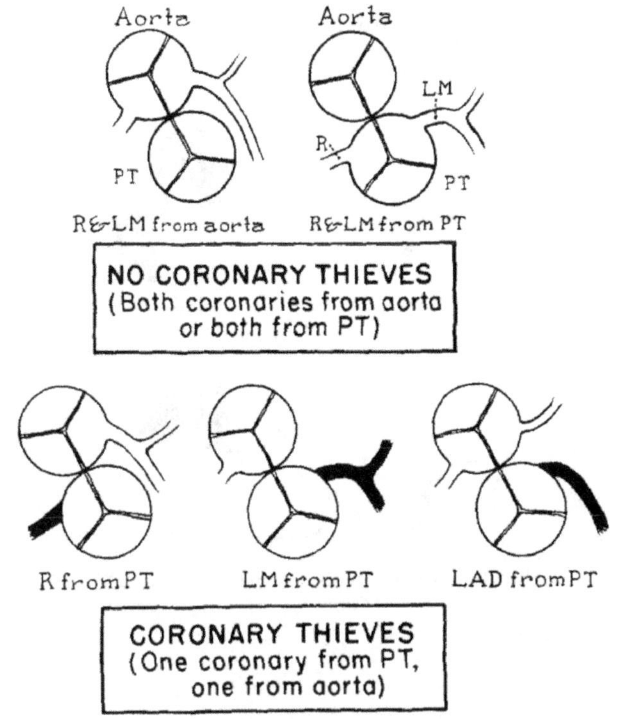

Fig. 2. Diagram showing the coronary anomalies not associated with the "coronary steal" phenomenon and those associated with this phenomenon. Abbreviations as in Fig. 1.

one) and the coronary artery attached to the PT (the LM).[7,8] At birth and during roughly the first 2 months of life, the systolic and diastolic pressures in the ascending aorta and PT are similar and consequently the LM coronary artery is perfused by blood within the PT. At about 2 months of life, the pressure in the PT falls so that by about 12 months of life the systolic pressure in the PT is about one fourth of that in the aorta. Survival is dependent on the development of collateral channels between the normally and abnormally arising coronary arteries, so that flow in the anomalous LM coronary artery is retrograde, it being entirely supplied by blood from the normally arising RCA. The anomalous artery "steals" blood from the normally arising artery (Fig. 2), placing considerable myocardium at risk of ischemia or necrosis (Fig. 3). It would appear that an extensive collateral system must develop for survival to occur. During the period of transition from antegrade to retrograde flow in the anomalously arising LM coronary artery, death is common.

Morphologic features. The heart is quite different in the infant dying with this anomaly compared to that of the patient surviving to adulthood. In the infant, the cardiac mass is increased (this anomaly provides the best evidence available that chronic myocardial ischemia causes an increase in cardiac mass) and the ventricular cavities are dilated. The area occupied by the mitral valve appears small in comparison to the entire left ventricular cavity. The left ventricular papillary muscles appear to arise in the left ventricle at about the junction of the cephalad and middle thirds of the wall. Normally, the papillary muscles tend to arise about the level of the middle and caudal thirds of the left ventricle. The arterolateral papillary muscle is much smaller than the posteromedial papillary muscle. Additionally, the anterolateral papillary muscle is scarred, often calcified, and in contrast, the myocardium of the posteromedial muscle is preserved. The endocardium of the left ventricle may be thickened so that it has the appearance of diffuse endocardial fibroelastosis. The margin of the anterior mitral leaflet is often thickened. The left atrium is dilated.

In contrast to the appearance in the infant heart,

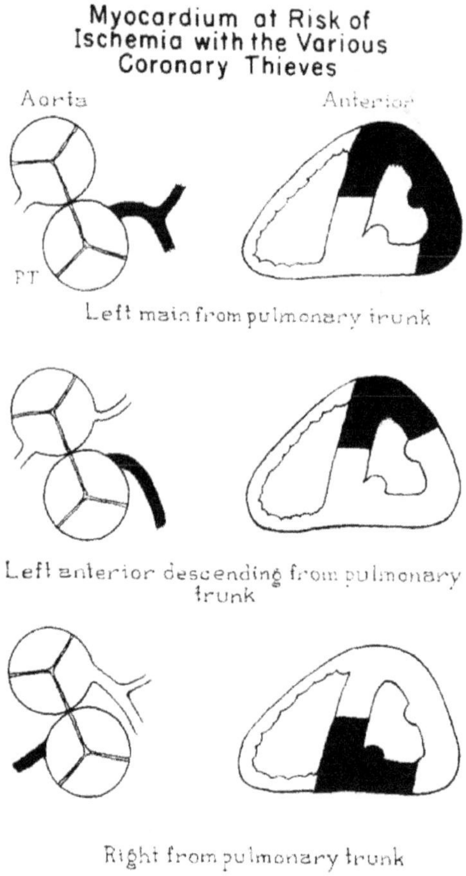

Fig. 3. Diagram showing the portion of left ventricular myocardium at risk of ischemia or necrosis when the left main, left anterior descending, or right coronary artery arises from the pulmonary trunk *(PT)*.

the survivors of this anomaly into adulthood have hearts which are distinguished primarily by the appearances of the epicardial coronary arteries. The right one is dilated and tortuous. The branches of the LM, in contrast, are straighter, not as dilated, but have a thinner wall (like a vein). Vascular channels connecting the RCA to the branches of the LM are visible on the surface of the heart. The mass of the heart is usually increased and the ventricular cavities are usually dilated. The anterolateral papillary muscle is usually scarred and it also contains calcific deposits. One of 10 adults (aged 15 to 54 years [mean 31]) reported by Moodie et al.[9] had extensive left ventricular calcific deposits. Left ventricular endocardial fibroelastosis, which is commonly observed in the infants at necropsy, is usually absent in the adults with this anomaly.

Symptoms of cardiac dysfunction. Symptoms of cardiac dysfunction occur in about 80% of infants in whom the LM arises from the PT, and the symptom complex was reported by Bland et al.[3] and has been substantiated by others.[10-19] In adults or in children surviving the first year of life, the symptoms complex is far more varied. Many patients with the adult form of anomalous LM arising from the PT are asymptomatic despite extremely active lives. A 29-year-old woman reported by Sabiston et al.[20] had had five full-term normal deliveries without difficulty. The 18-year-old boy reported by Harthorne et al.[16] was a star basketball player who eventually developed excessive dyspnea, chest pain, and finally syncope, only in association with the strenuous exertion of athletic endeavors. The 18-year-old boy reported by Jurishica[10] was a star football player.

The asymptomatic older patients with this anomaly were usually brought to medical attention by the detection of a precordial murmur (often a continuous one) on precordial examination, by the finding of an abnormal ECG showing ischemic changes, or by the occurrence of sudden unexpected death. The latter, unfortunately, is common. Of 14 adults aged 16 to 60 years (mean 36) with this anomaly reviewed by George and Knowlan,[11] 10 died suddenly and unexpectedly and of the 10, sudden death was the initial clinical manifestation of the coronary anomaly in eight. The sudden death was usually associated with sudden physical exertion.

Other reported symptoms in adults with this anomaly have included angina pectoris, exertional dyspnea, and syncope. Clinical features consistent with acute myocardial infarction have not been described, to my knowledge, in adults with this anomaly. Likewise, overt evidence of congestive heart failure is rare in adults, except possibly in those with clinical evidence of mitral regurgitation.[21,22]

Means of diagnosis. The definitive diagnosis of this anomaly is by angiography by injection of contrast material into the lumen of the right coronary artery (or aortic root) with drainage via collaterals into the LM branches and visualization of the connection of the LM to the PT. Although angiography is the only definitive test, other procedures provide important clues to the diagnosis. The presence of a precordial continuous murmur is very helpful. In infants the ECG showing ischemic myocardial changes (anterior wall) is most helpful.[19] In adults with this anomaly, unfortunately, the ECG is not as helpful. The ischemic changes in adults may or may not be present, and even if they are present they could be attributed to coronary narrowing from atherosclerosis. ECG evidence of left ventricular hypertrophy is common in adults with the anomaly.

The echocardiogram may provide clues to diagnosis. In each of three infants, Fisher et al.[23] demonstrated by cross-sectional echocardiography attachment of the LM coronary artery to the PT and markedly dilated poorly contracting left ventricles. Terai et al.,[24] also in an infant, demonstrated by cross-sectional echocardiography origin of the LM from the PT as well as a very large right coronary artery arising from the ascending aorta. Robinson et al.[26] cautioned that the only reliable echocardiographic finding in the anomaly was the actual demonstration of the LM arising from the PT, not the absence of identification of the origin of the LM from the aorta. King et al.,[27] by pulsed Doppler echocardiography, demonstrated in a 2-month-old infant bidirectional Doppler flow in the proximal portion of the PT. The late systolic flow pattern on the Doppler flow tracing indicated a left-to-right shunt through the LM arising from the PT. Whether echocardiography will be as useful in adults with this anomaly as in infants remains to be determined.

The presence of mitral regurgitation in a young person with ischemic changes on the ECG might suggest the presence of the coronary anomaly. Mitral regurgitation may be the dominant clinical feature of this coronary anomaly. Both Usman et al.[21] and Burchell and Brown[22] described a patient whose dominant clinical problem was mitral regurgitation.

Radionuclide angiography may be useful in distinguishing patients with origin of the LM from the PT from those with idiopathic dilated cardiomyopathy.[28] Origin of the LM from the PT cannot usually be seen by injecting contrast material into the PT. However, the LM can be seen arising from the PT if a balloon is inflated in the PT just distal to the site of contrast material injection.[29]

Operative treatment and results. A number of operative procedures have been utilized for treatment of this anomaly[5, 9, 14, 16, 19, 20, 23, 30-46]: (1) ligation of the LM coronary artery at its attachment to the PT; (2) obliteration of the LM ostium by covering it within the lumen of the PT with artificial or biologic material; (3) ligation of the LM artery or closure of its ostium plus insertion of a conduit, usually a reversed saphenous vein, from ascending aorta to left anterior descending coronary artery; (4) anastomosis of the LM to the ascending aorta either directly or via an artificial (polytetrafluoroethylene) or biologic graft, with closure of the site of origin of the LM from the PT; (5) division of the LM artery close to its ostium in the PT and direct anastomosis of a subclavian or common carotid artery to the LM in an end-to-end fashion. In the procedures in which a conduit has been interposed between the aorta and the LM coronary artery, the conduit has been located posterior to the PT, within the PT as a tunnel, and anterior to the PT. Despite the multiple different procedures utilized for treatment, the best one is unclear. Good results have been obtained with most of them.

An early operative procedure to correct this anomaly was a simple ligation of the LM coronary artery. This procedure has produced good long-term results in infants, children, and adults. Shrivastava et al.[41] followed two infants and two children (aged 6 and 7 years) for >10 years after simple LM ligation and all were asymptomatic postoperatively, although the ECG remained abnormal in two. Wilson et al.,[42] by polling many cardiovascular surgeons, collected 13 patients who had LM ligation only when they were aged 13 years or older. The mean age at last follow-up was 37 ± 9 years and the mean follow-up period was 9 years. Although there had been no deaths at operation or in the early postoperative period, three patients died later (2, 6, and 7 years after operation). These same authors also described results in 16 patients who had had LM ligation plus insertion of a saphenous vein between the ascending aorta and the LAD coronary artery at age 13 years or older. At a mean age of last follow-up of 38 ± 11 years and a mean of 5 ± 3 years after operation, there was only one death and that was in the early postoperative period. Wilson et al.[42] concluded that the probability of survival was similar following either LM ligation alone or LM ligation plus aorto-LAD grafting. About half the patients in both their two operative groups were improved symptomatically by the operation.

Moodie et al.[9] described operative results in 10 patients aged 15 to 54 years (mean 31) at the time of closure of the LM ostium from within the PT plus aorto-LAD grafting (six patients), isolated closure of the LM ostium from inside the PT (three patients), and transfer of the LM ostium with a cuff of PT directly to the ascending aorta (one patient). The 10 patients were followed 4 months to 16 years (mean 6 years): six were asymptomatic postoperatively, three were functional class II (each was class III preoperatively [New York Heart Association classification]), and one died late. Postoperative stress ECGs showed no evidence of myocardial ischemia in six of six patients and normal stress thallium tests in eight of eight patients.

The present commonly employed operative procedures for this anomaly—namely, LM ligation with aorto-LAD grafting or connection of the LM to the aorta either directly or via a graft—appear to have similar effects on the sizes of the collaterals between the branches of the RCA and the branches of the LAD and LC coronary arteries and the size of the RCA postoperatively. Early after operation and as long as 3 years postoperatively, the sizes of the collaterals and RCA postoperatively may be similar to their sizes preoperatively. By 3 years after operation, however, the collaterals are usually much smaller or have disappeared and the lumen of and the tortuosity of the RCA is much less than preoperatively. In a patient reported by Chaitman et al.,[37] however, who was evaluated at age 36 (over 8 years after LM ligation and aorto-LAD grafting via a saphenous vein), large collaterals were still present between the LM branches and the RCA.

These operations have variable effects on the degree of mitral regurgitation postoperatively if mitral regurgitation was present preoperatively. The valvular lesion may disappear or be unchanged or it may lessen postoperatively. If there is ECG evidence of left ventricular hypertrophy preoperatively, that condition usually persists after operation. Left ventricular function, however, is usually improved by operation. Bagger et al.[46] described a 19-year-old woman who had LM ligation and saphenous vein grafting between the aorta and LAD; evaluation 6 months postoperatively disclosed disappearance of the collaterals, normal left ventricular contractions compared to preoperative studies, a 100% increase in coronary sinus blood flow and a 128% increase during pacing, whereas preoperatively pacing did not increase the coronary sinus blood flow.

Right coronary artery from pulmonary trunk

Historic background. The first report of origin of the RCA from the PT was by Sir John Brooks, an anatomist, who studied two cadavers and postulated in 1885 that blood flow in the anomalously arising RCA was reversed: blood from the aorta entered the LM coronary artery, passed through collaterals to the RCA, and then drained into the PT.[47] Monckelberg[48] in 1914 studied at necropsy a 30-year-old man who had died shortly following an epileptic seizure and found the RCA anomaly. Schley[49] in 1925 described the anomaly in a 61-year-old man who died of syphilis. Jordan et al.[50] also found the anomaly in a patient at necropsy, as did Cronk et al.[51] The latter patient had lived 90 years before he died, shortly following seizures. These latter authors described severe atherosclerosis in the branches of the LM coronary artery and no atherosclerosis in the RCA, a finding which proves that the pressure in the RCA was venous and that in the left coronary arteries was arterial. Cronk et al.[51] also noted that the intramural coronary arteries in the right ventricular wall were numerous and in the left ventricular free wall they were relatively sparse. The left coronary artery (probably the LAD) had a maximal diameter of 20 mm and the RCA had a maximal diameter of 6 mm. The first patient with this anomaly who was treated operatively was reported by Tingelstad et al.[52] in 1972.

Frequency. This anomaly is far less common than is origin of the LM from the PT. In their 1962 book, Fontana and Edwards[4] found reports of only four necropsy cases of origin of the RCA from the PT, while at the same time finding reports of 58 necropsy cases of origin of the LM from the PT. From review of the necropsy reports at Yale–New Haven Hospital from 1952 to 1968, Ogden[53] found four cases of origin of the RCA from the PT and 39 cases of origin of the LM from the PT. By 1979, Lerberg et al.[54] found reports describing 14 patients with origin of the RCA from the PT and reports describing 140 patients with origin of the LM from the PT.

Flow in the anomalous artery. Flow in the anomalous artery, be it right, LM, LAD, or LC from the PT, should be similar and variable, depending on the patient's age. Although flow through the anomalously arising LM has been demonstrated to be antegrade early in life and retrograde after approximately a year (sometimes earlier) of life, antegrade flow has not been demonstrated in infancy when the RCA has arisen from the PT and the LM has arisen from the aorta. The reason of course is that diagnosis of origin of the RCA from the PT has not been made during infancy; indeed, the youngest child in whom this diagnosis has been established was 6 years old and that patient was described by Lerberg et al.[54] Retrograde flow through the anomalous RCA has been established both by angiogram and by visualization at operation.

Morphologic features. Whereas increase in ventricular mass, left ventricular scarring, anterolateral papillary muscle fibrosis and calcification, right ventricular and left ventricular dilatation, and diffuse left ventricular endocardial fibroelastosis (of variable degree) might be expected in cases of origin of the LM from the PT, none of these morphologic findings appear to be the consequence of origin of the RCA from the PT. Indeed, the only predictable morphologic finding is an increase in the size of the LM coronary artery and its branches and an increase (but less so) in the size of the RCA with thinning of its wall (compared to normal).

Clinical manifestations. This anomaly usually produces no symptoms of cardiac dysfunction and no evidence of myocardial ischemia. Of nine necropsy cases reported up to 1979 and summarized by

Lerberg et al.[54] one patient, a 2-year-old boy, was found dead in his crib without preceding evidence of any illnes. Another, an 11-year-old girl, had cardiac arrest, and another, a 72-year-old man, had evidence of chronic congestive cardiac failure. None of the three patients had another condition that could be responsible for their deaths. All six remaining necropsy patients were either free of clinical evidence of cardiac dysfunction or they had another cardiac disorder (aortic regurgitation or systemic hypertension or mitral stenosis) which could readily explain any cardiac dysfunction. These six patients were aged 30 to 90 years (mean 62). Five other patients up to 1979 had the anomaly diagnosed by angiography and each of them had operative therapy.[54] Their ages at operation were 11, 12, 25, 42, and 64 years, and three were female.[54-58] Three of them were asymptomatic and were found to have a continuous precordial murmur (left sternal border), one (age 64 years) presented with evidence of congestive cardiac failure,[56] and one (age 25 years) had cardiac arrest with successful resuscitation.[58] A year earlier, however, the latter patient had had one syncopal episode. Thus, anomalous origin of the RCA from the PT is a cause of cardiac arrest, and this fact by itself justifies operative intervention if this coronary anomaly is known to be present, even though the individual may be asymptomatic.

Recently, Mintz et al.[59] reported a 47-year-old man who had angina pectoris for 2 months. The resting ECG and the chest radiogram were normal. Thallium-201 myocardial perfusion scanning disclosed a decrease in perfusion in the 4-hour-study. Total anterograde LM coronary flow was 1440 to 1680 ml/min, but only 240 to 280 ml/min supplied the myocardium and the remainder passed to the PT via the RCA. Thus there was a 5:1 intercoronary shunt. This study was the first to quantitate the degree of the "coronary steal" in this anomaly (Fig. 2).

In contrast to its usefulness when the LM coronary artery arises from the PT, the ECG in origin of the RCA from the PT is usually of no benefit. Ischemic changes are usually absent and signs of ventricular hypertrophy are usually absent or only borderline. The chest radiogram usually shows mild enlargement of the cardiac silhouette, but the cardiac size may be entirely normal. Cross-sectional echocardiography may be useful for diagnosis. Origin of the RCA from the PT must be demonstrated—not absence of origin of the RCA from the aorta.[60] The finding of a large LM coronary artery or a large RCA by echocardiography might provide the initial suspicion of the pressure of this anomaly. Certain diagnosis is established by angiography, with injection of contrast material in the LM coronary artery arising from the aorta, and visualization of the RCA via collaterals from the LM branches and finally the appearance of contrast material in the PT.

Operative treatment and results. The operation of choice for this anomaly appears to be transsection of the RCA from the PT and direct anastomosis of the RCA to the aorta (end-to-side). Tingelstad et al.[52] were the first to report this technique. Their patient was a 12-year-old asymptomatic boy who was found to have a continuous precordial murmur. The left-to-right shunt from the LM to the RCA was calculated to have been 1.7 to 1. Others[53, 54, 56-61] have also successfully utilized this transsection technique. The patient operated on by Bregman et al.[58] had presented with cardiac arrest and was successfully resuscitated. The patient was asymptomatic 2 years postoperatively.

Left anterior descending coronary artery from pulmonary trunk.

At least eight patients have been reported in whom the LAD arose from the PT and both right and LC arteries arose from the aorta, and the findings in these patients were summarized by Roberts and Robinowitz.[62] At the time of their 1984 report, one patient (a 7-month-old girl) had died of an anterior wall acute myocardial infarct; the other seven (six women) were aged 18 to 55 years (mean 34). The patient reported by Roberts and Robinowitz[62] is the only male thus far described. Of the seven adults, six were asymptomatic, five with angina pectoris, one of whom also had an anterior wall acute myocardial infarct, and one with severe fatigue attributed to severe mitral regurgitation from papillary muscle dysfunction. The angina at some time in all five patients was stable, but three of the five had unstable angina just before cardiac operation. The age at onset of symptoms of myocardial ischemia in the six adults ranged from 18 to 37 years (mean 27). Precordial murmurs were described in five or six adults. (No information was provided in the "addendum case" of Donaldson et al.[63]) The murmur apparently was present only in systole in four patients, and also in diastole in two. The intensity of the murmurs was mentioned in three patients; it was "soft" in one, grade 2/6 in one, and grade 3/6 in one. Findings on the ECG at rest were described in five adults: four had poor R wave progression in leads V_1 to V_3 and at least two had ST-T-wave changes of ischemia in more than one lead. In one patient the ECG was normal. Exercise stress tests in two patients disclosed ST segment

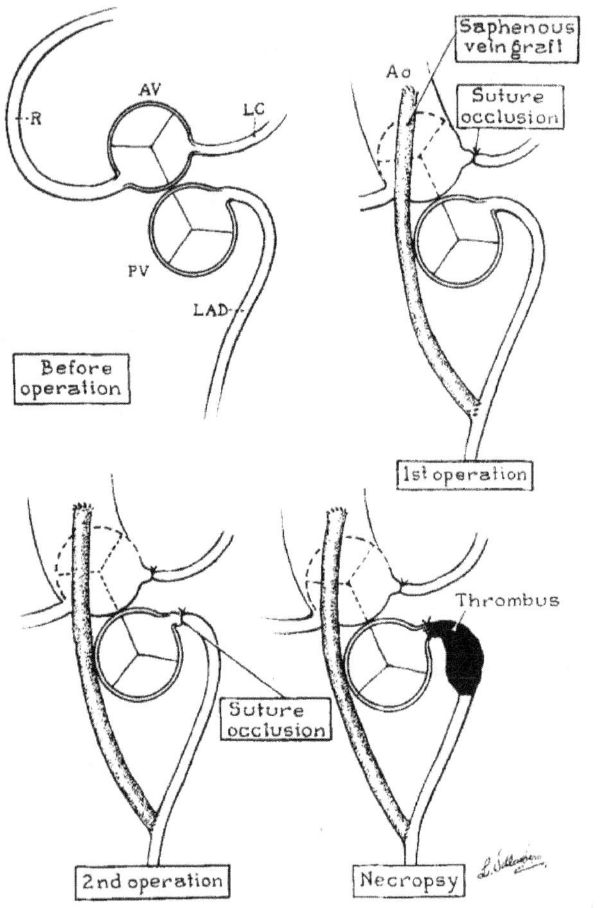

Fig. 4. Diagram showing sequence of events in a 32-year-old man in whom the left anterior descending *(LAD)* coronary artery arose from the pulmonary trunk. Before operation he was asymptomatic but had a precordial continuous murmur. At the first operation, the left circumflex *(LC)* coronary artery was inadvertently ligated rather than the LAD. At the second operation, performed 3 days after the first, a conduit was inserted between ascending aorta and LAD. The patient died suddenly soon after jogging 9 months after the cardiac operations. Obviously, if operation is to be performed for this anomaly, the anomalously arising artery must be clearly identified before ligation. *Ao* = aorta; *AV* = aortic valve; *LC* = left circumflex coronary artery; *PV* = pulmonic valve; *R* = right coronary artery. (From Roberts WC, and Robinowitz M: Am J Cardiol **54**:1381, 1984. Reproduced by permission.)

ischemic changes in each. Chest x-ray films in six of the seven adults disclosed normal-sized cardiac silhouettes in three and cardiac enlargement in three; the latter was mild in two and severe in one. Right-sided cardiac catheterization, performed in at least six patients, disclosed normal pressures in each and oxygen step-up in the PT in two. Coronary angiograpy with injection of contrast material in the right and LC coronary arteries in all seven adults disclosed that each of these two arteries in all seven patients was large, occasionally also tortuous, and that the LAD was filled by extensive collateral vessels from both the right and LC coronary arteries. Injection of contrast material into the PT did not cause filling of the LAD; when the LAD, however, was filled by injections into either the right or LC coronary artery, contrast material did enter the PT through the LAD, which was filled by collateral vessels.

Of the eight reported adults, operative treatment was carried out in six, four of whom preoperatively had angina; in two patients, the PT was opened and the ostium of the LAD was obliterated by sutures, and in two the LAD was ligated just proximal to its entrance into the PT and a reversed saphenous vein was inserted from the ascending aorta to the LAD. One patient, a 32-year-old asymptomatic man reported by Roberts and Robinowitz,[62] inadvertently had suture occlusion of the LC rather than of the LAD, with insertion of a saphenous vein from the aorta to the LAD at the first operation (Fig. 4). At the second operation 3 days later, the LAD was ligated proximally (Fig. 4). This patient died suddenly while jogging 9 months postoperatively. Of the five symptomatic patients who had operative treatment, angina disappeared in three and persisted in one. Two patients had repeat coronary and left ventricular angiography 24 and 36 months, respectively, after operation; in each, the right and LC coronary arteries were much smaller than they had been preoperatively, and the collateral vessels between the right and LC coronary arteries and the LAD coronary artery had disappeared. One patient had persistent angina postoperatively and the distal portions of both the right and LC coronary arteries (36 months postoperatively) were quite narrowed; the cause of narrowing was unclear. Left ventricular angiograms, performed in five adults, were normal in three, and in the other two the apical portion of the left ventricle was akinetic in one and aneurysmal in one. Repeat left ventricular angiography in these latter two patients disclosed better overall contractions in one and no change in one.

The presence of both subjective and objective evidence of myocardial ischemia in six of the eight reported adults and the disappearance of angina and of the collateral vessels between the two coronary arteries arising from the aorta and the LAD arising from the PT supports the view that operative treatment is proper for patients with this coronary anomaly. Whether LAD ligation alone is enough, or whether ligation plus insertion of a conduit between the aorta and LAD is preferable, is unclear. Direct connection of the LAD to aorta in this situation appears technically inadvisable. Four of the six patients in whom operation was performed had angina pectoris. Two patients were asymptomatic preoperatively. Obviously, no data are available on the advisability of operation in an asymptomatic person in whom the LAD arises from the PT, but it appears reasonable to believe that the operative therapy in this circumstance is proper. If an operation is to be performed, however, clear identification of the anomalous artery before ligation is mandatory.

Left circumflex coronary artery from the pulmonary trunk.

Effler et al.[64] mentioned an 8-year-old boy (their case No. 7) who by angiogram had a LC coronary artery attached to a pulmonary artery (which one was not mentioned); the correct diagnosis was not confirmed anatomically. Honey et al.[65] described a 13-year-old boy who had aortic isthmic coarctation, right aortic arch, bicuspid aortic valve, and origin of the LC coronary artery from the right main pulmonary artery. Chaitman et al.[66] described a 14-year-old asymptomatic girl in whom the LC apparently arose from the PT. Ott et al.[67] described an 8-year-old girl, also with a bicuspid aortic valve, in whom the LC coronary artery arose from the right main coronary artery. No adults have been reported with origin of the LC coronary artery from any pulmonary artery.

Accessory coronary artery from pulmonary trunk.

The most common accessory coronary artery arising from the PT is a conus artery. Origin of this small coronary artery from the PT is of no functional significance.

ORIGIN OF 1 OR 2 CORONARY ARTERIES FROM THE PULMONARY TRUNK WITHOUT ORIGIN OF A CORONARY ARTERY FROM THE AORTA

At least 12 patients with origin of both LM and right coronary arteries from the PT have been reported, and all died during the first month of life, usually in the first 1 or 2 days.[68-77] Thus, nearly all of these infants had patent ductus arteriosus. Most had other major anomalies of the heart or great arteries. At least two patients have been described in whom a single coronary artery arose from PT and no coronary artery arose from the aorta.[78,79] Feldt et al.[78] described a 7-year-old girl who had a ductus closed at age 6 and a ventricular septal defect (VSD) closed just before death. At necropsy, a single coronary arose for the PT and the mitral valve was stenotic. Monselise et al.[79] described a 1-year-old boy with a VSD and a single coronary artery arising from the PT. Survival in these two patients was made possible by the presence of the associated congenital anomalies which allowed systemic pressure in the PT.

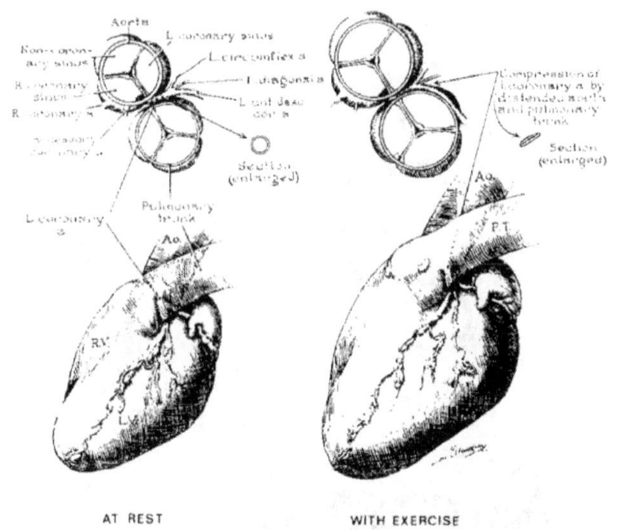

Fig. 5. Diagram showing a proposed mechanism by which origin of the left *(L)* main coronary artery *(a)* from the right sinus of Valsalva causes nonfatal or fatal cardiac dysfunction.

ANOMALOUS ORIGIN OF 1 OR MORE CORONARY ARTERIES FROM THE AORTA

Both *left main* and right coronary arteries from the *right* aortic sinus

Classification of the anomaly. This condition has been reviewed recently by Barth and Roberts.[80] Anomalous origin of the LM coronary artery from the right sinus of Valsalva can be classified into four major groups, according to the course taken by the LM in relation to the aorta and PT en route to the left side of the heart. The LM may course anterior to the PT, posterior to the aorta,[81] within the ventricular septum beneath the right ventricular infundibulum,[82] or between the aorta and PT (Fig. 5). When the LM passes anterior to the PT over the right ventricular infundibulum, symptoms of myocardial ischemia have not been reported unless significant coronary arterial narrowing due to atherosclerotic plaque was present. With the exception of the 12-year-old girl with this anomaly described by Murphy et al,[83] symptoms of myocardial ischemia have not been reported when the LM arises from the right sinus of Valsalva and courses posterior to the aorta.

Review of published reports. At least 43 necropsy patients have been reported with origin of the LM coronary artery from the right sinus of Valsalva, with coursing between the aorta and PT.[80,81,84-96] In nine, death was unrelated to the anomaly and symptoms of myocardial ischemia were absent during life. In the other 34 patients, death was of coronary origin. Of the 34 patients, 26 (76%) died

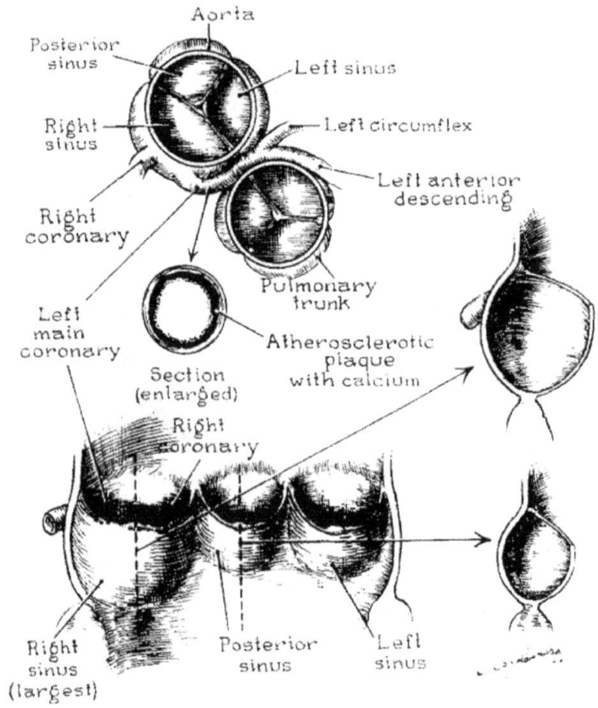

Fig. 6. Drawing of an anomalously arising left main coronary artery from the right sinus of Valsalva in an 81-year-old man (DCMEO No. 80-04-332) who never had evidence of cardiac dysfunction and who died of a noncardiac condition. The wall of the anomalously arising left main coronary artery is heavily calcified. (From Barth CW III, and Roberts WC: J Am Coll Cardiol **7**:366, 1986. Reproduced by permission.)

before age 20 years and the other eight (24%) died at ages ranging from 49 to 82 years (mean 64). Of the 26 patients who died young, 25 (96%) died suddenly during or shortly after vigorous exertion and one died of acute myocardial infarction, having survived for 19 hours after initial collapse, which likewise occurred shortly after exertion. Of the 14 patients where information was provided, 10 had had symptoms before the final collapse; there was exertional syncope in six, angina in four, and exertional dyspnea in one. Of the 26 young patients, 24 (92%) were male. At necropsy, 5 of the 26 patients had histologic evidence of myocardial necrosis; one patient apparently had atherosclerotic narrowing in the anomalous LM coronary artery.

Mechanism of death in older patients with the anomaly. Of the eight patients who died after age 20 years, seven were men. Four died of consequences of acute myocardial infarction: one died suddenly; one died of a noncardiac cause (alcoholism) (Fig. 6); the mode of death in the other two was not described. Symptoms of cardiac dysfunction were described in only one of the eight patients. Histologic evidence of myocardial necrosis or fibrosis was present in five, absent in one, and not discussed in two patients. Of the eight older patients, six apparently had significant coronary narrowing by atherosclerotic plaque in the abnormal and/or normally coursing arteries. One patient lacked the circumflex branch of the LM artery.

While it is clear from current necropsy information that this anomaly can cause sudden death at a young age, the role the anomaly plays in those who have survived past age 20 years is less clear. One of the two older patients reported by Barth and Roberts[80] appears to be the only one thus far reported in whom fatal myocardial ischemia could be attributed entirely to the coronary anomaly. Why this patient had fatal myocardial ischemia late in life after decades without symptoms is unclear. Possibly, the excessive cardiac weight (500 gm) was a factor. Why other older patients survive into the ninth decade free of symptoms of cardiac dysfunction is not clear either.

Pathogenesis of myocardial ischemia. The precise mechanism by which anomalous origin of the LM coronary artery from the right sinus of Valsalva with coursing between the PT and aorta causes myocardial ischemia is unclear. In each of the five patients reported by Barth and Roberts,[80] the normal RCA arose at an angle more or less perpendicular to the center of the aortic lumen, and it coursed directly away from the aorta; in contrast, the LM coronary artery arose from the aortic lumen at roughly a 180-degree angle to the center of the aorta. After takeoff, the anomalously arising LM was adherent to the wall of the aorta for roughly 1.5 cm as it coursed to the left side of the heart between the PT and aorta. Additionally, the ostium of the anomalously arising LM was slit-like, with the largest diameter in a cephalad-caudal direction; in contrast, the ostium of the normally arising RCA was circular and larger. The firmly anchored root of the PT appears to present a potential barrier against which the LM could be compressed by expansion of the aortic root that occurs during increased intra-aortic pressure associated with exertion. The LM coronary artery, of course, is equivalent to two arteries in the sense that it is responsible for supplying coronary blood flow to the major portion of the left ventricle; therefore significant reduction of flow through it is particularly perilous. While it is likely that the narrowed LM orifice has the potential to diminish flow through it, an actual reduction appears to be significant only during or immediately following exertion in those individuals without associated atherosclerosis.

Association of death with exertion. The association of death with exertion can be explained by three factors. (1) Myocardial oxygen requirements increase with exertion; therefore, any obstruction to coronary flow is more likely to result in myocardial ischemia. (2) It is likely that outward expansion of the roots of both the aorta and PT during exertion causes further compression of the ostial lumen of the LM. (3) The LM, as it courses between the aorta and PT, could be compressed against the root of the PT where it is firmly anchored to the infundibular septum when the aortic root and PT dilate during exertion. The fact that sudden exertional death and nonfatal myocardial ischemia have been seen in persons in whom the LM originates from the proximal RCA and then courses between the great arteries[81,85]—and who therefore do not have the abnormal oblique take-off of the LM nor the slit-like ostium in the right sinus of Valsalva—suggests that hemodynamic compression (hemodynamic vise) of the LM between the great arteries cannot be excluded as an additional mechanism of myocardial ischemia. Davia et al.[97] described a 14-year-old boy who had two "exertionally related myocardial infarctions" due to this anomaly, underwent surgical enlargement of the narrowed LM ostium, and is asymptomatic during heavy labor 9 years later. This case lends further support to the theory that the primary mechanism causing myocardial ischemia is related to the narrowed LM ostium.

Usefulness of exercise electrocardiography in diagnosis. The usefulness of stress electrocardiography in identifying the ischemic nature of this anomaly in young persons has received little attention. The fact that one patient reported by Barth and Roberts,[80] a 14-year-old boy, had a normal stress test 1 month before death prompted them to review previous experience with stress electrocardiography in young patients with isolated anomalous origin of the LM from the right sinus of Valsalva with coursing of the LM between the aorta and PT. Results of stress electrocardiography[6,81,91,98] in seven patients disclosed that three had abnormal stress ECGs (ECG evidence of ischemia or ventricular arrythmia) and four had normal stress ECGs. In three of the latter four, however, the test was not at maximal effort. Two of the seven, both of whom had normal submaximal stress electrocardiography, subsequently died suddenly. The other five patients had surgery. It is clear that the stress ECG, particularly that which is submaximal in effort, is not a reliable screening test for this anomaly in young patients who present with exertional syncope, angina, and even acute myocardial infarction.

Differential diagnosis and means of diagnosis. Young patients with this anomaly often present with exertional syncope, dizziness, and angina, but other cardiovascular abnormalities, such as hypertrophic cardiomyopathy and aortic valve stenosis, can present in a similar manner and therefore must be distinguished. The diagnostic approach taken with these young patients must take into account the fallibilities of the various noninvasive tests in identifying this potentially fatal coronary anomaly. The resting ECG is normal in almost all young persons with this anomaly and therefore it is not helpful. Physical examination may provide important clues to the noncoronary causes of these symptoms, i.e., murmurs and peripheral pulses characteristic for aortic stenosis or hypertrophic cardiomyopathy. Echocardiography also is helpful in assessing for or confirming aortic stenosis or hypertrophic cardiomyopathy. Liberthson et al.[99] reported a 54-year-old woman with angina pectoris in whom cross-sectional echocardiography identified anomalous origin of the LM coronary artery from the proximal RCA with coursing of the LM between the aorta and PT. Echocardiography, while potentially useful, has not been reported to have successfully identified origin of the LM directly from the right sinus of Valsalva. Continuous ambulatory electrocardiography may identify significant arrhythmias, but it provides no help in identifying the cause of the arrhythmias. If the noncoronary causes of exertional syncope and angina are not identified, then more extensive evaluation is dictated to exclude the possibility of anomalous origin of the LM. As has been demonstrated, stress electrocardiography does not always identify myocardial ischemia in young patients with this coronary anomaly who are at risk for sudden death, but it should be done and it should be carried to maximal effort if evidence of myocardial ischemia is not identified at lower levels of exercise. If stress electrocardiography is abnormal, then angiographic assessment of coronary anatomy is dictated.[100,101] If maximal stress electrocardiography is normal, then coronary angiography must still be considered in boys with clear cut exercise-induced symptoms. The usefulness of thallium stress electrocardiography for diagnosis of this anomaly is uncertain. The patient reported by Mustafa et al.[98] had normal thallium stress electrocardiography. Finally, in the specific case of exertional syncope at a young age, particularly in males, coronary angiography should be done after a second episode of syncope. Angiography should be considered, however, after a single episode if no other clear cause of exertional syncope is evident by noninvasive testing.

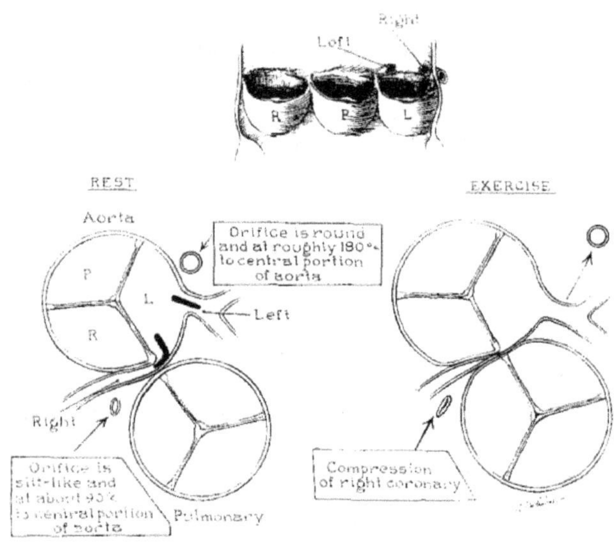

Fig. 7. Diagram showing mechanism by which origin of the right coronary artery arising from the left sinus of Valsalva might cause fatal or nonfatal cardiac dysfunction. (From Roberts WC, et al: Am J Cardiol **49**:863, 1982. Reproduced by permission.)

Management of patients with the anomaly. Once the origin of both LM and right coronary arteries from the right sinus with coursing of the LM between the great arteries has been diagnosed, at least in younger individuals, operative therapy appears warranted for the prevention of sudden death and for relief of exercise-induced symptoms of myocardial ischemia. Various operative approaches for revascularization have been described. Aortocoronary conduits, either saphenous vein or mammary artery, or both, to the LAD and LC coronary systems have resulted in relief of symptoms and in relief of objective evidence of myocardial ischemia in several patients.[99, 102, 103] Other surgical approaches have also been successful. Davia et al.[97] described a 14-year-old boy who had had two myocardial infarcts and subsequently underwent surgical enlargement of the narrowed LM coronary ostium by the extension of an incision from the ostium through the common wall of the aorta and the anomalous artery over the intercoronary commissure. He was free of symptoms and active 9 years later, despite the presence of mild aortic regurgitation due to the procedure. Four patients, aged 12 to 36 years, have undergone an operation of a similar nature to reestablish the normal anatomic location of the LM origin to the left sinus of Valsalva by incising along the course of the left sinus of Valsalva and joining the intima of the vessel to the aorta, resulting in a new ostium.[6, 98] No evidence of ischemia was present in a follow-up period of 10 to 36 months.

BOTH LEFT MAIN AND *RIGHT* CORONARY ARTERIES FROM THE *LEFT* AORTIC SINUS.

Origin of the RCA from the left sinus of Valsalva has until recently been considered a minor congenital anomaly of no clinical significance.

Frequency. This anomaly is missed probably as frequently at necropsy as it is observed. Its true occurrence at necropsy therefore is really not known. It appears, however, that this anomaly is more frequent than origin of both right and LM coronary arteries from the right sinus with subsequent coursing of the LM between the aorta and PT. At necropsy, I have seen five cases of origin of both LM arteries and RCAs from the right sinus and 16 cases of origin of both coronary arteries from the left sinus of Valsalva, with coursing of either the LM or RCA between the aorta and PT.

Angiographically, origin of both coronary arteries from the left sinus is more frequent than origin of both from the right sinus, because patients with the former are more likely to have evidence of myocardial ischemia. Liberthson et al.,[92] during the same time period, observed at coronary angiography nine patients in whom both LM and RCA arose from the right sinus and nine in whom both arose from the left sinus of Valsalva, with either the LM or the RCA passing between the aorta and PT.

Evidence of myocardial ischemia. With patients in whom both coronary arteries arise from the left aortic sinus with the RCA passing between the aorta and PT, it is unclear how many during life have evidence of myocardial ischemia and how many do not. Roberts et al.[104] collected reports describing at necropsy 26 patients with origin of both coronary arteries from the left sinus, and not a single patient had had symptoms of cardiac dysfunction and in none could death be attributed to the anomaly. In contrast, analysis of published data on 34 other patients in whom this congenital anomaly was detected by coronary angiography disclosed that at least 12 had had symptoms of cardiac dysfunction unassociated with significant coronary atherosclerosis or a noncoronary cardiac condition.[81, 92, 105-111] Of the 12, three had had acute myocardial infarcts, seven had angina pectoris, one had syncope, and one had nonfatal ventricular fibrillation. Of the 12 necropsy patients with this coronary anomaly reported by Roberts et al.[104] three died suddenly, two clearly during exertion, and two of them previously had had either angina or syncope. One of the three patients, a 23-year-old woman, became symptomatic only after she became a long-distance runner; she had frequent episodes of ventricular tachycardia. At necropsy, two of these three symptomatic patients had grossly visible left ventricular scars. Subsequently, Hanzlick and Stivers[112-114] reported a 26-year-old marathon runner who was training for the Iron-man Triathlon. He collapsed and died just past the finish line of a 13.5-mile race. This patient previously had had two episodes of abnormally severe dyspnea after long runs. Brandt et al.[111] reported a 35-year-old man who had at that age developed periodic substernal chest pain, one episode being acute myocardial infarction. He underwent operation with placement of a cephalic vein between the ascending aorta and the RCA. Doppler probe studies of this patient objectively confirmed that the coronary anomaly caused left ventricular functional impairment and that it impaired coronary artery reserve. Coronary reserve was returned to normal by the operation and the patient had been asymptomatic during the entire 9-month period after operation. Isner et al.[115] reported a 23-year-old man who developed severe chest pain after ingestion of a heavy meal, went to bed, and later was found dead in bed. This patient had had occasional episodes of chest pain before his sudden death.

Mechanism of myocardial ischemia. The mechanism of ischemia appears to be the same as in patients in whom both coronary arteries arise from the right sinus of Valsalva, just as long as one of the major coronary arteries courses between the aorta and PT. There are three possibilities: (1) the slit-like orifice of the anomalously arising coronary artery is compressed closed or nearly so as the aorta dilates with exertion; (2) the anomalous artery itself is compressed by the aorta and PT as it courses between these two arteries, which dilate with exertion; or (3) both factors 1 and 2 (Fig. 7). The upright nature of the slit-like orifice of the anomalous artery prevents blood within the aortic lumen from flowing into the RCA during ventricular diastole without a peculiar direction of flow. In a 60-year-old man with this coronary anomaly, Keren et al.[110] demonstrated angiographically significant narrowing of the RCA as it coursed between the two great arteries during ventricular *systole*.

Treatment. In contrast to the situation in which both coronary arteries arise from the right aortic sinus, therapy in the situation in which both coronary arteries arise from the left aortic sinus is not as clear-cut. In the former group of patients, operative intervention is indicated, even in the asymptomatic patient, to prevent fatal or nonfatal myocardial ischemia. In that situation, however, it is the LM coronary artery which has a slit-like orifice and which courses between the aorta and PT. The LM, of course, is not one but really two major coronary

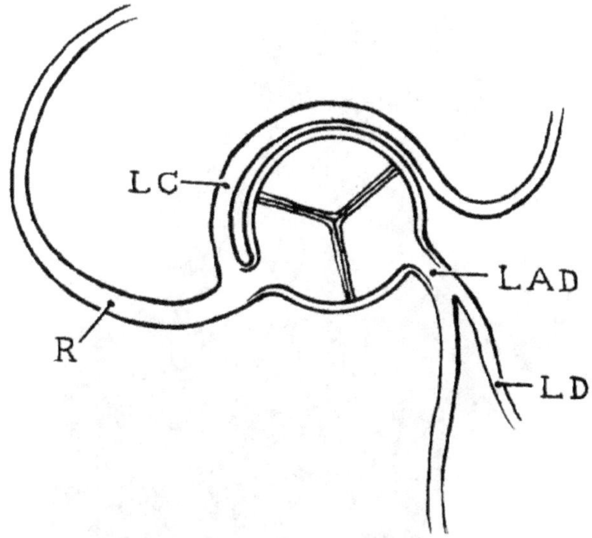

Fig. 8. Diagram showing origin of left circumflex *(LC)* coronary artery arising as the first branch of the right *(R)* coronary artery and then coursing posterior to the aorta before reaching the left atrioventricular sulcus. The left anterior descending *(LAD)* coronary artery arises from the left sinus of Valsalva. *LD* = left diagonal.

arteries. When both coronary arteries arise from the left aortic sinus, only one major coronary artery, the RCA, arises from a slit-like orifice and courses between the aorta and PT. In the latter situation, there appears no justification for operative intervention unless the patient has developed clinical signs of symptoms of myocardial ischemia. Sudden death as the initial manifestation of this coronary anomaly is extremely rare. Sudden death in almost all reported patients has been preceded by other symptoms of myocardial ischemia. If symptoms or signs of myocardial ischemia, however, have occurred, operative therapy is clearly warranted.

BOTH LEFT MAIN AND RIGHT CORONARY ARTERIES FROM THE POSTERIOR AORTIC SINUS.

To my knowledge, origin of both LM arteries and RCAs from the posterior sinus of Valsalva has never been reported.

BOTH RIGHT AND LEFT CIRCUMFLEX CORONARY ARTERIES FROM THE RIGHT AORTIC SINUS (OR ORIGIN OF THE LEFT CIRCUMFLEX FROM THE RIGHT CORONARY ARTERY) AND THE LEFT ANTERIOR DESCENDING CORONARY ARTERY FROM THE LEFT AORTIC SINUS

Initial description. The first description of this anomaly was by Antopol and Kugel[116] in 1933. These authors described four cases in adults (one a man; sex in other three not stated) at necropsy. In three the LC arose from the right sinus of Valsalva and in

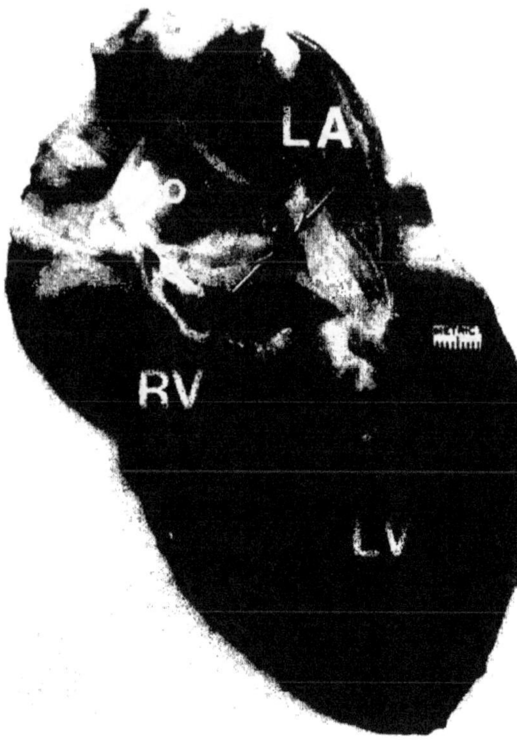

Fig. 9. Anteroposterior longitudinal view of the heart (SH No. A81-20) showing the course of an anomalously arising left circumflex coronary artery *(arrows)* between the aorta *(Ao)* and the left atrium *(LA)* before reaching the left atrioventricular sulcus. The left circumflex arose as the first branch of the right coronary artery. *RV* = right ventricle; *LV* = left ventricle.

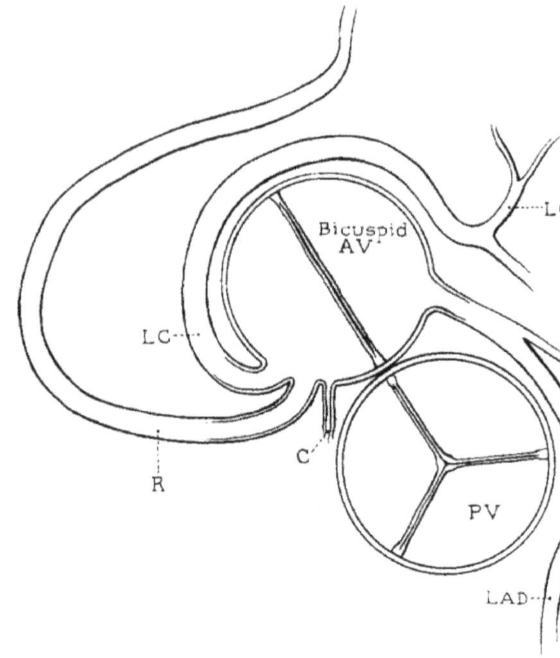

Fig. 10. Origin of left circumflex *(LC)* coronary artery directly from the right anterior aspect of the aorta with retroaortic coursing to the left atrioventricular sulcus in a 43-year-old man (No. A81-5757) who died of complications of severe coronary atherosclerosis. Although congenitally biscuspid, the aortic valve *(AV)* appeared to have functioned normally. *C* = conus coronary artery; *LAD* = left anterior descending coronary artery; *PV* = pulmonic valve; *R* = right coronary artery.

one, from the RCA. In all four, the RCA coursed retrograde to the aorta before reaching the left atrioventricular sulcus. The LAD arose from the left sinus of Valsalva, and it coursed directly to this usual location. The LM was absent. When, however, the LC arises as the first branch of the RCA, the initial portion of the RCA then is equivalent to the normal "LM" coronary artery[117] (Fig. 8). When the LC arises directly from the right sinus of Valsalva or as the first branch of the RCA, the LC always follows a retroaortic course to the left atrioventricular sulcus (Fig. 9).

Frequency. Origin of the LC from the right aortic sinus or from the RCA is the most common anomaly of coronary arterial origin. Among 600 hearts of patients aged 30 to 89 years (100 hearts in each of the six decades), White and Edwards[118] found two cases of this anomaly—both were men, one aged 76 and one aged 81 years. Thus there is a frequency of 1 per 300 adults at necropsy. Ogden[53] found this anomaly in 14 necropsy patients studied in a 16-year period at the Yale–New Haven Hospital. I have seen this anomaly at necropsy in 15 patients aged 22 to 71 years (mean 50) (11 men); 12 had no associated anomalies and three had valvular heart disease (rheumatic heart disease in two and a normally functioning bicuspid aortic valve in 1 [Fig. 10]). In 14 patients the coronary anomaly clearly was of no clinical significance; in one, a 22-year-old man who died suddenly while playing basketball, the anomaly may have been important. In eight patients the LC arose directly from the right aortic sinus and in seven patients it arose as the first branch of the RCA.

Of 2996 patients having selective coronary angiography, Page et al.[119] found that 20 (16 men) had origin of the LC from the right sinus of Valsalva or as the first branch of the RCA. In none of the 20 patients could cardiac dysfunction be attributed to the presence of this coronary anomaly (1 of the 20 also had origin of the LAD from the PT). Among 3750 coronary arteriograms reviewed by Chaitman et al.[105] 31 adults had anomalies of coronary origin, the most common (17 patients) being origin of the LC from the right sinus of Valsalva or as the first branch of the RCA. The sex of the 17 patients was not stated. Of 200 coronary angiograms reviewed by Ray et al.,[120] two—men aged 60 and 62 years—had

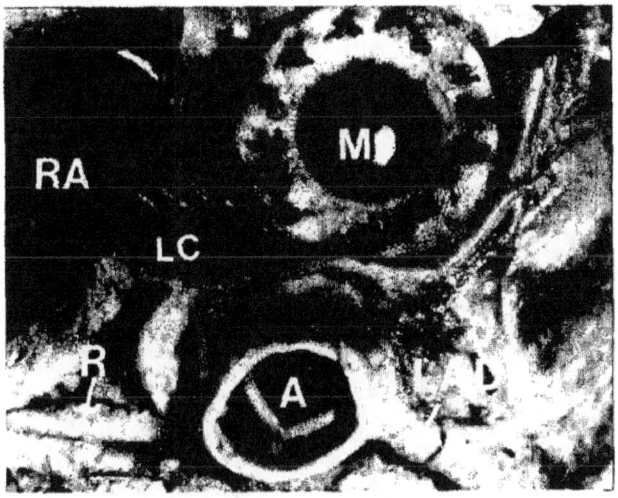

Fig. 11. Compression *(arrows)* of an anomalously arising left circumflex *(LC)* coronary artery from the right *(R)* coronary artery by the rings of prosthetic valves in both the aortic *(A)* and mitral *(M)* valve positions. *LAD* = left anterior descending coronary artery; *RA* = right atrium. (From Roberts WC, and Morrow AG: J Thorac Cardiovasc Surg **57**:834, 1969. Reproduced by permission.)

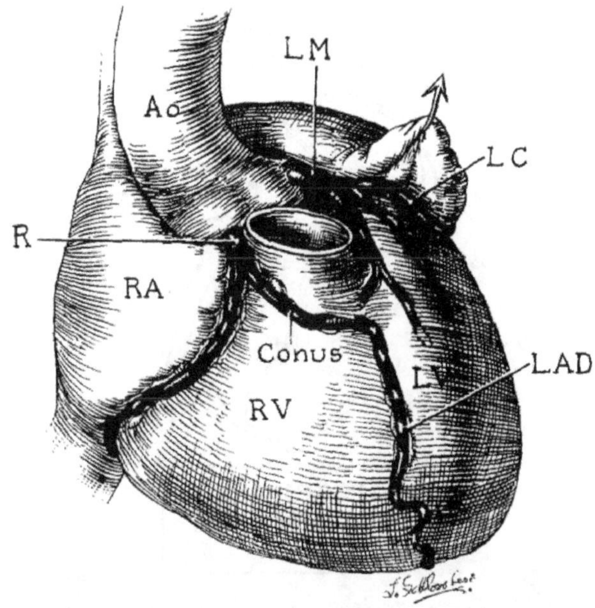

Fig. 12. Origin of the left anterior descending *(LAD)* from the right *(R)* coronary artery with coursing anterior to the right ventricular *(RV)* outflow tract in a 60-year-old man (No. A81-63) who died of consequences of severe coronary atherosclerosis. *Ao* = aorta; *LM* = left main; *LC* = left circumflex; *LV* = left ventricle; *RA* = right atrium. (From Robers WC, et al: AM HEART J **104**:638, 1982.)

origin of the LC from the RCA. Baltaxe and Wixson[121] reviewed 1000 consecutive coronary arteriograms performed mainly because of angina pectoris, and various coronary anomalies were found in nine; two of these, a 51-year-old woman and a 56-year-old man, had origin of the LC as the first branch of the RCA. Of 7000 patients having coronary angiograms, Kimbiris et al.[106] found anomalous aortic origin of one or more coronary arteries in 45; origin of the LC from the right sinus of Valsalva or as the first branch of the RCA was the most common of the five anomalies found, occurring in 26 patients (58%). The sex of the 26 patients was not stated. Of 21 cases of anomalous coronary origin reported by Liberthson et al.[122] (9 obtained at necropsy in a cardiovascular registry and 11 by selective coronary angiography), 11 had origin of the LC from the right sinus of Valsalva or as the first branch of the RCA. The mean age of the 11 patients was 54 years and eight were men.

Clinical significance. None, unless cardiac surgery is performed. If coronary perfusion during coronary bypass is limited to the artery arising from the left sinus of Valsalva, then the myocardium in the distribution of the LC coronary artery is not perfused. If perfusion is to the artery arising from the right sinus of Valsalva and if the LC arises as the first branch of the RCA, the tip of the perfusing cannula might be past the origin of the LC and again the myocardium dependent on the LC is deprived. If both right and LC coronary arteries arise from the right sinus of Valsalva, one artery would be deprived by cannulation of only one of the coronary ostia in this sinus. If this anomaly is present in the patient who has replacement of both mitral and aortic valves, the fixation rings of the prostheses may compress the lumen of the LC coronary artery which courses in a path between the prosthetic anuli[123] (Fig. 11).

BOTH RIGHT AND LEFT ANTERIOR DESCENDING FROM THE RIGHT AORTIC SINUS (OR LAD FROM THE RIGHT CORONARY ARTERY) AND LEFT CIRCUMFLEX CORONARY ARTERY FROM THE LEFT AORTIC SINUS.

This is a rare anomaly in hearts without other congenital anomalies of the heart or great anterior vessels. Several varieties have been recognized or are possible: (1) origin of the LAD from the right sinus or from the RCA with coursing to the left side of the heart anterior to the right ventricular infundibulum (Fig. 12); (2) origin of the LAD from the right sinus of Valsalva or directly from the RCA with coursing to the left side of the heart between the aorta and PT (to my knowledge, this pattern has not been observed but is theoretically possible); (3) origin of the LAD from the right aortic sinus or directly from the aorta with coursing to the left side of the heart in

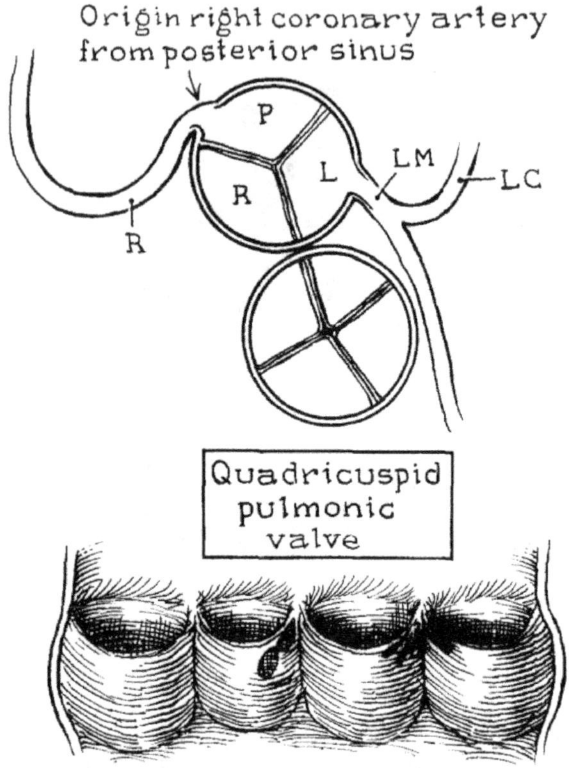

Fig. 13. Origin of the right *(R)* coronary artery from the posterior *(P)* aortic sinus in a 19-year-old man (DCMEO No. 83-09-602) who died suddenly while playing basketball. The pulmonic valve was quadricuspid. The cause of sudden death was not determined. Whether the coronary anomaly played a role in the sudden death is unclear.

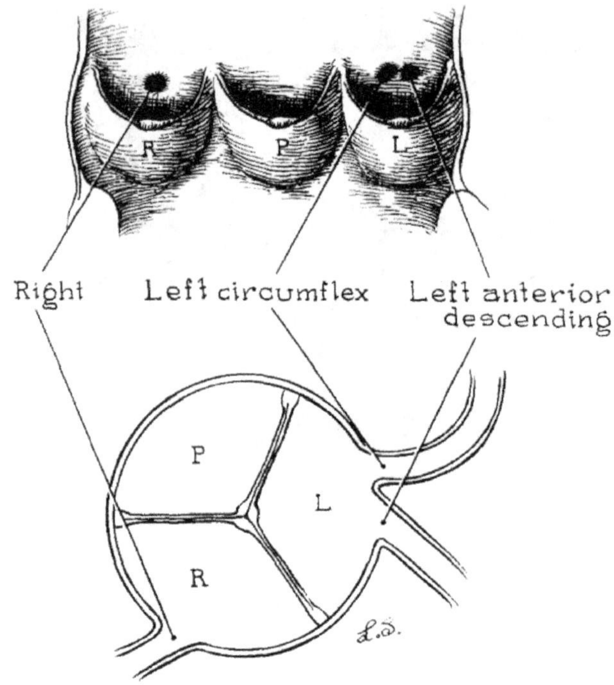

Fig. 14. Drawing of aorta showing origin of each of the left circumflex and left anterior descending coronary arteries from a separate ostium in the left *(L)* sinus of Valsalva. *R* = right and *P* = posterior sinus of Valsalva or cusp. (From Dicicco BS, et al: Am Heart J **104:**153, 1982.)

the ventricular septum beneath the right ventricular infundibulum.

RIGHT CORONARY ARTERY FROM THE POSTERIOR AORTIC SINUS AND THE LEFT MAIN CORONARY ARTERY FROM THE LEFT AORTIC SINUS.

This is an extremely rare anomaly in hearts without other congenital anomalies. Vlodaver et al.[124] found this anomaly in only one heart among their huge collection. That patient was a 72-year-old man who died from atherosclerotic coronary artery disease. I have seen this anomaly once (Fig. 13). The patient was a 19-year-old boy who died suddenly while playing basketball (DCMEO No. 83-09-602). It seemed unlikely that the anomaly was associated with the boy's sudden death because the heart weighed 450 gm, a weight which is clearly abnormal. The cause of the cardiomegaly, however, is unknown. I have observed one heart in which the ostium of the RCA was located just cephalad to the most cephalad extension of the commissures between the right and posterior aortic valve cusps (GT No. 85A-143). This patient was a 79-year-old man who died of consequences of atherosclerosis.

LEFT MAIN CORONARY ARTERY FROM THE POSTERIOR AORTIC SINUS AND RIGHT CORONARY ARTERY FROM THE RIGHT AORTIC SINUS.

To my knowledge this anomaly has not been reported in a patient without other anomalies of the heart or great vessels. I have examined a heart, however, in which the ostium of the LM coronary artery arose just above the commissure between the left and posterior aortic valve cusps (SGAH No. A82-1). The patient was a 54-year-old man who died from atherosclerotic coronary artery disease. The anomaly did not appear to have clinical significance.

BOTH LEFT ANTERIOR DESCENDING AND LEFT CIRCUMFLEX CORONARY ARTERIES FROM A SEPARATE OSTIUM IN THE LEFT AORTIC SINUS WITH THE RIGHT CORONARY ARTERY FROM THE RIGHT AORTIC SINUS.

This anomaly is fairly common. Ogden[53] found this anomaly in six necropsy patients in a 16-year period. I have observed it at necropsy in nine patients aged 35 to 82 years (mean 60) (seven men), all seen in a 7-year period. Two of the nine patients were reported previously[125] (Fig. 14). In none of the 9 patients was the anomaly of clinical significance. One of the nine patients was a 60-year-old man (A82-79) who also had congenitally bicuspid pulomonic and aortic valves; both LAD and LC arose from a separate ostium to the left of the raphe or in the location of the normal left aortic sinus of Valsalva (Fig. 15). Zumbo et al.[126] found this anomaly in 21 of 2089 hearts at necropsy.

ORIGIN OF ONLY 1 CORONARY ARTERY FROM THE AORTA WITHOUT ORIGIN OF A CORONARY ARTERY FROM THE PULMONARY TRUNK (SINGLE CORONARY OSTIUM IN AORTA)

History. According to Smith,[127] "single coronary artery" (a misnomer in my view—"single aortic coronary ostium without a pulmonary artery coronary ostium" is better) was first described in Banchi[128] in 1903.

Classification. Several authors have suggested classifications for single coronary ostium. Smith[127] in 1950 suggested three groups. (1) A single coronary artery that follows the course of the RCA with continuation into the LC which continues as the LAD, *or* a single LM which branches into the LAD and LC, the latter of which extends across the crux to form the RCA. (2) After its origin from a single aortic ostium, the main trunk branches quickly into a right and LM coronary artery or into a right, LAD, and LC coronary artery which reach their usual location a relatively short distance from the aortic ostium. (3) The single coronary artery branches so atypically that there is little similarity to the normal coursing of the three major (right, LAD, and LC) coronary arteries. In Smith's review of previously reported necropsy cases, there were nine in group one unassociated with other major cardiovascular anomalies (aged 33 to 66 years; six men), 15 in group 2 (aged 35 to 65; 10 men), and only two in group 3 (aged 22 and 38; one man). Smith actually found 15 patients in group 3 but 13 of them had various other congenital anomalies of the heart and great arteries.

Ogden and Goodyear[129] in 1970 suggested a classification employing five types subdivided by the letters "R" and "L" to indicate whether the single coronary ostium was in the right or left aortic sinus of Valsalva. These authors followed this letter by numbers 1 to 5 to indicate the pattern of anatomic distribution of the branches according to their initial divisions. In cases of single right coronary ostium, types 1 to 5, the letters "a," "b," and "c" were added to indicate the course of the branches. This classification has logic, but it is incomplete.

Lipton et al.[130] proposed a classification based on their angiographic studies, and it employed features

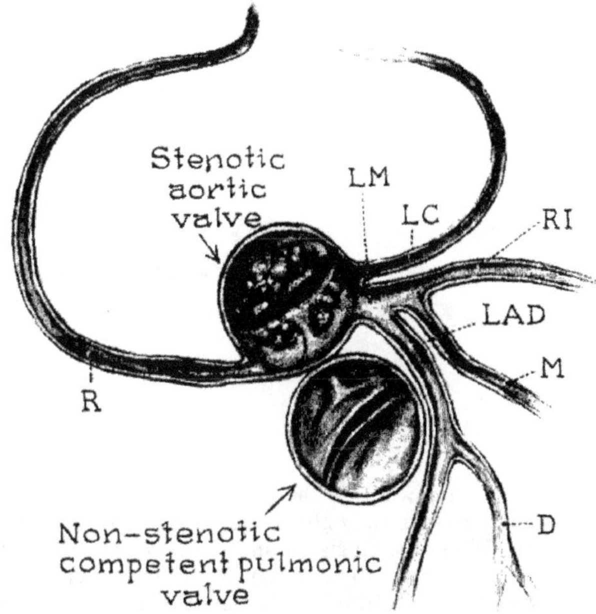

Fig. 15. Drawing showing origin of both left-sided coronary arteries directly from the left anterior side of the aorta in a 60-year-old man (No. A82-79) in whom both semilunar valves were congenitally bicuspid and the aortic valve was also stenotic. *D* = diagonal; *LAD* = left anterior descending; *LC* = left circumflex; *LM* = "left main"; *M* = marginal; *R* = right; *RI* = ramus intermedius.

of the classifications of both Smith[127] and Ogden and Goodyear.[129] These authors used the latter authors' "R" and "L" and "a" and "b" systems, but incorporated these letters into the three groups proposed by Smith. Thus, group 1 was designated R1 and L1; group 2 was designated R2-a and L2-a, R2-b and L2-b, and R2-p and L2-p; and group 3 included cases in which the LC and LAD arose separately from a single trunk arising from the right aortic sinus. The letter "a" indicated that the "transverse" branch from the single coronary artery passed "anterior" to the right ventricular infundibulum; "b" that it passed "between" the aorta and PT, and "p" that it passed retroaortic. This classification provides more easily memorable numbers and letters than that proposed by Ogden and Goodyear. I like this newer classification, but their group 3 is incomplete.

A purely descriptive classification of "single coronary artery" is presented in Table I.

Frequency. "Single coronary anomaly" is rare, particularly in the absence of other anomalies of the heart and great vessels. In 1968, Ogden (quoted by Ogden and Goodyear[129]) compiled 142 cases including 10 of his own. The male-to-female ratio was 1.4 to 1. The single coronary artery arose from the right aortic sinus in 70 cases (49%) and from the left aortic sinus in 64 cases (45%). Unfortunately, Ogden

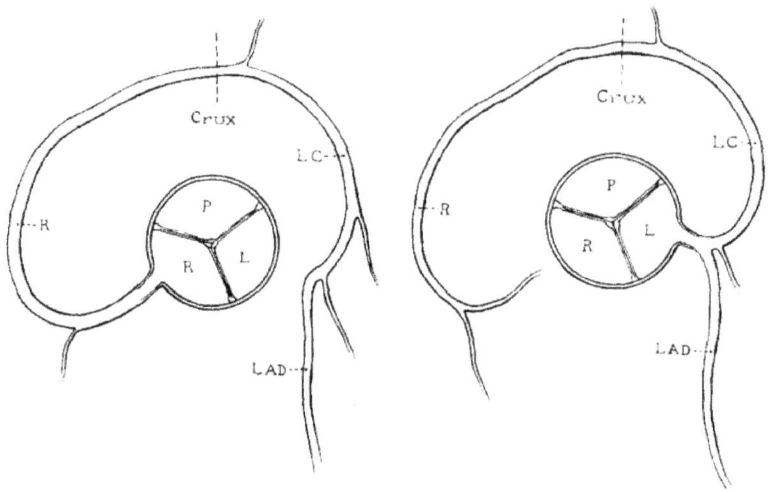

Fig. 16. Drawings of the two most common varieties of single coronary ostium. In one (*left*), the single ostium arises in the right aortic sinus and in the other (*right*), the single ostium arises in the left (*L*) aortic sinus. When the single coronary artery arises from the right aortic ostium, the right (*R*) coronary artery crosses the crux to continue as the left circumflex (*LC*), which in turn continues as the left anterior descending (*LAD*). When the single ostium is located in the left aortic sinus, the left main gives rise to the LAD and the LC, and LC crosses the crux to continue as the right coronary artery.

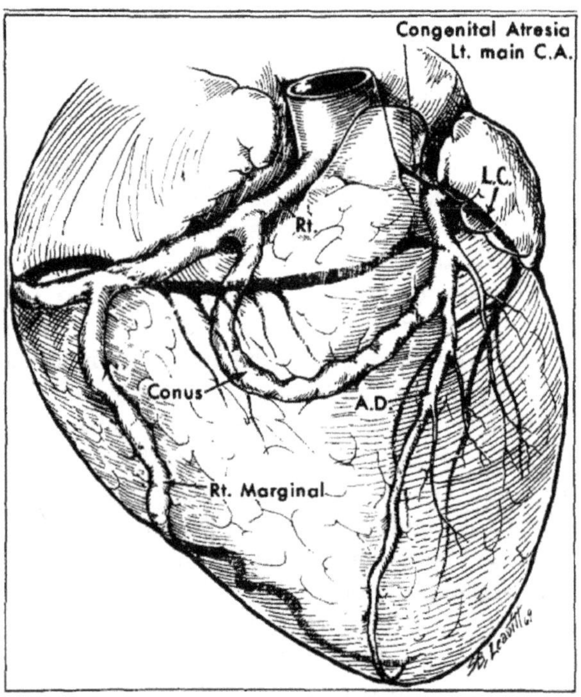

Fig. 17. Diagram of epicardial coronary arteries in a 60-year-old man (No. A69-61) who died suddenly as a consequence of severe coronary narrowing by atherosclerotic plaques but in whom the left *(Lt)* main coronary artery *(CA)* was congenitally atretic. This anomaly is equivalent to single coronary ostium with the single ostium in the right sinus of Valsalva. (From Fortuin NJ, and Roberts WC: Am J Med **50**:385, 1971. Reproduced by permission.)

included four cases in which a single LM coronary artery arose from the PT. The ages of the 142 patients ranged from 7 months to 20 years, and 41 (68%) of them had associated anomalies of the heart or great vessels; of the 82 patients aged 20 years or older, only five (6%) had associated anomalies of the heart or great arteries. Of the 46 cases with associated anomalies of the heart or great vessels, 17 (37%) had transposition of the great arteries, 10 (22%) had coronary artery fistula, and seven (15%) had bicuspid aortic valves; the remaining 12 patients (26%) had a variety of anomalies.

I have studied five adults at necropsy with single coronary ostium unassociated with other congenital cardiovascular defects. In two cases, both men, aged 39 and 73 years, a single LM pattern was present (Fig. 16). In one case, a 60-year-old man, the LM was congenitally atretic and the coronary pattern was of the single RCA type (Fig. 17). In one case, a 65-year-old man, the single artery arose in the left aortic sinus but the RCA coursed to the right between the aorta and PT after taking origin from the LM (Fig. 18). In the final case, a 69-year-old man with cardiovascular features of the Marfan syndrome but without the skeletal features of this syndrome, the single ostium was in the right aortic sinus with immediate origin of the LC with retroaortic course from the RCA and immediate origin of the LAD from the RCA, with coursing anterior to the right ventricular outflow tract.

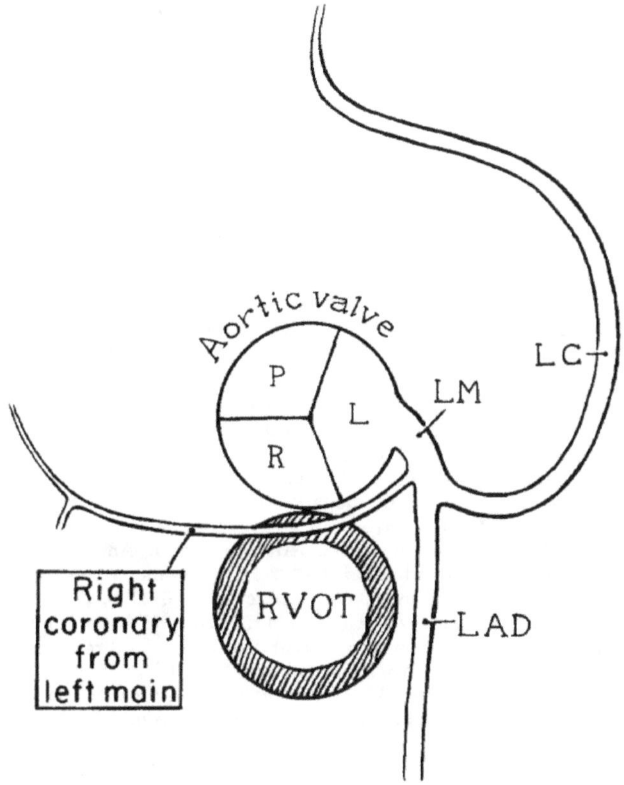

Fig. 18. Single coronary ostium with origin of the right coronary artery from the left main *(LM)* and coursing of the right coronary artery between aortic valve and right ventricular outflow tract *(RVOT)* on its way to the right atrioventricular sulcus in a 65-year-old man (DCVAH No. 84A-112) who never had signs or symptoms of cardiac dysfunction. *L* = left aortic sinus; *LAD* = left anterior descending; *LC* = left circumflex; *P* = posterior aortic sinus; *R* = right aortic sinus. (From Barbour DJ, and Roberts WC: Am J Cardiol **55**:609, 1985. Reproduced by permission.)

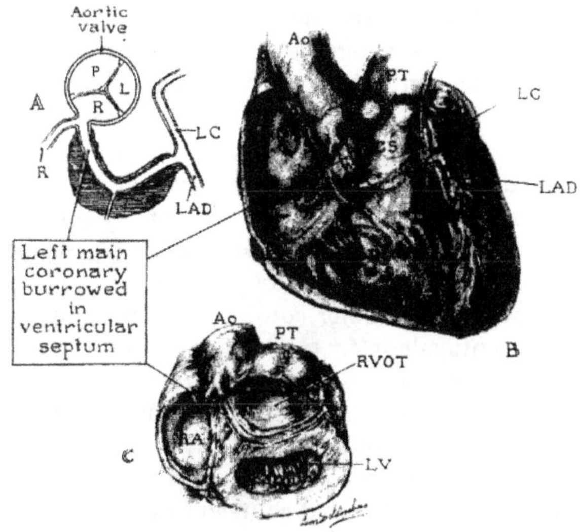

Fig. 19. Drawing of the heart in which the left main coronary artery arose from the right *(R)* aortic sinus and then the left main coursed behind the right ventricular outflow tract and within the crista supraventricular *(CS)* myocardium before entering the epicardium just anterior to the ventricular septum. The left main then divided into the left anterior descending *(LAD)* and left circumflex *(LC)* coronary arteries. This anomaly caused no cardiac dysfunction. *Ao* = ascending aorta; *L* = left aortic sinus; *LV* = left ventricle; *P* = posterior aortic sinus; *PT* = pulmonary trunk; *LV* = left ventricle; *R* = either right aortic sinus or right coronary artery; *RA* = right atrium; *RV* = right ventricle. (From Roberts WC, et al: Am Heart J **104**:303, 1982.)

Of the 142 cases analyzed by Ogden and Goodyear,[129] 31 (23%) had a single artery which did not branch (their type 1); 21 (15%) had two major branches with one coursing posterior to the aorta (type 2); 15 (11%) had two major branches with one branch coursing between the aorta and PT (type 3); 18 (13%) had two major branches with one branch coursing anterior to the PT (type 4); and seven patients (5%) had three major branches, all with origin of the single coronary artery in the right aortic sinus (type 5).

Of the 10 cases of single coronary artery diagnosed angiographically by Lipton et al.,[130] five had group 2R (a in one, b in two, and p in one), one had group 1L, and four had group 2L (b in three, and p in one). None of these 10 patients had other associated congenital cardiovascular anomalies; they ranged in aged from 39 to 64 years and eight were men.

Clinical significance. Although some patients have been described in whom symptoms of myocardial ischemia have occurred, the symptomatic patients nearly always have had associated atherosclerotic coronary disease, or valvular heart disease, or other major congenital anomalies of the heart or great arteries. Of course, severe atherosclerotic narrowing of the single coronary artery before it divides or narrowing of its ostium in the aorta may have particularly devastating consequences.

ORIGIN OF THE LM OR BOTH LAD AND LC CORONARY ARTERY FROM THE RCA WITH INTRAMYOCARDIAL COURSING TO THE LEFT SIDE OF THE HEART OF THE LM OR LAD IN THE VENTRICULAR SEPTUM BENEATH THE RIGHT VENTRICULAR INFUNDIBULUM.

At least 13 necropsy patients (10 men) have been described in whom a single aortic coronary ostium, located in the right aortic sinus, gave rise to the RCA. This in turn gave rise to the LM coronary artery, which coursed in the ventricular septum beneath the right ventricular infundibulum for about 5 cm before emerging in the epicardium just anterior to the ventricular septum where it gave off the LAD and LC branches (Fig. 19). These cases have been summarized by Roberts et al.[82] In none of the 13 patients was death, or myocardial dysfunction (if present) related to the coronary anomaly. These cases in which the LM coronary artery was in an intramyocardial location for about 5 cm indicate that tunneling of a major coronary artery—indeed, an artery equivalent to two major coronary arteries—has no functional significance in myocardium. Saner et al.[131] and Schulte et al.[132] reported single cases (a 73-year-old man and a 71-year-old woman) in whom the LAD arose either from the right aortic sinus or from the RCA and coursed in the ventricular septum beneath the right ventricular infundibulum before emerging just anterior to the ventricular septum. In neither patient had there been clinical evidence of myocardial ischemia.

REFERENCES

1. Abbott ME: Anomalous origin from the pulmonary arteries. *In* Osler W, editor: Osler's modern medicine, Its theories and practice. Philadelphia, 1908, Lea & Febiger, p. 420.
2. Abrikossoff A: Aneurysm des Linken Herzventrikels mit Abnromer Abganstelle der Linken Koronararterie von der Pulmonalis Bei Einem Funfmonatlichen Kinde. Virchows Arch Pathol Anat **203**:413, 1911.
3. Bland EF, White PD, Garland J: Congenital anomalies of the coronary arteries: Report of an unusual case associated with cardiac hypertrophy. Am Heart J **8**:787, 1933.
4. Fontana RS, Edwards JE: Congenital cardiac disease: A review of 357 cases studied pathologically. Philadelphia, 1962, W.B. Saunders Co., p. 291.
5. Thomas CS, Campbell WB, Alford WC Jr, Burrus GR, Stoney WS: Complete repair of anomalous origin of the left coronary artery in the adult. J Thorac Cardiovasc Surg **66**:439, 1973.
6. Donaldson RM, Raphael M, Radley-Smith R, Yacoub MH, Ross DN: Angiographic identification of primary coronary anomalies causing impaired myocardial perfusion. Cathet Cardiovasc Diagn **9**:237, 1983.
7. Edwards JE: Anomalous coronary arteries with special reference to arteriovenous-like communications. Circulation **17**:1001, 1958.
8. Edwards JE: The direction of blood flow in coronary arteries arising from the pulmonary trunk. Circulation **29**:163, 1964.
9. Moodie DS, Fyfe D, Gill CC, Cook SA, Lytle BW, Taylor PC, Fitzgerald R, Sheldon WC: Anomalous origin of the left coronary artery from the pulmonary artery (Bland-White-Garland syndrome) in adult patients: Long-term follow-up after surgery. Am Heart J **106**:381, 1983.
10. Jurishica AJ: Anomalous left coronary artery. Adult type. Am Heart J **54**:429, 1957.
11. George JM, Knowlan DM: Anomalous origin of the left coronary artery from the pulmonary artery in an adult. N Engl J Med **261**:993, 1959.
12. Lampe CFJ, Verheught APM: Anomalous left coronary artery. Adult type. Am Heart J **59**:769, 1960.
13. Liebman J, Hellerstein HK, Ankeney JL, Tucker A: The problem of the anomalous left coronary artery arising from the pulmonary artery in older children. Report of three cases. N Engl J Med **269**:486, 1963.
14. Talner NS, Halloran KH, Mahdavy M, Gardner TH, Hipona F: Anomalous origin of the left coronary artery from the pulmonary artery. A clinical spectrum. Am J Cardiol **15**:689, 1965.
15. Likar I, Criley JM, Lewis KB: Anomalous left coronary artery arising from the pulmonary artery in an adult. A review of the therapeutic problem. Circulation **33**:727, 1966.
16. Harthorne JW, Scannell JG, Dinsmore RE: Anomalous origin of the left coronary artery. Remediable cause of sudden death in adults. N Engl J Med **275**:660, 1966.
17. Wesselhoeft H, Fawcett JS, Johnson AL: Anomalous origin of the left coronary artery from the pulmonary trunk. Its clinical spectrum, pathology, and pathophysiology, based on a review of 140 cases with seven further cases. Circulation **38**:403, 1968.
18. Perry LW, Scott LP: Anomalous left coronary artery from pulmonary artery. Report of 11 cases; review of indications for and results of surgery. Circulation **41**:1043, 1970.
19. Askenazi J, Nadas AS: Anomalous left coronary artery originating from the pulmonary artery. Report of 15 cases. Circulation **51**:976, 1975.
20. Sabiston DC Jr, Floyd WL, McIntosh HD: Anomalous origin of the left coronary artery from the pulmonary artery in adults. Surgical management. Arch Surg **97**:963, 1968.
21. Usman A, Fernandez B, Uricchio JF, Nichols HT: Aberrant origin of left coronary artery combined with mitral regurgitation in an adult. Am J Cardiol **8**:130, 1961.
22. Burchell HB, Brown AL Jr: Anomalous origin or coronary artery from pulmonary artery masquerading as mitral insufficiency. Am Heart J **63**:388, 1962.
23. Fisher EA, Sepehri B, Lendrum B, Luken J, Levitsky S: Two-dimensional echocardiographic visualization of the left coronary artery in anomalous origin of the left coronary artery from the pulmonary artery. Pre- and postoperative studies. Circulation **63**:698, 1981.
24. Terai M, Nagai Y, Toba T: Cross-sectional echocardiographic findings of anomalous origin of left coronary artery from pulmonary artery. Br Heart J **50**:104, 1983.
25. Caldwell RL, Hurwitz RA, Girod DA, Weyman AE, Feigenbaum H: Two-dimensional echocardiographic differentiation of anomalous left coronary artery from congestive cardiomyopathy. Am Heart J **106**:710, 1983.
26. Robinson PJ, Sullivan ID, Kumpeng V, Anderson RH, MaCartney FJ: Anomalous origin of the left coronary artery from the pulmonary trunk. Potential for false negative diagnosis with cross sectional exhocardiography. Br Heart J **52**:272, 1984.
27. King DH, Danford DA, Huhta JC, Gutgesell HP: Noninvasive detection of anomalous origin of the left main coronary artery from the pulmonary trunk by pulsed Doppler echocardiography. Am J Cardiol **55**:608, 1985.
28. Gutgesell HP, Pinksy WW, DePuey EG: Thallium-201 myocardial perfusion imaging in infants and children; value in distinguishing anomalous left coronary artery from congestive cardiomyopathy. Circulation **61**:596, 1980.
29. Shem-Tov AA, Hegesh J, Schneeweiss A, Neufeld HN: Visualization of left coronary artery in anomalous origin of left coronary artery from pulmonary artery. Am Heart J **108**:621, 1984.
30. Sabiston DC Jr, Neill CA, Taussig HB: The direction of blood flow in anomalous left coronary artery arising from the pulmonary artery. Circulation **22**:591, 1960.
31. Rowe GG, Young WP: Anomalous origin of the coronary arteries with special reference to surgical treatment. J Thorac Cardiovasc Surg **39**:777, 1960.
32. Roche AHG: Anomalous origin of the left coronary artery from the pulmonary artery in the adult. Report of uneventful ligation in two cases. Am J Cardiol **20**:561, 1967.
33. Baue AE, Baum S, Blakemore WS, Zinsser HF: A later stage of anomalous coronary circulation with origin of the left coronary artery from the pulmonary artery. Coronary artery steal. Circulation **36**:878, 1967.

34. Reis RL, Cohen LS, Mason DT: Direct measurement of instantaneous coronary blood flow after total correction of anomalous left coronary artery. Circulation **39** and **40** (suppl I):229, 1969.
35. Somerville J, Ross DN: Left coronary artery from the pulmonary artery. Physiological considerations of surgical correction. Thorax **25**:207, 1970.
36. Neches WH, Mathews RA, Park SC, Lenox CC, Zuberbuhler JR, Siewers RD, Bahnson HT: Anomalous origin of the left coronary artery from the pulmonary artery. A new method of surgical repair. Circulation **50**:582, 1974.
37. Chaitman BR, Bourassa MG, Lesperance J, Grondin P: Anomalous left coronary artery from the pulmonary artery. An eight year angiographic follow-up after saphenous vein bypass graft. Circulation **51**:552, 1975.
38. Pinsky WW, Fagan LR, Mudd JGH, Willman VL: Subclavian–coronary artery anastomosis in infancy for the Blank-White-Garland syndrome. A three-year and five-year follow-up. J Thorac Cardiovasc Surg **72**:15, 1976.
39. Grace RR, Angelini P, Cooley DA: Aortic implantation of anomalous left coronary artery arising from pulmonary artery. Am J Cardiol **39**:608, 1977.
40. Wilson CL, Dlabal, PW, Holeyfield RW, Akins CW, Knauf DG: Anomalous origin of left coronary artery from pulmonary artery. Case report and review of literature concerning teenagers and adults. J Thorac Cardiovasc Surg **73**:887, 1977.
41. Shrivastava S, Castaneda AR, Moller JH: Anomalous left coronary artery from pulmonary trunk. Long-term follow-up after ligation. J Thorac Cardiovasc Surg **76**:130, 1978.
42. Wilson CL, Dlabal PW, McGuire SA: Surgical treatment of anomalous left coronary artery from pulmonary artery: Follow-up in teenagers and adults. Am Heart J **98**:440, 1979.
43. Donaldson RM, Raphael MJ, Yacoub MH, Ross DN: Hemodynamically significant anomalies of the coronary arteries. Surgical aspects. Thorac Cardiovasc Surg **30**:7, 1982.
44. Fisher J, McDonald G, Brinker J, Neill CA, Donahoo JS, Baughman KL: Transpulmonary artery correction of anomalous origin of the left coronary artery by saphenous vein graft. Cathet Cardiovasc Diagn **9**:373, 1983.
45. Savage RW, Glover MU, Utley JR: Reoperation for correction of anomalous origin of left coronary artery from the pulmonary artery with return of left ventricular function. Cathet Cardiovasc Diagn **10**:37, 1984.
46. Bagger JP, Vesterlund T, Nielsen TT: Cardiac metabolism and coronary hemodynamics before and after bypass surgery for anomalous origin of the left main coronary artery from the pulmonary trunk. Am J Cardiol **55**:864, 1985.
47. Brooks H St J: Two cases of an abnormal coronary artery of the heart arising from the pulmonary artery: with some remarks upon the effect of this anomaly in producing cirsoid dilation of the vessels. J Anat Physiol **20**:26, 1885 and 1886.
48. Monchelberg JG: Uber eine seltene Anomalie des Koronarterienabgangs. Zentralbl Herz Krankheiten **6**:441, 1914.
49. Schley J: Abnormer Ursprung der rechten Kranzarterie aus der Pulmonalis bei einem 61-jahringer Mann. Frankfurt Z Pathol **32**:1, 1925.
50. Jordan RA, DRy TJ, Edwards JE: Anomalous origin of the right coronary artery from the pulmonary trunk. Mayo Clin Proc **25**:673, 1950.
51. Cronk ES, Sinclair JG, Rigdon RH: An anomalous coronary artery arising from the pulmonary artery. Am Heart J **42**:906, 1951.
52. Tingelstad, JB, Lower RR, Eldredge WJ: Anomalous origin of the right coronary artery from the main pulmonary artery. Am J Cardiol **30**:670, 1972.
53. Ogden JA: Congenital anomalies of the coronary arteries. Am J Cardiol **25**:474, 1970.
54. Lerberg DB, Ogden JA, Zuberbuhler JR, Bahnson HT: Anomalous origin of the right coronary artery from the pulmonary artery. Ann Thorac Surg **27**:87, 1979.
55. Wald S, Stonecipher K, Baldwin BJ, Hutter DO: Anomalous origin of the right coronary artery from the pulmonary artery. Am J Cardiol **27**:677, 1971.
56. Eugstes GS, Oliva PB: Anomalous origin of the right coronary artery from the pulmonary artery. Chest **63**:294, 1973.
57. Achtel RA, Zaret BL, Iben AB, Hurley EJ: Surgical correction of congenital left coronary artery–main pulmonary artery fistula in association with anomalous right coronary artery. J Thorac Cardiovasc Surg **70**:46, 1975.
58. Bregman D, Brennan FJ, Singer A, Vinci J, Parodi EN, Cassarella WJ, Edie RN: Anomalous origin of right coronary artery from the pulmonary artery. J Thorac Cardiovasc Surg **72**:626, 1976.
59. Mintz GS, Iskandrian AS, Bemis CE, Mundth ED, Owens JS: Myocardial ischemia in anomalous origin of the right coronary artery from the pulmonary trunk. Proof of a coronary steal. Am J Cardiol **51**:610, 1983.
60. Worsham C, Sanders SP, Bulger BM: Origin of the right coronary artery from the pulmonary trunk: Diagnosis by two-dimensional echocardiography. Am J Cardiol **55**:232, 1985.
61. van Meurs-van Woezik H, Serruys PW, Reiber JH, Bos E, deVilleneuve VH: Coronary artery changes 3 years after reimplantation of an anomalous right coronary artery. Eur Heart J **5**:175, 1984.
62. Roberts WC, Robinowitz M: Anomalous origin of the left anterior descending coronary artery from the pulmonary trunk with origin of the right and left circumflex coronary arteries from the aorta. Am J Cardiol **54**:1381, 1984.
63. Donaldson RM, Thornton A, Raphael MJ, Sturridge MF, Emanuel RW: Anomalous origin of the left anterior descending coronary artery from the pulmonary trunk. Eur J Cardiol **10**:295, 1979.
64. Effler DB, Sheldon WC, Turner JJ, Groves LK: Coronary arteriovenous fistulae: Diagnosis and surgical management. Report of fifteen cases. Surgery **61**:41, 1967.
65. Honey M, Lincoln JCR, Osborne MP, de Bono DP: Coarctation of the aorta with right aortic arch. Report of surgical correction in 2 cases: One with associated anomalous origin of left circumflex coronary artery from the right pulmonary artery. Br Heart J **37**:937, 1975.
66. Chaitman BR, Bourassa MG, Lesperance J, Dominquez JLD, Saltiel J: Aberrant course of the left anterior descending coronary artery associated with anomalous left circumflex origin from the pulmonary artery. Circulation **52**:955, 1975.
67. Ott DA, Cooley DA, Pinsky WW, Mullins CE: Anomalous origin of circumflex coronary artery from right pulmonary artery. Report of a rare amonaly. J Thorac Cardiovasc Surg **76**:190, 1978.
68. Grayzel DM, Tennant R: Congenital atresia of the tricuspid orifice and anomalous origins of the coronary arteries from the pulmonary artery. Am J Pathol **10**:791, 1934.
69. Limbourg M: Uber den Ursprung der Kranzarterien des Herzens aus der Arteria pulmonalis. Beitr Pathol Anat **100**:191, 1937.
70. Williams JW, Johnson WS, Boulware JR Jr: Case of tetralogy of Fallot with both coronary arteries arising from pulmonary artery. J Fla Med Assoc **37**:561, 1951.
71. Swan WC, Werthammer S: Aberrant coronary arteries: Experiences in diagnosis with report of three cases. Ann Intern Med **42**:873, 1955.
72. Alexander RW, Griffith GC: Anomalies of the coronary arteries and their clinical significance. Circulation **14**:800, 1956.
73. Schulze WB, Rodin AE: Anomalous origin of both coronary arteries. Report of a case with discussion of teratogenic theories. Arch Pathol **72**:36, 1961.
74. Roberts WC: Anomalous origin of both coronary arteries from the pulmonary artery. Am J Cardiol **10**:595, 1962.
75. Blake HA, Manion WC, Mattingly TW, Baroldi G: Coronary artery anomalies. Circulation **390**:927, 1964.

76. Gonzales-Angulo A, Reyes HA, Wallace SA: Anomalies of the origin of coronary arteries (special reference to single coronary artery). Angiology **17**:96, 1966.
77. Kecton BR, Keenan DJM, Monro JL: Anomalous origin of both coronary arteries from the pulmonary trunk. Br Heart J **49**:397, 1983.
78. Feldt RH, Ongley PA, Titus JL: Total coronary arterial circulation from pulmonary artery with survival to age seven: Report of case. Mayo Clin Proc **40**:539, 1965.
79. Monselise MB, Vlodaver Z, Neufeld HN: Single coronary artery; origin from the pulmonary trunk in association with ventricular septal defect. Chest **58**:613, 1970.
80. Barth CW III, Roberts WC: Left main coronary artery originating from the right sinus of Valsalva and coursing between aorta and pulmonary trunk. J Am Col Cardiol **7**:366, 1986.
81. Cheitlin MD, DeCastro CM, McCallister HA: Sudden death as a complication of anomalous left coronary origin from the anterior sinus of Valsalva. A not so minor congenital anomaly. Circulation **50**:780, 1974.
82. Roberts WC, Dicicco BS, Waller BF, Kishel JC, McManus BM, Dawson SL, Hunsaker JC III, Luke JL: Origin of the left main from the right coronary artery or from the right aortic sinus with intramyocardial tunneling to the left side of the heart via the ventricular septum: The case against clinical significance of myocardial bridge or coronary tunnel. Am Heart J **104**:303, 1982.
83. Murphy DA, Roy DL, Sohal M, Chandler BM: Anomalous origin of left main coronary artery from anterior sinus of Valsalva with myocardial infarction. J Thorac Cardiovasc Surg **75**:282, 1978.
84. Sanes S: Anomalous origin and course of the left coronary artery in a child. Am Heart J **14**:219, 1978.
85. Nicod JL: Anomalie coronaire et mort subite. Cardiologia **20**:172, 1952.
86. Alexander RW, Griffith GC: Anomalies of the coronary arteries and their clinical significance. Circulation **14**:800, 1956.
87. Jokl E, McClellan JT, Ross GD: Congential anomaly of the left coronary artery in young athlete. JAMA **182**:174, 1962.
88. Jokl E, McClellan JT, Williams WC, Gouze FJ, Bartholomew RD: Congenital anomaly of left coronary artery in young athletes. Cardiologia **49**:253, 1966.
89. Benson PA, Lack AR: Anomalous aortic origin of the left coronary artery. Arch Pathol **86**:214, 1968.
90. Benson PR: Anomalous aortic origin of coronary artery with sudden death: Case report and review. Am Heart J **79**:254, 1970.
91. Pedal I: Aortale ursprungsanomalie einer koronararterie. Dtsch Med Wochenschr **101**:1601, 1976.
92. Liberthson RR, Dinsmore RE, Fallon JT: Abberant coronary artery origin from the aorta. Report of 18 patients, review of the literature and delineation of natural history and management. Circulation **59**:748, 1979.
93. Lynch P: Soldiers, sport and sudden death. Lancet **1**:1235, 1980.
94. Tsung SH, Huant TY, Change HH: Sudden death in young athletes. Arch Pathol Lab Med **106**:168, 1982.
95. Betend B, Gillet P, Moreau P, David L: Origine aortique anormale de l'artere coronaire gauche. A propos del la mort subite d'un adolescent. Arch Fr Pediatr **40**:479, 1983.
96. Topaz O, Edwards JE: Pathologic features of sudden death in children, adolescent, and young adults. Chest **87**:476, 1985.
97. Davia JE, Green DC, Cheitlin MD, DeCastro C, Brott WH: Anomalous left coronary artery origin from the right coronary sinus. Am Heart J **108**:165, 1984.
98. Mustafa I, Gula G, Radley-Smith R, Durrer S, Yacoub M: Anomalous origin of the left coronary artery from the anterior aortic sinus: A potential cause of sudden death. J Thorac Cardiovasc Surg **82**:297, 1981.
99. Liberthson RR, Zaman L, Weyman A, et al: Aberrant origin of the left coronary artery from the proximal right coronary artery: Diagnostic features and pre- and postoperative course. Clin Cardiol **5**:377, 1982.
100. Ishikawa T, Brandt PW: Anomalous origin of the left main coronary artery from the right anterior aortic sinus: Angiographic definition of anomalous course. Am J Cardiol **55**:770, 1985.
101. Kimbiris D: Anomalous origin of the left main coronary artery from the right sinus of Valsalva. Am J Cardiol **55**:765, 1985.
102. Moodie DS, Gill C, Loop FD, Sheldon WC: Anomalous left main coronary artery originating from the right sinus of Valsalva. Pathophysiology, angiographic definition and surgical approaches. J Thorac Cardiovasc Surg **80**:198, 1980.
103. Sacks JH, Londe SP, Rosenbluth A, Zalis EG: Left main coronary artery bypass for aberrant (aortic) intramural left coronary artery. J Thorac Cardiovasc Surg **73**:733, 1977.
104. Roberts WC, Siegel RJ, Zipes DP: Origin of the right coronary artery from the left sinus of Valsalva and its functional consequences: Analysis of 10 necropsy patients. Am J Cardiol **49**:863, 1982.
105. Chaitman BR, Lesperance J, Saltiel J, Bourassa MG: Clinical, angiographic, and hemodynamic findings in patients with anomalous origin of the coronary arteries. Circulation **53**:122, 1975.
106. Kimbiris D, Iskandrian AS, Segal BL, Bemis CE: Anomalous aortic origin of coronary arteries. Circulation **58**:606, 1978.
107. Thompson SI, Vieweg WVR, Alpert JS, Hagan AD: Anomalous origin of the right coronary artery from the left sinus of Valsalva with associated chest pain. Report of 2 cases. Cathet Cardiovasc Diagn **2**:397, 1976.
108. Benge W, Martins JB, Funk DC: Morbidity associated with anomalous origin of the right coronary artery from the left sinus of Valsalva. Am Heart J **99**:96, 1980.
109. Bloomfield P, Erhlich C, Folland ED, Bianco JA, Tow DE, Parisi AF: Anomalous right coronary artery: A surgically correctable cause of angina pectoris. Am J Cardiol **51**:1235, 1983.
110. Keren A, Tzivoni D, Stern S: Functional consequences of right coronary artery originating from left sinus of Valsalva (Letter). Am J Cardiol **51**:1241, 1983.
111. Brandt B III, Martins JB, Marcus ML: Anomalous origin of the right coronary artery from the left sinus of Valsalva. N Engl J Med **309**:596, 1983.
112. Hanzlick R, Stivers RR: Sudden death in a marathon runner with origin of the right coronary artery from the left sinus of Valsalva (Letter). Am J Cardiol **51**:1467, 1983.
113. Hanzlick RL, Stivers RR: Sudden death due to anomalous right coronary artery in a 26-year-old marathon runner. Am J Forensic Med Pathol **4**:265, 1983.
114. Hanzlick R, Stivers RR: Anomalous right coronary artery (Letter). Am J Forensic Med Pathol **5**:285, 1984.
115. Isner JM, Shen EM, Martin ET, Fortin RV: Sudden unexpected death as a result of anomalous origin of the right coronary artery from the left sinus of Valsalva. Am J Med **76**:155, 1984.
116. Antopol W, Kugel MA: Anomalous origin of the left circumflex coronary artery. Am Heart J **8**:802, 1933.
117. Roberts WC, Waller BF, Roberts CS: Fatal atherosclerotic narrowing of the right main coronary artery: Origin of the left arterior descending or left circumflex coronary artery from the right (the true "left main equivalent"). Am Heart J **104**:638, 1982.
118. White NK, Edwards JE: Anomalies of the coronary arteries: Report of four cases. Arch Pathol **45**:766, 1948.
119. Page HL Jr, Engel JH, Campbell WB, Thomas CS: Anomalous origin of the left circumflex coronary artery. Recognition, angiographic demonstration and clinical significance. Circulation **50**:768, 1974.
120. Ray PR, Saunders A, Sowton GE: Review of variations in origin of left circumflex coronary artery. Br Heart J **37**:287, 1975.

121. Baltaxe HA, Wixson D: The incidence of congenital anomalies of the coronary arteries in the adult population. Radiology **122**:47, 1977.
122. Liberthson RR, Dinsmore RE, Bharati S, Rubenstein JJ, Caulfeld J, Wheeler EO, Harthorne JW, Lev M: Aberrant coronary origin from the aorta. Diagnosis and clinical significance. Circulation **50**:774, 1974.
123. Roberts WC, Morrow AG: Compression of anomalous left circumflex coronary arteries by prosthetic valve fixation rings. J Thorac Cardiovasc Surg **57**:834, 1969.
124. Vlodaver Z, Neufeld HN, Edwards JE: Coronary arterial variations in the normal heart and in congenital heart disease. New York, 1975, Academic Press, Inc., p. 171.
125. DiCicco BS, McManus BM, Waller BF, Roberts WC: Separate aortic ostium of the left anterior descending and left circumflex coronary arteries from the left aortic sinus of Valsalva (absent left main coronary artery). AM HEART J **104**:153, 1982.
126. Zumbo O, Fani K, Jarmolych J, Daoud AS: Coronary atherosclerosis and myocardial infarction in hearts with anomalous coronary arteries. Lab Invest **14**:571, 1965.
127. Smith JC: Review of single coronary artery with report of 2 cases. Circulation **1**:1168, 1950.
128. Banchi A: Morfologia della arteriae coronariae cordis. Arch Ital Anat Embriol **3**:89, 1903.
129. Ogden JA, Goodyear AVN: Patterns of distribution of the single coronary artery. Yale J Biol Med **43**:11, 1970.
130. Lipton MJ, Barry WH, Obrez I, Silverman J, Wexler L: Isolated single coronary artery: Diagnosis, angiographic classification, and clinical significance. Radiology **130**:39, 1979.
131. Saner HE, Saner BD, Dykoski RK, Edwards JE: Origin of anterior descending coronary artery from right aortic sinus. Intramyocardial tunneling to the left side of the heart. Arch Pathol Lab Med **108**:642, 1984.
132. Schulte MA, Waller BF, Hull MT, Pless JE: Origin of the left anterior descending coronary artery from the right aortic sinus with intramyocardial tunneling to the left side of the heart via the ventricular septum: A case against clinical and morphologic significance of myocardial bridging. AM HEART J **110**:499, 1985.

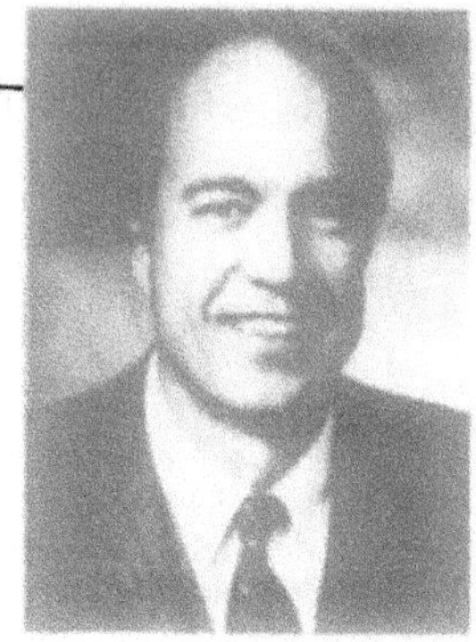

Sudden Cardiac Death: Definitions and Causes

The phrase "sudden death" has been used by lay and medical persons for nearly 450 years. It has many definitions. "Sudden death" might be a game played to break a tie or the extra minutes of play added to a tied game, the winning team being the first team to score. In medicine "sudden death" generally denotes death which is *nonviolent* or nontraumatic, which is *unexpected*, which is *witnessed* and which is *instantaneous* or occurs within a few minutes of an abrupt change in previous clinical state. In heart disease the word "cardiac" is usually placed between the words "sudden" and "death," and the phrase "sudden cardiac death" usually is applied to persons who die suddenly from atherosclerotic coronary artery disease.[1] Necropsy studies of persons dying suddenly from cardiac disease, however, disclose many causes of "sudden cardiac death," and, therefore, greater specificity is required in terms to prevent confusion (Figure). Of persons dying suddenly from cardiovascular disease, the cause may be *cardiac* or *noncardiac*. The cardiac causes may be subdivided into *coronary* and *noncoronary*. Of the coronary causes, atherosclerosis is, of course, by far the most common, and the term *atherosclerotic sudden coronary death* may be applied to them.[2–18] In young persons particularly, several *nonatherosclerotic* coronary conditions, mainly coronary anomalies, cause sudden death.[19–28] Of the cardiac but noncoronary causes of sudden death, the most common are cardiomyopathy, particularly hypertrophic cardiomyopathy,[29–39] and valvular heart disease, most commonly the conditions causing left ventricular outflow obstruction,[40–50] sometimes associated with prosthetic or bioprosthetic heart valves.[51] Also, there are noncardiac but vascular causes of sudden death.[52–55] Some cardiac arrhythmic causes of sudden death not necessarily associated with morphologic abnormalities, e.g., prolonged QT interval syndrome, do not appear in the accompanying figure.[19,56–59]

Some examples of the many causes of sudden cardiac death:

(1) A 13-year-old athletic boy, the son of a former professional football player, collapsed while jogging and died. He had always been asymptomatic. His brother, a year older, had died a year earlier also while jogging. M.M.'s electrocardiogram 6 months earlier was considered "abnormal" but his left ventricular pressure was normal and there was no obstruction to left ventricular outflow.

(2) A 17-year-old girl, who ran 40 miles weekly, suddenly collapsed and died just after crossing the finish line of a 3-mile race. She had been "healthy" all of her life.

(3) A 19-year-old male midshipman was always asymptomatic until he suddenly collapsed and died while sitting on a bench immediately after running around the track several times. On admission examination a year earlier, electrocardiogram had shown ventricular premature complexes and left-axis deviation. The heart was of normal size by chest roentgenogram. The blood pressure was 135/80 mm Hg.

(4) A 28-year-old woman, well all her life, suddenly collapsed and died while running for a bus.

(5) A 28-year-old man died suddenly while pushing a brick-loaded wheelbarrow. He had been well until 2 days earlier when he complained of "pain in his neck," but this did not prevent him from performing his usual construction job activities.

(6) A 33-year-old woman, a domestic, collapsed while at work and died immediately. She had been healthy all her life.

(7) A 44-year-old woman, a secretary, collapsed while walking in her office and died. She had been asymptomatic all her life but on routine examination several years earlier was found to have precordial murmurs (each grade 2/6) consistent with "aortic stenosis and regurgitation." Chest radiograph had shown mild cardiomegaly and electrocardiogram had shown left ventricular hypertrophy.

(8) A 44-year-old male taxicab driver was well until about 1 hour before death when he became enraged because his taxicab was bombarded by snowballs thrown by 3 youths. One snowball entered an open window and hit him in the face, knocking off his glasses. He immediately radioed the police, who arrived several minutes later and apprehended the youths. The police described the taxicab driver as "livid with rage" over the incident and advised him to leave the scene. Thirty minutes later he radioed his dispatcher that he was having breathing difficulties. He arrived at the dispatcher's office a few minutes later, collapsed, and died.

(9) A 60-year-old male school teacher had been well all his life except for recognized systemic hypertension until a

few minutes before death, when he became enraged when trying to prevent 2 students in the school gymnasium from fighting. He finally broke up the fight and, while walking away from the event minutes later, collapsed and died.

(10) An 81-year-old woman, who had had a pacemaker inserted for complete heart block 23 months earlier, collapsed and died while climbing a flight of stairs in her home. During the preceding 2 days, she had noted excessive fatigue, nausea and vomiting.

The cause of death in each of the above 10 patients was different and had not a necropsy been performed, the cause of death could not have been accurately predicted. Patient 1 had *hypertrophic cardiomyopathy*. Patient 2 had *congenital hypoplasia of both right and left circumflex coronary arteries with inadequate perfusion of the posterior wall of the left ventricle.*[19] Patient 3 had *origin of the left main coronary artery from the right sinus of Valsalva with coursing of the left main between the pulmonary trunk and ascending aorta.*[23] Patient 4 had *isolated coronary arterial dissection* involving the left anterior descending and left circumflex coronary arteries.[28] Patient 5 had extensive *cardiac sarcoidosis.*[35] Patient 6 had a *ruptured sinus of Valsalva aneurysm* (into the pericardial sac rather than into the right side of the heart).[60] Patient 7 had *congenital origin of the left main coronary artery from the pulmonary trunk.*[24] Patient 8 had *atherosclerotic coronary artery disease* with severe narrowing of each of the 3 major coronary arteries. Patient 9 had a large heart (550 g [normal ≤400 g]) from *systemic hypertension* but no significant coronary arterial narrowing or other recognized cause of sudden death.[61] Patient 10 had severe *coronary arterial atherosclerosis* with *acute myocardial infarction* complicated by *rupture of the left ventricular free wall* and hemopericardium. Tests of the pacemaker after death disclosed that it had functioned normally.

In any study discussing sudden death from cardiovascular disease, the word *sudden* needs defining. The World Health Organization has used a 24-hour definition of sudden, meaning, of course, death occurring within 24 hours of an abrupt change in previous clinical status.[62] When this definition of sudden is used, many cases of acute myocardial infarction are intermixed with cases of sudden atherosclerotic coronary death unassociated with myocardial necrosis. Because it takes over 6 hours for histologic evidence of myocardial necrosis to be apparent and because most persons who die suddenly do so within an hour of change in previous clinical status, the 6-hour definition for "sudden" when applied to "atherosclerotic sudden coronary death" more clearly separates the infarct cases from the noninfarct ones.[2,4,16,17]

Although the term sudden implies *unexpected*, in only a quarter of victims of atherosclerotic coronary artery disease is sudden death the initial manifestation of coronary artery disease, and therefore, truly unexpected. Sudden death in patients with angina pectoris or healed myocardial infarction is really not so unexpected. Likewise, in persons with hypertrophic cardiomyopathy and certain forms of valvular heart disease, death suddenly is always a shock but, in actuality, not so unexpected.

Although sudden death is usually reserved for *nonviolent* or nontraumatic deaths, various mentally or even physically traumatic events can precipitate sudden death.[63,64]

The term "sudden death" is often used for persons in hospitals who are found dead, most often in their beds. I try to reserve the term "sudden death" for persons who have fatal or nonfatal cardiac arrest *outside* the hospital or at least

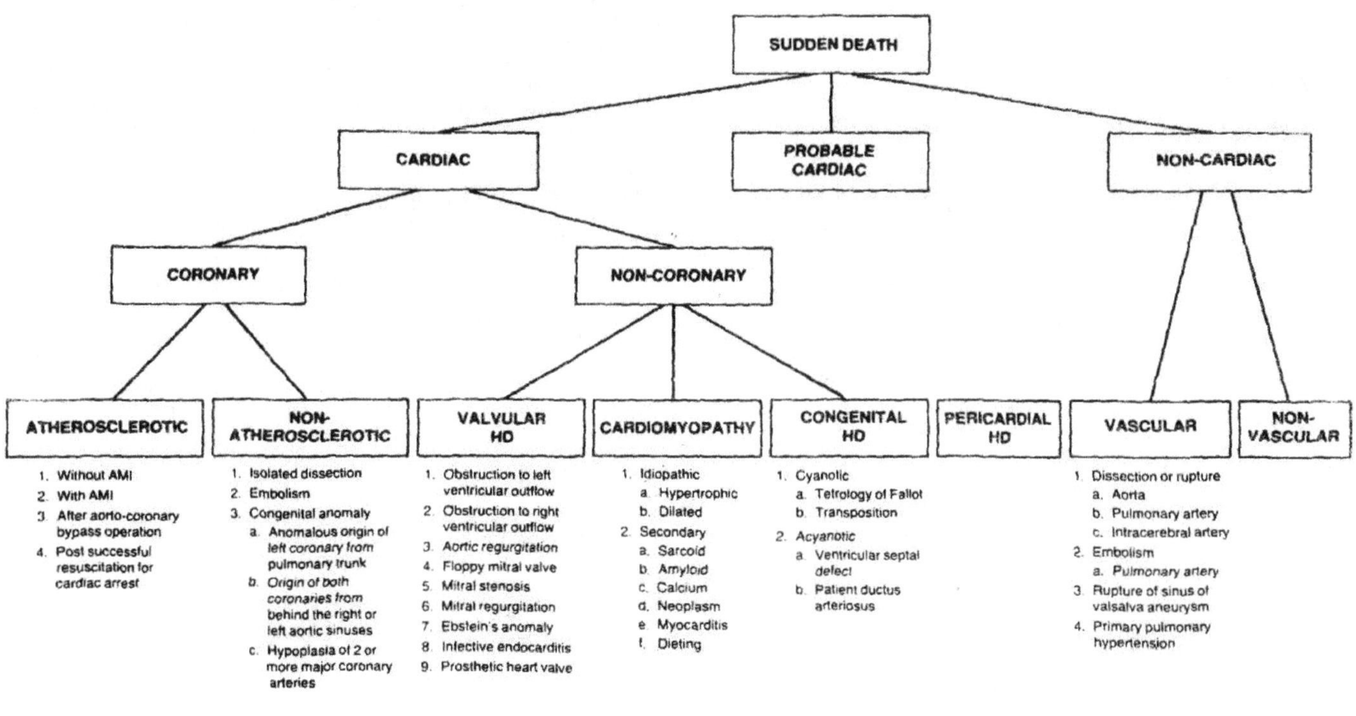

whose symptoms of cardiovascular dysfunction appear initially while outside a hospital. Some of these victims, of course, are rushed to hospitals, where fatal cardiac arrest occurs shortly after arrival.

I have examined many manuscripts that have used the phrase "sudden death" as a *cause* of death: "Patient so and so died of sudden death or patient so and so had sudden death but lived"! Obviously, the term "sudden death" should be used only as a *mode* of death or otherwise lawyers and editors will have a field day.

The use of the term "sudden death" in persons who are successfully resuscitated is not recommended. The use of the term *nonfatal cardiac arrest* (to contrast with *fatal cardiac arrest*) is preferable in this circumstance.

In summary, sudden cardiac death has many causes. Atherosclerotic coronary artery disease, obviously, is by far the most common cause of "sudden cardiac death," but the latter term is not synonmous with atherosclerotic coronary artery disease. "Sudden coronary death" is not ideal either because not all sudden coronary deaths are the result of atherosclerotic narrowing, but "sudden coronary death" is more precise than "sudden cardiac death." Sudden death is not always so *sudden*, or so *unexpected*, or *witnessed* and indeed it may be caused by or precipitated by mental or physical violence. Thus, greater precision is needed when discussing "sudden cardiac death."

William C. Roberts

William C. Roberts, MD
Editor in Chief

References

1. Eisenberg MS, Bergner L, Hallstrom AP, Cummins RO. *Sudden cardiac death. Sci Am 1986(May);254:37–43.*

2. Roberts WC, Buja LM. *The frequency and significance of coronary arterial thrombi and other observations in fatal acute myocardial infarction. A study of 107 necropsy patients. Am J Med 1972;52:425–443.*

3. Bulkley BH, Roberts WC. *Atherosclerotic narrowing of the left main coronary artery. A necropsy analysis of 152 patients with fatal coronary heart disease and varying degrees of left main narrowing. Circulation 1976;53:823–828.*

4. Roberts WC, Jones AA. *Quantitation of coronary arterial narrowing at necropsy in sudden coronary death. Analysis of 31 patients and comparison with 25 control subjects. Am J Cardiol 1979;44:39–45.*

5. Waller BF, Roberts WC. *Sudden death while running in conditioned runners aged 40 years or over. Am J Cardiol 1980;45:1292–1300.*

6. Brosius FC Jr, Blackbourne BD, Roberts WC. *Death in the disco. Chest 1980;78:321–323.*

7. Walker BF, Csere RS, Baker WP, Roberts WC. *Running to death. Chest 1981;79:346–349.*

8. Brosius FC III, Waller BF, Roberts WC. *Radiation heart disease. Analysis of 16 young (aged 33 to 50 years) necropsy patients who received over 3,500 rads to the heart. Am J Med 1981;70:519–530.*

9. Cabin HS, Roberts WC. *Fatal cardiac arrest during cardiac catheterization for angina pectoris: analysis of 10 necropsy patients. Am J Cardiol 1981;48:1–8.*

10. Roberts WC, Maron BJ. *Sudden death while playing professional football. Am Heart J 1981;102:1061–1063.*

11. McManus BM, Waller BF, Graboys TB, Mitchell JH, Siegel RJ, Miller HS Jr, Froelicher VF, Roberts WC. *Exercise and sudden death. Part I. Current Prob Cardiol 1981;6(9):1–89.*

12. McManus BM, Waller BF, Graboys TB, Mitchell JH, Siegel RJ, Miller HS Jr, Froelicher VF, Roberts WC. *Exercise and sudden death. Part II. Current Prob Cardiol 1982;6(10):1–57.*

13. Roberts WC, Curry RC Jr, Isner JM, Waller BF, McManus BM, Mariani-Constantini R, Ross AM. *Sudden death in Prinzmetal's angina with coronary spasm documented by angiography. Analysis of three necropsy patients. Am J Cardiol 1982;50:203–210.*

14. Warnes CA, Kishel JC, Roberts WC. *Fatal cardiac arrest during cardiac catheterization for angina pectoris. A marker of quadruple vessel disease. Chest 1983;84:631–632.*

15. Sprecher DL, Schaefer EJ, Kent KM, Gregg RE, Zech LA, Hoeg JM, McManus B, Roberts WC, Brewer HB Jr. *Cardiovascular features of homozygous familial hypercholesterolemia: analysis of 16 patients. Am J Cardiol 1984;54:20–30.*

16. Warnes CA, Roberts WC. *Sudden coronary death: relation of amount and distribution of coronary narrowing at necropsy to previous symptoms of myocardial ischemia, left ventricular scarring and heart weight. Am J Cardiol 1984;54:65–73.*

17. Warnes CA, Roberts WC. *Comparison at necropsy by age group of amount and distribution of narrowing by atherosclerotic plaque in 2995 five-mm long segments of 240 major coronary arteries in 60 men aged 31 to 70 years with sudden coronary death. Am Heart J 1984;108:431–435.*

18. Warnes CA, Roberts WC. *Sudden coronary death: comparison of patients with to those without coronary thrombus at necropsy. Am J Cardiol 1984;54:1206–1211.*

19. Maron BJ, Roberts WC, McAllister HA, Rosing DR, Epstein SE. *Sudden death in young athletes. Circulation 1980;62:218–229.*

20. Maron BJ, Epstein SE, Roberts WC. *Causes of sudden death in competitive athletes. JACC 1986;7:204–214.*

21. Roberts WC, Siegel RJ, Zipes DP. *Origin of the right coronary artery from the left sinus of Valsalva and its functional consequences: analysis of 10 necropsy patients. Am J Cardiol 1982;49:863–868.*

22. Roberts WC, Robinowitz M. *Anomalous origin of the left anterior descending coronary artery from the pulmonary trunk with origin of the right and left circumflex coronary arteries from the aorta. Am J Cardiol 1984;54:1381–1383.*

23. Barth CW III, Roberts WC. *Left main coronary artery originating from the right sinus of Valsalva and coursing between the aorta and pulmonary trunk. JACC 1986;7:366–373.*

24. Roberts WC. *Major anomalies of coronary arterial origin seen in adulthood. Am Heart J 1986;111:in press.*

25. Roberts WC, Silver MA, Sapala JC. *Intussusception of a coronary artery associated with sudden death in a college football player. Am J Cardiol 1986;57:179–180.*

26. Roberts WC. *Coronary embolism: a review of causes, consequences, and diagnostic considerations. Cardiovasc Med 1978;3:699–710.*

27. Waller BF, Dixon DS, Kim RW, Roberts WC. *Embolus to the left main coronary artery. Am J Cardiol 1982;50:658–660.*

28. Bulkley BH, Roberts WC. *Dissecting aneurysm (hematoma) limited to coronary artery. A clinicopathologic study of six patients. Am J Med 1973;55:747–756.*

29. Roberts WC, Ferrans VJ. *Pathologic anatomy of the cardiomyopathies. Idiopathic dilated and hypertrophic types, infiltrative types and endomyocardial disease with and without eosinophilia. Hum Pathol 1975;6:287–342.*

30. Maron BJ, Roberts WC, Edwards JE, McAllister HA, Foley DD, and Epstein SE. *Sudden death in patients with hypertrophic cardiomyopathy: characterization of 26 patients without functional limitation. Am J Cardiol 1978;41:803–810.*

31. Maron BJ, Lipson LC, Roberts WC, Savage DD, Epstein SE. *"Malignant" hypertrophic cardiomyopathy: identification of a subgroup of families with unusually frequent premature death. Am J Cardiol 1978;41:1133–1140.*

32. Maron BJ, Tajik AJ, Ruttenberg HD, Graham TP, Atwood GF, Victoria BE, Lie JT, Roberts WC. *Hypertrophic cardiomyopathy in infants: clinical features and natural history. Circulation 1982;65:7–17.*

33. Maron BJ, Roberts WC, Epstein SE. *Sudden death in hypertrophic cardiomyopathy: a profile of 78 patients. Circulation 1982;65:1388–1394.*

34. Maron BJ, Epstein SE, Roberts WC. *Hypertrophic cardiomyopathy: a common cause of sudden death in the young competitive athlete. Eur Heart J 1983;4:suppl F:135–144.*

35. Roberts WC, McAllister HA Jr, Ferrans VJ. *Sarcoidosis of the heart. A clinicopathologic study of 35 necropsy patients (group I) and review of 78 previously described necropsy patients (group II). Am J Med 1977;63:86–108.*

36. Virmani R, Bures JC, Roberts WC. *Cardiac sarcoidosis: a major cause of sudden death in young individuals. Chest 1980;77:423–428.*

37. Saffitz JE, Sazama K, Roberts WC. *Amyloidosis limited to small arteries causing angina pectoris and sudden death. Am J Cardiol 1983;51:1234–1235.*

38. Roberts WC, Waller BF. *Cardiac amyloidosis causing cardiac dysfunction: analysis of 54 necropsy patients. Am J Cardiol 1983;52:137–146.*

39. Saffitz JE, Ferrans VJ, Rodriquez ER, Lewis FR, Roberts WC. *Histiocytoid cardiomyopathy: a cause of sudden death in apparently healthy infants. Am J Cardiol 1983;52:215–217.*

40. Morrow AG, Fort L III, Roberts WC, Braunwald E. *Discrete subaortic stenosis complicated by aortic valvular regurgitation. Clinical, hemodynamic, and pathologic studies and the results of operative treatment. Circulation 1965;31:163–171.*

41. Roberts WC, Morrow AG. *Aortico-left ventricular tunnel. A cause of massive aortic regurgitation and of intracardiac aneurysm. Am J Med*

1965;39:662–667.
42. Roberts WC. *The structure of the aortic valve in clinically-isolated aortic stenosis. An autopsy study of 162 patients over 15 years of age.* Circulation 1970;42:91–97.
43. Roberts WC. The congenitally bicuspid aortic valve. A study of 85 autopsy cases. *Am J Cardiol 1970;26:72–83.*
44. Roberts WC. Anatomically isolated aortic valvular disease. The case *against its being of rheumatic etiology. Am J Med 1970;49:151–159.*
45. Roberts WC, Perloff JK, Constantino T. Severe valvular aortic stenosis in patients over 65 years of age. *A clinicopathologic study. Am J Cardiol* 1971;27:497–506.
46. Falcone MW, Roberts WC, Morrow AG, Perloff JK. Congenital aortic stenosis resulting from unicommissural valve. Clinical and anatomic features in twenty-one adult patients. *Circulation 1971;44:272–280.*
47. Roberts WC, Dangel JC, Bulkley BH. Non-rheumatic valvular cardiac disease. A clinicopathologic survey of 27 different conditions causing valvular dysfunction. Cardiovasc Clin 1973;5:333–446.
48. Maron BJ, Redwood DR, Roberts WC, Henry WL, Morrow AG, Epstein SE. Tunnel subaortic stenosis. Left ventricular outflow tract obstruction produced by fibromuscular tubular narrowing. Circulation 1976;54:404–416.
49. Roberts WC. Morphologic features of the normal and abnormal mitral valve. Am J Cardiol 1983;51:1005–1028.
50. Roberts WC. The 2 most common congenital heart diseases. Am J Cardiol 1984;53:1198.
51. Roberts WC. *The silver anniversary of cardiac valve replacement.* Am J Cardiol 1985;56:503–506.
52. Roberts WC. *The aorta: its acquired diseases and their consequences as* viewed from a morphologic perspective. In: Lindsay J Jr, Hurst JW, eds. The *Aorta. New York: Grune & Stratton, 1979:51–117.*
53. Roberts WC. Aortic dissection: anatomy, consequences, and causes. Am *Heart J 1981;101:195–214.*
54. Waller BF, Reis RL, McIntosh CL, Epstein SE, Roberts WC. The Marfan cardiovascular disease without the Marfan syndrome. Chest 1980;77:533–540.
55. Roberts WC, Honig HS. *The spectrum of cardiovascular disease in the* Marfan syndrome: a clinico-morphologic study of 18 necropsy patients and *comparison to 151 previously reported necropsy patients. Am Heart J* 1982;104:115–135.
56. Isner JM, Sours HE, Paris AL, Ferrans VJ, Roberts WC. *Sudden, unexpected death in avid dieters using the liquid-protein-modified-fast diet. Observations in 17 patients and the role of the prolonged QT interval.* Circulation 1979;60:1401–1412.
57. Siegel RJ, Cabeen WR Jr, Roberts WC. *Prolonged QT interval–ventricular tachycardia syndrome from massive rapid weight loss utilizing the liquid-protein-modified-fast diet: sudden death with sinus node ganglionitis and* neuritis. Am Heart J 1981;102:121–123.
58. Isner JM, Roberts WC, Heymsfield SB, Yager J. *Anorexia nervosa and* sudden death. Ann Intern Med 1985;102:49–52.
59. McManus BM, Fleury TA, Roberts WC. *Fatal catecholamine crisis in pheochromocytoma: curable cause of cardiac arrest.* Am Heart J 1981; 102:930–932.
60. Roberts WC. Congenital cardiovascular abnormalities usually "silent" until adulthood: morphologic features of the floppy mitral valve, valvular aortic stenosis, hypertrophic cardiomyopathy, sinus of Valsalva aneurysm, and the Marfan syndrome. In: Roberts WC, ed. Congenital Heart Disease in Adults. Philadelphia: FA Davis, 1979:407–453 (Cardiovasc Clin 10;[1]:-574).
61. Roberts WC. The hypertensive diseases. Evidence that systemic hypertension is greater risk factor to the development of other cardiovascular diseases than previously suspected. Am J Med 1975;59:523–532.
62. *Classification of atherosclerotic lesions. Report of a study group. WHO* Techn Rep Ser 1958 (No. 143).
63. Engel GL. *Sudden and rapid death during psychological stress.* Forklore or folk wisdom? Ann Intern Med 1971;74:771–782.
64. Engel GL. Psychologic stress, vasodepressor (vasovagal) syncope, and sudden death. Ann Intern Med 1978;89:403–412.

Idiopathic Dilated Cardiomyopathy: Analysis of 152 Necropsy Patients

WILLIAM C. ROBERTS, MD, ROBERT J. SIEGEL, MD,
and BRUCE M. McMANUS, MD, PhD

Certain clinical and cardiac necropsy findings are described in 152 patients aged 16 to 78 years (mean 45) with idiopathic dilated cardiomyopathy: 109 (72%) were men and 43 (28%) were women. Compared with the women, the men had a significantly ($p < 0.05$) shorter mean duration of chronic congestive heart failure (CHF) (43 vs 69 months), a higher percentage of habitual alcoholism (40 vs 24%) and a higher mean heart weight (632 vs 551 g). The male to female ratio among the 58 known alcoholics was 7.3:1 and among the 70 known nonalcoholics, 1.5:1 ($p < 0.05$). The mean duration of clinical evidence of CHF was similar among the known alcoholics and the known nonalcoholics (each 50 months). Of the 152 patients, 148 (97%) had clinical evidence of chronic CHF; in 114 patients it was the initial manifestation of idiopathic dilated cardiomyopathy, and in most it became intractable and caused death. The interval from onset of chronic CHF to death (known in 120 patients) ranged from 1 to 264 months (mean 54). Comparison of the 27 patients surviving >72 months after onset of chronic CHF to the 64 patients surviving ≤36 months disclosed a significantly higher frequency in the longer survival group of older patients, of women, of habitual alcoholics, of patients with chest pain syndromes, diabetes mellitus, pulmonary emboli, of patients treated with warfarin and of patients with larger hearts at necropsy. Each of the 4 patients without chronic CHF died suddenly and sudden death was the initial manifestation of idiopathic dilated cardiomyopathy in them. An additional 33 patients also died suddenly, but each of them previously had had chronic CHF. Of the 79 patients (of the 131 for whom information was available) with either pulmonary or systemic emboli or both, 67 (85%) had either right- or left-sided thrombi or mural endocardial plaques or both, whereas of the 52 patients without emboli, 36 (69%) had intracardiac thrombi or plaques ($p < 0.05$). Electrocardiograms in the last 6 months of life in 101 patients disclosed atrial fibrillation in 25; complete left (41 patients) or right (6 patients) bundle branch block or indeterminate intraventricular conduction delay (4 patients) in 51 patients; QRS voltage indicative of ventricular hypertrophy in 44 patients (left ventricular in 39 patients). The patients with left bundle branch block compared with those without had a significantly longer duration of CHF, (83 vs 43 months), larger mean heart weights (628 vs 590 g) and a higher frequency of grossly visible scars (44 vs 13%). The total 12-lead QRS amplitude in 35 men ranged from 74 to 250 mm (mean 147) (10 mm = 1 mV) and in the 14 women from 75 to 243 mm (mean 167). The hearts at necropsy in the women ranged from 360 to 860 g (mean 551) and in the men from 400 to 940 g (mean 632) ($p < 0.05$). Grossly visible left ventricular scars were observed in 22 (14%) patients. Histologic examination (96 patients) of sections of the ventricular myocardium disclosed interstitial or replacement fibrosis in 55 patients (57%), and inflammatory cell infiltrates in 5 patients.

(Am J Cardiol 1987;60:1340–1355)

Idiopathic dilated cardiomyopathy (IDC) is a well-recognized condition both clinically and morphologically. It is characterized by dilatation of both ventricular cavities and manifested clinically by chronic congestive heart failure (CHF), which usually becomes intractable and eventually fatal. Despite the relative frequency of this condition, few studies focusing on a large number of necropsy patients have been reported. Herein, we describe certain clinical and morphologic features in 152 necropsy patients fulfilling a rigorous definition of IDC.

Patients Studied

Criteria for inclusion: All 152 patients were older than 15 years of age, all had dilated right and left ventricular cavities and all had hearts of increased weight (>350 g in women and >400 g in men). None had narrowing of any of the epicardial coronary arteries of >75% in cross-sectional area, none had a significant congenital cardiac anomaly, none had an anatomically abnormal cardiac valve (except for minimal focal thickening of the margins of the anterior mitral leaflet), none had a defect in the atrial or ventricular septum other than possibly a valvular competent patent foramen ovale, none had an infiltrative myocardial disease (such as amyloid, sarcoid, iron, calcium or glycogen), none had a systemic disease other than possibly adult-onset diabetes mellitus, none had a neurologic disease, none had extensive cystic or interstitial pulmonary parenchymal disease and none had a major grossly visible abnormality of the pericardium. During the last 3 months of life, the systemic arterial systolic pressure was <140 mm Hg and the systemic arterial diastolic pressure was <90 mm Hg. Additionally, none had clinical evidence in the past of hypertrophic cardiomyopathy and none had other family members who had hypertrophic cardiomyopathy. Patients with complete heart block from birth were excluded, and patients who had received a drug known to be capable of causing a dilated cardiomyopathy, such as doxorubicin, were excluded. Patients with a history of habitual alcoholism were included and considered to have idiopathic dilated cardiomyopathy.

From the Pathology Branch, National Heart, Lung, and Blood Institute, National Institutes of Health, Bethesda, Maryland.
Manuscript received July 22, 1987, revised manuscript received and accepted August 18, 1987.

Address for reprints: William C. Roberts, MD, Building 10, Room 2N-258, National Institutes of Health, Bethesda, Maryland 20892.

Dr. Siegel's present address is Division of Cardiology, Department of Medicine, Cedars-Sinai Medical Center, Los Angeles, California.

Dr. McManus's present address is Cardiovascular Registry, Department of Pathology and Microbiology, University of Nebraska Medical Center, Omaha, Nebraska.

Selection of cases: All hearts and clinical and morphologic records of cases classified as IDC in the files of the Pathology Branch, National Heart, Lung, and Blood Institute, were reviewed. Of nearly 200 cases so classified, nearly 50 were eliminated from this study because they did not fulfill the aforementioned clinical and morphologic criteria. A total of 152 patients fulfilled the criteria and form the basis of this report. The clinical and necropsy records were reviewed in all 152 patients. Detailed data on the electrocardiograms recorded in the last 6 months of life were available in 101 of the 152 patients, and in 55 the electrocardiograms themselves were reexamined. All 152 hearts were examined initially by 1 of us (WCR) and most were examined later by RJS and BMM. All patients were studied at necropsy from 1959 through April 1981. The patients were studied clinically at 14 different hospitals, mainly those located in the Washington, DC, area, and the hearts were subsequently brought to one of us (WCR) for examination. In addition to the gross examination of each heart, at least 2 histologic sections of left ventricular wall extending from endocardium to epicardium and measuring ≥2 cm in circumferential length were examined in 96 of the 152 cases. A least 1 full-thickness histologic section of ventricular septum and right ventricular free wall also was examined in 80 and 88 of these 96 patients, respectively.

Statistics: Comparisons of all parametric data were made using the 2-tailed *t* test for independent samples when comparisons between 2 groups were made, and using a 1-way analysis of variance when comparisons among ≥3 groups were made. The level of significance was 0.05. Comparisons of nonparametric data were made using the chi-square method with a level of significance of 0.05. Correlations were tested using Spearman's rho and linear regression coefficients and calculated when deemed useful.

Clinical Findings

Age, race, sex and duration of congestive heart failure: The 152 patients ranged in age from 16 to 78

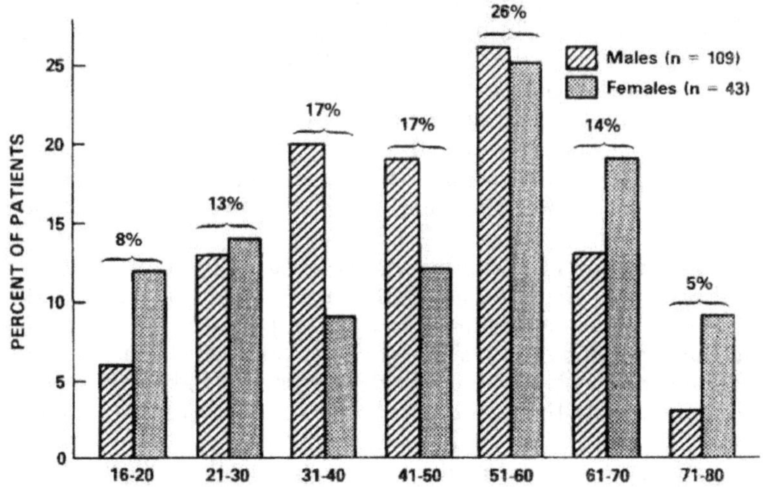

FIGURE 1. Bar graph showing the percent of patients with idiopathic dilated cardiomyopathy dying during various decades.

TABLE I Certain Clinical and Necropsy Characteristics of 152 Patients with Idiopathic Dilated Cardiomyopathy and Comparisons Between 109 Men and 43 Women

	Total (n = 152)	Men (n = 109)	Women (n = 43)	p Value
Age (yr) (mean)	16–78 (45)	16–73 (45)	16–78 (49)	NS
Black:white	90:47 (1.9:1)	63:36 (1.8:1)	27:11 (2.5:1)	NS
Duration (mo) CHF	0–240 (54)	6–204 (43)	1–240 (69)	<0.05
Pulmonary edema	34/86 (40%)	21/61 (34%)	13/25 (52%)	NS
Angina pectoris	15/105 (14%)	11/75 (15%)	4/30 (13%)	NS
Nonanginal chest pain	40/114 (35%)	29/82 (35%)	11/32 (34%)	NS
"AMI" (history)	25/113 (22%)	17/80 (21%)	8/33 (24%)	NS
Alcoholism	49/136 (36%)	40/99 (40%)	9/37 (24%)	NS
Emboli				
Pulmonary, clinical	49/126 (39%)	31/89 (35%)	18/37 (49%)	NS
Pulmonary, necropsy	39/101 (39%)	29/72 (40%)	10/29 (34%)	NS
Systemic, clinical	24/122 (20%)	20/88 (23%)	4/34 (12%)	NS
Pulmonary, necropsy	23/90 (26%)	19/65 (29%)	4/25 (16%)	NS
Mode of death				
Chronic CHF	81/139 (58%)	55/98 (56%)	26/41 (63%)	NS
Sudden	38/139 (27%)	28/98 (29%)	10/41 (24%)	NS
Pulmonary embolus	12/139 (9%)	8/98 (8%)	4/41 (10%)	NS
Other	8/139 (6%)	7/98 (7%)	1/41 (2%)	NS
Heart weight (g)	400–940 (605)	400–940 (632)	360–860 (551)	<0.05
Intracavitary thrombi (T) only	42/148 (28%)	30/105 (29%)	12/43 (28%)	NS
Endocardial plaques (P) only	32/148 (22%)	22/105 (21%)	10/43 (23%)	NS
Both T and P	37/148 (25%)	28/105 (27%)	9/43 (21%)	NS
Transmural LV scars (gross)	9/148 (6%)	9/105 (9%)	5/43 (12%)	NS
LV replacement fibrosis (microscopic only)	71/96 (73%)	50/74 (68%)	21/22 (95%)	<0.05

AMI = acute myocardial infarction; CHF = chronic congestive heart failure; LV = left ventricular; NS = not significant (p >0.05); SD = sudden death.

years (mean 45) (Figure 1). Of the 137 in whom race was known, 90 (66%) were black and 47 (34%) were white. Of the 152 patients, 109 (72%) were men and 43 (28%) were women. Comparison of various clinical and morphologic findings between the men and women is summarized in Table I. Of the 16 factors analyzed, 3 were significantly ($p < 0.05$) different between the 2 groups. Compared with women, men had a shorter mean duration of chronic CHF (43 vs 69 months), a higher percentage of habitual alcoholism (40 vs 24%) and a higher mean heart weight (632 vs 551 g).

Relation to pregnancy: Of the 43 women, the relation of onset of symptoms of chronic CHF to pregnancy was known in 39. In 13 (33%) of them, symptoms of CHF appeared either during pregnancy (2 patients) or within 12 months after delivery (11 patients). In 7 of the latter 11 patients, the onset of symptoms of cardiac dysfunction was within 3 months of delivery. Comparison of findings in the 13 women with onset of CHF in the peripartum period to those in 26 women in whom the onset of CHF was known not to be related to pregnancy disclosed only 1 statistically significant factor (Table II): the mean age of the peripartum patients was younger ($p < 0.001$) than that of the nonperipartum patients.

Habitual alcoholism: Information regarding habitual intake of alcohol was available in 128 of the 152 patients. At least 58 (45%) of the 128 patients were considered by their physicians to be "alcoholic." Comparison of 15 observations in the 58 known habitual alcoholics with those in the 70 nonalcoholic cases disclosed several factors to be significantly different (Table III). The male to female ratio among the alcoholics was 7.3:1 and in the nonalcoholics, 1.5:1 ($p < 0.05$). The mean duration of symptoms of CHF was the same (50 months); the mean heart weight (631 vs 593 g) was significantly ($p < 0.05$) greater in the alcoholics compared with the nonalcoholics, a reflection of the greater proportion of men in the alcoholic group.

Diabetes mellitus: Information regarding the presence or absence of diabetes mellitus was available in 110 of the 152 patients. Of that number, 8 patients (7%) (4 men, 4 women) had known diabetes mellitus beginning after age 35. Their ages at death ranged from 37 to 71 years (mean 55) and their ages at onset of diabetes from 36 to 64 years (mean 51). Two patients were treated with insulin and 4 with hypoglycemic agents; the type of diabetic treatment received in the other 2 patients is uncertain. Two of the 8 patients were habitual alcoholics. The duration of chronic CHF in the 8 patients ranged from 24 to 204 months (mean 105). At necropsy, 2 of the 8 patients had grossly visible left ventricular scars, and on histologic examination, none had abnormalities of the intramural coronary arteries.

Familial cardiomyopathy: At least 1 other family member had a similar fatal cardiac condition in 9 (6%) of the 152 patients. Of these 9 patients, at least 20 family members were affected by a similar cardiac condition, and all of the 20 affected relatives died before age 50 years, most before age 40 years. The 9 patients with familial dilated cardiomyopathy ranged in age from 17 to 58 years (mean 37); 7 were men and 2 were women. Only 2 were habitual alcoholics. The duration of the chronic CHF in 8 of the 9 patients ranged from 3 to 72 months (mean 46); the ninth patient had evidence of CHF for only 10 days. Six of the 9 patients died from chronic CHF and 3 died suddenly.

TABLE II *Idiopathic Dilated Cardiomyopathy in Women: Comparison of Findings in 13 Necropsy Patients with Onset in Peripartum Period to Those in 26 Necropsy Patients with Onset in Nonperipartum Period*

	Peripartum Onset (n = 13)	Nonperipartum Onset (n = 26)	p Value
Age (yr) (mean)	18–61 (32)	21–78 (57)	<0.001
Black:white	10:3	18:8	NS
Systemic hypertension	1 (8%)	8 (31%)	NS
Habitual alcoholism	2 (15%)	7 (27%)	NS
Duration CHF (mo) (mean)	2–264 (65)	1–240 (65)	NS
Embolic events	7 (54%)	18 (69%)	NS
Pulmonary	6 (46%)	13 (50%)	NS
Systemic	1 (8%)	5 (19%)	NS
Sudden death	3 (23%)	7 (26%)	NS
Heart weight (g) (mean)	370–770 (512)	360–810 (567)	NS
Transmural LV scars	1 (8%)	8 (31%)	NS
Intracardiac thrombi (only)	3 (23%)	8 (31%)	NS
Endocardial plaques (only)	3 (23%)	6 (22%)	NS
Both plaques and thrombi	2 (15%)	7 (27%)	NS
Either plaques or thrombi	8 (61%)	21 (81%)	NS

CHF = congestive heart failure; LV = left ventricular; NS = not significant.

TABLE III **Clinical and Necropsy Characteristics of 58 Alcoholic and 70 Nonalcoholic Patients with Idiopathic Dilated Cardiomyopathy**

	Alcoholic (n = 58)	Nonalcoholic (n = 70)	p Value
Age (yr) (mean)	21–78 (46)	16–75 (45)	NS
Male:female	51:7 (7.3:1)	42:28 (1.5:1)	<0.05
Black:white	37:14 (2.6:1)	34:29 (1.2:1)	NS
Duration (mo) CHF	0–144 (50)	1–168 (50)	NS
Pulmonary edema	9/33 (27%)	18/46 (39%)	<0.05
Angina pectoris	8/43 (19%)	7/59 (12%)	NS
"AMI" (history)	14/43 (32%)	8/61 (13%)	<0.05
Emboli			
Pulmonary, clinical	18/39 (46%)	24/59 (41%)	NS
Pulmonary, necropsy	16/36 (44%)	26/41 (63%)	<0.05
Systemic, clinical	12/41 (29%)	6/71 (8%)	<0.05
Systemic, necropsy	13/35 (37%)	8/38 (21%)	<0.05
Mode of death			
Chronic CHF	26/46 (57%)	39/67 (58%)	NS
Sudden death	14/46 (30%)	19/67 (28%)	NS
Pulmonary embolus	5/46 (11%)	5/67 (7%)	NS
Other	1/46 (2%)	4/67 (6%)	NS
Heart weight (g) (mean)	360–940 (631)	370–940 (593)	<0.05
Intracavitary thrombi (T) only	16/58 (28%)	18/70 (26%)	NS
Endocardial plaques (P) only	12/58 (21%)	14/70 (20%)	NS
Both T and P	16/58 (28%)	15/70 (21%)	NS
Transmural LV scars (gross)	8/58 (14%)	3/69 (4%)	NS
Replacement fibrosis (microscopic)	20/34 (59%)	19/31 (61%)	NS

AMI = acute myocardial function; CHF = congestive heart failure; LV = left ventricular; NS = not significant.

None of the 9 and none of the affected family members had evidence either clinically or morphologically of hypertrophic cardiomyopathy.

Congestive heart failure: Of the 152 patients, 148 (97%) had clinical evidence of chronic CHF; in 114 patients, it was the initial manifestation of their illness, and in most it became intractable and caused death. Good information on the interval from onset of chronic CHF to death was available in 120 of the 148 patients and it ranged from 1 to 264 months (mean 54) (Table I and Figure 2). From onset of CHF to death in these patients, 29 (24%) lived ≤12 months; 54 (45%), 13 to 60 months; 20 (17%) 61 to 120 months and 16 (14%), >120 months. These 120 patients were divided into 3 survival periods and 13 factors were compared (Table IV). Comparison of the 27 patients surviving >72 months after onset of chronic CHF to the 64 patients surviving ≤36 months disclosed a significantly ($p < 0.05$) higher frequency in the longer survival group of older patients, of women, of habitual alcoholics, of patients with chest pain syndromes, diabetes mellitus and pulmonary emboli, of patients treated with warfarin and of patients with bigger hearts at necropsy.

Sudden death: Each of the 4 patients without clinical evidence of chronic CHF died suddenly and unexpectedly and sudden death in them was the initial manifestation of IDC. All 4 were men aged 23 to 43 years (mean 31) with hearts weighing 480 to 780 g

TABLE IV Duration of Survival in Idiopathic Dilated Cardiomyopathy: Clinical and Necropsy Findings

	Duration (mo) of Survival			
	≤36	>36–72	>72	p value
Number of patients	64 (53%)	29 (24%)	27 (23%)	—
Age (yr) (mean)	16–75 (40)	20–71 (49)	16 –75 (51)	<0.05
Black:white	35/60(58%):25/60(42%)	16/27(59%):11/27(41%)	13/22(59%):9/22(41%)	NS
Male:female	49(77%):15(23%)	21(72%):8(28%)	13(48%):14(52%)	<0.05
Duration (mo) CHF (mean)	0–36 (15)	38–72 (58)	84–264 (131)	<0.05
Mode of death				
CHF	33 (52%)	17 (59%)	18 (67%)	<0.05
Sudden	12 (18%)	5 (17%)	3 (11%)	NS
Pulmonary emboli	6 (9%)	2 (7%)	4 (15%)	NS
Other	5 (7%)	4 (14%)	2 (7%)	NS
History				
Pulmonary edema	15 (21%)	9 (31%)	5 (36%)	<0.05
Angina pectoris	5 (7%)	4 (14%)	4 (20%)	<0.05
AMI	9 (14%)	5 (17%)	8 (33%)	<0.05
Hypertension	9 (14%)	2 (7%)	4 (17%)	NS
Diabetes mellitus	6 (8%)	3 (10%)	6 (26%)	<0.05
Emboli				
Pulmonary, clinical	21 (33%)	8 (28%)	13 (54%)	<0.05
Pulmonary, necropsy	23 (36%)	7 (24%)	9 (47%)	<0.05
Systemic, clinical	10 (16%)	6 (21%)	4 (17%)	NS
Systemic, necropsy	11 (17%)	4 (14%)	6 (32%)	NS
Warfarin therapy				
≥3 mo <12 mo	9 (14%)	5 (17%)	9 (33%)	<0.05
≥12 mo	3 (4%)	2 (7%)	6 (22%)	NS
Heart weight (g) (mean)	400–940 (586)	360–940 (615)	400–860 (625)	<0.05
LV scar				
Transmural	7 (11%)	3 (10%)	2 (7%)	NS
Subendocardial	9 (14%)	3 (10%)	5 (18%)	NS
Intracardiac				
Thrombi only	24 (36%)	7 (24%)	6 (22%)	NS
Plaques only	12 (18%)	3 (10%)	12 (44%)	<0.05
Both thrombi and plaques	14 (22%)	6 (21%)	7 (26%)	NS
Replacement fibrosis (microscopic)	7/25 (28%)	5/14 (36%)	3/18 (17%)	NS

Abbreviations as in Table III.

(mean 640). Three were habitual alcoholics. None had histories of systemic hypertension or evidence of diabetes mellitus. Thirty other patients died suddenly, but each of them previously had had CHF; of them, 19 had fatal cardiac arrest outside the hospital and the other 14 patients, while in the hospital.

Emboli: Information regarding the presence or absence of pulmonary or systemic emboli or both was available in 131 of the 152 patients, and of them 79 patients (60%) had either clinical or necropsy evidence or both of embolic events. Of the 79 patients, 40 (51%) had pulmonary emboli only, 13 (16%) had systemic emboli only and 26 (33%) had both. Thus, of the 79 patients, there were 66 (84%) with pulmonary emboli or infarcts and 39 (49%) with systemic emboli or infarcts. The manner in which the emboli were diagnosed, either clinically or morphologically or both, and their relation to intracardiac thrombi and to mural en-

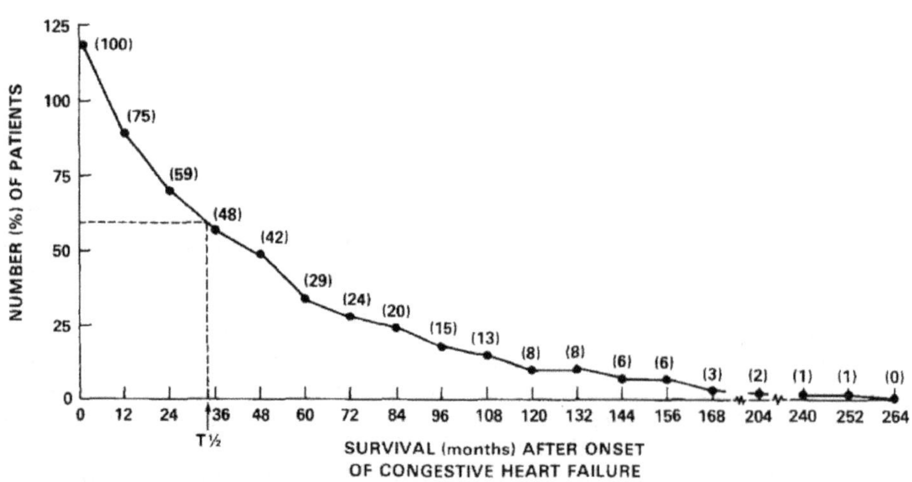

FIGURE 2. Cumulative survival of 118 patients with idiopathic dilated cardiomyopathy after onset of congestive heart failure. One-half of the patients were dead in <36 months ($T_{1/2}$).

TABLE V Frequency of Pulmonary and Systemic Emboli and Infarcts and Relation to Intracardiac Thrombi and Mural Endocardial Plaques in Idiopathic Dilated Cardiomyopathy

		Diagnosis																
Present	Pt	Clinically Only	Necropsy Only	Both	RV T Only	RV Plaques Only	Both	RAA T	RV or RAA T	Right-Sided T or Plaque	LV T Only	LV Plaques Only	Both	LAA T	LV or LAA T	Left-Sided T or Plaque	Either Right- or Left-Sided T or Plaque or Both	WS Rx
Pulmonary Emboli or Infarcts																		
+	66	19 (29%)	17 (20%)	30 (45%)	26 (39%)	8 (12%)	5 (8%)	20 (30%)	37 (56%)	45 (68%)	19 (29%)	11 (17%)	19 (29%)	10 (15%)	39 (59%)	50 (76%)	54 (82%)	12 (18%)
0	65	0	0	0	11 (17%)	4 (6%)	4 (6%)	15 (23%)	21 (32%)	26 (40%)	11 (17%)	14 (22%)	11 (17%)	11 (17%)	28 (43%)	45 (69%)	48 (74%)	11 (17%)
Systemic Emboli or Infarcts																		
+	39	15 (39%)	11 (28%)	13 (33%)	15 (22%)	7 (18%)	4 (10%)	13 (33%)	20 (51%)	29 (74%)	11 (28%)	8 (21%)	14 (36%)	6 (3%)	26 (66%)	34 (87%)	39 (100%)	10 (26%)
0	92	0	0	0	21 (23%)	5 (5%)	5 (5%)	20 (22%)	36 (39%)	40 (43%)	14 (15%)	22 (24%)	13 (14%)	13 (14%)	37 (40%)	59 (64%)	63 (68%)	13 (14%)
Total: Pulmonary or Systemic Emboli or Both																		
+	79	24 (30%)	20 (25%)	28* (35%)	29 (37%)	12 (15%)	6 (8%)	24 (30%)	41 (52%)	47 (59%)	33 (42%)	14 (18%)	28 (35%)	11 (14%)	64 (81%)	59 (75%)	67 (85%)	17 (22%)
0	52	0	0	0	8 (15%)	1 (27%)	3 (6%)	9 (17%)	15 (29%)	17 (33%)	9 (17%)	15 (29%)	8 (15%)	9 (17%)	20 (38%)	34 (65%)	36 (69%)	6 (12%)

* In an additional 2 patients with both pulmonary and systemic emboli, one was diagnosed clinically only and the other was diagnosed only at necropsy.
LAA = left atrial appendage; LV = left ventricular; RAA = right atrial appendage; RV = right ventricular; Rx = treatment; T = thrombus; WS = warfarin sodium.

docardial plaques (almost surely the result of organization of thrombi) are summarized in Table V. Comparison of the 66 patients with pulmonary emboli or infarcts to the 64 without disclosed a significantly higher frequency of right-sided intracardiac thrombi or endocardial plaques or both in the former (68 vs 40%, $p < 0.05$). Comparison of the 39 patients with systemic emboli or infarcts to the 92 without also disclosed a significantly higher frequency of left-sided intracardiac thrombi or endocardial plaques or both in the former (87 vs 64%, $p < 0.05$). Of the 79 patients with either pulmonary or systemic emboli or both, 67 (85%) had either right- or left-sided thrombi or mural endocardial plaques or both, whereas of the 52 without emboli, 36 (69%) had intracardiac thrombi or plaques ($p < 0.05$). The numbers of patients treated with warfarin sodium were not large enough to make meaningful conclusions.

Electrocardiographic findings: Electrocardiographic observations during the last 6 months of life were available in 101 of the 152 patients and the findings are summarized in Table VI. Of the 101 patients, 25 had atrial fibrillation, and findings in them are summarized in Table VII and compared with observations in 25 age- and sex-matched patients with sinus rhythm: no significant differences were noted with regard to race, history of habitual alcoholism, duration of chronic CHF or mode of death. The patients with atrial fibrillation had a lower frequency of embolic events (64 vs 80%) and a lower frequency of intracardiac thrombi (13 vs 18 patients). The frequency of atrial thrombi among the 2 groups of patients was identical. P-wave abnormalities (in addition to their absence in 25% of the patients) were present in 49 of the 101 patients; left only in 35, right only in 6 and both in 8.

Either left ventricular (38 patients) or right (5 patients) ventricular hypertrophy or both (1 patient) were observed electrocardiographically in 44 patients. Complete bundle branch block occurred in 51 patients: left in 41, right in 6 and indeterminate intraventricular conduction delay in 4. Comparison of 32 patients with complete left bundle branch block to 33 with left ventricular hypertrophy and 15 with neither bundle branch block nor left ventricular hypertrophy disclosed that the patients with left bundle branch block had an older mean age (55 vs 45 years vs 42 years [$p < 0.05$]), a longer mean duration of chronic CHF (83 vs 32 months vs 43 months [$p < 0.05$]), larger mean heart weights (628 vs 605 vs 590 g [$p < 0.05$]) and higher frequencies of grossly visible left ventricular scars (44 vs 21 vs 13% [$p < 0.05$]). These observations are summarized in Table VIII and in Figure 3.

In 49 patients in whom electrocardiograms were recorded in the last year of life and available for reexamination, the QRS amplitude in all 12 leads was measured (Table IX, Figure 4). The total 12-lead QRS amplitude in the 35 men (mean age 46 years) ranged from 74 to 250 mm (10 mm = 1 mV) (mean 147) and in the 14 women (mean age 54 years), from 75 to 243 mm (mean 167). The heart weights in the 35 men ranged from 400 to 940 g (mean 620), and in the 14 women, from 400 to 860 g (mean 602). The maximal width of the QRS complex in the 35 men averaged 0.104 second and in 19 patients (54%) was ≥0.12 second; the width in the 14 women averaged 0.122 second and in 11 (79%) patients it was ≥0.12 second. The mean PR interval and QT interval were identical in both men and women (0.19 and 0.39 second, respectively).

The mean 12-lead QRS amplitude among 18 patients with complete left bundle branch block, in 22 patients with electrocardiographic evidence of left ventricular hypertrophy and in 10 patients with neither left bundle branch block nor electrocardiographic left ventricular hypertrophy did not correlate with heart weight (Figure 3). Comparison of total 12-lead QRS amplitude in all 12 leads to heart weight within each group, however, disclosed a striking positive correlation between total 12-lead QRS amplitude and heart weight in the group with complete left bundle branch block (r = +0.81). Because the coefficient of determination was 0.66, approximately two-thirds of the total QRS amplitude in all 12 leads are presumed to be determined by heart weight in our patients with IDC and left bundle block branch. The correlation coefficients between total 12-lead QRS voltage and either voltage criteria of left ventricular hypertrophy or left bundle branch block or neither electrocardiographic criteria for left ventricular hypertrophy nor left bundle branch block were +0.09 and +0.15, re-

TABLE VI Electrocardiographic Findings in 101 Necropsy Patients with Idiopathic Dilated Cardiomyopathy*

	Number (= %)
Rhythm	
Sinus	76
Atrial fibrillation	25
QRS axis abnormality	50
Left (−30 to −90°)	43
Right (110 to 270°)	7
Atrial abnormality	49
Left†	35
Right‡	6
Both	8
Ventricular hypertrophy	44
Left§ only	38
Without strain pattern	21
With‖ strain pattern	17
Right§ only	5
Both	1
Conduction abnormality¶	
Prolonged (>0.20 s) P-R interval	23
Second degree atrioventricular block	1
Complete atrioventricular block	1
Complete bundle branch block	51
Left	41
Right	6
Indeterminant intraventricular conduction delay	4
Arrhythmias, episodic	
Atrial premature complexes	12
Ventricular premature complexes	41
Supraventricular tachycardia	7
Ventricular tachycardia	5
Low voltage (sum QRS in I, II + III ≤ 15 mm)	22
Myocardial damage pattern	38
A. Poor R-wave progression precordial leads**	22
B. Q wave II, III, aVF	7
C. Q wave I, AVL, V_{4-6}	2
D. Combinations A. + B. =	5
B. + C. =	2
Nonspecific ST-T wave changes	12

* Based on analysis of electrocardiograms in 55 patients and detailed reports in 46 patients.

† P terminal force in V_1 is equal to or more negative than −0.04 mm-s.

‡ P wave has height 2.5 mm in leads II, III or AVG.

§ Criteria of Chou.

‖ ST-segment depressed with upward convexity and final downward slope ends in an inverted T wave.

¶ Eleven patients had neither complete bundle branch block nor left ventricular hypertrophy.

** R wave in lead V_3 ≤4 mm.

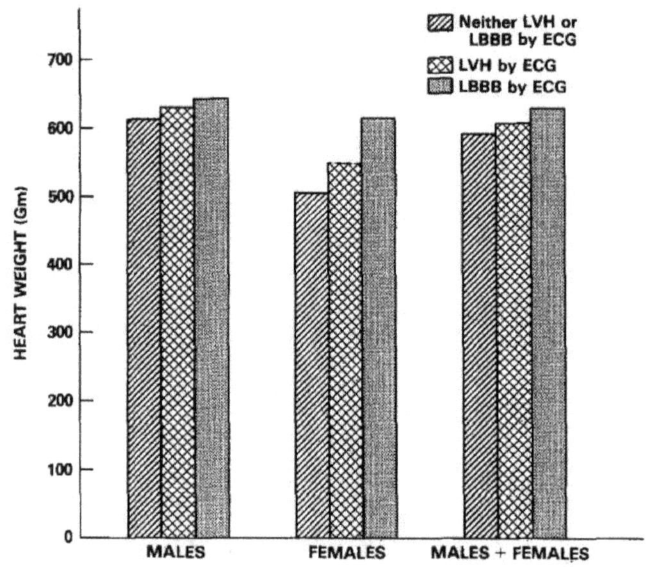

FIGURE 3. Bar graph showing relation of heart weight to electrocardiographic evidence of left ventricular hypertrophy (LVH) or left bundle branch block (LBBB) or neither in both sexes.

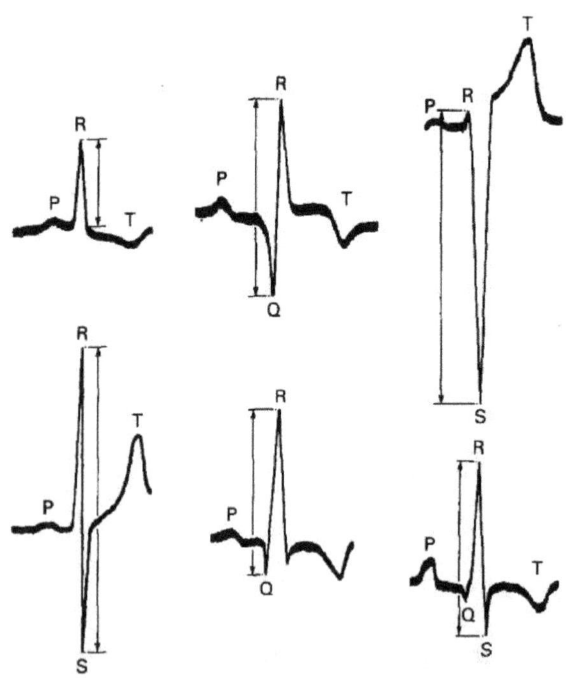

FIGURE 4. Various electrocardiographic QRS complexes showing how the voltage (in mm) was measured. Reproduced with permission from C.V. Mosby.[52]

TABLE VII Clinical and Necropsy Characteristics of 50 Patients with Idiopathic Dilated Cardiomyopathy: 25 with Atrial Fibrillation and 25 with Sinus Rhythm

	Sinus Rhythm (n = 25)	Atrial Fibrillation (n = 25)	p Value
Age (yr) (mean)	20–75 (49)	22–73 (53)	NS
Black:white	14:11 (56%:44%)	16:9 (64%:36%)	NS
Male:female	17:8 (68%:32%)	20:5 (80%:20%)	NS
Habitual alcoholism	12 (48%)	10 (40%)	NS
Duration (mo) CHF (mean)	8–168 (53)	1–264 (52)	NS
Mode of death			
CHF	17 (68%)	14 (60%)	NS
Emboli	3 (12%)	1 (4%)	NS
Sudden	4 (16%)	6 (26%)	NS
Other	1 (4%)	2 (8%)	NS
Emboli	20 (80%)	14 (64%)	NS
Pulmonary	15 (62%)	11 (44%)	NS
Systemic	10 (40%)	8 (32%)	NS
Electrocardiogram			
LV hypertrophy	3 (12%)	4 (16%)	NS
With strain	12 (48%)	2 (8%)	<0.01
Left BBB	9 (36%)	11 (44%)	NS
Right BBB	0	3 (12%)	NS
Heart weight (g)			
Total (mean)	400–940 (627)	370–770 (593)	NS
Male (mean)	440–940 (654)	390–760 (604)	NS
Female (mean)	400–860 (560)	370–770 (552)	NS
Cardiac thrombi			
RA-LA-RV-LV	10-6-12-15	10-6-6-7	<0.05
Thrombi only	7 (28%)	12 (48%)	NS
Mural plaque			
RA-LA-RV-LV	2-1-8-13	1-1-3-5	0.05
Plaque only	4 (16%)	4 (16%)	NS
Thrombi + plaque	11 (44%)	1 (4%)	0.001
Either:neither	22:3 (88%:12%)	17:8 (68%:32%)	NS
LV scars			
S:T	4:6	2:8	NS

BBB = bundle branch block; CHF = congestive heart failure; LA = left atrium; LV = left ventricular or left ventricle; NS = not significant; RA = right atrium; RV = right ventricle; S = subendocardial; T = transmural.

TABLE VIII Clinical and Necropsy Characteristics of Patients with Idiopathic Dilated Cardiomyopathy and Left Bundle Branch Block (BBB), Left Ventricular (LV) Hypertrophy or Neither by Electrocardiogram

	Left BBB (n = 32)	LV Hypertrophy (n = 33)	Neither (n = 15)
Ages (yr) (mean)	27–71 (55)	20–75 (45)	22–66 (42)
Male:female	21:11	27:6	8:7
Duration (mo) CHF (mean)	1–168 (83)	2–96 (32)	2–84 (43)
Heart weight (g) (mean)			
Male + female	400–860 (628)	400–870 (605)	370–940 (590)
Male only	400–860 (642)	400–870 (629)	410–940 (613)
Female only	460–800 (613)	440–650 (548)	370–680 (503)
Left ventricular scar			
Transmural (T):non-T	4:10 (12%:30%)	3:4 (9%:12%)	2:0 (13%:0)

spectively, indicating an insignificant relation between total 12-lead QRS amplitude and heart weight in these latter 2 groups.

Myocardial damage patterns unassociated with complete bundle branch block were observed by electrocardiogram in 38 (38%) of the 101 patients (Table VI). Thus, of the 50 patients without complete bundle branch block, 37 (76%) had myocardial damage patterns, including 22 with poor R-wave progression in the precordial leads, 7 with Q waves in leads II, III and aVF, 2 with Q waves in leads I, AVL and V_4 through V_6 and 7 with combinations of these 3. Comparison of the 38 patients to the 12 patients without a myocardial damage pattern on electrocardiogram (all 50 without complete bundle branch block) disclosed no significant differences in mean age, sex, mode of death, duration of CHF, frequency of chest pain syndromes, habitual alcoholism, diabetes mellitus, left ventricu-

TABLE IX Electrocardiographic Measurements in 35 Necropsy Men and in 14 Necropsy Women with Idiopathic Dilated Cardiomyopathy

Pt	Age (yr) at ECG	Days ECG to Death	Heart Weight (g)	QRS Voltage (mm) Leads All 12	I,II,III	A,L,F.	V_1–V_6	QRS Width (s)	P-R Interval (s)	Q-T Interval (s)	QRS Axis (degrees)	Ventricular Rate (beats/min)
Men												
1	19	30	550	97	16	14	67	0.08	0.16	0.40	+120	80
2	20	3	610	250	35	29	186	0.08	0.16	0.40	+30	75
3	21	30	460	113	13	6	94	0.14	0.16	0.36	−45	110
4	22	9	700	109	13	12	84	0.08	0.22	0.36	+45	105
5	27	10	700	219	46	46	127	0.08	0.16	0.36	+30	115
6	28	240	540	197	24	20	153	0.08	0.16	0.36	−20	80
7	28	120	460	196	43	36	117	0.08	0.20	0.50	−15	65
8	32	990	—	133	15	16	102	0.08	0.19	0.40	−30	80
	35	5	940	114	10	9	95	0.06	0.20	0.48	−15	120
9	35	3	870	152	18	17	117	0.08	0.24	—	−20	105
10	36	60	750	135	10	8	107	0.08	0.18	0.32	+40	90
11	36	350	730	149	26	22	101	0.12	0.16	0.40	120	80
12	38	60	400	90	18	14	58	0.12	—	0.36	−30	80
13	41	426	—	145	16	13	116	0.10	0.23	0.40	0	76
	42	3	500	131	13	14	104	0.11	0.24	0.40	−90	90
14	42	9	630	103	13	12	78	0.12	0.14	0.44	—	90
15	42	117	550	188	21	19	148	0.08	0.22	0.36	−45	100
16	45	840	—	148	20	21	107	0.13	0.22	0.36	−90	120
	47	60	620	159	19	15	125	0.13	0.21	0.40	−90	105
17	46	60	500	144	22	17	105	0.08	0.24	0.40	−60	75
18	47	180	550	148	14	12	122	0.09	0.24	0.36	+30	90
19	47	30	760	281	28	19	234	0.08	0.22	0.40	−40	80
20	48	240	650	172	25	20	127	0.09	0.18	0.40	−15	75
21	50	15	650	112	12	11	89	0.08	0.20	0.36	−60	100
22	51	45	—	179	20	17	142	0.08	0.16	0.56	−20	50
	51	20	500	115	20	18	77	0.10	0.16	0.52	−40	45
23	51	71	650	74	9	10	55	0.09	0.22	0.40	−110	80
24	53	450	—	103	13	10	80	0.12	0.23	0.41	—	58
	54	3	—	106	14	14	78	0.13	0.10	0.32	—	110
25	54	1,500	—	164	24	19	121	0.09	0.16	0.40	+40	75
	58	6	610	107	12	13	82	0.14	0.24	0.40	−60	105
26	56	20	830	202	50	44	108	0.12	0.20	0.42	—	—
27	53	1,100	—	179	33	27	119	0.14	0.12	0.36	−80	75
	56	80	460	136	18	17	101	0.14	0.16	0.36	−75	110
28	58	90	440	114	15	11	88	0.08	0.16	0.36	−40	115
29	59	10	690	146	12	13	123	0.16	0.24	—	−60	95
30	62	450	—	178	22	16	140	0.12	0.16	0.40	−15	120
	63	37	700	185	19	15	151	0.16	0.18	0.38	−30	100
31	62	60	600	141	21	15	105	0.12	0.20	0.40	−40	100
32	63	9	500	123	27	28	68	0.12	0.21	0.40	−70	72
33	67	1	—	137	6	3	128	0.16	—	0.44	0	70
34	70	210	—	128	25	27	76	0.13	—	0.40	−40	77
35	73	4	725	182	31	26	125	0.08	—	0.40	−30	70
Mean	46	64*	620	147	21	18	109	0.104	0.192	0.39		90
Women												
1	22	165	440	221	22	22	177	0.09	0.18	0.32	+60	90
2	32	12	650	195	18	17	160	0.08	0.16	0.36	+60	130
3	50	24	700	187	26	17	144	0.16	—	0.38	−45	75
4	51	270	570	75	16	13	46	0.06	—	0.36	−30	75
5	52	18	500	151	25	31	95	0.14	0.28	0.40	−80	110
6	53	20	400	155	18	17	120	0.08	0.18	0.42	0	70
7	54	900	—	154	15	13	126	0.13	0.20	0.36	+45	130
	57	9	550	108	12	8	88	0.14	0.22	0.40	+45	115
8	58	22	640	180	32	33	115	0.12	0.14	0.40	−40	110
9	58	180	—	196	55	54	87	0.18	0.22	0.40	−40	80
	58	30	860	241	48	48	145	0.20	0.24	0.44	−45	70
10	58	7	620	160	21	21	118	0.12	—	0.36	−70	120
11	59	15	750	243	25	18	200	0.14	0.20	0.42	−40	80
12	60	1	490	91	9	9	73	0.16	0.16	0.40	1	95
13	64	30	—	154	13	11	130	0.14	0.18	0.36	−60	90
14	75	7	650	182	28	26	128	0.08	0.21	0.40	−60	75
Mean	54	45*	602	167	22	21	124	0.122	0.195	0.39		93

* In the 9 patients with 2 ECGs analyzed, the mean utilizes the interval from the second ECG to death.
ECG = electrocardiogram.

TABLE X Hemodynamic Data in 26 Necropsy Patients with Idiopathic Dilated Cardiomyopathy

						Pressures (mm Hg)														
			Duration (mo)			RA					PAW							Thrombus		
Pt	Age (yr)	Sex	CHF	CHF → CC	CC → Death	a	v	m	RV (s/d)	PA (s/d)	a	v	m	LV (s/d)	SA (s/d)	CI	HW (g)	RV	LV	PE
1	17	M	36	9	27	9	8	5	26/10	26/14	20	22	16	100/14	100/60	4.1	585	0	+	0
2	18	F	5	2	3	—	—	—	—	36/22	—	—	—	80/25	80/40	—	—	0	0	+
3	20	M	46	4	2	10	8	5	26/7	26/12	10	12	9	102/13	115/60	3.0	610	0	0	+
4	22	M	12	1	11	—	—	—	—	—	—	—	—	100/26	100/50	—	600	+	+	+
5	26	M	16	4	12	9	4	2	17/13	17/10	8	12	5	110/10	110/75	1.4	700	0	+	0
6	26	M	4	1	3	—	—	—	—	27/14	—	—	14	100/12	100/60	1.4	460	0	0	0
7	26	M	5	4	1	—	—	13	—	45/20	—	—	32	—	—	1.5	—	0	+	—
8	29	F	108	103	5	—	—	—	90/-	90/-	—	—	32	90/25	90/60	—	460	0	+	+
9	30	M	5	3	2	18	17	13	70/22	70/26	26	22	18	150/28	140/70	1.5	410	0	0	+
10	32	M	96	84	12	2	3	2	26/2	24/17	—	—	22	120/27	120/70	—	550	+	+	+
11	37	F	23	22	5 days	16	18	17	51/23	51/37	—	—	28	—	—	—	—	0	0	+
12	37	M	36	22	14	AF	8	6	58/6	58/30	—	45	30	126/28	102/80	2.5	400	+	+	0
13	39	M	18	5	13	—	—	0	20/2	20/12	—	—	6	100/18	105/70	2.1	720	0	+	+
14	42	M	72	71	7 days	—	—	16	77/15	77/37	—	—	16	—	100/80	—	650	0	+*	+
15	42	M	30	25	5	30	27	23	40/20	43/32	—	—	35	—	100/60	1.6	550	+	+	0
16	42	M	24	11	13	—	—	7	55/10	55/30	—	—	35	95/35	95/60	1.6	510	0	0	+
17	47	M	12	6	6	9	6	5	45/7	45/20	26	38	25	85/25	85/60	1.5	550	0	+	+
18	48	M	60	48	12	—	—	—	45/8	45/30	—	—	30	85/30	85/55	—	—	0	+	0
19	49	M	48	41	7	AF	—	27	78/28	78/-	—	54	40	—	80/60	—	700	+	+	0
20	50	F	60	60	14 days	AF	30	25	74/24	70/40	—	45	36	100/30	110/75	1.1	700	+	+*	+
21	51	M	72	20	52	AF	10	9	50/9	52/24	—	—	15	120/20	120/75	1.85	570	0	0	0
22	55	M	60	59	1	AF	—	7	40/7	—	—	40	26	110/26	110/80	—	500	0	0	0
23	56	M	36	34	2	—	—	23	—	55/30	—	—	25	—	85/55	—	460	+	+	+
24	58	F	168	165	3	8	7	6	60/10	60/30	32	30	23	140/32	140/80	2.3	860	0	0	+
25	58	F	12	11	21 days	—	12	4	40/6	40/20	—	—	20	95/20	95/70	1.6	620	+	+*	+
26	62	F	62	24	1 day	—	—	4	55/24	55/35	—	—	25	108/23	110/90	2.4	760	0	0	+
27	63	M	—	—	5 days	AF	—	—	70/10	70/27	—	—	28	—	130/75	1.9	—	+	+	0
28	70	M	60	50	10	AF	—	4	60/10	60/20	—	9	7	150/8	150/60	—	580	+	+	+
Mean	41		44	33	8	12	12	11	51/12	50/25	20	30	28	108/23	106/67	2.0	587			

* Thrombus was not visualized on left ventricular angiogram performed 1 month or less before death.

a = a wave; AF = atrial fibrillation; CC = cardiac catheterization; CI = cardiac index (in liters/min/m^2); CHF = congestive heart failure; HW = heart weight; LV = left ventricle; m = mean; PA = pulmonary artery; PE = pulmonary emboli (at necropsy); Pt = patient; RA = right atrium; RV = right ventricle; SA = systemic artery; s/d = peak systole/end diastole; V = V wave.

lar hypertrophy on electrocardiogram or intracardiac thrombi. The frequencies of atrial fibrillation and grossly visible left ventricular scars, however, were different. Of the 38 patients with myocardial damage patterns on electrocardiogram, 1.0 (26%) had atrial fibrillation and 10 (26%) had left ventricular scars; in contrast, all 12 patients without myocardial damage patterns were in sinus rhythm and none had left ventricular scars.

Hemodynamic data: Cardiac catheterization data were available in 28 of the 152 patients (Table X). The mean atrial or ventricular end-diastolic pressures or both were elevated in all 28 patients. The right ventricular end-diastolic pressure was >6 mm Hg in 18 (82%) of 22 patients, the left ventricular end-diastolic pressure was >12 mm Hg in 18 (86%) of 21 patients and the mean pulmonary arterial wedge pressure was >12 mm Hg in 22 (85%) of 26 patients. The pulmonary arterial systolic pressure was >30 mm Hg in 20 (77%) of 26 patients, including 8 in whom this pressure was ≥60 mm Hg. Of the 28 patients who had cardiac catheterization, 17 had necropsy evidence of pulmonary emboli or infarcts, and 12 (71%) had pulmonary arterial systolic pressures >30 mm Hg, including 10 (59%) in whom this pressure was >50 mm Hg. A left ventricular to aortic peak systolic pressure gradient of 23 mm Hg was observed in 1 patient, and this patient at necropsy had a thrombus in the left ventricular outflow tract. The cardiac indexes were <2.5 liters/min/m^2 in 14 (82%) of 17 patients. Left ventricular angiograms in 18 patients disclosed global hypokinesia in all 18 and mitral regurgitation in 6 of 13 in whom it was mentioned. No significant correlation was observed between total duration of chronic CHF or duration of CHF from the time of catheterization to death and the pulmonary arterial systolic pressure ($r = +0.39$ and $r = -0.20$), but a significant correlation was observed between the total duration of CHF and the mean pulmonary arterial wedge pressure ($r = +0.65$) ($p < 0.002$). The left ventricular end-diastolic pressure did not correlate with heart weight ($r = -0.08$), total duration of CHF ($r = -0.14$) or duration of CHF from catheterization to death ($r = -0.17$).

Necropsy Findings

Heart weights and chamber sizes: The hearts at necropsy ranged in weight from 360 to 940 g (mean 615): in the women the range was from 360 to 860 g (mean 551) and in the men, from 400 to 940 g (mean 632) ($p < 0.05$). By definition, both right and left ventricular cavities were dilated in all patients (Figures 5 through 7). So were both atria. The frequency of intracavity thrombi and mural endocardial plaques have been described previously.

Ventricular scars: Grossly visible left ventricular or right ventricular scars or both (excluding isolated papillary muscle scars) were found in 22 (14%) patients: 21 scars involved, at some point, greater than the inner one-half of the myocardial wall, that is, transmural, and 1 was limited to the inner one-half, that is, subendocardial. The scars were small in 14 patients, moderate in 4 and large in 4. The scars involved left ventricular free wall in all 22 patients, the ventricular septum also in 20 and the right ventricular free wall in 5. The frequency of intraventricular thrombi and endocardial plaques was similar in the patients with and without grossly visible ventricular wall scars. The 22 patients with ventricular scars ranged in age from 17 to 67 years (mean 56), which is an average of 13 years older than the mean (43 years) of the 130 patients without grossly visible left ventricular scars ($p < 0.05$). Of these 22 patients, 21 had chronic CHF an average of 44 months, which is significantly ($p < 0.05$) less than the mean duration (65 months) of chronic CHF in the 99 patients in whom no grossly visible ventricular scars were present and information on the duration of chronic CHF was available. Of the 22 patients, 4 had clinical events during life considered to be compatible with "acute myocardial infarction." None, of course, had significantly (>75% in cross-sectional area) narrowed coronary arteries at necropsy. Of the 22 patients, 11 had histories of habitual alcoholism and 2 had adult-onset diabetes mellitus. Electrocardiograms, available in 21 of the 22 patients, disclosed voltage criteria for left ventricular hypertrophy in 6 (29%), complete bundle branch block in 9 (43%) and myocardial infarct or damage patterns in 6 (29%). The mean heart weight (available in 19 patients) in the patients

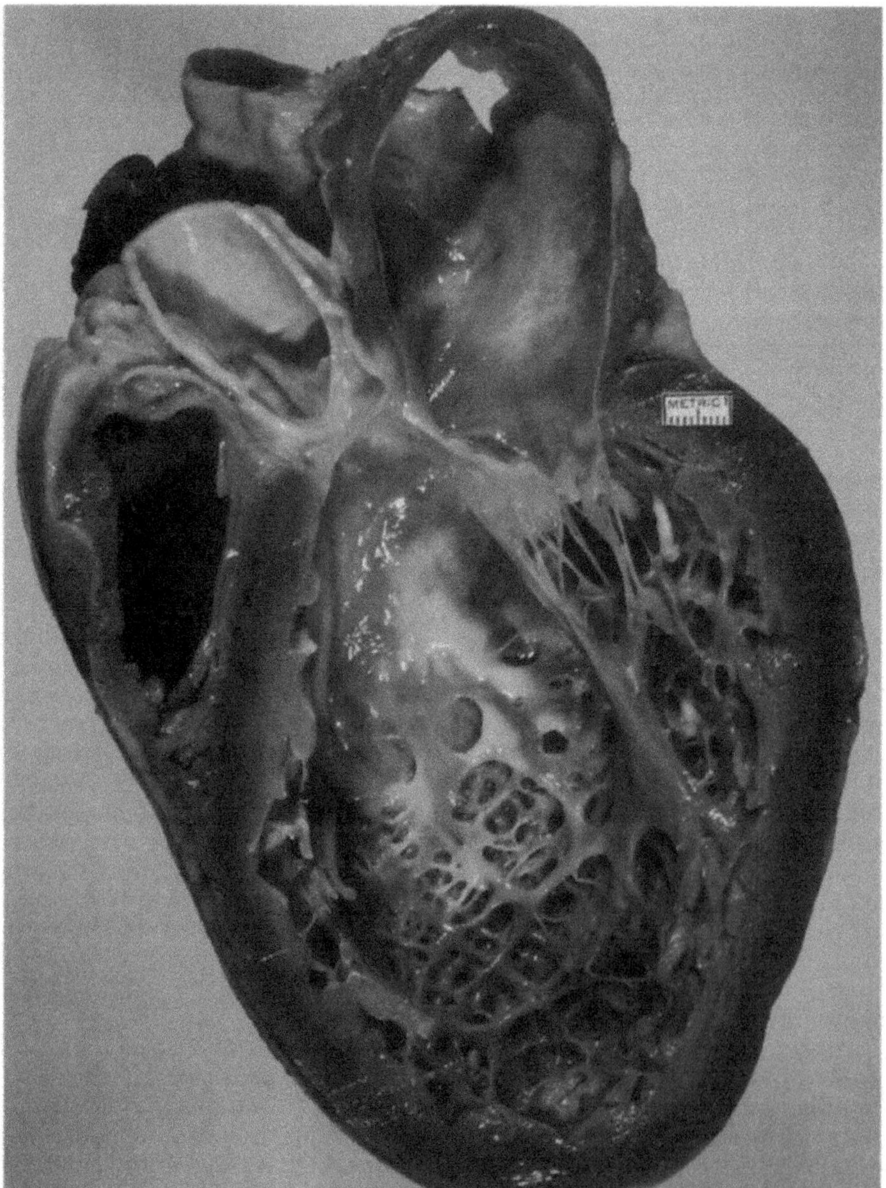

FIGURE 5. Longitudinal view of left side of the heart from a 54-year-old man (SH A81-57) with idiopathic dilated cardiomyopathy. Shown is the outflow portion of right ventricle and much of the left ventricle. The white plaques on the left ventricular aspect of the ventricular septum probably are residua of organization of thrombi. The mitral valve occupies a small portion of the very dilated left ventricular cavity. The heart weighed 920 g. Congestive heart failure had been present for 3.5 years.

with grossly visible scars was similar to that in the patients without (607 vs 615 g).

Histology of ventricular myocardium: A total of 1,422 histologic sections of myocardial wall from 96 patients were examined: 508 sections of left ventricle, 215 of ventricular septum, 355 of right ventricle and 344 of atrium. Additionally, 967 sections of cross-sections of major (right, left main, left anterior descending and left circumflex) epicardial coronary arteries were examined. The ventricular myocardium contained multiple patchy areas of replacement fibrosis in 29 (35%) of 83 sections of right ventricle and in 55 (57%) of 96 sections of left ventricle from the 96 patients. The replacement fibrosis often was accompanied by in-

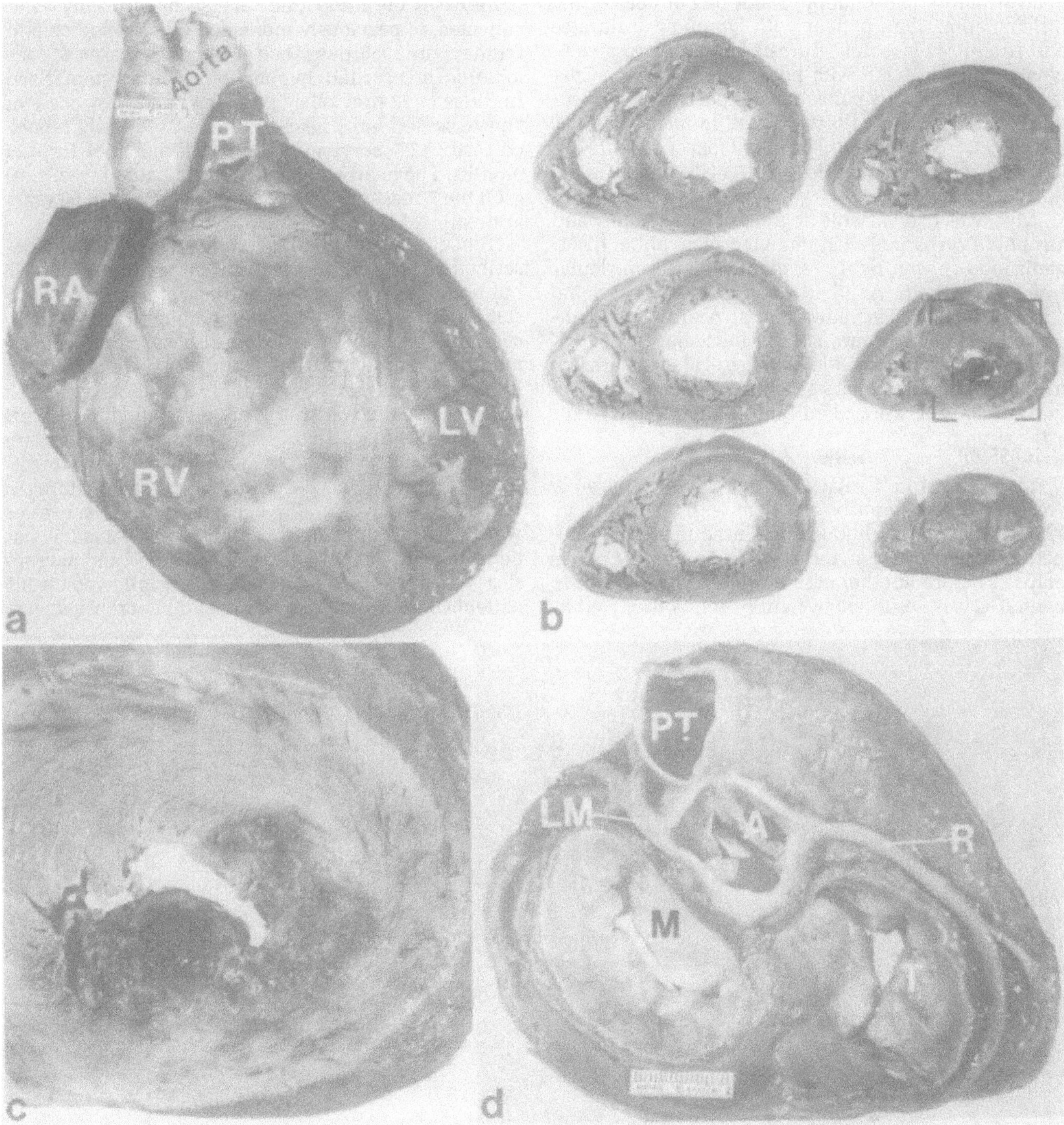

FIGURE 6. Heart from a 58-year-old woman (SH A78-7) with congestive heart failure for 10 years due to idiopathic dilated cardiomyopathy. *A*, exterior view of the heart. LV = left ventricle; PT = pulmonary trunk; RA = right atrium; RV = right ventricle. *B*, sections of the dilated cardiac ventricles after transverse sectioning. *C*, close-up view of the section shown in brackets in *B*. A thrombus is present. *D*, view of the mitral (M), tricuspid (T) and aortic (A) valves and of pulmonary trunk after removal of the atrial walls. R = right; LM = left main coronary arteries.

creased perivascular fibrous tissue and perimyocytic fibrosis in the left ventricle: it was present in 22 (23%) of 96 and 27 (28%) of 96 patients, respectively (Figure 8). In addition, in 13 (16%) of 83 sections of right ventricle and in 32 (33%) of 96 sections of left ventricle extensive subendocardial scarring was present. Interstitial inflammatory cell infiltrates were present in ventricular myocardium in 5 patients: 4 had prominent mononuclear infiltrates without associated myocardial necrosis and 1 had multiple small foci of necrotizing inflammation. One patient with lymphoid infiltrates and patchy replacement fibrosis had a progressive 5-week course of CHF with positive serology for Coxsackie B_3 virus. Tiny collections of perivascular "sentinal" mononuclear cells were seen in many patients. Seven (8%) of 83 patients had small foci of coagulation necrosis in the right ventricle and 11 (11%) of 96 in the left ventricle.

Myocytes had variable degrees of hypertrophy and atrophy. Two patients had small foci of myofiber disorganization in ventricular septum or left ventricular free wall or both. Another 2 patients had occasional calcified myocytes in ventricular myocardium and another 2 had subendocardial left ventricular foci of colliquative myocytolysis. Platelet aggregate was present in an intramural coronary artery in 1 patient. No infectious organisms were identified in any section.

Discussion

Josserand and Gallavardin[1] in 1901 apparently were the first to describe a patient with what appears to have been IDC, although they used the term "idiopathic hypertrophy of the heart." Another 24 years elapsed before another case of what appears to have been IDC was described by Laubry and Walser.[2] Whittle[3] in 1929 added another case. By 1944, Levy and Von Glahn[4] reported 10 necropsy cases of "cardiac hypertrophy of unknown cause" and they described the usual clinical features: "marked cardiac hypertrophy; occurrence of various types of arrhythmia; frequent emboli to the pulmonary and systemic circulations; rapidly progressive course after the onset of symptoms; and death from gradual cardiac failure or in sudden fashion." In 1955 Serbin and Chojnacki[5] reported 3 more cases of "idiopathic cardiac hypertrophy" and collected 46 previously published cases. Spodick and Littman[6] in 1958 described 8 necropsy cases of "idiopathic myocardial hypertrophy" and summarized findings in 72 previously published necropsy cases of "unexplained large hearts." Of the previously reported cases, 42% survived <12 months and 65% for <24 months. The heart weight in all but 1 patient was ≥400 g. Of the 72 cases, 62 (86%) were younger than 50 years at death.

Since 1958, numerous publications[7-47] have described various clinical features in patients with IDC, but none have focused on findings at necropsy. Massumi et al[11] in 1965 described clinical features of 50 cases of "primary myocardial disease" seen in a 41-month period; 13 died and necropsies were performed in 10. Goodwin[13] in 1970 studied 70 patients with IDC; 41 (55%) had died and the average duration from onset of symptoms to death was 3.5 years; necropsies were performed in 26 patients and all had heart weights ≥400 g. Hamby[14] in 1970 described clinical features in 100 cases; 44 died in a 5-year period, and necropsies were performed in 23. Shugoll et al[17] followed 50 patients for 3 to 72 months (mean 30); 10 died and necropsies were performed in 5. Hatle et al[22] followed up 106 patients for 2 to 12 years; 50 died and necropsies were

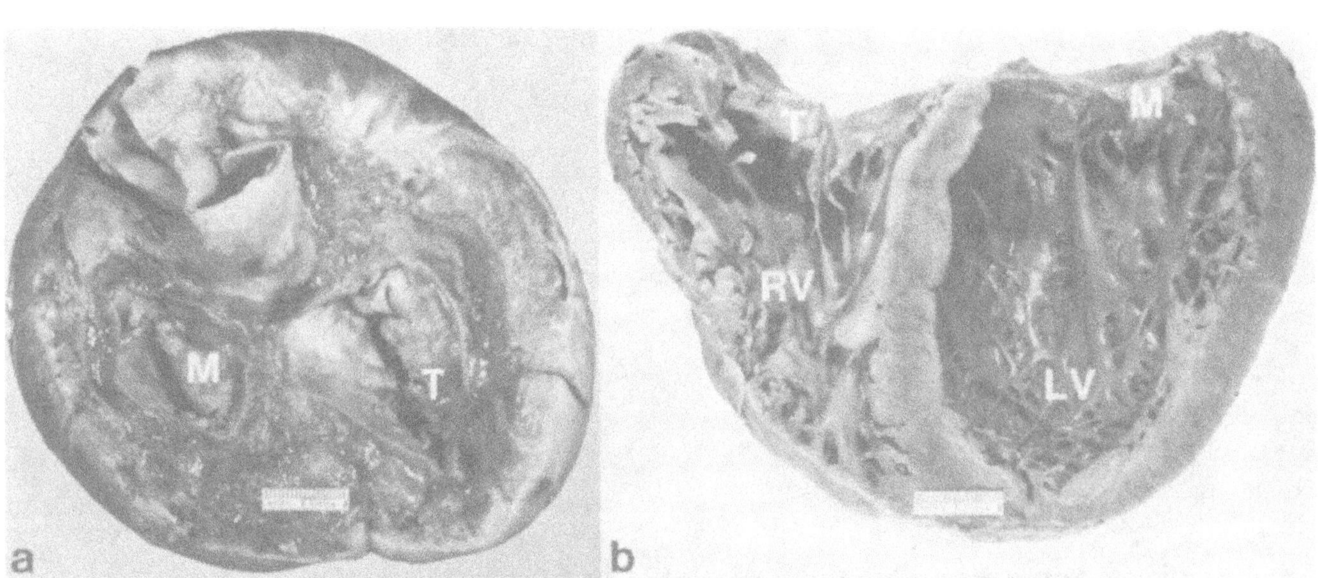

FIGURE 7. Heart (*A* and *B*) from a 34-year-old woman (DCGH 74A-65) with congestive heart failure for 5 years from idiopathic dilated cardiomyopathy. The mitral (M) anulus is only mildly dilated, whereas the tricuspid (T) valve anulus is considerably dilated, as are both ventricular cavities. The usual mechanism of tricuspid regurgitation in patients with idiopathic dilated cardiomyopathy is dilatation of the tricuspid valve anulus. In contrast, the usual mechanism of mitral regurgitation in idiopathic dilated cardiomyopathy is altered papillary muscle anchoring due to dilatation of the left ventricular cavity, mainly in its more central portion. The heart in this patient weighed 870 g.

TABLE XI Certain Reported Studies Since 1960 in Idiopathic Dilated Cardiomyopathy

	First Author	Year	No. Cases (males)	Period Patients Seen	Age Range (yr) (mean) When First Seen or When Studied	Age (yr) at Death (mean)	Race B	Race W	Range of Follow-up (mo) (mean)	Duration (mo) S → Death (mean)	History of Alcoholism	Peripartum (no. women)	Familial	Diabetes Mellitus	No. Having Coronary Angiography	No. Died in Follow-Up	No. Having Necropsy
1	Fowler et al[7,8]	1962	29 (25)	—1964	8–62 (36)	18–68 (45)	10	19	1–312 (—)	6–312 (120)	8/23	1 (4)	1	0	0	26	26
2	Dye et al[9,10]	1963	32 (32)	—	20–68 (43)	—	14	18	—48 (—)	— (44)	21	0 (0)	—	—	0	12	9
3	Massumi et al[11]	1965	50 (40)	1960–1963	20–79 (—)	28–79 (54)	45	5	—41 (—)	— (10)	30	— (10)	0	—	0	13	10
4	Alexander[12]	1966	83 (83)	1949–1960	19–67 (44)	— (47)	—	—	—	— (2)	24	0 (0)	—	—	0	27	—
5	Goodwin[13]	1970	70 (—)	—	—	—	—	—	—	— (42)	16	7 (—)	—	—	9	41	26
6	Hamby[14]	1970	100 (71)	1954–1968	20–61 (45)	— (45)	71	29	2–60 (15)	— (55)	40	— (29)	—	3	24	35	23
7	McDonald and Rahimtoola[15]	1971	48 (47)	1959–1969	21–57 (38)	—	42	6	0.2–108 (52)	— (45)	48	0 (1)	—	—	0	19	14
8	Demakis[16]	1971	27 (0)	—	—	—	—	—	12–252 (97)	—	0	27 (27)	0	—	0	13	—
9	Shugoll et al[17]	1972	50 (50)	—1961	22–50 (—)	—	46	4	3–72 (30)	12–108 (38)	31	0 (0)	0	—	23	10	5
10	Kreulen et al[18]	1973	33 (24)	—	20–69 (43)	—	—	—	—	—	7	— (9)	—	—	33	9	—
11	Feild et al[19]	1973	36 (23)	—	18–66 (46)	—	—	—	—56 (—)	3–144 (38)	5	— (13)	0	5	15	19	5
12	Damakis et al[20]	1974	57 (49)	1962–1970	23–50 (41)	—	47	10	4–96 (41)	— (36)	57	0 (8)	—	—	4	24	7
13	Bashour et al[21]	1975	65 (56)	1969–1974	21–66 (42)	—	—	—	— (21)	—	65	— (9)	—	—	—	—	—
14	Hatle et al[22,23]	1976	91 (—)	1962–1972	<10–>60 (—)	—	—	—	2–12 (—)	—	2	— (—)	5	0	81	50	36
15	Hess et al[24]	1976	30 (24)	—	— (43)	—	—	—	10–34 (24)	—	—	— (6)	—	—	30	8	—
16	Segal et al[25]	1978	115 (71)	1961–1976	1–65 (—)	1–65 (46)	37	78	60–192 (96)	— (74)	0	0 (44)	0	0	—	77	48
17	Shirey et al[26]	1980	113 (—)	—	—	—	—	—	—96 (60)	0.5–90 (25)	8	— (—)	—	12	113	44	—
18	Koide et al[27]	1980	36 (29)	1965–1978	(44 ± 13)	— (53)	—	—	1–216 (—)	— (53)	10	3 (7)	3	—	—	17	11
19	Convert et al[28]	1980	132 (110)	1969–1977	15–71 (46)	—	—	—	(40 ± 24)	<6–>36 (—)	77	— (22)	—	—	79	48	—
20	Fuster et al[29]	1981	104 (64)	1960–1973	— (49)	—	—	—	72–240 (132)	—	22	3 (40)	—	0	46	80	39
21	Lengyel and Kokeny[30]	1981	98 (88)	1973–1979	17–66 (41)	17–66 (40)	—	—	6–70 (18)	6–60 (13)	34	2 (10)	5	—	15	39	15
22	Engler et al[31]	1982	18 (—)	—	32–71 (54)	—	—	—	6–49 (25)	—	—	— (—)	—	—	18	—	—
23	Kuhn et al[32]	1982	258 (187)	1971–1980	8–68 (44)	(44 ± 10)	—	—	(36 ± 24)	(60 ± 36)	40	— (71)	—	—	258	69	18
24	Franciosa et al[33]	1983	87 (—)	1974–1981	—	—	—	—	1–41 (12)	(45 ± 43)	—	— (—)	—	—	22	30	—
25	Huang et al[34]	1983	35 (24)	1976–1980	22–72 (51)	—	—	—	4–74 (34)	—	—	— (11)	—	—	35	4	—
26	von Olshausen et al[35]	1984	60 (54)	1981–1982	18–60 (45)	—	—	—	1–18 (12)	—	—	—(6)	—	—	60	7	—
27	Meinertz et al[36,37]	1984	74 (—)	—	—	— (50)	—	—	2–21 (11)	(60 ± 37)	0	— (—)	—	—	74	19	—
28	Poll et al[38]	1984	11 (6)	1975–1983	27–74 (49)	—	—	—	— (21)—	—	—	—(5)	—	—	—	4	—
29	Unverferth et al[39,40]	1984	69 (49)	1979–1982	19–79 (45)	19–79 (45)			—12 (—)	(31 ± 46)	15	2 (20)	4	5	69	24	—
30	Wallis et al[41]	1984	50 (32)	1981–1983	11–68 (47)	—	—	—	1–26 (11)	—	—	— (18)	—	—	47	10	—
31	Holmes et al[42]	1985	15 (12)	1981–1983	34–66 (50)	—	—	—	6–21 (11)	—	3	1 (3)	0	0	5	5	—
32	Anderson et al[43,44]	1985	50 (33)	1981–1984	25–75 (50)	—	—	—	1–38 (19)	—	0	—	—	—	All > 30	11	—
33	Sanderson et al[45]	1985	20 (9)	—	— (34)	—	—	—	—	—	—	—	—	—	<9	—	—
34	Michels et al[46]	1985	169 (119)	1976–1982	<50	—	—	—	—	—	—	—	11	—	~80	—	—
35	O'Connell et al[47]	1986	69 (—)	—	— (44)	—	—	—	—	—	—	14 (—)	—	—	—	—	—

B = black; M = men; S = symptoms of cardiac dysfunction; W = white; — = no information available.

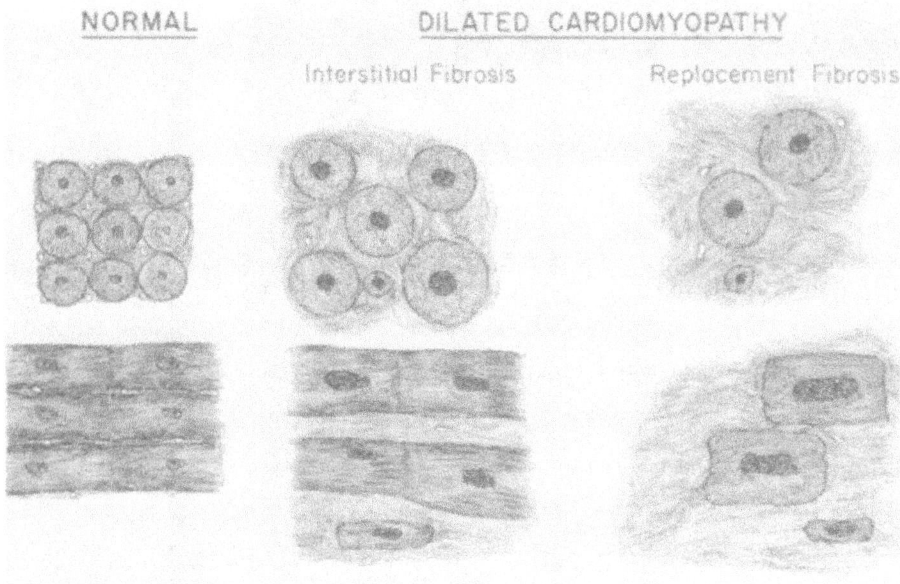

FIGURE 8. Diagram showing the various findings commonly observed in sections of left ventricular wall in the patients with idiopathic dilated cardiomyopathy. Some myocardial cells are larger than normal, others are smaller than normal and others have been replaced by fibrous tissue, which also is increased in the interstitium between the myocardial cells.

performed in 36. Segal et al[25] followed 115 patients with presumed IDC for a minimum of 5 years (median 8); 77 died and necropsies were performed in 48. Only 35 of the 48 had cardiomegaly at necropsy, an observation suggesting that some of the cases may not have been IDC. Shirey et al[26] studied 113 patients with IDC (only 48 of whom had CHF), following them up to 8 years (mean 5); 44 died but the number who had necropsy is unclear. Fuster et al[29] followed 104 patients from 6 to 20 years (median 11); 80 died and necropsy was performed in 39. Franciosa et al[33] followed 87 patients from 1 to 41 months (mean 12); 30 died but the number who had necropsy is unclear. These studies and many others are summarized in Table XI.

In contrast to the studies just mentioned, the starting point in the present study was the finding at necropsy of cardiac abnormalities fulfilling a rigorous definition of IDC. All 152 patients had hearts that were enlarged (>350 g in women and >400 g in men), all had dilated cardiac ventricular cavities, all had anatomically normal cardiac valves and pericardia, all had insignificant narrowing of the epicardial coronary arteries and none had an abnormality of a noncardiac body organ sufficient to cause the cardiac abnormalities. None during life had a systemic arterial indirect pressure >140/90 mm Hg during their last 3 months of life. Of the 148 patients with chronic CHF, the diagnosis of IDC was either made or suspected clinically. In the 4 patients whose initial manifestation of IDC was sudden death, diagnosis of IDC, of course, was not made until necropsy.

The findings in the present study are shown in detail in Tables I through X. This study provides the most extensive data for the natural history of IDC thus far presented. Clues to the cause of the IDC were not provided by this morphologically based study. Despite current interest in myocardial biopsy for identification of inflammatory myocardial injury in patients with IDC, this technique if applied shortly before death in the 152 patients included in this study probably would not have produced a diagnosis of "myocarditis" in a single patient. Our findings are in keeping with other observations regarding the infrequency of significant inflammatory cells in ventricular myocardium in patients with IDC.[48,49]

Although numerous reports have described electrocardiographic changes in patients with IDC (see references compiled by Perloff[50]), the present study is the first to describe total 12-lead QRS voltage in patients with IDC. A recent study by Odom et al[51] provided total 12-lead QRS voltage in a group of necropsy patients with no evidence of cardiac or pulmonary dysfunction or myocardial ischemia during life and all had normal-sized hearts at necropsy. Only 1 of the 30 subjects with normal-sized hearts had total 12-lead QRS voltage >175 mm (10 mm = 1 mV). The total 12-lead QRS voltage in 49 patients with IDC included in this study ranged from 75 to 250 mm (mean 153), a mean number within normal limits despite a mean heart weight for the group of >550 g. For comparison, Siegel and Roberts[52] determined total 12-lead QRS voltage in 50 patients aged 16 to 65 years with severe and fatal isolated aortic valve stenosis. The total 12-lead QRS voltage in these 50 patients ranged from 144 to 417 mm (mean 260), and the heart weights were similar to those in the present study of patients with IDC. In a study of total 12-lead QRS voltage in 30 patients with severe and fatal cardiac amyloidosis, Roberts and Waller[53] found total 12-lead QRS voltage to range from 60 to 199 mm (mean 104) despite a mean heart weight of the 30 patients of 532 g. Thus, by total 12-lead QRS voltage criteria, few IDC patients in the present study or patients with severe cardiac amyloidosis have "left ventricular hypertrophy" despite the occurrence of considerable cardiomegaly at necropsy.

References

1. Josserand E, Gallavardin L. *De l' a systolie progressive des jeunes sujets par myocardite subaigue primitive. Arch Gen Med 1901;6:513–548.*
2. Laubry C, Walser J. *Sur un cas d'insuffisance cardiaque primitive. Les*

myocardies. Bull Mem Soc Med Hop Paris 1925;49:409–418.
3. Whittle CH. "Idiopathic" hypertrophy of heart in young man. Lancet 1929;1:1354–1355.
4. Levy RL, Von Glahn WC. Cardiac hypertrophy of unknown cause. A study of the clinical and pathologic features in ten adults. Am Heart J 1944;28:714–741.
5. Serbin RA, Chojnacki B. Idiopathic cardiac hypertrophy. Report of 3 cases. N Engl J Med 1955;252:10–13.
6. Spodick DH, Littman D. Idiopathic myocardial hypertrophy. Am J Cardiol 1958;1:610–623.
7. Fowler NO, Gueron M, Rowlands DT Jr. Primary myocardial disease. Dis Chest 1962;41:593–602.
8. Fowler NO, Gueron M. Primary myocardial disease. Circulation 1965;32:830–836.
9. Dye CL, Rosenbaum D, Lowe JC, Behnke RH, Genovese PD. Primary myocardial disease: part I. Clinical features. Ann Intern Med 1963;58:426–441.
10. Dye CL, Genovese PD, Daly WJ, Behnke RH. Primary myocardial disease. Part II. Hemodynamic alterations. Ann Intern Med 1963;58:442–453.
11. Massumi RA, Rios JC, Gooch AS, Nutter D, De Vita VT, Datlow DW. Primary myocardial disease. Report of fifty cases and review of the subject. Circulation 1965;31:19–41.
12. Alexander CS. Idiopathic heart disease: I. Analysis of 100 cases, with special reference to chronic alcoholism. Am J Med 1966;41:213–228.
13. Goodwin JF. Congestive and hypertrophic cardiomyopathies. A decade of study. Lancet 1970;1:732–739.
14. Hamby RI. Primary myocardial disease. A prospective clinical and hemodynamic evaluation in 100 patients. Medicine 1970;49:55–78.
15. McDonald CD, Burch GE, Walsh JJ. Alcoholic cardiomyopathy managed with prolonged bed rest. Ann Intern Med 1971;74:681–691.
16. Demakis JG, Rahimtoola SH. Peripartum cardiomyopathy. Circulation 1971;44:964–968.
17. Shugoll GI, Bowen PJ, Moore JP, Lenkin ML. Follow-up observations and prognosis in primary myocardial disease. Arch Intern Med 1972;129:67–72.
18. Kreulen TH, Gorlin R, Herman MV. Ventriculographic patterns and hemodynamics in primary myocardial disease. Circulation 1973;47:299–308.
19. Feild BJ, Baxley WA, Russell RO Jr, Hood WP Jr, Holt JH, Dowling JT, Rackley CE. Left ventricular function and hypertrophy in cardiomyopathy with depressed ejection fraction. Circulation 47:1022–1031.
20. Demakis JG, Proskey A, Rahimtoola SH, Jamil M, Sutton GC, Rosen KM, Gunnar RM, Tobin JR Jr. The natural course of alcoholic cardiomyopathy. Ann Intern Med 1974;80:293–297.
21. Bashour TT, Fahdul H, Cheng TO. Electrocardiographic abnormalities in alcoholic cardiomyopathy. A study of 65 patients. Chest 1975;68:24–27.
22. Hatle L, Orjavik O, Storstein O. Chronic myocardial disease. I. Clinical picture related to long-term prognosis. Acta Med Scand 1976;199:399–405.
23. Hatle L, Stahe G, Storstein O. Chronic myocardial disease. II. Hemodynamic findings related to long-term prognosis. Acta Med Scand 1976;199:407–411.
24. Hess OM, Turina J, Goebel NH, Krayenbuhl HP. Clinical course of congestive cardiomyopathy. Schweiz Med Wochenschr 1976;106:1577–1579.
25. Segal JP, Stapleton JF, McClellan JR, Waller BF, Harvey WP. Idiopathic cardiomyopathy: clinical features, prognosis and therapy. Curr Probl Cardiol 1978;3:1–49.
26. Shirey EK, Proudfit WL, Hawk WA. Primary myocardial disease. Correlation with clinical findings, angiographic and biopsy diagnosis. Follow-up of 139 patients. Am Heart J 1980;99:198–207.
27. Koide T, Kato A, Takabatake Y, Iizuka M, Uchida Y, Ozeki K, Morooka S, Kakihana M, Serizawa T, Tanaka S, Ohya T, Momomura S, Murao S. Variable prognosis in congestive cardiomyopathy. Role of left ventricular function, alcoholism, and pulmonary thrombosis. Jpn Heart J 1980;21:451–463.
28. Convert G, Delaye J, Beaune J, Biron A, Gonin A. Prognosis of primary nonobstructive cardiomyopathies. Arch Mal Coeur 1980;73:227–237.
29. Fuster V, Gersh BJ, Giuliani ER, Tajik AJ, Brandenburg RO, Frye RL. The natural history of idiopathic dilated cardiomyopathy. Am J Cardiol 1981;47:525–531.
30. Lengyel M, Kokeny M. Follow-up study in congestive (dilated) cardiomyopathy. Acta Cardiol 1981;36:35–48.
31. Engler R, Ray R, Higgins CB, McNally C, Buxton WH, Bhargava V, Shabetai R. Clinical assessment and follow-up of functional capacity in patients with chronic congestive cardiomyopathy. Am J Cardiol 1982;49:1832–1837.
32. Kuhn H, Becker R, Fischer J, Curtius JM, Losse B, Hort W, Loogen F. Studies on the etiology, the clinical course and the prognosis of patients with dilated cardiomyopathy (DCM). Z Kardiol 1982;71:497–508.
33. Franciosa JA, Wilen M, Ziesche S, Cohn JN. Survival in men with severe chronic left ventricular failure due to either coronary heart disease or idiopathic dilated cardiomyopathy. Am J Cardiol 1983;51:831–836.
34. Huang SK, Musser JV, Denes P. Significance of ventricular tachycardia in idiopathic dilated cardiomyopathy: observations in 35 patients. Am J Cardiol 1983;51:507–518.
35. Von Olshausen K, Schäfer A, Mehmel HC, Schwarz F, Senges J, Kübler W. Ventricular arrhythmias in idiopathic dilated cardiomyopathy. Br Heart J 1984;51:195–201.
36. Meinertz T, Hofmann T, Kasper W, Treese N, Bechtold H, Stienen U, Pop T, Leitner E-RV, Andresen D, Meyer J. Significance of ventricular arrhythmias in idiopathic dilated cardiomyopathy. Am J Cardiol 1984;53:902–907.
37. Meinertz T, Treese N, Kasper W, Geibel A, Hofmann T, Zehender M, Bohn D, Pop T, Just H. Determinants of prognosis in idiopathic dilated cardiomyopathy as determined by programmed electrical stimulation. Am J Cardiol 1985;56:337–341.
38. Poll DS, Marchlinski FE, Buxton AE, Doherty JU, Waxman HL, Josephson ME. Sustained ventricular tachycardia in patients with idiopathic dilated cardiomyopathy; electrophysiologic testing and lack of response to antiarrhythmic drug therapy. Circulation 1984;70:451–456.
39. Unverferth DV, Mehegan JP, Magorien RD, Unverferth BJ, Leier CV. Regression of myocardial cellular hypertrophy with vasodilator therapy in chronic congestive heart failure associated with idiopathic dilated cardiomyopathy. Am J Cardiol 1983;51:1392–1398.
40. Unverferth DV, Magorien RD, Moeschberg ML, Baker PB, Fetters JK, Leier CV. Factors influencing the one-year mortality of dilated cardiomyopathy. Am J Cardiol 1984;54:147–152.
41. Wallis DE, O'Connell JB, Henkin RE, Costanzo-Nordin MR, Scanlon PJ. Segmental wall motion abnormalities in dilated cardiomyopathy: a common finding and good prognostic sign. JACC 1984;4:674–679.
42. Holmes J, Kubo SH, Cody RJ, Kligfield P. Arrhythmias in ischemic and nonischemic dilated cardiomyopathy: prediction of mortality by ambulatory electrocardiography. Am J Cardiol 1985;55:146–151.
43. Anderson JL, Lutz JR, Gilbert EM, Sorensen SG, Yanowitz FG, Menlove RL, Bartholomew M. A randomized trial of low-dose beta-blockade therapy for idiopathic dilated cardiomyopathy. Am J Cardiol 1985;55:471–475.
44. Anderson JL, Carlquist JF, Lutz JR, DeWitt CW, Hammond EH. HLA A, B and DR typing in idiopathic dilated cardiomyopathy: a search for immune response factors. Am J Cardiol 1984;53:1326–1330.
45. Sanderson JE, Koech D, David I, Ojiambo HP. T-lymphocyte subsets in idiopathic dilated cardiomyopathy. Am J Cardiol 1985;55:755–758.
46. Michels VV, Driscoll DJ, Miller FA Jr. Familial aggregation of idiopathic dilated cardiomyopathy. Am J Cardiol 1985;55:1232–1233.
47. O'Connell JB, Costanzo-Nordin MR, Subramanian R, Robinson JA, Wallis DE, Scanlon PJ, Gunnar RM. Peripartum cardiomyopathy: clinical, hemodynamic, histologic and prognostic characteristics. JACC 1986;8:52–56.
48. Cassling RS, Linder J, Sears TD, Waller BF, Rogler WC, Wilson JE, Kugler JD, Kay HD, Dillon JC, Slack JD, McManus BM. Quantitative evaluation of inflammation in biopsy specimens from idiopathically failing or irritable hearts: experience in 80 pediatric and adult patients. Am Heart J 1985;110:713–720.
49. Tazelaar HD, Billingham ME. Leukocytic infiltrates in idiopathic dilated cardiomyopathy. Am J Surg Pathol 1986;10:405–412.
50. Perloff JK. The cardiomyopathies: dilated and restrictive. Circulation 1981;63:1189–1198.
51. Odom H II, Davis JL, Dinh H, Baker BJ, Roberts WC, Murphy ML. QRS voltage measurements in autopsied men free of cardiopulmonary disease: a basis for evaluating total QRS voltage as an index of left ventricular hypertrophy. Am J Cardiol 1986;58:801–804.
52. Siegel RJ, Roberts WC. Electrocardiographic observations in severe aortic valve stenosis: correlative necropsy study to clinical, hemodynamic, and ECG variables demonstrating relation of 12-lead QRS amplitude to peak systolic transaortic pressure gradient. Am Heart J 1982;103:298–301.
53. Roberts WC, Waller BF. Cardiac amyloidosis causing cardiac dysfunction: analysis of 54 necropsy patients. Am J Cardiol 1983;52:137–146.

CONGENITAL CARDIOVASCULAR ABNORMALITIES USUALLY SILENT UNTIL ADULTHOOD

William C. Roberts, M.D.

Most congenital heart diseases are believed to consist of *defects* (absent tissue) in cardiac septa causing shunts, or *obstructions* (excess tissue) at or near valvular levels, or *anomalous connections* between arteries and veins or between arteries or veins and cardiac chambers, or *combinations* of these 3. A congenital cardiovascular malformation, however, may consist of an improperly formed tissue (abiotrophy) that functions normally or nearly normally at birth and during the early decades of life but later causes cardiac dysfunction. This chapter focuses on certain morphologic features in 6 of these conditions.

MITRAL VALVE PROLAPSE

Although recognized earlier,[1-4] delineation of the click–late systolic murmur syndrome as a consequence of mitral valve prolapse was not appreciated until the 1960s.[5-9] It is now apparent that the click–late systolic murmur is common, probably occurring in 5% or more of persons > 15 years of age.[10-12] Although generally not considered as such, the click–systolic murmur syndrome, probably in most persons, is a form of congenital heart disease, and, therefore, is the most common congenital heart disease. The auscultatory manifestations, however, are usually not evident until adulthood.

The click-murmur syndrome may be viewed from both auscultatory and morphologic standpoints as manifesting 3 stages (Fig. 1): (1) systolic click(s) only, (2) click(s) plus a mid to late systolic murmur, and (3) pansystolic murmur only. Although progression from stage 1 to 3 has been documented in relatively few patients, it appears likely that this is the natural sequence of events in some patients. In others, there may be no progression from stage 1, patients in stage 2 may revert to stage 1, patients in stage 1 may lose their click(s) altogether, and patients appearing in stage 3 (pansystolic murmur) may have had no documentation of stages 1 and 2. With rare exception, stages 1 and 2 are unassociated with symptomatic evidence of cardiac dysfunction. The exception includes patients with arrhythmias and/or chest pain. Patients in stage 3 may have congestive heart failure because of the asso-

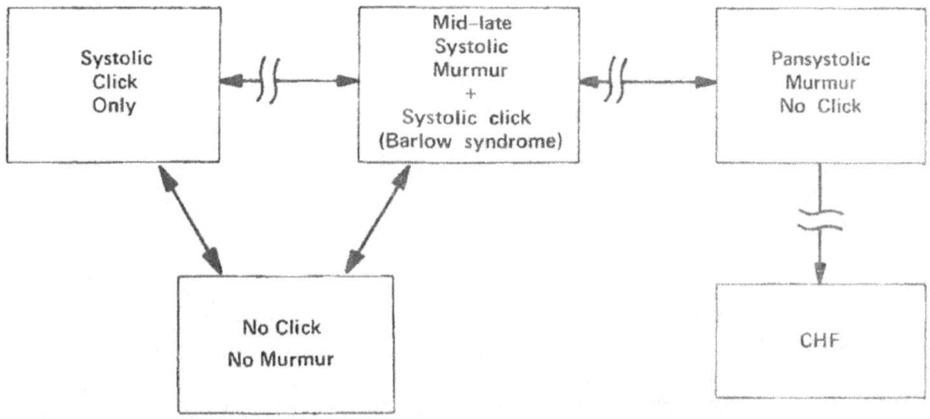

FIGURE 1. Diagram showing likely auscultatory progression in the prolapsing mitral valve syndrome. CHF = congestive heart failure. From Roberts WC, Glancy DB., Seningen RP, Maron BJ., Epstein SE. Prolapse of the mitral valve (floppy valve) associated with Ebstein's anomaly of the tricuspid valve. Am J Cardiol 1976; 377–382, with permission.

ciated severe mitral regurgitation. The stage 3 floppy mitral valve is the major cause of *pure* (no element of stenosis) *severe, isolated* (aortic valve normal anatomically and functionally) mitral regurgitation requiring valve replacement or repair.[13] As a consequence, there is considerable anatomic information available on the floppy mitral valve that produces a pansystolic murmur (stage 3) and causes severe mitral regurgitation.[13–35] In contrast, there is relatively little anatomic information available in patients with only a systolic click(s) (stage 1) or those with both a click(s) and a late systolic murmur (stage 2).

Several names applied to this syndrome describe to some extent what the valve looks like anatomically, thus the names "prolapsing posterior mitral leaflet," "prolapsing mitral valve," "billowing or ballooning mitral leaflet syndrome," "overshooting or hooded mitral valve," "floppy mitral valve," and "myxomatous or mucinous degeneration of the mitral valve." I prefer the term "mitral valve prolapse."

Defining mitral valve prolapse morphologically has not been easy. Pomerance[14] defined the entity as a ballooning deformity of the mitral leaflets, the affected portions of which were increased in area and protruded into the left atrium in ventricular systole. Waller and associates[13] also utilized either a focal or a diffuse increase in mitral area as a criterion but also required an increased length, either focal or diffuse, from basal attachment of the leaflet to its distal margin. Lucas and Edwards,[31] who prefer the term "floppy mitral valve," listed the following features for diagnosis: (1) interchordal hooding involving both the rough and the clear zones of the involved leaflet or leaflets, (2) height of the interchordal hooding > 4 mm, (3) interchordal hooding involving > 50% of the anterior leaflet or > 67% of the posterior leaflet.

Other useful anatomic findings in identifying mitral valve prolapse include the following: (1) *An increase in the transverse dimension of the leaflets such that the length of the mitral circumference measured on a line corresponding to the distal margin of the posterior leaflet is much larger than the circumference measured at the level of the mitral anulus.* In the normal valve, the 2 are the same. The result is analogous to an accordion not fully extended, or better, a skirt gathered at the waist. The leaflets of the opened mitral valve are flat or smooth (like the mucosa of the ileum), whereas those of the opened floppy mitral valve are undulating (like those of the duodenum or jejunum). (2) *Excessive thinning and lengthening of chordae tendineae.* Chordal elongation, however, is rare without concomitant leaflet elongation. The chordae also occasionally may be shorter than normal. (3) *Dilatation of the mitral anulus.* This does not occur to any significant degree in the absence of the mitral valve prolapse.[36] It appears that anular dilatation is the major cause of development of severe mitral regurgitation in the presence of mitral valve prolapse. (The other is rupture of chordae tendineae.) Normally, the mitral anulus in adults averages about 9 cm in circumference. In patients with left ventricular dilatation from any cause with or without mitral regurgitation, the circumference of the mitral anulus usually dilates slightly, usually to about 11 cm or < 25% above normal.[36] Among patients with mitral valve prolapse associated with severe mitral regurgitation, the circumference of the mitral anulus generally increases > 50% above normal or to circumferences of 14 to 18 cm.[13,36] When the anulus dilates to this extent, the leaflets may "stretch" or flatten transversely, and this stretching diminishes the amount of scalloping. In addition, the left ventricular dilatation may cause longitudinal stretching of the leaflets. The amount of scalloping in the stage 3 valves, therefore, appears to be less than that observed in the stage 2 valves. (4) *Focal thickening of mural endocardium of left ventricle behind the posterior mitral leaflet and the mitral chordae tendineae.* Salazar and Edwards[16] called these fibrous thickenings *"friction lesions"* to indicate that they are believed to result from friction between the overlying leaflets and chordae and the underlying left ventricular wall. Of the 102 necropsy cases with mitral valve prolapse studied by Lucas and Edwards,[31] 77 (75%) had these friction lesions, and in 3 (3%) the mural endocardial friction lesions had entraped the overlying chordae. These friction lesions are virtually specific for mitral valve prolapse. (5) *Fibrinous deposits on the atrial surface of the prolapsed portion of mitral leaflet and particularly at the angle formed between prolapsed leaflet and left atrial wall* (mitral valve–left atrial angle). These deposits in the angle may be a source of emboli.

Microscopically, the prolapsed mitral leaflet may or may not contain an excessive amount of acid mucopolysaccharide material. Both the normal and the prolapsed mitral leaflets consist of 2 elements, the fibrosa and the spongiosa. The *fibrosa* consists of fibrous tissue (collagen), and the *spongiosa,* of mucoid or myxomatous material high in acid mucopolysaccharide material. In most valve diseases, the fibrosa element proliferates and may entirely replace the spongiosa element. In the prolapsed mitral leaflet, the spongiosa element, the more central portion of the leaflet, may proliferate to a greater extent than the fibrosa element. The resulting proliferated myxoid or myxomatous stroma, however, does not appear abnormal, that is, degenerated. Thus, the term myxoid or myxomatous "degeneration" for this condition is not appropriate. The amount of fibrous tissue in the mitral leaflets in mitral valve prolapse also is usually increased but maybe its increase is a secondary phenomenon. The fibrosa element may be subdivided into 2 components, the *auricularis,* which normally is a thin layer forming the atrial or contact aspect of the leaflet, and the *ventricularis,* which normally is a relatively thick layer that covers the ventricular aspect of the leaflet. The atrial aspect of the prolapsed mitral leaflet often is focally thickened. This change probably is secondary to abnormal friction from contact between the prolapsed segment of the leaflet and its "opposite number," that is, the other leaflet, or between 2 prolapsed segments of the same leaflet.[25,26] The changes on the ventricular surface of the leaflet consist of connective tissue "pads" forming primarily in the interchordal segments, and this proliferation of fibrous tissue may extend into adjacent chordae tendineae and onto ventricular endocardium behind the posterior mitral leaflet.[16,26] The interchordal collections of fibrous tissue are considered responses to the tension and stretching that occur at the undersurface of a prolapsed leaflet or segment of leaflet.[26] This increase in fibrous tissue, particularly on the ventricular surface of the leaflet, has caused, I suspect, the floppy valve earlier to be considered rheumatic in origin.[25] Fibrin deposits also may occur on the atrial aspects of the prolapsed mitral leaflet, and they may not be found on gross examination.[14]

Ultrastructural studies of floppy mitral valves have disclosed alterations of the collagen fibers in the leaflets and in the chordae tendineae.[37] These changes have included fragmentation, splitting, swelling, and coarse granularity of the individual

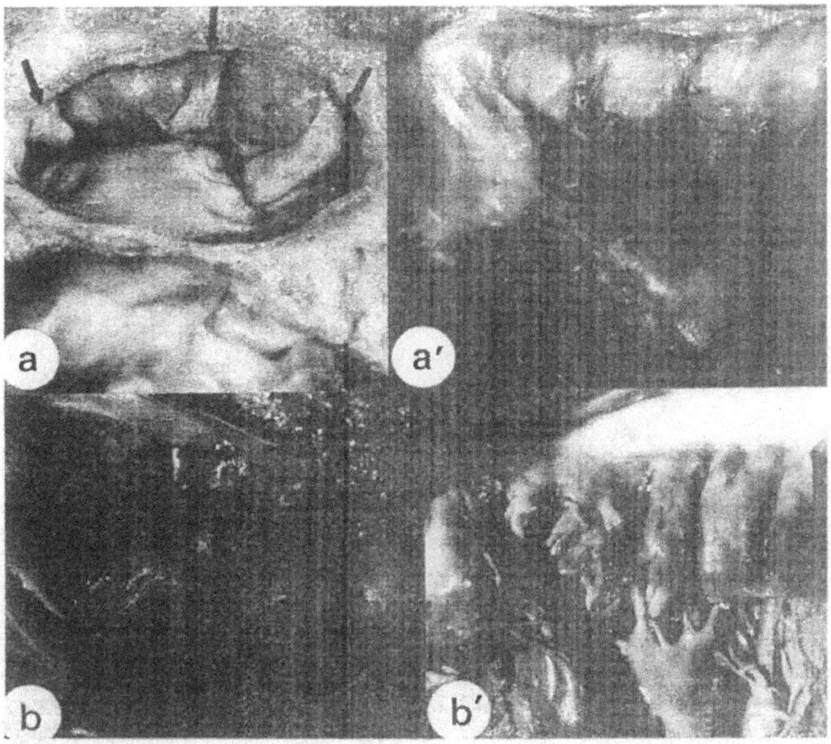

FIGURE 2. Mitral valves of 2 children, aged 9 and 13, who died of leukemia. Neither had symptoms of cardiac dysfunction. *a* and *a′*, Mitral valve as viewed from left atrium (*a*) and after opening (*a′*). Three areas of leaflet overlap (arrows) are present with the valve intact, and the orifice is competent. The leaflets are devoid of scallops and relatively smooth (*a′*). This child had 3 systolic clicks during life but no precordial murmur. *b* and *b′*, Mitral valve as viewed from left atrium (*b*) and after opening (*b′*). Both leaflets of this valve, in contrast to the valve above, are highly scalloped, causing the orifice to be incompetent. This child had a systolic click and a late systolic murmur. (The children whose valves are shown here were examined by Dr. John Barlow in Johannesburg, South Africa, and the auscultatory findings described above were those of Dr. Barlow. I am indebted to him for allowing me to photograph each of these hearts.) From Roberts WC. Congenital cardiovascular abnormalities usually "silent" until adulthood: Morphologic features of the floppy mitral valve, valvular aortic stenosis, discrete subvalvular aortic stenosis, hypertrophic cardiomyopathy, sinus of Valsalva aneurysm, and the Marfan syndrome. Cardiovasc Clin 1979; 10(1):409, with permission.

collagen fibers, and, in addition, spiraling and twisting of the fibers. Also, some elastic fibers are fragmented and contain cystic spaces. These alterations in the structure of the collagen may be more important than the accumulation of the acid mucopolysaccharide material in that they lead to focal weaknesses in the leaflets. The left ventricular systolic pressure exerted against these weakened areas may lead to prolapse or focal interchordal hooding. Although the actual prolapse of the mitral valve may be acquired and a consequence of the left ventricular systolic (closing) pressure, the focally weak areas of the leaflets are probably most often congenital in origin. This focal leaflet weakness may be analogous to the berry aneurysm of the cerebral artery—the weakness in the arterial wall is almost certainly congenital in origin, and the later bulging with or without rupture is acquired as a consequence of the high intra-arterial pressure. The frequency of mitral valve prolapse also may be higher in persons with elevated left ventricular systolic pressures compared with persons in whom this pressure is at normal levels.

Opportunities for structural study of a mitral valve associated with only a click(s) have been rare. I have studied 1 such valve (Fig. 2). (The child had been examined by John Barlow, M.D., of Johannesburg, South Africa.) The child, who had had no symptoms of cardiac dysfunction, died of leukemia and at necropsy had a perfectly competent mitral valve but 3 distinct foci where leaflet overlapped adjacent leaflet. The leaflets otherwise were smooth and, specifically, devoid of so-called scallops. There are no reported anatomic descriptions, to my knowledge, of mitral valves producing 1 or more systolic clicks without an associated precordial systolic murmur. Examination at necropsy of mitral valves of patients who during life had documentation of systolic click(s) plus a mid-late sytolic murmur (Barlow syndrome) also are infrequent (Figs. 3 and 4). Death in stage 2 as in stage 1 is usually from a noncardiac cause. In this stage, the most characteristic feature is leaflet scalloping, which represents excessive leaflet owing to an increase in the transverse or commissure-to-commissure dimension of the leaflet. The mitral anulus, as in stage 1, is not dilated. The chordae tendineae may or may not be elongated.

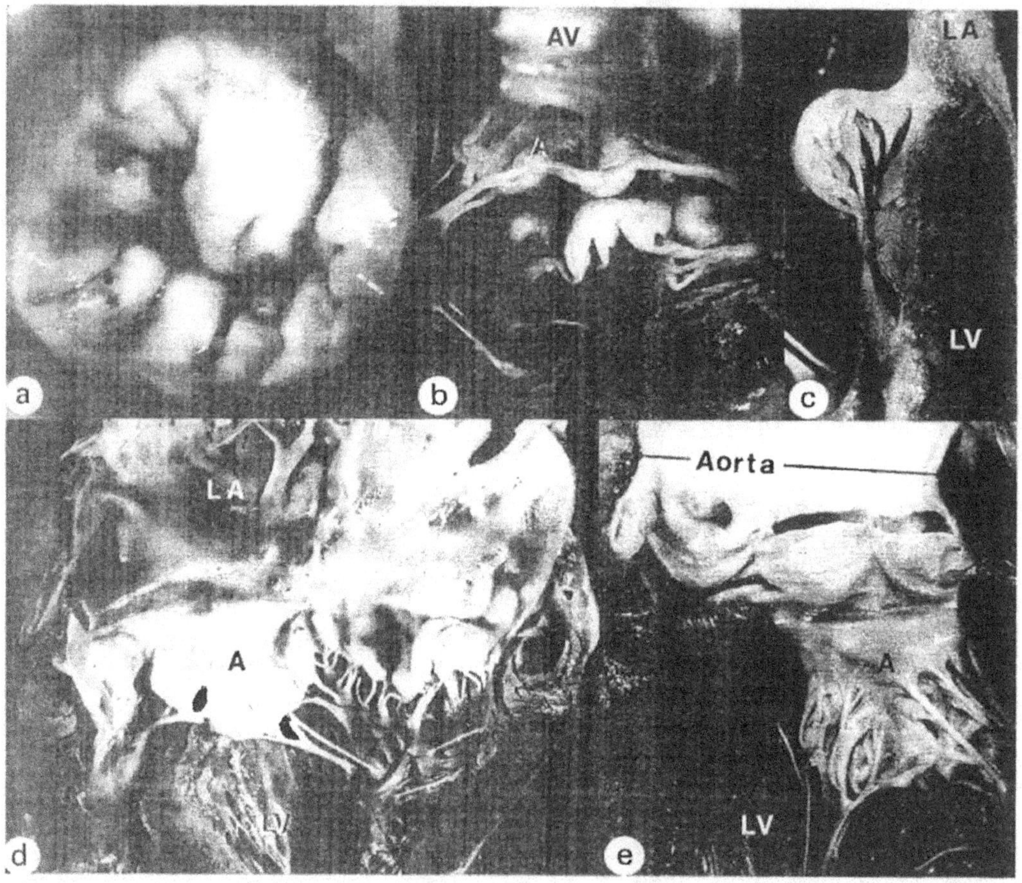

FIGURE 3. Floppy mitral valve in an 18-year-old girl who died of Ewing's sarcoma. She never had symptoms of cardiac dysfunction despite an active life. She had a mid-systolic click and a grade 3/6, ejection-type systolic murmur over the precordium, loudest over the apex. Necropsy revealed Ebstein anomaly of the tricuspid valve. The mitral leaflets shown are elongated transversely, but the chordae are not elongated. *a*, Mitral valve as viewed from left atrium showing market scalloping. *b*, Same valve as viewed from left ventricle (A = anterior mitral leaflet; AV = aortic valve). *c*, Longitudinal section of left atrium (LA), billowing posterior mitral leaflet, and left ventricle (LV). *d*, Opened mitral valve. *e*, View of anterior mitral leaflet (A) from the left ventricular (LV) aspect. The mitral leaflets and chordae tendineae contained excessive amounts of acid mucopolysaccharide material. From Roberts WC., Glancy DB., Sen-ingen RP., Maron BJ., Epstein SE. Prolapse of the mitral valve (floppy valve) associated with Ebstein's anomaly of the tricuspid valve. Am J Cardiol 1976; 38:377–382, with permission.

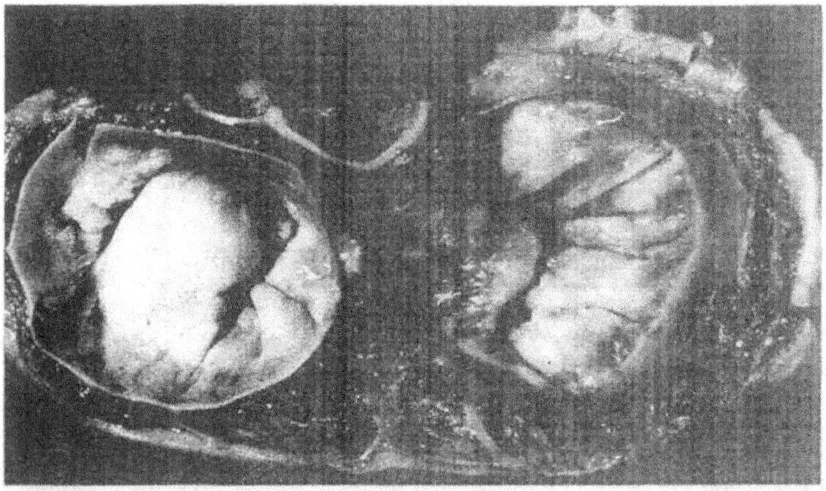

FIGURE 4. Floppy mitral valve (left) and floppy tricuspid valve (right) in a 51-year-old man who died suddenly at a dance. Although always asymptomatic, he was found to have a precordial systolic murmur when he was 36 years old. When evaluated about 1 year before death, he had a systolic murmur; echocardiogram disclosed the classic "hammocking" of the mitral leaflets during ventricular systole, and left ventricular angiography also showed "classic" mitral leaflet prolapse during ventricular systole.

At necropsy, at least ⅓ of the posterior mitral leaflet had prolapsed toward left atrium; several chordae tendineae to this prolapsed segment were thickened and a few were absent, indicating that rupture had occurred. The anterior mitral leaflet appeared normal from the left ventricular aspect, but from the left atrial aspect it was thickened as a result of abnormal contact by the large prolapsed segment of posterior leaflet. All chordae tendineae from the anterior leaflet were elongated, whereas those from the posterior leaflet were thickened. There was no clinical evidence of dysfunction of the tricuspid valve. Both atria were mildly dilated. The coronary arteries were normal in course and size and free of significant luminal narrowing. The myocardial free walls were free of foci of necrosis or fibrosis.

This case is an example of sudden death in a previously asymptomatic patient with classic auscultatory, echocardiographic, and left ventricular angiographic features of the systolic click-late systolic murmur syndrome. From Roberts WC. Congenital cardiovascular abnormalities usually "silent" until adulthood: Morphologic features of the floppy mitral valve, valvular aortic stenosis, discrete subvalvular aortic stenosis, hypertrophic cardiomyopathy, sinus of Valsalva aneurysm, and the Marfan syndrome. Cardiovasc Clin 1979; 10(1):411, with permission.

Just as the frequency of mitral valve prolapse varies clinically depending on the age and sex group being examined and in the clinical criteria employed for diagnosis (ausculatory, echocardiographic, angiographic), its frequency at necropsy is quite variable and the variation is determined by several factors: (1) age and sex group of population being examined; (2) type of institution where necropsy is performed (general hospital, referral hospital for cardiovascular disease, or medical examiner's [coroner's] office); (3) expertise in cardiovascular disease of the physician performing the necropsy or reporting the findings; (4) percent of total deaths having autopsies at the particular hospital; (5) presence or absence of evidence of cardiac disease before death; (6) whether the patient underwent mitral valve replacement or repair, and (7) whether the percentage of patients being examined had a high frequency of the Marfan syndrome, infective endocarditis, atrial septal defeat, and so on. No study better shows how bias alters the findings in necropsy studies than the one performed by Lucas and Edwards.[31] These investigators in 1 portion of their study determined the frequency of and complications of floppy mitral valves observed at necropsy in 1 community (nonreferral) hospital for adults. Of 1376 autopsies performed, 7.4%

or 102 patients at necropsy had morphologically floppy mitral valves. Their mean age at death was 69 ± 12 years; 62 (61%) were men and 40 (39%) were women. Of the 102 patients, mitral valve prolapse was the cause of death in only 2. Of the 102 patients, 1 cusp had prolapsed in 34 patients, and 2 cusps in 68. Only 18 had anatomic evidence of previous mitral regurgitation; 7, infective endocarditis: 7, ruptured chordae tendineae (without infection); 1, the Marfan syndrome; 3, secundum atrial septal defect. No patient died suddenly. In contrast, in the other portion of their study, these authors described complications in 69 necropsy patients whose hearts had been sent to Edwards for his opinion and interest. Among these 69 patients, 16 (23%) had died suddenly and unexpectedly; 19 (28%), had ruptured chordae tendineae (without infection); 7 (10%), infective endocarditis; 20 (29%), the Marfan syndrome; and 9 (13%), secundum type atrial septal defect. Thus, in contrast to their infrequency in their community hospital series, most cases submitted to their cardiovascular registry from other institutions had ruptured chordae, infective endocarditis, sudden unexpected and unexplained death, or the Marfan syndrome.

Two other necropsy studies can be compared with the community hospital series collected by Lucas and Edwards. Pomerance[14] collected from 1 general hospital 35 cases at necropsy of "ballooning deformity" of the mitral valve: 23 (66%) were men and 12 (34%) were women; their ages ranged from 51 to 98 years (mean 74). Death was attributed to mitral valve prolapse in only 4 patients (11%). One leaflet only had prolapsed in 12 patients and 2 leaflets in 23 (6%). Eight patients had anatomic evidence of mitral regurgitation, only 1 had atrial septal defect, 9 (26%) had anatomic evidence of tricuspid valve prolapse, 9 (26%) had mitral anular calcific deposits, and 13 (37%) had hearts of increased weight. Davies and associates[27] gathered 90 necropsy cases of the floppy mitral valve from 4 general hospitals. This number represented 4.5% of autopsies at the 4 hospitals during the time. Of the 90 patients, 44 (49%) were men and 46 (51%) were women; they ranged in age from $<$ 40 to 100 years. Death in 15 was attributed to mitral valve prolapse (the number dying suddenly was not mentioned). The prolapse involved 1 leaflet in 69 patients (77%) and both mitral leaflets in 21 (23%); 63 (70%) also had antomic evidence of tricuspid valve prolapse. Only 6 (7%) patients had dilated mitral anuli; only 3 (3%) had mitral anular calcium, and 8 had hearts weighing $>$ 300 g.

The frequency of mitral valve prolapse among patients undergoing mitral valve replacement for *isolated* (aortic valve function normal), *pure* (no element of stenosis), and *severe* mitral regurgitation is high—indeed, prolapse appears to be the most common etiology of isolated, pure, and severe mitral regurgitation. My associates and I[13] reviewed the records and operatively excised mitral valves of 97 patients (57 men) aged 32 to 78 years (mean 54), who underwent mitral valve replacement because of 3+/4+ or 4+/4+ mitral regurgitation as determined by left ventricular angiography. Of the 97 patients, the cause of the mitral regurgitation was leaflet prolapse in 60 (62%), papillary muscle dysfunction from coronary heart disease in 29 (30%), infective endocarditis involving apparently previously normal mitral valves in 5, and rheumatic heart disease in 3 patients. Of the 60 patients with mitral valve prolapse 13 had ruptured chordae tendineae, including all 4 patients with infective endocarditis superimposed on mitral valve prolapse.

The circumference of the mitral anulus in the patients with mitral valve prolapse without ruptured chordae was significantly larger than those in the patients in other groups and in 18 control subjects, both of which were normal. Likewise, the areas of the excised leaflets in the prolapsed valves were much larger than in the other groups and in the control subjects, both of which were normal. The product of the circumference (in cm) multiplied by the area (in cm squared) calculated for the normal valves ranged from 45 to 140 cm^3 (average 91). The average product was 150 cm^3 in the prolapsed valves with ruptured chordae, and 273 cm^3 in the prolapsed valves with intact chordae. The products were 87, 91, and 106 cm^3, respectively, in the valves regurgitant because of papillary muscle dysfunction, infective endocarditis, or rheumatic disease; these products did not differ from those of the normal valves.

The correct cause of the mitral regurgitation in the 97 patients was usually predictable from the history alone. Of the 29 patients with papillary muscle dysfunction from atherosclerotic coronary heart disease, all had clinical evidence of myocardial ischemia: history of acute myocardial infarction that had healed in 24, left ventricular aneurysm from a silent infarction in 1, and angina pectoris in 4. Of the 5 patients with mitral regurgitation secondary to infective endocarditis, 4 had well-documented episodes of infection that had been cured by antibiotic therapy; none had evidence of valvular dysfunction before the episode of infective endocarditis. Of the 3 patients with mitral regurgitation secondary to a rheumatic origin, 2 had a history of acute rheumatic fever, whereas this item was positive in only 5 of the other 94 patients. Clinical diagnosis of mitral valve prolapse was by a process of exclusion. Only 2 (3%) of the 60 patients had historical evidence of previous acute myocardial infarction, 5 (8%) had a history of acute rheumatic fever, and 4 (7%) had a history of active infective endocarditis. Compared with the 5 patients classified as having ruptured chordae tendineae on previously normal valves (4 of whom had a history of infective endocarditis), the 4 patients with healed infective endocarditis and mitral valve prolapse were older (mean age 61 years versus 42 years), had previous systolic murmurs of mitral regurgitation before the episode of infective endocarditis (4 of 4 versus 0 of 5), and had a longer mean duration of congestive heart failure (11 months versus 4 months). Thus, of the 60 patients with mitral valve prolapse, 51 (85%) had no historical evidence of myocardial ischemia, acute rheumatic fever, or infective endocarditis.

The origin of the mitral regurgitation also was suggested preoperatively by more objective means. All 29 patients with mitral regurgitation secondary to coronary artery disease had abnormal Q waves by electrocardiogram, whereas abnormal Q waves were present in only 4 of the 60 patients with mitral valve prolapse and in none of the 8 patients with mitral regurgitation from either infective endocarditis or rheumatic disease. Atrial fibrillation was significantly more common in the patients in whom the mitral regurgitation resulted from coronary artery disease: in 7 (24%) of these 29 patients, in only 4 (7%) of the 60 patients with mitral valve prolapse, and in 2 of the 8 patients with either infective endocarditis or a rheumatic origin. Of the 60 patients with mitral valve prolapse, 43 had M-mode echocardiograms, and in 32 (74%) mitral valve prolapse was demonstrated.[38] Of the 29 patients with coronary heart disease, M-mode echocardiograms were done in 22; only 2 (9%) demonstrated mitral valve prolapse. Of the 8 patients with mitral regurgitation from infective endocarditis or rheumatic etiology, 7 had echocardiograms; none demonstrated mitral valve prolapse. Left ventriculograms, performed in all 97 patients, indicated mitral valve prolapse in only 16 (27%) of the 60 patients with mitral valve prolapse and in none of the other 37 patients with other causes. Selective coronary angiograms were performed in 53 (55%) of the 97 patients. All 29 with mitral regurgitation secondary to coronary heart disease had significant (> 50% diameter reduction) coronary narrowing demonstrated angiographically in at least 2 of the 3 major coronary arteries. Of the 60 patients with mitral valve prolapse, coronary angiograms were performed in 23; only 3 (13%) had significant coronary arterial narrowing, limited in each to 1 (right) coronary artery. Auscultation and hemodynamic data at cardiac catheterization were not helpful in delineating the origin of the mitral regurgitation. None of the 97 patients—including the 60 classified as having mitral valve prolapse—had systolic clicks, and the systolic precordial murmurs in all 97 patients were holosystolic. The average pulmonary arterial, left atrial (or pulmonary aterial wedge), and left ventricular pressures were similar in the 97 patients irrespective of the origin of the mitral regurgitation. The systolic systemic arterial pressures, however, were significantly higher in the patients with mitral valve prolapse and ruptured chordae tendineae than in those with mitral valve prolapse and intact chordae tendineae.

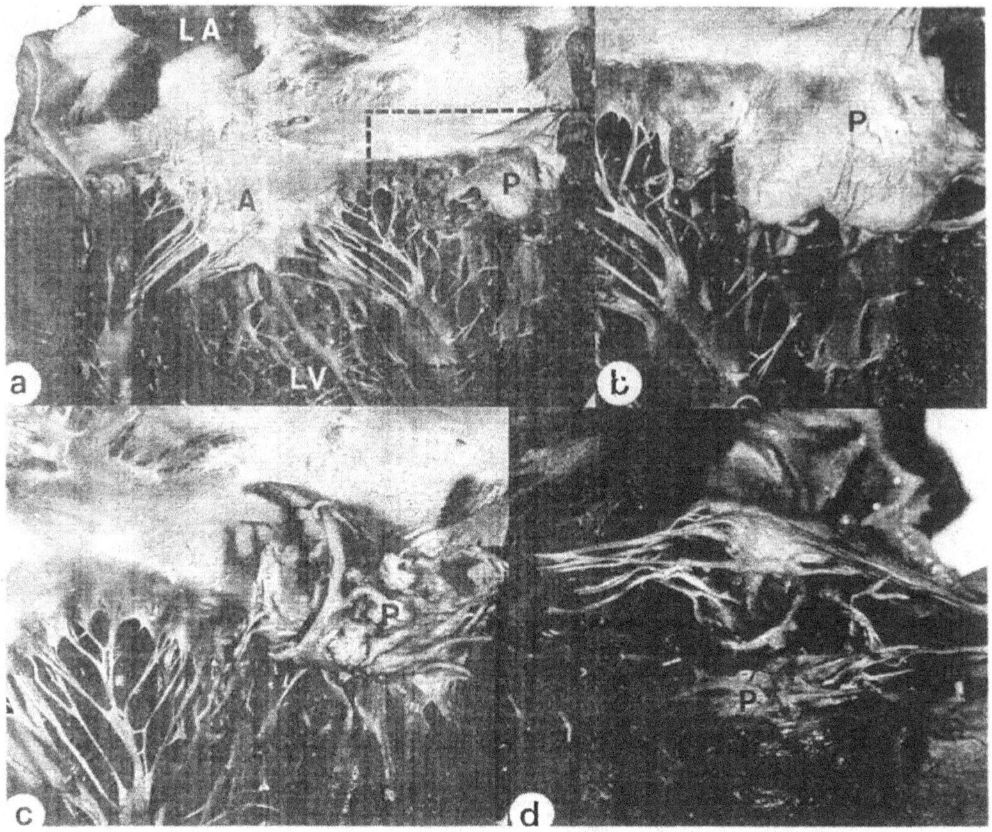

FIGURE 5. Floppy mitral valve in a 38-year-old man who had been well until 3 years before death, when he experienced a fairly abrupt onset of congestive heart failure. Cardiac catheterization at that time confirmed the presence of pure mitral regurgitation. His blood urea nitrogen at that time was 41 mg/dl. During the next 3 years, he developed severe systemic hypertension (240/140 mm Hg), severe anemia, severe azotemia (blood urea nitrogen = 230 mg/dl), and finally, fatal hemorrhagic cardiac tamponade. Necropsy revealed a large segment of posterior mitral leaflet, elongated and prolapsed into the left atrium. Most of the chordae tendineae from this prolapsed segment were ruptured. (The patient never had evidence of infective endocarditis.) The heart weighed 620 gm.

a, Opened left atrium (LA), mitral valve, left ventricle (LV), and prolapsed sement (P). The portion of mitral leaflets and chordae outside the boxed area is normal or near normal (A = anterior mitral leaflet). *b*, Closeup of atrial aspect of the prolapsed segment. *c*, Same view showing the prolapsed segment flipped back into left atrium, exposing its ventricular aspect. *d*, View of mitral valve from left ventricle. In this case, mitral prolapse may have been worsened by systemic hypertension; increased closing pressure on the mitral leaflets is created by the elevated systolic pressure. From Roberts WC. Congenital cardiovascular abnormalities usually "silent" until adulthood: Morphologic features of the floppy mitral valve, valvular aortic stenosis, discrete subvalvular aortic stenosis, hypertrophic cardiomyopathy, sinus of Valsalva aneurysm, and the Marfan syndrome. Cardiovasc Clin 1979; 10(1):417, with permission.

Mitral valve prolapse appears now to be a more common cause of rupture of mitral chordae tendineae than does infective endocarditis (Figs. 5 and 6). Among 25 patients having mitral valve replacement for pure mitral regurgitation associated with rupture of chordae tendineae, Jeresaty and associates[39] found mitral valve prolapse (based on "redundancy and marked hooding of the mitral leaflets") to be the cause of the chordal rupture in 23 (92%), only 1 of whom had had infective endocarditis. Four of the 25 patients had auscultatory and angiographic or echocardio-

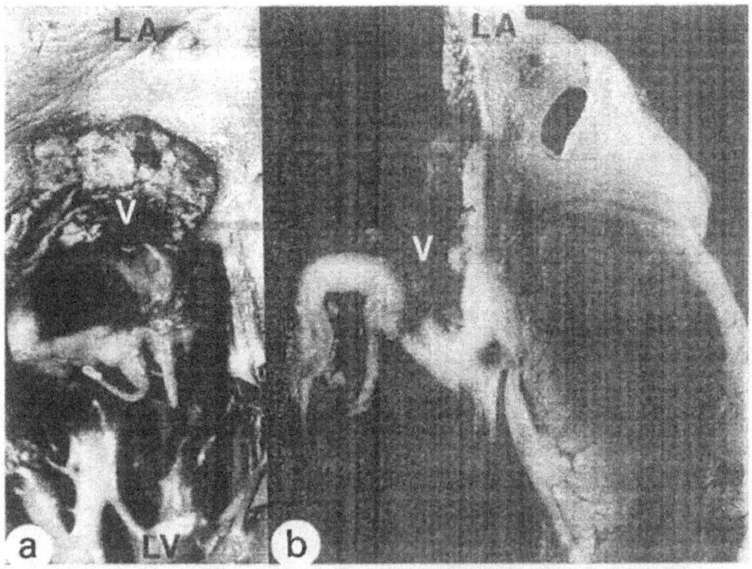

FIGURE 6. Floppy mitral valve with superimposed *Staphylococcus aureus* endocarditis in a 52-year-old man who was known to have a murmur of mitral regurgitation for 10 years. He was asymptomatic, however, until he developed typical clinical features of active infective endocarditis, which caused a fatal septic cerebral embolus. Necropsy revealed a portion of posterior mitral leaflet prolapsed toward left atrium (LA) and vegetative (V) material at the acute angle formed by the hooded posterior leaflet and mural endocardium of left atrium. (This junction is a common location of fibrin-platelet deposits in patients with prolapsed posterior mitral leaflets.) *a*, Closeup of hooded segment of posterior leaflet with the superimposed vegetation. *b*, Longitudinal section through left atrium, prolapsed and thickened posterior leaflet, and left ventricle (LV). From Roberts WC. Congenital cardiovascular abnormalities usually "silent" until adulthood: Morphologic features of the floppy mitral valve, valvular aortic stenosis, discrete subvalvular aortic stenosis, hypertrophic cardiomyopathy, sinus of Valsalva aneurysm, and the Marfan syndrome. Cardiovasc Clin 1979; 10(1):416, with permission.

graphic evidence of mitral valve prolapse before the chordal rupture. Among patients with ruptured chordae tendineae associated with mitral valve prolapse, sometimes it is actually difficult to identify ruptured chords. The term "rupture," however, is commonly applied to those leaflets where chordal insertions are no longer present but clearly chordae should be attached.

In addition to mitral regurgitation, rupture of chordae tendineae, and infective endocarditis, other complications of mitral valve prolapse include *mitral anular calcification* (Table 1, Fig. 7). Pomerance[14] observed mitral anular calcium in 9 (26%) of her 35 necropsy patients with mitral valve prolapse. The cause of the *arrhythmias* and *chest pain* is unclear.[40] There is no evidence of a myocardial or coronary arterial factor. Shrivastava and associates [26] have suggested that the friction between mitral chordae tendineae and the underlying left ventricular mural endocardium may be an arrhythmic stimulus. The cause of the *acute strokes* or *transient cerebral ischemic attacks* that occur in an occasional patient with mitral valve prolapse also is unclear. It has been suggested that the small fibrin-platelet thrombi occasionally seen at the mitral valve–left atrial angle are sources of emboli for either cerebral or myocardial ischemia.[31]

The cause of mitral valve prolapse, as alluded to earlier, almost certainly in most patients is congenital in origin, or at least the connective tissue of the mitral leaflets, chordae, and anulus appears to be congenitally defective. The finding of classic mitral valve prolapse at birth is certainly evidence for the congenital thesis (Fig. 8). The occurrence of mitral valve prolapse in certain clearly hereditary condi-

TABLE 1. Prolapsing Mitral Valve Complications

1. Mitral regurgitation
2. Calcification, mitral "anulus"
3. Rupture of chordae tendineae
   A. Infective endocarditis
   B. Noninfective ("spontaneous")
4. Infective endocarditis
5. Arrhythmias
6. Chest pain
7. Stroke (transient ischemic attacks)
8. Sudden death

From Roberts W C. Congenital cardiovascular abnormalities usually "silent" until adulthood: Morphologic features of the floppy mitral valve, valvular aortic stenosis, discrete subvalvular aortic stenosis, hypertrophic cardiomyopathy, sinus of Valsalva aneurysm, and the Marfan syndrome. Cardiovasc Clin 1979; 10(1):415, with permission.

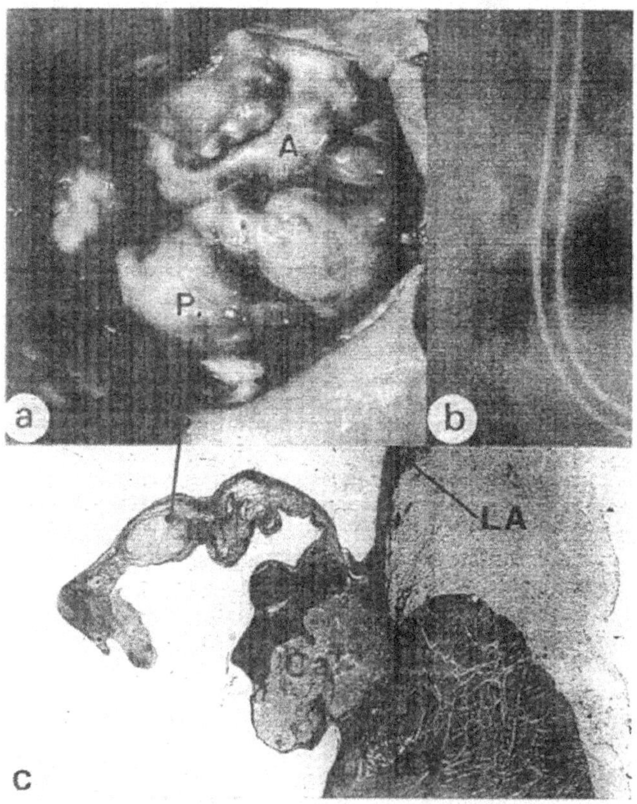

FIGURE 7. Floppy mitral valve and calcium in the mitral anulus of a 70-year-old woman who had a grade 3/6 murmur of mitral regurgitation, atrial fibrillation, and complete heart block. *a*, Mitral valve from left atrial aspect. (A, P. = anterior and posterior mitral leaflets, respectively.) *b*, Radiograph taken while the patient was alive shows a C-shaped deposit of calcium in the mitral anular area. Pacing wires are also visible. *c*, Photomicrograph through wall of left atrium (LA), prolapsed mitral leaflet, and left ventricle (LV). The calcium (Ca^{++}) in the anular area is apparent. From Roberts WC. Congenital cardiovascular abnormalities usually "silent" until adulthood: Morphologic features of the floppy mitral valve, valvular aortic stenosis, discrete subvalvular aortic stenosis, hypertrophic cardiomyopathy, sinus of Valsalva aneurysm, and the Marfan syndrome. Cardiovasc Clin 1979; 10(1):415, with permission.

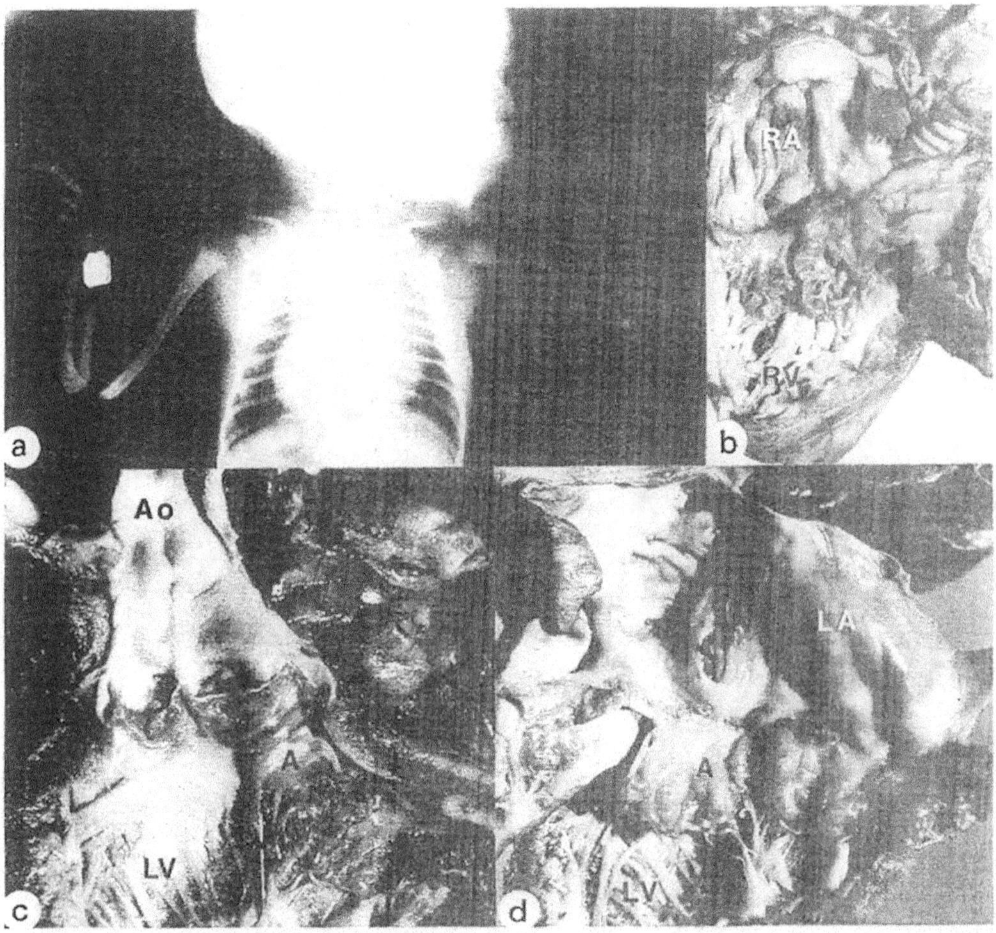

FIGURE 8. Congenital floppy mitral valve and floppy tricuspid valve in a 2-day-old boy who had long toes and fingers, a high-arched palate, and a grade 3/6 precordial systolic murmur typical of mitral regurgitation. The heart was enlarged (*a*), and he died of congestive cardiac failure. At necropsy, the intima of the ascending aorta (Ao) was wrinkled (*c*), suggesting that the underlying media was abnormal at this early stage. Shown here is the opened aorta, aortic valve, and left ventricle (LV) (A = anterior mitral leaflet). (*d*), Opened left atrium (LA), mitral valve, and left ventricle (LV). The mitral leaflets are considerably elongated in both longitudinal and transverse dimensions. The left atrium (LA) is dilated. *b*, The tricuspid valve leaflets also are elongated in both transverse and longitudinal dimensions (RA = right atrium; RV = right ventricle). From Roberts WC. Congenital cardiovascular abnormalities usually "silent" until adulthood: Morphologic features of the floppy mitral valve, valvular aortic stenosis, discrete subvalvular aortic stenosis, hypertrophic cardiomyopathy, sinus of Valsalva aneurysm, and the Marfan syndrome. Cardiovasc Clin 1979; 10(1):412, with permission.

tions, for example, the Marfan syndrome (Fig. 9), also is evidence of congenitally defective mitral tissue.

AORTIC-VALVE STENOSIS AND THE CONGENITALLY MALFORMED AORTIC VALVE

If papillary muscle dysfunction is excluded, valvular aortic stenosis is the most common fatal cardiac valve lesion, comprising 49% of 1010 personally studied necropsy patients > 15 years of age with valvular heart disease[34,41–49] (Table 2). Of the 495

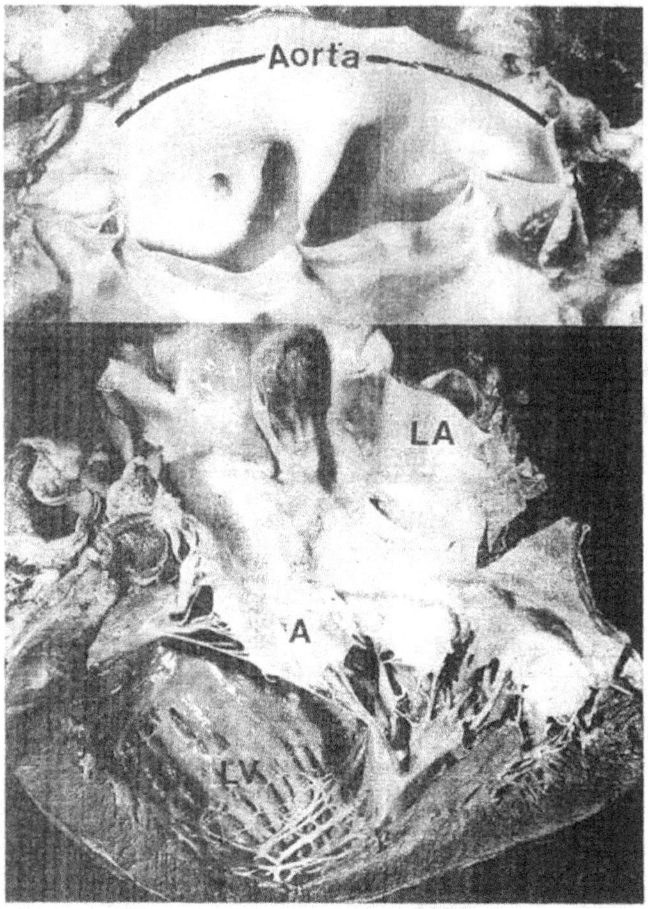

FIGURE 9. Floppy mitral valve—pure mitral regurgitation without aortic disease—in the Marfan syndrome in a 28-year-old man who died from severe mitral regurgitation. He had been well until age 24, when he developed exertional dyspnea and hemoptysis and was found to have cardiomegaly. Catheterization was performed at age 25, and the pressures (in mm Hg) were pulmonary artery, 19/10; right ventricle, 19/5; right atrial mean, 5; pulmonary arterial wedge mean, 10; and systemic artery, 130/80. The cardiac output was 2.3 L/min. He remained functionally class II for the next 3 years, but during his last year of life the congestive heart failure worsened and he became class IV. When examined 7 days before his death, he was quite ill. A grade 5/6 pansystolic precordial murmur, loudest over the apex, was audible. No diastolic murmur was present. The chest radiograph showed a big heart and severe kyphoscoliosis. Electrocardiogram showed sinus rhythm and left ventricular hypertrophy. He died of progressive heart failure.

At necropsy, the heart was huge (850 gm). Although the sinuses were dilated, the aorta was entirely normal histologically *(top)*. The mitral leaflets *(bottom)* were mildly thickened and elongated, and the mitral anulus was severely dilated (15 cm). Calcific deposits were present in the anulus behind the posterior mitral leaflet. The left atrium (LA) was quite dilated as was the left ventricle (LV) (A = anterior mitral leaflet). From Roberts WC. Congenital cardiovascular abnormalities usually "silent" until adulthood: Morphologic features of the floppy mitral valve, valvular aortic stenosis, discrete subvalvular aortic stenosis, hypertrophic cardiomyopathy, sinus of Valsalva aneurysm, and the Marfan syndrome. From Cardiovasc Clin 1979; 10(1):413, with permission.

TABLE 2. Functional and Anatomic Classification of Valvular Heart Disease in 1010 Necropsy Patients ≥ 15 Years of Age*

FUNCTIONAL CLASS	NO. (%) PATIENTS	ANATOMIC CLASS (NO. [%])				
		AV	MV	MV-AV	TV-MV	TV-MV-AV
1. Aortic Stenosis (AS)	292 (29)	256 (87.5)	0	35 (12.1)	0	1 (0.3)
2. Mitral Stenosis (MS)	189 (19)	0	117 (62)	40 (21)	13 (7)	19 (10)
3. MS + AS	152 (15)	0	0	120 (79)	0	32 (21)
4. Aortic Regurgitation (AR)	119 (12)	107† (90)	0	10 (8)	0	2 (2)
5. Mitral Regurgitation (MR)	97 (10)	0	85 (88)	8 (8)	1 (1)	3 (3)
6. MS + AR	65 (6)	0	52 (80)	0	0	13 (20)
7. MR + AR	45 (4)	0	0	39 (87)	0	6 (13)
8. AS + MR	23 (2)	0	0	21 (91)	0	2 (9)
9. Tricuspid stenosis + MS ± AS	28 (3)	0	0	0	4 (14)	24 (86)
TOTALS	1010 (100)‡	363 (36)	254 (25)	273 (27)	18 (2)	102 (10)

AV = aortic valve; MV = mitral valve; TV = tricuspid valve.

*Excludes patients with mitral regurgitation secondary to coronary heart disease (papillary muscle dysfunction), carcinoid heart disease, and hypertrophic cardiomyopathy and those with infective endocarditis limited to 1 or both right-sided cardiac valves. Tricuspid-valve regurgitation was present in many patients in most of the 9 functional groups. All patients were in functional class III or IV (New York Heart Association) and more than ½ had 1 or more cardiac operations.

†In many patients, the aortic valve cusps actually were normal and the regurgitation was the result of disease of the aorta (Marfan and Marfan-like syndromes, syphilis, systemic hypertension, healed aortic dissection)

‡The hearts in all 1010 patients were examined by, and classified by, W. C. Roberts.

TABLE 3. Configuration of Aortic Valve in Isolated Aortic Stenosis in Relation to Age

NO. VALVE CUSPS	≤ AGE 15 YEARS	AGE 16–65	> AGE 65 YEARS
1	60%	10%	0
2	20%	60%	10%
3	15%	25%	90%
Uncertain	5%	5%	0

From Roberts WC. Congenital cardiovascular abnormalities usually "silent" until adulthood: Morphologic features of floppy mitral valve, valvular aortic stenosis, discrete subvalvular aortic stenosis, hypertrophic cardiomyopathy, sinus of Valsalva aneurysm, and the Marfan syndrome. Cardiovasc Clin 1979; 10(1):418, with permission.

necropsy patients with aortic stenosis (with or without aortic regurgitation), the lesion was isolated in 59%, and in the other 41%, the mitral valve was stenotic or regurgitant or both.[34] The evidence is substantial that the cause of aortic stenosis, when associated with mitral valve disease, is rheumatic.[45,49] In contrast, the evidence is substantial that isolated (mitral valve anatomically normal) aortic stenosis (with or without associated aortic regurgitation) is nonrheumatic in origin.[34,41–49] This section focuses on patients with isolated aortic stenosis.

In contrast to what was generally believed 30 or so years ago,[50] at least 3 factors indicate that anatomically isolated aortic valve disease (actually either stenosis or pure regurgitation) is nonrheumatic in origin: (1) the low frequency (about 10%) of a positive history of acute rheumatic fever; (2) the absence of Achoff bodies; and, most importantly, (3) the frequency of an underlying congenital malformation of the aortic valve.

The structure of the aortic valve in aortic stenosis can be correlated to some extent with the age of the patient (Table 3).[48] In patients < 15 years old, the aortic valve most commonly (60%) is congenitally unicuspid and unicommissural, in patients 16 to 65 years of age, the valve is most commonly (60%) congenitally bicuspid, and in patients age > 65 years, the valve is most commonly (90%) tricuspid.[46] The stenosis is either due to, or superimposed on, the congenitally malformed aortic valve in virtually all patients < 15 years of age, and in at least 70% and possibly as high as 85% of patients aged 16 to 25 years.[43] A congenitally malformed, in this case congenitally bicuspid, valve appears to be the underlying condition in only about 10% of patients > age 65 years with aortic stenosis.

The unicommissural valve (Figs. 10 and 11), the only type of unicuspid valve observed in the aortic valve position, was described initially by Edwards in 1958.[51] Although this valve, like all other congenitally malformed aortic valves, tends to get progressively more stenotic with time,[47] the unicuspid aortic valve is almost certainly stenotic from the time of birth, whereas this usually is not the case with the congen-

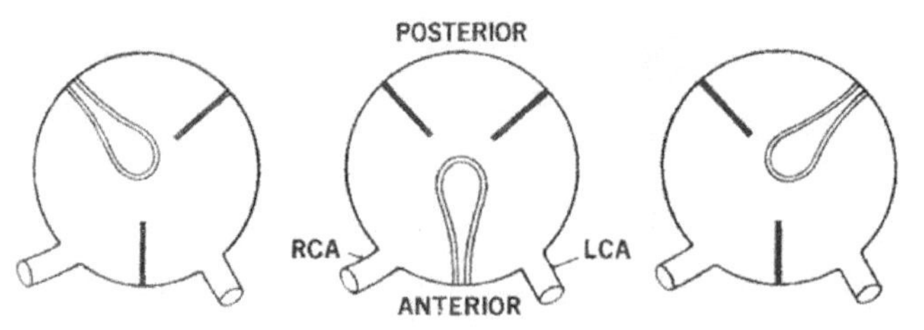

FIGURE 10. Location of the true commissure in congenitally unicommissural aortic valve stenosis. RCA, LCA = right and left coronary arteries, respectively. From Roberts WC. Congenital cardiovascular abnormalities usually "silent" until adulthood: Morphologic features of the floppy mitral valve, valvular aortic stenosis, discrete subvalvular aortic stenosis, hypertrophic cardiomyopathy, sinus of Valsalva aneurysm, and the Marfan syndrome. Cardiovasc Clin 1979; 10(1):418, with permission.

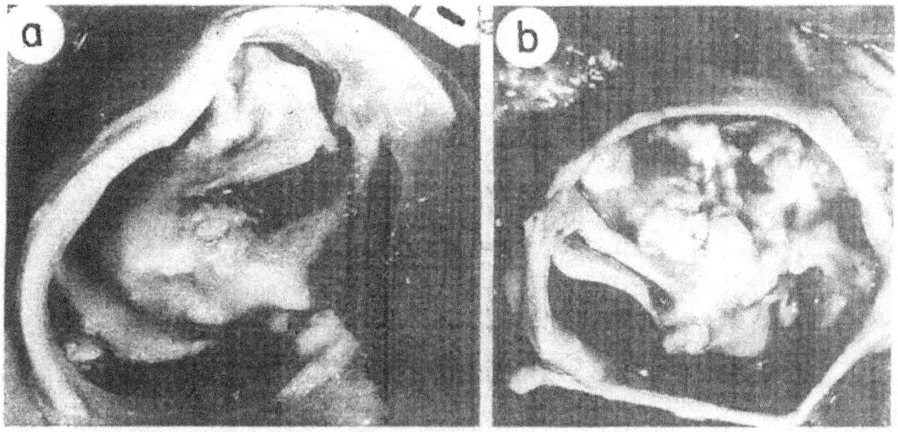

FIGURE 11. Congenitally unicommissural stenotic aortic valves in 2 men aged 28 years (*a*) and 48 years (*b*). From Roberts WC. Congenital cardiovascular abnormalities usually "silent" until adulthood: Morphologic features of the floppy mitral valve, valvular aortic stenosis, discrete subvalvular aortic stenosis, hypertrophic cardiomyopathy, sinus of Valsalva aneurysm, and the Marfan syndrome. From Cardiovasc Clin 1979; 10(1):419, with permission.

itally bicuspid valve. Actually, the fewer the number of aortic valve cusps and commissures, the greater the likelihood that the valve is stenotic from birth.

Next to the floppy mitral valve, the congenitally bicuspid aortic valve is the most frequent major congenital malformation of the heart or great vessels.[52] Although its exact frequency is uncertain, this malformation appears to occur in at least 1% of human births.[43] Osler[53] found 10 apparently normally functioning con-

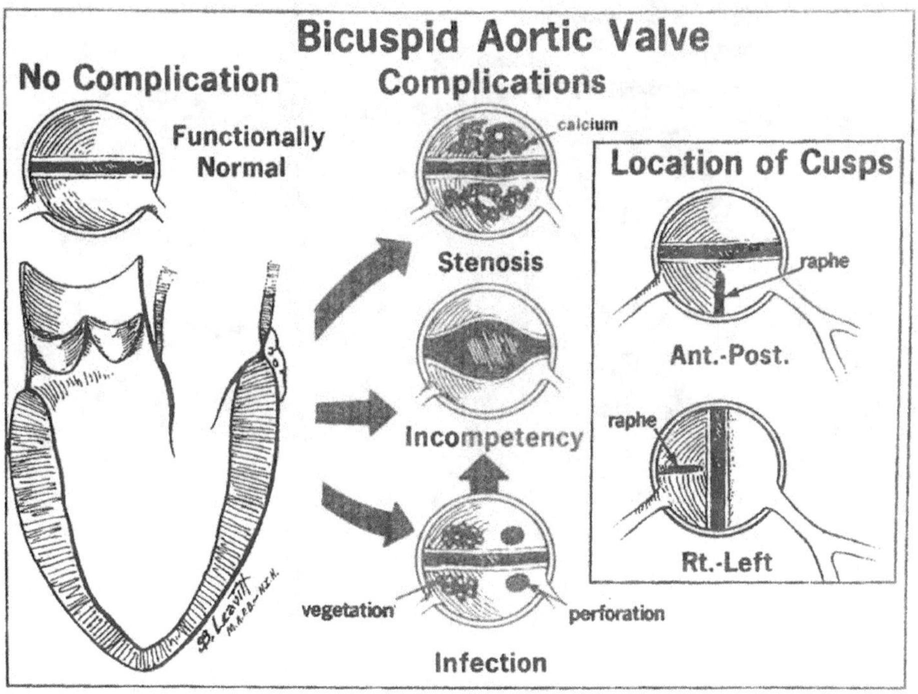

FIGURE 12. The congenitally bicuspid aortic valve. The location of the cusps and raphes and the acquired complications of the congenital malformation are depicted. From Roberts WC. Congenital cardiovascular abnormalities usually "silent" until adulthood: Morphologic features of the floppy mitral valve, valvular aortic stenosis, discrete subvalvular aortic stenosis, hypertrophic cardiomyopathy, sinus of Valsalva aneurysm, and the Marfan syndrome. Cardiovasc Clin 1979; 10(1):419, with permission.

genitally bicuspid aortic valves in 800 autopsies (750 of which were performed by him), a frequency of 1%. Eight additional patients had infective endocarditis involving congenitally bicuspid aortic valves. Thus, 18 (2%) of 800 had either normally functioning or infected congenitally bicuspid aortic valves. Grant and associates[54] found apparently normally functioning congenitally bicuspid aortic valves in 12 (1%) of 1350 necropsy patients. Osler,[53] Lewis and Grant,[55] and Grant and coworkers[54] do not appear to have appreciated that the biscuspid condition of this valve may underlie severe stenosis or calcification at this site. Thus, if congenitally bicuspid aortic valves that develop complications (stenosis or regurgitation with or without infection) are added to those that function normally during the entire lifetime, the frequency of congenitally bicuspid aortic valves may well be > 1% of the population.

Among the complications of the bicuspid condition of the aortic valve, stenosis is by far the most frequent; pure regurgitation is next,[56] and the latter lesion is most

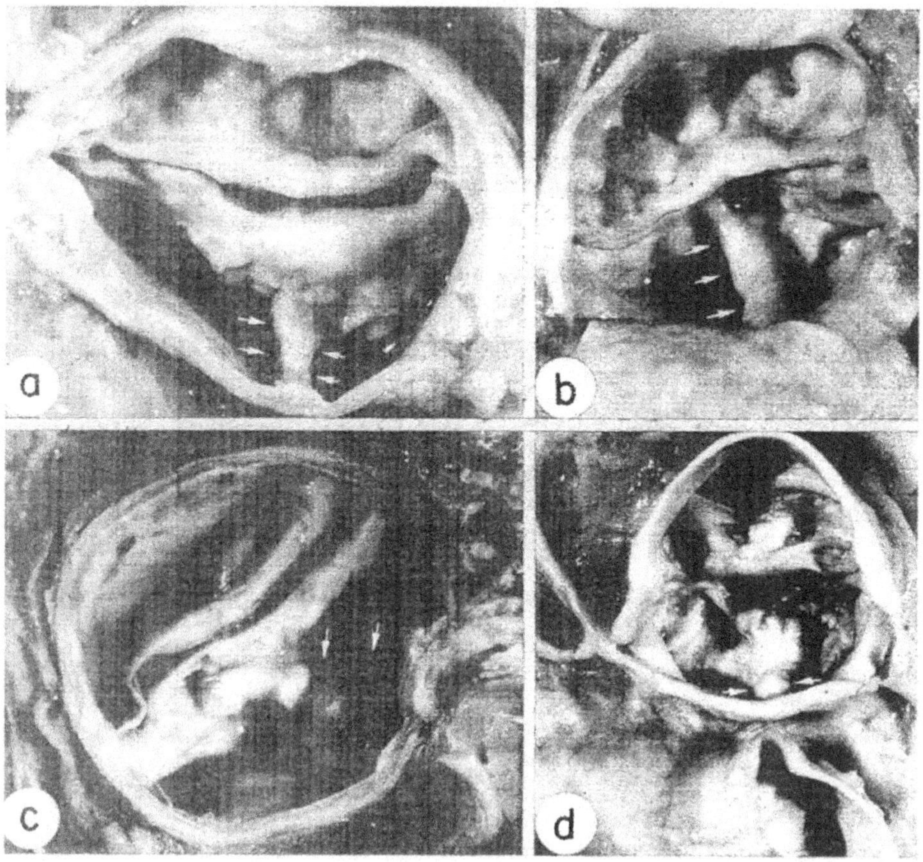

FIGURE 13. Calcified, stenotic, congenitally bicuspid aortic valves in 4 patients. The cusps are situated anteriorly and posteriorly, and the commissures right and left, respectively. Each of the valves has a raphe (white arrows) in the anterior cusp. *a*, Valve of a 61-year-old man. At catheterization 2 years before his death, the peak systolic gradient across the valve was 45 mm Hg when the cardiac index was 2.6 L/min/m^2. He had complete heart block secondary to destruction of the atrioventricular bundle by calcium. *b*, Valve of a 60-year-old man who suddenly collapsed on the street. Electrocardiogram recorded in the emergency room showed left bundle branch block. His only previous symptom of cardiac dysfunction was mild exertional dyspnea. *c*, Valve of a 75-year-old man who died after resection of an asymptomatic abdominal aortic aneurysm that had been discovered during a routine physical examination. A grade 3/6 murmur consistent with aortic stenosis had been heard, but he had no symptoms of cardiac dysfunction. *d*, Valve of a 51-year-old man. The peak systolic gradient across this valve was only 18 mm Hg, but it was severely incompetent. From Roberts,[43] with permission.

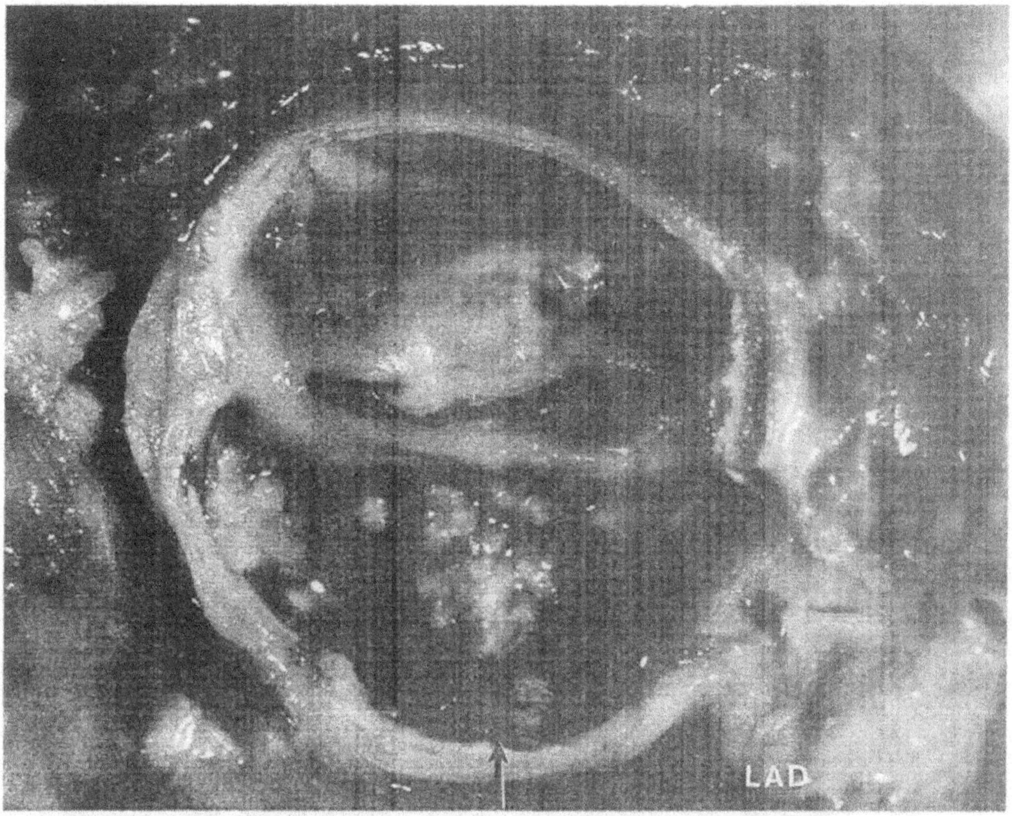

FIGURE 14. Congenitally bicuspid, stenotic aortic valve in an 87-year-old man who developed angina pectoris 1 year before his sudden death at home. He never had congestive heart failure or syncope. The 2 cusps are located anteriorly and posteriorly with a raphe (arrow), which is calcified, in the anterior cusp. In addition to the heavy deposits of calcium in the aortic valve, large calcific deposits also were present in the mitral anulus. Aortic stenosis had been diagnosed by physical examination 10 years before he died. LAD = left anterior descending coronary artery. From Roberts WC. Congenital cardiovascular abnormalities usually "silent" until adulthood: Morphologic features of the floppy mitral valve, valvular aortic stenosis, discrete subvalvular aortic stenosis, hypertrophic cardiomyopathy, sinus of Valsalva aneurysm, and the Marfan syndrome. Cardiovasc Clin 1979; 10(1):421, with permission.

FIGURE 15. Congenitally bicuspid aortic valve with superimposed *Staphylococcus aureus* endocarditis in a 30-year-old man. Before the onset of the infective endocarditis, the patient was asymptomatic, but before the infection the valve was already mildly stenotic and mildly calcified. Nail biting, to the point of bleeding, apparently was the source of the infection. At necropsy the heart weighed 560 gm. The infection of the aortic valve burrowed into the adjacent soft tissues (brackets), producing large "ring abscesses." Ring abscess caused complete right bundle branch block. There was extensive subendocardial and papillary muscle necrosis of the left ventricle, presumably the result of severely diminished cardiac output. The echocardiogram was recorded several days before death. The arrows in the ventricular septum of the echocardiogram designate the probable ring abscess. Ao = aorta; LA = left atrium; RV = right ventricle; LV = left ventricle; AML and PML = anterior and posterior mitral leaflets; VS = ventricular septum; MV = mitral valve; Endo = endocardium. From Roberts WC. Congenital cardiovascular abnormalities usually "silent" until adulthood: Morphologic features of the floppy mitral valve, valvular aortic stenosis, discrete subvalvular aortic stenosis, hypertrophic cardiomyopathy, sinus of Valsalva aneurysm, and the Marfan syndrome. Cardiovasc Clin 1979; 10(1):422, with permission.

frequently the result of its being the site of infective endocarditis[57] (Fig. 12). Among 200 patients with congenitally bicuspid aortic valves studied personally *at necropsy,* 157 (79%) had aortic stenosis (Figs. 13 and 14), 22 (11%) had pure aortic regurgitation (in 19 from infective endocarditis [Fig. 15]), and 21 (10%) had normally functioning bicuspid valves (Fig. 16, Table 4). The latter 21 patients died of noncardiac causes, and the presence of the congenitally bicuspid aortic valve was a surprise finding at necropsy (see Fig. 15). Other findings in these 200 patients are summarized in

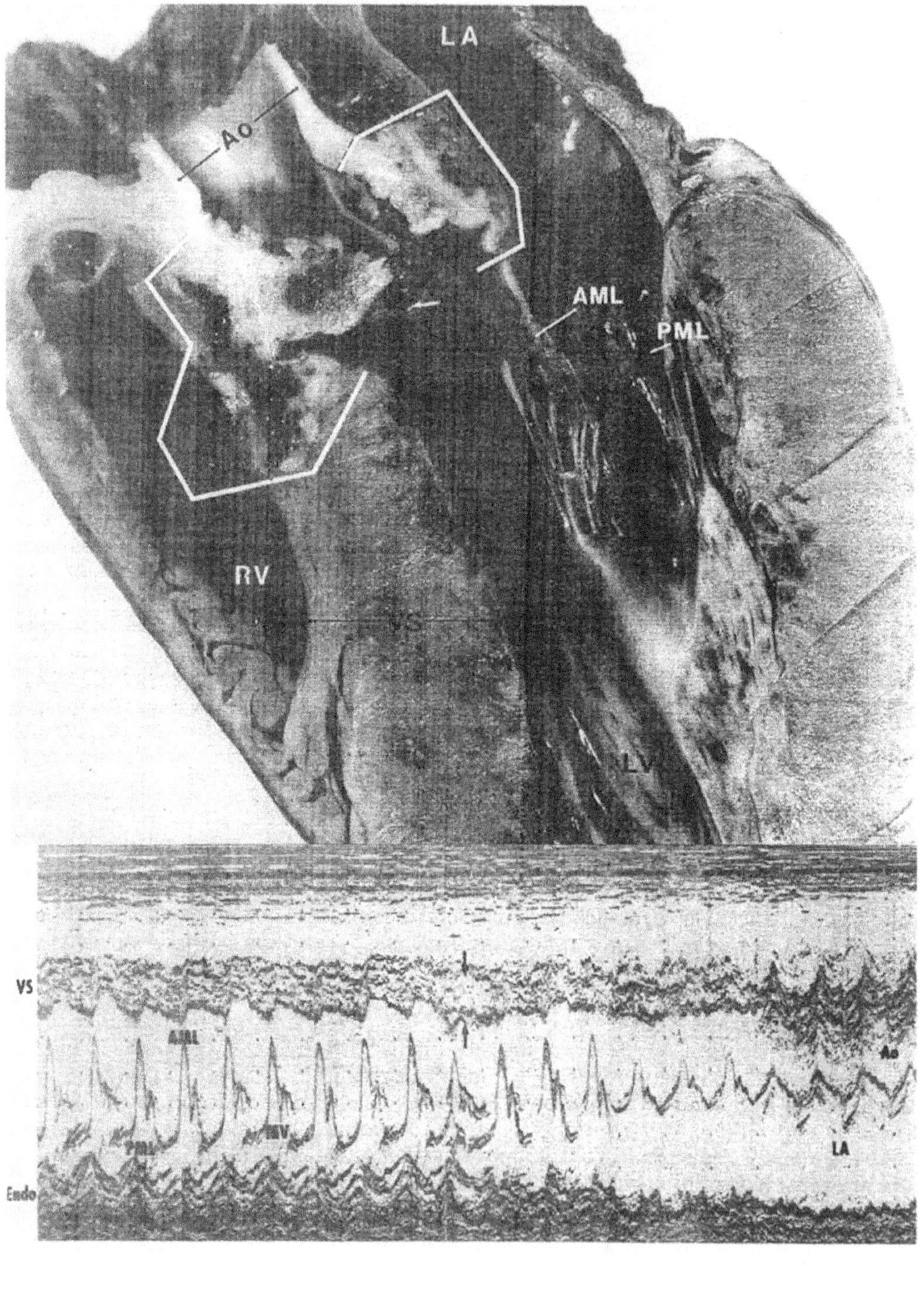

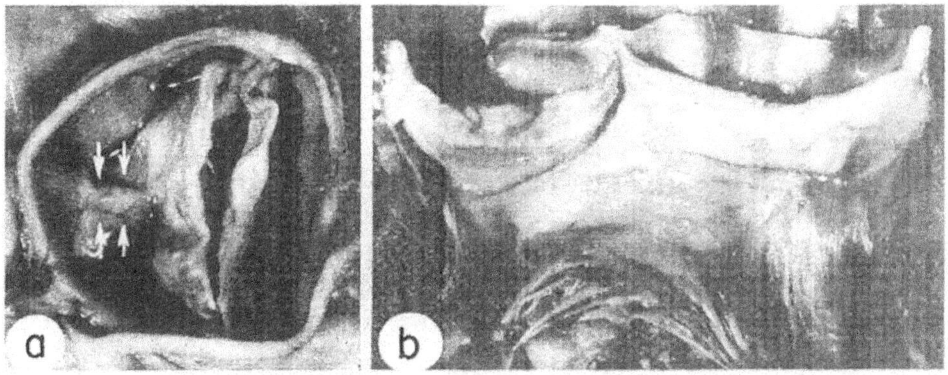

FIGURE 16. Functionally normal congenitally bicuspid aortic valve. *a*, The right cusp contains the raphe (arrows) and is the larger of the 2 cusps. *b*, Opened valve. From Roberts,[43] with permission.

Table 4. Of the 157 patients with aortic stenosis, calcific deposits were present on both aortic valve cusps in 155 (99%); the 2 patients without calcific deposits were < 30 years of age. Calcific deposits, in contrast, were rare in the patients with pure aortic regurgitation. Infective endocarditis occurred in 14 (9%) of the 157 patients with aortic stenosis and in 19 (86%) of the 22 with pure aortic regurgitation, and the infection was the prime cause of the regurgitation in all 19 patients. Of the 200 patients, 150 (75%) were males.

Congenitally bicuspid aortic valves also are observed commonly in patients having aortic valve replacement for *isolated* (mitral valve function normal) aortic stenosis with or without associated aortic regurgitation, and preoperative detection of the bicuspid valve is highly reliable by preoperative cross-sectional echocardiography.[58] Among 393 patients aged 17 to 74 years with aortic stenosis with or without aortic regurgitation having aortic valve replacement at the National Heart, Lung, and Blood Institute from 1962 to 1982, 28 (7%) had unicommissural, unicuspid aortic valves; 203 (52%) had congenitally bicuspid aortic valves; 101 (26%) had 3-cuspid aortic valves; and in 61 (15%) the number of cusps could not be determined by examination of the operatively excised valve. Subramanian and associates[59] determined the number of aortic valve cusps present in 338 patients (most aged 50 to 70 years) undergoing aortic valve replacement for isolated (I excluded their 36 patients with associated mitral stenosis or regurgitation) "pure" aortic stenosis during 4 different years (1965, 1970, 1975, and 1980). Of the 338 patients, 21 (6%) had unicommissural, unicuspid valves; 171 (51%) had congenitally bicuspid valves; 94 (28%) had tricuspid aortic valves; and in 14 patients (4%), the number of cusps present was not discernible.

Congenitally bicuspid aortic valves also are found commonly among patients undergoing aortic valve replacement for *isolated* (normal mitral valve function), pure (no element of stenosis) aortic regurgitation (Fig. 17), and the bicuspid status of the purely regurgitant aortic valve also is reliably detected by preoperative cross-sectional echocardiography.[60] In contrast to the stenotic bicuspid aortic valve in adults, calcific deposits are relatively infrequent in the purely regurgitant bicuspid aortic valve, and, when present, they are usually small.[61] The frequency of finding congenitally bicuspid vaortic valves in 190 patients aged 16 to 70 years having isolated aortic valve replacement for chronic, isolated (mitral valve function normal), pure (no element of AS) aortic regurgitation at the National Heart, Lung, and Blood Institute from 1962 through 1982 is summarized in Table 5.[56] Of the 190 patients, 21 (11%) had congenitally bicuspid aortic valves. Of the 21 patients, 14 (67%) never had infective endocarditis, and therefore the regurgitation was on the basis of the congenital malformation only; the other 7 (33%) had infective endocarditis super-

TABLE 4. Congenitally Bicuspid Aortic Valve: Observations in 200 Necropsy Patients > 15 Years of Age

COMPLICATION	NO. PTS.	SEX		AGE (YEARS) RANGE (AVG)	IE	C OF A	AV CA^{++}	AD	HEART WEIGHT (GM) RANGE (AVG)	AV OP
		M	F							
1. Stenosis*	157	117	40	16–87 (5.1)	14 (9%)	7	152 (97%)	4	270–1100	93 (59%)
2. Pure Regurgitation	22	19	3	20–55 (36)	19 (86%)	3	5 (23%)	0	390–1010 (641)	9 (41%)
3. None	21	14	7	23–73 (46)	0	1	3 (14%)	3	170–670 (342)	0
TOTALS	200	150 (75%)	50 (25%)	16–87 (49)	33 (16%)	11 (5%)	160	7 (3%)		102 (51%)

*LV-SA psg = 10–165 mm Hg (avg 81) (in 107 patients)

IF = infective endocarditis

AV = aortic valve

Op = operation

C of A = coarctation of aorta

AD = aortic dissection

LV-SA = left ventricular-systemic arterial

F = female

M = male

psg = peak systolic gradient

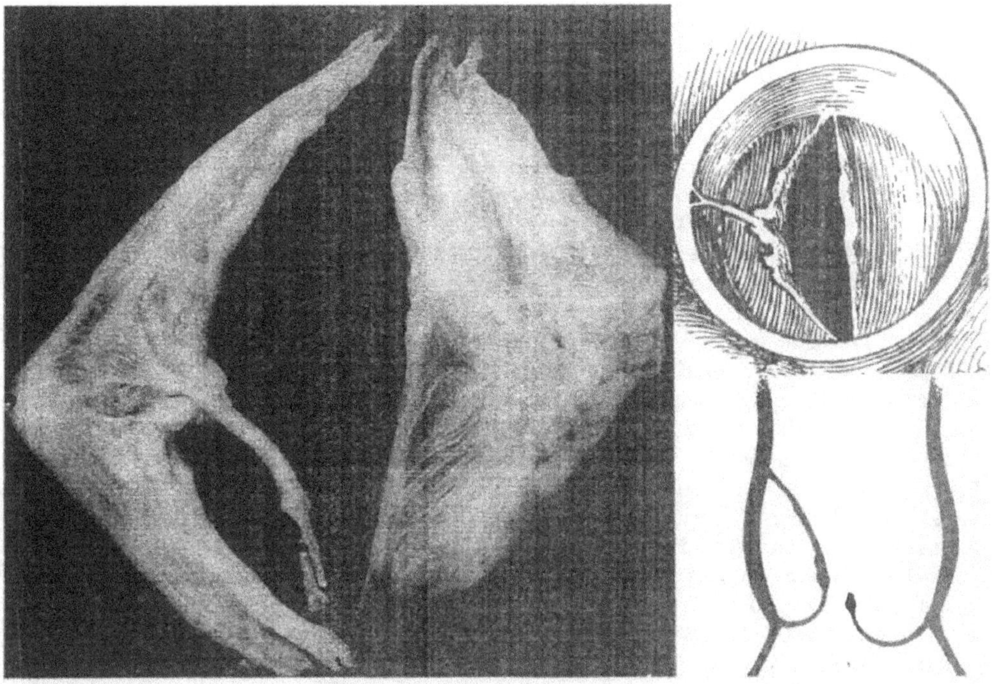

FIGURE 17. Purely incompetent congenitally bicuspid aortic valve in a 27-year-old man who was found to have aortic regurgitation at age 17; he developed exertional dyspnea at age 25. Just before valve replacement, simultaneous left ventricular and brachial arterial pressures were 125/25 and 126/54 mm Hg, respectively, when the cardiac index was 2.2 $L/min/m^2$. He died suddenly 13 months after valve replacement. The heart weighed 800 gm. Excised aortic valve is pictured at left. The drawing shows the supporting fibrous band that stretched from the margin in the midportion of 1 cusp to the aortic wall above 1 sinus of Valsalva (right). This patient is an example of pure severe aortic regurgitation of a congenitally bicuspid valve that was never the site of infective endocarditis. From Roberts,[43] with permission.

imposed on the bicuspid condition, and severe aortic regurgitation in each resulted primarily from the infection, which in each was healed by antibiotics. Olson and associates[62] also determined the frequency of bicuspid aortic valves in 145 patients having isolated aortic valve replacement for pure aortic regurgitation or severe regurgitation associated with only mild aortic stenosis. (The basis of the presence or absence of associated aortic stenosis was by "clinical" means, which apparently did

TABLE 5. Frequency of Congenitally Bicuspid Aortic Valve in Operatively Excised Aortic Valves in Patients Aged 17 to 74 Years with Clinically Isolated Aortic Stenosis with or without Associated Aortic Regurgitation

NO. VALVE CUSPS	NO. (%) PATIENTS
1	28 (7)
2	203 (52)
3	101 (26)
Uncertain	61 (5)
TOTAL	393 (100)

not mean hemodynamic studies.) Of the 145 patients, 49 (34%) had congenitally bicuspid aortic valves. Of these 49 patients, 41 (84%) apparently never had infective endocarditis, and the regurgitation primarily was on the basis of the bicuspid state of the valve; the other 8 (16%) had had infective endocarditis, which was the major cause of the regurgitation. Of the remaining 96 patients (66%), 94 (65% of total) had 3-cuspid aortic valves, and 2 (1% of total) had quadricuspid valves. Of the 94 patients with 3-cuspid aortic valves, the cause of the aortic regurgitation in 34 (36%) was "postinflammatory" (presumably rheumatic in at least 31—each of the aortic valve cusps in these patients was diffusely fibrotic with or without cuspal retraction and/or commissural fusion); associated with aortic root dilatation in 44 (47%) (idiopathic in 43 [98%] and syphilitic in 1 [2%]); associated with infective endocarditis in 12 (13%); and associated with ventricular septal defect in 4 (4%).

The reason 1 congenitally bicuspid aortic valve becomes stenotic, another purely regurgitant, and another the site of infective endocarditis is unknown. It is clear, however, that stenosis, regurgitation, and infection are complications of the bicupsid condition of the aortic valve, and none of them are present at birth. It appears likely that a congenitally bicuspid aortic valve becomes stenotic only as its cusps become fibrotic and calcified; neither cusp of a congenitally bicuspid aortic valve is severely thickened by fibrous tissue or calcific deposits at time of birth.

The frequency of development of stenosis or pure regurgitation at the site of a congenitally bicuspid aortic valve also is unknown. Lewis and Grant[55] concluded that vegetations develop at these sites in about 23% of adults (16 of 69) with congenitally bicuspid valves in patients with infective endocarditis involving the aortic valve. Of 31 patients with "subacute infective endocarditis" studied at necropsy by Lewis and Grant,[55] 8 (26%) had congenitally bicuspid aortic valves. Two (9%) of 22 patients studied at necropsy by Fulton and Levine[63] had congenitally bicuspid aortic valves. None of these investigators apparently was aware that congenitally bicuspid aortic valves also could become stenotic.

The mechanism by which a congenitally bicuspid aortic valve becomes stenotic or purely regurgitant is uncertain. There is no evidence that the valve is stenotic or regurgitant at birth. Likewise, there is no evidence that superimposed rheumatic fever or rheumatic heart disease is the cause of the stenosis or pure regurgitation. The explanation advanced by Edwards[64] is attractive. He proposed that it is not mechanically possible for a congenitally bicuspid aortic valve to open and close properly. The distances between the lateral attachments of normal aortic valvular cusps along their free margins are curved lines. The extra length allows the cusps to move freely during opening and closing of the valves. In contrast, the distances between the lateral attachments of congenitally bicuspid aortic valves along their free margins approach straight lines. If these distances were exactly straight lines, the valve could not open during ventricular systole. Consequently, at least 1 cusp is larger than the other. But the excessive length of 1 or both cusps of a congenitally bicuspid aortic valve produces abnormal contact between the cusps. This abnormal contact, in turn, causes focal fibrous thickening that with time becomes diffuse, and dystrophic calcification thereafter occurs. Thus, stenosis of a congenitally bicuspid aortic valve may be the result of trauma to these cusps produced by their abnormal contact with each other. Although this explanation is appealing, it does not explain why 1 congenitally bicuspid aortic valve becomes stenotic, another becomes entirely regurgitant with or without infection, and another remains free of complications.

Criteria for differentiating a bicuspid valve of congenital origin from a bicuspid valve of acquired origin have been debated (Fig. 18). No controversy has arisen in distinguishing a congenitally bicuspid aortic valve devoid of a raphe (false commissure or ridge) and of complications (stenosis, pure regurgitation or infection) from a tricuspid aortic valve also devoid of similar complications. Controversy had existed about the means of differentiating a congenitally bicuspid aortic valve with a raphe from an acquired bicuspid aortic valve resulting from fusion of 2 cusps at 1 true

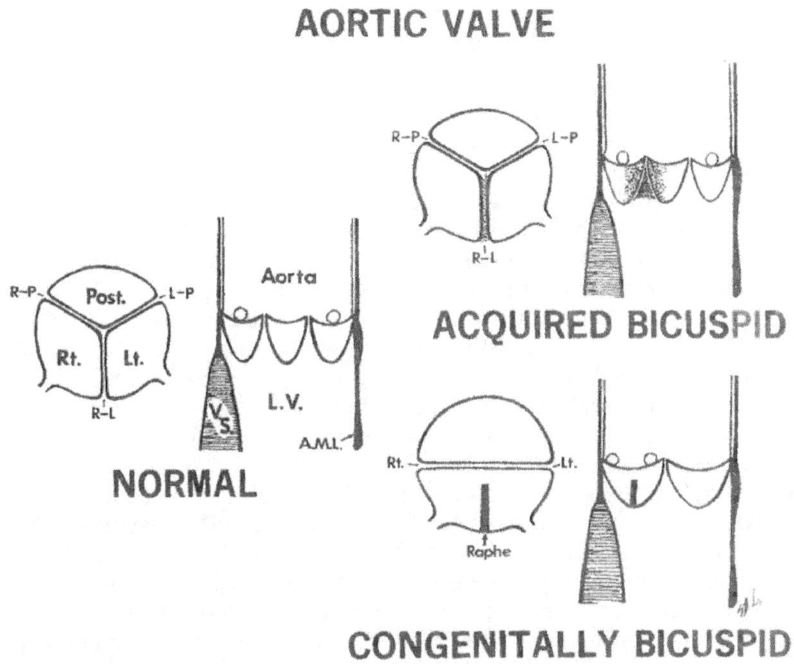

FIGURE 18. Diagram illustrating differences between bicuspid aortic valves of congenital origin as compared with the normal valve. The circumferential distances between each of the 3 commissures in a normally formed valve are similar. L-P = left-posterior; R-L = right-left, and R-P = right-posterior commissures; Rt., Lt., Post. = right, left, and posterior cusps, respectively; V.S. = ventricular septum; L.V. = left ventricular outflow tract; and A.M.L. = anterior mitral leaflet. In the acquired bicuspid valve, the circumferential distance between the commissures remains equal, as in a normal valve. The fused commissure is wide, the distal margins of each of the two fused cusps are still usually visible, and the most cephalad margin of the fused commissures is on the same horizontal level as the most cephalad margins of the 2 nonfused commissures. In the congenitally bicuspid valve, the raphe is generally narrow and rarely extends to the free margin of the conjoined cusp or to the cephalad level reached by the 2 true commissures. The circumferential distances between the 2 true commissures are greater than this distance between either true commissure and the raphe. The circumferential distance between the true commissures around the conjoined cusp, that is, the cusp with the raphe, is equal to or slightly greater than the circumferential distance between the true commissures around the cusp devoid of the raphe. From Roberts,[43] with permission.

commissure.* Osler,[53] from the study of 18 hearts (15 adults), listed the following characteristics of the congenitally bicuspid aortic valve, all recognizable by gross observation: (1) The raphe is located where normally the true commissure would be. (He stated between the right and left anterior aortic valve cusps, but that is the case only half the time.) (2) The length of the free margin of the cusp containing no raphe is shorter (by an average of 12% in his measurements on 7 hearts) than the length of the margin of the cusp containing a raphe, the "conjoint" cusp. (3) The free border of the conjoint cusp is straight or curled and free of nodular thickenings indicative of Corpora Arantii. (4) The border of attachment of the conjoint cusp, as viewed from

*The definition of a *commissure* differs depending on whether a semilunar or an atrioventricular cardiac valve is under consideration. The aortic valve commissure is the space between 2 lateral attachments on the aortic wall. Normally, each aortic valve cusp is an independent, nearly similarly sized unit, and adherence of 1 cusp to another at the narrow space (commissure) between the 2 cusps is abnormal. In contrast to a semilunar valve, the leaflets of an atrioventricular valve are continuous 1 with another. Thus, the commissures of the atrioventricular valves are the sites of connection between the unequal-sized leaflets, not the spaces between the cusps as in the case of semilunar valves.

the ventricular aspect, presents either the contour of a single semilunar cusp or a shallow groove, indicative of the junction of 2 cusps. (5) The raphe may be located on the aortic wall alone or may extend onto the cusps for variable distances, but in either case it usually divides the sinus of Valsalva into equal-sized units.

In 1923, Lewis and Grant[55] clarified several gross features of "unequivocally" congenitally bicuspid aortic valves and presented histologic criteria for differentiating bicuspid valves of "congenital" origin from those of "inflammatory" origin. In contrast to Osler, these authors found that fusion could occur not only between right and left anterior cusps but also between right anterior and posterior cusps. A raphe, dividing 1 of the 2 cusps, was observed "in about half the cases." The 2 cusps could be equal or unequal in size, but usually the conjoined cusp was larger, but not twice the size of the undivided cusp; or "the sub-divided cusp is larger than 1 normal cusp but smaller than 2 normal cusps." Lewis and Grant, however, considered gross distinction between congenital and acquired bicuspid aortic valves unreliable. Elastic tissue stains of transverse sections of congenital raphes disclosed them to consist mainly of elastic fibers; thus, the raphe histologically was similar to the media of the aorta. In contrast, transverse sections of 2 fused cusps at a true commissure disclosed that the fused commissure was devoid of elastic fibers and consisted of fibrous valvular tissue. Other investigators[65,66] confirmed these histoligic criteria. Koletsky[66] also pointed out that congenital raphes were devoid of vascular channels and of inflammatory cells, whereas both were seen in acquired, fused commissures.

Since Lewis and Grant described these histologic features, some morphologists have been reluctant to distinguish between congenital and acquired bicuspid aortic valves without microscopic examination of raphes. These histologic criteria, however, are helpful but not specific. In patients in whom some sections of a raphe show a structure like that of the aortic media, other sections of the same raphe may show only fibrous tissue. Also, the congenital raphe may lose its elastic fibers as the valvular cusps become fibrotic and calcified. The raphe appears to be the first portion of the congenitally bicuspid aortic valve to calcify, and these deposits destroy existing elastic fibers. Lewis and Grant and others who emphasized the importance of histologic distinction between congenital raphes and fused true commissures were unaware that calcific stenosis was a consequence of a congenitally bicuspid aortic valve. Once the valve is extensively scarred and calcified, histologic examination of the raphe is often fruitless. Furthermore, as Edwards[64] pointed out, in an occasional patient with a bicuspid aortic valve that must be assumed to be congenital, as in infants with aortic coarctation, the raphe not only may be fibrous, but may grossly have features suggesting fusion of 2 distinguishable, separate cusps.

It is well recognized that patients with aortic isthmic coarctation often have congenitally bicuspid aortic valves. Of 200 patients with aortic ischemic coarctation studied at necropsy by Abbott,[67] 27% had congenitally bicuspid aortic valves. Of 104 patients with aortic isthmic coarctation studied at necropsy by Reifenstein and associates,[68] 62% had congenitally bicuspid aortic valves. The finding in these 2 studies were summarized by Roberts.[69] These authors also pointed out that ascending aortic tears with or without dissection also were common (about 20%) in patients with aortic isthmic coarctation, but similar aortic lesions have an increased frequency among patients with congenitally bicuspid aortic valves unassociated with aortic isthmic coarctation.[70] It is less well appreciated that an occasional patient may present with clinical features of aortic stenosis but by aortogram be found to have aortic isthmic coarctation. Among 157 personally studied necropsy patients with stenotic congenitally bicuspid aortic valves, 7 (4%) had aortic isthmic coarctation (see Table 4).

Tricuspid aortic valves rarely appear to be stenotic at birth. If stenosis is present at birth and the aortic valve has 3 cusps, the stenosis is usually the result of a very small aortic "anulus" rather than the result of fusion of the cusps. Acquired stenosis of a 3-cuspid aortic valve, in contrast, is common. Of necropsy patients aged 16 to 65 years studied personally with clinically isolated aortic stenosis (with or without

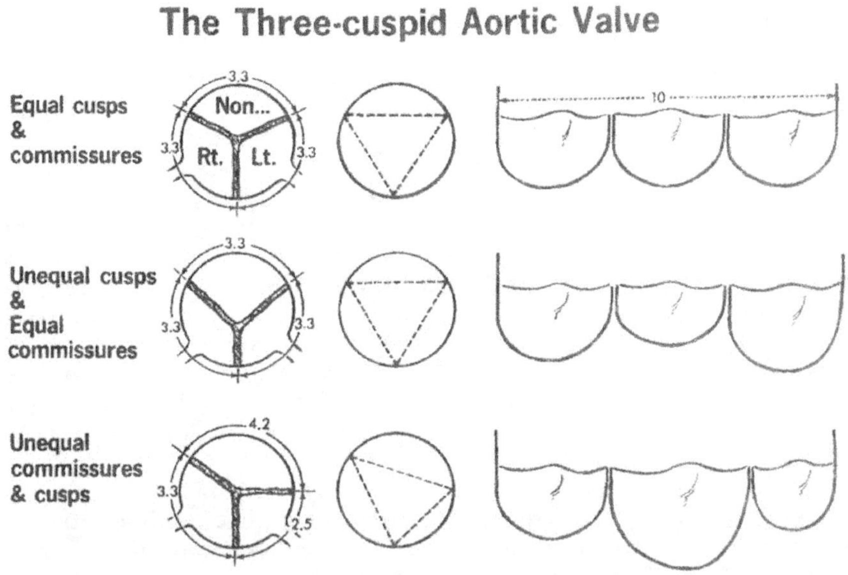

FIGURE 19. Diagrammatic portrayal of aortic valve cusps equal and unequal in size. *Top row,* The cusps of the aortic valve are equal in size, and the circumferential distances between the commissures are equal. The straight-line distances between the commissures (as indicated by the dashed lines in the center circle) also are equal. On the right, the aortic valve is opened. *Middle row,* Here the cusps are of unequal size, and they are made unequal by differing cephalocaudal lengths of the individual cusps. The distances between the commissures circumferentially around the aorta and the straight-line distances within the lumen of the aorta are similar to the normal shown in the top panel. *Bottom row,* Here the cephalocaudal lengths of the individual cusps differ, and the circumferential distances around the aorta and the straight-line distances within the lumen of the aorta between the commissures (lateral attachments) are different as well. From Roberts,[44] with permission.

regurgitation) (see Table 2), 25% had tricuspid valves, and among those aged > 65 years of age, 90% had tricuspid valves. In the age group 16 to 65 years, about 50% of these patients with clinically isolated aortic stenosis and 3-cuspid aortic valves also had diffuse fibrous thickening of the mitral leaflets. The associated diffuse mitral leaflet thickening is strong evidence that the etiology of the aortic stenosis in this group is rheumatic.[45] Also, nearly 75% of this group had positive histories of acute rheumatic fever, whereas 10% of the other group, that is, those with anatomically normal mitral valves with aortic stenosis, had positive histories. The etiology of the aortic stenosis in patients ≤ 65 years with 3-cuspid aortic valves and anatomically normal mitral valves is unsolved. Possibly, minor abnormalities in the sizes of the aortic valve cusps from birth set the stage for abnormal contact of the cusps with one another with resultant fibrosis and finally stenosis[71] (Fig. 19).

DISCRETE SUBAORTIC STENOSIS

Fixed or discrete subaortic stenosis most commonly is associated with other cardiovascular anomalies, but it also may be isolated.[72] This section is limited to its occurrence as an isolated lesion, and when this is the situation, symptoms of cardiac dysfunction commonly do not occur until adulthood. The average age of death is about 35 years.[73] Unlike valvular aortic stenosis, however, discrete subaortic stenosis is rare. In this condition, the discrete obstruction is located about 1 cm caudal to the bases of the aortic valve cusps,[48] and its location is discernible by cross-sectional echocardiography.[74] The obstruction is on a line corresponding to the site where the atrial septum inserts into the anterior mitral leaflet (Fig. 20). The obstruction, at least in adults, is produced by dense fibrous tissue—not really a "membrane"—that encircles the entire left ventricular outflow tract. The dense fibrous tissue may spread cephalad to the bases of the aortic valve cusps and caudally for about a centimeter. Because in discrete subaortic stenosis the obstruction is usually severe and located just below (1 cm) the bases of the aortic valve cusps, the aortic valve cusps are the site of the impact of the blood ejected through the discrete obstruction. As a consequence, the aortic valve cusps become thickened and thus are ideal sites for vegetations (Figs. 20 and 21). The consequence of cuspal thickening, with or without superimposed infective endocarditis, is development of aortic regurgitation, although never to a severe degree. As a result, nearly all adults with discrete subaortic stenosis have precordial diastolic murmurs of aortic regurgitation in addition to the systolic murmurs of left ventricular outflow obstruction.[75–76] The absence of aortic valve calcific deposits and the absence of dilatation of the ascending aorta in adults help to separate these patients before cardiac catheterization from patients with valvular aortic stenosis.

Although adequate data are not yet available, it is likely that discrete subaortic stenosis, on a percentage basis, is the most frequent cardiac condition to be complicated by infective endocarditis (Figs. 20 and 21), more common than that associated with the congenitally bicuspid and unicuspid aortic valve, the prolapsed aortic valve cusp associated with ventricular septal defect, or the floppy mitral valve.[77,78] The narrow jet of blood contacting 1 or more aortic valve cusps under high pressure and velocity provides the ideal circumstance for infective endocarditis to develop. Of 5 Newfoundland dogs with discrete subaortic stenosis dying naturally, 4 at necropsy had active infective endocarditis, which was the cause of death in each.[77] Among 7 patients with isolated discrete subaortic stenosis studied personally at necropsy, 4 had active infective endocarditis, fatal in each. Infective endocarditis complicating discrete subaortic stenosis may be difficult to diagnose clinically, at least before embolic events occur, and early diagnosis in this circumstance is essential to prevent severe damage to the aortic valve cusps. The high-pressure jet ejected through the discrete subaortic stenosis damages these cusps naturally, as already mentioned, but when infection is present, this damage by the jet is greatly accelerated and the cusps

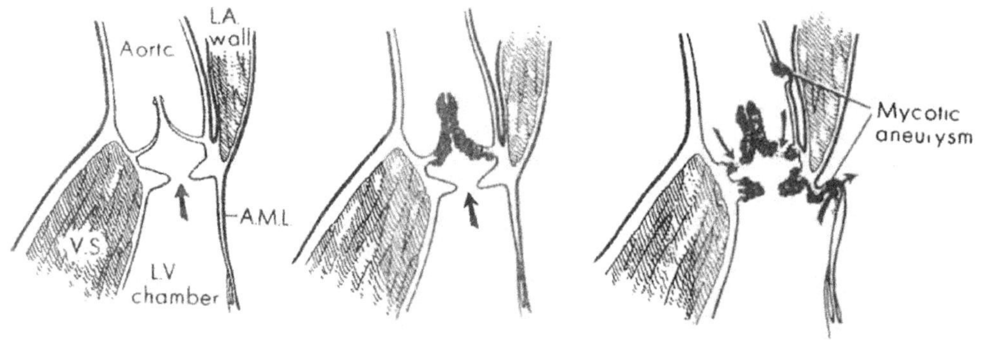

FIGURE 20. Diagram of aortic-valve region of the patient described in detail in Figure 21. Here the course of the pathologic process suggested by the necropsy findings is illustrated. The left diagram shows the discrete subvalvular obstruction before the development of bacterial endocarditis when the valve was traumatized by the jet of blood from below. The central diagram depicts the initial formation of bacterial vegetations, exclusively on the aortic valve cusps. As vegetations proliferated, the cusps ruptured (right diagram); the infection then extended to the discrete subvalvular fibrous band and the anterior mitral leaflet (A.M.L.), where a mycotic aneurysm formed immediately below the "membrane" where systolic pressure was highest. A second aneurysm in the wall of the ascending aorta resulted from the effects of a systolic jet through the valve. L.A. = left atrium; V.S. = ventricular septum; L.V. = left ventricle. From Morrow et al,[75] with permission.

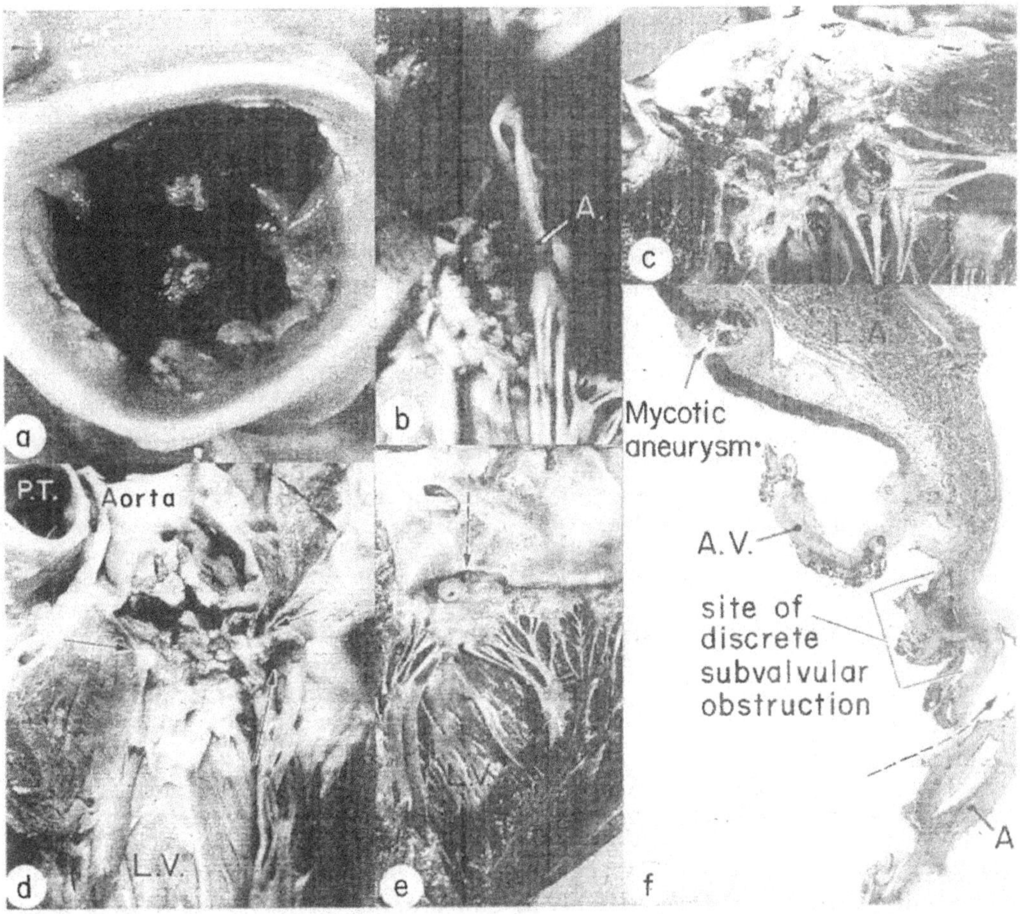

FIGURE 21. Alpha-hemolytic streptococcus endocarditis complicating congenitally discrete subaortic stenosis in a 28-year-old man. The infection, which appeared about 9 months before death, produced valvular aortic regurgitation. *a*, Aortic valve from above. *b*, Left ventricular outflow tract from below, showing vegetative material on the subvalvular "membrane" and adjacent anterior mitral leaflet (A.). *c*, Opened left ventricular outflow tract showing vegetations on each aortic cusp, on the subvalvular "membrane," and on the ventricular surface of anterior mitral leaflet. *d*, Longitudinal section showing the left ventricular outflow tract. The area of subaortic stenosis is apparent (between the solid arrows) and a mycotic aneurysm (dashed arrow) is seen in the anterior mitral leaflet. The mitral aneurysm is in the high-pressure portion of the left ventricle (L.V.), that is, below the discrete subvalvular obstruction. P.T. = pulmonary trunk. *e*, Opened mitral valve showing atrial aspect of the mycotic aneurysm (dashed arrow) on the anterior leaflet. *f*, Photomicrograph of section through aorta, left atrium (L.A.), aortic valve (A.V.) cusp, subvalvular "membrane," and anterior mitral leaflet (A.). A mycotic aneurysm is present in the ascending aorta (solid arrow) as well as in the anterior mitral leaflet (dashed arrow). Vegetations are present on the aortic valve cusp and on the subvalvular membrane. (Hematoxylin and eosin stain; × 2, reduced 15%.) From Morrow et al,[75] with permission.

are rapidly destroyed. In patients with destroyed aortic valve cusps and no discrete subaortic stenosis, the consequence is severe aortic regurgitation with progressive left ventricular dilatation and failure. In contrast, in patients with destroyed aortic valve cusps associated with discrete subaortic stenosis, severe aortic regurgitation is prevented by the subaortic obstruction, and, therefore, the aortic or systemic arterial diastolic pressure does not fall significantly despite an anatomically destroyed aortic valve. As a consequence, the left ventricle does not dilate and congestive cardiac failure may be absent. Because the aortic valve cusps in these patients are previously traumatized by the jet of blood traversing the discrete subaortic stenosis, the infection is superimposed on a previously abnormal valve. In this situation, the most common infecting organisms are alpha-streptococci, organisms of a relatively low virulence that are compatible with active infective endocarditis over a long period (many months) without antibiotic treatment.[78]

One reason to diagnose discrete subaortic stenosis before adulthood is to allow operative resection of the "membrane" so that cuspal damage is prevented.[72] Often, when operative treatment is delayed until adulthood, aortic valve replacement is required in addition to resection of the subaortic "membrane." Then survival becomes dependent on the "survival" of the valvular prosthesis or bioprosthesis, and, in addition, anticoagulants usually are required, with their inherent complications.

A recent anatomic observation in necropsy patients with discrete subaortic stenosis is the occurrence of severe thickening and luminal narrowing of the intramural coronary arteries located in the ventricular septum.[77] A similar finding has been observed in patients with hypertrophic cardiomyopathy (see below) and in patients wtih tunnel subaortic stenosis.[79]

HYPERTROPHIC CARDIOMYOPATHY

Probably no cardiovascular disease in recent years has engendered as much controversy or "professional" emotional display as has hypertrophic cardiomyopathy, a condition described originally in 1958 by Teare,[80] who applied the term "asymmetrical hypertrophy of the heart" to it. Subsequently, at least 57 other terms, including *"functional subaortic stenosis," "diffuse muscular subaortic stenosis," "idiopathic hypertrophic subaortic stenosis," "hypertrophic obstructive cardiomyopathy"* and *"asymmetric septal hypertrophy,"* have been applied. The terms that include the word "stenosis" or "obstruction" are inappropriate because obstruction is more often absent than present. The terms that emphasize asymmetry of the walls bordering the left ventricular cavity have served as useful purpose in emphasizing a frequent morphologic feature of this condition, but the ventricular septum may be thicker than the left ventricular free wall in some conditions other than hypertrophic cardiomyopathy, some patients with hypertrophic cardiomyopathy do not have asymmetric septal hypertrophy (i.e., septum thicker than free wall), and the free wall in hypertrophic cardiomyopathy is not always thickened.[81–87]

A major obstacle to understanding and discussing hypertrophic cardiomyopathy is lack of agreement among its students as to what it is. I once chaired a "fireside conference" on hypertrophic cardiomyopathy at a major scientific meeting, and we spent the entire 90-minute period attempting to define this entity. It is readily apparent that evidence of left ventricular outflow obstruction is not necessary for diagnosis of hypertrophic cardiomyopathy. The presence of asymmetric septal hypertrophy is not required for diagnosis because other conditions can cause the ventricular septum to be thicker than the left ventrciular free wall, and in some patients with hypertrophic cardiomyopathy the septum and free wall are of similar thicknesses.[81–87] Rapid upstroke of the arterial pulse, cardiomegaly, a systolic precordial murmur, and an abnormal electrocardiogram are usually present in these patients, but none of these are diagnostic or specific. Systolic anterior motion of the anterior mitral leaflet also is often present by echocardiogram, but any condition in which the left ventricular cavity is relatively small and the percentage of left ventricular volume ejected each beat is relatively high can also cause systolic anterior motion.[87] Thus, what is hypertrophic cardiomyopathy? It appears most reasonable simply to consider hypertrophic cardiomyopathy a condition characterized by (1) *hypertrophy of all or a portion of the walls of left ventricle,* that is, ventricular septum or free wall or both; (2)

nondilatation of the cavities of both cardiac ventricles, except in the presence of transmural ventricular wall necrosis or fibrosis[88]; (3) *absence of another cardiac condition that could produce left ventricular hypertrophy* (focal or diffuse) without ventricular cavity dilatation (such as systemic hypertension or valvular heart disease); (4) *presence of a normal or "supernormal" cardiac output and stroke volume,* except when associated with transmural cardiac ventricular necrosis or fibrosis; and (5) *absence of other states such as hyperthyroidism or pheochromocytoma that independently might increase cardiac output abnormally.* Atherosclerotic coronary heart disease, however, can coexist with hypertrophic cardiomyopathy.

Personal study of 177 patients with hypertophic cardiomyopathy at necropsy has disclosed certain predictable characteristic, although not absolutely specific, features of hypertrophic cardiomyopathy (Figs. 22 through 30, Table 6): (1) greater thickening of the ventricular septum than the left ventricular free wall (95%); (2) small or normal-sized left and right ventricular cavities (95%); (3) mural endocardial plaque, left ventricular outflow tract (75%) (mainly adults); (4) thickened mitral valve (75%) (mainly adults); (5) dilated atria (adults) (100%); (6) abnormal intramural coronary arteries (75%);[89,90] and (7) disorganization of myocardial fibers in the ventricular septum (95%).[91]

The chief morphologic abnormality in hypertrophic cardiomyopathy resides in the *ventricular septum.* As pointed out by Teare in his initial description of this con-

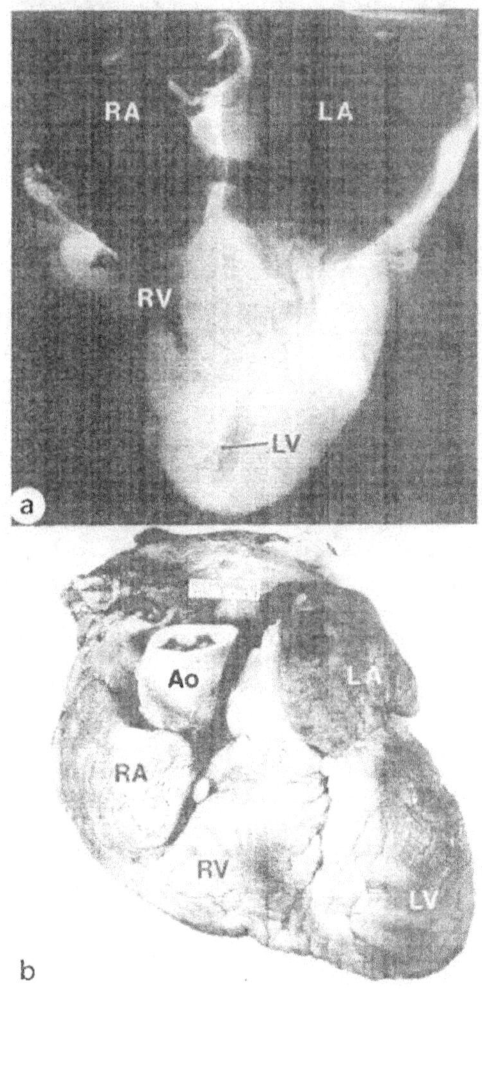

FIGURE 22. *a,* Radiograph of heart specimen and *b,* the heart itself in a 43-year-old woman with hypertrophic cardiomyopathy. Eleven years before she died, the peak systolic pressure gradient between left ventricle and aorta was 54 mm Hg at rest. She had periodic atrial fibrillation, chronic congestive cardiac failure, and an event compatible with cerebral embolus. The radiograph shows very dilated right (RA) and left (LA) atria, small-sized right (RV) and left (LV) ventricular cavities, and a ventricular septum thicker than the left ventricular free wall. The exterior view of the specimen also shows very prominent atria. Ao = aorta. From Roberts WC. Congenital cardiovascular abnormalities usually "silent" until adulthood: Morphologic features of the floppy mitral valve, valvular aortic stenosis, discrete subvalvular aortic stenosis, hypertrophic cardiomyopathy, sinus of Valsalva aneurysm, and the Marfan syndrome. Cardiovasc Clin 1979; 10(1):430, with permission.

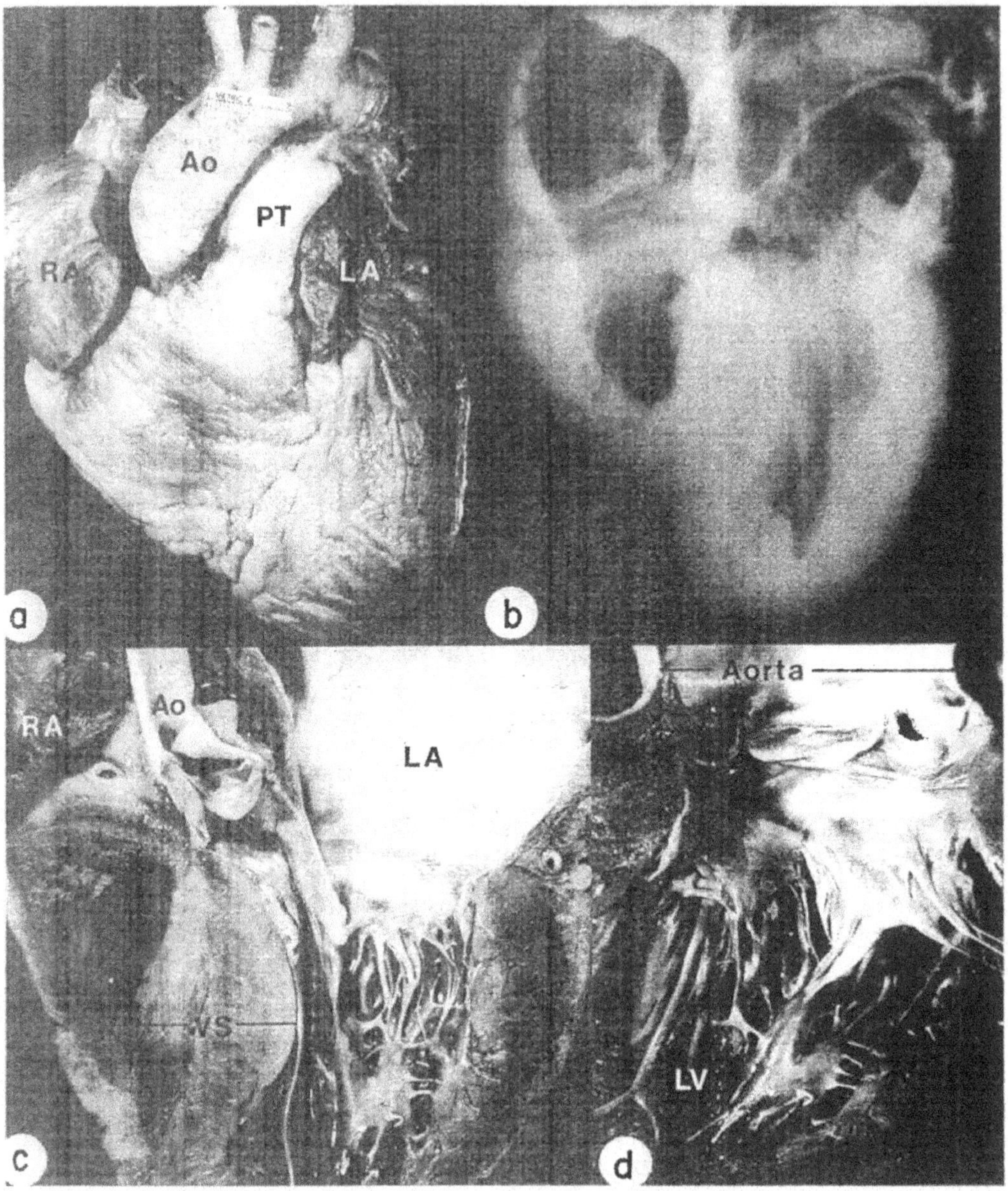

FIGURE 23. Heart of a 26-year-old man with hypertrophic cardiomyopathy. At catheterization 3 years before his death, a peak systolic pressure gradient of 30 mm Hg was present between left ventricle and brachial artery, and the gradient increased to 85 mm Hg with provocation (ouabain). The cardiac index was 2.1 L/min/m^2. At another catheterization done only 6 days before his sudden death, the gradient at rest was zero, and it rose to only 33 mm Hg when provoked (isoproterenol). The cardiac index was 2.0 L/min/m^2. The anatomic features of hypertrophic cardiomyopathy are demonstrated in these photographs. *a,* Exterior view; both right (RA) and left (LA) atria are dilated. AO = aorta; PT = pulmonary trunk. *b,* Radiograph of specimen showing the ventricular septum to be thicker than left ventricular free wall. *c,* Coronal section; the septum (VS) is clearly thicker than the left ventricular free wall, and an endocardial mural plaque is present in the left ventricular outflow tract in apposition to the anterior mitral leaflet. *d,* A closer view of the plaque and the thickened anterior mitral leaflet. From Roberts and Ferrans,[81] with permission.

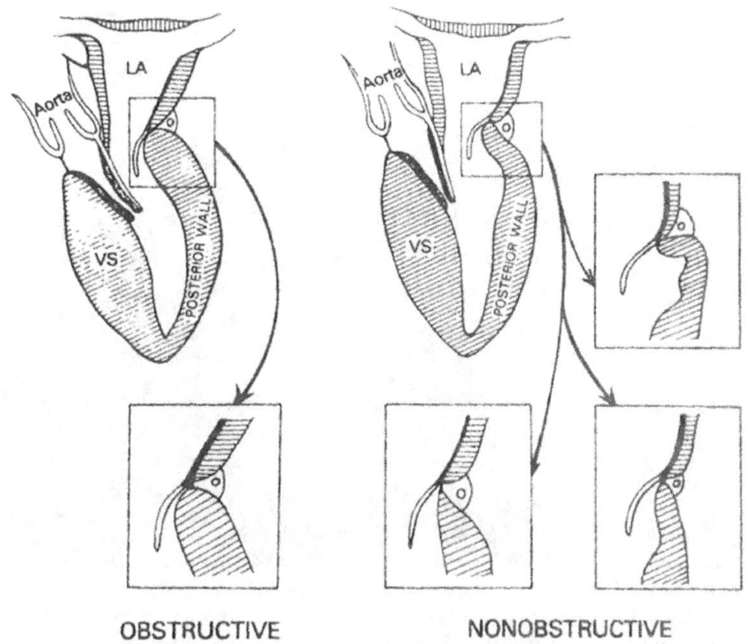

FIGURE 24. Diagram depicting the configuration and thickness of the posterolateral left ventricular free wall just behind the posterior mitral leaflet in the obstructive and nonobstructive types of hypertrophic cardiomyopathy. In the obstructive form, the most basal portion of free wall is rounded and thick. In the nonobstructive form, the most basal portion of left ventricular free wall is pointed and thin. In each type, the ventricular septum is much thicker than the left ventricular free wall. The mural endocardium in the left ventricular outflow tract and the anterior mitral leaflet in apposition to it are thickened. From Roberts and Ferrans,[82] with permission.

dition in 1958, the ventricular septum nearly always is thicker than the left ventricular free wall. Among our adult necropsy patients, the maximal thickness of ventricular septum averaged 3.0 cm, and the maximal thickness of left ventricular free wall, 1.8 cm.[81] The thickest portion of the septum is that part located about midway between aortic valve and left ventricular apex. This level corresponds approximately to the apex of right ventricle. Although in all our necropsy patients the ventricular septum was thicker than normal, the left ventricular free wall was usually but not always thicker than normal.

Although *ventricular asymmetry,* that is, a significant difference in maximal thickness of ventricular septum and left ventricular free wall, is a characteristic morphologic feature of hypertrophic cardiomyopathy, about 5% of our patients at necropsy with this condition had *ventricular symmetry,* that is, equal maximal thickness of the ventricular septum and left ventricular free wall. Thus, although asymmetric septal hypertrophy is a sensitive marker for hypertrophic cardiomyopathy, it is not specific for this condition.[87] Ventricular septa thicker than left ventricular free walls may occur in conditions causing thinning of the left ventricular free wall relative to the septum and in conditions causing thickening of the septum relative to the free wall. The most common cause of preferential free wall thinning is myocardial infarction, and the most common cause of preferential septal thickening is right ventricular systolic hypertension of any cause.

Among patients with hypertrophic cardiomyopathy, the thickness of the ventricular septum is not dependent on the presence of left ventricular outflow tract obstruction at rest, and, indeed, the thickness of the septum is similar in patients with outflow obstruction at rest and in those without outflow obstruction at rest.

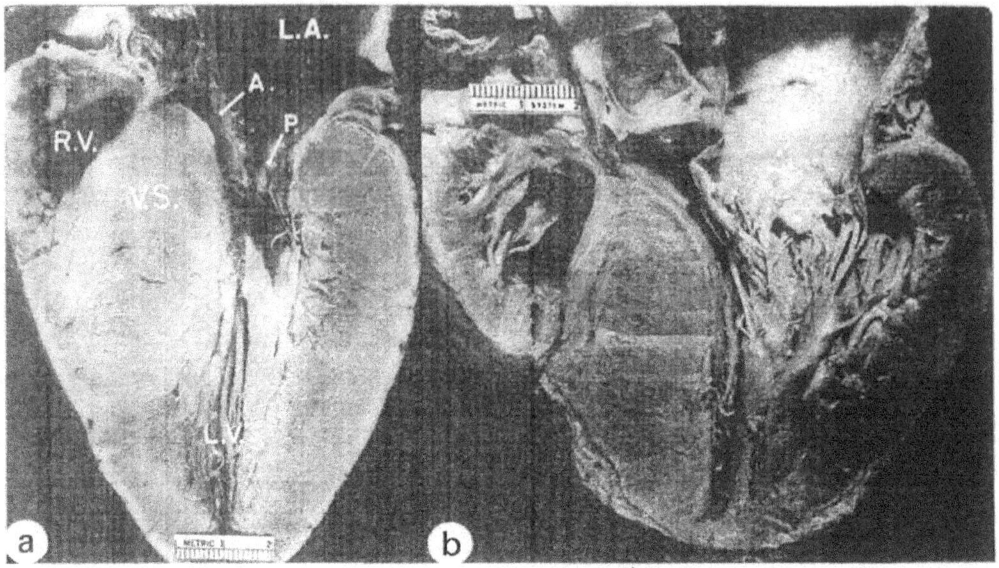

FIGURE 25. Hypertrophic cardiomyopathy in 2 patients. *a*, Left ventricular outflow obstruction in patient whose gradient at rest was 77 mm Hg. *b*, Patient with no gradient at rest. The posterobasal portion of left ventricular (L.V.) free wall in the first patient is rounded and thick; this portion of free wall in the second patient is more pointed and thin. The result is a larger left ventricular cavity in the basal portion in *b* than in *a* and, consequently, more room for the mitral valve. The ventricular septum (V.S.) in both patients, however, is severely thickened. A., P. = anterior and posterior mitral leaflets, respectively; R.V. = right ventricle. From Henry et al,[92] with permission.

FIGURE 26. Hypertrophic cardiomyopathy in a 16-year-old girl who was always asymptomatic and died suddenly while jogging. Her mother had hypertrophic cardiomyopathy, and 3 of her 4 siblings died suddenly. Hypertrophic cardiomyopathy had been demonstrated clinically in each of them. The present patient by echocardiograms had systolic anterior motion of the anterior mitral leaflet, an ejection fraction of 87%, and no evidence of left ventricular outflow obstruction. She had no precordial murmur. The electrocardiogram had shown narrow Q waves in II, III, and AVF. The heart weighed 310 gm, and the ventricular septum was twice as thick as the left ventricular free wall (19 to 9 mm). The left ventricular free wall was actually of normal thickness. RA = right atrium; RV = right ventricle; LA = left atrium; LV = left ventricle. From Roberts WC. Congenital cardiovascular abnormalities usually "silent" until adulthood: Morphologic features of the floppy mitral valve, valvular aortic stenosis, discrete subvalvular aortic stenosis, hypertrophic cardiomyopathy, sinus of Valsalva aneurysm, and the Marfan syndrome. Cardiovasc Clin 1979; 10(1):434, with permission.

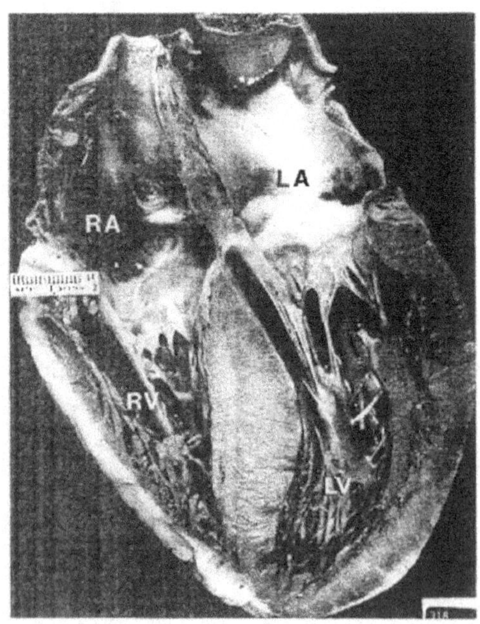

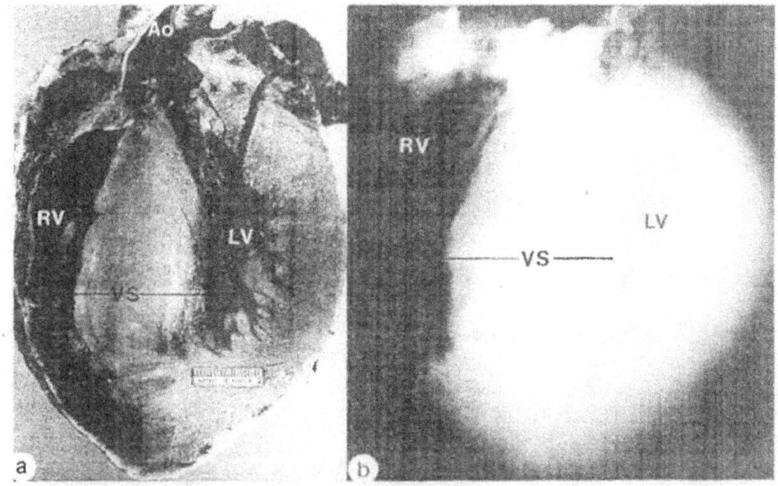

FIGURE 27. Hypertrophic asymmetric obstructive (right-sided) cardiomyopathy. This 18-year-old boy was first studied when he was asymptomatic at age 8; his brother had died suddenly at age 9 from hypertrophic cardiomyopathy (left-sided obstruction). At catheterization, no systolic pressure gradient was observed between the left ventricle and the systemic artery, but a systolic pressure gradient of 35 mm Hg was recorded between the right ventricle (56/5) and the pulmonary artery (21/9). An electrocardiogram showed right axis deviation, right ventricular hypertrophy, and a right ventricular conduction delay. The child remained asymptomatic until age 12, when he developed chest pain while playing football. Precordial pain recurred frequently thereafter and was precipitated by exertion of decreasing intensity so that he was forced to limit his activities to a sedentary level. When he was restudied at age 13, a grade 1/6 systolic ejection-type precordial murmur was heard, which was loudest along the left sternal border. Electrocardiogram now showed more severe right ventricular hypertrophy. Cardiac catheterization showed a peak systolic pressure gradient of 118 mm Hg between the right ventricle (135.7) and pulmonary artery (17/7), and there was no systolic gradient between the left ventricle (108/4) and the brachial artery (108/63 mm Hg). Resection of the right ventricular outflow myocardium with insertion of a patch at the right ventriculotomy was performed, and catheterization 7 months postoperatively showed virtually no systolic pressure gradient between the right ventricle (30/4 mm Hg) and the pulmonary artery (28/12). He was asymptomatic. Electrocardiograms now showed a right bundle branch block. This boy apparently remained asymptomatic until the day of death, when he felt faint while driving a car. He pulled over to the side of the road and collapsed. No anatomic explanation for death was revealed at necropsy. His heart weighed 660 gm. The right ventricular (RV) outflow tract was wide open. The ventricular septum (VS) was much thicker than the left ventricular (LV) free wall (1.0 compared with 1.9 cm), and the right ventricular wall was of normal thickness. The endocardium of the left ventricular outflow tract was not thickened, and the mitral valve was normal. Mild interstitial fibrosis involved the ventricular septum. *a*, A longitudinal section of the ventricles shows the disproportionate ventricular septal hypertrophy. The right ventricular cavity is larger than the left. Ao = aorta. *b*, The radiograph of the heart was taken before it was opened. From Roberts and Ferrans,[81] with permission.

Although examination of the septum in patients with hypertrophic cardiomyopathy is not helpful in separating patients *with* from those *without* left ventricular outflow obstruction at rest, examination of the basal portion of the left ventricular free wall (posterior or posterolateral portion) does permit delineation between these 2 groups of patients.[90] In the patients with the non-obstructive type of hypertrophic cardiomyopathy, this posterobasal portion is thinner than normal and often pointed like a bird's bill (Fig. 24). In the patients without obstruction at rest, the thickest portion of the left ventricular free wall is about midway between the base of posterior mitral leaflet and apex of left ventricle.

Another abnormality in the ventricular septum in patients with hypertrophic cardiomyopathy is focal *myocardial fiber disarray* or disorganization.[80,81,91] This abnor-

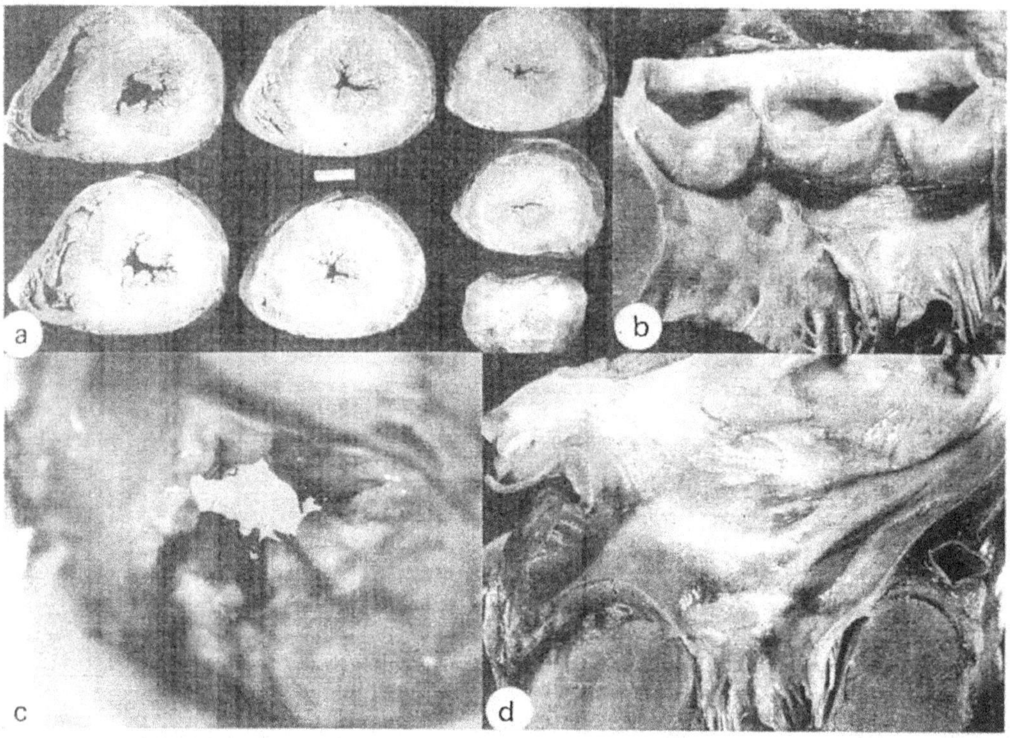

FIGURE 28. Hypertrophic cardiomyopathy in a 53-year-old man who died suddenly at home 6 weeks after onset of atrial fibrillation. Catheterization when he was asymptomatic (but had cardiomegaly) at age 46 disclosed a left ventricular to systemic arterial peak systolic gradient of 8 mm Hg at rest, and a gradient of 69 mm Hg with provocation (isoproterenol). Thereafter, he developed exertional dyspnea, dizziness, and angina. *a*, "Bread loaf" slices of cardiac ventricles. Although the echocardiogram had shown the ventricular septum to be thicker than left ventricular free wall during ventricular diastole, both were of similar thickness at necropsy (25 mm). *b*, Opened aortic valve showing thickening of the mural endocardium in apposition to the thickened anterior mitral leaflet. *c*, View of mitral leaflet from left atrium. Thickening of its leaflets is typical of hypertrophic cardiomyopathy. *d*, Opened left atrium and thickened mitral valve. The basal portion of left ventricular wall is rounded and thick. From Roberts WC. Congenital cardiovascular abnormalities usually "silent" until adulthood: Morphologic features of the floppy mitral valve, valvular aortic stenosis, discrete subvalvular aortic stenosis, hypertrophic cardiomyopathy, sinus of Valsalva aneurysm, and the Marfan syndrome. Cardiovasc Clin 1979; 10(1):436, with permission.

mality, described by Teare in 1958, occurs in about 95% of these patients depending on how "septal disorganization" is defined.[91] Small foci of groups of myocardial fibers not parallel to one another in the ventricular septum are common in normal developing and adult hearts. When, however, the definition of "septal disorganization" is rigid and quantitation of the amount of disorganization is introduced, about 90% of the patients with hypertrophic cardiomyopathy can be clearly delineated from persons with normal hearts or from patients with cardiac conditions other than hypertrophic cardiomyopathy. Studies by Maron and Roberts[91] have shown that among patients with hypertrophic cardiomyopathy nearly 90% had > 5% of the area of the ventricular septum showing myofiber disorganization. In contrast, among persons with normal hearts or heart conditions other than hypertrophic cardiomyopathy, < 5% and usually < 1% of the area of the ventricular septum showed myofiber disorganization.

Although "septal disorganization" of > 5% of the area of the ventricular septum occurs in about 90% of the patients with hypertrophic cardiomyopathy, about 10% of these patients have < 5% of the area of the septum showing disarray, and

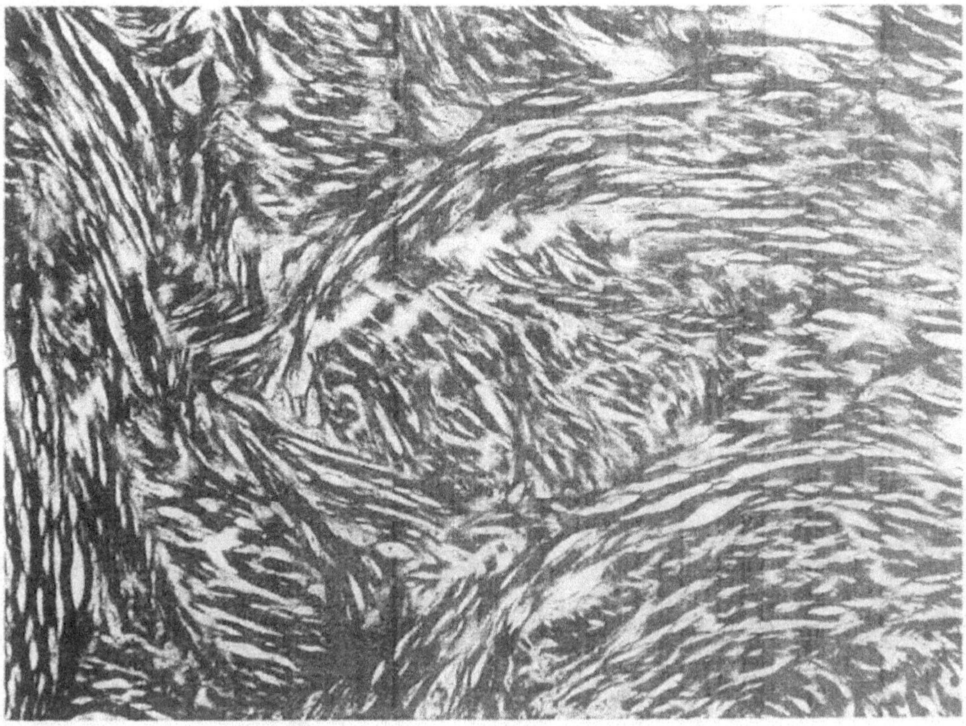

FIGURE 29. Photomicrograph of portion of ventricular septum in a 19-year-old man with hypertrophic cardiomyopathy showing the myocardial fiber disarray typical of this condition. (Masson stain; × 60 magnification.) From Roberts and Ferrans,[81] with permission.

of them a few patients have no disarray at all. Thus, like ventricular asymmetry, "septal disorganization" of > 5% of the area of the septum occurs in most patients with hypertrophic cardiomyopathy, but this abnormality may involve a smaller area of septum or, rarely, may be entirely absent.

Not only does disorganization of *myocardial fibers* occur, but, in addition, ultrastructural studies have shown disarray of *myofibrils* and *myofilaments* within individual cells.[93] Again, the abnormalities of myofibrils and myofilaments are not absolutely specific for hypertrophic cardiomyopathy, but when disorganization of these subcellular components is found in other cardiac conditions, the abnormal cells are in small numbers. The individual septal myocardial cells in hypertrophic cardiomyopathy also appear to have increased amounts of Z-band material and nonspecific changes of cellular hypertrophy and degeneration.

Myofiber disarray also occurs in the left and right ventricular free walls, but not to the extent observed in the ventricular septum.[91] Ultrastructural examination of the left and right ventricular free walls, however, has disclosed many bizarrely shaped, disorganized cells in the ventricular free walls of patients *without* obstruction, whereas the bizarrely shaped and disorganized myocardial fibers are less numerous in the ventricular free walls in the patients *with* obstruction.[91] Thus, the disorientation of groups of myocardial cells and the disarray of myofibrils and myofilaments within individual myocardial cells is not the result of left ventricular outflow obstruction or high intraventricular systolic pressures.

The functional or clinical significance of "septal disorganization" among patients with hypertrophic cardiomyopathy is not clear. Among patients studied at necropsy, those with high percentages of area of septum with disorganization were younger, had a higher frequency of premature death involving > 1 member of the same family, and had thicker ventricular septa than those with low percentages of area of the septum involved.[91] The presence or degree of left ventricular outflow

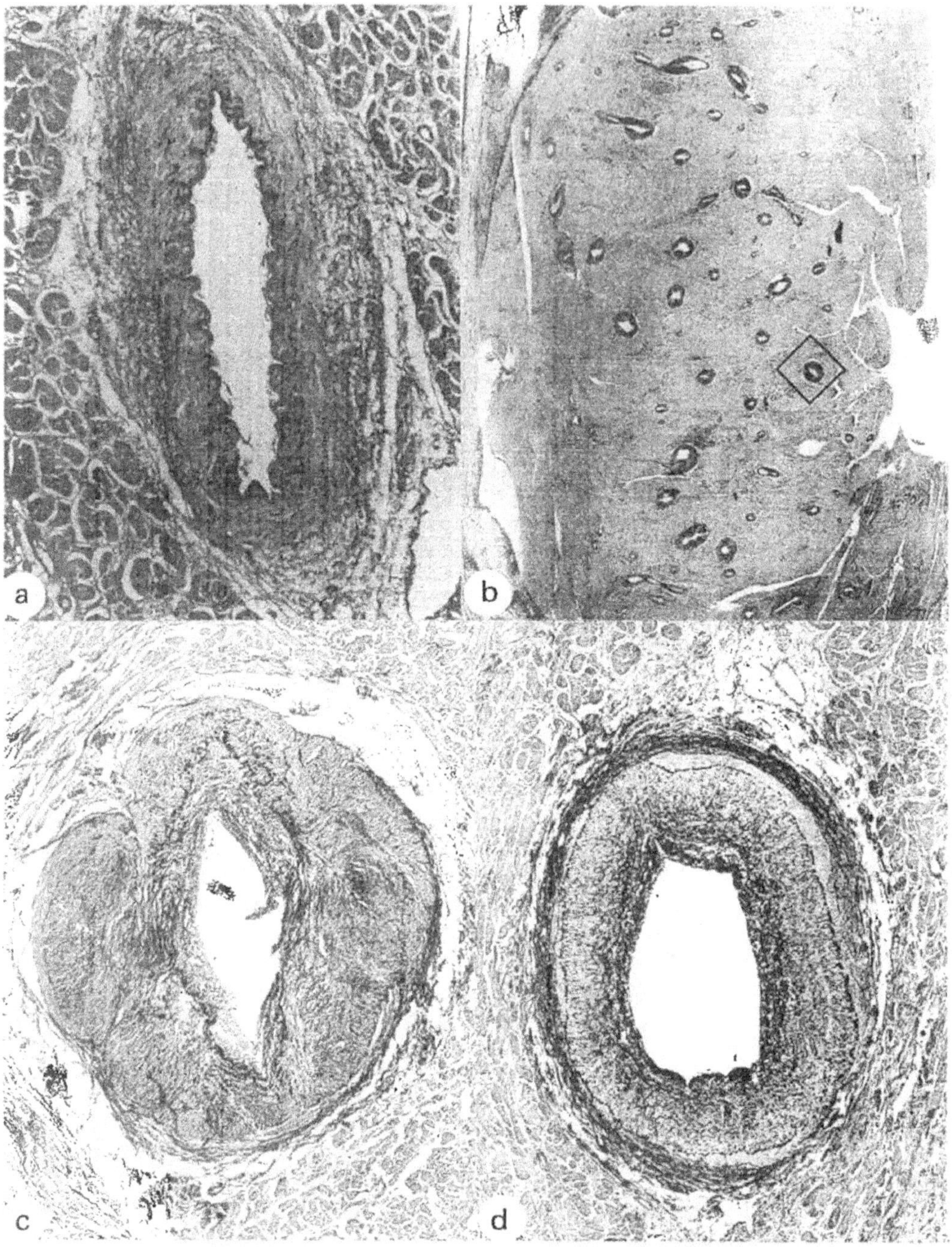

FIGURE 30. Intramural coronary arteries in ventricular septum in hypertrophic cardiomyopathy in 3 different patients. *a*, A normal artery (in a patient with hypertrophic cardiomyopathy) × 140. *b*, Low-power (× 4) photomicrograph of portion of ventricular septum showing marked prominence of the intramural coronary arteries in another patient. The arteries appear to be increased in number, size, and wall thickness. *c*, The artery enclosed by the box in *b* is shown here × 90. *d*, This artery, from another patient, has marked intimal thickening by fibroelastic proliferation, in contrast to the artery shown in *c*, which shows no delineation between intima and media. (Elastic van Gieson stains; reduced 18%) From Roberts WC. Congenital cardiovascular abnormalities usually "silent" until adulthood: Morphologic features of the floppy mitral valve, valvular aortic stenosis, discrete subvalvular aortic stenosis, hypertrophic cardiomyopathy, sinus of Valsalva aneurysm, and the Marfan syndrome. Cardiovasc Clin 1979; 10(1):438, with permission.

TABLE 6. Idiopathic Dilated (DC) and Hypertrophic (HC) Cardiomyopathies: Morphologic Differences

	DC	HC
1. Dilated ventricular cavities	+	0
2. Intracardiac thrombi	+	0
3. Asymmetric septal hypertrophy	0	+
4. Myocardial fiber disorientation	0	+
5. Endocardial plaque, LV outflow tract	0	+
6. Thickened mitral valve	0	+
7. Abnormal intramural coronary arteries	0	+
8. Ventricular scarring	0−+	+
9. Thickened ventricular walls	0−+	+
10. Increased cardiac weight	+	+
11. Dilated atrial cavities	+	+

From Roberts W C. Congenital cardiovascular abnormalities usually "silent" until adulthood: Morphologic features of floppy mitral valve, valvular aortic stenosis, discrete subvalvular aortic stenosis, hypertrophic cardiomyopathy, sinus of Valsalva aneurysm, and the Marfan syndrome. Cardiovasc Clin 1979; 10(1):430, with permission.

obstruction, length of symptoms of cardiac dysfunction, mode of death, arrhythmias, and so forth were not significantly different in the patients with high compared with those with low percentages of septal area involved by disorganization.

Another abnormality of ventricular septum in patients with hypertrophic cardiomyopathy is the presence of *abnormal intramural coronary arteries* in > 50% of the patients.[89,90] The abnormalities observed in the intramural coronary arteries in these patients are striking and consist of increased number and size of arteries with thickened walls and narrowed lumens. The thickening results from increased numbers of smooth-muscle cells and increased amounts of fibrous tissue in both the media and the intima. Also, mucoid deposits (acid mucopolysaccharide material) is increased. Like asymmetric ventricular septal thickening and septal disorganization, however, abnormality of the intramural coronary arteries is not specific for hypertrophic cardiomyopathy, but it is certainly more striking in hypertrophic cardiomyopathy than in most other conditions. Similar abnormality of the intramural coronary arteries may be observed in patients and in Newfoundland dogs with discrete subaortic stenosis,[77] in patients with tunnel subaortic stenosis,[79] in normal human fetuses,[94] and in newborns with aortic valve atresia.[95]

The significance of the changes in the intramural coronary arteries in patients with hypertrophic cardiomyopathy is unknown. Their presence or absence does not correlate with any analyzed clinical parameter including presence of, or degree of, left ventricular outflow tract obstruction, age, sex, presence of cardiac dysfunction including chest pain, or length of symptoms of cardiac dysfunction. The cause of the striking abnormalities of the intramural coronary arteries also is uncertain. In each of the 4 conditions in which this degree of abnormality has been observed, namely, hypertrophic cardiomyopathy, discrete and tunnel subaortic stenosis, and aortic-valve atresia, the septum is extremely thick, and movement of the septum during life as shown by echocardiogram is limited. It is possible that the severe septal thickening prevents adequate expansion of these arteries during ventricular diastole so that flow through them during this phase of the cardiac cycle is greatly reduced. The fibrous-smooth muscle cell response, in turn, may serve to obliterate the unused lumen. This explanation, however, does not explain the large size of these arteries. It is possible that the proliferation of the smooth-muscle cells in the walls of these arteries represents a response to the same stimulus that is causing severe hypertrophy and abnormal configuration of many striated myocardial cells.

A fourth abnormality of the ventricular septum in adults with hypertrophic cardiomyopathy is the occurrence of a *fibrous plaque on the mural endocardium of the outflow portion of the septum.*[81] This fibrous thickening is located in direct apposition to the ventricular aspect of the anterior mitral leaflet and is the result of contact between the valvular and mural endocardium. The mural plaque, in other words, is the *anatomic equivalent of the "systolic anterior motion"* of the anterior mitral leaflet observed on echocardiogram in hypertrophic cardiomyopathy and occasionally in other conditions. The obstruction in hypertrophic cardiomyopathy when present almost certainly begins at a level corresponding to the distal margin of the anterior mitral leaflet and with the caudal margin of the septal endocardial plaque. The mural endocardial septal plaque is present more frequently and is thicker in the patients with obstruction at rest compared with those without obstruction at rest.

It appears that hypertophic cardiomyopathy is primarily a disease of the ventricular septum and that the morphologic abnormalities in it are apparent at the gross, microscopic, and ultrastructural levels. Other portions of the heart, however, are affected in hypertrophic cardiomyopathy but it seems likely that these other abnormalities are secondary to the abnormalities of the ventricular septum. These other abnormalities include *decreased ventricular cavity size* or at least lack of ventricular cavity dilatation, *increased atrial cavity size,* varying degrees of interstitial and replacement *myocardial fibrosis* (particularly in the ventricular septum), *thickening of the posterior* as well as the anterior *mitral leaflet,* and, in the elder patients, *calcification of the mitral anulus.*

The cause of the relatively small sizes of the ventricular cavities in hypertrophic cardiomyopathy is unclear. The septum, being on the average about twice normal thickness, surely occupies space normally represented by cavity. Furthermore, the ventricular free walls, on the average about ⅓ thicker than normal, also probably compromise slightly the intracavitary space. Additionally, the greater thickness of the septum makes this structure relatively noncompliant (as demonstrated by its absent or minimal movement on echocardiogram). Although the left ventricular free wall in hypertrophic cardiomyopathy (by echocardiogram) usually contracts vigorously (in contrast to the septum), it appears to have little capacity to distend outwardly. Whatever the explanation, ventricular cavity size is rarely enlarged in these patients. Those with dilated ventricular cavities (about 15% of personally studied necropsy patients) have either unscarred left and/or right ventricular free walls of normal thickness or scarred ventricular free walls of less than normal thickness.[88] Left ventricular dilatation also may occur after operative septotomy-septectomy in hypertrophic cardiomyopathy.[96]

The impression of ventricular cavity size as observed at necropsy in patients with hypertrophic cardiomyopathy may be somewhat misleading because the cavity at necropsy in patients with hypertrophic cardiomyopathy represents the size at the end of ventricular systole.[97] This information was derived by comparing the left ventricular free wall thickness at necropsy to that measured by echocardiogram during life. The thickness at necropsy corresponds to the thickness during ventricular systole, not diastole, as observed by echocardiogram.

In contrast to the ventricular cavities, the atrial cavities in hypertrophic cardiomyopathy, at least in adults, are always dilated. The dilatation appears to be a response to difficulty in filling the relatively small ventricular cavities.

Not only is the anterior mitral leaflet thickened, but often (more frequently in the patients with outflow obstruction) the posterior mitral leaflet is also. The *thickening of both mitral leaflets* is probably the consequence of the small left ventricular cavity. The mitral valve resides in the left ventricle, which, being small, causes abnormal contact of the leaflets with themselves and also causes the anterior leaflet to contact the septum. In the patients without obstruction, the basal portion of the left ventricular cavity is larger than in the patients with obstruction because of the thinning of the basal portion of free wall posteriorly and laterally. The focal fibrous thickening of the posterior mitral leaflet probably results from abnormal contact during ventricular systole because there is not enough room in the ventricular cavity to easily accommodate the leaflets and chordae. The ventricle and mitral leaflets in this respect may be regarded as being similar to an accordian. The mitral leaflet thickening in hypertrophic cardiomyopathy is somewhat analogous to that which occurs normally as a consequence of aging. With aging, the left ventricular cavity becomes smaller, presumably in response to the lowered cardiac output; the mitral leaflets thicken; the left ventricular muscle becomes less compliant; and the left atrium dilates in response to increased work required to fill the small left ventricle. Similar mechanisms appear to be accelerated in hypertrophic cardiomyopathy.

Most patients with hypertrophic cardiomyopathy have some degree of *mitral regurgitation.* It is not related to anular dilatation because the mitral anulus in this condition is not dilated. Furthermore, the leaflet thickening, in and of itself, is not extensive enough to cause valvular regurgitation. The most likely explanation appears to be abnormal bending of the papillary muscles, particularly the anterolateral one.[98] These structures may be bent abnormally by the bulging ventricular septum with resulting excessive tension on the chordae tendineae preventing closure of the mitral orifice. Although they are usually present in the papillary muscles in hypertrophic cardiomyopathy, focal scars cannot account for the regurgitation. Although it is usually mild in hypertrophic cardiomyopathy, mitral regurgitation may be the predominant clinical feature of this condition. Despite its advocacy by some investigators,[99,100] mitral valve replacement in hypertrophic cardiomyopathy is hazardous and, in my view, rarely warranted.[101] The exception is the patient with severe mitral regurgitation from superimposed infective endocarditis, a condition not rare in patients with hypertrophic cardiomyopathy. The small left ventricular cavity is rarely capable of freely accommodating a prosthesis, and the mitral regurgitation in patients with hypertrophic cardiomyopathy, except when due to valvular damage from infective endocarditis, nearly always either disappears or is strikingly lessened by adequate partial septectomy-septotomy.

SINUS OF VALSALVA ANEURYSM

Each of the 3 sinuses of Valsalva dilates as a normal consequence of aging, and this "senile-type dilatation" is greater in persons with enlarged hearts (from systemic hypertension) than in those with normal-sized hearts.[71] In addition to aging and systemic hypertension, there are at least 3 other causes of dilatation of each of the 3 sinuses of Valsalva, namely, the Marfan[102] and Marfan-like syndromes,[103] syphilis,[104] and ankylosing spondylitis.[105] A congenital type of dilatation of all 3 aortic sinuses unassociated with other congenital anomalies of the heart or great vessels also has been recorded,[106] but its occurrence, if indeed of congenital origin, must be unique.

In contrast to the common occurrence of dilatation of all 3 aortic sinuses, aneurysmal dilatation of only 1 or 2 of the 3 sinuses is quite unusual. The most common cause is probably infective endocarditis with spread of the infection into adjacent structures and formation of 1 or more ring abscesses.[107] Aneurysmal dilatation of only 1 aortic sinus unassociated with infective endocarditis is extremely rare. Generally, in this circumstance, the localized aneurysmal dilatation is attributed to a congenital absence of media in the wall of the aorta behind a sinus of Valsalva[108] (Figs. 31 to 33). The wall of aorta behind the sinus may rupture, and when this occurs, aortic regurgitation into either right ventricle or right atrium is the usual consequence (see Fig. 32). Less commonly, the sinus aneurysm may obstruct right ventricular outflow or cause a conduction disturbance.[109–112]

The basic defect in patients with aneurysms involving only 1 or 2 of the 3 aortic-valve sinuses is an absence of a portion of, or all of, the media in the wall of aorta behind the sinus (see Fig. 31). Just because the media is deficient, however, does not

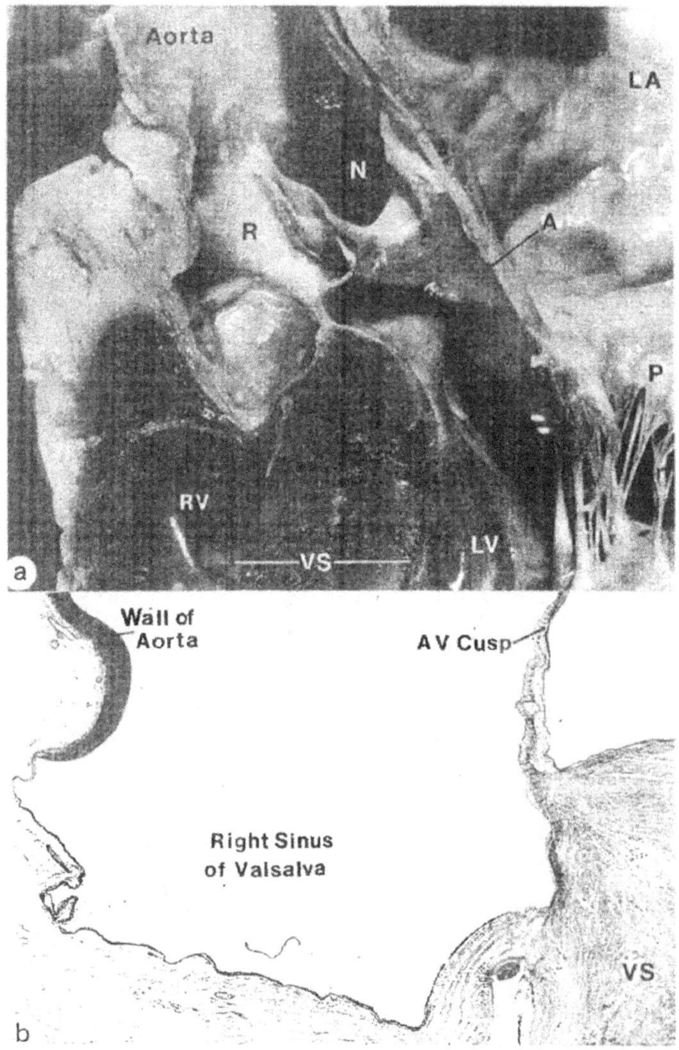

FIGURE 31. Unruptured sinus of Valsalva aneurysm in an 82-year-old man who died of cancer. An unexpected finding at necropsy was aneurysmal dilatation of the right sinus of Valsalva. The right sinus was 2.5 cm deep and held 15 ml of fluid, whereas the left and noncoronary sinuses of Valsalva were only 1.5 cm deep and held only 5 ml of fluid.

a, Longitudinal section of heart showing the aneurysmal dilatation of the right (R) sinus of Valsalva. N = noncoronary sinus of Valsalva; A, P = anterior and posterior mitral leaflets, respectively; LA = left atrium; LV = left ventricle; VS = ventricular septum. *b*, Histologic section of wall of right sinus of Valsalva showing the absence of aortic media in the caudal portion of the aneurysm. AV = aortic valve. From Fishbein, et al,[110] with permission.

assure the appearance of an aortic sinus aneurysm. When a deficiency of aortic media occurs, the wall involved most commonly (about 70% of patients) is that behind the right anterior cusp; occasionally (about 29%) it is the portion behind the posterior cusp; and virtually never (< 1%), that portion behind the left anterior cusp.[113] The explanation for these differences is uncertain.

Whether or not a sinus of Valsalva aneurysm is ever present from birth is uncertain; most likely, the aneurysm is acquired, presumably the result of the aortic pressure. The higher the aortic pressure (for example, in patients with coarctation of the aortic isthmus), the more likely is an aortic sinus aneurysm to develop. The youngest child described with isolated sinus of Valsalva aneurysm was 4 years old.[114]

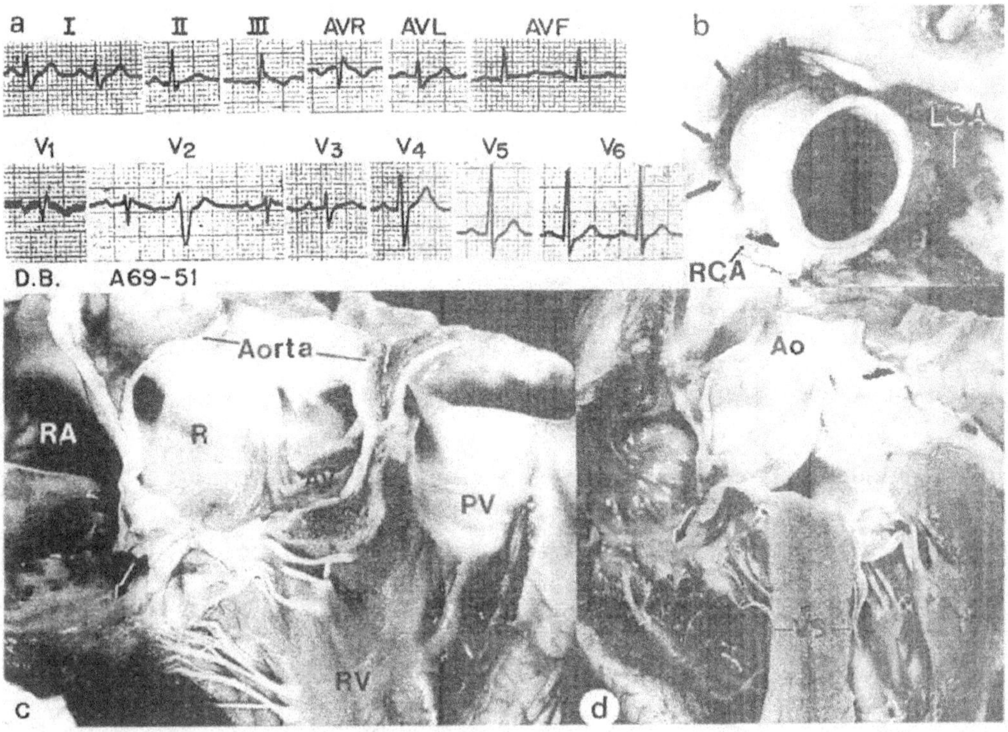

FIGURE 32. Rupture of right (R) sinus of Valsalva aneurysm into right ventricle (RV) in a 31-year-old woman who had been well until about 60 days before death, when exertional dyspnea appeared. Eighteen days before death, she developed acute pulmonary edema and a murmur of aortic regurgitation. She died of progressive congestive cardiac failure. *a*, An electrocardiogram taken several days before her death. At necropsy, the heart weighed only 300 gm. *b*, an aneurysm of the right sinus of Valsalva was present and bulged to the right (arrows). LCA, RCA = left and right coronary arteries, respectively. *c*, Opened right ventricle (RV) and wall of aorta behind right (R) sinus of Valsalva showing the aneurysm that had ruptured (arrow) into the right atrium (RA) anatomically and into the right ventricle functionally. AV = aortic valve; PV = pulmonic valve. *d*, In this view, the anterior half of the heart has been removed; the ruptured (arrow) aneurysm's relation to the right side of the heart and to the ventricular septum (VS) is apparent. Ao = aorta. From Roberts WC. Congenital cardiovascular abnormalities usually "silent" until adulthood: Morphologic features of the floppy mitral valve, valvular aortic stenosis, discrete subvalvular aortic stenosis, hypertrophic cardiomyopathy, sinus of Valsalva aneurysm, and the Marfan syndrome. Cardiovasc Clin 1979; 10(1):441, with permission.

Although the aneurysm itself may or may not be congenital, the deficiency in aortic media behind the sinus must be congenital.[110]

Both the natural history and the frequency of media-deficient aortic sinus wall are uncertain. The number of persons with a media-deficient aortic sinus wall in whom a sinus aneurysm develops is uncertain, as is the frequency of rupture of a developed sinus aneurysm (Fig. 34). Among 78 cases of sinus of Valsalva aneurysm collected from publications by Kieffer and Winchell,[115] 59 (76%) had ruptured and 19 (24%) had not. In some of the cases included by these authors, however, the aneurysms involved all 3 sinuses, and therefore they were probably associated with the Marfan syndrome. Among 7 hearts with aneurysm of 1 aortic sinus studied at necropsy by Edwards and Burchel,[108] 4 aneurysms had ruptured and 3 had not. Of 6 single (1 of 3 sinuses involved) aortic sinus aneurysms studied personally at necropsy, 6 had ruptured and 1[110] was unruptured. The latter patient was 82 years old (see Fig. 31); the ages in the 6 patients with ruptured aneurysms ranged from 31 to

FIGURE 33. Rupture of right sinus of Valsalva aneurysm into pericardial sac in a 33-year-old woman who had been well until she died suddenly while house cleaning. At necropsy the pericardial sac was filled with blood. *a*, The right sinus of Valsalva is exteriorly round, and a rupture (arrow) is visible in its right lateral wall. Extravasation was into the pericardial space only and not into a cardiac chamber. An = aneurysm; Ao = aorta; PT = pulmonary trunk; RA = right atrium; RV = right ventricle: *b*, The anterior portion of the heart has been removed again showing the right (R) sinus of Valsalva aneurysm. A = anterior mitral leaflet; LV = left ventricle; VS = ventricular septum. From Roberts WC. Congenital cardiovascular abnormalities usually "silent" until adulthood: Morphologic features of the floppy mitral valve, valvular aortic stenosis, discrete subvalvular aortic stenosis, hypertrophic cardiomyopathy, sinus of Valsalva aneurysm, and the Marfan syndrome. Cardiovasc Clin 1979; 10(1):442, with permission.

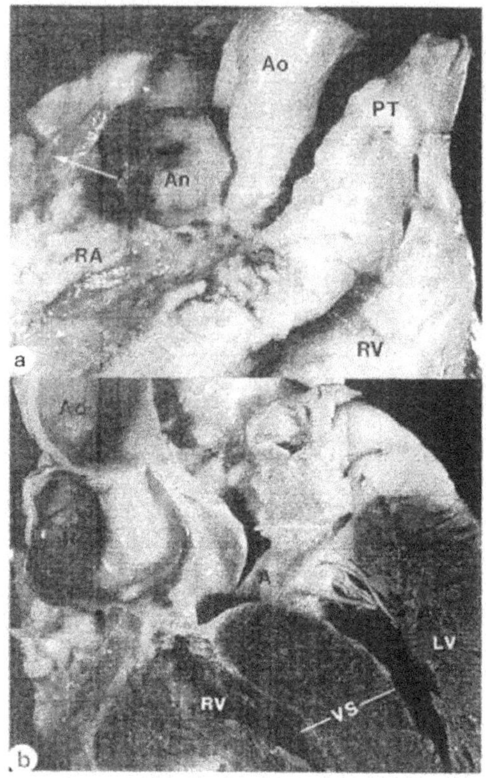

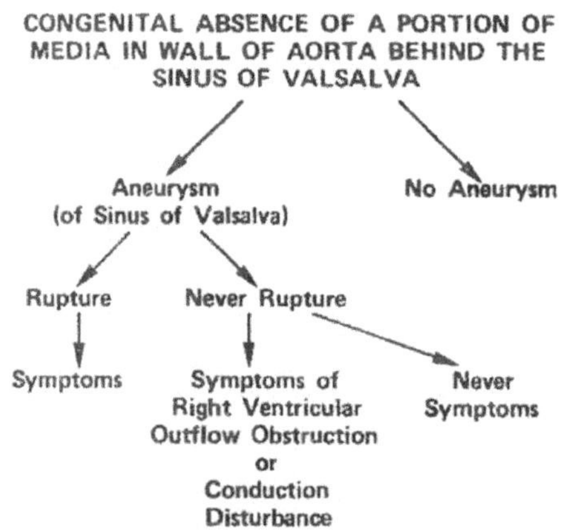

FIGURE 34. Diagram showing possible outcome in patients with congenital absence of a portion of media in aortic wall behind sinus of Valsalva. If no aneurysm occurs, the congenital defect will go unrecognized. If an aneurysm does occur, it may or may not rupture. Rupture will virtually always produce clinical symptoms and signs of cardiac dysfunction. If rupture does not occur, symptoms will usually be present only if there is right ventricular outflow obstruction or conduction disturbances. From Roberts WC. Congenital cardiovascular abnormalities usually "silent" until adulthood: Morphologic features of the floppy mitral valve, valvular aortic stenosis, discrete subvalvular aortic stenosis, hypertrophic cardiomyopathy, sinus of Valsalva aneurysm, and the Marfan syndrome. Cardiovasc Clin 1979; 10(1):442, with permission.

TABLE 7. Clinical and Necropsy Observations in 18 Personally Studied Patients with the Marfan Syndrome

PT	Age (yr)	Race	Sex	Marfan Features: MS	Marfan Features: Ocular	Marfan Features: FH	Ht (cm)	Wt (kg)	CHF	Murmur (0–6/6): AR	Murmur (0–6/6): MR	Indirect SAP (mm Hg): S	Indirect SAP (mm Hg): D
Fusiform Aneurysm of Ascending Aorta													
1	15	W	M	+	+	?	193	68	+	3	3	140	0
2	20	W	M	+	0	+	198	49	0	3	3	220	70
3[a]	21	B	M	+	+	+	203	—	0	1	0	130	80
4	21	B	M	+	+	+	147	67	+	4	3	160	60
5	26	W	M	+	0	+	198	—	+	5	0	110	40
6	31	W	M	+	+	+	183	45	+	2	4	135	40
7	35	W	F	+	+	+	158	50	+	3	0	110	40
8	36	B	F	+	0	+	185	49	+	3	0	100	40
9	38	B	F	+	+	+	173	50	+	3	4	140	20
10	38	B	M	+	0	+	191	59	0	3	0	115	55
11	41	B	M	+	+	—	193	82	+	5	0	150	50
12	47	W	M	+	+	+	187	64	+	4	2	140	40
13	48	W	F	+	0	+	179	54	+	3	0	150	40
Dissection of Aorta													
14	43	W	M	+	+	0	193	86	0	0[b]	0	210	100
15	49	B	F	+	+	+	173	47	0	0[b]	3	110	70
16	52	B	F	+	+	0	178	72	0	0[b]	0	180	100
Isolated Mitral Regurgitation													
17	28	W	M	+	+	+	175	59	+	0	5	130	80
18	35	W	F	+	+	0	184	66	+	0	4	120	80
Total or Mean	34	10 W 8 B	11 M 7 F	18	13	13	173	60	12	13	9	142	56

Abbreviations: AA = ascending aorta; AAR = ascending aortic replacement (graft); AR = aortic regurgitation; AV = aortic valve; AVR = aortic valve replacement; Ca^{++} = calcium; CAD = coronary heart disease; CHF = congestive heart failure; C of A = aortic isthmic coarctation; CMN = cystic medial necrosis; CV = cardiovascular; d = end-diastole; F = female; FH = family history of Marfan syndrome; Ht = height; IE = infective endocarditis; LVP = left ventricular pressure; M = male; MR = mitral regurgitation; MS = musculoskeletal; MV = mitral valve; PDA = patent ductus arteriosus; PV = pulmonic valve; RCT = ruptured chordae tendineae; s = peak systole; SAP = systemic arterial pressure; TV = tricuspid valve; Yr = years; Wt = weight.

(Reproduced from Roberts and Honig, with permission.)

49 years (mean 38). An additional patient, a 57 year-old woman, had a congenitally bicuspid aortic valve, with rupture of 1 of the 2 sinus walls into the right side of the heart.[116] These figures indicate that among reported cases of aortic sinus aneurysm, rupture is more common than nonrupture, but the data are probably considerably biased in favor of ruptured aneurysms. The unruptured sinus aneurysm, for example, may be missed at necropsy. The unruptured aneurysm, with few exceptions, produces no evidence of cardiac dysfunction; and, therefore, at necropsy there may be no clinical sign or symptom to alert the pathologist to the presence of an aortic sinus aneurysm. Furthermore, incidental necropsy findings, which is what an unruptured aortic sinus aneurysm usually represents, are infrequently reported. Thus, it is likely that the frequency of unruptured aortic sinus aneurysm is considerably greater than has been reported.

An unruptured single aortic sinus aneurysm on rare occasion may produce evidence of cardiac dysfunction. Kerber and associates[109] described clinical and operative findings in a 62-year-old man who had evidence of right ventricular outflow obstruction as the result of an aortic sinus aneurysm's bulging into the crista supraventricularis. Complete heart block also has been described in a patient with unruptured aortic sinus aneurysm.[112] The latter patient, however, also had calcific aortic stenosis, and thus it is not certain that the sinus aneurysm was responsible for the conduction defect.

Rupture of the sinus of Valsalva aneurysm, obviously, is the most frequent complication of aneurysm involving only 1 of the 3 aortic sinuses. Rupture rarely occurs before adulthood. Like all conditions affecting the aorta and the aortic valve, it is more common in males than females, about 4 to 1. Death occurs suddenly if the rupture is into the pericardial space rather than into a cardiac cavity (see Fig. 33).

TABLE 7. (*Continued*)

Direct LVP (s/d)	SAP (s/d)	AR (0-4+)	Operation AAR	AVR	Other	Heart Weight (gm)	Aortic Tears	CMN AA	Circumference Valve Anuli (cm) TV	MV	PV	AV	Prolapse TV	MV	RCT MV	Ca^{++} MV Anulus	Associated CV Lesions
—	—	—	0	0	0	730	0	+	16	16	8	12	+	+	+	0	0
170/20	170/65	3+	0	0	+	900	0	+	12	10	7	8	0	+	+	+	C of A
—	—	—	0	0	0	460	+	+	14	13	8	9	+	0	0	0	0
136/18	158/62	4+	+	+	+	700	+	+	12	13	9	9	0	0	0	+	0
—	—	3+	+	0	0	725	+	+	14	12	9	16	0	0	0	0	0
—	—	—	0	0	+	700	0	+	14	16	9	12	+	+	+	+	IE
120/25	120/50	4+	+	+	0	375	+	+	9	9	7	9	0	0	0	0	PDA
—	130/38	4+	0	0	0	750	+	+	14	13	10	10	0	0	0	0	0
—	—	—	+	0	0	750	+	+	14	15	9	18	0	+	+	0	IE
—	140/65	3+	0	0	0	520	+	+	13	10	9	14	0	0	0	0	0
110/35	110/35	3+	+	+	0	750	0	+	11	12	7	9	0	0	0	0	0
108/24	108/39	4+	+	+	0	830	+	+	—	—	—	—	0	0	0	0	CAD
150/12	150/40	3+	+	+	0	520	0	+	12	11	8	12	0	0	0	0	0
—	—	—	0	0	+[d]	500	0	0	12	9	8	8	0	0	0	0	0
—	—	—	0	0	0	480	0	0	12	14	8	9	0	+	0	0	0
—	—	—	0	+[c]	+	700	0	0	11	10	8	9	0	0	0	0	0
—	130/80	—	0	0	0	830	0	0	13	17	9	8	+	+	+	+	0
100/14	100/75	0	0	0	0	555	0	0	12	17	7	9	0	+	0	+	0
128/21	132/55	9	7	6	5	654	8	13	13	13	8	11	4	7	5	5	5

a = Daughter of patient #9.

b = Not present before the dissection but appeared afterward.

c = The aortic dissection, which occurred 8 years before death, was operatively plicated at the time. Severe AR developed thereafter due to the dissection to the aortic root and AVR was done 3 days before death, the consequence of excessive bleeding.

d = Aortic dissection, 14 days before death, was plicated 13 days before death, which resulted from rupture of the aorta into the pericardial sac.

Death usually occurs, however, within a year after rupture with regurgitation into a cardiac chamber (see Fig. 32). Death most commonly is the result of congestive cardiac failure.

THE MARFAN SYNDROME

The Marfan syndrome generally involves the bones, joints, eyes, heart, and blood vessels. The extremities are long and thin (dolichostenomelia), the ligments and joint capsules are redundant, the lenses are dislocated (ectopia lentis), the ascending aorta often is dilated, and one or both left-sided cardiac valves frequently are regurgitant. Cardiovascular disease is by far the most common cause of death in patients with the Marfan syndrome. Of 18 personally studied necropsy patients fulfilling McKusick's criteria for this syndrome (Table 7), all died from cardiovascular disease and death in each was premature (mean age = 34 years [range 15 to 52]).[102] Of 56 deceased patients with this syndrome studied during life by Murdoch and associates,[117] cardiovascular disease was the cause of death in 52 (93%), and the mean age at death was 32 years. Of the 151 previously reported necropsy patients wtih the Marfan syndrome, the mean age at death was 23 years and ranged from stillbirth to 65 years (Table 8). (The 91 articles in which these 151 patients were described are listed in the article by Roberts and Honig.[102])

A variety of cardiovascular lesions has been observed in the great arteries and hearts of patients with the Marfan syndrome. The personally studied 18 necropsy patients with this syndrome readily separated into 3 groups on the basis of their

TABLE 8. Observations in 151 Previously Reported Necropsy Patients with the Marfan Syndrome (for References, See Roberts and Honig[102])

CV CATEGORY	NO. PTS.	AGES (YR) RANGE (MEAN)	M:F (%:%)	NO. AGE ≤ 15 YEARS	AR	CA	P	T	CV OP
1. Fusiform ascending aortic aneurysm	53 (35%)	7 mo–62 (28)	30:23 (57:43)	8 (15%)	40/42 (95%)	5 (9%)	4 (7%)	2 (4%)	5 (9%)
2. Aortic dissection	57 (38%) (healed = 14)	13–52 (27	35:21 (63:37)	4 (7%)	3/30 (10%)	5 (9%)	10 (18%)	3 (5%)	4 (7%)
3. Mitral regurgitation without #1 or # 2	33 (22%)	2 mo–65 (12)	15:16 (48:52)	24 (73%)	1 (3%)	0	1 (3%)	0	2 (6%)
4. Miscellaneous (not #1, #2 or #3)	8 (5%)	Stillborn–35 (14)	3:4	4	0	0	0	0	2
TOTALS	151 (100%)	Stillborn–65 (23)	83:64 (56:44)	40 (26%)	—	10 (7%)	15 (10%)	5 (3%)	13 (9%)

AR = aortic regurgitation; CA = coarctation of aorta; CV = cardiovascular; F = female; M = male; mo = month; No. = number, P = pregnancy; Pts = patients; T = trauma, Op = operation.

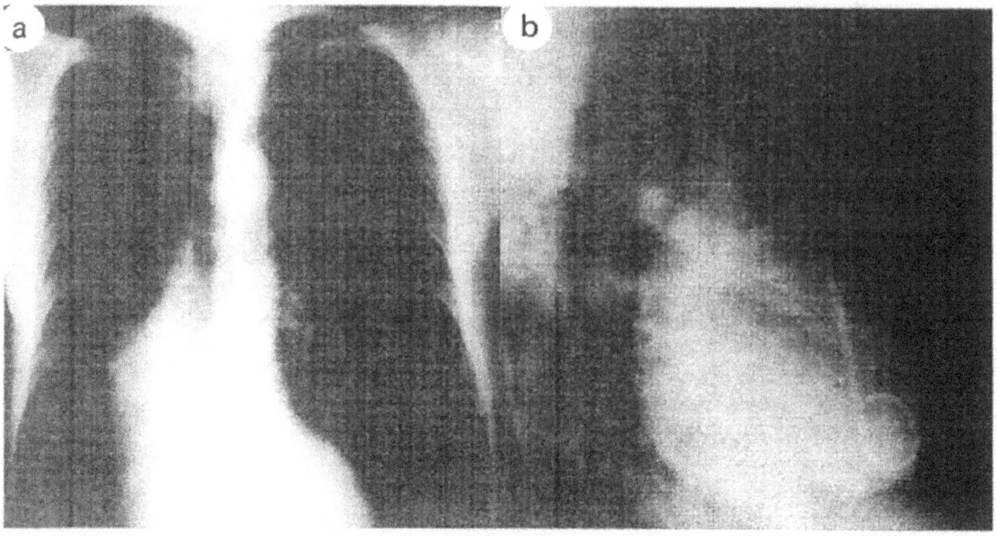

FIGURE 35. Chest radiograph (*a*) and aortogram (*b*) in a 38-year-old man with Marfan syndrome. A large aortic "root" aneurysm is present. (See Figure 36 for additional findings in this patient.) From Roberts WC. Congenital cardiovascular abnormalities usually "silent" until adulthood: Morphologic features of the floppy mitral valve, valvular aortic stenosis, discrete subvalvular aortic stenosis, hypertrophic cardiomyopathy, sinus of Valsalva aneurysm, and the Marfan syndrome. Cardiovasc Clin 1979; 10(1):443, with permission.

cardiovascular lesions. Group I included 13 patients with *fusiform aneurysms of the ascending aorta* (Figs. 35 to 37). All 13 patients had aortic regurgitation, and 6 also had associated mitral regurgitation. In each, the aneurysm involved the sinus and the proximal tubular portions of ascending aorta; 2 also had fusiform aneurysms in the descending thoracic aorta. Histologic study of the wall of the ascending aorta disclosed the typical lesion of this syndrome, that is, massive loss of elastic fibers and increased amounts of mucoid material in the media. Group II included 3 patients with *dissection* of the entire aorta (Fig. 38). Before dissection, the aorta in each was of normal size, and, histologically, the wall of aorta was normal. None of these 3 patients had either aortic or mitral regurgitation before the aortic dissection. Two, however, had had systemic hypertension. Group III included 2 patients with isolated mitral regurgitation with floppy mitral leaflets and markedly dilated mitral anuli. In each, the aortic lumen was of normal size and its wall was normal histologically.

In contrast to the predominant occurrence of fusiform ascending aortic aneurysm in the personally studied patients (13 of 18) and the relatively infrequent occurrence of aortic dissection (3 of 18), aortic dissection was the most frequent gross cardiovascular abnormality observed in the previously reported necropsy patients with the Marfan syndrome (57 [38%] of 151 patients), followed by aortic root aneurysm without dissection (53 [38%] patients), then mitral regurgitation without aortic root aneurysm or dissection (33 [22%] patients); and finally, 8 patients (5%) did not have aortic dissection or root aneurysm or mitral regurgitation and were placed in a miscellaneous group (see Table 8). Analysis of the previously reported necropsy patients disclosed that those with either fusiform ascending aortic aneurysm or aortic dissection had similar mean ages (28 and 27 years), males were slightly more frequent in both groups (3:2), and only 10% of the 110 patients were aged $\leq$ 15 years (see Table 8). In contrast, the 33 previously reported necropsy patients with isolated or predominant mitral regurgitation and the 8 patients classified as miscellaneous had a much younger mean age (12 and 14 years), virtually equal numbers of males and females, and a very high percentage of patients aged $\leq$ 15 years (nearly 70%) (see Table 8). Sisk and associates[118] observed similar findings in 15 patients with the Marfan syndrome diagnosed $<$ 15 years of age.

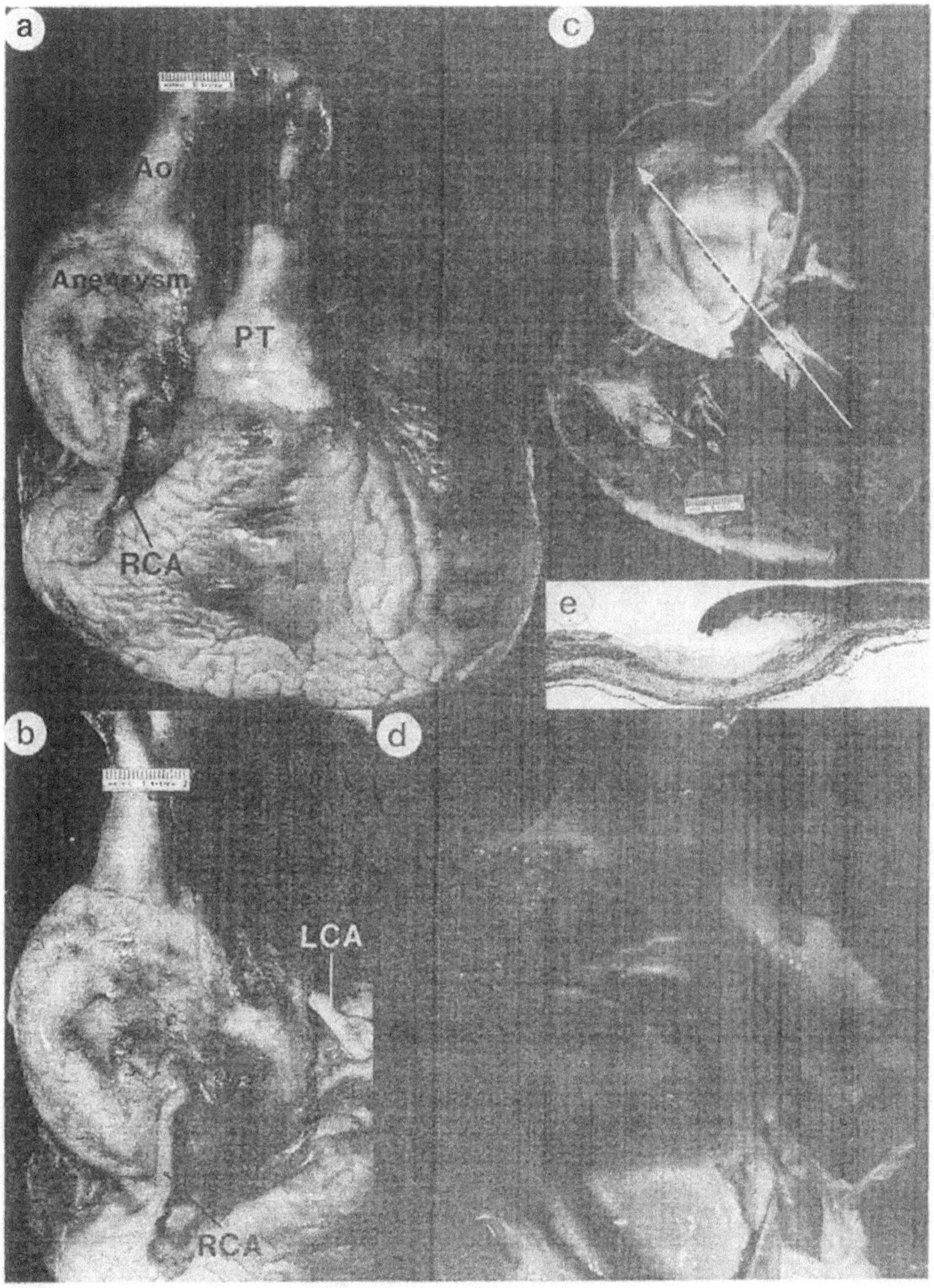

FIGURE 36. The Marfan syndrome with rupture of ascending aortic aneurysm in a 38-year-old black man. The patient was known to have a murmur of aortic regurgitation (aortic pressure 115/55 mm Hg) but there was no evidence of congestive heart failure. He died suddenly at home, and at necropsy the pericardial space was filled with blood and a tear was present in a large aneurysm involving all three sinuses of Valsalva and the proximal tubular portion of ascending aorta. *a*, View of heart shows the size of the aneurysm in comparison with the sizes of other structures. Ao = aorta; PT = pulmonary trunk; RCA = right coronary artery. *b*, A closer view of the large aneurysm with the coronary arteries arising from it. LCA = left coronary artery. *c*, The anterior half of the heart and aorta have now been removed. The dashed line depicts the direction of the blood ejected from the left ventricle. The arrow points to the rupture site in the wall of the aneurysm. The right lateral wall is the site of the rupture. VS = ventricular septum. *d*, Closeup of interior lining of aortic aneurysm at site of rupture.

As in all my 13 patients with fusiform ascending aortic aneurysms (or "anulaortic ectasia"), evidence of aortic regurgitation was present in almost all (95%) of the previously reported necropsy patients with fusiform ascending aortic aneurysm. As an indication of the severity of the aortic regurgitation in the reported patients with fusiform ascending aortic aneurysm, the average indirect peak systolic systemic arterial pressure in the 29 (of the 53) patients in whom this information was available was 146 mm Hg (range 100 to 195), and the average end-diastolic systemic arterial pressure was 43 mm Hg (range 0 to 90), yielding an average pulse pressure of just over 100 mm Hg (range 40 to 170). Of the 29 patients with fusiform root aneurysms and reported blood pressure measurements, 18 (62%) had systemic arterial systolic pressures < 140 mm Hg, 26 (90%) had systemic diastolic pressures < 60 mm Hg, and 23 (79%) had pulse pressures > 60 mm Hg.

In contrast to their frequent recording in the reported necropsy patients with fusiform ascending aortic aneurysms, blood pressure values *before the dissection occurred* were virutally unreported in the 57 previously reported necropsy patients with aortic dissection (see Roberts and Honig[102]). Nevertheless, evidence of the presence of aortic regurgitation before the aortic dissection was rare. The reason that aortic regurgitation before dissection is rare in the patients with aortic dissection is because dissection is infrequent in the patients with fusiform ascending aortic aneurysm, and it is the latter which primarily is responsible for the severe aortic regurgitation (in the absence of healed dissection). With few exceptions, aortic dissection in patients with the Marfan syndrome tends to affect the previously normal-sized aorta or the aorta only slightly dilated. None of 13 personally studied necropsy patients with fusiform ascending aortic aneurysm had aortic dissection, and none of 3 personally studied patients with dissection of the entire aorta had evidence of fusiform ascending aortic aneurysm or aortic regurgitation before the dissection. Of the reported patients with aortic dissection, those with dilated ascending aortas over a long period of time usually had healed dissections, and the dilatation in them appeared to be the result of aneurysm of the false channel. In at least 14 of the 57 previously reported patients with aortic dissection, the dissection had healed (see Roberts and Honig[102]).

The reason that fusiform ascending aortic aneurysm occurs in some patients with the Marfan syndrome and aortic dissection in others appears to lie in the status of the aortic media. In each of the 13 personally studied necropsy patients with fusiform aneurysm of the ascending aorta, histologic study of the wall of the aorta disclosed severe degrees of "cystic medial necrosis." In contrast, none of 3 patients with dissection involving the entire aorta had cystic medial necrosis by histologic examination. Furthermore, in 44 of the 53 previously reported necropsy patients with fusiform ascending aortic aneurysm, cystic medial necrosis was described, and in the other 9 patients, its presence or absence was simply not mentioned. It was not mentioned as being absent in any patient, and in those in whom photomicrographs were illustrated, the degree of cystic medial necrosis was nearly always severe. Among the 57 previously reported necropsy patients with aortic dissection, cystic medial necrosis was described as being present in 35 and as being absent in 7.[102] In the patients, however, in whom photomicrographs of aorta were illustrated, the degree of cystic medial necrosis was usually minimal or mild, and rarely was the degree of

---

Several healed incomplete tears are present in the wall of the aneurysm, and these have been confused with aortic dissection. *e*, Photomicrograph through 1 of the aortic tears showing massive degeneration of elastic fibers. From Roberts WC. Congenital cardiovascular abnormalities usually "silent" until adulthood: Morphologic features of the floppy mitral valve, valvular aortic stenosis, discrete subvalvular aortic stenosis, hypertrophic cardiomyopathy, sinus of Valsalva aneurysm, and the Marfan syndrome. Cardiovasc Clin 1979; 10(1):444, with permission.

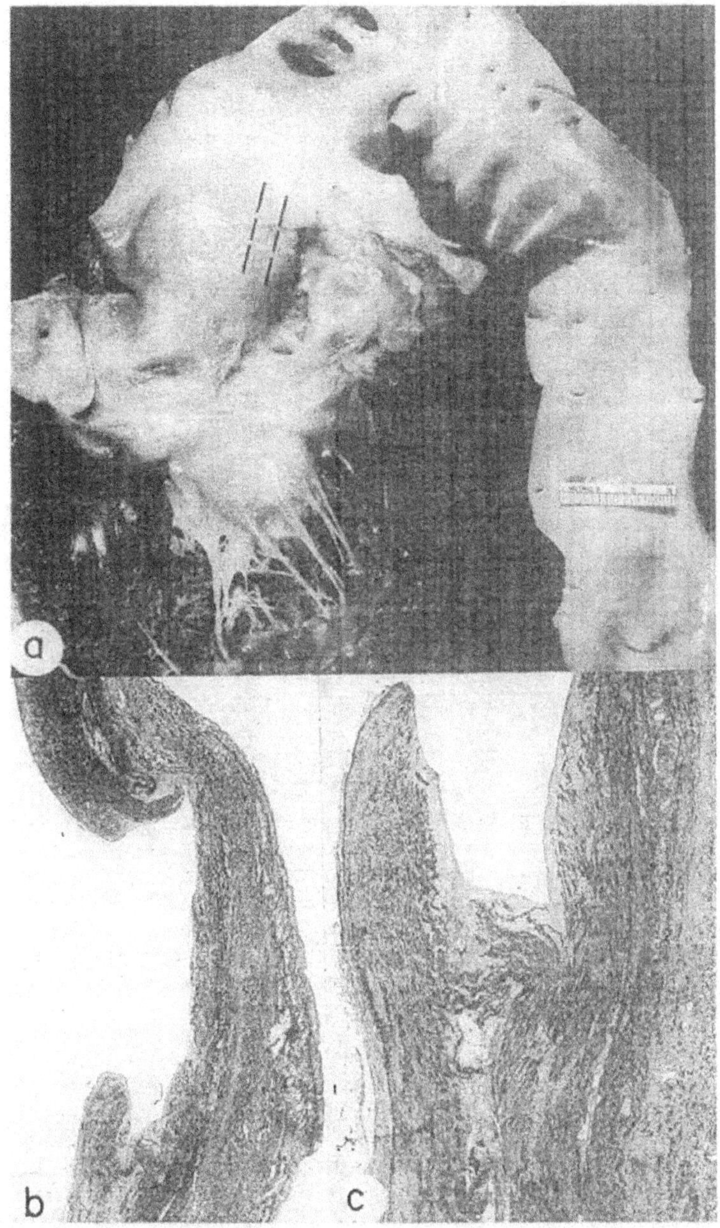

FIGURE 37. The Marfan syndrome. This 21-year-old man had the typical skeletal and optic features of this syndrome but had always been asymptomatic. He was found dead in his parked car after playing in a band for several hours. At necropsy the pericardiac sac was filled with blood. *a*, Evidence of a through-and-through rupture is visible in the ascending aorta just above the aortic valve. In addition, several partial ruptures or tears are also present in the ascending aorta. *b*, A histologic section of one tear (shown between dashed lines in *a*). *c*, A closeup of an adjacent section of *b* reveals severe degeneration of elastic fibers of the media. (Elastic tissue stains; *b*, × 7 and *c*, × 18 magnification.) From Roberts WC. Congenital cardiovascular abnormalities usually "silent" until adulthood: Morphologic features of the floppy mitral valve, valvular aortic stenosis, discrete subvalvular aortic stenosis, hypertrophic cardiomyopathy, sinus of Valsalva aneurysm, and the Marfan syndrome. Cardiovasc Clin 1979; 10(1):446, with permission.

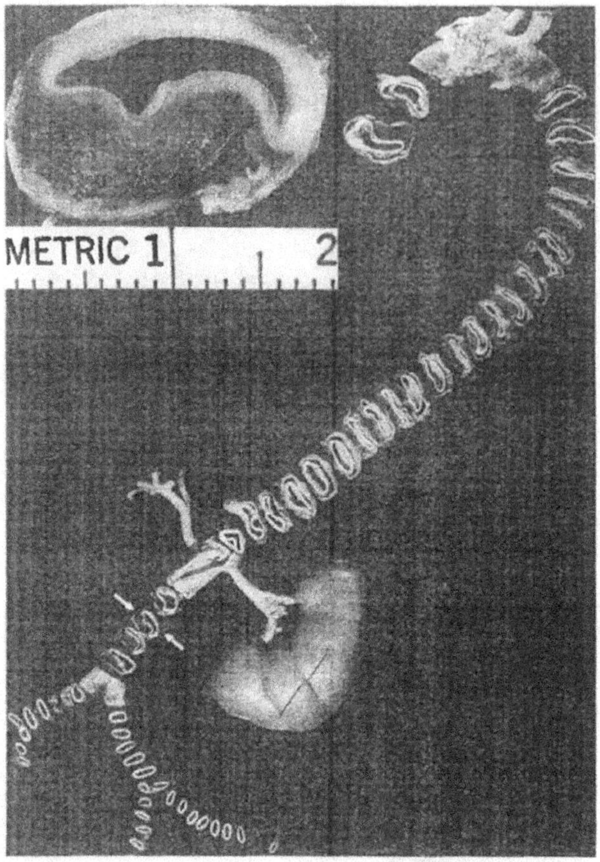

FIGURE 38. Aorta in a 43-year-old man known to have Marfan syndrome. He died 15 days after the sudden onset of typical clinical features of aortic dissection. Before the aortic dissection, there was no precordial murmur. At necropsy, except for the acute dissection, there was no enlargement of the aorta, and except at the site of the entrance into the false channel, there were no tears in the aorta. Shown here is the complete aorta with both true and false channels and a hematoma in the false channel of the abdominal portion. A closeup of the transverse section indicated by arrows is shown in the upper left. Histologically, there was no evidence of elastic fiber degeneration in the media of aorta. The heart weighed 500 gm, and neither ventricle was dilated. Thus, although this patient had both aortic dissection and Marfan syndrome, the typical histologic aortic medial lesion of this syndrome was absent. Therefore, it is more likely that the systemic hypertension was a more important contributing factor to the aortic dissection. From Roberts WC. Congenital cardiovascular abnormalities usually "silent" until adulthood: Morphologic features of the floppy mitral valve, valvular aortic stenosis, discrete subvalvular aortic stenosis, hypertrophic cardiomyopathy, sinus of Valsalva aneurysm, and the Marfan syndrome. Cardiovasc Clin 1979; 10(1):447, with permission.

cystic medial necrosis as severe as that observed routinely in the patients with fusiform ascending aortic aneurysm.

Thus, the aortic media appears to be quite different in the patients with fusiform ascending aortic aneurysm and in those with aortic dissection, particularly when the latter involves the entire aorta. In the patients with fusiform ascending aortic aneurysm, there are usually "massive" degeneration or loss of the elastic fibers of the media and increased quantities of collagen and mucoid material. The increased quantities of collagen would appear to prevent longitudinal aortic dissection. The aortic media in the patients with aortic dissection, in contrast, tends to be normal or to have only a mild degree of cystic medial necrosis, just as in patients with aortic dissection and systemic hypertension who do not have the Marfan syndrome.[119–121]

Two of the 3 personally studied patients with aortic dissection had evidence of diastolic systemic hypertension, whereas none of the other 16 patients had diastolic hypertension.

In none of the previous reports describing necropsy patients with the Marfan syndrome was the degree of cystic medial necrosis graded.[102] In 1970, however, Carlson and associates[119] graded the severity of cystic medial necrosis from 1 to 4 among patients with systemic hypertension and among others with normotension. They found that the frequency of cystic medial necrosis increased progressively from 10% in the first 2 decades of life to 60 and 64% in the seventh and eighth decades, respectively. The frequency and extent of cystic medial necrosis were higher in the hypertensive than in the normotensive patients of similar age. Schlatmann and Becker[120] confirmed the observation that certain degrees of cystic medial necrosis are observed in the normal aorta and that the degrees of cystic medial necrosis increase with age. Schlatmann and Becker[121] also compared the ascending aortic media in patients with dilated aortas with those in patients with complete or incomplete dissection and found only quantitative differences between the normal aging aorta and the overtly abnormal aorta. Thus, these newer observations regarding the frequency, extent, and significance of cystic medial necrosis must be taken into account when evaluating its presence in patients with the Marfan syndrome. Probably many of the Marfan patients with aortic dissection have no more cystic medial necrosis than might be expected for the patient's age or level of systemic arterial pressure.

The term "cystic medial necrosis," incidentally, has certain defects because "cysts" are relatively infrequent and "necrosis" is difficult to identify. Furthermore, the striking histologic aortic lesion, when full blown, is massive degeneration of elastic fibers, and this feature is ignored by the term "cystic medial necrosis." When Gsell[122] in 1928 first used the term "medionecrosis" and a year later Erdheim,[123,124] the term "cystic medial necrosis," stains for elastic fibers were apparently infrequently employed and loss or degeneration of elastic fibers may be difficult to appreciate on hematoxylin-eosin–stained sections.

When elastic fibers disappear from the aortic wall in this condition, the space previously occupied by them appears to be replaced by collagen fibrils and mucoid material. Although the increased acid mucopolysaccharide material has been considered an inherent defect in this condition, it is just as reasonable to believe that this material serves simply as "a filler" for the lost elastic fibers. Normally, the media of aorta in the ascending portion contains approximately 58 elastic lamellae.[125] It is not clear whether or not the numbers of the elastic lamellae are normal or decreased at the time of birth in the patients with the Marfan syndrome. Whether normal or decreased, however, fusiform ascending aortic aneurysm, with or without tears, has not been described in newborns with this syndrome. Thus, it appears that although the composition of the aortic media may be defective at birth, the aneurysms form later, presumably the consequence of the intra-aortic pressure's effect on an inherently weak wall. The possible consequences of the inherently or congenitally weakened aortic media are shown in Figure 39.

Although most fusiform aneurysms in the Marfan syndrome involve the ascending aorta (both sinus and tubular portions), aneurysm also may involve the descending thoracic aorta (as it did in 2 personally studied patients) and, as reported by others,[102] the abdominal aorta. Because the numbers of elastic fibers in the abdominal aorta are only about ½ of those present in the ascending aorta with intermediate numbers in between, and because the major histologic finding in the medial portion of the aneurysmal wall is massive loss of elastic fibers, it is logical, of course, that the ascending aorta is the most common location of fusiform aneurysm in the Marfan syndrome. The ascending portion also moves ("stretches") the most with each heart beat ("hypermobile aorta"),[126] and this factor also may play a role in this preferential location of aneurysms in this syndrome.

Although dissection limited to the ascending aorta has been considered by some to be characteristic of the Marfan syndrome, the descending thoracic and abdominal aortas are often involved in the dissection in these patients. In each of 3 personally studied patients with aortic dissection, the dissection involved the entire aorta. In the 36 (of 57) previously reported necropsy patients with aortic dissection, the location of the dissection was described: it involved the entire aorta or at least down to the abdominal aorta in 19 (53%), in 5 (14%) it extended to the aortic isthmus; in 7 (19%) it appeared to involve only the ascending portion; and in 5 (14%) it involved only the descending thoracic aorta with or without involvement of the abdominal portion.[102] When the dissection is limited to ascending aorta, there may be confusion with rupture of a fusiform aneurysm without actual longitudinal dissection. In at least 2 previously reported necropsy patients, the authors described dissection limited to the ascending aorta, but the description was far more typical of rupture of a fusiform aneurysm without dissection.[102] Dissection, however, may occur in the descending thoracic and abdominal aorta without dissection in the ascending portion but with a fusiform aneurysm in the ascending portion.

Certain conditions superimposed on the Marfan syndrome appear to predispose the fusiform ascending aortic aneurysm to rupture or to further dilation (thereby worsening or initiating aortic regurgitation) and the aorta to dissect. Of 16 personally studied patients with aortic fusiform ascending aneurysm or dissection, 1

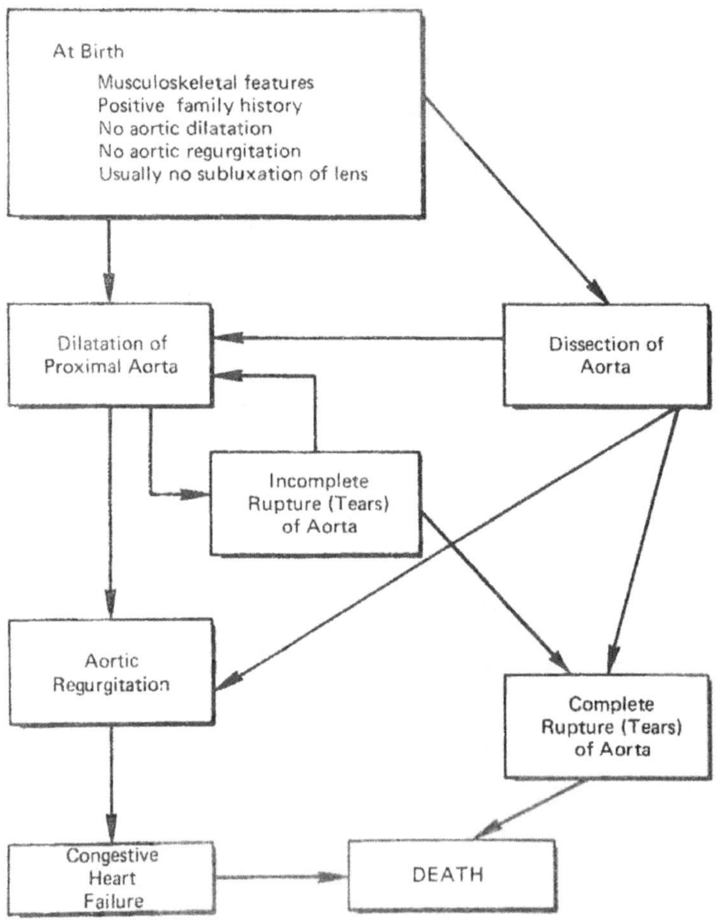

FIGURE 39. The Marfan syndrome. Schema of development of the aortic complications. From Roberts WC. Congenital cardiovascular abnormalities usually "silent" until adulthood: Morphologic features of the floppy mitral valve, valvular aortic stenosis, discrete subvalvular aortic stenosis, hypertrophic cardiomyopathy, sinus of Valsalva aneurysm, and the Marfan syndrome. Cardiovasc Clin 1979; 10(1):448, with permission.

had *coarctation of the aorta*, and of the 110 previously reported necropsy patients with fusiform aneurysm or dissection, 10 had aortic isthmic coarctation, but in each the degree of aortic narrowing appeared to be mild.[102] Fourteen (13%) of the 110 previously reported necropsy patients with either fusiform ascending aortic aneurysm or dissection were *pregnant* or in labor only a short period before the fatal catastrophic event occurred, and 1 (3%) of the 33 patients with isolated mitral regurgitation was pregnant.[102] Some type of *trauma* may have predisposed the aorta to rupture or to further dilation in 5 previously reported necropsy patients with either fusiform ascending aortic aneurysm or dissection.[102]

Although the major consequence of fusiform ascending aortic aneurysm in the Marfan syndrome is aortic regurgitation (100% of 13 personally studied patients and 95% of 42 previously reported patients where this information was recorded), rupture of the anuerysm, of course, is also a danger. This event occurred in 2 of 13 personally studied patients and in at least 14 (25%) of the 57 previously reported necropsy patients with aortic dissection.[102] Thus, treatment of Marfan patients with fusiform ascending aortic aneurysms must be directed at elimination or prevention of aortic regurgitation and at prevention of aneurysmal rupture, not at prevention of dissection, because the latter is an infrequent complication in such patients.

Mitral regurgitation also is frequent in patients with the Marfan syndrome. At least 6 factors may be important in causing the mitral regurgitation: (1) dilatation of mitral anuli; (2) floppiness or prolapse of mitral leaflets and/or elongation of chordae tendineae; (3) calcification of mitral anuli; (4) rupture of mitral chordae tendineae; (5) infective endocarditis; and (6) papillary muscle dysfunction. Of these 6 factors, numbers 1, 2, 3, and 5 appear most important in causing severe degrees of mitral regurgitation. Of the 18 personally studied necropsy patients, 9 had mitral regurgitation, isolated in 2 and combined with aortic regurgitation in 7. Of these 9 patients, 4 had floppy mitral valves, whereas none of the 9 patients without mitral regurgitation had floppy valves. The "floppiness" involved the posterior mitral leaflet in all 4 patients. Of the 9 patients with mitral regurgitation, the circumference of the mitral anulus ranged from 10 to 17 cm (mean = 15; normal = 9), and of the 9 patients without mitral regurgitation, the circumference ranged from 9 to 13 cm (mean 11). Thus, the mean circumference of the mitral anulus in the 9 patients with mitral regurgitation was dilated 67% over normal (15 compared with 9), and that in the 9 patients without mitral regurgitation, only 22% over normal (12 compared with 9). Thus, both mitral leaflet prolapse and anular dilatation play significant roles in causing mitral regurgitation in these patients.

Calcification of the mitral anulus is known to cause or at least to be associated with mitral regurgitation. The degree of regurgitation produced by this mechanism alone, however, is nearly always mild or minimal, and, in addition, the mitral anuli in non-Marfan patients with mitral anular calcification are nearly always of normal or near-normal circumference.[35] Of the 18 personally studied necropsy patients, 5 had mitral anular calcific deposits: all 5 had associated mitral regurgitation, but, in addition, 4 had prolapsing mitral leaflets and in 4 the circumference of the mitral anulus was quite dilated (range 13 to 17 cm [mean = 15]). Evidence for rupture of mitral chordae tendineae was found in 5 of 9 personally studied patients with, and in none of the 9 patients without, mitral regurgitation. Two of these 5 patients had histories of infective endocarditis that had healed. All 5 patients with evidence of mitral chordal rupture had prolapsing mitral leaflets, and 4 had dilated mitral anuli (range 15 to 17 cm [mean = 16]).

The role played by "papillary muscle dysfunction" in causing mitral regurgitation in these patients is less clear. Among the 18 personally studied patients, the left ventricle was dilated in each and the left ventricular mass was increased in each. The hearts of the 18 patients ranged in weight from 375 to 850 gm (mean = 654). In 13 of the 18 patients, the mitral leaflets were increased in length from their basal attachments to their distal margins. This "stretching" probably in part was the result of the elongation (apex to base) of the left ventricular cavities, resulting primarily from the associated aortic regurgitation. The resulting left ventricular dilatation may have altered the normal angulation between the papillary muscles and mitral leaflets.[35] Whether or not mitral regurgitation was increased in any patient by this mechanism, however, is uncertain.

In contrast to fusiform ascending aortic aneurysm and dissection, which generally become manifest after childhood, mitral valve abnormalities in the Marfan syndrome may be present at birth. I have studied at necropsy the heart of a 2-day-old child who at birth was found to have a loud murmur typical of mitral regurgitation and at necropsy, floppy mitral and tricuspid valve leaflets (see Fig. 8). Although this child had the typical musculoskeletal features of the Marfan syndrome, the eyes were not examined and there was no family history of the Marfan syndrome in other family members; therefore, this child was not included among the 18 personally studied necropsy patients because the definition of the syndrome was not fulfilled. Nevertheless, it is likely that the child did have the Marfan syndrome. Others[102] also have described abnormalities of the mitral or tricuspid valves in patients < 1 year of age with the Marfan syndrome.

Although most reports describing necropsy observations in patients with the Marfan syndrome have not mentioned the status of the mitral or tricuspid valves, it must be recalled that the floppy or prolapsing mitral valve was not recognized clinically until 1963[5] and at necropsy not until a year or so later. Thus, morphologic descriptions of floppy or prolapsing mitral or tricuspid valves would not be expected in the Marfan patients until about 1965, and most of the detailed reported necropsy descriptions were before that date. Nevertheless, it is now clear that prolapse of 1 or both mitral leaflets is common at necropsy in the Marfan syndrome and that clicks, late systolic murmurs, and echocardiographic evidence of prolapse are common in these patients.[127,128] Spangler and associates[127] found mitral valvular abnormalities by echocardiogram in 16 (62%) of 26 patients with the Marfan syndrome, and late or pansystolic apical murmurs and/or clicks or both in 16 (62%). Of 50 consecutive patients with the Marfan syndrome examined and reported by Pyeritz and McKusick,[128] 24 (48%) had mid-systolic clicks with or without late systolic murmurs, and 29 (58%) had echocardiographic evidence of mitral valve prolapse. Although necropsy studies demonstrate abnormalities of the aorta with or without aortic regurgitation to be the most frequent cardiovascular abnormality in the Marfan syndrome, recent clinical and echocardiographic studies show that mitral valve dysfunction is even more common. Even among the previously reported necropsy patients aged $\leq$ 15 years, however, mitral regurgitation was the most frequent type of cardiovascular dysfunction (see Table 8).[102] The mitral regurgitation on rare occasion may require operative treatment early in life. Pifarre and associates[129] reported severe mitral regurgitation requiring mitral valve replacement in a 21-month-old-girl with the Marfan syndrome.

Relatively little information on the circumference of the mitral and tricuspid valve anuli has been provided in the previously reported necropsy patients with the Marfan syndrome with or without mitral regurgitation. Of the reported patients with mitral regurgitation, the mitral or tricuspid anular circumference was described as "increased" in several patients.[102] In the 21-year old man with severe mitral regurgitation reported by Van Buchem,[130] the mitral anulus was reported to be 18 cm and the tricuspid anulus, 23 cm in circumference. These are the largest anular circumferences encountered.

Marfan patients with fusiform ascending aortic aneurysms, of course, also may have mitral valvular abnormalities with or without mitral regurgitation. Seven of 13 personally studied patients with fusiform ascending aortic aneurysms had mitral regurgitation, but none of the 3 patients with aortic dissection had mitral regurgitation. Of the 53 previously reported necropsy patients with fusiform ascending aortic root aneurysms, at least 9 (17%) had anatomic mitral valve abnormalities, but only 1 definitely had evidence of mitral regurgitation and that patient was only 7 months old, by far the youngest of any of the reported patients with aortic root aneurysm and the Marfan syndrome.[102] Of the 57 reported necropsy patients with aortic dissection, 9 (16%) had anatomic abnormalities of the mitral valve with mitral regurgitation in at least 3.[102]

The Marfan syndrome may be associated with mitral anular calcification at a young age.[102] Mitral anular calcific deposits were described in 5 of the 151 previously reported necropsy patients with the Marfan syndrome, and their ages ranged from 15 to 35 years (mean 27) (102); 3 were female and 2 were male; only 2 definitely had evidence of mitral regurgitation.

Infective endocarditis involving the mitral valve was described in 6 and possibly 7 of the 151 previously reported necropsy patients with the Marfan syndrome.[102] Five of the 6 definite cases were among the 33 patients in the mitral regurgitation group (see Table 8). In 5 patients, the infection was active: the infecting bacterium was alpha-streptococcus in 4 and *Staphylococcus aureus* in 1. In all 7 patients, the infection involved the mitral valve, and in 1, also the aortic valve. Thus, the mitral valve is the usual site of vegetations when infective endocarditis occurs in patients with the Marfan syndrome.[131] The floppy or prolapsing valve, of course, is the one most likely to be the site of infection. Because rupture of chordae tendineae is a frequent complication of infection involving the mitral valve, the degree of mitral regurgitation resulting from the infection can be severe.[132]

Of the 8 previously reported necropsy patients with the Marfan syndrome classified in the miscellaneous group (see Table 8), 3 died from pulmonary infections, 2 from rupture of abdominal aortic aneurysms, 2 from consequences of ventricular septal defect, and 1 was stillborn.[102] Except for the 2 with ventricular septal defect, the other 6 appeared to have had normal hearts and normal ascending aortas.

Although the above discussion concerned only patients with typical features of the Marfan syndrome, the cardiovascular features described in them also occur, of course, in patients without skeletal or ocular features of this syndrome or histories of this syndrome in other family members.[103] In addition, the characteristic histologic features in the wall of ascending aorta also have been observed in the aorta of patients with congenitally malformed aortic valves, particularly the bicuspid condition,[133] and in patients with aortic stenosis when superimposed on a congenitally malformed valve.[133,134]

REFERENCES

1. Griffith JP. Mid-systolic and late systolic mitral murmurs. Am J Med Sci 1982; 104:285.
2. Levine SA, Thompson WP. Systolic gallop rhythm. A clinical study. New Engl J Med 1935; 213:1021–1025.
3. Brigden W, Lathan A. Mitral incompetence. Br Heart J 1953; 15:55.
4. Reid JVO. Mid-systolic clicks. S Afr Med J 1961; 35:353.
5. Barlow, JB, Pocock WA, Marchand P, Denny M. The significance of late systolic murmurs. Am Heart J 1963; 66:443–452.
6. Segal BL, Likoff W. Late systolic murmur of mitral regurgitation. Am Heart J 1964; 67:757–763.
7. Barlow JB, Bosman DK. Aneurysmal protrusion of the posterior leaflet of the mitral valve. An auscultatory-electrocardiographic syndrome. Am Heart J 1965; 71:166–178.
8. Criley JM, Lewis KB, Humphries JO, Ross RS. Prolapse of the mitral valve: clinical and cine-angiocardiographic findings. Br Heart J 1966; 28:488–496.
9. Barlow JB, Bosman CK, Pocock WA, Marchand P. Late systolic murmurs and non-ejection (mid-late) systolic clicks. An analysis of 90 patients. Br Heart J 1968; 30:208–218.
10. Markiewicz W, Stoner J, London E, Hunt SA, Popp RL. Mitral valve prolapse in one hundred presumably healthy young females. Circulation 1976; 53:464–473.
11. Procacci PM, Savran SV, Schreiter SL, Bryson AL. Prevalence of clinical mitral-valve prolapse in 1169 women. N Engl J Med 1976; 294:1086–1088.
12. Savage DD, Garrison RJ, Devereux RB, Castelli WP, Anderson SJ, Levy D, McNamara PM, Stokes J III, Kannel WB, Feinleib M. Mitral valve prolapse in the general population. I. Epidemiologic features of the Framingham study. Am Heart J 1983; 106:571–576.

13. Waller BF, Morrow AG, Maron BJ, Del Negro AA, Kent KM, McGrath FJ, Wallace RB, McIntosh CL, Roberts WC. Etiology of clinically isolated severe, chronic, pure mitral regurgitation: analysis of 97 patients over 30 years of age having mitral valve replacement. Am Heart J 1982; 104:276–288.
14. Pomerance A. Ballooning deformity (mucoid degeneration) of atrioventricular valves. Br Heart J 1969; 31:343–351.
15. Sherman EB, Char F, Dungan WT, Campbell GS. Myxomatous tranformation of the mitral valve producing mitral insufficiency. Floppy valve syndrome. Am J Dis Child 1970; 119:171.
16. Salazar AE, Edwards JE. Friction lesions of ventricular endocardium. Relation to chordae tendineae of mitral valve. Arch Pathol 1970; 90:364–376.
17. McCarthy LJ, Wolf PL. Mucoid degeneration of heart valves: "Blue valve syndrome." Am J Clin Pathol 1970; 54:582.
18. Davis RH, Schuster B, Knoebel SB, Fisch C. Myxomatous degeneration of the mitral valve. Am J Cardiol 1971; 28:449–455.
19. Edwards JE. Mitral insufficiency resulting from "overshooting" of leaflets. Circulation 1971; 43:606–612.
20. Kern WH, Tucker BL. Myxoid changes in cardiac valves: pathologic, clinical, and ultrastructural studies. Am Heart J 1972; 84:294–301.
21. McKay R, Yacoub MH. Clinical and pathological findings in patients with "floppy" valves treated surgically. Circulation 1973; 47:III63.
22. Ranganathan N, Silver MD, Robinson TI, Kostuk WJ, Felderhof CH, Patt NL, Wilson JK, Wigle ED. Angiographic-morphologic correlation in patients with severe mitral regurgitation due to prolapse of the posterior mitral valve leaflet. Circulation 1973; 48:514–518.
23. Marshall CE, Shappell SD. Sudden death and the ballooning posterior leaflet syndrome: detailed anatomic and histochemical investigation. Arch Path 1974; 98:134–138.
24. Hill HB, Davies MJ, Braimbridge MV. The natural history and surgical management of the redundant cusp syndrome (floppy mitral valve). J Thorac Cardiovasc Surg 1974; 67:519.
25. Guthrie RB, Edwards JE. Pathology of the myxomatous mitral valve: nature, secondary changes and complications. Minn Med 1976; 59:637–647.
26. Shrivastava S, Guthrie RB, Edwards JE. Prolapse of the mitral valve. Mod Concepts Cardiovasc Dis 1977; 46:57–61.
27. Davies MJ, Moore BP, Baimbridge MV. The floppy mitral valve. Study of incidence, pathology, and complications in surgical necropsy, and forensic material. Br Heart J 1978; 40:468–481.
28. Rippe J, Fishbein MC, Carabello B, Angoff GA, Sloss L, Collins JJ Jr, Alpert JS. Primary myxomatous degeneration of cardiac valves. Clinical, pathological, haemodynamic, and echocardiographic profile. Br Heart J 1980; 44:621–629.
29. Olsen EGJ, Al-Rufaie HK. The floppy mitral valve: study of pathogenesis. Brit Heart J 1980; 44:674–683.
30. Ringer M, Feen DJ, Drapkin M. Mitral valve prolapse: jet stream causing mural endocarditis. Am J Cardiol 1980; 45:383–385.
31. Lucas RV Jr, Edwards JE. The floppy mitral valve. Curr Probl Cardiol 1982; 7(4):1–48 (July).
32. King DB, Clark MA, Baba N, Kilman JW, Wooley CF. Myxomatous mitral valves: collagen dissolution as the primary defect. Circulation 1982; 66:288–296.
33. Chesler E, King RA, Edwards JE. The myxomatous mitral valve and sudden death. Circulation 1983; 67:632–639.
34. Roberts WC. Morphologic features of the normal and abnormal mitral valve. Am J Cardiol 1983; 51:1005–1028.
35. Kolibash AJ, Bush CA, Fontana MB, Ryan JM, Kilman J, Wooley CF. Mitral valve prolapse syndrome: analysis of 62 patients aged 60 years and older. Am J Cardiol 1983; 52:534–539.
36. Bulkley BH, Roberts WC. Dilatation of the mitral anulus. A rare cause of mitral regurgitation. Am J Med 1975; 59:457–463.
37. Renteria VG, Ferrans VJ, Jones M, Roberts WC. Intracellular collagen fibrils in prolapsed ("floppy") human atrioventricular valves. Lab Invest 1976; 35:439–443.
38. Waller BF, Maron BJ, Del Negro AA, Gottdiener JS, Roberts WC. Frequency and significance of M-mode echocardiographic evidence of mitral valve prolapse in clinically isolated pure mitral regurgitation. Analysis of 65 patients having mitral valve replacement. Am J Cardiol 1984; 53:139–147.

39. Jeresaty RM, Edwards JE, Chawla SK. Mitral valve prolapse and ruptured chordae tendineae. Am J Cardiol 1985; 55:138–142.
40. Savage DD, Levy D, Garrison RJ, Castelli WP, Kliglield P, Devereux RB, Anderson SJ, Kannel WB, Feinleib M. Mitral valve prolapse in the general population. 3. Dysrhythmias: the Framingham study. Am Heart J 1983; 106:582–586.
41. Roberts WC, Morrow AG. Congenital aortic stenosis produced by a unicommissural valve. Br Heart J 1965; 27:505–510.
42. Roberts WC, Elliott LP. Lesions complicating the congenitally bicuspid aortic valve. Anatomic and radiographic features. Radiologic Clin North Am 1968; 6:409–421.
43. Roberts WC. The congenitally bicuspid aortic valve. A study of 85 autopsy cases. Am J Cardiol 1970; 26:72–83.
44. Roberts WC. The structure of the aortic valve in clinically-isolated aortic stenosis. An autopsy study of 162 patients over 15 years of age. Circulation 1970; 42:91–97.
45. Roberts WC. Anatomically isolated aortic valvular disease. The case against its being of rheumatic etiology. Am J Med 1970; 49:151–159.
46. Roberts WC, Perloff JK, Costantino T. Severe valvular aortic stenosis in patients over 65 years of age. A clinicopathologic study. Am J Cardiol 1971; 27:497–506.
47. Falcone MW, Roberts WC, Morrow AG, Perloff JK. Congenital aortic stenosis resulting from unicommissural valve; Clinical and anatomic features in twenty-one adult patients. Circulation 1971; 44:272–280.
48. Roberts WC. Valvular, subvalvular, and supravalvular aortic stenosis: morphologic features. Cardiovasc Clin 1973; 5:97–126.
49. Roberts WC, Virmani R. Aschoff bodies *at necropsy* in valvular heart disease. Evidence from an analysis of 543 patients over 14 years of age that rheumatic heart disease, at least anatomically, is a disease of the mitral valve. Circulation 1978; 57:803–807.
50. Karsner HT, Koletsky S. Calcific Disease of the Aortic Valve. Philadelphia: JB Lippincott, 1947:111.
51. Edwards JE. Pathologic aspects of cardiac valvular insufficiences. Arch Surg 1958; 77:634.
52. Roberts WC. The 2 most common congenital heart diseases. Am J Cardiol 1984; 53:1198.
53. Osler W. The bicuspid condition of the aortic valves. Trans Assoc Amer Physicians 1886; 2:185–192.
54. Grant RT, Wood JE, Jones TD. Heart valve irregularies in relation to subacute bacterial endocarditis. Heart 1928; 14:247–261.
55. Lewis T, Grant RT. Observations relating to subacute infective endocarditis. Part 1. Notes on the normal structure of the aortic valve. Part 2. Bicuspid aortic valves of congenital origin. Part 3. Bicuspid aortic valves in subacute infective endocarditis. Heart 1923; 10:21–99.
56. Roberts WC, Morrow AG, McIntosh CL, Jones M, Epstein SE. Congenitally bicuspid aortic valve causing severe, pure aortic regurgitation without superimposed infective endocarditis. Analysis of 13 patients requiring aortic valve replacement. Am J Cardiol 1981; 47:206–209.
57. Arnett EN, Roberts WC. Active infective endocarditis: a clinicopathologic analysis of 137 necropsy patients. Curr Probl Cardiol 1976; 1:1–76 (October).
58. Bradenburg RO, Jr, Tajik AJ, Edwards WD, Reeder GS, Shub C, Seward JB. Accuracy of 2-dimensional echocardiographic diagnosis of congenitally bucuspid aortic valve. Echocardiographic-anatomic correlation in 115 patients. Am J Cardiol 1983; 51:1469–1473.
59. Subramanian R, Olson LJ, Edwards WD. Surgical pathology of pure aortic stenosis: a study of 374 cases. Mayo Clin Proc 1984; 59:683–690.
60. Stewart WJ, King ME, Gillam LD, Guyer DE, Weyman AE. Prevalence of aortic valve prolapse with bicuspid aortic valve and its relation to aortic regurgitation: a cross-sectional echocardiographic study. Am J Cardiol 1984; 54:1277–1282.
61. Roberts WC, Byram MT. Frequency and extent of clacific deposits in purely regurgitant *aortic* valves. Analysis of 252 operatively excised valves. Am J Cardiol 1985; in press.
62. Olson LJ, Subramanian R, Edwards WD. Surgical pathology of pure aortic insufficiency: a study of 225 cases. Mayo Clin Proc 1984; 59:835–841.
63. Fulton MN, Levine SA. Subacute bacterial endocarditis, with special reference to the valvular lesions and previous history. Am J Med Sci 1932; 183:60–77.
64. Edwards JE. The congenital biscupid aortic valve. Circulation 1961; 23:485–488.
65. Bishop LF Jr, Trubek M. Bicuspid aortic valve. A differential study between inflammatory and congenitial origin. J Tech Meth 1936; 15:111–131.

66. Koletsky S. Congenital bicuspid aortic valves. Arch Intern Med 1941; 67:129–176.
67. Abbott ME. Coarctation of the aorta of the adult type. II. A statistical study and historical retrospect of 200 recorded cases, with autopsy, of stenosis or obliteration of the descending arch in subjects above the age of two years. Am Heart J 1928; 3:392, 574.
68. Reifenstein GH, Levine SA, Gross RE. Coarctation of the aorta. A review of 104 autopsied cases of "adult type," 2 years of age or older. Am Heart J 1947; 33:146.
69. Roberts WC. Cardiac valvular residua and sequelae after operation for congenital heart disease. Am Heart J 1983; 106:1181–1187.
70. Larson E, Edwards WD. Risk factors for aortic dissection. A necropsy study of 161 cases. Am J Cardiol 1984; 53:849–855.
71. Silver MA, Roberts WC. Detailed anatomy of the normally functioning aortic valve in hearts of normal and increased weight. Am J Cardiol 1985; 55:454–461.
72. Wright GB, Keane JF, Nadas AS, Bernhard WF, Castaneda AR. Fixed subaortic stenosis in the young: medical and surgical course in 83 patients. Am J Cardiol 1983; 52:830–835.
73. Fontana RS. Edwards JE. Congenital Cardiac Disease. A Review of 357 Cases Studied Pathologically. Philadelphia: WB Saunders, 1962:291.
74. Motro M, Schneeweiss A, Shem-Tov A, Vered Z, Hegesh J, Neufeld HN, Rath S. Two-dimensional echocardiography in discrete subaortic stenosis. Am J Cardiol 1984; 53:896–898.
75. Morrow AG, Fort L III, Roberts WC, Braunwald E. Discrete subaortic stenosis complicated by aortic valvular regurgitation. Clinical, hemodynamic, and pathologic studies and the results of operative treatment. Circulation 1965; 31:163–171.
76. Reis RL, Peterson LM, Mason DT, Simon AL, Morrow AG. Congenital fixed subvalvular aortic stenosis. An anatomical classification and correlations with operative results. Circulation 1971; 43 & 44 (Suppl):I-11–I-18.
77. Muna WFT, Ferrans VJ, Pierce JE, Roberts WC. Discrete subaortic stenosis in Newfoundland dogs: association of infective indocarditis. Am J Cardiol 1978; 41:746–754.
78. Arnett EN, Roberts WC. Pathology of active infective endocarditis. A necropsy analysis of 192 patients. Thorac Cardiovasc Surg 1982; 30:327–335.
79. Maron BJ, Redwood DR, Roberts WC, Henry WL, Morrow AG, Epstein SE. Tunnel subaortic stenosis. Left ventricular tract obstruction produced by fibromuscular tubular narrowing. Circulation 1976; 54:404–416.
80. Teare D. Asymmetrical hypertrophy of the heart in young adults. Br Heart J 1958; 20:1–18.
81. Roberts WC, Ferrans VJ. Pathologic anatomy of the cardiomyopathies. Idiopathic dilated and hypertrophic types, infiltrative types, and endomyocardial disease with and without eosinophilia. Human Pathol 1975; 6:287–342.
82. Maron BJ, Edwards JE, Ferrans VJ, Clark CE, Lebowitz EA, Henry WL, Epstein SE. Congenital heart malformations associated with disproportionate ventricular septal thickening. Circulation 1975; 52:926–932.
83. Maron BJ, Clark CE, Henry WL, Fukuda T, Edwards JE, Mathews EC, Redwood DR, Epstein SE. Prevalence and characteristics of disproprotionate ventricular septal thickening in patients with acquired or congenital heart disease: echocardiographic and morphologic findings. Circulation 1977; 55:489–496.
84. Maron BJ, Savage DD, Clark CE, Henry WL, Vlodaver Z, Edwards JE, Epstein SE. Prevalence and characteristics of disproportionate ventricular septal thickening in patients with coronary artery disease. Circulation 1978; 57:250–256.
85. Maron BJ, Edwards JE, Epstein SE. Disproportionate ventricular septal thickening in patients with systemic hypertension. Chest 1978; 73:466–470.
86. Isner JM, Falcone MW, Virmani R, Roberts WC. Cardiac sarcoma causing "ASH" and simulating coronary heart disease. Am J Med 1979; 43:1234–1237.
87. Maron BJ, Epstein SE. Hypertrophic cardiomyopathy. Recent observations regarding the specificity of three hallmarks of the disease: asymmetric septal hypertrophy, septal disorganization and systolic anterior motion of the anterior mitral leaflet. Am J Cardiol 1980; 45:141–154.
88. Maron BJ, Epstein SE, Roberts WC. Hypertrophic cardiomyopathy and transmural myocardial infarction without significant atherosclerosis of the extramural coronary arteries. Am J Cardiol 1979; 43:1086–1102.
89. McReynolds RA, Roberts WC. The intramural coronary arteries in hypertrophic cardiomyopathy (abstract). Am J Cardiol 1975; 35:120.

90. Maron BJ, Wolfson JK, Epstein SE, Roberts WC. The intramural coronary arteries in hypertrophic cardiomyopathy. Am J Cardiol 1985; in press
91. Maron BJ, Roberts WC. Hypertrophic cardiomyopathy and cardiac muscle cell disorganization revisited: relation between the two and significance. Am Heart J 1981; 102:95–110.
92. Henry WL, Clark CE, Roberts WC, Morrow AG, Epstein SE. Differences in distribution of myocardial abnormalities in patients with obstructive and non-obstructive asymmetric septal hypertrophy (ASH). Echocardiographic and gross anatomic findings. Circulation 1974; 50:447–455.
93. Ferrans VJ, Morrow AG, Roberts WC. Myocardial ultrastructure in idiopathic hypertrophic subaortic stenosis. A study of operatively excised left ventricular outflow tract muscle in 14 patients. Circulation 1972; 45:769–792.
94. Maron BJ, Verter J, Kapur S. Disproportionate ventricular septal thickening in the developing normal human heart. Circulation 1978; 57:520–526.
95. Roberts WC, Perry LW, Chandra RS, Myers GE, Shapiro SR, Scott LP. Aortic valve atresia: a new classification based on necropsy study of 73 cases. Am J Cardiol 1976; 37:753–756.
96. Merrill WH, Henry WL, Maron BJ, Epstein SE, Morrow AG. Echocardiographic assessment of the left ventricle following myotomy and myectomy for idiopathic hypertrophic subaortic stenosis (IHSS) (abstract). Am J Cardiol 1978; 41:435.
97. Maron BJ, Henry WL, Roberts WC, Epstein SE. Comparison of echocardiographic and necropsy measurements of ventricular wall thicknesses in patients with and without disproportionate septal thickening. Circulation 1977; 55:341–345.
98. Epstein SE, Henry WL, Clark CE, Roberts WC, Maron BJ, Ferrans VJ, Redwood DR, Morrow AG. Asymmetric septal hypertrophy. Ann Intern Med 1974; 81:650–680.
99. Cooley DA, Leachman RD, Wukasch DC. Diffuse muscular subaortic stenosis: surgical treatment. Am J Cardiol 1973; 31:1–6.
100. Cooley DA, Grace RR, Wukasch DC, Leachman RD. Replacement and/or repair of the mitral valve as treatment of idiopathic hypertrophic subaortic stenosis. Cardiovasc Diseases Bull Texas Heart Inst 1976; 3:381–393.
101. Roberts WC. Operative treatment of hypertrophic obstructive cardiomyopathy. The case against mitral valve replacement. Am J Cardiol 1973; 32:377–381.
102. Roberts WC, Honig HS. The spectrum of cardiovascular disease in the Marfan syndrome: a clinico-morphologic study of 18 necropsy patients and comparison to 151 previously reported necropsy patients. Am Heart J 1982; 104:115–135.
103. Waller BF, Reis RL, McIntosh CL, Epstein SE, Roberts WC. Marfan cardiovascular disease without the Marfan syndrome. Fusiform ascending aortic aneurysm with aortic and mitral valve regurgitation. Chest 1980; 77:533–540.
104. Roberts WC. Left ventricular outflow tract obstruction and aortic regurgitation. In: Edwards JE, Lev M, Abell MR, eds. The Heart. Baltimore: Williams & Wilkins, 1974:110–175.
105. Bulkley BH, Roberts WC. Ankylosing spondylitis and aortic regurgitation. Description of the characteristic cardiovascular lesion from study of eight necropsy patients. Circulatio 1973; 48:1014–1027.
106. Pomerance A, Davies MJ. Congenital aneurysms of all three sinuses of Valsalva. J Pathol Bact 1965; 89:607–610.
107. Arnett EN, Roberts WC. Valve ring abscess in active infective endocarditis. Frequency, location, and clues to clinical diagnosis from the study of 95 necropsy patients. Circulation 1976; 54:140–145.
108. Edwards JE, Burchell HB. Specimen exhibiting the essential lesion in aneurysm of the aortic sinus. Proc Staff Meetings Mayo Clin 1956; 31:407–412.
109. Kerber RE, Ridges JD, Kriss JP, Silverman JF, Anderson ET, Harrison DC. Unruptured aneurysm of the sinus of Valsalva producing right ventricular outflow obstruction. Am J Med 1972; 53:775–783.
110. Fishbein MC, Obma R, Roberts WC. Unruptured sinus of Valsalva aneurysm. Am J Cardiol 1975; 35:918–922.
111. Warnes CA, Maron BJ, Jones M, Roberts WC. Asymptomatic sinus of Valsalva aneurysm causing right ventricular outflow obstruction before and after rupture. Am J Cardiol 1984; 54:1383–1384.
112. Duras PF. Heart block with aneurysm of the aortic sinus. Br Heart J 1944; 6:61–65.

113. Sakakibara S, Konno S. Congenital aneurysm of the sinus of Valsalva. Anatomy and classification. Am Heart J 1962; 63:405–424.
114. Fowler REL, Bevel HH. Aneurysms of the sinus of Valsalva. Pediatrics 1951; 8:340–348.
115. Kieffer SA, Winchell P. Congenital aneurysms of the aortic sinuses with cardioartic fistula. Dis Chest 1960; 38:79–96.
116. Roberts WC. Aneurysm (redundancy) of the atrial septum (fossa ovale membrane) and prolapse (redundancy) of the mitral valve. Am J Cardiol 1984; 54:1153–1154.
117. Murdoch JL, Walker BA, Halpern BL, Kuzma JW, McKusick VA. Life expectancy and causes of death in the Marfan syndrome. N Engl J Med 1972; 286:804–808.
118. Sisk HE, Zahka KG, Pyeritz RE. The Marfan syndrome in early childhood: analysis of 15 patients diagnosed at less than 4 years of age. Am J Cardiol 1983; 52:353–358.
119. Carlson RG, Lillehei CW, Edwards JE. Cystic medial necrosis of the ascending aorta in relation to age and hypertension. Am J Cardiol 1970; 25:411–415.
120. Schlatmann TJM, Becker AE. Histologic changes in the normal aging aorta: implications for dissecting aortic aneurysm. Am J Cardiol 1977; 39:13–20.
121. Schlatmann TJM, Becker AE. Pathogenesis of dissecting aneurysm of aorta. Comparative histopathologic study of significance of medial changes. Am J Cardiol 1977; 39:21–26.
122. Gsell O: Wandnekrosen der Aorta als selbstandige Erkrandkung and ihre Beziehung zur Spontanruptur. Vichows Arch Path Anat Physiol 1928; 270:1–36.
123. Erdheim J. Medionecrosis aortae idiopathica. Virchows Arch Path Anat Physiol 1929; 273:454–479.
124. Erdheim J. Medionecrosis aortae idiopathica cystica. Virchows Arch Path Anat Physiol 1930; 276:187–229.
125. Wolinsky H, Glagov S. A lamellar unit of aortic medial structure and function in mammals. Cir Res 1967; 20:99.
126. Benchimol A, Dresser KB, Neese TC. Hypermobility of the aorta in Marfan's syndrome. Angiology 1972; 23:103–104.
127. Spangler RD, Nora JJ, Lorfscher RH, Wolfe RR, Okin JT. Echocardiography in Marfan's syndrome. Chest 1976; 69:72–78.
128. Pyeritz RE, McKusick VA. The Marfan syndrome: diagnosis and management. N Engl J Med 1979; 300:772–777.
129. Pifarre R, Caralps JM, Sinha SN. Mitral valve replacement for regurgitation in an infant with Marfan's syndrome. J Thorac Cardiovasc Surg 1974; 67:233–236.
130. Van Buchem FSP. Cardiovascular disease in arachnodactyly. Acta Med Scand 1958; 161:197–205.
131. Bowers D, Lim DW. Subacute bacterial endocarditis and Marfan's syndrome. Canad Med Assoc J 1962; 86:455–458.
132. Roberts WC, Braunwald E, Morrow AG. Acute mitral regurgitation secondary to ruptured chordae tendineae. Clinical, hemodynamic, and pathologic considerations. Circulation 1966; 33:58–70.
133. Edwards ED, Leaf DS, Edwards JE. Dissecting aortic aneurysm associated with congenital bicuspid aortic valve. Circulation 1978; 57:1022.
134. Roberts WC. Aortic dissection: anatomy, consequences and causes. Am Heart J 1981; 101:195–214.

CARDIAC VALVULAR RESIDUAE AND SEQUELAE AFTER CARDIOVASCULAR OPERATIONS*

William C. Roberts, M.D.

This chapter focuses on valvular abnormalities that remain after operations for congenital anomalies of the heart (residuae) and on changes occurring later in congenitally malformed cardiac valves subjected to direct operative manipulation to relieve stenosis and/or regurgitation (sequelae).

RESIDUAE

MITRAL VALVE

Mitral Valve Prolapse

1. **WITH SECUNDUM TYPE ATRIAL SEPTAL DEFECT.** In about a third of patients with secundum type atrial septal defect, auscultatory and/or echocardiographic evidence of mitral valve prolapse is present.[1] The frequency of mitral valve prolapse in these patients increases with age.[2] Liberthson and associates[2] in a retrospective review of 498 patients with secundum atrial septal defect found a 0.4% incidence of severe mitral valve prolapse in 213 patients < age 21 years, 2% in 187 patients aged 21 to 49 years, and 15% in 98 patients ≥ 50 years. Calcification of the mitral anulus, a recognized complication of mitral valve prolapse, occurs in a higher frequency of adults with uncorrected secundum-type atrial septal defect than adults of similar age and sex without atrial septal defect.

What will happen to the mitral valve several decades after operative closure of secundum-type atrial septal defect remains to be determined. Whether or not the frequency of mitral valve prolapse with or without mitral anular calcification will be similar in patients having secundum-type atrial septal defect closed in the first or second decade of life compared with the patients of similar age and sex not having the atrial septal defect closed early in life or not at all remains to be seen.

Why the frequency of mitral valve prolapse is increased in patients with secundum atrial septal defect is uncertain. Of patients with mitral valve prolapse associated with secundum-type atrial septal defect and examined at necropsy, the prolapse involved only the posterior leaflet and then only a portion of it. The posterior leaflet is continuous with the free wall of left atrium and not with the atrial septum. The anterior mitral leaflet, in contrast, is continuous with the atrial septum which, of course, with atrial septal defect is deficient. Nevertheless, prolapse of the anterior mitral leaflet has not been reported, to my knowledge, in a patient with secundum-type atrial septal defect.

I have not observed or seen reported dilatation of the mitral anulus in association with secundum-type atrial septal defect with or without associated mitral valve prolapse. Anular dilation is a recognized complication of mitral valve prolapse and the most common mechanism of severe mitral regurgitation with mitral valve prolapse.[3]

The prolapsed mitral valve, of course, has a greatly increased tendency to be the site of infective endocarditis, a rarity in isolated atrial septal defect.[4] Whether this tendency is still increased after closure of atrial septal defect is uncertain.

A variety of mitral valve abnormalities other than mitral valve prolapse has been observed at necropsy in patients with secundum atrial septal defect. Of 16 hearts of adults with uncorrected secundum atrial septal defect examined by Davies,[5] 15 had thickening of the posterior half of the anterior mitral leaflet and fusion and fibrous thickening of chordae attached to this portion of anterior leaflet.

2. WITH EBSTEIN ANOMALY OF THE TRICUSPID VALVE. Several patients with Ebstein anomaly of the tricuspid valve have been observed to have prolapse of the mitral valve.[6] The reason for the association is unclear. Although the Ebstein-type tricuspid valve in 1 way is directly opposite the prolapsed valve in that the former is displaced downward into the ventricle rather than displaced backward toward the atrium, the Ebstein valve, nevertheless, has some features in common with the prolapsed valve. These features include severe elongation and increased area of the leaflets, particularly the anterior 1, and marked dilatation of the anulus.

Mitral valve prolapse has been observed in patients with the Ebstein anomaly of the tricuspid valve both with and without a defect in the atrial septum.[6] Thus, the mitral valve prolapse cannot be attributed in this circumstance to some relation with secundum-type atrial septal defect or valvular competent or incompetent patent foramen ovale.

In patients with corrected transposition of the great arteries and Ebstein anomaly of the left-sided tricuspid valve, the frequency of prolapse of the right-sided mitral valve is not recognized to be increased.

3. WITH THE MARFAN AND MARFAN-LIKE SYNDROME. It is well recognized that mitral valve prolapse is common in patients with the Marfan syndrome[7] and in patients with the characteristic anulo-ectatic deformity of the ascending aorta unassociated with the skeletal, ocular, and familial features of the Marfan syndrome.[8] The mitral valve in this circumstance often is associated with massive anular dilatation and often with anular calcific deposits. Severe mitral regurgitation may appear sometime after operations to eliminate aortic regurgitation and/or to excise an aneurysmally dilated ascending aorta.

4. WITH HYPERTROPHIC CARDIOMYOPATHY. Several patients with hypertrophic cardiomyopathy associated with mitral valve prolapse have been described.[9] The small left ventricular cavity and the frequently observed elevation of the left ventricular closing pressure in these patients likely are important factors.

Mitral Valve Cleft

Partial atrioventricular canal is a syndrome that consists of more than 1 of the following components:[10] (1) defect in the lowermost portion of the atrial septum (primum-type atrial septal defect); (2) cleft in the anterior leaflet of the mitral valve; (3) anomalous insertion of some chordae tendineae onto the ventricular septum; (4) ventricular septal defect; and (5) partial or complete absence of the septal tricuspid valve leaflet. Of the 5 components, the 2 nearly universely present are a cleft in the anterior mitral leaflet and anomously inserting chordae from the anterior mitral leaflet. The occurrence of these latter 2 components in the absence of a primum-type atrial septal defect, of course, is quite rare, but recently Di Segni and Edwards[11] described 20 necropsy patients with a cleft in the anterior mitral leaflet unassociated with a primum-type atrial septal defect; the ventricular septum was intact in 9 and contained a defect in the other 11.

The cleft in the anterior mitral leaflet extends from the leaflet's margins varying distances into the leaflet itself. The complete cleft subdivides the anterior leaflet into 2 more or less equal-sized components by extending all the way from margin to "anulus." The complete cleft is far less common than is the partial cleft, which does not extend as far as the "anulus." With either the partial or complete cleft, anomalous chordae tendineae connect the ventricular surface of both components of the clefted anterior mitral leaflet to the crest of the ventricular septum.

Most patients having primum-type atrial septal defect have either no mitral regurgitation or only a mild degrees of mitral regurgitation.[12] In this circumstance, some surgeons have left the cleft in the anterior mitral leaflet unclosed when the defect in the atrial septum was closed, and others have closed the cleft by direct suture. When the mitral regurgitation, however, is of moderate to severe degree in partial atrioventricular canal, there is a much greater tendency to close the leaflet cleft. A recommendation was made by Edwards[13] in 1960 to cut the anomalous chordae that extended from the clefted leaflet to the ventricular septum, but this recommendation has not been acted on.

Irrespective of whether the cleft is closed or the anomalously inserting chordae are severed, how will the malformed mitral valve function many years after closure of the primum-type atrial septal defect? The answer to this question, of course, is not yet available. It is unlikely, however, that such a malformed mitral valve will stay completely competent during a full lifetime.

Among patients with varying degrees of mitral regurgitation before closure of the primum-type atrial septal defect, the mitral regurgitation usually disappears immediately after the atrial septal defect is closed irrespective of the extent, that is, partial or complete, of the cleft in the anterior mitral leaflet. Irrespective of whether or not the leaflet cleft is closed, mitral regurgitation usually disappears after closure of the primum atrial septal defect. Of 35 patients having closure of the primum atrial septal defect, suture closure of the mitral cleft, and cardiac catheterization an average of 11 months postoperative, 7 (20%) had mitral regurgitation, mild in 5 and severe in 1.[12] The latter 2 had a second mitral operation.

It appears likely that patients with partial atrioventricular canal having closure of the primum atrial septal defect in early life will require mitral valve replacement several decades later. Systemic hypertension, which, of course, increases the closing pressure of the mitral valve, probably accelerates development of mitral regurgitation late postoperatively. Results of left ventricular angiography > 10 years after closure of the primum-type atrial septal defect are not available.

Another potential problem after closure a primum-type atrial septal defect is development of left ventricular outflow obstruction owing to the anomalously inserting chordae tendineae from the clefted anterior mitral leaflet to the ventricular septum. Of 99 patients with partial atrioventricular canal followed by Taylor and Somerville[14] after closure of the primum atrial septal defect and elimination of the mitral cleft, 3 patients developed severe, fixed subaortic obstruction postoperatively. Excluding the 1 patient who had had mitral valve replacement at the first operation, 1 had the peak systolic pressure gradient increase postoperatively from 15 to 80 mm Hg, and in the second this gradient increased from 21 to 120 mm Hg (in 11 years). These observations suggest that severing of some anomalously inserting chordae may be proper at the time of closure of the primum atrial septal defect, particularly if some left ventricular outflow tract obstruction is present preoperatively.

Other Mitral Valve Abnormalities

1. WITH ANOMALOUS ORIGIN OF THE LEFT MAIN CORONARY ARTERY FROM THE PULMONARY TRUNK. Most individuals with this coronary anomaly have some degree of mitral regurgitation, which, on occasion, may be the dominant or presenting clinical manifestation of this condition.[15] The mitral valve moorings in this anomaly are usually abnormal in that the stumps of both left ventricular papillary muscles tend to arise near the junctions of the basal and mid portions of the left ventricular wall rather than at or near the junction of the mid and apical thirds of the wall.[15] Additionally, by the time clinical manifestations are apparent in patients with anomalous origin of the left coronary artery from the pulmonary trunk, the left ventricular papillary muscles, particularly the anterior 1, are scarred, calcified, and atrophied. Furthermore, scars, either subendocardial or transmural or both, are present in other portions of the left ventricular free wall. Additionally, by the time these patients present clinically, the left ventricular cavity is considerably dilated and its endocardium, diffusely thickened (endocardial fibroelastosis). Thus, despite operative procedures that establish direct connection of the anomalous coronary artery to the aorta and/or prevent run off from the coronary artery into the pulmonary trunk, mitral regurgitation is already present and the left ventricular myocardium, considerably damaged.

Thus, in a long-term survivor of operations for this coronary anomaly, mitral regurgitation will probably remain a significant problem.

2. WITH COMPLETE TRANSPOSITION OF THE GREAT ARTERIES. A number of abnormalities of the mitral valve have been described in patients with transposition of the great arteries.[16] Because long-term survivors of operative interventions for transposition of the great arteries are not yet available to examine, whether or not these commonly observed mitral anomalies will eventually become clinical problems are unknown.

3. WITH "PURE" PULMONIC-VALVE STENOSIS. Although of no apparent clinical importance, I have observed considerable diffuse mitral leaflet and chordal thickening in 2 necropsy patients who during life have evidence only of pulmonic-valve stenosis. Whether these observations are unique or common is unclear, and if they are of any clinical relevance remains uncertain.

4. WITH SUPRAVALVULAR AORTIC STENOSIS. A variety of mitral abnormalities has been observed in patients with supravalvular aortic stenosis.[17] Their clinical significance with time remains to be established.

TRICUSPID VALVE

Real and Potential Damage After Closure of Ventricular Septal Defect

Closure of a perimembranous or "high" ventricular septal defect requires manipulation of the septal and anterior tricuspid valve leaflets. On occasion, 1 or more chordae must be severed to manipulate the patch into position. All these maneuvers cause the leaflet to be denuded of endothelial cells, and the subsequent healing process can lead to leaflet thickening. The greater the thickening, the greater the chance of eventual tricuspid regurgitation, which, of course, has a greater chance of occurring if the right ventricular systolic pressure remains elevated or, for some reason, is acquired after ventricular septal defect closure. A left-to-right shunt via the ventricular septal defect preoperatively also can produce a "jet lesion" on the tricuspid valve, which in itself may be a nidus for further damage.

AORTIC VALVE

Bicuspid or Unicuspid Valve

1. WITH AORTIC ISTHMIC COARCTATION. Abbott[18] called attention to the frequency of a congenitally bicuspid aortic valve in patients with the usual type (isthmic or periductal) coarctation of the aorta. Her figure was 15% (Table 1). Reifenstein and associates[19] found a higher percentage (see Table 1). The figure probably is higher than reported by either of these 2 major authors. The biscuspid valve is not the only kind of malformed aortic valve found in patients with coarctation of the aorta. A unicuspid valve also has been observed.[20-22] Whatever the correct percentage, it is clear that patients who have coarctation of the aorta severe enough to warrent resection of the coarcted segment (and even those without functional narrowing but with an anatomic indentation, so called pseudocoarctation) have a high frequency of aortic valve malformations, most commonly the bicuspid condition.

Bicuspid aortic valves, of course, whether isolated or associated with coarctation of the aorta, are prone to 3 major complications:[23] (1) aortic valve stenosis, (2) pure aortic regurgitation unassociated with superimposed infective endocarditis,[24] and (3) infective endocarditis causing aortic regurgitation and/or embolic complications.[4] Thus, patients having resection of coarctation of the aorta must be followed carefully for development of a complication, and, of course, should receive prophylactic antibiotic protection for dental or other operative procedures.

Another potential complication of coarctation of the aorta with or without resection of the coarcted segment is rupture of the aorta with or without dissection (Table 2). This complication usually occurs proximal to the aortic isthmus and may occur in patients with resected coarctation of the aorta but with a normally functioning aortic valve.[18,25] There is evidence that the medial wall of the ascending and transverse aorta is abnormal in patients with coarctation of the aorta and that tears in this wall occur far more frequently from a percentage standpoint in patients with bicuspid compared with those with tricuspid (normally formed) aortic valves.[26]

2. WITH INTERRUPTION OF THE AORTIC ARCH. Virtually all patients with interruption of the aortic arch have a congentially bicuspid aortic valve.[27] Because results of operative treatment of patients with this complex anomaly (reanastomosis of ascending to descending aorta, closure of ventricular septal defect, and closure of the persistent patent ductus arteriosus) are poor, no long-term survivors are available for study at this time.

Tricuspid Aortic Valve

1. WITH AORTIC REGURGITATION ASSOCIATED WITH VENTRICULAR SEPTAL DEFECT. About 5% of patients with isolated ventricular septal defect develop aortic regurgitation before the ventricular septal defect is closed, and at operation some of these patients do not have a direct procedure performed on the aortic valve. If 1 or 2 of the 3 cusps prolapsed enough, however, to produce aortic

TABLE 1. Reported Frequency of Congenitally Bicuspid Aortic Valves (BAV) in Necropsy Patients With Aortic Isthmic Coarctation (AIC)

FIRST (YEAR)	NO. PTS WITH AIC	AGES (YEARS) (MEAN)	NO. MALES	NO. (%) PTS WITH BAV	NO. AORTIC DISSECTION OR RUPTURE			ACTIVE IE OR AORTITIS	LOCATION OF VEGETATION		
					TOTAL	WITH BAV	WITHOUT BAV		AV ONLY	AIC ONLY	MV ONLY
Abbott (1928) (1791–1928)	200	3–92 (34)	147/195 (75%)	50[a]/183 (27%)	38 (19%)	17 (45%)	21 (55%)	13 (7%)		13	
Reifenstein (1947) (1928–1947)	104	3–76 (35)	87 (84%)	58[b]/93 (62%)	24 (23%)	10 (42%)	14 (58%)	23 (22%)	15[c]	6	2[d]

[a]Includes 4 cases in which the biscuspid condition was believed to be acquired. Additionally, 73 patients were considered to have acquired valvular lesions.

[b]Includes 3 cases of bicuspid aortic valves stated to be of "acquired origin" and 11 patients with aortic valve stenosis considered by the reporters to be of rheumatic origin.

[c]Aortic valve known to be bicuspid in 11 of the 12 in whom the number of aortic valve cusps was described.

[d]One of these 2 patients had a congenitally bicuspid aortic valve.

AV = aortic valve

MV = mitral valve

IE = infective endocarditis

TABLE 2. Reported Frequency of Aortic Dissection (AD) (or Tears) in Patients With Aortic Isthmic Coarctation

FIRST AUTHOR (YEAR)	NO. PTS C OF A	AGES (YEARS) (MEAN)	NO. MALES	NO. AD OR RUPTURE	BICUSPID AORTIC VALVE		
					TOTAL	WITH AD	WITHOUT AD
Abbott (1928) (1791–1928)	200	3–92 (34)	147/195 (75%)	38 (19%)	46/183 (25%)	17 (37%)	29
Reifenstein (1947) (1928–1947)	104	3–76 (35)	87 (84%)	24 (23%)	47/93 (51%)	10 (21%)	14

regurgitation before closure of the ventricular septal defect, it is likely that the basic support of the aortic valve is inadequate to prevent development of further aortic regurgitation in the future. Of course, the prolapsed cusp that is resuspended is not likely to remain adequately suspended during a full lifetime. The occasional patient with aortic regurgitation with ventricular septal defect requires aortic valve replacement with all of the ensuing complications that that procedure entails.

Closure of any ventricular septal defect via an aortotomy incision requires much manual manipulation of the aortic valve cusps whether or not previously associated with aortic regurgitation, and the manipulation necessitates debridement of the cuspal endothelial cells. Healing of the debrided surfaces may lead to excessive fibrous thickening, which eventually may lead to development of aortic regurgitation.

2. WITH DISCRETE SUBAORTIC STENOSIS. The site of left ventricular outflow obstruction in patients with discrete subaortic stenosis is about 1 cm below the bases of each of the 3 aortic valve cusps.[28] Because the degree of stenosis in isolated descrete subaortic stenosis is usually severe, the blood exiting the discrete obstruction has an extremely high velocity and contacts the aortic valve cusps with enormous impact. The anatomic consequence of these "jet lesions" is fibrous thickening of the aortic valve cusps. Because a significant percentage of patients with discrete subaortic stenosis are not diagnosed until late childhood or adulthood, a considerable amount of damage may be done to the aortic valve cusps by the time that diagnosis is established.[29] Additionally, because vegetations in infective endocarditis tend to form at sites of jet lesions, patients with discrete subaortic stenosis have a very high frequency of infective endocarditis, which, of course, may produce additional damage to the cusps.[28,29] Despite extreme destruction of the aortic valve cusps by infective endocarditis in this setting, aortic regurgitation is never severe because significant quantities of blood cannot regurgitate through the discrete subaortic obstruction.

If the aortic valve is not sufficiently damaged to require replacement at the time of operative treatment of the discrete subaortic stenosis, it is likely that many of these patients will subsequently require aortic valve replacement because of the combined damage done to the valve by the preoperative jet lesions and by the healing process resulting from manual manipulation of the aortic valve during the operative procedure to relieve the discrete subaortic stenosis.

3. WITH TUNNEL SUBAORTIC STENOSIS. In this condition, more than 1 level of obstruction to left ventricular outflow exists.[30] One or more levels of obstruction exist below the aortic valve, and other levels of obstruction may be present at or above the aortic valve. The aortic valve in this circumstance may be prone to damage similar to that described in patients with discrete subaortic stenosis.

4. WITH OBSTRUCTIVE HYPERTROPHIC CARDIOMYOPATHY. Operative relief of the left ventricular outflow tract obstruction in hypertrophic cardiomyopathy usually is performed via an aortotomy and insertion through it of various incising and excising instruments into the ventricular septum for varying distances below the aortic valve.[31] The procedure requires considerable manipulation of the aortic valve cusps, and this contact may lead to excessive fibrosis during healing of the denuded cuspal surfaces. Aortic regurgitation, severe enough to require aortic valve replacement, now has been reported in a 51-year-old man with obstructive hypertrophic cardiomyopathy and partial septotomy and septectomy 15 years earlier.[32] Preoperatively, aortic valve function had been normal, and the aortic valve cusps were normal at the first operation. Evidence of aortic regurgitation appeared for the first time 12 years after the initial operation, and it progressively worsened thereafter. I fear that this complication will increase significantly with time.

5. WITH TETRALOGY OF FALLOT. I have never understood why aortic regurgitation is rare (< 1%) in patients with tetralogy of Fallot when the aortic valve appears to be so poorly supported, being located directly above the ventricular septal defect and overriding both ventricular chambers. In patients with isolated ventricular septal defect, in contrast, the aortic valve appears to be much better supported and yet aortic regurgitation is far more common. The ventricular septal defect in tetralogy of Fallot is a communication between the right ventricle and aorta, not really 1 between the 2 ventricles as in isolated ventricular septal defect. As a consequence, the ventricular septal defect in tetralogy of Fallot is closed by a patch that lies roughly horizontal, whereas in isolated ventricular septal defect the patch lies roughly vertical. Blood ejected from the left ventricle after closure of the ventricular septal defect in tetralogy of Fallot courses in a far more S-shaped pattern than in the normal heart because flow just below the aortic valve (or just above the patch) is more or less horizontal. Thus, flow just below the aortic valve in patients with tetralogy of Fallot in whom the verticular septal defect has been closed must be considerably more turbulent than normal. The combination of this unusually positioned if not poorly supported aortic valve and the subvalvular turbulent flow in tetralogy of Fallot after ventricular septal defect closure potentially at least could lead to aortic regurgitation many years after operative repair.

6. WITH PERSISTENT TRUNCUS ARTERIOSUS. In this condition, the truncal valve lies immediately above the ventricular septal defect and usually half of it overrides the right ventricle and the other half, the left ventricle. Although the truncal valve may contain 2, 4, 5, or 6 cusps, most commonly it contains 3. Because all blood ejected from the heart in truncus arteriosus crosses the truncal valve, its size and that of the trunk itself is quite large. After operation in this condition, the truncal valve, of course, becomes the aortic valve and the persistent trunk, the ascending aorta, but the amount of blood crossing this valve becomes half that before operation. Although regurgitation occurs in some truncal valves preoperatively, possibly aortic regurgitation will occur late postoperatively because of inability of the previously dilated trunk to contract sufficiently, plus the relatively poor support of its semilunar valve in a fashion similar to that described for the aortic valve in tetralogy of Fallot.

SEQUELAE

PULMONIC VALVE

In Pulmonic Valve Stenosis with Intact Ventricular Septum

In patients with pulmonic valve stenosis with intact ventricular septum severe enough to warrent operative or balloon[33] valvulotomy, the peak right ventricular systolic pressure is always very high.[34] After valvulotomy, this pressure falls to normal or near-normal levels. Although the valvulotomy may relieve the obstruction and drastically lower the peak right ventricular systolic pressure, the pulmonic valve cusp—most commonly a domed central orificed valve with 3 rudimentary commissures—remains abnormal and the valve orifice is incompetent. As long as the opening and the closing pressures on this valve remain low and the tricuspid valve is competent, it is unlikely that pulmonic stenosis can recur or that pulmonic regurgitation will become a problem late postoperatively. If, however, pulmonary hypertension develops because of an acquired pulmonary parenchymal or vascular condition and/or because of an acquired disease affecting the left side of the heart, pulmonic regurgitation, of course, could become a clinical problem, particularly if tricuspid regurgitation develops because of right ventricular systolic hypertension.

In Valvular and/or Subvalvular Pulmonic Stenosis with Ventricular Septal Defect (Tetralogy of Fallot)

In patients with tetralogy of Fallot, the right ventricular outflow obstruction may be below or at the pulmonic valve or at both levels. When the valve itself is stenotic, the degree of stenosis at this site is usually less than at the subvalvular level, the pulmonic valve is usually 3-cuspid (75%) or bicuspid (25%), and the cusps are virtually never as thick or have a domed configuration as occurs in patients with pulmonic stenosis with intact ventricular septum. Valvulotomy is often achieved by excising portions of 1 or more cusps, or by inserting a widening patch that extends into the pulmonary trunk and over most or all of the infundibulum, the wall of which has been partially excised. Both partial cuspal incision and insertion of a right ventricular outflow patch, of course, produce some degree of pulmonic regurgitation. In this circumstance, the pulmonic regurgitation should not be a problem if the pressure in the pulmonary trunk remains low and the tricuspid valve remains competent.

Any damaged valve, including the stenotic pulmonic valve that has undergone either valvulotomy or partial excision, has an increased likelihood for development of infective endocarditis. As long as the right ventricular systolic pressure remains low, however, this "increased likelihood," although greater than that for a normal pulmonic valve, is, nevertheless, extremely low.

AORTIC VALVE

In Aortic Valve Stenosis

When aortic valve stenosis causes symptoms during the first decade of life, the severe degrees of obstruction can usually be relieved by valvulotomy. Aortic stenosis in early life is associated with a malformed valve with thickened cusps and often a small "anulus." The success of valvulotomy is usually dependent on the number of cusps present, their degree of thickening and the size of the "anulus." The unicuspid unicommissural configuration is the most common 1 observed in patients with aortic stenosis dying in the first year of life.[35] After age 10 and until age 65 years, the bicuspid valve is the most common 1 encountered.[23] Valvulotomy in the presence of a unicuspid unicommissural valve virtually assures the development of some degree of aortic regurgitation postoperatively because commissures are not widened, the cusp itself is incised.[21;22] Thus, in this circumstances, aortic regurgitation is the price for relief of the AS. With the bicuspid or tricuspid valvular configuration, commissurotomy is the procedure performed and aortic regurgitation in this circumstance is less likely to develop or if present not to be of major significance, at least early.

Irrespective of whether aortic regurgitation develops, or the aortic stenosis is completely relieved when operations are performed for aortic stenosis in the first decade or 2 of life, the peak systolic pressure in the left ventricular cavity remains relatively high when compared to the right ventricular peak systolic pressure after relief of pulmonic stenosis. As a consequence, the malformed aortic valve, although completely or significantly relieved of stenosis, continues to be traumatized by these pressures and redevelopment of aortic stenosis or worsening of incompletely relieved aortic stenosis is an inevitable consequence. Additionally, these malformed valves continue to possess the increased potential for development of infective endocarditis. It is most likely that all infants and children having valvulotomy or commissurotomy for aortic stenosis in the first 2 decades of life will require aortic valve replacement sometime later.

REFERENCES

1. Betriu A, Wigle ED, Felderhot CH, McLoughlin MJ. Prolapse of the posterior leaflet of the mitral valve associated with secundum atrial septal defect. Am J Cardiol 1975; 35:363–369.
2. Liberthson RR, Boucher CA, Fallon JT, Buckley MJ. Severe mitral regurgitation: a common occurrence in the aging patient with secundum atrial septal defect. Clin Cardiol 1981; 4:229–232.
3. Waller BF, Morrow AG, Maron BJ, Del Negro AA, Kent KM, McGrath FJ, Wallace RB, McIntosh CL, Roberts WC. Etiology of clinically isolated, severe, pure mitral regurgitation: analysis of 97 patients over 30 years of age having mitral valve replacement. Am Heart J 1982; 104:276–288.
4. Arnett EN, Roberts WC. Pathology of active infective endocarditis: a necropsy analysis of 192 patients. Thorac Cardiovasc Surgeon 1982; 30:327–335.
5. Davies MJ. Mitral valve in secundum atrial septal defects. Br Heart J 1981; 46:126–128.
6. Cabin HS, Roberts WC. Ebstein's anomaly of the tricuspid valve and prolapse of the mitral valve. Am Heart J 1981; 101:177–180.
7. Waller BF, Reis RL, McIntosh CL, Epstein SE, Roberts WC. The Marfan cardiovascular disease without the Marfan syndrome. Chest 1980; 77:533–540.
8. Roberts WC, Honig HS. The spectrum of cardiovascular disease in the Marfan syndrome: a clinico-morphologic study of 18 necropsy patients and comparison to 151 previously reported necropsy patients. Am Heart J 1982; 104:115–135.
9. Chandraratna PAN, Tolentino AO, Mutucumarana W, Gomez L. Echocardiographic observations on the association between mitral valve prolapse and asymmetric septal hypertrophy. Circulation 1977; 55:622–626.
10. Roberts WC. Morphologic features of the normal and abnormal mitral valve. Am J Cardiol 1983; 51:1005–1028.
11. Di Segni E, Edwards JE. Cleft anterior leaflet of the mitral valve with intact septa. A study of 20 cases. Am J Cardiol 1983; 51:919–926.
12. Goldfaden DM, Jones M, Morrow AG. Long-term results of repair of incomplete persistent atrioventricular canal. J Thorac Cardiovasc Surg 1981; 82:669–673.
13. Edwards JE. The problem of mitral insufficiency caused by accessory chordae tendineae in persistent common atrioventricular canal. Mayo Clinic Proceed 1960; 35:299–305.
14. Taylor NC, Somerville J. Fixed subaortic stenosis after repair of ostium primum defects. Br Heart J 1981; 45:689–697.
15. Noren GR, Raghib G, Moller JH, Amplatz K, Adams P Jr, Edwards JE. Anomalous origin of the left coronary artery from the pulmonary trunk with special reference to the occurrence of mitral insufficiency. Circulation 1964; 30:171–179.
16. Layman TE. Edwards JE. Anomalies of the cardiac valves associated with complete transposition of the great vessels. Am J Cardiol 1967; 19:247–255.
17. Becker AE, Becker MJ, Edwards JE. Mitral valvular abnormalities associated with supravalvular aortic stenosis. Observations in 3 cases. Am J Cardiol 1972; 29:90–94.
18. Abbott ME. Coarctation of the aorta of the adult type. II. A statistical study and historical retrospect of 200 recorded cases, with autopsy, of stenosis or obliteration of the descending arch in subjects above the age of two years. Am Heart J 1928; 3:392–421, 574–618.
19. Reifenstein GH, Levine SA, Gross RE. Coarctation of the aorta. A review of 104 autopsied cases of "adult type," 2 years of age or older. Am Heart J 1947; 33:146–168.

20. Edwards JE. Pathologic aspects of cardiac valvular insufficiencies. AMA Arch Surg 1958; 77:634–649.
21. Roberts WC, Morrow AG. Congenital aortic stenosis produced by a unicommissural valve. Brit Heart J 1965; 27:505–510.
22. Falcone MW, Roberts WC, Morrow AG, Perloff JK. Congenital aortic stenosis resulting from a unicommissural valve. Clinical and anatomic features in twenty-one adult patients. Circulation 1971; 44:272–280.
23. Roberts WC. The congenitally bicuspid aortic valve. A study of 85 autopsy cases. Am J Cardiol 1970; 26:72–83.
24. Roberts WC, Morrow AG, McIntosh CL, Jones M, Epstein SE. Congenitally bicuspid aortic valve causing severe, pure aortic regurgitation without superimposed infective endocarditis. Analysis of 13 patients requiring aortic valve replacement. Am J Cardiol 1981; 47:206–209.
25. Edwards WD, Leaf DS, Edwards JE. Dissecting aortic aneurysm associated with congenital biscuspid aortic valve. Circulation 1978; 57:1022–1025.
26. Roberts WC. Aortic dissection: anatomy, consequences, and causes. Am Heart J 1981; 101:195–214.
27. Roberts WC, Morrow AG, Braunwald E. Complete interruption of the aortic arch. Circulation 1962; 26:39–59.
28. Morrow AG, Fort L III, Roberts WC, Braunwald E. Discrete subaortic stenosis complicated by aortic valvular regurgitation. Clinical, hemodynamic, and pathologic studies and the results of operative treatment. Circulation 1965; 31:163–171.
29. Roberts WC. Congenital cardiovascular abnormalites usually "silent" until adulthood: morphologic features of the floppy mitral valve, valvular aortic stenosis, hypertrophic cardiomyopathy, sinus of Valsalva aneurysm, and the Marfan syndrome. Cardiovasc Clin 1979; 10(1):407–453.
30. Maron BJ, Redwood DR, Roberts, WC, Henry WL, Morrow AG, Epstein SE. Tunnel subaortic stenosis. Left ventricular outflow tract obstruction produced by fibromuscular tubular narrowing. Circulation 1976; 54:404–416.
31. Morrow AG. Hypertrophic subaortic stenosis—operative methods utilized to relieve left ventricular outflow obstruction. J Thorac Cardiovasc Surg 1978; 76:423–430.
32. Wiener MW, Vondoenfoff LJ, Cohen J. Aortic regurgitation first appearing 12 years after successful septal myectomy for hypertrophic obstructive cardiomyopathy. Am J Med 1982; 72:157–160.
33. Pepine CJ, Gessner IH, Feldman RL. Percutaneous balloon valvuloplasty for pulmonic valve stenosis in the adult. Am J Cardiol 1982; 50:1442–1445.
34. Roberts WC, Shemin RJ, Kent KM. Frequency and direction of interatrial shunting in valvular pulmonic stenosis with intact ventricular septum and without left ventricular inflow or outflow obstruction. An analysis of 127 patients treated by valvulotomy. Am Heart J 1980; 99:142–148.
35. Moller JH, Nakib A, Eliot RS, Edwards JE. Symptomatic congenital aortic stenosis in the first year of life. J Pediat 1966; 69:728–734.

Qualitative and Quantitative Comparison of Amounts of Narrowing by Atherosclerotic Plaques in the Major Epicardial Coronary Arteries at Necropsy in Sudden Coronary Death, Transmural Acute Myocardial Infarction, Transmural Healed Myocardial Infarction and Unstable Angina Pectoris

William C. Roberts, MD

The amounts of narrowing of the 4 major (left main, left anterior descending, left circumflex and right) epicardial coronary arteries by atherosclerotic plaques were compared in 4 subsets of coronary patients. Of the 129 patients studied at necropsy, an average of 2.7 of the 4 arteries was narrowed >75% in cross-sectional area at some point (0.7/4 in controls), and the group with unstable angina pectoris (3.2/4) had more narrowing than did the groups with sudden coronary death (2.8/4), acute myocardial infarction (2.7/4) and healed myocardial infarction (2.3/4). Each of the 4 major epicardial coronary arteries was divided into 5-mm long segments and a histologic section was prepared and stained by the Movat method of each of the 6,461 segments in the 129 patients and in the 1,849 segments in the 40 control subjects. In the 129 patients, 35% of the 5-mm segments were narrowed 75 to 100% in cross-sectional area (3% in controls) and the group with unstable angina had the highest percent (48%) of segments severely narrowed compared to the groups with sudden coronary death (36%), acute myocardial infarction (34%) and healed myocardial infarction (31%). Thus, of the 4 subsets of patients with fatal coronary artery disease studied at necropsy, those with unstable angina pectoris had the most severe and extensive coronary artherosclerosis.

(Am J Cardiol 1989;64:324–328)

From the Pathology Branch, National Heart, Lung, and Blood Institute, Bethesda, Maryland. Manuscript received May 4, 1989, and accepted May 19.

Address for reprints: William C. Roberts, MD, Building 10, Room 2N258, National Institutes of Health, Bethesda, Maryland 20892.

Ten years ago my colleagues and I began examining at necropsy the 4 major epicardial coronary arteries in what we have called a *quantitative* manner. The left main, left anterior descending, left circumflex and right coronary arteries are excised from the heart intact and divided into 5-mm segments. A histologic section was then prepared from each segment. Using this approach, we have examined in the same manner and with similar control subjects the major epicardial coronary arteries in patients with sudden coronary death;[1] transmural acute myocardial infarction;[2] transmural healed myocardial infarction with noncardiac death,[3] with chronic and eventually fatal congestive heart failure without left ventricular aneurysm[4] and with left ventricular aneurysm;[5] and in patients with unstable angina pectoris dying at cardiac catheterization or shortly after coronary artery bypass grafting.[6] This article summarizes these previous studies and, in turn, compares the results of the previous separate studies in these various subsets of coronary patients.

METHODS

Patients: A total of 129 necropsy patients, each of whom had had a coronary event, were studied (Tables I and II). They included 27 patients with transmural (involving greater than the inner half of the left ventricular wall) acute myocardial infarction, which by history and by histologic examination was between 1 and 30 days old; 49 patients with transmural healed myocardial infarction with death either from progressive congestive heart failure ("ischemic cardiomyopathy") without left ventricular aneurysm (9 patients) or from a noncardiac condition (18 patients) or those with left ventricular aneurysm (22 patients); 22 patients with clinically isolated, unstable angina pectoris (without historical evidence at any time of acute myocardial infarction or congestive heart failure) and death within 7 days of an aortocoronary bypass operation or death during a cardiac catheterization procedure; and 31 patients who died suddenly, i.e., within 6 hours after onset of chest pain, which if

TABLE I Number of Major (Right, Left Main, Left Anterior Descending and Left Circumflex) Coronary Arteries Narrowed >75% in Cross-Sectional Area by Atherosclerotic Plaque in Fatal Coronary Artery Disease

Coronary Event	Pts (n)	Mean Age (yrs)	No. of Four Arteries/Pt >75%↓ in CSA by Plaque				
			4	3	2	1	Mean
Sudden coronary death	31	47	3	20	6	2	2.8
Acute myocardial infarction	27	59	3	14	10	0	2.7
Healed myocardial infarction							
Asymptomatic	18	66	0	7	7	4	2.2
Chronic CHF without aneurysm	9	63	0	3	5	1	2.2
Left ventricular aneurysm	22	61	1	12	6	3	2.5
Angina pectoris/unstable	22	48	10	8	3	1	3.2
Total (%)	129	56	17 (13)	64 (50)	37 (29)	11 (8)	2.7
Controls (%)	40	52	0 (0)	5 (5)	12 (13)	21 (23)	0.7

CHF = congestive heart failure; CSA = cross-sectional area.

present, began outside the hospital, who never had evidence of congestive cardiac failure, and who at necropsy had >75% cross-sectional area narrowing of at least 1 of the 4 major coronary arteries and no ventricular wall myocardial coagulation necrosis. Patients with associated primary valvular, congenital or pericardial heart diseases, hypertrophic cardiomyopathy or other myocardial diseases not secondary to coronary artery disease (CAD) and patients who had had a cardiac operation (other than the unstable angina group) were excluded.

The coronary arteries in all 129 patients were studied in similar fashion. The hearts were fixed for at least 1 day in formalin. The 4 major epicardial coronary arteries were then excised intact, x-rayed and fixed for at least another day. Following decalcification (if necessary), each of the 4 major coronary arteries were cut transversely to their longitudinal axes into approximately 5-mm long segments and each segment was labeled sequentially from either its aortic ostium or from its origin from the left main. Of the coronary arteries, the average length (in cm) of the right was 11; left main, 1; left anterior descending, 10; and left circumflex, 6. The 5-mm segments were labeled, processed in alcohol and xylene, dehydrated and embedded in paraffin. Then 2 histologic sections were cut and stained from each paraffin block. The Movat stain was used on 1 histologic section, and all determinations of luminal narrowing were based on examination of the Movat-stained sections. The degrees of narrowing were based on histologic examination of each cross-section magnified 25 to 50 times. The judgment regarding the degree of luminal narrowing of each 5-mm segment was based on the degree of luminal obliteration within the luminal circle bordered by the internal elastic membrane. The circle was visually subdivided into 4 equally sized quadrants. The percent of narrowing in each 5-mm segment was determined as follows: 0 to 25, 26 to 50, 51 to 75 and 76 to 100%. The observations in the patients with CAD were compared to controls, all of whom died from noncardiac causes, mainly acute leukemia. None of the control subjects had evidence of cardiac dysfunction or myocardial ischemia during life, all had had normal (<140/90 mm Hg) systemic arterial pressures and all had normal sized (<350 g in women and <400 g in men) hearts at necropsy.

RESULTS

Qualitative studies: Table I summarizes the number of major (right, left main, left anterior descending and left circumflex) epicardial coronary arteries narrowed >75% in cross-sectional area by atherosclerotic plaque alone in the patients with fatal CAD. Among the 129 patients, 516 major epicardial coronary arteries were examined and of them 345 (67%) were narrowed at some point 76 to 100% in cross-sectional area by atherosclerotic plaque. In contrast, of 40 control subjects, 160 major epicardial coronary arteries were examined and of them 60 (38%) were narrowed at some point >75% in cross-sectional area by plaque. Among the 129 coronary patients, only 11 (8%) had a single coronary artery severely (>75% in cross-sectional area) narrowed (controls = 23%); 37 (29%) had 2 arteries so narrowed (controls = 13%); 64 (50%) had 3 arteries severely narrowed (controls = 5%) and 17 patients (13%) had all 4 major arteries so narrowed (controls = 0). Thus, of the 4 major coronary arteries in the coronary patients an average of 2.7 were narrowed >75% in cross-sectional area by plaque and among the control subjects, 0.7 of 4.

The number of major coronary arteries severely narrowed by atherosclerotic plaque among the various subsets of coronary patients was relatively similar except for the unstable angina patients (Table I). Among the 31 *sudden coronary death* patients, an average of 2.8 of the 4 major arteries were narrowed severely; this is virtually identical to that of the 27 patients with *transmural acute myocardial infarction*, all of whom died in a coronary care unit. Only 2 of the 31 sudden death victims and none of the 27 acute myocardial infarction victims had only a single coronary artery ("1-vessel disease") severely narrowed.

The *healed myocardial infarction* group was divided into 3 subgroups. One consisted of patients who had had an acute myocardial infarct that healed; thereafter there was never clinical evidence of myocardial isch-

TABLE II Amounts of Cross-Sectional Area Narrowing of Each 5-mm Segment of the Four Major (Right, Left Main, Left Anterior Descending and Left Circumflex) Epicardial Coronary Arteries by Atherosclerotic Plaques in Subjects with Fatal Coronary Artery Disease

Subgroup	Pts (n)	Mean Age (yrs)	No. 5-mm Segments	Percent Segments Narrowed 0–25%	26–50%	51–75%	76–100%		Mean Score	Mean % Narrowing/ 5-mm Segments
Sudden coronary death	31	47	1,564	7	23	34	36		2.98	67
Acute myocardial infarction	27	59	1,403	5	23	38	34		3.01	68
Healed myocardial infarction										
Asymptomatic	18	66	924	11	23	35	31		2.87	64
Chronic CHF without aneurysm	9	63	529	11	23	37	29	31%	2.78	61
LV aneurysm	22	61	992	4	21	42	33		3.03	68
Angina pectoris	22	48	1,049	11	12	29	48		3.12	70
Total	129	56	6,461	8	21	36	35		2.98	67
Controls	40	52	1,849	31	44	22	3		1.97	32

CHF = congestive heart failure; LV = left ventricular.

emia and they died from a noncardiac cause, usually cancer. Nevertheless, the average number of major coronary arteries severely narrowed at necropsy was 2.2 of 4. Another subgroup consisted of patients who had chronic congestive heart failure in the absence of left ventricular aneurysm after healing of an acute myocardial infarction. They might be called the *ischemic cardiomyopathy* group. Their average number of major coronary arteries severely narrowed also was 2.2 of 4. The other subgroup of healed myocardial infarction patients had a true left ventricular aneurysm. The average number of major coronary arteries severely narrowed in them was 2.5 of 4.

The final subgroup consisted of 22 patients with *unstable angina pectoris.* Nineteen of them had had coronary artery bypass grafting procedures within 7 days of death and the other 3 had cardiac arrest during cardiac catheterization. Preoperatively, all had normal left ventricular function and none had a clinically apparent acute myocardial infarct or congestive heart failure at any time. The average number of major coronary arteries severely narrowed by plaque was 3.2 of 4, and 10 of the 22 patients had severe narrowing of the left main coronary artery as well as severe narrowing of the other 3 major arteries ("4-vessel disease").

Quantitative studies: The results of the quantitative studies are summarized in Table II. A total of 6,461 five-mm segments were sectioned and examined histologically. The sections were stained by the Movat method to delineate the internal elastic membrane. The findings in the 129 coronary patients were compared to those in 1,849 five-mm segments from the 40 control subjects. In each coronary subgroup the 5-mm segments from each of the 4 major coronary arteries were pooled together; thus by this approach the amount of narrowing in an individual patient is not discernible. The percent of 5-mm segments narrowed 76 to 100% in cross-sectional area by atherosclerotic plaque was 35 for the coronary patients and 3 for the control subjects; the percent narrowed 51 to 75% was 36 for the coronary patients and 22 for the control subjects. Thus, 71% of the 5-mm segments in the coronary patients were narrowed >50% in cross-sectional area by atherosclerotic plaque. For the control subjects it was 25%. In contrast, only 29% of the 5-mm segments in the coronary patients were narrowed <50% and only 8% even approached normal, i.e., narrowed 25% or less in cross-sectional area. In contrast, 75% of the 5-mm segments in the control subjects were narrowed <50% and 31% of them were normal or nearly normal. Thus, in the coronary patients 92% of the 6,461 five-mm segments of the 4 major epicardial coronary arteries were narrowed >25% in cross-sectional area by atherosclerotic plaque.

Among the various subsets of coronary patients, those with *sudden coronary death* and *acute myocardial infarction* had similar percentages of 5-mm segments narrowed 76 to 100% in cross-sectional area by plaque (36 and 34%, respectively); patients with *healed myocardial infarction* as a group had the least severe narrowing (31% of segments narrowed >75%), and the patients with *unstable angina pectoris* had the most severe narrowing (48% of the 5-mm segments were narrowed >75% by plaque).

In an attempt to provide a single number for the amount of coronary arterial narrowing in each patient, a score system was used. A segment narrowed 0 to 25% in cross-sectional area was assigned a score of 1; a segment narrowed 26 to 50% = 2; a segment narrowed 51 to 75% = 3, and 1 narrowed 76 to 100% = 4. The mean score for all 129 patients or for each of the 6,461 five-mm coronary segments was 3.0 and that for the 40 control subjects or 1,849 five-mm segments, 2.0. Again, the unstable angina patients had the most extensive coronary narrowing by this approach.

In all of the aforementioned quantitative coronary arterial studies the amount of cross-sectional area luminal narrowing by atherosclerotic plaque in the right, left anterior descending and left circumflex coronary arteries was similar if the 5-mm segments in each of the 3 longest coronary arteries were pooled together from a number of patients. This statement might be best understood by examining a single subset of coronary patients with fatal CAD. Among the 27 patients with fatal transmural acute myocardial infarction, a total of 1,358 five-mm long segments were analyzed from the right, left anterior descending and left circumflex coronary arteries, and the percentage of segments narrowed 0 to 25, 26 to 50, 51 to 75 and 76 to 100% was similar at each of these 4 categories of cross-sectional area narrowing in each of these 3 major epicardial coronary arteries. The same findings were observed in the patients with sudden coronary death, healed myocardial infarction and unstable angina pectoris.

In a single patient, however, the percent of 5-mm long coronary segments severely (>75% in cross-sectional area) narrowed by atherosclerotic plaque in 1 major epicardial coronary artery may be greater or lesser than that of another major coronary artery. If the segments from 1 coronary artery (e.g., right), however, were pooled together from several patients with fatal CAD and compared to pooled 5-mm segments from another coronary artery (e.g., left anterior descending) from several patients with fatal CAD, the percentage of segments narrowed at each of the 4 categories of cross-sectional area narrowing in each artery was similar.

DISCUSSION

The information derived at necropsy quantitating the severity and extent of atherosclerosis in the 4 major epicardial coronary arteries in fatal CAD is potentially useful clinically in 2 areas: in interpreting degrees of coronary narrowing by angiography during life, and in deciding which of the major coronary arteries needs a conduit at the time of coronary artery bypass grafting.

Without coronary angiography neither coronary bypass nor angioplasty would be done. The only way during life to obtain information on the status of the epicardial coronary arteries is angiography, and, therefore, this procedure revolutionized diagnosis of CAD just as aortocoronary bypass grafting revolutionized therapy of CAD. But angiography—as good as it is—has certain deficiencies. Angiography is a luminogram and a narrowed segment is compared to a less narrowed segment, which is assumed to be normal. The angiogram does not delineate the internal elastic membrane of the artery, and, therefore, the artery's true lumen remains uncertain.

The aforementioned coronary quantitative studies[1-5] demonstrated that in fatal CAD 92% of the 5-mm long segments of the 4 major epicardial coronary arteries were narrowed >25% in cross-sectional area by atherosclerotic plaque. Thus, only 8% of the 5-mm segments even approached normal and virtually none was normal. Thus, at least in fatal CAD, and probably also in live patients with symptomatic myocardial ischemia, it is infrequent that an angiographically severely narrowed segment of a coronary artery can be compared to a segment of coronary artery that is actually normal. In patients with symptomatic myocardial ischemia, the coronary angiogram measures degrees of narrowing by comparing severely narrowed segments to segments that are simply less narrowed but by no means normal. Accordingly, coronary angiograms in patients with symptomatic myocardial ischemia usually underestimate the degrees of luminal narrowing.[7,8]

The unit of measuring degrees of narrowing by angiography is different than the unit of measurement at necropsy. In the anatomic quantitative studies presented herein, the unit was *cross-sectional area* narrowing. The unit of angiography is *diameter* narrowing. In general, a 75% cross-sectional area narrowing is equivalent to a 50% diameter reduction, and, therefore, a ≥50% diameter reduction during life has generally been considered the cutoff point between clinically significant and clinically insignificant coronary narrowing.

The second potential use of the information derived from these quantitative studies at necropsy is the appreciation that the atherosclerotic process in patients with symptomatic myocardial ischemia is usually diffuse and severe. Therefore, more rather than fewer aortocoronary conduits provide a higher frequency of relief or improvement in symptoms of myocardial ischemia, in improvement in results of exercise testing and in prolonging life. Among patients surviving ≤60 days or >60 days after aortocoronary bypass operations, the amount of severe narrowing in the *nonbypassed native* coronary arteries is usually similar to that in the *bypassed native* coronary arteries.[9] From study at necropsy of 102 patients dying either early (≤60 days) or late (2.5 to 108 months [mean 35]) after bypass operations, Waller and I[9] found that the bypassed and nonbypassed native coronary arteries had similar degrees of severe luminal narrowing by atherosclerotic plaques. Specifically, in 213 (94%) of the 226 bypassed native arteries and in 73 (91%) of 80 nonbypassed native arteries the lumens were narrowed >75% in cross-sectional area by atherosclerotic plaque. The reason the native arteries were not bypassed was not that they were too small or severely narrowed distally, but because by angiogram the lumens were judged not to be sufficiently narrowed to warrant the insertion of a conduit. Thus, if 2 of the major coronary arteries are severely narrowed by angiogram and the third major artery is "insignificantly" narrowed and if a bypass operation is to be done, the insertion of a conduit in all 3 major coronary arteries could be reasonably argued. There is, of course, potential danger in inserting a conduit in an artery insignificantly narrowed, but, nevertheless, it may be more advantageous to err on the side of too many conduits than too few. At necropsy, "3-vessel disease" is far more frequent than "2-vessel disease" and even when only 2 of the 3 major arteries at necropsy are narrowed >75% in cross-sectional area, the third one is usually narrowed 51 to 75% in cross-sectional area. Thus, an appreciation of the diffuse nature of coronary atherosclerosis in fatal CAD and probably also in symptomatic myocardial ischemia encourages the tilt toward more rather than fewer conduits at coronary bypass operations.

A possible criticism of the 5-mm segment approach to quantifying coronary arterial narrowing is that the epicardial coronary arteries were fixed in an unphysiologic pressure state, namely a zero pressure state, rather than at a systemic arterial diastolic pressure. In an attempt to take into account the unphysiologic fixation state, the degrees of narrowing were conservatively judged, that is, if a segment was more or less in between 2 quadrants (51 to 75% and 76 to 100%), the lesser degree of narrowing was always chosen. Second, in any segment in which a portion of wall was collapsed by the fixation process, the degree of narrowing was determined as if the segment was expanded. Most important, the segments narrowed the most, i.e., >75% in cross-sectional area, were affected the least by the fixation process. Irrespective of whether or not the histologic technique used in this study is perfect or imperfect, the same technique was used in all subsets of coronary patients and also in all control subjects, and, therefore, the comparison data are highly reliable. Irrespective of whether or not the degree of luminal narrowing should be slightly greater or slightly less than that determined by this technique, it is clear that the atherosclerotic process is a diffuse one in nearly all patients with fatal CAD. The accuracy of the technique determining degrees of cross-sectional area narrowing by estimating from stained histologic sections magnified about 40 times is similar (≤5%) to that determined by planimetry.[10]

Another possible concern of the quantitative data is its applicability to living patients with symptomatic or other clinical evidence (e.g., positive exercise test) of myocardial ischemia. It is my view that the major difference in coronary arterial narrowing occurs at the stage of conversion from the asymptomatic to the symptomatic myocardial ischemia state and that there is relatively little difference in degrees of coronary narrowing between the symptomatic and the fatal states. Support for this view can be obtained by the presence of severe and extensive coronary narrowing on the angiogram during life, and by studying the coronary tree at necropsy in patients who had a coronary event and who died later from a noncardiac cause. Although data from the latter situation are minimal, the degrees of coronary narrowing at necropsy are similar to that in other patients with fatal symptomatic myocardial ischemia. Finally, among the subsets of coronary patients described herein, those with unstable angina pectoris had by far the worst degrees of coronary narrowing and the subjects in this group were the only ones in whom their natural course was interrupted by an iatrogenic event, namely coronary artery bypass grafting (within a week of death).

REFERENCES

1. Roberts WC, Jones AA. Quantitation of coronary arterial narrowing at necropsy in sudden coronary death. Analysis of 31 patients and comparison with 25 control subjects. *Am J Cardiol 1979;44:39–45.*

2. Roberts WC, Jones AA. Quantification of coronary arterial narrowing at necropsy in acute myocardial infarction: analysis and comparison of findings in 27 patients and 22 controls. *Circulation 1980;61:786–790.*

3. Virmani R, Roberts WC. Non-fatal healed transmural myocardial infarction and fatal non-cardiac disease. Qualification and quantification of coronary arterial narrowing and of left ventricular scarring in 18 necropsy patients. *Br Heart J 1981;45:434–441.*

4. Virmani R, Roberts WC. Quantification of coronary arterial narrowing and of left ventricular myocardial scarring in healed myocardial infarction with chronic, eventually fatal, congestive cardiac failure. *Am J Med 1980;68:831–838.*

5. Cabin HS, Roberts WC. True left ventricular aneurysm and healed myocardial infarction. Clinical and necropsy observations including quantification of degrees of coronary arterial narrowing. *Am J Cardiol 1980;46:754–763.*

6. Roberts WC, Virmani R. Quantification of coronary arterial narrowing in clinically-isolated unstable angina pectoris. An analysis of 22 necropsy patients. *Am J Med 1979;67:792–799.*

7. Arnett EN, Isner JM, Redwood DR, Kent KM, Baker WP, Ackerstein H, Roberts WC. Coronary artery narrowing in coronary heart disease: comparison of cineangiographic and necropsy findings. *Ann Intern Med 1979;91:350–356.*

8. Isner JM, Kishel J, Kent KM, Ronan JAJ, Ross AM, Roberts WC. Accuracy of angiographic determination of left main coronary arterial narrowing. Angiographic-histologic correlative analysis in 28 patients. *Circulation 1981;63:1056–1064.*

9. Waller BF, Roberts WC. Amount of narrowing by atherosclerotic plaque in 44 nonbypassed and 52 bypassed major epicardial coronary arteries in 32 necropsy patients who died within 1 month of aortocoronary bypass grafting. *Am J Cardiol 1980;46:956–962.*

10. Isner JM, Wu M, Virmani R, Jones AA, Roberts WC. Comparison of coronary arterial luminal narrowing determined by visual inspection of histologic sections under magnification among three independent observers and comparison to that obtained by video planimetry. An analysis of 559 five-millimeter segments of 61 coronary arteries from eleven patients. *Lab Invest 1980;42:566–570.*

MORPHOLOGIC FEATURES

Charles Stewart Roberts
William Clifford Roberts

Since 1958, numerous publications have described various morphologic cardiac findings in patients with hypertrophic cardiomyopathy (HCM).[1-39] Although it was Teare in 1958 who first described certain characteristic features of the heart in HCM,[40] earlier descriptions were suggestive of this condition.

In 1869, Liouville and Hallopeau each reported a patient probably having HCM.[41,42] Both authors noted striking hypertrophy of the ventricular septum, and each considered the left ventricular outflow tract to be obstructed by the hypertrophied septal muscle; Hallopeau also noted thickening of the anterior mitral leaflet in his 69-year-old patient.

In 1907, Schmincke described severe hypertrophy of the ventricular septum in the hearts of 2 women, aged 50 and 56 years.[43] In addition to the thickening of the septum, the left ventricular free wall in each patient was severely hypertrophied. Schmincke considered the ventricular septal hypertrophy to be primary and of congenital origin, leading to obstruction to left ventricular ejection and to secondary hypertrophy of the left ventricular free wall. He further speculated that the latter, in turn, aggravated the degree of obstruction, thereby initiating a vicious cycle.

In 1910, Bernheim described a syndrome of right-sided congestive cardiac failure in 10 patients with left ventricular hypertrophy of various causes.[44] Proper function of the right ventricle was thought to be impeded by severe hypertrophy of the ventricular septum, which protruded into the right ventricular outflow tract. It has been suggested that some of Bernheim's cases were examples of HCM.[45] Because of the marked left ventricular dilatation in 9 of the 10 hearts described, a finding rarely seen in adults with HCM, it seems unlikely that the cases described by Bernheim were examples of this disease.

After Schmincke's report in 1907,[43] a period of nearly 50 years elapsed before another report of the structural abnormalities of the disease appeared. In 1952, Davies described a family in whom many members had heart disease, a history of sudden death, and systolic precordial murmurs.[46] At necropsy, the heart in one patient showed "diffuse subaortic stenosis" associated with left ventricular hypertrophy. He described an area of fibrosis 4 cm^2 in the left ventricular outflow tract opposite the anterior mitral leaflet, a lesion suggestive of HCM.

In 1957, Brock operated on a 63-year-old woman thought to have valvular aortic stenosis and systemic hypertension.[47] At operation, however, the aortic valve was normal, and no obstruction to left ventricular outflow was encountered by dilating instruments, despite direct pressure tracings showing subvalvular obstruction. The patient died shortly after operation, and necropsy showed a hypertrophied, nondilated left ventricle and no subaortic fibrous stricture.

Although the cases reported by Liouville,[41] Hallopeau,[42] Schmincke,[43] Davies,[46] and Brock[47] are probably examples of HCM, the comparative thicknesses of the ventricular septum and left ventricular free wall and other features of HCM were not described in any of them. Thus, it can only be presumed that these patients had HCM. The first unequivocal description of HCM was by Teare from London, and the report appeared in the *British Heart Journal* in January of 1958.[40] Although Brock's clinical report was published in *Guy's Hospital Reports* in the final quarterly issue of 1957,[47] Teare's article had been received by the journal office in January of 1957, that is, *before* Brock had operated on his patient. Therefore, it seems fair to credit Teare with the first detailed anatomic description and to credit Brock with the first description of the functional nature of this entity.

Teare described gross and histologic cardiac findings in 9 patients, aged 14 to 45 years (mean 26), 2 women and 7 men, 8 of whom died suddenly. Although Teare did not give measurements of the thicknesses of the ventricular septum and left ventricular free wall, he clearly indicated that the septum was thicker than the left ventricular free wall and, indeed, called the condition "asymmetrical hypertrophy of the heart." He considered the localized septal hypertrophy to be a "benign tumor" or "hamartoma." He observed on histologic examination a "bizarre arrangement of muscle bundles" and "considerable variation in size" of the myocardial fibers in the ventricular septum. Teare also noted similar disordered arrangement of muscle bundles in the adjacent anterior free wall of the left ventricle. In one patient, the posterior left ventricular free wall "appeared thinner than normal," and histologic examination showed normal arrangement and uniform size of the myocardial fibers. Although one of Teare's 9 patients underwent valvulotomy for suspected mitral stenosis (this was the only patient in his study who did not die suddenly), there were no descriptions of the mitral valve, no mention of mural endocardial thickening in the left ventricular outflow tract, and no comments regarding the sizes of the various cardiac chambers. This report, however, established HCM as a distinct entity and described the peculiar arrangement of and variation in size of the fibers in the ventricular septum.

DEFINITION

Probably no cardiovascular disease in recent years has engendered as much controversy or "professional" emotional display as has HCM. Since Teare applied the term "asymmetrical hypertrophy of the heart" to HCM, at least 57 other terms, including "functional subaortic stenosis," "diffuse muscular subaortic stenosis," "idiopathic hypertrophic subaortic stenosis," "hypertrophic obstructive cardiomyopathy," and "asymmetric septal hypertrophy" have been applied.[48] Terms that include the word "stenosis" or "obstruction" are inappropriate because obstruction is more often absent than present. Terms that emphasize asymmetry of the walls bordering the left ventricular cavity have served a useful purpose in emphasizing a frequent morphologic feature of this condition, but the ventricular septum may be thicker than the left ventricular free wall in some conditions other than HCM, and some patients with HCM do not have asymmetric septal hypertrophy (i.e., septum thicker than free wall), and the free wall in HCM is not always thickened.

A major obstacle to understanding and discussing HCM is the lack of agreement among its students as to what it is. It is readily apparent that evidence of left ventricular outflow obstruction is not necessary for a diagnosis of HCM. The presence of asymmetric septal hypertrophy is not required for diagnosis because other conditions can cause the ventricular septum to be thicker than the left ventricular free wall, and in many patients with HCM the septum and free wall are of similar thicknesses. Rapid upstroke of the arterial pulse, cardiomegaly, a systolic precordial murmur, and an abnormal electrocardiogram are usually present, but none of these are diagnostic or specific. Systolic anterior motion of the anterior mitral leaflet also is often present by echocardiogram, but any condition in which the left ventricular cavity is relatively small and the percentage of left ventricular volume ejected each beat is relatively high can also cause systolic anterior motion. Thus, what is HCM? It appears most reasonable simply to consider HCM a condition characterized by: (1) hypertrophy of all or a portion of the walls of left ventricle, that is, ventricular septum or free wall or both; (2) dilated right and left atria; (3) nondilatation of the cavities of both cardiac ventricles, except in the presence of transmural ventricular wall necrosis or fibrosis or complete heart block; (4) absence of another cardiac condition that could produce left ventricular hypertrophy (focal or diffuse) without ventricular cavity dilatation, such as systemic hypertension or valvular heart disease; (5) presence of a normal or "supernormal" cardiac output and stroke volume; and (6) absence of other states such as hyperthyroidism or pheochromocytoma that independently might increase cardiac output abnormally. Atherosclerotic coronary artery disease can coexist with HCM.

Personal study of 220 patients with HCM at necropsy has disclosed certain predictable, grossly visible, characteristic, although not absolutely specific, features of HCM (Table 1): (1) dilated atria (100%); (2) increased heart weight (95%); (3) nondilated left ventricle (79%); (4) thickened mitral valve (75%); (5) mural endocardial plaque in the left ventricular outflow tract in apposition to the anterior mitral leaflet (72%); (6) greater maximal thickness of the ventricular septum than that of the left ventricular free wall (69%); and (7) grossly visible left ventricular scarring (42%), usually in the absence of significant narrowing of the epicardial coronary arteries. The hearts in

TABLE 1. CARDIAC MORPHOLOGIC FEATURES OF HYPERTROPHIC CARDIOMYOPATHY: FINDINGS IN 220 NECROPSY CASES

	Cardiac Operation		
Characteristics	**0 (n = 145)**	**+ (n = 75)**	**Total (n = 220)**
1. Dilated atria	145 (100%)	75 (100%)	220 (100%)
2. Increased heart weight*	138 (95%)	72 (96%)	210 (95%)
3. Nondilated left ventricle	118 (81%)	56 (76%)	174 (79%)
4. Thickened mitral valve	90/137 (66%)	64/68 (94%)	154/205 (75%)
5. Fibrous plaque, left ventricular outflow	83/137 (61%)	66/71 (93%)	149/208 (72%)
6. Ventricular septum > left ventricle	102/142 (72%)	46/73 (63%)	148/215 (69%)
7. Gross left ventricular fibrosis	60/145 (41%)	32/73 (44%)	92/218 (42%)

* Adult women >350 g; adult men >400 g.

no 2 patients with HCM are alike. Almost invariably, the atria are dilated and the heart weight is increased, but the remaining 5 gross characteristics are variable.

MORPHOLOGIC FEATURES

A chief morphologic abnormality in HCM resides in the ventricular septum. As pointed out by Teare in his initial description of this condition in 1958, the ventricular septum usually is thicker than the left ventricular free wall. Among our adult necropsy patients, the maximal thickness of ventricular septum was usually about 3.0 cm and that of the left ventricular free wall, about 2.0 cm. The thickest portion of the septum is that part located about midway between aortic valve and left ventricular apex. This level corresponds approximately to the apex of right ventricle. Although in nearly all our necropsy patients the ventricular septum was thicker than normal, the left ventricular free wall was usually, but not always, thicker than normal.

Although ventricular asymmetry, that is, a significant difference in maximal thickness of ventricular septum and left ventricular free wall, is a characteristic morphologic feature of HCM, about 30% of our patients at necropsy had ventricular symmetry, that is, equal maximal thicknesses of the ventricular septum and left ventricular free wall. Thus, although asymmetric septal hypertrophy is a sensitive marker for HCM, it is not specific for this condition. Ventricular septa thicker than left ventricular free walls may occur in conditions causing thinning of the left ventricular free wall relative to the septum and in conditions causing thickening of the septum relative to the free wall. The most common cause of preferential free wall thinning is myocardial infarction, and the most common cause of preferential septal thickening is right ventricular systolic hypertension of any cause.

Among patients with HCM, the thickness of the ventricular septum is not dependent on the presence of left ventricular outflow tract obstruction at rest, and indeed, the thickness of the septum is similar in patients with and without outflow obstruction at rest. Although examination of the septum in patients with HCM is not helpful in separating patients *with* from those *without* left ventricular outflow obstruction at rest, examination of the basal portion of the left ventricular free wall (posterior or posterolateral portion) does permit delineation between these two groups of patients. In patients with the nonobstructive type of HCM, this posterobasal portion is thinner than normal and is often pointed like a bird's bill. In patients without obstruction at rest, the thickest portion of the left ventricular free wall is about midway between the base of posterior mitral leaflet and apex of the left ventricle.[14]

Another abnormality in the ventricular septum in patients with HCM is focal myocardial fiber disarray or disorganization. This abnormality, described initially by Teare, occurs in about 95% of these patients, depending on how "septal disorganization" is defined. Small foci of groups of myocardial fibers not parallel to one another in the ventricular septum are common in normal developing and adult hearts. When, however, the definition of "septal disorganization" is rigid and quantitation of the amount of disorganization is introduced, about 90% of the patients with HCM can be clearly delineated from persons with normal hearts or from patients with cardiac conditions other than HCM. Studies by Maron and associates have shown that, among patients with HCM, nearly 90% had > 5% of the area of the ventricular septum showing myofiber disorganization.[15,20,22,26] In contrast, among persons with normal hearts or heart conditions other than HCM, < 5% and usually < 1% of the area of the ventricular septum showed myofiber disorganization.

Although "septal disorganization" of > 5% of the area of the ventricular septum occurs in about 90% of the patients with HCM, about 10% of these patients have < 5% of the area of the septum showing disarray, and of them a few patients have no disarray at all. Thus, like ventricular asymmetry, "septal disorganization" of > 5% of the area of the septum occurs in most patients with HCM, but this abnormality may involve a smaller area of septum or, rarely, may be entirely absent.

Not only does disorganization of myocardial fibers occur, but in addition, ultrastructural studies have shown disarray of myofibrils and myofilaments within individual cells.[4] Again, the abnormalities of myofibrils and myofilaments are not specific for HCM, but when disorganization of these subcellular components is found in other cardiac conditions, the abnormal cells are found in small numbers. The individual septal myocardial cells in HCM also appear to have increased amounts of Z-band material and nonspecific changes of cellular hypertrophy and degeneration.

Myofiber disarray also occurs in the left and right ventricular free walls, but not to the extent observed in the ventricular septum. Ultrastructural examination of the left and right ventricular free walls, however, has disclosed many bizarrely shaped, disorganized cells in the ventricular free walls of patients *without* obstruction, whereas the bizarrely shaped and disorganized myocardial fibers are less numerous in the ventricular free walls in the patient *with* obstruction.[4] Thus, the disorientation of groups of myocardial cells and the disarray of myofibrils and myofilaments within individual myocardial cells are not the result of left ventricular outflow obstruction or high intraventricular systolic pressures.

The functional or clinical significance of "septal disorganization" among patients with HCM is not clear. Among patients studied at necropsy, those with high percentages of area of septum with disorganization were younger, had a higher frequency of premature death involving >1 member of the same family, and had thicker ventricular septa than those with low percentages of area of involved septum.[20] The presence or degree of left ventricular outflow obstruction, length of symptoms of cardiac dysfunction, mode of death, arrhythmias, and so forth were not significantly different in patients with high than in those with low percentages of septal area involved by disorganization.

Another abnormality of ventricular septum in patients with HCM is the presence of abnormal intramural coronary arteries in >50% of the patients.[12,34] The abnormalities observed in the intramural coronary arteries in these patients are striking and consist of increased number and size of arteries with thickened walls and narrowed lumens. The thickening results from increased numbers of smooth-muscle cells and increased amounts of fibrous tissue in both the media and the intima. Moreover, mucoid deposits (acid mucopolysaccharide material) are increased. Like asymmetric ventricular septal thickening and septal disorganization, however, abnormality of the intramural coronary arteries is not specific for HCM, but it is certainly more striking in HCM than in other conditions. Similar abnormality of the intramural coronary arteries may be observed in patients and in Newfoundland dogs with discrete subaortic stenosis,[49] in patients with tunnel subaortic stenosis,[50] in normal human fetuses,[22] and in newborns with aortic valve atresia.[51]

The significance of the changes in the intramural coronary arteries in patients with HCM is unknown. Their presence or absence does not correlate with any analyzed clinical parameter, including presence or degree of left ventricular outflow tract obstruction, age, sex, presence of cardiac dysfunction or ischemia including chest pain, or length of symptoms of cardiac dysfunction. The cause of the striking abnormalities of the intramural coronary arteries also is uncertain. In each of the four conditions in which this degree of abnormality has been observed, namely, HCM, discrete and tunnel subaortic stenosis, and aortic valve atresia, the septum is extremely thick, and movement of the septum during life is limited, as shown by echocardiogram. It is possible that the severe septal thickening prevents adequate expansion of these arteries during ventricular diastole, so flow through them during this phase of the cardiac cycle is greatly reduced. The fibrous-smooth muscle cell response, in turn, may obliterate the unused lumen. This hypothesis, however, does not explain the large size of these arteries. It is possible that the proliferation of the smooth-muscle cells in the walls of these arteries represents a response to the same stimulus that causes severe hypertrophy and abnormal configuration of many striated myocardial cells.

Another abnormality of the ventricular septum in adults with HCM is the occurrence of a fibrous plaque on the mural endocardium of left ventricle in apposition to the anterior mitral leaflet (Figs. 1 to 4). This fibrous thickening is the result of contact between the valvular and mural endocardium. The mural plaque, in other words, is the anatomic equivalent of "systolic anterior motion" of the anterior mitral leaflet observed on echocardiogram in HCM and occasionally in other conditions. The obstruction in HCM, when present, almost certainly begins at a level corresponding to the distal margin of the anterior mitral leaflet and with the caudal margin of the septal endocardial plaque. The mural endocardial septal plaque is present more frequently and is thicker in patients with obstruction at rest than in those without obstruc-

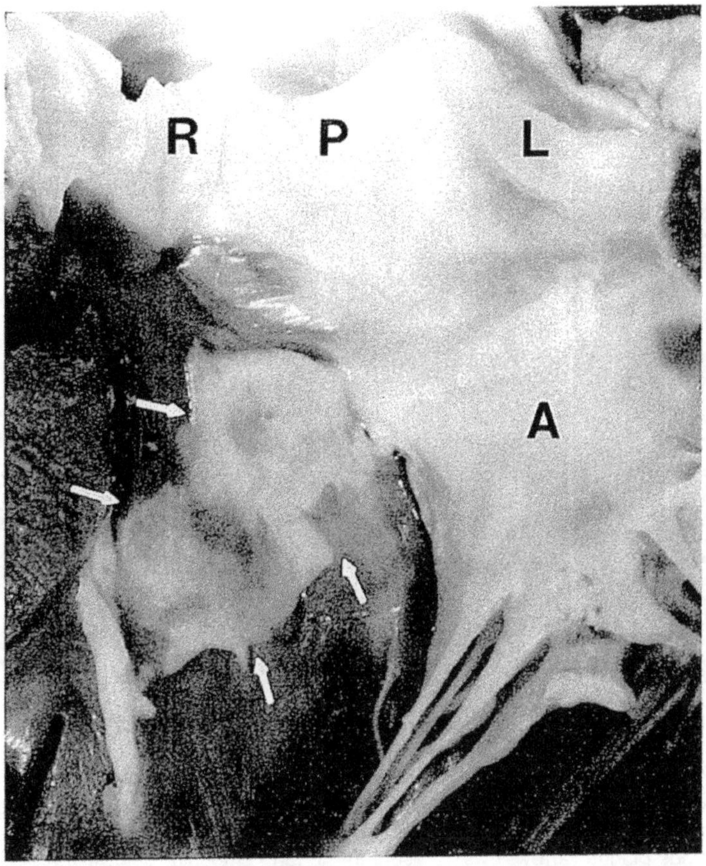

Fig. 1. Opened left ventricular outflow tract and aortic valve of a 14-year-old adopted boy who died suddenly during a basketball game. Sudden death was his first symptom of hypertrophic cardiomyopathy. He was known, however, to have had a precordial murmur, and an echocardiogram had shown systolic anterior motion of the anterior mitral leaflet. At necropsy, the heart weighed 410 g. Neither ventricular cavity was dilated, and both atria were dilated. A mural endocardial fibrous plaque (arrows) was present in the left ventricular outflow tract in apposition to the anterior mitral leaflet (A). The anterior mitral leaflet was mildly thickened by fibrous tissue. R, Right; P, posterior; L, left aortic valve cusp.

tion at rest. The mural outflow plaque, however, is often absent (Figs. 5 to 11).

It appears that HCM is primarily a disease of the ventricular septum, and the morphologic abnormalities in it are apparent at the gross, microscopic, and ultrastructural levels. Other portions of the heart, however, are affected in HCM, but it seems likely that these other abnormalities are secondary, at least in part, to the abnormalities of the ventricular septum. These other abnormalities include decreased ventricular cavity size or at least lack of ventricular cavity dilatation, increased atrial cavity size, varying degrees of interstitial and replacement myocardial fibrosis (Fig. 12), particularly in the ventricular septum, thickening of the posterior as well as the anterior mitral leaflet, and in elderly patients, calcification of the mitral anulus.

The cause of the relatively small sizes

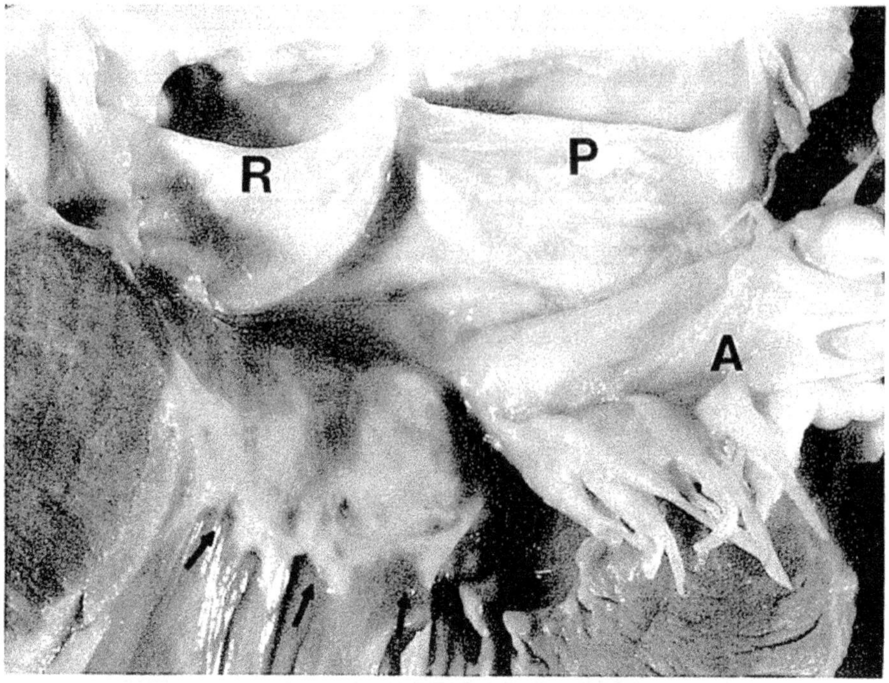

Fig. 2. Opened left ventricular outflow tract and aortic valve of a 56-year-old man who died suddenly in bed shortly after awaking. Sudden death was his first and only symptom of hypertrophic cardiomyopathy. On routine physical examination to obtain a commercial pilot's license, he was found to have a precordial murmur. Echocardiogram had disclosed the maximal thickness of the ventricular septum to be greater than that of the left ventricular free wall, and the ventricles were not dilated. At necropsy, the heart weighed 670 g, and a mural fibrous plaque (arrows) was present in the left ventricular outflow tract in apposition to the anterior mitral leaflet (A), which was thickened by fibrous tissue. R, Right and P, posterior aortic valve cusp.

of the ventricular cavities in HCM is unclear. The septum, being on average about twice normal thickness, surely occupies space normally represented by cavity. Furthermore, the ventricular free walls, on average about one third thicker than normal, also probably compromise the intracavitary space slightly. Additionally, the greater thickness of the septum makes this structure relatively noncompliant, as shown by its absent or minimal movement on echocardiogram. Although the left ventricular free wall in HCM (by echocardiogram) usually contracts vigorously, in contrast to the septum, it appears to have little capacity to distend outwardly. Whatever the explanation, ventricular cavity size is infrequently enlarged in these patients. Those with dilated ventricular cavities have either unscarred left or right ventricular free walls of normal thickness or scarred ventricular free walls of less than normal thickness. Left ventricular dilatation also may occur after operative septotomy-septectomy in HCM.

The impression of ventricular cavity size, as observed at necropsy in patients with HCM, may be misleading because the cavity at necropsy in patients with

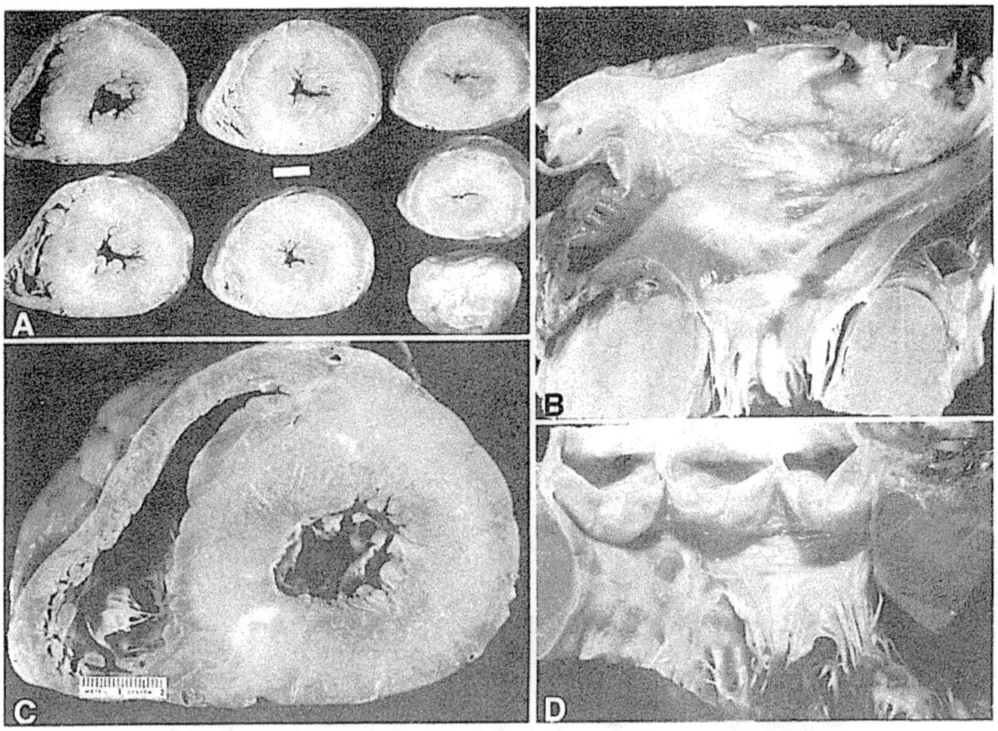

Fig. 3. Heart of a 53-year-old man who died suddenly at home. At age 33, he was found to have labile systemic hypertension. At age 45, although still asymptomatic, cardiac catheterization disclosed an 8-mm Hg peak systolic pressure difference between left ventricle (150/10 mm Hg) and radial artery (142/73 mm Hg) and a 69-mm Hg gradient with provocation. Symptoms of cardiac dysfunction (dyspnea) began at age 47, when his indirect systemic arterial pressure was 170/110 mm Hg. Episodes of dizziness and angina occurred in his fifties. Atrial fibrillation appeared 6 weeks before his sudden death. At necropsy, the heart weighed 750 g. *A,* Transverse sections of the cardiac ventricles disclosed no cavity dilatation, and the septum and left ventricular free wall were of similar thickness. *B,* View of the opened and dilated left atrium and of the atrial aspect of the anterior mitral leaflet, which is thickened. *C,* View of the cardiac base at the level of the distal margins of the mitral leaflets; a small scar is present in the septum posteriorly. *D,* Opened left ventricular outflow tract showing a mural endocardial fibrous plaque in apposition to the thickened anterior mitral leaflet.

HCM represents the size at the end of ventricular systole. This information was derived by comparing the left ventricular free wall thickness at necropsy to that measured by echocardiogram during life. The thickness at necropsy corresponds to the thickness during ventricular systole, not diastole, as observed by echocardiogram.[14]

In contrast to the ventricular cavities, the atrial cavities in HCM, at least in adults, are always dilated. The dilatation appears to be a response to difficulty in filling the relatively small ventricular cavities.

Not only is the anterior mitral leaflet thickened, but often, more frequently in patients with outflow obstruction, the posterior mitral leaflet is also. The thickening of both mitral leaflets is probably

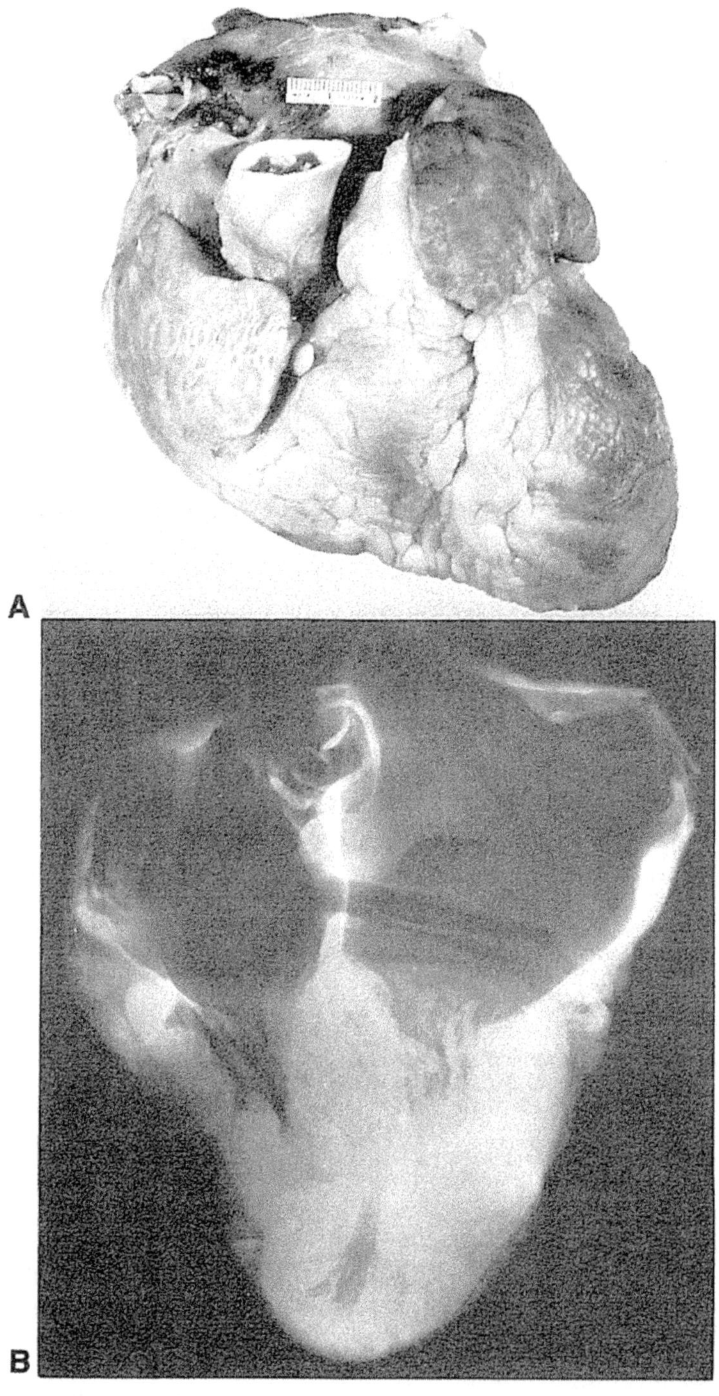

Fig. 4. Photograph of heart anteriorly (*A*) and radiograph of the heart specimen (*B*) of a 43-year-old woman who died of progressive congestive heart failure. At cardiac catheterization when 33 years old, she had a 54-mm Hg peak systolic pressure gradient at rest between the left ventricle (146/18 mm Hg) and a systemic artery (92/56 mm Hg). Both her mother and 2 siblings died of hypertrophic cardiomyopathy. She had had evidence of congestive heart failure for many years and atrial fibrillation for at least 6 years. At necropsy, the heart weighed only 310 g, but the patient weighed only 40 kg. Both atria were huge, and neither ventricular cavity was dilated. A mural endocardial plaque was present in the left ventricular outflow tract in apposition to the thickened anterior mitral leaflet. The maximal thickness of both ventricular septum and left ventricular free wall was similar.

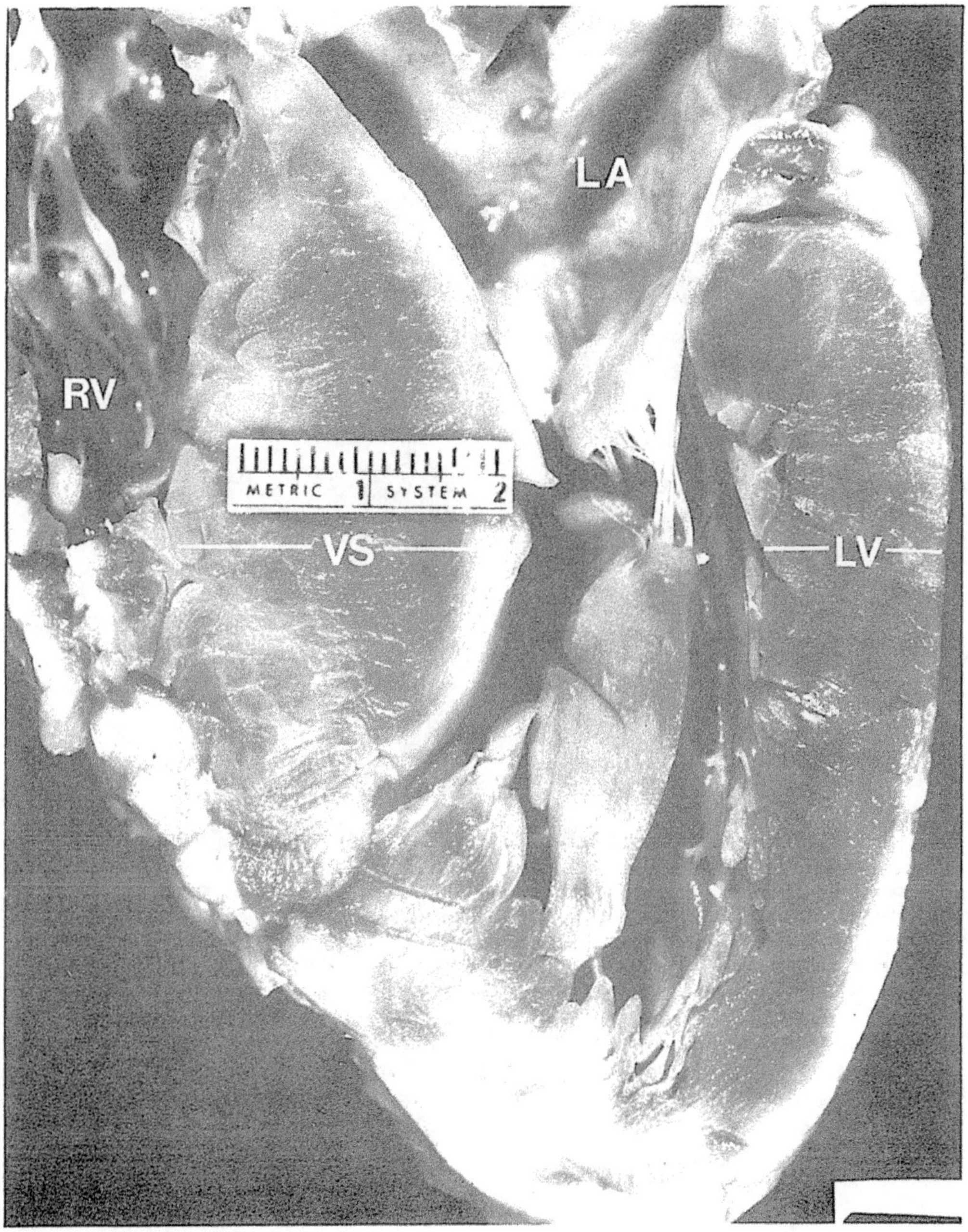

Fig. 5. Longitudinal view of the heart of a 12-year-old girl who died suddenly. Sudden death was her first and last symptom of hypertrophic cardiomyopathy, which was not known to have been present clinically. At necropsy, the heart weighed 275 g. Both atria were dilated; both ventricles were slightly dilated. The maximal thickness of the ventricular septum (VS) was 26 mm and that of the left ventricular (LV) free wall 14 mm. The mitral valve was normal, and no mural endocardial plaque was present in the left ventricular outflow tract. LA, Left atrium; RV, right ventricle.

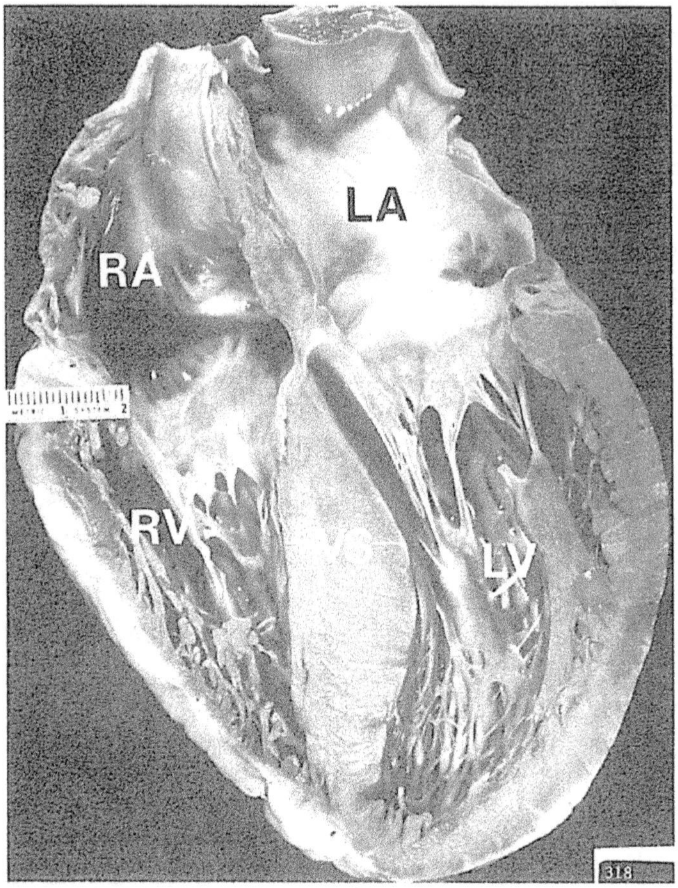

Fig. 6. Longitudinal cut of the heart of a 16-year-old girl who died suddenly while jogging. Her mother had symptomatic (angina) hypertrophic cardiomyopathy, nonobstructive, and she was 45 years old. A maternal aunt had died at 3 months of age; 3 siblings had died at 4, 10, and 13 years of age, and all had documented hypertrophic cardiomyopathy. The child whose heart is shown here had been asymptomatic, but by echocardiogram, the ventricular septum was 14 mm thick, and the left ventricular free wall was 8 mm thick. Systolic anterior motion of the anterior mitral leaflet had been present. The photograph shows that all 4 cavities are dilated, the ventricular septum (VS) is much thicker than the left ventricular (LV) free wall, and the mitral valve is normal. No endocardial mural plaque was present in the left ventricular outflow tract. LA, Left atrium; RA, right atrium; RV, right ventricle.

the consequence of the small left ventricular cavity. The mitral valve resides in the left ventricle, which, being small, causes abnormal contact of the leaflets with themselves and also causes the anterior leaflet to contact the septum. In the patients without obstruction, the basal portion of the left ventricular cavity is larger than in the patients with obstruction because of the thinning of the basal portion of free wall posteriorly and laterally. The focal fibrous thickening of the posterior mitral leaflet probably results from abnormal contact during ventricular systole because there is not enough room in the ventricular cavity to accom-

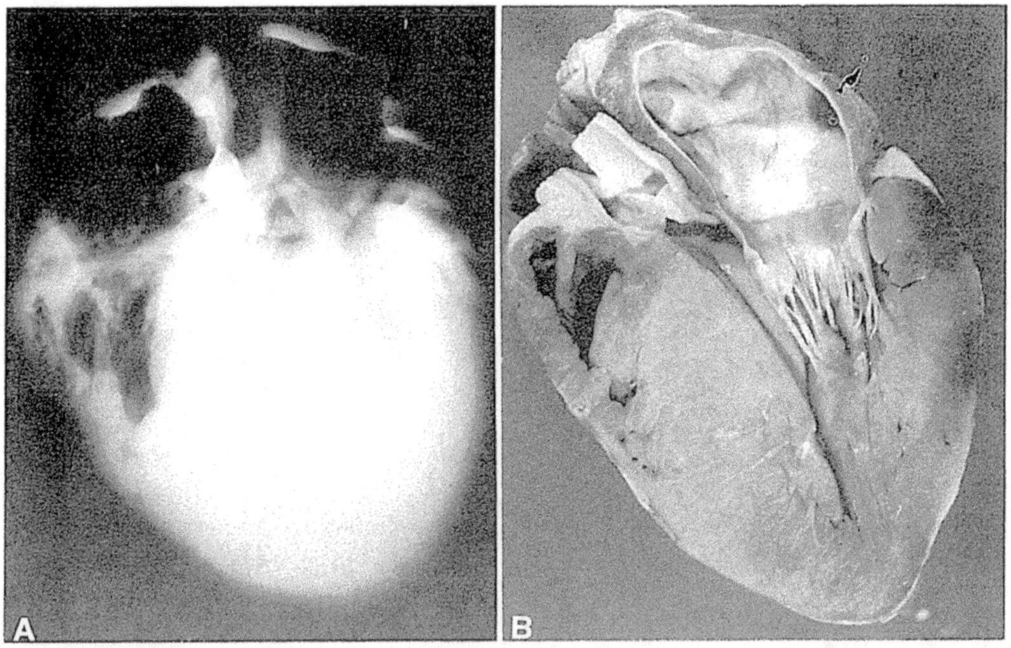

Fig. 7. Radiograph of heart specimen (*A*) and longitudinal cut of heart (*B*) of a previously asymptomatic 18-year-old woman who died suddenly at home shortly after running up some stairs. Her father, a paternal uncle, and a sister had hypertrophic cardiomyopathy. On echocardiogram, the ventricular septum was 35 mm thick, and the left ventricular free wall, 8 mm thick. Systolic anterior motion of the anterior mitral leaflet was absent. The heart weighed 490 g. The radiograph shows the small ventricular cavities and the massiveness of the ventricular myocardium. The right view shows the septum (35 mm) to be much thicker than the left ventricular free wall (10 mm), the mitral leaflets to be normal, and the absence of a left ventricular mural endocardial plaque in apposition to the anterior mitral leaflet.

modate the leaflets and chordae easily. The ventricle and mitral leaflets in this respect may be regarded as similar to an accordion. The mitral leaflet thickening in HCM is analogous to that which occurs normally as a consequence of aging. With aging, the left ventricular cavity becomes smaller, presumably in response to increased work required to fill the small left ventricle. Similar mechanisms appear to be accelerated in HCM.

Most patients with HCM have some degree of mitral regurgitation. It is not related to annular dilatation because the mitral anulus in this condition is not dilated. Furthermore, the leaflet thickening, in and of itself, is not extensive enough to cause valvular regurgitation. The most likely explanation appears to be abnormal bending of the papillary muscles, particularly the anterolateral one. These structures may be bent abnormally by the bulging ventricular septum, with resulting excessive tension on the chordae tendineae preventing closure of the mitral orifice. Although they are usually present in the papillary muscles in HCM, focal scars cannot account for the regurgitation. Although it is usually mild in HCM, mitral regurgitation may be the dominant clinical feature of this condition. Despite its advocacy by some in-

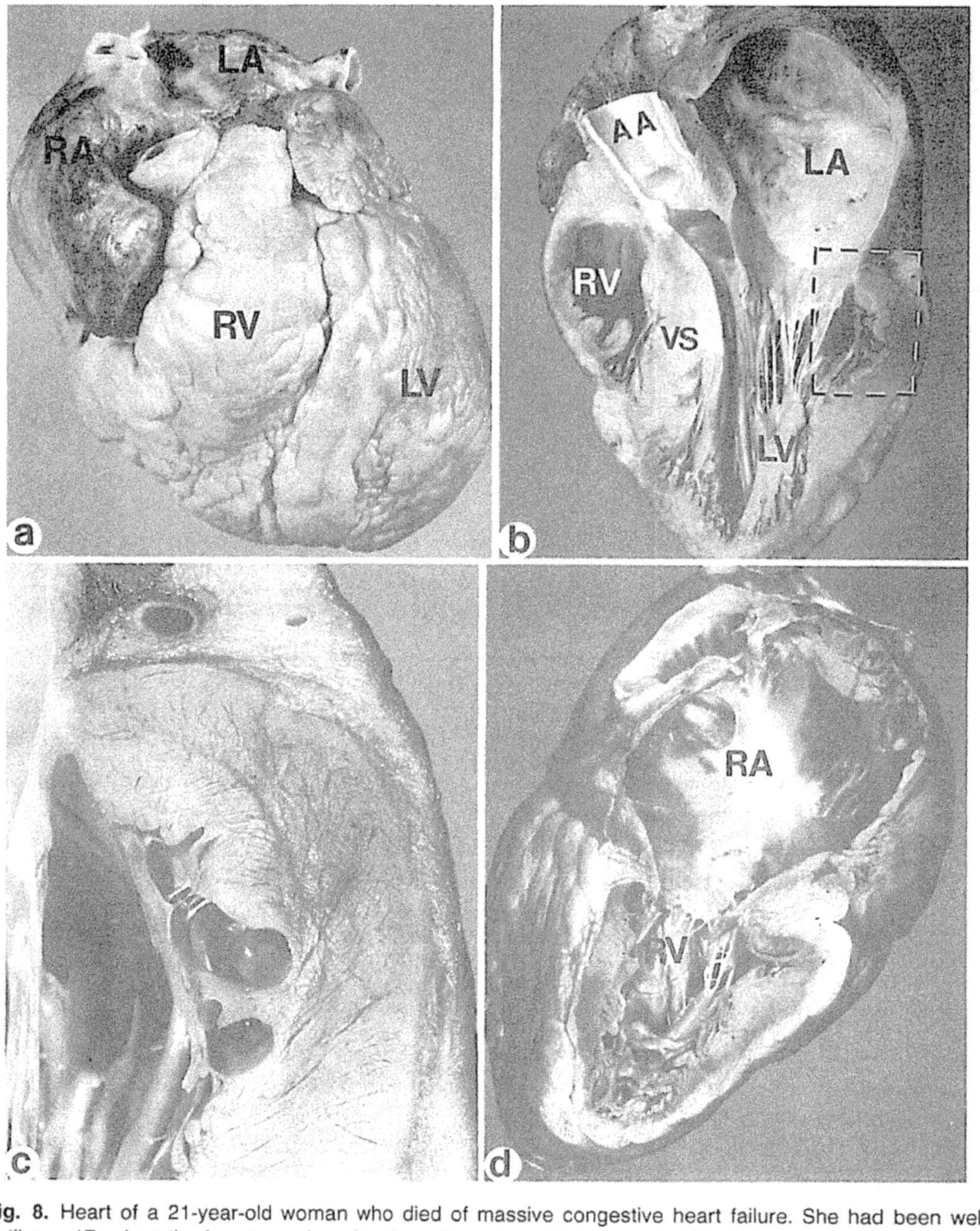

Fig. 8. Heart of a 21-year-old woman who died of massive congestive heart failure. She had been well until age 17, when the heart was found to be enlarged and the electrocardiogram to be abnormal. Echocardiogram showed the ventricular septum (26 mm) to be thicker than the left ventricular free wall (11 mm) and the ventricular cavities to be of normal size. Systolic anterior motion of the anterior mitral leaflet was present, and the left atrial diameter was 48 mm. At 2 cardiac catheterizations, no peak systolic outflow pressure gradient was present either at rest or on provocation. Atrial fibrillation appeared about a year before death. No other family members had hypertrophic cardiomyopathy. At necropsy, the heart weighed 410 g. *a,* Exterior view; both the right (RA) and the left atrium (LA) are dilated; extensive adipose tissue covers the right (RV) and the left ventricle (LV). *b,* Longitudinal view of the heart; the ventricular septum (VS) is thicker than the left ventricular free wall; the left atrium is dilated, and the ascending aorta (AA) is of normal size. *c,* A close-up of the rectangular, dotted area in *b;* when the free wall behind the posterior mitral leaflet is thinner (0.8 cm) than the free wall more caudally, left ventricular outflow obstruction is nearly always absent. *d,* Longitudinal view of the dilated right atrium and the right ventricle.

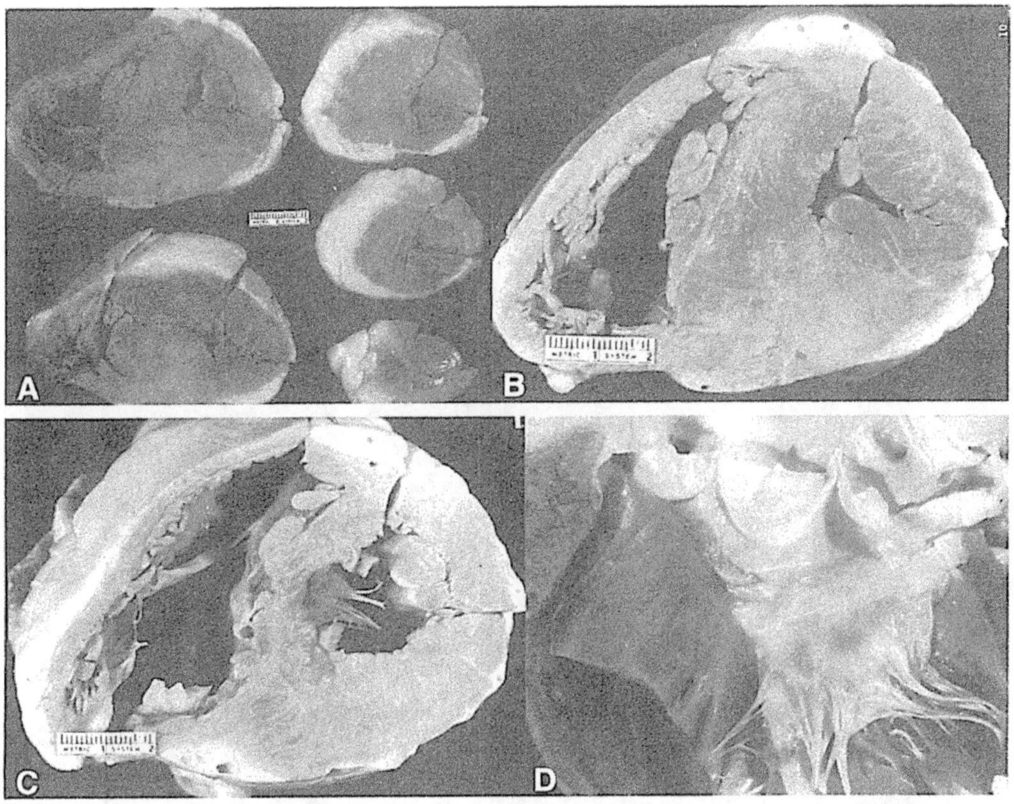

Fig. 9. Heart of a 26-year-old woman who died suddenly outside the hospital. Several family members also had hypertrophic cardiomyopathy. At necropsy, the heart weighed approximately 500 g. *A*, Transverse sections of the ventricles showing the cavities to be of normal size and the septum to be thicker than the left ventricular free wall. *B*, Close-up of a section not shown in *A*. *C*, Basal section showing the septum at this level to be thinner than the left ventricular free wall. *D*, Opened left ventricular outflow tract and aortic valve showing the mitral valve to be normal and the absence of a mural endocardial outflow plaque. The ventricular septum in this patient was thicker in the apical half than in the basal half.

vestigators,[52-55] mitral valve replacement in HCM is potentially hazardous and rarely warranted.[6] The exception is the patient with severe mitral regurgitation from superimposed infective endocarditis, a condition not rare in patients with HCM. The small left ventricular cavity makes mitral valve replacement difficult, and the small cavity may prevent a prosthesis or bioprosthesis in the mitral position from functioning properly. Furthermore, the mitral regurgitation in patients with HCM, except when due to valvular damage from infective endocarditis, nearly always either disappears or is strikingly lessened by adequate partial septectomy and septotomy.

GROSS MORPHOLOGIC DIFFERENCES BY AGE AND SEX

Patients with HCM can die in any decade of life. Figure 13 presents the ages of

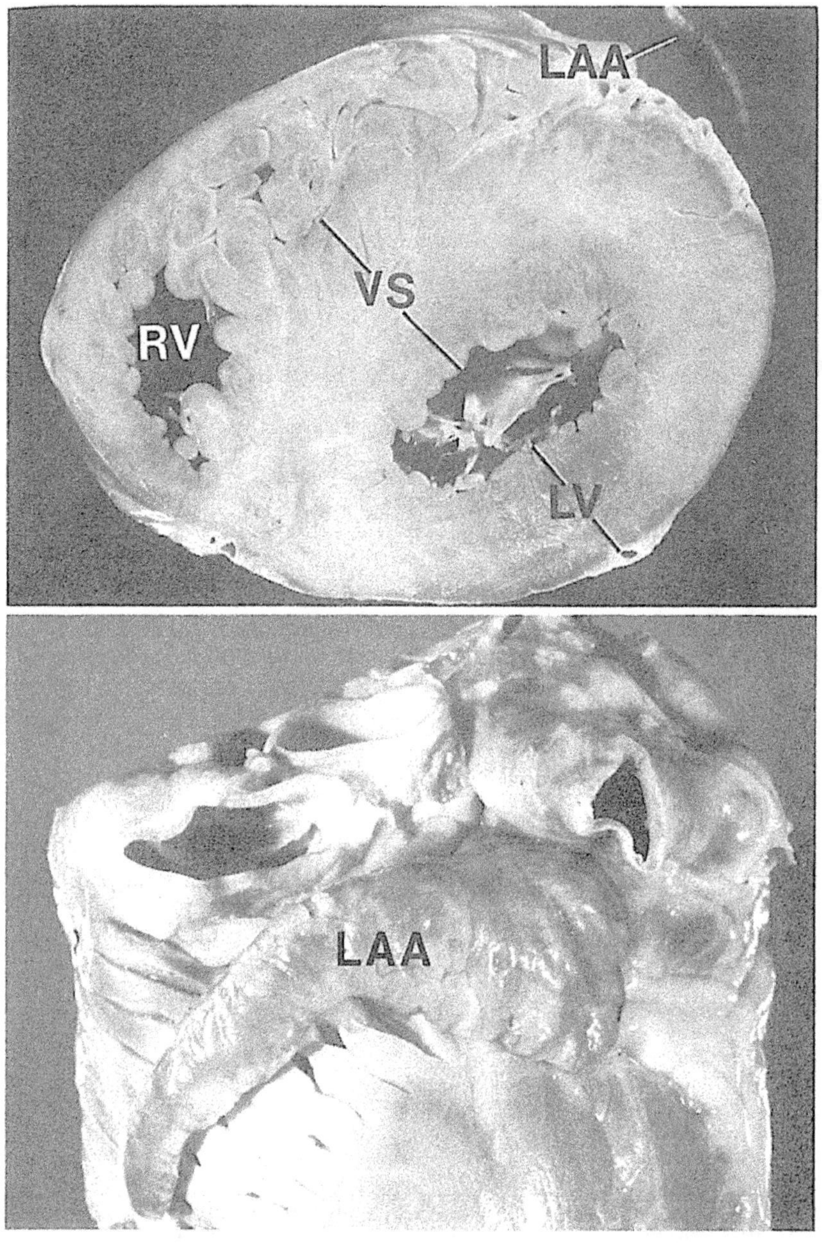

Fig. 10. Heart of a 28-year-old man in whom sudden death was the first and only manifestation of hypertrophic cardiomyopathy, which was not diagnosed clinically. At necropsy, the heart weighed 970 g. *A*, Transverse section of the ventricles at the level of the margins of the mitral leaflets; the septum is 35 mm, and the left ventricular free wall is 20 mm thick; the mitral valve is normal, and the mural endocardium of the left ventricular outflow tract is normal. LAA, Left atrial appendage; LV, left ventricular wall; VS, ventricular septum; RV, right ventricular cavity. *B*, View of the dilated left atrial appendage, which has a tail-like appearance.

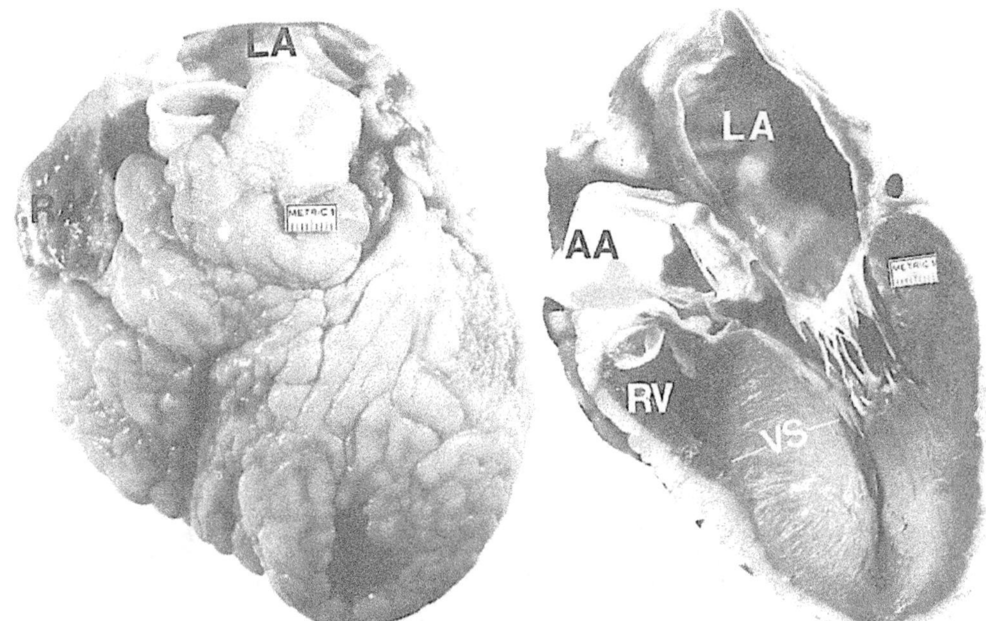

Fig. 11. Heart of a 38-year-old woman who died suddenly at home. At least 6 other members of her family also had hypertrophic cardiomyopathy. She had had episodic chest pain since age 18; by age 36, she was having 20 to 30 episodes of chest pain daily. At catheterization on 3 occasions, no left ventricular outflow obstruction was present. By echocardiogram, systolic anterior motion of the anterior mitral leaflet was absent. At necropsy, the heart weighed 460 g. *A*, Exterior of the heart showing considerable subepicardial fat. RA, Right atrium; LA, left atrium. *B*, Longitudinal view of the heart. The septum measures about 25 mm, and the left ventricular free wall is about 19 mm in maximal thickness. Neither ventricular cavity is dilated, but right and left atria are dilated. The mitral valve is normal, and there is no thickening of mural endocardium in the left ventricular outflow tract. AA, Ascending aorta; RV, right ventricle; VS, ventricular septum.

death by decade of the 220 patients studied in the Pathology Branch of the National Heart, Lung, and Blood Institute. In the first 2 decades of life, a higher percentage of the necropsied patients were male, whereas most necropsy patients over 60 years of age were women. Between 20 and 60 years of age, the percentage of males and females among necropsied patients was similar.

Among the 220 patients studied at necropsy, 145 had not had a cardiac operation, and 75 had undergone such a procedure. The 145 patients with unoperated HCM were separated into 3 groups according to the age of death (Table 2). In the 118 patients who died from ages 11 to 70 years, the diagnosis of HCM at necropsy was not difficult. In the 13 extremely young (age ≤ 10 years) and in the 14 oldest patients (age >70 years), however, diagnosis of HCM both clinically and at necropsy was usually difficult. Tables 3 and 4 present clinical and morphologic findings in the 13 patients ≤ 10 years of age and the 14 patients >70 years of age at death, respectively.

In all 13 patients who died at <10 years of age (see Table 3; Figs. 14 to 16), the heart at necropsy was increased in

TABLE 2. CLINICAL AND CARDIAC MORPHOLOGIC CHARACTERISTICS IN 3 DIFFERENT AGE GROUPS OF 145 NECROPSY PATIENTS WITH UNOPERATED HYPERTROPHIC CARDIOMYOPATHY

Group	Age (yr)	Number of Patients	Age (yr) Range (mean)	Males/ females	Heart weight (g) Range (mean)	VS > LV	Fibrous Plaque, LVOT	Thickened MV	Dilated LV Cavity	Gross Fibrosis LV/VS	Epicardial CAD
I	≤10	13	0.2–9	8/5	28–670 (190) (male = 256) (female = 57)	9/13 (69%)	2/13 (15%)	3/13 (23%)	4/13 (31%)	0/13 (0)	0/13 (0)
II	11–70	118	11–70 (35)	63/55	250–1250 (559) (male = 606) (female = 506)	82/115 (71%)	69/110 (63%)	73/110 (66%)	22/118 (19%)	53/118 (45%)	9/114 (8%)
III	>70	14	71–87 (79)	3/11	265–710 (468) (men = 558) (women = 443)	11/14 (79%)	12/14 (86%)	14/14 (100%)	1/14 (7%)	7/14 (50%)	7/14 (50%)
	TOTALS or MEAN	145	(36)	74/71	(526) (men = 574) (women = 476)	102/142 (72%)	83/137 (61%)	90/137 (66%)	27/145 (19%)	60/145 (41%)	16/141 (11%)

CAD, Significant coronary artery disease; LV, left ventricular or left ventricle; OT, outflow tract; MV, mitral valve; VS, ventricular septum.

TABLE 3. CLINICAL AND CARDIAC MORPHOLOGIC CHARACTERISTICS OF 13 PATIENTS AGED ≤10 YEARS WITH HYPERTROPHIC CARDIOMYOPATHY

Case	Age	Sex	LV-SA PSG at rest (mm Hg)	HCM Diagnosed During Life	FH of HCM	Mode of Death	Heart Weight (g)	VS > LV	Fibrous Plaque, LVOT	Thickened MV	Dilated LV Cavity	Gross Fibrosis LV/VS	MFD in VS
1	1 mo	M	—	0*	0	Operation†	—	+	0	0	0	0	—
2	1 mo	M	—	0*	0	CHF	80	0	+	+	0	0	+
3	2 mo	M	—	0*	—	Unknown	50	+	0	+	0	0	+
4‡	2 mo	F	0	0*	0	CHF	62	+	0	0	+§	0	+
5	2 mo	F	—	+	0	Sudden	28	+	0	0	0	0	—
6	6 mo	F	—	0*	0	Sudden	80	0	0	0	0	0	+
7	7 mo	F	100	+	0	Procedure∥	—	+	+	+	0	0	—
8	9 mo	F	—	+	0	Pneumonia	—	+	0	0	0	0	+
9	12 mo	M	—	0*	0	CHF	270	+	0	0	0	0	+
10	18 mo	M	0	0*	0	Unknown	—	+	0	0	+	0	—
11	7 yr	M	0	0*	0	Sudden	227	+	0	0	+	0	+
12	9 yr	M	0	0*	0	Sudden	240	0	0	0	+#	0	+
13	9 yr	M	0	+	0	Sudden	670	0	0	0	0	0	—

* Heart disease diagnosed, but not hypertrophic cardiomyopathy.

† This patient underwent operative ligation of the left main coronary artery for presumed anomalous origin from the pulmonary trunk; no coronary anomaly was found at necropsy.

‡Case reported by Maron, B. J., et al.: Am. Heart J., *101*:857, 1981.

§ This patient had complete heart block from birth and the cavity dilatation may have resulted from the conduction disturbance.

∥ Right ventricular wall perforated during endomyocardial biopsy producing hemopericardium.

\# Left ventricular cavity normal in size at angiogram several months before death.

CHF, Congestive heart failure; F, female; FH, family history; HCM, hypertrophic cardiomyopathy; LV, left ventricle or left ventricular; LVOT, left ventricular outflow tract; M, male; MFD, myocardial fiber disorganization; MV, mitral valve; PSG, peak systolic gradient; SA, systemic artery; VS, ventricular septum; +, present or positive; 0, absent or negative; —, no information available.

TABLE 4. CLINICAL AND CARDIAC MORPHOLOGIC CHARACTERISTICS OF PATIENTS >70 YEARS OF AGE WITH HYPERTROPHIC CARDIOMYOPATHY WITHOUT A CARDIAC OPERATION

Case	Age (yr)	Sex	HCM diagnosed in Life	SH	FH of HCM	Mode of Death	Heart Weight (g)	VS > LV	Thickness VS	Thickness LV	Fibrous Plaque, LVOT	Thickened MV	MAC (0–4)	Dilated LV Cavity	Gross Fibrosis, LV/VS	No. 4 CAs >75% in CSA
1	71	M	0	+	0	NC (C)	710	+	3.5	2.5	0	+	0	0	+	1
2	71	F	+(e)	+	0	CHF	475	+	2.5	1.4	+	+	0	0	0	1
3	73	F	+	—	+	NC (C)	430	0	0.6	1.1	0	+	0	+	+*	0
4	74	F	0	—	0	NC (C)	360	+	2.1	1.5	+	+	1	0	0	0
5	74	F	+	+	0	CHF	650	+	3.7	2.5	+	+	4	0	+	0
6	76	F	+(e)	0	0	Sudden	510	+	1.8	1.4	+	+	2	0	0	1
7	78	M	0	+	0	NC	450	+	—	—	+	+	0	0	+	0
8	79	F	0	0	0	Sudden	430	+	2.5	1.8	+	+	4	0	+	2
9	81	F	0	0	0	NC	265	0	1.2	1.2	+	+	0	0	0	0
10	82	F	+(e)	—	0	Sudden	310	+	2.0	1.5	+	+	2	0	0	1
11	83	F	+(e)	—	0	CHF†	450	+	3.0	2.0	+	+	0	0	0	0
12	84	M	0	0	0	Operation‡	515	0	2.0	2.0	+	+	1	0	+	3
13	86	F	0	+	0	Sudden	520	+	3.0	2.0	+	+	0	0	+	0
14	87	F	+(e)	—	0	NC (C)	470	+	2.5	2.0	+	+	4	0	0	1

* Involves nearly all the ventricular septum.

† Patient also had active infective endocarditis involving the mitral valve.

‡ Patient died shortly after thoracotomy for planned pericardiectomy for suspected pericardial constriction.

NC, Noncardiac; C, cancer; CHF, congestive heart failure; CAs, major epicardial coronary arteries; CSA, cross-sectional area; e, echocardiogram; F, female; FH, family history; HCM, hypertrophic cardiomyopathy; LV, left ventricle; LVOT, left ventricular outflow tract; M, male; MAC, mitral annular calcium; MV, mitral valve; SH, systemic hypertension by history; VS, ventricular septum; +, present or positive; 0, absent or negative; —, no information available.

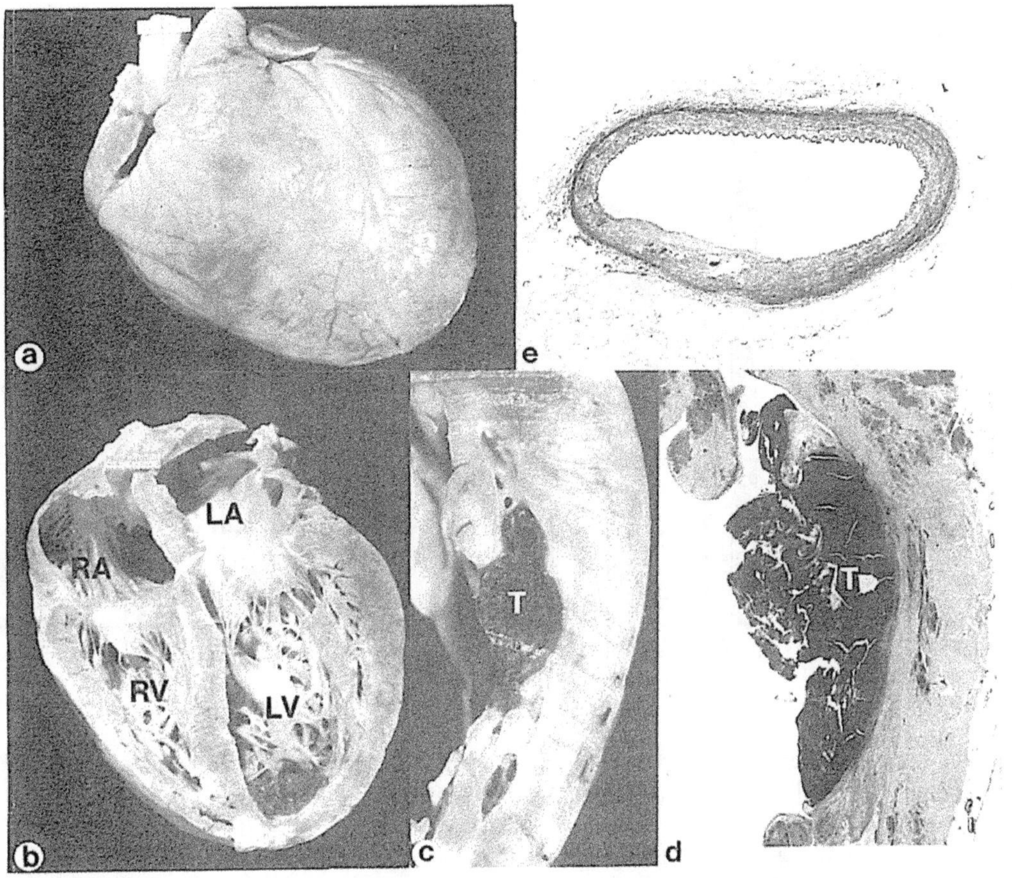

Fig. 12. Heart of a 19-year-old woman who died of progressive congestive heart failure. Her mother and a brother had evidence of hypertrophic cardiomyopathy. At cardiac catheterization when asymptomatic at age 11, the left ventricular cavity was normal in size by angiogram, and a small (<30 mm Hg) pressure gradient was present on provocation, but not at rest. Exertional dyspnea began at age 12 and slowly progressed thereafter. Two months before death, she had acute pulmonary edema. A month before death, echocardiogram disclosed the left ventricular cavity to be 57 mm in transverse diameter in end-diastole and 50 mm in end-systole; the left atrium was 42 mm, and the ejection fraction was 30%. The maximal thickness of the ventricular septum and left ventricular free wall were similar. *a*, Heart from the anterior view. *b*, Four-chamber view showing a dilated right (RV) and left (LV) ventricle and a lesser dilated right (RA) and left (LA) atrium. *c*, Longitudinal view of severely scarred left ventricular free wall with a superimposed thrombus (T). *d*, Photomicrograph of a portion of the wall shown in *c;* only a few islands of myocardial cells remain. *e*, Left main coronary artery; all major epicardial coronary arteries were normal.

weight. The thickness of the septum was greater than that of the left ventricular free wall in 9 patients (69%), a percentage similar to that in the other age groups. A fibrous plaque in the left ventricular outflow tract, however, was present in only 2 patients (15%), and the mitral valve was thickened in only 3 patients (23%). Furthermore, the left ventricle at necropsy was dilated in 4 patients (31%). No patient had a grossly visible left ventricular or septal scar. In

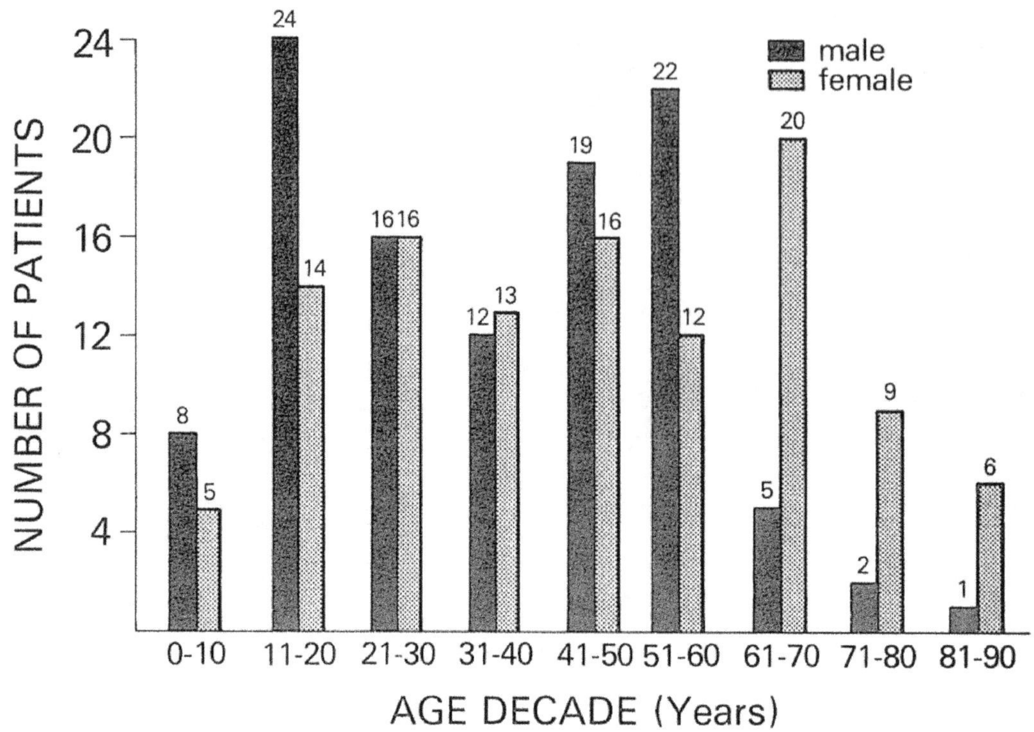

Fig. 13. Ages by decade and sex of the 220 patients with hypertrophic cardiomyopathy studied at necropsy in the Pathology Branch of the National Heart, Lung, and Blood Institute.

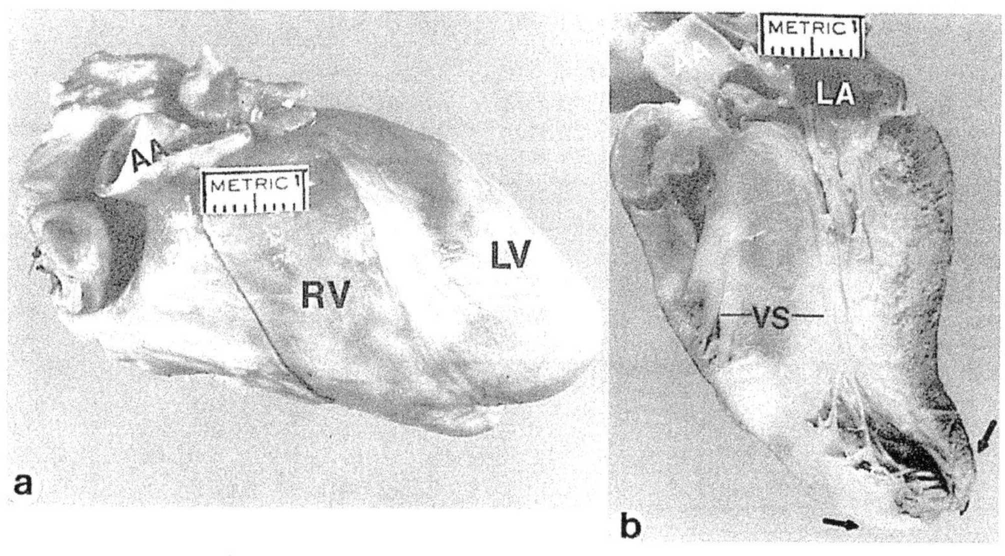

Fig. 14. Heart of a 2-month-old boy who died suddenly. Echocardiogram shortly before death disclosed the ventricular septum to be thicker than the left ventricular free wall, possible systolic anterior motion of the anterior mitral leaflet, hyperdynamic ventricles, and a dilated left atrium. *a*, Exterior of the heart; AA, ascending aorta; LV, left ventricle; RV, right ventricle. *b*, Longitudinal view of the heart showing the ventricular septum (VS) to be thicker than the left ventricular free wall, a thickened mitral valve, but no mural endocardial plaque in the left ventricular outflow tract; LA, left atrium.

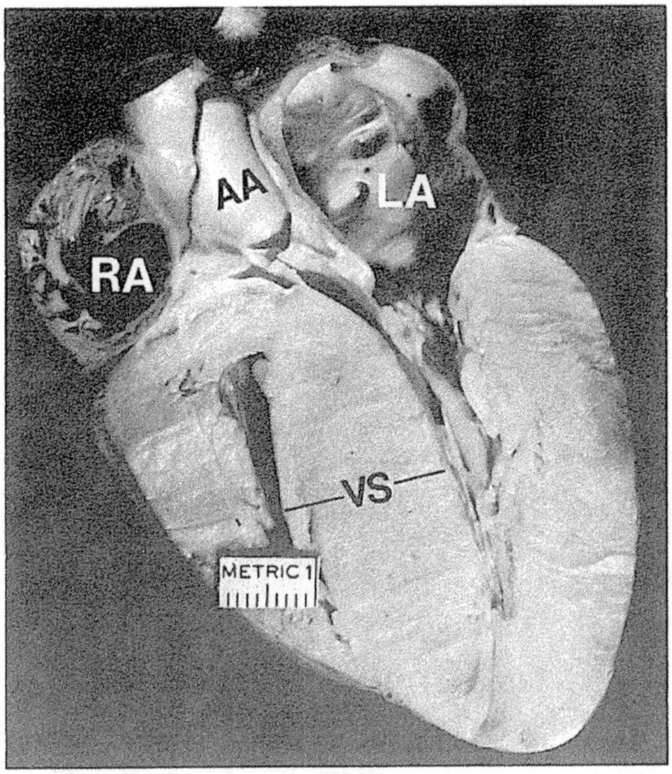

Fig. 15. Longitudinal view of heart of a 7.5-year-old boy who began having grand mal seizures at the age of 4 months and was found to have an enlarged heart with poor ventricular contractions and an abnormal electrocardiogram. A grade 3/6 systolic precordial murmur was recorded. He was found dead in bed. At necropsy, the heart weighed 230 g. Shown here is a longitudinal cut showing the ventricular septum (VS) to be thicker than the left ventricular wall and a dilated right (RA) and left atrium (LA). The mitral valve is normal, and the mural endocardial in apposition to the anterior leaflet is normal. AA, Ascending aorta.

only 4 patients was the diagnosis of HCM made during life, although all 13 were considered clinically to have heart disease.

Of the 14 patients >70 years of age at death, only 3 (21%) were men (Table 4). Diagnosis of HCM was made in 7 of these 14 patients during life. Only 1 patient had a family history of HCM, and 5 had had systemic hypertension. All but 2 patients had a heart of increased weight; the mean increase, however, was not as great as that in the patients aged 11 to 70 years. The maximal thickness of the ventricular septum was greater than that of the left ventricular free wall in 11 patients (79%). The mitral valve was thickened in all 14 patients. A fibrous plaque was present in the left ventricular outflow tract in 12 patients (86%), and the left ventricular cavity was of normal or smaller-than-normal size in 13 patients (93%). Gross left ventricular fibrosis was present in 7 of the 14 elderly patients, and 7 had significant narrowing of 1 or more major epicardial coronary arteries.

In the necropsied patients with HCM aged 11 to 70 years, the numbers of males and females were similar. Heart weight was increased in 113 patients (96%); 71%

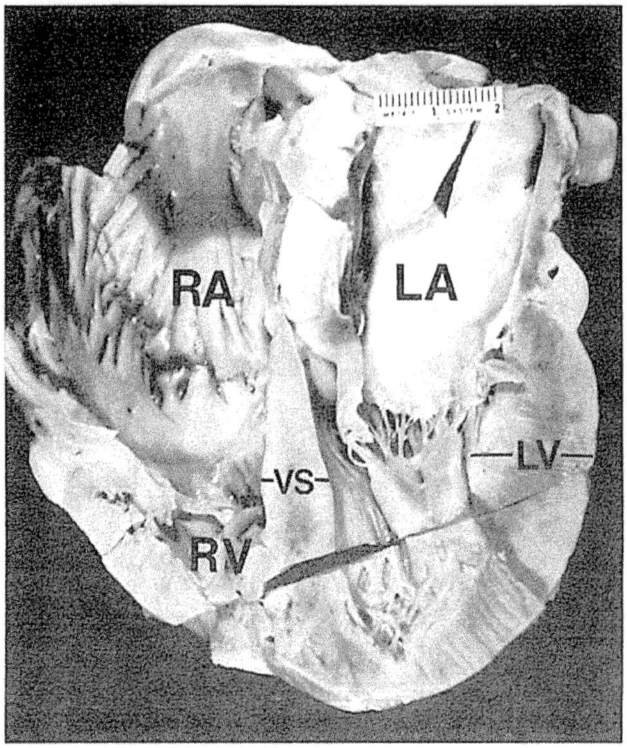

Fig. 16. Four-chamber view of the heart of a 9-year-old boy. He was well until about 1 year before death, when evidence of congestive heart failure appeared, and it rapidly progressed. At catheterization, the following pressures in mm Hg were recorded: right ventricle, 90/27; pulmonary artery 90/60; left ventricle, 90/34, and femoral artery, 105/60. At angiogram, the left ventricular cavity was of normal size, but it contracted poorly. He died suddenly. At necropsy, the heart weighed 240 g. Both the right (RA) and left (LA) atrium are enormously dilated. The ventricular septum (VS) is thinner than the left ventricular (LV) free wall. Neither right (RV) nor left ventricle (LV) is dilated. The 4 valves are normal, and no endocardial mural plaque is present in the left ventricular outflow tract. The cause of the severe pulmonary hypertension is unclear, but it may have been the result of the extremely depressed left ventricular function.

had a septum thicker than the left ventricular free wall; 66% had a thickened mitral valve, and 63% had a fibrous endocardial plaque in the left ventricular outflow tract. The left ventricular cavity was of normal or smaller-than-normal size in 96 patients (81%), and gross left ventricular fibrosis was present in 53 patients (45%). Only 8% of these 113 patients had 1 or more major epicardial coronary arteries severely (>75% decrease in cross-sectional area lumen) narrowed.

OBSTRUCTIVE VERSUS NONOBSTRUCTIVE TYPES

The 145 patients with unoperated HCM were separated into 3 groups (Table 5): those in whom a left ventricular outflow tract gradient was present at rest (group I), absent (group II), and unknown (group III) (cardiac catheterization not performed). Certain morphologic features of the obstructive type (group I) were different from those of the nonob-

TABLE 5. COMPARISON OF CLINICAL AND CARDIAC MORPHOLOGIC CHARACTERISTICS IN 145 UNOPERATED NECROPSY PATIENTS WITH HYPERTROPHIC CARDIOMYOPATHY IN WHOM A LEFT VENTRICULAR OUTFLOW TRACT PRESSURE GRADIENT WAS PRESENT, ABSENT, OR UNKNOWN

Group	LVOT Gradient	Number of Patients	Ages (yr) Range (mean)	M/F	Heart weight (g) Range (mean)	VS > LV	Fibrous Plaque, LVOT	Thickened MV	Dilated LV Cavity	Gross Fibrosis LV/VS	Epicardial CAD
I	Present	32	0.2–70 (43)	11/21	310–1250 (613) (male = 736) (female = 546)	25/32 (78%)	31/32 (97%)	31/32 (97%)	2/32 (6%)	15/32 (47%)	7/32 (22%)
II	Absent	33	0.2–54 (31)	18/15	62–1065 (507) (male = 560) (female = 446)	21/33 (64%)	15/32 (47%)	15/32 (47%)	13/33 (39%)	15/33 (45%)	2/33 (6%)
III	Unknown	80	0.1–87 (35)	45/35	28–1200 (499) (male = 539) (female = 450)	56/77 (73%)	37/73 (51%)	44/73 (60%)	12/80 (15%)	30/80 (38%)	7/76 (9%)
TOTALS or MEAN		145	(36)	74/71	28–1250 (526) (male = 574) (female = 476)	102/142	83/137	90/137	27/145	60/145 (41%)	16/141 (11%)

LVOT, Left ventricular outflow tract; M, male; F, female; VS, ventricular septum; LV, left ventricular or left ventricle; MV, mitral valve; CAD, coronary artery disease.

structive type (group II). The mean heart weights of male and female patients with left ventricular outflow tract gradients were greater than in patients without a gradient, and disproportionately thickened septa also were more common (78% versus 64%). A thickened mitral valve and a fibrous plaque in the left ventricular outflow tract were present in 31 (97%) of 32 patients with a gradient and in 15 (47%) of 32 patients without a gradient. A dilated left ventricular cavity was found more frequently in patients without a gradient (39% versus 6%). The frequency of gross left ventricular fibrosis was similar in both groups, but epicardial coronary artery disease occurred in a higher percentage of patients with the obstructive type.

Cardiac catheterization was not done in 80 of the 145 patients with unoperated HCM. This group presumably included both obstructive and nonobstructive types, and as expected, the frequency of disproportionately thickened septa, fibrous plaque in the outflow tract, thickened mitral valve, and nondilated left ventricular cavity were between those of groups I and II.

CARDIAC MORPHOLOGIC FEATURES AFTER OPERATIVE TREATMENT

Of the 220 necropsy patients with HCM, 75 underwent operative treatment: partial septal myectomy in 66 (Fig. 17); septal myotomy alone in 4; and mitral valve replacement in 7. The patients were separated into 3 groups according to length of survival after operation (Table 6). Thirty-seven patients survived ≤ 60 days; 15 patients, 61 days to 42 months; and 23 patients, >42 months. The average age of death for all 75 patients was 47 years. In the patients who died ≤ 60 days after operation, a disproportionately high number were women, and the mean left ventricular outflow tract gradient preoperatively was higher than in those who survived longer periods. A fibrous plaque in the left ventricular outflow tract and a thickened mitral valve were present in $>90\%$ of patients who underwent operation. An impressive morphologic change after operation was dilation of the left ventricular cavity. Only 2 of 52 patients who died ≤ 42 months after operation had dilated left ventricular cavities, whereas 16 (73%) of 22 patients who survived >42 months after operation had dilated left ventricular cavities.

SUMMARY

The morphologic features of 220 patients with HCM are described. The major gross morphologic features of HCM, in order of decreasing frequency, are as follows: (1) dilated atria (100%); (2) increased heart weight (95%); (3) nondilated left ventricle (79%); (4) thickened mitral valve (75%); (5) fibrous endocardial mural plaque, left ventricular outflow tract (72%); and (6) a ventricular septum thicker than the left ventricular free wall (69%). Gross left ventricular fibrosis occurred in 42% of the patients and rarely was a consequence of associated narrowing of an epicardial coronary artery disease. HCM may cause death in any decade of life. The diagnosis of HCM in the extremely young (age ≤ 10 years) and the extremely old (age >70) is more difficult clinically and at necropsy than in the intermediate age group. Patients with the obstructive type of HCM usually have larger hearts, a higher frequency of a fibrous plaque in the left ventricular outflow tract, and a higher frequency of a thickened mitral valve than those without obstruction. Left ventricular cavity dilation is present in about 20% of patients with HCM and is a result of either operation (with survival >42 months) or extensive left ventricular wall scarring.

TABLE 6. CLINICAL AND CARDIAC MORPHOLOGIC CHARACTERISTICS OF 75 NECROPSY PATIENTS WITH HYPERTROPHIC CARDIOMYOPATHY WHO HAD CARDIAC OPERATIVE TREATMENT

Group	Survival After Operation	Number of Patients	Age (yr) Range (mean)	Males/ females	LV-SA PSG at Rest (mm Hg) Range (mean)	Cardiac Operation		
						Septal Myotomy	Septal Myectomy	MVR
I	≤60 days	37	18–69 (48)	13/24	0–162 (70)	0	32	5
II	61 days–42 mo	15	22–72 (47)	8/7	0–130 (50)	2	13	0
III	>42 mo	23	21–81 (47)	13/10	0–130 (48)	2	21	2
TOTAL		75	18–81 (47)	34/41	0–162 (61)	4	66	7

Interval 0 to Death Range (mean)	Heart weight (g) Range (mean)	VS > LV	Fibrous Plaque, LVOT	Thickened MV	Dilated LV Cavity	Gross Fibrosis LV/VS	Epicardial CAD
0–57 days (6)	290–1070 (582) (men = 733) (women = 500)	23/37 (62%)	31/35 (89%)	32/35 (91%)	2/37 (5%)	12/37 (32%)	10/37 (27%)
2–39 months (20)	450–870 (603) (men = 678) (women = 517)	10/15 (67%)	15/15 (100%)	15/15 (100%)	0/15 (0)	6/15 (40%)	4/15 (27%)
47–204 months (111)	550–1150 (718) (men = 717) (women = 718)	13/21 (62%)	20/21 (95%)	17/18 (94%)	16/22 (73%)	14/21 (67%)	4/22 (18%)
0–204 months (38)	290–1150 (628)	46/73 (63%)	66/71 (93%)	64/68 (94%)	18/74 (24%)	32/73 (44%)	18/74 (24%)

MVR, Mitral valve replacement; 0, cardiac operation; PSG, peak systolic gradient; SA, systemic artery; LV, left ventricular or left ventricle; VS, ventricular septum; LVOT, left ventricular outflow tract; CAD, coronary artery disease.

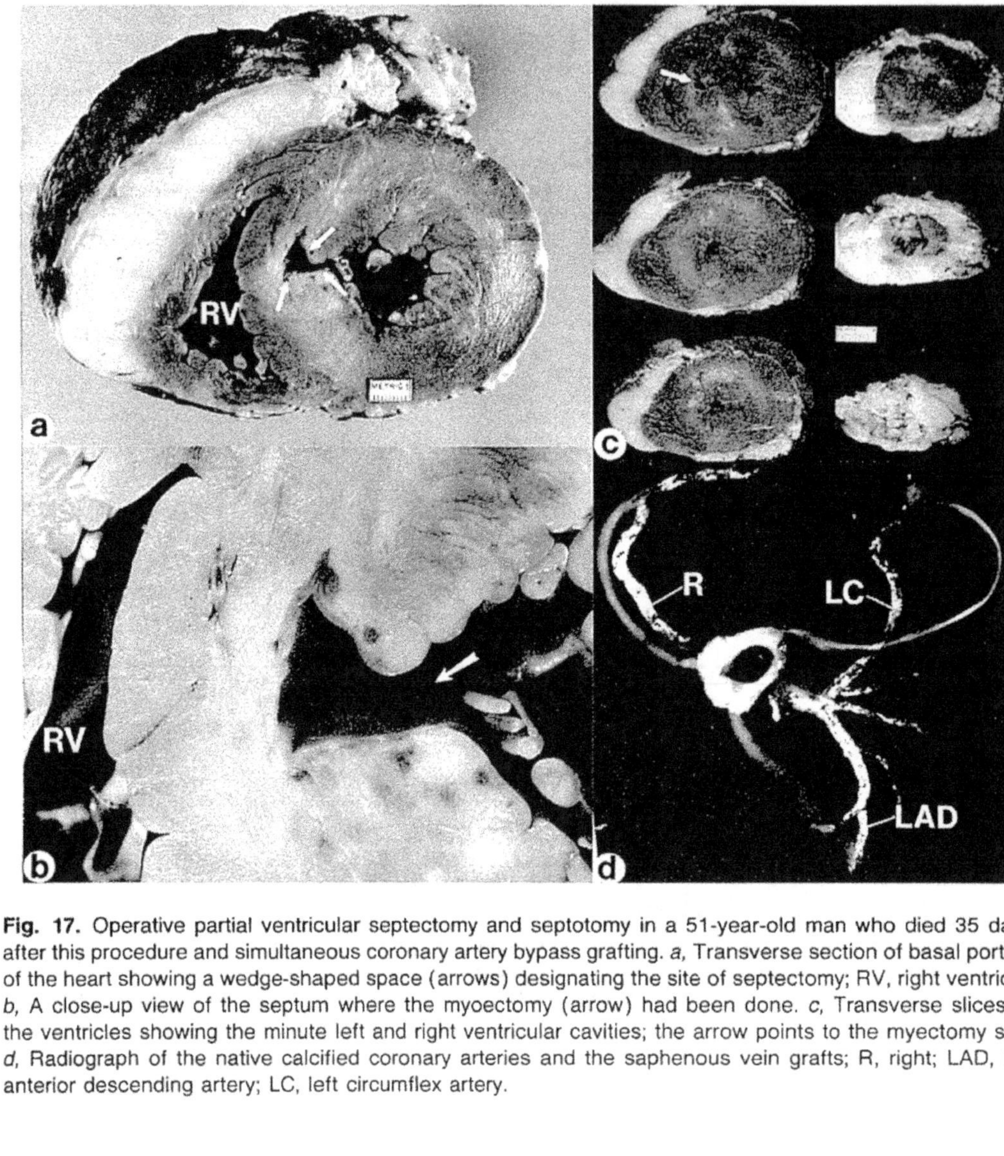

Fig. 17. Operative partial ventricular septectomy and septotomy in a 51-year-old man who died 35 days after this procedure and simultaneous coronary artery bypass grafting. *a,* Transverse section of basal portion of the heart showing a wedge-shaped space (arrows) designating the site of septectomy; RV, right ventricle. *b,* A close-up view of the septum where the myoectomy (arrow) had been done. *c,* Transverse slices of the ventricles showing the minute left and right ventricular cavities; the arrow points to the myectomy site. *d,* Radiograph of the native calcified coronary arteries and the saphenous vein grafts; R, right; LAD, left anterior descending artery; LC, left circumflex artery.

REFERENCES

1. Menges, H., Jr., Brandenburg, R.O., and Brown, A.L., Jr.: The clinical, hemodynamic, and pathologic diagnosis of muscular subvalvular aortic stenosis. Circulation, *24:*1126, 1961.
2. Ewy, G.A., et al.: Muscular subaortic stenosis: clinical and pathologic observations in an elderly patient. Am. J. Cardiol., *22:*126, 1968.
3. Buja, L.M., and Roberts, W.C.: Pulmonary parenchymal ossific nodules in idiopathic hypertrophic subaortic stenosis. Am. J. Cardiol., *25:*710, 1970.
4. Ferrans, V.J., Morrow, A.G., and Roberts, W.C.: Myocardial ultrastructure in idiopathic hypertrophic subaortic stenosis: a study of operatively excised left ventricular outflow tract muscle in 14 patients. Circulation, *45:*769, 1972.
5. Roberts, W.C.: Valvular, subvalvular and supravalvular aortic stenosis: morphologic features. Cardiovasc. Clin., *5:*104, 1973.
6. Roberts, W.C.: Operative treatment of hypertrophic obstructive cardiomyopathy. Am. J. Cardiol., *32:*377, 1973.

7. Roberts, W.C., and Ferrans, V.J.: Morphologic observations in the cardiomyopathies. *In* Myocardial Disease. Edited by N.O. Fowler. New York, Grune & Stratton, 1973, p. 59.
8. Roberts, W.C., and Ferrans, V.J.: Pathological aspects of certain cardiomyopathies. Circulation, *34/35* (Suppl. 2): 128, 1974.
9. Maron, B.J., et al.: Differences in distribution of myocardial abnormalities in patients with obstructive and nonobstructive asymmetric septal hypertrophy (ASH): light and electron microscopic findings. Circulation, *50:*436, 1974.
10. Roberts, W.C., and Ferrans, V.J.: Pathologic anatomy of the cardiomyopathies: idiopathic dilated and hypertrophic types, infiltrates types, and endomyocardial disease with and without eosinophilia. Hum. Pathol. *6:*287, 1975.
11. Epstein, S.E., et al.: Asymmetric septal hypertrophy. Ann. Intern. Med., *81:*650, 1974.
12. McReynolds, R.A., and Roberts, W.C.: The intramural coronary arteries in hypertrophic cardiomyopathy. (Abstract.) Am. J. Cardiol., *35:*154, 1975.
13. Maron, B.J., et al.: Asymmetric septal hypertrophy in childhood. Circulation, *53:*9, 1976.
14. Maron, B.J., Henry, W.L., Roberts, W.C., and Epstein, S.E.: Comparison of echocardiographic and necropsy measurements of ventricular wall thicknesses in patients with and without disproportionate septal thickening. Circulation, *55:*341, 1977.
15. Maron, B.J., et al.: Prevalence and characteristics of disproportionate ventricular septal thickening in patients with acquired or congenital heart diseases. Circulation, *55:*489, 1977.
16. Maron, B.J., et al.: Left ventricular outflow tract obstruction due to systolic anterior motion of the anterior mitral leaflet in patients with concentric left ventricular hypertrophy. Circulation, *57:*528, 1978.
17. Spray, T.L., et al.: A discussion of hypertrophic cardiomyopathy. Am. Heart J., *95:*511, 1978.
18. Maron, B.J., et al.: Sudden death in patients with hypertrophic cardiomyopathy: characterization of 26 patients without functional limitation. Am. J. Cardiol., *41:*803, 1978.
19. Maron, B.J., et al.: "Malignant" hypertrophic cardiomyopathy: identification of a subgroup of families with unusually frequent premature death. Am. J. Cardiol., *41:*1133, 1978.
20. Maron, B.J., and Roberts, W.C.: Quantitative analysis of cardiac muscle cell disorganization in ventricular septum of patients with hypertrophic cardiomyopathy. Circulation, *59:*689, 1979.
21. Maron, B.J., Epstein, S.E., and Roberts, W.C.: Hypertrophic cardiomyopathy and transmural myocardial infarction without significant atherosclerosis of the extramural coronary arteries. Am. J. Cardiol., *43:*1086, 1979.
22. Maron, B.J., et al.: Quantitative analysis of cardiac muscle cell disorganization in the ventricular septum: comparison of fetuses and infants with and without congenital heart disease and patients with hypertrophic cardiomyopathy. Circulation, *60:*685, 1979.
23. Isner, J.M., Maron, B.J., and Roberts, W.C.: Comparison of amount of myocardial cell disorganization in operatively excised septectomy specimens with amount observed at necropsy in 18 patients with hypertrophic cardiomyopathy. Am. J. Cardiol., *46:*42, 1980.
24. Waller, B.F., Maron, B.J., Epstein, S.E., and Roberts, W.C.: Transmural myocardial infarction in hypertrophic cardiomyopathy. Chest, *79:*461, 1981.
25. Maron, B.J., Connor, T.M., and Roberts, W.C.: Hypertrophic cardiomyopathy and complete heart block in infancy. Am. Heart J., *101:*857, 1981.
26. Maron, B.J., and Roberts, W.C.: Hypertrophic cardiomyopathy and cardiac muscle cell disorganization revisited: relation between the two and significance. Am. Heart J., *102:*95, 1981.
27. Waller, B.F., Maron, B.J., Morrow, A.G., and Roberts, W.C.: Hypertrophic cardiomyopathy mimicking pericardial constriction or myocardial restriction. Am. Heart J., *102:*790, 1981.
28. Maron, B.J., et al.: Hypertrophic cardiomyopathy in infants: clinical features and natural history. Circulation, *65:*7, 1982.
29. Maron, B.J., Roberts, W.C., and Epstein, S.E.: Sudden death in hypertrophic cardiomyopathy: a profile of 78 patients. Circulation, *65:*1388, 1982.
30. Ciro, E., Maron, B.J., and Roberts, W.C.: Coexistence of asymmetric and symmetric left ventricular hypertrophy in a family with hypertrophic cardiomyopathy. Am. Heart J., *104:*643, 1982.
31. Maron, B.J., et al.: Systolic anterior motion of the posterior mitral leaflet: a previously unrecognized cause of dynamic subaortic obstruction in patients with hypertrophic cardiomyopathy. Circulation, *68:*282, 1983.
32. Warnes, C.A., Maron, B.J., and Roberts, W.C.: Massive cardiac ventricular scarring in first-degree relatives with hypertrophic cardiomyopathy. Am. J. Cardiol., *54:*1377, 1984.
33. Wigle, E.D., et al.: Hypertrophic cardiomyopathy. The importance of the site and the extent of hypertrophy: a review. Prog. Cardiovasc. Dis., *28:*1, 1985.
34. Maron, B.J., Wolfson, J.K., Epstein, S.E., and Roberts, W.C.: Intramural ("small vessel") cor-

onary artery disease in hypertrophic cardiomyopathy. J. Am. Coll. Cardiol., *8*:545, 1986.

35. Ross, E.M., et al.: Impaired left ventricular systolic and diastolic function without left ventricular dilatation associated with papillary muscle calcification in hypertrophic cardiomyopathy. Am. J. Cardiol., *57*:488, 1986.
36. Roberts, W.C.: Congenital cardiovascular abnormalities usually "silent" until adulthood: morphologic features of the floppy mitral valve, valvular aortic stenosis, discrete subvalvular aortic stenosis, hypertrophic cardiomyopathy, sinus of Valsalva aneurysm, and the Marfan syndrome. *In* Adult Congenital Heart Disease. Edited by W.C. Roberts. Philadelphia, F.A. Davis, 1987, p. 407.
37. Maron, B.J., et al.: Hypertrophic cardiomyopathy: interrelations of clinical manifestations, pathophysiology, and therapy. N. Engl. J. Med., *316*:780, 1987.
38. Unverferth, D.V., et al.: Regional myocyte hypertrophy and increased interstitial myocardial fibrosis in hypertrophic cardiomyopathy. Am. J. Cardiol. *59*:932, 1987.
39. Motamed, H.E., and Roberts, W.C.: Frequency and significance of mitral anular calcium in hypertrophic cardiomyopathy: analysis of 200 necropsy patients. Am. J. Cardiol., *60*:877, 1987.
40. Teare, D.: A symmetrical hypertrophy of the heart in young adults. Br. Heart J., *20*:1, 1958.
41. Liouville, H.: Rétrécissement cardiaque sous aortique. Gazette Med. Paris, *24*:161, 1869.
42. Hallopeau, M.: Rétrécissement ventriculo-aortique. Gazette Med. Paris, *24*:683, 1869.
43. Schmincke, A.: Ueber linkseitige muskulose Conusstenosen. Dtsch. Med. Wochenschr., *33*:2082, 1907.
44. Bernheim, P.I.: De L'asystolie veineuse dans l'hypertrophie du coeur gauche par sténose concomitante du ventricle droit. Rev. Med., *30*:785, 1910.
45. Braunwald, E., et al.: Idiopathic hypertrophic subaortic, stenosis. American Heart Association Monograph No. 10. New York, American Heart Association, 1984, p. 1.
46. Davies, L.G.: Familial heart disease. Br. Heart J., *14*:206, 1952.
47. Brock, R.: Functional obstruction of the left ventricle (acquired aortic subvalvular stenosis). Guy's Hosp. Rep., *106*:221, 1957.
48. Maron, B.J., and Epstein, S.E.: Hypertrophic cardiomyopathy: a discussion of nomenclature. Am. J. Cardiol., *43*:1242, 1979.
49. Muna, W.F.T., Ferrans, V.J., Pierce, J.E., and Roberts, W.C.: Discrete subaortic stenosis in Newfoundland dogs: association of infective endocarditis. Am. J. Cardiol., *41*:746, 1978.
50. Maron, B.J., et al.: Tunnel subaortic stenosis: left ventricular outflow tract obstruction produced by fibromuscular tubular narrowing. Circulation, *54*:406, 1976.
51. Roberts, W.C., et al.: Aortic valve atresia: a new classification based on necropsy study of 73 cases. Am. J. Cardiol., *37*:753, 1976.
52. Ellis, J.G., Terneny, O.J., Winters, W.L., and Leachman, R.D.: Critical role of the mitral valve leaflet in hypertrophic subaortic stenosis and amelioration of the disease by mitral valve replacement. Chest, *59*:378, 1971.
53. Cooley, D.A., Leachman, R.D., and Wukasch, D.C.: Diffuse muscular subaortic stenosis: surgical treatment. Am. J. Cardiol., *31*:1, 1973.
54. Cooley, D.A., Grace, R.R., Wukasch, D.C., and Leachman, R.D.: Replacement and / or repair of the mitral valve as treatment of idiopathic hypertrophic subaortic stenosis. Cardiovasc. Dis., *3*:381, 1976.
55. McIntosh, C.L., and Maron, B.J.: Current operative treatment of obstructive hypertrophic cardiomyopathy. Circulation, *78*:487, 1988.

Coronary "Lesion," Coronary "Disease," "Single-Vessel Disease," "Two-Vessel Disease": Word and Phrase Misnomers Providing False Impressions of the Extent of Coronary Atherosclerosis in Symptomatic Myocardial Ischemia

Coronary arterial angiography in patients with symptomatic myocardial ischemia generally discloses a significant narrowing in 1 or more of the 4 major (right, left main, left anterior descending and left circumflex) epicardial coronary arteries. The degree of narrowing is determined by measuring the transverse dimension of the opacified narrowed lumen and comparing this dimension to an adjacent lumen which is considered to be angiographically normal or nearly so. Thus, if the luminal diameter of the narrowing is 1 mm and the diameter of the adjacent lumen is 3 mm, the diameter reduction is considered to be about 70%. This degree of narrowing frequently is described as a "70% lesion" and the artery containing the "lesion" is spoken of as being "diseased." If only 1 of the 4 major coronary arteries contains a "significant lesion" (most commonly considered to be a narrowing >50% in diameter), then the patient is described as having "1-vessel or single vessel disease." If >1 major epicardial coronary artery contains a "lesion" >50% in diameter, the patient is considered to have "multivessel disease." If 2 arteries contain a "significant lesion" then the patient is spoken of as having "2-vessel disease"; if 3 arteries contain a "significant lesion," then the phrase "3-vessel disease" is applied. If 4 arteries contain "significant lesions," the phrase "4-vessel disease" has rarely been applied. Most commonly in this circumstance the patient is spoken of as having "left main disease," meaning that the lumen of the left main coronary artery is narrowed >50% or >70% in diameter. Whenever, however, the lumen of the left main coronary artery is narrowed >50% or >70% in diameter, the lumens of the other 3 major coronary arteries also are narrowed to a similar extent, and, therefore, the phrase "4-vessel disease" is usually applicable in this circumstance.[1]

I have problems with the use of the words "lesion" and "disease" in the above described circumstances, and also problems with the phrases "1-vessel disease," "2-vessel disease," and "3-vessel disease." The reason for concern is that the word "lesion" implies the presence of abnormality at one site and the absence of abnormality at another site. Numerous necropsy studies in patients >30 years of age with fatal coronary artery disease, irrespective of the type of fatal coronary event, have disclosed that the atherosclerotic process, in essentially all patients, is diffuse and extensive.[2] Furthermore, intravascular ultrasonic imaging in patients with symptomatic myocardial ischemia also has shown that the coronary atherosclerotic process is diffuse and extensive. Thus, the diffuse nature of coronary atherosclerosis as observed at necropsy in patients with fatal coronary artery disease also has been confirmed to be present during life. It no longer can be surmised, therefore, that the diffuse nature of coronary atherosclerosis is limited to patients with fatal coronary artery disease. Furthermore, the same diffuse process of coronary atherosclerosis is observed at necropsy in patients with previous symptomatic myocardial ischemia but who died from a non-cardiac cause.[3]

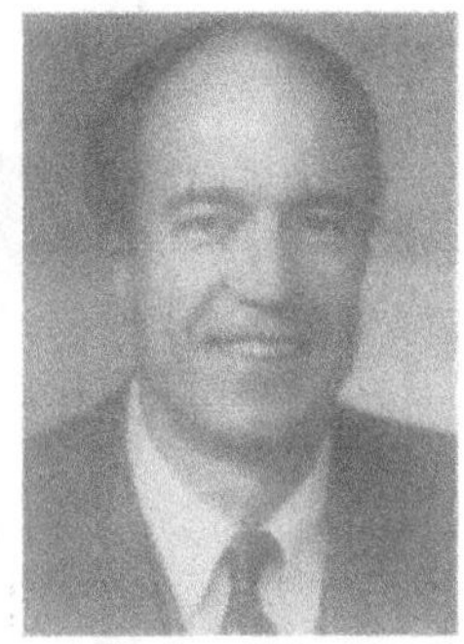

Thus, the word "lesion" to describe an angiographic narrowing is not incorrect, but its implication, that "lesions" are not present elsewhere in that artery or in another artery, is incorrect. I prefer the use of the word "narrowing" to describe angiographic luminal reductions because lesions are present in all segments of the epicardial artery. Some "lesions" result in luminal narrowings ≤25% in diameter; others result in narrowings 26 to 50% in diameter; others 51 to 75%, and still others produce narrowings of 76 to 100%. The continual use of the word "lesion" instead of the words "significant narrowing" leads many to believe that coronary atherosclerosis in persons with symptomatic myocardial ischemia is a focal process, and this belief is incorrect.

The word "disease" is not correct when applied to a "significant narrowing." "Disease" is a word to be applied to the general condition which, in this case of course, is "atherosclerosis." The word "disease" is incorrectly applied when describing the most severely narrowed site in the artery. Thus, neither the word "lesion" nor "disease" is correct because the condition is not limited to a single location in any one artery.

The phrases "single-vessel disease" (1-vessel disease), "double-vessel disease" (2-vessel disease), "triple-vessel disease" (3-vessel disease) are not ideal because they

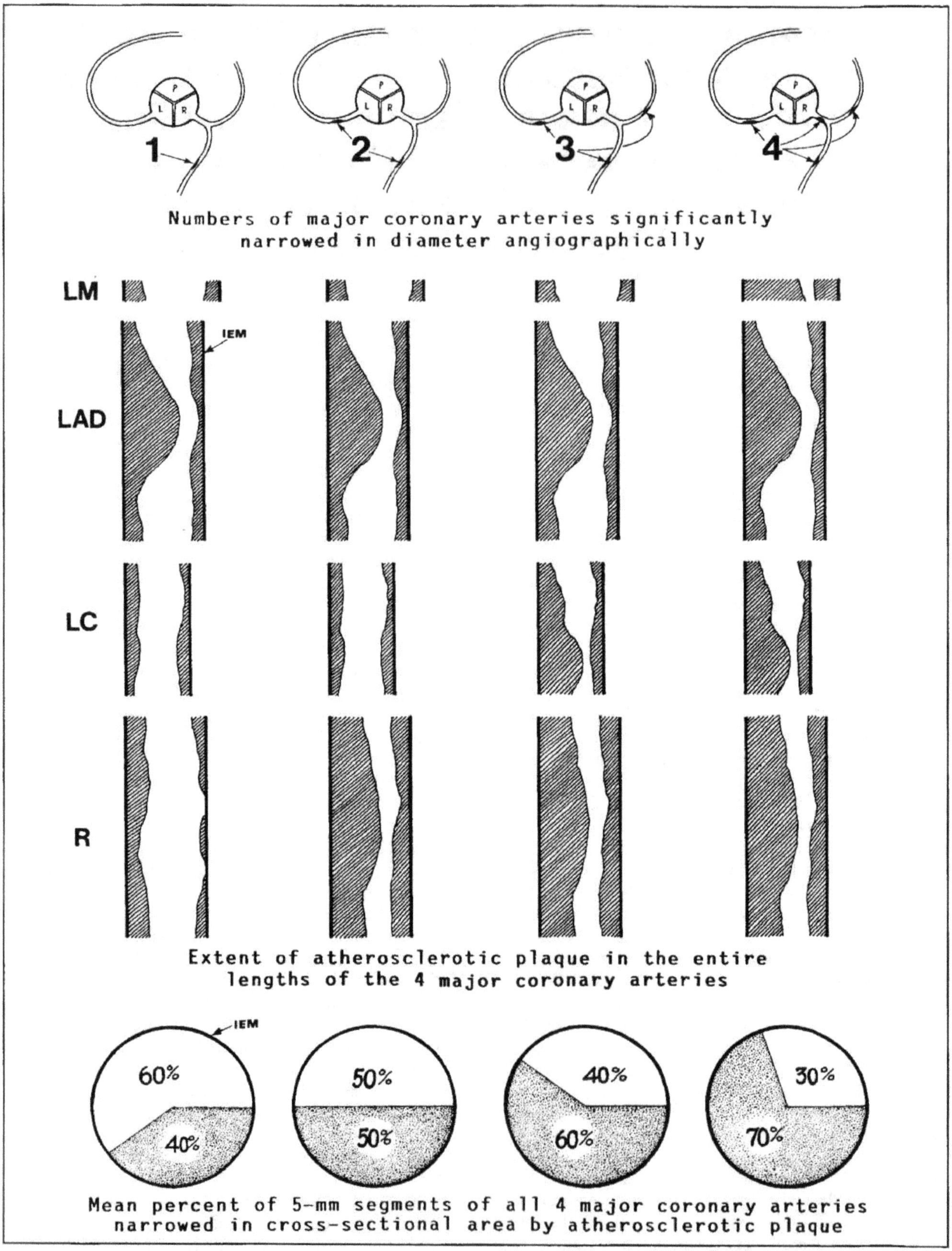

FIGURE 1. Diagram showing numbers of coronary arteries significantly narrowed by angiogram (*top*), the amounts of plaque in the entire lengths of the 4 major (left main [LM], left anterior descending [LAD], left circumflex [LC], and right [R]) epicardial coronary arteries (*middle*), and a cross-sectional area view (*bottom*) of the average amount of plaque in each 5-mm segment of the entire lengths of the 4 major coronary arteries according to the numbers of major arteries significantly narrowed by angiogram.

imply that the atherosclerotic process involves some and spares other coronary arteries. In persons over 30 years of age with symptomatic myocardial ischemia, a "significant narrowing" by angiography occasionally is limited to a single major coronary artery, but the other major coronary arteries are not "free of disease"; they simply have atherosclerotic plaques which reduce the luminal diameter <50% (or whatever definition is selected for "significant narrowing"). The significant narrowing or narrowings represent only the sites of the largest atherosclerotic plaques; the other sites also contain plaques, but they are smaller ones, and consequently produce less luminal narrowing. Whenever any plaque in a coronary artery is large enough to cause "significant narrowing" at any site, it is best to assume that all portions of the epicardial coronary arteries also contain plaque. Thus, if 1 major epicardial coronary artery is significantly narrowed (the narrowing may be shorter in length than 1 cm) and the lengths of the right (10 cm), left anterior descending (10 cm), left circumflex (6 cm), and left main (1 cm) coronary arteries are placed together, all 27 cm contain atherosclerotic plaques of varying sizes (Figure 1). The sites of "significant narrowing" merely represent the largest mountains in the 27-cm chain. Even in the patient with "significant narrowing" of a single major coronary artery, the amount of plaque present in all 4 major coronary arteries as a proportion of the total potential lumen (that enclosed by the internal elastic membrane) of all 4 arteries probably represents about 40% (Figure 1). In the patient with significant narrowing by angiogram of 2 major coronary arteries, the other major arteries always contain plaque in each of their 5-mm long segments. In this circumstance, the amount of plaque present in all 4 major arteries, as a proportion of the total potential lumen, probably represents at least 50%. In the patient with significant narrowing by angiogram of 3 major arteries (right, left anterior descending, left circumflex), the amount of plaque present in all 4 major arteries, as a proportion of the total potential lumen, probably represents at least 60%. In the patient with significant narrowing by angiogram of all 4 major coronary arteries, the amount of plaque present in all 4 arteries, as a proportion of the total potential lumen, probably represents at least 70%. Thus, the more arteries containing a "significant narrowing" at any site in the artery, the greater the amount of total plaque in that artery and in the "insignificantly narrowed" arteries.

Not only are virtually all 5-mm long segments of the 4 major epicardial coronary arteries sites of atherosclerotic plaque in patients with symptomatic or fatal myocardial ischemia, but a certain threshold of total luminal narrowing appears to be required to produce fatal or non-fatal myocardial ischemia. By study of each 5-mm long segment of each of the 4 major epicardial coronary arteries in various subsets of coronary patients, the lumens in about a third of the entire lengths of the 4 arteries are narrowed >75% in cross-sectional area by plaque and another third are narrowed 51–75% in cross-sectional area by plaque.[2] Although some patients with fatal coronary events have considerably less quantities of plaque in the coronary arteries, others have considerably more quantities of plaque, to such an extent at times that <20% of the potential lumen of the 4 major coronary arteries is not obliterated by plaque.

Thus, coronary atherosclerosis in patients with fatal or symptomatic myocardial ischemia is *a diffuse and extensive process*. Knowledge that the plaque deposits are extensive and diffuse might cause some to question the rationale of coronary bypass or coronary angioplasty. These procedures, however, have proved their value irrespective of the extent of the atherosclerotic process. Nevertheless, the extensive nature of the process suggests that only a fine line separates adequate myocardial oxygenation from inadequate myocardial oxygenation and that small structural alterations can produce large functional differences. Because such large amounts of coronary plaque are required before evidence of myocardial ischemia results, it is possible that relatively small changes in our dietary habits could have relatively large effects on the sizes of plaques in our coronary arteries.

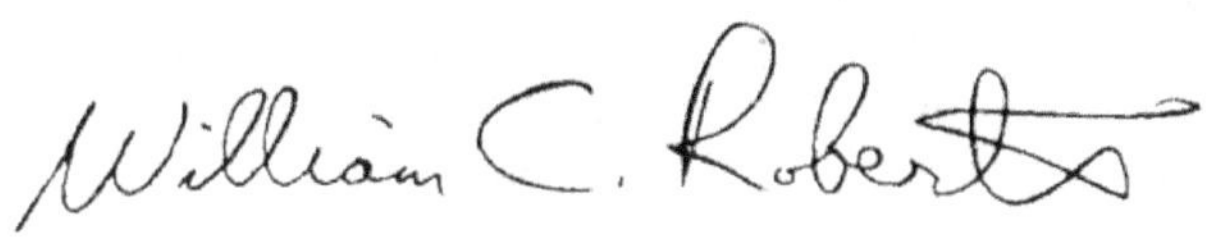

William Clifford Roberts, MD
Editor in Chief

1. Bulkley BH, Roberts WC. Atherosclerotic narrowing of the left main coronary artery. A necropsy analysis of 152 patients with fatal coronary heart disease and varying degrees of left main narrowing. *Circulation 1976;53:823–828.*
2. Roberts WC. Qualitative and quantitative comparison of amounts of narrowing by atherosclerotic plaques in the major epicardial coronary arteries at necropsy in sudden coronary death, transmural acute myocardial infarction, transmural healed myocardial infarction and unstable angina pectoris. *Am J Cardiol 1989;64:324–328.*
3. Virmani R, Roberts WC. Non-fatal healed transmural myocardial infarction and fatal non-cardiac disease. Qualification and quantification of coronary arterial narrowing and of left ventricular scarring in 18 necropsy patients. *Br Heart J 1981;45:434–441.*

Preventing and arresting coronary atherosclerosis

William Clifford Roberts, MD *Dallas, Texas*

Atherosclerosis is the biggest killer in the Western world. Approximately 45% of the inhabitants in this portion of the planet will die from its consequences. In the United States alone an estimated 7 million people have symptomatic myocardial ischemia resulting from coronary atherosclerosis, and countless more have consequences of its attacks on the aorta and the peripheral arteries. The sad thing about atherosclerosis is that in most of us it is preventable. It is estimated that only one in 500 people has the genetic form, namely heterozygous familial hypercholesterolemia. Thus the rest of us, 499 of 500 people, determine ourselves whether we will have sufficient quantities of atherosclerotic plaques to narrow our arterial lumens sufficiently to cause organ ischemia or infarction. This chapter reviews atherosclerosis, with a focus on that involving the coronary arteries, by asking seven questions. (1) How much atherosclerosis is present in the coronary arteries in patients with myocardial ischemia? (2) What do coronary atherosclerotic plaques consist of in patients with symptomatic myocardial ischemia? (3) What acute lesions occur in the coronary arteries in patients with symptomatic myocardial ischemia, and how frequently do they occur in the three acute coronary events, unstable angina pectoris (UAP), acute myocardial infarction (AMI), and sudden coronary death (SCD)? (4) How many *direct* atherosclerotic risk factors exist? (5) What factors indicate that cholesterol causes atherosclerosis? (6) How can symptomatic atherosclerosis be prevented or, if present, arrested? (7) How can normal cholesterol levels be prevented from rising, and how can elevated levels be lowered to normal?

From the Baylor Cardiovascular Institute, Baylor University Medical Center.

Received for publication Oct. 28, 1994; accepted Dec. 14, 1994.

Reprint requests: William C. Roberts, MD, Baylor Cardiovascular Institute, Baylor University Medical Center, 3500 Gaston Ave., Dallas, TX 75246.

AM HEART J 1995;130:580-600.

0002-8703/95/$3.00 + 0 **4/1/65062**

HOW MUCH ATHEROSCLEROSIS IS PRESENT IN THE CORONARY ARTERIES IN PATIENTS WITH SYMPTOMATIC MYOCARDIAL ISCHEMIA?

The amount of coronary arterial narrowing observed at necropsy in patients with UAP, AMI, and SCD is generally enormous, and certain evidence suggests that patients with symptomatic myocardial ischemia have as much plaque as do those with fatal myocardial ischemia. From study of 80 patients at autopsy with these three coronary events, an average of 2.9 of the four major (right, left main, left anterior descending, and left circumflex) coronary arteries were severely (>75% decrease in cross-sectional area) narrowed at some point, and no significant differences were observed among the three coronary subsets.[1, 2] Patients with UAP had a much higher frequency of severe narrowing of the left main coronary artery (10 [45%] of 22 patients compared with those with AMI (three [11%] of 27 patients and SCD (three [10%] of 31 patients).[1, 2]

A more sophisticated approach to determining degrees of luminal narrowing is to examine the entire lengths of the four major epicardial coronary arteries. One technique involves incising each of the four major coronary arteries transversely at 5 mm intervals and then preparing a histologic section from each 5 mm segment. Normally the total length of the four major arteries is approximately 27 cm (right = 10 cm, left main = 1 cm, left anterior descending = 10 cm, and left circumflex = 6 cm), and thus approximately 55 five-millimeter–long segments are available for examination from each heart. Of the 4016 five-millimeter–long segments studied in the 80 previously mentioned patients, 38% were narrowed 76% to 100% in cross-sectional area by plaque alone (control 3%); 34% were narrowed 51% to 75% (control 22%); 20% were narrowed 26% to 50% (control 44%); and only 7% were narrowed 25% or less (control 31%).[1, 2] Similar degrees of narrowing by plaque alone in all four categories of narrowing were observed in the groups with AMI and SCD; patients with UAP had significantly more severe coronary narrowing than the other two groups.[1, 2]

Thus in general patients with fatal UAP have more extensive severe narrowing by plaque alone of the four major epicardial coronary arteries than patients with either AMI or SCD, and patients with UAP compared with the other two groups have a significantly higher frequency of severe narrowing of the left main coronary artery. The good news is that it takes a huge quantity of plaque before overt myocardial ischemia occurs; the bad news is that despite the requirement for huge quantities of plaque before problems occur, nearly half of us in the Western world eventually have these huge quantities of plaque.

WHAT DO CORONARY ATHEROSCLEROTIC PLAQUES CONSIST OF IN PATIENTS WITH SYMPTOMATIC MYOCARDIAL ISCHEMIA?

Until recently no detailed information was available concerning the composition of atherosclerotic plaques in the epicardial coronary arteries of patients with fatal coronary events. With the use of a computerized morphometric system, Kragel et al.[3, 4] determined the various components of atherosclerotic plaques in histologic sections prepared from 1438 five-millimeter–long segments of the four major epicardial coronary arteries in 37 patients with fatal coronary artery disease. The dominant component of the coronary atherosclerotic plaques in all three subsets of patients was fibrous tissue, composing approximately 80% of the plaques in each subset; extracellular lipid (pultaceous debris) and calcium each made up approximately 5% of the plaques, and several miscellaneous components composed the remainder of the plaques. The cellular component of the fibrous tissue occupied a larger portion of plaque in the patients with UAP and SCD, and the acellular (dense) component of fibrous tissue occupied a larger portion of the plaque in the group with AMI. In all three subsets the amount of dense fibrous tissue increased as plaque size increased (or as lumen size decreased), and the amount of cellular fibrous tissue decreased as plaque size increased.

Plaques in women had a higher percent of cellular fibrous tissue and a lower percent of acellular fibrous tissue than did those of men in a similar age group.[5] Plaques in saphenous veins used as aortocoronary conduits became similar to those in the native coronary arteries in the same patients at approximately 7 years after the bypass operation, and the dominant component of the plaques at this point also was fibrous tissue.[6]

WHAT ACUTE LESIONS OCCUR IN THE CORONARY ARTERIES IN PATIENTS WITH SYMPTOMATIC MYOCARDIAL ISCHEMIA, AND HOW FREQUENTLY DO THEY OCCUR IN THE THREE ACUTE CORONARY EVENTS?

In recent years considerable effort has been directed toward understanding the acute coronary events that may be responsible for the development of UAP, AMI, and SCD. From angiographic, angioscopic, and autopsy studies it has been speculated that plaque rupture and hemorrhage with overlying intraluminal thrombus, which are the acute lesions usually responsible for AMI, are also responsible for UAP and possibly SCD. Kragel et al.[7] examined 3101 five-millimeter–long segments of 268 epicardial coronary arteries from 67 patients with fatal coronary events. The frequency of *intraluminal thrombus* was similar in the groups with UAP and SCD (29% in each) and significantly lower than that in the group with AMI (69%). The thrombus was nonocclusive in all patients with UAP and in 5 of 6 patients with SCD, but it was nonocclusive in only four of 22 patients with AMI. The composition of the nonocclusive and occlusive thrombi also was different, that is, the nonocclusive thrombus consisted mainly of platelets, and the occlusive thrombus consisted mainly of fibrin. *Plaque rupture* was found in 33 (49%) of 67 patients. Its frequency was insignificantly different in the groups with UAP (36%) and SCD (19%); in both groups the frequency was significantly lower than in the group with AMI (75%). *Plaque hemorrhage* was observed in 27 (40%) of 67 patients, and its frequency was significantly lower in the groups with UAP (21%) and SCD (19%) compared with that in the group with AMI (63%). Multiple small vascular channels were present in 60 (90%) of 67 patients and with an insignificantly different frequency in each of the three groups of patients.

Thus comparison of findings from examination of a histologic section from each of 3101 five-millimeter–long segments of 268 major epicardial coronary arteries from 67 patients with fatal coronary artery disease disclosed that the frequency of three acute coronary lesions (intraluminal thrombus, plaque rupture, and plaque hemorrhage) was similar in patients with UAP and SCD and significantly higher in patients with a fatal first transmural AMI.

HOW MANY *DIRECT* ATHEROSCLEROTIC RISK FACTORS EXIST?

Several factors have been considered to predispose to atherosclerosis including elevated low-density lipoprotein (LDL) cholesterol and low levels of high-density lipoprotein (HDL) cholesterol, systemic hypertension, cigarette smoking, family history of atherosclerotic disease, obesity, diabetes mellitus, and male sex.[8] The key word in the question posed is *direct*, which can be defined in many ways. If this word is used to mean that this risk factor must be present for atherosclerosis to occur, all but one of these factors can be eliminated. Atherosclerosis of severe degree may occur in individuals with normal blood pressures, in nonsmokers, in nonobese persons, in those with normal glucose metabolism, and in women. Thus these factors are indirect and may worsen the atherosclerotic process, but in the absence of the direct factor they do not cause atherosclerosis. This section examines each of these atherosclerotic risk factors to ask whether it is a direct or independent factor.

Elevated serum (or plasma) total cholesterol, LDL cholesterol, and low HDL cholesterol. In my view the only absolute, unequivocal, independent atherosclerotic risk factor is an elevated serum total or LDL cholesterol, a low HDL cholesterol level, or both.[9] What constitutes an elevated total cholesterol level is debated. If an elevated level is that minimal level above which atherosclerotic events occur, then that level would be approximately 150 mg/dl (3.9 mmol/L). If it is the level where the risk of atherosclerotic events is substantially increased compared with lower levels, then that level would be approximately 200 mg/dl. Irrespective of which level is chosen, the higher the level is, the greater is the risk of an atherosclerotic event. From study of more than 350,000 men, Stamler et al.[10] clearly demonstrated that the higher the serum total cholesterol level is, the greater is the risk of an atherosclerotic event. The Framingham study,[11] involving approximately 5000 residents of that Massachusetts community, also showed that the higher the total and LDL cholesterol levels are and the lower the HDL cholesterol level is, the greater the risk is of having an atherosclerotic event. International epidemiologic studies[12] have shown that populations with serum total cholesterol levels less than 150 mg/dl for decades have a near absence of atherosclerotic events. A certain critical serum total cholesterol level is necessary before an atherosclerotic event can occur, and this critical level appears to be approximately 150 mg/dl. As the level increases above this value, the risk of an atherosclerotic event increases roughly proportional to the level and to the amount of time that this level has been present.[13]

In adults in the United States the mean plasma HDL level in men is 45 mg/dl and in women, 55 mg/dl.[14] Data, especially from Framingham, Massachusetts, have shown that high levels of HDL are associated with decreased risk and that low levels are associated with increased risk of atherosclerotic events.[11, 15] The evidence is convincing that high HDL is good and low HDL is bad. But what is the risk of a serum HDL level of 20 mg/dl, if the LDL-cholesterol is less than 100 mg/dl and the serum total cholesterol is less than 150 mg/dl? The answer is no risk. Is an HDL of 100 mg/dl protective when the total cholesterol is 300 (ratio = 3) and LDL cholesterol is near 200 mg/dl? The answer is probably no. Whether the HDL-cholesterol is an independent risk factor, that is, independent of the LDL-cholesterol level, is not yet clear. It is reasonable to view a low HDL-cholesterol as an additive atherosclerotic risk factor if the LDL-cholesterol is elevated, but not as an additive atherosclerotic risk factor if the LDL-cholesterol is low. Mautner et al.[16] studied a 72-year-old man who had had a coronary bypass operation at age 60 and who during his last 17 years of life had 30 fasting lipoprotein analyses; the serum total cholesterol averaged 70, the LDL cholesterol 45, the triglycerides 45, and the HDL cholesterol 1 mg/dl. Thus severe atherosclerosis occurred despite low LDL and total cholesterol levels and virtually absent HDL cholesterol. The total cholesterol-HDL cholesterol ratio in that patient was 70!

Systemic hypertension. In experimental animals given atherogenic diets (high fat, high cholesterol), those previously made hypertensive have more atherosclerotic plaques than do the normotensive animals. Hypertensive persons with total and LDL-cholesterol levels similar to those in normotensive persons have a higher frequency of atherosclerotic events compared with normotensive subjects. These two facts have supported the contention that systemic hypertension is an atherosclerotic risk factor. Most studies describing benefits of antihypertensive therapy have not demonstrated a reduction in coronary or peripheral atherosclerotic events by such therapy. No evidence exists that systemic hypertension accelerates atherosclerosis if the serum total cholesterol level is less than 150 mg/dl. It appears that systemic hypertension is a cholesterol-dependent risk factor, because the serum total cholesterol must be greater than 150 mg/dl before hypertension has the ability to accelerate atherosclerosis, and therefore hypertension is not an independent atherosclerotic risk factor.

Although evidence implicating systemic hypertension as a direct atherosclerotic risk factor is lacking, systemic hypertension clearly is the major risk factor for development of stroke and aortic dissection.[17] These two lesions are not atherosclerotic-dependent. The prime effect of hypertension is on the media of arteries, causing this arterial layer to tear, dissect, or rupture. Atherosclerosis is an intimal process, and only indirectly is the media affected.

Cigarette smoking. Although it is incompatible with good health, cigarette smoking does not in and of itself produce atherosclerotic plaques. In populations where serum total cholesterol levels are less than 150/mg/dl, atherosclerotic events are rare, even when cigarette smoking is widespread. In Japan cigarette smoking is common, but atherosclerotic events are relatively uncommon. The average serum total cholesterol in adults in Japan is approximately 170 mg/dl, which is not a level associated with a high frequency of atherosclerotic events. Many Japanese adults have serum total cholesterol levels less than 150 mg/dl. In populations where the average serum total cholesterol level in adults is greater than 200 mg/dl, such as the United States, smoking cigarettes appears to accelerate atherosclerosis, but this acceleration appears to be a cholesterol-dependent phenomenon.

Family history. When atherosclerotic events occur in persons younger than 55 years of age, it generally means (1) that the affected individuals have serum total cholesterol levels considerably higher than persons of similar age and sex without atherosclerotic events, and (2) that the affected individuals have total cholesterol levels much higher than those found in older individuals with atherosclerotic events. In persons with untreated familial hypercholesterolemia of the *heterozygous* type, the serum total cholesterol level is usually 300 to 400 mg/dl, and these individuals usually have atherosclerotic events when they are 31 to 50 years of age.[18, 19] In untreated individuals with familial hypercholesterolemia of the *homozygous* variety, the serum total cholesterol is usually greater than 800 mg/dl, and these individuals usually have atherosclerotic events before they are 20 years of age.[18, 19] Thus individuals who have atherosclerotic events before the age of 50 years generally have higher total LDL cholesterol levels than do individuals who have atherosclerotic events later in life, and the genetic forms of hyperlipidemia are primarily in these younger groups. An atherosclerotic event occurring in a young person simply denotes very high serum total cholesterol levels, and it is the cholesterol level, not the patient's age or the presence of atherosclerotic events in other family members, that is the villain.

Severe obesity. In general, obese persons have higher total and LDL-cholesterol levels than do nonobese persons of similar age and sex.[20] This fact is of course not surprising, because obese persons eat more fat than do nonobese persons. Although few exist to study, I am not aware that obese adults with serum total cholesterol levels less than 150 mg/dl have any risk of development of atherosclerotic events. Thus obesity is a cholesterol-dependent risk factor, not an independent risk factor.

Diabetes mellitus. Juvenile diabetic patients clearly have more atherosclerotic plaques and a higher frequency of atherosclerotic events than do nondiabetic patients of similar age and sex.[21, 22] But the juvenile diabetics usually have higher serum total and LDL-cholesterol and lower HDL-cholesterol levels than do their nondiabetic counterparts. Likewise adult-onset diabetics have more atherosclerosis and a higher frequency of atherosclerotic events than do nondiabetics of similar age and sex.[23] Moreover, the adult-onset diabetics have higher serum total and LDL-cholesterol, triglyceride, and lower HDL-cholesterol levels than do their nondiabetic counterparts.[24] No evidence exists that diabetics who have serum total cholesterol levels less than 150 mg/dl have an increased frequency of atherosclerotic events compared with nondiabetic counterparts with similar cholesterol levels. Indeed, no evidence exists that diabetics with low serum total cholesterol levels have atherosclerosis of any significance. Thus diabetes mellitus also appears to be a cholesterol-dependent risk factor.

Male sex. As many women as men die from atherosclerotic events. The average age of death from atherosclerotic coronary artery disease in men (without angioplasty or bypass) is 60 years; in women it is 68 years.[25, 26] Men have higher total and LDL serum cholesterol levels earlier in life than do women, but later in life women have higher levels than do men.[27] Neither men nor women, however, have atherosclerotic events unless the total cholesterol level is greater than 150 mg/dl, and the higher the level is, the greater is the chance of an event, and the earlier the event occurs irrespective of sex. Thus it is the person's blood cholesterol level, not the sex, that determines whether an atherosclerotic event occurs. Therefore male sex cannot be viewed as an independent atherosclerotic risk factor.

WHAT FACTORS INDICATE THAT CHOLESTEROL CAUSES ATHEROSCLEROSIS?

Although the relation between cholesterol and atherosclerosis has been discussed for nearly 90

Table I. Deciles of serum total cholesterol and 6-year coronary artery disease mortality rate in 356,222 primary screenees (all men 35 to 37 years of age in 1973 to 1975) of the Multiple Risk Factor Intervention Trial*

Decile	*Serum TC (mg/dl)* Range	Mean	*CAD mortality rate (rate/1000)*	*Relative risk*
1	≤167	153	3.2	1.0
2	168-181	175	3.3	1.1
3	182-192	187	4.1	1.3
4	193-202	198	4.2	1.3
5	203-212	208	5.4	1.7
6	213-220	216	5.8	1.8
7	221-231	226	6.9	2.2
8	232-244	238	7.4	2.3
9	245-263	253	9.1	2.9
10	≥264	290	13.1	4.1

*Modified from Stamler et al., JAMA 1986;256:2823-8.
TC, serum total cholesterol; *CAD*, coronary artery disease.

years, only in recent years has sufficient evidence accumulated to indicate without reasonable doubt that cholesterol plays a major role in the development of atherosclerotic plaques. This section reviews the various factors linking cholesterol to atherosclerosis:

1. Feeding high-cholesterol diets to certain animals produces atherosclerotic plaques similar to those in human beings. The initial connection between cholesterol and atherosclerotic plaques began in 1912, when Anitschkow[28, 29] reported finding atherosclerotic plaques similar to those occurring in humans in rabbits fed diets high in cholesterol. (This was the same year that James Herrick[30] first reported that acute myocardial infarction could be diagnosed clinically and that it was not always immediately fatal.) Subsequently atherosclerotic plaques were produced also in other animals (guinea pig, chicken, monkey) by feeding them high-cholesterol diets.[29] Anitschkow, from his experiment, laid down the dictum that increased cholesterol in the blood was the inciting cause of atherosclerosis. It is not possible to produce atherosclerosis in a carnivore (dog, cat, lion, tiger) no matter how much fat or cholesterol is provided, unless the thyroid gland is excised before the atherogenic diet is initiated. Feeding humans a diet high in fat and cholesterol obviously readily produces atherosclerotic plaques. This fact suggests that humans basically are herbivores.

2. Cholesterol is found in both experimentally induced atherosclerotic plaques in nonhuman animals and in plaques in human beings. Three main types of lipid accumulate in atherosclerotic lesions: free sterols (almost exclusively cholesterol), cholesterol esters (mainly cholesteryl linoleate, oleate, and palmitate), and phospholipids (mainly phosphatidylcholine and spingomyelines).[31] All three lipids are insoluble in water. These lipids make up approximately 95% of the total lipids in both normal intima and in atheromatous plaques. The lipids present in small amounts include triacylglycerols, fatty acids, and lysophospholipids. Cholesterol esters are nearly absent in newborn intima, but they are a major part of atherosclerotic plaques.[31] Triglycerides are lowest in newborn intima, and they never become a major component of plaques, although they rise to 6% in the gruel-like material of plaques.[31]

3. Atherosclerotic plaques large enough to produce clinical problems occur only in persons with serum or plasma total cholesterol levels greater than 150 mg/dl for long periods of time. Most native African, Latin American, and oriental populations have a low frequency of coronary atherosclerosis.[12, 32] Their diets are low in saturated fat, cholesterol, and animal protein. Most adults in these populations have serum total cholesterol levels less than 150 mg/dl. Fatal atherosclerotic vascular disease in the United States is rare in anyone with a serum total cholesterol level less than 150 mg/dl for many years. In the United States, however, only 5% of the population older than 40 years of age has a serum or plasma total cholesterol level less than 150 mg/dl.[33]

4. The higher the blood total cholesterol level is, the greater is the chance of having symptomatic and fatal atherosclerotic disease. Although the Framingham,[34] the "Seven Countries,"[12, 32] and the Israeli[35] studies have demonstrated that persons with higher serum total cholesterol levels have higher incidences of atherosclerotic disease than do persons of similar age and sex with lower levels, in my view the best study demonstrating the relation between serum total cholesterol level and symptomatic or fatal atherosclerotic disease is the Multiple Risk Factor Intervention Trial (MRFIT)[10] (Table I). The reason is that MRFIT involved more than 350,000 persons, whereas the seven-country study involved just more than 12,000 men from each of seven nations and the Framingham study, 5127 persons. The 356,222 persons without clinical evidence of coronary artery disease sampled in the MRFIT study were divided into deciles on the basis of their serum total cholesterol levels. The 6-year coronary-artery-disease mortality rate per 100 persons increased as the serum total cholesterol level increased. This study shows dramatically that the serum total cholesterol level is a quantity and that the greater the quantity is, the greater is the risk of symptomatic and fatal coronary artery disease.

Persons with enormously elevated (6 to 10 times normal) LDL cholesterol levels usually die of consequences of atherosclerosis in the first 2 decades of life.[11, 12, 36, 37] These individuals have familial hypercholesterolemia of the homozygote variety. They inherit two mutant genes at the LDL receptor locus, one from each parent, and approximately one in 1 million persons have this abnormality. The heterozygous variety of familial hypercholesterolemia has a twofold increase in blood LDL levels, and these individuals often have fatal heart attacks in their 30s and 40s. Approximately one in every 500 persons among most ethnic groups throughout the world have familial hypercholesterolemia of the heterozygous variety. Both the homozygous and heterozygous varieties of familial hypercholesterolemia provide strong evidence that persons with severe elevations of serum LDL and total cholesterol levels have both symptomatic and fatal coronary artery disease at much earlier ages than do persons with lower levels.

5. The higher the serum total and LDL cholesterol levels are, the greater is the extent of the atherosclerotic plaques. The International Atherosclerosis Project quantified the extent of coronary and aortic atherosclerotic plaques at necropsy in 23,207 persons in 14 countries.[38] The extent of the atherosclerotic plaques differed markedly among populations, and the mean serum total cholesterol level correlated positively with the severity of the atherosclerotic plaques. The severity of the atherosclerotic plaques in aorta also correlated positively with the percent of dietary calories from fat.[39]

6. Lowering the blood total cholesterol and LDL cholesterol levels decreases the chances of fatal or nonfatal atherosclerotic disease. Two studies, the Lipid Research Clinics-Coronary Primary Prevention Trial (LRC-CPPT) (cholestyramine)[40-43] and the Helsinki Primary Prevention Trial (gemfibrozil),[44-45] provided evidence that lowering the blood total and LDL cholesterol levels reduces the frequency of fatal and nonfatal coronary artery disease. Both studies were randomized, double-blind, placebo-controlled, multicenter, primary prevention trials analyzed by the intention-to-treat method.

The LRC trial included 3806 men 35 to 59 years of age (mean 48 years) at entry with plasma total cholesterol levels ≥265 mg/dl (after dieting); half the subjects received cholestyramine (24 gm a day) and the other half, placebo (24 gm a day). All subjects underwent follow-up for a minimum of 7 years and up to 10 years (mean 7.4 years). The cholestyramine group (1899 men) had average total and LDL cholesterol reductions at the end of the first year of 18% (292 → 239 mg/dl) and 28% (216 → 159 mg/dl), respectively, and by the end of the seventh year of 12% (292 → 257 mg/dl) and 19% (216 → 175 mg/dl), respectively. In contrast, the placebo group (1907 men), also on a cholesterol-lowering diet, had average total and LDL cholesterol reductions at the end of the first year of 6% (292 → 275 mg/dl) and 8% (216 → 199 mg/dl), respectively, and by the end of the seventh year of 5% (292 → 277 mg/dl) and 9% (216 → 198 mg/dl), respectively. The primary end points, fatal coronary artery disease or nonfatal acute myocardial infarction, were reduced 19%, which is the difference in the cumulative 7-year incidence of the primary end point, which was 7% in the cholestyramine group (133 of 1899 men) and 8.6% (164 of 1907 men) in the placebo group, or the difference in the cumulative rate of cardiac end points at 7 years of 70 of 1000 in the cholestyramine group and 86 of 1000 in the placebo group. In addition, other cardiovascular events also decreased in the cholestyramine group compared with the placebo group: *positive exercise test results* fell 25% (260[14.9%] vs 345 [19.8%]); *angina pectoris* fell 18% (235[12.4%] vs 287 [15.1%]); and need for *coronary artery bypass grafting* fell 17% (93 [4.9%] vs 122 [5.9%]).

The Helsinki trial included 4081 men 40 to 55 years of age (mean 47 years) at entry with serum non-HDL cholesterol greater than 200 mg/dl. The mean serum total cholesterol for the 4081 men was 290 mg/dl, and the mean HDL cholesterol was 48 mg/dl. Half of the subjects received gemfibrozil (1.2 gm/day) and the other half, placebo (1.2 gm/day). All subjects underwent follow-up for a minimum of 5 years. The gemfibrozil group had average total and LDL cholesterol reductions during both the first 2 years and during the last 3 years of study of 9% (270 → 245 mg/dl) and 9% (189 → 173 mg/dl), respectively. The HDL cholesterol rose during both the first 2 years and the last 3 years of study by 9% (47 → 52 mg/dl). In contrast, the placebo group, also on a cholesterol-lowering diet, had no change in either serum total (270 → 273 mg/dl) or LDL cholesterol (48 → 47 mg/dl) during the entire 5 years of the trial. The primary end points, fatal coronary artery disease or nonfatal acute myocardial infarction, were reduced 34%, which is the difference between the 2.7% incidence of primary end points in the gemfibrozil group (56 in 2051 men) and the 4.1% incidence in the placebo group (84 in 2030 men), or the difference in the cumulative rate of cardiac end points at 5 years of 27 of 1000 in the gemfibrozil group and 41 of 1000 in the placebo group.

Thus both the LRC and Helsinki primary prevention trials demonstrate that lowering the blood total and LDL cholesterol levels reduces the incidence of

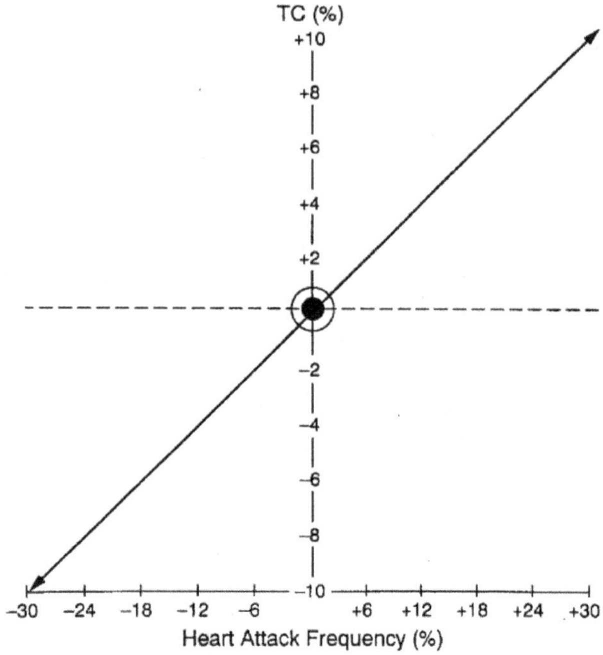

Fig. 1. Effect of increasing or decreasing serum total cholesterol level on frequency of fatal coronary artery disease or nonfatal acute myocardial infarction. These data are derived primarily from Helsinki heart study. For every 10% decrease in serum total cholesterol, there is 30% decrease in heart attack frequency. The reverse also is true. For every 10% increase in serum total cholesterol, there is 30% increase in frequency of heart attack.

fatal and nonfatal coronary artery disease. The trials, when analyzed by the intention-to-treat method, showed that every 1% reduction in serum total cholesterol resulted in a 2% reduction in heart attack frequency during a 5- to 7-year period. If the trials had been analyzed by comparison of those who actually took the drugs in the prescribed amounts with those who did not take the drugs, the studies would have shown at least a 3% reduction in heart attack frequency for every 1% reduction in serum total cholesterol (Fig. 1).

7. Atherosclerotic plaques may regress or fail to progress when high total and LDL cholesterol levels are lowered. Several experimental studies in animals have shown that atherosclerotic plaques regress when blood lipid levels fall after atherogenic diets are eliminated.[46] Several studies, most published this decade, in humans have demonstrated that lipid-lowering retards the rate of progression of angiographically demonstrated coronary arterial narrowing, causes reduction in size of atherosclerotic plaques, or both, (Fig. 2) as indicated by increased luminal diameters, and it usually decreases the frequencies of recurrences of atherosclerotic events.[47-62] For plaque progression to cease, it appears that the serum total cholesterol needs to be lowered to the 150 mg/dl area. In other words the serum total cholesterol must be lowered to that of the average pure vegetarian. Because relatively few persons are willing to abide by the vegetarian lifestyle, lipid-lowering drugs are required in most to reach the 150 mg/dl level.

In summary, seven factors provide evidence that elevation of the blood total (specifically the LDL) cholesterol level is the cause of atherosclerosis. There no longer is any controversy about cholesterol's role in atherosclerosis. In my view physicians should provide a clear and united voice to the public regarding the dangers of elevation of the blood LDL cholesterol level. Every person needs to know his or her serum or plasma total cholesterol level, and if it is elevated, every attempt should be made to lower it. The most effective means of improving the health of the largest percent of Americans is for each to lower his or her LDL cholesterol level.

HOW CAN SYMPTOMATIC ATHEROSCLEROSIS BE PREVENTED OR, IF PRESENT, ARRESTED?

To prevent symptomatic or fatal atherosclerosis in those persons whose serum total cholesterol is approximately 150 mg/dl, this level must be prevented from rising, and to prevent symptomatic or fatal atherosclerosis in those persons with elevated serum total cholesterol levels, the level must be reduced to the 150 mg/dl area. The best news about atherosclerosis is that it can be prevented in 499 of 500 persons by keeping the total cholesterol in the 150 mg/dl area and that it can be arrested by lowering an elevated level to the 150 mg/dl level.

The mean serum total cholesterol of umbilical blood of newborns is approximately 75 mg/dl (1.9 mmol/L). Within 2 weeks of life that value rises to a mean of 150 mg/dl (3.9 mmol/L) and remains at that level until approximately age 20 years, when it gradually starts to rise. The average serum total cholesterol level in the United States in persons 20 to 74 years of age is 215 mg/dl, and the average in persons in coronary care units with acute myocardial infarction is 225 mg/dl.[63] Men have higher levels earlier in life, and women, in later life. Nearly 50% of women in the United States older than 60 years of age have serum total cholesterol levels greater than 240 mg/dl (>6.2 mmol/L), and 25% of the U. S. population 20 to 74 years of age have serum total cholesterol levels greater than 240 mg/dl; 5% have levels greater than 265 mg/dl (>6.9 mmol/L).[27]

HOW CAN NORMAL SERUM CHOLESTEROL LEVELS BE PREVENTED FROM RISING, AND HOW CAN ELEVATED LEVELS BE LOWERED TO NORMAL?

To keep a normal cholesterol level normal and to return an elevated level to normal, dietary intake of cholesterol, fat, and total calories must be restricted or one or more lipid-lowering drugs must be administered, or both.

Cholesterol intake. The average adult in the United States consumes approximately 500 mg of cholesterol daily. To picture 500 mg, hardly a calorie, a toothpick may be useful. The average toothpick weighs approximately 100 mg, so we consume the equivalent of five toothpicks of cholesterol daily. Dietary cholesterol, of course, is derived exclusively from animals and their products, so limiting their intake automatically reduces the intake of cholesterol. Nearly 50% of the direct cholesterol consumed by adults in the United States comes from the visible and nonvisible eggs eaten, so giving up eggs eliminates nearly half of our direct cholesterol intake. Bovine muscle ("beef") accounts for nearly 30% of our direct cholesterol intake, so giving up these two items along with other bovine products (butter, cheese, milk) essentially eliminates the direct cholesterol intake problem. Men and women in the United States consume similar amounts of cholesterol, but through slightly different sources: men consume more meat, and women more cheese. Cholesterol contents of most flesh eaten by human beings is similar in amounts of cholesterol. A 100 gm portion of muscle from cows, pigs, deer, chicken, turkey, and fish each contains approximately 85 mg of cholesterol, and thus switching from one flesh to another has little impact on cholesterol intake. Fish is advantageous in that it contains relatively little fat, whereas the muscle of cows and pigs, at least those raised in the United States, is laden with fat.

Fat intake. Most adults in the United States consume more than 100 gm of fat daily; many consume more than 150 gm daily. None of us should consume more than 75 gm of fat daily—the equivalent of a deck of cards—and ideally men should consume no more than 60 gm and women no more than 50 gm of fat daily. There are two problems, of course, with fat: (1) all fats possess a saturated component, and (2) all fats are high in calories. All fatty acids contain a polyunsaturated component, a monounsaturated component, and a saturated component. A polyunsaturated fat is one in which polyunsaturated component is dominant, and the remainder is divided between the monounsaturated and saturated components; a monounsaturated fat is one in which the monounsaturated component is dominant. The saturated fatty acids (coconut oil, palm kernel oil, beef fat) raise the serum total cholesterol level, and the polyunsaturated (safflower, cottonseed, corn, sesame, soybean, fish oils) and monounsaturated (olive, peanut, avocado) fatty acids either lower the level or have a neutral effect on the total cholesterol level. The reason the saturated fat component is so dangerous is that it is essentially converted into cholesterol as it is broken down in the body. Thus for an individual who consumes 120 gm of fat daily, usually approximately 40 gm of that is saturated, and when that 40 gm enters the body, it is essentially converted into cholesterol. The saturated fat can be identified by its being solid at room temperature; the polyunsaturated and monounsaturated fats are soft or liquid at room temperature. All three fatty acids are very high in calories (9 calories/gm).

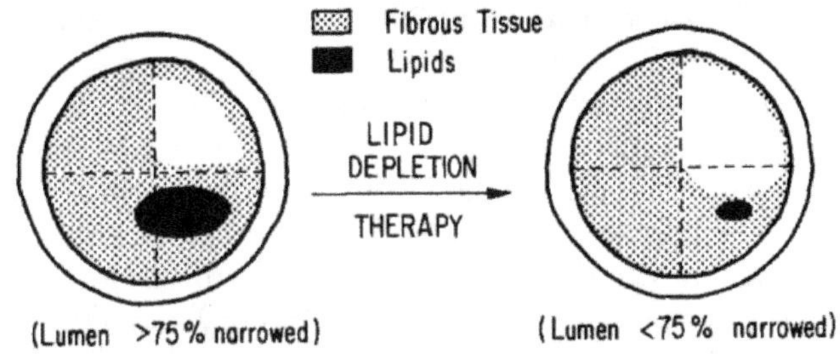

Fig. 2. Mechanism of plaque regression. *Left*, Drawing of coronary artery that is narrowed >75% in cross-sectional area by atherosclerotic plaque. Most of the plaque consists of fibrous tissue, and it is unlikely that fibrous tissue is reversible. Lipid portion, however, may shrink if serum total and LDL cholesterol levels are substantially reduced, probably down to the 150 mg/dl area. If lipid portion shrinks, lumen may widen as is shown in *right* portion of diagram. Unless lumen is narrowed >75%, flow is not reduced. Thus opening lumen so that it is <75% narrowed in cross-sectional area is as if there is no narrowing at all. Small reductions in plaque mass, in other words, may lead to large increases in lumen size.

Although there are many sources of fat in contrast to the relatively few sources of direct cholesterol, a major source (approximately 30%) is flesh, primarily because of the way cattle are raised in the United States. Cows for slaughter in the United States are placed in feed lots their last 4 to 6 months of life, and there they are fed 20 to 25 pounds of various grains and soybeans each day. The purpose of this heavy feeding is to make the animals fat so that they taste better when cooked. Then once they are fat enough, we kill the cows, and then they kill us! This cycle is the merry-go-round of unhealthiness.

Fast-food restaurants. One of the easiest means of rapidly acquiring a heavy dose of fat and cholesterol is the fast-food restaurant.[64, 65] In the United States $5 of every $10 spent on restaurant food is spent at a fast-food restaurant. More than 160,000 fast-food restaurants are available in the United States, and more than $70,000,000,000 (10 zeros) are spent at them each year. The fast-food restaurants outnumber the traditional restaurants in the United States. One of five persons in the United States visits a fast-food restaurant every day, and four of five every month. Fast-food restaurants are located in hospitals, zoos, military bases, college campuses (including dormitories), museums, airports, naval ships and boats, bus stations, amusement parks, private-office and state-government buildings, and department stores. Mobile (restaurants on wheels) fast-food restaurants visit neighborhoods, playgrounds, and beaches. More than 50% of the population of the United States lives within 3 minutes of a McDonald's. McDonald's alone has employed more than 8 million workers, 7% of the U. S. work force, and it has replaced the U.S. Army as America's largest job-training organization. McDonald's alone is the world's largest owner of commercial real estate.

The *FAST FOOD GUIDE* by Jacobson and Fritschner[66, 67] has detailed the amounts of calories, fat, sodium, sugar, and other "nutrients" in the foods and liquids sold by the 15 largest fast-food chains in the United States. The champion hamburger at the moment is *Carl's Double Western Bacon Cheeseburger*, which contains 1030 calories, 14 teaspoons of fat, and 1800 mg of sodium. This dandy is truly the coronary artery bypass special! It is quickly followed by *Jack in the Box Ultimate Cheeseburger* and the *Burger King Double Whopper with Cheese*. The *Burger King Chicken Sandwich*, the bird champ, contains nearly 700 calories, 9 teaspoons of fat, and 1415 mg of sodium. *Carl's Jr. Carl's Fish Sandwich*, the champ of the fish, contains 560 calories, 7 teaspoons of fat, and 1220 mg of sodium. Arby's 5-ounce french fries contain nearly 500 calories. The *Dairy Queen Health Blizzard, regular*, the champ of shakes and malts, contains 820 calories, 8 teaspoons of fat, 410 mg of sodium, and 14 teaspoons of sugar. *Taco Bell Taco Salad with shell*, the salad champion, contains 905 calories, 14 teaspoons of fat, and 910 gm of sodium. Thus these fast foods lead to quick plaques!

Mexican food. And the Mexican foods are no better.[68, 69] A *Chicken Burrito* dinner (cheese-topped flour tortilla stuffed with chicken and refried beans) contains enough sodium for 1.5 days. A *Chile Relleno* dinner (cheese-stuffed, deep-fried pepper, topped with cheese and red sauce) contains as much saturated fat as 27 slices of bacon and is much fattier than a cup of Häagen-Dazs Exträäs Cookie Dynamo ice cream. Two *Crispy Chicken Tacos* (crisp corn tortillas stuffed with chicken, cheese, lettuce, and tomato) with refried beans and rice amount to 1042 calories, 36% of which come from fat, a total of 42 gm of fat including 13 gm of saturated fat and 2260 mg of sodium. Two *Soft Chicken Tacos* with refried beans and rice are just as bad: 1022 calories, 38% of which come from fat; a total of 43 gm of fat including 15 gm of the saturated variety, and 2690 mg of sodium. Two *Chicken Enchiladas* (chicken and cheese in an oil-dipped corn tortilla) total 1264 calories, 40% of which come from fat; a total of 57 gm of fat, 19 gm of which are saturated, plus 2855 mg of sodium! Two *Beef Enchiladas* with beans and rice amount to 1253 calories, 42% of which come from fat, a total of 58 gm of fat, 16 gm being saturated, plus 2880 mg of sodium. The appetizers and side dishes are not much better. The *Mexican Rice* (¾ cup), sautéd in oil or shortening before it is cooked in sodium-soaked chicken broth, is 15% fat, and *Refried Pinto Beans* (¾ cup) contains nearly 40% more calories than the rice, and 39% of the 375 calories come from fat. The only dish considered decent enough to recommend is *chicken fajitas* but without the beans, sour cream, and guacamole. Unlike Chinese or Italian restaurant food, it is tough to make Mexican dishes less fatty and less salty.

Foods and liquids consumed in 1 day in the United States. The total quantity of calories, fat, and cholesterol eaten by American adults each day is mind-boggling. As estimated by Parker[70] 10 years ago and summarized elsewhere,[71] our daily oral intake includes some of the following (this was in 1984 when the U. S. population was 236 million, not 260 million like today): approximately 815 billion calories of food are consumed, roughly 200 billion more than we need to maintain a moderate level of activity enough extra calories to feed everyone in Mexico, a country in 1984 of 80 million people). Approximately 100 million cows live in the United States, and nearly 100,000 of them are herded into slaughterhouses, where they leave 60 million pounds of red meat and nearly 4 million square feet of hide. Every day approximately 250,000 hogs and 17,700 lambs and sheep are butchered. More than 4 million pounds of bacon are eaten every day. Every day approximately 1.5 million pounds of lard (hog fat) and 47 million hot dogs (smoked sausage of beef or beef and pork) are eaten daily. McDonald's restaurants serve the equivalent of 2250 head of cattle daily.

Dairy cows in the United States produce 47 million gallons of milk daily, 19 of which are used as *liquid milk*, and the rest as cheese, yogurt, and other dairy products. We eat 12.5 million pounds of cheese, including 85,000 pounds of blue cheese, 700 pounds of cream cheese, 650,000 pounds of Swiss, cheese and 5.8 million pounds of cheddar cheese. Americans eat 170 million eggs and 12 million chickens every day!

Americans smoke 85 million packs of cigarettes. If one cigarette deducts 5.5 minutes of life from the smoker, collectively, Americans shorten their lives by 18,000 years every day. We fill 85,000 bushels with cigarette butts. Four thousand children and teenagers take up smoking each day.

Excessive body weight. The tremendous quantity of fat consumed in the United States displays itself by the largeness of our society. In 1990 60% of Americans 18 years of age and older were considered overweight, and 30% were frankly obese (>20% above ideal body weight). No society has ever been as overweight as the present U. S. one. And the percent overweight continues to increase.[72] Adults in the United States in 1993 gained 155 million pounds. A survey in 1991 showed an average weight loss of 10 pounds for adults in the United States; in 1993 a similar poll showed an average gain of 2.1 pounds. Four national surveys between 1960 and 1991 of 6000 to 13,000 adults in the United States showed that 33% were overweight (>120% of desirable weight) during the last survey (1988 to 1991). Overweightness frequency increased 8% between the 1976 to 1980 and the 1988 to 1991 surveys. The mean body weight during this approximate 10-year period increased 8 pounds (3.6 kg)! For the first time in 15 years, neither losing weight nor stopping smoking was the number 1 New Year's resolution in 1994. Instead, people are most concerned with managing their personal finances better. According to the National Cattlemen's Association, beef production is increasing: 23 billion pounds in carcass weight in 1993 and an increase to nearly 24 billion in 1994. Per capita beef consumption in the United States, as measured by retail weight, lags behind chicken by 68.7 to 65.6 pounds. Beef consumption, however, if measured by "boneless edible weight," leads chicken consumption by a wide margin, 62.2 to 48.0 pounds.

There is no better monitor for fat consumption than body weight. The first road to health is the maintenance of ideal or near ideal body weight. The more we weigh, the sooner we die.[73] All of us can identify the exception, such as Sir Winston Churchill, but he was an exception. Physicians need to set the example here. And losing weight is so difficult! A pound of body fat contains approximately 3500 calories. To lose 1 pound of fat, 3500 more calories must be burned than consumed. One pound can be lost each week by burning 500 more calories each day than consumed. Because walking or running a mile each consumes about 400 calories, combining exercise with reduced calorie consumption may speed weight reduction.

Table II. Calories needed daily to sustain ideal body weight

Height (inches)	*Ideal body weight (pounds)*	*Activity level*			
		+	++	+++	++++
Women					
59	95	1045	1235	1425	1710
60	100	1100	1300	1500	1800
61	105	1155	1365	1575	1890
62	110	1210	1430	1650	1980
63	115	1265	1495	1725	2070
64	120	1320	1560	1800	2160
65	125	1375	1625	1875	2250
66	130	1430	1690	1950	2340
67	135	1485	1755	2025	2430
68	140	1540	1820	2100	2520
69	145	1595	1885	2175	2610
70	150	1650	1950	2250	2700
71	155	1705	2015	2325	2790
72	160	1760	2080	2400	2880
Men					
62	118	1298	1534	1770	2124
63	124	1364	1612	1860	2232
64	130	1430	1690	1950	2340
65	136	1496	1768	2040	2448
66	142	1562	1846	2130	2556
67	148	1628	1924	2220	2664
68	154	1694	2002	2310	2772
69	160	1760	2080	2400	2880
70	166	1826	2158	2490	2988
71	172	1892	2236	2580	3096
72	178	1958	2314	2670	3204
73	184	2024	2392	2760	3204
74	190	2090	2470	2850	3420
75	196	2156	2548	2940	3528
76	202	2222	2626	3030	3636

Calculating the percentage of calories from fat and the grams of fat consumed daily to maintain an ideal body weight. To help maintain or achieve an ideal or near ideal body weight, it is useful to know how many calories are permissible each day.[74] Most adults in the Western world need from 11 to 18 calories per pound per day to sustain an ideal weight: 11 for the near sedentary individual (+), 13 for the moderately active (++), 15 for the moderate exerciser or physical laborer (+++), and 18 for the extremely active exerciser of physical worker (++++). Table II lists the calories needed in both women and men at the various activity levels to maintain an ideal body weight, and Table III lists the maximal grams of fat allowed with

Table III. Maximal grams of fat allowed with four different percent-of-calories-from-fat diets

Daily calorie intake	Maximum grams of fat allowed for ideal body weight with four different percent-of-calories-from-fat diets			
	15%	*20%*	*25%*	*30%*
1200	20	27	33	40
1300	22	29	36	43
1400	23	31	39	47
1500	25	33	42	50
1600	26	36	44	53
1700	28	38	47	57
1800	30	40	50	60
1900	31	42	53	63
2000	33	44	56	67
2100	35	47	58	70
2200	36	49	61	73
2300	38	51	64	77
2400	40	53	67	80
2500	41	56	69	83
2600	43	58	72	87
2700	45	60	75	90
2800	46	62	77	93
2900	48	64	80	96
3000	50	67	83	100

four different percentage-of-calories-from-fat diets. Because I am 6-feet-tall and like to weigh no more than 170 pounds and am moderately active (++), I need approximately 2300 calories daily: a 30%-of-calories-from-fat diet for me would be 690 calories from fat (2300 × 0.30); at 20% fat, 460 calories, (2300 × 0.20) and at 10% fat, 230 calories (2300 × 0.10). Given the new food-labeling regulations, which provide grams of fat on food labels, it is better to calculate the grams of fat rather than the percentage of calories from fat in each of the various percentage-of-calories-from-fat diets. Thus the maximal grams of fat I should consume can easily be determined by dividing by 9 (the number of calories in 1 gm of fat) the number of calories derived from fat were I to consume a 30% (690 ÷ 9 = 75 gm), a 20% (460 ÷ 9 = 50 gm), or a 10% (230 ÷ 9 = 25 gm) calories-from-fat diet. Total calories is the important factor from the standpoint of body weight, but fat calories or fat grams is the important item from the standpoint of atherosclerotic disease. If all of us consumed no more than 25 gm of fat daily, none of us would have atherosclerosis of clinical significance, but unfortunately few of us are pure vegetarians, a near requirement to maintain a 25 gm fat intake. At 50 gm of fat daily (a little <2 ounces) our risk of significant atherosclerotic disease also is small. At 75 gm it is greater. If the quantity could be closer to 50 gm of fat daily, our arteries would be cleaner, and then atherosclerosis and excessive body weight would not be so prevalent. Unfortunately most American adults consume more than 100 gm of fat daily, many of us more than 140 gm. Our body weights are increased, and our risk for having significant atherosclerosis is enormous.

Flesh consumption. If clinically significant atherosclerosis is to be prevented or arrested, the amount of fat consumed must be diminished. An easy way to decrease fat consumption is to decrease flesh consumption. The ideal of course is a pure vegetarian-fruit diet that provides no more than approximately 10% of calories from fat. Not many persons in the Western world are desirous, however, of becoming vegetarians (either pure [vegans] or ovolacto-type), but that should be our goal. For atherosclerotic health to improve, however, at least the quantity of flesh consumed must be decreased. With 21 meals a week, we must make more of them meatless. The type of flesh consumed also must be altered. Bovine and porcine muscle are the most heavily laden with fat, and therefore their quantity must be decreased the most. In general, the higher the grade of meat is, the more fat it contains. Regardless of the grade or cut, the fat of all red meats is predominantly saturated (approximately 45% of the fat), and only 2% of the fat is polyunsaturated. Ground beef contributes more saturated fat to the average American diet than any other single food. The fat-ladened skin of chickens and turkeys must be avoided. Fish is the preferred flesh because it contains relatively little fat (and because its consumption has the least unfavorable effects on our environment.)[75-82] Fish also contains some potentially favorable fatty acids in contrast to that in the muscle of cows, pigs, chickens, turkeys, sheep, etc. Additionally, we need to avoid snacks between meals, because many of them are laden with fat and calories, and desserts, except on special occasions. Calories just before bedtime are rarely fat- or calorie-friendly.

Characteristics of carnivores and herbivores. Human beings basically are not carnivores.[83] If several characteristics of carnivores and herbivores are compared, human beings clearly have more characteristics of herbivores than carnivores. The appendages of carnivores contain claws; those of herbivores, hands or hoofs. The teeth of carnivores are sharp; those of herbivores, mainly flat (for grinding). The intestinal tract of carnivores is short; that of herbivores is long. (The small intestine of humans is 26 feet long!) Carnivores lap fluids; herbivores sip them. Carnivores cool their bodies by panting; herbivores, by sweating.

Carnivores make their own vitamin C; herbivores obtain their vitamin C from their diet. Most human beings believe themselves to be carnivores (we eat flesh), but fundamentally our characteristics more closely resemble the herbivores. Foods intended for *homo sapiens* probably are only three: starches (rice, corn, potatoes, beans, and pasta), vegetables, and fruits.

Diseases infrequent in vegetarians. Human beings who eat exclusively a vegetarian-fruit diet for many decades (assuming that consumption of the fatty acids high in saturated fat are avoided—coconut oil, palm kernel oil) infrequently have the diseases so commonly observed in human meat eaters.[77] Diseases very uncommon in vegetarians include *atherosclerosis*; *systemic hypertension* (at least 60 of the 160 million persons in the United States older than 20 years of age have systemic arterial pressures >140/90 mm Hg); *cancer of the breast and colon*, and possibly *cancer of the prostate gland*; *diabetes mellitus* (with onset after age 50 years); *obesity; peptic ulcer, appendicitis, diverticulitis*, and *irritable bowel syndrome*; *osteoporosis* and *osteoarthritis*; *gallstones* and *kidney stones*; and *salmonellosis* and *trichinosis*.

Diets and diseases of our stone-age ancestors. Most diseases that vegetarians do not get were apparently also rare or very uncommon among our stone age or Paleolithic ancestors and also among the few remaining groups of hunters-gatherers still living on Earth. Eaton et al.[81, 84] have made some observations about our stone-age ancestors, and some are summarized as follows[85]:

Lack of genetic change. The gene pool has changed little since anatomically modern human beings, *Homo sapiens sapiens*, became widespread approximately 30,000 years ago. From a genetic standpoint current humans are still late Paleolithic preagricultural hunters-gatherers. We have stone age bodies in an atomic age. Our genetic makeup was selected, over geologic eras, ultimately to fit the lifestyle of Paleolothic humans.

Enormous environmental change. The increasing industrialized affluence of the last 200 years has affected health both beneficially and adversely. Improved housing, sanitation, and medical care have ameliorated the impact of infection and trauma, the chief causes of death from the Paleolithic era until 1900. The result is that average life expectancy is now approximately double what it was for preagricultural humans. Concomitantly, the past century has accelerated the biologic estrangement that has increasingly differentiated humans from other mammals for more than 2 million years. In today's Western nations we have little need for exercise, but we consume foods quite different from those available to other mammals and expose ourselves to such harmful agents as alcohol and tobacco. We have crossed an epidemiologic boundary and entered a watershed in which disorders such as atherosclerosis, systemic hypertension, obesity, diabetes mellitus, and certain cancers have become common in contrast to their rarity or near nonexistence among remaining preagricultural humans.

The late Paleolithic lifestyle. The period 35,000 to 20,000 years ago is the last time period during which the collective human gene interacted with bioenvironmental circumstances typical of those for which it had been originally selected. Thus the diet, exercise patterns, and social adaptions of that time have continuing relevance today.

Nutrition. The dietary requirement of all stone age persons were met exclusively by uncultivated vegetables and wild game. The amount of protein was great, probably 33% of calories, compared with the current American diet, which derives 12% of its calories from protein. Because game animals are lean, Paleolithic people ate much less fat than Americans and Europeans do today. Stone Age people ate more polyunsaturated than saturated fat. Their cholesterol intake equaled or exceeded that now common in industrialized nations. Stone Age people ate much more dietary fiber than do most Americans. They obtained far more potassium than sodium from their food (as do all other mammals). Because they had no domesticated animals, they had no dairy foods; despite this fact, their calcium intake far exceeded that consumed today.

Physical exercise. The hunter-gatherer way of life generated high levels of physical and aerobic fitness. Strength and stamina were characteristic of both sexes at all ages. The hunters-gatherers were stronger and more muscular than succeeding agriculturalists.

Alcohol. Alcoholic beverages were infrequently consumed, and those available, all products of natural fermentation, were far less potent than present-day distilled liquors. Solitary, addictive drinking apparently did not occur.

Tobacco. Tobacco was practically unavailable until agriculture appeared in the Americas approximately 5000 years ago. Pipes and cigars were the only methods used for smoking until approximately 1850, when cigarettes first appeared. The major impact of tobacco abuse is a postcigarette phenomenon.

Effects of changes in lifestyle on disease prevalence. The three chief killers of the Stone Age humans were childbirth and diseases of infancy, infection (particularly parasitism), and trauma.

Obesity. Stone Age human beings were lean, and leanness today in the Western world is nearly the exception. Most food today is calorically concentrated in comparison with the wild game and uncultivated fruits and vegetables that constituted the Paleolithic diets. In eating a given volume, enough to create a feeling of fullness, Paleolithic humans consumed fewer calories than those consumed in a similar volume in the Western world today. Most beverages consumed today provide a significant caloric load. Paleolithic human beings, in contrast, drank water. Energy expenditure, that is, calories burned by modern human beings, is much less than by the Stone Age humans.

Atherosclerosis. Present-day preliterate societies have little or no atherosclerosis. Like our Paleolithic ancestors, they rarely use tobacco, are normotensive, have low serum total cholesterol levels, and are physically active. The adverse changes that occur in atherosclerotic risk factors when people from societies with little such disease become westernized recapitulate the patterns observed for other diseases of civilization. The present-day remaining hunter-gatherers and the other remaining preliterates (rudimentary horticulturists, simple agriculturists, and pastoralists) consume diets low in total fat with more polyunsaturated than saturated fatty acids (a higher polyunsaturated than saturated fat ratio) but with an amount of cholesterol similar to that in the current American diet (500 mg). Because the fibrinolytic activity of blood and platelet aggregation are enhanced by physical activity but decreased by cigarette smoking, obesity, and hypercholesterolemia, the preliterate peoples also have more such activity and less platelet aggregation than do average Westerners.

Systemic hypertension. There are still several cultures on earth whose members do not have essential hypertension and whose blood pressure does not rise with age. When people living in these remaining preliterate cultures, however, adopt a Western lifestyle, either by migration or acculturation, they first have a tendency for their blood pressure to rise with age and then an increasing tendency to have systemic hypertension. The diets of these normotensive preliterates are low in sodium, high in potassium, high in calcium, and low to absent in alcohol.

Diabetes mellitus. Obesity and maturity-onset diabetes are among the first disorders to appear when unacculturated people undergo economic development. The overall prevalence of noninsulin-dependent diabetes among adults in industrialized countries ranges from 3% to 10%, but among unacculturated native populations it is 0% to 2%. The most powerful risk factor to diabetes is obesity, and excessive weight gain is virtually absent in preliterate societies. Obese people have reduced numbers of cellular insulin receptors, a relative tissue resistance to insulin, and higher blood insulin levels than lean people. Conversely, high-level physical fitness, characteristic of aboriginal persons, is associated with an increased number of insulin receptors and better insulin binding, both of which enhance the body's sensitivity to insulin. Diets containing ample amounts of nonnutrient fiber and complex carbohydrates lower both fasting and postprandial blood glucose levels, and these types of diets are the rule among technologically primitive societies but the exception in Western nations.

Thus the message from Eaton et al.[81, 84] is this: we need to eat and exercise like the Stone Age people. If we do, our health will improve substantially, and our medical bills will decrease substantially.

Effectiveness or noneffectiveness of various diets in lowering the total and low-density lipoprotein cholesterol levels. The effectiveness of diet in lowering our total and LDL-cholesterol levels is nearly directly dependent on the percent of calories from fat in the diet. The average American adult consumes a diet containing nearly 40% of the calories from fat, one third of which is of the saturated variety. The most commonly prescribed diet by physicians in the United States is the National Cholesterol Education Program Step 2 diet, which is a 30%-of-calories-from-fat diet with saturated fat less than 7% and cholesterol less than 200 mg/day.[86] This diet, however, is relatively ineffective in reducing the total and LDL-cholesterol levels. With this diet, which is a 25% reduction in percent of calories from fat, the average serum total cholesterol is reduced by only 5% (e.g., 240 → 228 mg/dl [6.2 → 5.9 mmol/L], and the average serum LDL-cholesterol also is reduced an average of 5% (e.g., 160 → 152 mg/dl [4.1 → 3.9 mmol/L]).[87, 88] Some individuals lower their serum total and LDL cholesterol by up to 30% by this modest diet, and in other patients the serum cholesterol levels actually increase by up to 20%. The average change, however, is a 5% decrease. A reduction in the percent of calories from fat from 40% to 20% (The American Heart Association phase III diet) decreases the serum total cholesterol by approximately 20% (e.g., 240 → 192 mg/dl [6.2 → 5.0 mmol/L] and the LDL-cholesterol also about 20% (e.g., 160 → 128 mg/dl [4.1 → 3.3 mmol/L]).[89] Most Americans, however, are not willing to reduce their percent of calories from fat to the 20% level. A reduction of the percent of calories from fat from 40% to 10% can reduce the serum total cholesterol level in persons without familial hypercholesterolemia to the 150 mg/dl (3.9 mmol/L) area, a level achieved for practical purposes only by those following a vegetarian-fruit diet, but a level where atherosclerotic plaques do not form and where those present shrink in size. Incidently, the diet of the Japanese historically has consisted of a 10%-of-calories-from-fat diet, and significant atherosclerosis has seldom been observed.[12] Today the Japanese are consuming a diet averaging approximately 23% of calories from fat, and the consequence has been a significant increase in the frequency of symptomatic atherosclerosis. Thus for diets to be very effective in lowering the serum total and LDL-cholesterol levels, the percentage of calories from fat must be reduced to 20% and ideally to 10%.

If all adults in the United States were to reduce their percentage of calories from fat by 25% (40% → 30% of calories from fat), the frequency of symptomatic and fatal atherosclerosis and the extent of atherosclerosis would decrease for the population. For an individual, however, the percentage of calories from fat must be reduced to approximately 20% before the risk of a first or subsequent atherosclerotic event will be substantially reduced. And in individuals who have already had an atherosclerotic event, in whom the challenge is to decrease the chances of a subsequent atherosclerotic event, a reduction of 50% of the percentage of calories from fat (and also of direct cholesterol) is necessary to significantly reduce the risk of a further event. For Americans who have consumed approximately 40% of their calories from fat for 40 years to suddenly reduce that percentage by half is a burden most are not willing to tackle. Thus lipid-lowering drugs have a major role in cholesterol lowering in the United States.

Lipid-lowering drugs. For persons with familial hypercholesterolemia, diet alone will not be adequate to lower the total and LDL-cholesterol levels sufficiently to substantially reduce the risk of having an atherosclerotic event. Furthermore for persons who have had an atherosclerotic event, lipid-lowering drug therapy is recommended, unless the person is willing to reduce the percent of calories from fat to approximately 10%.[90] Additionally, for persons with very high serum total and LDL-cholesterol levels not produced by an identifiable cause such as a drug (e.g., diuretic), hepatic disease, renal disease, or hypothyroidism and unassociated with an atherosclerotic event, a lipid-lowering drug may be required if diet therapy is ineffective.

Primary prevention. Except for the person with familial hypercholesterolemia, the first and ideally the only step required to lower the total and LDL-cholesterol levels adequately is diet, followed by diet, and then more diet. Each succeeding step of diet means further lowering of the quantity of fat and cholesterol consumed. If the diet alone does not lower the total and LDL-cholesterol levels adequately, the lipid-lowering (altering) drugs are useful.

Secondary prevention. In my view persons who have had an atherosclerotic event should be on one or more cholesterol-lowering drugs irrespective of the serum or plasma lipid levels, because whatever the levels are in those with events, they are too high.[90] This recommendation is not made lightly, because approximately 7 million persons in the United States alone have symptomatic myocardial ischemia, and many others have limb or cerebral ischemia from atherosclerosis. Nevertheless there is increasing evidence that lipid-lowering medicines after heart attacks may be even more beneficial than aspirin, β blockers, angiotensin-converting-enzyme inhibitors, and calcium antagonists in preventing subsequent atherosclerotic events. Furthermore lipid-lowering drugs, if they can bring the serum total cholesterol down to the 150 mg/dl area and the LDL-cholesterol level to less than 100 mg/dl, can prevent or at least retard atherosclerotic progression and produce some regression. Neither lack of progression nor initiation of regression, however, appears to occur unless the serum total cholesterol is lowered to the range enjoyed by pure or nearly pure vegetarians. The use of lipid-lowering drugs, of course, does not negate the use of a low-cholesterol, low-fat diet, because each appears to work synergistically. Even in patients who refuse to follow the low-cholesterol, low-fat diet, however, the lipid-lowering drugs nevertheless produce substantial reductions in the serum cholesterol levels[87] and decrease the chances of first and subsequent events (Fig. 3).

In November 1994 the results of the Scandinavian Simvastatin Survival Study (4S) was published,[91] and this study is the best of the secondary prevention trials so far. The 4S study involved 4444 Scandinavian adult men and women who had had either an acute myocardial infarction that had healed (80%) or angina pectoris (20%) with serum total cholesterol levels from 212 to 309 mg/dL (5.5 to 8.0 mmol/L). The

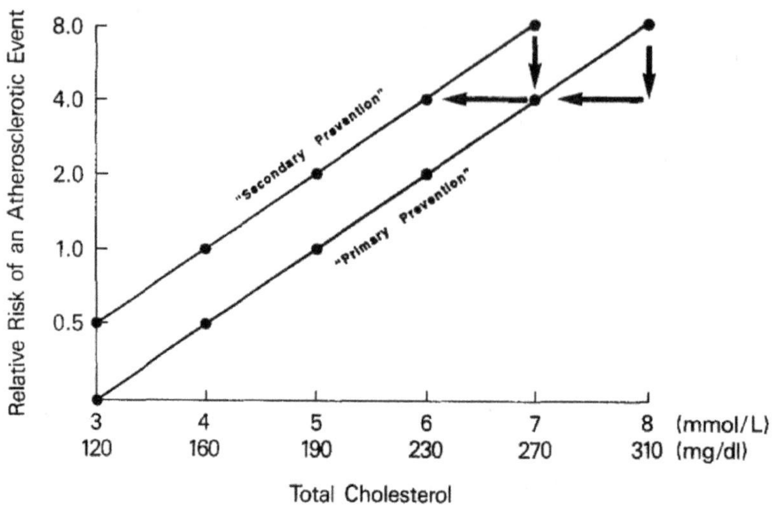

Fig. 3. Effects of serum total cholesterol reduction on risk of first or subsequent atherosclerotic event. "Average risk" refers to primary prevention—person has not had atherosclerotic event. "High risk" refers to secondary prevention—person has had atherosclerotic event. Occurrence of event shifts line to left. Nevertheless wherever serum total cholesterol level is, reduction of that level by approximately 40 mg/dl (or 1 mmol/L) reduces relative risk of atherosclerotic event (either a first one or a subsequent one) in half. Thus large benefits result from reducing serum total cholesterol.

double-blind, randomized, placebo-controlled study was continued until 440 patients had died. One half of the patients were treated with simvastatin (20 mg [63%] or 40 mg [37%] daily) and one half with matching placebo. During the 5 years of the study in the treatment group, the serum total cholesterol fell 28%, the LDL cholesterol fell 38%, and the HDL cholesterol rose 8%. During the study period total mortality in the treatment group fell 30% (256 [placebo] vs 182 [simvastatin]), coronary mortality fell 42% (189 [placebo] vs 111 [simvastatin]), and noncardiovascular mortality was similar in both treatment and placebo groups. The risk of coronary death and nonfatal acute myocardial infarction fell 34%, the risk of survival without an atherosclerotic event was reduced 26%, and the need for coronary angioplasty or bypass was reduced 37% in the treatment group compared with the control group. This latter 37% reduction was in five Scandinavian countries where these procedures are performed far less frequently per capita than in the United States. Thus this percent reduction of need for these procedures, if applied to the United States, would probably be much higher and the cost savings substantial. No patient was lost to follow-up in the entire study, and only 10% of patients in the treatment group discontinued taking simvastatin. In summary, the 4S study provides substantial justification for initiating lipid-lowering drug therapy (and low-cholesterol, low-fat dieting) after onset of either acute myocardial infarction or angina pectoris. The study also shows that noncardiovascular mortality is not increased by simvastatin therapy.

Types of lipid-lowering drugs. The first-line lipid-lowering drugs in my view should be the 3-hydroxy-3-methyglutaryl coenzyme A (HMG-CoA) reductase inhibitors (the statins), because they are the best LDL-cholesterol-lowering drugs, they are the only lipid-lowering drugs that can be taken only once a day, because they are well tolerated, and because they have few side effects. Four statin drugs are presently available in the United States, and more than 70% of patients taking them are taking only one tablet daily; few patients are taking the maximal recommended doses of these drugs. Equivalent doses would be 10 mg simvastatin = 20 mg lovastatin = 20 mg provastatin = 40 mg fluvastatin.[92] Not only do these drugs lower the serum LDL-cholesterol and total cholesterol, but they raise the serum HDL-cholesterol (approximately 6%) and lower the triglyceride level (approximately 20%). Side effects of the statins at the low doses are extremely uncommon.

Niacin, a vitamin taken in high doses, generally approximately 1.5 gm daily, may be thought of as a poor person's HMG-CoA reductose inhibitor, because it too has favorable effects on all four lipoproteins. Niacin is the best HDL-cholesterol raiser of the lipid-lowering agents. Its side effects, flushing, itching, and head pounding, limit its use in most patients.

Gemfibrozil, the only fibrate available in the United States, lowers the triglyceride level more effectively than any of the other lipid-lowering drugs, but it has only modest effect on the LDL-cholesterol, and not infrequently it raises rather than lowers the LDL-cholesterol level.

Cholestyramine and *colestipol*, the bile-acid resins, are the safest of the lipid-altering drugs, but these medicines must be taken in huge amounts (approximately 30,000 mg/day) to have the same effects on LDL-cholesterol as do the smaller doses of the statin drugs. Furthermore these drugs raise the triglyceride level, and they have small (4% ↑) effects on the HDL cholesterol.

Probucol, an antioxidant, has not been demonstrated to prevent or retard atherosclerosis, and it is rarely used now in the United States. This drug also lowers (23% ↓) the HDL-cholesterol, has no effect on the triglyceride level, and its LDL-cholesterol lowering is only modest. Other antioxidants, vitamin E, C, and A, have yet to be shown either to prevent or to retard atherosclerosis.

Because the most common cause of ventricular arrhythmias and congestive heart failure is atherosclerotic coronary artery disease, the lipid-lowering drugs by their ability to diminish progression and initiate atherosclerotic regression may be the best antiarrhythmic and anticongestive heart failure agents, at least prophylactically.[93, 94]

A major problem with the lipid-lowering drugs is compliance. Approximately 50% of persons who started taking these drugs quit taking them within a year, and this rate holds true whether the drug is easily tolerated, like the statins, or has disturbing side effects such as niacin or the bile-acid resins.

Another problem with lipid-lowering drugs is that most of the persons needing them are not on them, because they have not been prescribed. Probably no more than 1 million of the 7 million persons with symptomatic myocardial ischemia in the United States are taking one or more lipid-lowering agents, and no more than 1 million of the 40 million persons in the United States with serum total cholesterol levels greater than 240 mg/dl are taking one or more lipid-lowering agents.

Getting cardiologists interested in lipid-lowering drugs. Most cardiologists appear to be hesitant in prescribing lipid-lowering drugs to their patients, even those who have had one or more atherosclerotic events. Several surveys have shown that cardiologists rank only slightly above general internists, general practitioners, and the general public in considering "cholesterol" of major importance for development of atherosclerosis. It takes few fingers to name prominent cardiologists around the world who have become recognized as lipid experts or who have a major interest in lipids. Yet the data show that cholesterol causes atherosclerosis. When high cholesterol levels are lowered, clinical atherosclerotic events decrease, and the amounts of atherosclerotic plaque deposited in arteries decrease. Although there are many exceptions, cardiologists in general have relatively little interest in cholesterol and its role in atherosclerosis. Why might this be the case?[95]

1. Cardiologists as a group are not completely convinced of the important role of cholesterol in atherosclerosis. Most patients seen by cardiologists have serum total cholesterol levels greater than 200 mg/dl (>5.2 mmol/L), and there is not much difference in the cholesterol levels in those patients with and those without overt evidence of myocardial ischemia. Thus the actual serum total cholesterol is not very helpful in the United States in separating patients with myocardial ischemia from those without myocardial ischemia. Furthermore nearly half the patients with angiographic evidence of significant coronary arterial narrowing have serum total cholesterol levels less than 200 mg/dl (<5.2 mmol/L). (Most of the latter group, however, have relatively low LDL cholesterol levels.) It is impossible to get excited about cholesterol if one is not convinced of its importance!

2. Cardiologists view cholesterol management as unexciting. Cholesterol management is long-term. Witnessed changes in outcome are rarely apparent. It is similar to the management of systemic hypertension. Cardiologists are certainly convinced of the importance of lowering elevated blood pressure, but as a group cardiologists are not interested in the management of systemic hypertension. The same goes for the management of hypercholesterolemia. Its management is relatively boring compared with the excitement of treating patients with chest pain, arrhythmias, overt congestive heart failure, heart block, etc. Cardiology focuses primarily on management of acute events, the management of which is exciting. Dramatic changes in outcome in response to therapies (drugs and procedures) are witnessed. Lowering of cholesterol or blood pressure levels do not, in contrast, produce overt changes in the patients' symptoms or appearances. Cardiologists also tend to be more excited by the acute lesions in coronary arteries than by the masses of plaque in the coronary arteries.

3. Cardiologists avoid cholesterol management because they know that successful management requires expert knowledge of nutrition, of cholesterol-lowering drugs, and a change in their own lifestyles. Cardiologists as a group are uncomfortable when nutrition is the topic. Cardiologists are not calorie counters or grocery-store shoppers. Housewives know more about calories, fats, and carbohydrates than do many cardiologists. Cardiologists as a group are not experts on lipid-lowering drugs. Cardiologists, in contrast, are comfortable with nitroglycerin, digitalis, β blockers, calcium antagonists, angiotensin-converting-enzyme inhibitors, antiarrhythmic agents, thrombolytic agents, aspirin, heparin, warfarin, and vasopressors, but not lipid-lowering and antioxidant agents. I am afraid that we all tend to dismiss as unimportant that which we do not understand well or are not interested in.

4. *Cardiologists are a bit confused by the recommendations of the lipid experts regarding whom to treat and whom not to treat with diet and lipid-lowering agents.* The recommendations do change. The first U. S. recommendations, however, appeared in January 1988,[8] and the second U. S. recommendations appeared in June 1993,[86] so the argument that the recommendations are "always changing" is not valid. The recommendations may intermix primary and secondary prevention, but the importance of therapy in secondary prevention is more emphasized in the June 1993 recommendation than previously. Patients who have had atherosclerotic events should be clearly separated from those who have not, because management of the two is entirely different. I too believe that the recommendations can be simplified a bit.

5. *Cardiologists resent being excluded from important roles in the cholesterol-lowering world.* The adult-lipid-expert committee in the United States is composed almost entirely of persons whose subspecialty in medicine is endocrinology and metabolism. Only one cardiologist is a member of the recent adult-lipid-expert panel in the United States.[86] I suspect that cardiologists as a group are a bit uncomfortable in a situation where they are not the dominant players. Leaders in the lipid world are not physicians whose training had focused on cardiology. Yet in the real world it is the cardiologists who see patients who have had atherosclerotic events. In other words lipidologists dominate primary prevention, that is, treating persons with lipid disorders before atherosclerotic events. Cardiologists, however, because they see persons who have or have had atherosclerotic events, are the dominant forces of secondary prevention. In my view all of these patients should be on a low-fat, low-cholesterol diet, and with few exceptions, should be taking one or more lipid-lowering drugs. Cardiologists simply have no choice but to become better informed about these diets and these drugs.

6. *Cardiologists view the lipid-lowering drugs as too expensive.* Compared with what? In the United States in 1993, approximately $20 billion was spent on coronary bypass alone, and probably approximately half that much was spent on coronary angioplasty procedures. The lipid-lowering drugs are cheap and cost-effective in comparison. If every person in the United States with symptomatic myocardial ischemia was given a 20 mg tablet of lovastatin daily, the cost would be approximately $3 billion a year, and I suspect the benefit would be substantial.

7. *Cardiologists consider cholesterol-lowering drugs to have too many side effects with too high risk/benefit ratios.* The presently used lipid-lowering drugs are some of the safest of all drugs available. The EXCEL study[96, 97] showed the side effects of a 20 mg tablet of lovastatin daily to be no more than that of placebo! The bile-acid resins have no systemic effects, although the quantity of them required to provide good cholesterol lowering is high. Although enormously effective, the unpleasant side effects of niacin are considerable. Thus compared with the toxic effects of atherosclerosis, the lipid-lowering drugs, in contrast, are essentially nontoxic.

8. *Cardiologists view cholesterol management as financially unrewarding.* Certainly in comparison to the financial rewards resulting from the various cardiologic procedures, lipid-lowering endeavors are time-consuming, often discouraging, and financially of relatively little benefit. Additionally, some cardiologists consider lipid management the purview of the referring physicians.

Thus because secondary prevention is in the hands of cardiologists and because cholesterol lowering has proven benefit after atherosclerotic events, cardiologists must increase their knowledge of and use of low-fat, low-cholesterol diets and lipid-lowering agents.

Retail costs of lipid-lowering drugs. Several physicians have mentioned to me that their patients cannot afford the lipid-lowering drugs. Their patients, however, seem able to afford the far more expensive procedures, angioplasty and bypass, that help relieve at least temporarily the acute consequences of severe narrowings in the coronary and peripheral arterial systems. If the 12-ounce steaks were eliminated or reduced drastically in size, there would be plenty of change left over to purchase any of the lipid-lowering agents that have been proven to decrease recurrences of atherosclerotic events and to decrease progression and cause some regression in persons who have already had atherosclerotic events. The

Table IV. Retail costs of four 3-hydroxy-3-methylglutaryl coenzyme A (HMG-CoA) reductase inhibitors in the Dallas/Fort Worth, Tex., area, September 1994

Product (mg/day)	*A ($)*	*B ($)*	*C ($)*	*D ($)*	*E ($)*	*F ($)*	*Mean cost/ month ($)*	*Cost mg/ day ($)*	*LDL (%↓)*	*Cost/dose/day for 1% LDL↓ ($)*
Fluvastatin (20)	36.39	30.92	31.69	31.12	32.89	34.81	32.97	1.10	−18	0.06
Lovastatin (10)	39.96	38.78	34.19	37.69	38.78	37.79	37.86	1.26	−19	0.07
Pravastatin (10)	54.59	46.98	47.39	35.84	49.62	56.91	48.55	1.61	−20	0.08
Simvastatin (5)	49.79	46.68	48.19	46.29	46.98	48.86	47.79	1.59	−24	0.07
Fluvastatin (40)	39.79	33.98	35.19	35.34	35.72	38.71	36.46	1.21	−24	0.05
Lovastatin (20)	53.39	50.74	52.69	50.84	47.49	52.21	51.22	1.71	−27	0.06
Pravastatin (20)	51.29	49.72	54.29	46.95	51.97	49.44	50.61	1.68	−25	0.07
Simvastatin (10)	50.29	48.92	50.19	48.21	49.68	51.23	49.75	1.65	−33	0.05
Fluvastatin (80) (40 bid)	79.58	67.96	70.38	70.68	71.44	77.42	72.92	2.43	−35	0.07
Lovastatin (40)	93.79	94.68	99.49	91.24	82.69	89.71	91.93	3.06	−30	0.10
Lovastatin (40) (20 bid)	118.18	98.79	107.89	97.53	94.27	106.99	103.94	3.46	−34	0.10
Pravastatin (40)	99.49	82.84	84.29	86.89	88.54	81.11	87.19	2.91	−34	0.09
Pravastatin (40) (20 bid)	102.58	97.78	108.58	93.68	103.94	102.99	101.59	3.38	—	—
Simvastatin (20)	99.59	85.98	97.59	87.77	84.49	86.39	90.29	3.01	−36	0.08
Lovastatin (80) (40 bid)	181.18	185.97	178.99	194.09	188.76	189.99	186.51	6.22	−40	0.16
Simvastatin (40)	101.29	91.62	102.29	92.43	91.97	93.25	95.47	3.18	−41	0.08

bid, Twice daily; *LDL*, low-density lipoprotein cholesterol; —, no information available.

lipid-lowering agents appear to be better than aspirin, β blockers, and other agents for decreasing subsequent atherosclerotic events in persons who have already had an event. The retail costs (the prices the patients pay) of the four presently available statin drugs in one metropolitan area in the United States in 1 month of 1994 are tabulated in Table IV.[98]

SUMMARY

The good news about coronary atherosclerosis is that it takes an awful lot of plaque before symptoms of myocardial ischemia occur. The bad news is that despite the need for large quantities of plaque for symptoms to occur, nevertheless nearly half of us in the United States eventually have the necessary quantity. Atherosclerosis is infrequently hereditary in origin. Most of us get atherosclerosis because we consume too much fat, cholesterol, and calories. The consequence is an elevated (>150 mg/dl) serum total cholesterol level, and the higher the number is above 150, the greater is the quantity of plaque deposited in our arteries. If the serum total cholesterol level can be prevented from rising to more than 150 mg/dl, plaques are not laid down; if elevated levels are lowered to 150 mg/dl, further plaque does not form, and parts of those present may vanish. A fruit-vegetarian-starch diet is necessary as a rule to achieve the 150 mg/dl level in most adults. Lipid-lowering drugs are required in the patients with familial hypercholesterolemia and in most patients with atherosclerotic events. The best news about atherosclerosis is that it can be prevented in those without the hereditary form, and it can be arrested by lowering elevated serum total (and LDL) cholesterol to the 150 mg/dl level.

REFERENCES

1. Roberts WC. Qualitative and quantitative comparison of amounts of narrowing by atherosclerotic plaques in the major epicardial coronary arteries at necropsy in sudden coronary death, transmural acute myocardial infarction, transmural healed myocardial infarction and unstable angina pectoris. Am J Cardiol 1989;64:324-8.
2. Roberts WC, Kragel AH, Gertz SD, Roberts CS. Coronary arteries in unstable angina pectoris, acute myocardial infarction, and sudden coronary death. Am Heart J 1994;127:1588-93.
3. Kragel AH, Reddy SG, Wittes JT, Roberts WC. Morphometric analysis of the composition of atherosclerotic plaques in the four major epicardial coronary arteries in acute myocardial infarction and in sudden coronary death. Circulation 1989;80:1747-56.
4. Kragel AH, Reddy SG, Wittes JT, Roberts WC. Morphometric analysis of the composition of coronary arterial plaques in isolated unstable angina pectoris with pain at rest. Am J Cardiol 1990;66:562-7.
5. Mautner SL, Lin F, Mautner GC, Roberts WC. Comparison in women versus men of composition of atherosclerotic plaques in native coronary arteries and in saphenous veins used as aortocoronary conduits. J Am Coll Cardiol 1993;21:1312-8.
6. Mautner SL, Mautner GC, Hunsberger SA, Roberts WC. Comparison of composition of atherosclerotic plaques in saphenous veins used as aortocoronary conduits with plaques in native coronary arteries in the same men. Am J Cardiol 1994;70:1380-7.
7. Kragel AH, Gertz SD, Roberts WC. Morphologic comparison of frequency and types of acute lesions in the major epicardial coronary ar-

teries in unstable angina pectoris, sudden coronary death and acute myocardial infarction. J Am Coll Cardiol 1991;18:801-8.
8. The Expert Panel. Report of the National Cholesterol Education Program Expert Panel on detection, evaluation, and treatment of high blood cholesterol in adults. Arch Intern Med 1988;148:36-69.
9. Roberts WC. Atherosclerotic risk factors—are there ten or is there only one? Am J Cardiol 1989;64:552-4.
10. Stamler J, Wentworth D, Neaton JD, for the MRFIT Research Group. Is relationship between serum cholesterol and risk of premature death from coronary heart disease continuous and graded? Findings in 356,222 primary screenees of the Multiple Risk Factor Intervention Trial (MRFIT). JAMA 1986;256:2823-8.
11. Castelli WP, Garrison RJ, Wilson PWF, Abbott RD, Kalousdian S, Kannel WB. Incidence of coronary heart disease and lipoprotein cholesterol levels: the Framingham study. JAMA 1986;256:2835-8.
12. Keys A. Seven Countries: a Multivariate Analysis of Death and Coronary Heart Disease. Cambridge, Massachusetts: Harvard University Press, 1980:381.
13. Hoeg JM, Feuerstein IM, Tucker EE. Detection and quantitation of calcific atherosclerosis by ultrafast computed tomography in children and young adults with homozygous familial hypercholesterolemia. Arterioscler Thromb 1994;14:1066-74.
14. The Lipid Research Clinics Program Epidemiology Committee. Plasma lipid distributions in selected North American populations: the Lipid Research Clinics Program Prevalence Study. Circulation 1979;60:427-39.
15. Gordon T, Castelli WP, Hjortland MC, Kannel WB, Dawber TR. High density lipoprotein as a protective factor against coronary heart disease. Am J Med 1977;62:707-14.
16. Mautner SL, Sanchez JA, Rader DJ, Mautner GC, Ferrans VJ, Fredrickson DS, Brewer HB Jr, Roberts WC. The heart in Tangier disease: severe coronary atherosclerosis with near absence of high-density lipoprotein cholesterol. Am J Clin Pathol 1992;98:191-8.
17. Roberts WC. Frequency of systemic hypertension in various cardiovascular diseases. Am J Cardiol 1987;60:1E-8E.
18. Goldstein JL, Brown MS. Regulation of low-density lipoprotein receptors: implications for pathogenesis and therapy of hypercholesterolemia and atherosclerosis. Circulation 1987;76:504-7.
19. Brown MS, Goldstein JL. A receptor-mediated pathway for cholesterol homeostasis. Science 1986;232:34-47.
20. Garrison RJ, Castelli WB. Weight and 30-year mortality of men in the Framingham study. Ann Intern Med 1985;106:1006-9.
21. Crall FV Jr, Roberts WC. The extramural and intramural coronary arteries in juvenile diabetes mellitus: analysis of nine necropsy patients aged 19 to 38 years with onset of diabetes before age 15 years. Am J Med 1978;64:221-30.
22. Mautner SL, Lin F, Roberts WC. Composition of atherosclerotic plaques in the epicardial coronary arteries in juvenile (type I) diabetes mellitus. Am J Cardiol 1992;70:1264-8.
23. Waller BF, Palumbo PJ, Lie JT, Roberts WC. Status of the coronary arteries at necropsy in diabetes mellitus with onset after age 30 years: analysis of 229 diabetic patients with and without clinical evidence of coronary heart disease and comparison to 183 control subjects. Am J Med 1980;69:498-506.
24. Cowie CC, Howard BV, Harris MI. Serum lipoproteins in African Americans and whites with non-insulin-dependent diabetes in the US population. Circulation 1994;90:1185-93.
25. Roberts WC, Potkin BN, Solus DE, Reddy SG. Modes of death, frequency of healed and acute myocardial infarction, number of major epicardial coronary arteries severely narrowed by atherosclerotic plaque, and heart weight in fatal atherosclerotic coronary artery disease: analysis of 889 patients studied at necropsy. J Am Coll Cardiol 1990;15:196-203.
26. Roberts WC, Kragel AH, Potkin BN. Ages at death and sex distribution in age decade in fatal coronary artery disease. Am J Cardiol 1990; 66:1379-81.
27. The Lipid Research Clinics Program Epidemiology Committee. Plasma lipid distribution in selected North American populations: the Lipid Research Clinics Program Prevalence Study. Circulation 1979;60:427-39.
28. Anitschkow NN. Lesions of organs under lipid infiltration. Proc Med Soc Petersburg 1912;80:1.
29. Anitschkow NN. A history of experimentation on arterial atherosclerosis in animals. In: Blumenthal HT, ed. Cowdry's arteriosclerosis. A Survey of the Problem. 2nd ed. Springfield, Illinois: Charles C Thomas, 1967:21-44.
30. Herrick JB. Clinical features of sudden obstruction of the coronary arteries. JAMA 1912;59:2015-9.
31. Small DM. Progression and regression of atherosclerotic lesions: insights from lipid physical biochemistry. Arteriosclerosis 1988;8:103-29.
32. Keys A, ed. Coronary heart disease in seven countries. Circulation 1970;41,42(suppl I):I-1-211.
33. The Lipid Research Clinics Population Studies Data Book. Vol 1. The Prevalence Study. Aggregate distributions of lipids, lipoproteins and selected variables in 11 North American Populations. NIH Publication No 80-1527, July 1980:1-136.
34. Castelli WP. The epidemiology of coronary heart disease: the Framingham study. Am J Med 1984;76:4-12.
35. Brunner D, Weisbort J, Meshulam N, Schwartz S, Gross J, Saltz-Rennert H, Altman S, Loebl K. Relation of serum total cholesterol and high-density lipoprotein cholesterol percentage to the incidence of definite coronary events: twenty-year follow-up of the Donolo-Tel Aviv prospective coronary artery disease study. Am J Cardiol 1987;59:1271-6.
36. Sprecher DL, Schaefer EJ, Kent KM, Gregg RE, Zech LA, Hoeg JM, McManus B, Roberts WC, Brewer HB Jr. Cardiovascular features of homozygous familial hypercholesterolemia: analysis of 16 patients. Am J Cardiol 1984;54:20-30.
37. Roberts WC. Extreme hypercholesterolemia = malignant atherosclerosis. Am J Cardiol 1984;54:242-3.
38. McGill HC Jr, ed. The geographic pathology of atherosclerosis. Baltimore: Williams & Wilkins, 1968:193.
39. Newman WP, Freedman DS, Voors AW, Gard PD, Srinivasan SR, Cresanta JL, Williamson GD, Webber LS, Berenson GS. Relation of serum lipoprotein levels and systolic blood pressure to early atherosclerosis: the Bogalusa Heart Study. N Engl J Med 1986;314:138-44.
40. The Coronary Primary Prevention Trial: design and implementation. The Lipid Research Clinics Program. J Chronic Dis 1979;32:609-31.
41. The Lipid Research Clinics Coronary Primary Prevention Trial results. I. Reduction in incidence of coronary heart disease. Lipid Research Clinics program. JAMA 1984;251:351-64.
42. The Lipid Research Clinics Coronary Primary Prevention Trial results II. The relationship of reduction in incidence of coronary heart disease to cholesterol lowering. Lipid Research Clinics Program. JAMA 1984;251:365-74.
43. Roberts WC. Reducing the blood cholesterol level reduces the risk of heart attack. Am J Cardiol 1984;53:649.
44. Frick MH, Elo O, Haapa K, Heinonen OP, Heinsalmi P, Helo P, Huttunen JK, Kaitaniemi P, Koskinen P, Manninen V, Maenpaa H, Malkonen M, Manttari M, Norola S, Pasternack A, Pikkarainen J, Romo M, Sjoblom T, Nikkila EA. Helsinki Heart Study: primary-prevention trial with gemfibrozil in middle-aged men with dyslipidemia. Safety of treatment, changes in risk factors, and incidence of coronary heart disease. N Engl J Med 1987;317:1237-45.
45. P. Huttunen JK, Kaitaniemi P, Koskinen P, Manninen V, Maenpaa H, Malkonen M, Norola S, Pasternack A, Pikkarainen J, Roma M, Sjoblom T, Nikkila EA. The Helsinki Heart Study: basic design and randomization procedure. Eur Heart J 1987;8(suppl I):1-29.
46. Armstrong ML, Megan MB. Lipid depletion in atheromatous coronary arteries in rhesus monkeys after regression diets. Circ Res 1972;30:675-80.
47. Duffield RGM, Lewis B, Miller NE, Jamieson CW, Brunt JNH, Colchester ACF. Treatment of hyperlipidaemia retards progression of symptomatic femoral atherosclerosis: a randomized controlled trial. Lancet 1983;2:639-41.
48. Brensike JF, Levy RI, Kelsey SF, Passamani ER, Richardson JM, Loh IK, Stone NJ, Aldrich RF, Battaglini JW, Moriarty DJ, Fisher MR, Friedman L, Friedwald W, Detre KM, Epstein SE. Effects of therapy with cholestyramine on progression of coronary arteriosclerosis: results of the NHLBI type II coronary intervention study. Circulation 1984;69:313-24.

49. Levy RI, Brensike JF, Epstein SE, Kelsey SF, Passamani ER, Richardson JM, Stone NJ, Aldrich RF, Battaglini JW, Moriarty DJ, Fisher ML, Friedman L, Friedewold W, Detre KM. The influence of changes in lipid values induced by cholestyramine and diet on progression of coronary artery disease: results of the NHLBI type II coronary intervention study. Circulation 1984;69:325-36.
50. Blankenhorn DH, Nessim SA, Johnson RL, Sanmarco ME, Azen SP, Cashin-Hemphill L. Beneficial effects of combined colestipol-niacin therapy on coronary atherosclerosis and coronary venous bypass grafts. JAMA 1987;257:3233-40.
51. Ornish D, Brown SE, Scherwitz LW, Billings JH, Armstrong WT, Ports TA, McLanahan SM, Kirkeeide RL, Brand RJ, Gould KL. Can lifestyle changes reverse coronary artery disease? The Lifestyle Heart Trial. Lancet 1990;336:129-33.
52. Kane JP, Malloy MJ, Ports TA, Phillips NR, Diehl JC, Havel RJ. Regression of coronary atherosclerosis during treatment of familial hypercholesterolemia with combined drug regimens. JAMA 1990; 264:3007-12.
53. Cashin-Hemphill L, Mack WJ, Pogoda MJ, Sanmarco ME, Azen SP, Blankenhorn DH. Beneficial effects of colestipol-niacin on coronary atherosclerosis. JAMA 1990;264:3013-7.
54. Buchwald H, Varco RL, Matts JF, Long JM, Fitch LL, Campbell GS, Pearce MB, Yellin AE, Edmiston WA, Smirk RD Jr, Sawin HS Jr, Campos CT, Hansen BJ, Tuna N, Karnegis JN, Sanmarco ME, Amplatz K, Casteneda-Zuniga WR, Hunter DW, Bissett JK, Weber FJ, Stevenson JW, Leon AS, Chalmer TC, and the POSCH group. Effect of partial ileal bypass surgery on mortality and morbidity from coronary heart disease in patients with hypercholesterolemia. Report of the Program on the Surgical Control of the Hyperlipidemias (POSCH). New Engl J Med 1990;323:946-55.
55. Brown G, Albers JJ, Fisher LD, Schaefer SM, Lin J-T, Kaplan C, Zhao X-Q, Bisson BD, Fitzpatrick VF, Dodge HT. Regression of coronary artery disease as a result of intensive lipid-lowering therapy in men with high levels of apolipoprotein B. New Engl J Med 1990;323:1289-98.
56. Brown BG, Zue-Qiao X, Sacco DE, Albers JJ. Lipid lowering and plaque regression: new insights into prevention of plaque disruption and clinical events in coronary disease. Circulation 1993;87:1781-91.
57. Schuler G, Hambrecht R, Schlierf G, Niebauer J, Hauer K, Neumann J, Hoberg E, Drinkmann A, Bacher F, Grunze M, Kubler W. Regular physical exercise and low-fat diet: effects on progression of coronary artery disease. Circulation 1992;86:1-11.
58. Watts GF, Lewis B, Brunt JNH, Lewis ES, Coltart DJ, Smith LDR, Mann JI, Swan AV. Effects on coronary artery disease of lipid-lowering diet, or diet plus cholestyramine, in the St Thomas' Atherosclerosis Regression Study (STARS). Lancet 1992;339:563-9.
59. Blankenhorn DH, Azen SP, Kramsch DM, Mack WJ, Cashin-Hemphill L, Hodis HN, DeBoer LWV, Mahrer PR, Masteller MJ, Vailas LI, Alaupovic P, Hirsch LJ, and the MARS Research Group. Coronary angiographic changes with lovastatin therapy. The Monitored Atherosclerosis Regression Study (MARS). Ann Intern Med 1993;119:969-76.
60. Waters D, Higginson L, Gladstone P, Kimball B, LeMay M, Boccuzzi SJ, Lespérance J—the CCAIT Study Group. Effects of monotherapy with an HMG-CoA reductase inhibitor on the progression of coronary atherosclerosis as assessed by serial quantitative arteriography. The Canadian Coronary Atherosclerosis Intervention Trial. Circulation 1994;89:959-68.
61. Haskell WL, Alderman EL, Fair JM, Maron DJ, Mackey SF, Superko HR, Williams PT, Johnstone IM, Champagne MA, Krauss RM, Farquhar JW. Effects of intensive multiple risk factor reduction on coronary atherosclerosis and clinical cardiac events in men and women with coronary artery disease: the Stanford Coronary Risk Intervention Project (SCRIP). Circulation 1994;89:975-89.
62. MAAS investigators. Effect of simvastatin on coronary atheroma: the Multicentre Anti-Atheroma Study (MAAS). Lancet 1994;344:633-8.
63. Sempos CT, Cleeman JI, Carroll MD, Johnson CL, Bachorik PS, Gordon DJ, Burt VL, Briefel RR, Brown CD, Lippel K, Rifkind BM. Prevalence of high blood cholesterol among US adults: an update based on guidelines from the second report of the National Cholesterol Education Program Adult Treatment Panels. JAMA 1993;269:3009-13.
64. Roberts WC. Fast Foods and quick plaques. Am J Cardiol 1987;59:721-3.
65. Roberts WC. More on fast foods and quick plaques. Am J Cardiol 1992;70:268-70.
66. Jacobson MF, Fritschner S. Fast Food Guide. New York: Workman Publishing, 1986:225.
67. Jacobson MF, Fritschner S. The Completely Revised and Updated Fast-Food Guide. 2nd ed. New York: Workman Publishing, 1991:333.
68. Hurley J, Schmidt S. Mexican food: oilé. Nutrition Action Healthletter 1994 (July/August);21:1,4-7.
69. Roberts WC. Mexican Food: oilé. Am J Cardiol 1994;74:974-5.
70. Parker T. In one day. Boston: Houghton Mifflin, 1984:94.
71. Roberts WC. In one day in the USA. Am J Cardiol 1986;58:193-4.
72. Kuczmarski RJ, Flegal KM, Campbell SM, Johnson CL. Increasing prevalence of overweight among US adults. The National Health and Nutrition Examination Surveys, 1960-1991. JAMA 1994;272:205-11.
73. Manson JE, Stampfer MJ, Henneken CH, Willett WC. Body weight and longevity: a reassessment. JAMA 1987;257:353-358.
74. Roberts WC. Calculating the percentage of calories from fat and the grams of fat consumed daily to maintain an ideal body weight. Am J Cardiol 1994;73:719-20.
75. Lappé FM. Diet For a small planet. Tenth Anniversary Edition. New York: Ballantine Books, 1982:496.
76. Harris M. Cows, pigs, wars and witches: the riddles of culture. New York: Vintage Books, 1974:238.
77. Trowell HC, Burkitt DP, eds. Western diseases: their emergence and prevention. Cambridge, Mass.: Harvard University Press, 1981:456.
78. Ferguson D, Ferguson N. Sacred cows at the public trough. Bend, Oregon: Maverick Publications, 1983:250.
79. McDougall JA. McDougall's medicine: a challenging second opinion. Piscataway, N.J.: New Century Publishers, Stillpoint, 1985:307.
80. Robbins J. Diet For a New America. Walpole, New Hampshire: 1987:423.
81. Eaton SB, Konner M, Shostak M. The Paleolithic prescription. New York: Harper and Row, 1988:306.
82. Rifkin J. Beyond beef: the rise and fall of the cattle culture. New York: Dutton, 1992:353.
83. Roberts WC. We think we are one, we act as if we are one, but we are not one. Am J Cardiol 1990;66:896.
84. Eaton SB, Konner M, Shostak M. Stone agers in the fast lane: chronic degenerative diseases in evolutionary perspective. Am J Med 1988;84:739-49.
85. Roberts WC. Stone agers in the atomic age: lessons from the paleolithic life-style for modern man. Am J Cardiol 1988;61:1365-66.
86. Expert panel on detection, evaluation, and treatment of high blood cholesterol in adults. Summary of the Second Report of the National Cholesterol Education Program (NCEP) Expert Panel on Detection, Evaluation, and Treatment of High Blood Cholesterol in Adults (Adult Treatment Panel II). JAMA 1993;269:3015-23.
87. Hunninghake DB, Stein EA, Dujovne CA, Harris WS, Feldman EB, Miller VT, Tolbert JA, Laskarzewski PM, Quiter E, Held J, Taylor AM, Hopper S, Leonard SB, Brewer BK. The efficacy of intensive dietary therapy alone or combined with lovastatin in outpatients with hypercholesterolemia. N Engl J Med 1993;328:1213-9.
88. Roberts WC. The ineffectiveness of a commonly recommended lipid-lowering diet in significantly lowering the serum total and low-density lipoprotein cholesterol levels. Am J Cardiol 1994;73:623-4.
89. Grundy SM, Nix D, Whelan MF, Franklin L. Comparison of three cholesterol-lowering diets in normolipidemic men. JAMA 1986;256:2351-5.
90. Roberts WC. Lipid-lowering therapy after an atherosclerotic event. Am J Cardiol 1989;64:693-5.
91. Scandinavian Simvastatin Survival Study Group. Randomised trial of cholesterol lowering in 4444 patients with coronary heart disease: the Scandinavian Simvastatin Survival Study (4S). Lancet 1994;344:1383-94.
92. Illingworth DR, Tobert JA. A review of clinical trials comparing HMG-CoA reductase inhibitors. Clinical Therapeutics 1994;16:366-85.
93. Roberts WC. The best antiarrhythmic agent will be a lipid-lowering agent. Am J Cardiol 1990;66:1402.
94. Roberts WC. The best anti-heart failure agent will be a lipid-lowering agent. Am J Cardiol 1993;71:628.

95. Roberts WC. Getting cardiologists interested in lipids. Am J Cardiol 1993;72:744-5.
96. Bradford RH, Shear CL, Chremos AN, Dujovne C, Franklin FA, Hesney M, Higgins J, Langendorfer A, Pool JL, Schnaper H, Stephenson WP. Expanded Clinical Evaluation of Lovastatin (EXCEL) study: design and patient characteristics of a double-blind, placebo-controlled study in patients with moderate hypercholesterolemia. Am J Cardiol 1990;66:44B-55B.
97. Bradford RH, Shear CL, Chremos AN, Dujovne C, Downton M, Franklin FA, Gould AL, Hesney M, Higgins J, Hurley DP, Langendorfer A, Nash DT, Pool JL, Schnaper H. Expanded Clinical Evaluation of Lovastatin (EXCEL) study results. I. Efficiency in modifying plasma lipoproteins and adverse event profile in 8245 patients with moderate hypercholesterolemia. Arch Intern Med 1991;151:43-9.
98. Roberts WC. Retail costs of the -statin lipid-lowering drugs. Am J Cardiol 1994;74:1181.

Relation of Weights of Operatively Excised Stenotic Aortic Valves to Preoperative Transvalvular Peak Systolic Pressure Gradients and to Calculated Aortic Valve Areas

William C. Roberts, MD, MACC, Jong M. Ko, BA
Dallas, Texas

OBJECTIVES The purpose of this study was to correlate the weights of operatively excised stenotic aortic valves to preoperative transvalvular peak systolic gradients and to calculated aortic valve areas.

BACKGROUND No previous publication has correlated the weights of stenotic aortic valves to the transvalvular gradients or to the calculated aortic valve areas.

METHODS We weighed operatively excised stenotic aortic valves in 324 adults who had undergone preoperative left-sided cardiac catheterization.

RESULTS As the weights of the operatively excised stenotic aortic valves increased (from <1 g to >6 g), the average transvalvular peak systolic pressure gradients progressively increased. For any valve weight, in general, the women had higher average transvalvular gradients ($p \leq 0.005$) and lower average valve areas ($p \leq 0.008$) than did the men. Correlation between aortic valve weight and transvalvular gradient improved further when gender was taken into account.

CONCLUSIONS Preoperative transvalvular peak systolic pressure gradients across stenotic aortic valves correlate better with the weights of the operatively excised valves than do the calculated valve areas. (J Am Coll Cardiol 2004;44:1847–55) © 2004 by the American College of Cardiology Foundation

Recently, we reported weights of operatively excised stenotic unicuspid, bicuspid, and tricuspid aortic valves in 499 adults and their relation to age, gender, body mass index (BMI), and presence or absence of concomitant coronary artery bypass grafting (CABG) (1). No previous studies have compared weights of stenotic aortic valves to transvalvular pressure gradients across them or to calculated aortic valve areas. Such is the purpose of this study.

See page 1856

METHODS

From January 1998 through June 2003 (65 months), a total of 1,272 patients had one or more cardiac valves or portions of cardiac valves submitted to the surgical pathology unit of the Department of Pathology of Baylor University Medical Center (Fig. 1). After elimination of the 33 patients with active infective endocarditis, the 6 who had isolated tricuspid valve replacement, the 444 who had mitral valve replacement or repair, and the 58 who had combined mitral and aortic valve replacements, 731 patients who had isolated aortic valve replacement remained. Of them, 151 had the valve replacement for pure aortic regurgitation (no element of valve stenosis) and 580 for aortic valve stenosis (with or without some associated aortic regurgitation). Of the 580 patients with stenotic aortic valves, the operatively excised valve was weighed by one of us (W.C.R.) in 575 patients; of them, 251 were eliminated from this study because cardiac catheterization was not performed before aortic valve replacement, the data obtained at cardiac catheterization was not available to us, or the left-sided cardiac hemodynamic data was missing or incomplete. The present study is limited to the 324 patients who had isolated aortic valve replacement to excise a stenotic aortic valve, had peak left ventricular (LV) to systemic arterial peak systolic pressure gradients ≥10 mm Hg, had calculated aortic valve areas obtained at cardiac catheterization before the aortic valve replacement, and had the operatively excised stenotic aortic valve weighed.

Each operatively excised cardiac valve arrived at the surgical pathology unit in a container filled with formaldehyde. The valve was removed from the container, placed on absorbing paper to absorb excess formaldehyde, and then weighed on an Ohaus scale (Ohaus Corp., Florham Park, New Jersey), which has an accuracy to 0.01 g. The age and gender of each patient were obtained from the patient identification label pasted on the container submitted from the operating room. The type of dysfunction of the operatively excised aortic valve was determined initially by gross inspection of the valve, and confirmation that the valve was stenotic was obtained from the cardiac catheterization report. The interval from the cardiac catheterization to aortic valve replacement was <3 months (usually <1 week) in 312 (96%) of the 324 patients, from >3 to 6 months in

From the Baylor Heart & Vascular Institute and the Departments of Pathology and Medicine, Baylor University Medical Center, Dallas, Texas.

Manuscript received December 18, 2003; revised manuscript received April 16, 2004, accepted April 27, 2004.

Abbreviations and Acronyms

BMI = body mass index
CABG = coronary artery bypass grafting
LV = left ventricular

5 patients, from >6 to 12 months in 6 patients, and 14 months in 1 patient. Most of the pertinent clinical information, including age, gender, BMI, whether or not concomitant CABG was performed, was obtained from the Baylor University Medical Center Apollo Advance Cardiovascular Data Integration system. In the 26 patients in whom cardiac catheterization was not performed at Baylor University Medical Center, the record room chart was reviewed to obtain the pertinent hemodynamic data.

Statistical analysis was performed by using SigmaStat Version 2.0 (SPSS Inc., Chicago, Illinois). Parametric tests were used for the analysis of the data that passed the assumption tests of normality and equal variance: for continuous variables, the unpaired *t* test was performed for two variable comparisons and one-way analysis of variance for more than two variable comparisons. When the data did not pass the assumption tests, nonparametric tests (i.e., Mann-Whitney rank-sum test for two variable comparisons and Kruskal-Wallis one-way analysis of variance on ranks test for more than two continuous variable comparisons) were used. The correlation coefficient (r) was obtained by using either the parametric Pearson product moment test or the nonparametric Spearman rank order test. A value $p < 0.05$ was considered to be statistically significant. The study protocol was approved by the Institutional Review Board of Baylor University Medical Center.

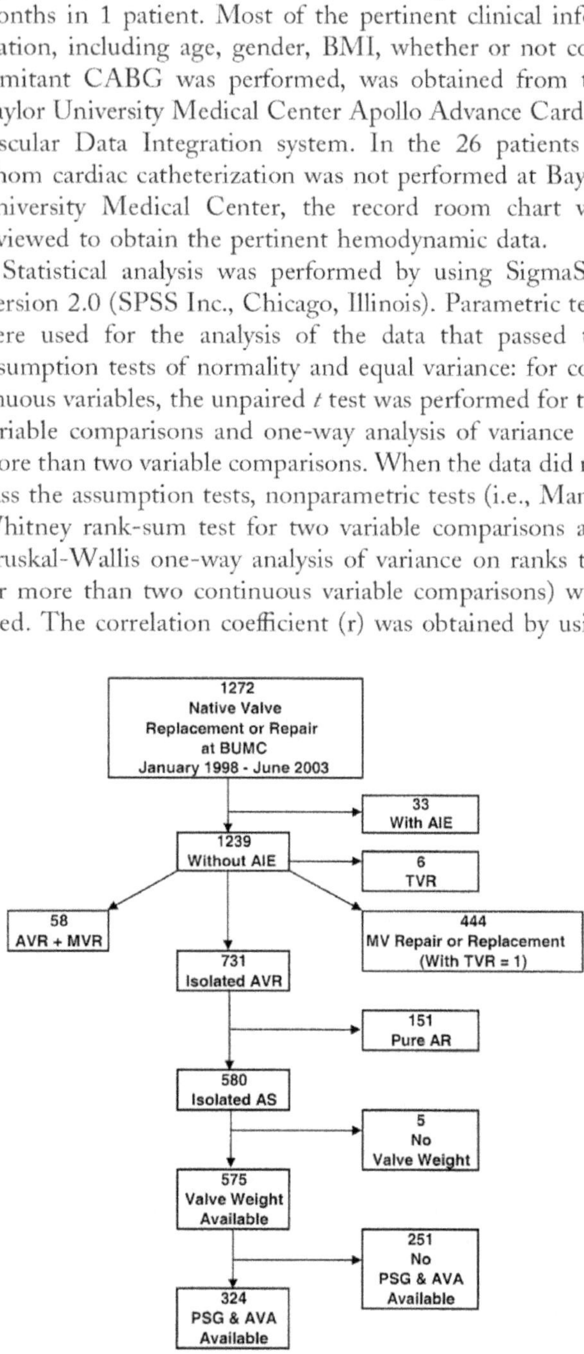

Figure 1. Algorithm showing breakdown of the 1,272 patients having valve replacement or repair at Baylor University Medical Center (BUMC) in a 65-month period and the origin of the 324 cases included in the present study. AIE = active infective endocarditis; AR = aortic regurgitation; AS = aortic stenosis; AVA = aortic valve area; AVR = aortic valve replacement; MV = mitral valve; MVR = mitral valve replacement; PSG = peak systolic gradient; TVR = tricuspid valve replacement.

RESULTS

The weights of the operatively excised stenotic aortic valves ranged from 0.69 to 11.30 g (mean 2.72 g), a 16-fold difference between the smallest and the largest (Table 1). The ages, BMIs, LV to aortic peak systolic pressure gradients, calculated aortic valve areas, whether or not concomitant CABG was performed, and ejection fractions are summarized for both men and women according to the aortic valve weights in Table 1. The transvalvular peak systolic pressure gradients in both men and women increased as the valve weights increased ($p < 0.001$, Kruskal-Wallis one-way analysis of variance on ranks test) (Table 1), the calculated aortic valve areas also decreased as the valve weights increased ($p \leq 0.002$, Kruskal-Wallis one-way analysis of variance on ranks test), but the changes were not as impressive (Table 1). The men in general had higher valve weights than did the women ($p < 0.001$, Mann-Whitney rank-sum test), lower transvalvular gradients ($p \leq 0.005$, unpaired *t* test), and higher valve areas ($p \leq 0.008$, unpaired *t* test) (Table 1).

The valve weights, gradients, and valve areas in both men and women according to aortic valve structure (unicuspid, bicuspid, or tricuspid) are summarized in Table 2. The fewer the number of aortic valve cusps, the heavier the valves were, the greater the peak transvalvular gradients, and the smaller the valve areas.

Valve weights, gradients, and valve areas were not significantly different (by Kruskal-Wallis one-way analysis of variance on ranks test) in patients ≤40 years, 41 to 70 years, and 71 to 90 years of age (Table 3). Valve weights, gradients, and mean areas varied relatively little in patients with BMIs <25 kg/m^2, 25 to 30 kg/m^2, and >30 kg/m^2 (Table 4).

Compared with the 166 patients having coronary bypass, the 158 patients not having concomitant bypass grafting had heavier valves ($p < 0.001$, Mann-Whitney rank-sum test), higher transvalvular peak pressure gradients ($p = 0.045$, Mann-Whitney rank-sum test), but similar valve areas (Table 5).

Valve weights, gradients, and areas were insignificantly different (by either Kruskal-Wallis one-way analysis of variance on ranks test or one-way analysis of variance) when women were compared with women and men with men with LV ejection fractions ≤35%, 36% to 45%, and >45% (Table 6).

The relation of aortic valve weight to transvalvular peak systolic gradient for each of the 201 men is illustrated in Figure 2 and in the 123 women, in Figure 3. The relation of aortic valve weight to aortic valve area in each of the 201 men is shown in Figure 4 and in each of the 123 women in Figure 5.

Table 1. Ages, BMI, and Concomitant Coronary Artery Bypass, LV to Aortic PSG, and AV Areas in Seven AV Weight Groups in Men and Women

AV Weight (g)	No. of Patients	Ages (yrs) Range (Average)	BMI (kg/m^2) Range (Average)	AV Weights (g) Range (Average)	LV-Aorta PSG (mm Hg) Range (Average)	AV Area (cm^2) Range (Mean)	Coronary Bypass	UAV or BAV	Ejection Fraction (%) No.	Ejection Fraction (%) Range (Mean)	Ejection Fraction (%) No. (%) ≤ 40	Ejection Fraction (%) No. (%) >40
Men												
≤1	0	—	—	—	—	—	—	—	—	—	—	—
>1–2	41	47–90 (72)	19–37 (27)	1.16–2.00 (1.64)	11–81 (36)	0.27–1.43 (0.86)	27 (66%)	11 (27%)	37	15–78 (48)	13 (35%)	24 (65%)
>2–3	60	29–87 (69)	20–43 (29)	2.01–3.00 (2.58)	15–97 (45)	0.42–2.25 (0.89)	32 (53%)	24 (40%)	52	10–85 (51)	14 (27%)	38 (73%)
>3–4	50	37–84 (69)	17–40 (27)	3.03–4.00 (3.40)	20–100 (56)	0.20–1.63 (0.75)	26 (52%)	30 (60%)	44	15–80 (53)	7 (16%)	37 (84%)
>4–5	29	42–87 (69)	18–45 (28)	4.01–4.84 (4.40)	20–108 (64)	0.32–1.06 (0.67)	11 (38%)	25 (86%)	26	15–70 (53)	5 (19%)	21 (81%)
>5–6	12	49–90 (70)	24–36 (28)	5.03–5.93 (5.60)	50–116 (71)	0.40–0.88 (0.60)	3 (25%)	10 (83%)	10	20–65 (43)	4 (40%)	6 (60%)
>6	9	38–84 (58)	21–38 (28)	6.24–11.30 (7.92)	35–141 (87)	0.39–1.23 (0.71)	2 (22%)	8 (89%)	8	15–70 (51)	2 (25%)	6 (75%)
Subtotal	201 (62%)	29–90 (69)	17–45 (28)	1.16–11.30 (3.27)	11–141 (52)	0.20–2.25 (0.79)	101 (50%)	108 (54%)	177	10–85 (51)	45 (25%)	132 (75%)
Women												
≤1	10	55–85 (74)	21–44 (30)	0.69–0.95 (0.83)	15–62 (28)	0.34–1.28 (0.83)	7 (70%)	2 (20%)	9	30–70 (47)	4 (44%)	5 (56%)
>1–2	73	19–88 (71)	17–51 (29)	1.02–1.99 (1.46)	10–119 (49)	0.18–1.49 (0.72)	40 (55%)	14 (19%)	66	15–80 (56)	9 (14%)	57 (86%)
>2–3	29	30–87 (70)	18–50 (28)	2.04–3.00 (2.42)	26–113 (63)	0.27–1.09 (0.58)	15 (52%)	12 (41%)	23	30–80 (54)	4 (17%)	19 (83%)
>3–4	10	47–85 (73)	17–35 (26)	3.14–4.00 (3.42)	53–131 (85)	0.23–0.78 (0.51)	3 (30%)	9 (90%)	9	45–75 (53)	0	9 (100%)
>4–5	1	83	29	4.27	53	0.75	0	1 (100%)	1	50	0	1 (100%)
>5–6	0	—	—	—	—	—	—	—	—	—	—	—
>6	0	—	—	—	—	—	—	—	—	—	—	—
Subtotal	123 (38%)	19–88 (71)	17–51 (29)	0.69–4.27 (1.82)	10–131 (53)	0.18–1.49 (0.68)	65 (53%)	38 (31%)	108	15–80 (55)	17 (16%)	91 (84%)

AV = aortic valve; BAV = bicuspid aortic valve; BMI = body mass index; LV = left ventricular; No. = number; PSG = peak systolic gradient; UAV = unicuspid aortic valve.

Table 2. Ages, BMI, Concomitant Coronary Bypass, and AV Weights in Men Versus Women According to AV Structure

Valve Structure	No. of Patients	Ages (yrs)	BMI (kg/m^2)	AV Weights (g)	LV-Aorta PSG (mm Hg) Range (Average)	AV Area (cm^2) Range (Mean)	Coronary Bypass	Ejection Fraction (%) No.	Ejection Fraction (%) Range (Mean)	Ejection Fraction (%) No. (%) ≤40	Ejection Fraction (%) No. (%) >40
Men											
Unicuspid	8 (4%)	29–51 (44)	21–42 (30)	2.89–8.00 (4.98)	26–141 (64)	0.48–1.82 (0.91)	0	7	15–74 (51)	1 (14%)	6 (86%)
Bicuspid	100 (50%)	37–90 (67)	17–42 (28)	1.20–11.30 (3.74)	13–121 (56)	0.30–1.63 (0.76)	48 (48%)	92	10–78 (51)	24 (26%)	68 (74%)
Tricuspid	93 (46%)	42–90 (74)	19–43 (28)	1.16–6.60 (2.63)	11–100 (47)	0.20–2.25 (0.82)	53 (57%)	78	15–85 (50)	20 (26%)	58 (74%)
Women											
Unicuspid	1 (1%)	33	26	1.35	65	0.88	0	—	—	—	—
Bicuspid	37 (30%)	19–85 (68)	18–42 (27)	0.79–4.27 (2.35)	16–131 (66)	0.23–1.09 (0.59)	12 (32%)	31	20–70 (51)	4 (13%)	27 (87%)
Tricuspid	85 (69%)	30–88 (73)	17–51 (30)	0.69–3.14 (1.60)	10–119 (48)	0.18–1.49 (0.71)	53 (63%)	77	15–80 (57)	13 (17%)	64 (83%)

Abbreviations as in Table 1.

Table 3. Gender, BMI, Concomitant Coronary Artery Bypass, AV Weights, LV to Aortic PSG, and AV Areas in Three Age Groups

Ages (yrs)	Gender	No. of Patients	BMI (kg/m^2) Range (Average)	AV Weights (g) Range (Average)	LV-Aorta PSG (mm Hg) Range (Average)	AV Area (cm^2) Range (Mean)	Coronary Bypass	UAV or BAV	Ejection Fraction (%) No.	Ejection Fraction (%) Range (Mean)	Ejection Fraction (%) No. (%) ≤40	Ejection Fraction (%) No. (%) >40
≤40	Men	4	25–42 (32)	2.90–8.00 (5.40)	31–141 (66)	0.65–1.63 (1.03)	0	4 (100%)	4	15–64 (50)	1 (25%)	3 (75%)
	Women	4	25–31 (27)	1.30–2.76 (1.87)	37–75 (55)	0.40–1.09 (0.80)	0	3 (75%)	2	58–60 (59)	0 (0%)	2 (100%)
41–70	Men	99	17–45 (29)	1.16–9.04 (3.28)	11–116 (54)	0.20–1.90 (0.82)	45 (45%)	71 (72%)	88	10–78 (51)	23 (26%)	65 (74%)
	Women	47	18–51 (31)	0.87–4.00 (1.75)	11–131 (55)	0.28–1.49 (0.72)	16 (34%)	18 (38%)	42	20–77 (55)	6 (14%)	36 (86%)
71–90	Men	98	18–43 (27)	1.20–11.30 (3.18)	14–121 (50)	0.27–2.25 (0.76)	56 (57%)	33 (34%)	86	15–85 (52)	19 (22%)	67 (78%)
	Women	72	17–44 (27)	0.69–4.27 (1.86)	10–119 (52)	0.18–1.28 (0.64)	49 (68%)	17 (24%)	63	15–80 (54)	13 (21%)	50 (79%)

Abbreviations as in Table 1.

Table 4. Gender, Ages, Concomitant Coronary Artery Bypass, AV Weights, LV to Aortic PSG, and AV Areas in Three BMI Groups

BMI (kg/m^2)	Gender	No. of Patients	Ages (yrs) Range (Average)	AV Weights (g) Range (Average)	LV-Aorta PSG (mm Hg) Range (Average)	AV Area (cm^2) Range (Mean)	Coronary Bypass	UAV or BAV	Ejection Fraction (%) No.	Ejection Fraction (%) Range (Mean)	Ejection Fraction (%) No. (%) ≤40	Ejection Fraction (%) No. (%) >40
<25	Men	53	45–90 (73)	1.15–9.04 (3.23)	17–121 (54)	0.20–1.82 (0.71)	29 (55%)	25 (47%)	45	15–78 (49)	12 (27%)	33 (73%)
	Women	34	58–88 (75)	0.90–4.00 (1.94)	11–105 (57)	0.23–1.10 (0.57)	17 (50%)	11 (31%)	29	15–80 (50)	9 (31%)	20 (69%)
25–30	Men	93	38–87 (71)	1.20–11.30 (3.33)	11–141 (51)	0.39–1.43 (0.79)	50 (54%)	52 (56%)	86	10–85 (51)	22 (26%)	54 (74%)
	Women	51	30–85 (71)	0.76–4.27 (1.79)	10–119 (48)	0.18–1.28 (0.70)	28 (54%)	20 (39%)	43	15–80 (56)	7 (16%)	36 (84%)
>30	Men	55	29–84 (63)	1.23–7.70 (3.21)	15–116 (52)	0.44–2.25 (0.89)	22 (39%)	31 (56%)	47	15–80 (53)	9 (19%)	38 (81%)
	Women	38	19–84 (68)	0.69–4.00 (1.75)	12–131 (57)	0.27–1.49 (0.74)	20 (51%)	8 (21%)	35	25–75 (56)	3 (9%)	32 (91%)

Abbreviations as in Table 1.

Table 5. Ages, BMI, AV Weights, LV to Aortic PSG, and AV Areas in Patients Without Versus Patients With Concomitant Coronary Artery Bypass Grafting

Coronary Bypass	Gender	No. of Patients	Ages (yrs) Range (Average)	BMI (kg/m^2) Range (Average)	AV Weights (g) Range (Average)	LV-Aorta PSG (mm Hg) Range (Average)	AV Area (cm^2) Range (Mean)	UAV or BAV	Ejection Fraction (%) No.	Ejection Fraction (%) Range (Mean)	Ejection Fraction (%) No. (%) ≤40	Ejection Fraction (%) No. (%) >40
0	Men	100	29–90 (66)	18–45 (28)	1.21–11.30 (3.64)	11–141 (55)	0.20–1.82 (0.79)	60 (60%)	84	10–80 (55)	13 (15%)	71 (85%)
	Women	58	19–85 (66)	18–51 (28)	0.74–4.27 (1.98)	10–131 (55)	0.23–1.28 (0.67)	26 (45%)	50	15–80 (56)	5 (10%)	45 (90%)
+	Men	101	51–90 (72)	17–43 (27)	1.16–8.30 (2.91)	13–121 (49)	0.30–2.25 (0.80)	48 (48%)	93	15–85 (47)	32 (34%)	61 (66%)
	Women	65	52–88 (75)	17–50 (29)	0.69–3.25 (1.68)	16–119 (52)	0.18–1.49 (0.68)	12 (18%)	58	20–80 (55)	12 (21%)	46 (79%)

Abbreviations as in Table 1.

Table 6. Gender, Age, BMI, Concomitant Coronary Artery Bypass, AV Weights, LV to Aortic PSG, and AV Areas in Three Ejection Fraction Groups

Ejection Fraction (%)	Gender	No. of Patients	Age (yrs)	BMI (kg/m^2) Range (Average)	AV Weights (g) Range (Average)	LV-Aorta PSG (mm Hg) Range (Average)	AV Area (cm^2) Range (Mean)	Coronary Bypass	UAV or BAV
≤35	Men	34	39–90 (70)	17–35 (27)	1.16–8.30 (3.17)	11–121 (45)	0.30–1.43 (0.80)	27 (73%)	18 (53%)
	Women	10	58–83 (72)	20–30 (24)	0.76–2.19 (1.47)	10–94 (41)	0.39–1.28 (0.65)	7 (70%)	4 (40%)
36–45	Men	22	50–88 (69)	21–42 (28)	1.19–5.55 (3.01)	19–93 (49)	0.41–1.28 (0.80)	13 (59%)	14 (64%)
	Women	17	48–87 (73)	17–44 (27)	0.90–4.00 (2.09)	22–105 (56)	0.23–1.01 (0.57)	9 (53%)	5 (29%)
>45	Men	121	29–90 (69)	18–45 (28)	1.24–11.30 (3.35)	15–141 (53)	0.27–2.25 (0.82)	53 (44%)	67 (55%)
	Women	81	19–88 (71)	17–51 (30)	0.69–4.27 (1.78)	11–131 (55)	0.18–1.49 (0.72)	42 (52%)	22 (27%)

The ejection fractions were obtained from cardiac catheterization in 190 patients, 34 from echocardiogram, and 61 from an unspecified source.
Abbreviations as in Table 1.

Of the 324 patients, only 13 had moderate (3+ of 4+) or severe (4+ of 4+) aortic regurgitation, and the data in these 13 patients are tabulated in Table 7. Although these patients were considered to have moderate or severe aortic regurgitation after cardiac catheterization, only three had dilated LV cavities, and these were the three with low LV ejection fractions.

DISCUSSION

The present study shows that the peak systolic pressure gradients across stenotic aortic valves correspond reasonably well with the weights of the operatively excised stenotic aortic valves in adults when gender is considered (Figs. 2 and 3). Although the average transvalvular peak systolic pressure gradients were similar in both men and women (approximately 52 mm Hg), the mean weights of the stenotic aortic valves in the men were nearly twice (1.8 ×) those is the women. Thus, for any given weight, the peak systolic pressure gradients across stenotic aortic valves were greater in the women than in the men. The smallest valves belonged to the women, and the largest ones to the men (Table 1).

No previous attempts have been made to estimate the valve weight from the transvalvular peak pressure gradient. The present data suggest that in women, each 1-mm Hg peak systolic pressure gradient represents about 35 mg of stenotic aortic valve, and in men each 1-mm Hg peak gradient represents about 65 mg of stenotic aortic valve. Thus, a 53-mm Hg peak systolic gradient across a stenotic aortic valve in a woman calculates into a 1.80-g valve, and a 52-mm Hg transvalvular peak gradient across a stenotic aortic valve in a man translates into a 3.27-g valve.

The peak systolic transvalvular gradients correlated better with valve weights than did the valve areas. In the men, as the valve weights progressively increased from >1 to >6 g, the average transvalvular peak systolic pressure gradients progressively increased from an average of 36 to 87 mm Hg (Fig. 2), whereas the valve areas decreased from 0.86 to 0.71 cm^2 (Fig. 4). In the women, as the valve weights progressively increased from <1 to 4 g, the transvalvular peak systolic pressure gradients progressively increased from 28 to 85 mm Hg (Fig. 3), whereas the valve areas decreased from 0.83 to 0.51 cm^2 (Fig. 5).

Although valve area is used in many medical centers as the gold standard of valve stenosis (2–4), the present study—the first to correlate either transvalvular peak systolic pressure gradient or the calculated aortic valve area with valve weight—demonstrates that the peak systolic transvalvular pressure gradient is more indicative of the degree of valvular obstruction than is the calculated valve area, particularly in the patients with low transvalvular peak systolic pressure gradients.

We are well aware that the gradient across a stenotic valve is dependent on flow across that valve. Several publications have discussed patients with "low gradient-severe aortic stenosis," but in none of these reports has the operatively excised valve been illustrated, described, or weighed (5–11). The peak systolic gradient across a stenotic aortic valve is, of course, a direct measurement. The aortic valve area, in contrast, is

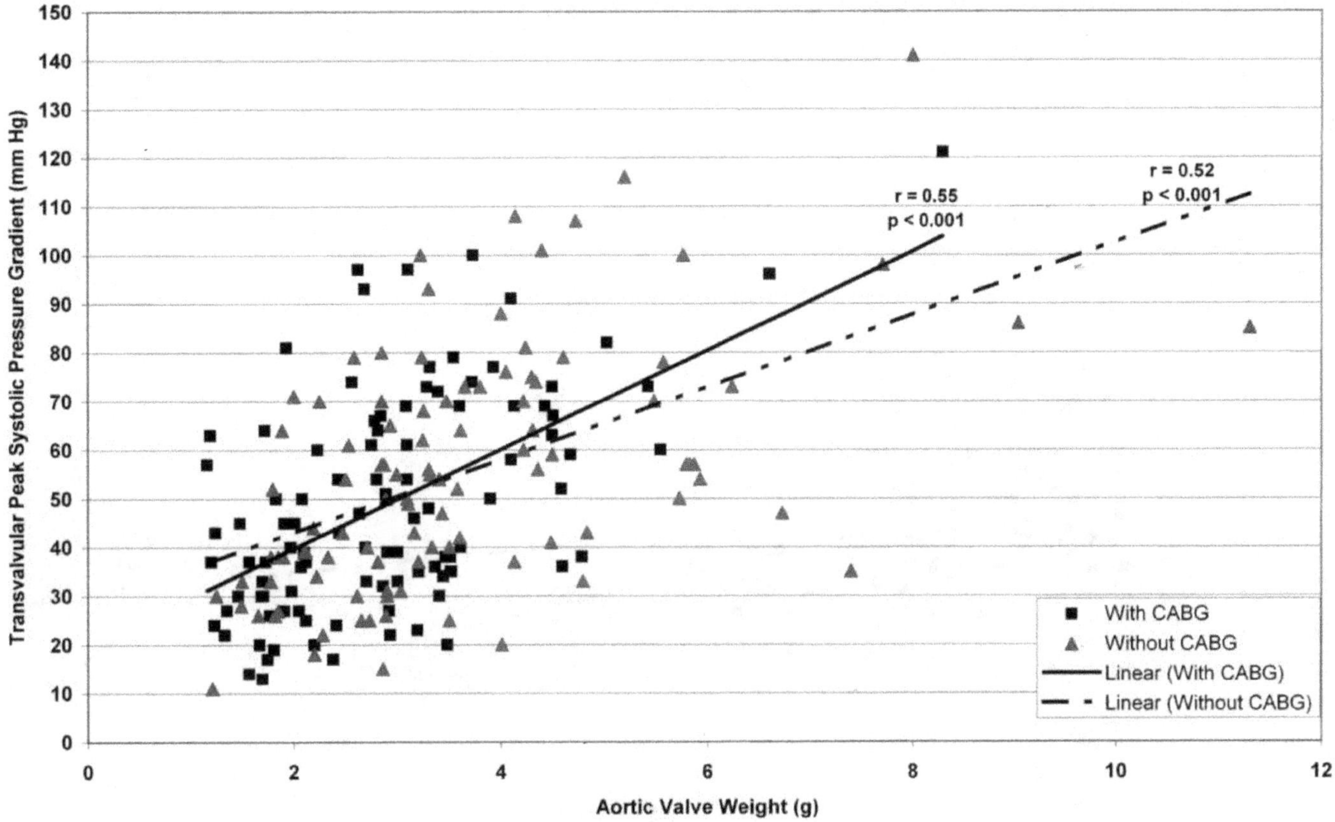

Figure 2. Relation of weights (g) of the operatively excised stenotic aortic valves to preoperative transvalvular peak systolic pressure gradients (mm Hg) in the 201 men. CABG = coronary artery bypass grafting.

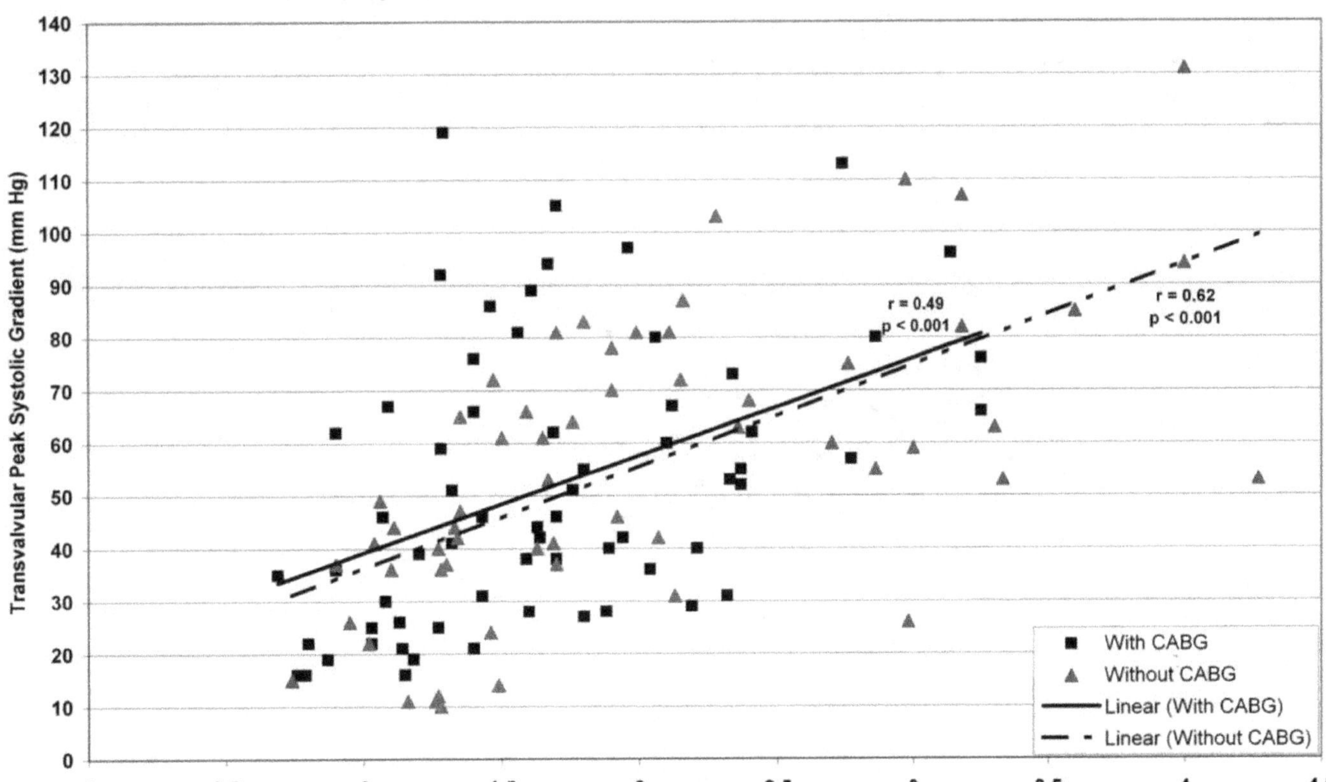

Figure 3. Relation of weights (g) of the operatively excised stenotic aortic valves to preoperative transvalvular peak systolic pressure gradients (mm Hg) in the 123 women. CABG = coronary artery bypass grafting.

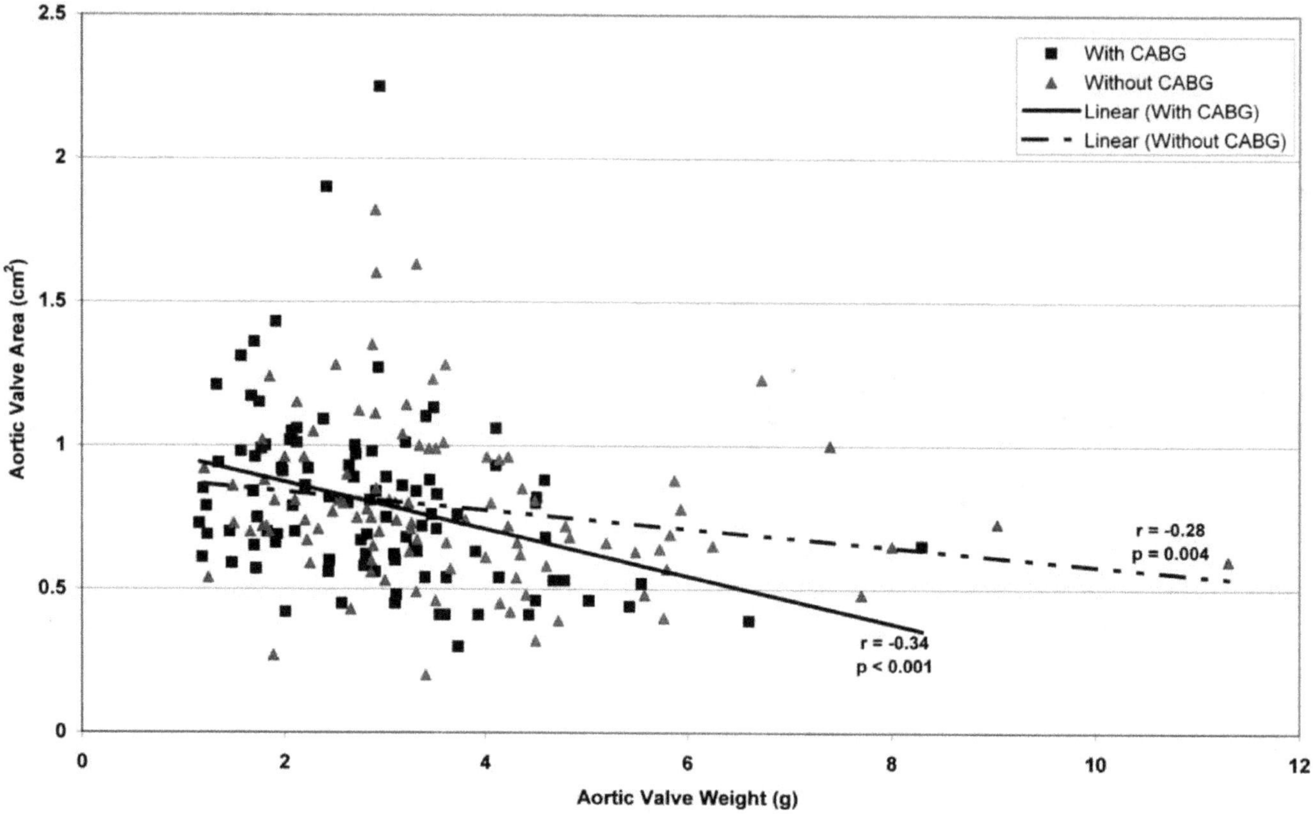

Figure 4. Relation of weights (g) of the operatively excised stenotic aortic valves to preoperative aortic valve area (cm^2) in the 201 men. CABG = coronary artery bypass grafting.

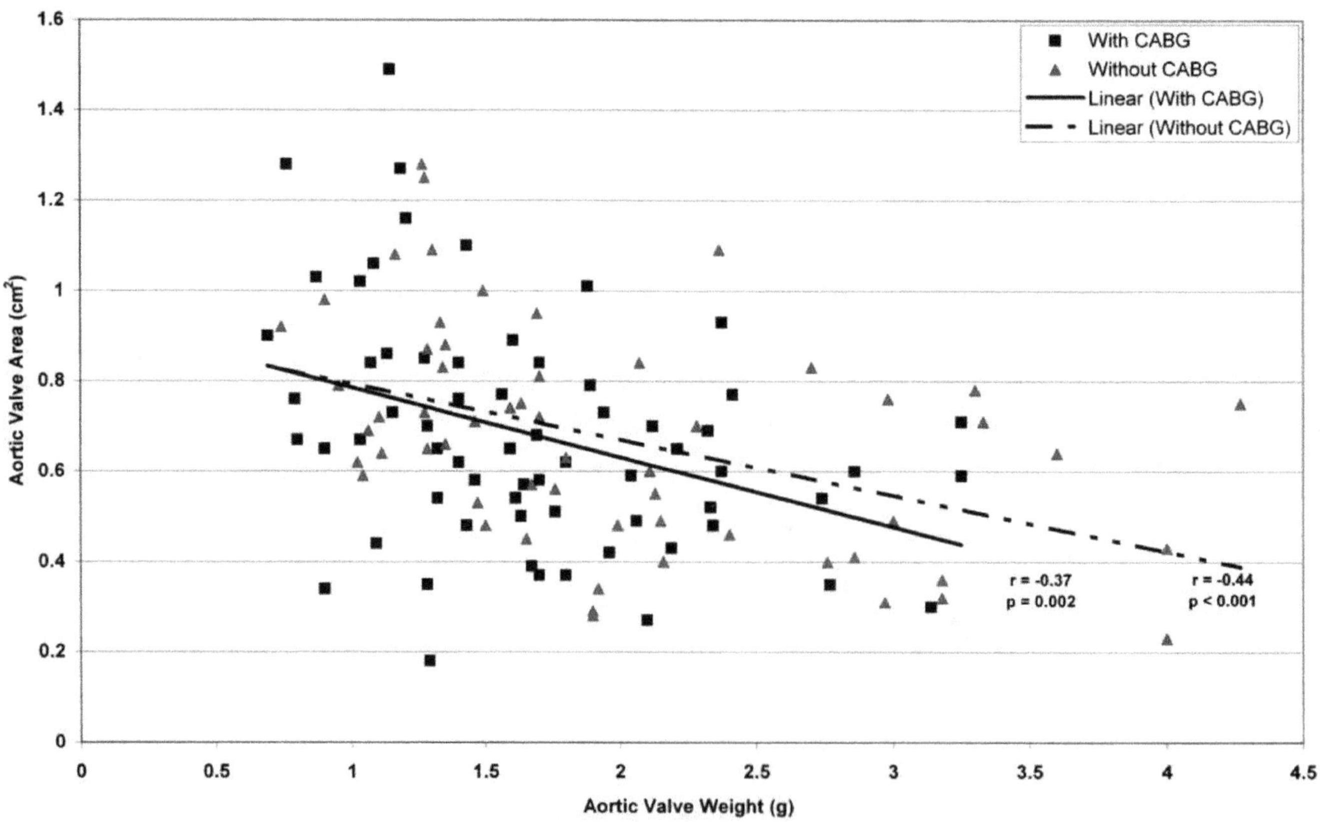

Figure 5. Relation of weights (g) of the operatively excised stenotic aortic valves to preoperative aortic valve area (cm^2) in the 123 women. CABG = coronary artery bypass grafting.

Table 7. Clinical Findings on 13 Patients With Moderate or Severe AR

	Age (yrs)	Gender	AR (3+/4+, 4+/4+)	LV Pressure (s/d) (mm Hg)	Aortic Pressure (s/d) (mm Hg)	LV-Ao PSG (mm Hg)	AV Area (cm^2)	Ao Pulse Pressure (mm Hg)	Cardiac Output (l/min)	EF (%)	Dilated LV Cavity	Number of Coronary Arteries Narrowed >50%	CABG	Body Weight (lbs)	Height (in.)	BMI (kg/m^2)	Number of Cusps	Valve Weight (g)
1	42	M	4	160/34	145/58	15	1.35	87	—	50	0	0	0	240	67	38	2	2.86
2	73	M	4	203/34	178/58	25	1.12	120	6.3	50	0	0	0	207	71	29	3	2.73
3	60	M	3	176/31	150/73	26	0.72	77	4.0	30	+	0	0	146	68	22	3	1.82
4	75	M	3	173/29	143/71	30	1.60	72	6.1	70	0	0	0	174	72	24	3	2.90
5	29	M	4	194/38	163/64	31	0.85	99	5.6	50	0	0	0	300	71	42	1	2.90
6	39	M	3	155/19	114/64	35	1.00	50	—	15	+	0	0	176	70	25	1	7.39
7	62	M	3	151/16	113/50	38	0.81	63	4.8	50	0	0	0	192	70	28	2	1.90
8	43	M	3	173/22	126/67	47	1.23	59	7.7	70	0	0	0	235	71	33	2	6.72
9	77	M	3	179/33	129/59	50	0.8	79	4.9	40	+	0	0	234	76	29	2	3.09
10	68	M	3	209/35	145/76	64	0.57	69	—	60	0	1	+	227	70	33	2	1.72
11	47	M	4	185/23	121/52	64	0.66	69	5.0	75	0	0	0	208	68	32	1	3.61
12	83	F	4	183/23	172/51	11	1.08	121	2.6	55	0	0	0	136	63	24	3	1.16
13	30	F	4	187/37	145/79	42	0.84	66	4.9	60	0	0	0	144	64	25	3	2.07

Ao = aorta; AR = aortic regurgitation; CABG = coronary bypass grafting; EF = ejection fraction; s/d = peak systolic/end diastolic; other abbreviations as in Table 1.

indirect and calculated from the cardiac output, the heart rate, the systolic LV ejection period, a constant (44.3), and the square root of the mean transvalvular gradient. The major message of this study is that care must be taken in concluding that "severe" stenosis can or does occur in the absence of a large peak systolic pressure gradient across the valve. The data herein support the view that a low gradient—irrespective of flow—means non-severe stenosis, and that the valve area calculation is, or can be, very unreliable in patients with low peak systolic gradients across stenotic aortic valves.

The positive features of the present study are the fact that a large group of patients were analyzed, that all valves were weighed by the same person, and that all cases analyzed were seen over a relatively short period (65 months). The negative feature of this study is the fact that the cardiac catheterizations were performed by numerous cardiologists and that the standards of each probably varied, and that most (98%) of the ejection fractions were estimated rather than calculated.

Reprint requests and correspondence: Dr. William C. Roberts, Baylor Heart & Vascular Institute, Baylor University Medical Center, 3500 Gaston Avenue, Dallas, Texas 75246. E-mail: wc.roberts@baylorhealth.edu.

REFERENCES

1. Roberts WC, Ko JM. Weights of operatively excised stenotic unicuspid, bicuspid, and tricuspid aortic valves and their relation to age, sex, body mass index, and presence or absence of concomitant coronary artery bypass grafting. Am J Cardiol 2003;92:1057–65.
2. Cannon SR, Richards KL, Crawford M. Hydraulic estimation of stenotic orifice area: a correction of the Gorlin formula. Circulation 1985;71:1170–8.
3. Burwash IG, Thomas DD, Sadahiro M, et al. Dependence of Gorlin formula and continuity equation valve areas on transvalvular volume flow rate in valvular aortic stenosis. Circulation 1994;89:827–35.
4. Cannon JD Jr., Zile MR, Crawford FA Jr., Carabello BA. Aortic valve resistance as an adjunct to the Gorlin formula in assessing the severity of aortic stenosis in symptomatic patients. J Am Coll Cardiol 1992; 20:1517–23.
5. Brogan WC III, Grayburn PA, Lange RA, Hillis LD. Prognosis after valve replacement in patients with severe aortic stenosis and a low transvalvular pressure gradient. J Am Coll Cardiol 1993;21:1657–60.
6. deFilippi CR, Willett DL, Brickner ME, et al. Usefulness of dobutamine echocardiography in distinguishing severe from nonsevere valvular aortic stenosis in patients with depressed left ventricular function and low transvalvular gradients. Am J Cardiol 1995;75: 191–4.
7. Connolly HM, Oh JK, Schaff HV, et al. Severe aortic stenosis with low transvalvular gradient and severe left ventricular dysfunction: result of aortic valve replacement in 52 patients. Circulation 2000;101: 1940–6.
8. Monin J-L, Monchi M, Gest V, Duval-Moulin A-M, Dubois-Rande J-L, Gueret P. Aortic stenosis with severe left ventricular dysfunction and low transvalvular pressure gradients: risk stratification by low-dose dobutamine echocardiography. J Am Coll Cardiol 2001;37:2101–7.
9. Schwammenthal E, Vered Z, Moshkowitz Y, et al. Dobutamine echocardiography in patients with aortic stenosis and left ventricular dysfunction: predicting outcome as a function of management strategy. Chest 2001;119:1766–77.
10. Nishimura RA, Grantham JA, Connolly HM, Schaff HV, Higano ST, Holmes DR Jr. Low-output, low-gradient aortic stenosis in patients with depressed left ventricular systolic function: the clinical utility of the dobutamine challenge in the catheterization laboratory. Circulation 2002;106:809–13.
11. Grayburn PA, Eichhorn EJ. Dobutamine challenge for low-gradient aortic stenosis. Circulation 2002;106:763–5.

Pericardial heart disease: its morphologic features and its causes

WILLIAM CLIFFORD ROBERTS, MD

Probably no serious disease is so frequently overlooked by the practitioner. Post-mortem experience shows how often pericarditis is not recognized or goes on to resolution and adhesion without attracting notice. —WILLIAM OSLER (1892) (1)

Clinically, pericardial heart disease is one of the more infrequent types of cardiac diseases, but morphologically, it is common. Nevertheless, many publications have appeared on clinical aspects of pericardial disease and surprisingly few have focused on its morphologic features. This report focuses on morphologic features of pericardial heart disease.

Although the term "pericarditis" is applied to many, indeed most, pericardial disorders, relatively few of the disorders actually are associated with inflammatory-cell reaction, and therefore probably most do not warrant the designation "pericarditis." Fibrinous deposits without inflammatory cells, as occur in most patients with uremia, for example, do not justify a diagnosis of "pericarditis." The presence of inflammatory cells in the pericardia rather than an acute clinical course or a pericardial friction rub should determine whether the term "pericarditis" is appropriate. "Pericardial heart disease" is a better general term.

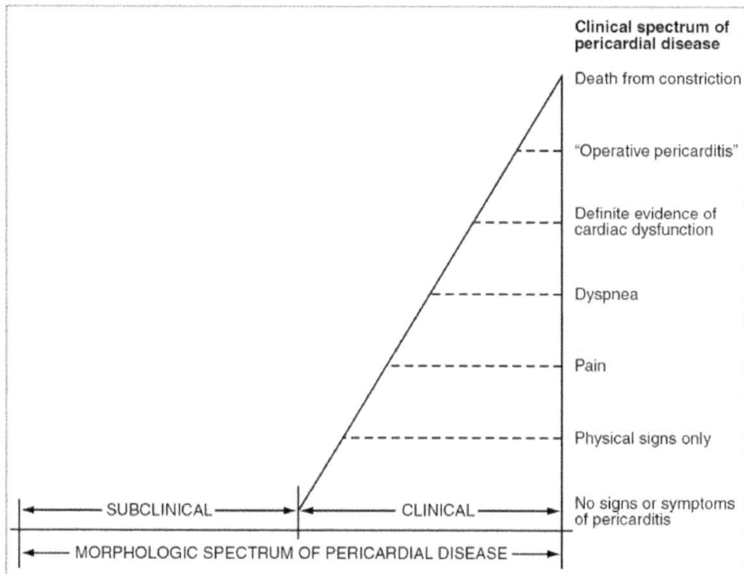

Figure 1. The clinical and morphologic spectrum of pericardial heart disease.

CLINICAL AND MORPHOLOGIC SPECTRUM

Although its exact frequency from either clinical or necropsy standpoints is not certain, pericardial heart disease, as Osler emphasized, is observed more frequently at necropsy than during life. Pericardial heart disease has been found clinically in <1% of patients admitted to one large general hospital (2) and in about 5% of consecutive necropsies at another large general hospital (3). These figures were produced in the era before cardiac catheterization or operation, renal dialysis, or widespread use of antibiotics. The clinical and necropsy frequencies of pericardial heart disease in recent years are unknown. Better diagnostic tools, particularly echocardiography, and prolonged longevity in many systemic illnesses have almost certainly increased the clinical recognition of pericardial heart disease in recent years.

Nevertheless, as shown in *Figure 1*, pericardial heart disease is more often subclinical than clinical. Even when clinical manifestations are present, evidence of myocardial constriction is uncommon. Myocardial constriction from pericardial disease may result from pericardial effusion without pericardial thickening, from pericardial thickening without pericardial fluid, or from both effusion and thickening. As shown in *Figures 2* and *3*, among patients with "pericardial" constriction (in actuality, it is the myocardium that is constricted, not the pericardium), the larger the amount of pericardial fluid, the thinner the pericardia and, conversely, the thicker the pericardia, the smaller the amount of pericardial fluid.

The type of clinical presentation of pericardial heart disease, i.e., acute or chronic, does not necessarily correlate with the type of morphologic derangement. The person with a thick constricting pericardium (obvious evidence of chronic disease) may present clinically with an acute picture (*Figure 4*). Probably more often than not, however, the clinical course follows the morphologic picture.

NORMAL PERICARDIUM

The normal *parietal pericardium* (fibrous sac or fibrous pericardium), the bag that encloses the heart, consists of a 1-mm-thick layer of dense collagen (fibrous layer) with sparse interspersed

From the Baylor Heart and Vascular Institute and the Departments of Pathology and Internal Medicine, Baylor University Medical Center, Dallas, Texas.

Corresponding author: William Clifford Roberts, MD, Baylor Heart and Vascular Institute, 621 North Hall Street, Dallas, Texas 75226 (e-mail: wc.roberts@BaylorHealth.edu).

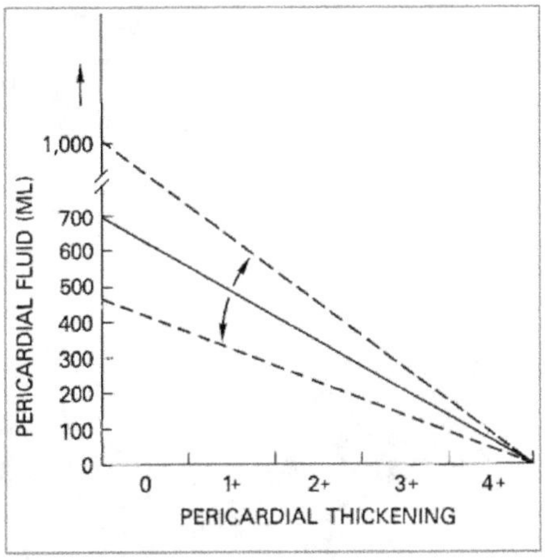

Figure 2. Pericardial fluid accumulation is, in general, not proportional to pericardial thickening: the more the pericardial fluid, the less the pericardial thickening and vice versa. The dashed lines on either side of the uninterrupted line indicate that the latter may be shifted by an acute or chronic course. Less fluid is needed to produce tamponade if the fluid accumulation is rapid than if it is slow. Likewise, less pericardial thickening is needed to produce constriction if the thickening occurs rapidly as opposed to slowly.

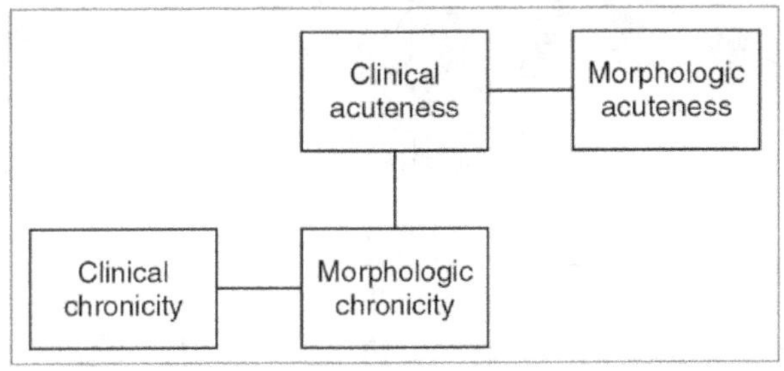

Figure 4. Relationship between the clinical and morphologic features in pericardial heart disease. Although clinical and morphologic acuteness and clinical and morphologic chronicity often go together, a chronic morphologic process can present acutely.

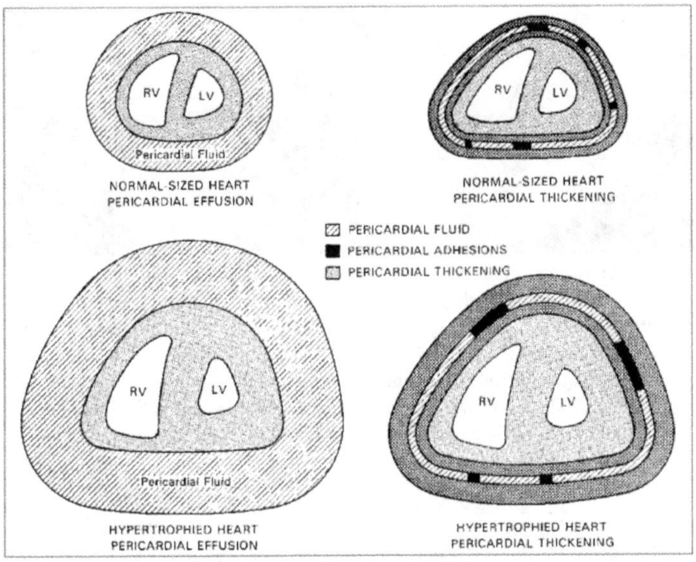

Figure 3. More pericardial fluid or thicker pericardia is necessary to constrict a hypertrophied heart than a normal-sized one. RV indicates right ventricle; LV, left ventricle.

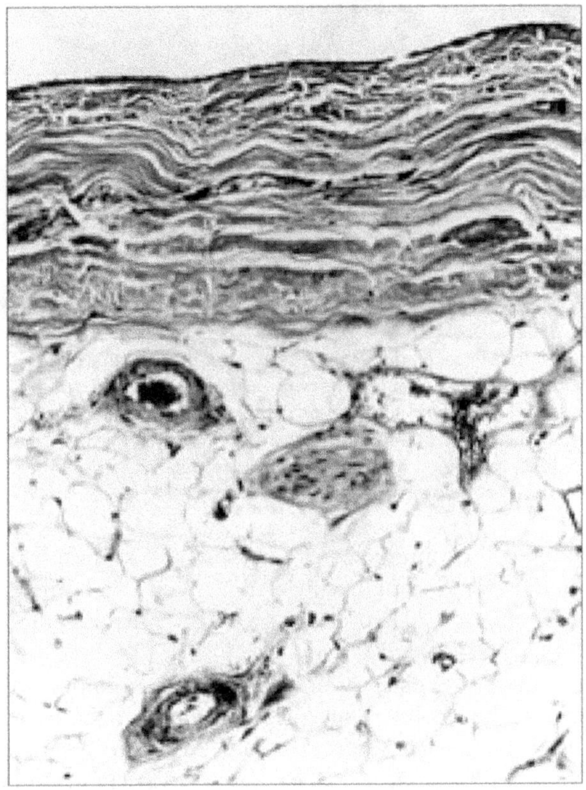

Figure 5. Normal parietal pericardium. A single layer of mesothelial cells covers the layer of dense fibrous tissue on the cardiac side. On the mediastinal side of the fibrous layer is adipose tissue, and in it are located vascular channels and nerves. Masson stain, ×185.

elastic fibrils, and it is covered by a layer of mesothelial cells (serous layer) *(Figure 5)*. The *visceral pericardium* (epicardium or serous pericardium) is the surface of the heart itself and consists of a thin (<1 mm) layer of loose fibrous tissue covered by mesothelial cells (serous layer). The serous layer of parietal pericardium is continuous with the serous layer of visceral pericardium at or near sites of attachment of the great vessels to the heart. The portion of epicardium that covers the vessels is arranged in the form of 2 tubes: the ascending aorta and pulmonary trunk are enclosed in the first *(arterial mesocardium)*, and the superior and inferior venae cavae and the 4 pulmonary veins are enclosed in the second *(venous mesocardium)*. The attachment of the latter to the parietal pericardium is in the shape of an inverted U, and the cul-de-sac enclosed between the limbs of the U lies behind the left atrium and is known as the *oblique sinus*. The passage between the venous and arterial mesocardia, i.e., that between the aorta and pulmonary trunk anteriorly and the atria posteriorly, is the *transverse sinus*.

The flask-shaped bag of parietal pericardium is closed at its neck by fusion with the adventitia of the great vessels; its base is attached to the tendinous and muscular portions of the left-sided diaphragm. It is also attached to the posterior surface of the sternum by the *superior* (to manubrium) and *inferior* (to xiphoid process) *pericardiosternal ligaments*. Between the left main pulmonary artery and subjacent pulmonary vein is a triangular fold of visceral pericardium known as the *ligament of the left vena cava*, a remnant of the lower part of the left superior vena cava. The sinus node is located near the attachment of the parietal pericardium to the superior vena cava, and consequently it may be "irritated" by a pericardial process, producing an arrhythmia or a conduction disturbance.

Electron microscopic studies of the normal parietal pericardium show that the tissue is composed of 3 layers: 1) the serosa, consisting of a surface layer of mesothelial cells and a narrow submesothelial space, 2) the fibrosa, containing variously oriented layers of collagen fibrils and small elastic fibers, and 3) the epipericardial connective tissue, containing mainly large coarse bundles of collagen and forming part of the pericardiosternal

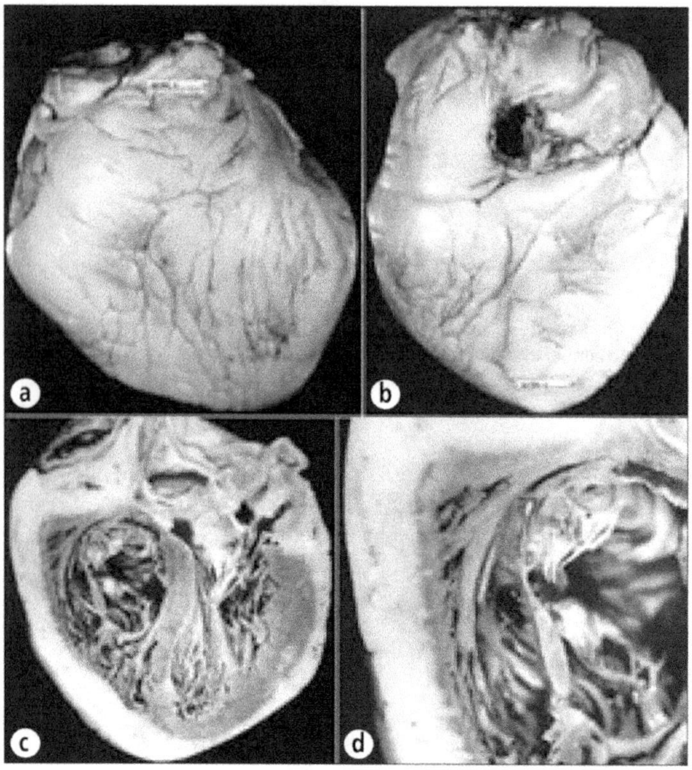

Figure 6. Massive increase in subepicardial adipose tissue in an 82-year-old man with idiopathic hemochromatosis. The myocardium was completely covered by fat. The heart weighed 500 gm. **(a)** Anterior view. **(b)** Posterior view. **(c)** Longitudinal section showing the thickness of fat compared with the thickness of the myocardial wall. **(d)** Close-up view of the right ventricular wall. The cause of the massive subepicardial adiposity in this patient is not certain.

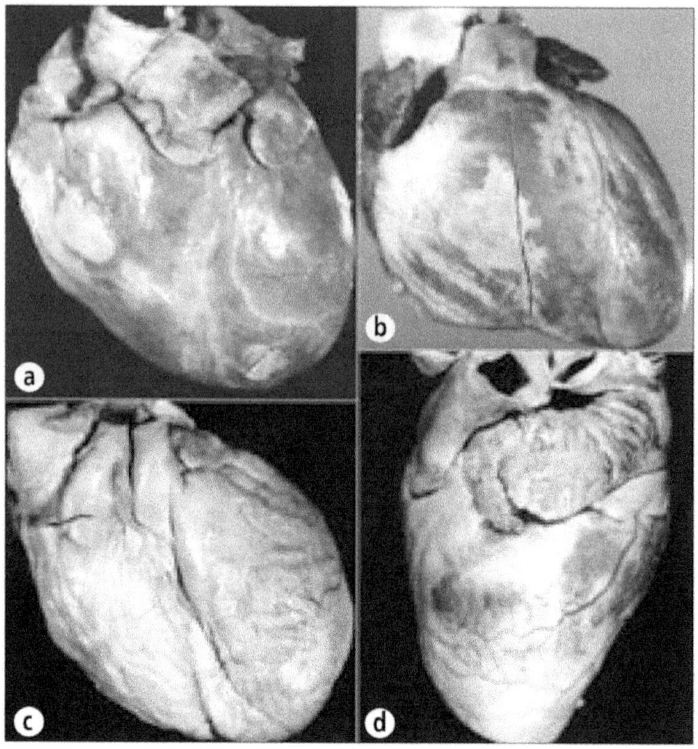

Figure 7. Epicardial collagen plaques (soldier's plaques, milk spots) in the hearts of 4 different patients. **(a)** Collagen plaques are present over the right ventricle and over the left ventricular apex. **(b)** A discrete collagen plaque is visible over the right ventricle. **(c)** Virtually the entire right ventricle and pulmonary trunk are covered by a collagen plaque. **(d)** The lateral view shows the collagen plaques just beneath the left atrial appendage and over the left ventricular apex. Note that the subepicardial adipose tissue is relatively sparse in the 4 patients. When more subepicardial fat is present, epicardial collagen plaques are less likely to form.

ligament (4). Scanning electron microscopic studies show the mesothelial cells to contain single cilia covered with microvilli. The latter appear to bear friction and to increase the surface area for fluid transport.

Beneath the visceral pericardium is either myocardium or adipose tissue. The amount of subepicardial adipose tissue increases, up to a point, with age. Large quantities are rare in persons under 10 years of age and over 90 years of age. The deposits are largest in the atrioventricular sulci and, next, around the anterior and posterior descending coronary arteries. At times, the entire surface of the heart is covered by fat *(Figure 6)*. In general, the amount of subepicardial adipose tissue is proportional to the amount of fat present in other body tissues (5, 6). At times, however, considerable quantities of subepicardial adipose tissue are present in persons of normal body weight, and the amount may not be excessively increased in persons of huge body weight (>135 kg [300 lb]). Corticosteroid therapy causes the amount of subepicardial tissue to increase (7, 8). In persons with debilitating diseases such as malignant neoplasms or chronic starvation, the subepicardial fat may atrophy, giving it a watery, gelatinous appearance.

When subepicardial adipose tissue is excessive, strands of fat cells also extend into adjacent myocardium. This occurrence is most frequent in the walls of the right ventricle and right atrium. The fat may extend through the myocardial wall and infiltrate the endocardium. Although they had no hemodynamic documentation, many writers in the 1800s believed that excessive subepicardial adipose tissue could cause cardiac dysfunction. Osler, writing in 1892, stated that excessive subepicardial fat "occasionally leads to dangerous or even fatal impairment of the contractile power of the heart" (1). Sudden nontraumatic death in the late 1800s was often attributed to a "fatty heart."

Although normally the serous layer of parietal pericardium contacts the serous layer of visceral pericardium, up to 50 mL of fluid, which has a chemical composition similar to that of serum, normally is present in the pericardial sac (9). The pericardial fluid, in essence, serves as a "lubricating oil" to diminish the amount of friction between the moving heart and the adjacent tissues.

In the adipose tissue beneath the visceral pericardium and on the mediastinal aspect of the parietal pericardium are located vascular channels, including arteries, veins, and lymphatics, and also nerves. None of these structures is located within the fibrosa component of the parietal pericardium. The arteries of the pericardium arise from the internal mammary artery and its musculophrenic branch and from the descending thoracic aorta. Branches of the vagus and phrenic nerves and from the sympathetic trunk supply the pericardium.

Normally, the visceral pericardium is translucent and the underlying subepicardial tissue or myocardium is readily visible. In many individuals, the epicardium is focally white *(Figure 7)*, and then the underlying structures are obscured. These foci (variously called milk spots, soldiers' spots, tendinous patches, and maculae tendineae) most commonly are present over the anterior surface of the right ventricle, often are multiple, and increase in incidence and size with age and with cardiac enlargement. His-

Table 1. Morphologic classification of pericardial heart disease

Primary morphologic component	Potential for constriction
1. Fibrin	0
2. Fluid	+
A. Serous	
B. Blood	
C. Lymph	
3. Purulent matter	+
4. Fibrous tissue	+
5. Neoplasm	+
6. Granuloma	+
7. Calcium	+
8. Cholesterol	+

tologically, these foci consist of dense collagen, occasionally with underlying small collections of mononuclear cells (lymphocytes). Consequently, they may most appropriately be called "collagen plaques." They are usually absent in the first decade of life and nearly always present by the sixth decade.

When the right ventricle is enlarged, the collagen plaques over its anterior surface may be quite prominent and presumably result from contact of the beating heart with the undersurface of the sternum. In conditions producing considerable enlargement of the right atrium—for example, atrial septal defect, chronic lung disease, or cardiomyopathy—the collagen plaques may occur over the right atrium (10). In kyphoscoliosis, the plaques often are found on the posterior surface of the heart, presumably due to contact with the vertebral bodies during cardiac motion. In conditions that cause left ventricular enlargement, particularly systemic hypertension and left ventricular outflow tract obstruction, collagen plaques often are present over the apex of the left

Table 2. Etiologic and morphologic classifications of pericardial heart disease

	Morphologic							
Etiologic	Fibrinous	Effusion	Infective	Fibrous	Neoplastic	Granulomatous	Calcific	Cholesterol
1. Idiopathic	++	+	0	++	0	0	++	++
2. Infective								
A. Pyogenic (purulent)	+	+	++	+	0	0	0	0
B. Tuberculous	+	+	+	++	0	++	+	+
C. Viral or "acute benign nonspecific"	++	0	+	+	0	0	0	0
D. Parasitic	+	+	++	+	0	+	+	0
E. Fungal	+	+	++	+	0	+	+	0
3. Associated with systemic disease								
A. Collagen disease								
1. Rheumatic fever	++	0	0	0	0	0	0	0
2. Rheumatoid arthritis	+	0	0	++	0	+	0	+
3. Systemic lupus erythematosus	+	+	0	++	0	0	0	0
4. Scleroderma	+	0	0	++	0	0	0	0
B. Renal disease	++	+	0	+	0	0	0	0
C. Thyroid disease	0	+	0	0	0	+	+	++
D. Sarcoidosis	0	0	0	0	0	++	0	0
4. Associated with other diseases of the heart or aorta								
A. Acute myocardial infarction	++	0	0	+	0	0	0	0
B. Ascending aortic aneurysm	+	++	0	0	0	0	0	0
5. Traumatic and iatrogenic								
A. Penetrating and nonpenetrating injury	+	++	0	++	0	0	0	+
B. Cardiac catheterization	++	+	0	0	0	0	0	0
C. Cardiac operation and postpericardiotomy syndrome	+	+	+	++	0	0	0	0
D. Resuscitation	+	+	0	++	0	0	0	0
E. Radiation	+	+	0	++	0	0	0	0
F. Drugs and hypersensitivity states	++	+	0	0	0	0	0	0
G. Talc	+	0	0	+	0	++	0	0
6. Neoplastic	+	+	0	0	++	0	0	0
7. Congenital								
A. True and false (diverticulae) cysts	–	–	–	–	–	–	–	–
B. Complete and partial absence	–	–	–	–	–	–	–	–

Table 3. Etiology of fibrinous pericardial heart disease

1. Acute myocardial infarction
2. Iatrogenesis and trauma
   A. Cardiovascular operation
   B. Complications of catheterization
   C. Irradiation
   D. Chemical agents
   E. Penetrating and nonpenetrating injury
3. Infectious agents
4. Idiopathy ("acute benign nonspecific")
5. Neoplasm
6. Association with systemic disease
   A. Renal disease ("uremia")
   B. Collagen disease
      1. Acute rheumatic fever
      2. Rheumatoid arthritis
      3. Systemic lupus erythematosus
   C. Hypersensitivity states and drug induction

ventricle. Plaques in this location may be anatomic expressions of the "point of maximal impulse" and result from contact of the left ventricular apex with the undersurface of the anterior ribs during ventricular systole. In patients with large amounts of subepicardial adipose tissue, collagen plaques may be less numerous, presumably since the epicardial fat acts as a cushion or absorbing vehicle for the underlying myocardium.

MORPHOLOGIC RESPONSES OF THE PERICARDIA TO INJURY

Although pericardial disease has many causes, the morphologic reaction of the pericardia to injury is rather limited. The pericardium reacts to acute injury by exuding *fluid*, *fibrin*, or *cells* or combinations of these three. The type of fluid and/or cells exuded is determined by the cause of the pericardial disease. There is no pericardial reaction to either serous fluid or to blood in the pericardial sac. If, however, the lipid component of pooled lysed erythrocytes is injected into the pericardial sac, a fibrinous reaction may result and fibrous or even cholesterol pericardial heart disease may develop (11). Blood in the pericardial space of injured pericardia, however, may lead to fibrous pericardial adhesions. Isolated injury to the serosal pericardia of rabbits without associated bleeding causes only a fibrinous reaction; if blood is injected after the serosal injury, pericardial adhesions may result (12). Deposits of fibrin alone on the pericardial surfaces apparently cause no permanent reaction.

If microorganisms enter the pericardial space or tissues, the reaction appears to depend on the type of infecting organism. Viruses, the presumed cause of "acute benign pericarditis," generally produce only a transient pericardial reaction, which usually resolves (13). Acid-fast organisms produce a mononuclear cell reaction and generally go on to cause severe fibrous thickening of the pericardia. Pyogenic organisms cause a violent polymorphonuclear cell reaction that also may progress to fibrous thickening with or without constriction.

General morphologic responses to injury are listed in *Tables 1* and *2*. Although their occurrence in pure form is unusual, the

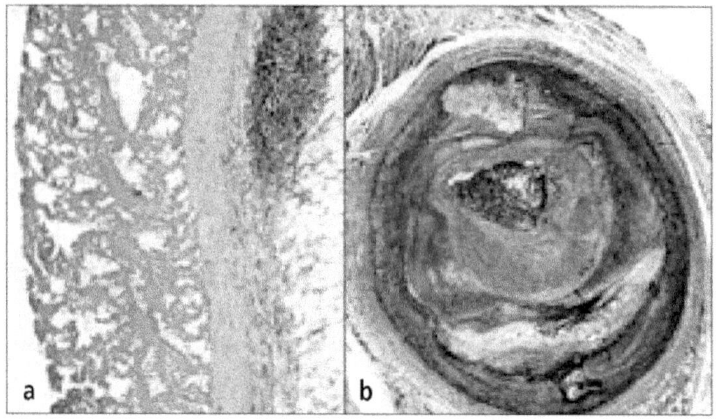

Figure 8. Diffuse fibrinous pericarditis from acute myocardial infarction. This 56-year-old man developed a precordial friction rub on day 6 following infarction and died on day 16. **(a)** A deposit of fibrin covers the mildly thickened epicardium. **(b)** The left circumflex coronary artery is completely occluded by both atherosclerotic plaque and thrombus. Hematoxylin-eosin stain, ×28 (a); Movat stain, ×14 (b).

recognition of the dominant morphologic component is useful in determining the cause of pericardial heart disease in any particular patient. The causes of each of the primary morphologic components are discussed more thoroughly in the remainder of this report.

FIBRINOUS PERICARDIAL HEART DISEASE

Fibrin deposits on the pericardial surfaces are observed commonly at necropsy. The deposits may be focal or diffuse, and they may or may not be associated with an increased quantity of pericardial fluid. Every type of pericardial disease probably is associated with fibrinous deposits at one time, and probably most cases resolve without residua. Fibrinous deposits are not capable by themselves of causing myocardial constriction. There are 6 general causes of fibrinous pericardial heart disease (*Table 3*).

Acute myocardial infarction

Fibrinous pericardial heart disease probably occurs in most patients with transmural acute myocardial infarction (*Figure 8*). The deposits may be limited to the visceral and parietal pericardium immediately overlying the area of transmural necrosis or may spread to involve the pericardial surfaces diffusely. The mechanism of development of diffuse fibrinous pericardial heart disease in these patients is not clear but may be related to the presence of an associated serosanguineous effusion. The parietal pericardium may adhere to the underlying visceral pericardium at the site of the transmural acute myocardial infarction. If the pericardial adherence occurs before the left ventricular free wall ruptures (as a consequence of the infarction), extravasation of blood into the pericardial space may be prevented and a false left ventricular aneurysm may result (14, 15) (*Figure 9*).

Iatrogenesis and trauma

Cardiac surgery probably is the most common cause of pericardial heart disease today. Whenever the mesothelial cells of the pericardia are "rubbed off," a fibrinous reaction ensues. As the injured pericardia heal, the fibrin disappears and the 2 serous layers of pericardium remain adherent by fibrous adhesions. Despite this adherence, the parietal pericardium rarely is thickened by operative intervention. Obviously, blood and its products enter

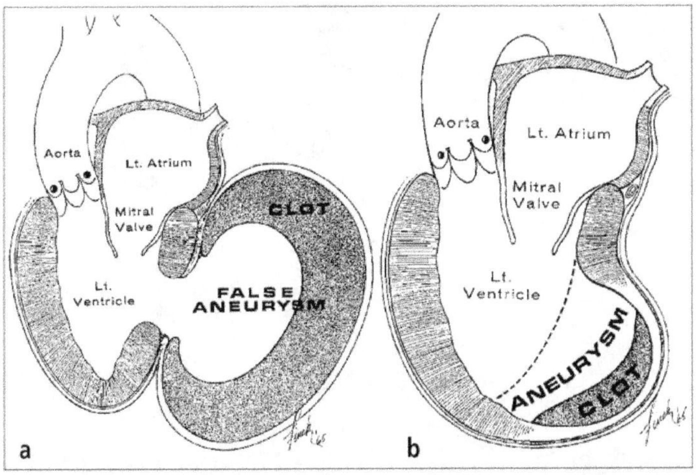

Figure 9. **(a)** False vs **(b)** true left ventricular aneurysms with adherent parietal pericardia. The wall of the false aneurysm is parietal pericardium, which had adhered to the epicardium before the left ventricle ruptured. In the true aneurysm, the parietal pericardium adheres to the scarred left ventricular myocardium, but the actual wall of the aneurysm had been myocardium at one time.

the pericardial space during any cardiac operation, and organization of the blood products may be more responsible for the eventual fibrous pericardial obliteration (12). Perforation of a cardiac wall by a *catheter* may lead to a pericardial reaction similar to that produced by cardiac surgery (16). Blunt or penetrating trauma also may cause a fibrinous pericardial reaction, which on rare occasion may progress to constriction (17).

Irradiation to the mediastinum and *chemical agents* initially cause a fibrinous pericardial reaction that also may heal by fibrous obliteration (18).

Infectious agents

Infectious agents are discussed under infective (purulent) pericardial heart disease.

Idiopathy

Although abundant clinical information is available on "acute benign pericarditis," morphologic information on this entity is lacking because of its self-limited character and rare association with "pericardial constriction" (19). A viral etiology of this entity has been implicated on the basis of "viral shedding," a rise in viral titers and the presence of lymphocytes and virus in aspirated pericardial fluid (20). However, a virus has never to my knowledge been observed ultrastructurally in pericardium, although viral antigen has been located in pericardium by immunofluorescence (21).

Neoplasm

A fibrinous pericardial reaction is common whenever the pericardium is infiltrated by a neoplasm, but the fibrin deposits are of minor consequence in this circumstance.

Association with systemic disease

"*Uremic pericarditis*," at least initially, always is fibrinous and is found at necropsy in >50% of patients with fatal acute or chronic renal disease (22). Its cause remains unclear. The term "uremic pericarditis" is a misnomer because injection of neither urea nitrogen nor creatinine into the pericardial space results in a fibrinous pericardial reaction. Furthermore, "uremic pericarditis" may occur in patients with chronic renal disease whose levels of urea nitrogen and creatinine have been made normal for long periods by frequent dialysis (23, 24). Usually the amount of pericardial fluid is increased in patients with renal failure in addition to the fibrinous pericardial deposition. On occasion, the pericardia may become quite thick by fibrous proliferation, leading to constriction with or without associated serous or hemorrhagic effusion (25, 26).

Acute rheumatic fever usually is associated with a subclinical fibrinocellular cell reaction (27, 28). This pericardial reaction appears to resolve because evidence of previous pericardial disease is rarely observed at necropsy in patients with rheumatic heart disease. Calcific pericardial deposits also may occur in patients with rheumatic heart disease, but they too are rare and, when present, are focal and never associated with myocardial constriction.

In the precorticosteroid era, fibrinous pericardial heart disease occurred in about 60% of patients with *systemic lupus erythematosus* (7, 8). Today, a fibrous obliterative pericardial reaction is observed more commonly (8). A fibrinous pericardial reaction also is observed at necropsy in about 40% of patients with *rheumatoid arthritis* (29).

The morphologic features of pericardial disease resulting from *hypersensitivity states* and *drug reactions* are not certain, but it is presumed that the reaction is of a fibrinous type.

Table 4. Etiology of effusion (>50 mL) into pericardial space

Etiology
Serous effusion
1. Congestive cardiac failure
2. Hypoalbuminemia
3. Irradiation
Bloody effusion (hematocrit >10%)
1. Iatrogenesis
A. Cardiac operation
B. Cardiac catheterization
C. Trauma (penetrating and nonpenetrating)
D. Anticoagulant agents
E. Chemotherapeutic agents
2. Neoplasm
3. Trauma
4. Acute myocardial infarction
5. Cardiac rupture
6. Rupture of ascending aorta or major pulmonary artery
7. Coagulopathy
A. Thrombocytopenia
B. Hypoprothrombinemia
C. Other (hemophilia, Gaucher's disease, etc.)
8. Renal disease
Lymphatic or chylous effusion
1. Neoplasm
2. Iatrogenesis
A. Cardiothoracic surgery
3. Congenital condition
4. Idiopathy ("primary chylopericardium")
5. Nonneoplastic obstruction of pulmonary hilum or superior vena cava

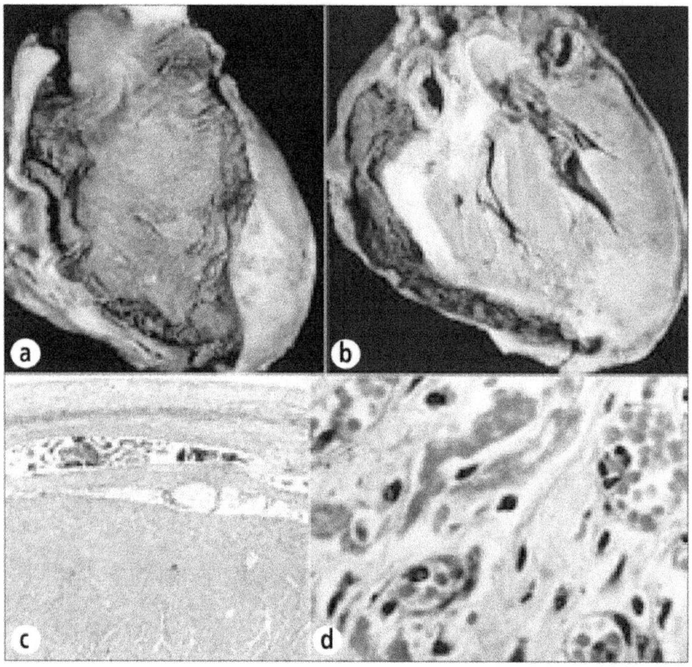

Figure 10. Hemorrhagic pericardial heart disease in chronic renal disease. This 26-year-old woman had renal failure and pericardial effusion on admission 3 weeks before death. Pericardiocentesis was performed twice, but cardiac tamponade progressed. At necropsy, 800 mL of hemorrhagic fluid was present and the pericardia were diffusely thickened and covered by fibrin deposits and blood clots. **(a)** Exterior view of the heart anteriorly. **(b)** Longitudinal section of the heart. The pericardial space over the left ventricle is obliterated. **(c)** Photomicrograph showing adherence of the parietal pericardium to underlying visceral pericardium over the left ventricle. **(d)** Close-up portion of the epicardium showing many vascular channels, the presumed source of the hemorrhagic pericardial effusion. Phosphotungstic acid hematoxylin, ×7.5 (c); hematoxylin-eosin stain; ×628 (d).

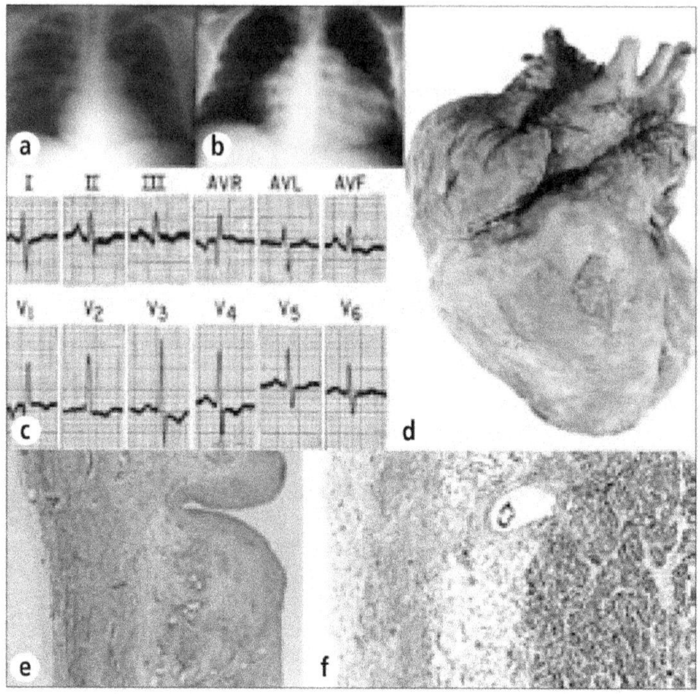

Figure 11. Hemorrhagic pericardial heart disease in a 30-year-old man with Gaucher's disease and pulmonary hypertension (from Gaucher cells plugging pulmonary capillaries). Chest radiographs **(a)** 2 months before death and **(b)** day of death, demonstrating marked enlargement of the cardiac silhouette. About 750 mL of blood was present in the pericardial sac. **(c)** Electrocardiogram recorded 1 hour before death. **(d)** Exterior of the heart showing diffuse fibrinous pericarditis and marked enlargement of the right atrium and ventricle. **(e)** Thickened parietal pericardium containing large vascular channels. **(f)** Thickened visceral pericardium. The cause of the hemorrhagic pericardial effusion was not determined. Periodic acid-Schiff stain, ×22 (e), ×33 (f).

EFFUSION INTO PERICARDIAL SAC

Excessive (>50 mL) effusion into the pericardial sac is extremely common, probably far more common than generally appreciated, because the amounts rarely are measured accurately at necropsy. Serous effusions up to 200 mL, as occur commonly in patients with congestive cardiac failure or hypoalbuminemia, may be overlooked entirely at necropsy.

The amount of pericardial fluid necessary to cause ventricular constriction is highly variable and dependent on several factors: 1) the time period required to accumulate the fluid, 2) the amount of thickening of the underlying or overlying pericardia, 3) the amount of muscle mass (weight) of the cardiac ventricles, and 4) the blood volume. The more rapidly fluid accumulates, the greater the chance that myocardial dysfunction (constriction) will result. Fluid volumes many times the normal amount may be present without myocardial constriction if the accumulation is slow (Figure 2). The greater the thickness of the parietal or visceral pericardia or both, the smaller the amount of fluid needed to produce signs or symptoms of constriction. The thicker the ventricular walls, the greater the amount of fluid required for constriction. More fluid is required, for example, to constrict the hypertensive ventricle than the normotensive ventricle (see Figure 3).

The effusions can be serous, bloody, or lymphatic/chylous (*Table 4*).

Serous effusions

Serous effusions are most common in patients with congestive cardiac failure and hypoalbuminemia (30). Irradiation (usually >4000 cGy) to the mediastinum may produce a large effusion with tamponade (31).

Bloody effusions

Bloody effusions most commonly result from acute myocardial infarction, rupture of the heart or aorta (32), neoplasms, cardiac operations or other procedures, drugs that alter clotting mechanisms (33), and chronic renal disease (34). That renal disease may be associated with large bloody effusions is largely unappreciated (35); this circumstance may occur in the natural history of renal disease (*Figure 10*) as well as that prolonged by chronic dialysis. Gaucher's disease also may be associated with large pericardial effusions (36, 37) (*Figure 11*). Hemopericardium always is an ominous sign because malignancy is one of its more common causes. Hemorrhages into the epicardium are common in patients with thrombocytopenia (*Figure 12*).

Lymphatic and chylous effusion

Most reports concerning lymph or chyle within the pericardial space concern isolated patients because this condition is rare (38). *Chylopericardium*, i.e., milky effusion, most commonly results from obstruction or injury of the thoracic duct (39). At other times, its cause is not discernible but, nevertheless, hemipericardiectomy and ligation of pericardial lymphatics may result in disappearance

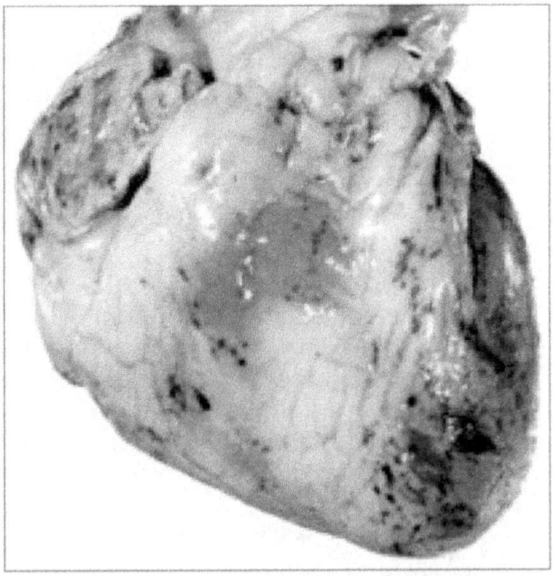

Figure 12. Focal epicardial hemorrhages in hypothrombocytopenia. The anterior surface of the heart shows focal hemorrhages in a 56-year-old man with acute myelogenous leukemia. The epicardial hemorrhages seen here are typical of those observed in many patients with severe hypothrombocytopenia from any cause. This man's platelet count 2 days before death was 500 per mm^3.

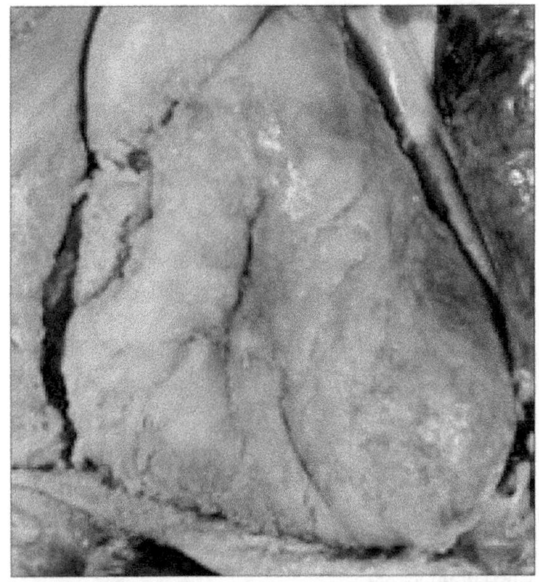

Figure 13. Purulent pericarditis in the exterior of the heart in a 56-year-old man with squamous cell carcinoma arising in the floor of the mouth. He developed a neoplastic abscess cavity in the left posterior mediastinum, and it opened into the esophagus, bronchus, left pleural cavity, and pericardial sac. *Candida albicans* was cultured from the purulent material in the pericardial sac.

of the chylous effusion (38). Lymphangiomatous hamartoma (cystic hygroma) of the mediastinum associated with a communication between the thoracic duct and pericardial space (40) also has caused chylopericardium. Chylous fluid may accumulate rapidly and even lead to tamponade (38, 41). Lymphopericardium, i.e., clear fluid, which is even less common than chylopericardium, usually results from pericardial lymphangiomas that may be part of generalized lymphangiectasia (42).

INFECTIVE (PURULENT) PERICARDIAL HEART DISEASE

Infective pericarditis is the presence of pus, microorganisms, or both in the pericardial sac or tissues. Nontuberculous infective pericarditis is infrequent. In the preantibiotic and prethoracic surgical eras, the infection was usually spread from the lung, pleura, mediastinum, or abdomen or was a complication of a generalized septicemia. Today, the most common predisposing factors are cardiothoracic operations, immunosuppressive therapy, trauma, rupture of the esophagus into the pericardial sac secondary to neoplasm *(Figure 13)*, and infective endocarditis with rupture of a ring abscess, septic coronary embolus, or rupture of a myocardial abscess (43) *(Figure 14)*.

The expected increase in frequency of purulent pericarditis with the advent of cardiothoracic operations has been offset by the widespread use of antibiotics and the decrease in bacterial infections in general. Indeed, purulent pericarditis is less frequent today than in the past (44). The occurrence of infective pericarditis as a consequence of infective endocarditis is not widely appreciated (45). In a review by Buchbinder and Roberts of 1284 patients with fatal infective endocarditis, 172 (13%) had pericarditis at necropsy. The pericarditis in this circumstance need not be purulent (45). Figure 14 shows several mechanisms of formation of pericarditis in patients with infective endocarditis.

The organisms responsible for nontuberculous infective pericarditis have changed considerably since the introduction

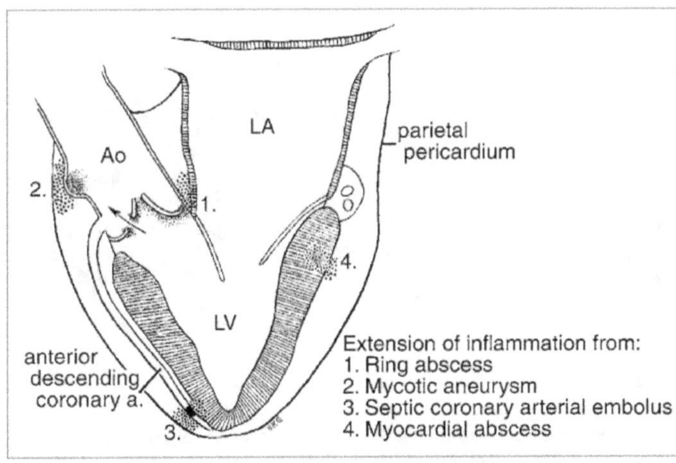

Figure 14. Schematic portrayal of the pathogenesis of pericarditis in infective endocarditis. Ao indicates aorta; LV, left ventricle; LA, left atrium.

of antibiotics, cardiothoracic surgery, and immunosuppression. In the preantibiotic era, a gram-positive bacterium was responsible in 80% and a gram-negative bacterium in 4% of cases *(Table 5)*. These figures were from the study by Cabot of 186 necropsy patients with purulent pericarditis (28). In a later study from the same hospital (Massachusetts General) of 26 patients with purulent pericarditis, gram-positive bacteria were responsible in 42%, gram-negative bacteria in 39%, and fungi in 19% of cases (43) (Table 5). In none of Cabot's patients were fungi the causative agent. Furthermore, the types of gram-positive bacteria causing infective pericarditis have changed considerably. Streptococcus and pneumococcus were most common in the preantibiotic era and staphylococcus in the recent antibiotic era (Table 5).

Purulent pericarditis with or without antibiotic treatment has a poor prognosis. It nearly always indicates a widespread infection of the mediastinum and lung. Although tamponade and

Table 5. Organisms responsible for nontuberculous infective pericardial heart disease

	Preantibiotic era (1896–1919)*	Early antibiotic era (1949–1959)†	Antibiotic era (1960–1974)‡
I. Gram-positive			
Staphylococcus aureus	14	7	8
Staphylococcus epidermidis	3	0	0
Staphylococcus (species unspecified)	4	0	0
Streptococcus	39	1	1
Pneumococcus	33	0	2
II. Gram-negative			
Escherichia coli	3	1	0
Klebsiella pneumoniae	1	0	0
Hemophilus influenzae	0	0	2
Neisseria meningitidis	0	0	1
III. Multiple bacteria	7	0	0
IV. Fungi	0	0	5
V. Unspecified or unproved	9	2	7§
VI. Negative cultures	73	0	0
Totals	186	11	26

*From Cabot (28).
†From Boyle et al (44).
‡From Rubin and Moellering (43).
§All of these may be gram-negative organisms.

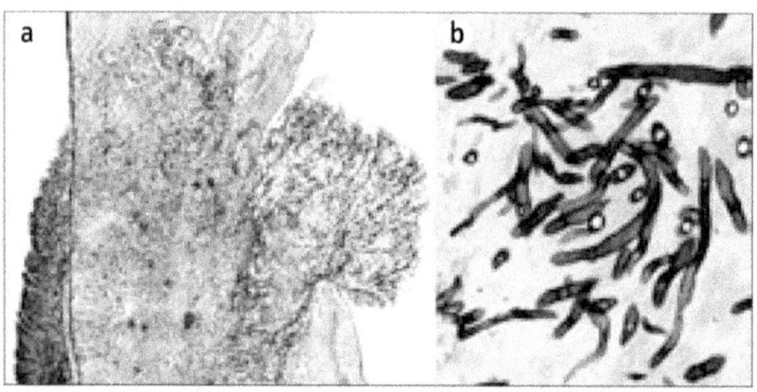

Figure 15. *Candida tropicalis* pancarditis in a 7-year-old girl with acute lymphocytic leukemia and a 21-month illness. The child never had signs or symptoms of cardiac disease but died of disseminated candidiasis. **(a)** Section of the right atrial wall with fungi extending from the epicardium through the myocardium into the endocardium. **(b)** Close-up of *Candida* organisms. Methenamine silver stain, ×12 (a), ×520 (b).

constriction may occur, drainage of the pericardial pus usually is not lifesaving because the infective process is so extensive.

Although *parasites* can infect pericardium, all are rare. About 100 patients with amebic pericarditis have been reported, and in each spread was from a hepatic abscess (46). Before actual perforation into the pericardial space, amebic pericarditis is described classically as "anchovy-sauce" pus, but *Entamoeba histolytica* organisms are infrequently found in it (46). A rapid course to constriction may occur. Pericardial involvement by toxoplasmosis and echinococcosis is extremely rare, and cases of pericardial involvement by dracunculosis have been reported (47).

Fungal pericarditis has increased in frequency with the use of immunosuppressive agents. Although usually granulomatous, fungal pericarditis may be purulent. *Coccidioides immitis* has been found in pericardium, and clinical evidence of pericarditis occurs in about 15% of patients with pulmonary coccidioidomycosis (48). Pericarditis occurred in 2% of 470 necropsied patients with actinomycosis (49), but sulfur granules were rare. Pericardial calcific deposits may occur in patients who react to histoplasmosis but not to other fungal antigens, but acute pericarditis has not been reported in patients with histoplasmosis. Pericardial candidiasis has been observed in patients with leukemia receiving immunosuppressive drugs (*Figure 15*).

Pericarditis has been seen in association with several *viral* diseases, including infectious mononucleosis, atypical pneumonia, mumps, measles, smallpox, and influenza. Although viral titers may rise, morphologic confirmation of a viral etiology is lacking.

Pericarditis probably is most frequent from Coxsackie viruses (50). Biopsy of parietal pericardium, however, has not revealed intracellular virions, although viral antigens may be present. Indeed, almost no morphologic information is present on viral pericarditis in humans.

FIBROUS PERICARDIAL HEART DISEASE

Fibrous pericardial heart disease is thickening of the pericardia or the presence of adhesions between the visceral and parietal pericardia or both. Either the thickening or the adhesions may be focal or diffuse. The thickening may involve both visceral and parietal pericardia or only one of them. The collagen plaque, for example, is a form of fibrous pericardial heart disease with focal thickening, usually limited to the epicardium. Pericardial thickening may occur in the absence of pericardial adhesions, adhesions may occur in the absence of pericardial thickening, or the two may occur together. When pericardial adhesions are diffuse, the pericardial space is obliterated, and this circumstance has been called "*obliterative pericarditis*."

"Obliterative pericarditis" may occur in the absence of thickening of the parietal pericardium. Obviously, since its space no longer is present, pericardial effusion, by definition, cannot be present in the patient with "obliterative pericarditis." A pericardial effusion may be present in patients with focal pericardial adhesions or in patients with diffuse pericardial thickening with either no adhesions or only focal adhesions.

There are many causes of pericardial thickening and pericardial adhesions. The most common are listed in *Table* 6.

Healing of hemopericardium (of any cause)

As mentioned earlier, in and of itself the presence of blood within the pericardial sac leaves no residua. However, the presence of blood superimposed on injured pericardial surfaces (mesothelial layer "rubbed off," for example) generally leads to adhesions between the pericardia with or without thickening of the pericardia. After cardiac operations, the pericardia adhere to each other by fibrous adhesions. In this circumstance, it is presumed that manipulation of the pericardia at operation damaged the pericardial surfaces. The healing of these damaged surfaces by organization of the blood products presumably accounts for the development of the pericardial adhesions. The adherence of the 2 layers therefore

Table 6. Etiology of fibrous (adhesive) pericardial heart disease

1. Healing of hemopericardium (of any cause) in the presence of serosal injury
   A. Cardiac operation
   B. Trauma—blunt and penetrating
2. Irradiation
3. Association with another disease
   A. Renal disease
   B. Rheumatoid arthritis
   C. Systemic lupus erythematosus
   D. Scleroderma
4. Infectious agent
5. Idiopathy

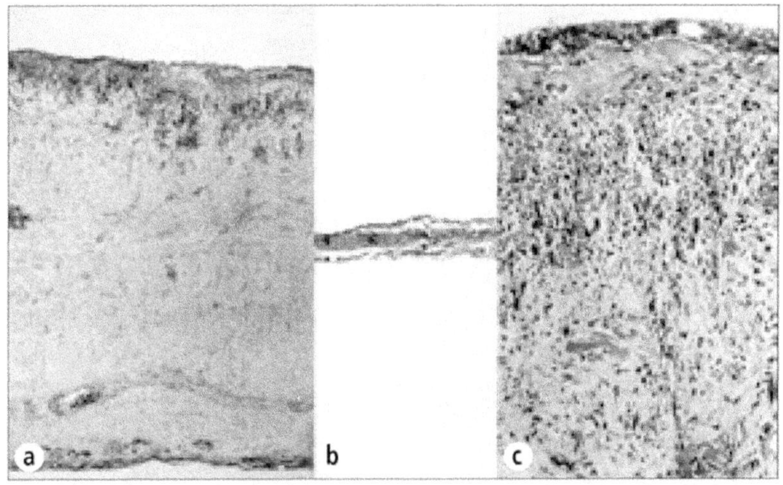

Figure 16. Radiation pericarditis. Stage IIIB Hodgkin's disease was diagnosed in this 54-year-old man, and he then received radiation therapy to the mediastinum. Eighteen months later, he developed recurrent pericardial effusion and signs of pericardial constriction, including elevated venous pressure and congestive cardiac failure. He underwent pericardiectomy, and at operation the pericardial sac contained about 150 mL of fluid. The parietal and visceral pericardia were focally adherent by fibrinous adhesions. After excision of the anterior portion of parietal pericardium, which was up to 1.0 cm in thickness, the central venous pressure dropped from 15 to 8 cm of water. The patient had an uneventful recovery and no further symptoms of myocardial constriction. **(a)** Section of parietal pericardium showing diffuse fibrous thickening with fibroblast proliferation. Plasma cells and lymphocytes are present. **(b)** Section of normal pericardium for comparison. **(c)** Higher-power view of parietal pericardium in this patient showing fibroblasts, lymphocytes, and plasma cells. These changes are characteristic of radiation pericarditis. Hematoxylin-eosin stain, ×27 (a and b), ×160 (c).

represents an "overreaction" of the healing process. After a cardiotomy, the parietal pericardium is not thickened. Blunt external trauma from, for example, resuscitation may produce a similar reaction. Nonpenetrating blunt trauma may also simply "bruise" the pericardial surfaces, producing a focal fibrinous reaction that may resolve or go on to fibrous adhesions if blood exudes into the pericardial space at the site of the contusion.

Irradiation

Radiation always produces injury, and repair of that injury may cause fibrous proliferation (18). Although the endocardium, myocardium, and pericardium may be injured by high-dose irradiation, the portion of the heart most frequently damaged is the pericardium. Experimentally, mediastinal irradiation to rabbits (in a dosage equivalent to 4000 cGy to the mediastinum of humans) initially produces a polymorphonuclear reaction in the pericardia followed in 1 or 2 days by a mononuclear reaction (51). Damage to the endothelial cells of both lymphatic and blood capillaries leads to luminal obstruction of these channels, which in turn leads to pericardial effusion. The pericardia also are thickened by fibrous tissue, but its mechanism of development is not certain.

Mediastinal irradiation in high doses in humans, with resulting pericardial injury, occurs primarily in patients with Hodgkin's disease (18, 52, 53), because it is the most common mediastinal tumor irradiated in sufficient doses to cause cardiac disease (*Figure 16*). Pericardial injury probably occurs in most patients receiving ≥4000 cGy to the mediastinum. Fibrous thickening of the pericardia combined with pericardial effusion (usually serous) has been the most frequent consequence of this irradiation. Clinical evidence of cardiac dysfunction resulting from pericardial disease occurs in about 5% of patients with Hodgkin's disease treated with high-dose mediastinal irradiation (31). Cardiac tamponade may occur, usually a result of combined pericardial effusion and fibrous thickening of the parietal pericardium (54). The coronary arteries lying in the subepicardial adipose tissue also may be damaged by irradiation, with resulting coronary arterial luminal narrowing and symptomatic or fatal ischemic heart disease (52, 53).

A diagnostic dilemma occurs in patients who have mediastinal irradiation for a tumor and then develop evidence of pericardial effusion. Is the pericardial effusion radiation induced or is it due to contiguous spread of the neoplasm to the pericardium? It is of some value to know that pericardial effusion of sufficient magnitude to be detected by echocardiogram commonly is found after mediastinal irradiation, that it may lead to pericardial tamponade, and that the peak evidence of the pericardial reactions appears from 2 to 8 months after radiation therapy, although a wide range of time from irradiation to onset of pericardial symptoms has been reported.

Association with another disease

Although fibrinous pericarditis is the most common type of pericardial involvement in patients with chronic renal disease, fibrous thickening of the pericardia with or without associated fibrous adhesions or pericardial effusion also may occur in patients not treated with dialysis (Figure 10). Fibrous pericardial heart disease, however, appears to be more frequent in patients on chronic dialysis than in patients with chronic renal disease not treated in this fashion.

At necropsy, nearly 50% of patients with rheumatoid arthritis have fibrous obliterative pericardial heart disease and, rarely, calcific or cholesterol pericardial disease (55). Usually, no functional consequence results from the obliterative pericardial heart disease.

Among 36 patients with *systemic lupus erythematosus* (SLE) studied at necropsy (7, 8), 19 had pericardial heart disease: fibrinous in 4, purulent in 2, and fibrous in 13. Before corticosteroids were introduced, the fibrinous type was the most common seen in patients with SLE. Among patients with SLE treated with

Table 7. Etiology of constrictive pericardial heart disease in the USA treated by pericardiectomy

Type of pericardial heart disease	Totals*
Idiopathic	213 (68%)
Tuberculous	63 (20%)
Traumatic	6 (2%)
Rheumatic	2 (1%)
Neoplastic	3 (1%)
Pyogenic	4 (1%)
Irradiation	4 (1%)
Postcardiotomy	2 (1%)
Rheumatoid arthritis	2 (1%)
Viral	1 (0%)
Acute nonspecific	14 (4%)
Total	314 (100%)

*Includes patients seen from 1930 to 1969 and included in 6 different studies.

corticosteroids, the fibrous type is the most common. Among 19 SLE patients with pericardial heart disease at necropsy, none had evidence of myocardial dysfunction as a consequence of the pericardial involvement. Eleven of the 19 had pericardial friction rubs. In patients with SLE, pericardial heart disease serves as an excellent marker of the presence of associated endocarditis: endocarditis was present at necropsy in 18 of the 19 SLE patients with and in none of the 17 SLE patients without pericardial disease.

Although uncommon clinically, pericardial heart disease is common at necropsy in patients with scleroderma (56). The fibrous obliterative type is the most common form in scleroderma. The fibrinous type, seen less commonly, may result from associated renal failure rather than scleroderma per se (56). Among the scleroderma patients I studied at necropsy, a third had pericardial involvement, fibrous in each.

Infectious agent

See the section on infective (purulent) pericardial heart disease.

Idiopathy

Fibrous pericardial disease of unknown etiology is the most common "cause" today of "chronic constrictive pericarditis" (*Table 7*) (57). In a report of 137 patients undergoing pericardiectomy because of "constrictive pericarditis," no cause was found on histologic study of the excised pericardia in 106 (77%) (58).

An interesting entity called "occult constrictive pericardial disease" has been described. This syndrome consists of nonspecific symptoms of fatigue, dyspnea, and chest pain in patients, most of whom had a history of pericarditis in the past. They had abnormal hemodynamics at cardiac catheterization until they were challenged by an infusion of 1 L of warm saline. They then developed hemodynamic findings characteristic of constrictive pericarditis. These findings were absent in control patients with heart disease similarly challenged with volume expansion. Pericardiectomy relieved the symptoms and altered the hemodynamic findings in response to saline infusion in all patients. The pericardium was abnormal in all subjects.

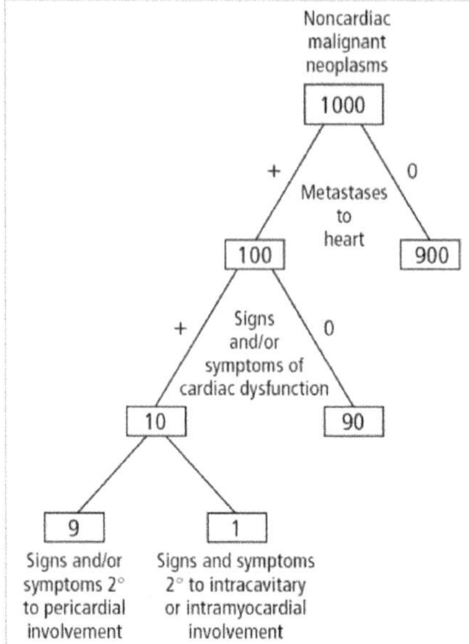

Figure 17. The frequency of pericardial involvement in malignant neoplasms.

Administration of procainamide, methysergide, or practolol has been well documented to result in constrictive pericarditis. One wonders whether a significant percentage of patients who have "idiopathic constrictive pericarditis" may have developed it as a complication of drug therapy.

NEOPLASTIC PERICARDIAL HEART DISEASE

As seen in *Figure 17*, the heart is involved in approximately 10% of patients with malignant neoplasms, and 85% of the patients with cardiac involvement have neoplastic involvement of the pericardium (59). Furthermore, only about 10% of patients with cardiac involvement have clinical evidence of cardiac disease, and in 90% of those the clinical dysfunction is the result of pericardial involvement, usually constriction by either pericardial effusion or neoplastic thickening of pericardia or both. The most common neoplasms in absolute numbers with cardiac metastases are lung (in men) and breast (in women), followed by leukemia and lymphoma (*Table 8*). Nearly any tumor, however, may metastasize to the heart. Among patients with carcinoma of the breast or lung, about 10% have neoplastic involvement of the heart (59). Because spread of these 2 tumors to the heart appears to be by direct extension, the pericardia virtually always are involved.

Among specific malignant neoplasms, the ones with the highest percentage of metastases to the heart are melanoma (70%) (60), leukemia (37%) (61), and lymphoma (24%) (62). As with the tumors that spread by direct extension, melanoma, leukemia, and lymphoma invade the pericardia in 85% of the patients with cardiac metastases, and spread of these neoplasms appears to be by the hematogenous routes.

Although pericardial effusions, often bloody, are frequent in patients with cardiac metastases, pericardial effusions also are common in patients with malignant neoplasms without cardiac metastases (59, 62). Pericardial effusions (>50 mL) were recorded in 17% of 48 patients with cardiac lymphoma and in 14% of 148 patients with lymphoma but without cardiac metastases (62). In both groups, the effusions were serous and probably the result of

Table 8. Etiology of neoplastic pericardial heart disease

1. Metastatic
   A. Lung
   B. Breast
   C. Lymphoma
   D. Leukemia
   E. Miscellaneous
2. Primary
   A. Benign
      1. Teratoma
      2. Fibroma
      3. Lipoma
      4. Angioma
   B. Malignant
      1. Mesothelioma
      2. Sarcoma
         a. Differentiated
         b. Undifferentiated

Table 9. Etiology of granulomatous pericardial heart disease

1. Infectious agent
   A. Tuberculosis
   B. Fungus
   C. Parasite
2. Cholesterol
   A. Idiopathy
   B. Association with another condition
      1. Hypothyroidism
      2. Rheumatoid arthritis
      3. Tuberculosis
      4. Hypercholesterolemia
3. Iatrogenesis
   A. Talc
   B. Other foreign body
4. Sarcoidosis

hypoalbuminemia (<3.5 gm/dL), which was present in 95% of the 196 necropsy patients with lymphoma (62).

Pericardial heart disease may occur in patients with malignant neoplasms who do not have involvement of the heart (including pericardia) by neoplasm. Varying types of the disease were present in 21% of 48 patients with cardiac lymphoma and in 7% of 148 patients with lymphoma but without metastases to the heart (62).

Symptoms and signs in patients with cardiac metastases often are attributed to cardiac involvement by the neoplasm, but this may not be justified. Dyspnea, for example, was present in 27% of 48 patients with and in 52% of 148 patients without cardiac lymphoma (62). Likewise, precordial or substernal chest pain (6%), precordial murmurs (35%), and ventricular gallops (5%) were present in the same frequencies among patients with lymphoma irrespective of the presence or absence of cardiac metastases (62). Surprisingly, electrocardiographic abnormalities were present in identical frequency among patients with lymphoma with and without cardiac tumor deposits: 62% in each of the 2 groups (62).

Primary pericardial neoplasms are extremely rare, and about half of them are benign (59). The most common is teratoma (63). Although usually histologically benign, teratoma can produce fatal compression of a cardiac chamber. Hemangioma, leiomyofibroma, lipoma, and fibroma are other "benign" pericardial neoplasms. The hemangioma may rupture to cause hemorrhagic pericardial effusion with or without tamponade.

Among the primary malignant pericardial neoplasms, mesothelioma is by far the most frequent. It may totally encase the heart, resulting in fatal myocardial constriction.

GRANULOMATOUS PERICARDIAL HEART DISEASE

Infectious agent

Among the causes of granulomatous pericarditis (*Table 9*), tuberculosis is by far the most important. Pericardial involvement by tuberculosis was described initially by Rokitansky in 1852, and it was he who noted the "association with, and dependence upon, an earlier tuberculous lesion" (64). Since that time there has been much debate over whether "primary" tuberculous pericarditis is a separate clinicopathologic entity or whether it is the recognizable result of an earlier resolved or inactive primary lesion.

The frequency of tuberculous pericarditis has diminished in recent years, presumably paralleling the reduction in incidence of pulmonary tuberculosis. Osler observed tuberculosis in 215 (22%) of 1000 necropsies, and 7 (3%) of the 215 had pericardial involvement (65). Subsequent studies (66) have shown pericarditis to be present at necropsy in 8% of patients with pulmonary tuberculosis.

The pathogenesis of pericardial involvement by tuberculosis is not clear. Pericardial disease probably results from early dissemination following a primary infection. The infection appears to reach the pericardium either from the blood (miliary) or, more commonly, by retrograde lymphatic spread from infected mediastinal glands. The pericardial infection rarely arises from direct spread from the lung or pleura.

Four stages of tuberculous pericarditis have been described (67). The *fibrinous* stage is characterized by diffuse deposits of fibrin associated with a granulomatous reaction. This stage is observed rarely, and there is some debate as to whether it can resolve or whether it always goes on to the second stage, which is characterized by *effusion* into the pericardial sac. The effusions, which may be massive (>2000 mL), usually are serous or serosanguineous but may be bloody or turbid. Many lymphocytes may be present in the effusion, but tuberculous organisms are uncommonly observed morphologically in the fluid or cultured from it.

By stage 3, the parietal pericardium is considerably thickened by both fibrous tissue and granulomas, and most of the fluid has resolved. If the parietal pericardium becomes markedly thickened, myocardial *constriction* may occur, and this is considered stage 4. By this time, the pericardial space may be completely obliterated by diffuse fibrous adhesions. Eventually the granulomas apparently can be replaced entirely by fibrous tissue and, if observed morphologically at this point, the pericardial disease would have

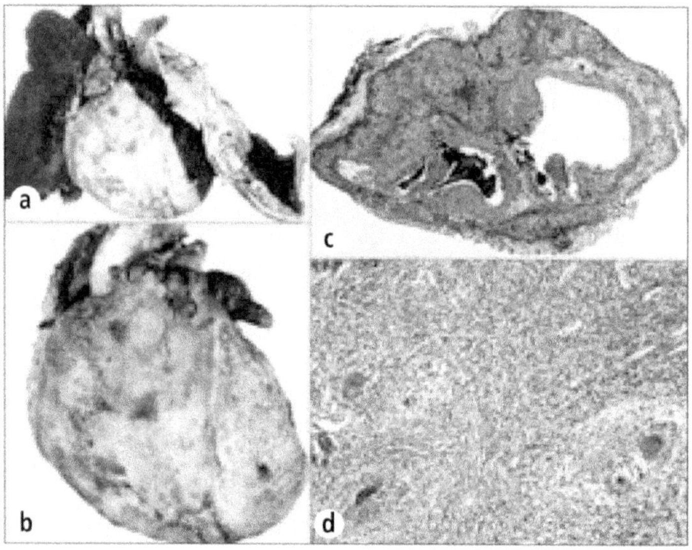

Figure 18. Tuberculous pericarditis in a 45-year-old dyspneic man whose chest radiograph showed complete loss of volume of the left lung and massive left pleural effusion. Congestive cardiac failure and respiratory insufficiency led to death. At necropsy, the entire left lung was collapsed, and the left hemithorax was filled with pus. The left pleura was markedly thickened and focally calcified. No granulomas or foci of caseation necrosis were observed in either lung or in the hilar lymph nodes. **(a)** Heart and lungs showing loss of left lung, cardiomegaly (600 gm), and diffuse pericarditis. **(b)** Closer view of the exterior of the heart showing fibrinous exudate covering the entire myocardial surface. **(c)** Section of the left atrial appendage showing complete involvement of the epicardium by caseating granulomas and giant cells. Fibrinous pericardial exudate also covers most of its surface. **(d)** High-power view of granulomas covering the left atrial appendage. No acid-fast organisms were found. Hematoxylin-eosin stain, ×5 (c); periodic acid-Schiff stain, ×80 (d).

to be called idiopathic rather than granulomatous (tuberculosis). Calcific deposits with or without bone formation may occur in the markedly thickened pericardia. Progression from stage 3 to stage 4 may occur despite antituberculous therapy.

Tuberculous pericarditis by no means always progresses to the constrictive fibrous stage *(Figure 18)*. Heimann and Binder (68) described 31 patients with granulomatous pericarditis; none had constriction and all had tuberculous hilar lymph nodes. Among patients with "chronic" constrictive pericarditis, however, tuberculosis remains an important cause, accounting for nearly 10% of the cases in the USA (Table 7). In some areas of the world, a tuberculous cause of constrictive pericarditis is more common than a nontuberculous cause. Among 61 patients with constrictive pericarditis undergoing pericardiectomy in India, the etiology was tuberculous in 37 (61%) and nontuberculous in 24 (39%) (69).

Fungi and parasites are rare causes of granulomatous pericarditis.

Cholesterol

So-called cholesterol pericarditis always produces a granulomatous reaction; it is discussed separately below.

Iatrogenesis

The sprinkling of *talc* in the pericardial space, a procedure introduced in the early 1940s (70, 71) as a form of treatment for coronary heart disease, produces an extensive granulomatous reaction resulting in obliteration of the pericardial space (72) *(Figure 19)*. A similar type of granulomatous reaction occurs in the lungs of persons who intravenously inject drugs intended

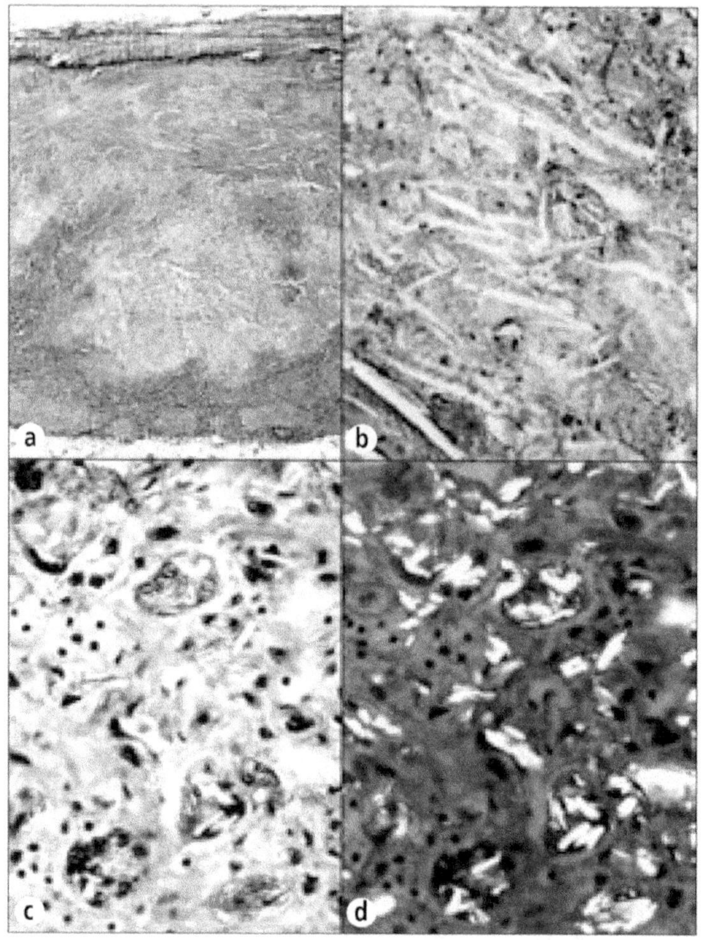

Figure 19. Talc-induced granulomatous pericarditis in a 92-year-old woman who was stated to have had angina pectoris beginning at age 63. At age 67, she underwent talcum-powder sprinkling on her pericardium (Beck or Thompson procedure). Immediately preoperatively, she was in congestive heart failure with atrial fibrillation and a slow ventricular response. At necropsy, an old healed anterolateral apical infarct was present, but no myocardial necrosis was observed. The striking finding, however, was a diffuse fibrous and granulomatous pericarditis secondary to talc with complete obliteration of the pericardial space. **(a)** Section of parietal pericardium showing large foci of acellular debris containing multiple cholesterol clefts. **(b)** Higher-power view showing cholesterol clefts and talc. **(c)** Multinucleated foreign-body giant cells with intracellular talc granules. A few mononuclear cells are present. **(d)** Same field as (c) with polarization showing highly refractile talc particles both intracellularly and extracellularly. Hematoxylin-eosin stain, ×23 (a), ×250 (b), ×480 (c, d).

for oral use because virtually every tablet contains talc (73). A foreign-body type of granulomatous reaction results from deposition of starch granules within the pericardial space, a minor complication of cardiac operations (74).

Sarcoidosis

Not generally recognized as a cause of pericarditis because clinical evidence of pericardial involvement is rare and focal, noncaseating pericardial granulomas are observed at necropsy in patients with sarcoidosis (75). Among 35 patients with cardiac sarcoidosis studied at necropsy by Roberts and associates (75), 12 (34%) had granulomas involving epicardium *(Figure 20)*. None, however, had clinical signs. In addition, another patient had obliterative fibrous pericardial heart disease causing no clinical signs. Only 3 patients had excessive pericardial fluid measured at necropsy, but it was <300 mL in each.

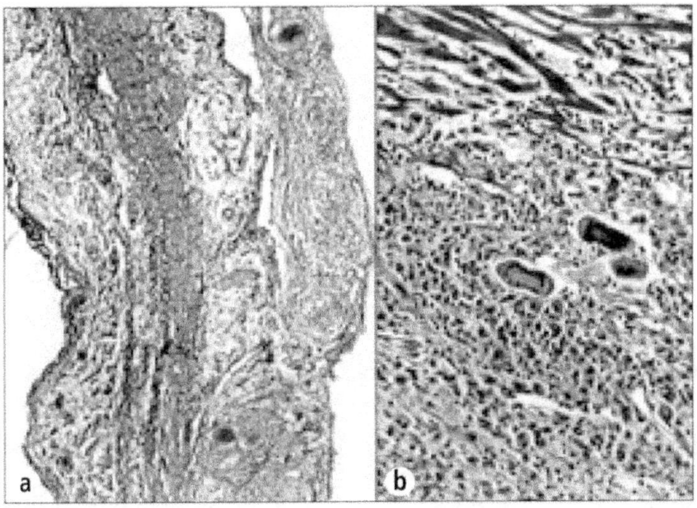

Figure 20. Sarcoidosis of the pericardium in a 47-year-old woman who was well until 16 months before death, when exertional dyspnea appeared. Thereafter, there was clinical evidence of recurring pleural and pericardial effusions. She died of progressive respiratory insufficiency. At necropsy, both lungs were extensively infiltrated by noncaseating granulomas devoid of microorganisms. Grossly, the pericardium and myocardium contained no focal lesions except in the left ventricular papillary muscles. On histologic examination, however, noncaseating granulomas were found in the **(a)** parietal pericardium and **(b)** visceral pericardium. In addition to the noncaseating granulomas in the papillary muscle, similar microscopic-sized granulomas were observed in the walls of all 4 cardiac chambers. Hematoxylin-eosin stain, ×80 (a), ×220 (b).

Table 10. Etiology of calcific pericardial heart disease

1. Idiopathy
2. Tuberculosis
3. Infection
4. Rheumatic fever
5. Trauma

CALCIFIC PERICARDIAL HEART DISEASE

The occurrence of calcific deposits in pericardia constitutes calcific pericardial heart disease. The calcific deposits may vary in size from microscopic, i.e., visible only by histologic examination, to massive, i.e., encircling all or most of the heart and readily visible by radiographic examination. Calcific deposits appear to represent the end stage of organization of a pericardial process and in themselves are not indicative of any specific etiology. Histologic examination of calcified pericardia rarely provides specific diagnoses. Conditions predisposing to calcific pericardial heart disease are listed in *Table 10*. The etiology is based on historical data or an associated abnormality rather than on specific pericardial alteration. There is strong suggestive evidence that large calcific pericardial deposits represent "burnt out" pericardial tuberculosis.

At times, huge calcific deposits may be present in the pericardia without evidence of myocardial constriction or other myocardial dysfunction (76) *(Figure 21)*. For myocardial constriction to occur, the calcific deposits must encircle both ventricles *(Figure 22)*. Localized bands of calcium, however, may cause cardiac dysfunction. The occurrence of a large band of calcium transversing the right ventricular conus has led to right ventricular outflow obstruction. An anular band of calcium in the right or left atrioventricular sulcus may delay or inhibit ventricular filling and consequently simulate tricuspid or mitral stenosis.

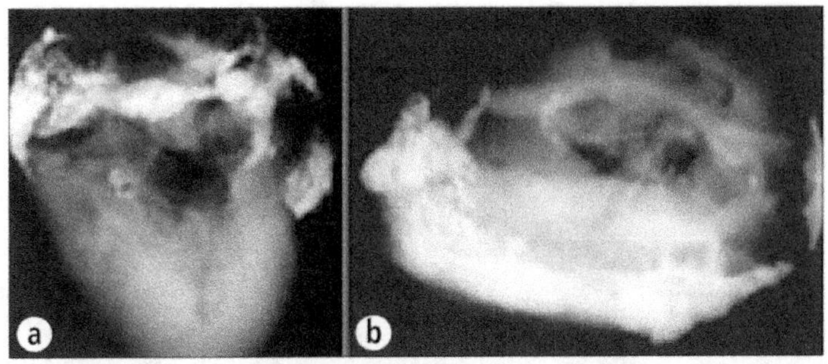

Figure 21. Calcific pericardial heart disease in a 78-year-old man, an alcoholic with cirrhosis, esophageal varices, and chronic pancreatitis, who died of a gastrointestinal hemorrhage. No evidence of cardiac dysfunction was ever present clinically. At necropsy the pericardial space was obliterated by fibrous adhesions. The adherence of the parietal to the visceral pericardium could not be separated over the right atrioventricular sulcus. The cardiac chambers, valves, and coronary arteries were normal. The right atrioventricular sulcus was extensively infiltrated by calcific deposits. Radiographs of the heart specimen at necropsy: **(a)** anteroposterior view; **(b)** cephalad caudal view. Calcific deposits also are present in the mitral anulus.

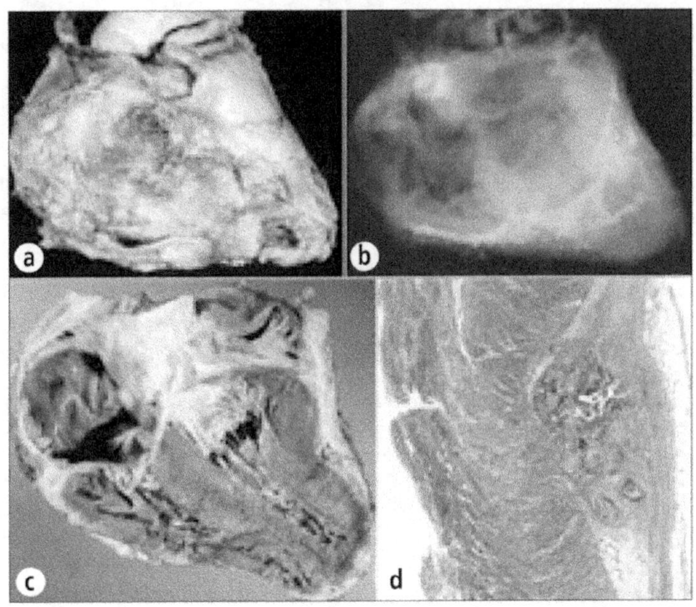

Figure 22. Calcific constrictive pericardial heart disease in a 68-year-old man who had had pericardiectomies for relief from constriction 15 and 7 years before death. Terminally, evidence of myocardial constriction reappeared. Chylous ascites secondary to obstruction of the thoracic duct by carcinoid tumor also were present. At necropsy, the heart weighed 530 gm. Diffuse obliterative constrictive pericarditis was present, and the remaining parietal pericardium was bound down to the epicardium by fibrous tissue. The inferior and superior venae cavae were enlarged, and the right atrium and pulmonary trunk were dilated. Yellow intimal streaks were seen in the pulmonary arteries, suggesting pulmonary arterial hypertension. Histologic sections showed fibrous thickening with calcific deposits of the pericardia with occasional collections of lymphocytes, plasma cells, and histiocytes, but no granulomas. The intrapulmonary arteries had thickened walls. No granulomas were found in the lungs. The cause of the pericardial constriction was never determined. **(a)** Exterior of the heart. **(b)** Radiograph of the heart showing residual calcific deposits over the ventricles. **(c)** Longitudinal section of the heart showing right atrial dilatation and right ventricular hypertrophy. **(d)** Section of left ventricle compressed by overlying calcific deposit. Hematoxylin-eosin stain, ×3.

CHOLESTEROL PERICARDIAL HEART DISEASE

Clinically, cholesterol pericardial heart disease most often is characterized by slowly developing, nonconstricting large effu-

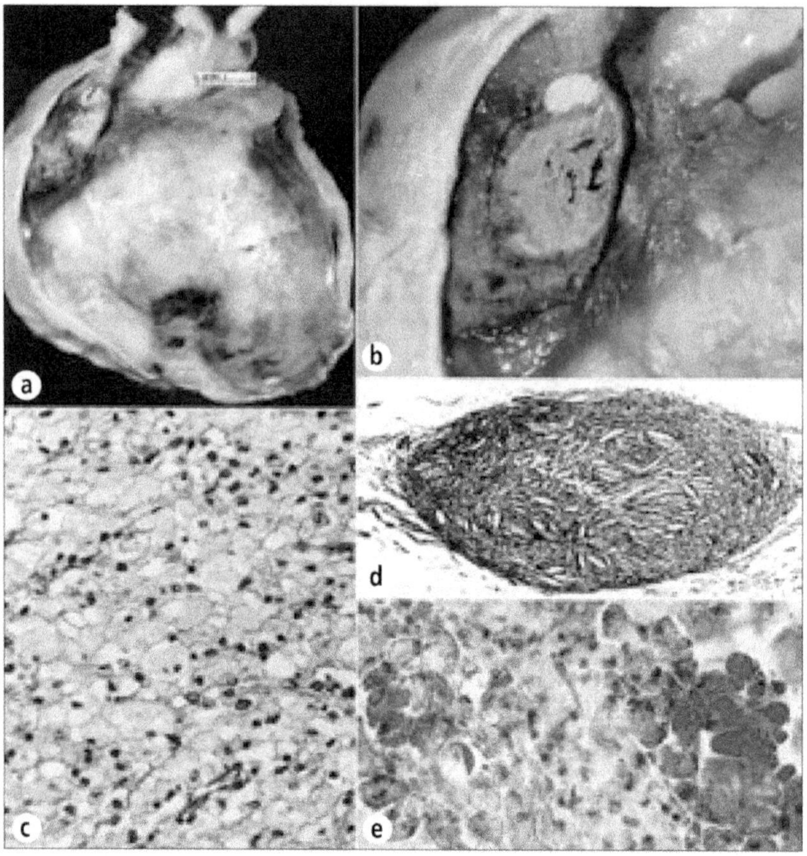

Figure 23. Cholesterol pericardial heart disease in a 34-year-old woman with hypothyroidism. She was short and stocky and had enlarged earlobes, bilateral hypoplastic fourth toes, receding hairline, small tongue, and no menstruation. She had orthopnea, pedal edema, and hypoactive deep tendon reflexes. Chest radiograph showed a globular-shaped cardiac silhouette and clear lung fields, and angiogram showed an 18-mm-thick pericardial effusion. Despite diuresis, the pedal edema persisted. Pleuritic-type anterior chest pain appeared, and a 15-mm paradoxic pulse pressure was measured. Pericardiocentesis produced 500 mL of cloudy golden-colored fluid. The polyethylene catheter was left in place and over the next 5 days, 2 L of fluid was removed. Fluid cholesterol was 165 mg/dL; serum cholesterol was 355 mg/dL. The patient improved after pericardiocentesis but became anuric following aortography and died. **(a)** Exterior surface of the heart and pericardium showing thickening of the parietal pericardium and focal deposits of cholesterol (yellow) over the right ventricle. **(b)** View of thickened parietal pericardium over the right atrial appendage and an epicardial cholesterol deposit. **(c)** Foam cells in the cholesterol deposit shown in (b). **(d)** Cholesterol granuloma in the pericardium showing cholesterol clefts and a foreign body reaction. **(e)** Frozen section of epicardial deposits stained for lipid. The foam cells stain strongly for lipid. Hematoxylin-eosin stain, ×400 (c), ×50 (d); oil-red O stain, ×400 (e).

sions (77). Although the pericardial fluid may be turbid or clear, cholesterol crystals give the effusion a "gold paint" appearance. The parietal and visceral pericardia may become markedly thickened; histologic examination shows giant cells containing cholesterol clefts, mononuclear cells including foam cells, and fibrous tissue *(Figure 23)*.

Cholesterol pericardial heart disease may be seen in many different conditions *(Table 11)* but is most common in patients with *hypothyroidism*, *rheumatoid arthritis*, and *tuberculosis* (77).

The cause of the increased cholesterol content of the pericardial fluid in these patients is not clear, but several theories have been presented: 1) that necrosis of superficial cells of the pericardia liberates intracellular cholesterol, 2) that lysis of erythrocytes following hemopericardium yields the cholesterol, and 3) that pericardial inflammation decreases lymphatic drainage of pericardia, causing decreased reabsorption of cholesterol, with ultimate precipitation and crystallization (77). The cholesterol crystals then incite a vigorous cellular reaction, enhancing fluid production and pericardial thickening. Chronic exudation and diminished reabsorption of cholesterol might increase its concentration and allow crystallization. The total lipid content of the pericardial fluid, however, is approximately the same as that of serum.

Table 11. Etiology of cholesterol pericardial heart disease

1. Idiopathy
2. Association with another condition
   A. Hypothyroidism
   B. Rheumatoid arthritis
   C. Tuberculosis
   D. Hypercholesterolemia (from any cause)

In patients with hypothyroidism, the primary effusion may contain sufficient cholesterol to incite a local pericarditis, which then further increases the cholesterol concentration as less is reabsorbed. Large effusions with resulting high levels of cholesterol are produced. In these patients, the pericarditis appears to be a secondary phenomenon whereas cholesterol pericardial heart disease in euthyroid patients must be associated with an actual pericardial inflammation for the cholesterol to accumulate. Experimental studies have shown that small amounts of blood in the presence of pericardial damage from any cause will produce dense adhesions; this phenomenon probably accounts for cases of constriction in cholesterol pericardial disease.

CONGENITAL ANOMALIES OF THE PERICARDIUM

Congenital anomalies include cysts and *absence of all or portions of parietal pericardia*. These cases are rare. Cysts can be true or false. The true ones are located within the pericardial sac but have no communication with it; the false ones, or diverticulae, are protrusions of parietal pericardium and consequently have direct communication with it. Of 72 cysts reported by Wychulis and associates (78), 88% were true and 12% were false. The cysts are thin-walled and translucent, are lined by endothelial cells, contain watery yellow fluid, usually are attached by a thick fibrous pedicle, and most commonly are located in the right cardiophrenic angle *(Figure 24)*. In one series, the cysts ranged in size from 2 to 16 cm in largest diameter. Although they can be multilobulated, 99% are unilobular. The fluid within the cysts is similar to normal pericardial fluid. The cysts produce signs or symptoms of cardiac dysfunction in 25% of the patients and no evidence of dysfunction in the other 75%. The larger the size, the more likely symptoms will result. The mechanism of formation of pericardial cysts is not clear. Failure of the pericardial mesenchymal lacunae to unite with the pericardial coelom has been suggested (79).

Absence of, or defects in, parietal pericardium may be classified into 3 major types (80): 1) heart and left lung in a com-

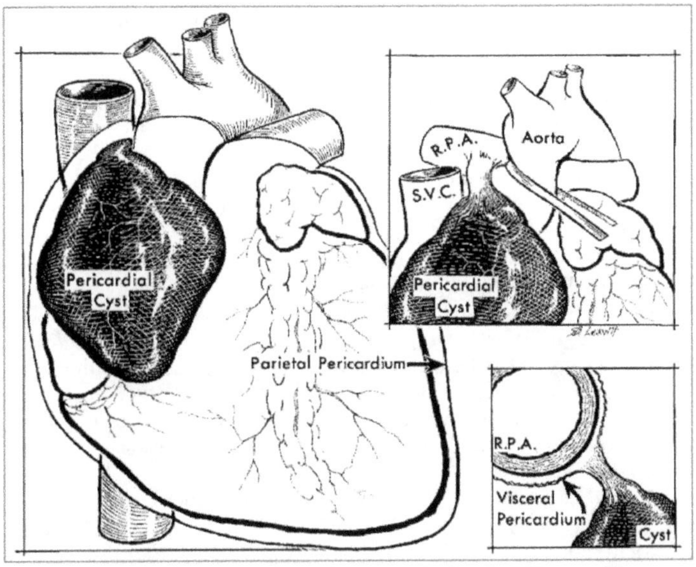

Figure 24. Pericardial cyst, an incidental necropsy finding in a 75-year-old woman. The cyst, which contained serous fluid, overlay the right atrium and arose from a pedicle attached to the right main pulmonary artery (RPA). SVC indicates superior vena cava.

mon cavity (60%), 2) defect or foramen in parietal pericardium providing communication between pericardial sac and pleural sac (20%) (nearly always the left one) and 3) totally absent or rudimentary parietal pericardium (20%). These defects may be associated with anomalies of the heart (30%), lungs, pleura, peritoneum, or kidney and are more common in males. Cardiac enlargement occurs in about half of the patients, and commonly the heart is displaced to the left and abnormally mobile. Total absence of parietal pericardium usually produces no functional disturbance. Partial absence, however, may result in herniation of the entire heart or a part of the left atrium through the defect or allow direct extension of a lung infection to the pericardium via the defect.

Complete absence of the parietal left pericardium over the left side of the heart presents a clinical syndrome that is usually diagnostic. It consists of a physical finding of left ventricular enlargement and hypertrophy (apical impulse forceful and displaced to the left), a systolic ejection murmur at the base, an electrocardiogram that shows right axis deviation (as in the normal individual assuming the left lateral decubitus position), and a chest radiograph that shows levo position of the heart. This condition may be confused with a cardiomyopathy. Partial absence of the partial pericardium has been confused with a diagnosis of congenital heart disease with the prominent left atrial appendage misinterpreted as enlargement of the pulmonary trunk.

DIFFERENTIAL DIAGNOSIS

Constrictive pericardial heart disease—from pericardial effusion, thickened pericardia, or both—may be confused with a number of conditions (*Table 12*). An occasional patient with idiopathic dilated cardiomyopathy or extensive cardiac amyloidosis has been subjected in the past to thoracotomy because of suspected pericardial constriction. Echocardiography, of course, makes it easier to differentiate pericardial heart disease from these other conditions.

Table 12. Differential diagnosis of constrictive pericardial heart disease

1. Congestive cardiac failure from other causes
   - A. Idiopathic cardiomyopathy
     1. Ventricular dilated type
     2. Hypertrophic type
   - B. Mitral stenosis or left atrial tumor
   - C. Pulmonary heart disease
   - D. Restrictive heart disease
     1. Amyloid
     2. Endomyocardial fibrosis
   - E. Tricuspid stenosis or right atrial tumor
2. Hepatic cirrhosis
3. Mediastinal neoplasm
4. Obstruction (usually by thrombus) of portal vein, hepatic vein, or vena cava

SUMMARY

An ideal classification of pericardial heart disease would take into account clinical, etiologic, and morphologic features of this condition, but a single classification combining these 3 components is lacking. Pericardial heart disease is relatively uncommon clinically. When present at necropsy, it usually had not been recognized during life. The term "pericarditis" is inaccurate because most pericardial diseases are noninflammatory. Morphologically, chronic pericardial heart disease symptoms are present; however, few patients develop evidence of cardiac dysfunction (constriction). When pericardial "constriction" occurs, it is the result of increased pericardial fluid or increased pericardial tissue or both. Increased fluid is treated by drainage; increased tissue is treated by excision. In most patients with chronic constrictive "pericarditis," the etiology is not apparent even after histologic examination of pericardia.

1. Osler W. *The Principles and Practice of Medicine. Designed for the Use of Practitioners and Students of Medicine*. New York: Appleton Co, 1892:1079.
2. Reeves RL. Cause of acute pericarditis. *Am J Med Sci* 1953;225:34.
3. Griffith GC, Wallace L. The etiology of pericarditis. *Am Heart J* 1949;37:636.
4. Ishihara T, Ferrans VJ, Jones M, Boyce SW, Kawanami O, Roberts WC. Histologic and ultrastructural features of normal parietal pericardium. *Am J Cardiol* 1980;46:744–753.
5. Shirani J, Berezowski K, Roberts WC. Quantitative measurement of normal and excessive (cor adiposum) subepicardial adipose tissue, its clinical significance, and its effect on electrocardiographic QRS voltage. *Am J Cardiol* 1995;76:414–418.
6. Shirani J, Roberts WC. Clinical, electrocardiographic and morphologic features of massive fatty deposits ("lipomatous hypertrophy") in the atrial septum. *J Am Coll Cardiol* 1993;22:226–238.
7. Bulkley BH, Roberts WC. The heart in systemic lupus erythematosus and the changes induced in it by corticosteroid therapy. A study of 36 necropsy patients. *Am J Med* 1975;58:243–264.
8. Roberts WC, High ST. The heart in systemic lupus erythematosus. *Curr Probl Cardiol* 1999;24:1–56.
9. Ferrons VJ, Roberts WC. Pathology of pericardial effusion. In Reddy PS, Leon DF, Shaver JA, eds. *Pericardial Disease*. New York: Raven Press, 1982:77–92.
10. Just H, Mattingly TW. Interatrial septal defect and pericardial disease. Coincidence or causal relationship? *Am Heart J* 1968;76:157–167.
11. Ehrenhaft JL, Taber RE. Hemopericardium and constrictive pericarditis. *J Thorac Surg* 1952;24:355.

12. Cliff WJ, Grobéty J, Ryan GB. Postoperative pericardial adhesions. The role of mild serosal injury and spilled blood. *J Thorac Cardiovasc Surg* 1973;65: 744–750.
13. Swan WGA. Acute non-specific pericarditis. *Br Heart J* 1960;22:651–659.
14. Roberts WC, Morrow AG. Pseudoaneurysm of the left ventricle. An unusual sequel of myocardial infarction and rupture of the heart. *Am J Med* 1967;43: 639–644.
15. Gobel FL, Visudh-Arom K, Edwards JE. Pseudoaneurysm of the left ventricle leading to recurrent pericardial hemorrhage. *Chest* 1971;59:23–27.
16. Peter R, Whalen R, Orgain E, McIntosh H. Postpericardiotomy syndrome as a complication of percutaneous left ventricular puncture. *Am J Cardiol* 1966;17:86–90.
17. Goldstein S, Yu PN. Constrictive pericarditis after blunt chest trauma. *Am Heart J* 1965;69:544–550.
18. Brosius FC III, Waller BF, Roberts WC. Radiation heart disease. Analysis of 16 young (aged 15 to 33 years) necropsy patients who received over 3,500 rads to the heart. *Am J Med* 1981;70:519–530.
19. Rabiner SF, Spector LS, Gripstein CB, Schlecker AA. Chronic constrictive pericarditis as a sequel to acute benign pericarditis—report of a case. *N Engl J Med* 1954;251:425–428.
20. Hirschman SZ, Hammer GS. Coxsackie virus myopericarditis. A microbiological and clinical review. *Am J Cardiol* 1974;34:224–232.
21. Burch GE, Colcolough HL. Progressive Coxsackie viral pancarditis and nephritis. *Ann Intern Med* 1969;71:963–970.
22. Wacker W, Merrill JP. Uremic pericarditis in acute and chronic renal failure. *JAMA* 1954;156:764–765.
23. Schupak E, Merrill JP. Experience with long-term intermittent hemodialysis. *Ann Intern Med* 1965;62:509–518.
24. Abella R, Blondeel NJ, Roguska J, Walker C, Simon NM, Del Greco F. Periodic dialysis in terminal uremia. *JAMA* 1967;199:362–368.
25. Reyman TA. Subacute constrictive uremic pericarditis. *Am J Med* 1969;46: 972–975.
26. Lindsay J Jr, Crawley IS, Callaway GM Jr. Chronic constrictive pericarditis following uremic hemopericardium. *Am Heart J* 1970;79:390–395.
27. Moschcowitz E. Pathogenesis of constrictive pericardium. *JAMA* 1953;153: 194–198.
28. Cabot RC. *Facts on the Heart*. Philadelphia: WB Saunders Co, 1926:781.
29. Cathcart ES, Spodick DH. Rheumatoid heart disease. A study of the incidence and nature of cardiac lesions in rheumatoid arthritis. *N Engl J Med* 1962;266:959–964.
30. Sagrista-Sauleda J, Angel J, Sanchez A, Permanyer-Miralda G, Soler-Soler J. Effusive-constrictive pericarditis. *N Engl J Med* 2004;350:469–475.
31. Martin RG, Ruckdeschel JC, Chang P, Byhardt R, Bouchard RJ, Wiernik PH. Radiation-related pericarditis. *Am J Cardiol* 1975;35:216–220.
32. Roberts WC. Aortic dissection: anatomy, consequences, and causes. *Am Heart J* 1981;101:195–214.
33. Fell SC, Rubin IL, Enselberg CD, Hurwitt ES. Anticoagulant-induced hemopericardium with tamponade: its occurrence in the absence of myocardial infarction or pericarditis. *N Engl J Med* 1965;272:670–674.
34. Beaudry CB, Nakamoto S, Kolff WJ. Uremic pericarditis and cardiac tamponade in chronic renal failure. *Ann Intern Med* 1966;64:990–995.
35. Buja LM, Friedman CA, Roberts WC. Hemorrhagic pericarditis in uremia. Clinicopathologic studies in six patients. *Arch Pathol* 1970;90:325–330.
36. Roberts WC, Fredrickson DS. Gaucher's disease of the lung causing severe pulmonary hypertension with associated acute recurrent pericarditis. *Circulation* 1967;35:783–789.
37. Harvey PKP, Jones MC, Anderson EG. Pericardial abnormalities in Gaucher's disease. *Br Heart J* 1969;31:603–606.
38. Naef AP. Primary chylopericardium: its surgical treatment. *Dis Chest* 1956;30: 160–167.
39. Hawker RE, Cartmill TB, Celermajer JM, Bowdler JD. Chylous pericardial effusion complicating aorta-right pulmonary artery anastomosis. *J Thorac Cardiovasc Surg* 1972;63:491–494.
40. Pereira WM, Kalil RA, Prates PR, Nesralla IA. Cardiac tamponade due to chylopericardium after cardiac surgery. *Ann Thorac Surg* 1988;46:572–573.
41. Miller SW, Pruett HJ, Long A. Fatal chylopericardium caused by hamartomatous lymphangiomatosis. *Am J Med* 1959;24:951–956.
42. Offerijns FGJ, van der Veen KJ, Durrer D, Ziedses des Plantes BG. Lymphopericardium with hypoproteinemia, intestinal loss of protein, and congenital defects of lymphatic system. *Circulation* 1969;39:116–120.
43. Rubin RH, Moellering RC Jr. Clinical, microbiologic and therapeutic aspects of purulent pericarditis. *Am J Med* 1975;59:68–78.
44. Boyle JD, Pearce JL, Guze LB. Purulent pericarditis: review of literature and report of 11 cases. *Medicine* 1961;40:119–144.
45. Buchbinder NA, Roberts WC. Left-sided valvular active infective endocarditis. A study of forty-five necropsy patients. *Am J Med* 1972;53:20–35.
46. Ibarra-Pérez C, Green L, Calvillo-Juárez M, Vargas de la Cruz J. Diagnosis and treatment of rupture of amebic abscess of the liver into the pericardium. *J Thorac Cardiovasc Surg* 1972;64:11–17.
47. Kinare SG, Parulkar GB, Sen PK. Constrictive pericarditis resulting from dracunculosis. *Br Med J* 1962;1:845–846.
48. Chapman MG, Kaplan L. Cardiac involvement in coccidioidomycosis. *Am J Med* 1957;23:87–98.
49. Louria DB, Gordon RE. Pericarditis and pleuritis cased by a recently discovered microorganism, *Waksmania rosea*. *Am Rev Respir Dis* 1960;81:83–88.
50. Gibbons JE, Goldbloom RB, Dobell ARC. Rapidly developing pericardial constriction in childhood following acute nonspecific pericarditis. *Am J Cardiol* 1965;15:863–867.
51. Fajardo LF, Stewart JR. Experimental radiation-induced heart disease. I. Light microscopic studies. *Am J Pathol* 1970;59:299–316.
52. McReynolds RA, Gold GL, Roberts WC. Coronary heart disease after mediastinal irradiation for Hodgkin's disease. *Am J Med* 1976;60:39–45.
53. Harvey LAC, DeMaio SJ, Roberts WC. Radiation-induced cardiovascular disease including stenosis of coronary ostium, coronary and carotid arteries, and aortic valve. *BUMC Proceedings* 1994;7(3):33–36.
54. Morton DL, Kagan AR, Roberts WC, O'Brien KP, Holmes EC, Adkins PC. Pericardiectomy for radiation-induced pericarditis with effusion. *Ann Thorac Surg* 1969;8:195–208.
55. Arthur A, Oskvig R, Basta LL. Calcified rheumatoid constrictive pericarditis with cardiac failure treated by pericardiectomy. *Chest* 1973;64:769–771.
56. McWhorter JE IV, LeRoy EC. Pericardial disease in scleroderma (systemic sclerosis). *Am J Med* 1974;57:566–575.
57. Conti CR, Friesinger GC. Chronic constrictive pericarditis. Clinical and laboratory findings in 11 cases. *Johns Hopkins Med J* 1967;120:262–274.
58. Wychulis AR, Connolly DC, McGoon DC. Surgical treatment of pericarditis. *J Thorac Cardiovasc Surg* 1971;62:608–617.
59. Roberts WC. Neoplasms involving the heart, their simulators, and adverse consequences of their therapy. *BUMC Proceedings* 2001;14:358–376.
60. Glancy DL, Roberts WC. The heart in malignant melanoma: A study of 70 autopsy cases. *Am J Cardiol* 1968;21:555–571.
61. Roberts WC, Bodey GP, Wertlake PT. The heart in acute leukemia. A study of 420 autopsy cases. *Am J Cardiol* 1968;21:388–412.
62. Roberts WC, Glancy DL, De Vita VT Jr. Heart in malignant lymphoma (Hodgkin's disease, lymphosarcoma, reticulum cell sarcoma and mycosis fungoides). A study of 196 autopsy cases. *Am J Cardiol* 1968;22:85–107.
63. Van Buren PC, Roberts WC. Cholesterol pericarditis and cardiac tamponade with congenital hypothyroidism in adulthood. *Am Heart J* 1990;119: 697–700.
64. Rokitansky CK. *A Manual of Pathological Anatomy*, 4th ed. London: The Sydenham Society, 1852:137.
65. Osler W. Tuberculous pericarditis. *Am J Med Sci* 1893;105:20–37.
66. Woods JA. Tuberculous pericarditis: a study of forty-one cases with special reference to prognosis. *Am Heart J* 1951;42:737–745.
67. Peel AAF. Tuberculous pericarditis. *Br Heart J* 1948;10:195–207.
68. Heimann HL, Binder S. Tuberculous pericarditis. *Br Heart J* 1940;2: 165–176.
69. Das PB, Gupta RP, Sukumar IP, Cherian G, John S. Pericardiectomy: indications and results. *J Thorac Cardiovas Surg* 1973;66:58–70.
70. Thompson SA, Raisbeck MJ. Cardio-pericardiopexy. The surgical treatment of coronary arterial disease by the establishment of adhesive pericarditis. *Ann Intern Med* 1942;16:495–520.
71. Schildt P, Stanton E, Beck CS. Communications between the coronary arteries produced by the application of inflammatory agents to the surface of the heart. *Ann Surg* 1943;118:34–45.
72. Eiseman B, Seeling MG, Womack NA. Talcum powder granuloma: a frequent and serious postoperative complication. *Ann Surg* 1947;126:820–832.
73. Arnett EN, Battle WE, Russo JV, Roberts WC. Intravenous injection of talc-containing drugs intended for oral use: a cause of pulmonary granulomatosis and pulmonary hypertension. *Am J Med* 1976;60:711–718.

74. Osborne MP, Paneth M, Hinson KFW. Starch granules in the pericardium as a cause of the post-cardiotomy syndrome. *Thorax* 1974;29:199–203.
75. Roberts WC, McAllister HA Jr, Ferrans VJ. Sarcoidosis of the heart. A clinicopathologic study of 35 necropsy patients (group I) and review of 78 previously described necropsy patients (group II). *Am J Med* 1977;63: 86–108.
76. Mathewson FAL. Calcification of the pericardium in apparently healthy people. Electrocardiographic abnormalities found in tracings from apparently healthy persons with calcification of the pericardium. *Circulation* 1955;12: 44–51.
77. Brawley RK, Vasko JS, Morrow AG. Cholesterol pericarditis. Considerations of its pathogenesis and treatment. *Am J Med* 1966;41:235–248.
78. Wychulis AR, Connolly DC, McGoon DC. Pericardial cysts, tumors, and fat necrosis. *J Thorac Cardiovasc Surg* 1971;62:294–300.
79. Lillie WI, McDonald JR, Clagett OT. Pericardial coelomic cysts and pericardial diverticula. A concept of etiology and report of cases. *J Thorac Surg* 1950;20:494–504.
80. Moore RL. Congential deficiencies of the pericardium. *Arch Surg* 1925;11: 765–777.

Causes of Pure Aortic Regurgitation in Patients Having Isolated Aortic Valve Replacement at a Single US Tertiary Hospital (1993 to 2005)

William Clifford Roberts, MD; Jong Mi Ko, BA;
Timothy Richard Moore, MD; William Hampton Jones III, MD

Background—The causes of aortic regurgitation (AR) severe enough to warrant aortic valve replacement (AVR) have received little attention in the last 20 years.

Methods and Results—We analyzed the causes of pure AR in 268 patients >20 years of age having isolated AVR at Baylor University Medical Center from 1993 to 2005 that was unassociated with mitral stenosis, mitral valve replacement, or a previous operation involving a cardiac valve or ascending aorta. In 122 patients (46%), the AR resulted from a problem with the aortic valve: congenital malformation unassociated with infective endocarditis, 66 patients (54%); infective endocarditis, 46 patients (38%; 15 with bicuspid valves); probable rheumatic heart disease, 8 patients (6%); and miscellaneous, 2 patients (2%). In the other 146 patients (54%), the AR was the consequence of a condition affecting the ascending aorta: dissection, 28 patients (19%); the Marfan syndrome or its forme fruste variety, 15 patients (10%); aortitis, 12 patients (8%), and in the remaining 91 patients (62%), the cause of the AR was not determined. This latter group was the oldest (mean age 66 years), 83 (91%) had hypertension, 26 (29%) had small calcific deposits in the valve cusps, and 46 (51%) had simultaneous coronary artery bypass grafting.

Conclusions—The causes of pure AR severe enough to warrant isolated AVR are diverse. The most common category in this study was "cause unclear." ***(Circulation*. 2006;114:422-429.)**

Key Words: bypass ■ calcium ■ coronary disease ■ hypertension ■ regurgitation

In contrast to aortic stenosis, which essentially has 3 causes (congenital, atherosclerotic, and rheumatic),[1-3] pure aortic regurgitation (AR; no element of aortic stenosis) has multiple causes, some of which directly affect the aortic valve and others of which are due to problems with the aorta without direct involvement of the aortic valve. Furthermore, unlike aortic stenosis, which essentially is always a slowly progressing chronic condition, AR may develop acutely (acute AR) or over a prolonged period (chronic AR). This report analyzes the causes of pure AR in patients having isolated aortic valve replacement (AVR) at Baylor University Medical Center (Dallas, Texas) from 1993 to 2005.

Clinical Perspective p 429

Methods

Since March 1993, all operatively excised cardiac valves and aortas submitted to the surgical pathology division of the department of pathology have been examined and described by one of us (W.C.R.). Additionally, the preoperative cardiac catheterization and echocardiographic data, and often pertinent clinical records and operative notes, on most of these patients have been obtained.

The present study was limited to patients who, before AVR, had either no gradient or a negative gradient between peak systolic left ventricular and peak systolic aortic pressures or at least a transvalvular peak systolic pressure gradient of ≤10 mm Hg. Patients with associated mitral valve disease that required mitral replacement or repair or insertion of an annular ring, patients ≤20 years of age at the time of AVR, patients with a previous operation involving the ascending aorta or a cardiac valve, and patients with associated ventricular septal defect or discrete subaortic stenosis or hypertrophic cardiomyopathy were excluded. Mild degrees of mitral regurgitation preoperatively did not exclude patients from inclusion in the present study.

Most operatively excised valves and most operatively excised aortas were weighed (all by W.C.R.) on an Ohaus scale (Ohaus Corporation, Florham Park, NJ) accurate to 2 decimal places. All operatively excised valves and most aortas were photographed. The valves that contained vegetations were sectioned and processed in

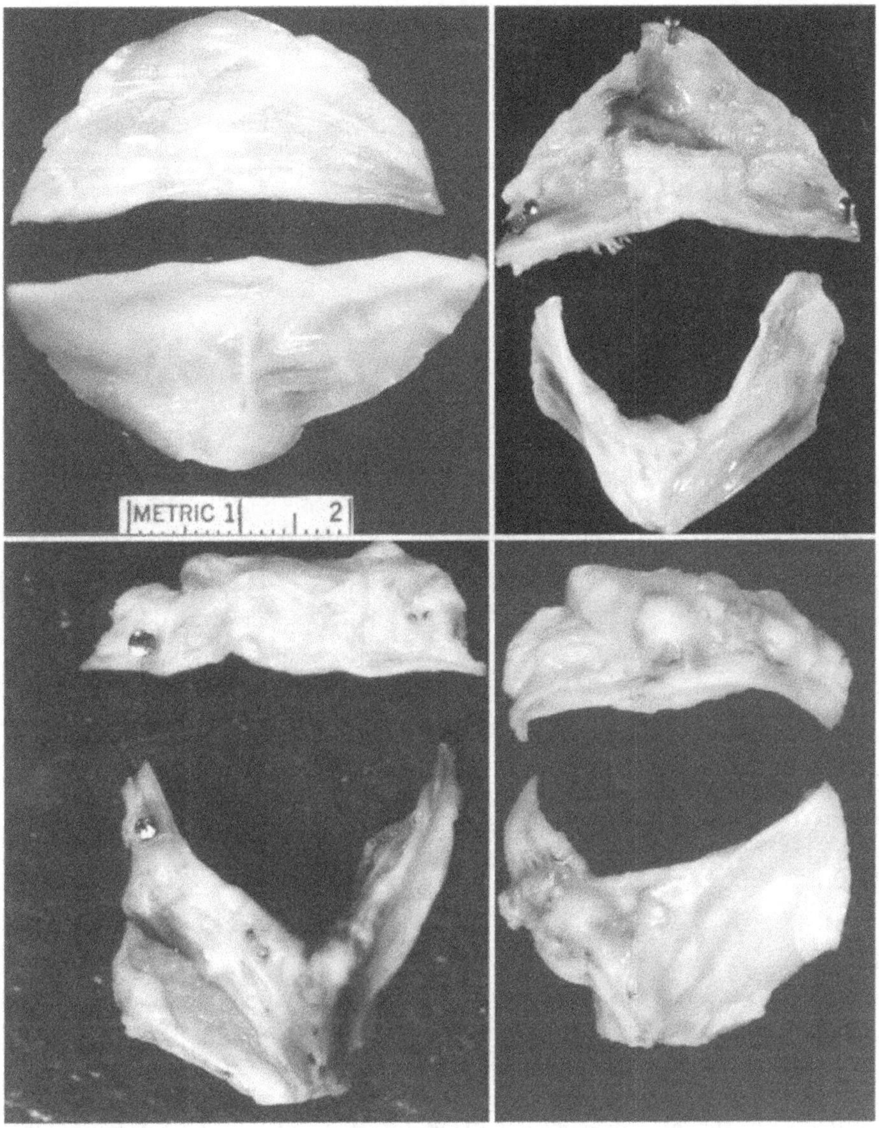

Figure 1. Congenitally bicuspid aortic valves unassociated with infective endocarditis in 4 men. Upper left, Age 53 years. The valve was devoid of calcific deposits and weighed 1.69 g. Upper right, Age 56 years. The valve weighed 1.65 g. Lower left, Age 66 years. The valve weighed 1.05 g. Lower right, Age 71 years. The valve weighed 2.43 g. The last 3 valves had calcific deposits on both cusps, mainly in their raphe.

alcohols and xylene, and sections were cut and stained, one with hematoxylin-eosin and another with the Gram method. All aortas were also processed for histological study and, after they were cut, were stained, one with hematoxylin-eosin and another by the Movat method.

The study protocol was approved by the Institutional Review Board of Baylor University Medical Center.

The authors had full access to the data and take full responsibility for its integrity. All authors have read and agree to the manuscript as written.

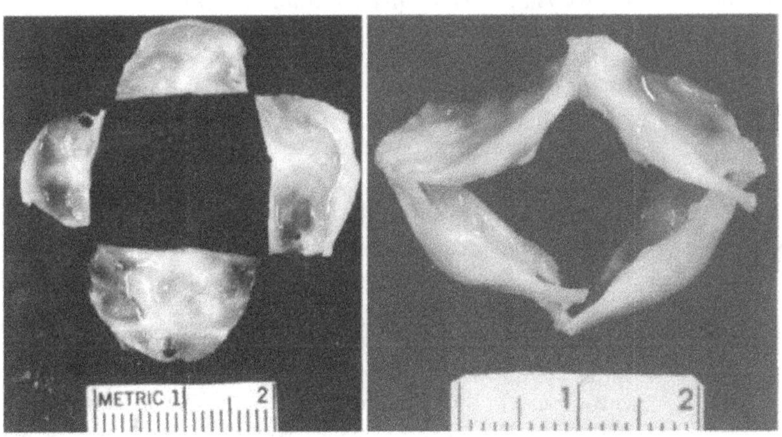

Figure 2. Congenitally quadricuspid aortic valves in 2 women. Left, Age 79 years. The valve weighed 0.57 g. Right, Age 53 years. The valve weighed 1.13 g.

TABLE 1. Causes of AR in Patients Having Isolated AVR at Baylor University Medical Center (1993–2005)

Cause of AR	Total	Ages at Operation, Range (Mean), y	M	F	Acute	Chronic	SH	Coronary Artery Bypass Grafting	Portions of Ascending Aorta		
									Excised	Examined Histologically	CMN (3+, 4+)
Valve (122 [46%])											
Congenital malformation without Infective endocarditis											
Bicuspid	59 (22%)	22–77 (55)	49	10	0	59	39 (66%)	18 (31%)	22	22	11
Quadricuspid	2 (1%)	53–79 (66)	0	2	0	2	0	1 (50%)	0	0	0
Tricuspid	5 (2%)	33–48 (40)	3	2	0	5	2 (40%)	0	1	1	0
Infective endocarditis	46 (17%)	21–82 (45)	31	15	27	19	29 (63%)	7 (15%)	6	4	0
Rheumatic?	8 (3%)	25–63 (47)	6	2	0	8	6 (75%)	2 (25%)	0	0	0
Miscellaneous	2 (1%)	24–42 (33)	1	1	0	2	2 (100%)	1 (50%)	0	0	0
Nonvalve (146 [54%])											
Aortic dissection	28 (10%)	25–78 (58)	20	8	21	7	22 (79%)	5* (17%)	28	20	5
Marfan or forme fruste	15 (6%)	21–71 (47)	9	6	0	15	10 (67%)	1† (7%)	15	13	13
Aortitis	12 (4%)	35–82 (66)	5	7	0	12	10 (83%)	5 (42%)	12	12	12
Cause unclear	91 (34%)	50–84 (66)	58	33	0	91	83 (91%)	46 (51%)	7	7	0
Total	268 (100%)	21–84 (57)	182 (68%)	86 (32%)	48 (18%)	220 (82%)	203 (76%)	86 (32%)	91 (34%)	76	41

SH indicates systemic hypertension; M, male; F, female; CMN, cystic medial necrosis; and BAV, bicuspid aortic valve.
Cystic medial necrosis is used here to refer to the magnitude of loss of elastic fibers in the aorta's media.
*Four other patients had CABG due to extension of the aortic dissection into a coronary artery.
†One additional patient had CABG due to extension of the aortic dissection into a coronary artery.
‡No. of cases with aortic valve weight.

Results

The study included all patients having AVR for pure AR who met the above criteria and had AVR from March 24, 1993, to March 31, 2005. A total of 268 patients aged 21 to 84 years (mean 57 years) met the above criteria, and the findings in these patients are summarized in Table 1. The 268 patients were divided into 2 major groups: those in whom the AR was secondary to a problem with the valve (n=122, 46%) and those in whom the AR was secondary to a problem with the ascending aorta (nonvalve; n=146, 54%). Of the 268 patients, 48 (18%) had acute AR, which in 27 was due to active infective endocarditis and in 21 to acute aortic dissection; the remaining 220 patients had chronic AR.

Hemodynamic or echocardiographic data were available in 235 (88%) of the 268 patients: One hundred thirty-seven patients had both cardiac catheterization data and echocardiographic data available; 40 other patients had only cardiac catheterization data available, and 58 others had only echocardiographic data available. Of the 177 patients with hemodynamic data from cardiac catheterization, 67 (38%) had transvalvular peak systolic pressure gradients that varied from 1 to 10 mm Hg.

Of the 268 operatively excised aortic valves, the valve was weighed in 226 patients, and its weight ranged from 0.48 to 2.99 g (mean 1.22 g) in the men and from 0.31 to 2.50 g (mean 0.81 g) in the women. Of the 91 patients in whom portions of ascending aorta were resected, the resected specimens were weighed on the same scales in 63 (69%) and ranged from 0.40 to 60 g (median 13 g) in the men and from 0.40 to 37 g (median 13 g) in the women. Whether the ascending aorta was resected was determined by its size, by its appearance, and by the operator. Of the latter 63 patients, the aorta weighed ≤4 g in 13 patients and >4 g in 50 patients.

Valve Problem

Congenital Malformation of the Aortic Valve Unassociated With Infective Endocarditis

This group included 59 patients with congenitally bicuspid aortic valves (Figure 1), 2 with quadricuspid valves (Figure 2), and 5 with tricuspid valves (Figure 3). At operation in each of the latter 5 patients, 1 or 2 of the 3 aortic valve cusps was described as being prolapsed such that the free margins of the cusps did not coapt with each other at the same cephalad level. Examination of the operatively excised valves in these 5 patients did not disclose cuspal inequality but indeed similar-sized cusps. In other words, examination of the operatively excised valves in these 5 patients did not allow us to determine or predict which cusps had prolapsed. In 19 (32%) of the 59 patients with congenitally bicuspid aortic valves, the ascending aorta was dilated, and a large portion (>4 g) of it was resected. Histological study of the

TABLE 1. Continued

BAV	Calcium Deposits on AV Cusps	Aortic Valve Weight (g), Range (Mean) Men	Women
59	31	0.52–2.99 (1.42)	0.68–1.80 (1.24)
0	0	. . .	0.57–1.13 (0.85)
0	0	1.11–1.40 (1.23)	0.34–0.66 (0.50)
15	8	0.77–2.31 (1.53)	0.44–2.50 (0.98)
0	3	1.10–2.45 (1.81)	1.31–1.83 (1.57)
0	0	0.55	. . .
3	4	0.51–1.19 (0.81)	0.37–0.90 (0.59)
0	2	0.73–1.01 (0.94)	0.35–0.85 (0.66)
0	2	0.63–0.79 (0.70)	0.35–0.70 (0.54)
0	26	0.48–2.13 (1.08)	0.31–1.74 (0.73)
77 (29%)	76/263 (29%)	0.48–2.99 (1.22) 151‡	0.31–2.50 (0.81) 75‡

resected aorta showed severe loss of medial elastic fibers in 11 cases (58%).

Infective Endocarditis

In 46 patients, the cause of the pure AR was infective endocarditis (Figure 4), which was active in 27 patients (59%) and healed in 19 (41%). Each of the 27 patients with active infective endocarditis had an acute onset of AR, whereas each of the 19 patients with healed infective endocarditis had chronic AR. Of these 46 patients, 15 (33%) had the infection superimposed on a 2-cuspid aortic valve, and in the other 31 patients (67%), the infection involved a 3-cuspid aortic valve.

Probable Rheumatic Heart Disease

In 8 patients, the pure AR was attributed to rheumatic heart disease (Figure 5). Each of the 3 cusps in each of these 8 patients was quite thickened, mainly by fibrous tissue, but in 3 of the 8 patients, the cusps also contained small calcific deposits. Cardiac catheterization in 5 of these 8 patients disclosed small (2 to 9 mm Hg) peak systolic pressure gradients between left ventricle and aorta. None of these 8 patients had hemodynamic or echocardiographic evidence of mitral stenosis, although mild mitral regurgitation was present in several of them.

Miscellaneous

Two patients had 3-cuspid aortic valves that were mildly and focally thickened by fibrous tissue. No abnormalities of the aorta were described. One patient, a 24-year-old woman, had the Behçet syndrome with multiple noncardiovascular problems. The other patient, a 42-year-old obese woman, took phentermine-fenfluramine, and the AR was believed to be related to that medication. Histologically, however, no features of the phentermine-fenfluramine (carcinoid) valve lesion were evident.

Aortic (Nonvalve) Problem

Aortic Dissection With Tear in Ascending Aorta

In 28 patients, the AR was secondary to aortic dissection, acute in 21 (75%) and healed in 7 (25%; Figure 6). Portions of ascending aorta were excised in all 21 cases with acute dissection and were weighed in 10 cases; the resected aorta weighed from 0.40 to 51 g (median 13 g). Histologically, the number of patients with a clear loss of medial elastic fibers was 3. In 7 with healed dissection, the 6 resected aortas weighed from 11 to 60 g (mean 38 g); histologically, the media contained a normal number of elastic fibers in 5 and were severely deficient in elastic fibers in 2 patients.

The Marfan Syndrome and Forme Fruste Varieties of It

Pure AR was attributed to the Marfan syndrome in 15 patients. The resected ascending aorta weighed from 6 to 24 g (mean 13 g); portions of the resected aortas in 13 cases submitted for histological study showed massive loss of medial elastic fibers with normal intima and adventitia, which resulted in an aortic wall that was thinner than normal, and each of them had intima-media tears, without dissection in 14 and with dissection in 1.

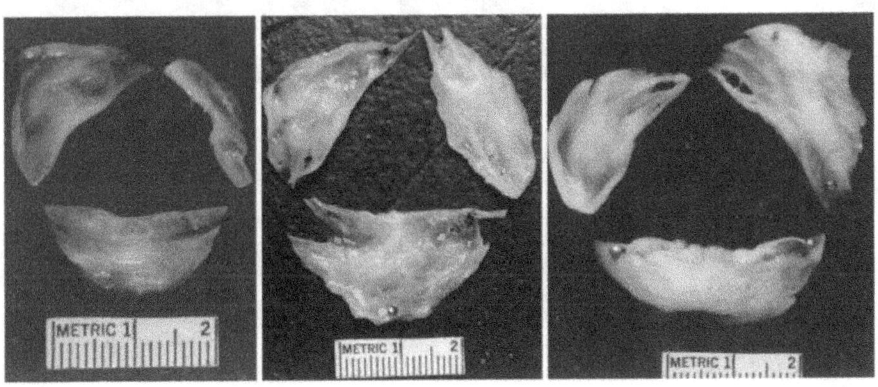

Figure 3. Congenitally malformed tricuspid aortic valves. Left, In a 33-year-old woman, the valve weighed 0.34 g. Middle, In a 44-year-old man, the valve weighed 1.11 g. Right, In a 33-year-old man, the valve weighed 1.19 g. Which of these cusps were attached more caudally than normal was not discernible after the cusps had been excised.

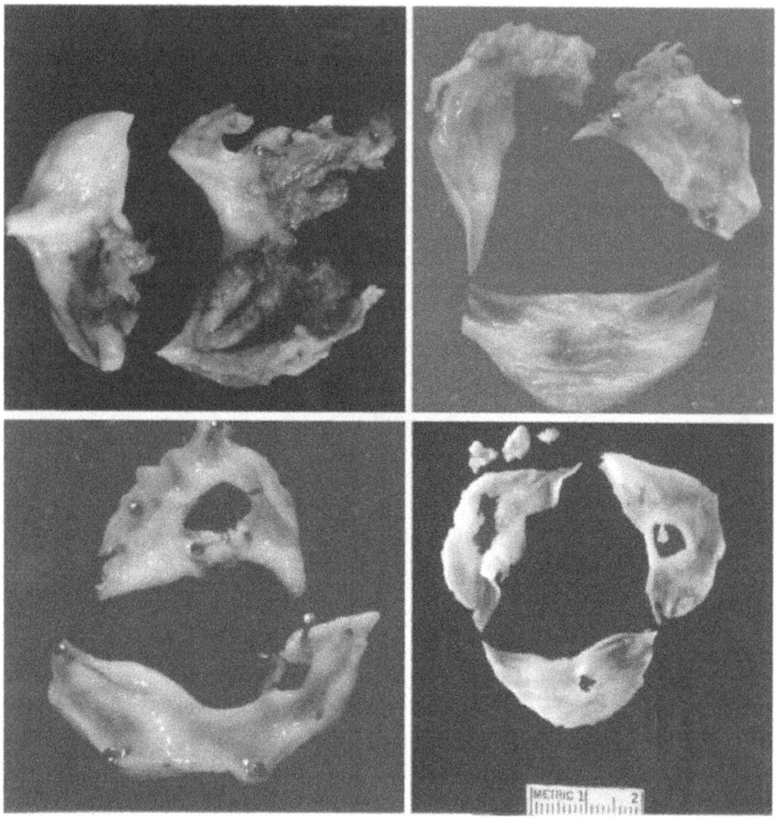

Figure 4. Infective endocarditis. Upper left, Acute infection in a bicuspid valve in a 41-year-old man. Upper right, Acute infection in a tricuspid valve in a 40-year-old man. The valve weighed 1 g. Lower left, Healed infection with cuspal perforations in a bicuspid valve in a 27-year-old man. The valve weighed 0.86 g. Lower right, Healed infection with cuspal perforations in a tricuspid valve in a 69-year-old man. The valve weighed 0.96 g.

Diffuse Aortitis

The AR was secondary to diffuse aortitis of the ascending aorta in 12 patients (Figure 7): granulomatous in 3 and nongranulomatous in 9. Eight (aged 42 to 82 years [mean 67 years]) of the latter 9 patients had typical histological features of syphilis; the ninth, aged 35 years, was believed to have Takayasu arteritis. In the 3 patients with granulomatous aortitis, its cause was not determined. The only difference between these 2 types of aortitis was the presence of multinucleated giant cells in 1 group and their absence in the other group. In both groups, both the intima and the adventitia were considerably thickened, mainly by fibrous tissue. The resected ascending aorta weighed from 0.40 to 25 g (median 18 g). Of these 12 patients, 8 were ≥65 years of age.

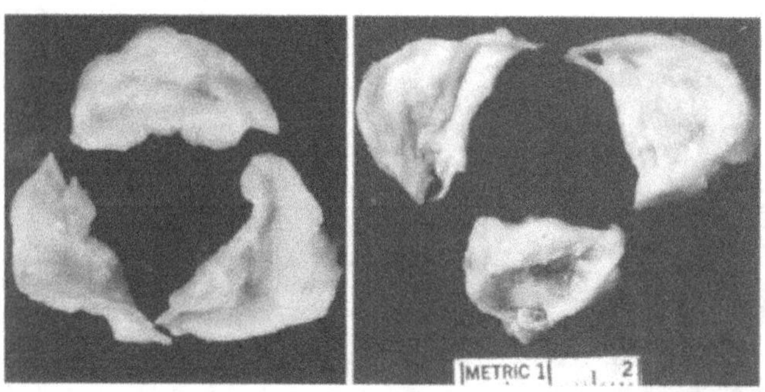

Figure 5. Probable rheumatic heart disease. Left, Tricuspid valve in a 60-year-old man. The valve weighed 2.06 g. Right, Tricuspid valve in a 55-year-old man. The valve weighed 1.52 g. The cusps in both patients are thickened by fibrous tissue.

Cause Unclear

Each patient in this group had 3-cuspid aortic valves (Figure 8). Seven, aged from 51 to 81 years (mean 67 years), had a portion of the ascending aorta excised (weight 1 to 31 g [median 12 g]), but 3 were small biopsies. In all 7, the aorta histologically was normal. Most of them had mildly dilated aortas, probably the result of aging alone. Of these 91 patients, 83 (91%) had either a history of systemic hypertension or a directly or indirectly measured peak systolic systemic pressure >140 mm Hg. Of these 91 patients, 46 (51%) also had coronary artery bypass grafting at the time of AVR.

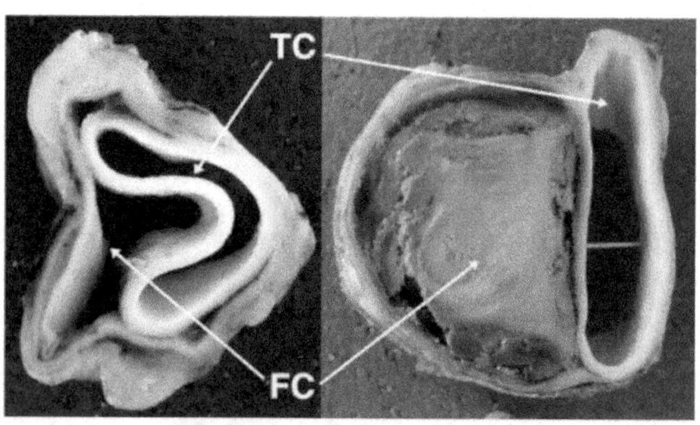

Figure 6. Aortic dissection. Left, Cross section of a portion of ascending aorta in an acute dissection in a 42-year-old man. The partition between the false channel (FC) and the true channel (TC) buckled into the lumen of the TC. Right, Cross section of a portion of ascending aorta in a healed dissection in a 79-year-old man. The FC is filled with a thrombus and is larger than the TC.

Discussion

The present study describes causes of pure (no element of stenosis) AR in 268 patients having isolated AVR unassociated with mitral stenosis or mitral valve replacement. The patients were divided into 2 groups: those in whom the cause of the AR was a problem with the valve (46%) and those in whom the cause was a problem with the aorta (54%). Hemodynamic or echocardiographic data were available in 235 patients (88%). All excised valves and ascending aortas were examined by the same physician (W.C.R.), who has been examining operatively excised aortic valves for 45 years.

Several findings in the present study were surprising to the authors, the main one being the high frequency with which we were unable to determine the cause of the AR, an occurrence in 91 patients (34% of the total or 62% of the 146 patients in whom the AR was considered the consequence of a problem with the aorta). The ages of these 91 patients were among the oldest of any of the groups, namely, 50 to 84 years (mean 66 years), and all 91 had tricuspid aortic valves. Although probably all had some degree of dilatation of the ascending aorta, mainly due to aging,[4] only 4 had significant portions of the ascending aorta resected, and in each of them, it was histologically normal. Of these 91 patients, at least 83 (91%) had either a transvalvular peak systolic aortic pressure >140 mm Hg, an end-diastolic aortic pressure >90 mm Hg, or both. It appears reasonable to believe that the systemic hypertension in some way caused or at least contributed to the AR in these patients. The operatively excised aortic valve cusps contained small calcific deposits in 26 (29%) of these 91 patients, but the valve weights were relatively small- (mean 0.73 g in women and 1.08 g in men). Almost certainly, some of these 91 patients had a cardiac operation primarily because of severe coronary artery disease; 46 (51%) of these 91 patients had CABG. Nevertheless, the degree of AR appears to have been similar in the patients with versus those without simultaneous coronary bypass. In 79 of these 91 patients, the degree of AR was classified by either aortic angiography or echocardiography; the AR was severe in 67 (85%) and mild to moderate in 12 (15%).

That systemic hypertension can cause AR severe enough to warrant AVR has been debated. Waller and colleagues[5] in 1982 described 4 patients with severe AR from systemic hypertension (without aortic dissection) who underwent AVR, and they reviewed previously reported patients with systemic hypertension and pure AR. Of their 4 patients, the systemic arterial pressures ≈1 month postoperatively remained elevated in 2 of the 3 survivors. Among previous reports describing precordial murmurs consistent with AR in patients with systemic hypertension, Waller and colleagues found 7 studies that analyzed 79 patients with AR associated with systemic hypertension, and 17 had severe AR with evidence of considerable heart failure. In 11 of the 17 patients, systemic hypertension appeared to be the only reasonable cause of the AR. Barlow and Kincaid-Smith[6] studied 100 patients with systemic hypertension and peak systolic pressures >180 mm Hg; 9 had diastolic blowing murmurs consistent with AR. Their report and reports of others pointed out that among hypertensive patients, the higher the systemic arterial pressure, the greater the chance that AR would develop. Among patients with similar levels of systemic arterial pressure, older patients had a higher frequency of AR than did younger patients. Of patients of similar age and with similar blood pressures, those with systemic hypertension of longer duration had a higher frequency of AR than did those with hypertension of shorter duration. Among the few patients with severe AR due to systemic hypertension, arterial diastolic pressure is usually >60 mm Hg; nevertheless, the pulse pressure is high (often >100 mm Hg).

Another finding, not unexpected, was the high frequency of a congenitally bicuspid aortic valve, which occurred in 77 (29%) of the 268 patients, including 74 (61%) of the 122 patients in whom the AR was a consequence of a valve problem and 3 (2%) of the 146 patients in whom the AR appeared to be the consequence of a problem with the aorta. All 3 of the latter patients were among the 28 patients with aortic dissection. Thus, 11% of the patients in whom the AR resulted from aortic dissection had a congenitally bicuspid aortic valve. Of the 74 patients with a congenitally bicuspid aortic valve, the AR in 59 (80%) was in patients who had never had a clinical event compatible with active or healed infective endocarditis and 15 (33%) were in the 46 patients in whom the AR appeared to result from active or healed infective endocarditis superimposed on a congenitally bicuspid aortic valve. Small calcific deposits were present in 34 (44%) of the 77 congenitally bicuspid aortic valves. The calcific deposits usually were localized to the raphe. Although its high frequency in patients with aortic valve stenosis is well appreciated, the bicuspid aortic valve as a cause of pure AR—at least, when unassociated with infective endocarditis—is less well appreciated. Indeed, that a bicuspid aortic valve could cause AR severe enough to warrant AVR in the absence of active or healed infective endocarditis was not described initially until 1981.[7]

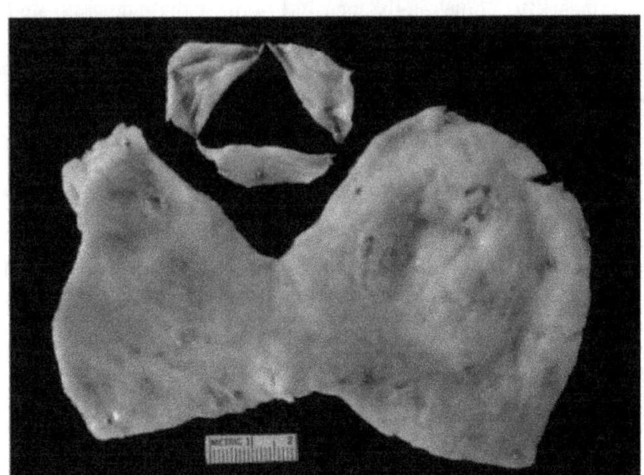

Figure 7. Diffuse aortitis. Valve and a portion of an ascending aorta in a 69-year-old man with syphilis. The aortic wall is thickened, and the intimal surface is 100% involved by the process. The tricuspid aortic valve is essentially normal and weighed 0.63 g.

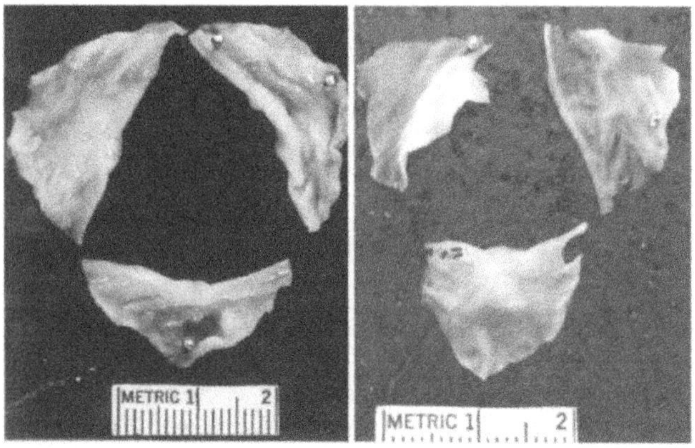

Figure 8. Cause of AR unclear. Left, Valve in a 74-year-old man. The valve weighed 1.08 g. Right, Valve in a 56-year-old woman. The valve weighed 0.31 g. The cusps are focally but minimally thickened.

In addition to the findings of a congenitally bicuspid aortic valve in 77 patients, 7 other patients had congenitally malformed aortic valves. Two had quadricuspid valves, and 5 had tricuspid aortic valves. In each of the latter 5 patients, 1 or 2 of the 3 cusps was attached more caudally than usual such that the free margins of these cusps did not coapt with the normally attached cusp(s), which resulted in prolapse. The prolapsed cusp, however, was usually similar in size to the nonprolapsed cusps, just attached more caudally. That a tricuspid aortic valve can be congenitally malformed or malpositioned is not a well-recognized cause of AR.

Portions of the ascending aorta were resected in 91 (34%) of the 268 patients, and in 63 of them, the excised portion of aorta was weighed (range 0.40 to 60 g [median 13 g] in men and 0.40 to 37 g [median 13 g] in women); in 13 patients (21%), the excised portion of aorta weighed ≤4 g, and in the other 50 patients, it weighed >4 g. Ascending aortas having features of the Marfan syndrome, aortitis (usually syphilis), and acute or healed dissection were excised. Patients having AR secondary to congenitally bicuspid aortic valves unassociated with infective endocarditis often (22 [37%] of 59 patients) had portions of the aorta excised, and the aortas histologically usually had evidence of loss of medial elastic fibers.

There are few reported studies to which the present data can be compared. Roberts and colleagues[7] in 1981 briefly described causes of pure AR in 177 patients, aged 18 to 70 years, having AVR at the National Heart, Lung, and Blood Institute from 1963 to 1979. Of the 177 patients fulfilling the same criteria as in the present study, these authors attributed the AR to rheumatic heart disease in 94 patients (53%); to infective endocarditis in 41 (23%; bicuspid aortic valve in 7 and tricuspid valve in 34); to the Marfan syndrome or its forme fruste variety in 15 (8%); to a congenitally bicuspid aortic valve unassociated with infective endocarditis in 13 (7%)[7]; to syphilis in 9 (5%); to aortic dissection in 2 (1%); and to trauma in 1 (<1%). Thus, there were no patients in whom the AR was attributed to an unclear cause.

Olson and colleagues[8] in 1984 described 221 patients with "clinically pure aortic insufficiency" having AVR at the Mayo Clinic during the 4 years of 1965, 1970, 1975, and 1980. In contrast to the present study, however, these authors included patients who also had simultaneous mitral valve replacement (80 patients [36%]) or who were aged <20 years (8 patients), and none had the presence of pure AR confirmed by hemodynamic data, angiography, or echocardiography. Rheumatic heart disease was the most frequent cause of "clinically pure" AR in their patient population (100 [45%] of 221 patients). The second most common cause was "idiopathic aortic dilatation" (43/221 [19%]). We suspect that their group of "idiopathic aortic dilatation" would have been similar to our group classified as "cause unclear." The Mayo clinic study did not provide information on blood pressure, and therefore, the frequency of hypertension in this group is not known. Their third most common cause of AR was congenitally bicuspid aortic valve unassociated with either infective endocarditis or aortic dissection (42/221 [19%]). Infective endocarditis was next (21/221 [10%], 9 of whom had a bicuspid aortic valve). Other causes included the Marfan syndrome (4 patients), aortic dissection (3 patients, each of whom had a bicuspid aortic valve), ankylosing spondylitis (3 patients), indeterminate (2 patients), and syphilis (1 patient). Their study did not include any information regarding coronary artery bypass grafting or resection of the ascending aorta, and there was no information regarding preoperative echocardiographic or hemodynamic data.

No previous studies have weighed operatively excised purely regurgitant aortic valves. Table 2 shows the range and mean weights of the purely regurgitant aortic valves in the present study and the weights for comparative

TABLE 2. Comparison of Aortic Valve Weight (g) in Patients Having Isolated AVR for Pure AR Versus Aortic Stenosis (With or Without Associated AR)*

	Bicuspid		Tricuspid	
	Men	Women	Men	Women
AR	0.52–2.99 (1.39)	0.68–1.80 (1.24)	0.48–2.45 (1.06)	0.31–1.83 (0.70)
No. of cases with aortic valve weight	45	9	86	55
AS†	0.89–11.30 (3.57)	0.73–4.97 (2.30)	1.03–6.60 (2.40)	0.45–4.81 (1.56)
No. of cases with aortic valve weight	237	104	181	152

*Patients with infective endocarditis were excluded.
†Data from Roberts et al.[3]

purposes of operatively excised stenotic aortic valves-(with or without associated AR).[3] In both groups, the mean weights were heavier in the men than in the women. The mean weights of the purely regurgitant valves ranged from 39% to 54% of the mean weights of the stenotic valves. The normal aortic valve in adults weighs ≈0.5 g.[9]

Disclosures

None.

References

1. Roberts WC, Ko JM. Weights of operatively-excised stenotic unicuspid, bicuspid, and tricuspid aortic valves and their relation to age, sex, body mass index, and presence or absence of concomitant coronary artery bypass grafting. *Am J Cardiol*. 2003;92:1057–1065.
2. Roberts WC, Ko JM. Frequency by decades of unicuspid, bicuspid, and tricuspid aortic valves in adults having isolated aortic valve replacement for aortic stenosis, with or without associated aortic regurgitation. *Circulation*. 2005;111:920–925.
3. Roberts WC, Ko JM, Hamilton C. Comparison of valve structure, valve weight, and severity of the valve obstruction in 1849 patients having isolated aortic valve replacement for aortic valve stenosis (with or without associated aortic regurgitation) studied at 3 different medical centers in 2 different time periods. *Circulation*. 2005;112:3919–3929.
4. Roberts WC. Morphological features of the elderly heart. In: Tresch D, Aronow WS. 2nd ed. *Cardiovascular Disease in the Elderly Patient*. New York, NY: Marcel Dekker; 1999:17–42.
5. Waller BF, Zoltick JM, Rosen JH, Katz NM, Gomes MN, Fletcher RD, Wallace RB, Roberts WC. Severe aortic regurgitation from systemic hypertension (without aortic dissection) requiring aortic valve replacement. *Am J Cardiol*. 1982;49:473–477.
6. Barlow J, Kincaid-Smith P. The auscultatory findings in hypertension. *Br Heart J*. 1960;22:505–514.
7. Roberts WC, Morrow AG, McIntosh CL, Jones M, Epstein SE. Congenitally bicuspid aortic valve causing severe, pure aortic regurgitation without superimposed infective endocarditis. *Am J Cardiol*. 1981;47: 206–209.
8. Olson LJ, Subramanian R, Edwards WD. Surgical pathology of pure aortic insufficiency: a study of 225 cases. *Mayo Clin Proc*. 1984;59:835–841.
9. Silver MA, Roberts WC. Detailed anatomy of the normally functioning aortic valve in hearts of normal and increased weight. *Am J Cardiol*. 1985;55:454–461.

CLINICAL PERSPECTIVE

In the first 30 years of aortic valve replacement (AVR) for pure aortic regurgitation (AR), the cause of the AR was usually readily apparent. We reviewed causes of pure AR among 268 patients having AVR from 1993 to 2005. To our surprise, despite examining the operatively excised valves and occasionally portions of ascending aorta and the medical records, the cause of the AR was clear in 177 patients (66%) and unclear in 91 (34%). The frequency of simultaneous coronary bypass was much less in the clear-cause group than in the unclear-cause group (40/177 [23%] versus 46/91 [51%]).

Some observations on mitral and aortic valve disease

William Clifford Roberts, MD, and Jong Mi Ko, BA

SOURCES FOR MORPHOLOGIC STUDIES

Before 1960, the only source for studying the heart was the autopsy. The early years of cardiac valve replacement provided a rich source of necropsy "material" until valve techniques and artificial heart valves became more refined. In the 1950s and 1960s, most physicians attributed valvular heart disease in adults to rheumatic heart disease. During the 1960s and 1970s, many thousands of patients with rheumatic heart disease underwent replacement of one or more cardiac valves. By the 1980s, most of this rheumatic heart disease pool of patients had undergone operation; in addition, the frequency of rheumatic fever and subsequently rheumatic heart disease had dropped dramatically. By the 1970s, the congenitally malformed aortic valve was found to be frequent in adults with aortic stenosis (AS), and mitral valve prolapse (MVP) was being recognized as a common cause of pure (no associated stenosis) mitral regurgitation (MR). By the 1990s, the frequency of autopsies in US hospitals had dropped enormously compared with the 1950s, and operatively excised cardiac valves were becoming the major source of anatomic study. Although established by the 1980s, cardiac transplantation was rarely performed in patients with valvular heart disease.

Table 1. Functional and anatomic classification of valvular heart disease in 1010 necropsy patients aged ≥15 years*

Functional class	Patients (%)	Anatomic class				
		AV	MV	MV-AV	TV-MV	TV-MV-AV
1. Aortic stenosis (AS)	292 (29%)	256 (88%)	0	35 (12%)	0	1 (0.3%)
2. Mitral stenosis (MS)	189 (19%)	0	117 (62%)	40 (21%)	13 (7%)	19 (10%)
3. MS + AS	152 (15%)	0	0	120 (79%)	0	32 (21%)
4. Aortic regurgitation (AR)†	119 (12%)	107 (90%)	0	10 (8%)	0	2 (2%)
5. Mitral regurgitation (MR)	97 (10%)	0	85 (88%)	8 (8%)	1 (1%)	3 (3%)
6. MS + AR	65 (6%)	0	52 (80%)	0	0	13 (20%)
7. MR + AR	45 (4%)	0	0	39 (87%)	0	6 (13%)
8. AS + MR	23 (2%)	0	0	21 (91%)	0	2 (9%)
9. Tricuspid stenosis + MS ± AS	28 (3%)	0	0	0	4 (14%)	24 (86%)
Totals	1010 (100%)‡	363 (36%)	254 (25%)	273 (27%)	18 (2%)	102 (10%)

*Excludes patients with mitral regurgitation secondary to coronary heart disease (papillary muscle dysfunction), carcinoid heart disease, hypertrophic cardiomyopathy, and those with infective endocarditis limited to one or both right-sided cardiac valves. Tricuspid valve regurgitation was present in many patients in most of the nine functional groups. All patients were in functional class III or IV (New York Heart Association), and more than half had one or more cardiac operations.

†In many patients, the aortic valve cusps were normal or nearly normal and the regurgitation was the result of disease of the aorta (the Marfan and Marfan-like syndrome, syphilis, systemic hypertension, healed aortic dissection).

‡The hearts in all 1010 patients were examined and classified by WCR.

From Roberts WC, 1987 (1); reproduced with permission from Roberts WC, 1983 (39).

AV indicates aortic valve; MV, mitral valve; TV, tricuspid valve.

FREQUENCY OF VARIOUS VALVULAR DISORDERS IN NECROPSY STUDIES

Roberts (1) personally studied 1010 hearts at necropsy in patients with fatal valvular heart disease *(Table 1)*. All had died between 1955 and 1980 and the specimens were retrieved from a number of different hospitals, most of which were located in the Washington, DC, area. As shown in Table 1, these cases were given both a *functional* (valve stenosis ± regurgitation or pure regurgitation [no element of stenosis]) and an *anatomic* classification. A number of these patients had only one dysfunctional valve but in addition had one or more anatomically abnormal valves (normal function). (A valve may be anatomically abnormal yet function normally.) AS was the most common functional

From the Baylor Heart and Vascular Institute and the Departments of Pathology and Medicine (Cardiology), Baylor University Medical Center, Dallas, Texas.

Corresponding author: William C. Roberts, MD, Baylor Heart and Vascular Institute, Baylor University Medical Center, 621 North Hall Street, Dallas, Texas 75226 (e-mail: wc.roberts@BaylorHealth.edu).

Table 2. Type of valvular dysfunction in patients* having aortic valve replacement and/or mitral valve replacement or repair at Baylor University Medical Center at Dallas (1993–2006)

Valve dysfunction	Patients (%)
1. Aortic stenosis (AS)	985 (53%)
2. Mitral stenosis (MS)	129 (7%)
3. MS + AS	54 (3%)
4. Aortic regurgitation (AR)†	326 (17%)
5. Mitral regurgitation (MR)*	313 (17%)
6. MS + AR	10 (<1%)
7. MR + AR	28 (1%)
8. AS + MR	27 (1%)
9. Tricuspid stenosis + MS + AS	0
Totals	1872 (100%)‡

*Excludes patients with mitral regurgitation secondary to coronary heart disease (papillary muscle dysfunction), carcinoid heart disease, hypertrophic cardiomyopathy, and those with infective endocarditis limited to one or both right-sided cardiac valves. Tricuspid valve regurgitation was present in many patients in most of the nine functional groups.

† In many patients, the aortic valve cusps were normal or nearly normal and the regurgitation was the result of disease of the aorta (the Marfan and Marfan-like syndrome, syphilis, systemic hypertension, healed aortic dissection).

‡The operatively excised valves in the 1872 patients were examined and classified by WCR.

disorder (29%); in 35 (12%) of these 292 patients, the mitral leaflets were diffusely thickened (rheumatic heart disease) but there was no clinical evidence of mitral dysfunction. Most of the 256 patients with AS and anatomically normal mitral valves had congenitally unicuspid or bicuspid aortic valves.

Mitral stenosis (MS) was the next most common functional valve disease, but 72 (38%) of these 189 patients also had anatomic involvement of one or more other cardiac valves. All patients with MS, whether isolated or associated with a functional disorder of another cardiac valve, had the valvular disease attributed to rheumatic heart disease.

Combined MS and AS was the third most common functional valvular disease (15%), and 32 (21%) of these 152 cases also had anatomic disease of the tricuspid valve leaflets. The purely regurgitant lesions (aortic regurgitation [AR], MR, or both) were less common. Tricuspid stenosis of rheumatic etiology occurred in only 3% of the 1010 cases, and all had associated MS with or without associated AS. No other large series of patients with valvular heart disease studied at necropsy has been reported in the last 25 years, and it is unlikely that such a large series, all studied by a single physician, will be accumulated in the future because of the low autopsy rates in most hospitals today and because few specimens are retained indefinitely after autopsy.

CHANGING FREQUENCY OF VARIOUS VALVULAR DISORDERS IN RECENT DECADES IN THE WESTERN WORLD

Today the most frequently studied operatively excised valve is the stenotic aortic valve, followed by a portion of posterior mitral leaflet in patients with MR excised secondary to MVP *(Table 2)*. Operatively excised purely regurgitant aortic valves with or without excision of portions of ascending aorta are also common. Purely regurgitant mitral valves that are replaced usually yield only anterior mitral leaflets as specimens; the posterior leaflet is usually not excised. Tricuspid valves are rarely excised today.

The remainder of this article discusses specific mitral and aortic valvular disorders.

AORTIC STENOSIS (± REGURGITATION)

Frequency and causes

If systemic hypertension is not considered, AS is the second most common potentially fatal or fatal heart disease after coronary heart disease. There are three major causes of AS: *atherosclerosis* (formerly called degenerative), *congenitally malformed valves*, and *rheumatic heart disease.*

That atherosclerosis is a cause of AS is derived primarily from five pieces of evidence:

1. Patients with familial homozygous hyperlipidemia (serum total cholesterol levels >800 mg/dL from birth) usually develop calcific deposits on the aortic aspects of their aortic valve cusps early in life, usually by the teenage years (2).
2. Progression of AS can be slowed by lowering total and low-density lipoprotein cholesterol levels by statins (3).
3. Patients >65 years of age with AS involving a three-cuspid aortic valve (unassociated with mitral valve disease) usually have extensive atherosclerosis involving the major epicardial coronary arteries and usually other systemic arterial systems (4).
4. Serum total cholesterol levels and concomitant coronary bypass grafting tend to be higher in patients with AS involving three-cuspid aortic valves than in patients of similar age and sex without AS or with congenitally bicuspid aortic valves (5).
5. Histologic study of three-cuspid stenotic aortic valves demonstrates features similar to those in atherosclerotic plaques (2).

The unicuspid aortic valve appears to be stenotic from birth (6, 7). The congenitally bicuspid valve, however, is infrequently stenotic at birth but becomes stenotic as calcific deposits form on the aortic aspects of the cusps (8). Rheumatic heart disease never involves the aortic valve anatomically without also involving the mitral valve (9). Although the mitral valve may be diffusely abnormal anatomically, its function can be normal. Consequently, a patient with rheumatic heart disease can present initially with only aortic valve dysfunction, and therefore rheumatic heart disease has to be considered a cause of functionally isolated AS (± AR) or pure AR (9).

Valve structure

In patients with isolated AS (± AR) (only cardiac valve anatomically abnormal) the aortic valve may be unicuspid, bicuspid, tricuspid, or quadricuspid. The congenitally *unicuspid valve* is of two types: acommissural and unicommissural (7, 10). The acommissural valve, which represents <10% of the unicuspid valves, has a central orifice and no distinct commissures. The

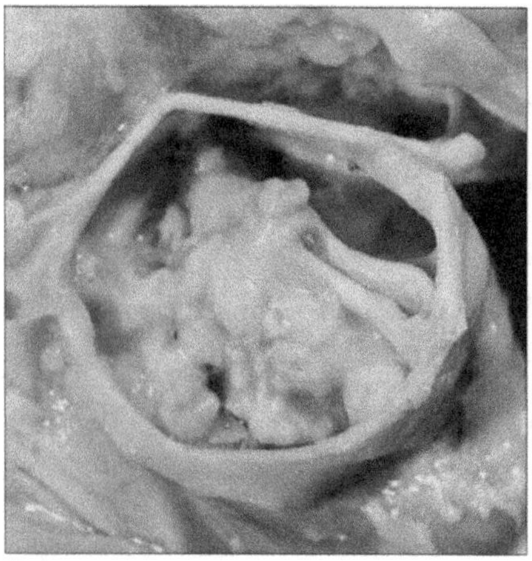

Figure 1. Aortic stenosis. *Congenitally unicuspid unicommissural aortic valve* in a 48-year-old man. The heart weighed 750 g. Reproduced with permission from Falcone MW et al, 1971 (7).

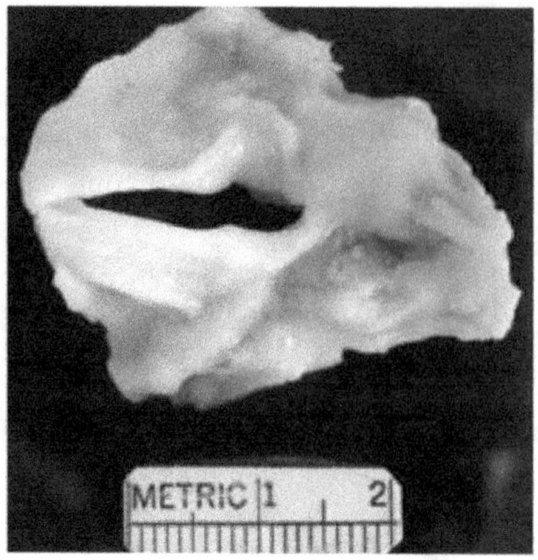

Figure 2. Aortic stenosis. Operatively excised *unicuspid unicommissural aortic valve* in a 41-year-old man. The valve weighed 5.42 g. The mean transvalvular pressure gradient was 51 mm Hg.

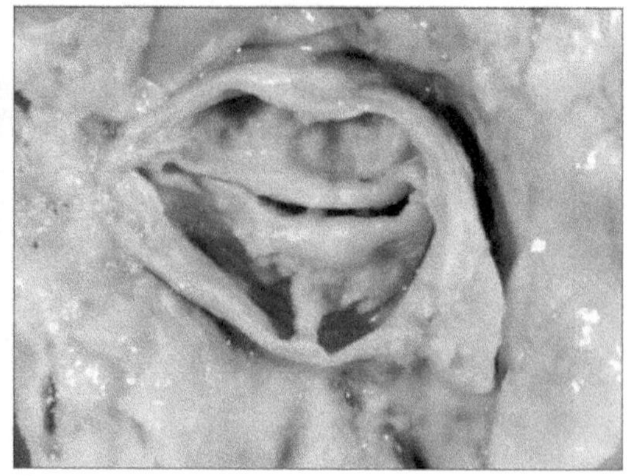

Figure 3. Aortic stenosis. *Congenitally bicuspid aortic valve* in a 61-year-old man. At catheterization 2 years before his death, the peak systolic transvalvular pressure gradient was 45 mm Hg when the cardiac index was 2.6 L/min/m². He had complete heart block secondary to destruction of the atrioventricular bundle by calcium. The heart weighed 700 g.

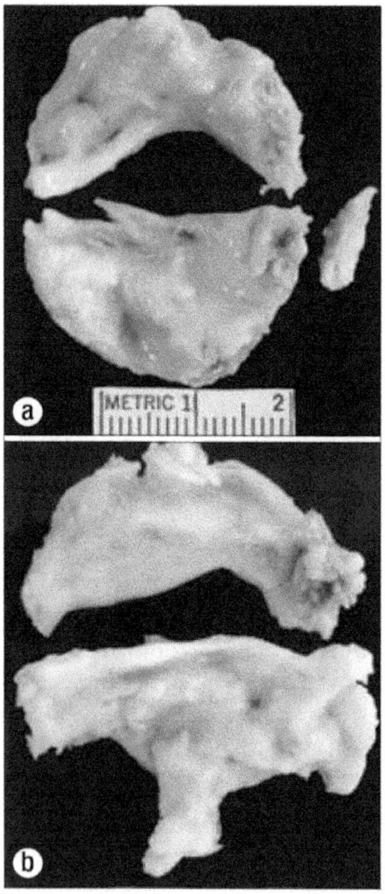

Figure 4. Aortic stenosis. Two operatively excised *congenitally bicuspid aortic valves.* **(a)** Valve in a 60-year-old man with severe heart failure. The valve weighed 4.65 g. **(b)** Valve in a 66-year-old man. The valve weighed 4.79 g and the peak systolic transvalvular gradient was 84 mm Hg.

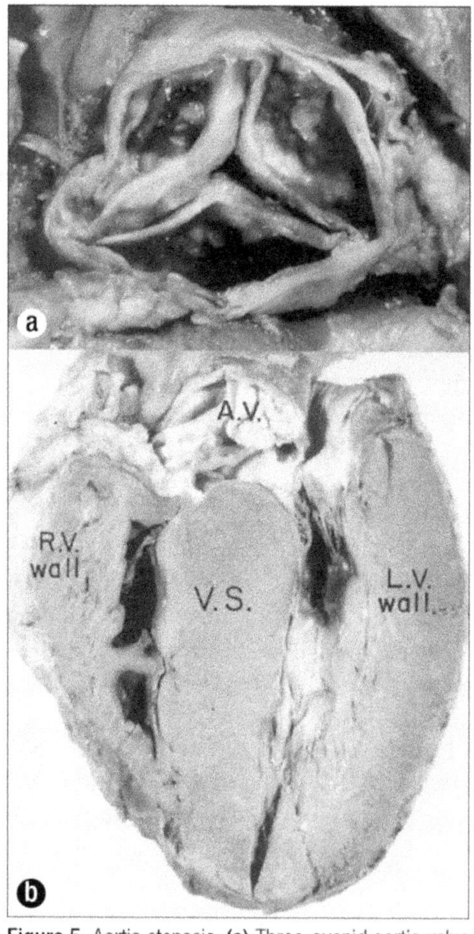

Figure 5. Aortic stenosis. **(a)** Three-cuspid aortic valve and **(b)** longitudinal section of the heart in an 89-year-old man whose heart weighed 440 g. None of the three aortic valve commissures are fused. The mitral annulus contains calcific deposits. Reproduced with permission from Roberts WC et al, 1971 (4).

unicommissural valve, which constitutes most of the unicuspid valves, has one commissure and usually two other rudimentary commissures (raphae) and a vertical orifice extending from the only true commissure *(Figures 1 and 2)* (9).

The *congenitally bicuspid valve (Figures 3 and 4)* of course has two cusps, and they are usually of slightly unequal size in both cuspal surface area and weight. Usually one of the two cusps contains a raphe in its central portion. Often the raphe cusp has free margins that are V-shaped with the apex of the V pointing to the raphe, producing a concave configuration. The nonraphe cusp in this circumstance commonly has a convex configuration that fits nicely into the concave shape of the raphe cusp such that associated regurgitation is absent or minimal. These bicuspid valves with a concave configuration of the raphe cusp and a convex appearance of free margin of the nonraphe cusp are often confused with tricuspid valves with fusion of one of three commissures. In other bicuspid valves the free margins of both cusps are relatively straight.

The *tricuspid aortic valve* is common in older patients with AS (atherosclerotic origin) and in patients in whom the AS is of rheumatic etiology. (These latter patients always have mitral leaflets that are diffusely fibrotic [with or without focal calcific deposits], or at least the margins of both leaflets are everywhere thickened by fibrous tissue.) In patients with AS of rheumatic etiology, one or more of the three commissures are often fused and the cusps may be either diffusely or focally fibrotic with or without commissural fusion or calcific deposits. The stenotic tricuspid aortic valve in older persons contains calcific deposits on the aortic surfaces, usually involving the sites of cuspal attachments, and the commissures characteristically are not fused *(Figure 5)*. Thus, operative excision produces three cusps, none of which is attached to another *(Figure 6)*. Older patients with AS often

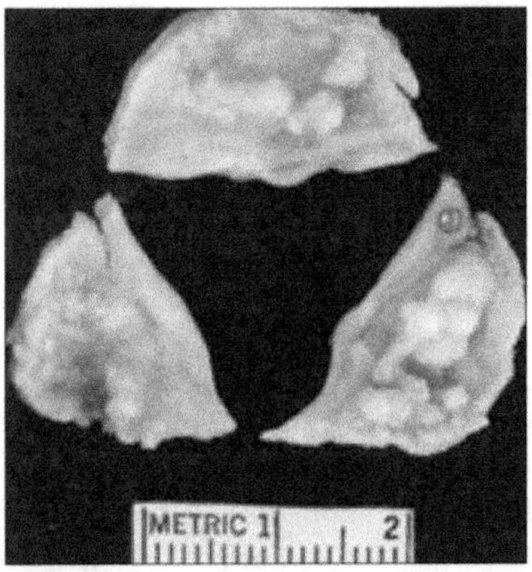

Figure 6. Aortic stenosis. Operatively excised aortic valve in a 70-year-old man. The valve weighed 1.69 g, the peak systolic transvalvular gradient was 55 mm Hg, and left ventricular function was normal (ejection fraction = 60%).

also have calcified mitral anomaly. *Figure 7* shows how calcium might develop in both the aortic valve and the mitral annulus.

The *quadricuspid aortic valve* is rare (12). When present and if dysfunctional, the dysfunction is usually pure AR. AS with a quadricuspid valve is exceedingly rare, seen by Roberts (13) in 1 of 1118 operatively excised stenotic aortic valves.

Necropsy studies of patients with isolated aortic stenosis (± AR) and never a cardiac operation—natural history

During a 32-year period at the National Institutes of Health (NIH), Roberts collected (mainly from hospitals in the Washington, DC, area) the hearts of 192 adults (aged 16–99 years) with isolated AS; none of them had ever had a cardiac operation (unpublished data). Of the 192 patients, 139 (72%) were men and 53 (28%) were women *(Table 3)*. The average age of the men was 61 years, and that of the women, 71 years, the same average ages of death as in coronary heart disease. The weight of the hearts was 610 ± 135 g (normal, <400 g) in the men and 486 ± 111 g (normal, <350 g) in the women. The aortic valve was congenitally unicuspid in 17 patients (9%), congenitally bicuspid in 89 patients (46%), and tricuspid in 86 (45%) *(Table 4)*. Other observations in these 192 patients are shown in Tables 3 and 4.

Table 3. Findings at necropsy in unoperated isolated aortic valve stenosis in men vs women (n = 192)

Variable	Men (n = 139)		Women (n = 53)	
Age (years): range (mean)	16–99 (61)		32–90 (71)	
Symptomatic	103/129 (80%)		41/49 (84%)	
Total cholesterol (mg/dL)	206 ± 63		161± 26	
Severity of stenosis				
1+	24 (17%)		7 (13%)	
2+	22 (16%)		9 (17%)	
3+	93 (67%)		37 (70%)	
Coronary narrowing				
0	73 (53%)		20 (38%)	
≥1	66 (47%)		33 (62%)	
Mitral annular calcium				
0	101 (73%)		23 (43%)	
1+–3+	38 (27%)		30 (57%)	
Heart weight (g)	610 ± 135		486 ± 111	
Aortic valve				
Unicuspid	16 (12%)	59%	1 (2%)	45%
Bicuspid	66 (47%)		23 (43%)	
Tricuspid	57 (41%)		29 (55%)	
Left ventricular				
Fibrosis	57 (41%)		13 (25%)	
Necrosis	13 (9%)		5 (9%)	

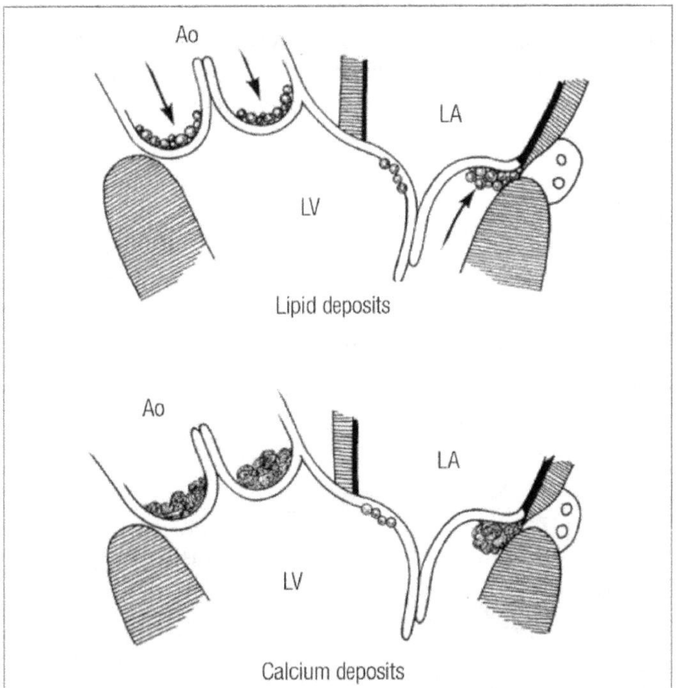

Figure 7. Aortic valve and mitral annular calcium. Commonly calcific deposits are present in the aortic valve cusps, mitral annulus, and epicardial coronary arteries. Roberts has referred to this condition as "the senile cardiac calcification syndrome" (11). The cause of the deposits is speculative, but atherosclerosis seems to be the most reasonable. In younger individuals lipid deposits are usually present on the aortic aspects of the aortic valve cusps and on the ventricular aspects of the posterior mitral leaflet and, to a much lesser extent, on the ventricular aspect of the anterior mitral leaflet. The lipid in these locations is usually both intracellular and extracellular. Degeneration of the lipid probably leads to the calcific deposits in these locations.

Weights of operatively excised stenotic aortic valves

The weight of operatively excised stenotic aortic valves is useful in quantitating the severity of the stenosis because the weight is determined primarily by the quantity of calcific deposits and the larger the calcific deposits, the greater the transvalvular pressure gradient (13–24). Roberts and colleagues (22) reported weights in 1849 operatively excised stenotic valves in patients aged 21 to 91 years without concomitant mitral valve replacement or mitral stenosis. These authors found that the weight of the stenotic valves varied inversely with the number of aortic valve cusps (14). The unicuspid valves were the heaviest, the bicuspid valves the next heaviest, and the tricuspid aortic valves, the lightest. The men had heavier valves than did the women *(Figure 8)*, and the younger patients had heavier valves than did the older patients. The mean weights of the valves were similar in patients whose body mass index was <25, 25–30, and >30 kg/m^2. Mean valve weights also were heavier in the patients

Table 4. Underlying structure of the aortic valve in unoperated patients studied at necropsy with isolated aortic valve stenosis with or without associated aortic regurgitation (n = 192)

Variable	Unicuspid (n = 17) [9%]	Bicuspid (n = 89) [46%]	Tricuspid (n = 86) [45%]
Age (years): range (mean)	25–73 (46)	16–87 (62)	36–99 (64)
Males	16 (94%)	66 (74%)	57 (66%)
Symptomatic	15 (88%)	73/84 (87%)	57/78 (73%)
Total cholesterol (mg/dL)	216	203	173
Mode of death			
Sudden (outside hospital)	1 (6%)	15 (17%)	11 (13%)
Sudden (inside hospital)	1 (6%)	13 (15%)	6 (7%)
Nonsudden (cardiac)	14 (82%)	47 (53%)	45 (52%)
Vascular	0	2 (2%)	4 (5%)
Noncardiovascular	1 (6%)	12 (14%)	20 (23%)
Severity of stenosis			
1+	1 (6%)	11 (12%)	19 (22%)
2+	0	14 (16%)	17 (20%)
3+	16 (94%)	64 (72%)	50 (58%)
Coronary narrowing			
0	15 (88%)	57 (64%)	41 (48%)
≥1	2 (12%)	32 (36%)	45 (52%)
Mitral annular calcium			
0	12 (71%)	72 (81%)	40 (47%)
1+–3+	5 (29%)	17 (19%)	46 (53%)
Heart weight (g) (mean)	617	578	573
Left ventricular			
Fibrosis	8/15 (53%)	34/88 (39%)	28/85 (33%)
Necrosis	1/16 (6%)	8/87 (9%)	9/85 (11%)

who *did not* undergo simultaneous coronary artery bypass grafting than in those who did.

Table 5 shows various clinical findings in the 1849 patients whose stenotic aortic valves were studied by Roberts and colleagues (22). The patients underwent aortic valve replacement at three different institutions: NIH from 1963 to 1989, Georgetown University Medical Center (GUMC) from 1969 to 1992, and Baylor University Medical Center (BUMC) from 1993 to 2004. All 1849 operatively excised stenotic valves were examined and classified by WCR. Patients having simultaneous mitral valve replacement or mitral stenosis were excluded. The valves excised at NIH and at GUMC from 1963 to 1992 were heavier than the valves excised at BUMC from 1993 to 2004: men 4.05 ± 1.91 (NIH), 4.36 ± 1.83 (GUMC), and 3.11 ± 1.51 g (BUMC); women 2.80 ± 1.26 (NIH), 3.02 ± 1.26 (GUMC), and 1.89 ± 0.87 g (BUMC).

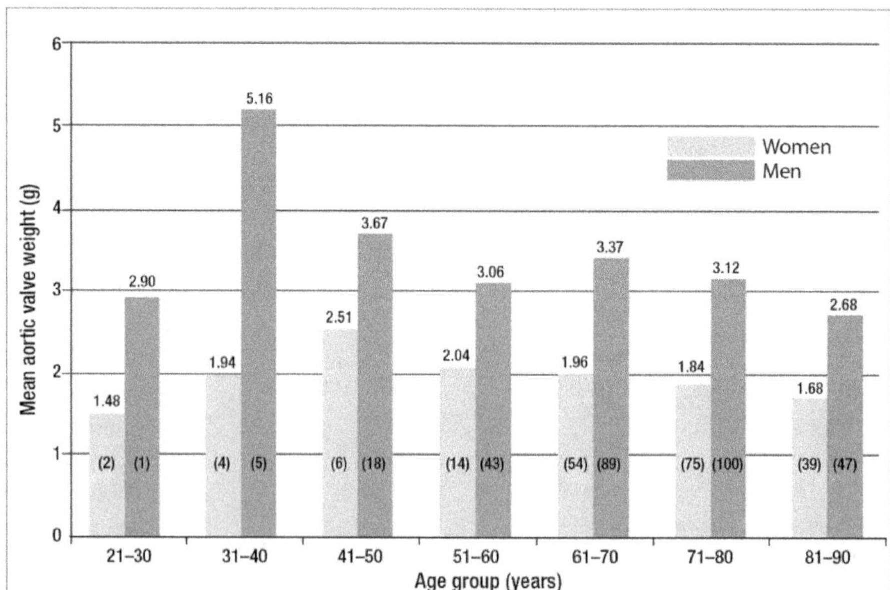

Figure 8. Aortic valve weights in men and women in each of 7 decades. All had aortic stenosis. Reproduced with permission from Roberts WC and Ko JM, 2003 (14).

Not only did the valve weights vary according to valve structure (unicuspid > bicuspid > tricuspid), but often there was variation in individual cusps among patients with bicuspid valves and among patients with tricuspid valves (15, 16). Of 200 operatively excised stenotic congenitally bicuspid valves, the two cusps in 152 patients (76%) differed in weight by >0.2 g, and in 48 patients (24%) the cusps were of similar weight (≤0.2 g difference) (15). In 161 of the 200 patients, a raphe was present in one of the two cusps: the raphe and nonraphe cusps differed in weight in 120 patients (74%) with the raphe cusps being heavier in 89 patients (55%), lighter in 31 patients (19%), and of similar weight in 41 (26%). Of the 39 patients without a raphe in one cusp, in 32 patients (82%) the two cusps were of different (>0.2 g) weight and in 7 patients (18%), similar in weight (≤0.2 g).

Of 260 operatively excised stenotic three-cuspid aortic valves, all three cusps differed (by >0.1 g) in weight in 71 patients (27%); all three cusps were similar (≤0.1 g difference) in weight in 33 patients (13%), and in 156 patients (60%) one cusp differed from either of the other two cusps which were similar in weight (16).

Why might cusps of operatively excised stenotic valves differ in weight? The most likely explanation seems to be that the cusps differ in size, that is, in surface area, from birth. The cusp with the largest surface area has, of course, a larger area on which calcium can be deposited, and the weight of a cusp is determined primarily by the amount of calcium deposited on its aortic surface.

Relation of aortic valve weight to transvalvular peak systolic pressure gradient

The best determinant of the magnitude of obstruction in patients with AS has been debated. Determinants considered have been aortic valve area or index, mean transvalvular systolic gradient, and peak transvalvular systolic gradients. Roberts and Ko (17) compared the weights of operatively excised stenotic

Table 5. Data in patients having isolated aortic valve replacement for aortic stenosis (± aortic regurgitation) at three different medical centers

Variable	NIH (1963–1989)	GUMC (1969–1992)	BUMC (1993–2004)
Valve structure			
Unicuspid			
Men	84/342 (25%)	56/255 (22%)	36/601 (6%)
Women	14/110 (13%)	24/145 (17%)	12/356 (4%)
Bicuspid			
Men	158/342 (46%)	129/255 (50%)	316/601 (53%)
Women	53/110 (48%)	68/145 (47%)	153/356 (43%)
Tricuspid			
Men	47/342 (14%)	63/255 (25%)	242/601 (40%)
Women	28/110 (25%)	48/145 (33%)	186/356 (52%)
Indeterminate			
Men	53/342 (15%)	7/255 (3%)	7/601 (1%)
Women	15/110 (14%)	5/145 (3%)	5/356 (1%)
Age (years): range (mean ± SD)			
Men	21–82 (54 ± 12)	24–88 (64 ± 11)	25–91 (69 ± 12)
Men ≥65	62/331 (19%)	124/251 (49%)	424/601 (71%)
Women	33–86 (57 ± 11)	22–89 (67 ± 12)	27–91 (70 ± 11)
Women ≥65	27/104 (26%)	94/142 (66%)	273/356 (77%)
Gender			
Men	342/452 (76%)	255/400 (64%)	601/957 (63%)
Women	110/452 (24%)	145/400 (36%)	356/957 (37%)
Aortic valve weight (g): range (mean ± SD)			
Men	0.70–10.2 (4.05 ± 1.91)	1.20–11.0 (4.36 ± 1.83)	0.89–11.30 (3.11 ± 1.51)
Women	0.55–5.50 (2.80 ± 1.26)	0.40–6.70 (3.02 ± 1.26)	0.45–4.97 (1.89 ± 0.87)
Left ventricular to aortic peak systolic gradient (mm Hg): range (mean ± SD)			
Men	10–145 (69 ± 30)	10–160 (69 ± 25)	10–141 (52 ± 23)
Women	10–165 (76 ± 34)	30–170 (81 ± 32)	10–133 (54 ± 28)
Aortic valve area (cm^2): range (mean ± SD)			
Men	0.20–1.90 (0.66 ± 0.32)	0.27–1.97 (0.75 ± 0.31)	0.20–1.90 (0.78 ± 0.26)
Women	0.23–1.10 (0.53 ± 0.21)	0.20–1.30 (0.57 ± 0.21)	0.18–1.49 (0.67 ± 0.22)
Cardiac index ($L/min/m^2$): range (mean ± SD)			
Men	1.10–5.00 (2.58 ± 0.72)	1.00–7.30 (2.87 ± 0.93)	–
Women	1.60–4.50 (2.68 ± 0.69)	1.60–6.20 (2.79 ± 0.81)	–
Simultaneous coronary bypass			
Men	21/238 (9%)	77/198 (39%)	332/601 (55%)
Women	6/74 (8%)	29/118 (25%)	167/356 (47%)

Reproduced with permission from Roberts WC et al, 2005 (22).

BUMC indicates Baylor University Medical Center; GUMC, Georgetown University Medical Center; NIH, National Institutes of Health.

aortic valves to peak transvalvular systolic pressure gradient and to aortic valve area. The results of these studies in 201 men and in 123 women with isolated AS are shown in *Table 6*. In both men and women the weights of the stenotic aortic valves increased significantly as the peak left ventricular-to-aortic systolic gradient increased, but valve weight had essentially no relation to aortic valve area. Women had significantly lower valve weights, with peak gradients similar to those in men. In men with valve weights from 1 to 2 g, the peak transvalvular gradient averaged 36 mm Hg and the valve areas, 0.86 cm^2; in the men with valve weights >6 g, the peak gradients averaged 87 mm Hg, whereas the valve was 0.71 cm^2. In women with valve weights ≤1 g, the peak gradient averaged 28 mm Hg and valve area, 0.83 cm^2; in women whose valve weighed from >3 to 4 g, the peak gradients averaged 85 mm Hg, and the valve area, 0.51 cm^2 (Table 6).

Relatively few operatively excised aortic valves in adults with AS are ≥5 g, and those reaching that weight are usually congenitally malformed. Of unicuspid valves, 37 (30%) of 124 valves in men and 5 (11%) of 44 in women reached this weight; of bicuspid valves, 96 (18%) of 521 valves in men and 4 (2%) of 236 valves in women reached this weight (unpublished data). In contrast, only 15 (4%) of 361 tricuspid valves in men and only 2 (0.7%) of 281 valves in women reached this weight. Of 1038 operatively excised stenotic aortic valves in men, 161 (16%) were ≥5 g, and of 571 valves in women, only 13 (2%) reached this weight. Seven operatively excised stenotic valves weighed ≥10 g: all were in men and all seven were either unicuspid or bicuspid and the peak pressure gradient across them ranged from 80 to 143 mm Hg (average, 101) (unpublished data).

Associated coronary arterial narrowing

Patients with operatively excised congenitally unicuspid and bicuspid valves have significantly less epicardial coronary arterial narrowing than do patients with tricuspid aortic valves *(Table 7)*. Concomitant coronary artery bypass grafting also varies according to the era during which the aortic valve replacement was done and the institution where it was done. Also, criteria for performing coronary artery bypass grafting in patients having aortic valve replacement have changed with time.

Relation to left bundle branch block and/or complete heart block

At one time, patients with AS and left bundle branch block or complete heart block were believed to have these conduction disturbances because of associated severe coronary arterial narrowing from atherosclerosis. Study at necropsy, however, of many patients with combined AS and left bundle branch block or complete heart block has indicated that the conduction disturbance was due not to associated coronary narrowing but to destruction of the left bundle branches or the atrioventricular bundle by calcific deposits that had extended caudally from the aortic valve (Roberts, unpublished data). Most of these patients had congenitally malformed aortic valves—not tricuspid valves—and severe degrees of hemodynamic obstruction as a result of the heavy calcific deposits.

Table 6. Age, body mass index, concomitant coronary artery bypass, left ventricular to aortic peak systolic gradients, and aortic valve areas in seven aortic valve weight groups in men and in women

AV weight (g)	No. of patients	Age (years): range (average)	BMI (kg/m²): range (average)	AV weights (g): range (average)	LV–aorta PSG (mm Hg): range (average)	AV area (cm²): range (mean)	Coronary bypass	UAV or BAV	Ejection fraction (%)			
									No.	Range (mean)	No. (%) ≤40	No. (%) >40
Men												
≤1	0	–	–	–	–	–	–	–	–	–	–	–
>1–2	41	47–90 (72)	19–37 (27)	1.16–2.00 (1.64)	11–81 (36)	0.27–1.43 (0.86)	27 (66%)	11 (27%)	37	15–78 (48)	13 (35%)	24 (65%)
>2–3	60	29–87 (69)	20–43 (29)	2.01–3.00 (2.58)	15–97 (45)	0.42–2.25 (0.89)	32 (53%)	24 (40%)	52	10–85 (51)	14 (27%)	38 (73%)
>3–4	50	37–84 (69)	17–40 (27)	3.03–4.00 (3.40)	20–100 (56)	0.20–1.63 (0.75)	26 (52%)	30 (60%)	44	15–80 (53)	7 (16%)	37 (84%)
>4–5	29	42–87 (69)	18–45 (28)	4.01–4.84 (4.40)	20–108 (64)	0.32–1.06 (0.67)	11 (38%)	25 (86%)	26	15–70 (53)	5 (19%)	21 (81%)
>5–6	12	49–90 (70)	24–36 (28)	5.03–5.93 (5.60)	50–116 (71)	0.40–0.88 (0.60)	3 (25%)	10 (83%)	10	20–65 (43)	4 (40%)	6 (60%)
>6	9	38–84 (58)	21–38 (28)	6.24–11.30 (7.92)	35–141 (87)	0.39–1.23 (0.71)	2 (22%)	8 (89%)	8	15–70 (51)	2 (25%)	6 (75%)
Women												
≤1	10	55–85 (74)	21–44 (30)	0.69–0.95 (0.83)	15–62 (28)	0.34–1.28 (0.83)	7 (70%)	2 (20%)	9	30–70 (47)	4 (44%)	5 (56%)
>1–2	73	19–88 (71)	17–51 (29)	1.02–1.99 (1.46)	10–119 (49)	0.18–1.49 (0.72)	40 (55%)	14 (19%)	66	15–80 (56)	9 (14%)	57 (86%)
>2–3	29	30–87 (70)	18–50 (28)	2.04–3.00 (2.42)	26–113 (63)	0.27–1.09 (0.58)	15 (52%)	12 (41%)	23	30–80 (54)	4 (17%)	19 (83%)
>3–4	10	47–85 (73)	17–35 (26)	3.14–4.00 (3.42)	53–131 (85)	0.23–0.78 (0.51)	3 (30%)	9 (90%)	9	45–75 (53)	0	9 (100%)
>4–5	1	83	29	4.27	53	0.75	0	1 (100%)	1	50	0	1 (100%)
>5–6	0	–	–	–	–	–	–	–	–	–	–	–
>6	0	–	–	–	–	–	–	–	–	–	–	–

Reproduced with permission from Roberts WC and Ko JM, 2004 (17).

AV indicates aortic valve; BAV, bicuspid aortic valve; BMI, body mass index; LV, left ventricular; PSG, peak systolic gradient; UAV, unicuspid aortic valve.

PURE AORTIC REGURGITATION

There are two major causes of pure (no element of stenosis) AR: 1) conditions affecting primarily the valve, and 2) conditions affecting the aorta and only secondarily causing the valve to be incompetent. Roberts and Ko (25) recently reviewed the cause of pure AR in 268 patients having isolated aortic valve replacement at BUMC from 1993 to 2005. As shown in *Table 8*, conditions affecting primarily the valve were the cause of the AR in 122 patients (46%), and nonvalve conditions were the cause in 146 patients (54%). Among the former, the *congenitally bicuspid valve* unassociated with infective endocarditis was the problem in 59 patients, 22 (37%) of whom had resection of portions of the dilated ascending aorta. Eleven of the 22 patients with resected aortas had severe loss of medial elastic fibers. Infective endocarditis was the cause in 46 patients, 15 (33%) of whom had congenitally bicuspid aortic valves. Thus, of the 122 with valve conditions causing the AR, 74 (61%) had congenitally bicuspid aortic valves. Why one congenitally bicuspid aortic valve becomes stenotic (8, 26), another has pure regurgitation without superimposed infective endocarditis (27), another becomes severely dysfunctional only when

Table 7. Frequency of concomitant coronary artery bypass grafting among patients having isolated aortic valve replacement for aortic stenosis at three different institutions*

Valve structure	NIH (1963–1989) (n = 259)	GUMC (1969–1992) (n = 308)	BUMC (1993–2007) (n = 1351)
Unicuspid	2/61 (3%)	13/55 (24%)	13/83 (16%)
Bicuspid	13/140 (9%)	42/162 (26%)	280/646 (43%)
Tricuspid	10/58 (17%)	47/91 (52%)	390/622 (63%)

*Excludes cases in which the number of valve cusps was unclear (indeterminate).

BUMC indicates Baylor University Medical Center; GUMC, Georgetown University Medical Center; NIH, National Institutes of Health.

Table 8. Causes of aortic regurgitation in patients having isolated aortic valve replacement at Baylor University Medical Center (1993–2005)

Causes of aortic regurgitation	Total	Age (years) at operation: range (mean)	M	F	Acute	Chronic	SH	CABG	Portions of ascending aorta			BAV	Calcium deposits on AV cusps	Aortic valve weight (g): range (mean)	
									Excised	Examined histologically	CMN (3+, 4+)			Men	Women
Valve (n = 122; 46%)															
Congenital malformation without infective endocarditis															
Bicuspid	59 (22%)	22–77 (55)	49	10	0	59	39 (66%)	18 (31%)	22	22	11	59	31	0.52–2.99 (1.42)	0.68–1.80 (1.24)
Quadricuspid	2 (1%)	53, 79 (66)	0	2	0	2	0	1 (50%)	0	0	0	0	0	—	0.57, 1.13 (0.85)
Tricuspid	5 (2%)	33–48 (40)	3	2	0	5	2 (40%)	0	1	1	0	0	0	1.11–1.40 (1.23)	0.34, 0.66 (.050)
Infective endocarditis	46 (17%)	21–82 (45)	31	15	27	19	29 (63%)	7 (15%)	6	4	0	15	8	0.77–2.31 (1.53)	0.44–2.50 (0.98)
Rheumatic?	8 (3%)	25–63 (47)	6	2	0	8	6 (75%)	2 (25%)	0	0	0	0	3	1.10–2.45 (1.81)	1.31, 1.83 (1.57)
Miscellaneous	2 (1%)	24, 42 (33)	1	1	0	2	2 (100%)	1 (50%)	0	0	0	0	0	0.55	—
Nonvalve (n = 146; 54%)															
Aortic dissection	28 (10%)	25–78 (58)	20	8	21	7	22 (79%)	5* (17%)	28	20	5	3	4	0.51–1.19 (0.81)	0.37–0.90 (0.59)
Marfan or forme fruste	15 (6%)	21–71 (47)	9	6	0	15	10 (67%)	1† (7%)	15	13	13	0	2	0.73–1.01 (0.94)	0.35–0.85 (0.66)
Aortitis	12 (4%)	35–82 (66)	5	7	0	12	10 (83%)	5 (42%)	12	12	12	0	2	0.63–0.79 (0.70)	0.35–0.70 (0.54)
Etiology unclear	91 (34%)	50–84 (66)	58	33	0	91	83 (91%)	46 (51%)	7	7	0	0	26	0.48–2.13 (1.08)	0.31–1.74 (0.73)
Total	268 (100%)	21–84 (57)	182 (68%)	86 (32%)	48 (18%)	220 (82%)	203 (76%)	86 (32%)	91 (34%)	76	41	77 (29%)	76/263 (29%)	0.48–2.99 (1.22) 151‡	0.31–2.50 (0.81) 75‡

*Four other patients had CABG due to extension of the aortic dissection into a coronary artery.

†One additional patient had CABG due to extension of the aortic dissection into a coronary artery.

‡Number of cases with aortic valve weight.

Reproduced with permission from Roberts WC et al, 2006 (25).

AV indicates aortic valve; BAV, bicuspid aortic valve; CABG, coronary artery bypass grafting; CMN, "cystic medial necrosis" (magnitude of loss of elastic fibers in the aorta's media); F, female; M, male; SH, systemic hypertension.

infective endocarditis appears (28), and some function normally an entire lifetime is unclear (8). Of 85 patients, aged 15 to 79 years, with congenitally bicuspid aortic valves studied at autopsy by Roberts (8), 61 valves (72%) were stenotic, 2 (2%) had pure regurgitation without superimposed infective endocarditis, 9 (11%) had AR because of infective endocarditis, and 13 (15%) functioned normally during the patients' 23 to 59 years of life (mean, 45).

Rheumatic heart disease is a relatively infrequent cause of pure AR in patients with normally functioning mitral valves (9). All such patients (by our definition of rheumatic heart disease) have diffuse fibrosis of the mitral leaflets or at least diffuse thickening of the margins of these leaflets. In this circumstance mitral valve function would be normal despite the anatomic abnormality.

Infective endocarditis more commonly involves a three-cuspid aortic valve than a two-cuspid one because the tricuspid valve is so much more common than the bicuspid valve (28).

Rheumatoid arthritis is a rare cause of AR. The anatomic abnormality is specific for this condition and consists of rheumatoid nodules within the aortic valve cusps (29, 30).

Conditions affecting the ascending aorta and causing it to dilate cause AR more commonly than those conditions

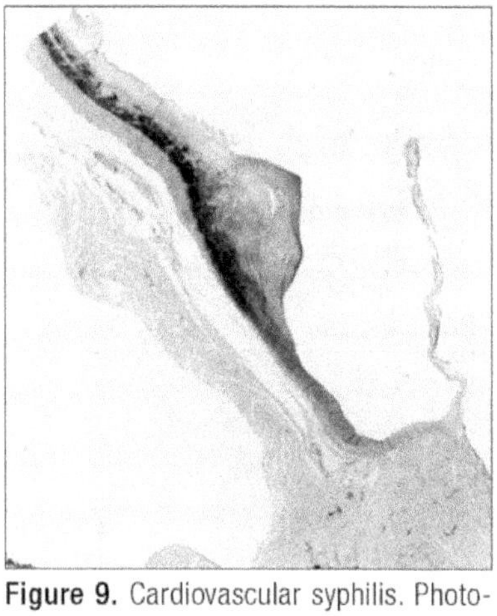

Figure 9. Cardiovascular syphilis. Photomicrographs of an aortic valve cusp, sinus portion of aorta (behind the cusp), and proximal tubular portion of ascending aorta, which is thickened by intimal and adventitial fibrous tissue. Many medial elastic fibers have been destroyed. The location of the process in the tubular portion of the aorta with sparing of the sinus portion of the aorta is characteristic of cardiovascular syphilis. Elastic tissue stain, ×4.5.

affecting primarily the aortic valve. Of 146 patients having pure AR and isolated aortic valve replacement, the cause of the AR was not determined after examination of the operatively excised aorta and aortic valve (25). Many of these patients had *systemic hypertension* but only mild dilation of the aorta, and all had normal or nearly normal three-cuspid aortic valves. It is likely that systemic hypertension in some way played a role in the AR (31, 32).

Aortic dissection usually produces acute AR due to the splitting of the aortic media behind the aortic valve commissures, resulting in prolapse of one or more cusps toward the left ventricular cavity (33).

Diffuse thickening of the tubular portion of the central ascending aorta with sparing of the aortic wall behind the sinuses is characteristic of *cardiovascular syphilis* (34). These patients generally undergo a cardiovascular operation because of diffuse aneurysmal dilatation of the tubular portion of ascending aorta, not as a rule because of severe AR. *Granulomatous (giant cell) aortitis* grossly mimics cardiovascular syphilis but is far less common. During the past 10 years, 15 patients have had resection of aneurysmally dilated syphilitic aortas with or without simultaneous aortic valve replacement at BUMC (unpublished). The characteristic histologic feature of cardiovascular syphilis is extensive thickening of the aortic wall due to fibrous thickening of the intima and adventitia *(Figure 9)*. The medial elastic fibers and smooth-muscle cells are also replaced focally by scars due to narrowings in the vasa vasora. Focal collections of plasma cells and lymphocytes are present in the adventitia. Giant cell aortitis is similar to syphilitic aortitis except for the presence of multinucleated giant cells.

The AR in patients with *the Marfan syndrome* and forme fruste varieties of it is the result of severe dilatation of the sinus portion and proximal tubular portion of the aorta (35). The consequence of the "aortic root" dilatation is stretching of the aortic valve cusps in roughly a straight line between the commissures, leading to a wide-open central regurgitant stream. In contrast to cardiovascular syphilis, the aortic wall in the Marfan syndrome is thinner than normal due to the massive loss of medial elastic fibers and lack of thickening of either the intima or the adventitia.

Ankylosing spondylitis causes AR by involving both the valve cusps and the portion of aorta behind and adjacent to the lateral attachments of the aortic valve cusps (36, 37). About 5% of patients with this form of arthritis develop AR. The bases of the aortic valve cusps become densely thickened by fibrous tissue, which is also present on the ventricular aspect of the anterior mitral leaflet and on the left ventricular aspect of the membranous ventricular septum. Varying degrees of heart block may result from this subaortic deposit of dense fibrous tissue. The AR associated with ankylosing spondylitis is usually severe, with diastolic pressures in both the aorta and the left ventricle often being similar. The histologic appearance of the aorta in ankylosing spondylitis is similar to that in syphilitis, but the syphilitic process never extends onto the aortic valve cusps or into the subvalvular area and rarely involves the wall of aorta behind the sinuses.

A diagram of the various conditions affecting the aortic valve is shown in *Figure 10*.

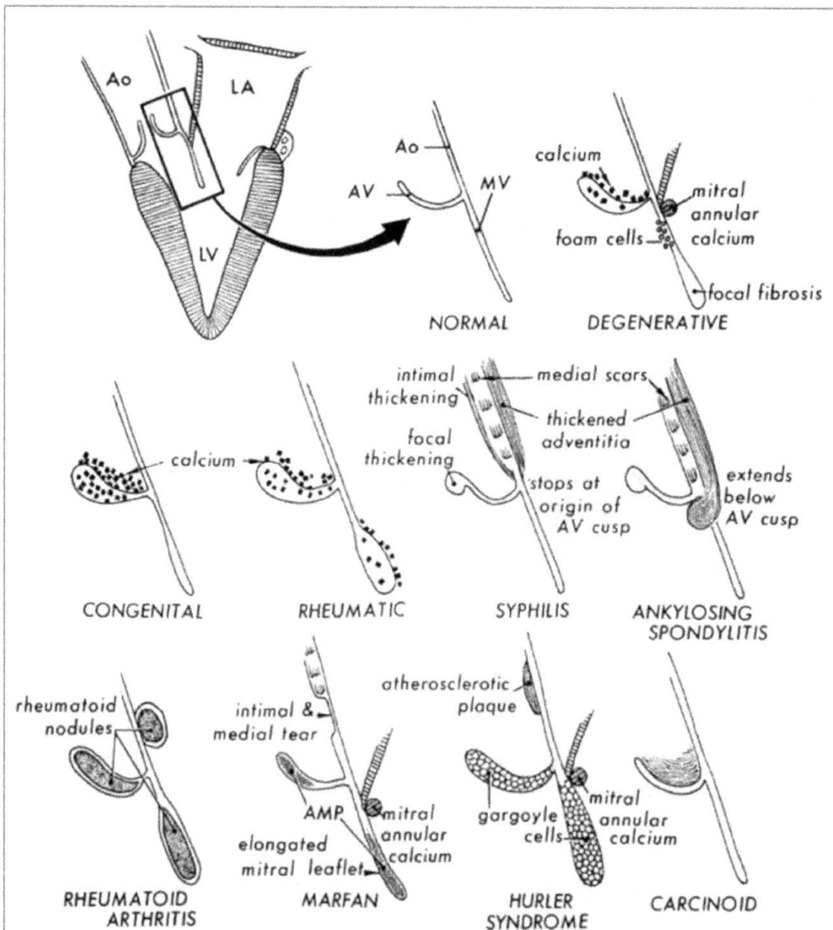

Figure 10. Some of the conditions affecting the aorta or aortic valve or mitral valve. Reproduced with permission from Roberts WC and Perloff JK, 1972 (38).

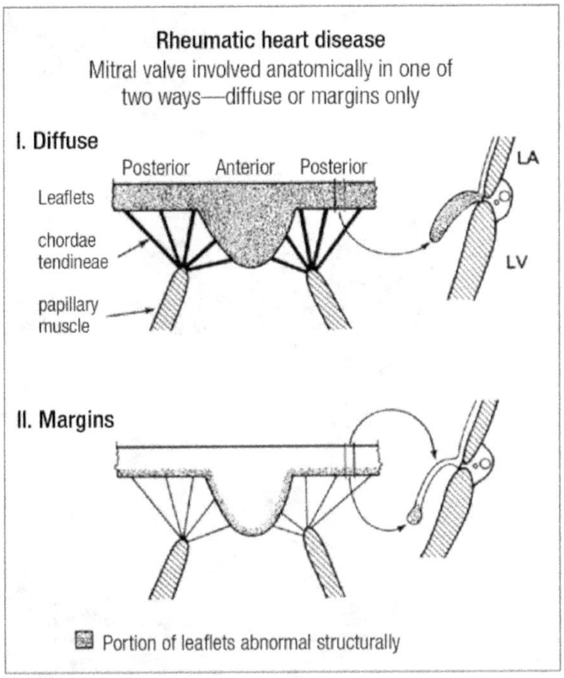

Figure 11. The two types of anatomic involvement of the mitral valve in rheumatic heart disease.

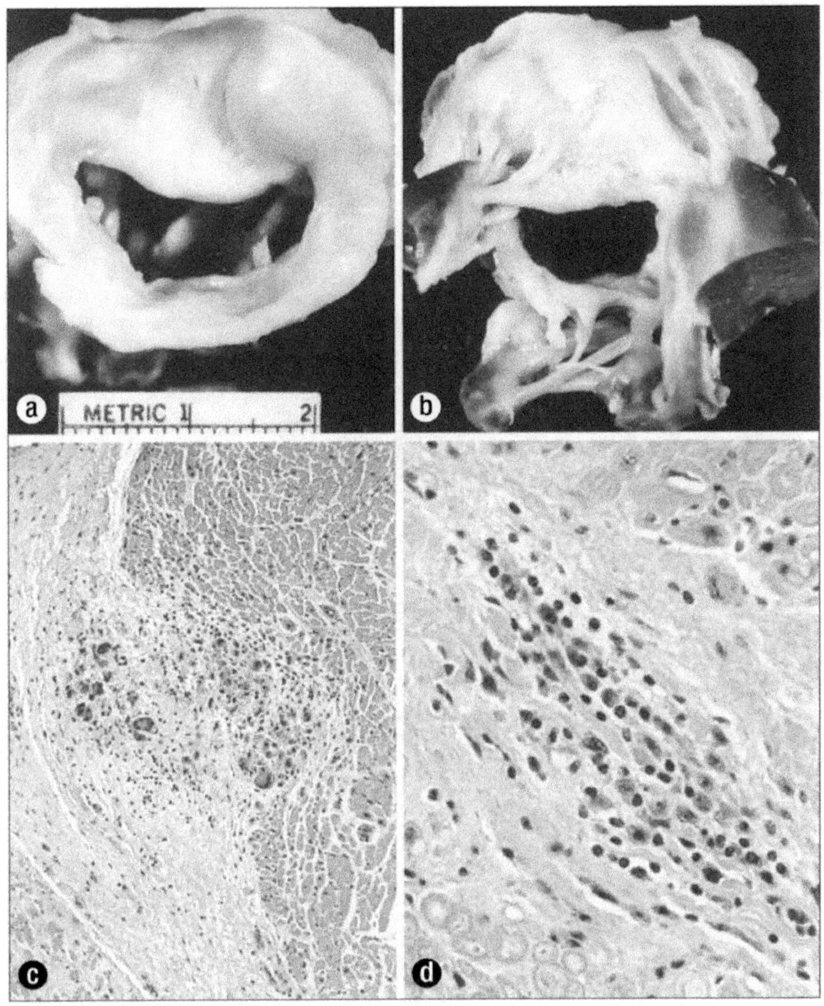

Figure 12. Acute rheumatic fever and mitral stenosis. Excised mitral valve in a 23-year-old Indian woman with mitral stenosis (13 mm Hg mean diastolic pressure gradient between pulmonary artery wedge and left ventricle) and regurgitation. She had had acute rheumatic fever initially at age 7 years and recurrence of migratory polyarthritis at age 22. During the early postoperative course after mitral valve replacement, she had swelling and pain in one knee and one ankle and erythema about two joints. Shown are the excised valves viewed from **(a)** the left atrium and **(b)** the left ventricle and **(c, d)** Aschoff bodies, which were numerous in both excised left ventricular papillary muscles. Hematoxylin and eosin stain, ×110 (c), ×400 (d). Reproduced with permission from Virmani R and Roberts WC, 1977 (41).

MITRAL STENOSIS

Of the 1010 patients aged ≥15 years with functionally severe valvular cardiac disease studied at necropsy by Roberts up to 1980, 434 (44%) had MS (1). MS occurred alone in 189 (44%) patients and in combination with other functional valve lesions in the other 245 patients (56%). MS was of rheumatic etiology in all 434 patients.

Rheumatic heart disease may be viewed as a disease of the mitral valve; other valves also may be involved both anatomically and functionally, but anatomically the mitral valve is always involved (38, 39) *(Figure 11). Aschoff bodies* have never been reported in hearts without anatomic disease of the mitral valve (39). Of the first 543 patients with severe valvular heart disease that Roberts and Virmani (40) studied at necropsy, 11 (2.7%) had Aschoff bodies, and all had anatomic mitral valve disease. The 11 patients ranged in age from 18 to 68 years (mean, 38), and 9 had a history of acute rheumatic fever; 9 had MS with or without dysfunction of one or more other cardiac valves; 1 had isolated AR; and 1 had both AR and MR. All 11 had diffuse fibrous thickening of the mitral leaflets, and all but one had diffuse anatomic lesions of at least two other cardiac valves. Thus, among patients with chronic valve disease, Aschoff bodies, the only anatomic lesion pathognomic of rheumatic heart disease, usually indicate diffuse anatomic lesions of one or more cardiac valves, and the most common hemodynamic lesion is MS ± MR.

Although rare at necropsy in patients with fatal chronic valve disease, Aschoff bodies are fairly common in the heart of patients having mitral commissurotomy for MS. Among 481 patients having various valve operations, Aschoff bodies were found by Virmani and Roberts (41) in 40 (21%) of 191 operatively excised left atrial appendages, in 4 (2%) of 273 operatively excised left ventricular papillary muscles, and in 1 (6%) of 17 patients in whom both appendage and papillary muscle were excised. Of these 45 patients with Aschoff bodies, 44 had MS *(Figure 12)* and only one, a 10-year-old boy, had pure MR. Sinus rhythm was present preoperatively in 38 (84%), and atrial fibrillation in 7 (16%).

Not only is rheumatic heart disease a disorder of the cardiac valves, it may also affect mural endocardium, epicardium, and myocardium. The atrial walls virtually always have increased amounts of fibrous tissue in both the myocardial interstitium and in the mural endocardium, atrophy of some and hypertrophy of other myocardial cells, and hypertrophy of smooth muscles in the mural endocardium. In all patients with rheumatic MS, the leaflets are diffusely thickened either by fibrous

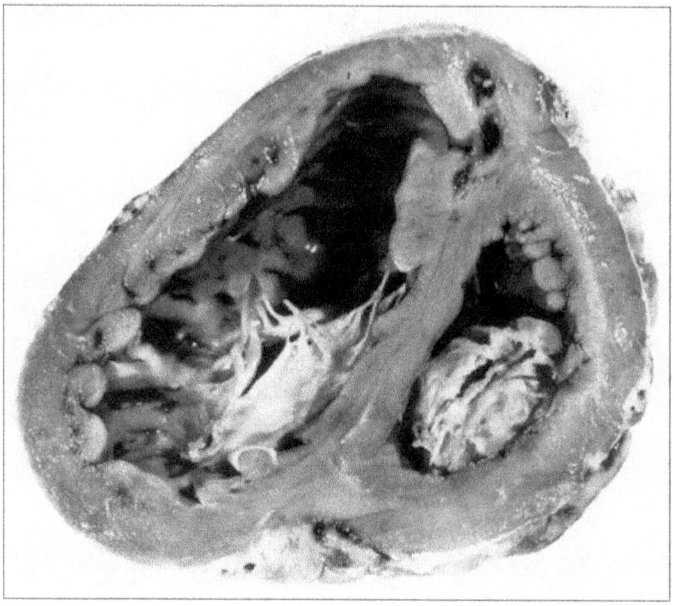

Figure 13. Mitral stenosis. Heart in a 16-year-old boy who had acute rheumatic fever at age 6 years and chronic heart failure beginning at age 10. He had severe mitral stenosis and tricuspid valve regurgitation. At cardiac catheterization 10 hours before death, the right ventricular pressure was 100/20 and the left ventricular pressure, 100/10 mm Hg. By left ventricular angiogram, the left ventricular cavity was of normal size and there was no mitral regurgitation. At necropsy, the heart weighed 450 g (patient weight, 43 kg). The right ventricular cavity was greatly dilated, and both ventricular walls were of similar thickness. Both mitral and tricuspid valve leaflets were diffusely thickened and free of calcific deposits. No Aschoff bodies were found. Reproduced with permission from Roberts WC, 1983 (39).

tissue or calcific deposits or both, the two commissures are usually fused, and the chordae tendineae are usually (but not always) thickened and fused *(Figures 13 and 14).*

The amount of calcium in the leaflets of stenotic mitral valves varies considerably *(Figure 15).* Generally, the calcific deposits are more frequent and in larger quantities in men than in women, in older than in younger patients, and in those with higher vs those with lower pressure gradients between the left atrium and left ventricle (Figure 14). The rapidity with which calcium develops also varies considerably: it is present at a younger age in men than in women. Lachman and Roberts (42) determined the presence or absence and the extent of calcific deposits in operatively excised stenotic mitral valves in 164 patients aged 26 to 72 years. The amount of calcific deposits in the stenotic mitral valves correlated with *sex* and the *mean transvalvular pressure gradient (Figure 16),* but it did not correlate with the patients' age (after 25 years), cardiac rhythm, pulmonary arterial or pulmonary arterial wedge pressure, previous mitral commissurotomy, presence of thrombus in the body or appendage of left ventricle, or the presence of disease in one or more other cardiac valves. Of the 164 patients, radiographs of the operatively excised valve showed no calcific deposits in 14 and only minimal deposits in 43. Of these 57 patients, however, 37 had moderate or severe MR. The remaining 20 in an earlier era would have been ideal or nearly ideal candidates for mitral commissurotomy (43).

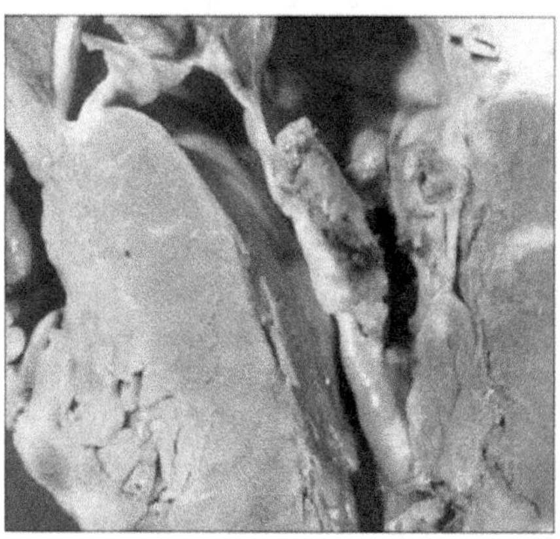

Figure 14. Mitral stenosis. Longitudinal view of a very narrow and thickened mitral valve in a 55-year-old man with equal peak systolic pressures in the right and left ventricles and no associated mitral regurgitation during cannulation of the aorta for planned mitral valve replacement. Both anterior and posterior mitral leaflets are heavily calcified. Reproduced with permission from Roberts WC, 1983 (39).

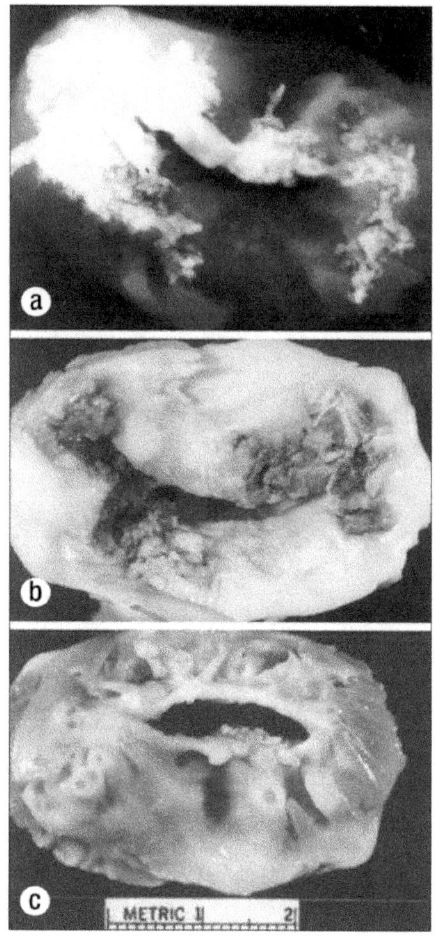

Figure 15. Mitral stenosis. Operatively excised heavily calcified stenotic mitral valve in a 57-year-old man with combined mitral stenosis (12 mm Hg mean transvalvular diastolic gradient) and aortic stenosis. **(a)** Radiograph of the excised valve. **(b)** View of valve from the left atrial aspect. Thrombi are present near and at the commissures. **(c)** View from the left ventricular aspect. The orifice is severely narrowed.

A major complication of MS is *thrombus formation in the left atrial cavity.* The thrombus may be limited to the atrial appendage (by far most common) or be located in both the appendage and body of the left atrium. Left atrial "body" thrombus was observed in 5% of the 1010 necropsy patients with fatal valvular heart disease studied by Roberts, and all had severe MS (unpublished data). Left atrial "body" thrombus was not found in any of the 165 patients with pure MR. All patients with left atrial "body" thrombus had atrial fibrillation. In contrast, of 46 patients with MS who had cardiotomy at the National Heart, Lung, and Blood Institute and had thrombus in the left atrial "body," 42 (91%) had atrial fibrillation and 4 (9%) had sinus rhythm. *Thrombus appears to occur in the body of the left atrium only in patients with MS, and atrial fibrillation in the absence of MS is incapable of forming thrombus in the left atrial body.*

Calcific deposits on the mural endocardium of the left atrium almost certainly are indicative of previous organization of left

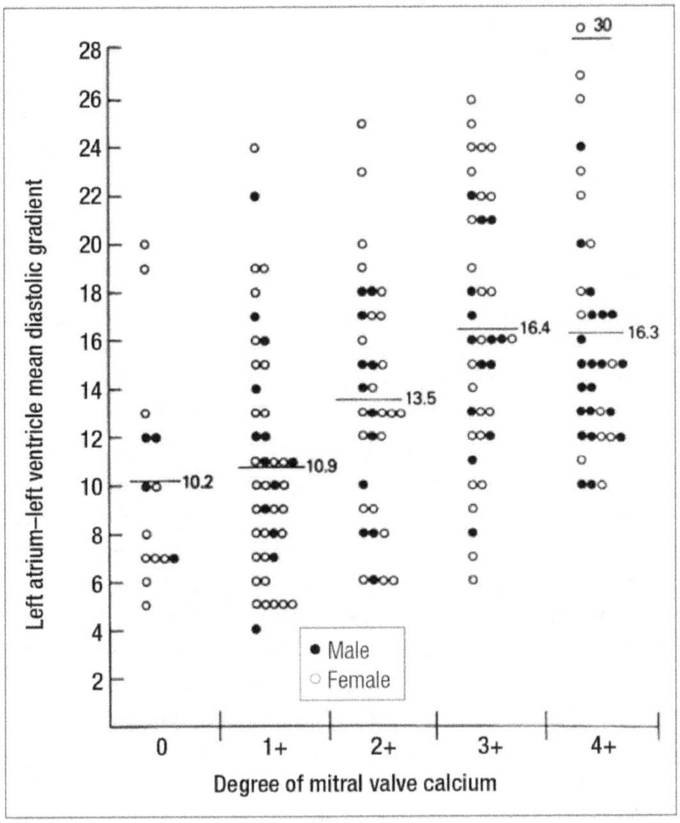

Figure 16. Mitral stenosis. Comparison of the relation of the mean left atrial–left ventricular diastolic gradient to the quantity of mitral valve calcium graded by radiograph of the operatively excised mitral valve. The greater the quantity of mitral calcium, the greater the transvalvular gradient. Reproduced with permission from Lachman AS and Roberts WC, 1978 (42).

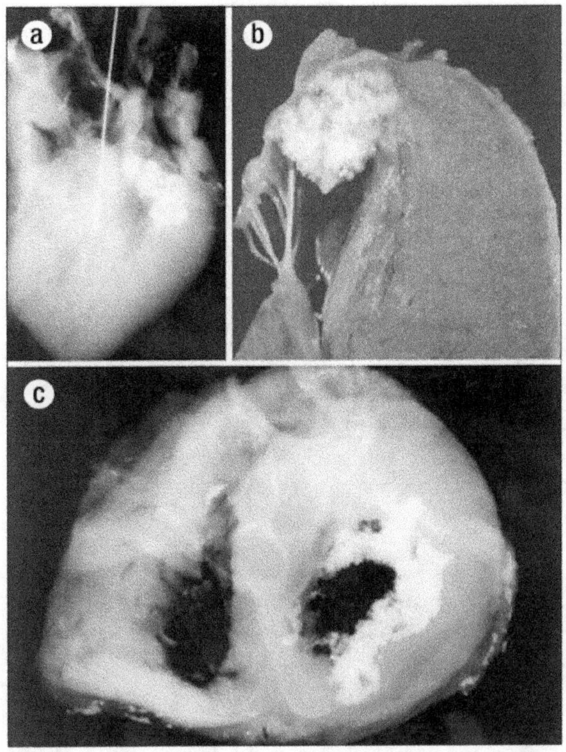

Figure 17. Mitral annular calcium. Heavily calcified mitral annulus in a 71-year-old woman with previous second-degree heart block and a pacemaker for 23 months. She died of acute myocardial infarction complicated by rupture of the left ventricular free wall. **(a)** Radiograph of the heart at necropsy showing mitral annular calcium and the pacemaker leads. **(b)** Longitudinal section showing heavy calcific deposits behind the posterior mitral leaflet. **(c)** Radiograph of the base of the heart (after removing its apical one-half) showing the circumferential extent of the mitral annular calcific deposits. Reproduced with permission from Roberts WC et al, 1973 (34).

atrial thrombi (44). Histologically, the "calcific thrombi" also contain cholesterol clefts and are identical to atherosclerotic plaques. The observation that left atrial thrombi can organize into lesions identical to atherosclerotic plaques supports the view that atherosclerotic plaques may in part be the result of organization of thrombi.

Nonrheumatic causes of MS include *congenital anomalies* (38, 39); *large mitral annular calcific deposits associated with left ventricular outflow obstruction* (45, 46) *(Figure 17); neoplasms* (particularly myxoma) protruding through the mitral orifice (47); *large vegetations from active infective endocarditis* (48); and of course a mechanical prosthesis or bioprosthesis used to replace a native mitral valve (49).

Histologic examination of sections of stenotic mitral valves when stained for elastic fibers shows the mitral leaflet to have lost most or all of its spongiosa element such that the leaflet itself consists entirely or nearly entirely of the fibrosa element. The leaflet (as are the chordae) is outlined by an elastic fibril (which stains black by an elastic tissue stain), and covering it on both atrial and ventricular aspects is dense fibrous tissue containing focally some vascular channels. Similar dense fibrous tissue surrounds the chordae, and the chordae themselves appear normal.

Patients with MS usually have distinct pulmonary vascular changes secondary to the pulmonary venous and arterial hypertension. These anatomic changes consist of thickening of the media of the muscular and elastic pulmonary arteries and focal intimal fibrous plaques. Plexiform lesions never occur in the lungs as a result of MS. The alveolar septa also thicken due to dilatation of the capillaries, proliferation of lining alveolar cells, and some increase of alveolar septal fibrous tissue.

PURE MITRAL REGURGITATION

Pure MR (no element of MS) is the most common dysfunctional cardiac valve disorder, and, in contrast to MS, it has many different causes. If patients with MR due to left ventricular dilatation from any cause (ischemic cardiomyopathy, idiopathic dilated cardiomyopathy, anemia, etc.) are excluded, the most common cause of MR treated operatively in the Western world today is *MVP (Figures 18 and 19)*. This condition, which was described initially in the 1960s by Barlow and colleagues (50) and by Criley and colleagues (51), is now recognized to occur in approximately 5% of adults, and, if one considers this condition a congenital deficiency of mitral tissues—which we do—it is the most common congenital cardiovascular disease. Among 97 patients having mitral valve replacement for pure MR from 1968 to 1981 at the National Heart, Lung, and Blood Institute, MVP was responsible in 60 patients (62%), papillary muscle dysfunction from coronary heart disease in 29 (30%), infective endocarditis in 5 (5%), and possibly rheumatic disease in 3 (3%) (52).

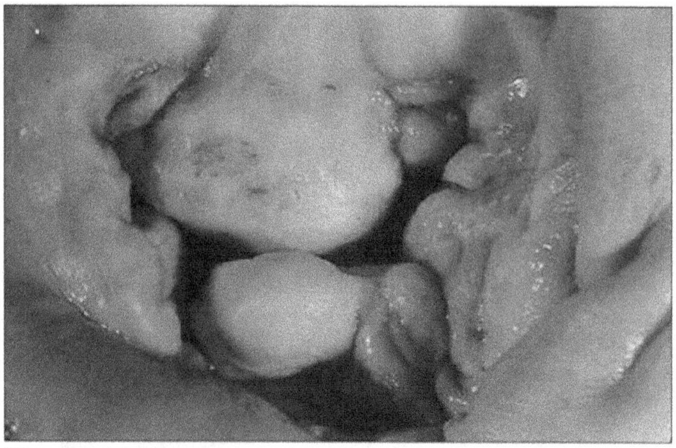

Figure 18. Mitral valve prolapse. View from above shows prolapse of both anterior and posterior cusps in a man who died from consequences of an acute myocardial infarction.

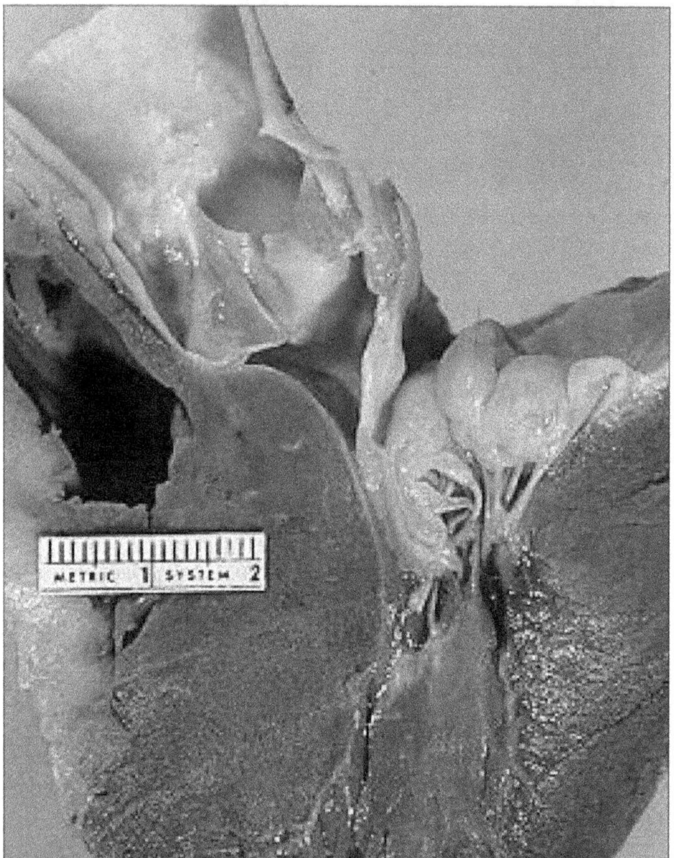

Figure 19. Mitral valve prolapse. View of prolapsed posterior leaflet in a 74-year-old woman who during life was found to have a precordial murmur but never had symptoms of cardiac dysfunction.

Although several authors have attempted to do so, defining MVP has not been easy (1). The following have proved useful in separating the valve affected by MVP from mitral valves affected by other conditions:

1. *Focal lengthening of the posterior and/or anterior mitral leaflets from their site of attachment to their distal margins.* Normally, the length of the posterior leaflet from its attachment to distal margin is about 1 cm. In MVP, this leaflet focally is often as long as the anterior leaflet (52).
2. *Elongation and thinning of chordae tendineae.*
3. *Focal thickening of the posterior and/or anterior leaflet.* This finding is particularly prominent on the portion of leaflet that prolapses toward or into the left atrium during ventricular systole. The atrial surface is uniformly smooth. The thickening of the leaflet produces a spongy feel.
4. *Increase in area, either focally or diffusely, of one or both mitral leaflets* (52).
5. *Loss of chordae tendineae on the ventricular aspect of the posterior mitral leaflet.* It is rare to actually see a ruptured chorda, but what is seen are areas where chordae should be attached but none are there. They presumably ruptured in the past and with time were matted down on the leaflets' ventricular aspect, giving this surface a "bumpy" appearance and feel. Chordae are nearly uniformly missing (previously ruptured) in portions of posterior mitral leaflet excised during mitral valve repair or during replacement. Indeed, MVP appears to be by far the most common cause of ruptured chordae tendineae. Infective endocarditis is the next most frequent cause (53).
6. *Dilatation of the mitral annulus.* Annular dilatation is probably the major cause of development of severe MR in the presence of MVP (52, 54). (The other is rupture of chordae tendineae.) Normally, the mitral annulus in adults averages about 9 cm in circumference. In patients with left ventricular dilatation from any cause, with or without MR, the mitral circumference usually dilates slightly, usually to about 11 cm or <25% above normal (55). Among patients with MVP associated with severe MR, this annular circumference generally increases >50% to 12 to 18 cm. Acute rupture of chordae tendineae may occur in patients with MVP in the absence of mitral annular dilatation.
7. *An increase in the transverse dimension of the mitral leaflets such that the length of the mitral circumference measured on a line corresponding to the distal margin of the posterior leaflet is much larger than the circumference measured at the level of the mitral annulus* (52). In the normal mitral valve, the two are the same. It is analogous to a skirt gathered at the waist. The leaflets of the opened normal mitral valve are flat or smooth on the atrial aspect (like the mucosa of the ileum) whereas those of the opened floppy mitral valve are undulating (like those of the duodenum or jejunum).
8. *Focal thickening of mural endocardium of the left ventricle behind the posterior mitral leaflet.* Salazar and Edwards (56) called these fibrous thickenings "friction lesions" to indicate that they are believed to result from friction between the overlying leaflets and chordae and the underlying left ventricular wall. Lucas and Edwards (57) observed these "friction lesions" in 77 (75%) of 102 necropsy cases of MVP, and Dollar and Roberts (58) found them in 23 (68%) of 34 necropsy cases of MVP.
9. *Fibrinous deposits on the atrial surface of the prolapsed portion of mitral leaflet and particularly at the angle formed between the prolapsed leaflet and left atrial wall* (mitral valve–left atrial angle). These fibrin deposits may be a source of emboli.

Histologically, the MVP valve is distinctive. Elastic tissue stains reveal that the mitral leaflet and chordae are surrounded by a single thick elastic fibril. The underlying leaflet generally—

Table 9. Reported necropsy cases of mitral valve prolapse

First author, year (reference)	Number with MVP	Age (years)	Male/female	MVP cause of death	No. of mitral leaflets prolapsed 1/2	MR	RCT	IE	SD	MS	ASD*	MAC	HW increased	DMA
Pomerance, 1969 (60)	35†	51–98 (mean 74)	23/12	4	12/23	8	2‡	2	1	0	1	9	13	–
Davies, 1978 (61)	90§	<40–100	44/46	6	69/21	23	–	9	13	0	0	3	8‖	6
Lucas, 1982 (57)	102¶	69 ± 12	62/40	4	34/68	18	7‡	7	0	1	3	–	–	–
Lucas, 1982 (57)	69**	–	–	–	–	–	19‡	7	16	20	9	–	–	–
Dollar, 1991 (58)	56**	16–70 (mean 48)	33/23	29	50/6	32	18‡	0	15	2	4	12	30††	40

*Secundum type atrial septal defect.
†Thirty cases from a single hospital (1% of autopsies).
‡Unassociated with infective endocarditis.
§Cases acquired from four different hospitals (4.5% of autopsies).
‖Heart weight >300 g.
¶Cases seen in a single community hospital (7% of autopsies).
**Cases "whose hearts had been sent to Edwards or Roberts for his opinion and interest."
††Heart weight >350 g in women and >400 g in men.
ASD indicates atrial septal defect; DMA, dilated mitral annulus; HW, heart weight; IE, infective endocarditis; MAC, mitral annular calcium; MR, mitral regurgitation; MS, the Marfan syndrome; MVP, mitral valve prolapse; RCT, ruptured chordae tendineae; SD, sudden death; –, no information available.

but not always—contains an excessive amount of the spongiosa element, and this causes the leaflet itself to be a bit thicker than normal. Most of the leaflet thickening, however, is due to superimposed fibrous tissue on both its atrial and ventricular aspects. The covering on the atrial side of the leaflet contains numerous elastic fibrils, whereas that on the ventricular aspect contains few or no elastic fibrils. Often on the ventricular aspect, previously ruptured and now "matted" chordae tendineae are covered by fibrous tissue. The spongiosa element within the leaflet itself appears normal—just increased in amount—and therefore the phrase "mucoid degeneration" appears inappropriate.

Ultrastructural studies of mitral valves grossly characteristic of MVP have disclosed alterations of the collagen fibers in the leaflets and in the chordae tendineae (59). These changes have included fragmentation, splitting, swelling, and course granularity of the individual collagen fibers, and also spiraling and twisting of the fibers. These alterations in the structure of the collagen are probably far more important than the excess acid mucopolysaccharide material in the leaflet in that they lead to focal weakness of the leaflets and chordae and their subsequent elongation. The left ventricular systolic pressure exerted against these weakened areas may account for the prolapse.

Just as the frequency of MVP varies clinically depending on the age and sex group being examined and in the clinical criteria employed for diagnosis (auscultatory, echocardiographic, angiographic), its frequency at necropsy is quite variable and the variation is determined by several factors: 1) age and sex group of the population being examined; 2) type of institution where necropsy is performed (general hospital, referral hospital for cardiovascular disease, or medical examiner's [coroner's] office); 3) expertise in cardiovascular disease of the physician performing the necropsy or reporting the findings; 4) percentage of total deaths having autopsies at the particular hospital; 5) presence or absence of evidence of cardiac disease before death; 6) whether the patient underwent mitral valve replacement or repair; and 7) whether the percentage of patients being examined had a high frequency of the Marfan syndrome, infective endocarditis, atrial septal defect, and so on.

No study shows better how bias alters the finding in necropsy studies than the one performed by Lucas and Edwards *(Table 9)* (57). These investigators, in one portion of their study, determined the frequency of and complications of floppy mitral valves observed at necropsy in one community (nonreferral) hospital for adults. Of 1376 autopsies performed, 7% or 102 patients had morphologically floppy mitral valves at necropsy. Their mean age at death was 69 ± 12 years; 62 (61%) were men and 40 (39%) were women. Of the 102 patients, MVP was the cause of death in only four. Of the 102 patients, one leaflet had prolapsed in 34 patients and two leaflets in 68. Only 18 had anatomic evidence of previous MR; 7 had infective endocarditis; 7 had ruptured chordae tendineae (without infection); 1 had the Marfan syndrome; and 3 had secundum atrial septal defect. No patient died suddenly. In contrast, in the other portion of their study, these authors described complications in 69 necropsy patients whose hearts had been sent to Edwards for his opinion and interest. Among these 69 patients, 16 (23%) had died suddenly and unexpectedly; 19 (28%) had ruptured chordae tendineae (without infection); 7 (10%) had infective endocarditis; 20 (29%) had the Marfan syndrome; and 9 (13%) had secundum-type atrial septal defect. Thus, in contrast to their infrequency in their community hospital series, most cases submitted to their cardiovascular registry from other institutions had ruptured chordae, infective endocarditis, sudden unexpected and unexplained death, or the Marfan syndrome.

The earlier studies by Pomerance (60) and by Davies and colleagues (61) can also be compared to the community hospital series of Lucas and Edwards (57) *(Table 9)*. The study by

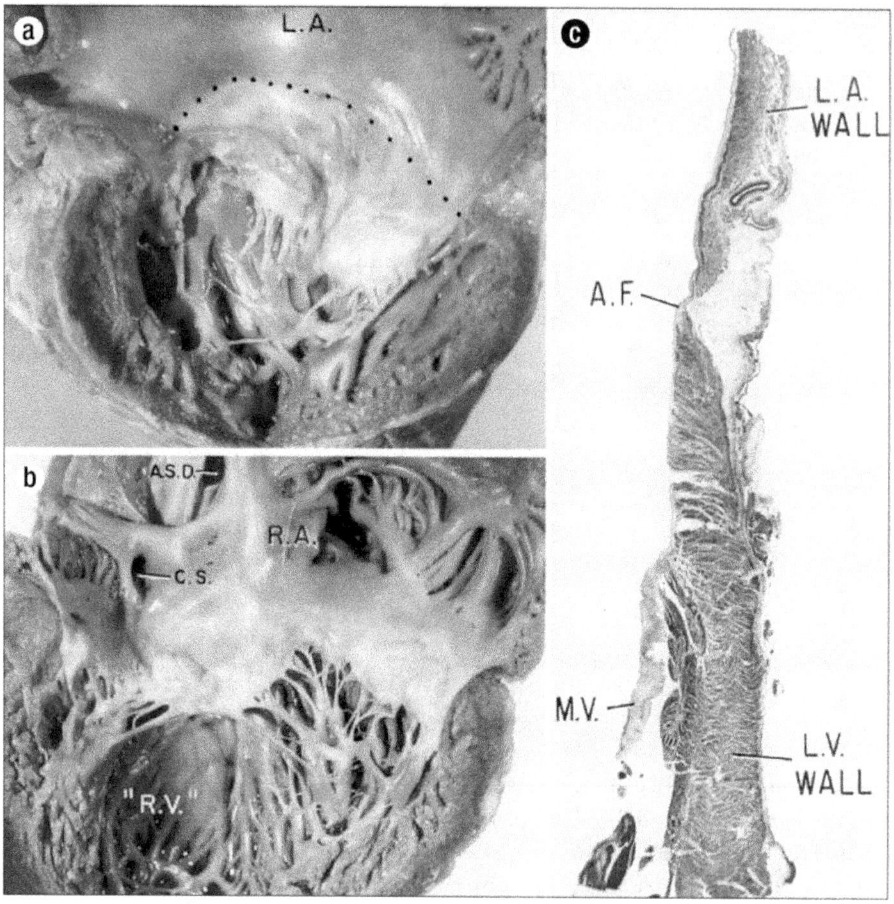

Figure 20. Corrected transposition of the great arteries and Ebstein's anomaly of the left-sided atrioventricular valve in a 38-year-old woman who was cyanotic from birth and in heart failure periodically all of her life. She also had severe pulmonic valve stenosis and ventricular septal defect. She died shortly after operative insertion of a conduit between the left subclavian and left main pulmonary arteries. **(a)** Opened left atrium (LA) and anatomic right ventricle. The normal annulus is shown by the dotted line. **(b)** Opened right atrium (RA) and anatomic left ventricle (RV). ASD indicates atrial septal defect; CS, ostium of coronary sinus. **(c)** Histologic section of left atrial and left ventricular (LV) walls showing the normal annulus fibrosis (AF) and insertion of the mitral valve (MV) considerably caudal to the annulus and directly across from the ventricular wall. Verhoeff-von Gieson stain, ×4. Reproduced with permission from Berry WB et al, 1964 (67).

Dollar and Roberts (58) is comparable to the study of Lucas and Edwards and their selected cases. These authors studied at necropsy 56 patients, aged 16 to 70 years (mean, 48), and compared findings in the 15 who died suddenly and unexpectedly with the other 41 who did not. Compared with the 34 patients without associated congenital heart disease and with non-MVP conditions capable in themselves of being fatal, the 15 patients who died suddenly with isolated MVP were younger (mean age, 39 vs 52 years), were more often women (67% vs 26%), had a lower frequency of MR (7% vs 38%), and were less likely to have ruptured chordae tendineae (29% vs 67%).

The frequency of atrial fibrillation is different in patients with MVP and those with MS immediately before a mitral valve replacement or "repair." Among 246 patients aged 21 to 84 years (mean, 61; men, 66%) who had mitral valve repair or replacement for MR secondary to MVP, Berbarie and Roberts (62) found only 37 patients (15%) (mean age, 60) with atrial fibrillation and 209 patients (88%) with sinus rhythm. In contrast, of 104 patients aged 33 to 80 years (12% men) with rheumatic MS severe enough or symptomatic enough to warrant mitral valve replacement, Sims and Roberts (63) found atrial fibrillation by electrocardiogram immediately preoperatively in 47 (45%) and sinus rhythm in 57 (55%).

Other causes of pure mitral regurgitation

Cleft anterior mitral leaflet. Partial atrioventricular "defect" includes a spectrum of five anatomic anomalies (64). Some patients have all five and others have only one or two. The five are the following: 1) defect in the lowermost portion of the atrial septum, so-called primum atrial septal defect; 2) defect in, or absence of, the posterobasal portion of the ventricular septum; 3) cleft anterior mitral leaflet; 4) anomalous chordae tendineae from the anterior mitral leaflet to the crest of the ventricular septum; and 5) partial or complete absence of the septal tricuspid valve leaflet. There are at least four potential functional consequences of these five anatomic anomalies: 1) shunt at the atrial level, 2) shunt at the ventricular level, 3) MR, and 4) obstruction to left ventricular outflow. Well over 95% of patients with partial atrioventricular defect have a primum-type atrial septal defect, and most of those without a primum defect have a shunt at the ventricular level. The occurrence of MR from a cleft in the anterior mitral leaflet unassociated with a defect in either atrial or ventricular septa is rare, but such has been the case in several reported patients (65).

Left-sided atrioventricular valve regurgitation associated with corrected transposition of the great arteries. Corrected transposition is an entity that has produced much confusion (66, 67). Corrected transposition and complete transposition are quite different; the only thing they have in common is the word "transposition." Complete transposition is essentially one defect: the great arteries are transposed, so that the aorta arises from the right ventricle and the pulmonary trunk from the left ventricle. In corrected transposition, the great arteries also are transposed, but in addition, the ventricles, atrioventricular valves, epicardial coronary arteries, and conduction system are inverted. Patients with complete transposition die because they have inadequate communications between the two circuits. Patients with corrected transposition theoretically should be able to live a full lifespan, but usually this is not the case because associated defects—namely, ventricular septal defect or regurgitation of the left-sided atrioventricular valve or both—cause the heart to function abnormally. The left-sided valve anatomically is a tricuspid valve (in the case of the situs solitus heart), and its most frequent abnormality is the Ebstein-type abnormality *(Figure 20)*. Although most patients with corrected transpo-

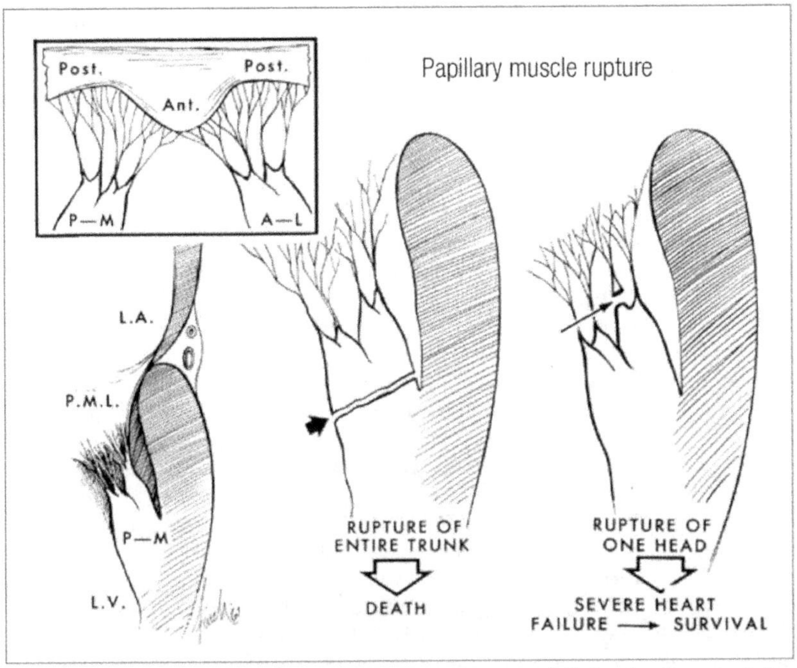

Figure 21. Papillary muscle rupture secondary to acute myocardial infarction. Representation of the possible consequences of papillary muscle rupture during acute myocardial infarction. Rupture of the entire trunk is incompatible with survival (left). With rupture of an apical "head" (right), survival depends on the extent to which function of the left ventricle has been impaired by the infarct. With severely impaired left ventricular function, the additional burden of even modest MR may be intolerable. If the left ventricle is less severely compromised, survival is possible for weeks or months, but heart failure will almost invariably develop. Modified with permission from Morrow AG et al, 1968 (72).

sition present with excessive pulmonary blood flow because of the left-to-right shunt via the ventricular septal defect, an occasional patient with corrected transposition has no defect in the cardiac septa and has evidence of pure "MR," occasionally mistaken for other causes of MR (68).

Infective endocarditis. The most common cardiac valve affected by infective endocarditis is the aortic valve, and the mitral valve is most commonly affected by vegetations growing down the anterior mitral leaflet from the regurgitant aortic valve causing mitral leaflet damage and chordal rupture (69, 70). Infection isolated to the mitral valve is far less common, and when this situation occurs the vegetations are on the atrial aspects of the mitral leaflets (71).

Coronary heart disease. The MR in patients with coronary heart disease is due to myocardial infarction, which may acutely cause necrosis of one or more left ventricular papillary muscles (usually the posteromedial one) with or without rupture of the entire muscle or, far more commonly, rupture of a portion of the "tip" of the papillary muscle (38, 72, 73) *(Figure 21).* Rupture, either partial or complete, of a papillary muscle during acute myocardial infarction is a far less common cause of acute MR than is necrosis of a papillary muscle and the free wall beneath it. When it occurs late after acute myocardial infarction, the MR is usually the result of dilatation of the left ventricular cavity and severe scarring of a papillary muscle, which tends to pull the mitral leaflets laterally, preventing proper coaptation of the two mitral leaflets during ventricular systole.

Cardiomyopathy. Most patients with idiopathic dilated cardiomyopathy (74), ischemic cardiomyopathy (75, 76), and hypertrophic cardiomyopathy (77) have MR at some time in their course. The first two conditions of course are associated with dilatation of the left ventricular cavity primarily in a lateral or right-to-left direction—not in a caudal-cephalad direction—and the consequence is abnormal papillary muscle "pull" on the mitral leaflets during ventricular systole with resulting incomplete coaptation of the mitral leaflets. Evidence that mitral annular dilatation is the prime cause of MR in patients with dilated cardiomyopathy is lacking (55). The cause of MR in patients with hypertrophic cardiomyopathy is entirely different from that in patients with dilated cardiomyopathy and results at least in part in anterior movement of the anterior mitral leaflet toward the ventricular septum during ventricular systole (77). Patients with chronic anemia, e.g., sickle cell anemia, usually also have MR from papillary muscle fibrosis and left ventricular cavity dilatation (78).

1. Roberts WC. Congenital cardiovascular abnormalities usually silent until adulthood. In Roberts WC, ed. *Adult Congenital Heart Disease.* Philadelphia: FA Davis, 1987:631–691.
2. Sprecher DL, Schaefer EJ, Kent KM, Gregg RE, Zech LA, Hoeg JM, McManus B, Roberts WC, Brewer HB Jr. Cardiovascular features of homozygous familial hypercholesterolemia: analysis of 16 patients. *Am J Cardiol* 1984;54(1):20–30.
3. Moura LM, Ramos SF, Zamorano JL, Barros IM, Azevedo LF, Rocha-Gonçalves F, Rajamannan NM. Rosuvastatin affecting aortic valve endothelium to slow the progression of aortic stenosis. *J Am Coll Cardiol* 2007;49(5):554–561.
4. Roberts WC, Perloff JK, Costantino T. Severe valvular aortic stenosis in patients over 65 years of age. A clinicopathologic study. *Am J Cardiol* 1971;27(5):497–506.
5. Stephan PJ, Henry AC 3rd, Hebeler RF Jr, Whiddon L, Roberts WC. Comparison of age, gender, number of aortic valve cusps, concomitant coronary artery bypass grafting, and magnitude of left ventricular-systemic arterial peak systolic gradient in adults having aortic valve replacement for isolated aortic valve stenosis. *Am J Cardiol* 1997;79(2):166–172.
6. Roberts WC, Morrow AG. Congenital aortic stenosis produced by a unicommissural valve. *Br Heart J* 1965;27:505–510.
7. Falcone MW, Roberts WC, Morrow AG, Perloff JK. Congenital aortic stenosis resulting from a unicommissural valve. Clinical and anatomic features in twenty-one adult patients. *Circulation* 1971;44(2):272–280.
8. Roberts WC. The congenitally bicuspid aortic valve. A study of 85 autopsy cases. *Am J Cardiol* 1970;26(1):72–83.
9. Roberts WC. Anatomically isolated aortic valvular disease. The case against its being of rheumatic etiology. *Am J Med* 1970;49(2):151–159.
10. Roberts WC, Ko JM. Clinical and morphologic features of the congenitally unicuspid acommissural stenotic and regurgitant aortic valve. *Cardiology* 2007;108(2):79–81.
11. Roberts WC. The senile cardiac calcification syndrome. *Am J Cardiol* 1986;58(6):572–574.
12. Hurwitz LE, Roberts WC. Quadricuspid semilunar valve. *Am J Cardiol* 1973;31(5):623–626.
13. Roberts WC, Ko JM, Filardo G, Henry AC, Hebeler RF Jr, Cheung EH, Matter GJ, Hamman BL. Valve structure and survival in *sexagenarians* having aortic valve replacement for aortic stenosis (± aortic regurgitation) with versus without coronary artery bypass grafting at a single US medical center (1993 to 2005). *Am J Cardiol* 2007;100(8):1286–1292.

14. Roberts WC, Ko JM. Weights of operatively-excised stenotic unicuspid, bicuspid, and tricuspid aortic valves and their relation to age, sex, body mass index, and presence or absence of concomitant coronary artery bypass grafting. *Am J Cardiol* 2003;92(9):1057–1065.
15. Roberts WC, Ko JM. Weights of individual cusps in operatively-excised congenitally bicuspid stenotic aortic valves. *Am J Cardiol* 2004;94(5):678–681.
16. Roberts WC, Ko JM. Weights of individual cusps in operatively-excised stenotic three-cuspid aortic valves. *Am J Cardiol* 2004;94(5):681–684.
17. Roberts WC, Ko JM. Relation of weights of operatively excised stenotic aortic valves to preoperative transvalvular peak systolic pressure gradients and to calculated aortic valve areas. *J Am Coll Cardiol* 2004;44(9):1847–1855.
18. Roberts WC, Ko JM. Frequency by decades of unicuspid, bicuspid, and tricuspid aortic valves in adults having isolated aortic valve replacement for aortic stenosis, with or without associated aortic regurgitation. *Circulation* 2005;111(7):920–925.
19. Roberts WC, Ko JM, Matter GJ. Isolated aortic valve replacement without coronary bypass for aortic valve stenosis involving a congenitally bicuspid aortic valve in a nonagenarian. *Am J Geriatr Cardiol* 2006;15(6):389–391.
20. Roberts WC, Ko JM, Garner WL, Filardo G, Henry AC, Hebeler RF Jr, Matter GJ, Hamman BL. Valve structure and survival in *octogenarians* having aortic valve replacement for aortic stenosis (± aortic regurgitation) with versus without coronary artery bypass grafting at a single US medical center (1993 to 2005). *Am J Cardiol* 2007;100(3):489–495.
21. Roberts WC, Ko JM, Filardo G, Henry AC, Hebeler RF Jr, Cheung EH, Matter GJ, Hamman BL. Valve structure and survival in *septuagenarians* having aortic valve replacement for aortic stenosis (± aortic regurgitation) with versus without coronary artery bypass grafting at a single US medical center (1993 to 2005). *Am J Cardiol* 2007;100(7):1157–1165.
22. Roberts WC, Ko JM, Hamilton C. Comparison of valve structure, valve weight, and severity of the valve obstruction in 1849 patients having isolated aortic valve replacement for aortic valve stenosis (with or without associated aortic regurgitation) studied at 3 different medical centers in 2 different time periods. *Circulation* 2005;112(25):3919–3929.
23. Roberts WC, Ko JM, Filardo G, Henry AC, Hebeler RF Jr, Cheung EH, Matter GJ, Hamman BL. Valve structure and survival in *quinquagenarians* having aortic valve replacement for aortic stenosis (± aortic regurgitation) with versus without coronary artery bypass grafting at a single US medical center (1993 to 2005). *Am J Cardiol* 2007;100(10):1584–1591.
24. Roberts WC, Ko JM, Filardo G, Kitchens BL, Henry AC, Hebeler RF Jr, Cheung EH, Matter GJ, Hamman BL. Valve structure and survival in *quadragenarians* having aortic valve replacement for aortic stenosis (± aortic regurgitation) with versus without coronary artery bypass grafting at a single US medical center (1993 to 2005). *Am J Cardiol* 2007;100(11):1683–1690.
25. Roberts WC, Ko JM, Moore TR, Jones WH 3rd. Causes of pure aortic regurgitation in patients having isolated aortic valve replacement at a single US tertiary hospital (1993 to 2005). *Circulation* 2006;114(5):422–429.
26. Roberts WC. The structure of the aortic valve in clinically isolated aortic stenosis: an autopsy study of 162 patients over 15 years of age. *Circulation* 1970;42(1):91–97.
27. Roberts WC, Morrow AG, McIntosh CL, Jones M, Epstein SE. Congenitally bicuspid aortic valve causing severe, pure aortic regurgitation without superimposed infective endocarditis. Analysis of 13 patients requiring aortic valve replacement. *Am J Cardiol* 1981;47(2):206–209.
28. Roberts WC, Oluwole BO, Fernicola DJ. Comparison of active infective endocarditis involving a previously stenotic versus a previously nonstenotic aortic valve. *Am J Cardiol* 1993;71(12):1082–1088.
29. Carpenter DF, Golden A, Roberts WC. Quadrivalvular rheumatoid heart disease associated with left bundle branch block. *Am J Med* 1967;43(6):922–929.
30. Roberts WC, Kehoe JA, Carpenter DF, Golden A. Cardiac valvular lesions in rheumatoid arthritis. *Arch Intern Med* 1968;122(2):141–146.
31. Waller BF, Zoltick JM, Rosen JH, Katz NM, Gomes MN, Fletcher RD, Wallace RB, Roberts WC. Severe aortic regurgitation from systemic hypertension (without aortic dissection) requiring aortic valve replacement: analysis of four patients. *Am J Cardiol* 1982;49(2):473–477.
32. Waller BF, Kishel JC, Roberts WC. Severe aortic regurgitation from systemic hypertension. *Chest* 1982;82(3):365–368.
33. Roberts WC. Aortic dissection: anatomy, consequences, and causes. *Am Heart J* 1981;101(2):195–214.
34. Roberts WC, Dangel JC, Bulkley BH. Nonrheumatic valvular cardiac disease: a clinicopathologic survey of 27 different conditions causing valvular dysfunction. *Cardiovasc Clin* 1973;5(2):333–446.
35. Roberts WC, Honig HS. The spectrum of cardiovascular disease in the Marfan syndrome: a clinico-morphologic study of 18 necropsy patients and comparison to 151 previously reported necropsy patients. *Am Heart J* 1982;104(1):115–135.
36. Bulkley BH, Roberts WC. Ankylosing spondylitis and aortic regurgitation. Description of the characteristic cardiovascular lesion from study of eight necropsy patients. *Circulation* 1973;48(5):1014–1027.
37. Roberts WC, Hollingsworth JF, Bulkley BH, Jaffe RB, Epstein SE, Stinson EB. Combined mitral and aortic regurgitation in ankylosing spondylitis. Angiographic and anatomic features. *Am J Med* 1974;56(2):237–243.
38. Roberts WC, Perloff JK. Mitral valvular disease. A clinicopathologic survey of the conditions causing the mitral valve to function abnormally. *Ann Intern Med* 1972;77(6):939–975.
39. Roberts WC. Morphologic features of the normal and abnormal mitral valve. *Am J Cardiol* 1983;51(6):1005–1028.
40. Roberts WC, Virmani R. Aschoff bodies at necropsy in valvular heart disease. Evidence from an analysis of 543 patients over 14 years of age that rheumatic heart disease, at least anatomically, is a disease of the mitral valve. *Circulation* 1978;57(4):803–807.
41. Virmani R, Roberts WC. Aschoff bodies in operatively excised atrial appendages and in papillary muscles. Frequency and clinical significance. *Circulation* 1977;55(4):559–563.
42. Lachman AS, Roberts WC. Calcific deposits in stenotic mitral valves. Extent and relation to age, sex, degree of stenosis, cardiac rhythm, previous commissurotomy and left atrial body thrombus from study of 164 operatively-excised valves. *Circulation* 1978;57(4):808–815.
43. Roberts WC, Lachman AS. Mitral valve commissurotomy versus replacement. Considerations based on examination of operatively excised stenotic mitral valves. *Am Heart J* 1979;98(1):56–62.
44. Roberts WC, Humphries JO, Morrow AG. Giant right atrium in rheumatic mitral stenosis. Atrial enlargement restricted by mural calcification. *Am Heart J* 1970;79(1):28–35.
45. Hammer WJ, Roberts WC, deLeon AC. "Mitral stenosis" secondary to combined "massive" mitral anular calcific deposits and small, hypertrophied left ventricles. Hemodynamic documentation in four patients. *Am J Med* 1978;64(3):371–376.
46. Theleman KP, Grayburn PA, Roberts WC. Mitral "annular" calcium forming a complete circle "O" causing mitral stenosis in association with a stenotic congenitally bicuspid aortic valve and severe coronary artery disease. *Am J Geriatr Cardiol* 2006;15(1):58–61.
47. Roberts WC. Neoplasms involving the heart, their simulators, and adverse consequences of their therapy. *Proc (Bayl Univ Med Cent)* 2001;14(4):358–376.
48. Roberts WC, Ewy GA, Glancy DL, Marcus FI. Valvular stenosis produced by active infective endocarditis. *Circulation* 1967;36(3):449–451.
49. Roberts WC, Bulkley BH, Morrow AG. Pathologic anatomy of cardiac valve replacement: a study of 224 necropsy patients. *Prog Cardiovasc Dis* 1973;15(6):539–587.
50. Barlow JB, Pocock WA, Marchand P, Denny M. The significance of late systolic murmurs. *Am Heart J* 1963;66:443–452.
51. Criley JM, Lewis KB, Humphries JO, Ross RS. Prolapse of the mitral valve: clinical and cine-angiocardiographic findings. *Br Heart J* 1966;28(4):488-496.
52. Waller BF, Morrow AG, Maron BJ, Del Negro AA, Kent KM, McGrath FJ, Wallace RB, McIntosh CL, Roberts WC. Etiology of clinically isolated, severe, chronic, pure mitral regurgitation: analysis of 97 patients over 30 years of age having mitral valve replacement. *Am Heart J* 1982;104(2 Pt 1):276–288.

53. Roberts WC, Braunwald E, Morrow AG. Acute severe mitral regurgitation secondary to ruptured chordae tendineae: clinical, hemodynamic, and pathologic considerations. *Circulation* 1966;33(1):58–70.
54. Roberts WC, McIntosh CL, Wallace RB. Mechanisms of severe mitral regurgitation in mitral valve prolapse determined from analysis of operatively excised valves. *Am Heart J* 1987;113(5):1316–1323.
55. Bulkley BH, Roberts WC. Dilatation of the mitral anulus. A rare cause of mitral regurgitation. *Am J Med* 1975;59(4):457–463.
56. Salazar AE, Edwards JE. Friction lesions of ventricular endocardium. Relation to chordae tendineae of mitral valve. *Arch Pathol* 1970;90(4):364–376.
57. Lucas RV Jr, Edwards JE. The floppy mitral valve. *Curr Probl Cardiol* 1982;7(4):1–48.
58. Dollar AL, Roberts WC. Morphologic comparison of patients with mitral valve prolapse who died suddenly with patients who died from severe valvular dysfunction or other conditions. *J Am Coll Cardiol* 1991;17(4):921–931.
59. Rentería VG, Ferrans VJ, Jones M, Roberts WC. Intracellular collagen fibrils in prolapsed ("floppy") human atrioventricular valves. *Lab Invest* 1976;35(5):439–443.
60. Pomerance A. Ballooning deformity (mucoid degeneration) of atrioventricular valves. *Br Heart J* 1969;31(3):343–351.
61. Davies MJ, Moore BP, Braimbridge MV. The floppy mitral valve. Study of incidence, pathology, and complications in surgical, necropsy, and forensic material. *Br Heart J* 1978;40(5):468–481.
62. Berbarie RF, Roberts WC. Frequency of atrial fibrillation in patients having mitral valve repair or replacement for pure mitral regurgitation secondary to mitral valve prolapse. *Am J Cardiol* 2006;97(7):1039–1044.
63. Sims JB, Roberts WC. Comparison of findings in patients with versus without atrial fibrillation just before isolated mitral valve replacement for rheumatic mitral stenosis (with or without associated mitral regurgitation). *Am J Cardiol* 2006;97(7):1035–1038.
64. Braunwald E, Ross RS, Morrow AG, Roberts WC. Differential diagnosis of mitral regurgitation in childhood: clinical pathological conference at the National Institutes of Health. *Ann Intern Med* 1961;54:223–242.
65. Barth CW 3rd, Dibdin JD, Roberts WC. Mitral valve cleft without cardiac septal defect causing severe mitral regurgitation but allowing long survival. *Am J Cardiol* 1985;55(9):1229–1231.
66. Schiebler GL, Edwards JE, Burchell HB, Dushane JW, Ongley PA, Wood EH. Congenital corrected transposition of the great vessels: a study of 33 cases. *Pediatrics* 1961;27(5 Suppl):849–888.
67. Berry WB, Roberts WC, Morrow AG, Braunwald E. Corrected transposition of the aorta and pulmonary trunk: clinical, hemodynamic and pathologic findings. *Am J Med* 1964;36:35–53.
68. Roberts WC, Ross RS, Davis FW Jr. Congenital corrected transposition of the great vessels in adulthood simulating rheumatic valvular disease. *Bull Johns Hopkins Hosp* 1964;114:157–172.
69. Buchbinder NA, Roberts WC. Left-sided valvular active infective endocarditis. A study of forty-five necropsy patients. *Am J Med* 1972;53(1):20–35.
70. Arnett EN, Roberts WC. Active infective endocarditis: a clinicopathologic analysis of 137 necropsy patients. *Curr Probl Cardiol* 1976;1(7):2–76.
71. Fernicola DJ, Roberts WC. Clinicopathologic features of active infective endocarditis isolated to the native mitral valve. *Am J Cardiol* 1993;71(13):1186–1197.
72. Morrow AG, Cohen LS, Roberts WC, Braunwald NS, Braunwald E. Severe mitral regurgitation following acute myocardial infarction and ruptured papillary muscle. Hemodynamic findings and results of operative treatment in four patients. *Circulation* 1968;37(4 Suppl):II124–II132.
73. Barbour DJ, Roberts WC. Rupture of a left ventricular papillary muscle during acute myocardial infarction: analysis of 22 necropsy patients. *J Am Coll Cardiol* 1986;8(3):558–565.
74. Roberts WC, Siegel RJ, McManus BM. Idiopathic dilated cardiomyopathy: analysis of 152 necropsy patients. *Am J Cardiol* 1987;60(16):1340–1355.
75. Virmani R, Roberts WC. Quantification of coronary arterial narrowing and of left ventricular myocardial scarring in healed myocardial infarction with chronic, eventually fatal, congestive cardiac failure. *Am J Med* 1980;68(6):831–838.
76. Ross EM, Roberts WC. Severe atherosclerotic coronary arterial narrowing and chronic congestive heart failure without myocardial infarction: analysis of 18 patients studied at necropsy. *Am J Cardiol* 1986;57(1):51–56.
77. Klues HG, Maron BJ, Dollar AL, Roberts WC. Diversity of structural mitral valve alterations in hypertrophic cardiomyopathy. *Circulation* 1992;85(5):1651–1660.
78. Berezowski K, Mautner GC, Roberts WC. Scarring of the left ventricular papillary muscles in sickle-cell disease. *Am J Cardiol* 1992;70(15):1368–1370.

"Repaired" Tetralogy of Fallot Mimicking Arrhythmogenic Right Ventricular Cardiomyopathy (Another Phenocopy)

Betsy Ann George, MD[a,d], Jong Mi Ko, BA[d], Forrester Dubus Lensing, MD[b], Johannes Jacob Kuiper, MD[a,d], and William Clifford Roberts, MD[a,c,d,*]

Described is a 41-year-old man who at age 6 had partial resection of an obstructed right ventricular outflow tract with insertion of a patch and closure of a ventricular septal defect (tetralogy of Fallot). At age 41, cardiac transplantation was performed because of right ventricular outflow patch aneurysm, numerous episodes of ventricular tachycardia, and chronic heart failure, all features of the familial form of arrhythmogenic right ventricular cardiomyopathy (ARVC). Additionally, the patient had bundle branch block and epsilon waves on electrocardiogram, other features of ARVC. The case is described to introduce the concept of *acquired* ARVC, because the patient had many of the clinically recognized features of familial ARVC. **(Am J Cardiol 2011; 108:326–329)**

Arrhythmogenic right ventricular cardiomyopathy (ARVC) is characterized by localized thinning of the right ventricular (RV) wall with the localized portion consisting mainly of fibrofatty tissue.[1–3] The thinning of the RV wall commonly leads to aneurysm formation.[2] ARVC also is characterized by the presence of epsilon waves, bundle branch block, late potentials, and ventricular tachyarrhythmias on the electrocardiogram. ARVC has been recognized exclusively as a familial disease with autosomal dominant inheritance.[1,2] In this report, we introduce the concept of acquired ARVC in a patient who was operatively treated for tetralogy of Fallot and later developed features of ARVC.

Case Description

A 41-year-old man, born on October 10, 1969, had a right Blalock-Taussig shunt placed in 1974, at 4 years of age, for tetralogy of Fallot. In 1976, at age 6, he underwent widening of the RV outflow tract using a Dacron patch (4.5 × 3 cm) and closure of a large (2 × 3 cm) subaortic ventricular septal defect. Preoperatively, the peak systolic pressure gradient between the right ventricle and pulmonary trunk had been 85 mm Hg. The patch extended through the nonobstructive pulmonary valve, and 2 of its 3 cusps were excised. The Blalock-Taussig shunt was ligated. Immediately after operation, the peak systolic RV pressure was 70 mm Hg and that in the pulmonary trunk 35 mm Hg. The peak systolic left ventricular pressure was 100 mm Hg.

The patient thereafter was asymptomatic until 26 years of age, when he had his first episode of ventricular tachycardia (VT). Transthoracic echocardiogram performed at age 26 revealed a peak systolic pressure gradient between the right ventricle and pulmonary trunk of 25 mm Hg, marked RV dilatation, a mildly dilated left ventricular cavity, severely depressed right and left ventricular ejection fractions, and severe pulmonary regurgitation. An electrophysiologic study at the time disclosed sustained monomorphic VT with left bundle branch block morphology and superior axis. Mapping disclosed the VT to involve the RV infundibulum (that myocardium between the residual pulmonary valve and tricuspid valve) in a counterclockwise activation pattern. Radiofrequency ablation failed to terminate the VT, and it resulted in acute lengthening of the cycle length from 375 to 420 ms. The VT was then terminated with ventricular burst pacing. Repeat stimulation did not induce further VT. The patient was placed on atenolol and propafenone.

At 27 years of age, 8 months later, the patient had runs of VT again, and a second electrophysiologic study was done. Again, the inducible VT was mapped to involve the RV infundibulum but this time in a bidirectional activation pattern. A total of 23 linear and point radiofrequency ablations were made, and on several occasions the VT was terminated. Nevertheless, the VT was still inducible. Ablation prolonged the cycle length from 380 to 450 ms.

For several years thereafter, the patient was lost to follow-up. He started using alcohol and marijuana heavily. He quit taking all medications. At 36 years of age, he presented again to the hospital with chest pain, which was preceded by a viral gastroenteritis. His troponin level was 25 ng/ml. An electrocardiogram showed sinus tachycardia, a QRS duration of 200 ms, right bundle branch block, and nonspecific ST-T changes. Cardiac catheterization disclosed normal coronary arteries, normal mean pulmonary arterial pressures, no RV outflow obstruction, and no shunts. Transthoracic echocardiogram showed severely depressed RV and left ventricular function. Magnetic resonance imaging disclosed marked dilatation of the RV outflow tract (Figure 1). An automated internal cardiac defibrillator with a biventricular pacing device was implanted.

At 40 years of age, the patient began experiencing multiple episodes of automated internal cardiac defibrillator firings and symptoms of severe heart failure (Table 1).

Departments of [a]Internal Medicine (Division of Cardiology), [b]Radiology, and [c]Pathology and [d]The Baylor Heart and Vascular Institute, Baylor University Medical Center, Dallas, Texas. Manuscript received January 27, 2011; revised manuscript received and accepted March 7, 2011.

*Corresponding author: Tel: 214-820-7911; fax: 214-820-7533.

E-mail address: wc.roberts@baylorhealth.edu (W.C. Roberts).

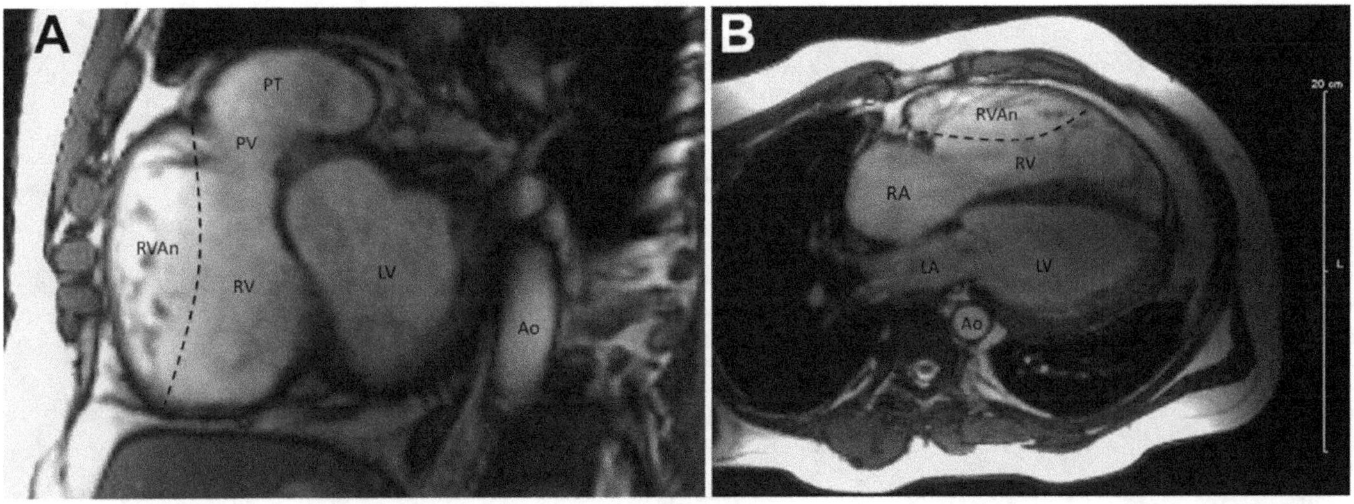

Figure 1. Parasagittal *(A)* and axial *(B)* white blood magnetic resonance imaging scans demonstrating marked right ventricular (RV) dilatation, RV aneurysm (RVAn), left ventricle (LV), left atrium (LA), right atrium (RA), pulmonaric valve (PV), pulmonary trunk (PT), and aorta (Ao).

Table 1
Hemodynamic data late after operative "correction" of tetralogy of Fallot

Variable	Date of Study			
	June 5, 2006	February 3, 2010	August 20, 2010	October 27, 2010
Right atrium (mean) (mm Hg)	10	8	16	11
Right ventricle (mm Hg)	36/15	41/12	45/19	38/5
Pulmonary artery (mm Hg)	34/7	34/5	33/13	35/10
Pulmonary capillary wedge (mean) (mm Hg)	—	9	16	14
Left ventricle (mm Hg)	96/31	—	—	—
Aorta (mm Hg)	91/61	—	—	—
Cardiac index (L/min/m^2)	1.69	2.64	2.48	1.59

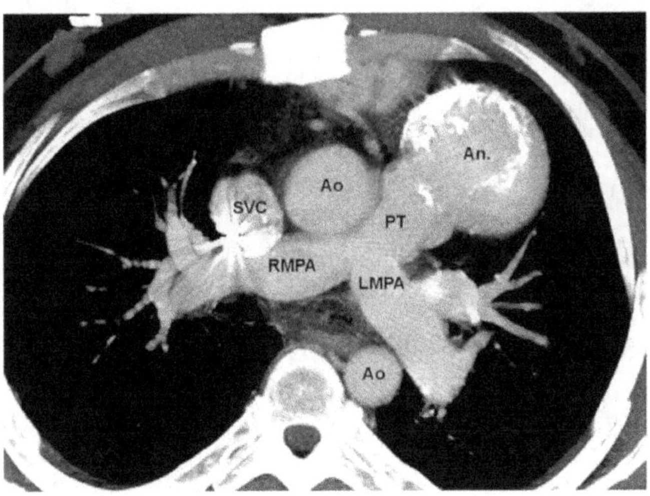

Figure 2. Axial contrast-enhanced computed tomographic scan demonstrating right ventricular (RV) outflow tract aneurysm (An) with heavy calcific deposits in its wall and synthetic graft repair. Ao = aorta; LMPA = left main pulmonary artery; PT = pulmonary trunk; RMPA = right main pulmonary artery; SVC = superior vena cava.

Cardiac computed tomography disclosed again severe dilatation of the RV outflow tract and heavy calcific deposits in its wall (Figure 2). Electrocardiogram now showed epsilon waves in the right precordial leads, T-wave inversions, and complete right bundle branch block (Figure 3). In February 2010, chronic inotropic therapy was initiated. The patient stopped using alcohol and marijuana completely. Six months later, when hospitalized for severe heart failure, runs of monomorphic nonsustained VT were demonstrated (Figure 4). On November 7, 2010, heart transplantation was performed.

The RV outflow patch was aneurysmal and bulged anteriorly (Figure 5). X-ray revealed a heavily calcified RV outflow tract. The ventricular septal defect was well closed, and a few calcific deposits were present in the closing patch. Both ventricles were dilated. The left ventricular wall had focal scars. The endocardium at the apex of the left ventricle was thickened by white fibrous tissue. The epicardial coronary arteries were wide open and free of plaque.

Comments

The modified International Task Force criteria for the diagnosis of ARVC were published in April 2010.[4] Our patient fulfilled 4 of the 6 major criteria and 1 of the 6 minor criteria: regional RV akinesia and a fractional area change ≤33%, thinning of a large portion of RV wall (by a patch), epsilon waves in the right precordial leads, inducible nonsustained VT of left bundle branch block morphology with superior axis, and inverted T waves in leads V_1 to V_4 in the presence of a complete right bundle branch block. Thus, the patient had criteria of ARVC but in an *acquired* way, after surgical resection of a large portion of the RV outflow tract.

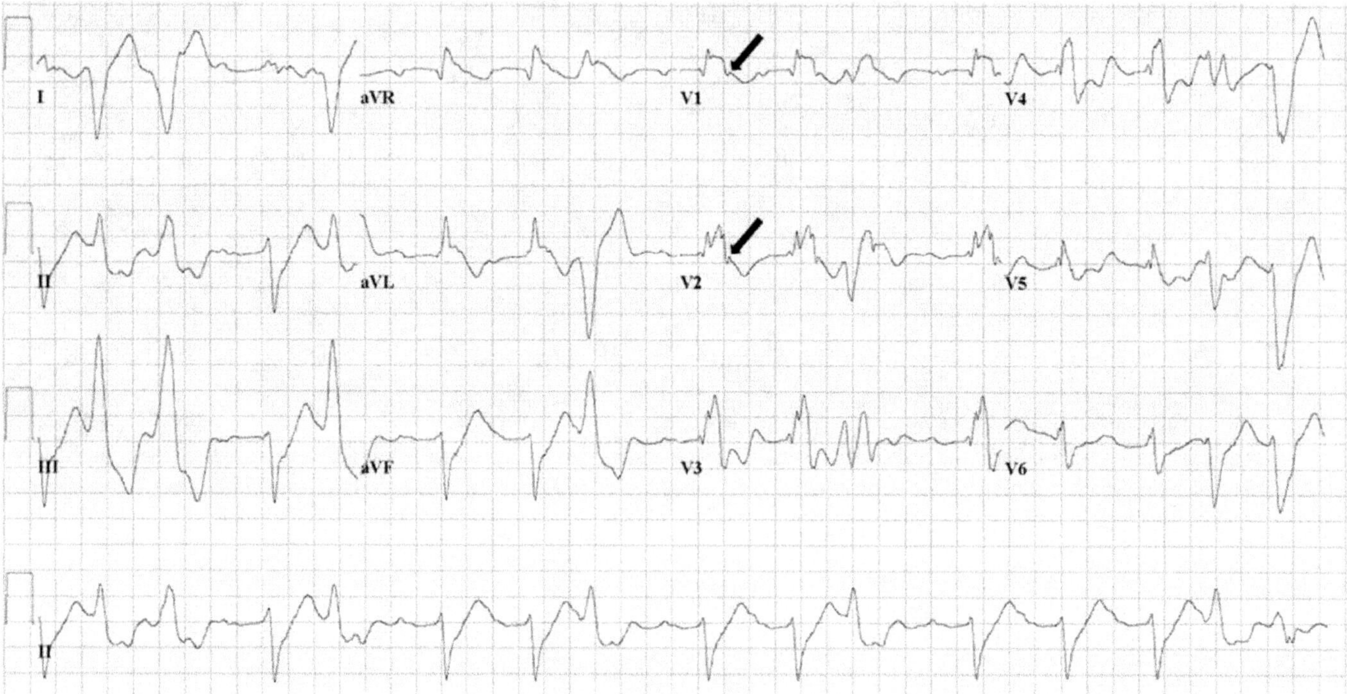

Figure 3. Electrocardiogram depicting epsilon waves *(arrows)* in the right precordial leads and inverted T waves in leads V_1 to V_4 with the presence of a complete right bundle branch block.

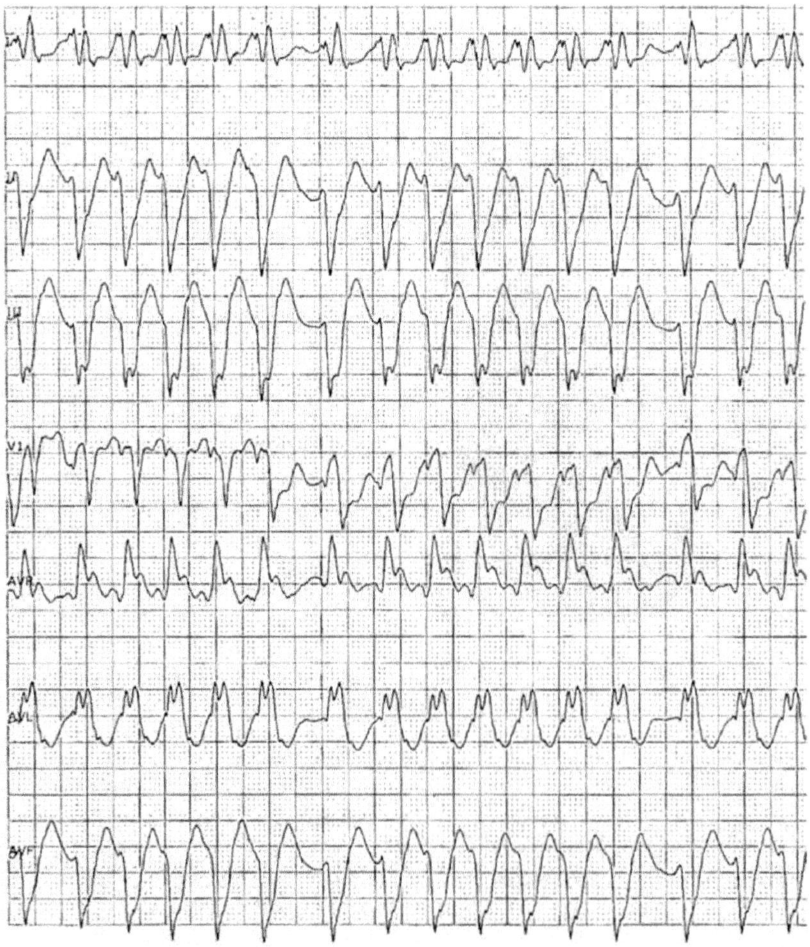

Figure 4. Nonsustained ventricular tachycardia (VT) of left bundle branch morphology with superior axis.

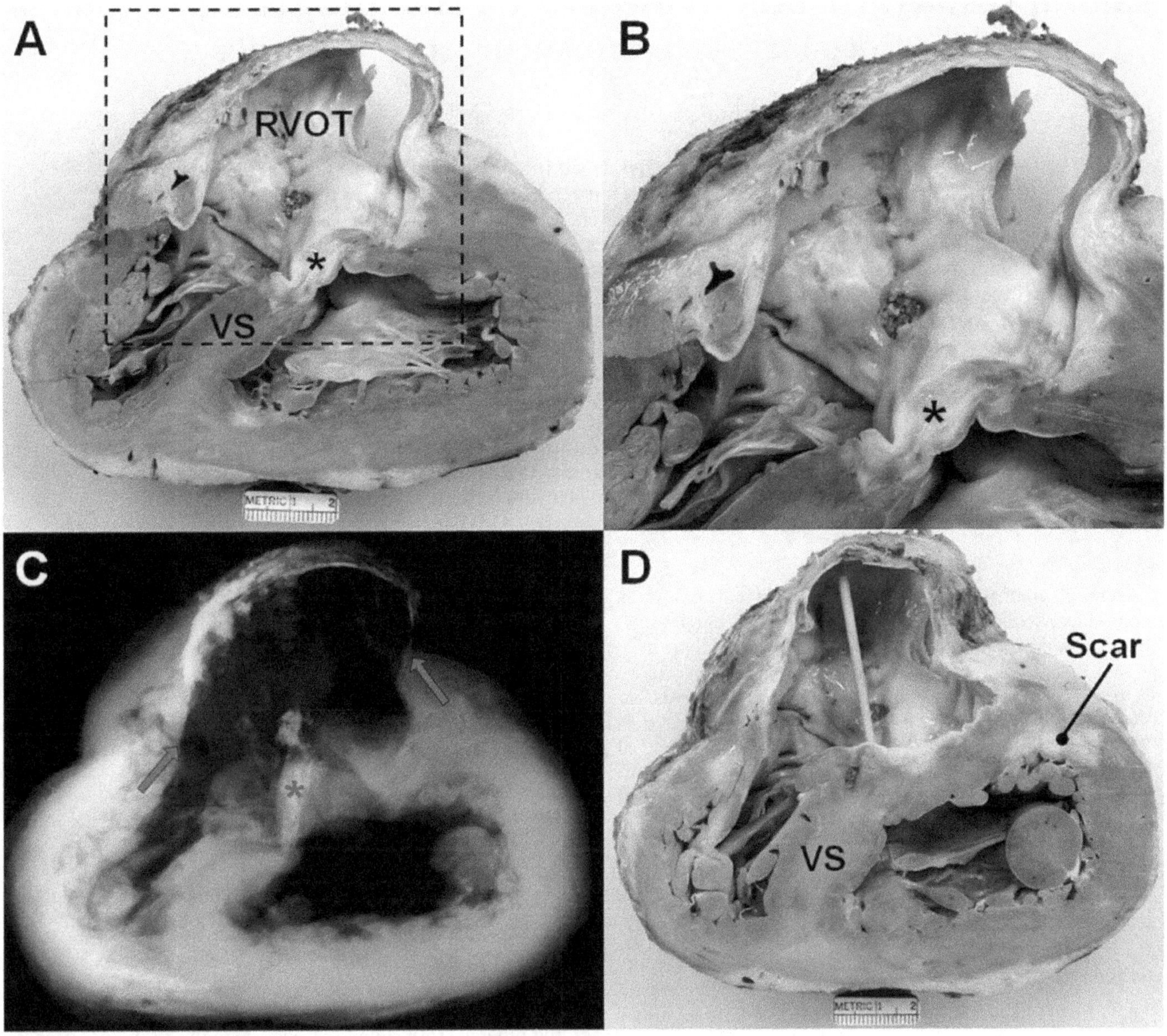

Figure 5. Heart. *(A,B)* View portraying right ventricular (RV) outflow patch aneurysm and marked dilatation of both ventricles. *(C)* X-ray showing a heavily calcified RV outflow tract (RVOT) aneurysm *(arrows)* and a well-closed ventricular septal defect *(asterisk)* with a few calcific deposits in the closing patch. *(D)* The left ventricular wall showing focal scar. VS = ventricular septum.

One reviewer suggested that the repeated and aggressive ablations in the electrophysiologic studies possibly contributed to the morphologic findings and to the repeated ventricular arrhythmias.

Aneurysmal development of the RV outflow tract after patch widening for RV outflow obstruction of course has been reported previously.[5] Additionally, the development of calcium deposits within the RV outflow patch also is most unusual but has been reported previously.[6]

1. Basso C, Thiene G, Corrado D, Angelini A, Nava A, Valente M. Arrhythmogenic right ventricular cardiomyopathy: dysplasia, dystrophy, or myocarditis? *Circulation* 1996;94:983–991.
2. Basso C, Corrado D, Marcus FI, Nava A, Thiene G. Arrhythmogenic right ventricular cardiomyopathy. *Lancet* 2009;373:1289–1300.
3. Roberts WC, Ko JM, Kuiper JJ, Hall SA, Meyer DM. Some previously neglected examples of arrhythmogenic right ventricular dysplasia/cardiomyopathy and frequency of its various reported manifestations. *Am J Cardiol* 2010;106:268–274.
4. Marcus FI, McKenna WJ, Sherrill D, Basso C, Bauce B, Bluemke DA, Calkins H, Corrado D, Cox MG, Daubert JP, Fontaine G, Gear K, Hauer R, Nava A, Picard MH, Protonotarios N, Saffitz JE, Sanborn DM, Steinberg JS, Tandri H, Thiene G, Towbin JA, Tsatsopoulou A, Wichter T, Zareba W. Diagnosis of arrhythmogenic right ventricular cardiomyopathy/dysplasia: proposed modification of the Task Force criteria. *Circulation* 2010;121:1533–1541.
5. Saffitz JE, McIntosh CL, Roberts WC. Massive right ventricular outflow tract aneurysm after ventriculotomy for subvalvular pulmonic stenosis associated with peripheral pulmonary arterial stenoses. *Am J Cardiol* 1983;51:1460–1462.
6. Ross EM, McIntosh CL, Roberts WC. "Massive" calcification of a right ventricular outflow parietal pericardial patch in tetralogy of Fallot. *Am J Cardiol* 1984;54:691–692.

Natural History, Clinical Consequences, and Morphologic Features of Coronary Arterial Aneurysms in Adults

William Clifford Roberts, MD[a,b,*]

Clinical and morphologic features are described in 20 adults (15 men) aged 17 to 85 years (mean 56) who at necropsy were found to have ≥1 aneurysm in ≥1 of their 3 major (right, left anterior descending, and left circumflex) epicardial coronary arteries. Of the 34 coronary aneurysms in the 20 patients (single in 10 patients, ≥2 in 10 patients), 27 (79%) contained intra-aneurysmal thrombi, and in each, the thrombus severely narrowed the lumen. Additionally, atherosclerotic plaque was present in the aneurysmal wall in all 27 aneurysms containing thrombi and also in the major coronary arteries uninvolved by aneurysm. The causes of the aneurysms in the 16 patients with intra-aneurysmal thrombi were therefore considered atherosclerotic. In the other 4 patients, with 7 aneurysms, none contained intra-aneurysmal thrombus or atherosclerotic plaque, and the aneurysms were considered congenital. Clinical diagnosis of coronary aneurysm was not made in any of the 20 patients, but none had proper imaging studies during life. Despite the coronary aneurysms and the associated luminal narrowing, only 8 patients (40%) had left ventricular wall scarring or necrosis or clinical evidence of myocardial ischemia. Proper therapy remains ill defined. **(Am J Cardiol 2011;108:814–821)**

Although atherosclerosis commonly involves the aorta, a common consequence of that involvement is aneurysmal dilatation, most commonly involving the abdominal portion, and significant narrowing or total occlusion of the aorta by this process is rare. In contrast, when atherosclerosis involves the coronary arteries, a common consequence is severe narrowing or total obstruction leading to myocardial ischemia and/or infarction, and aneurysmal dilatation involving these arteries is rare. Indeed, examination of several cardiac pathology books disclosed either no or minimal mention of coronary arterial aneurysm.[1–7] This report describes clinical and morphologic features in 20 adults with coronary arterial aneurysm observed personally during a 24-year period.

Methods

All hearts were initially examined by the author (W.C.R.), and most were reexamined all together at a later time. The hearts were submitted to W.C.R.'s cardiac pathology laboratory from 12 different medical institutions: 6 from 1 institution, 3 from another, 2 from another, and 1 each from 9 different institutions. The 20 cases were seen by W.C.R. during a 24-year period (1975 to 1999). The hearts were received after fixation in formaldehyde. After excising extraneous tissues, the hearts were weighted, described, and either photographed or illustrations prepared.

To be included in this study, ≥1 of the major epicardial coronary arteries (left anterior descending, left circumflex, and right) had to be focally dilated. The diameter of the aneurysm had to be ≥2 times the diameter of the right and left main coronary arteries in the first centimeter of their courses. Patients with previous cardiac surgery or percutaneous coronary intervention were excluded. Clinical records were obtained from the submitting institutions.

Results

Pertinent clinical and morphologic data for each of the 20 patients are listed in Table 1, and several hearts are illustrated in Figures 1 to 11.

The 20 patients ranged in age at death from 17 to 85 years: the 5 women from 17 to 85 years (mean 63) and the 15 men from 37 to 84 years (mean 56). Of the 20 patients, 10 (50%) had a single aneurysm in a single coronary artery; the other 10 (50%) had ≥1 aneurysm in ≥2 major coronary arteries. Of the latter 10 patients, 6 had aneurysms involving 2 major coronary arteries, and 4 patients had aneurysms in 3 major coronary arteries (right, left anterior descending, and left circumflex [excluding the left main]). Thus, the 20 patients had 34 coronary aneurysms: left anterior descending in 12, left circumflex in 9, and right in 13.

Intra-aneurysmal thrombi were present in 16 patients (80%), and 4 patients (20%) had no thrombi within coronary aneurysms. Of the total 34 coronary aneurysms in the 20 patients, 27 (79%) contained thrombi and 7 (21%) did not. Of the 34 aneurysms, 33 were fusiform (the entire wall was involved), and 1 (case 2) was saccular (only a portion of the wall was involved). In the latter patient, the aneurysm ruptured and led to fatal hemopericardium.

Maximal luminal narrowing at the coronary aneurysm, nearly entirely by thrombus, with some underlying atherosclerotic plaque was >75% in cross-sectional area in 28 aneurysms (82%) and zero or <25% in 6 aneurysms (18%).

[a]Baylor Heart and Vascular Institute of Baylor University Medical Center, Dallas, Texas; and [b]Pathology Branch, National Heart, Lung, and Blood Institute, National Institutes of Health, Bethesda, Maryland. Manuscript received April 14, 2011; revised manuscript received and accepted May 1, 2011.

*Corresponding author: Tel: 214-820-7911; fax: 214-820-7533.

E-mail address: wc.roberts@baylorhealth.edu (W.C. Roberts).

Table 1
Clinical and morphologic cardiac data in 20 necropsy patients with ≥1 aneurysm in ≥1 epicardial native coronary artery

Case	Age (Years)	Gender	CA With Aneurysm (n)	Coronary Aneurysm		Maximal Diameter (cm) First 1 cm of RCA or LMCA	Intra-Aneurysmal Thrombus	Maximal Luminal Narrowing at Aneurysm (CSA)	Atherosclerosis in Aneurysmal Wall	Maximal Narrowing of Nonaneurysmal CAs
				Diameter (cm)	Length (cm)					
1	17	F	LAD (1)	1.5	1.8	0.4	0	0	0	0
2	37	M	LC (1)	3.0	Saccular	0.5	0	0	0	0
3	41	M	R (1)	1.0	1.0	0.4	+	>75%	+	>75%
4	41	M	LAD (1)	1.0	1.5	0.4	+	>95%	+	>75%
5	41	M	R (2)	2.0	4.0	0.5	+	>95%	+	>75%
			LAD (2)	1.5	4.0		0	0	+	26%–50%
			LC (1)	1.5	3.0		0	0	+	26%–50%
6	42	M	LAD (1)	2.0	4.0	0.5	+	>75%	+	51%–75%
7	50	M	R (1)	1.0	2.0	0.4	+	>95%	+	>75%
			LC (1)	0.9	1.5		+	>95%	+	
8	54	M	R (1)	1.5	8.0	0.5	+	>75%	+	>75%
			LAD (1)	1.5	4.0		+	>75%	+	
9	55	M	R (1)	1.5	3.0	0.4	+	>95%	+	>75%
10	56	M	R (1)	1.3	2.2	0.4	+	>95%	+	>75%
			LAD (1)	2.3	3.0		+	>95%	+	
11	61	M	R (1)	2.0	3.5	0.4	+	>95%	+	>75%
12	65	M	R (1)	1.1	7.0	0.5	0	51–75%	+	>75%
			LAD (1)	1.0	1.5		0	51–75%	+	
13	68	M	LAD (1)*	1.5	2.0	0.5	+	>75%	+	>75%
			LC (1)*	2.0	2.0		+	>75%	+	
14	68	F	R (1)	2.5	2.2	0.6	+	>95%	+	>75%
15	70	M	R (1)	5.0	7.0	0.5	+	>75%	+	>75%
			LAD (1)	2.0	3.0		+	>75%	+	>75%
			LC (1)	4.0	3.0		+	>75%	+	>75%
16	70	M	LC (1)†	2.5	9.0	0.5	0	0	0	<25%
17	72	F	R (2)	1.3	3.0	0.4	+	>75%	+	>75%
			LAD (1)	1.3	2.0		+	>75%	+	>75%
			LC (1)	1.4	2.0		+	>75%	+	>75%
18	74	F	R (1)	2.0	4.0	0.5	+	>75%	+	>75%
			LC (1)	2.0	2.5		+	>75%	+	
19	84	M	R (1)	8.0	10.0	0.7	+	>75%	+	>75%
			LAD (1)	5.0	3.5		+	>75%	+	>75%
			LC (1)	6.0	2.5		+	>75%	+	>75%
20	85	F	LAD (1)	1.5	2.0	0.4	+	>75%	+	>75%

*Also involved the distal LMCA.
†Dominate artery: went to the crux.
AAA = abdominal aortic aneurysm; AMI = acute myocardial infarction; AP = angina pectoris; C = cardiac; CA = coronary artery; CHF = chronic heart failure; CSA = cross-sectional area; DA = descending aorta; F = female; Fib = fibrosis; LAD = left anterior descending coronary artery; LC = left circumflex coronary artery; LMCA = left main coronary artery; LV = left ventricle; M = male; N = necrosis; R = right; RCA = right coronary artery; RV = right ventricle; SD = sudden death; SH = systemic hypertension; V = vascular; — = no information available.

Atherosclerotic plaques, usually calcified ones, were present in 31 (91%) of the 34 aneurysms in the 20 patients and were absent in 3 (9%) of the 34 aneurysms.

Of the 20 patients, 16 (80%) had ≥1 major epicardial coronary artery narrowed >75% in cross-sectional area by atherosclerotic plaque. Among these 16 patients with 48 major coronary arteries (left anterior descending, left circumflex, and right), 38 (79%) of the 48 arteries were narrowed >75% in cross-sectional area by atherosclerotic plaque alone. Of the 3 major coronary arteries in these 16 patients (excluding the left main), an average of 2.3 of the 3 arteries were narrowed >75% in cross-sectional area by plaque alone.

The heart weight in the 5 women ranged from 310 to 490 g (mean 400) and in the 14 men from 380 to 910 g (mean 503).

Grossly visible left ventricular scars were present in 8 patients (40%), and in 3 others (15%), grossly visible foci of necrosis (acute myocardial infarction) were present.

Clinically, 7 patients (35%) had clinical events in which acute myocardial infarction was diagnosed, 2 of whom also had angina pectoris. One other patient who did not have a myocardial infarct clinically had angina pectoris. Three patients (15%) had evidence of chronic heart failure. Eight patients (40%) died suddenly, and death in each was attributed to coronary heart disease.

Table 1
(*continued*)

Number of Major CAs ↓ >75% in CSA by Plaque	Heart Weight (g)	Left Ventricular Wall		Clinically							Cause of Death			Dilated	
		N	Fib	AP	AMI	CHF	SD	SH	DAA	AAA	C	Non-C, V	Non-C, Non-V	RV	LV
0	—	0	0	0	0	0	+	0	0	0	+	0	0	0	0
0	420	0	0	0	0	0	+	0	0	0	+	0	0	0	0
3	510	0	+	0	0	0	+	+	0	0	+	0	0	+	+
2	380	0	0	0	0	0	+	0	0	0	+	0	0	0	0
1	375	+	+	0	+	0	+	0	0	0	+	0	0	+	+
0	500	0	0	0	0	0	0	+	+	0	0	+	0	0	0
3	460	0	+	0	0	0	+	—	0	0	+	0	0	0	+
3	400	0	+	0	+	+	+	0	0	0	+	0	0	+	+
3	450	+	0	+	+	0	0	+	0	+	+	0	0	+	+
3	510	0	+	+	0	0	0	+	0	+	0	0	+	0	+
1	380	0	+	0	+	0	0	0	0	0	0	0	+	+	+
2	910	0	+	0	+	+	0	+	0	0	+	0	0	+	+
3	560	0	+	0	0	0	0	+	0	0	0	0	+	+	+
2	490	0	0	0	0	0	0	+	0	+	0	0	+	0	0
3	750	+	0	0	0	0	0	+	0	0	0	0	+	0	0
0	420	0	0	0	0	0	0	+	0	0	0	0	+	0	0
3	390	0	0	0	0	0	+	+	0	0	+	0	0	0	0
2	390	0	0	0	0	0	0	+	0	0	0	0	+	0	0
3	—	0	+	+	+	+	0	+	0	0	+	0	0	0	+
2	420	+	0	0	+	0	0	+	0	0	+	0	0	+	+

Of the 20 patients, 12 (60%) died from cardiac disease (including the 8 who died suddenly outside the hospital), 1 (5%) of noncoronary vascular disease, and 7 (35%), of noncardiac and nonvascular causes.

Discussion

The present study summarizes clinical and morphologic findings in 20 patients with ≥1 aneurysm in ≥1 of the major epicardial coronary arteries. Ten patients (50%) had a single aneurysm in a single coronary artery, and the other 10 had 2 or 3 major coronary arteries containing aneurysms. Of the 34 aneurysms in the 20 patients, 27 (79%) contained thrombus, which in most cases severely narrowed the lumens. The residual lumen in all 27 cases was eccentrically located and adjacent to the atherosclerotic, partially calcified, wall. Of the 16 patients with thrombus in ≥1 coronary aneurysm, all but 1 had severe luminal narrowing by atherosclerotic plaque in the coronary artery containing the aneurysm as well as in the major coronary arteries not containing aneurysms. The largest coronary aneurysm in diameter was 8 cm, and this was also the longest (10 cm).

Of the 7 coronary aneurysms not containing intra-aneurysmal thrombus, 3 had none or insignificant quantities of atherosclerotic plaque within the aneurysms or in the non-aneurysmal portion of the artery containing the aneurysm or in the coronary arteries not containing an aneurysm. Thus, the cause of the coronary aneurysm in them was considered nonatherosclerotic, probably congenital in origin. Three other patients without thrombus in coronary aneurysm had insignificant atherosclerosis in the major coronary arteries; only 1 without intra-aneurysmal thrombus had severe coronary atherosclerosis. One patient without intra-aneurysmal thrombus had a large saccular aneurysm that ruptured, leading to fatal hemopericardium. The other 33 aneurysms were fusiform.

Despite the severe narrowing by intra-aneurysmal thrombus or by atherosclerotic plaque, only 8 patients (40%) had grossly visible left ventricular scars, and only 3 had grossly

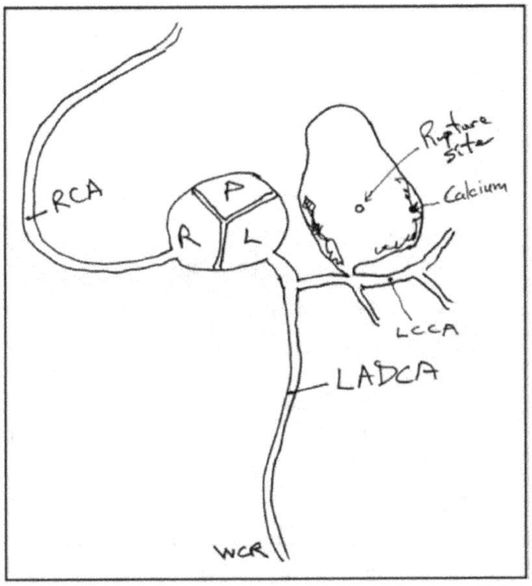

Figure 1. Case 2: diagram of the major coronary arteries in a 37-year-old man who collapsed at home. Necropsy disclosed hemopericardium and a large saccular aneurysm arising from the left circumflex coronary artery (LCCA). A perforation was present in the aneurysm. Calcific deposits were present in the basal portion of the wall of the aneurysm. The right coronary artery (RCA) and the left anterior descending coronary artery (LADCA) were free of atherosclerotic plaques. Cusps of the aortic valve: L = left; P = posterior; R = right.

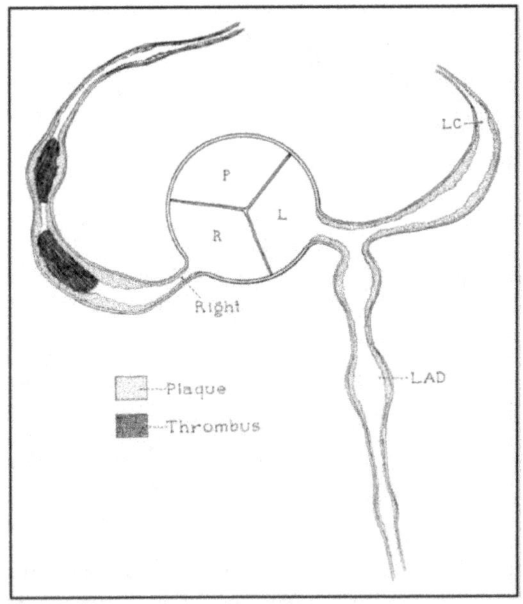

Figure 2. Case 5: diagram of the coronary arteries in a 41-year-old man with coronary aneurysms in the right, left anterior descending (LAD), and left circumflex (LC) coronary arteries. The 2 in the right contain large thrombi. He died from acute aortic dissection. Cusps of the aortic valve: L = left; P = posterior; R = right.

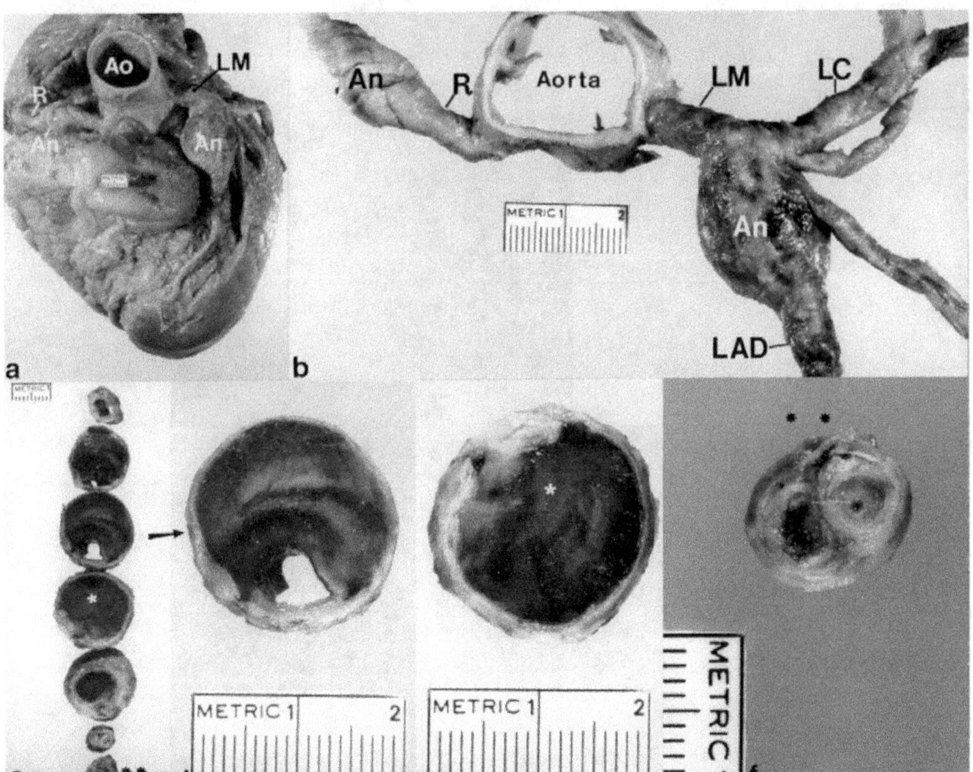

Figure 3. Case 10: the heart in a 56-year-old man with an aneurysm (An) in the right (R) and left anterior descending (LAD) coronary arteries. He died from cancer. *(a)* Anterior view of the heart showing the 2 aneurysms. *(b)* View of the R, left main (LM), and LAD coronary arteries showing the 2 aneurysms. The R and LM coronary arteries just after their origins from the aorta (Ao) are much smaller in diameter than either coronary aneurysm. *(c)* Cross sections of the LAD coronary artery with intra-aneurysmal thrombus. *(d)* Cross section of 1 section. The lumen is severely narrowed by intra-aneurysmal thrombus. *(e)* Another cross section of the same aneurysm. *(f)* Small coronary segment distal to the aneurysm. Its lumen is occluded by complicated plaque plus thrombus. LC = left circumflex.

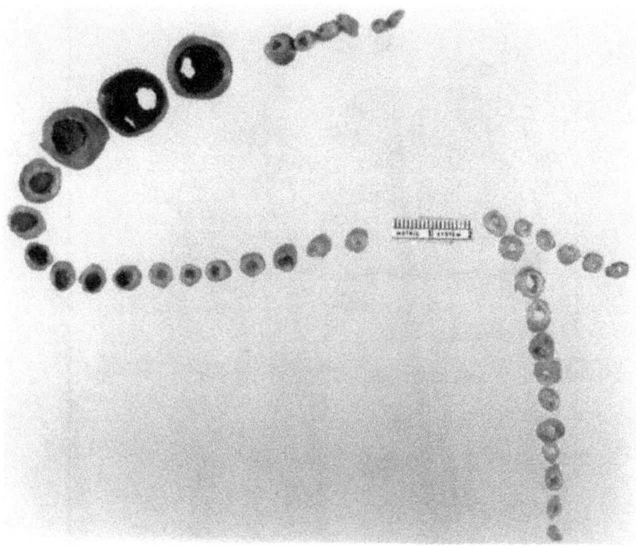

Figure 4. Case 11: coronary arteries in a 61-year-old man who died from complications of cancer. These cross sections of coronary arteries show a large aneurysm filled with thrombus in the distal right coronary artery.

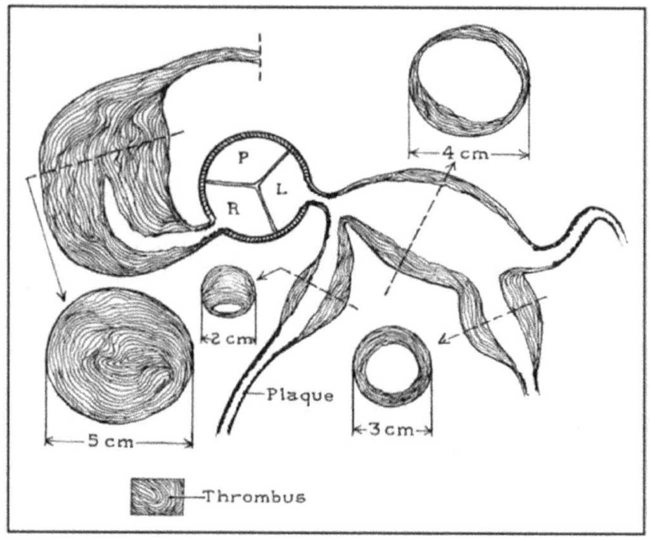

Figure 6. Case 15: diagram of coronary arterial aneurysms in a 70-year-old man who died from a gastrointestinal condition. Necropsy disclosed very large aneurysms in the right, left anterior descending, and left circumflex coronary arteries and in 1 of its obtuse marginal branches. Thrombus is present in each aneurysm and occludes the lumen of the right coronary artery. Cusps of the aortic valve: L = left; P = posterior; R = right.

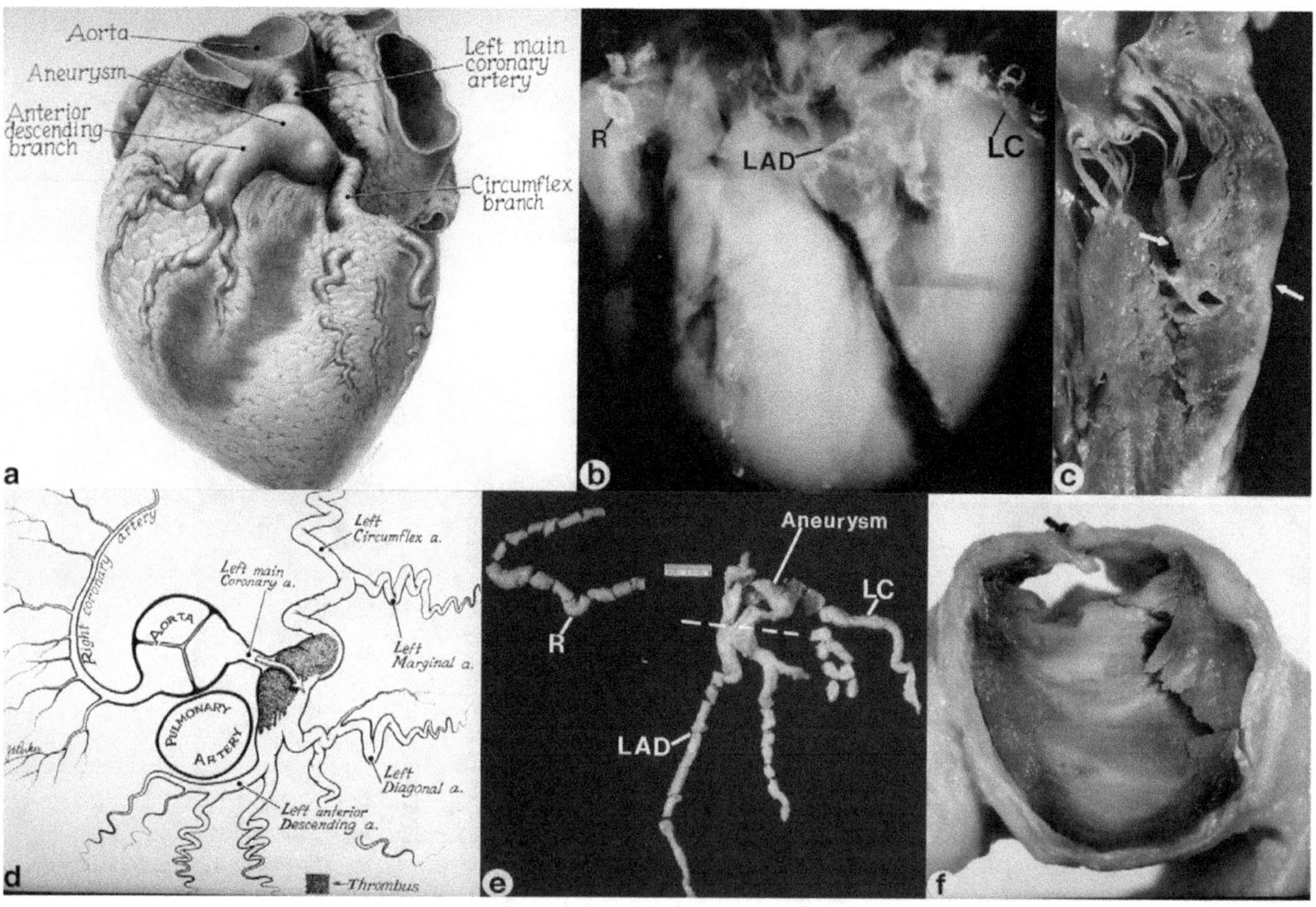

Figure 5. Case 13: heart in a 68-year-old man with a large aneurysm with intra-aneurysmal thrombus involving the proximal portion of the left anterior descending (LAD) and left circumflex (LC) coronary arteries *(a,d)*. The walls of the coronary arteries are focally calcified *(b)*. *(c)* A transmural scar *(between the arrows)* in the posterior wall of left ventricle. *(e)* View of the coronary arteries after their removal from the heart. *(f)* Cross section through the LAD aneurysm showing the large intra-aneurysmal thrombus.

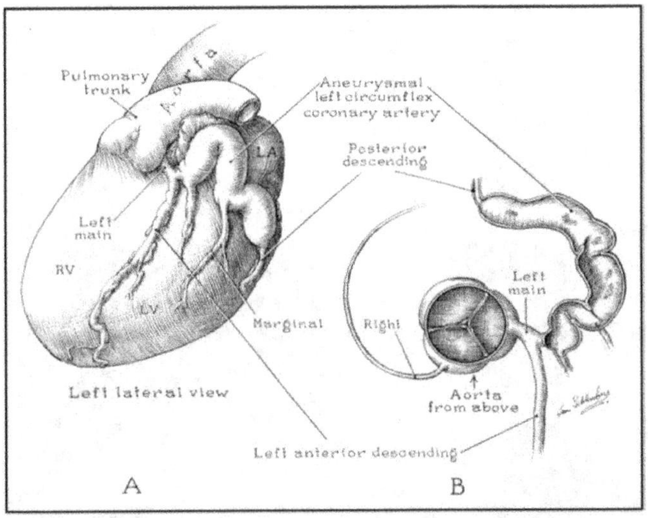

Figure 7. Case 16: diagram showing a large long aneurysm involving the left circumflex coronary artery in a 70-year-old man who died from a noncardiovascular condition (trauma). The coronary aneurysm is devoid of thrombus. LA = left atrium; LV = left ventricle; RV = right ventricle.

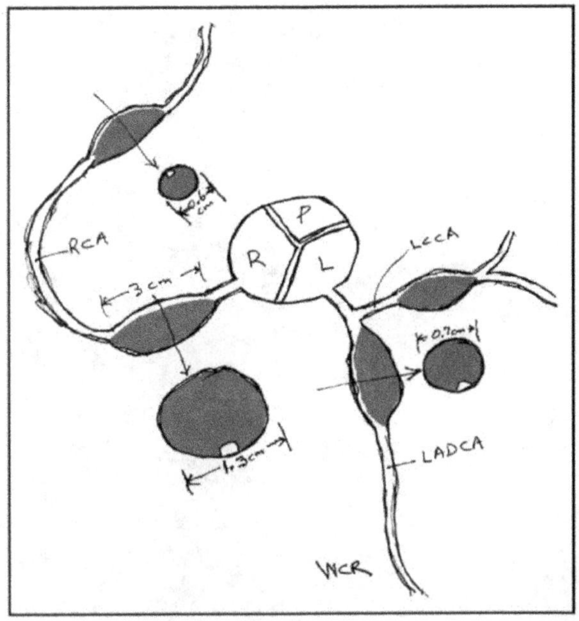

Figure 8. Case 17: diagram of coronary arteries in a 72-year-old woman who died suddenly and unexpectedly outside the hospital. She had never had clinical evidence of myocardial ischemia previously. Necropsy disclosed fusiform aneurysms filled with thrombi in each of the 3 major coronary arteries, including 2 aneurysms in the right coronary artery (RCA). At the sites of aneurysms, cross sections show thrombi filling most of the lumen, and the only residual opening is eccentric, adjacent to the artery's wall. LADCA = left anterior descending coronary artery; LCCA = left circumflex coronary artery. Cusps of the aortic valve: L = left; P = posterior; R = right.

visible foci of left ventricular necrosis, including 1 of the 8 with left ventricular scarring.

Only 3 patients had a diagnosis of angina pectoris, and 7 had a diagnosis of acute myocardial infarction during life. Three patients had evidence of chronic heart failure. Eight died suddenly outside the hospital. A diagnosis of coronary

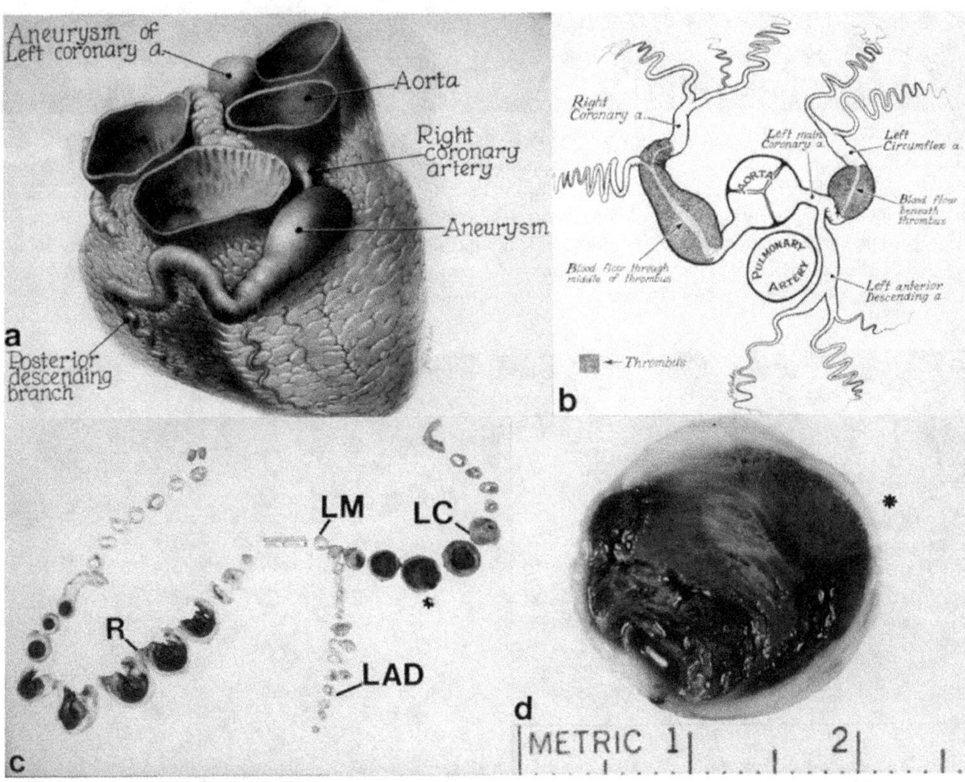

Figure 9. Case 18: coronary aneurysms of the left circumflex (LC) and right (R) coronary arteries in a 74-year-old woman who died from a noncardiovascular condition (chronic obstructive pulmonary disease). *(a)* Diagram of the heart. *(b)* Diagram of the coronary arteries showing that both coronary aneurysms contained thrombi. *(c)* Cross sections of the right R, left main (LM), left anterior descending (LAD), and LC coronary arteries. *(d)* Cross section of the LC coronary aneurysm showing its lumen to be virtually occluded by thrombus.

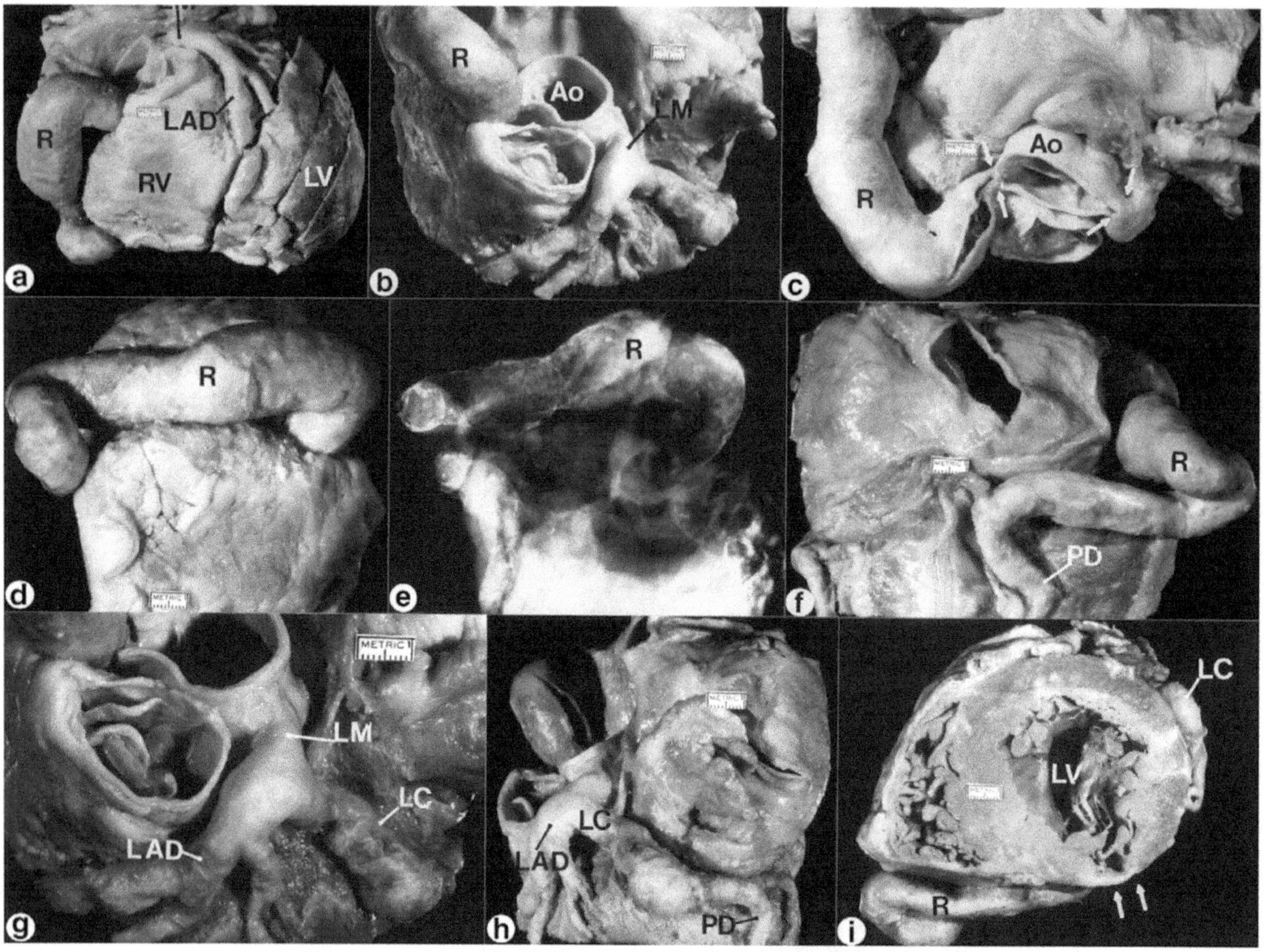

Figure 10. Case 19: heart in an 84-year-old man, who had a myocardial infarction at 80 years of age, showing a huge aneurysm involving nearly all the right (R) coronary artery, with smaller aneurysms involving the distal left main (LM) and proximal portions of the left anterior descending (LAD) and left circumflex (LC) coronary arteries. He died from pneumonia. *(a)* View of the anterior portion of the heart. Note the huge size of the R coronary artery. *(b)* View from above. *(c)* Another view of the aneurysm in the R coronary artery. *(d)* Still another view. *(e)* X-ray showing calcific deposits in the R coronary artery. *(f)* Distal portion of the right coronary artery and its posterior descending (PD) branch. i View of the left-sided coronary aneurysms. *(h)* Still another view. *(i)* Cross section of the cardiac ventricles showing transmural scars *(arrows)* in the left ventricular wall. Ao = aorta; LV = left ventricle; RV = right ventricle.

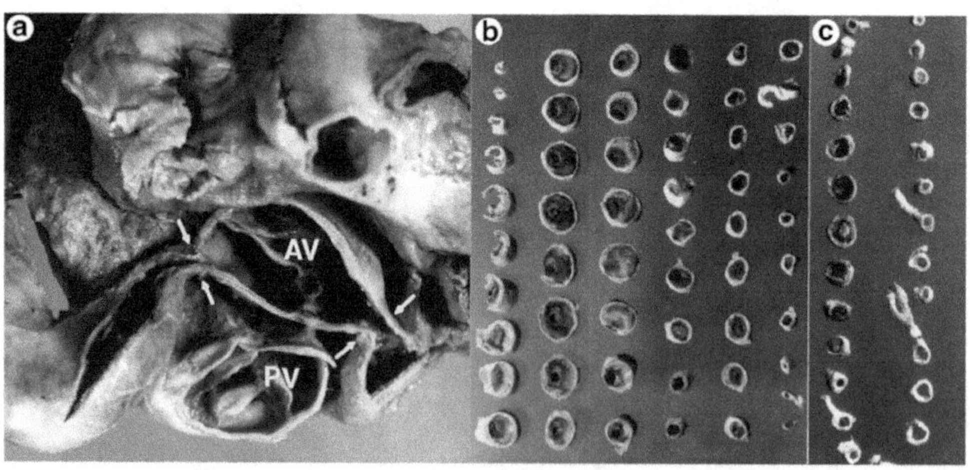

Figure 11. Case 19: *(a)* View of both coronary arteries from above showing that the most proximal portions of the right and left main coronary arteries *(between the arrows)* are of normal size. *(b)* Cross sections of the right coronary artery showing its lumen to be filled with thrombus. *(c)* Cross sections of the left anterior descending coronary artery. Again, the aneurysm is filled with thrombus. AV = aortic valve; PV = pulmonary valve.

aneurysm was not made in any patient during life. However, none had coronary angiographic or computed tomographic studies during life.

The cause of death was considered cardiac in 12 patients, 8 of whom died suddenly outside the hospital, and 4 others had fatal acute myocardial infarction within a hospital. Another patient died from noncoronary vascular causes, and 7 died from neither coronary nor noncoronary vascular causes. At necropsy, 3 patients were found to have abdominal aortic aneurysms, and 1 other patient had a saccular aneurysm of the descending thoracic aorta. At least 13 of the 20 patients had a history of systemic hypertension.

In the past 30 years, numerous reports on coronary artery aneurysm have been published. Most have been single case studies of "giant" coronary aneurysms diagnosed by computed tomography, magnetic resonance imaging, echocardiography, coronary angiography, and even routine chest radiography.[8–13] Many have been in patients with Kawasaki disease.[14] Most of the latter patients were aged <5 years, and they were excluded from the present study. (The youngest patient in the present study was 17 years of age.)

The largest reported necropsy study was that by Virmani et al[8] of 52 patients. Their patients ranged in age from 5 months to 80 years and included 14 patients in whom they attributed coronary aneurysms to inflammation (mean age 14 years) and 38 patients in whom the aneurysms were attributed to atherosclerosis (mean age 38 years). Of their 38 patients with atherosclerotic aneurysms, "20 (53%) had histories of ischemic heart disease." The coronary aneurysms involved a single coronary artery in 31 patients (82%) and >1 artery in 7 patients (18%). The data from their study were obtained from autopsy protocols and clinical records, not from examination of the hearts themselves.

When a coronary aneurysm is diagnosed during life, the best therapeutic course to follow has not been determined. In patients without evidence of myocardial ischemia the best course may be to do nothing unless the aneurysm is truly giant in size, such that rupture is a potential consequence. Because thrombi are present in most adults with coronary aneurysms, anticoagulation may be justified. In patients with symptomatic myocardial ischemia and ≥1 large coronary aneurysm, operative intervention has been the most common therapeutic option.[15] However, what is the proper operative procedure? Some surgeons have simply placed a bypass conduit distal to the coronary aneurysm with or without placing a ligature at both the proximal and distal ends of the coronary aneurysm. Percutaneous coronary intervention in those circumstances appears less appealing (to me).

The positive feature of the present study was that all cases were studied by the same individual, namely the author, who has been studying hearts for 50 years. Most of the hearts were photographed and/or illustrated. The major deficiency of this study is that none of the coronary aneurysms were diagnosed clinically, and no echocardiographic, computed tomographic, magnetic resonance imaging, or coronary angiograms were available in any patient. The coronary aneurysms were surprise necropsy findings in all 20 patients. With autopsy rates in hospital deaths now about 5%, the "material" illustrated in the present study will be far less available in the future.

1. Hudson REB. Cardiovascular Pathology, Volume 1. Baltimore, Maryland: Williams & Wilkins, 1965:630–631.
2. Gould SE, Ioannides G. Diseases of the coronary vessels. In: Gould SE, ed. Pathology of the Heart and Blood Vessels. 3rd ed. Springfield, Illinois: Charles C. Thomas, 1968:557–558.
3. Davies MJ, Robertson WB. Diseases of the coronary arteries. In: Pomerance A, Davies MJ, eds. Pathology of the Heart. London, United Kingdom: Blackwell Scientific, 1975:114–115.
4. Olsen EGJ. The Pathology of the Heart. 2nd ed. Baltimore, Maryland: University Park Press, 1980:308.
5. Baroldi G. Diseases of the coronary arteries. In: Silver MD, ed. Cardiovascular Pathology, Volume I. New York, New York: Churchill Livingstone, 1983:362–364.
6. Virmani R, Robinowitz M, Darcy TP. Coronary vasculitis. In: Virmani R, Atkinson JB, Fenoglio JJ, eds. Cardiovascular Pathology. Philadelphia, Pennsylvania: W.B. Saunders, 1991:180–185.
7. Davies MJ, Mann JM. Part B: acquired diseases of the heart. In: Davies MJ, Mann JM. The Cardiovascular System. New York, New York: Churchill Livingstone, 1995:64–65.
8. Virmani R, Robinowitz M, Atkinson JB, Forman MB, Silver MD, McAllister HA. Acquired coronary arterial aneurysms: an autopsy study of 52 patients. *Hum Pathol* 1986;17:575–583.
9. Meinert D, Mohammed Z. MRI of congenital coronary artery aneurysm. *Br J Radiol* 2000;73:322–324.
10. Pahlavan PS, Niroomand F. Coronary artery aneurysm: a review. *Clin Cardiol* 2006;29:439–443.
11. Nichols L, Lagana S, Parwani A. Coronary artery aneurysm. A review and hypothesis regarding etiology. *Arch Pathol Lab Med* 2008;132: 823–828.
12. Johnson PT, Fishman EK. CT angiography of coronary artery aneurysms: detection, definition, causes, and treatment. *AJR Am J Roentgenol* 2010;195:928–934.
13. Shambrook JS, Chowdhury R, Brown IW, Peebles CR, Harden SP. Cross-sectional imaging appearances of cardiac aneurysms. *Clin Radiol* 2010;65:349–357.
14. Sudo C, Monobe Y, Yashiro M, Sadakane A, Uehara R, Nakamura Y. Case-control study of giant coronary aneurysms due to Kawasaki disease: the 19th nationwide survey. *Pediatr Int* 2010;52:790–794.
15. Harandi S, Johnston SB, Wood RE, Roberts WC. Operative therapy of coronary arterial aneurysm. *Am J Cardiol* 1999;83:1290–1293.

Prophylactic Replacement of a Dilated Ascending Aorta at the Time of Aortic Valve Replacement of a Dysfunctioning Congenitally Unicuspid or Bicuspid Aortic Valve

Recently, I examined a beautifully excised severely stenotic congenitally bicuspid aortic valve in a 64-year-old man who, at the same operation, had undergone excision of the ascending aorta, which, by preoperative imaging studies, had a maximal diameter of 4.3 cm. Histologically, the wall of the aorta was normal. Although the aortic valve replacement (AVR) was clearly appropriate, was excision of the ascending aorta justified on a prophylactic basis? I would argue that the latter should be reconsidered.

Before the 1990s, relatively few patients with stenotic or purely regurgitant congenitally malformed aortic valves also underwent concomitant resection of the dilated ascending aorta. During the 1990s, some prominent and persuasive cardiac surgeons began advocating prophylactic concomitant ascending aortic resection in these circumstances, mainly for 3 reasons. First, to prevent postoperative dilation of the ascending aorta in a previously normal sized aorta or to prevent additional dilation in an already dilated aorta; second, to prevent aortic dissection, which is recognized to occur more commonly in patients with congenitally unicuspid and bicuspid aortic valves than in patients with tricuspid aortic valves[1,2]; and, finally, to prevent rupture of the ascending aorta late postoperatively. The latter reason was because it is recognized that the media of the ascending aorta in patients with congenitally bicuspid aortic valves can be depleted of certain elements (elastic fibers, smooth muscle cells, collagen) and can be repleted with certain other elements (mucopolysaccharide material) compared to the aorta's structure in adults with tricuspid aortic valves[3] (except in those patients with the Marfan syndrome and the forme fruste variety of it,[4] cardiovascular syphilis,[5–7] and ankylosing spondylitis,[8] and giant-cell aortitis[9]).

But how often do these potential aortic complications (additional dilation, dissection, rupture) occur in patients who have had AVR because of a dysfunctioning congenitally malformed aortic valve (either unicuspid or bicuspid) without concomitant resection of the dilated ascending aorta? The answer is infrequently. The best data (largest number of patients and longest follow-up) supporting that view comes from an analysis of 1,286 patients (1,180 [92%] with aortic stenosis [AS], 85 [7%] with aortic regurgitation [AR], and 20 [1%] aortic valve dysfunction type not stated) who had undergone AVR at the Mayo Clinic from 1960 to 1995 because of a dysfunctioning bicuspid aortic valve, without concomitant resection of the ascending aorta, irrespective of its size.[10] The mean age at operation was 58 years (72% men). The follow-up period was 0 to 38 years (median 12). During that postoperative period (excluding the 36 who died early [2.8%] and the 26 lost to follow-up [2.6%]), documented aortic dissection occurred in 13 (1%) and additional aortic dilation (ascending aorta diameter reached ≥5.0 cm or >1.0 from that at the time of AVR) occurred in 127 (9.9%). Additionally, 11 (0.08%) of the 1,227 patients not dying early or lost to follow-up later underwent resection of the ascending aorta; in 9 of the 11, however, it was at the time of replacement of a malfunctioning mechanical prosthesis or a bioprosthesis in the aortic valve position.

Although 151 events affecting the ascending aorta occurred during the long follow-up period, 127 (84%) consisted of dilation of the aorta, something that can occur after any aortotomy, irrespective of the structure of the aortic valve, and dilation of the ascending aorta after an aortotomy in and of itself infrequently produces clinical consequences. Indeed, the 15-year all-cause survival was greater in the patients with "enlarged" aortas than in those with normal-size aortas at the time of AVR (56% vs 50%). Although the ascending aorta was later excised in 11 patients, that aortic resection probably would not have been done in 9 if excision of a dysfunctioning prosthesis or bioprosthesis had not been required. Additionally, aortotomy, performed with isolated AVR, causes proliferation of fibrous tissue around the aorta, making the aorta thicker than normal, and the resulting thicker wall almost surely is more difficult to rupture than an aortic wall of normal or less than normal thickness. Furthermore, any type of interruption of the wall of ascending aorta (be it for insertion of a saphenous vein conduit or arterial cannula or incision for AVR or for resection of an aortic tear in aortic dissection) increases the risk of late dissection or rupture, be it in patients with unicuspid, bicuspid or tricuspid aortic valves.[11]

Similar long-term follow-up after isolated AVR in patients with dysfunctioning tricuspid aortic valves without concomitant resection of ascending aorta was recently presented by Gaudino et al.[12] They described 93 consecutive patients (mean age 67 years; 74% men) undergoing isolated AVR for AS at their institution (Catholic University Rome) from January 1990 to December 2000. Preoperatively, the maximal diameter of the ascending aorta ranged from 5.0 to 5.9 cm (mean 5.6). The diagnosis of tricuspid aortic valve was confirmed in each patient at operation by visual inspection. The ascending aorta was neither replaced nor plicated. The 92 patients surviving the operation were followed up for a mean of 14.7 ± 4.8 years. During that period, 16 patients died (17%). In no case was death attributed to an aortic event. Indeed, no patient during the long follow-up experienced an acute ascending aortic rupture, dissection, or pseudoaneurysm formation. Also, during the follow-up, no patient required reoperation for thoracic aortic complications. Additionally, the diameter of the ascending aorta during the 10 years after AVR changed insignificantly (56 ± 2 mm preoperatively vs 57 ± 11 mm at the end of follow-up). The mean expansion rate of the ascending aorta was 0.3 ± 0.2 mm/year. Patients with connective tissue disorders such as the Marfan syndrome were excluded from their study. The report by Gaudino et al[12] included the largest number of patients with dilated ascending aortas and stenotic 3-cuspid aortic valves undergoing AVR alone and followed up for ≥10 years. The frequency of late ascending aortic complications is lacking in patients who have had combined AVR for dysfunctioning unicuspid, bicuspid, or tricuspid aortic valves and resection of the dilated ascending aortas with similarly long (10 to 15 years) follow-up.

Adding ascending aortic resection to AVR usually significantly increases the operative mortality. Data from the Society of Thoracic Surgeons database indicate that ascending aortic resection increases the operative risk by a factor of 2.78 compared to AVR alone.[13] I agree with McKeller et al[10] from the Mayo Clinic who stated: "The widespread adoption of an aggressive attitude toward [aortic] root replacement, therefore, may create more problems than it solves."

Another recent report also provides some evidence that prophylactic resection of the ascending aorta is probably performed too frequently (unnecessarily) in patients undergoing AVR for dysfunctioning congenitally malformed aortic valves.[14] The evidence is provided by a histologic study of operatively excised dilated (>4.5-cm) aortas in patients undergoing AVR for dysfunctioning unicuspid or bicuspid aortic valves. My colleagues and I examined histologically the operatively excised ascending aortas in 58 patients undergoing AVR for AS involving a congenitally unicuspid or bicuspid aortic valve and in 38 patients undergoing AVR for pure AR involving a bicuspid aortic valve.[14] All 96 patients by preoperative imaging studies had ascending aortas with diameters >4.5 cm. We found that dividing the patients into those with AS and those with pure AR, something that had not been done previously, was helpful in predicting whether the structure of the ascending aorta was likely to be normal, in which case its resection probably was not indicated, or abnormal, in which case its resection probably was indicated. In the 58 patients with AS, the structure of the aortic media was normal or nearly normal (consistent with aging) in all 14 patients with unicuspid aortic valves and in 39 (87%) of the 44 patients with bicuspid valves. In contrast, of the 38 patients with purely regurgitant congenitally bicuspid aortic valves (none had unicuspid valves), the aortic media was normal in 20 (53%) and abnormal in 18 (47%). These findings suggest that among patients with preoperative imaging studies showing the ascending aorta to have a diameter >4.5 cm, it is unlikely the ascending aorta requires resection if the congenitally malformed aortic valve is stenotic. However, aortic resection will be necessary in about 1/2 of the patients with purely regurgitant congenitally bicuspid valves. Unfortunately, among the patients with pure AR, no preoperative features were found to distinguish those with normal from those with abnormal aortic media histologically (judged exclusively by the degree, if any, of the loss of medial elastic fibers).

In summary, it is likely that too many dilated ascending aortas are being excised prophylactically in patients with aortic valve dysfunction involving a congenitally unicuspid or bicuspid aortic valve. The rates of late postoperative occurrence of aortic dissection and/or rupture are extremely low, and additional dilation of the ascending aorta after AVR infrequently produces deleterious clinical events. The histologic structure of the dilated ascending aorta is usually normal in patients with stenotic congenitally unicuspid or bicuspid aortic valves. In contrast, the aortic histologic structure is often (about 50%) abnormal in patients with dilated ascending aortas and purely regurgitant congenitally bicuspid aortic valves.

William Clifford Roberts, MD
Baylor Heart and Vascular Institute
Baylor University Medical Center
Dallas, Texas

1. Roberts CS, Roberts WC. Dissection of the aorta associated with congenital malformation of the aortic valve. *J Am Coll Cardiol* 1991;17:712–716.
2. Roberts CS, Roberts WC. Morphologic aspects of aortic dissection. In: Ernst CB, Stanley JC, eds. *Current Therapy in Vascular Surgery*. Philadelphia: B.C. Decker; 1991:245–151.
3. Fazel SS, Mallidi HR, Lee RS, Sheehan MP, Liang D, Fleishman D, Herfkens R, Mitchell RS, Miller DC. The aortopathy of bicuspid aortic valve disease has distinctive patterns and usually involves the transverse aortic arch. *J Thorac Cardovasc Surg* 2008;135:901–907.
4. Roberts WC, Honig HS. The spectrum of cardiovascular disease in the Marfan syndrome: a clinico-morphologic study of 18 necropsy patients and comparison to 151 previously reported necropsy patients. *Am Heart J* 1982;104:115–135.
5. Roberts WC, Ko JM, Vowels TJ. Natural history of syphilitic aortitis. *Am J Cardiol* 2009;104:1578–1587.
6. Roberts WC, Bose R, Ko JM, Henry AC, Hamman BL. Identifying cardiovascular syphilis at operation. *Am J Cardiol* 2009;104:1588–1594.
7. Roberts WC, Lensing FD, Kourlis H Jr, Ko JM, Newberry JW, Smerud MJ, Burton EC, Hebeler RF Jr. Full blown cardiovascular syphilis with aneurysm of the innominate artery. *Am J Cardiol* 2009;104:1595–1600.
8. Bulkley BH, Roberts WC. Ankylosing spondylitis and aortic regurgitation. Description of the characteristic cardiovascular lesion from study of eight necropsy patients. *Circulation* 1973;48:1014–1027.
9. Roberts WC, MacGregor RR, DeBlanc HJ Jr, Beiser GD, Wolff SM. The prepulseless phase of pulseless disease, or pulseless disease with pulses: a newly recognized cause of cardiac disease, monoclonal gammopathy and "fever of unknown origin." *Am J Med* 1969;46:313–324.
10. McKeller SH, Michelena HI, Li Z, Schaff HV, Sundt TM III. Long-term risk of aortic events following aortic valve replacement in patients with bicuspid aortic valves. *Am J Cardiol* 2010;106:1626–1633.
11. Muna WF, Spray TL, Morrow AG, Roberts WC. Aortic dissection after aortic valve replacement in patients with valvular aortic stenosis. *J Thorac Cardiovasc Surg* 1977;74:65–69.
12. Gaudino M, Anselmi A, Morelli M, Pragliola C, Tsiopoulos V, Glieca F, Possati G. Aortic expansion rate in patients with dilated post-stenotic ascending aorta submitted only to aortic valve replacement: long-term follow-up. *J Am Coll Cardiol* 2011;58:581–584.
13. Rankin JS, Hammill BG, Ferguson TB Jr, Glower DD, O'Brien SM, DeLong ER, Peterson ED, Edwards FH. Determinants of operative mortality in valvular heart surgery. *J Thorac Cardiovasc Surg* 2006;131:547–557.
14. Roberts WC, Vowel TJ, Ko JM, Filardo G, Hebeler RF Jr, Henry AC, Matter GJ, Hamman BL. Comparison of the structure of the aortic valve and ascending aorta in adults having aortic valve replacement for aortic stenosis versus for pure aortic regurgitation and resection of the ascending aorta for aneurysm. *Circulation* 2011;123:896–903.

Aortic Medial Elastic Fiber Loss in Acute Ascending Aortic Dissection

William Clifford Roberts, MD[a,b,c,*], Travis James Vowels[a,g], Benjamin Lee Kitchens[h], Jong Mi Ko, BA[a], Giovanni Filardo, PhD, MPH[e,f], Albert Carl Henry, MD[d], Baron Lloyd Hamman, MD[d], Gregory John Matter, MD[d], and Robert Frederick Hebeler, Jr., MD[d]

The cause of acute aortic dissection continues to be debated. One school of thought suggests that underlying aortic medial cystic necrosis is the common denominator. The purpose of the present study was to determine if there was loss and, if so, how much loss of medial elastic fibers in the ascending aorta in patients with acute aortic dissection with the entrance tear in the ascending aorta. We examined operatively excised ascending aortas in 69 patients having acute dissection with tears in the ascending aorta. Patients with previous aortotomy, healed dissection, and connective tissue disorders were excluded. The 69 patients' ages ranged from 31 to 88 years (mean 56); 49 were men and 20 were women. Loss of aortic medial elastic fibers was graded as 0 (no loss), 1+ (trace), 2+ (mild), 3+ (moderate), and 4+ (full thickness loss). Of these 69 patients, 56 (82%) had 0 or 1+ elastic fiber loss; 13 patients (18%), 2+ to 4+ loss including 4 with 2+, 6 with 3+, and 2 with 4+. Nearly all patients (97%) had a history of systemic hypertension and/or had received antihypertensive drug therapy. In conclusion, most patients (82% in this study) having acute aortic dissection with entrance tears in the ascending aorta have normal numbers or only trace loss of aortic medial elastic fibers. Thus, underlying abnormal ascending aortic structure uncommonly precedes acute dissection. **(Am J Cardiol 2011;108:1639–1644)**

Numerous publications have appeared in the last 50 years describing operative procedures and their results in patients having operative therapy for acute dissection involving the ascending aorta.[1–10] Far fewer studies have been published on results of examination of the operatively resected portion of the ascending aorta.[11–21] The present report focuses on aortic medial elastic-fiber structure in 69 patients having portions of the ascending aorta operatively resected because of acute dissection involving the ascending aorta with or without involvement of other portions of the aorta.

Methods

Surgical pathology files of the cardiovascular laboratory—a part of the pathology department of Baylor University Medical Center at Dallas—were searched for patients having operatively resected portions of the ascending aorta with or without excision or repair of the aortic valve for acute dissection involving the ascending aorta with or without involvement of other portions of aorta. From May 1994 through June 2010, a period of 194 months (16.2 years), 119 specimens labeled as aortic dissection were received in the surgical pathology section and each was examined and described by 1 of us (W.C.R.). After the examination and description of the submitted specimen, histologic sections of all aortas were prepared: ≥1 paraffin section was stained by the Movat method.[22] All histologic sections were examined initially by W.C.R. to prepare the surgical pathology report and later, all together, as part of the present report. Total lengths (centimeters) of the sections of the aorta on each Movat-stained slide were measured and recorded.

Degree of loss of elastic fibers in the aortic media from examination of the Movat-stained slides was graded 0 to 4+; grade 0 or 1+ represented no loss or minimal loss or mild fragmentation of elastic fibers; grade 4 represented complete loss of elastic fibers in some full-thickness portions of media; grades 2 and 3 were intermediate (Figure 1).

Ascending aortas in 19 necropsy cases were selected to serve as controls for this study. None had cardiac valve disease or dilated ascending aortas. The 19 ranged in age from 28 to 82 years (mean 61); 10 were women and 9 were men. Twelve had died from cardiac causes (coronary artery disease events in 10, amyloidosis in 1, and lymphocytic myocarditis in 1) and 7 from noncardiac and nonvascular causes. Sections of ascending aorta perpendicular and parallel to the long axis were prepared from each control subject. In each of the 19 cases, 1 section was stained by hematoxylin and eosin, another by

[a]Baylor Heart and Vascular Institute and [b]Departments of Pathology, Internal Medicine ([c]Division of Cardiology), and [d]Cardiothoracic Surgery, Baylor University Medical Center, Dallas, Texas; [e]Institute for Health Care Research and Improvement, Baylor Health Care System and [f]Department of Statistical Science, Southern Methodist University, Dallas Texas; [g]Senior, University of Texas at Austin, Austin, Texas; [h]Junior, University of Texas School of Medicine at San Antonio, Texas. Manuscript received September 9, 2011; revised manuscript received and accepted September 10, 2011.

The study was funded by Baylor Health Care System Foundation, Dallas, Texas.

*Corresponding author: Tel: 214-820-7911; fax: 214-820-7533.

E-mail address: wc.roberts@baylorhealth.edu (W.C. Roberts).

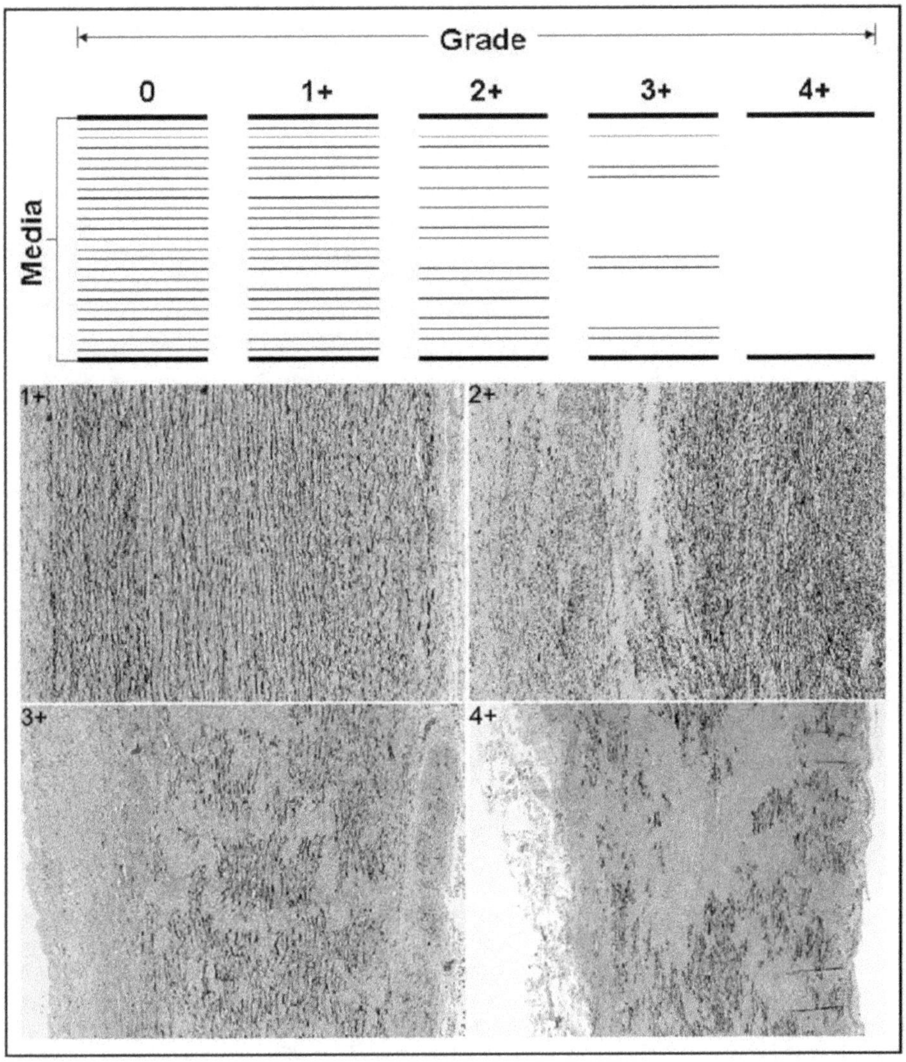

Figure 1. Diagram showing grading system used in this study. *(Top)* Diagram showing 0 to 4+ loss of medial elastic fibers. The internal *(top dark line)* and external *(bottom dark line)* elastic membranes and elastic fibers in the media *(lighter lines)* are represented. (See text for explanation.) *(Bottom)* Photographs (100×) and stained by Movat stain show medial elastic fiber loss 1+ *(mid left)* to 4+ *(lower right)*. (Reproduced with permission from W.C. Roberts and the publisher of *Circulation* 2011;123:896–903.)

Movat stain, and another by elastic-van Gieson methods. Lengths of the aorta examined histologically were measured in centimeters.

Clinical records including admission note and/or discharge summary, echocardiographic and cardiac catheterization reports, and operative records were sought from all patients' medical charts and/or from the Baylor University Medical Center Apollo cardiovascular database (Apollo Advance C/S 4.2.13, LUMEDX Corp., Oakland, California).

Included in the present study were 69 patients who had resection of portions of the ascending aorta and initiating tears in the ascending aorta. Excluded from this study were 50 patients: 5 who had an acute aortic dissection in the operating room at the time of coronary artery bypass grafting or aortic valve replacement; 4 patients who had acute dissection involving the ascending aorta late postoperatively after coronary artery bypass grafting and/or aortic valve replacement; 6 patients who had a tear in the descending thoracic aorta (isthmic area) and acute retrograde dissection of the ascending aorta; and 35 patients who had healed (chronic) aortic dissection irrespective of the location of the initial aortic entrance site, including 20 patients who had a previous aortotomy of the ascending aorta. Also excluded were patients with genetically mediated conditions such as Marfan syndrome and Loeys-Dietz syndrome. None of the 69 patients included in the present study had a previous aortotomy, and all had dissection entrance sites in the ascending aorta and dissection afterward with operative resection of portions of the ascending aorta.

Descriptive statistics (percentage, mean ± SD) were used to describe patients included in the study. A Cox proportional hazards model (without covariates) was used to assess the unadjusted association of loss of medial elastic fibers (2+, 3+, or 4+) and mortality. Unadjusted survival curves and survival estimates were computed using the Kaplan–Meier method.

This study was approved by the institutional review board at Baylor University Medical Center.

Table 1
Characteristics of patients with acute aortic dissection with tears in ascending aorta

Variable	Elastic Fiber Loss		p Value*
	0–1+ (n = 56)	2+–4+ (n = 13)	
Ages (years), range (mean ± SD) [median]	31–88 (59 ± 14) [60]	34–66 (45 ± 10) [45]	0.003
Men	38 (68%)	11 (85%)	0.234†
	31–77 (56 ± 13) [56]	34–66 (44 ± 9) [44]	
Women	18 (32%)	2 (15%)	
	43–88 (65 ± 13) [68]	46, 63	
Race			0.381
White	34 (61%)	10 (77%)	
Black	14 (25%)	3 (23%)	
Hispanic	4 (7%)	0	
Other or unclear	4 (7%)	0	
Systemic hypertension by history or antihypertension therapy	51 (91%)	13 (100%)	0.268
Previous resection, abdominal aortic aneurysm	3 (5%)	0	0.397
Body mass index (kg/m^2) (n = 65)	18.9–46.4 (28.9 ± 6.8) [27.7]	20.9–42.1 (29.5 ± 6.9) [28.1]	0.947
Men	19.8–46.4 (29.8 ± 7.0) [28.3]	20.9–42.1 (30.7 ± 7.0) [29.6]	
≤25	9 (26%)	3 (30%)	
26–30	14 (40%)	3 (30%)	
>30	12 (34%)	4 (40%)	
Women	18.9–44.7 (27.1 ± 6.4) [26.8]	21, 26.6	
≤25	7 (41%)	1 (50%)	
26–30	6 (35%)	1 (50%)	
>30	4 (24%)	0	
Aortic valve (n = 49)			0.797
Replaced	20 (54%)	7 (58%)	
"Repaired"	17 (45%)	5 (41%)	
Number aortic valve cusps (n = 56)			0.3559
2	3 (7%)	2 (15%)	
3	40 (93%)	11 (85%)	
Weight (g) of excised aortic valves (n = 17)	0.38–1.75 (0.77 ± 0.43) [0.67]	0.39–0.93 (0.68 ± 0.20) [0.69]	0.675
Bicuspid	0.53, 1.52, 1.75	0.77	—
Tricuspid	0.38–0.81 (0.60 ± 0.15) [0.66]	0.39–0.93 (0.66 ± 0.22) [0.66]	0.587
Coronary bypass	7‡ (13%)	0	0.181
Weight of excised ascending aorta (g) (n = 66)	0.4–59.5 (16.59 ± 11.52) [13.4]	6.14–30 (17.37 ± 9.73) [14.9]	0.834
With bicuspid valve	27.5–51 (35.50 ± 7.75) [28]	25.05	—
With tricuspid valve	0.4–59.5 (15.42 ± 11.30) [13.2]	6.14–30 (16.60 ± 9.73) [14.6]	0.764
Lengths (cm) of ascending aorta examined	4–19 (10 ± 4) [10.5]	4–21 (14 ± 5) [14]	0.063
Men	4–19 (10 ± 4) [10.5]	4–21 (14 ± 5) [14]	0.057
Women	6–16 (11 ± 3) [12]	8, 17	0.824
Intimal plaque, ascending aorta	7 (13%)	2 (15%)	0.785
Died: days after operation (n = 30)			0.115
≤30	19 (79%)	3 (50%)	
	0–28 (5 ± 7) [3]	2, 8, 13	
>30	5 (21%)	3 (50%)	
	58–2,418 (712 ± 1,004) [141]	150, 445, 2,060	
Days in hospital postoperatively in patients living >30days	4–48 (14 ± 11) [10]	5–63 (16 ± 18) [10]	0.548

* The p values accounted for multiple comparisons.
† The p value accounts for gender versus elastic fiber loss comparison.
‡ One of the 7 patients had bypass because of coronary artery disease; the other 6 had bypass because the dissection or tear involved the left and/or right coronary ostia.

Results

Findings in the 69 patients are presented in Table 1. Qualitative comparison of degree of loss of medial elastic fibers at the initial examination of the Movat-stained sections to the re-examination of the Movat-stained sections showed only minimal discrepancies: some cases called normal at the initial examination were occasionally called 1+ on re-examination or vice-versa; sections classified as 2+ or 3+ or 4+ initially were classified similarly on re-examination. Photomicrographs of typical acute dissection are shown in Figure 2.

Examination of Movat-stained and elastic-van Gieson–stained sections of aorta in the 19 control subjects disclosed no discrepancies in degree of medial elastic fiber loss or lack thereof between the 2 stains in any subject. Degree of elastic fiber loss in all 19 control subjects was zero or 1+. Specifically, no subject had 2+, 3+, or 4+ elastic fiber loss. Lengths of ascending aorta examined from the Movat-stained sections ranged from 4 to 16 cm (mean 10).

At the time of the operation the mean age of the 49 men was 53 years and that of the 20 women was 64 years (Table

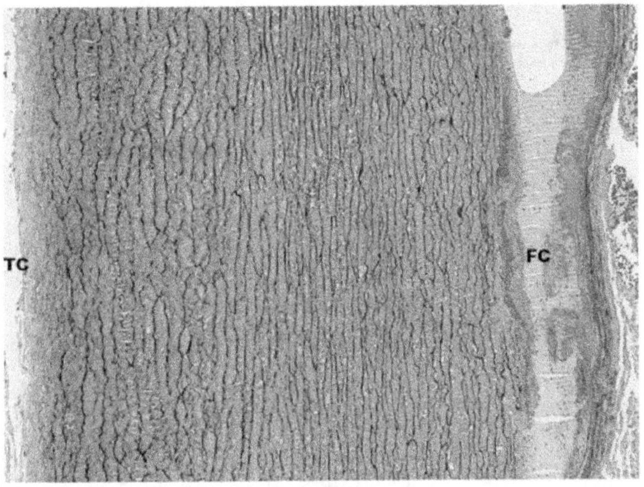

Figure 2. Photomicrograph of a typical aortic dissection in a 57-year-old man. The tear was in the ascending aorta and the dissection traveled retrograde into the aorta behind the sinuses of Valsalva and anterograde to the common iliac arteries. The true lumen (TC) *(left)* and the false channel (FC) *(right)* are visible. The dissection is located in the very outer media. The black-staining medial elastic fibers are few in number in the outer wall of the false channel. Because the outer wall is so much thinner than the partition of media between the true lumen and false channel, rupture exteriorly is very common but rupture of the false channel back into the true lumen is very rare. Medial elastic fiber loss in this patient was graded 1+/4+ (Movat stain, 100×).

1). Nearly 2/3 were white. Thirty of the 69 patients (43%) have died: 22 (32%) within 30 days of the operative procedure and 8 (12%) >30 days later. Of the 47 surviving >30 days, stay in the hospital after operation ranged from 4 to 63 days (mean 15, median 10). By history, 92% of patients (59 of 64) had systemic hypertension, 70% (40/57) were on antihypertensive therapy, and 97% (64/66) had a history of hypertension or were on antihypertensive therapy. Body mass indexes (BMIs; kilograms per square meter) ranged from 18.9 to 46.4 (mean 29.0, median 27.7) and 20 of 64 patients (31%) had BMI <25 kg/m^2. Only 1 of the 69 patients was documented to have atherosclerotic coronary artery narrowing. Seven patients, however, had coronary bypass, 6 because of dissection or tears involving the origin of the right (5 patients) or left main (1 patient) coronary artery. The aortic valve was replaced in 27 patients (39%) and "repaired" in another 22 patients (32%). At least 5 patients were described at operation or by the surgical pathologist (W.C.R.) as having congenitally bicuspid aortic valves. The operatively excised 3-cuspid valves (13 patients) weighed 0.38 to 0.93 g (mean 0.62), and the congenitally bicuspid valves (4 patients) weighed from 0.53 to 1.75 g (mean 1.14). The aortic valve was replaced with a bioprosthesis in 3 patients, a mechanical prosthesis in 19, and a homograft in 5 patients (Table 2).

Operatively excised aortas ranged in weight from 0.4 to 59 g (mean 17, median 14) and in 50 patients (76%) weighed >10 g. Lengths of ascending aorta examined in the Movat-stained slides (those stained for elastic fibers) ranged from 4 to 21 cm (mean 11, median 12). Losses of elastic fibers in the media of sections of ascending aorta were 0 (24 patients, 35%), 1+ (32 patients, 46%), 2+ (5 patients, 7%), 3+ (6 patients, 9%), and 4+ (2 patients, 3%). Atherosclerotic plaques were present in the ascending aorta in 9 patients (13%). Of the 5 patients with bicuspid aortic valves, aortic medial elastic fiber loss was 0 in 1, 1+ in 2, and 3+ in 2. A typical example of aortic dissection is shown in Figure 2.

Unadjusted association between loss of medial elastic fibers and mortality was not significant (hazard ratio 0.95, 95% confidence interval 0.39 to 2.34, log-rank p = 0.91). Survival curves are shown in Figure 3. Survival was assessed by the Social Security Death Index.

Discussion

The present study focused on 69 patients who had acute aortic dissection with entrance tears in the ascending aorta and operative resection of a portion of ascending aorta with or without replacement or repair of the native aortic valve. The purpose was to determine if the elastic fiber structure of the media of the ascending aorta was normal or abnormal. Examination of 4 to 21 cm (mean 12) of aorta stained for elastic fibers (Movat stain) showed that 56 of the 69 patients (81%) had normal or nearly normal numbers of medial elastic fibers and that only 13 (19%) had focal loss (2+ to 4+) of medial elastic fibers. The 2+ to 4+ losses of elastic fibers are considered changes greater than that expected by aging alone.[13]

Why did the study of histologic sections of ascending aorta focus only on medial elastic fibers when the wall of the ascending aorta also contains smooth muscle cells, collagen, and some mucoid material? The reason is that examination of the elastic fiber structure is easily discernible and interpretation is highly reproducible. Grading of degree of medial elastic fiber loss when examined initially (when preparing the surgical pathology report) and then again altogether when re-examining sections for the present study showed no discordant interpretations. A few patients considered to have 0 elastic fiber loss initially were graded 1+ on re-examination and vice-versa; all cases graded 2+, 3+, or 4+ initially were graded similarly on re-examination. When medial elastic fibers are lost, it appears they are replaced by fibrous tissue and by small deposits of mucoid material, suggesting that medial elastic fibers serve as a good marker of other changes in the aortic media.

The phrases "idiopathic cystic medionecrosis," "cystic medionecrosis," or simply "medionecrosis" were first used by Erdheim[23,24] in 1929 and subsequently have often been used to describe aortic medial histologic lesions in patients with acute aortic dissection. Indeed, there is a widely held perception that medial cystic necrosis is the chief predisposing cause of acute aortic dissection. However, as pointed out by Hirst and Gore,[12] Erdheim studied only 2 patients, describing the aorta histologically in meticulous detail, but each of his 2 patients had rupture of a nondissecting aneurysm of the ascending aorta, not aortic dissection!

Erdheim's terms, as pointed out by Hirst and Gore,[12] Schlatmann and Becker,[13] and Roberts,[17] are not ideal because the terms are inappropriate: "cystic" refers to cysts, which are generally considered to have true linings (not so in the aortic media); "necrosis" is extremely difficult to determine but almost surely is the result, when it occurs, of intraluminal arterial pressure compressing the adjacent me-

Table 2
Mortality rate of patients having operative treatment for acute ascending aortic dissection with or without concomitant aortic valve replacement or repair

Died Postoperatively	Concomitant AVR Using						
	Mechanical Prosthesis (n = 19)	Bioprosthesis (n = 3)	Homograft (n = 5)	Any Type of Substitute Valve (n = 27)	Concomitant AV Repair (n = 22)	Without AVR or Repair (n = 20)	Total (n = 69)
≤30 days	5	2	3	10	5	7	22 (32%)
>30 days	3	0	1	4	2	2	8 (12%)
Total	8 (42%)	2 (67%)	4 (80%)	14 (52%)	7 (32%)	9 (45%)	30 (44%)

AV = aortic valve; AVR = aortic valve replacement.

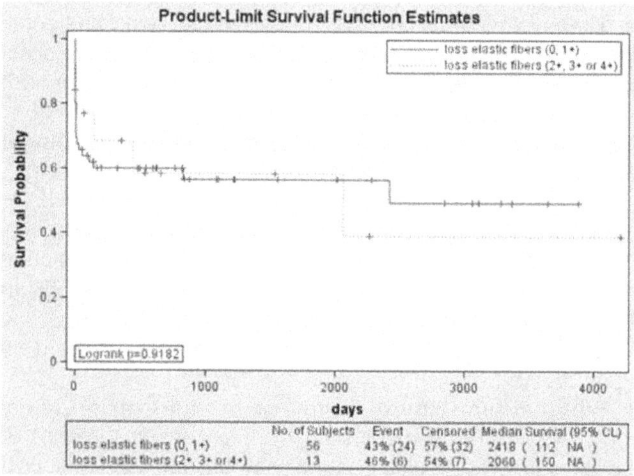

Figure 3. Unadjusted (Kaplan–Meier) curves depicting long-term survival by loss of medial elastic fiber. CL = confidence limit; NA = not available.

dia—something occurring after, not before, acute dissection. We believe that focusing on medial elastic fibers alone provides the most accurate and reproducible description of the aortic media in patients with acute aortic dissection, and that the phrase "cystic medionecrosis," as emphasized by Schlatmann and Becker,[14] should be abandoned and no longer used to indicate a pathologic condition that underlies acute aortic dissection.

A near universal finding in our 69 patients was systemic hypertension: by history in 92% (59/64), by antihypertensive therapy in 70% (40/57), and by history and/or antihypertensive therapy in 97% (64/66). Many others, of course, have emphasized the frequency of systemic hypertension in patients with acute aortic dissection.[25–29] Frequency of systemic hypertension increases as body weight increases[30]: 73% of the men (33/45) had BMI >25 kg/m^2, including 36% whose BMI was >30 kg/m^2; 58% of the women (11/19) had BMI >25 kg/m^2, including 21% whose BMI was >30 kg/m^2. African-Americans have a higher frequency of systemic hypertension than do European-Americans[31]: there was a larger percentage of African-Americans in our study than are present in the general population (25% vs 13%). Certain activities that cause a sudden increase in systemic arterial pressure have precipitated acute aortic dissection, e.g., cocaine inhalation.[32] As pointed out by Carlson et al,[33] the incidence of cystic medial necrosis (basophilic discoloration of hematoxylin–eosin stains, medial cysts, elastic fiber interruption with or without "retraction") of the ascending aorta is higher in hypertensive than normotensive subjects of comparable ages.

Patients with congenitally bicuspid aortic valves have a higher frequency of aortic dissection with tears in the ascending aorta than do patients with tricuspid aortic valves[34]: ≥9% of our patients (5/56) had congenitally bicuspid valves: loss of medial elastic fibers in them was 0 in 1, 1+ in 2, and 3+ in 2 patients. The bicuspid valves were heavier than the tricuspid valves (mean 1.14 vs 0.62 g).

Acute aortic dissection generally occurs in patients younger than those with acute coronary syndrome.[25–29] In 1 large study the average age of death in men from coronary heart disease not treated by revascularization was 61 years and that in women was 71 years.[35] In contrast, in our 69 dissection patients, mean age at operation in the 49 men was 53 years and that in the 20 women was 64 years. Had not the operative procedure been performed, death almost certainly would have rapidly followed.

Atherosclerosis appears to be unrelated to acute aortic dissection.[36] Only 9 of our patients had atherosclerotic plaques in the ascending aorta and in each the plaques were small. In addition, atherosclerotic narrowing of ≥1 major coronary artery was documented in only 1 of our 69 patients.

The positive features of the present study are the following: (1) all histologic sections were examined and medial elastic fiber loss graded initially for the surgical pathology report and later all together by the same investigator (W.C.R.); (2) lengths of the ascending aorta examined histologically were recorded for the first time in dissection patients; (3) reproducibility of the histologic grading system was nearly 100%; (4) weights of resected portions of dissected ascending aorta were recorded for the first time; (5) weights of operatively excised valves were recorded; (6) data on BMI were recorded; and (7) a relatively long follow-up after operative treatment was available.

The present study has limitations: (1) although preoperative computed tomography was performed in many patients (65%), most were performed at the referring hospital and the results—other than the presence of aortic dissection—of most are not known to us; (2) different quantities of aorta were available for examination, although ≥4 cm of aorta was examined histologically in all patients; and (3) aortic valve structure (unicuspid, bicuspid, tricuspid) was not known in 19% of patients (it was known in 81% of patients.).

1. Fann JI, Smith JA, Miller DC, Mitchell RS, Moore KA, Grunkemeier G, Stinson EB, Oyer PE, Reitz BA, Shumway NE. Surgical management of aortic dissection during a 30-year period. *Circulation* 1995; 92:113–121.
2. Von Segesser LK, Lorenzetti E, Lachat M, Niederhäuser U, Schönbeck M, Vogt PR, Turina MI. Aortic valve preservation in acute type A dissection: is it sound? *J Thorac Cardiovasc Surg* 1996; 111: 381–391.
3. Bachet J, Goudot B, Dreyfus GD, Brodaty D, Dubois C, Delentdecker P, Guilmet D. Surgery for acute type A aortic dissection: the hospital Foch experience (1977–1998). *Ann Thorac Surg* 1999; 67: 2006–2009.
4. David TE, Armstron S, Ivanov J, Barnard S. Surgery for acute type A aortic dissection. *Ann Thorac Surg* 1999; 67: 1999–2001.
5. Leyh RG, Schmidtke C, Bartels C, Sievers HH. Valve-sparing aortic root replacement (remodeling/reimplantation) in acute type A dissection. *Ann Thorac Surg* 2000; 70: 21–24.
6. Sabik JF, Lytle BW, Blackstone EH, McCarthy PM, Loop FD, Cosgrove DM. Long-term effectiveness of operations for ascending aortic dissections. *J Thorac Cardiovasc Surg* 2000; 119: 946–962.
7. Westaby S, Saito S, Katsumata T. Acute type A dissection: conservative methods provide consistently low mortality. *Ann Thorac Surg* 2002; 73: 707–713.
8. Elefteriades JA. Natural history of thoracic aortic aneurysms: indications for surgery, and surgical versus nonsurgical risks. *Ann Thorac Surg* 2002; 74: 1877–1880.
9. Lai DT, Robbins RC, Mitchell RS, Moore KA, Oyer PE, Shumway NE, Reitz BA, Miller DC. Does profound hypothermic circulatory arrest improve survival in patients with acute type A aortic dissection? *Circulation* 2002;106:218–228.
10. Tan ME, Morshuis WJ, Dossche KM, Kelder JC, Waanders FG, Schepens MA. Long-term results after 27 years of surgical treatment of acute type A aortic dissection. *Ann Thorac Surg* 2005; 80: 523–529.
11. Gore I, Seiwert VJ. Dissecting aneurysm of the aorta; pathological aspects; an analysis of eighty-five fatal cases. *AMA Arch Pathol* 1952; 53: 121–141.
12. Hirst AE, Gore I. Editorial: Is cystic medionecrosis the cause of dissecting aortic aneurysm? *Circulation* 1976; 53: 915–916.
13. Schlatmann TJ, Becker AE. Histologic changes in the normal aging aorta: implications for dissecting aortic aneurysm. *Am J Cardiol* 1977; 39: 13–20.
14. Schlatmann TJM, Becker AE. Pathogenesis of dissecting aneurysm of aorta. Comparative histopathologic study of significance of medial changes. *Am J Cardiol* 1977; 39: 21–26.
15. Kunita Y. A pathological study of dissecting aneurysm in individuals under forty years of age including a case of a 13 years old boy. *Acta Pathol Jpn* 1978; 28: 253–263.
16. Leonard JC, Hasleton PS. Dissecting aortic aneurysm: a clinicopathological study. *Q J Med* 1979;189:55–76.
17. Roberts WC. Aortic dissection: anatomy, consequences, and causes. *Am Heart J* 1981;101:195–214.
18. Larson EW, Edwards WD. Risk factors for aortic dissection: a necropsy study of 161 cases. *Am J Cardiol* 1984; 53: 849–855.
19. Lindsay J Jr, Hurst JW. Clinical features and prognosis in dissecting aneurysm of the aorta. A re-appraisal. *Circulation* 1967; 35: 880–888.
20. McManus BM, Cassling RS, Soundy TJ, Wilson JE, Sears TD, Rogler WC, Buehler BA, Wolford JF, Duggan MJ, Byers PH, Fleming WH, Sanger WG. Familial aortic dissection in the absence of ascending aortic aneurysms: a lethal syndrome associated with precocious systemic hypertension. *Am J Cardiovasc Pathol* 1986;1:55–67.
21. Mészáros I, Mórocz J, Szlávi J, Schmidt J, Tornóci L, Nagy L, Szép L. Epidemiology and clinicopathology of aortic dissection. *Chest* 2000; 117: 1271–1278.
22. Movat HZ. Demonstration of all connective tissue elements in a single section; pentachrome stains. *AMA Arch Pathol* 1955; 60 :289–295.
23. Erdheim J. Medionecrosis aortae idiopathica. *Virchows Arch Pathol Anat*1929; 273: 454–479.
24. Erdheim J. Medionecrosis aortae idiopathica cystica. *Virchows Arch Pathol Anat* 1930; 276: 187–229.
25. Spittell PC, Spittell JA, Joyce JW, Tajik AJ, Edwards WD, Schaff HV, Stanson AW. Clinical features and differential diagnosis of aortic dissection: experience with 236 cases (1980 through 1990). *Mayo Clin Proc* 1993; 68: 642–651.
26. Hagan PG, Nienaber CA, Isselbacher EM, Bruckman D, Karavite DJ, Russman PL, Evangelista A, Fattori R, Suzuki T, Oh JK, Moore AG, Malouf JF, Pape LA, Gaca C, Sechtem U, Lenferink S, Deutsch HJ, Diedrichs H, Marcos y Robles J, Llovet A, Gilon D, Das SK, Armstrong WF, Deeb GM, Eagle KA. The International Registry of Acute Aortic Dissection (IRAD): new insights into an old disease. *JAMA* 2000; 283: 897–903.
27. Januzzi JL, Isselbacher EM, Fattori R, Cooper JV, Smith DE, Fang J, Eagle KA, Mehta RH, Nienaber CA, Pape LA; International Registry of Aortic Dissection (IRAD). Characterizing the young patient with aortic dissection: results from the international registry of aortic dissection (IRAD). *J Am Coll Cardiol* 2004; 43: 665–669.
28. Clouse WD, Hallett JW, Schaff HV, Spittell PC, Rowland CM, Ilstrup DM, Melton LJ. Acute aortic dissection: population-based incidence compared with degenerative aortic aneurysm rupture. *Mayo Clin Proc* 2004;79:176–180.
29. Olsson C, Thelin S, Ståhle E, Ekbom A, Granath F. Thoracic aortic aneurysm and dissection: increasing prevalence and improved outcomes reported in a nationwide population-based study of more than 14,000 cases from 1987 to 2002. *Circulation* 2006; 114: 2611–2618.
30. Wilson PW, D'Agostino RB, Sullivan L, Parise H, Kannel WB. Overweight and obesity as determinants of cardiovascular risk: the Framingham experience. *Arch Intern Med* 2002; 162: 1867–1872.
31. Morris RC Jr, Sebastian A, Forman A, Tanaka M, SchmidlinO. Normotensive salt sensitivity: effects of race and dietary potassium. *Hypertension* 1999; 33: 18–23.
32. Barth CW III, Bray M, Roberts WC. Rupture of the ascending aorta during cocaine intoxication. *Am J Cardiol* 1986; 57: 496.
33. Carlson RG, Lillehei CW, Edwards JE. Cystic medial necrosis of the ascending aorta in relation to age and hypertension. *Am J Cardiol* 1970; 25: 411–415.
34. Roberts CS, Roberts WC. Dissection of the aorta associated with congenital malformation of the aortic valve. *J Am Coll Cardiol* 1991; 17: 712–716.
35. Roberts WC, Potkin BN, Solus DE, Reddy G. Mode of death, frequency of healed and acute myocardial infarction, number of major epicardial coronary arteries severely narrowed by atherosclerotic plaque, and heart weight in fatal atherosclerotic coronary artery disease: analysis of 889 patients studied at necropsy. *J Am Coll Cardiol* 1990; 15: 196–203.
36. Achneck H, Modi B, Shaw C, Rizzo J, Albornoz G, Fusco D, Elefteriades J. Ascending thoracic aneurysms are associated with decreased systemic atherosclerosis. *Chest* 2005;128:1580–1586.

Cardiac Findings at Necropsy in Patients With Chronic Kidney Disease Maintained on Chronic Hemodialysis

William C. Roberts, MD, Marc A. Taylor, MD, and Jamshid Shirani, MD

Abstract: Studies of multiple hearts at necropsy are lacking in patients who have been on chronic hemodialysis for chronic kidney disease (CKD). We studied at necropsy 120 patients who had been treated with hemodialysis for more than 1 year (mean, 5.25 ± 4.33 yr). Their ages ranged from 24 to 81 years (mean, 53 yr); 91 (76%) were men. Calcific deposits were present in the heart at necropsy in 74 (62%) patients: in the epicardial coronary arteries in all 74 (62%); in the mitral annular region in 52 (42%) patients, and in the aortic valve cusps in 42 (35%) patients. The frequency and quantity of the cardiac calcific deposits were significantly greater in the older compared with the younger patients, and in those with longer durations of hemodialysis compared with those with shorter durations. Despite the calcific deposits, which were sometimes huge, only 47 (39%) patients had 1 or more coronary arteries narrowed more than 75% in cross-sectional area by atherosclerotic plaques, apparently no patient had clinical evidence of mitral stenosis, and 9 patients had clinical evidence of aortic valve stenosis. Thus, we found that CKD treated with hemodialysis is a major producer of cardiac calcific deposits, some of which can be massive. Only a minority of the calcific deposits, however, appeared to lead to cardiac dysfunction or myocardial ischemia during life.

(*Medicine* 2012;91: 165–178)

Abbreviations: CKD = chronic kidney disease, CT = computed tomography.

INTRODUCTION

Calcific deposits have been described in the heart in many patients with chronic kidney disease (CKD) irrespective of whether they received hemodialysis or not.[12–15,19,23,27,29–32,35,38,39,48,49,51] Except for a few patients studied at necropsy with CKD treated with hemodialysis 50 or so years ago,[3,24,26,28,31,50] the cardiac calcific deposits in patients with CKD have been demonstrated mainly by imaging studies, including echocardiography, computed tomography (CT), and magnetic resonance imaging. In this report we describe necropsy findings in 120 patients aged 20 years or more with CKD treated with hemodialysis for more than 1 year. Our purpose is simply to demonstrate via gross photographs the magnitude of the cardiac calcific deposits and their clinical consequences.[1,2,4,5,7–9,17,18,21,22,25,33,34,37,40,41,45,53,55] Another purpose is to determine the causes of death in these CKD patients, something probably given inadequate attention in the past.[6,10,16,52]

From the Pathology Branch (WCR, MAT, JS), National Heart, Lung, and Blood Institute, National Institutes of Health, Bethesda, Maryland, and Baylor Heart and Vascular Institute (WCR), Baylor University Medical Center, Dallas, Texas.

Dr. Taylor's current address: Florida Cardiovascular Institute, 509 South Armenia, Tampa, FL 33609. Dr. Shirani's current address: St. Luke's Hospital & Health Network, Heart and Vascular Center, 801 Ostrum Street, Bethlehem, PA 18015.

This study was supported by the National Heart, Lung, and Blood Institute, Intramural Program, National Institutes of Health, Bethesda, MD; and the Baylor Health Care System Foundation, Dallas, TX.

The authors have no conflicts of interest to disclose.

Figure 14 can be viewed in color online at http://www.md-journal.com.

Reprints: William C. Roberts, MD, Baylor Heart and Vascular Institute, Baylor University Medical Center, 3500 Gaston Avenue, Suite H-030, Dallas, TX 75246 (e-mail: wc.roberts@baylorhealth.edu).

ISSN: 0025-7974

DOI: 10.1097/MD.0b013e318256e076

STUDY DESIGN AND METHODS

Patients, Sources, and Study Criteria

We searched the files of the Pathology Branch, National Heart, Lung, and Blood Institute, National Institutes of Health for all cases coded as having had "hemodialysis." We found 156 such cases and examined their records. We excluded patients who had hemodialysis for 1 year or less (15 cases), patients who had peritoneal dialysis for more than 6 months in their last year of life (6 cases), patients lacking adequate clinical information (12 cases), and patients aged 15 years or younger at the onset of hemodialysis (3 cases). The remaining 120 patients are the focus of the present study. All patients were aged 20 years or more at death, all were maintained on chronic hemodialysis for more than 1 year, none had chronic peritoneal dialysis during their last year of life, all had clinical records available for our examination, all of their hearts were submitted to the Pathology Branch, and all of their hearts were examined by us—initially by WCR, and later most were examined by MAT and JS and reexamined by WCR.

From 1973 to 1992, 1–13 cases were seen annually (Figure 1). The 120 hearts had been submitted from 12 different institutions and medical centers including 24 hearts from the District of Columbia Veterans Administration Hospital, 21 from Washington Hospital Center (Washington, DC), 20 from the Georgetown University Hospital (Washington, DC), 18 from Howard University Hospital (Washington, DC), 18 from the District of Columbia Medical Examiner's Office, 10 from the George Washington University Hospital (Washington, DC), 4 from the District of Columbia General Hospital, and 1 each from 5 different local and nonlocal medical centers.

Examination of the Hearts

The submitted hearts were cleaned of extraneous material, weighed on accurate scales (Mettler P1210 or Mettler PM2000, Mettler Instrument Corporation, Hightstown, NJ) and usually a radiograph of the heart was made in a Hewlett-Packard Faxitron Series 43805N machine using a voltage of 30–50 Kev and an exposure time of 30–60 seconds. All hearts were classified and coded by us (WCR). They were then opened in a manner dependent on the pathology believed to be present.[42] After thorough gross study of the heart itself, sections were taken of the left ventricular free wall for histologic examination. The clinical and necropsy records from the submitting hospital also were reviewed.

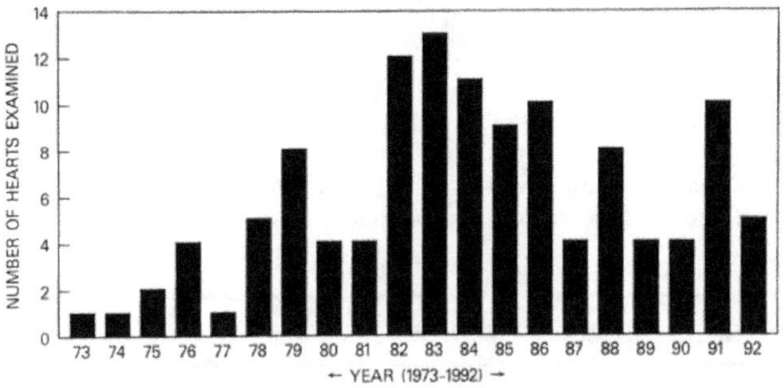

FIGURE 1. Number of patients studied during each of the years from 1973 through 1992.

Statistical Analysis

Results are reported as mean ± standard deviation for continuous variables, and frequencies for noncontinuous variables. The Student t test was used to assess the significance of differences between 2 age groups (patients aged ≤50 yr and those aged >50 yr) and between 2 ranges of hemodialysis duration (>1–4 yr and >4–22 yr), and to compare patients with or without heavy calcific deposits in the hearts. A significant difference was defined as $p < 0.05$.

RESULTS

Patient Age and Duration of Hemodialysis

The patients at death ranged in age from 24 to 81 years (mean, 53 yr); only 5 were younger than 31 and only 1 patient was older than 80 years (Table 1). The patients were maintained on hemodialysis for >12–264 months (mean, 63 mo): two-thirds were treated with hemodialysis for more than 2 years; 38 (32%) for more than 5 years, and 12 (10%) for more than 10 years (Table 2).

Causes of Chronic Kidney Disease

Systemic hypertension and diabetes mellitus were responsible for CKD in 70 (58%) of the 120 patients (Table 3). In 10 (8%) patients the etiology was primary glomerular disease, and in 15 (12%) patients the etiology was uncertain.

Clinical and Laboratory Findings

Clinical and laboratory findings are presented in Table 4. Two patients had primary and 15 patients had secondary hyperparathyroidism. Systemic hypertension was present in 107 (90%); diabetes mellitus in 36 (30%); and peripheral vascular disease in 19 (16%), including 11 who had lower extremity amputation. Angina pectoris occurred in at least 31 (26%)

TABLE 1. Age Distribution of 120 Adults With Chronic Kidney Disease Treated With Hemodialysis for >1 Year

	Age (yr)	No. (%)
	24–30	5 (4)
	31–40	19 (16)
	41–50	25 (21)
	51–60	26 (22)
	61–70	27 (23)
	71–80	17 (14)
	81	1 (<1)
Total	**24–81**	**120 (100)**

TABLE 2. Duration of Hemodialysis in 120 Adults With Chronic Kidney Disease

	Duration (yr)	No. (%)
	>1–2	40 (34)
	>2–3	19 (16)
	>3–4	10 (8)
	>4–5	13 (11)
	>5–6	6 (5)
	>6–7	2 (<2)
	>7–8	8 (7)
	>8–9	5 (4)
	>9–10	5 (4)
	>10–11	1 (<1)
	>11–12	2 (<2)
	>12–13	3 (<3)
	>13–14	1 (<1)
	>14–15	1 (<1)
	>15–16	1 (<1)
	>16–17	1 (<1)
	>17	2 (<2)
Total	**>1–22**	**120 (100)**

TABLE 3. Etiology of Chronic Kidney Disease in 120 Adults

Etiology	No. (%)
Systemic hypertension	41 (34)
Diabetes mellitus	29 (24)
Systemic disease	4 (3)
Systemic vasculitis	2
Systemic lupus erythematosus	1
Alport syndrome	1
Primary glomerular disease	10 (8)
Acute glomerulonephritis	2
Chronic glomerulonephritis	4
Crescentic glomerulonephritis	1
Membranous glomerulonephritis	1
Membranoproliferative glomerulonephritis	1
Rapidly progressive glomerulonephritis	1
Miscellaneous causes	21 (18)
Adult polycystic kidney disease	7
Heroin nephropathy	3
Trauma	2
Primary hyperparathyroidism	2
Chronic pyelonephritis	2
AIDS nephropathy	1
Renal cell carcinoma	1
Acute tubular necrosis	1
Obstructive uropathy	1
Analgesic nephropathy	1
Uncertain	15 (12)
Total	**120 (100)**

TABLE 4. Clinical and Laboratory Findings in 120 Adults

Variable	No. (%)
Age, yr; range (mean)	24–81 (53 ± 13)
White/black	37 (31)/83 (69)
Men/women	91 (76)/29 (24)
Duration of hemodialysis, yr; range (mean)	>1–22 (5.25 ± 4.33)
>1–5	82 (68)
>5–10	26 (22)
>10	12 (10)
Blood pressure, mm Hg; range (mean)	
Peak systolic	90–260 (172 ± 36)
End diastolic	40–140 (98 ± 21)
Systemic hypertension (history)	107 (90)
Diabetes mellitus	36 (30)
Angina pectoris	31 (26)
Acute myocardial infarction (history)	17 (14)
Chronic heart failure (history)	34 (29)
Peripheral vascular disease (history)	18 (15)
Cerebrovascular disease (history)	11 (9)
Laboratory tests: range (mean)	
Blood	
Urea nitrogen (mg/dL)	22–179 (77 ± 33)
Hematocrit (%)	9–44 (25 ± 6)
Serum	
Creatinine (mg/dL)	2.1–17.7 (9.7 ± 3.7)
Glucose (mg/dL)	37–500 (137 ± 77)
Total cholesterol (mg/dL)	90–268 (164 ± 51)
Total protein (g/dL)	2–4.8 (3.4 ± 0.6)
Calcium (mg/dL)	5.5–12 (9.0 ± 1.5)
Phosphorus (mg/dL)	2.5–14.5 (5.7 ± 2.2)
Surgery for pericardial disease	18 (15)
Renal transplantation	24 (20)

patients; 17 (14%) had a history of acute myocardial infarction, and 34 (29%) had signs and symptoms of chronic heart failure. Renal transplantation was done in 24 (20%) patients after years of chronic hemodialysis.

During life acute myocardial infarction was diagnosed in 17 of the 120 patients. Of these 17 patients, at necropsy 5 had foci of necrosis (acute myocardial infarction) in the left ventricular wall, and each of the 5 also had foci of fibrosis (healed myocardial infarction). Four additional patients with a clinical history of acute myocardial infarction had grossly visible left ventricular scars but no necrosis. Thus, 9 (53%) of the 17 patients with histories compatible with myocardial infarction had at necropsy evidence of either left ventricular wall necrosis or fibrosis or both. Of the 32 patients with either left ventricular necrosis or fibrosis or both at necropsy, only 9 (28%) had a history of acute myocardial infarction during life.

Causes of Death

Cardiac causes accounted for the death of 36 (30%) patients, most of whom (21 patients) died as a direct consequence of atherosclerotic coronary artery disease (Table 5). Vascular events and infections, other than active infective endocarditis, caused death in 15 (13%) and 17 (14%) patients, respectively. In 22 (17%) patients, the cause of death was uncertain. In 20 patients, death occurred during or at the termination of a hemodialysis treatment. The clinical features and the cardiac morphologic findings in these 20 patients are shown in Table 6. At least 1 major epicardial coronary artery was narrowed more than 75% in cross-sectional area by atherosclerotic plaque in 11 patients, 4 of whom had healed and 3 of whom had acute myocardial infarcts. Two had large bloody pericardial effusions that caused fatal cardiac tamponade.

TABLE 5. Causes of Death in 120 Adults

Cause of Death		No. (%)
I. Cardiac		36/120 (30)
A. Atherosclerotic coronary artery disease		21/36
1. Sudden death	7/21	
2. Acute myocardial infarct	11/21	
3. Ischemic cardiomyopathy	1/21	
4. Complications of coronary angioplasty or coronary artery surgery	2/21	
B. Cardiac tamponade		5/36
C. Active infective endocarditis		8/36
1. Mitral valve only	4/8	
2. Aortic valve only	3/8	
3. Both mitral and aortic valves	1/8	
D. Other cardiac causes		2/36
1. Giant cell myocarditis	1/2	
2. Cardiomegaly and left ventricular failure of uncertain etiology	1/2	
II. Vascular		16/120 (13)
A. Cerebrovascular accident		5/16
B. Aortic dissection		4/16
C. Hemorrhage		5/16
D. Pulmonary embolism		1/16
E. Peripheral vascular disease (complication of leg amputation)		1/16
III. Noncardiac and nonvascular		47/120 (40)
A. Infection (other than infective endocarditis)		17/47
1. Septicemia and/or infection of the dialysis arteriovenous fistula	11/17	
2. Soft tissue infection	2/17	
3. Pneumonia/empyema	3/17	
4. Perinephric abscess	1/17	
B. Metabolic derangement/volume overload		13/47
C. Opiate overdose		6/47
D. Trauma		5/47
E. Other		6/47
1. Rejection of renal transplant	2/6	
2. Cancer	2/6	
3. Following leg amputation	1/6	
4. Perforation of duodenal ulcer	1/6	
IV. Etiology unclear		22/120 (17)
A. Sudden death		15/22
1. During hemodialysis	7/15	
2. Outside hospital	8/15	
B. Circumstances of death unknown		7/22

TABLE 6. Clinical and Cardiac Morphologic Findings in 20 Patients With Chronic Kidney Disease Who Died During Hemodialysis

Patient	Age (yr)	Sex	Dialysis (mo)	Cause of Renal Disease	SH	DM	Sepsis	HW (g)	LVW		CA >75% in CSA by Plaque*	Dilated (1–3+)		AS	Pericardium		
									Fi	N		RV	LV		Diffuse Fibrinous	Diffuse Fibrous	Effusion
1	40	M	60	ATN	+	0	0	580	0	0	0	+	+	0	0	0	0
2	43	M	36	DM	+	+	0	565	0	0	0	+	+	0	0	0	0
3	44	M	96	SH	+	0	0	600	0	0	0	0	0	0	0	0	0
4	52	M	90	SH	+	0	0	780	0	0	+	+	+	0	0	0	0
5	58	M	72	SH	+	+	0	825	0	0	+	+	+	0	0	+	0
6	59	M	36	SH	+	0	+	580	0	0	+	+	+	0	0	+	0
7	59	M	108	DM	+	+	0	510	0	+	+	0	0	0	0	+	0
8	64	M	18	DM	+	+	0	660	+	+	+	++	++	0	0	0	0
9	64	M	192	–	+	0	+	550	0	0	+	++	+	0	0	0	0
10	66	M	30	DM	0	+	+	375	+	0	+	0	0	0	+	0	0
11	71	M	48	DM	+	+	0	440	0	0	0	0	0	+	+	0	0
12	72	M	58	DM	+	+	0	440	0	0	0	0	0	0	0	0	0
13	76	M	228	GN	+	0	0	500	0	0	+	+	+	+	+	0	0
Subtotal	(59)	13	(82)		12	7	3	(570)	2	2	8	8	8	2	3	3	0
14	43	F	13	SLE		0	0	385	0	0	0	0	0	0	0	0	0
15	47	F	24	SH	+	0	0	650	+	+	+	0	0	0	0	0	0
16	51	F	120	SH	+	+	0	590	+	0	+	0	0	+	+	0	+†
17	52	F	180	–	0	0	0	580	0	0	0	0	0	+	0	+	0
18	58	F	0	DM	+	+	0	500	0	0	+	+	0	0	0	+	0
19	62	F	13	SH	+	0	0	590	0	0	0	0	0	0	0	0	+†
Subtotal	(54)	7	(62)		6	2	0	(540)	2	1	3	1	0	2	1	2	2
Total	(57)		(75)		18	9	3	(560)	4	3	11	9	8	4	4	5	2

Abbreviations: AS = aortic stenosis, ATN = acute tubular necrosis, CA = coronary artery, CSA = cross-sectional area, DM = diabetes mellitus, Fi = fibrosis, GN = glomerulonephritis, HW = heart weight, LV = left ventricle, LVW = left ventricular wall, N = necrosis, RV = right ventricle, SH = systemic hypertension, SLE = systemic lupus erythematosus.

*At least 1 coronary artery was narrowed more than 75% in cross-sectional area by atherosclerotic plaque.

†Bloody effusion.

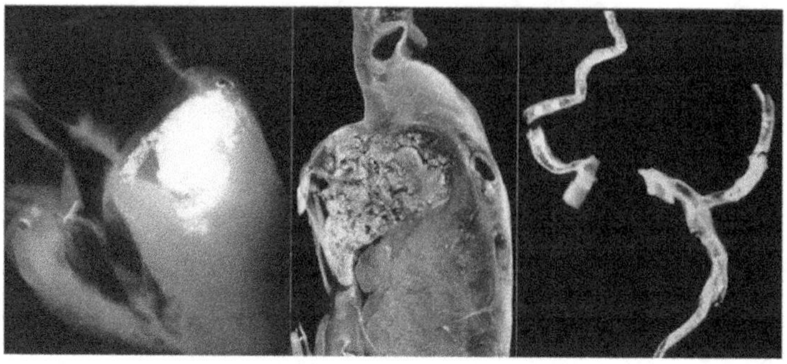

FIGURE 2. Portions of the heart of a 42-year-old man who had developed post-streptococcal glomerulonephritis at age 19 and was on chronic hemodialysis during the next 23 years. He worked regularly until 3 weeks before death when he was hospitalized because of massive upper gastrointestinal bleeding secondary to ruptured esophageal varicies. His hospital course was complicated by splenic vein thrombosis requiring splenectomy and persistent sepsis following total gastrectomy. None of the portable chest radiographs before death showed cardiac calcific deposits. At necropsy, the heart weighed 450 g. The amount of calcium in the mitral annular region was massive, and it formed a circle "O" around the mitral annulus (left). The calcium beneath the posterior mitral leaflet extended through the myocardium in a transmural fashion and into the subepicardial adipose tissue (left). The posterior mitral leaflet was made totally immobile by the massive calcific deposits (middle). Smaller calcific deposits were present on the aortic aspects of each of the 3 aortic valve cusps. Extensive calcific deposits were present in the major epicardial coronary arteries (right). The ventricular myocardium was free of foci of fibrosis and necrosis. The lumens of all epicardial coronary arteries were narrowed less than 50% in cross-sectional area. One year before death the serum total cholesterol was 123 mg/dL. Necropsy also showed cirrhosis, type uncertain. *Left:* Radiograph of the heart specimen showing massive calcific deposits in the mitral annular region and focal calcific deposits in epicardial coronary arteries. *Middle:* Longitudinal section of a portion of the wall of left atrium, posterior mitral leaflet with massive calcific deposits beneath it, and a portion of left ventricular free wall. The calcium at this site extended nearly through the myocardial wall, and in other sites calcium extended through the entire left ventricular free wall and into the subepicardial adipose tissue. *Right:* Radiograph of the major epicardial coronary arteries after excision from the heart. Numerous calcific deposits were present in these arteries.

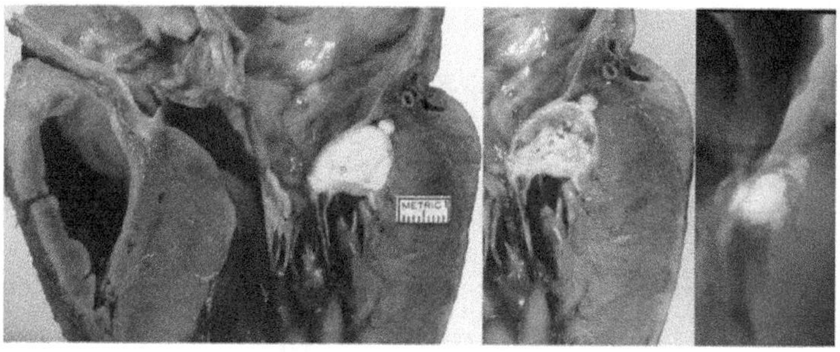

FIGURE 3. Mitral annular area in a 72-year-old woman treated with hemodialysis for 3 years. The mitral annular region contained a large calcific deposit, whereas the aortic valve was devoid of calcific deposits. The coronary arteries contained only small calcific deposits. The ventricular walls were devoid of foci of fibrosis and necrosis.

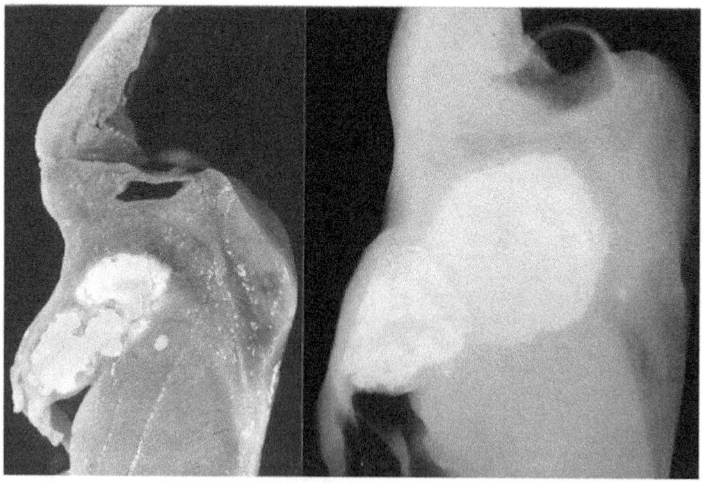

FIGURE 4. Mitral annular calcium which had partially "dissolved" in a 47-year-old woman who was known to have systemic hypertension since age 18 years. There was also extremely heavy calcific deposits in the aortic valve, all major epicardial coronary arteries, and in the aorta. A transmural scar was present in the posterior left ventricular wall.

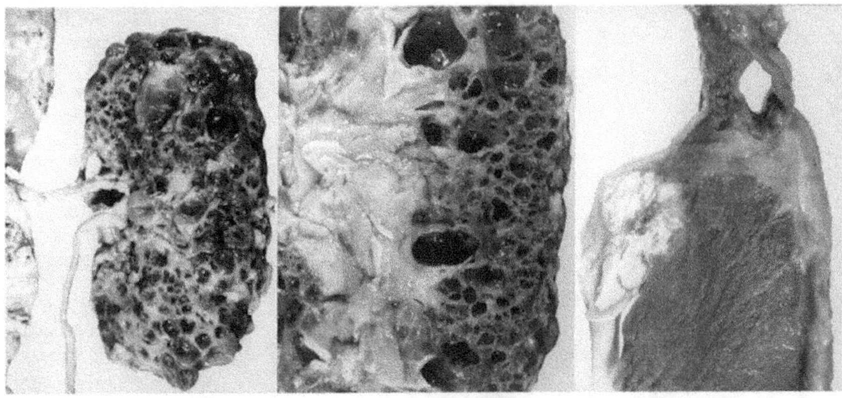

FIGURE 5. Kidney and mitral annular region in a 65-year-old man with polycystic kidney disease who had been on hemodialysis since age 57.[11] He had heavy calcific deposits in the mitral annular region, in the aortic valve causing aortic stenosis, in all of the major epicardial coronary arteries with severe narrowing of 2 of them (without resulting myocardial fibrosis or necrosis), and in the aorta. The heart weighed 765 g.

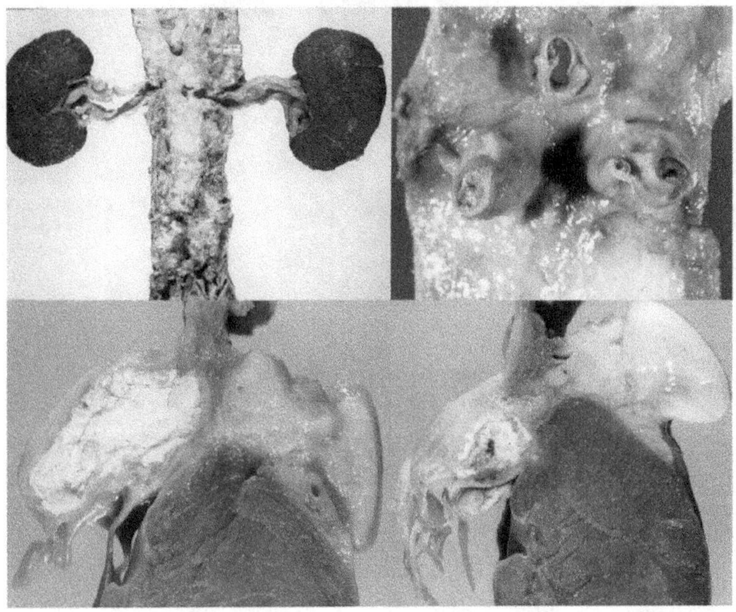

FIGURE 6. Portion of aorta and heart in a 52-year-old man who had hypertension since age 22 and had been on hemodialysis since age 43. The heart weighed 780 g. *Upper left:* Severely calcified abdominal aorta. *Upper right:* Adventitia side of aorta showing severe narrowing of both renal arteries. *Lower left* and *lower right:* Two views of posterior mitral leaflet and adjacent wall of left atrium and left ventricle showing heavy calcium behind the leaflet (mitral annular calcium). All major coronary arteries were heavily calcified. The aortic valve cusps contained small calcific deposits on their aortic surfaces.

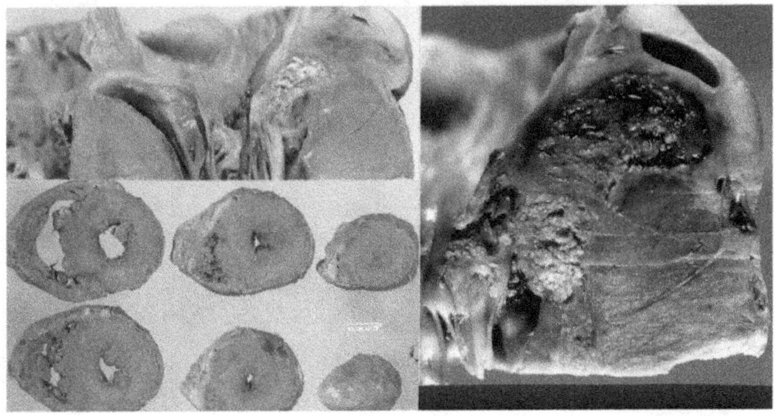

FIGURE 7. This patient was a 55-year-old woman with long-standing chronic renal failure secondary to congenitally hypoplastic kidneys. Treatment with hemodialysis was started at age 48 (7 yr before death) and continued until death. At age 52 years a bilateral nephrectomy was performed because of severe systemic hypertension. Seven days before death she received a cadaver renal transplant. Three days before death blood cultures became positive for *Staphylococcus aureus.* On the day of death she developed complete heart block. The heart at necropsy weighed 360 g. Massive calcific deposits were present in the mitral annulus, and vegetations were present on the mitral leaflets. The infection had burrowed into the mitral annular calcium producing an abscess. *Upper left:* Longitudinal view of left ventricle exposing the mitral valve and the heavy calcific deposit in the mitral annulus. *Right:* Close-up view showing the infection in the area of the mitral annular calcium. *Lower left:* Transverse views of the ventricles showing severe concentric left ventricular hypertrophy without cavity dilatation or foci of fibrosis or necrosis.

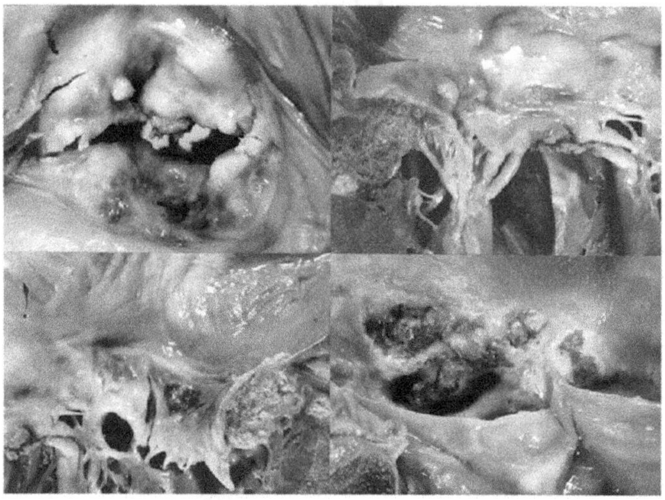

FIGURE 8. This 53-year-old man had glomerulonephritis and had been on hemodialysis since age 42. He was known to have systemic hypertension for many years. He had a parathyroidectomy at age 43 years and, clinically, in recent years, had evidence of pericarditis and supraventricular and ventricular arrhythmias. At age 51, he had an episode of *Streptococcus viridans* sepsis without evidence of infective endocarditis. Although no precordial murmurs were heard, Doppler echocardiography suggested mitral, aortic, and tricuspid regurgitation. At necropsy, the heart weighed 790 g. A thrombus was present in the right atrial appendage. All 4 cardiac chambers were markedly dilated. Scars were present and focal in both anterior and posterior walls of left ventricle. The right coronary artery was occluded near its aortic ostium, but the left main, left anterior descending, and left circumflex coronary arteries were narrowed less than 50% in cross-sectional area by atherosclerotic plaque. Massive calcific deposits were present in the mitral annular region, and focal calcific deposits were present on both mitral leaflets and on the aortic aspect of the pulmonic valve cusp. Radiograph of the base of the heart specimen showed massive calcium in all of the major epicardial coronary arteries as well as huge deposits in the mitral annular region. *Upper left:* Mitral valve from the left atrial aspect. Focal calcific deposits were present on both leaflets. *Upper right:* The mitral valve here is open, showing considerable thickening of the leaflets and attached chordae tendineae and heavy calcium in the mitral annulus. *Lower left:* Another portion of mitral leaflet, considerably thickened by fibrous tissue in addition to the heavy calcium in the mitral annulus. *Lower right:* A portion of the opened aortic valve and large plaque immediately above 1 of the cusps. This plaque was colored brown, a finding commonly observed in patients on hemodialysis for long periods.

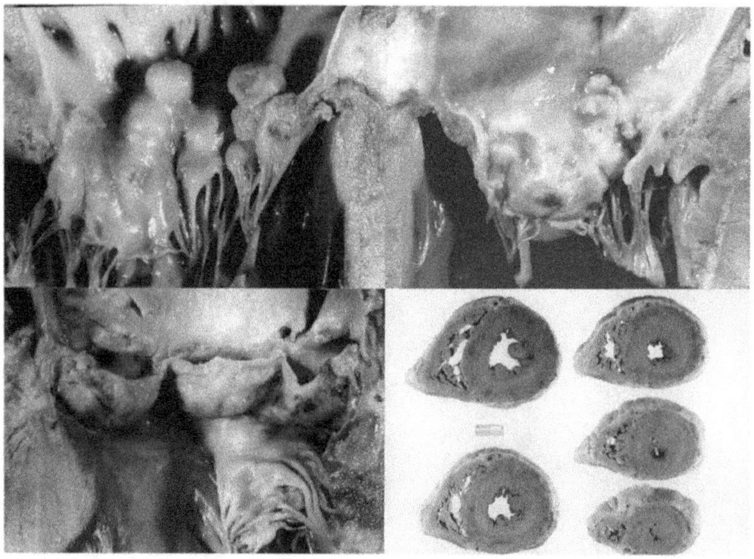

FIGURE 9. The patient whose heart is shown here was a 44-year-old man who was on hemodialysis for 9 years. His blood pressure was 180/100 mm Hg. At one time he had meningitis and infective endocarditis. At necropsy, the heart weighed 595 g. *Upper left:* Close-up view of the tricuspid valve. Aneurysms protruded toward the right atrium. Heavy calcific deposits were present in the tricuspid valve annular region. *Upper right:* View of atrial aspect of anterior mitral leaflet showing focal calcific deposits in it and in the mitral annular region. *Lower left:* Opened aortic valve showing its thickened cusps containing focal calcific deposits. *Lower right:* Cross-sections of the cardiac ventricles showing severe concentric left ventricular hypertrophy.

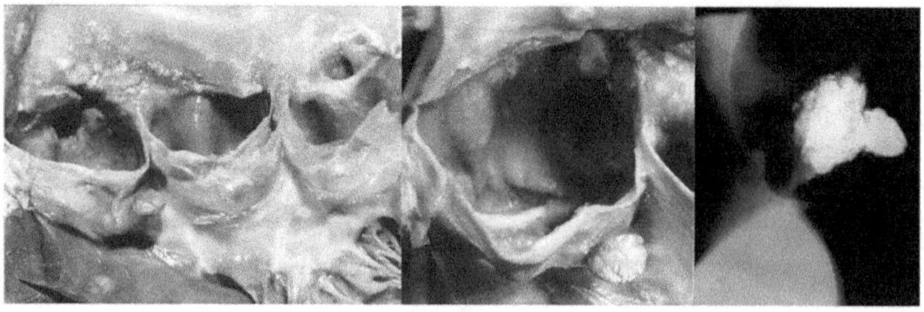

FIGURE 10. Opened aortic valve showing a single calcific deposit on the right cusp in a 73-year-old man with minimal mitral annular calcium (1+/4+), but heavy calcium in the epicardial coronary arteries. The heart weighed 540 g and the left anterior descending coronary artery was severely narrowed. He had been on hemodialysis for several years.

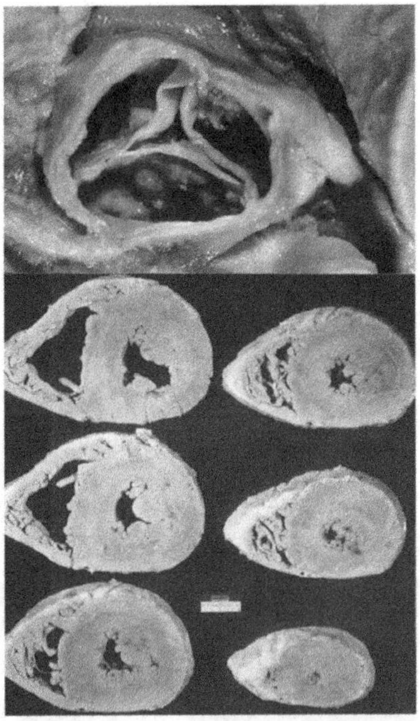

FIGURE 11. Stenotic aortic valve *(upper)* and hypertrophied left ventricle *(lower)* in a 71-year-old man who had been on chronic hemodialysis since age 67. He died suddenly during hemodialysis. He was known to have diabetes mellitus and systemic hypertension since age 52 years. The heart weighed 440 g, and the pericardial space was obliterated by fibrous adhesions. The aortic valve contained heavy calcific deposits on the aortic aspects of each cusp, and 2 cusps were partially fused at commissures. Calcific deposits were also present in the coronary arteries and in the mitral annular region.

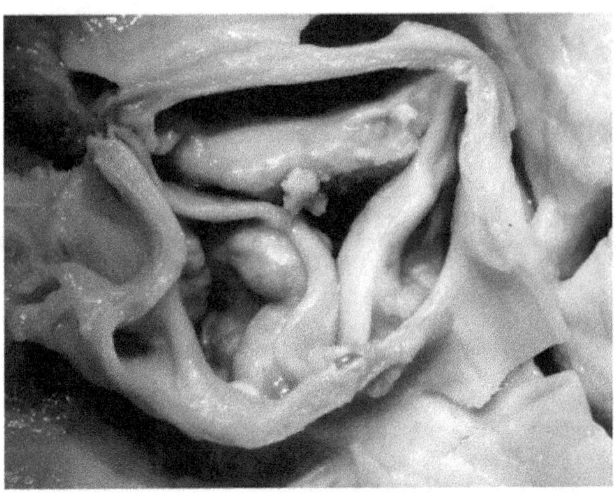

FIGURE 12. Heavily calcified stenotic aortic valve in a 52-year-old woman who had been on hemodialysis since age 37. The peak systolic transaortic valve pressure gradient was 85 mm Hg. She had fatal cardiac arrest immediately following hemodialysis. She also had severe mitral annular calcium. The left ventricular wall was severely hypertrophied but its cavity was not dilated. The ventricular wall was free of foci of fibrosis and necrosis. The major coronary arteries were virtually free of plaques. Each kidney weighed about 50 g.

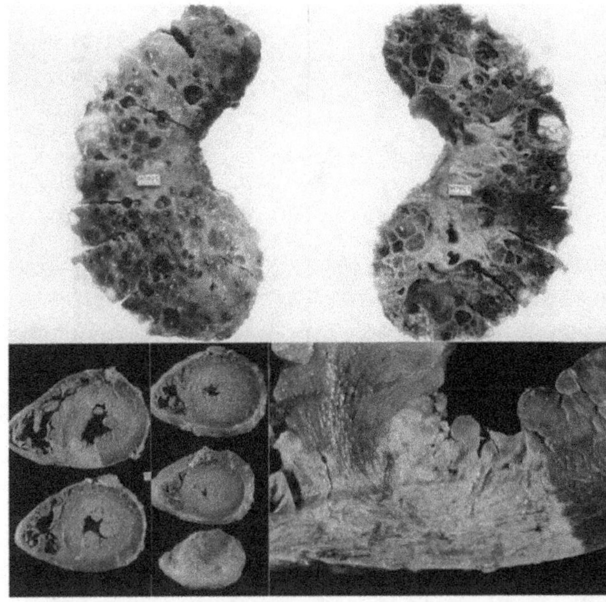

FIGURE 13. Polycystic kidneys *(upper),* severely hypertrophied left ventricular wall *(lower left),* and magnification of acute myocardial infarct *(lower right)* in the posterobasal portion of the left ventricular free wall in a 74-year-old man who had been on hemodialysis since age 57. The acute infarct, which also involved the right ventricular wall, was not diagnosed clinically. He died early postoperatively after herniorrhaphy. Although all major coronary arteries contained atherosclerotic plaque diffusely, only the right was severely narrowed.

Necropsy Findings

The heart weight ranged from 350 to 1010 g (mean, 600 g) (Figures 2–17; Table 7). The left and/or right ventricle was dilated in 61 (51%) patients. At least 1 of the 4 major (left main, left anterior descending, left circumflex, and right) epicardial coronary arteries was narrowed more than 75% in cross-sectional area at some point by atherosclerotic plaque in 47 (39%) patients. Gross, histologic, and radiographic examination of the hearts revealed calcific deposits in the epicardial coronary arteries in 74 (62%) patients, in the aortic valve in 42 patients, in

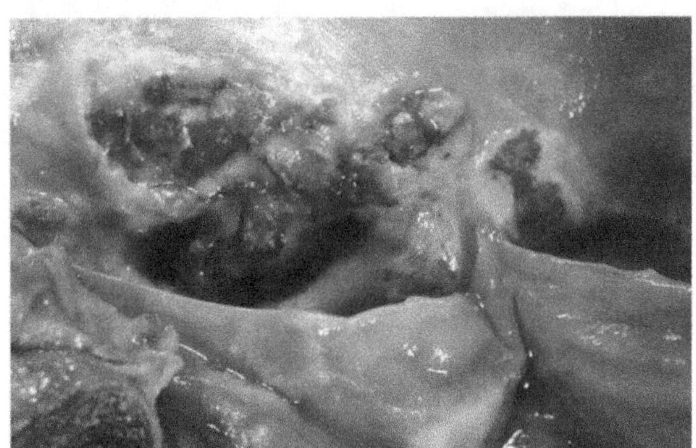

FIGURE 14. Opened aortic valve in a 53-year-old man showing a large calcific deposit at the sinotubular junction, a common finding in patients with chronic renal disease with or without chronic hemodialysis. [This figure can be viewed in color online at http://www.md-journal.com.]

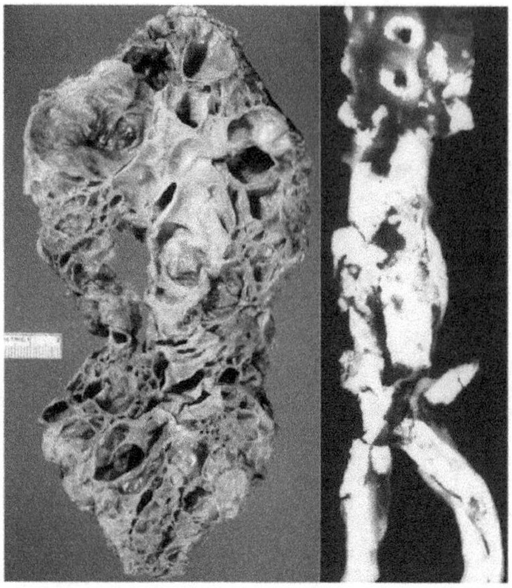

FIGURE 15. Polycystic kidney *(left)* and massively calcified abdominal aorta and common iliac arteries *(right)* in a 64-year-old man who had known systemic hypertension since age 19 and was on chronic hemodialysis since age 54 years. At age 58 he had a pericardial window placed for pericardial tamponade. At age 60 he had parathyroidectomy for chronic hypercalcemia. A brother and sister (twins) also had polycystic kidneys. The heart weighed 365 g, and the left ventricular wall was free of foci of necrosis or fibrosis despite heavily calcified coronary arteries. Neither the aortic valve nor the mitral valve (or annulus) contained calcium.

the mitral valve annulus in 52 patients, and in myocardium in 4 patients. As a result of the calcific deposits in the aortic valve, 9 (8%) patients had aortic valve stenosis. All 9 patients with aortic stenosis had 3-cuspid aortic valves. In 9 patients calcific deposits also were found in other parts of the heart (pulmonic valve, tricuspid valve, papillary muscle, or chordae tendineae).

Heavy atherosclerotic lesions with calcific deposits were present in most aortas examined. Many aortic atherosclerotic lesions had a brownish discoloration (iron).

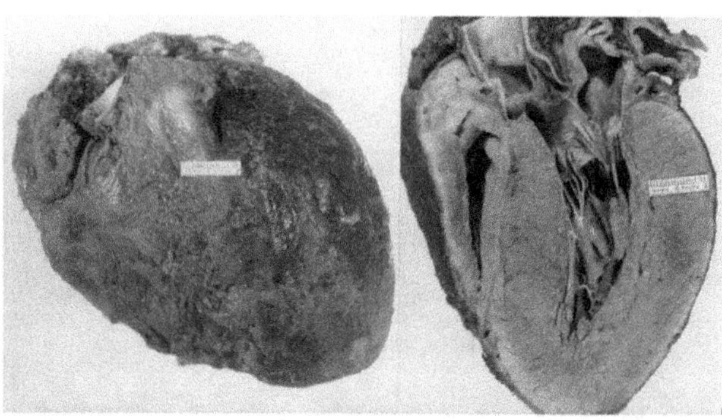

FIGURE 16. Heart of a 31-year-old man, a former heroin addict, who developed chronic renal failure at age 24 and was treated with chronic hemodialysis from age 25. He died of tamponade secondary to a hemorrhagic pericardial effusion. The heart weighed 710 g and the pericardial surfaces contained diffuse fibrin deposits of blood *(left)*. The cardiac ventricular walls were severely hypertrophied. The cardiac valves and coronary arteries were free of calcific deposits, and the only deposits in the aorta were in its isthmic portion.

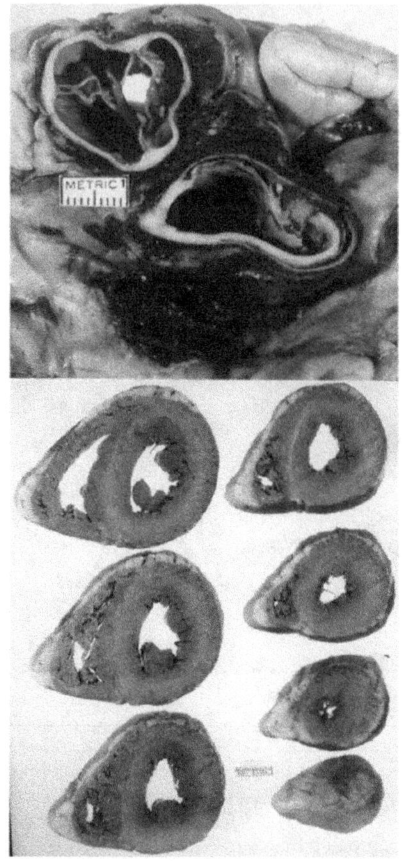

FIGURE 17. Tear and dissection in ascending aorta *(upper)* and sections of the hypertrophied left ventricle *(bottom)* in a 30-year-old man with fatal cardiac tamponade from rupture of the ascending aorta. He had Alport syndrome and had been on hemodialysis for 3 years.

Features of Patients by Duration of Hemodialysis

We observed significant differences in right and left ventricular cavity sizes and the amount of calcific deposits in the heart between patients on hemodialysis for 4 years or less and those on hemodialysis for more than 4 years (Table 8). (The 4-year cutoff point was arbitrary.) Compared to the group with the shorter duration, more patients in the group with the longer duration had dilated right (41% vs. 65%, $p < 0.05$) or left (39% vs. 67%, $p < 0.05$) ventricles, and more had calcific deposits in the epicardial coronary arteries (53% vs. 72%, $p < 0.05$), aortic valve (19% vs. 57%, $p < 0.001$), or mitral valve annulus (29% vs. 63%, $p = 0.03$). In addition, calcific aortic valve stenosis was found in only 1 patient who was on hemodialysis for 48 months or less, but was found in 8 patients on hemodialysis for more than 48 months (<1% vs. 16%, $p < 0.01$).

Features of Patients by Age

Several significant differences were observed between patients aged 50 years or younger and those aged more than 50 years (Table 9). The older patients had a lower frequency of diabetes mellitus compared to the younger group (20% vs. 37%, $p < 0.05$), and a higher frequency of atherosclerotic coronary artery disease (46% vs. 28%, $p = 0.03$) and calcific deposits in epicardial coronary arteries (68% vs. 53%, $p = 0.04$), aortic valve (43% vs. 22%, $p = 0.01$), and mitral valve annulus (52%

TABLE 7. Cardiac Morphologic Findings in 120 Adults

Variable			No. (%)
1. Heart weight, g; range (mean)			350–1010 (600 ± 140)
Men (mean)			623 ± 137
Women (mean)			520 ± 94
2. Epicardial fat increased			40/72 (56)
3. Dilated ventricular cavity			
Left			61 (51)
Right			61 (51)
4. Left ventricular wall			32 (27)
Fibrosis only (n = 20)			
Necrosis only (n = 4)			
Both fibrosis and necrosis (n = 8)			
5. No. of coronary arteries narrowed >75% in cross-sectional area by plaque			
0			73 (61)
1			15 (12.5)
2			16 (13)
3			15 (12.5)
4			1 (1)
6. Coronary artery narrowed >75% in cross-sectional area by plaque			
Left main			2 (2)
Left anterior descending			35 (29)
Left circumflex			26 (22)
Right			33 (27)
7. Pericardium			
Diffuse fibrinous			20 (17)
Diffuse fibrous			35 (29)
Effusion			16 (13)
Bloody (n = 13)			
Serous (n = 3)			
8. Aortic valve stenosis			9 (8)
9. Calcific deposits			
Coronary arteries			74 (62)
Heavy	(3+)	22 (19)	
Moderate	(2+)	7 (5.5)	
Mild	(1+)	45 (37.5)	
None		46 (38)	
Mitral valve annulus			52 (43)
Heavy	(3+)	23 (19)	
Moderate	(2+)	11 (9)	
Mild	(1+)	18 (15)	
None		68 (57)	
Aortic valve			42 (35)
Heavy	(3+)	8 (7)	
Moderate	(2+)	15 (12)	
Mild	(1+)	19 (16)	
None		78 (65)	
Myocardium			4 (3)
Other parts of the heart			9 (8)
Tricuspid valve		2	
Pulmonic valve		3	
Both tricuspid and pulmonic valve		2	
Papillary muscle		1	
Chordae tendineae		1	

vs. 31%, $p = 0.02$). More patients in the older group died of cardiovascular causes (51% vs. 30%, $p < 0.001$) and during hemodialysis treatment (21% vs. 10%, $p < 0.05$). Renal transplantation had been performed more in the younger group (19 patients [39%]) than the older group (5 patients [7%]).

TABLE 8. Clinical and Morphologic Findings by Duration of Hemodialysis in 120 Adults

	Duration of Hemodialysis (yr)	
Finding	>1–4 (n = 69) No. (%)	>4–22 (n = 51) No. (%)
Age, yr (mean)	55 ± 13	53 ± 14
Black/white	46 (67)/23 (37)	37 (73)/14 (27)
Men/women	51 (74)/18 (26)	40 (78)/11 (22)
Systemic hypertension (history)	60 (87)	47 (92)
Diabetes mellitus (history)	20 (29)	16 (31)
Angina pectoris (history)	19 (28)	12 (24)
Acute myocardial infarct (history)	11 (16)	6 (12)
Chronic heart failure	22 (32)	12 (24)
Laboratory tests (mean)		
Blood:		
Urea nitrogen (mg/dL)	79 ± 34	73 ± 31
Hematocrit (%)	25 ± 6	25 ± 5
Serum:		
Creatinine (mg/dL)	9.5 ± 3.6	10.0 ± 3.8
Total cholesterol (mg/dL)	178 ± 51	144 ± 47
Total protein (g/dL)	6.6 ± 0.8	6.6 ± 1.1
Albumin (g/dL)	3.3 ± 0.6	3.5 ± 0.6
Glucose (mg/dL)	146 ± 99	126 ± 33
Calcium (mg/dL)	9.0 ± 1.5	9.1 ± 1.5
Phosphorous (mg/dL)	6.2 ± 2.6	5.2 ± 1.7
Blood pressure, mm Hg (mean)		
Peak systolic	171 ± 40	173 ± 33
End diastolic	95 ± 24	102 ± 18
Heart weight, g (mean)	560 ± 120	640 ± 160
Pericardial disease		
Diffuse fibrinous	12 (17)	8 (16)
Diffuse fibrous	20 (29)	15 (29)
Pericardial effusion	7 (10)	9 (17)
Dilated ventricle		
Right	28 (41)*	33 (65)*
Left	27 (39)*	34 (67)*
Left ventricular		
Fibrosis	19 (28)	11 (22)
Necrosis	10 (14)	6 (12)
≥1 Coronary artery >75% ↓ in cross-sectional area by plaque	60 (87)	36 (71)
Coronary artery >75% ↓ in cross-sectional area by plaque		
Left main	1 (1)	1 (2)
Left anterior descending	22 (32)	13 (26)
Left circumflex	16 (23)	10 (20)
Right	20 (29)	13 (25)
Calcific deposits		
Coronary arteries	37 (54)*	37 (72)*
Heavy (3+)	9 (13)	13 (25)
Moderate (2+)	5 (7)	2 (4)
Mild (1+)	23 (33)	22 (43)
Aortic valve	30 (43)*	47 (92)*
Heavy (3+)	2 (3)*	13 (25)*
Moderate (2+)	5 (7)	12 (24)
Mild (1+)	23 (33)	22 (28)
Mitral valve anulus	20 (29)*	31 (61)*
Heavy (3+)	8 (12)	15 (29)
Moderate (2+)	6 (8.5)	5 (10)
Mild (1+)	6 (8.5)	11 (22)
Aortic valve stenosis	1 (1)*	8 (16)*
Increased epicardial fat	23/36 (64)	17/36 (47)
Cause of death		
Cardiovascular	26 (38)	25 (49)
Infection (other than infective endocarditis)	9 (13)	8 (16)
Death during hemodialysis	9 (13)	11 (22)
Renal transplantation	14 (20)	10 (20)

*$p < 0.05$.

TABLE 9. Clinical and Cardiac Morphologic Findings by Age at Death in 120 Adults

Finding	Age at Death (yr) ≤50 (n = 49) No. (%)	>50 (n = 71) No. (%)
Men/women	39 (80)/10 (20)	52 (73)/19 (27)
Black/white	38 (78)/83 (69)	45 (63)/26 (37)
Duration of hemodialysis, mo (mean)	52 ± 47	66 ± 52
Systemic hypertension (history)	42 (86)	65 (92)
Diabetes mellitus (history)	10 (20)	26 (37)
Angina pectoris	11 (22)	20 (28)
Acute myocardial infarct (history)	7 (14)	10 (14)
Chronic heart failure (history)	16 (32)	18 (25)
Laboratory tests (mean)		
Blood:		
Urea nitrogen (mg/dL)	79 ± 38	75 ± 28
Hematocrit (%)	24 ± 6	25 ± 6
Serum:		
Creatinine (mg/dL)	9.5 ± 4.2	9.8 ± 3.4
Total cholesterol (mg/dL)	169 ± 60	160 ± 45
Total protein (g/dL)	6.6 ± 0.6	6.6 ± 1.2
Albumin (g/dL)	3.5 ± 0.5	3.3 ± 0.7
Calcium (mg/dL)	8.8 ± 1.3	9.2 ± 1.6
Phosphorous (mg/dL)	5.7 ± 2.0	5.7 ± 2.4
Blood pressure, mm Hg (mean)		
Peak systolic	178 ± 36	168 ± 36
End diastolic	150 ± 20*	93 ± 21
Heart weight, g (mean)	603 ± 134	594 ± 147
Pericardial disease		
Diffuse fibrinous	6 (12)	14 (20)
Diffuse fibrous	14 (29)	21 (30)
Pericardial effusion	6 (12)	10 (41)
Dilated ventricle		
Right	28 (57)	33 (46)
Left	28 (57)	33 (46)
Left ventricular		
Fibrosis	10 (20)	20 (28)
Necrosis	6 (12)	10 (14)
≥1 Coronary artery >75% ↓ in cross-sectional area by plaque	14 (28)*	33 (46)*
Coronary artery >75% ↓ in cross-sectional area by plaque		
Left main	0	2 (3)
Left anterior descending	11 (22)	24 (34)
Left circumflex	7 (14)	19 (27)
Right	9 (18)*	24 (34)*
Calcific deposits		
Coronary arteries	26 (53)	48 (56)
Heavy (3+)	8 (16)	14 (20)
Moderate (2+)	3 (6)*	4 (6)*
Mild (1+)	15 (31)	30 (42)
Aortic valve	11 (22)*	31 (44)*
Heavy (3+)	3 (6)	5 (7)
Moderate (2+)	4 (8)	11 (15)
Mild (1+)	4 (8)	15 (21)
Mitral valve anulus	15 (31)*	37 (52)*
Heavy (3+)	11 (23)	12 (17)
Moderate (2+)	0	11 (15)
Mild (1+)	4 (8)	14 (20)
Aortic valve stenosis	2 (4)	7 (10)
Increased epicardial fat	19/32 (59)	21/40 (52)
Cause of death		
Cardiovascular	15 (30)*	36 (51)*
Infection (other than infective endocarditis)	9 (18)	8 (11)
Death during hemodialysis	5 (10)*	15 (21)*
Renal transplantation	19 (39)*	5 (7)*

*p < 0.05.

TABLE 10. Clinical and Cardiac Morphologic Findings by Calcium Deposits in 120 Adults

	Mild Calcium Deposits (n = 64) No. (%)	Heavy Calcium Deposits (n = 56) No. (%)
Calcium score†	≤2	>2
Range (mean)	0–2 (0.5)	3–12 (5.5)
Age, yr	51 ± 14*	58 ± 12*
Black/white	50 (78)*/14(22)*	33 (59)*/23(41)*
Men/women	48 (75)/16 (25)	43 (77)/13 23
Duration of hemodialysis, mo (mean)	44 ± 36*	78 ± 58*
Blood urea nitrogen (mg/dL) (mean)	74 ± 35	80 ± 29
Serum creatinine (mg/dL) (mean)	9.7 ± 3.8	9.7 ± 3.7
Serum calcium (mg/dL) (mean)	8.6 ± 1.4*	9.5 ± 1.4*
Blood pressure, mm Hg (mean)		
Peak systolic	117 ± 37	165 ± 35
End diastolic	103 ± 20*	92 ± 21*
Heart weight, g (mean)	596 ± 127	600 ± 146
Left ventricular		
Fibrosis	16 (25)	14 (25)
Necrosis	6 (9)	10 (18)
≥1 Coronary artery >75% ↓ in cross-sectional area of plaque	18 (28)*	29 (52)*
Aortic stenosis	0*	9 (16)*

*p < 0.05.

†Calcium score=sum of scores for calcific deposits in the aortic valve, mitral anulus, major epicardial coronary arteries (absent + 0, mild = 1, moderate = 2, severe = 3, each) and myocardium, tricuspid valve, pulmonic valve, papillary muscle, or chordae tendineae (absent = 0 or present = 1, each).

Calcium Score

A 0–3+ score was devised for quantifying calcium in the epicardial coronary arteries, aortic valve, and mitral valve anulus (Table 10). In addition, a score of 1 was given to calcium present in myocardium, pulmonic valve, tricuspid valve, papillary muscle, or chordae tendineae. Comparing the 64 patients with low calcium scores (range, 0–2; mean, 0.5) and the 56 patients with high scores (range, 3–12; mean, 5.5), we found that the latter group was older (mean age, 58 vs. 51 yr; $p = 0.001$), was on hemodialysis for longer periods of time (mean duration, 78 mo vs. 44 mo; $p = 0.0001$), had higher mean serum calcium levels (9.5 mg/dL vs. 8.6 mg/dL, $p < 0.05$), and had a higher prevalence of atherosclerotic coronary artery disease (52% vs. 28%, $p = 0.03$).

Infective Endocarditis

Eight patients were found to have active infective endocarditis at necropsy (Table 11).

DISCUSSION

The present necropsy study included 120 patients who were on hemodialysis for more than 1 year because of CKD. Probably

TABLE 11. Clinicopathologic Findings in 8 Patients With Active Infective Endocarditis While on Chronic (>1 yr) Maintenance Dialysis

Patient	Age (yr)	Sex	Cause of Renal Failure	Duration of Hemodialysis (yr)	SH	DM	Valve Infected	Organism	HW (g)	Dilated (1–3+) LV	Dilated (1–3+) RV	Calcific Deposits (1–3+) AV	MA	CA	Myocardium	Other	AS	MS	No. of Major Epicardial CA >75% in CSA	LVW Fi	LVW N
1	44	M	SH	9	+	0	MV	*S. aureus*	595	0	0	++	+++	+	0	0	+	0	0	0	+
2	50	M	DM	3	+	+	MV	*S. aureus*	520	+	++	+	+++	+	0	0	0	0	2	0	0
3	55	F	SH	7	+	0	MV	*S. aureus*	360	0	0	+	+++	+	0	0	0	0	0	0	0
4	58	F	—	4	+	0	MV	*S. aureus*	590	0	0	0	++	0	0	0	0	0	0	0	+
5	73	F	Analgesic	5	+	0	MV	*S. aureus*	450	0	0	+	+++	+	0	0	0	0	0	0	0
6	44	M	SH	9	+	0	MV+AV	*S. aureus*	595	0	0	++	+++	+	0	0	0	0	0	0	0
7	53	F	SH	8	+	0	AV	a-*Streptococcus*	450	0	0	0	+++	0	0	0	0	0	0	0	0
8	73	M	Vasculitis	2	0	0	AV	*S. aureus*	465	+	+	0	0	+	0	0	0	0	0	0	0
Total or (mean)				(5)	6	1			(505)	2	2	5	7	6	0	0	1	0	—	0	2

Abbreviations: See Table 6. AV = aortic valve, MA = mitral anulus, MS = mitral stenosis, MV = mitral valve.

the most impressive finding in the heart was the extensive calcific deposits, most common in the epicardial coronary arteries (62%, 74/120), mitral annular region (43%, 52/120), and aortic valve cusps (35%, 42/120). Despite the impressive appearance of the cardiac calcific deposits, only a minority appeared to lead to cardiac dysfunction or myocardial ischemia. For example, only 47 (39%) had narrowing more than 75% in cross-sectional area of 1 or more major (right, left main, left anterior descending, left circumflex) epicardial coronary arteries, and only 32 (27%) had acute or healed myocardial infarcts. Additionally, even though 23 (44%) of the 52 patients with mitral annular calcium had very heavy calcific deposits in that region of the heart, none appeared to have evidence of clinically significant mitral stenosis or regurgitation as a consequence of those calcific deposits.[20,44] Furthermore, only 8 (19%) of the 42 patients with calcium deposits in the aortic valve cusps had deposits heavy enough at this site to clearly lead to aortic valve stenosis.[43] Or, to approach the cardiac calcific "syndrome" from the opposite aspect, 46 (38%) of the 120 patients had no calcific deposits in the epicardial coronary arteries, 68 (57%) had no calcium in the mitral annular region, and 78 (65%) patients had no calcium in the aortic valve cusps.

The duration of chronic hemodialysis (>1–4 yr vs. >4 yr) had a significant effect on the frequency and extent of calcific deposits in all 3 cardiac sites: epicardial coronary arteries, mitral annular region, and aortic valve cusps (see Table 8). Patients treated with hemodialysis for the longer periods had more frequent and more extensive cardiac calcific deposits. The mean serum total cholesterol and systemic arterial pressures were similar in the groups with shorter and longer durations of hemodialysis. Age also had an effect on the frequency and extent of cardiac calcific deposits. Compared to patients aged 50 years or less, those aged more than 50 years had more frequent and more extensive calcific deposits in the coronary arteries, mitral annular region, and aortic valve (see Table 9).

Calcific deposits were found at necropsy in 1 or both right-sided cardiac valves in 7 (6%) patients, but in none was there evidence of valvular regurgitation or stenosis.

Calcific atherosclerotic plaques were also extremely common in the aorta and in its branches. Many of the calcific deposits had a brownish tint to them, an almost distinguishing feature of calcific deposits in patients with CKD with or without hemodialysis in the time period (1973–1992) in which these patients were studied.

Comparing the patients with and without mitral annular calcium disclosed some significant differences between the 2 groups. Those with mitral annular calcium were older (mean age, 58 ± 12 yr vs. 52 ± 14 yr; p = 0.01), had a longer duration of hemodialysis (mean, 72 ± 56 mo vs. 52 ± 43 mo; p = 0.03), and had a much greater frequency of aortic stenosis (8 cases vs. 1 case, p = 0.0003).

Coronary arterial disease may be both under- and overdiagnosed in patients with CKD on hemodialysis. During life, acute myocardial infarction was diagnosed in 17 (14%) of the 120 patients but only 5 of them had left ventricular necrosis (infarction) at necropsy, although each of these 5 had left ventricular wall scars (healed myocardial infarcts). Four additional patients with a clinical history of acute myocardial infarction in the past had grossly visible left ventricular scars, but no necrosis. Thus, only 9 (53%) of the 17 patients with histories of acute myocardial infarction had evidence of either left ventricular wall necrosis or fibrosis or both. Of the 32 patients who at necropsy had evidence of myocardial infarction (necrosis only in 4, fibrosis only in 20, and both in 7), only 9 (28%) had a history compatible with acute myocardial infarction during life. Parfrey and colleagues[35] commented on the low prevalence of symptomatic coronary arterial diseases in dialysis patients: only 26 (17%) of their 153 nondiabetic dialysis patients had symptoms of myocardial ischemia. Roig and associates[46] and Rostand and colleagues[47] found that symptoms of myocardial ischemia far exceeded the frequency of significant coronary narrowing on angiogram in their chronic dialysis patients, thus overestimating the prevalence of significant coronary arterial disease. Of 14 hemodialysis patients with coronary calcium detected by CT reported by Goodman et al,[18] none had angina pectoris or a history of myocardial infarction.

A weakness of the present study is the lack of a control group. We considered using the 15 patients who were on hemodialysis for less than 1 year, but comparison to the 120 patients on hemodialysis for more than 1 year did not seem particularly useful. More importantly, 10 of the 15 patients were on hemodialysis for less than 1 month, mainly for *acute* renal failure, not chronic renal failure. In other words, the patients on hemodialysis for less than 1 year were quite different from those who were on hemodialysis for more than 1 year for *chronic* renal failure. Another potential control group was the group of necropsy patients with severe CKD who had not undergone chronic hemodialysis or renal transplantation. Unfortunately, such patients were few in our files. Hujairi et al,[23] however, found necropsy data (1966–1975) among patients with CKD: arterial ± valvular calcific deposits were present in 44 (79%) of the 56 dialyzed patients and in 8 (44%) of the 18 nondialyzed patients in their study. Moreover, a number of echocardiographic[4,9,13,33,36,37,54] and CT imaging[5,18,23,32,39,41] studies in the last 20 years have demonstrated a very high frequency of calcific deposits in the epicardial coronary arteries, mitral annulus, and aortic valve cusps in patients with CKD with and without hemodialysis. Most of the echocardiographic studies focused on the left ventricular cavity dimensions, wall thicknesses, and ejection fractions. In contrast, most CT studies focused on the presence and quantity of calcific deposits in the epicardial coronary arteries, with relatively little focus on these deposits in the mitral annulus region or aortic valve cusps.

In conclusion, in the current study we demonstrate via gross photographs the magnitude of cardiac calcific deposits and their clinical consequences in patients with CKD treated with hemodialysis. We found that CKD treated with hemodialysis is a major producer of cardiac calcific deposits, some of which can be massive. Only a minority of the calcific deposits, however, appeared to lead to cardiac dysfunction or myocardial ischemia during life.

REFERENCES

1. Abrahms C, D'Cruz I, Kathpalia S. Abnormalities in the mitral valve apparatus in patients undergoing long-term hemodialysis: autopsy and echocardiographic correlation. *Arch Intern Med.* 1982;142: 1796–1800.
2. Arora KK, Lacy JP, Schacht RA, Martin DG, Gutch CF. Calcific cardiomyopathy in advanced renal failure. *Arch Intern Med.* 1975;135:603–605.
3. Barber ND, Nakamoto S, McCormack LJ, Kolff WJ. Pathologic anatomy of 13 patients after prolonged periodic hemodialysis. *Trans Amer Soc Artif Int Organs.* 1963;9:21–27.
4. Bazzi C, Arrigo G, Luciani L, Casazza F, Saviotti M, Malaspina D, Bonucci E, Ballanti P, Amaducci S, Lattuada P, Manna G, Pozzi F, D'Amica G. Clinical features of 24 patients on regular hemodialysis treatment (RDT) for 16-23 years in a single unit. *Clin Nephrol.* 1995;44:96–107.
5. Bellasi A, Ferramosca E, Muntner P, Ratti C, Wildman RP, Block GA, Raggi P. Correlation of simple imaging tests and coronary artery calcium measured by computed tomography in hemodialysis patients. *Kidney Int.* 2006;70:1623–1628.
6. Bleyer AJ, Russell GB, Satko SG. Sudden and cardiac death rates in hemodialysis patients. *Kidney Int.* 1999;55:1553–1559.
7. Castro L, Hofling B, Hassler R, Hillebrand G, Land W, Kreuzer E, Kemes B, Gurland HJ, Erdmann E. Progression of coronary and valvular heart disease in patients on dialysis. *Trans Am Soc Artif Intern Organs.* 1985;31:647–650.
8. Cheung AK, Sarnak MJ, Yan G, Dwyer JT, Heyka RJ, Rocco MV, Teehan BP, Levey AS, and The Hemodialysis (HEMO) Study. Atherosclerotic cardiovascular disease risks in chronic hemodialysis patients. *Kidney Int.* 2000;58:353–362.
9. Covic A, Goldsmith DJA, Georgescu G, Venning MC, Ackrill P. Echocardiographic findings in long-term, long-hour hemodialysis patients. *Clin Nephrol.* 1996;45:104–110.
10. Degoulet P, Legrain M, Reach I, Aime F, Devries C, Rojas P, Jacobs C. Mortality risk factors in patients treated by chronic hemodialysis. Report of the Diaphane Colloborative Study. *Nephron.* 1982;31:103–110.
11. Evandoff GV, Thompson CS, Foley R, Weinman EJ. Spectrum of gas within the kidney: emphysematous pyelonephritis and emphysematous pyelitis. *Am J Med.* 1987;83:149–154.
12. Foley RN, Parfrey PS, Sarnak MJ. Clinical epidemiology of cardiovascular disease in chronic renal disease. *Am J Kidney Dis.* 1998;32:S112–S119.
13. Forman MB, Virmani R, Robertson RM, Stone WJ. Mitral anular calcification in chronic renal failure. *Chest.* 1984;85:367–371.
14. Fox CS, Larson MG, Vasan RS, Guo C-Y, Parise H, Levy D, Leip EP, O'Donnell CJ, D Agostino RB, Benjamin EJ. Cross-sectional association of kidney function with valvular and annular calcification: the Framingham Heart Study. *J Am Soc Nephrol.* 2006;17:521–527.
15. Fried LF, Katz R, Cushman M, Sarnak M, Shlipak MG, Kuller L, Newman AB. Change in cardiovascular risk factors with progression of kidney disease. *Am J Nephrol.* 2009;29:334–341.
16. Gold CH. The mortality rate and causes of death in black patients on chronic haemodialysis. *S Afr Med J.* 1980;58:611–614.
17. Goldsmith DJA, Covic A, Sambrook PA, Ackrill P. Vascular calcification in long-term haemodialysis patients in a single unit: a retrospective analysis. *Nephron.* 1997;77:37–43.
18. Goodman WG, Goldin J, Kiuzon BD, Yoon C, Gales B, Sider D, Wang Y, Chung J, Emerick A, Greaser L, Elashoff RM, Salusky IB. Coronary-artery calcification in young adults with end-stage renal disease who are undergoing dialysis. *N Engl J Med.* 2000;342:1478–1483.
19. Goodman WG, London G on behalf of the Vascular Work Group. Vascular calcification in chronic kidney disease. *Am J Kidney Dis.* 2004;43:572–579.
20. Hammer WJ, Roberts WC, deLeon AC Jr. "Mitral stenosis" secondary to combined "massive" mitral anular calcific deposits and small, hypertrophied left ventricles: hemodynamic documentation in four patients. *Am J Med.* 1978;64:371–376.
21. Himmelfarb J, Apa Ikizler T. Hemodialysis. *N Engl J Med.* 2010;363: 1833–1845.
22. Honkanen E, Kauppila L, Wikstrom B, Rensma PL, Krzesinski J-M, Aasarod K, Verbeke F, Jensen PB, Mattelaer P, Volck B on behalf of the CORD study group. Abdominal aortic calcification in dialysis patients: results of the CORD study. *Nephrol Dial Transplant.* 2008;23: 4009–4015.
23. Hujairi NMA, Afzali B, Goldsmith DJA. Cardiac calcification in renal patients: what we do and don't know. *Am J Kidney Dis.* 2004;43:234–243.
24. Ibels LS, Alfrey AC, Huffer WE, Craswell PW, Anderson JT, Weil R III. Arterial calcification and pathology in uremic patients undergoing dialysis. *Am J Med.* 1979;66:790–796.

25. Ikram H, Lynn KL, Bailey RR, Little PJ. Cardiovascular changes in chronic hemodialysis patients. *Kidney Int.* 1983;24:371–376.

26. Kuzela DC, Huffer WE, Conger JD, Winter SD, Hammond WS. Soft tissue calcification in chronic dialysis patients. *Am J Pathol.* 1977;86:403–424.

27. Levey AS, Beto JA, Coronado BE, Eknoyan G, Foley RN, Kasiske BL, Klag MJ, Mailous LU, Menske CL, Meyer KB, Parfrey PS, Pfeffer MA, Wenger NK, Wilson PWF, Wright JT Jr. Controlling the epidemic of cardiovascular disease in chronic renal disease: what do we know? What do we need to learn? Where do we go from here? *Am J Kidney Dis.* 1998;32:853–906.

28. Lindner A, Charra B, Sherrard DJ, Scribner BH. Accelerated atherosclerosis in prolonged maintenance hemodialysis. *N Engl J Med.* 1974;290:697–701.

29. London GM, Guerin AP, Marchais SJ, Metivier F, Pannier B, Adda H. Arterial media calcification in end-stage renal disease: impact on all-cause and cardiovascular mortality. *Nephrol Dial Transplant.* 2003;18:1731–1740.

30. Maher ER, Curtis JR. Calcific aortic stenosis in chronic renal failure. *Lancet.* 1985;2:1007.

31. Meema HE, Oreopoulos DG, deVeber GA. Arterial calcifications in severe chronic renal disease and their relationship to dialysis treatment, renal transplant, and parathyroidectomy. *Radiology.* 1976;121:315–321.

32. Moe SM, O'Neill KD, Fineberg N, Persohn S, Ahmed S, Garrett P, Meyer CA. Assessment of vascular calcification in ESRD patients using spiral CT. *Nephrol Dial Transplant.* 2003;18:1152–1158.

33. Nestico PF, DePace NL, Kotler MN, Rose LI, Brezin JH, Swartz C, Mintz GS, Schwartz AB. Calcium phosphorus metabolism in dialysis patients with and without mitral anular calcium. Analysis of 30 patients. *Am J Cardiol.* 1983;51:497–500.

34. Okuno S, Ishimura E, Kitatani K, Fujino Y, Kohno K, Maeno Y, Maekawa K, Yamakawa T, Imanishi Y, Inaba M, Nishizawa Y. Presence of abdominal aortic calcification is significantly associated with all-cause and cardiovascular mortality in maintenance hemodialysis patients. *Am J Kidney Dis.* 2007;49:417–425.

35. Parfrey PS, Foley RN. The clinical epidemiology of cardiac disease in chronic renal failure. *J Am Soc Nephrol.* 1999;10:1606–1615.

36. Parfrey PS, Harnett JD, Barre PE. The natural history of myocardial disease in dialysis patients. *J Am Soc Nephrol.* 1991;2:2–12.

37. Parfrey PS, Harnett JD, Griffiths SM, Taylor R, Hand J, King A, Barre PE. The clinical course of left ventricular hypertrophy in dialysis patients. *Nephron.* 1990;55:114–120.

38. Qunibi WY. Reducing the burden of cardiovascular calcification in patients with chronic kidney disease. *J Am Soc Nephrol.* 2005;16:S95–S102.

39. Qunibi WY, Nolan CA, Ayus JC. Cardiovascular calcification in patients with end-stage renal disease. A century-old phenomenon. *Kidney Int.* 2002;62:S73–S80.

40. Raggi P, Ali O. Phosphorus restriction and control of coronary calcification as assessed by electron beam tomography. *Curr Opin Nephrol Hypertens.* 2002;11:391–395.

41. Raggi P, Boulay A, Chasan-Taber S, Amin N, Dillon M, Burke SK, Chertow GM. Cardiac calcification in adult hemodialysis patients. A link between end-stage renal disease and cardiovascular disease? *J Am Coll Cardiol.* 2002;39:695–701.

42. Roberts WC. Examining the precordium and the heart. *Chest.* 1970;57: 567–571.

43. Roberts WC, Ko JM, Hamilton C. Comparison of valve structure, valve weight, and severity of the valve obstruction in 1849 patients having isolated aortic valve replacement for aortic valve stenosis (with or without aortic regurgitation) studied at 3 different medical centers in 2 different time periods. *Circulation.* 2005;112:3919–3929.

44. Roberts WC, Perloff JK. Mitral valvular disease. A clinicopathologic survey of the conditions causing the mitral valve to function abnormally. *Ann Intern Med.* 1992;77:939–975.

45. Roberts WC, Waller BF. Effect of chronic hypercalcemia on the heart: an analysis of 18 necropsy patients. *Am J Med.* 1981;71:371–384.

46. Roig E, Betriu A, Castaner A, Magrina J, Sanz G, Navarro-Lopez F. Disabling angina pectoris with normal coronary arteries in patients undergoing long-term hemodialysis. *Am J Med.* 1981;71:431–434.

47. Rostand SG, Kirk KA, Rutsky EA. Dialysis-associated ischemic heart disease: insights from coronary angiography. *Kidney Int.* 1984;25:653–659.

48. Ryan TP, Fisher SG, Elder JL, Winters PC, Beckett W, Tacci J, Sloand JA. Increased cardiovascular risk associated with reduced kidney function. *Am J Nephrol.* 2009;29:620–625.

49. Schwarz U, Buzello M, Ritz E, Stein G, Raabe G, West G, Mall G, Amann K. Morphology of coronary atherosclerotic lesions in patients with end-stage renal failure. *Nephrol Dial Transplant.* 2000;15:218–223.

50. Sokol A, Gral T, Edelbaum N, Rosen V, Rubini ME. Correlation of autopsy findings and clinical experience in chronically dialyzed patients. *Trans Amer Soc Artif Int Organs.* 1967;13:51–57.

51. Terman DS, Alfrey AC, Hammond WS, Donndelinger T, Ogden DA, Holmes JH. Cardiac calcification in uremia: a clinical, biochemical and pathologic study. *Am J Med.* 1971;50:744–755.

52. Weiner DE, Tighiouart H, Amin MG, Stark PC, Macleod B, Griffith JL, Salem DN, Levey AS, Sarnak MJ. Chronic kidney disease as a risk factor for cardiovascular disease and all-cause mortality: a pooled analysis of community-based studies. *J Am Soc Nephrol.* 2004;15:1307–1315.

53. Yanagi S, Teragaki M, Tahara A, Itagane H, Akioka K, Yasuda M, Oku H, Takeuchi K, Takeda T, Ueda M. Extensive specifically localized myocardial calcium deposition in a hemodialysis patient. *Jpn Circ J.* 1992;56:27–31.

54. Yildiz A, Oflaz H, Pusuroglu H, Marcanoglu F, Genchallac H, Akkaya V, Alp Igizler T, Sever MS. Left ventricular hypertrophy and endothelial dysfunction in chronic hemodialysis patients. *Am J Kidney Dis.* 2003;41:626–623.

55. Zazgornik J, Balcke P, Giesenbach G, Kaiser W, Stockenhuber F. Myocardial calcinosis associated with hemodialysis. *Am J Cardiol.* 1987;60:421–422.

Effect of Coronary Bypass and Valve Structure on Outcome in Isolated Valve Replacement for Aortic Stenosis

William Clifford Roberts, MD[a,b,d,*], Carey Camille Roberts[d,g], Travis James Vowels[d,h], Jong Mi Ko, BA[d], Giovanni Filardo, PhD, MPH[e,f], Baron Lloyd Hamman, MD[c], Gregory John Matter, MD[c], Albert Carl Henry III, MD[c], and Robert Frederick Hebeler, Jr., MD[c]

Reports differ regarding the effect of concomitant coronary artery bypass grafting (CABG) in patients who undergo aortic valve replacement (AVR) for aortic stenosis (AS), and no reports have described the effect of aortic valve structure in patients who undergo AVR for AS. A total of 871 patients aged 24 to 94 years (mean 70) whose AVR for AS was their first cardiac operation, with or without first concomitant CABG, were included. Patients who underwent mitral valve procedures were excluded. In comparison with the 443 patients (51%) who did not undergo CABG, the 428 (49%) who underwent concomitant CABG were significantly older, were more often male, had lower transvalvular peak systolic pressure gradients and larger valve areas, had lower frequencies of congenitally malformed aortic valves, had lighter valves by weight, had higher frequencies of systemic hypertension, and had longer stays in the hospital after AVR. Early and late (to 10 years) mortality were similar by propensity-adjusted analysis in patients who did and did not undergo concomitant CABG. Congenitally unicuspid or bicuspid valves occurred in approximately 90% of those aged 21 to 50, in nearly 70% in those aged 51 to 70 years, and in just over 30% in those aged 71 to 95 years. Unadjusted and adjusted survival was significantly higher in patients with unicuspid or bicuspid valves compared to those with tricuspid valves. In conclusion, although concomitant CABG had no effect on the adjusted probability of survival, the type of aortic valve (unicuspid or bicuspid vs tricuspid) significantly affected the unadjusted and adjusted probability of survival. **(Am J Cardiol 2012;109:1334–1340)**

Adults with isolated (no mitral valve disease) aortic stenosis (AS) (with or without aortic regurgitation) frequently have associated narrowing of ≥1 major (right, left main, left anterior descending, or left circumflex) epicardial coronary arteries. In reported patients who undergo aortic valve replacement (AVR) for AS, the effect of concomitant coronary artery bypass grafting (CABG) on early and late mortality has been variable. The aim of this study was to compare among patients with isolated AS the outcomes of AVR in patients with versus without CABG and also the effect of aortic valve structure (unicuspid or bicuspid vs tricuspid) on the probability of long-term survival after AVR for AS.

Methods

The surgical pathology files of the cardiovascular laboratory, a part of the pathology department at Baylor University Medical Center (BUMC) in Dallas, were searched for patients having operatively excised aortic valves without simultaneous replacement of the mitral valve or evidence of mitral stenosis. From January 2002 through June 2010 (102 months [8.5 years]), a total of 1,040 operatively excised stenotic aortic valves were submitted to the cardiovascular laboratory at BUMC. Each was described, and the surgical report was prepared by W.C.R. and photographed by J.M.K. The valve structure in each was determined by W.C.R from examination of the operatively excised aortic valve. This study was approved by the Institutional Review Board at BUMC on May 5, 2010, and the requirement for individual patient consent was waived.

Included in the present study were 871 adults whose AVR for AS was their first cardiac operation, with or without first simultaneous CABG. Patients who underwent isolated AVR for AS and later in a second operation underwent CABG or vice versa were excluded.

Clinical records, including admission note, discharge summary, echocardiographic and cardiac catheterization reports, and operative records, were sought from the patients' medical charts and/or BUMC Apollo cardiovascular database (Apollo Advance c/s version 4.2.13; LUMEDX Corporation, Oakland, California). (The Apollo system became operational at BUMC in January 2002.)

Echocardiographic and hemodynamic data were obtained from the cardiovascular computer database. Whether simultaneous CABG was performed at the time

Departments of [a]Internal Medicine (Division of Cardiology), [b]Pathology, and [c]Cardiothoracic Surgery and the [d]Baylor Heart and Vascular Institute, Baylor University Medical Center; [e]Institute for Health Care Research and Improvement, Baylor Health Care System; [f]Department of Statistical Science, Southern Methodist University, Dallas Texas; [g]University of Georgia, Athens, Georgia; and [h]University of Texas at Austin, Austin, Texas. Manuscript received December 5, 2011; revised manuscript received and accepted December 8, 2011.

*Corresponding author: Tel: 214-820-7911; fax: 214-820-7533.

E-mail address: wc.roberts@baylorhealth.edu (W.C. Roberts).

Table 1
Frequency of concomitant coronary artery bypass grafting in patients who underwent isolated aortic valve replacement for aortic stenosis (n = 871)

Variable	Coronary Artery Bypass Grafting		p Value
	Yes (n = 428 [49%])	No (n = 443 [51%])	
Age group (years)			<0.001
21–50	12 (3%)	54 (12%)	
51–70	139 (32%)	201 (45%)	
71–95	277 (65%)	188 (42%)	
Gender			<0.001
Male	289 (68%)	233 (53%)	
Female	139 (32%)	210 (47%)	
Race			0.953
White	354 (83%)	367 (83%)	
Black	24 (6%)	22 (5%)	
Hispanic	16 (4%)	19 (4%)	
Other or unknown	34 (8%)	35 (8%)	
Number of major coronary arteries narrowed ≥50%	(n = 205)	(n = 272)	<0.001
0	32 (16%)*	246 (90%)	
1	60 (29%)	20 (7%)	
2	68 (33%)	5 (2%)	
3	34 (17%)	1 (<1%)	
4	11 (5%)	0	
LV-aorta peak systolic gradient (mm Hg) (n = 475), range (mean) [median]	10–119 (46) [41]	11–154 (54) [52]	<0.001
Aortic valve area (cm^2) (n = 474), mean ± SD	0.85 ± 0.31	0.76 ± 0.25	0.008
Aortic valve structure			<0.001
Unicuspid	11 (3%)	49 (11%)	
Bicuspid	142 (33%)	243 (55%)	
Tricuspid	275 (64%)	151 (34%)	
Aortic valve weight (g)			<0.001
Unicuspid, range (mean) [median]	1.20–4.78 (2.89) [2.71]	1.19–7.15 (3.47) [3.28]	
Bicuspid, range (mean) [median]	0.67–18.38 (3.11) [2.62]	0.81–9.68 (3.11) [2.91]	
Tricuspid, range (mean) [median]	0.43–6.40 (2.00) [1.84]	0.55–5.63 (2.11) [1.98]	
Systemic hypertension by history	324 (76%)	292 (66%)	0.015
Body mass index (kg/m^2)			0.872
≤25	148 (35%)	140 (32%)	
>25–30	156 (37%)	136 (31%)	
>30–40	104 (24%)	141 (32%)	
>40	18 (4%)	22 (5%)	
Range (mean ± SD)	15–69 (28 ± 6)	15–61 (29 ± 6)	
Days in hospital postoperatively in patients living >30 days, range (mean) [median]	3–53 (10) [8]	3–71 (8) [6]	0.001
Died ≤30 days postoperatively	29/427 (7%)	18/437 (4%)	0.179
Ascending aorta replaced	11 (3%)	26 (6%)	0.159
Implanted valve type			<0.001
Mechanical	64 (16%)	140 (32%)	
Bioprosthetic	355 (84%)	289 (67%)	
Ross procedure	1 (<1%)	6 (1%)	

* These patients had significant narrowing of a branch of ≥1 major coronary artery.

of AVR was also obtained from either the computer database or from the medical records. Information regarding the death of any patient was obtained from 3 sources: (1) the medical records in the deaths during the hospitalization at the time of AVR, (2) the Society of Thoracic Surgeons National Database, and (3) the Social Security Death Index for posthospitalization deaths. Echocardiographic data preoperatively were available for 426 patients (49%). Cardiac catheterization data preoperatively were available for 561 patients (64%).

Means, standard deviations, and percentages were calculated to describe the study cohort (n = 871). Differences in demographic, clinical, and morphologic details were tested using Wilcoxon's tests (for continuous variables) or chi-square tests (for categorical variables). Bonferroni's correction was used to account for multiplicity. Unadjusted p values, odds ratios, hazard ratios, 95% confidence intervals (CIs), and log-rank statistics were estimated to describe 30-day and long-term mortality. Kaplan-Meier plots were used to describe unadjusted survival in patients who underwent concomitant CABG compared to those who did not and in patients with unicuspid or bicuspid valves compared to those with tricuspid valves.

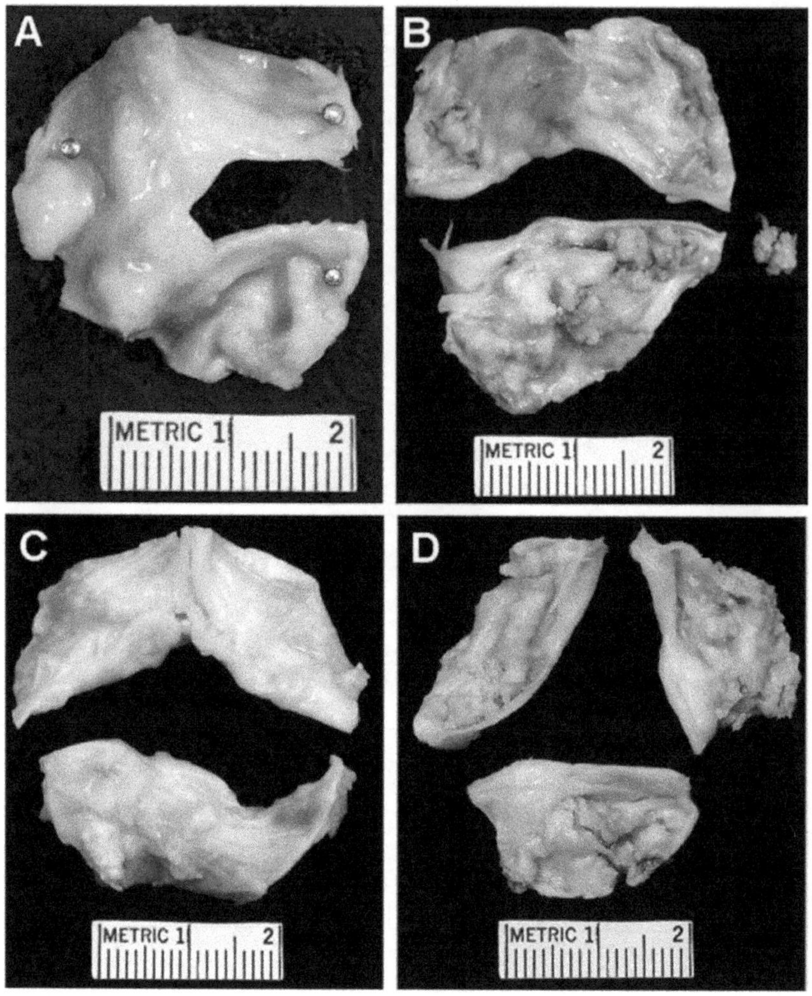

Figure 1. Photographs of operatively excised stenotic aortic valves in 4 patients. *(A)* Congenitally unicuspid unicommissural valve in a 66-year-old patient. *(B)* Congenitally bicuspid valve in an 81-year-old man. *(C)* Congenitally bicuspid valve in a 58-year-old man. *(D)* Tricuspid aortic valve in a 79-year-old woman. CABG was performed also in patients whose valves are shown in *(B)* and *(D)*. Valve weights were 2.48 g *(A)*, 3.55 g *(B)*, 3.19 g *(C)*, and 2.71 g *(D)*.

A propensity score approach was used to assess the adjusted association between undergoing concomitant CABG (vs not) and 30-day and long-term mortality.[1,2] To estimate the propensity score, we used a logistic regression model with receiving concomitant CABG (vs not) as the dependent variable and age, gender, race, body mass index, aortic valve structure, valve weight, systemic hypertension, ascending aorta replaced, and type of implanted valve as independent variables. Restricted cubic splines were used for all continuous variables.[3,4] Multiple imputation via predictive mean matching was used to account for missing data regarding the independent variables in this model.[1] Estimates from the aforementioned propensity model were then used to adjust the effect of concomitant CABG on 30-day mortality in a logistic regression model and on long-term mortality in a Cox proportional-hazards model. Possible effect modification by gender and age was investigated for the 2 models and ruled out. The Grambsch and Therneau test statistic was used to test for proportionality of hazards in the Cox model.[5]

The same approach, controlling for the same confounding factors except that valve structure was replaced by concomitant CABG, was used to assess the adjusted association between valve structure (unicuspid or bicuspid vs tricuspid valve structure) and 30-day and long-term mortality.

Statistical analyses were performed using SAS version 9.2 (SAS Institute Inc., Cary, North Carolina) and R software version 2.12.1 (R Project for Statistical Computing, Vienna, Austria).

Results

Demographic, clinical, and morphologic findings in the 871 patients included in the present study and their comparison between those with versus without concomitant CABG are listed in Table 1. Of the 871 patients, 428 (49%) underwent concomitant CABG, and 443 (51%) did not. In comparison to the group that did not undergo CABG, those who underwent concomitant CABG were significantly older, were more often male, had lower transvalvular peak systolic pressure gradients and larger valve areas, had higher frequencies of tricuspid aortic

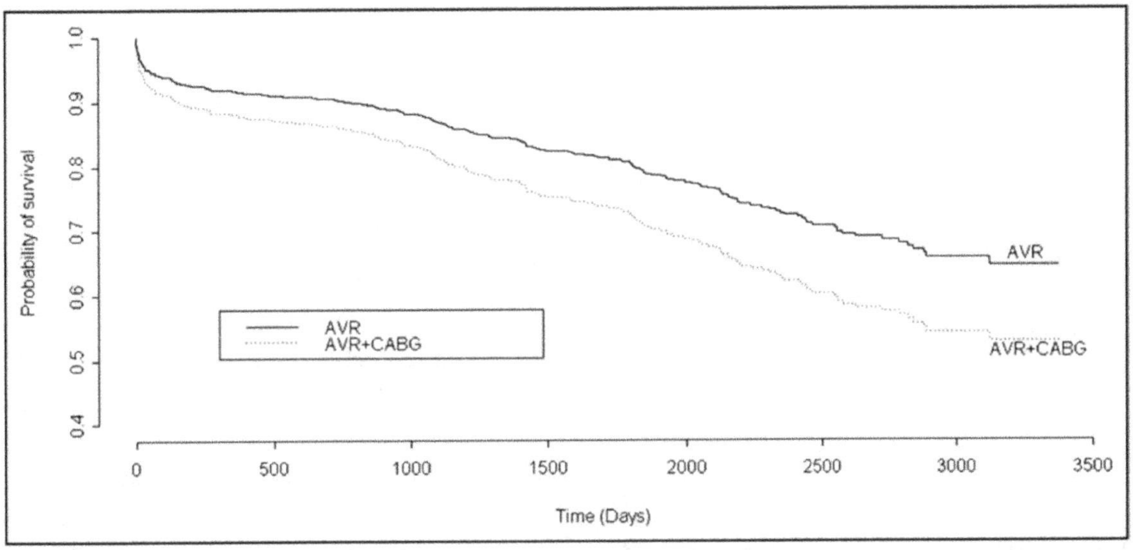

Figure 2. Unadjusted (Kaplan-Meier) curves depicting the probability of long-term survival in the patients who underwent compared to those who did not undergo concomitant coronary artery bypass grafting with the aortic valve replaced for stenosis (unadjusted hazard ratio 1.46, 95% CI 1.12 to 1.91, log-rank p = 0.005).

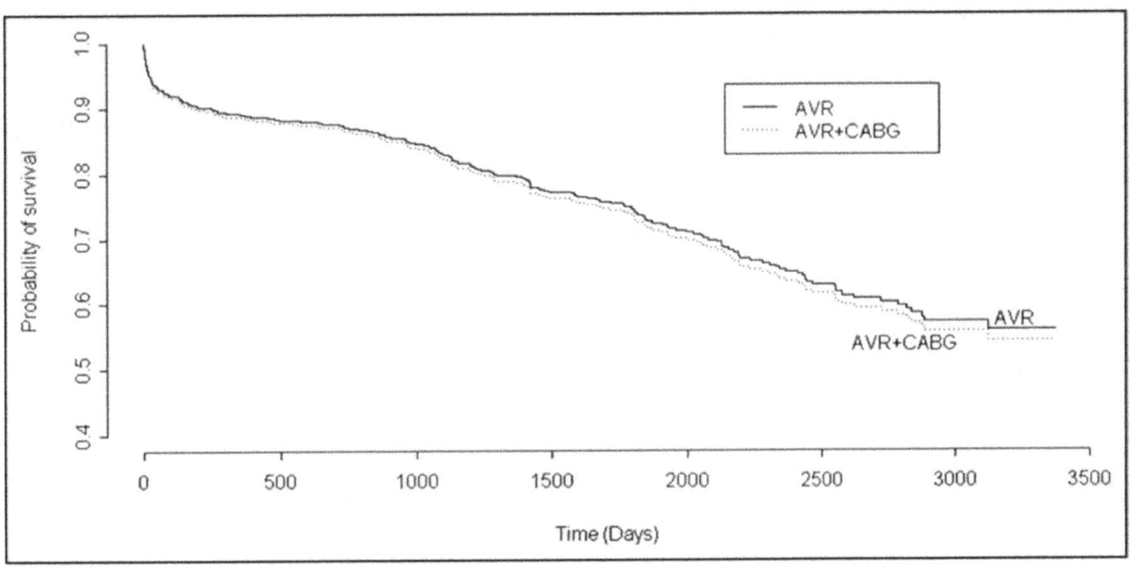

Figure 3. Adjusted (proportional-hazards model) curves depicting no significant difference in long-term survival in those who underwent compared to those who did not undergo concomitant coronary artery bypass grafting. The propensity-adjusted model included the following risk factors: age, gender, race, body mass index, aortic valve structure, valve weight, systemic hypertension, ascending aorta replaced, and type of implanted valve (adjusted hazard ratio 1.01, 95% CI 0.74 to 1.34, adjusted p = 0.976).

valves and lower frequencies of congenitally malformed aortic valves (Figure 1), had lighter aortic valves by weight, had higher frequencies of systemic hypertension, and had longer stays in the hospital after AVR (Table 1). Unadjusted early mortality (30 days) was not significantly (odds ratio 1.59, 95% CI 0.89 to 2.85) different between those who underwent (29 deaths [7%]) and those who did not undergo (18 deaths [4%]) simultaneous CABG. The length of stay for patients surviving >30 days and long-term survival (up to 10-year follow-up) were significantly higher in those who underwent concomitant CABG (median length of stay 8 days vs 6 days for patients who did not undergo concomitant CABG, p = 0.001; unadjusted hazard ratio for survival 1.46, 95% CI 1.12 to 1.91, log-rank p = 0.005). The unadjusted survival curves are depicted in Figure 2. However, after adjustment for possible confounders (age, gender, race, body mass index, aortic valve structure, valve weight, systemic hypertension, ascending aorta replaced, and type of implanted valve), neither early mortality (30 days; adjusted odds ratio 1.69, 95% CI 0.87 to 3.29) nor long-term mortality (10-year follow-up; adjusted hazard ratio 1.01, 95% CI 0.74 to 1.34) was different between those who did and did not undergo simultaneous CABG. The adjusted long-term survival curves are depicted in Figure 3.

Table 2
Comparison of aortic valve structure in patients who underwent isolated aortic valve replacement for aortic stenosis with or without concomitant coronary artery bypass grafting (n = 871)

Variable	Aortic Valve Structure			p Value
	Unicuspid (n = 60 [7%])	Bicuspid (n = 385 [44%])	Tricuspid (n = 426 [49%])	
Age group (years)				<0.001
21–50	31 (52%)	29 (8%)	6 (1%)	
51–70	24 (40%)	206 (54%)	110 (26%)	
71–95	5 (8%)	150 (39%)	310 (73%)	
Gender				0.169
Male	36 (60%)	252 (65%)	234 (55%)	
Female	24 (40%)	133 (35%)	192 (45%)	
Race				0.274
White	47 (78%)	324 (84%)	350 (82%)	
Black	2 (3%)	12 (3%)	32 (8%)	
Hispanic	4 (7%)	18 (5%)	13 (3%)	
Other	7 (12%)	31 (8%)	31 (7%)	
Coronary artery bypass grafting	11 (18%)	142 (37%)	275 (65%)	<0.001
Number of major coronary arteries narrowed ≥50%	(n = 29)	(n = 212)	(n = 236)	<0.001
0	23 (79%)	143 (67%)	102 (43%)	
1	3 (10%)	34 (16%)	52 (22%)	
2	2 (7%)	23 (11%)	49 (21%)	
3	1 (3%)	8 (4%)	26 (11%)	
4	0	4 (2%)	7 (3%)	
LV-aorta peak systolic gradient (mm Hg) (n = 475), range (mean) [median]	20–154 (64) [63]	11–130 (55) [51]	11–119 (45) [41]	<0.001
Aortic valve area (cm^2) (n = 474), mean ± SD	0.80 ± 0.34	0.78 ± 0.25	0.83 ± 0.30	0.139
Aortic valve weight (g), range (mean) [median]	1.19–7.15 (3.37) [3.17]	0.67–18.38 (3.11) [2.79]	0.43–6.40 (2.04) [1.92]	<0.001
Systemic hypertension by history	27 (45%)	260 (68%)	329 (77%)	<0.001
Body mass index (kg/m^2)				0.863
≤25	24 (41%)	119 (31%)	145 (34%)	
>25–30	21 (36%)	130 (34%)	141 (33%)	
>30–40	13 (22%)	111 (29%)	121 (29%)	
>40	1 (2%)	22 (6%)	17 (4%)	
Range (mean ± SD)	17–44 (27 ± 5)	16–66 (29 ± 7)	15–69 (29 ± 6)	
Days in hospital postoperatively in patients living >30 days, range (mean) [median]	3–32 (7) [6]	3–43 (8) [6]	3–71 (10) [8]	<0.001
Died ≤30 days postoperatively	0/59	20/380 (5%)	27/425 (6%)	0.222
Ascending aorta replaced	9 (15%)	25 (6%)	3 (1%)	<0.001
Implanted valve type				<0.001
Mechanical	41 (68%)	118 (31%)	53 (12%)	
Bioprosthetic	17 (28%)	264 (69%)	371 (87%)	
Ross procedure	2 (3%)	3 (<1%)	2 (<1%)	

The valve structure in the 871 patients is listed in Table 2. The 426 patients (49%) with tricuspid aortic valves, compared to the 445 patients (51%) with either congenitally unicuspid or bicuspid valves, were significantly older (p <0.001), had much higher frequencies of concomitant CABG (p <0.001), had higher likelihoods of having ≥1 major epicardial coronary artery being narrowed >50% in diameter on angiogram (p <0.001), had lower transvalvular peak systolic pressure gradients (p <0.001), had lighter aortic valves by weight (p <0.001), had higher frequencies of systemic hypertension (p <0.001), had more days in the hospital after AVR (p <0.001), and had higher late (>30 days) mortality rates after AVR. Unadjusted early mortality (30 days) was not significantly (odds ratio 1.16, 95% CI 0.56 to 2.42) different between patients with unicuspid or bicuspid versus tricuspid valves. Both unadjusted and adjusted survival, however, were significantly higher in patients with unicuspid or bicuspid valves compared to patients with tricuspid aortic valves (adjusted hazard ratio 0.70, 95% CI 0.50 to 0.97; Figures 4 and 5).

Coronary angiographic data were available for 477 of the 871 patients (55%). Compared to the 278 patients (58%) in whom none of the major coronary arteries was narrowed to this degree, the 199 patients (42%) with ≥1 coronary artery narrowed >50% were significantly older (p = 0.012), were more often male (p = 0.005), had much higher frequencies of concomitant CABG (p <0.001), had smaller peak systolic transvalvular pressure gradients (p = 0.010) and larger valve areas (p = 0.002), had higher frequencies of tricuspid aortic valves and lower frequencies of congenitally malformed valves (p <0.001), and had smaller aortic valves by weight (p = 0.030).

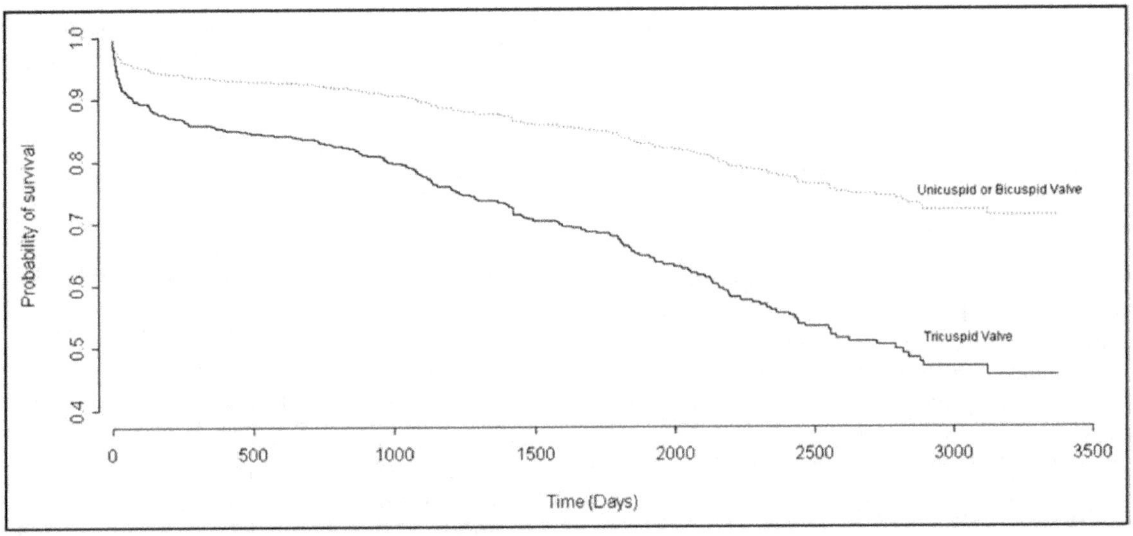

Figure 4. Unadjusted (proportional-hazards model) curves depicting significantly different survival in patients with unicuspid or bicuspid valves compared to those with tricuspid valves, all of whom underwent AVR (unadjusted hazard ratio 0.43, 95% CI 0.32 to 0.57, unadjusted $p < 0.001$).

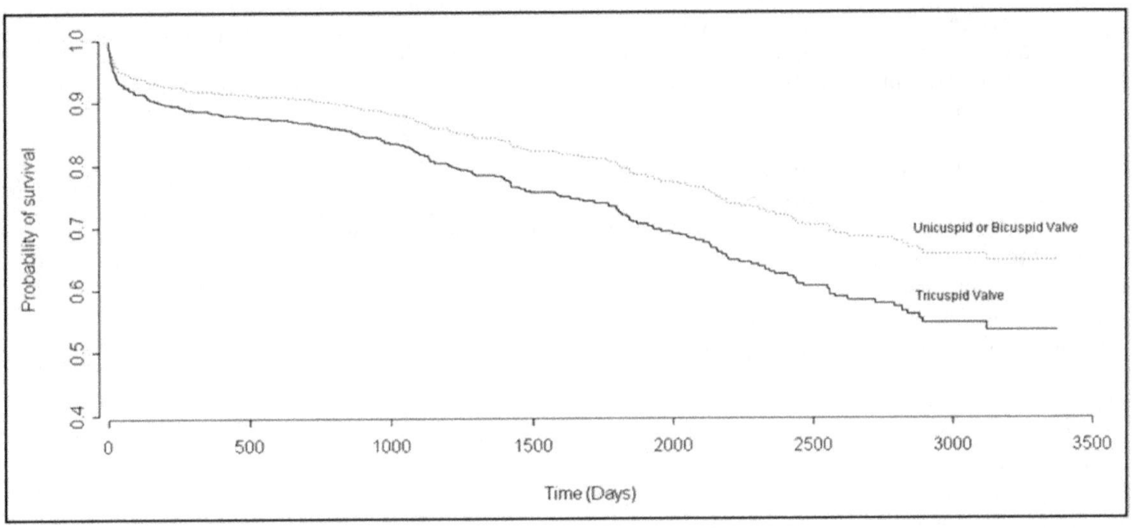

Figure 5. Adjusted (proportional-hazards model) curves depicting significantly different survival in those with unicuspid or bicuspid aortic valves compared to those with tricuspid valves, all of whom underwent AVR (adjusted hazard ratio 0.70, 95% CI 0.50 to 0.97, adjusted $p = 0.031$). The propensity-adjusted model included the following risk factors: age, gender, race, body mass index, concomitant CABG, valve weight, systemic hypertension, ascending aorta replaced, and type of implanted valve.

Discussion

The present study of patients who underwent AVR for AS (with or without aortic regurgitation) examined whether simultaneous CABG (vs not) and aortic valve structure (unicuspid or bicuspid vs tricuspid) affected short- and long-term survival. Although the patients who underwent simultaneous CABG compared to those who did not were significantly older, were more often male, had smaller transvalvular peak systolic pressure gradients and larger valve areas, most often had tricuspid aortic valves and much less frequently congenitally malformed valves, had higher frequencies of systemic hypertension, and had longer hospital stays, the adjusted probability of long-term survival was no different in those with versus without concomitant CABG. The unadjusted p value regarding the association between concomitant CABG (vs not) and long-term survival was 0.005, while the adjusted p value was 0.976.

None of the previously published reports of patients who underwent AVR for AS with or without simultaneous CABG focused on the structure of stenotic aortic valve.[6–13] In the present study, aortic valve structure was determined by the same investigator (W.C.R.) from examination of the operatively excised valve. We found in a previous study that congruence between cardiac surgeons and cardiac pathologists regarding aortic valve structure is virtually 100% when the structure of the aortic valve is tricuspid but that it is only 56% in the case of congenitally bicuspid valves and only 15% in the case of unicuspid valves.[14] Thus, uniformity of determination of valve structure results in far more accurate information compared to valve structure determined by several different surgeons, each of whom may have varying expertise in describing aortic valve structure or even mentioning valve structure in the operative note. Additionally, the intervals between AVR and dictation of the operative note were quite variable among surgeons, whose memories also might be quite variable.[14] The present study found that among the 426 patients with tricuspid aortic valves, 65% underwent concomitant CABG, whereas among the 60 patients with unicuspid valves and the 385 with congenitally bicuspid valves, concomitant CABG was far less frequently performed (18% and 37%, respectively). Both unadjusted and adjusted survival was significantly better in the patients with unicuspid or bicuspid aortic valves compared to those with tricuspid aortic valves.

A bit surprising to many students of aortic valve disease was the relatively high frequency of the congenitally malformed valves in all 3 age groups examined. Among the 66 patients aged 21 to 50 years, 60 (91%) had congenitally malformed aortic valves (unicuspid in 31 and bicuspid in 29); of the 340 patients aged 51 to 70 years, 230 (68%) had congenitally malformed valves (unicuspid in 24 and bicuspid in 206); and of the 465 patients aged 71 to 95 years, 155 (33%) had congenitally malformed valves (unicuspid in 5 and bicuspid in 150).

That CABG was significantly more frequent in the group with tricuspid aortic valves partly supports the view that AS in older patients with tricuspid aortic valves is the result of "atherosclerosis" involving the aortic valve. Patients with rheumatic heart disease were presumably excluded from the present study on the basis of having excluded all patients with mitral stenosis and those who underwent any operative procedure on the mitral valve (either repair or replacement).

There were limitations to the present study. Echocardiographic and hemodynamic data were not available in all patients. Not all patients with narrowing >50% in diameter of ≥1 major coronary artery underwent CABG. Many patients who underwent concomitant CABG and AVR would not have undergone AVR unless ≥1 of the coronary arteries had not been quite narrowed by preoperative angiogram. A major strength of the present study is that it is the first to compare long-term survival after AVR for AS (with or without aortic regurgitation) according to the underlying valve structure (unicuspid, bicuspid, or tricuspid).

1. Harrell FE Jr. Regression Modeling Strategies: With Application to Linear Models, Logistic Regression, and Survival Analysis. *New York, New York: Springer-Verlag*; 2001.
2. D'Agostino RB Jr. Propensity score methods for bias reduction in the comparison of a treatment to a non-randomized control group. *Stat Med* 1998;17:2265–2281.
3. Filardo G, Hamilton C, Hamman B, Ng HK, Grayburn P. Categorizing BMI may lead to biased results in studies investigating in-hospital mortality after isolated CABG. *J Clin Epidemiol* 2007;60:1132–1139.
4. Filardo G, Hamilton C, Hamman B, Grayburn P. Obesity and stroke after cardiac surgery: the impact of grouping body mass index. *Ann Thorac Surg* 2007;84:720–722.
5. Grambsch PM, Therneau T. Proportional hazards tests and diagnostics based on weighted residuals. *Biometrika* 1994;81:515–526.
6. Jones EL, Weintraub WS, Craver JM, Guyton RA, Shen Y. Interaction of age and coronary disease after aortic valve replacement: implications for valve selection. *Ann Thorac Surg* 1994;58:378–385.
7. Akins CW. Long-term results with the Medtronic-Hall valvular prosthesis. *Ann Thorac Surg* 1996;61:806–813.
8. Litmathe J, Boeken U, Feindt P, Gams E. Concomitant CABG procedures in elderly patients undergoing aortic valve replacement. *Z Kardiol* 2003;92:947–952.
9. Gillinov AM, Garcia MJ. When is concomitant aortic valve replacement indicated in patients with mild to moderate stenosis undergoing coronary revascularization? *Curr Sci* 2005;7:101–104.
10. Kuduvalli M, Grayson AD, Au J, Grotte G, Bridgewater B, Fabri BM. A multi-centre additive and logistic risk model for in-hospital mortality following aortic valve replacement. *Eur J Cardiothorac Surg* 2007;31:607–613.
11. Kobayashi KJ, Williams JA, Nwakanma L, Gott VL, Baumgartner WA, Conte JV. Aortic valve replacement and concomitant coronary artery bypass: assessing the impact of multiple grafts. *Ann Thorac Surg* 2007;83:969–978.
12. Gulbins H, Malkoc A, Ennker J. Combined cardiac surgincal procedures in octogenarians: operative outcome. *Clin Res Cardiol* 2008;97: 176–180.
13. Likosky DS, Sorensen MJ, Dacey LJ, Baribeau YR, Leavitt BJ, DiScipio AW, Hernandez F Jr, Cochran RP, Quinn R, Helm RE, Charlesworth DC, Clough RA, Malenka DJ, Sisto DA, Sardella G, Olmstead EM, Ross CS, O'Connor GT. Long-term survival of the very elderly undergoing aortic valve surgery. *Circulation* 2009;120:127–133.
14. Roberts WC, Vowels TJ, Ko JM. Comparison of interpretations of valve structure between cardiac surgeon and cardiac pathologist among adults having isolated aortic valve replacement for aortic valve stenosis (± aortic regurgitation). *Am J Cardiol* 2009;103: 1139–1145.

Formulating an Answerable Question, Displaying Data, Illustrating, Writing, Reviewing, and Editing Manuscripts for Publication in Medical Journals

William Clifford Roberts, MD[a,*]

"In our instruction, we have tried to emphasize that a manuscript can be grammatically and semantically perfect and still be worthless if it is not scientifically valid. So we stress, first, clinical reasoning and analysis of experimental design and data, scientific validity, logical organization, and coherent development, and only then attention to the prose – grammar, semantics, conciseness, lucidity, readability, style."

—Selma and Lois DeBakey

Qualifications for Preparing a Manuscript on Writing, Reviewing, and Editing

Before describing some aspects of writing, reviewing, and editing medical manuscripts, it seems reasonable to give my qualifications for doing so. Since my first publication in a peer-reviewed medical journal in 1961, I have subsequently authored a number of articles each year.[1] I have been editor in chief of *The American Journal of Cardiology* (*AJC*) since June 1982 and of *The Baylor University Medical Center (BUMC) Proceedings* since 1994. During these 30 years with the *AJC*, 61,000 manuscripts have passed across my desk, and during the 17 years with the *BUMC Proceedings*, 1,500 manuscripts. As editor, I have tried to put my stamp, so to speak, on the editorial pages of both journals: by writing periodic editorials in one (*AJC*) and a column (Facts and Ideas from Anywhere) in the other (*BUMC Proceedings*).[2–4] I have written a number of editorials on writing and editing,[5–36] and several of these will be highlighted in the remainder of this piece.

Formulating an Answerable Question

When considering a potential clinical topic for investigation and later publication in a medical journal, the first step is to formulate a precise question which is answerable. Sometimes it takes considerable thought to formulate the question properly. The key is to have something to report. Does the message add to the present knowledge base, or does it simply confirm a previous observation or describe it better than before?

Order of Manuscript Preparation

Every author probably creates a manuscript a bit differently. First, I prepare the *tables* and *figures* and try to make them final before a single word of the manuscript is written. Next, I write the *title*. Next, the *abstract* (summary); writing it early on forces me to focus on the manuscript's important points. Then, during each revision, the abstract can be tweaked a bit. Next is the *introduction*, which I try to make a single paragraph that provides specifically the purpose of the manuscript. Then the *methods* and *results*, which should be in exquisite detail. These 2 sections are the heart of the manuscript. Some journals put these in a smaller font than that used in other portions of the manuscript. That move is not logical, in my view. If anything, the methods and results should be in a larger font than the rest of the manuscript. Then the *discussion*, which, in essence, focuses on how the results should be interpreted. Finally, the *references*; their selection, accuracy of recording, and formulation according to the style of the journal are clues to the scholarship of the authors.

Preparing the Tables

Tables 1 and 2 are good examples. Table 1 summarizes data in several large multicenter studies, and there is only 1 line across per study. Tables with a lot of words in them usually are unsatisfactory. Table 2 illustrates a study involving a limited number of patients. This table shows how each patient receives only 1 line across. If the number of patients studied is ≤30, individual patient data can be provided. There should be some logical order for listing the patients, such as by increasing age or order of the figures, as done in Table 2. I prefer to spell out the variables (parameters) to be analyzed. It is better to put the percent sign after the number rather than in the variable column. The units of measurement in the variable column are best placed in parentheses. Vertical lines are best avoided.

Finding the Masterful Figure[27]

When examining a new manuscript (or a published article), after reading the title, the authors' names, and abstract, I immediately go to the figures, seeking the one figure that provides the message of the manuscript. With my own publications, I spend more time in developing the figures and tables than I do in writing the manuscripts. I believe that the graphic or tabular presentation of the data carries more impact than the written text, which in essence simply describes the findings and interpretations of the graphs and figures.

I was pleased years ago to acquire Edward R. Tufte's *Visual Display of Quantitative Information* (Graphics Press, Cheshire, Connecticut, 1983). Contained in the 187-page book are numerous data graphics that display measured quantities by combined use of points, lines, coordinates,

[a]Baylor Heart and Vascular Institute and the Departments of Internal Medicine (Division of Cardiology) and Pathology, Baylor University Medical Center, Dallas, Texas. Manuscript received and accepted February 29, 2012.

*Corresponding author: Tel: 214-820-7911; fax: 214-820-7500.

E-mail address: wc.roberts@baylorhealth.edu (W.C. Roberts).

Table 1
Cardiovascular outcome studies with lipid-lowering agents in the first decade of the 21st century

Study	Year	Journal	Subjects	Diagnosis	Age (yrs)	Length of Study (yrs)	Agents Comparison	Events			Mean LDL-C (mg/dl)			
											Patients		Controls	
								Patients	Control	Relative Risk Reduction	Baseline	End	Baseline	End
MIRACL	2001	*JAMA*	3,086	ACS	Mean 65	0.31	A 80 vs P	14.80%	17.40%	↓ 16%	124	72	124	135
HPS	2002	*Lancet*	20,526	CAD, PVD, DM	40–80	5	S 40 vs P	7.60%	9.10%	↓ 17%	131	90	131	129
ASCOT-LLA	2003	*Lancet*	10,305	SH	40–79	Median 3.3*	A 10 vs P	1.90%	3.00%	↓ 31%	133	90	133	126
PROVE-IT	2004	*NEJM*	4,162	ACS	Mean 58	Mean 2	A 80 vs PRA 40	19.70%	22.30%	↓ 14%	106	62	106	95
CARDS	2004	*Lancet*	3,838	DM	40–75	Median 3.9[?]	A 10 vs P	9.40%	13.40%	↓ 37%	117	81	117	120
A to Z	2004	*JAMA*	4,497	ACS	Mean 61	0.5–2	S 40 to S 80 vs P to S 20	14.40%	16.70%	↓ 11%†	112	66	111	81
TNT	2005	*NEJM*	10,001	CAD, PVD	Mean 61	Median 4.9	A 80 vs A 10	8.70%	10.90%	↓ 22%	97	77	98	97
IDEAL	2005	*JAMA*	8,888	MI	<80	Median 4.8	A 80 vs S 20	9.3%[?]	10.4%[?]	↓ 11%†	122	81	121	104
SPARCL	2006	*NEJM*	4,731	Stroke, TIA	Mean 63	Median 4.9	A 80 vs P	11.20%	13.10%	↓ 16%	133	43	134	129
SEAS	2008	*NEJM*	1,873	AS	Mean 67	Median 4.3	S 40 + E 10 vs P	35.30%	38.20%	↓ 9%†	140	75	139	134
JUPITER	2008	*NEJM*	17,802	Healthy	Mean 66	Median 1.9[?]	R 20 vs P	0.02%	0.03%	↓ 47%	108	55	108	109

This table is an example showing a number of multicenter studies, but each study involves only 1 line across. It takes thought to produce a table which is crisp and clean. Reproduced with permission from the author and the publisher (Elsevier) from Roberts WC. Evaluating lipid-lowering trials in the twenty-first century. *Am J Cardiol* 2009;103:1325–1328.

A = atorvastatin; ACS = acute coronary syndrome; AS = aortic stenosis; CAD = coronary artery disease; DM = diabetes mellitus; *JAMA* = *Journal of the American Medical Association*; LDL-C = low-density-lipoprotein cholesterol; MI = myocardial infarction; *NEJM* = *New England Journal of Medicine*; P = placebo; PRA = pravastatin; PVD = peripheral vascular disease; R = rosuvastatin; S = simvastatin; SH = systemic hypertension; TIA = transient ischemic attack.

* Stopped early - Study planned for 5 years.

† Not significant.

Table 2

Pertinent clinical findings in the patients with bicuspid aortic valves and dysfunctioning mitral valves with replacement of both

Case No. (Fig. No.)	Age (years)	Sex	AVR to Discharge (days)	AVR to Death (days)	CABG	AS	AR	MS	MR	IE	RHD	IMR	MVP	MAC	Pre-op AF	BMI (kg/m^2)
1 (2)	53	F	5	Alive (5264)	0	+	0	+	0	0	+	0	0	0	0	34
2	50	M	9	3704	+	+	0	+	0	0	+	0	0	0	0†	27
3 (3)	46	M	4	2534	0*	+	0	+	0	0	+	0	0	0	+	26
4 (4)	74	F	13	4856	0	+	0	+	0	0	+	0	0	0	+	21
5 (5)	71	M	12	Alive (1162)	+	+	0	+	0	0	0	0	0	+	0	35
6 (6)	84	F	18	3858	+	+	0	0	+	0	0	+	0	0	0	29
7 (7)	77	M	7	867	+	+	0	0	+	0	0	+	0	0	0†	22
8 (8)	58	F	6	Alive (1301)	0	+	0	0	+	0	0	0	0	0	0	42
9 (9)	68	M	6	1540	0	+	0	0	+	0	0	0	+	0	0	23
10 (10)	67	M	6	Alive (1267)	0	+	0	0	+	0	0	0	+	0	0†	24
11 (11)	66	M	7	472	0	+	0	0	+	0	0	0	+	0	0	27
12	48	M	56	Alive (6096)	+	0	+	0	+	0	0	0	+	0	+	–
13 (12)	66	M	6	Alive (1252)	0	0	+	0	+	+	0	0	0	0	0	23
14 (13)	47	M	5	674	0	0	+	0	+	+	0	0	0	0	0	36
15	24	M	14	Alive (2017)	0	0	+	0	+	+	0	0	0	0	0	20
16 (14)	50	M	11	Alive (1127)	0	0	+	0	+	+	0	0	0	0	0	23

This is an example of an individual data table showing the findings in each of 16 patients but only 1 line across for each patient. The patients are listed by figure number. Reproduced with permission from the author and the publisher (Elsevier) from Roberts WC, Janning KG, Vowels TJ, Ko JM, Hamman BL, Hebeler RF Jr. Presence of a congenitally bicuspid aortic valve among patients having combined mitral and aortic valve replacement. *Am J Cardiol* 2012;109:263–271.

AF = atrial fibrillation; AR = aortic regurgitation; AS = aortic stenosis; AVR = aortic valve replacement; BMI = body mass index; CABG = coronary artery bypass grafting; IE = infective endocarditis; IMR = ischemic mitral regurgitation; MAC = mitral annular calcium; MR = mitral regurgitation; MS = mitral stenosis; MVP = mitral valve prolapse; RHD = rheumatic heart disease.

* Previous resection of aortic isthmus coarctation.

† Developed atrial fibrillation postoperatively after double valve replacement.

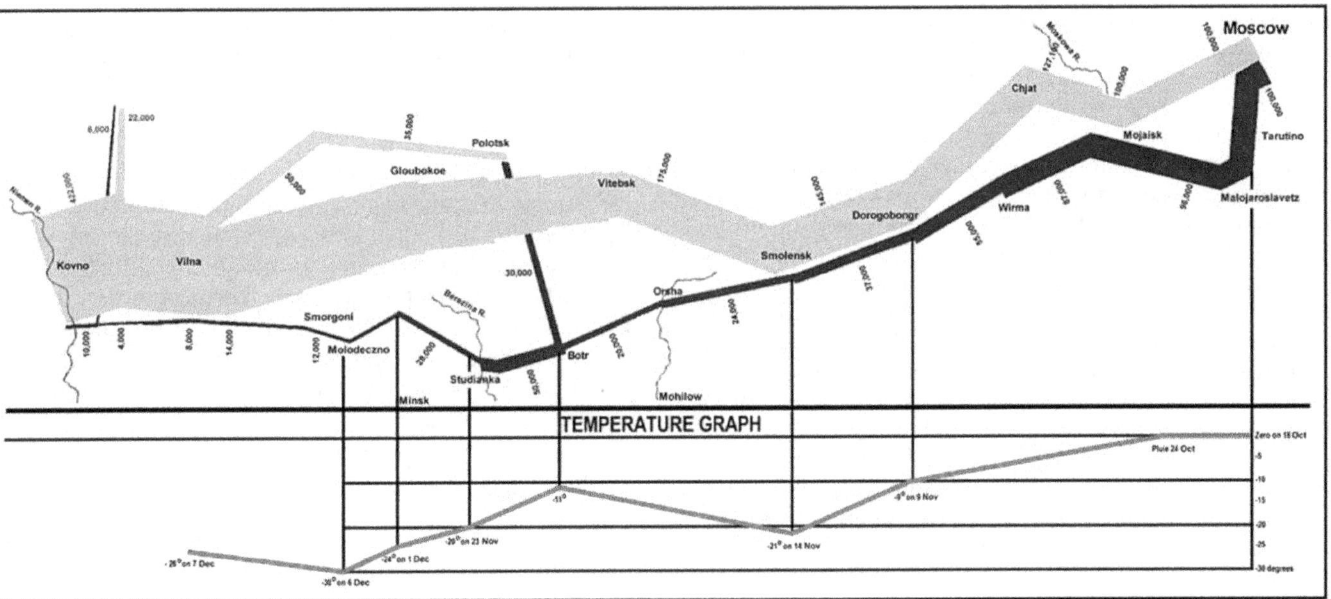

Figure 1. This illustration by Charles Joseph Minard (1781-1870), a French engineer, was reproduced by Edward R. Tufte in his 1983 book entitled *Visual Display of Quantitative Information*. Drawn in 1869, it shows the terrible fate of Napoleon Bonaparte's campaign into Russia. On the left, beginning at the Polish-Russian border near the Niemen River, the number of soldiers when the campaign began in June 1812 was 420,000. When the troops reached Moscow in September 1812 the number of soldiers was down to 100,000, and the city was deserted and sacked. The retreat in the bitterly cold winter is shown by the darker lower band. The widths of the bands indicate the size of the army at each place on the map. As they crossed the Berezina River (just to the left of the center of the graph), about half of the soldiers were lost, and when they finally reached the point where the march had begun, there were only 10,000 soldiers. Six variables are plotted: the size of the army, its location on a 2-dimensional surface, the direction of the army's movement, and the temperature of various dates during the retreat. It may well be the best statistical graphic ever drawn.

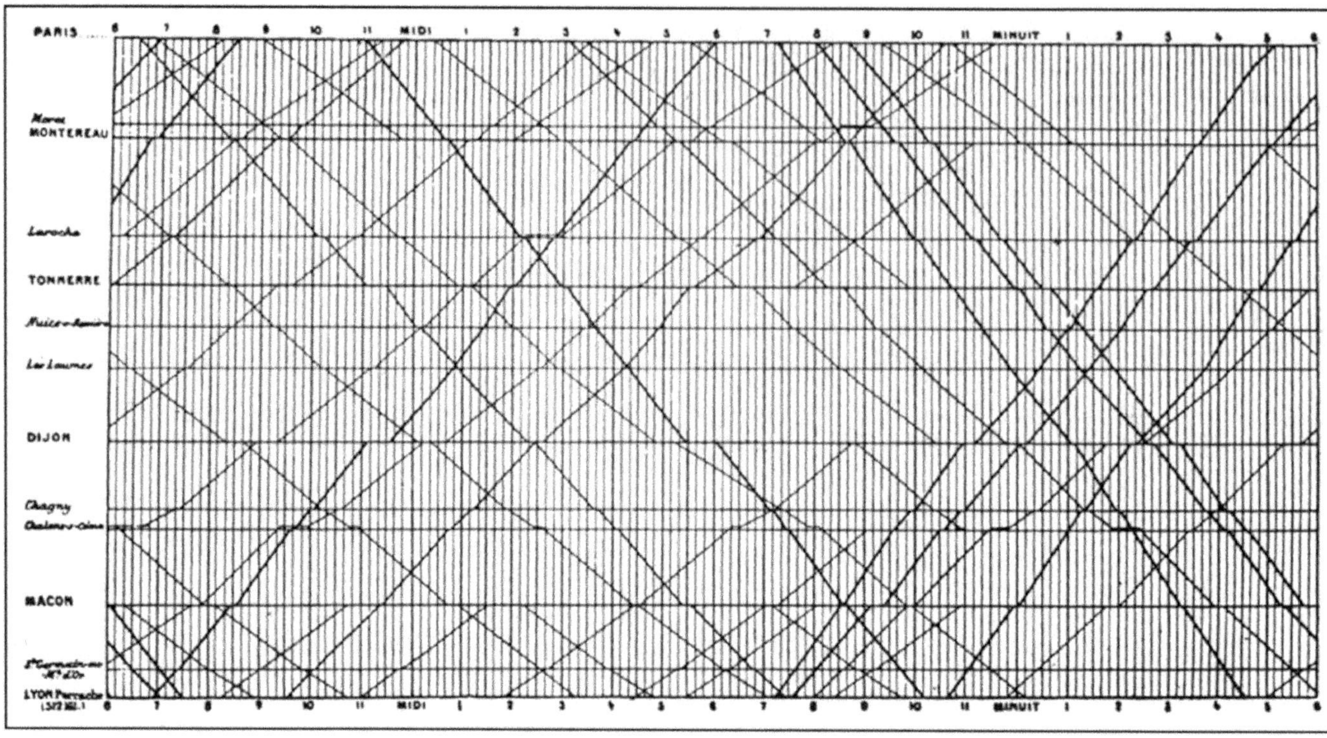

Figure 2. This diagram also comes from Tufte's book. It illustrates the train schedule from Paris to Lyon. Each of the spaces between the vertical lines represents 10 minutes. If one boarded the 6:30 AM train from Paris, it would arrive in Lyon just after 7:20 PM, or over 12 hours later. Other times of departing and arriving are also illustrated.

numbers, symbols, shading, sometimes color, and a few words. As pointed out by Tufte, the use of abstract pictures to statistical graphics—length and area to show quantity, time series, scatter plots, and multivariant displays—was not invented until 1750 to 1800, long after logarithms, Cartesian coordinates, calculus, and the basics of probability theory. As Tufte emphasized, modern data graphics do much more than simply substitute for statistical tables. They serve as instruments for reasoning about quantitative information. Often the most effective way to describe, explore, and summarize a set of numbers is to look at pictures. Of methods for analyzing and communicating statistical information, well-designed data graphics usually are the simplest and most powerful. According to Tufte, who presently is professor emeritus of political science and statistics and computer science at Yale University, each year somewhere between 900 billion and 2,000 billion images of statistical graphics are published, and some of them appear in cardiology journals. Two of Tufte's graphics are illustrated in Figures 1 and 2. Each of these graphics tells a huge story in a very simplified but sophisticated manner (see legends).

The Article's Title[25]

Although it is the most frequently read part of a manuscript, the title too often is given too little attention by authors. Whenever I write an article, the first words put on paper are those of the article's title. Then, with each revision of the manuscript, the title is carefully reexamined and usually reworded such that it is changed several times before the final typing of the manuscript. Focusing on the title requires careful focusing on the actual contents of the manuscript, because the title should be a precise description of those contents. I change the titles of most *AJC* manuscripts returned to authors for response to comments of reviewers and editors. The change in some may be the deletion or addition of only 1 or 2 words; in others, the change may be extensive.

What constitutes a good title? Above all, the title should be descriptive of the manuscript's contents. This description should not be in general terms but in as specific and precise terms as possible. The title should be devoid of excessive words but sufficient in words to adequately describe the manuscript's contents. The title should have a smooth flow. The message of the manuscript should not be in the title, which ideally should arouse the reader's curiosity so that he or she will go past it into the manuscript's text. If the manuscript's message is in the title, the curiosity may be immediately satisfied and the next article then sought. Subtitles should be avoided. Subtitles often are more specific than the main title, and therefore, they deserve to be the main title or at least incorporated into the main title. A minor factor against use of subtitles is that they often are omitted when the article is later referenced. Titles of experimental studies should include the animal species when the manuscript involves nonhuman animals. Titles as questions should be avoided. Abbreviations in titles should be avoided. Occasionally, the use of italics for 1 or 2 words in a title provides useful emphasis. Cardiologic titles are of many types, but common recurring ones include comparison of . . . , usefulness of . . . , association of . . . , effect of . . . , efficacy of . . . , evaluation of . . . , importance of . . . , influence of . . . , limitations of . . . , relation of . . . , results of . . . , analysis of . . . , and value of . . . .

The Abstract: The Manuscript's Bottom Line[18]

After the title, the next most frequently read portion of the manuscript is the summary (abstract). But is the summary given the same attention by authors as that given by readers? I think not. The summary, I suspect, tends to be written by many authors just before the final typing of the manuscript. Thus, when written last, the summary tends to be disjointed, as it attempts to tie together the important points of the paper. When written first, the summary serves as an outline. Moreover, by being done last, the summary may not receive the thoughtful deliberation given other portions of the manuscript.

Because the summary is so important to a manuscript, I suggest that an author write this portion *first* (after the title) rather than last. By doing so, one may focus better on the number of points the particular manuscript is trying to make. If the manuscript has essentially only 1 point, the summary can be particularly crisp and short; if >1 point, it serves as an outline of the points to be made. After the point or points of the manuscript are clearly in focus, the remainder of the paper can more readily build a case to demonstrate the validity of each point. The summary needs to be given the same emphasis and importance by authors as it receives from readers.

The Discussion

This is the only portion of the manuscript that I outline before writing. In general, the first paragraph provides a brief summary of the major finding, and then a discussion of previous publications on the same topic including what is different about the present study compared to previous publications. Does the present study provide new information or simply confirm that provided by previous publications? Then some comments on the strengths and limitations of the present study. A summary at the end of the discussion is usually unnecessary.

The References[16]

References are an important part of a manuscript. Their selection is an indicator of the authors' knowledge of and regard for work preceding their own, and their accuracy of recording is a clue to the quality of the authors' own work. Some authors tend to support statements in their manuscripts by multiple references, but often when this is done, some references do not support the statement for which they are being used. Other authors provide few references and open themselves to criticism for not giving sufficient credit to their predecessors. Should the initial or latest work on the subject be cited, or simply the present authors' previous work on the subject? A middle course between "too many" and "too few" references appears most reasonable. In the *AJC*, the number of references, except in reviews, is generally limited to ≤30.

An occasional criticism by reviewers of manuscripts is that their work was not cited. Accordingly, the reviewer may feel slighted and may react by being overcritical. References to an individual increase the chances, however, that that person will be selected to review the manuscript in question. I certainly look at the references cited when deciding to whom to send a manuscript for review. When reading a published or unpublished paper on which they too have contributed information, many authors and readers review the list of references cited. I am reminded of a story regarding 2 prominent authors. The late *William F. Buckley, Jr.*, and *John Kenneth Galbraith* habitually exchanged their most recently published books with each other. Galbraith upon receiving Buckley's latest book immediately turned to the title page, anticipating a note from his friend. Finding none, Galbraith then turned to the references, and beside the first citation of one of Galbraith's books, Buckley had written, "Hi, John, Bill."

Some manuscripts contain too many references and too little data. That a publication has been read during the preparation of a manuscript is not justification for its being cited as a reference. References should be carefully selected, and they should support the statements or comments to which they are attributed. And, just as a good paragraph should have no unnecessary sentences and a good sentence no unnecessary words, a manuscript should have no unnecessary references. Each reference, like each paragraph or sentence, should have a meaningful purpose.

Many errors are made in recording references. Examine any 10 references in a medical journal, and usually at least 1, often more, will contain an error. I suspect that inaccurately recorded references are found most frequently in manuscripts containing inadequately recorded data. Therefore, both as an editor and a reader, I examine the references in manuscripts: names are often misspelled, initials preceding the last name are often wrong, and "Junior" or "III" occasionally is omitted; titles often are recorded inaccurately and subtitles are frequently omitted; volume numbers, page numbers, and year of publication may be erroneously recorded. A major source of errors in references is recording a reference listed in another publication without actually reading that publication. In this way, previous recording errors are propagated in subsequent publications.

The following procedures have proved useful to me in diminishing errors in recording references for my own manuscripts:

1. *Each reference initially is recorded on a 3 × 5 inch card in print rather than script to prevent subsequent misinterpretation when typed.* All authors, full title with subtitle, volume, inclusive page numbers, and month and year of publication are recorded on these cards. Recording both the month as well as the year of publication allows chronologic listing of references published in the same year on the same subject.
2. *The senior or established author must check references recorded by young or relatively new investigators to ensure accuracy.*

3. *References are recorded only from the original publication.* To cite a reference from a previously published reference list without checking the original publication is poor research. A medical publication should never be referenced without reading it!
4. *References are typed only once, and that is in final form in the final manuscript directly from the 3 × 5 cards on which they are originally recorded.* The cards are numbered in pencil in the order in which they appear. Having each reference on a separate card allows the author to change the order without altering the entire typed format.
5. *The typed list of references is carefully proofed from the original 3 × 5 cards by the recorder of the references on the cards.* This person can read his or her handwriting better than anyone else. More typographic errors are made in typing references than any other portion of a manuscript. Therefore, the single typing of references from the original reference cards prevents errors which occur from multiple typing.
6. *The references in the galley proofs are checked against the original 3 × 5 reference cards.*

References listed in the *AJC* and in the *BUMC Proceedings* are complete in that the names of all authors, subtitles as well as primary titles, and inclusive page numbers are required. References submitted to these 2 journals in another format suggest that the manuscript has been submitted previously to another journal, which rejected it, or that the authors are not sensitive students of medical publications. With text pages at a premium, why are all authors, all titles, and inclusive page numbers required in the *AJC* and *BUMC Proceedings*? By listing all authors, all titles, and inclusive page numbers (rather than just the first page number of the article), the authors of the manuscript are virtually required to check the original article, and this checking increases the likelihood that the entire reference is recorded accurately. Supplying all authors' names assists an editor in the selection of possible manuscript reviewers. (The last author is likely to be a member of the journal's editorial board or more prominent than is the first author.) Listing inclusive page numbers prevents confusion of a reference to a previously published manuscript versus one to an abstract, which is virtually never >1 page. To diminish the space occupied by references without diminishing their accuracy or usefulness, the font size utilized for references in both the *AJC* and the *BUMC Proceedings* is small.

The method just described is a bit old fashioned in our present high-tech era. EndNote, a software program setup specifically for organizing references, is used by many investigators today.

In summary, references are a reflection of a manuscript's quality and should be selected carefully, recorded accurately, and prepared in the style of the journal to which the manuscript is submitted.

Abbreviations in Medical Journals[15]

Most medical journals allow some abbreviations. I favor limited numbers of appropriate abbreviations for 2 reasons: (1) *abbreviations save space and therefore permit more articles to be published*, and (2) *abbreviations, if limited to commonly used terms, decrease rather than increase reading time.* I prefer to limit abbreviations to the terms appearing in the manuscript's title. An article appearing in the *AJC* years ago was entitled "Left Ventricular Response to Isometric Exercise and Its Value in Predicting Change in Ventricular Function After Mitral Valve Replacement for Mitral Regurgitation." The phrase "left ventricular" (occupying 16 spaces) appeared 38 times, "mitral regurgitation" (20 spaces) 28 times, and "mitral valve replacement" (24 spaces) 12 times. Spelling out these 3 phrases would have occupied 1,456 spaces, but by abbreviating each ("LV," "MVR," and "MR"), only 168 spaces were used, and 24 single-column lines were saved—an average of nearly 8 column lines per page. In the same article, "LV" was used on other occasions: "LV mass," "LV ejection fraction," "LV peak systolic pressure," LV end-diastolic pressure, etc. Another article, entitled "Relation Between the Site of Origin of Ventricular Tachycardia and Relative Left Ventricular Myocardial Perfusion and Wall Motion," used the phrase "ventricular tachycardia" (23 spaces) 57 times and the phrase "left ventricular" 42 times. Spelling out these 2 phrases would have occupied 1,983 spaces, but the abbreviations occupied only 198 spaces, and 33 single-column lines were saved, an average of >8 column lines per printed page.

Abbreviations need, in general, to be limited to commonly recognized terms. Recently, I examined a manuscript which used the abbreviation "LVT," indicating "left ventricular thrombus." "LVT" is not a commonly recognized abbreviation, and therefore I changed it to "LV thrombus," abbreviating "left ventricular" throughout but not "thrombus." (The most commonly used phrase in cardiologic journals is "left ventricular"; hence, the abbreviation "LV" is highly useful. Note that "LV" most commonly signifies "left ventricular," not "left ventricle," which is far less commonly used.).

Not only must abbreviations be limited to commonly used terms, but also they must be appropriate, in that each letter in a phrase must stand for a single word. It is inappropriate to use a single letter for 1 word in a phrase and then >1 letter for a second word in the same phrase. Specifically, it is inappropriate to abbreviate "hypertrophic cardiomyopathy" as "HCM." The proper abbreviation is "HC." The commonly used abbreviations for the coronary arteries, namely, "RCA," "LAD," and "LCx," are not consistent. If "CA," the abbreviation for "coronary artery," is used after "right" to read "RCA," then it should be used after "left anterior descending" to read "LADCA" and after "left circumflex" to read "LCCA." It is inappropriate to abbreviate 2 syllables in "left circumflex" and not follow the same principle for "left anterior descending." It is best to abbreviate "left anterior descending" as "LAD" and "left circumflex" as "LC" (omitting the "x"), but not abbreviate "right coronary artery." It might best be labeled as "right."

Exceptions to the abbreviation principle of 1 letter per word occur when a single word is abbreviated. The correctly used abbreviations for "electrocardiogram" ("ECG"), "atrioventricular" ("AV"), and "radionuclide angiography" or "angiocardiography" ("RNA") are really inappropriate, but each is so ingrained that they have become appropriate.

It might be best to use certain terms universally to prevent confusion when abbreviating. The term "mitral regurgitation" is better than the term "mitral insufficiency" for several reasons; one is that it allows the abbreviation "MR," which prevents its confusion with "MI," which might stand for "myocardial infarction" or "myocardial infarct." Although it would be consistent with the rule of parallelism to abbreviate "coronary heart disease" as "CHD," this might produce confusion with "congenital heart disease," and therefore it might be preferable to allow "CAD" to signify both "coronary heart disease" and "coronary artery disease." To use the terms "interatrial septal defect" and "interventricular septal defect" is undesirable, because each implies that extra atrial and extra ventricular septal defects also exist. The prefix "inter" should be discarded: there is only 1 atrial septum and 1 ventricular septum, thus, "atrial septal defect" ("ASD") and "ventricular septal defect" ("VSD"), not "IASV and IVSD." The ventricular septum should be labeled "VS," not "IVS."

After first appearing in both summary and introduction, the phrase to be abbreviated should be spelled out and thereafter abbreviated consistently throughout the manuscript.

As an editor, I want maximal data per page. Abbreviations help achieve that goal. The use of numerals in the text (except when they begin a sentence or 2 are placed together in a sentence), and symbols for less than (<) and greater than (>), and the percent sign (%), also save space and make reading faster.

Making Clinical Studies Involving Many Patients Useful to the Single Patient[29]

"Doctoring" centers on the single patient, the one-to-one relationship. Yet, most clinical studies published in medical journals involve many patients. How can articles in medical journals be presented such that practitioners can fit their single patients into a large clinical study? Two suggestions:

1. *Keep patient populations as homogenous as possible.* I was surprised when becoming editor of the *AJC* how heterogenous were some patient populations included in various studies. An example: a manuscript on the effects of ≥1 drug on ventricular tachycardia typically might include 80 patients with coronary artery disease, 25 patients with idiopathic dilated cardiomyopathy, 5 patients with mitral valve prolapse, 4 patients who earlier had had valve replacement for aortic valve disease, 3 with hypertensive heart disease, 5 who earlier had tetralogy of Fallot repaired, and 10 patients without structural heart disease. The results of the study were pooled together so that it was impossible to know whether or not the results were similar in each of the various conditions associated with the ventricular tachycardia. In these circumstances, I have asked authors to limit their studies to the 80 patients with ventricular tachycardia associated with coronary artery disease, often with a comment that when the numbers of patients with the other conditions were large enough, another manuscript focusing on that group would be welcomed.

   Another area where heterogenous populations are likely to be found is in studies describing the effects of ≥1 drug in patients with heart failure. A study might include 20 patients in whom the chronic heart failure was associated with coronary artery disease (ischemic cardiomyopathy), 10 patients with idiopathic dilated cardiomyopathy, 3 with pure mitral regurgitation, 2 who earlier had had aortic valve replacement for reasons unspecified, 4 with hypertensive heart disease, and 2 in whom the etiology of the heart failure was not determined. In this circumstance, I would ask the authors to limit their study to the patients with heart failure associated with coronary artery disease and with idiopathic cardiomyopathy and to eliminate from their study the small numbers of patients in the other etiologic groups.
2. *Provide individual patient data rather than pooled data.* Many manuscripts submitted to medical journals report on 10 or so patients, and surprisingly, despite the small numbers, the data are pooled. In studies involving ≤30 patients, it is preferable to present the pertinent data on each patient. To present individual patient data in studies involving 30 patients, however, much care must be exerted in formulating a table. With rare exception, no patient should occupy more than 1 line across. Each column must ask a precise question that is answerable by either a number or a positive sign "+" (positive or present), a zero "0" (negative or absent), or a dash "—" (no information available or not applicable). Writing within the body of a table usually indicates that a precise question has not been formulated in the heading and that the table needs additional work.

Tables presenting individual patient data allow the reader to know the extent of missing data points in each patient. When data are pooled, missing data points usually cannot be detected. Presenting individual patient data tables allows the reader to insert his or her single patient more readily into a study. Of course, individual patient variability is more readily detected by presentation of individual patient data.

Thus, keep study populations as homogenous as possible, and display individual patient data when reporting ≤30 patients.

The "Hot Eye" and the "Cold Eye"[24]

For many years, I submitted manuscripts to medical journals for publication immediately after the final draft had been typed. Before the final typing, I would check the manuscript carefully for accuracy, clarity and precision of meaning, conciseness of expression, and errors in grammar, punctuation, and spelling. Then, when the manuscript was returned from the journal's editor for revision after the usual 1- to 2-month review process, I was surprised on reexamining the manuscript that I was often able to detect some minor inaccuracy or able to

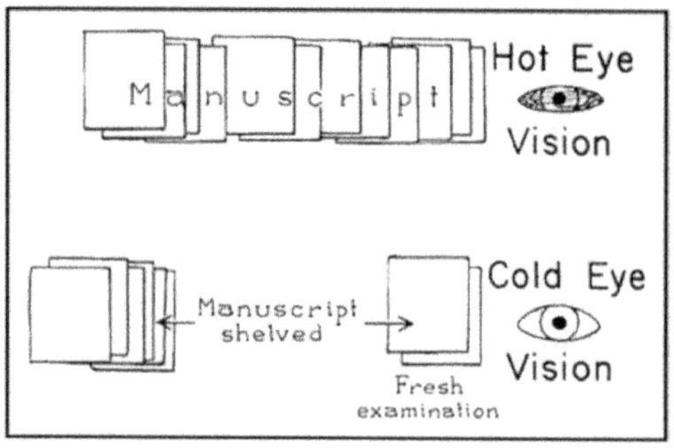

Figure 3. The diagram here shows the difference between examining a manuscript continuously (hot eye) versus examining a manuscript and then not seeing it for awhile, which allows one to essentially see the manuscript with a fresh eye (cold eye). Reproduced with permission from the author (Dr. Roberts) and the publisher (Elsevier) from *Am J Cardiol.*[24]

delete 1 or more paragraphs that did not now seem so pertinent or more precisely describe a method, result, or idea.

The answer, I believe, has to do with the "hot eye"–"cold eye" concept. Before initial submission of the manuscript, 1 draft was followed by another without essentially any cooling-off period between the various manuscript drafts. The manuscript in this circumstance may be thought of as being examined with a "hot eye" (Figure 3). Return of the manuscript to the author after the 1- to 2-month review process provides a needed cooling-off period for the authors, so that now the manuscript can be reexamined with a "cold eye." This first reexamination allows authors to identify previously unrecognized errors; unwarranted conclusions; flawed reasoning; exaggerated statements; redundancies; needless words, sentences, and paragraphs; and grammatical and spelling errors. I am convinced that this cooling-off period provides such an opportunity for manuscript improvement that even manuscripts in which both reviewers and editor have found few or no faults usually are returned to the authors for reexamination.

One reason almost any editor or reviewer can find defects in the work of almost any other writer, however talented, is that they view the manuscript with a "cold eye" because they have not seen it before. The cooling-off period provided for authors by the review process allows the authors to review their manuscripts more like an editor or reviewer—with a "cold eye." I suspect that all of our manuscripts would be improved if we shelved them for a week or so before our final check preceding the final typing for initial submission to a medical journal.

Getting the Manuscript Accepted: Think Like a Lawyer and Cover the Flanks[11]

A manuscript might be viewed as a legal brief in which an author presents logical arguments supporting the contention that he or she has created and proven a new concept. Reviewers in a way are like lawyers who attempt to find flaws in the authors' contentions. Finding such flaws often casts doubt on other claims by the author. Indeed, the finding by reviewers or the editor of *omissions of mention* can be a major stumbling block preventing the acceptance of a manuscript.

A manuscript's quality may be compared to the game of tic-tac-toe, in which 2 players in turn fill in 9 compartments, 1 at a time, with X's and O's (Figure 4). The best manuscript fills in all the blocks, covers all the bases, and, in addition, lines up 3 X's in a row, signifying focus, clarity, and positivity. A row of O's indicates that the manuscript provides an essentially negative observation. A manuscript also can have all the blocks filled in but no symbols lined up in a row, indicating a lack of clarity and focus. The worst paper fails to fill in 1 or more compartments with either symbol (omissions of mention), and none line up in a row, an indication that the authors failed to mention all the points necessary to prove their case and to focus the points properly.

Clarity and Conciseness in Writing

The wonderful book entitled *The Elements of Style* by Strunk and White[37] contains the following paragraph: "Vigorous writing is concise. A sentence should contain no unnecessary words, a paragraph no unnecessary sentences, for the same reason that a drawing should have no unnecessary lines and a machine no unnecessary parts. This requires not that the writer make all his sentences short or that he avoid all detail and treat his subjects only in outline, but that every word tell."

There are many good books on writing, word selection, and editing. I have 3 bookshelves of them in my home. I particularly like the ones listed in Table 3. *The Elements of Style* is a must for anyone trying to advance in the academic arena. Likewise, the Fowler and Gowers books serve a similar purpose. I am very fond of the chapter on clutter in Zinsser's book. James Jackson Kilpatrick, who became editor of the Richmond, Virginia, newspaper at age 26, wrote *The Writer's Art*, in which he gives numerous examples of good and bad writing. Most dictionaries have chapters on grammar.

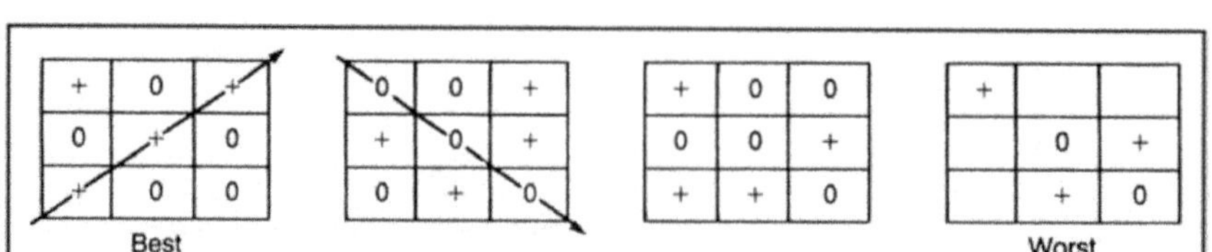

Figure 4. This figure displays the tic-tac-toe concept of manuscript writers thinking like a lawyer and covering their flanks (see text). Reproduced with permission from the author (Dr. Roberts) and the publisher (Elsevier) from *Am J Cardiol.*[11]

Table 3
Books on writing, words, and editing

- DeBakey, Lois. *The Scientific Journal: Editorial Policies and Practices: Guidelines for Editors, Reviewers, and Authors*. St. Louis, Missouri: Mosby, 1976:129.
- Huth, Edward J. *How to Write and Publish Papers in the Medical Sciences*. Philadelphia, Pennsylvania: ISI Press, 1982:203.
- Allbutt, Thomas C. *Notes on the Composition of Scientific Papers*. London, United Kingdom: The Keynes Press (British Medical Association), 1984: 161.*
- Strunk, William Jr. *The Elements of Style With Revisions, an Introduction, and a New Chapter on Writing by E. B. White*. New York, New York: Macmillan, 1959:71.
- Fowler, H. W. *A Dictionary of Modern English Usage*. 2nd ed., revised by Ernest Gowers. New York, New York: Oxford University Press, 1965:725.
- Bernstein, Theodore M. *The Careful Writer: A Modern Guide to English Usage*. New York, New York: Atheneum, 1965:487.
- Bernstein, Theodore M. *Miss Thistlebottom's Hobgoblins: The Careful Writer's Guide to the Taboos, Bugbears and Outmoded Rules of English Usage*. New York, New York: Simon & Schuster, 1971:260.
- Gowers, Ernest. *The Complete Plain Words*. Revised ed., by Bruie Fraser. London, United Kingdom: Her Majesty's Stationery Office, 1973:241.
- Bernstein, Theodore M. *Dos, Don'ts & Maybes of English Usage*. New York, New York: Times Books, 1977:250.
- Zinsser, William. *On Writing Well: An Informal Guide to Writing Nonfiction*. 2nd ed. New York, New York: Harper & Row, 1980:187.
- Kilpatrick, James J. *The Writer's Art*. Kansas City, Missouri: Andrews, McMeel & Parker, 1984:254.
- Morris, William, Editor. *The Heritage Illustrated Dictionary of the English Language, Volumes I and II*. Boston, Massachusetts: Houghton Mifflin, 1969:1550.
- Woolf, Henry Bosley, Editor-in-Chief. *Webster's New Collegiate Dictionary*. Springfield, Massachusetts: Merriam, 1977:1536.
- Chapman, Robert L, Reviser. *Roget's International Thesaurus*. 4th ed. New York, New York: Thomas Y. Crowell, 1979:1317.

These are books on writing, words, and editing that have appealed particularly to me (W.C.R.).
* This is a reproduction of the third edition, appearing in 1923.

Oft-Repeated Requests to Authors from an Editor of a Medical Journal[31]

Before manuscripts are published in the *AJC*, nearly all have been reviewed by 2 reviewers and by me. If the manuscript looks acceptable for publication—pending revision by the author(s)—I dictate a rather lengthy letter stipulating the requirements for acceptance. Many conditional acceptance letters contain oft-repeated requests to authors, and 8 of them are the following: *(1) Limit the study to the patients whose cardiovascular disease was caused by only 1 or 2 conditions, and eliminate the small numbers of patients in whom multiple different disease states caused the heart disease. (2) Eliminate the present tables displaying pooled data and in their place provide a single table listing the pertinent data in each study patient but no more than 1 line across for any patient. (3) Decrease the length of the manuscript, particularly the discussion and introduction portions. (4) Try not to repeat data in the tables again in the text. (5) Limit the number of abbreviations to commonly recognized cardiologic phrases and preferably to those phrases in the manuscript's title. (6) Prepare the references in the style of the journal. (7) Crop the figures. (8) Read the instructions to authors, and, even more important, study a recent issue of the journal so that you clearly understand its style before submitting a revision.*

Reviewing Manuscripts: Occasionally a Test of Character[9]

One of the least appreciated tasks performed by members of the medical community is their reviewing of manuscripts submitted to them by editors of medical journals. Reviewing a manuscript can be a test of character. A manuscript sent to a reviewer often concerns a subject about which the reviewer has contributed information, or a subject he or she is currently investigating. Thus, the reviewer may be asked to evaluate work done by someone else on a subject of personal interest. In this situation, the reviewer and author might well be described as competitors. Furthermore, the reviewer is asked not only to evaluate the author's work but also to provide suggestions for improving it free of charge. Medicine and science appear to be one of the few areas in which competitors consult one another for free advice. Can you imagine Ford Motor Company asking General Motors Corporation or vice versa to provide suggestions for improving the quality of a newly designed automobile—without remuneration? Occasionally, a reviewer may be asked to evaluate the manuscript of an author for whom he has no fondness, either for professional or personal reasons, or conversely, to evaluate the manuscript of an author for whom he has an especially high personal regard. In either case, the reviewer may be less than objective and the review less than ideal.

Detecting prejudice (conscious or otherwise) in a review is a continuing challenge for editors. To help meet this challenge, I have requested that authors submitting manuscripts to the *AJC* provide in the covering letters names of potentially objective and nonobjective reviewers so that predictable or possible conflicts might be avoided.[9] In this professionally competitive and human atmosphere in which we all reside, the consistently objective reviewer deserves our appreciation and admiration.

Reviews of Classic Books and Ineptness of Reviewers: Lessons for Judges of Medical Manuscripts[26]

A manuscript submitted to the *AJC* generally receives 2 reviews. On the review form, the recommendations available to the reviewer are "definitely accept," "probably accept," "definitely reject," and "probably reject." The most frequent recommendations from 2 reviewers of the same manuscript are "probably accept" from 1 and "probably reject" from the other; next, both recommend "probably accept," and next, both recommend "probably reject." Rarely do both recommend "definitely accept" or "definitely reject." On occasion, the same manuscript receives a "definitely accept" recommendation from 1 reviewer and a "definitely reject" from the other reviewer. When this situation occurs, the reputation and experience of both reviewers are carefully weighed, and the reasons for their respective recommendations are analyzed. Unfortunately, when this situation exists, both reviewers may be major forces in the same area of specialization. Thus, when a manuscript reviewed by 2 leaders receives opposing recommendations, the reviewer recommending "definitely reject" may be upset if the manuscript is accepted, and the reviewer who recommended "definitely accept" may be upset if the manuscript is rejected. Obviously, the same manuscript cannot be both "terrible" and "excellent." Does this particular example illustrate more about the reviewers than it does about the manuscript? How can 2 experts have such opposite reactions to the same subject matter? If 2 experts disagree so sharply, how meaningful are recommendations, similar or divergent, from reviewers who are not major forces or leaders in their area of expertise?

It is clear to me that no one—including editors—has a monopoly on correct decisions when it comes to degrees of quality of our manuscripts. With these conflicting recommendations from experts in mind, I was delighted to acquire years ago the book *Rotten Reviews: A Literary Companion*, edited by Bill Henderson (Pushcart Press 1986:93). The book contains excerpts from 175 scathing notices about a number of famous books and poems published up to 1961. While researching for his book, Henderson was impressed by the balance, intelligence, and fairness of most reviews and emphasized that truly malicious reviews were rare. He found, however, striking examples of inability of reviewers to appreciate quality or the lack thereof in books they evaluated. Often, reviewers went into spasms of appreciation for books of slight value: "Martin Tupper (1810 – 1889) has won for himself the vacant throne waiting for him amidst the immortals, and has been adopted by the suffrage of mankind and the final decrees of publishers into the same rank with Wordsworth, Tennyson and Browning (The Spectator - 1866)." Even bad reviews sometimes were appreciated. When the Concord, Massachusetts, public library banned *Huckleberry Finn*, Mark Twain exulted: "That will sell 25,000 books for sure!"

Rotten Reviews is filled with examples of how great writers can be wrong about other great writers, a reason for some humility in those of us passing judgments on works of others. It was Henry James who called *Wuthering Heights* (1847) by Emily Bronte "a crude and morbid story" and said of Charles Dickens's great novel *Our Mutual Friend* that "we are convinced that it is one of the chief conditions of his genius not to see beneath the surface of things. . . . We are aware that this definition confines him to an inferior rank." It was Emile Zola who said of Charles Baudelaire's *Les Fleus du Mal* (1857), "In a hundred years the histories of the French literature will only mention (this work) as a curio." It was Gertrude Stein who called Ezra Pound "a village explainer, excellent if you were a village, but if you were not, not." It was Ralph Waldo Emerson who said of Jane Austen, "I am at a loss to understand why people hold Miss Austen's novels at so high a rate, which seem to me vulgar in tone, sterile in artistic invention, imprisoned in the wretched conventions of English society, without genius, wit, or knowledge of the world. Never was life so pinched and narrow. The one problem in the mind of the writer . . . is marriageableness. . . . Suicide is more respectable." And Edmund Wilson on W.H. Auden: "Mr. Auden himself has presented the curious case of a poet who writes an original poetic language in the most robust English tradition but who seems to have been arrested in the mentality of an adolescent schoolboy."

And virtually every reviewer had a field day with Walt Whitman and Herman Melville. On Walt Whitman's *Drum-Taps* (1865), Henry James wrote, "Mr. Whitman's attitude seems monstrous. It is monstrous because it pretends to persuade the soul while it slights the intellect; because it pretends to gratify the feelings while it outrages the taste. . . . Our hearts are often touched through a compromise with the artistic sense, but never in direct violation of it." Robert Louis Stevenson: "Whitman, like a shaggy dog, just unchained, scouring the beaches of the world and baying at the moon." Peter Bayne: "Incapable of true poetical originality, Whitman had the cleverness to invent a literary trick, and the shrewdness to stick to it." And Francis Fisher Browne: Whitman's "lack of a sense of poetic fitness, his failure to understand the business of a poet, is clearly astounding."

A few reviewers' comments on Herman Melville: "*Redburn* was a stupid failure, *Mardi* was hopelessly dull, *White Jacket* was worse than either; and, in fact was such a very bad book, that, until the appearance of *Moby Dick* we had set it down at the very ultimatum of weakness to which the author could attain. It seems, however, that we were mistaken. In bombast, in caricature, in rhetorical artifice—generally as clumsy as it is ineffectual—and in low attempts at humor, each of his volumes has been an advance upon its predecessors." Another reviewer: "The captain's ravings and those of Mr. Melville are such as would justify a *writ de lunatic* against all parties." And another: "a huge dose of hyperbolical slang, maudlin sentimentalism and tragic-comic bubble and squeak." Still another: "This sea novel is a singular medley of naval observation, magazine article writing, satiric reflection upon the conventionalisms of civilized life and rhapsody run mad." Herman Melville, who was in his early 30s when he wrote *Moby-Dick*, was so upset by the reviews of his 4 books that he went 40 years before writing his fifth and final book in his last year of life. The manuscript was found 5 months after his death in 1891. Its title was *Billy Budd*.

Criticism, of course, serves a useful function, but not all criticisms are justified. Not all changes in manuscripts to pacify critics produce improvements in manuscripts. No one has a monopoly on justifiable criticisms or on the correctness of the decision to accept or reject a manuscript. The power to pass judgment on the works of others is a power which should generate humility, not arrogance. "Writers" (investigators), notes Saul Bellow, "seldom wish other writers [investigators] well." Thus, recommendations of reviewers have complex origins, and these must be taken into consideration when evaluating the quality of a manuscript.

Reducing Flaws in the Review Process of Manuscripts Submitted to Medical Journals[34]

Before providing suggestions to reduce flaws in the review process, let me mention some advantages and disadvantages of it. Some *advantages*: Clearly, the review process improves the reporting of medical science and in this way is useful to authors, to editors, to reviewers, to readers, to themselves, and consequently to patients. Most reviewers are impartial, and most are good at detecting inconsistencies, incongruities, omissions, commissions, and inadvertent errors; inadequate descriptions or characterizations of the populations studied; improper study designs; outdated methods; poor figures and tables; inappropriate or exaggerated conclusions; and poor syntax. Correction of these deficiencies obviously improves manuscripts. Reviewing a manuscript makes the reviewer read more critically than he or she might do otherwise; it thus improves his or her own database and theoretically makes him or her a better investigator, teacher, and physician. Another infrequently mentioned advantage of the review process is that it makes authors more careful in their preparation of manuscripts, because they need to "cover their flanks," so to speak, to persuade reviewers and editors that their manuscripts are of high quality. And reviewers also provide "ammunition" for editors, making the declining of manuscripts, particularly ones from a very prominent investigators or friends, a bit easier.

Some *disadvantages*: The review process, of course, is time consuming and expensive; delays publication; is often biased; is relatively poor at detecting plagiarism, deceit, and intentional errors (fraud); and, on occasion, the suggestions provided (if carried out) do not improve the scientific quality or the readability of manuscripts. Not all reviewers are experts in the subjects of the manuscripts they are asked to review. The process can exhaust the better reviewers. And the worst manuscripts usually get the most reviews because they move from one rejection to another until they are accepted for publication by some journal.

Now to *suggestions*, directed mostly to editors, for reducing flaws in the review process:

1. *Give careful thought to who would be the best reviewers of a manuscript.* The expertise of the review is dependent on the expertise of the reviewer.
2. *Request that authors give names of potential out-of-city reviewers whom they believe will provide* **non-biased** *critical reviews of their work.* Editors have no monopoly on the correct picking of reviewers! Reviewers and recommendations by authors are usually relatively similar to those recommended by editors.
3. *Request of authors also the names of potential out-of-city reviewers whom they believe will provide* **biased** *(unfair) reviews of their work, and honor those requests.*
4. *Refrain from sending many manuscripts to hypercritical potential reviewers to whom no manuscript or work (other than their own) is quite good enough.* Likewise, reviewers with obvious conflicts of interest or those who abuse the review process (acquiring ideas or protecting their own investigations) should be avoided.
5. *Don't overwork the exceptional reviewers.* These particularly helpful reviewers tend to review for multiple journals, and their energies can be depleted by excessive reviewing. Consider saving them for the most controversial or potentially controversial manuscripts.
6. *Refrain from regularly sending manuscripts that initially receive mixed recommendations to third reviewers.* Discussion of these manuscripts with associate editors and colleagues saves additional reviews.
7. *Compose the editorial board in a meritorious fashion, including individuals proved to be conscientious and prompt reviewers,* not just prominent investigators or chiefs of prominent departments or divisions.
8. *Decline extremely poor manuscripts without outside review, thus saving the time and energy of reviewers for more worthwhile manuscripts.*
9. *Refrain from sending some types of manuscripts for review*, or at least have no requirement that all submissions be sent for outside review, for example, readers' comments (letters to the editor), debates, pros-and-cons, symposia, and case reports.
10. *Don't substitute reviewers for editors.* All manuscripts need the editor-in-chief's opinion. Authors deserve it. I edit originally submitted manuscripts before returning them to authors for their revisions.
11. *Reduce the reviewing of a previously declined manuscript by another journal by sending the previous reviews and responses to them, the manuscript originally sent to the journal that rejected it, and the revised manuscript to the new journal.* This option has been used by *AJC* since 1982, and it usually prevents the necessity of starting the review process anew.
12. *Refrain, except in unusual circumstances, from sending revised manuscripts back to 1 or more reviewers of the originally submitted manuscript for reevaluation.*
13. *Remember the golden rule of reviewing. Frequent* authors are usually *frequent* reviewers, but the 2 hats are worn at different times. When authors submit manuscripts to a journal, their patience for delay in receiving the "acceptance" or "rejection" decision often is short. When these same authors, however, become reviewers, their patience for delay often appears to be much longer. Reviewers need to treat authors as they would like to be treated when they are authors.
14. *Do the reviewing process on-line, or, if not, convert accordingly.* On-line reviewing improves efficiency; reviews are returned more quickly, authors receive decisions more quickly, and so on, than when transferring paper.
15. *Forget blind reviewing, whereby the names and institutions of the authors are not supplied to the reviewers.* This system was tried at *AJC* for 6 months, and a few reviewers resented not knowing for sure the names of the authors of the manu-

scripts they were asked to review. Giving authors, however, the option of requesting blind reviews and giving reviewers the option of signing their reviews are reasonable and improve the transparency of the process.

16. *Keep the final decision on manuscripts in the hands of the editor-in-chief.* Reviewers serve to provide suggestions to both authors and editors on means to improve the quality of manuscripts. Reviewers should not replace editors, whose charge is to decide, among other things, which manuscript to accept and which to reject and, if acceptable, in what form.
17. *Continuously update the reviewer files.* Ask periodically editorial board members, among others, for names to be added to the journal's reviewer files. Get investigators involved in the reviewing process of others early in their careers. The young are often more critical than the old, and they generally have more time to do the reviews.
18. *Emphasize to authors the importance of following the journal's instructions to authors.* Study the journal's format before submitting the manuscript! An editor's patience can be tested by not doing so. And, if a manuscript is declined by one journal, make sure that the previous reviewers' comments are responded to by altering the manuscript before sending it to the next journal. Not doing so is an insult to the review process.
19. *Befriend the publisher.* Work in parallel as much as possible. Minimize surprises on both sides. The process works more smoothly when there is a friendly relationship between editor and publisher.
20. *Peer review also follows publication by publication of readers' comments and other discussions* (such as journal clubs, medical meetings, and media).
21. *Thank reviewers for particularly outstanding reviews.* Occasionally publish their reviews alongside the manuscripts reviewed.

In summary, as many have pointed out, peer review is imperfect, being subjective, frequently biased, and not reliable at detecting many imperfections or even fraud, but nevertheless, the review process improves most manuscripts, and there is no substitute for it. Reviewing manuscripts of others is unselfish, honorable, altruistic, and poorly rewarded, but it is absolutely essential to keep the reporting of scientific investigations to high standards. All of us benefit by having others make suggestions for improving our manuscripts.

Franz J. Ingelfinger's Comment on Peer Review

The following comment was made by Dr. Ingelfinger, former editor of *The New England Journal of Medicine*, in an article published in *The American Journal of Medicine* in May 1974: "The conventional reviewing system of American biomedical journals determines where and when an author may publish, and hence may affect his career. Yet the system's effectiveness in validating reports, or the cost of such validation, has been little studied. Problems are inadequate review, unrealistic editorial expectation of what reviewers can do, and bias. Expert reviewers frequently disagree. Thus, concurrence between 2 reviewers of each of some 500 papers submitted to *The New England Journal of Medicine* was only moderately better than a chance result. Costs of the reviewing system include time and effort involved; the possible violation of confidentiality, and occasional suppression of the novel advance. . . . Despite deficiencies, the reviewing system is important to maintain standards. It could be improved if studies of its operation were carried out, if reviewers were better indoctrinated, if the workload of reviewers were lessened, if reviews were signed, and if the reviewing process were more rewarding to reviewers."

Speeding Up the Manuscript-Reviewing Process[10]

All reviewers for the *AJC* are asked to send their reviews to the editor within 3 weeks. (Some journals ask for a 2-week interval.) When this time period is met by each reviewer, authors can be notified that their manuscript is accepted or rejected within a month. Although this time sequence operates well for most manuscripts submitted to the *AJC*, some reviewers fail to return their reviews to the editor for several additional weeks. A delay by 1 reviewer in actuality translates into a delay by both reviewers.

How can a reviewer decrease the length of time between receipt of a manuscript and its return to the editor? One procedure is to *examine the manuscript briefly the day it arrives.* In this way, the subject of the manuscript can be reflected upon for several days before the review is actually prepared. If the manuscript concerns a subject of considerable interest to a colleague, the colleague can be consulted the day the manuscript arrives. Some reviewers appear to wait 3 or 4 weeks before initially examining the manuscript. If a manuscript is particularly poor, cursory examination on the day it arrives is often sufficient to advise rejection. It surely makes the editor's job easier when there is little delay in providing a negative decision to an author.

In summary, let us try to review other authors' manuscripts as promptly as we want our own manuscripts reviewed. (The golden rule of manuscript reviewing.).

Revising Manuscripts After Studying Reviewers' Comments[33]

When examining a manuscript submitted to the *AJC*, I often sense that it had earlier been sent to another journal which had declined it. This suspicion is usually prompted by observing that the submitted manuscript was not formatted according to the *AJC*'s instructions to authors (e.g., the abstract is structured rather than nonstructured, names of all authors and full inclusive pages are not provided for every reference, subheadings are retained in the methods, results and discussion sections, etc.) Occasionally, a reviewer will indicate that "I earlier reviewed this manuscript for another journal, and the authors made no attempt to alter their manuscript in response to my suggestions." Such behavior on the part of authors is an affront to the review process. A rejection by one journal is not a ticket to ignore the comments of the reviewers or to refrain from revising the man-

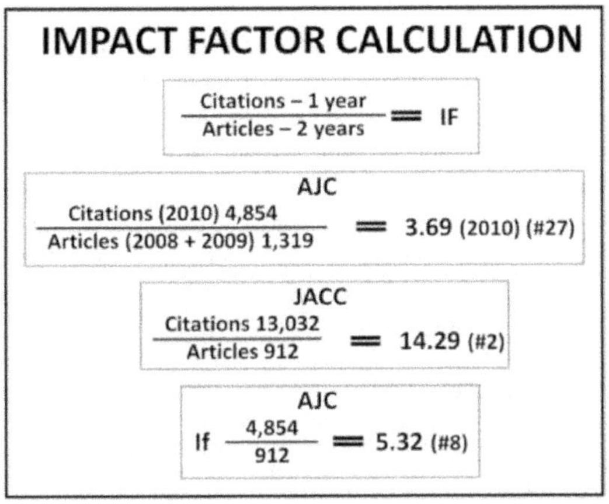

Figure 5. This illustration shows how the IF is calculated. The *AJC* had an IF in 2010 of 3.69, which was 27th on the list. If, however, the number of articles published in the *AJC* was 400 less in the 2-year period, such that they were the same number as in *JACC*, the IF would jump to 8th, namely, 5.32 or thereabouts. The diagram shows how the denominator number can alter the IF considerably.

uscript appropriately before sending it to another journal. Reviewers serve authors unselfishly, and authors must respect their objective comments by revising their manuscripts accordingly before sending their manuscripts to other journals.

I have on several occasions reacted inappropriately to reviews of *my own* manuscripts, thinking, "The reviewers didn't really understand the manuscript or appreciate its quality" or "The reviewers didn't really read the manuscript" or "Their comments were not appropriate or applicable to my manuscript." Nearly always after further reflection on the comments of reviewers, I have realized that their criticisms, although not always stated in a beautifully articulate manner, were in actuality quite useful. Many reviewers, especially our best investigators, today are burdened with too many manuscripts to review. The busier the potential reviewer, the less time he or she has to spend on a review. Most, I suspect, dictate their reviews and spend little time editing the reviews once prepared. Thus, reviews are not like manuscripts. They are not edited multiple times but are performed relatively quickly and, as a consequence, sentence structure is not always the best, and paragraphs are not always well developed. As a result, it is important for authors after receiving reviewers' comments to try to "smell out" what the reviewer is really getting at by his or her words. It's the intent of the reviewer, not his or her actual words, which is important for an author to perceive. That might take several readings of the reviews to sense what the reviewer feels is wrong or inappropriate or unsupported in another's manuscript.

In conclusion, we all need to be grateful for reviews of our manuscripts and more appreciative of those who spent time reviewing our work. We must respond to reviewers' comments by revising our manuscripts appropriately, whether they are returned to the journal where the manuscript was originally submitted or submitted to an entirely different journal for the first time.

The Impact Factor and the Eigenfactor™[35]

The Science Edition of the *Journal Citation Reports* ranks the "cardiac and cardiovascular system" journals by their impact factors (IFs). The 2010 list included the names of 114 cardiovascular journals and among several items their total citations through 2010, their latest IFs, the number of articles published in each journal in 2010, the Eigenfactor™ score, and the Article Influence™ Score.

Ninety (79%) of the 114 journals published <200 articles in 2010, and only 6 journals, >400 articles in 2010: *Annals of Thoracic Surgery*, 608; *AJC*, 604; *Circulation*, 549; *Journal of Thoracic and Cardiovascular Surgery*, 492; *American Journal of Physiology–Heart and Circulatory Physiology*, 490, and the *Journal of the American College of Cardiology* (*JACC*), 456. Only 7 (6%) of the 114 journals through 2010 had >20,000 total citations: *Circulation*, 151,020; *JACC*, 69,405; *Circulation Research*, 42,343; *AJC*, 36,401; the *American Journal of Physiology–Heart and Circulatory Physiology*, 29,457, and the *European Heart Journal* (*EHJ*), 26,311. The *American Heart Journal* started in 1926 (total citations 19,976), *Circulation* began in

Table 4
Eigenfactor.org rankings of cardiovascular journals in 2010 and comparison to the impact factor (see text for details)

Journal	Price/Eigenfactor™	IF (Rank)	Citable Articles 2010	Total Cites
1. *Circulation*	$1,137	14.43 (1)	549	151,020
2. *Journal of the American College of Cardiology*	$2,118	14.29 (2)	456	69,405
3. *American Journal of Cardiology*	$3,883	3.68 (27)	604	36,401
4. *Circulation Research*	$6,198	9.50 (4)	322	42,343
5. *American Heart Journal*	$9,734	5.05 (13)	320	19,976
6. *Journal of Thoracic and Cardiovascular Surgery*	$9,939	3.61 (28)	492	19,274
7. *American Journal of Physiology–Heart and Circulatory Physiology*	$11,836	3.88 (25)	490	29,457
8. *Journal of Heart and Lung Transplantation*	$13,804	3.42 (34)	185	6,798
9. *Cardiovascular Research*	$20,753	6.05 (9)	275	18,421
10. *European Heart Journal*	$20,753	10.05 (3)	275	4,346
Nature Reviews Cardiology		7.47 (5)	57	1,011
Progress in Cardiovascular Disease	$201,412	4.84 (14)	53	1,883
Current Problems in Cardiology	$329,376	3.44 (33)	12	413
Heart	$53,038	4.71 (18)	287	12,289
International Journal of Cardiology	$150,967	6.80 (6)	295	11,529

1952 (total citations 151,020), the *AJC* began in 1958 (total citations 36,401), the *JACC* began in 1983 (total citation 69,405), and the *EHJ* started in 1980 (total citations 26,311). Major cardiologic societies' official journals virtually always have more cites than those of independent journals.

The IF is calculated as follows: citations to "citable articles" (excludes editorials and letters to the editor [readers' comments in the *AJC*]) in a single year of articles published in the previous 2 years divided by the number of citable articles published in the same 2-year period (Figure 5). If a journal had an IF of 3 in 2010, then its articles published in 2008 and 2009 each received an average of 3 citations.

The IF in 2010 for the 114 journals was ≤2 in 57 journals (50%), >2 to 5 in 44 (39%); >5.0 to ≤10.0 in 10 (9%), and >10.0 in 3 (3%). Despite the *AJC*'s publishing the largest number of articles of any cardiology journal and being the fourth most cited cardiovascular journal, the *AJC* ranked only 27th among the IF category (Table 4). The *AJC* published 623 articles in 2008 and 623 in 2009. The *AJC*'s IF for 2010 was derived by dividing the number of cites from these 2 previous years (total 4,854) by the number of articles published in the 2 previous years (total 1,319), the result being 3.68. Of the 26 journals with higher IFs than the *AJC* in 2010, none published as many articles as did the *AJC*, and only 3 had more citations. Indeed, of the 26 journals with higher IFs, 11 (42%) published <100 articles in 2010, 9 (35%) published 101 to 300, and only 4 (15%) published >300 articles (*Circulation*, 549; the *American Journal of Physiology–Heart and Circulatory Physiology*, 490; *JACC*, 456; and *Circulation Research*, 322).

Methods to improve a journal's IF: First, *publish many guidelines*, surely the most frequently referenced articles. Essentially, only official journals of major cardiovascular societies publish guidelines! Thus, *Circulation* (the official journal of the American Heart Association), *JACC* (the official journal of the American College of Cardiology Foundation), and the *EHJ* (the official journal of the European Society of Cardiology) are the journals publishing guidelines, and these 3 have the highest IFs of all cardiovascular journals. Generally, guidelines are published simultaneously in both *Circulation* and *JACC*, thus benefiting both journals from the citations.

Second, *publish many reviews*, another frequently referenced type article. *Nature Reviews Cardiology* published only 57 articles in 2010, had only 440 cites the 2 previous years, and its 2010 IF was 7.47; *Progress in Cardiovascular Disease* published only 53 articles in 2010, had 1,883 cites with a resulting IF of 4.84; and *Current Problems in Cardiology* published only 12 articles in 2010 and had 413 cites, yielding an IF of 3.44, not much different from the IF of the *AJC* (3.68), which published 50 times as many articles. The *AJC* also publishes few reviews.

Third, *publish relatively few articles* each year. The larger the number of articles published, the larger the denominator, which lessens the IF (Figure 5). The *EHJ*, the journal with the third highest IF, published 275 articles in 2010, 329 (55%) fewer than in the *AJC*. *Heart* published 287 articles in 2010, 317 fewer than in the *AJC* the same year, and its IF (4.71) was ranked 22% higher than that of the *AJC*. And the most overt example of all, *Current Problems in Cardiology*, published only 12 articles in 2010, 50 times fewer than the *AJC*, and its IF was similar to that of the *AJC*.

Fourth, *publish large numbers of references*. The larger the number of references published, the greater the likelihood that one's own journal will be referenced. (The *AJC* generally limits the number of references in articles to ≤30.).

Fifth, *require authors to reference generously the journal to which their manuscript is submitted*. I recently received a cover letter where the author indicated that most of the references in his manuscript were to articles previously published in the *AJC*. I presume that his mentioning that fact was to increase the possibility of acceptance of his manuscript. (I do not check which journals are referenced in manuscripts submitted to the *AJC*.) I understand, however, that some editors do encourage authors to reference generously the journals they edit.

Sixth, *have a large readership audience*. There are far more cardiologists than cardiac surgeons. The latter groups' journals have relatively small circulations compared to the cardiology journals, which, in general, have much larger potential audiences. The society-owned *Journal of Thoracic and Cardiovascular Surgery* and the *Annals of Thoracic Surgery* had IFs in 2010 of 3.61 and 3.56, respectively; they published 492 and 608 articles, respectively, and had 19,274 and 27,678 total citations, respectively. The 3 large society-owned cardiology journals (*Circulation*, *JACC*, and *EHJ*) each published fewer articles in 2010 than did either of the 2 aforementioned cardiovascular surgical journals and had far more total cites (151,020, 69,405, and 26,311) and the highest IFs (14.43, 14.29, and 10.05). Some of the general medical journals (*New England Journal of Medicine*, *The Lancet*, and *JAMA*) have huge audiences and huge IFs (53, 34, and 33, respectively).

The Eigenfactor™ score and Article Influence™ Score rank journals much as Google ranks Web sites. The Eigenfactor™ algorithms use the structure of the entire network, not just citation information, to evaluate the importance of each journal. Eigenfactor.org reports both journal prices and citation influence. Although the Eigenfactor™ score and Article Influence™ Score, both free and searchable, do not incorporate price information directly, the Cost-Effectiveness Search ranks journals by a measure of the value per dollar that they provide (Table 4).

In summary, the IF obviously has value, but its importance, in my view, is not great enough to alter the operation of any scientific journal. The IF can be spuriously manipulated, and doing so diminishes considerably its value and also that of its manipulators. The IF in a way is like unadjusted versus adjusted data. A factor such as the number of original articles published yearly in a journal is underrated, whereas reviews are overrated. Whether or not a journal publishes guidelines is not included in the analysis. The potential size of the readership for a journal seems underrated in some instances and overrated in others. And whether a journal is an official organ of a major society or not is a nonfactor for calculating the IF, while at the same time, it is probably the most important variable of all. Metrics, putting a number on things, is a tough and complicated business. The IF is a major attempt to measure quality of scientific journals by a single number, and that is a useful endeavor.

I have become intrigued by the Eigenfactor™. It ranks cardiovascular journals in a much more logical fashion, in my view, than does the IF. It provides a 5-year analysis of articles published and citations rather than a 2-year evaluation, and it does not include self-citations in its analyses. Although the method of calculating the Eigenfactor™ has been well described and available to all, one needs to be a mathematician to understand it, and I am not that. Nevertheless, I suspect that the Eigenfactor™ will be a major metric in the future for evaluating the quality of scientific journals.

Alkaline Paper and Preserving the Record[32]

The paper used for articles published in many of our major medical journals including *The New England Journal of Medicine, JAMA, Circulation, The American Heart Journal,* and the *AJC*, is acidic, and therefore, these pages will crumble and blow away as dust within about 50 years. In contrast, if these journals had been published on acid-free (alkaline) paper, the articles would be preserved for 500 years, maybe longer, depending on how they were stored. So why do these journals, which record our scientific record, use the nonpermanent paper?

Nearly 80 million books in North American research libraries and an estimated 1,000 million books in libraries worldwide are threatened with destruction because they were printed on acidic paper. In most university libraries in the United States, about 30% of the volumes are brittle such that just 1 reading or 1 xerographic or 1 microfilming of the pages causes them to shatter irreparably. At the New York Public Library, over 35 of 88 miles of bookshelves contain over 2.5 million dying books. An estimated 25% of the 24 million books in the Library of Congress are not circulated because the pages crack when folded, and every year, 77,000 more books in the collection become equally brittle. The collection of the National Library of Medicine contains about 5 million items—books, journals, technical reports, manuscripts, microfilms, and pictorial materials—and about 12% of the print volumes are brittle. It is estimated that 92% of the post-1800 holdings of the library were printed on acidic paper. Seventy percent of books and journals printed in the 20th century are not usable.

The oldest material in libraries and archives are not the most endangered ones, because acid was not introduced into the papermaking process until about 1850. With the coming of the industrial revolution and the increase in literacy in the mid-19th century, the demand for paper skyrocketed. The result was that the hand-processed rag stock was largely abandoned in favor of wood pulp churned out by newly perfected machines. The wood pulp was of 2 types. *Mechanical* wood pulp is that produced by grinding up logs or shredding and grinding wood chips, and it contains lignin, which is the primary noncellulosic component in trees, and it causes paper to darken upon exposure to light and to degrade relatively quickly by oxidation and hydrolysis. (Newsprint has a high lignin content.) Because mechanical wood pulp contains lignin and other impurities, paper containing it has a relatively short lifespan. *Chemical* wood pulp is pulp produced by cooking wood chips in chemicals (to remove impurities). Depending on what chemicals are added in subsequent processing, the resulting paper can be either acidic or alkaline. Unfortunately, until recent years, the most common chemical added was aluminum sulfate, an acid salt. In the late 1930s, it was discovered that it was the acid, primarily sulfuric acid derived from the aluminum sulfate or alum, in the paper that caused it to be unstable and to degenerate. By 1910, however, it was also learned that papers containing alkaline fillers, calcium carbonate for example, were quite stable and therefore permanent.

Preservation of the present print heritage is the major problem facing most libraries today. The National Library of Medicine now invests the equivalent of 1/3 of its acquisition budget to "clean up" the backlog of embrittled material. Microfilming of the brittle books is about the only currently available recourse, but this process does not save the book. Currently, the National Library of Medicine is microfilming about 25,000 volumes a year as part of its preservation program. Another preservation technique, which also treats 1 book at a time, consists of placing the book in a water-based solution, but this technique requires removal of the book's binding and is even more expensive than microfilming. In yet another process, which takes hours, each page is sprayed by hand with a base that neutralizes the acid. Electronic document storage and retrieval using digital optical discs as the storage medium is being developed, but thus far this method of preserving the record is not ideal. Most discs have a lifetime of about 10 years, shorter than that of acid paper!

The prevention of future paper embrittlement is actually easy. The answer is simply to use acid-free (alkaline) paper for all future publications. Progress is being made rapidly toward that goal. In January 1987, the first meeting took place of the National Library of Medicine's Permanent Paper Task Force, consisting of 34 members representing publishers, paper manufacturers, printers, editors, writers, and librarians. (I was pleased to be the only physician on that task force.) In January 1987, only 4% of the 3,050 titles of *Index Medicus* were published on acid-free paper. By October 1991, nearly 50% of the titles of *Index Medicus* were known to be published on acid-free paper! It is estimated that slightly over 50% of the paper produced for United States print is now alkaline paper. Alkaline paper is smoother and stronger than acidic paper, and the type printed on it is usually sharper and easier to read than type on acidic paper. Acid-free paper also is price comparable in quality weights and grades to acidic paper.

In March 1989, nearly 100 distinguished authors and major publishing figures gathered at the New York Public Library to pledge their commitment to the preservation of the printed word. They signed a landmark declaration of book preservation calling for the use of acid-free paper for all first printings of quality hardcover trade books. A major impetus toward conversion to acid-free paper has come from the federal government of the United States. In October 1990, the 101st Congress passed Public Law 101–423, which requires "the use of acid free permanent papers for publications of enduring value produced by the Government Printing Office or produced by Federal grant or contract." This law has had a rapid impact on paper producers in North America because of the enormity of the United States governmental printer. Subsequently, most states in the United States have passed similar laws or resolutions in their statehouses.

There is a view that publishing in the foreseeable future will be by electronic means rather than by print means, and therefore, it will not be necessary to preserve our previous print record or to prevent the deterioration of our future print publications. Although electronics someday may be dominant, most experts still believe that paper publishing will remain the dominant type for years to come.

In summary, the most productive period of human beings on planet earth has been the past 160 years (since 1850), and most publications during that period have been on acid paper, and therefore they have vanished or soon will vanish into dust. The next 160 years surely will be an even more productive period for humankind, and that record of accomplishment must be prevented from slowly burning into ashes. It is easy to prevent such an outcome. Simply printing our records on alkaline paper will allow our writings to remain permanently for future generations. A good quantity of toilet paper and paper towels now consist of acid-free paper. Surely if some of our toilet paper can be alkaline, most of our medical publications, including all our peer-reviewed journals, can use a paper of at least similar quality.

Author, Editor, Advertiser, Publisher, and Printer[13]

Occasionally I hear a physician complain about the number of advertising pages in medical journals. The number of medical journals, however, would be few and very expensive were it not for the ads. If there were no advertisements, a year's subscription to the *AJC* instantly would be approximately twice its present cost and later, as the number of subscribers diminished because of the journal's high price, even more. Although few physicians pick up a medical journal to read ads, there would be few journals to pick up were ads not present. Thus, physicians must appreciate the enormous contribution of advertisers to their education.

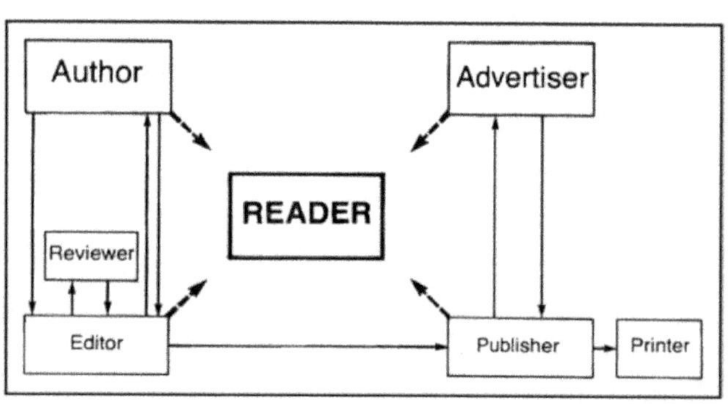

Figure 6. This illustration shows how author, editor, advertiser, and publisher are all working to produce something that is useful for the reader. Reproduced with permission from the author (Dr. Roberts) and the publisher (Elsevier) from *Am J Cardiol*.[14]

All elements of a medical journal focus on providing the reader the best available information in the most presentable form (Figure 6). The 2 key elements in publishing medical articles are the authors (investigators) and advertisers. Among his many responsibilities, the publisher acquires the ads; the more ads acquired, the more editorial pages are provided. The publisher provides the editor with editorial pages based on several factors, a major one being the projected number of ads to be acquired over a specified period. Without the advertisements, the number of editorial pages would diminish enormously, and the patient would be the ultimate loser.

Writing Versus Editing[21]

For many years, my professional fate was determined by what I wrote and had published in medical journals. One of the hardest lessons for me to learn during that long period was that the creating, "packaging," and publishing of new ideas really never got easier. Although the focusing and writing got easier, standards continued to improve, and therefore, the amount of time and energy—both physical and mental—expended continued to be about the same for each major published investigation. This period of trying to go to work every day with a new idea was obviously challenging, but enormously rewarding and fulfilling. To have a position that stretches one's potential to the fullest and to be paid for it is certainly one of life's greatest blessings.

After a lengthy (25-year) production period, the editorship of a major cardiovascular journal was offered. Again, a mentally and physically "stretching" position, but, unlike writing, one that involves not creating new ideas, but determining which ones of those created, and, to some extent, in what form, reach the cardiovascular community. Editing, however, is quite different from writing. Writing is relatively lonely and selfish. One's time must be enormously protected to create new ideas and publish them. Editing, in contrast, is relatively social and unselfish in that it requires much communication with authors, publishers, and readers. But after many years in the other role, the change to editorship was surprisingly easy to make. Of the 2, however, editing is much easier than writing, judging is much easier than creating; it is the creator who will provide the significant change, and deservedly so, not the judge of the creator's work.

1. Roberts WC, Roberts CS. William Clifford Roberts, MD: an interview by Charles Stewart Roberts, MD. *Am J Cardiol* 2007;100:338–390.
2. Roberts WC. *Facts and Ideas from Anywhere*. Armonk, New York: Futura, 2000:172.
3. Roberts WC. *Facts and Ideas from Anywhere 2000–2005*. Dallas, Texas: Baylor Health Care System, 2006:180
4. Roberts WC. *Facts and Ideas from Anywhere 2006–2010*. Dallas, Texas: Baylor Health Care System, 2011:212
5. Roberts WC. A few words from the journal's second editor. *Am J Cardiol* 1982;50:A3.
6. Roberts WC. Blind reviews. *Am J Cardiol* 1982;50:A5.
7. Roberts WC. Brief reports. *Am J Cardiol* 1982;50:A3.
8. Roberts WC. The editorial board. *Am J Cardiol* 1982;50:A3.
9. Roberts WC. Reviewing manuscripts: occasionally a test of character. *Am J Cardiol* 1982;50:A3.

10. Roberts WC. Speeding up the manuscript review process. *Am J Cardiol* 1982;50:A3.
11. Roberts WC. Getting the manuscript accepted: think like a lawyer and cover the flanks. *Am J Cardiol* 1983;51:A3.
12. Roberts WC. Paper accepted/abstract rejected or vice versa: differences in the grading of abstracts and the reviewing of manuscripts. *Am J Cardiol* 1983;51:A3.
13. Roberts WC. Author-editor-reviewer: how the triumvirate is working at the *AJC*. *Am J Cardiol* 1983;51:A9–A10.
14. Roberts WC. Author-advertiser: their dependency on one another. *Am J Cardiol* 1983;51:A3.
15. Roberts WC. Abbreviations in the *AJC*. *Am J Cardiol* 1983;51:A9–A10.
16. Roberts WC. References: a clue to scholarship. *Am J Cardiol* 1983; 51:A9–A10.
17. Roberts WC. Changes in the *AJC* since June 1982. *Am J Cardiol* 1983;51:A9–A10.
18. Roberts WC. The summary: the manuscript's bottom line. *Am J Cardiol* 1983;52:A3.
19. Roberts WC. Studying the "instructions to authors" before final typing of a manuscript for submission to a medical journal. *Am J Cardiol* 1984;52:398.
20. Roberts WC. Editorial board changes. *Am J Cardiol* 1984;54:704.
21. Roberts WC. Writing versus editing. *Am J Cardiol* 1984;54:934.
22. Roberts WC. A suggestion to lighten the load of manuscript reviewing. *Am J Cardiol* 1985;55:247.
23. Roberts WC. Brief reports in the AJC in 1984. *Am J Cardiol* 1985; 55:870.
24. Roberts WC. The "hot eye" and the "cold eye." *Am J Cardiol* 1985; 55:1663.
25. Roberts WC. The article's title. *Am J Cardiol* 1985;56:210–212.
26. Roberts WC. Reviews of classic books and ineptness of reviewers: lessons for judges of medical manuscripts. *Am J Cardiol* 1987;59:922–923.
27. Roberts WC. The search for the masterful figure. *Am J Cardiol* 1987; 60:633–634.
28. Roberts WC. Publishing manuscripts faster than abstracts. *Am J Cardiol* 1987;60:1133.
29. Roberts WC. Making clinical studies involving many patients useful to the single patient. *Am J Cardiol* 1990;65:1408.
30. Roberts WC. Comparison of the four major USA cardiology journals in 1990: a look at 51 kilograms (112 pounds) of journals and over 15,000 editorial pages. *Am J Cardiol* 1991;67:551–554.
31. Roberts WC. Oft-repeated requests to authors from an editor of a cardiology journal. *Am J Cardiol* 1991;68:1121–1122.
32. Roberts WC. Alkaline paper and preserving the record. *Am J Cardiol* 1991;68:1729–1732.
33. Roberts WC. Revising manuscripts after studying reviewers' comments. *Am J Cardiol* 2006;98:989.
34. Roberts WC. Reducing flaws in the review process of manuscripts submitted to medical journals for publication. *Am J Cardiol* 2009;103: 891–892.
35. Roberts WC. Piercing the impact factor and promoting the Eigenfactor. *Am J Cardiol* 2011;108:896–898.
36. Roberts WC. Some realities of present-day cardiologic journal publishing in the USA. *Cardiology* 1987;74:254–262.
37. Strunk W Jr. The Elements of Style with Revisions, an Introduction, and a New Chapter on Writing by E. B. White. New York, New York: Macmillan; 1959:71.

Acute Aortic Dissection With Tear in Ascending Aorta Not Diagnosed Until Necropsy or Operation (for Another Condition) and Comparison to Similar Cases Receiving Proper Operative Therapy

William Clifford Roberts, MD[a,b,c,*], Travis James Vowels, BBA[c,d], Jong Mi Ko, BA[c] and Joseph Manuel Guileyardo, MD[b]

Acute aortic dissection (AD) with a tear in ascending aorta (AA) is recognized to masquerade occasionally as another condition, and therefore the proper diagnosis is never made or made too late. During a recent 3-year period (2009 to 2011) at Baylor University Medical Center at Dallas, 30 patients with acute AD with tear in AA were diagnosed: 23 (77%) were diagnosed clinically and underwent proper urgent operative therapy; the remaining 7 (23%) with AD with tear in AA were not diagnosed until operation (for another condition) or necropsy or retrospectively by review of antemortem computed tomographic scan after death. The number of patients with AD from tear in AA whose cardiac condition was not diagnosed clinically and who died in the hospital but did not have an autopsy is unclear. Because the autopsy rate in most United States hospitals, including Baylor University Medical Center, is now <5%, many cases of AD are probably not diagnosed and thus its frequency is being underestimated. In conclusion, ≥7 of 30 patients (23%) with acute AD with a tear in AA were not diagnosed until necropsy or operation (for another condition) or retrospectively by computed tomography during a 3-year period at a large tertiary medical center showing that this condition continues to be underdiagnosed, and when not diagnosed correctly is usually rapidly fatal. Because the autopsy rate today is so low, the percentage not diagnosed clinically is probably >23%. **(Am J Cardiol 2012;110:728–735)**

It is well known that acute aortic dissection (AD) can masquerade as another condition or that the correct diagnosis can be delayed.[1–8] In a recent 36-month period at Baylor University Medical Center (BUMC) at Dallas, 30 patients with acute AD with tear in ascending aorta (AA) were diagnosed: 23 of them went immediately to the operating room where proper operative therapy was carried out; 4 others underwent operative therapy for another condition (coronary bypass in 3 and closure of atrial septal defect in 1) and the presence of AD with tear in the AA was not recognized until operation or necropsy; and 3 others died suddenly in the hospital (hemopericardium) without operation and the AD was a surprise finding at autopsy. A review of those 30 cases is the purpose of this report to call attention again to the frequency of underdiagnosis of this condition.

Methods

The surgical pathology files of BUMC were searched for patients having resection of the AA for acute AD with a tear in the AA over a 3-year period (2009 to 2011), and the necropsy files of BUMC were searched during the same 3-year period for patients having fatal AD with a tear in AA. The aortas in all patients having operative resection for AD with a tear in AA were examined initially by W.C.R. who provided the report (10 of the 23 operative cases during this 3-year period were included in a study of 69 patients with AD studied during a 16-year period[9]). The hearts and aortas in the patients initially found to have AD with a tear in AA at autopsy were studied initially by J.M.G. and W.C.R. The photographs of the heart and aorta were taken by J.M.K.

The clinical records including admission history and physical, discharge summary, echocardiographic reports, cardiac catheterization reports, computed tomographic (CT) and coronary angiographic studies, operative records, and autopsy records were sought from the patients' medical charts at BUMC.

Results

Three groups of patients were analyzed. The largest group consisted of 23 patients who were diagnosed clinically as having AD with tear in AA and they rapidly underwent proper operative replacement of the AA (Table 1).

The second largest group consisted of 4 patients (numbers 1 to 4) in whom the diagnosis of AD with tear in AA was not suspected clinically but all 4 underwent a cardiac operation for another condition (coronary artery bypass grafting in 3 and closure of a secundum atrial septal defect

Departments of [a]Internal Medicine (Division of Cardiology), [b]Pathology, and the [c]Baylor Heart and Vascular Institute, Baylor University Medical Center, Dallas, Texas; [d]First Year Medical Student, The University of Texas Medical School at Houston, Houston, Texas. Manuscript received March 5, 2012; revised manuscript received and accepted April 17, 2012.

*Corresponding author: Tel: 214-820-7911; fax: 214-820-7533.

E-mail address: wc.roberts@baylorhealth.edu (W.C. Roberts).

Table 1

Clinical findings in 23 patients having operative therapy for acute aortic dissection with tear in ascending aorta over a three-year period (2009 to 2011) at Baylor University Medical Center

Patient Number	1	2	3	4	5	6	7	8	9	10	11	12	13*	14	15	16	17	18†	19	20	21	22	23
Age (years)	34	35	38	42	45	47	52	52	53	55	59	64	68	70	70	72	72	73	74	74	74	75	82
Gender	M	F	M	M	F	F	M	F	M	M	M	M	F	M	M	M	M	M	M	F	F	F	M
On admission																							
Chest pain	+	+	+	+	+	+	+	+	+	+	+	+	+	+	+	+	0	0	+	+	0	0	+
Back pain	0	+	+	0	+	+	0	0	0	0	+	0	0	0	0	0	+	0	0	0	0	+	0
Neck pain	0	0	+	0	0	+	+	0	0	0	0	+	0	0	0	0	0	+	0	0	0	0	0
Extremity																							
Weakness	0	0	0	0	0	0	0	0	0	0	0	0	+ (L)	0	0	0	0	0	0	0	+ (L)	0	+ (L)
Numbness	0	0	+ (A, L)	+ (L)	0	0	0	0	0	0	0	0	0	+ (A)	0	+ (L)	+ (A, L)	0	0	0	0	+ (L)	0
Hypertension‡	+	+	+	+	+	+	+	+	+	+	+	+	+	+	+	+	+	+	+	+	+	+	+
Highest BP (mm Hg)																							
Systolic	200	170	130	130	135	210	80	110	205	110	110	130	175	185	105	200	120	125	95	135	150	135	115
Diastolic	110	80	50	65	65	100	50	80	100	60	55	70	80	105	55	60	55	55	55	85	60	60	70
Troponin (ng/ml)	<0.03	0.06	—	0.06	—	<0.02	<0.02	—	0.09	<0.03	—	<0.05	0.16	<0.02	2.19	0.09	<0.02	<0.02	0.04	<0.02	<0.02	<0.02	—
Precordial murmur	0	0	0	0	+ (1/6)	0	0	0	0	0	0	0	0	0	0	+ (3/6)	+	0	0	0	0	+ (3/6)	—
BMI (kg/m^2)	30.0	27.4	24.7	24.8	21.5	44.0	26.6	22.0	29.1	24.4	41.4	23.6	23.4	23.5	28.2	34.9	27.1	37.8	31.1	44.7	26.6	21.0	31.2
Computed tomography	+	+	+	+	+	+	+	+	+	+	+	+	+	+	0	+	+	+	+	+	+	+	+
Echocardiogram	0	0	0	0	+	0	0	0	+	0	0	0	0	+	+	0	0	0	+	0	0	0	0
Chest radiograph	+	+	0	+	+	+	+	0	+	+	0	0	0	+	+	0	+	0	+	+	+	0	0
Interval (hours)																							
Symptom onset to admission	1	1	—	1	13	3	1	1	340	1	1	1	2	340	1	1	3	1	1	1	1	1	—
Admission to operation	3	6	5	7	5	16	3	5	15	6	8	7	5	42	15	2	3	6	17	13	3	10	—
Hemopericardium	0	+	0	0	0	0	+	+	0	0	0	+	0	0	+	0	+	0	+	0	0	0	+
AMEFL (0–4+)	1	0	3	0	0	0	4	0	0	0	0	1	0	0	0	0	0	2	0	0	1	1	3
Portion of aorta dissected																							
Ascending	+	+	+	+	+	+	+	+	+	+	+	+	+	+	+	+	+	+	+	+	+	+	+
Arch	+	+	+	+	+	+	+	+	+	+	+	+	0	+	+	+	+	+	+	0	+	+	0
Descending	+	0	+	+	+	+	+	+	+	+	+	0	0	0	+	+	+	+	+	0	+	+	0
Abdominal	+	0	+	+	+	+	+	+	+	+	+	0	0	0	0	+	+	0	0	0	+	0	0

— = no information available or not applicable; + = positive or present; 0 = negative or absent; A = arm; AMEFL = Aortic medial elastic fiber loss; BMI = body mass index; BP = blood pressure; F = female; L = leg; M = male.

* Patient had coronary artery bypass grafting (×3) 7 days before presentation.

† Patient had abdominal aortic aneurysm resection 5 years before presentation.

‡ By history or antihypertensive treatment.

Table 2
Clinical and morphologic findings in 7 patients seen over a three-year period (2009 to 2011) at Baylor University Medical Center with acute aortic dissection with tear in ascending aorta not diagnosed until necropsy or at operation for another condition

Patient Number	1*	2*	3*§	4†	5‡	6‡	7‡
Age (years)	57	74	82	52	54	75	76
Gender	man	woman	woman	woman	man	woman	woman
On admission							
Chest pain	+	+	0	+	+	+	0
Back pain	0	0	0	0	0	+	0
Neck pain	0	0	0	0	0	+	0
Extremity							
Weakness	0	+ (legs)	0	0	+	0	0
Numbness	+ (arm)	0	0	0	0	+ (legs)	0
Systemic hypertension$^{\mu}$	+	+	+	+	+	+	+
Highest blood pressure (mm Hg)	130/85	120/70	190/85	150/90	135/60	130/50	255/110
Troponin (ng/ml)	0.07	<0.03	0.10	—	<0.02	0.20	<0.02
Precordial murmur	0	0	0	+	0	+	0
Body mass index (kg/m^2)	23.7	37.0	17.9	17.4	36.7	23.3	16.1
Bruce stress test	+	0	0	0	+	0	0
Computed tomogram	0	0	0	0	0	+	+
Echocardiogram	0	0	0	+	0	0	0
Chest radiograph	+	+	0	0	+	+	+
Coronary angiogram	+	+	+	0	0	0	0
Interval							
Symptom onset to admission (hours)	12	1	1	—	1	1	72
Admission to operation	1 day	2 days	2 hours	1 day	—	—	—
Operation to death (days)	12	12	alive	10	—	—	—
Admission to death	13 days	14 days	alive	11 days	66 hours	10 hours	37 hours
Heart weight (g)	415	580	—	340	595	380	310
Left ventricular wall							
Necrosis	+	0	—	+	0	0	0
Fibrosis	0	0	—	0	0	0	0
Left ventricular cavity dilated	0	0	—	+	+	0	0
Hemopericardium (ml)	+ (300)	0	0	0	+ (750)	+ (600)	+ (600)
Aortic medial elastic fiber loss (0–4+)	0	—	2	4	0	0	1
Portion of aorta dissected							
Ascending	+	+	+	+	+	+	+
Arch	+	+	0	+	+	+	+
Descending thoracic	+	+	0	+	+	+	+
Abdominal	—¶	+	0	—¶	—¶	+	—¶
Illustrated in figure(s)	1 and 2	3	—	4	5	6	7

Abbreviations as in Table 1.
* Aortic dissection not diagnosed preoperatively and cardiac operation performed for coronary artery bypass grafting.
† Aortic dissection not diagnosed preoperatively and cardiac operation performed for closure of atrial septal defect.
‡ Aortic dissection not diagnosed before death from hemopericardium.
§ Patient presented with severe dyspnea and cardiac catheterization showed multivessel coronary disease, moderate aortic insufficiency, and a dilated ascending aorta. She subsequently underwent elective coronary bypass operation during which her ascending aortic dissection was discovered.
$^{\mu}$ By history or antihypertensive treatment.
¶ Necropsy limited to chest only.

[ASD] in 1) and AD was diagnosed at operation in 2 (patients 2 and 3) and at necropsy in the other 2 (patients 1 and 4; Table 2). Review of the clinical and morphologic features of the latter 2 cases strongly suggested that the AD was indeed present before operation but masqueraded as a coronary event or ASD, respectively. The patient with the ASD presented initially with acute dyspnea, echocardiogram disclosed the ASD, and her symptoms were attributed to the ASD rather than the AD. The initial operative incision was a right thoracotomy. The AA was noted to be quite large after median sternotomy. Details of cases 1, 2, and 4 are presented in the legends to Figures 1 to 4. Details of case 3 are presented in the footnotes of Table 2.

The smallest group consisted of 3 patients (numbers 5 to 7 [Table 2]) who died 66, 10, and 37 hours, respectively, after admission to the hospital. Antemortem CT scans, done in 2 of the 3 patients, on retrospective examination (after the autopsy) did show features typical of AD with tear in AA. Details of these 3 cases (numbers 5 to 7) are presented in the legends to Figures 5 to 7.

Discussion

This article describes findings in 30 patients with AD with tear in AA diagnosed at a single tertiary hospital in a 3-year period (2009 to 2011). The diagnosis was established

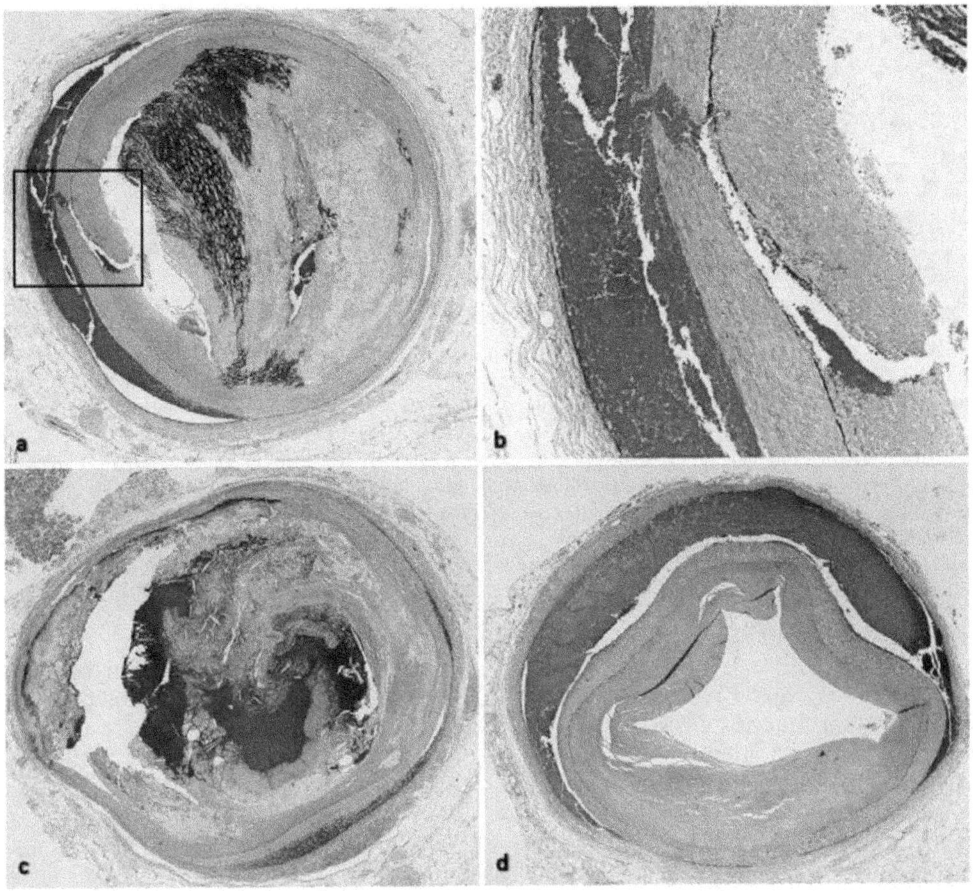

Figure 1. (Patient number 1.) Photomicrographs of right coronary artery in a 57-year-old man who was hospitalized because of substernal chest pain and left arm numbness. A stress test was positive and coronary angiography disclosed insignificant narrowing of the left main, left anterior descending, and left circumflex coronary arteries but severe (99%) narrowing of the right coronary artery. Angioplasty resulted in a coronary dissection and coronary bypass was performed with insertion of a saphenous venous conduit from the aorta to distal right coronary artery. Bleeding occurred postoperatively and re-exploration was performed. He was discharged 6 days postoperatively but 6 days thereafter while at home he suddenly died. Hemopericardium was found at autopsy. *(a, b)* Photomicrographs of right coronary artery at the site of the angioplasty. The crack extends through the intimal plaque and into the outer media. *(c)* Another area where plaque has been cracked with thrombus formation and hemorrhage into the plaque. *(d)* Further downstream showing a large false channel in the outer media. Movat stains: ×20 *(a, c, and d)*; ×100 *(b)*.

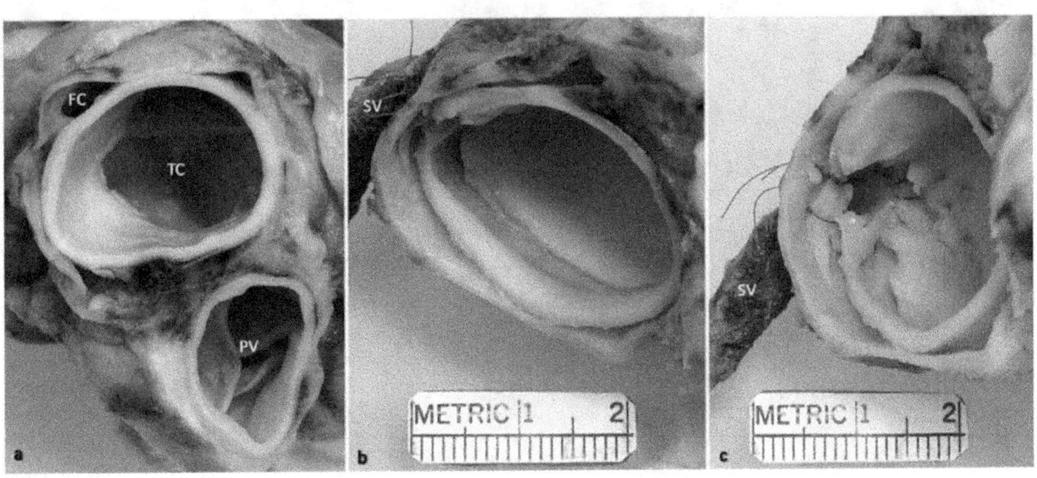

Figure 2. (Patient number 1.) Aorta. *(a)* View from above showing the true channel (TC) and false channel (FC) in the aorta. *(b)* View of aorta at the site of the large intimal–medial tear which is at the site of the insertion of the saphenous venous conduit (SV). *(c)* Another view at the site of the tear. It appears that some of the sutures used for the anastomosis are sewn directly into the outer partition of the false channel. PV = pulmonic valve.

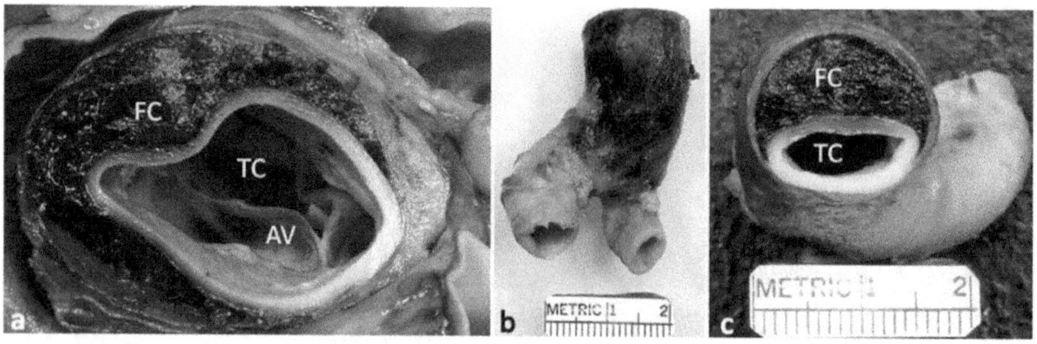

Figure 3. (Patient number 2.) Photographs of ascending aorta *(a)* and abdominal aorta *(b, c)* in a 74-year-old woman who developed severe substernal chest pain while in her physician's office. The pain was considered anginal in type and urgent coronary angiography was performed and it showed virtual total occlusion of the right coronary artery. Immediate median sternotomy was performed for coronary bypass and visualization of the ascending aorta disclosed the presence of acute aortic dissection. Thus, coronary bypass and resection of ascending aorta were performed 12 days before death. The postoperative period was characterized by excessive bleeding prompting return to the operating room, progressive hypotension, and multiorgan "failure." The reason the patient visited the physician in the first place was increasing claudication which was attributed to a previous aortic dissection with tear in descending thoracic aorta. Necropsy however showed a tear in the operatively excised ascending aorta. Thrombus in the false channel was similar in ascending aorta, thoracic aorta, and abdominal aorta. The thrombus in the false channel of the abdominal aorta compressed the true channel in this portion of aorta probably accounting for the claudication. No healed dissection was found. *(a)* Photograph of thrombus in the false channel in ascending aorta. *(b)* Exterior of the distal aorta and proximal portion of the 2 common iliac arteries. *(c)* Cross section of abdominal aorta. AV = aortic valve. Other abbreviations as in Figure 2.

clinically in 23 patients and they underwent urgent and proper operative therapy. In the other 7 patients, AD with tear in AA was never diagnosed clinically: 3 had narrowing of ≥1 major epicardial coronary artery and went for planned coronary bypass; the remaining patient went for closure of an ASD and the AA was noted to be quite dilated. Diagnosis of AD was not made until necropsy in 2 patients and at operation in the other 2. The remaining 3 patients never had AD diagnosed clinically and died suddenly in the hospital of ruptured aorta with hemopericardium. Retrospective examination of the antemortem CT study, however, disclosed features characteristic of AD in 2 of these 3 patients. Thus, 7 of 30 patients (23%) with AD with tear in AA were not diagnosed clinically and 5 of these 7 did not receive proper operative therapy.

According to Bonser and colleagues,[8] missing the diagnosis of AD with tear in AA usually (90%) results in death within 30 days and delay of diagnosis leads to an

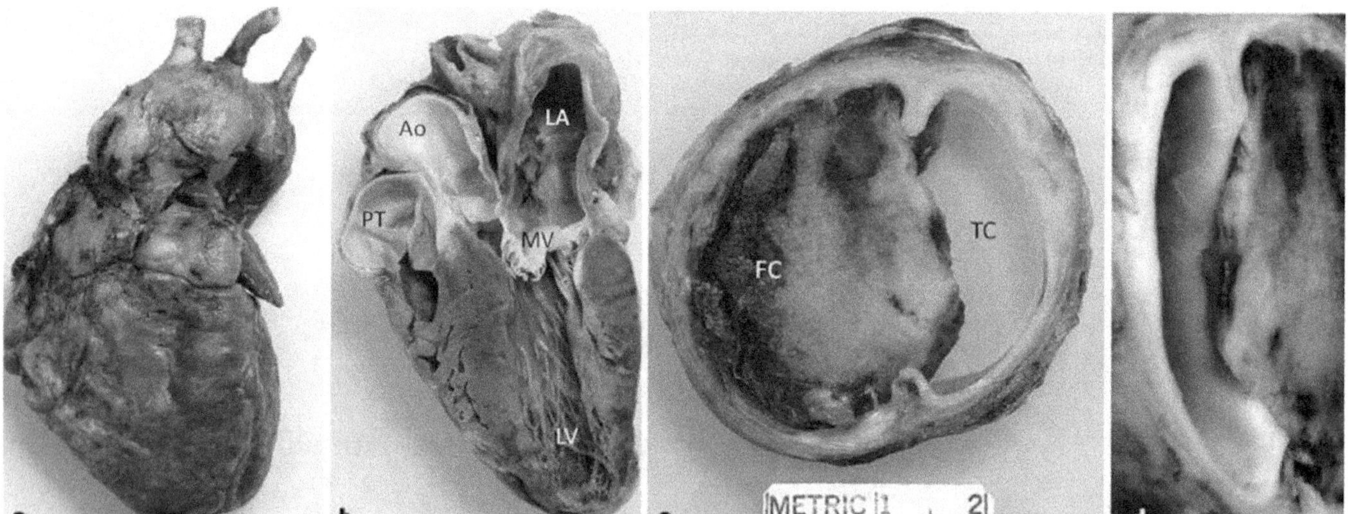

Figure 4. (Patient number 4.) Heart *(a, b)* and aorta *(c, d)* in a 52-year-old woman asymptomatic at the time, who was referred for an echocardiogram 56 days before death because of a precordial murmur. It confirmed the presence of an atrial septal defect, fossa ovale type. On the day of hospitalization, 10 days before death, she developed some chest pain of unclear type and underwent an operative procedure to close the atrial septal defect that same day. There was difficulty in weaning the patient from cardiopulmonary bypass. ST-segment elevation was present at the end of operation but gradually declined, and an intra-aortic balloon pump was inserted. The entire 10-day postoperative period was characterized by hypotension and evidence of extremely depressed pump function (loss of consciousness, respiratory insufficiency, and ischemic necrosis of fingers bilaterally). *(a)* View of the heart anteriorly. The ascending aorta and arch portions are dilated and irregular. *(b)* Longitudinal view showing aorta (Ao), left atrium (LA), mitral valve (MV), necrotic wall of left ventricle (LV), and pulmonary trunk (PT). *(c)* Cross section of ascending aorta with a large thrombus in the false channel. The tear is between the 2 interior dimensions of the intimal–medial wall. *(d)* Better view of the tear in ascending aorta. The organizing thrombus in the false channel and the smoothness of the margins of the aortic tear strongly suggest that the aortic dissection predated the operation to close the atrial septal defect. Other abbreviations as in Figure 2.

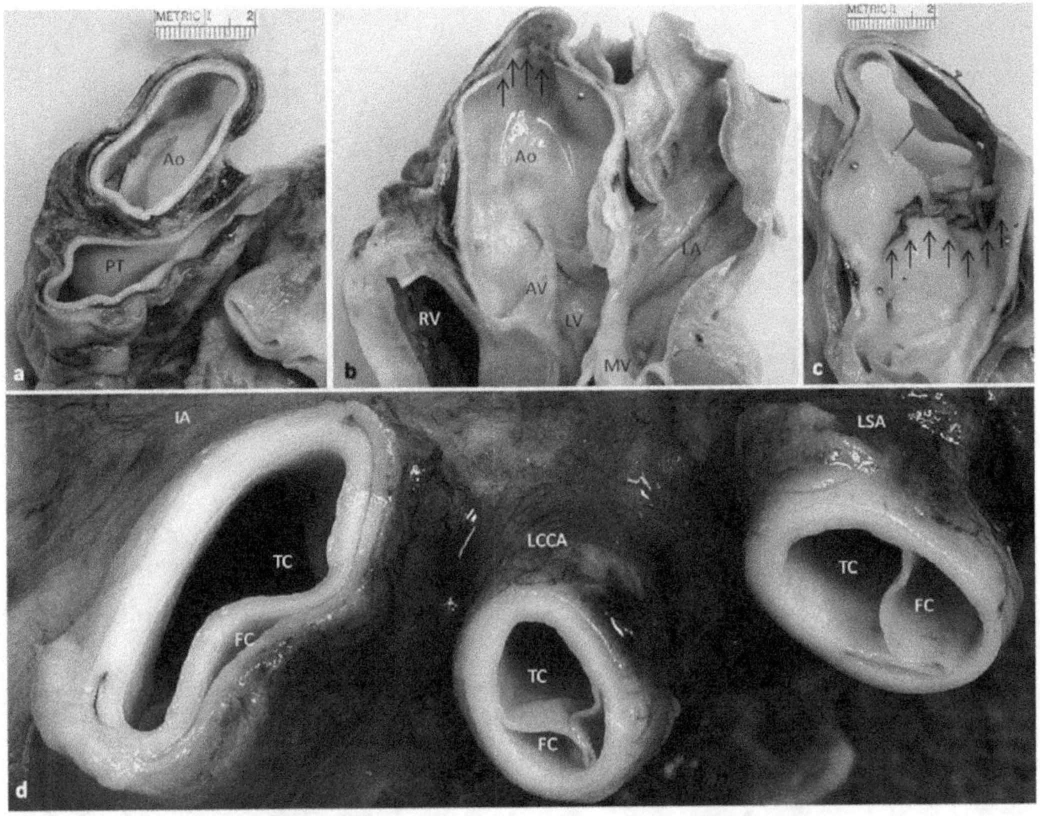

Figure 5. (Patient number 5.) Heart *(a–c)* and aortic arch *(d)* in a 54-year-old man who developed substernal chest pain and extreme generalized weakness before admission. He died suddenly during a stress test while in the hospital 66 hours after admission. *(a)* Extravasated blood in the adventitia of aorta and pulmonary trunk. *(b)* Longitudinal view of heart exposing the aorta, aortic valve, left atrium, mitral valve, left ventricle, and right ventricle (RV). The tear is in the distal portion of ascending aorta *(arrows)*. *(c)* Close-up view of the tear *(arrows)* in ascending aorta. *(d)* View of the 3 arch arteries from above showing the true channel and false channel in each. IA = innominate artery; LCCA = left common carotid artery; LSA = left subclavian artery. Other abbreviations as in Figures 2, 3, and 4.

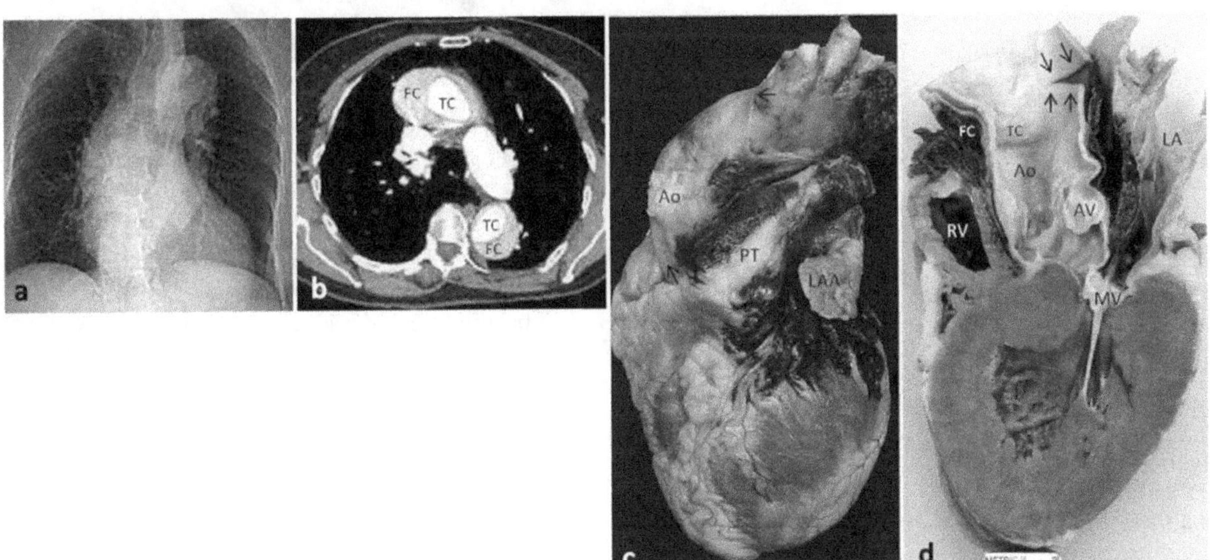

Figure 6. (Patient number 6.) Chest radiograph *(a)* and computed tomographic angiogram of the chest *(b)* and heart *(c, d)* in a 75-year-old woman who developed chest, back, and neck pain and bilateral lower extremity numbness before hospitalization and died 10 hours after admission. Although computed tomographic study was performed, the diagnosis of acute aortic dissection with tear in ascending aorta was not made until necropsy. *(a)* Chest radiograph showing an enlarged cardiac silhouette. *(b)* Computed tomographic angiogram showing an extensive aortic dissection with large thrombus in the false channel of the ascending and descending thoracic aorta. *(c)* View of the heart from the front. Extravasated blood is in the adventitia of the aorta, pulmonary trunk, and the base of the heart. The ascending aorta is dilated *(arrows)*. *(d)* Longitudinal view showing the tear in the aorta *(arrows)* and extravasated blood surrounding the aorta, invading the wall of the left atrium, and, sparsely, the wall of the right ventricle. LAA = left atrial appendage. Other abbreviations as in Figures 2, 3, 4, and 5.

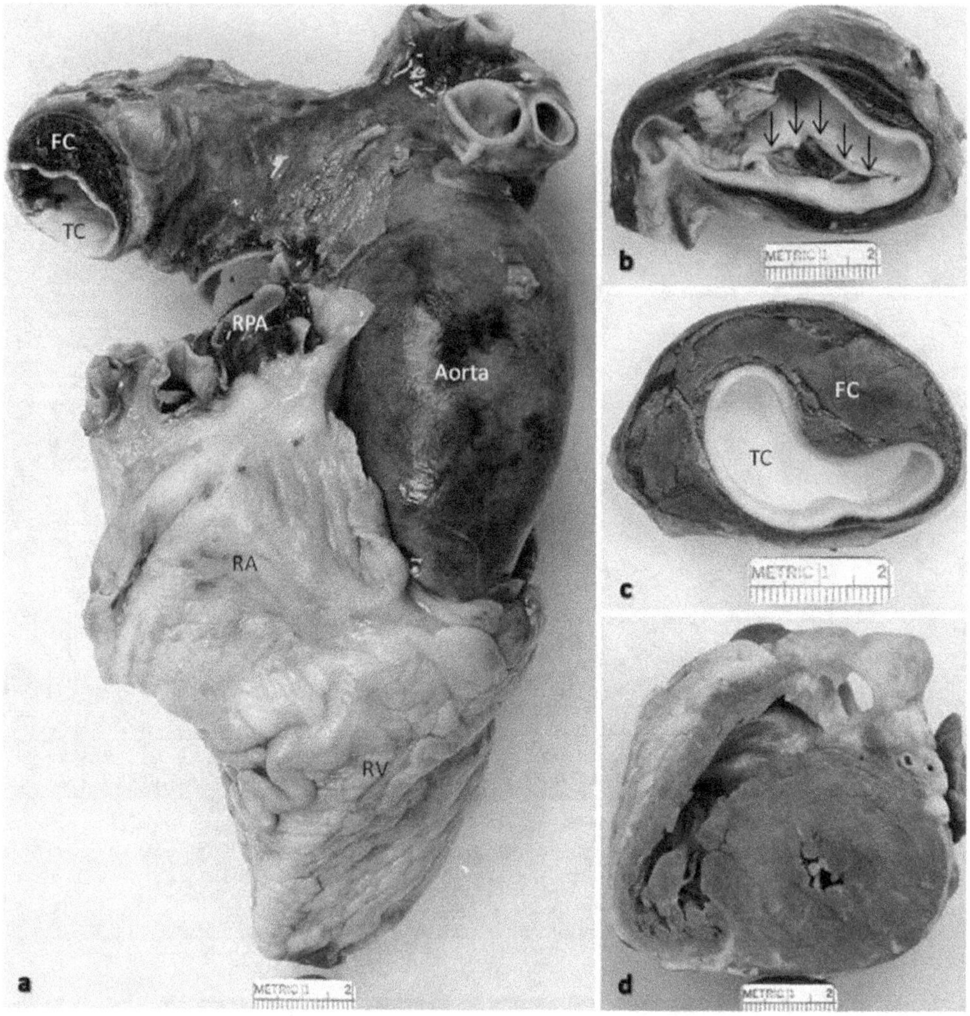

Figure 7. (Patient number 7.) Heart *(a, d)* and aorta *(a–c)* in a 76-year-old woman who was hospitalized for fever, dyspnea, and poor food intake for 3 days. During her 37 hours in the hospital computed tomographic scan was done which showed "atherosclerotic plaques" in the aorta. She died suddenly and a large hemopericardium was found. Retrospective examination of the computed tomographic scan disclosed that it had features more characteristic of aortic dissection. *(a)* View of the heart and aorta from the right side. The heart is small (310 g) and the ascending aorta is huge. The false channel is filled with clotted blood and is larger than the true channel. The right pulmonary artery (RPA) contains extravasated blood in the adventitia. *(b)* Portion of aorta showing the intimal–medial tear *(arrows)*. *(c)* Cross section of descending thoracic aorta. The true channel is compressed by the clot in the false channel. *(d)* Cross section of left ventricle showing a minute cavity and no myocardial lesions. RA = right atrium. Other abbreviations as in Figures 2 and 5.

untreated mortality of 1% to 2% per hour after onset of symptoms. As stated so well by Hagan and colleagues[6] in 2000: "Acute aortic dissection presents with a wide range of manifestations, and classic findings are often absent. A high clinical index of suspicion is necessary . . ." Spittell and colleagues[3] found that only 66 of 113 patients (58%) with AD with tear in AA studied at necropsy at the Mayo Clinic had the correct antemortem diagnosis. Once suspected, definitive imaging (computed tomography [with or without angiography], transthoracic and/or transesophageal echocardiography, and/or magnetic resonance imaging) is required for confirmation.

The frequency that AD with tear in AA is misdiagnosed or not diagnosed in patients admitted to hospitals is actually unclear because autopsy rates in most United States hospitals in recent times have fallen to such low levels (<10% of hospital deaths). At BUMC there are approximately 130 to 175 hospital deaths each month and about 3% have a hospital autopsy each month. In the present study during the 3-year period, AD with tear in AA was diagnosed clinically in 23 patients, all of whom had rapid operative intervention, and in the other 7, the diagnosis of AD with tear in AA was not made until necropsy (5 patients) or operation (2 patients). The 2 numbers missing of course are the number diagnosed clinically and not operated on and the number not diagnosed clinically and died and no autopsy was performed (Figure 8). Thus, it is likely that the frequency of misdiagnosis of acute AD with tear in AA is higher than previously suggested.

A weakness of this study, and, indeed, of all studies on this topic, is that the frequency of acute AD with tear in AA is unknown in patients dying in the hospital and not having a necropsy or an operation (for AD or for another condition [usually coronary bypass]).

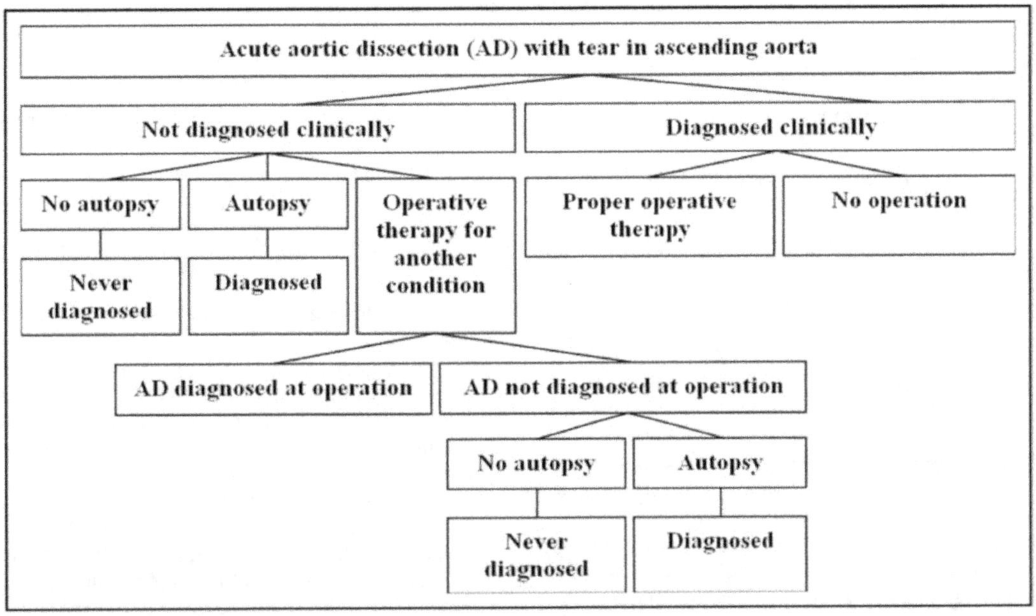

Figure 8. Flow chart of means of diagnosis of patients with aortic dissection with tear in ascending aorta.

1. Slater EE, DeSanctis RW. The clinical recognition of dissecting aortic aneurysm. *Am J Med* 1976;60:625–633.
2. Roberts WC. Aortic dissection: anatomy, consequences, and causes. *Am Heart J* 1981;101:195–214.
3. Spittell PC, Spittell JA Jr, Joyce JW, Tajik AJ, Edwards WD, Schaff HV, Stanson AW. Clinical features and differential diagnosis of aortic dissection: experience with 236 cases (1980 through 1990). *Mayo Clin Proc* 1993;68:642–651.
4. Rosman HS, Patel S, Borzak S, Paone G, Retter K. Quality of history taking in patients with aortic dissection. *Chest* 1998;114:793–795.
5. Scholl FG, Coady MA, Davies R, Rizzo JA, Hammond GL, Kopf GS, Elefteriades JA. Interval or permanent nonoperative management of acute type A aortic dissection. *Arch Surg* 1999;134:402–406.
6. Hagan PG, Nienaber CA, Isselbacher EM, Bruckman D, Karavite DJ, Russman PL, Evangelista A, Fattori R, Suzuki T, Oh JK, Moore AG, Malouf JF, Pape LA, Gaca C, Sechtem U, Lenferink S, Deutsch HJ, Diedrichs H, Marcos y Robles J, Llovet A, Gilon D, Das SK, Armstrong WF, Deeb GM, Eagle KA. The International Registry of Acute Aortic Dissection (IRAD): new insights into an old disease. *jama* 2000;283:897–903.
7. Olin JW, Fuster V. Acute aortic dissection: the need for rapid, accurate, and readily available diagnostic strategies. *Arterioscler Thromb Vasc Biol* 2003;23:1721–1723.
8. Bonser RS, Ranasinghe AM, Loubani M, Evans JD, Thalji NM, Bachet JE, Carrel TP, Czerny M, Di Bartolomeo R, Grabenwöger M, Lonn L, Mestres CA, Schepens MA, Weigang E. Evidence, lack of evidence, controversy, and debate in the provision and performance of the surgery of acute type A aortic dissection. *J Am Coll Cardiol* 2011;58:2455–2474.
9. Roberts WC, Vowels TJ, Kitchens BL, Ko JM, Filardo G, Henry AC, Hamman BL, Matter GJ, Hebeler RF. Aortic medial elastic fiber loss in acute ascending aortic dissection. *Am J Cardiol* 2011;108:1639–1644.

Natural History of Adults With Congenitally Malformed Aortic Valves (Unicuspid or Bicuspid)

William Clifford Roberts, MD, Travis James Vowels, BBA, and Jong Mi Ko, BA

Abstract: Appreciation of the frequency of the congenitally malformed aortic valve has come about during the last 50 years, a period during which aortic valve replacement became a predictably successful operation. Study of patients at necropsy with either a congenitally unicuspid (1 true commissure) or bicuspid (2 true commissures) valve in whom no aortic valve operation has been performed has not been conducted during these 50 years, to our knowledge. We studied 218 patients at necropsy with congenitally malformed aortic valves: 28 (13%) had a unicuspid valve and 190 (87%), a bicuspid valve. Their ages at death ranged from 21 to 89 years (mean, 55 yr), and 80% were men. Of the 218 adults, the aortic valve functioned normally during life in 54 (25%) and abnormally in 164 (75%): aortic stenosis in 142 (65%), pure aortic regurgitation without superimposed infective endocarditis (IE) in 2 (1%), and IE superimposed on a previously normally functioning aortic valve in 20 (9%). IE occurred in a total of 31 (14%) of the 218 patients: involving a previously normally functioning valve in 20 (65%) and a previously stenotic valve in 11 (35%). Of the 218 patients, at least 141 (65%) died as a consequence of aortic valve disease (124 patients) or ascending aortic tears with or without dissection (17 patients). An estimated 1% of the population, maybe higher in men, has a congenitally malformed aortic valve. Data from this study suggest that about 75% of them will develop a major complication. Conversely, and encouragingly, about 25% will go through life without a complication.

(*Medicine* 2012;91: 287–308)

Abbreviations: AR = aortic regurgitation, AS = aortic stenosis, CABG = coronary artery bypass grafting, IE = infective endocarditis, NHLBI = National Heart, Lung, and Blood Institute.

INTRODUCTION

The frequency of the congenitally malformed aortic valve at birth remains unclear but the best estimates are that it is present in 1% of live births,[22,50,58] probably a bit higher in males. That frequency translates into 3,130,000 persons in the United States having a congenitally malformed aortic valve. If systemic hypertension is excluded, complications of the malformation of this valve may be the second most common cardiac cause of death (after coronary heart disease) if untreated.

The frequency of the malformed aortic valve has not been properly appreciated until relatively recent decades. Paul Dudley White, the most prominent cardiologist in the United States in the first half of the 20th century, wrote in the 4th edition (1951) of his book *Heart Disease*, "Serious congenital aortic valve lesions, stenosis and atresia, are very rare, but congenital bicuspid aortic valves are found occasionally and are likely to be the site of subacute bacterial endocarditis…".[101] Paul Wood, the most prominent cardiologist in the United Kingdom during his lifetime, wrote in the 3rd edition (1968) of his book *Diseases of the Heart and Circulation*, "Apart from its association with [aortic] coarctation, bicuspid aortic valve is clinically important for four reasons: 1) it may leak spontaneously or as a result of acquired hypertension; 2) about one-quarter of all cases become infected sooner or later; 3) an associated weakness of the sinuses of Valsalva may lead to aneurysmal dilatation or rupture; 4) an insidious sclerosing process may lead to calcified aortic stenosis in middle age…".[103] And in the 3rd edition (1968) of *Pathology of the Heart and Blood Vessels* edited by S. E. Gould, only 2 of 1162 pages were devoted to aortic stenosis (AS), and bicuspid aortic valve was mentioned in only 1 of 9 paragraphs.[28] It is notable that successful aortic valve replacement had been a reality for 8 years, since 1960.[48]

The congenitally bicuspid aortic valve has captured the interest of many prominent physicians and one illustrious artist.[98,99] Leonardo da Vinci (1452–1519) appears to have been the first to draw and publish a congenitally bicuspid aortic valve and indeed to appreciate its clear difference from a tricuspid aortic valve.[34] Sir James Paget (1814–1899) described at necropsy 3 patients with stenotic bicuspid aortic valves.[52] Sir Thomas Peacock (1812–1882) also described and illustrated 3 patients studied at necropsy with stenotic congenitally bicuspid aortic valves.[54] A number of reports followed (Table 1), describing mainly patients studied at necropsy with valvular AS.[1,2,6,7,9,10,12–15,17,18,20,24,25,29,31,33,35,37–41,47,50,52,54,56,57,91,92,100] Many authors considered the AS to be the result of rheumatic heart disease,[2,7,9,13–15,17,18,29,31,33,37,57] but several authors provided illustrations of the stenotic aortic valve showing it clearly to be a congenitally bicuspid valve.[2,6,7,9,12,14,18,20,24,33,40,54,91,92] Roberts in 1970 provided a strong case against a rheumatic etiology for AS in patients with anatomically normal mitral valves.[59,60] Maude Abbott (1868–1940) demonstrated that most patients (about 75%) with coarctation of the aorta have congenitally bicuspid aortic valves,[1] and many authors later supported that view.[6,26,57,58,92] Roberts and colleagues[82] opined that 100% of patients with complete interruption of the aortic arch have bicuspid aortic valves. Authors after 1950 describing patients with AS commonly described and illustrated underlying congenitally bicuspid valves (see Table 1).[6,10–12,20,24,32,36,49,55,58–61,64,92]

Although Carl Rokitansky (1804–1878) had earlier identified bacteria in vegetations in patients with infective endocarditis (IE), Osler (1849–1919) in his 1885 Gulstonian Lectures[51] called

From the Departments of Internal Medicine (Division of Cardiology) and Pathology (WCR), and Baylor Heart and Vascular Institute (WCR, TJV, JMK), Baylor University Medical Center, Dallas, Texas.
Travis James Vowels is currently a medical student at The University of Texas Medical School at Houston, Houston, Texas.
This work was supported by the Baylor Heart and Vascular Institute, Cardiovascular Research Review Committee, the Cardiovascular Research Fund of the Baylor Health Care System Foundation.
The authors have no conflicts of interest to disclose.
Reprints: Dr. William Clifford Roberts, Baylor Heart and Vascular Institute, Baylor University Medical Center, 3500 Gaston Avenue, Dallas, TX (e-mail: wc.roberts@baylorhealth.edu).

ISSN: 0025-7974
DOI: 10.1097/MD.0b013e3182764b84

TABLE 1. Reported Necrospy Cases (Before 1970) of Aortic Stenosis and/or Bicuspid Aortic Valves in Adults Without Anatomic Disease of the Mitral Valve

Year of Publication	Author(s) (Reference)	Number of Cases						Etiology of Aortic Valve Disease
		Total	Bicuspid Aortic Valve	Aortic Stenosis	Infective Endocarditis	Coarctation of Aorta	Photos (BAV)*	
1844	Paget[52]	6	3	3	0	0	0	C
1865	Peacock[54]	3	3	3	0	0	+(3/3)†	C
1886	Osler[50]	18	18	6‡	8	0	0	C
1904	Mönckeberg[47]	32	0	32	0	0	0	D
1923	Lewis, Grant[39]	13	13	0	13	0	0	C
1926	Cabot[9]	28	2	23	5	0	+(2/3)	R
1926	Clawson, Bell, Hartzell[14]	13	—	13	6	0	+(1/1)	R
1928	Wauchope[100]	52	52	0	7	2	0	C
1928	Abbott[1]	200	51	0	13	200§	0	C
1931	Christian[13]	21	0	21	0	0	0	R
1931	Margolis, Ziellessen, Barnes[40]	42	20	42	0	0	+(3/4)¶	U
1933	Laws, Levine[37]	11	—	11	2	0	0	R
1934	McGinn, White[41]	35	4	35	1	0	0	U
1934	Bishop, Bishop, Trubek[7]	9	9	2	1	1	+(2/2)	R
1935	Gibbs[25]	12	0	12	0	0	0	A
1936	Sohval, Gross**[24,91]	15	1	15	0	0	+(1/4)	NR
1937	Gross[29]	16	2	16	—	—	+	R
1938	Lesnick, Schlesinger[38]	17	0	17	0	0	0	NR
1938	Clawson, Noble, Lufkin[15]	132	0	97	0	0	0	R
1939	Dry, Willius[18]	15	1	15	0	0	+(2/4)	R
1940	Cohen, Gray, Nash, Fink[17]	7	1	7	0	0	0	R
1941	Koletsky[35]	7	7	4	1	1	0	C
1945	Reich[56]	22	0	22	0	0	0	—
1947	Karsner, Koletsky[33]	119	16	119	0	0	+(2/8)	R
1947	Reifenstein, Levine, Gross[57]	104	58	11	23	104	0	C, R
1948	Horan, Barnes[31]	100	—	100	6	0	0	R
1952	Anderson, Kelsey, Edwards[2]	49	—	49	0	0	+(2/4)||	C, R
1953	1953 Campbell, Kauntze[12]	4	4	4	0	0	+(4/4)#	C
1955	Smith, Matthews[92]	27	20	27	0	7	+(2/2)	C
1959	Bacon, Matthews[6]	28	28	19	0	4	+(6/6)	C
1961	Edwards[20]	10	8	9	0	0	+(8/10)	C
1968	Campbell[10]	46	16	46	0	0	0	C

Abbreviations: A = atherosclerotic, C = congenital, D = degenerative, NR = non-rheumatic, R = rheumatic, U = uncertain.

*The second number in this vertical column represents the number of gross illustrations of the aortic valve.

†Drawings.

‡Osler described only 1 of these 6 cases as having aortic stenosis ("The two segments from their position obstruct and narrow the orifice") but the description of the valves make it likely that the orifices were stenotic.

§Rupture of ascending aorta in 33 and cerebral hemorrhage in 25.

||One of the 2 is unicuspid.

¶One of the 3 is unicuspid.

#Three of the 4 are unicuspid. All are drawings.

**Clinical features in the cases were reported by Friedberg and Sohval.

attention to the congenitally bicuspid aortic valve's extreme propensity to be the site of IE. Whether Osler realized that stenosis was also a complication of the bicuspid condition is less clear; if he did, he did not write about that possibility. Mensah and Friesinger[44] believed that Osler missed entirely "the link" between the bicuspid valve and AS. The reason they suggested was that the average age of death in the United States in 1900 was 47 years, and most patients with stenosis superimposed on a bicuspid aortic valve are older than that. Osler described 18 patients with congenitally bicuspid aortic valves that he studied at autopsy, and although the aortic valve "was invariably thickened and the seat of sclerotic changes," clear AS was seen in only 1 of the 18 patients. During the 20th century a number of other authors stressed the frequent connection between IE and the congenitally malformed aortic valve.[3–5,8,22,23,58,63]

That pure aortic regurgitation (AR) without superimposed IE may be a consequence of the bicuspid condition was not reported, to our knowledge, until 1981 when Roberts and colleagues[83] described 13 such patients who had undergone aortic valve replacement. Today, the bicuspid valve without superimposed IE is recognized as one of the most common causes of pure (no element of stenosis) AR severe enough to warrant aortic valve replacement.[65,80,83,88]

An association between aortic valve disease and "cystic medial necrosis" of the ascending aorta appears to have been first described by McKusick (1921–2008) and colleagues[43] in 1957. Although the structure of the valve was not known in their 4 cases, the severity of stenosis and the lack of associated mitral valve disease makes congenital malformation of the aortic valve highly likely, and that association has been reported often since then.[30,42,86,88,95,97,104] Not only is the ascending aorta dilated in patients with stenotic and/or purely regurgitant congenitally bicuspid aortic valves, but tears in the ascending aorta with or without dissection also is a recognized complication.[86,88] Roberts and Roberts[86] found aortic dissection to be 5 times more frequent in patients with bicuspid compared to those with tricuspid aortic valves. Although the ascending aorta may be dilated in patients with AS or pure AR, Roberts and associates[88] found that aortic-medial-elastic-fiber loss was absent or minimal in 90% of their patients undergoing aortic valve replacement for stenotic unicuspid or bicuspid aortic valves, but in only

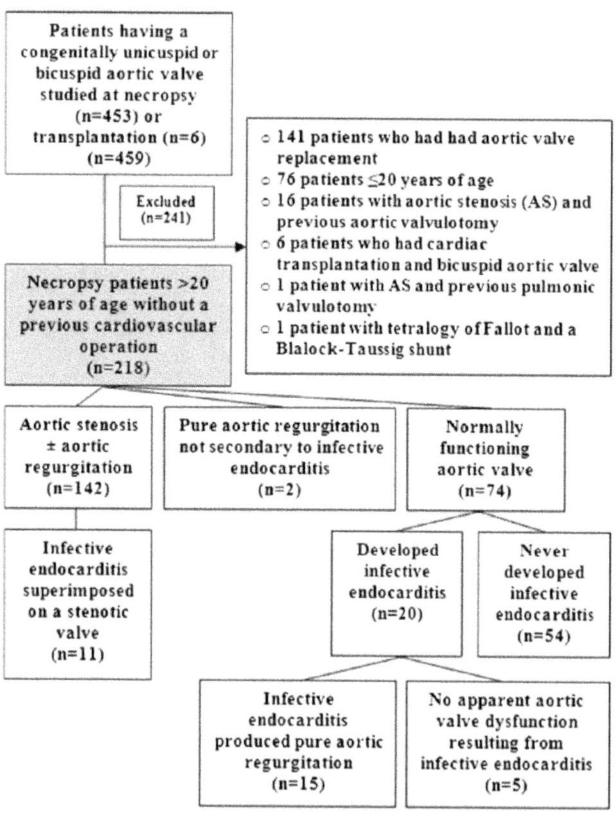

FIGURE 1. Flow chart showing our experience with patients having a congenitally malformed aortic valve. Of the total 453 patients with unicuspid or bicuspid aortic valves studied at necropsy, 241 (53%) were eliminated from this analysis mainly because of an operative intervention on the aortic valve. (In addition, we have examined 276 operatively excised congenitally unicuspid and 1330 operatively excised congenitally bicuspid aortic valves, but these 1606 cases were not included in the present analysis.)

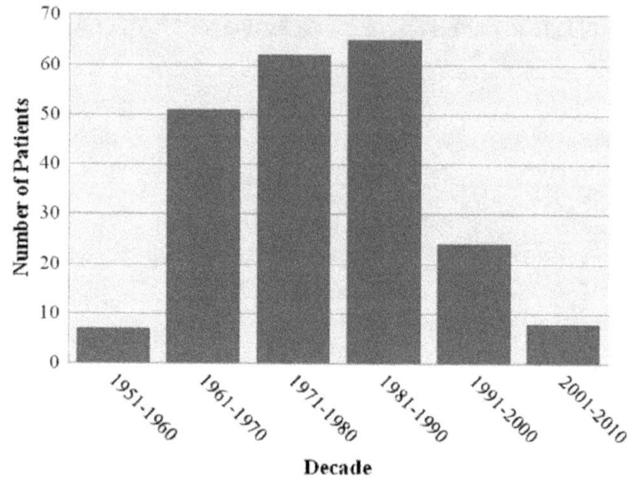

FIGURE 2. Decades during which the 218 patients were studied.

50% of patients with purely regurgitant bicuspid aortic valves. This observation suggests that the type of aortic valve dysfunction may be a major determinant of whether the ascending aorta needs to be resected at the time of aortic valve replacement, an occurrence that has become quite common in the last 2 decades.[95,96,104]

To our knowledge, the concept of the unicuspid aortic valve was first proposed by Edwards[19] (1911–2008) in 1958. He described a unicuspid unicommissural stenotic aortic valve as having only 1 true commissure and a slit-like orifice resembling an exclamation point. He opined that the unicuspid unicommissural aortic valve was stenotic from the time of birth, and that this valve structure was the structure most commonly seen in infants and very young children with severe AS. In contrast, he believed that the bicuspid aortic valve was not stenotic at birth but became so as fibrous tissue and calcific deposits developed on its cusps. Several reports on consequences of the unicuspid unicommissural aortic valve followed.[21,70,78,81,88] Probably most surgeons and pathologists call the unicuspid unicommissural aortic valve a congenitally bicuspid valve.[87] In 2007, Roberts and associates[71] described 4 patients whose operatively excised stenotic aortic valves had no true commissures and similar degrees of "commissural" fusion resulting in a central symmetrical triangular-shaped orifice. The authors called the valve congenitally unicuspid acommissural.

In the last 20 years most morphologic studies of stenotic, purely regurgitant, and infected congenitally malformed aortic valves have been of operatively excised valves, because the frequency of autopsy in patients dying in hospitals in the United States has dropped to <10% in most institutions, and operative intervention is now common and usually successful.[48,53,66–80,88,90,93,94] Nevertheless, multiple studies of operatively excised valves have demonstrated that the unicuspid ones contain the most calcium and therefore are the heaviest and the most stenotic,[69] that the bicuspid valves are the next most calcified, and that the stenotic tricuspid valves have the least calcific deposits and therefore are the lightest and the least stenotic.[66,69,70,72,78,84] Additionally, these studies have shown that men have significantly heavier valves than women, and that the stenotic valves are far heavier than the purely regurgitant valves with or without superimposed active IE.[66,69,70,72,78,80,88]

Although the natural history of patients having congenitally unicuspid or bicuspid aortic valves has received attention during the last 50 years, most reports included some patients

TABLE 2. Comparison of Various Variables Among Patients With Unicuspid vs Bicuspid Aortic Valves (n = 218)

Variable	Total, n = 218 (100%)	Aortic Valve Structure: Unicuspid, n = 28 (13%)	Bicuspid, n = 190 (87%)
Age at death (years)			
Mean ± SD [median]	55 ± 15 [57]	48 ± 15 [53]*	56 ± 15 [57]*
(Range)	(21–89)	(25–77)	(21–89)
Gender†			
Men	169 (80%)	26 (93%)	143 (78%)
Women	43 (20%)	2 (7%)	41 (22%)
Aortic valve function (before infective endocarditis)			
Normal	74 (34%)	0	74 (39%)
Stenosis	142 (65%)	27 (96%)	115 (61%)
Pure regurgitation	2 (1%)	1 (4%)	1 (<1%)
Infective endocarditis‡			
Active	25 (11%)	2 (7%)	23 (12%)
Healed	6 (3%)	1 (4%)	5 (3%)
Infective endocarditis superimposed on a:			
Previously normally functioning valve	20 (9%)	0	20 (11%)
Previously stenotic valve	11 (5%)	3 (11%)	8 (4%)
Previously purely regurgitant valve	0	0	0
Heart weight (g)			
Mean ± SD [median]	558 ± 162 [530]	603 ± 143 [605]§	551 ± 164 [520]§
(Range)	(170–1050)	(320–880)	(170–1050)

*-*p - value = 0.0109.

†Data missing on 6 patients.

‡Of the 25 patients with active infective endocarditis, 16 had a normally functioning aortic valve prior to infection and 9 had a previously stenotic valve; of the 6 patients with healed infective endocardititis, 4 had a previously normal aortic valve and 2 had infection superimposed onto a stenotic valve.

§-§p - value = 0.1428.

TABLE 3. Comparison of Various Variables According to Type of Function of the Congenitally Malformed Aortic Valve (n = 218)

Variable	Aortic Valve Function Prior to Infective Endocarditis: Normal, n = 74 (34%)	Stenosis, n = 142 (65%)	Pure Regurgitation, n = 2 (1%)
Age at death (years)			
Mean ± SD [median]	48 ± 16 [48]*	59 ± 14 [59]*	32, 42
(Range)	(21–82)	(23–89)	
Gender†			
Men	57 (78%)	110 (80%)	2
Women	16 (22%)	27 (20%)	0
Valve structure			
Unicuspid	0	27 (19%)	1
Bicuspid	74	115 (81%)	1
Infective endocarditis			
Active	16 (22%)	9 (6%)	0
Healed	4 (5%)	2 (1%)	0
Aortic valve orientation			
Anterior/posterior	43/63 (68%)	62/89 (70%)	1
Right/left	20/63 (32%)	27/89 (30%)	0
Raphe present	46/57 (81%)	66/78 (85%)	1
Heart weight (g)			
Mean ± SD [median]	477 ± 148 [450]‡	598 ± 152 [573]‡	470, 920
(Range)	(170–1010)	(300–1050)	

-, ‡-‡p - value = <0.0001.

†Data missing on 6 patients.

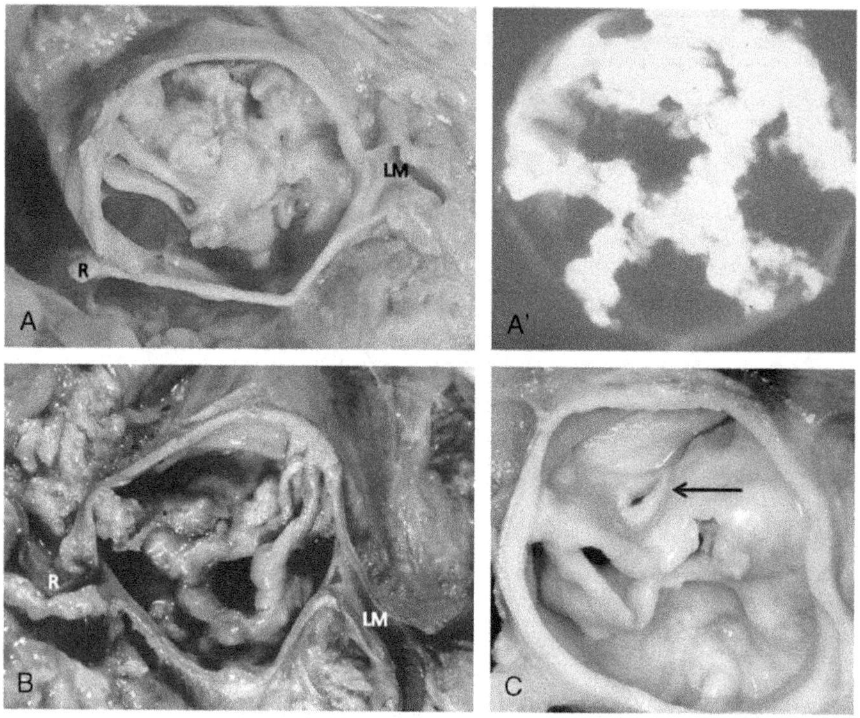

FIGURE 3. Unicuspid aortic valves in 3 patients. A and A′ (radiograph), Valve of a 48-year-old man who had been well until 5 months before death when signs and symptoms of heart failure began and progressed. Terminally, he developed pneumonia, which prevented cardiac catheterization and cardiac valve replacement. The heart weighed 750 g. LM = left main coronary artery; R = right coronary artery. B, Valve of a 31-year-old man who had been a splendid 3-letter athlete and had won his country club golf championship several days before dying quickly of severe acute heart failure. The heart failure was the first he had ever had. The peak systolic pressure difference between left ventricle and aorta was 11 mm Hg. The patient also had considerable AR with similar diastolic pressures in both left ventricle and aorta (50 and 60 mm Hg respectively). He was deemed too sick to undergo aortic valve replacement in 1969. His heart at necropsy weighed 880 g. C, Valve of a 26-year-old man who died suddenly while dancing in a disco. According to some friends, he had no known medical ailments and was not taking any medications. Prior to the sudden collapse there were apparently no complaints of feeling ill. The heart weighed 760 g. A cuspal perforation (arrow) is present, suggesting previous IE that had healed.

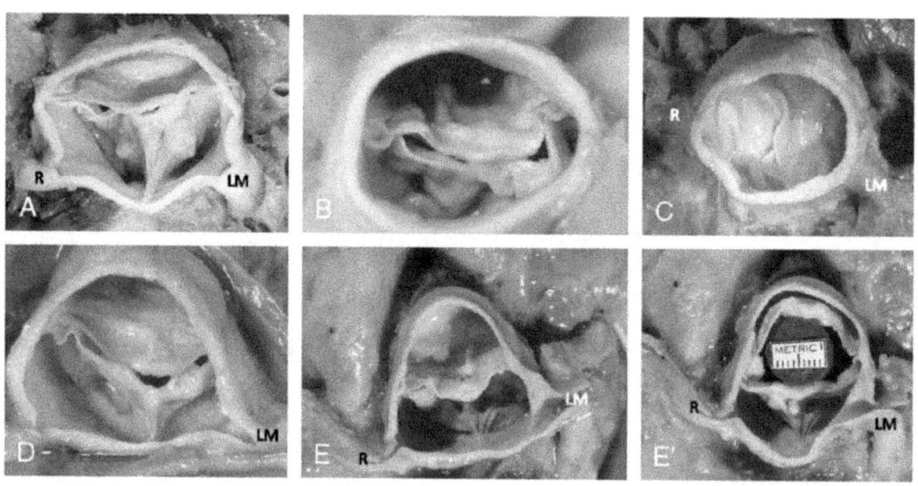

FIGURE 4. Congenitally bicuspid normally functioning aortic valves in 5 different patients, none of whom had clinical evidence of aortic valve disease. In 4 of the 5 patients the cusps are situated anterior-to-posterior, and in 1 patient (C), right-to-left. A, Valve in a 36-year-old man who died suddenly while watching television. He was a habitual alcoholic and he had a fatty liver that weighed 2900 g. The heart weighed 405 g and the coronary arteries were clean. The right coronary artery was dominant. He was found dead by fellow residents in a shelter home. LM = left main coronary artery; R = right coronary artery. B, Valve in a 63-year-old man who had undergone 2 coronary bypass grafting operations. The second operation was performed 17 days before death. The heart weighed 590 g. There are a few calcific deposits on each cusp but each cusp was freely mobile. C, Valve in a 60-year-old man who died of cancer of the pancreas. His heart weighed 470 g and he had systemic hypertension. D, Valve in a 71-year-old woman who died from Parkinson disease. She was cachexic. The heart weighed 290 g. E and E′, Valve shown in both ventricular diastole (E) and ventricular systole (E′) in a 72-year-old woman who died after a fall. The heart weighed 300 g. Small calcific deposits were present in each cusp.

who also had aortic valve replacement or repair, and thus their "natural history" was interrupted by this therapeutic event, or they included only children or young adults, or patients were followed not until death, but just for a few years.[11,16,22,32,45,46,55,89] In the present report we focus on 218 patients with congenitally malformed aortic valves all studied at necropsy by the same investigator (WCR) during the last 50 years. Our purpose is to determine the natural history of patients with this valvular abnormality without operative intervention on the aortic valve at any time.

METHODS

The cases included in the current study came from 37 different institutions including 34 cases from the National Heart, Lung, and Blood Institute (NHLBI), Bethesda, MD; 133 cases from 12 different hospitals in the Washington, DC, area, including 31 from Georgetown University Hospital; 27 from medical institutions in Dallas, TX, and the remaining 24 from 22 different medical centers excluding those in the Washington, DC, and Dallas, TX, areas. The cases from the Washington, DC, area were obtained as follows: WCR gave a conference for nearly 25 years on cardiovascular pathology at 11 or 12 hospitals each month (at Georgetown University Hospital weekly) and after conference the specimens were brought to the Pathology Branch, NHLBI, and described and photographed. Both the reports and photographs were sent to the submitting institutions. Some specimens were received via mail from more distant institutions. All hearts were examined and classified by WCR, and most were photographed or drawn or both.

The clinical records were provided by the Clinical Center of the National Institutes of Health (34 cases) or Baylor University Medical Center at Dallas (16 cases) or by the submitting hospital. Cardiac catheterization and echocardiographic data were sought in all patients. The symptomatic status of each patient was determined from the clinical records. The severity of the aortic valve dysfunction, if present, was determined by the cardiac catheterization reports for patients having that procedure. For the few cases with echocardiograms, we used that examination to determine severity, and if a patient had both an echocardiogram and a left-sided cardiac catheterization, we used the catheterization data. Photographs of stenotic aortic valves in patients in whom cardiac catheterization had been performed were compared to valves in patients in whom no cardiac catheterization was performed to show that the degrees of severity by anatomic examination were similar. All patients included were aged >20 years at the time of death. We excluded patients who had undergone aortic valvulotomy, aortic valve replacement, or replacement of another cardiac valve. Additionally, patients with mitral stenosis irrespective of the structure of the aortic valve were excluded. Patients with diffuse fibrous thickening of the mitral valve leaflets irrespective of the function of the mitral valve

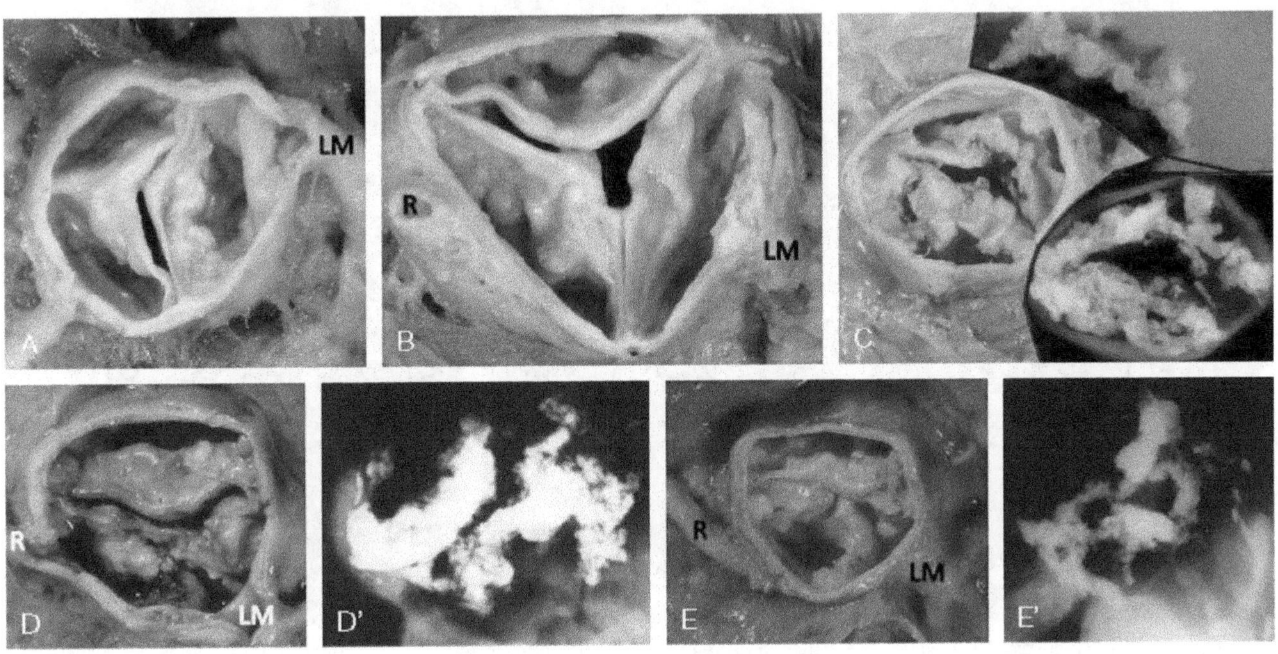

FIGURE 5. Stenotic bicuspid aortic valves in 5 patients, all of whom had undergone cardiac catheterization. The 2 cusps in the valve shown in (A) are located right and left, and all of the others are located anterior and posterior. Heavy calcific deposits are present in each valve. A, Valve belonging to a 65-year-old woman who died from cancer of the breast. She never had evidence of cardiac dysfunction. The heart at necropsy weighed 410 g. The transvalvular peak systolic pressure gradient was 25 mm Hg. LM = left main coronary artery. B, Valve in a 77-year-old man who had evidence of severe heart failure. The peak transvalvular systolic pressure gradient was 50 mm Hg. The left main coronary artery was severely narrowed, and the left ventricular ejection fraction was 40%. The heart weighed 570 g and the left ventricular wall was free of foci of necrosis and fibrosis. R = right coronary artery. C, Valve in a 37-year-old man who died suddenly in a cardiac clinic of a major hospital. He had periodic chest pain and exertional dyspnea for nearly 2 years. The peak transvalvular systolic pressure gradient was 50 mm Hg. Not only was the aortic valve heavily calcified, but also the mitral annulus was as well. The coronary arteries were insignificantly narrowed. D and D′, Heavily calcified aortic valve in a 67-year-old man who had severe angina pectoris and a 72 mm Hg peak systolic pressure gradient across the aortic valve. He had cardiac arrest the night before planned aortic valve replacement. At necropsy, the heart weighed 680 g and the heart was devoid of foci of necrosis and fibrosis. E and E′, Heavily calcified valve in a 61-year-old man who died suddenly. Earlier, the peak transvalvular systolic pressure gradient was 100 mm Hg. The heart weighed 530 g.

also were excluded. The origin of the 218 patients included in the present study is shown in the flow chart of Figure 1. The decades in which the patients were studied at necropsy are shown in Figure 2.

Means, standard deviations, and percentages were calculated to describe the study cohort. Differences in demographic, clinical, and morphologic details were tested using a 2-tailed t-test with equal variance in Microsoft Excel 2007 (Microsoft, Redmond, WA).

RESULTS

Frequency of Unicuspid and Bicuspid Aortic Valves

Of the 218 patients, 28 (13%) had unicuspid aortic valves and 190 (87%) had bicuspid aortic valves (Table 2). The men (80% of the total) at death ranged in age from 21 to 89 years (mean, 54 ± 15 yr) and the women (20% of the total), from 21 to 87 years (mean, 59 ± 15 yr). Of the 28 unicuspid valves, 26 (93%) were in men and 2 (7%) were in women; of the 190 bicuspid aortic valves, 78% were in men and 22% were in women. Thus, of the congenitally malformed aortic valves in men, 85% were bicuspid and 15% were unicuspid; in the women, 95% were bicuspid and 5% were unicuspid.

Age and Race

The ages of patients with unicuspid and bicuspid aortic valves differed significantly ($p < 0.02$): 48 ± 15 years in the unicuspid group and 56 ± 15 years in the bicuspid group (Table 2). The mean age of patients with stenotic valves was greater than that of patients with normally functioning valves before IE occurred (age 59 ± 14 yr vs. 48 ± 16 yr, respectively; $p < 0.0001$) (Table 3). Of the total patients, 89% were white, 8% were black, and 3%, other.

Aortic Valve Function

Of the 28 patients with unicuspid valves, 27 (96%) were stenotic and 1 (4%) was purely regurgitant (no apparent evidence of stenosis) (Figure 3, Table 3). Of the 190 bicuspid valves, 74 (39%) appeared to have functioned normally (until IE appeared and caused AR in 15 [20%] of the 74 patients) (Figure 4); 115 (61%) were clearly stenotic as judged morphologically (Figures 5–8); and 1 (<1%) was purely regurgitant without evidence at any time of IE. Thus, none of the 28 unicuspid valves appeared to have functioned normally, whereas 74 (39%) of the bicuspid valves (at least before IE altered that status) appeared to have functioned normally; only 2 valves (1 unicuspid, 1 bicuspid) were purely regurgitant (neither having

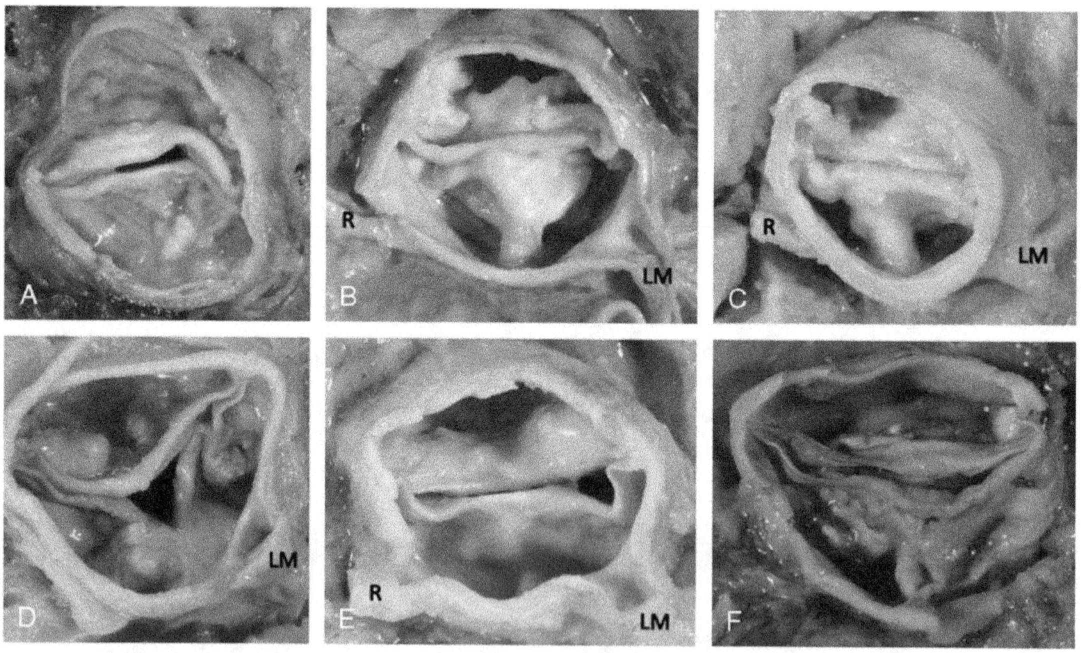

FIGURE 6. Stenotic bicuspid aortic valves in 6 patients, none of whom had undergone cardiac catheterization. At autopsy, the left ventricular walls in each were free of foci of necrosis and fibrosis. The cusps in each of these 6 patients are located anterior and posterior. A, Valve in a 69-year-old woman who died suddenly while driving. Necropsy disclosed a tear in the ascending aorta and an aortic dissection limited to the ascending and arch portions. The heart weighed 400 g. Both right and left circumflex coronary arteries were narrowed by atherosclerotic plaque. B, Valve in a 57-year-old woman in whom aortic valve stenosis was never diagnosed clinically. She presented to the hospital in severe pulmonary edema, and precordial examination did not disclose a murmur because of the chest noise. The coronary arteries were insignificantly narrowed. LM = left main coronary artery; R = right coronary artery. C, Valve in a 56-year-old woman who died suddenly after running up a flight of stairs. Previously she had fainted on 2 occasions during exertion, the first time was 10 months before she died. She never went to a physician and was not known to have medical problems. At autopsy, the heart weighed 380 g. D, Valve in a 62-year-old man who had nonfatal cardiac arrest 5 months before death and severe acute heart failure beginning 14 days before death, which progressively worsened. The patient weighed >135 kg and had considerable pulmonary hypertension (pulmonary artery pressure was 70/30 mm Hg). He also developed ventricular tachycardia. His heart weighed 900 g. E, Valve in a 48-year-old man who died suddenly while eating. At autopsy, there was no evidence of aspiration. The heart weighed 540 g. F, Valve in a 56-year-old man who had evidence of heart failure during his last 3 years of life. He died suddenly. The heart weighed 670 g and the coronary arteries were devoid of atherosclerotic plaques.

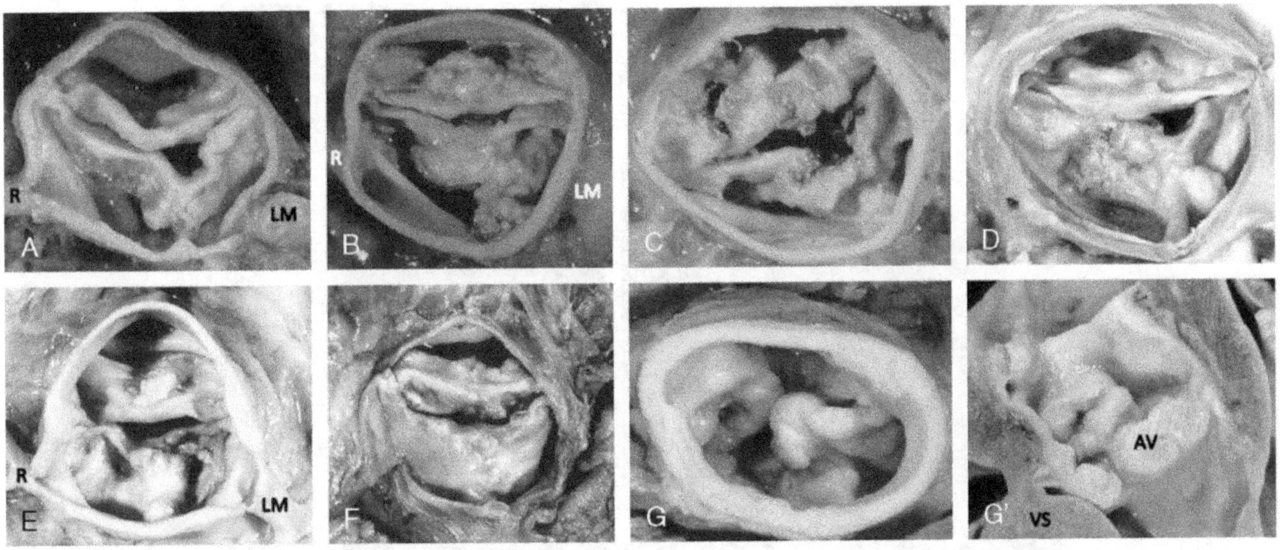

FIGURE 7. Stenotic aortic valves in 7 patients, none of whom had cardiac catheterization but all of whom had morphologic evidence of severe aortic valve stenosis. A, Valve in a 66-year-old man who died suddenly but also had severe coronary disease. A healed myocardial infarct was present in the left ventricular wall. LM = left main coronary artery; R = right coronary artery. B, Valve in an 81-year-old man who also had considerable coronary disease, a healed left ventricular myocardial infarct, and severe angina pectoris. The heart weighed 750 g. C, Valve in a 60-year-old man who died of heart failure. Heavy calcific deposits were found in the aortic valve cusps, the mitral valve annulus, and the major epicardial coronary arteries. At necropsy, he had both a healed and an acute myocardial infarct. His coronary arteries were severely narrowed. His heart weighed 1050 g. D, Valve in a 64-year-old woman who developed exertional dyspnea 4 months before death and the heart failure progressed. At necropsy the coronary arteries were essentially devoid of atherosclerotic plaques and there were no foci of necrosis or fibrosis in the ventricular walls. The heart weighed approximately 500 g. Additionally, the patient had evidence of pulmonary fibrosis. E, Heart in a 51-year-old man who died suddenly while taking a shower. At necropsy, the heart weighed 800 g, the coronary arteries were devoid of plaques, and the ventricular walls were free of foci of necrosis or fibrosis. F, Valve in a 69-year-old woman who had evidence of heart failure intermittently for 2 years but never chest pain or syncope. She was hospitalized for evaluation and found to have AS but she refused to have cardiac catheterization or operation and died of worsening heart failure. At necropsy, the aortic valve, mitral annulus, and epicardial coronary arteries were heavily calcified. The coronary arteries were severely narrowed but the left ventricular wall was devoid of foci of necrosis or fibrosis. G and G′, Aortic valve from above and from the side in a 23-year-old man who died suddenly while walking home after playing tennis for 2 hours. The heart weighed 590 g and a small scar was present near the apex of the left ventricle. The coronary arteries were devoid of plaques. AV = aortic valve; VS = ventricular septum.

IE). Thirty-four percent of the men and 37% of the women had normally functioning aortic valves; 65% of the men and 63% of the women had stenotic valves, and 2 men and no women had intrinsically purely regurgitant valves.

Frequency of IE

Of the 25 patients with active IE, 16 (64%) involved a previously normally functioning aortic valve (Figures 9–13) and 9 (36%), a previously stenotic valve (Figures 14–18, Table 4).

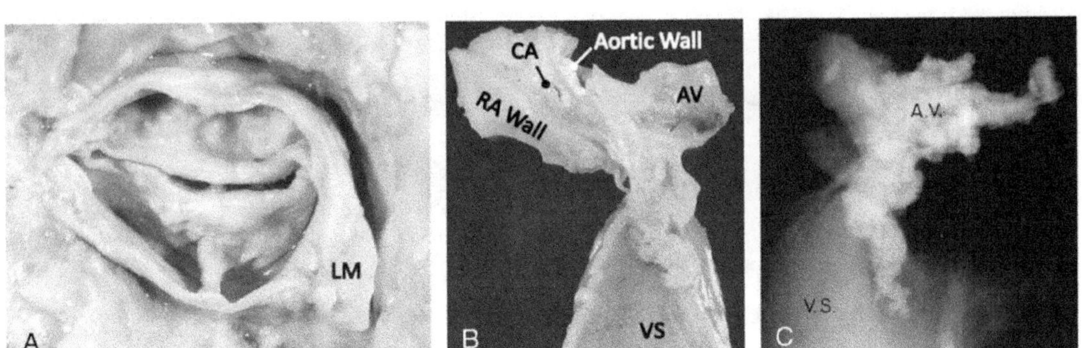

FIGURE 8. Stenotic bicuspid aortic valve. A, Aortic valve from above in a 59-year-old man who died of heart failure. The left ventricular peak systolic pressure gradient across the aortic valve was 45 mm Hg by catheterization. A raphe is present in the anterior cusp. LM = left main coronary artery. B, Longitudinal section through the right atrial (RA) wall, coronary artery (CA), aortic valve (AV), and ventricular septum (VS) showing heavy calcific deposits in the aortic valve and in the apex of the muscular ventricular septum obliterating the AV bundle and also the left bundle branch. C, Radiograph of the same longitudinal section showing heavy calcific deposits again in the aortic valve, membranous ventricular septum, and in the area of the AV bundle and left bundle branch. An electrocardiogram showed complete heart block.

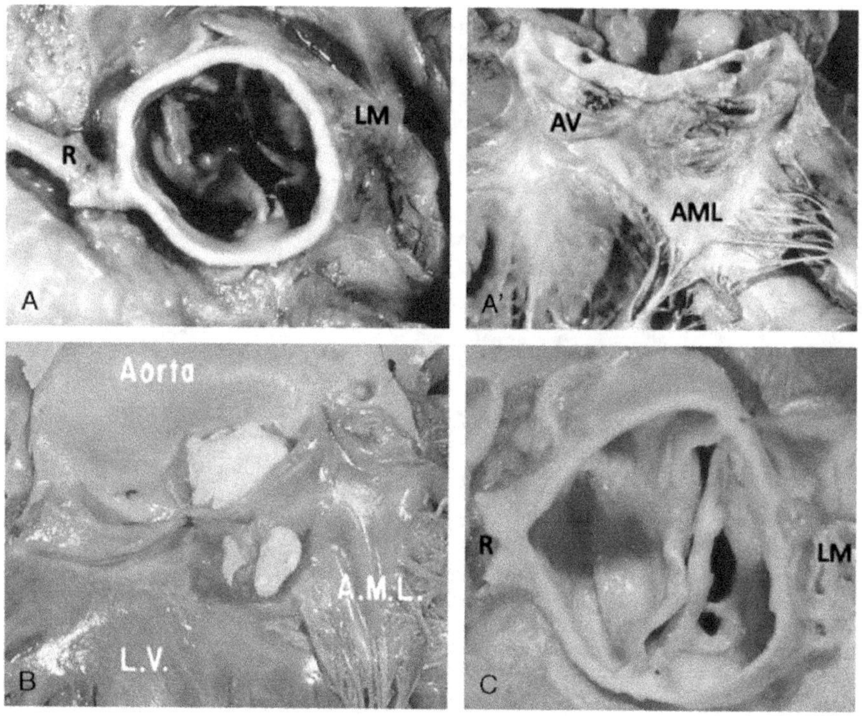

FIGURE 9. Infective endocarditis involving a bicuspid valve. A and A′, Aortic valve from above and after opening showing perforations in each of the 2 cusps and vegetative material on the ventricular surface of each cusp and bordering the perforations. The patient was a 39-year-old man who died suddenly on the golf course. His heart weighed 1010 g and he had evidence of severe AR. In addition to evidence of both active and healed infection on the aortic valve, several chordae tendineae from the mitral valve had ruptured due to dislodgment of vegetative material from the aortic valve. The ventricle, despite its severe dilatation, was devoid of foci of necrosis and fibrosis in its wall. Three months before his sudden death he underwent cardiac catheterization. The left ventricular pressure was 140/20 and simultaneous aortic pressure, 140/38 mm Hg. AML = anterior mitral leaflet; AV = aortic valve; LM = left main coronary artery; R = right coronary artery. B, Valve opened in a 33-year-old man who had had IE that healed and left severe AR thereafter. Cotton has been placed in the posterior (noncoronary) cusp. One of the 2 cusps was perforated by the infection, and heart failure was the consequence. He died of severe heart failure, becoming emaciated. The heart weighed 430 g. No foci of ventricular wall necrosis or fibrosis were present at autopsy. LV = left ventricle. C, Valve in a 47-year-old man who had active IE in the past that had healed. He died suddenly from a skull fracture when a horse kicked him in the head. In addition to the bicuspid aortic valve he had a congenitally bicuspid pulmonic valve that had functioned normally. His heart weighed 590 g. The regurgitation was due mainly to the perforations in 1 of the 2 cusps.

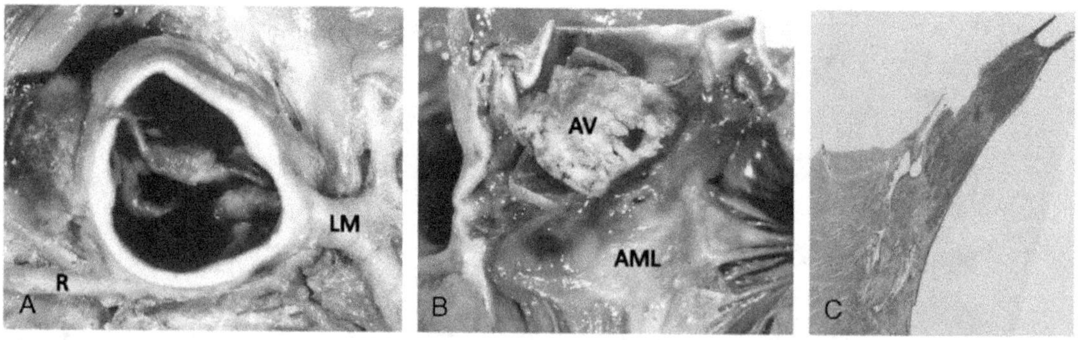

FIGURE 10. Active IE superimposed on a congenitally bicuspid valve. A, Valve from above in a 22-year-old man, an opiate addict who developed *Staphylococcus epidermidis* endocarditis several weeks before death. The cusps are located anterior and posterior. The infection involves mainly the anterior cusp which is perforated by the vegetative material. LM = left main coronary artery; R = right coronary artery. B, Longitudinal view of the vegetation that has spread to the aortic wall causing a ring abscess in it. AML = anterior mitral leaflet; AV = aortic valve. C, Photomicrograph of a histology section of a left ventricular papillary muscle that is completely necrotic. The epicardial coronary arteries were entirely normal. The patient developed severe AR with resulting severe heart failure. At necropsy, the heart weighed 670 g. A mycotic aneurysm also developed in the membranaceous portion of the ventricular septum protruding into the right side of the heart. (Hematoxylin and eosin stain, 5× magnification.)

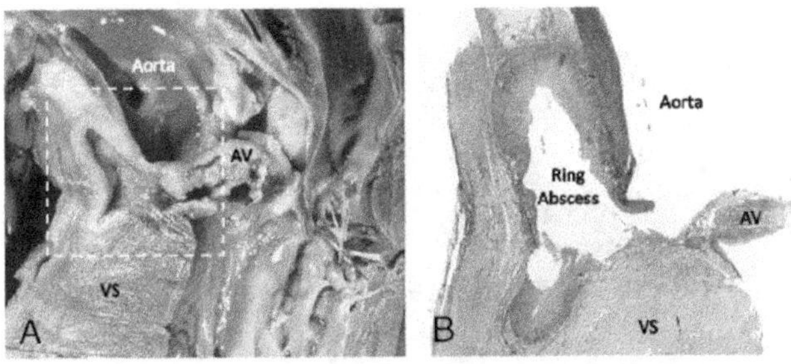

FIGURE 11. Active IE superimposed on a previously normally functioning bicuspid aortic valve. A, Longitudinal view of an aortic valve showing massive destruction of the cusps with a ring abscess adjacent to the aorta within the ventricular septum in a 41-year-old man. The valve was made severely incompetent by the infection. AV = aortic valve; VS = ventricular septum. B, Photomicrograph showing an incompetent aortic valve cusp, wall of aorta and ring abscess that separates the aorta from the left ventricle. VS = ventricular septum. The valve cusps were oriented right and left. This patient developed alpha streptococcus IE following a dental procedure approximately 2 months before the onset of symptoms or approximately 4 months before death. During the infection he developed evidence of severe AR. When hospitalized 20 days before death his blood pressure was 100/0 mm Hg and he was in pulmonary edema. He died the night before scheduled aortic valve replacement, which almost certainly would have been fruitless. His heart weighed 500 g. The residual aortic valve cusps contained minimal calcific deposits. (Movat stain, 5 × magnification.)

Additionally, 6 patients had both histories of and morphologic residual damage from active IE that had healed. Of the 31 total cases of IE, 3 (10%) involved a unicuspid valve (3 [11%] of the

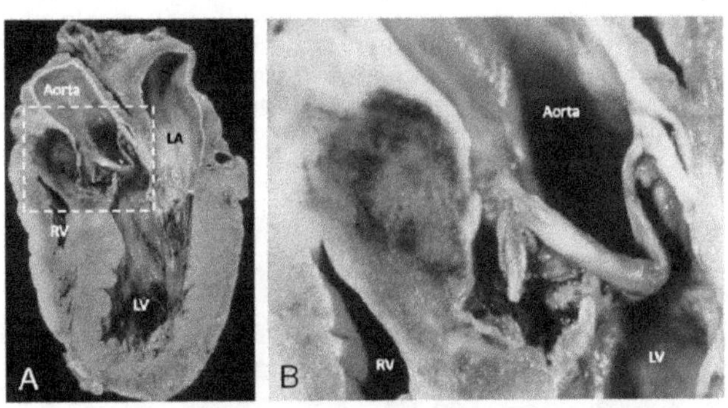

FIGURE 12. Active IE involving a bicuspid aortic valve that had probably functioned normally before the infection. A, Longitudinal view of a heart showing a huge ring abscess anteriorly in a 36-year-old woman who had multiple myeloma and Turner syndrome. LA = left atrium; LV = left ventricle; RV = right ventricle. B, Close-up of the ring abscess. The cusps are slightly thickened by fibrous tissue and were oriented right and left. The patient was in her usual state of health until approximately 6 weeks before death, when she developed abdominal pain and was found to have a large spleen. A bone marrow biopsy was done and it was consistent with multiple myeloma. Several days before death she lost consciousness and was hospitalized. Blood cultures grew alpha streptococcus. She died shortly thereafter. At autopsy, the cardiac infection was limited to the aortic valve and adjacent para-aortic areas. The spleen weighed 1850 g and the liver, 2600 g. The heart weighed 460 g and was devoid of myocardial lesions except in the area adjacent to the aortic valve.

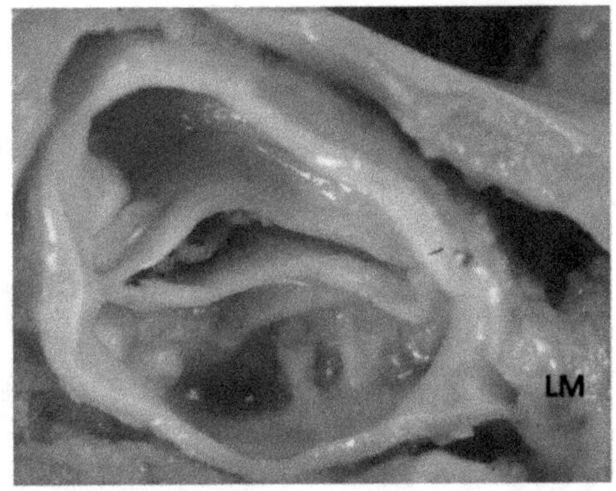

FIGURE 13. Active IE involving a normally functioning bicuspid aortic valve. View of the aortic valve from above showing vegetation between the 2 cusps but no vegetative material on the aortic aspect of either cusp. The patient was a 52-year-old man who had undergone bone marrow transplantation 1 month before death because of myelodysplastic syndrome. After the bone marrow transplant he never left the hospital. Infective endocarditis was never diagnosed clinically. Necropsy disclosed vegetation on each of the 2 cusps of the bicuspid valve, and the cusps were located anterior and posterior. The heart weighed 610 g. LM = left main coronary artery.

28 unicuspid valves) and 28 (90%) involved a bicuspid valve (28 [15%] of the 190 bicuspid valves). Of the 31 cases, 26 (84%) were men (15% of total men), and 5 (16%) were women (12% of total women). Various clinical and morphologic findings in the 31 patients with active and healed IE are summarized in Table 4.

Hemodynamic Data

Of the 218 patients, hemodynamic data were available in 36 patients (17%): 34 had AS, with peak transvalvular gradients ranging from 11 to 148 mm Hg (mean, 69; median, 69 mm Hg).

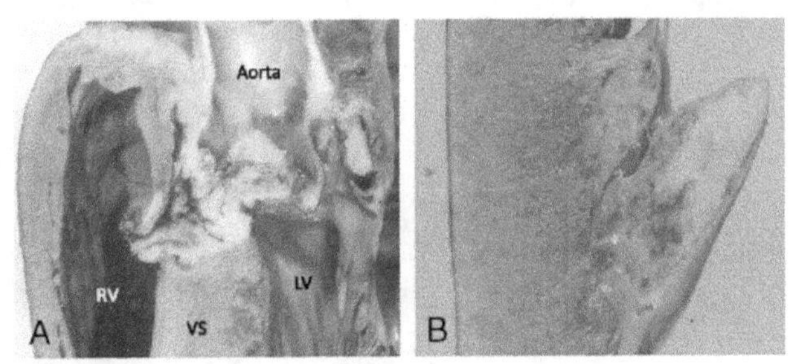

FIGURE 14. Active IE. A, Longitudinal cut of the aortic valve and adjacent structures showing severe destruction of the aortic valve cusps and large ring abscesses both anteriorly burrowing into the right ventricle (RV) and posteriorly pushing toward the left atrium in a 30-year-old man who was a habitual fingernail biter to the extent that his fingernail area would bleed. X-ray of the heart at necropsy showed calcific deposits in the aortic valve. LV = left ventricle. VS = ventricular septum. B, A left ventricular papillary muscle that is necrotic due to extremely diminished profusion of the left ventricle. The epicardial coronary arteries were normal. The patient was hospitalized 16 days before death because of fever, chills, malaise, and myalgia. Several blood cultures grew *Staphylococcus aureus*. He developed several signs typical of active IE. An electrocardiogram showed right bundle branch block, and an echocardiogram suggested a bicuspid aortic valve. The heart at autopsy weighed 560 g.

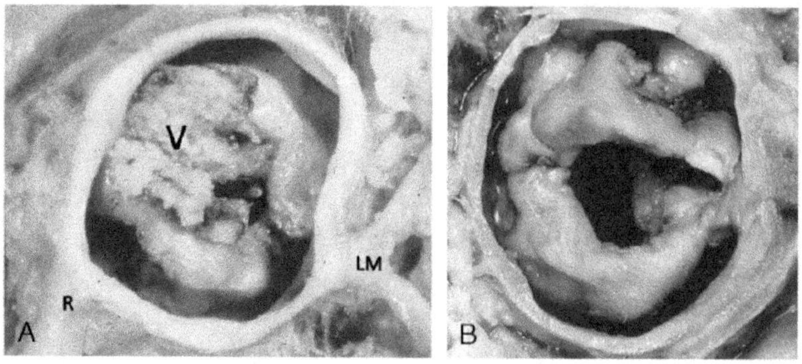

FIGURE 15. Active IE superimposed on a stenotic unicuspid unicommissural aortic valve. A, View of the valve from above showing vegetation (V) further narrowing the orifice. LM = left main coronary artery; R = right coronary artery. B, View of the valve after excising the vegetation showing the underlying stenotic valve with heavy calcific deposits. The patient was a 35-year-old man, an opiate addict who became ill 6 weeks before death, including the last 4 weeks in a hospital. Despite septic emboli in the kidneys and spleen, blood cultures throughout his hospitalization were negative. At necropsy, the heart weighed 550 g.

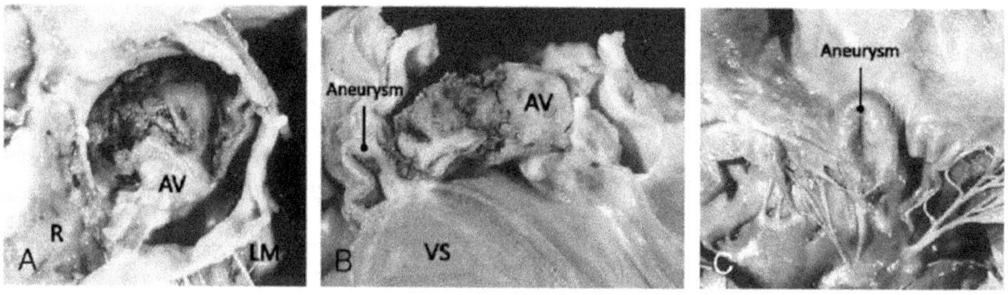

FIGURE 16. Active IE superimposed on a stenotic bicuspid aortic valve. A, Aortic valve from above showing vegetation superimposed on the right cusp of a congenitally bicuspid aortic valve in a 67-year-old man who was known to have AS and had some evidence of heart failure for at least a year before his final illness, which was rapidly progressing heart failure. Calcific deposits are present in both right and left cusps but the vegetative material involves the right cusp much more than the left. AV = aortic valve; LM = left main coronary artery; R = right coronary artery. B, Longitudinal section across the aortic valve showing the large vegetation involving mainly the right cusp with rather heavy calcific deposits in the left cusp. A ring abscess is also present in the base of the aorta. VS = ventricular septum. C, View of the tricuspid valve, right atrium, and right ventricle showing an aneurysm of the membranaceous ventricular septum bulging into the right side of the heart. Blood cultures were all positive for alpha hemolytic streptococcus, and the patient was treated with penicillin. During the infection his electrocardiogram changed from prolonged P-R interval to complete heart block. Not only did he have evidence of AS, but mitral regurgitation also developed during the infection. This is an example of IE superimposed on a heavily calcified stenotic aortic valve. The infection rapidly spread to the soft tissue both above and below the valve creating a ring abscess of the aorta and an aneurysm of the membranaceous ventricular septum.

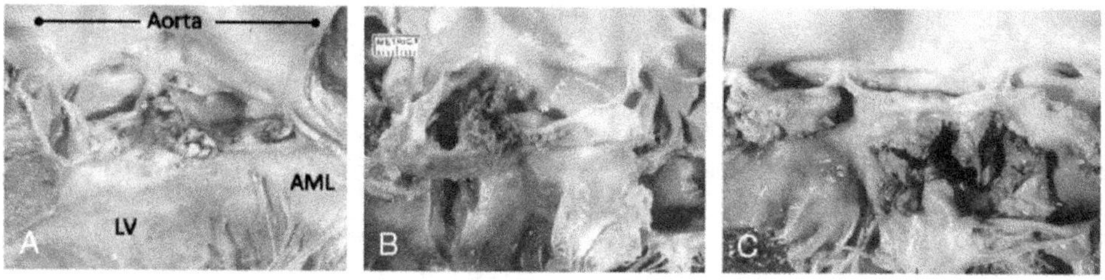

FIGURE 17. Active IE: opened aortic valves exposing vegetations that have destroyed the 2 aortic valve cusps to varying degrees. A, Valve in a 35-year-old man who had alpha streptococcus IE with a ring abscess and severe AR. This patient was an opiate addict who probably had infection in the past that healed because the heart at necropsy weighed 760 g. The cusps are located anterior and posterior, and a raphe is present in the anterior cusp. The infection caused severe AR. AML = anterior mitral leaflet; LV = left ventricle. B, Valve in a 60-year-old man. The cusps are located anterior and posterior, and vegetative material is particularly heavy in the area of the raphe. This patient had the triad of active IE, meningitis, and pneumonitis. The vegetative material had burrowed into the aortic wall causing a large ring abscess and complete heart block. The patient was a habitual alcoholic. The last episode of IE produced acute symptoms beginning 7 days before death. Blood cultures grew *Streptococcus pneumoniae*. Complete heart block developed 2 days before death. Six months before death he had undergone cardiac catheterization because of severe AR: an 11 mm Hg peak transvalvular pressure gradient and severe AR were found. C, Bicuspid valve in a 45-year-old man with pre-existing aortic valve stenosis who was hospitalized 12 days before death because of confusion, fever, and leukocytosis. Echocardiogram showed vegetation on the aortic valve, and blood cultures grew *Streptococcus milleri*. Computed tomogram (CT) disclosed multiple cerebral infarcts. The patient weighed >135 kg. At autopsy, the heart weighed 920 g. The 2 aortic valve cusps were calcified. The vegetative material had burrowed into the right ventricular cavity. Emboli were present in the brain. Additionally, there was diffuse fibrinous pericarditis. Both left ventricular papillary muscles were necrotic in the absence of significant coronary disease. Both aortic valve cusps were perforated by the vegetation.

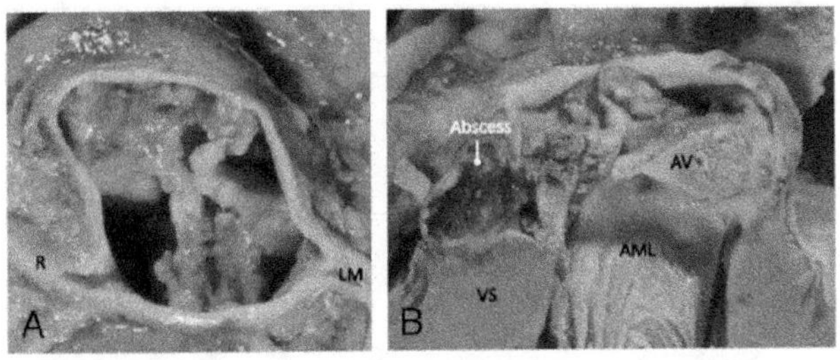

FIGURE 18. Active IE superimposed on a heavily calcified stenotic bicuspid aortic valve. A, Valve from above with vegetative material involving the cuspal margins with underlying heavy calcific deposits. The cusps are located right and left. LM = left main coronary artery; R = right coronary artery. B, Longitudinal cut of the aortic valve area showing destruction by vegetative material of 1 cusp with extension into the ventricular septum (VS) producing a large ring abscess. The aortic valve (AV) is heavily calcified and was quite stenotic. At autopsy, the heart weighed 850 g. The patient was a 54-year-old man who was known to have a precordial murmur for at least 10 years. He developed exertional dyspnea 2 years before death. Cardiac catheterization 2 months before death disclosed severe AS. The aortic valve could not be crossed by the catheter, and he was discharged to have his carious teeth extracted before planned aortic valve replacement. He developed alpha streptococcus endocarditis with onset of symptoms 23 days before death. While being treated on the ward he had sudden fatal cardiac arrest. Both left ventricular papillary muscles were necrotic. AML = anterior mitral leaflet.

TABLE 4. Patients Having Infective Endocarditis (IE) on a Unicuspid or Bicuspid Aortic Valve (n = 31)

	Infective Endocarditis	
Variable	Active n = 25 (81%)	Healed n = 6 (19%)
Unicuspid aortic valve	2	1
Bicuspid aortic valve	23	5
Aortic valve function before IE		
Normal	16	4
Stenosis ± regurgitation	9	2
Pure regurgitation	0	0
Aortic valve function after IE		
Normal	5	0
Stenosis ± regurgitation	9	2
Pure regurgitation*	11	4
Predisposing factors		
Intravenous opiate use	5	0
Alcoholism	4	1
Dental procedure	4	1
Stepped on a nail	1†	0
Habitual fingernail biter	1	0
Heart block		
First degree	1	0
Right bundle branch	1	0
Complete	2	0
Infected aneurysm		
Cerebral	3	0
Aorta	4	2

*The 15 patients with pure aortic regurgitation as a result of infective endocarditis had normally functioning aortic valves prior to infection.

†Patient is also an alcoholic.

TABLE 5. Men With Bicuspid Aortic Valves and Coronary Artery Bypass Grafting (n = 12)

Patient	Aortic Valve Function*	Age (Years)	Total Number of CABG Procedures	Total Number of Distal Anastamoses	Interval From Last (First) CABG to Death (Months)	Heart Weight (g)	Cause of Cardiac Death
1	Normal	43	1	3	0	530	CABG
2	Normal	62	1	4	<1	470	CABG
3	Normal	63	1	4	110	690	CAD-IC
4	Normal	63	2	—	<1 (—)	590	CABG
5	Normal	69	1	2	108	700	CAD-IC
6	Normal	71	2	7	<1 (84)	650	CABG
7	Stenotic	49	1	2	96	525	CAD-IC
8	Stenotic	53	2	3	0 (132)	460	CABG
9	Stenotic	56	1	2	17	475	AS-SD
10	Stenotic	58	1	—	2	—	CABG
11	Stenotic	68	1	4	17	550	CAD-IC
12	Stenotic	69	2	4	48 (132)	760	CAD-SD

Abbreviations: AS = aortic stenosis, CABG = coronary artery bypass grafting, CAD = coronary artery disease, IC = ischemic cardiomyopathy, SD = sudden death, — = no information available.

*Prior to infective endocarditis.

TABLE 6. Causes or Modes of Death in Patients Studied at Necropsy Having a Unicuspid or Bicuspid Aotic Valve (n = 218)

Variable	Aortic Valve Function Prior to Infective Endocarditis			Total	
	Normal n = 74 (34%)	Stenosis n = 142 (65%)	Pure Regurgitation n = 2 (1%)	n = 218 (100%)	
Cardiac					
Aortic valve disease					
Heart failure	0	62		62	
Infective endocarditis					
Active	16*	9		25	
Healed	4†	2‡		6	124
Sudden	0	21	1§	22	(57%)
Cardiac catheterization	0	7		7	
Anesthesia induction for aortic valve replacement	0	1		1	
Ruptured sinus of Valsalva aneurysm	1	0		1	
Coronary artery disease					
Acute myocardial infarction	2	5		7	
Ischemic cardiomyopathy	3	2		5	25
Sudden	3	4		7	(11%)
Early post coronary bypass¶	4	2		6	
Other					
Hypertrophic cardiomyopathy (sudden)	1	0		1	
SUBTOTAL	34	115	1	150 (69%)	
Non-cardiac vascular					
Ascending aortic tear (±dissection)	12**	4	1	17	
Cerebrovascular accident	0	1		1	
Pulmonary embolism	1	0		1	
Early postop after vascular surgery	0	3‖		3	
SUBTOTAL	13	8	1	22 (10%)	
Non-cardiac non-vascular					
Cancer	14	3		17	
Suicide	2	0		2	
Trauma	3#	0		3	
Renal failure	1	3		4	
Pancreatitis (alcoholism)	1	0		1	
Gastrointestinal hemorrhage	0	1		1	
Food aspiration	0	1		1	
Hypothermia	0	1		1	
Cirrhosis	1	0		1	
Parenchymal lung disease	1	1		2	
Parkinson's disease	1	0		1	
Early postop after bowel surgery	0	2		2	
SUBTOTAL	24	12	0	36 (17%)	
Cause unclear					
Sudden death outside hospital, cause unclear	2	0		2	
Unknown	1	7		8	
SUBTOTAL	3	7	0	10 (5%)	

*The aortic valve appeared to have been normal before the active infective endocarditis (IE) appeared. Of the 16 patients, all but 1 died of the active infection; the remaining patient developed IE after a bone marrow transplant for myelodysplastic syndrome, and the aortic valve appeared funtionally normal despite the infection.

†The IE caused perforation in 1 or both aortic valve cusps in 3 of these 4 patients leading to severe aortic regurgitation (AR) in each. The remaining patient had no cuspal perforations, but had a prolapsed aortic valve, several ruptured chords of anterior mitral leaflet, and a saccular aneurysm of ascending aorta causing residual AR from IE; he died suddenly; he also had coarctation of the aorta.

‡The degree of stenosis probably was worsened by the superimposed IE which healed in each.

§Patient had massive cardiomegaly: heart weight 920 g. Of the 218 patients, 5 (2%) had hearts weighing >900 g. One had AR secondary to healed cuspal perforation from IE; 3 others had severely stenotic aortic valves, and of these 3, 1 had superimposed IE.

‖One patient died 1 day after resection of abdominal aortic aneurysm; 1 patient died 3 days after femoral-popliteal bypass grafting; 1 patient died 6 hours after axillo-femoral bypass grafting.

¶A total of 12 patients (6%) had coronary artery bypass grafting (CABG): 6 died within 2 months of the last CABG operation and are included here; of the other 6 patients having had CABG, all died late: 2 with ischemic cardiomyopathy (IC) and a normally functioning aortic valve; 2 with IC and a stenotic aortic valve; 1 died suddenly secondary to aortic stenosis, and 1 with a stenotic aortic valve died suddenly secondary to coronary artery disease.

#One patient, a habitual alcoholic, died from injuries in a single-car accident; the other 2 from broken necks from falls. None had significant coronary disease.

**One patient died during operative repair of ascending aortic dissection, and another, 3 weeks after operative repair for dissection.

The peak transvalvular gradient was ≤50 mm Hg in 12 patients (35%) and >50 mm Hg in 22 patients (65%). Neither of the 2 patients with normally functioning aortic valves had a gradient across the valve. The heart weights in the patients with hemodynamically confirmed AS ranged from 410 to 880 g (mean, 629; median, 655 g).

Coronary Artery Bypass Grafting

Twelve (6%) (all men) of the 218 patients had coronary artery bypass grafting (CABG), in 4 patients on 2 occasions (Table 5). In none of the 16 CABG operations on those 12 patients was a procedure performed on the aortic valve. At necropsy, the bicuspid aortic valve appeared to have functioned normally in 6, and to be stenotic in the other 6. Two of the latter 6 had CABG twice. The presence of AS in these latter 6 patients was either not diagnosed at the time of CABG or the degree of AS was not considered severe enough to warrant aortic valve replacement at the time of CABG.

Causes of Death

Causes of death are divided into 4 major groups: cardiac, noncardiac vascular, noncardiac and nonvascular, and cause unclear (Table 6). Of the 218 patients, death was attributed to aortic valve disease in 124 patients (57%), to the consequences of coronary arterial atherosclerosis in 25 (11%), and to hypertrophic cardiomyopathy in 1. Thus, death was attributed to cardiac disease in 150 (69%) of the 218 patients. Death in 22 patients (10%) was attributed to noncardiac vascular causes, and in 36 patients (17%) to neither cardiac nor vascular causes. Among the 22 patients with noncardiac vascular causes of death, 17 (8% of the total) died of tears in the ascending aorta with resulting fatal hemopericardium; 14 had tears with dissection and 3 had tears without dissection[86] (Table 7; Figure 19).

Reasons Aortic Valve Operation Was Not Performed

We considered the reasons an aortic valve operation was not performed in these patients (Table 8). Of the 131 patients with AS without superimposed IE, 25 patients (19%) died suddenly outside the hospital, and most of them previously were asymptomatic. Another 32 patients (24%) died before 1970, a period when aortic valve replacement essentially was limited to only those with severe symptoms and severe AS. Most patients with acute IE were not operated on because their physicians believed aortic valve replacement to be fruitless in the circumstances.

Heart Weight and Its Relation to Aortic Valve Structure, Valve Function, and Sex

Heart weight data were available in 178 (82%) of the 218 patients (Tables 2, 3, and 9). The mean heart weights were greater in patients with unicuspid aortic valves than in those with bicuspid aortic valves (603 ± 143 g vs. 551 ± 164 g, respectively; $p = 0.14$); in patients with stenotic compared to those with normally functioning valves (598 ± 152 g vs. 477 ± 148 g, respectively; $p < 0.0001$); and in men compared to women (586 ± 156 g [270–1050 g] vs. 433 ± 136 g [170–730], respectively; $p < 0.0001$).

Orientation of the 2 Cusps and Presence of a Raphe Among Patients With Bicuspid Valves and Relation to Valve Complication

In 69% of the valves, 1 cusp was located anterior, and the other posterior, such that both coronary arteries arose from the anterior cusp; in 31% of cases, 1 cusp was right and the other, left, such that 1 coronary artery arose from 1 cusp and the other

TABLE 7. Patients Studied at Necropsy Having a Unicuspid or Bicuspid Aortic Valve and Tear in Ascending Aorta (n = 17)

Patient	Aortic Valve Function*	Age (Years)	Gender	Heart Weight (g)	Number of Aortic Valve Cusps	Aortic Valve Orientation	Raphe Present	SH
Aortic Tear With Dissection								
1	Normal	21	M	450	2	A/P	+	+
2	Normal	30	M	410	2	A/P	+	—
3†	Normal	48	M	—	2	A/P	+	+
4	Normal	52	M	530	2	A/P	+	+
5†	Normal	57	M	—	2	A/P	+	+
6	Normal	62	M	690	2	A/P	0	—
7	Normal	67	M	—	2	R/L	+	+
8	Normal	69	F	—	2	A/P	+	0
9	Normal	71	F	430	2	A/P	+	—
10	Regurgitant	32	M	470	1	—	—	—
11	Stenotic	25	M	610	1	—	—	—
12	Stenotic	69	F	400	2	A/P	0	—
13	Stenotic	70	M	390	2	R/L	+	+
14	Stenotic	82	M	590	2	A/P	+	+
Aortic Tear Without Dissection								
15	Normal	21	M	450	2	A/P	+	—
16	Normal	32	F	310	2	A/P	+	—
17	Normal	32	M	510	2	A/P	0	—

Abbreviations: — = no information available or not applicable, 0 = absent, + = present, A/P = anterior/posterior, R/L = right/left, SH = systemic hypertension by history.

*Prior to infective endocarditis.

†Patient had operative intervention for acute aortic dissection.

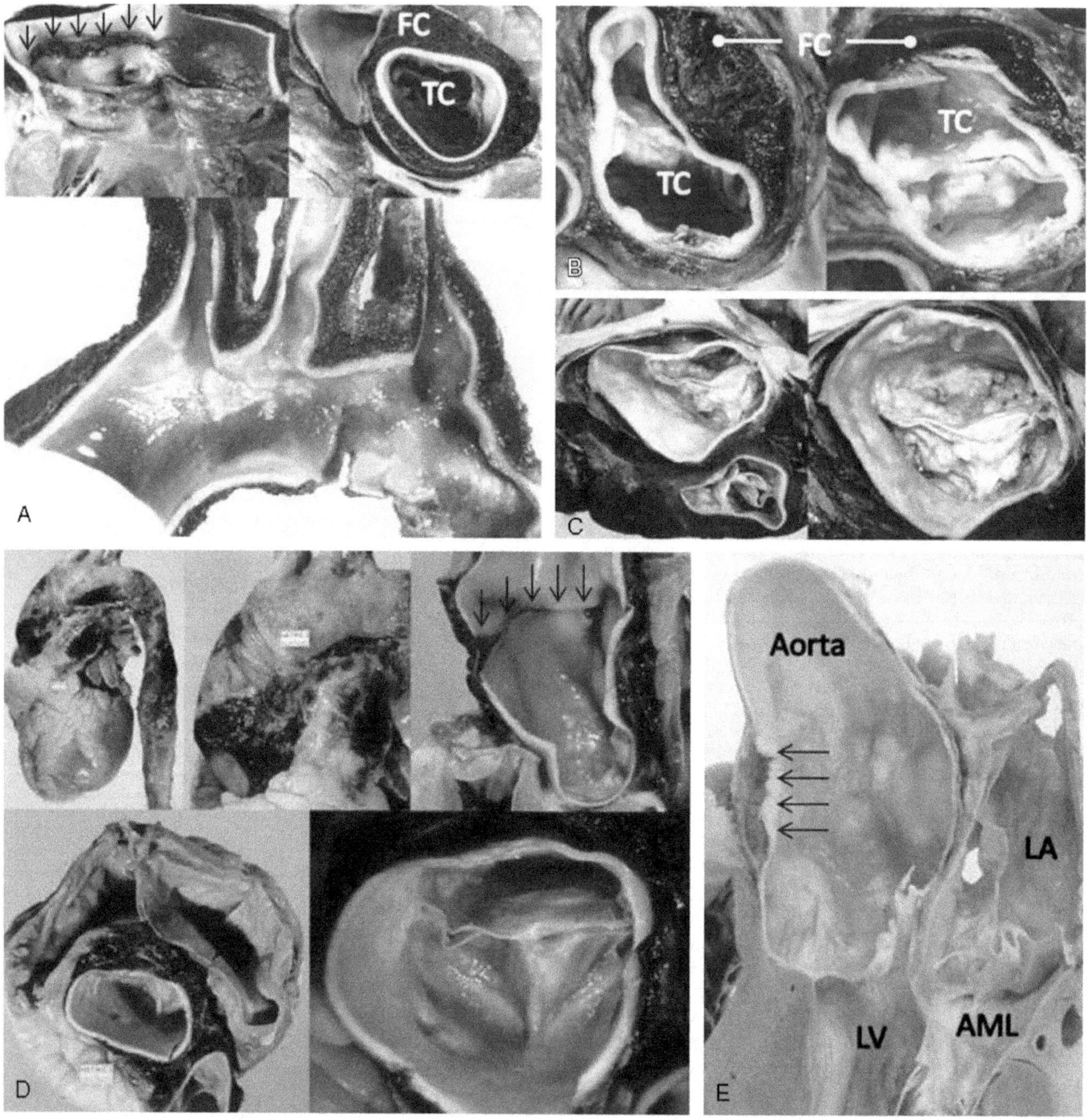

FIGURE 19. Acute aortic dissection with tear (arrows) in ascending aorta in 5 patients with congenitally bicuspid aortic valves. All patients died from rupture of the false channel (FC) into the pericardial sac. A, Views of the opened bicuspid aortic valve and a transverse tear just above that with hematoma in the false channel of ascending aorta and in the false channel of each of the arch arteries and in a portion of descending thoracic aorta. This woman had Turner syndrome. The aortic valve had functioned normally. The heart weighed 310 g. The medial dissection of aorta extended into its adventitia and then into the adventitia of the pulmonary trunk, which shares a common adventitia with the aorta. TC = true channel. B, Two views of hematoma in the false channel just above the aortic valve (left) and at the level of the aortic valve (right). The true channel is indented by the hematoma in the false channel. The bicuspid valve is calcified and stenotic. The heart weighed 385 g. C, Stenotic bicuspid valve with a hematoma in the false channel and fatal rupture into the pericardial sac. The valve is stenotic. Symptoms of the acute dissection began 36 hours before death. The dissection was limited to ascending aorta. A large tear was present in the distal ascending aorta. The heart weighed 585 g. D, Bicuspid valve that functioned normally in a 69-year-old woman who developed chest and neck pain a few hours before dying suddenly in the hospital. The dissection was limited to ascending aorta. The dissection extended into the adventitia of aorta and then into the adventitia of pulmonary trunk. E, Longitudinal view of ascending aorta, left atrium (LA), and left ventricle (LV) showing a false channel in the anterior of the aorta just above the 1 aortic valve commissure. The patient had an aortic isthmus coarctation that had been resected earlier in life. The proximal ascending aorta had a diameter of 8.5 cm. The heart weighed 690 g. The bicuspid aortic valve was devoid of calcium and appeared to have functioned normally. AML = anterior mitral leaflet.

TABLE 8. Reasons Patients With Aortic Stenosis or Pure Aortic Regurgitation Did Not Undergo Aortic Valve Replacement (Excludes 74 Patients With Normally Functioning Aortic Valves With or Without Superimposed Infective Endocarditis)

Variable	AS (n = 142)	AR Without IE (n = 2)
Not diagnosed during life	43	1
Active infective endocarditis	9	0
Diagnosed clinically but		
Died before 1962 (before AVR established)	5	0
Severe heart failure/too sick to have AVR	23	0
Another condition preventing AVR	8	0
AVR planned but died before operation	10	1
Refused AVR	7	0
Refused cardiac catheterization	1	0
Death in the cardiac catheterization lab	7	0
AS not severe enough to warrant AVR or severity of AS not appreciated clinically	12	0
Reason unclear/died suddenly	5	0
Unknown	12	0

Abbreviations: AR = aortic regurgitation, AS = aortic stenosis, AVR = aortic valve replacement, IE = infective endocarditis.

TABLE 9. Comparison of Heart Weights According to Gender, and Structure and Function of the Congenitally Malformed Aortic Valve (n = 178*)

Variable	Heart Weight (g) Mean ± SD [Median] (Range), Number (%) of Enlarged Hearts†
Total	
Men (n = 146)	586 ± 156 [570] (270–1050), n = 127 (87%)
Women (n = 32)	433 ± 136 [413] (170–730), n = 21 (66%)
Valve structure	
Unicuspid	
Men (n = 23)	607 ± 144 [610] (320–880), n = 21 (91%)
Women (n = 1)	510, n = 1 (100%)
Bicuspid	
Men (n = 123)	582 ± 159 [550] (270–1050), n = 106 (86%)
Women (n = 31)	431 ± 138 [410] (170–730), n = 20 (65%)
Aortic valve function	
Aortic stenosis	
Men (n = 95)	622 ± 149 [610] (320–1050), n = 88 (93%)
Women (n = 20)	491 ± 130 [478] (300–730), n = 17 (85%)
Pure aortic regurgitation secondary to IE	
Men (n = 12)	583 ± 175 [545] (405–1010), n = 12 (100%)
Women (n = 3)	350, 400, 460, n = 2 (67%)
Unassociated with IE	
Men (n = 2)	920, 470, n = 2 (100%)
Women (n = 0)	—
Functionally normal	
Men (n = 37)	487 ± 120 [470] (270–700), n = 25 (68%)
Women (n = 9)	314 ± 81 [310] (170–430), n = 2 (22%)
Infective endocarditis	
Active	
Men (n = 21)	571 ± 147 [540] (375–920), n = 20 (95%)
Women (n = 4)	363 ± 93 [375] (240–460), n = 2 (50%)
Healed	
Men (n = 4)	670 ± 245 [620] (430–1010), n = 4 (100%)
Women (n = 1)	510, n = 1 (100%)

— = not applicable.

*Heart weights were only available in 178 (82%) of the 218 patients included in this study.

†Hearts weighing >350 g in women and >400 g in men.

coronary artery from the other cusp (Tables 3 and 10). A raphe (false commissure) was present in at least 83%: if the configuration of the cusps was anterior and posterior, the raphe, if present, was always in the anterior cusp; if the cusps were configured right and left, the raphe, if present, was always in the right cusp.

Associated Congenital Cardiovascular Anomalies

Six patients had aortic isthmic coarctation, with operative excision in 2 early in life; 5 patients had a congenitally bicuspid pulmonic valve, and 1 had a quadricuspid pulmonic valve, all of which functioned normally and otherwise were structurally normal; 1 patient had a parachute mitral valve or single papillary muscle syndrome (Shone syndrome); 2 patients had Turner syndrome; and 4 had a congenital coronary anomaly (Table 11). None of the coronary anomalies was clinically important.

DISCUSSION

We describe here the findings in 218 patients studied at necropsy with congenitally unicuspid (n = 28) or bicuspid (n = 190) aortic valves. Of the 4 major complications of this congenital anomaly—valve stenosis, pure valve regurgitation, valve infection, and aortic dilatation—most (142 [65%]) had AS including 27 (96%) of the 28 patients with unicuspid valves and 115 (61%) of the 190 patients with bicuspid valves. Of the 17 with pure AR, 15 developed it as a consequence of IE and 2 as a consequence of the aortic valve malformation without superimposed IE; of these 17 patients, 1 had a unicuspid valve and 16 (94%) had a bicuspid valve. Possibly the most intriguing observation in this study was the finding of 59 patients (27%) (aged 21–82 yr; mean, 51 ± 16 yr) with congenitally bicuspid valves that appeared to have functioned normally during their entire lifetimes. Although 31 (14%) of the 218 patients developed IE at some time, the infection was superimposed on an already stenotic valve in 11, and on a previously normally functioning valve in 20. Of the latter 20 patients, 15 developed AR as a consequence of IE; of the other 5, all of whom died during the active infection, none apparently had AR during life as a consequence of IE.

Although several studies have discussed the natural history of AS, particularly of congenital origin,[11,16,21,22,32,45,46,55,58,59,84,89] to our knowledge only 4 reports have described the natural history of patients with bicuspid aortic valve. Roberts[58] in 1970 described at necropsy 85 patients in whom he found a congenitally bicuspid aortic valve, but only 42 (19% of 218) of them are included in the present study because the other 43 patients underwent operative therapy for AS (n = 40) or pure AR (n = 3). Nevertheless, as far as we know it was the first study to separate the patients into those with AS, pure AR, and IE. Nearly all of the AS patients had severe AS (peak transvalvular gradient ranging from 12 to 165 mm Hg [mean, 92 mm Hg]).

Fenoglio and colleagues[22] in 1977 described 152 patients with congenitally bicuspid aortic valves studied at autopsy. Of their 43 patients with AS, 23 (53%) had "died with congestive heart failure or during attempted surgical repair of the stenotic aortic valve." Therefore, their "natural history" was also interrupted by this iatrogenic event, namely aortic valve surgery. Nevertheless, their study is the closest to the present study, and some similarities and differences are shown in Table 12. The percentage of patients with AS and pure AR, for reasons unclear, is quite different between the 2 studies. It appears that their study was based on examination of observations recorded in autopsy reports prepared by a number of different prosectors.

TABLE 10. Comparison of Various Variables Among Patients With Bicuspid Aortic Valves Oriented Right to Left vs Anterior to Posterior (n = 153)

	Aortic Valve Orientation	
Variable	**Right/Left, n = 47 (31%)**	**Anterior/Posterior, n = 106 (59%)**
Age at death (years)		
Mean ± SD [median]	53 ± 16 [57]*	56 ± 15 [59]*
(Range)	(23–82)	(21–89)
Gender†		
Men	38 (84%)	79 (75%)
Women	7 (16%)	26 (25%)
Aortic valve function (before infective endocarditis)		
Normal	20 (43%)	43 (41%)
Stenosis	27 (57%)	62 (58%)
Pure regurgitation	0	1 (1%)
Infective endocarditis		
Active	11 (23%)	7 (7%)
Healed	2 (4%)	3 (3%)
Infective endocarditis superimposed on a:		
Previously normally functioning valve	10 (21%)	7 (7%)
Previously stenotic valve	3 (6%)	3 (3%)
Previously purely regurgitant valve	0	0
Heart weight (g)		
Mean ± SD [median]	545 ± 163 [505]‡	535 ± 165 [510]‡
(Range)	(320–1010)	(170–1050)

*-*p - value = 0.27

† Data missing on 3 patients.

‡-‡p - value = 0.76.

TABLE 11. Patients Studied at Necropsy Having a Unicuspid or Bicuspid Aortic Valve and Other Congenital Cardiovascular Malformations (n = 19)

Congenital Abnormality	Aortic Valve Function*	Age (Years)	Gender	Number of AV Cusps	Aortic Valve Orientation	Raphe Present	Infective Endocarditis		Heart Weight (g)
							Active	Healed	
Coarctation of aorta									
1†,‡	Normal	21	M	2	A/P	+	0	0	450
2	Normal	30	M	2	A/P	+	0	0	410
3	Normal	36	M	2	A/P	+	+	0	500
4	Stenotic	39	M	2	—	—	0	0	1000
5†	Normal	46	M	2	A/P	0	0	+	650
6	Normal	62	M	2	A/P	0	0	0	690
Coronary anomalies									
Hypoplasia									
RCA and LMCA									
7	Stenotic	26	M	1	—	—	0	0	760
High takeoff									
LMCA									
8	Normal	29	M	2	A/P	+	+	0	500
LMCA and RCA									
9	Normal	40	M	2	A/P	+	0	0	320
RCA									
10	Normal	52	M	2	—	—	+	0	610
Pulmonic valve									
Bicuspid									
11	Stenotic	34	M	1	—	—	0	0	570
12	Stenotic	37	M	2	R/L	+	0	0	860
13	Stenotic	47	F	2	R/L	+	0	0	340
14	Normal	47	M	2	R/L	+	0	+	590
15	Stenotic	66	M	2	R/L	+	0	0	—
Quadricuspid									
16	Normal	57	F	2	A/P	0	0	0	—
Shone syndrome									
17	Normal	30	M	2	R/L	+	0	0	395
Turner syndrome									
18	Normal	32	F	2	A/P	+	0	0	310
19	Normal	36	F	2	R/L	+	+	0	460

Abbreviations: — = not applicable or no information available, 0 = absent, + = present, A/P = anterior/posterior, AV = aortic valve, LMCA = left main coronary artery, RCA = right coronary artery, R/L = right/left.

*Prior to infective endocarditis.

†Early operative intervention for isthmic coarctation.

‡Patient also has a separate left main and circumflex coronary ostia.

TABLE 12. Comparison of the Present Necropsy Study to the Earlier Study (1977) by Fenoglio et al

Aortic Valve Function (After Infective Endocarditis)	Fenoglio Series (n = 152)	Roberts Series (n = 218)
Aortic stenosis	43 (28%)	142 (65%)
Age (year) (mean)	28–89 (55)	23–89 (59)
Men	40 (93%)	110 (77%)
Infective endocarditis		
Acute	5 (12%)	9 (6%)
Healed	4 (9%)	2 (1%)
Coarctation of aorta	5 (12%)	1 (1%)
Heart weight (g) (mean)	320–900 (603)	300–1050 (598)
Unicuspid aortic valves	0	27 (19%)
Aortic valve calcium	43 (100%)	142 (100%)
Pure aortic regurgitation	61 (40%)	17 (8%)
Age (year) (mean)	21–69 (35)	22–52 (37)
Men	61 (100%)	14 (82%)
Infective endocarditis		
Acute	28 (46%)	11 (65%)
Healed	19 (31%)	4 (24%)
Coarctation of aorta	6 (10%)	1 (6%)
Heart weight (g) (mean)	310–1300 (611)	350–1010 (569)
Unicuspid aortic valves	0	1 (6%)
Aortic valve calcium	25 (41%)	4 (24%)
Functionally normal	48 (32%)	59 (27%)
Age (year) (mean)	20–81 (48)	21–82 (51)
Men	41 (85%)	45 (76%)
Infective endocarditis*		
Acute	5 (10%)	5 (8%)
Healed	0	0
Coarctation of aorta	7 (15%)	4 (7%)
Heart weight (g) (mean)	200–675 (386)	170–700 (453)
Unicuspid aortic valves	0	0
Aortic valve calcium	7 (15%)	15 (25%)

*Infective endocarditis on a previously normally functioning aortic valve resulting in no valvular dysfunction.

Mills and associates[46] in 1978 described 41 patients with "non-invasive" evidence of a bicuspid aortic valve and followed them for 5–25 years (mean, 11 yr). Two patients underwent an aortic valve operation for severe AS; 2 developed pure AR; 3 developed IE resulting in AR in 2 and death in 1; 5 developed mild AS; 3 died (none as a consequence of aortic valve disease); and the clinical status did not change in the remaining 26.

The study by Michelena and colleagues[45] in 2008 from the Mayo Clinic was an analysis of 212 asymptomatic patients (mean age, 32 ± 20 yr) in whom a bicuspid aortic valve was found by echocardiogram. Survival 20 years after diagnosis was 90% ± 3%. The natural history centered on the status (operated, unoperated, dead, symptomatic, asymptomatic) 20 years after diagnosis.

We found only 1 study that included any natural history information on patients with unicuspid aortic valves, the study by Falcone and colleagues[21] in 1971 who described at necropsy 21 patients with stenotic unicuspid aortic valves, 3 of whom had undergone an aortic valve operation. Their ages (17 males) ranged from 16 to 62 years (mean, 44 yr). The transvalvular peak gradients (13 patients) ranged from 15 to 158 mm Hg (mean, 87 mm Hg). The heart weights ranged from 400 to 800 g (mean, 590 g).

Today, most congenitally malformed aortic valves are encountered by echocardiogram, computed tomography, or magnetic resonance imaging and not at operation or autopsy.[62] Although prophylactic use of antibiotics to prevent infectious endocarditis has not been recommended,[102] the identification of a congenitally malformed aortic valve allows patients and physicians to have a heightened awareness for symptoms that may suggest valve infection. Further, noninvasive imaging can help determine the need for, and proper timing of, valve surgery, and can identify aortic dilatation, which often occurs without causing symptoms. Because aortic valve malformations may occur in families, the finding in 1 family member should probably suggest a search in other family members.[27]

It is also well to keep in mind that another malformation of the aortic valve, namely aortic valve atresia, is the worst known cardiac condition because it allows the shortest lifespan. Indeed, aortic valve atresia is the most common cause of death in the first week of life.[85]

Some positive features of the present study include the following: 1) a large number of unoperated cases were collected during the 50 years in which aortic valve commissurotomy and replacement operations were available; 2) all cases were studied by a single investigator (WCR) and data were not simply retrieved from autopsy protocols prepared by a variety of physicians with varying expertise in cardiovascular disease; 3) most of the patients appeared to have had severe AS or AR; and 4) natural history data were presented on patients with unicuspid aortic valves.

Deficiencies or limitations of the present study include the following: 1) hemodynamic and echocardiographic data were available in a minority of patients; 2) 12 (6%) of the 218 patients studied had had CABG but no aortic valve surgery (possibly considered a "contaminant"); and 3) despite an extensive examination of a large number of patients, all studied at necropsy, the reason that some patients with bicuspid valves developed AS, some developed IE, a few developed AR without superimposed IE, and some (59 [31%] of the 190 with bicuspid valves) never developed an aortic valve complication, was not forthcoming.

Conclusion

In conclusion, the current study highlights several important findings in patients with congenitally malformed aortic valves. A patient with a unicuspid or bicuspid aortic valve 1) may go through life without ever developing dysfunction of the valve (27% of the total); 2) will most likely develop AS as a result of the congenital malformation (65% of the total); 3) is most likely male (80% of the total); 4) appears to be highly susceptible to IE (14% of the total); 5) is at a relatively high risk of developing aortic dissection or tears in the ascending aorta (8% of the total); and 6) is at an increased risk of dying from complications related to the aortic valve (57% of the total).

REFERENCES

1. Abbott ME. Coarctation of the aorta of the adult type. II. A statistical study and historical retrospect of 200 recorded cases, with autopsy, of stenosis or obliteration of the descending arch in subjects above the age of two years. *Am Heart J.* 1928;3:574–628.
2. Anderson MW, Kelsey JR Jr, Edwards JE. Clinical and pathological considerations in cases of calcific aortic stenosis. *JAMA.* 1952;149:9–15.

3. Arnett EN, Roberts WC. Active infective endocarditis: a clinicopathologic analysis of 137 necropsy patients. *Curr Probl Cardiol*. 1976;1:1–76.

4. Arnett EN, Roberts WC. Valve ring abscess in active infective endocarditis. Frequency, location, and clues to clinical diagnosis from the study of 95 necropsy patients. *Circulation*. 1976;54:140–145.

5. Arnett EN, Roberts WC. Pathology of active infective endocarditis: a necropsy analysis of 192 patients. *Thorac Cardiovasc Surg*. 1982;30:327–335.

6. Bacon APC, Matthews MB. Congenital bicuspid aortic valves and the aetiology of isolated aortic valvular stenosis. *Q J Med*. 1959;28:545–560.

7. Bishop LF, Bishop LF Jr, Trubek M. Aortic stenosis of inflammatory origin with a differential study of the acquired or congenital origin of a bicuspid aortic valve. *Am J Med Sci*. 1934;188:506–510.

8. Buchbinder NA, Roberts WC. Left-sided valvular active infective endocarditis. A study of forty-five necropsy patients. *Am J Med*. 1972;53:20–35.

9. Cabot RC. *Facts on the Heart*. Philadelphia: WB Saunders; 1926.

10. Campbell M. Calcific aortic stenosis and congenital bicuspid aortic valves. *Br Heart J*. 1968;30:606–616.

11. Campbell M. The natural history of congenital aortic stenosis. *Br Heart J*. 1968;30:514–526.

12. Campbell M, Kauntze R. Congenial aortic valvular stenosis. *Br Heart J*. 1953;15:179–194.

13. Christian HA. Aortic stenosis with calcification of the cusps. A distinct clinical entity. *JAMA*. 1931;97:158–161.

14. Clawson BJ, Bell ET, Hartzell TB. Valvular diseases of the heart. With special reference to the pathogenesis of old valvular defects. *Am J Pathol*. 1926;2:193–234.

15. Clawson BJ, Noble JF, Lufkin NH. The calcified nodular deformity of the aortic valve. *Am Heart J*. 1938;15:58–76.

16. Cohen LS, Friedman WF, Braunwald E. Natural history of mild congenital aortic stenosis elucidated by serial hemodynamic studies. *Am J Cardiol*. 1972;30:1–5.

17. Cohen L, Gray I, Nash PI, Fink H. Calcareous aortic stenosis; report of nine cases with autopsy findings. *Ann Intern Med*. 1940;13:2091–2103.

18. Dry TJ, Willius FA. Calcareous disease of the aortic valve. A study of two hundred twenty-eight cases. *Am Heart J*. 1939;17:138–157.

19. Edwards JE. Pathologic aspects of cardiac valvular insufficiencies. *AMA Arch Surg*. 1958;77:634–649.

20. Edwards JE. Calcific aortic stenosis: pathologic features. *Proc Staff Meet Mayo Clin*. 1961;36:444–451.

21. Falcone MW, Roberts WC, Morrow AG, Perloff JK. Congenital aortic stenosis resulting from a unicommissural valve. Clinical and anatomic features in twenty-one adult patients. *Circulation*. 1971;44:272–280.

22. Fenoglio JJ Jr, McAllister HA Jr, DeCastro CM, Davia JE, Cheitlin MD. Congenital bicuspid aortic valve after age 20. *Am J Cardiol*. 1977;39:164–169.

23. Fernicola DJ, Roberts WC. Clinicopathologic features of active infective endocarditis isolated to the native mitral valve. *Am J Cardiol*. 1993;71:1186–1197.

24. Friedberg CK, Sohval AR. Nonrheumatic calcific aortic stenosis. *Am Heart J*. 1939;17:452–469.

25. Gibbs AJ. Aortic stenosis: its etiology and morbid anatomy. *Guy's Hosp Rep*. 1935;85:275–288.

26. Glancy DL, Morrow AG, Simon AL, Roberts WC. Juxtaductal aortic coarctation. Analysis of 84 patients studied hemodynamically, angiographically and morphologically after age 1 year. *Am J Cardiol*. 1983;51:537–551.

27. Glick BN, Roberts WC. Congenitally bicuspid aortic valve in multiple family members. *Am J Cardiol*. 1994;73:400–404.

28. Gould SE. *Pathology of the Heart and Blood Vessels*. 3rd ed. Springfield, IL: Charles C Thomas; 1968.

29. Gross L. So-called congenital bicuspid aortic valve. *Arch Pathol*. 1937;23:350–362.

30. Guntheroth WG. A critical review of the American College of Cardiology/American Heart Association practice guidelines on bicuspid aortic valve with dilated ascending aorta. *Am J Cardiol*. 2008;102:107–110.

31. Horan MJ Jr, Barnes AR. Calcareous aortic stenosis and coronary artery disease. *Am J Med Sci*. 1948;215:451–455.

32. Hossack KF, Neutze JM, Lowe JB, Barratt-Boyes BG. Congenital valvular aortic stenosis. Natural history and assessment for operation. *Br Heart J*. 1980;43:561–573.

33. Karsner HT, Koletsky S. *Calcific Disease of the Aortic Valve*. Philadelphia: JB Lippincott; 1947.

34. Keele KD. *Leonardo da Vinci on Movement of the Heart and Blood*. London: Harvey and Blythe; 1952.

35. Koletsky S. Congenital bicuspid aortic valves. *Arch Intern Med*. 1941;67:129–176.

36. Lander SR, Taylor JE, Roberts WC. Observations on the heart—congenitally bicuspid stenotic aortic valves in octogenarians. *Am J Geriatr Cardiol*. 1999;8:304–306.

37. Laws CL, Levine SA. Clinical notes on rheumatic heart disease with special reference to the cause of death. *Am J Med Sci*. 1933;186:833–849.

38. Lesnick G, Schlesinger MJ. Calcareous aortic valve stenosis. With particular reference to its etiology. *Am Heart J*. 1938;16:43–50.

39. Lewis T, Grant RT. Observations relating to subacute infective endocarditis. *Heart*. 1923;10:21–99.

40. Margolis HM, Ziellessen FO, Barnes AR. Calcareous aortic valvular disease. *Am Heart J*. 1931;6:349–374.

41. McGinn S, White PD. Clinical observations on aortic stenosis. *Am J Med Sci*. 1934;188:1–15.

42. McKusick VA. Association of congenital bicuspid aortic valve and Erdheim's cystic medial necrosis. *Lancet*. 1972;1:1026–1027.

43. McKusick VA, Logue RB, Bahnson HT. Association of aortic valvular disease and cystic medial necrosis of the ascending aorta. *Circulation*. 1957;16:188–194.

44. Mensah GA, Friesinger GC. Calcific aortic valve stenosis and the congenitally bicuspid aortic valve: did Osler miss the link? *Am J Cardiol*. 1996;77:417–419.

45. Michelena HI, Desjardins VA, Avierinos JF, Russo A, Nkomo VT, Sundt TM, Pellikka PA, Tajik AJ, Enriquez-Sarano M. Natural history of asymptomatic patients with normally functioning or minimally dysfunctional bicuspid aortic valve in the community. *Circulation*. 2008;117:2776–2784.

46. Mills P, Leech G, Davies M, Leatham A. The natural history of a non-stenotic bicuspid aortic valve. *Br Heart J*. 1978;40:951–957.

47. Monckeberg JG. Der normale histologische Bau und die Sklerose der Aortenklappen. *Virchows Arch Pathol Anat Physiol*. 1904;176:472–514.

48. Morrow AG, Austen G, Braunwald E. The surgical treatment of calcific aortic stenosis: operative methods and the results of the pre- and postoperative hemodynamic assessments. *Ann Surg*. 1963;158:936–951.

49. Morrow AG, Roberts WC, Ross J Jr, Fisher RD, Behrendt DM, Mason DT, Braunwald E. Obstruction to left ventricular outflow. Current concepts of management and operative treatment. *Ann Intern Med*. 1968;69:1255–1286.

50. Osler W. The bicuspid condition of the aortic valve. *Trans Assoc Am Physicians*. 1886;1:185–192.

51. Osler W. The Gulstonian Lectures, on malignant endocarditis. *Br Med J*. 1885;1:467–470.

52. Paget J. On obstructions of the branches of the pulmonary artery. *Med Chir Trans*. 1884;27:162–188.

53. Passik CS, Ackerman DM, Pluth JR, Edwards WD. Temporal changes in the causes of aortic stenosis: a surgical pathologic study of 646 cases. *Mayo Clin Proc*. 1987;62:119–123.

54. Peacock TB. *On Malformations, & c., of the Human Heart With Original Cases*. London: John Churchill; 1865.

55. Peckham GB, Keith JD, Evans JR. Congenital aortic stenosis: some observations on the natural history and clinical assessment. *Can Med Assoc J*. 1964;91:639–643.

56. Reich NE. Calcific aortic valve stenosis: a clinicopathologic correlation of 22 cases. *Ann Intern Med*. 1945;22:234–251.

57. Reifenstein GH, Levine SA, Gross RE. Coarctation of the aorta. A review of 104 autopsied cases of the "adult type," 2 years of age or older. *Am Heart J*. 1947;33:146–168.

58. Roberts WC. Tzhe congenitally bicuspid aortic valve. A study of 85 autopsy cases. *Am J Cardiol*. 1970;26:72–83.

59. Roberts WC. The structure of the aortic valve in clinically isolated aortic stenosis. An autopsy study of 162 patients over 15 years of age. *Circulation*. 1970;42:91–97.

60. Roberts WC. Anatomically isolated aortic valvular disease. The case against its being of rheumatic etiology. *Am J Med*. 1970;49:151–159.

61. Roberts WC. The 2 most common congenital heart diseases. *Am J Cardiol*. 1984;53:1198.

62. Roberts WC. Living with a congenitally bicuspid aortic valve. *Am J Cardiol*. 1989;64:1408–1409.

63. Roberts WC, Buchbinder NA. Healed left-sided infective endocarditis: a clinicopathologic study of 59 patients. *Am J Cardiol*. 1977;40:876–888.

64. Roberts WC, Dangel JC, Bulkley BH. Non-rheumatic valvular cardiac disease: a clinicopathologic survey of 27 different conditions causing valvular dysfunction. *Cardiovasc Clin*. 1973;5:333–446.

65. Roberts WC, Day PJ. Electrocardiographic observations in clinically isolated, pure, chronic, severe aortic regurgitation: analysis of 30 necropsy patients aged 19 to 65 years. *Am J Cardiol*. 1985;55:432–438.

66. Roberts WC, Ko JM. Weights of operatively-excised stenotic unicuspid, bicuspid, and tricuspid aortic valves and their relation to age, sex, body mass index, and presence or absence of concomitant coronary artery bypass grafting. *Am J Cardiol*. 2003;92:1057–1065.

67. Roberts WC, Ko JM. Weights of individual cusps in operatively-excised congenitally bicuspid stenotic aortic valves. *Am J Cardiol*. 2004;94:678–681.

68. Roberts WC, Ko JM. Weights of individual cusps in operatively-excised stenotic three-cuspid aortic valves. *Am J Cardiol*. 2004;94:681–684.

69. Roberts WC, Ko JM. Relation of weights of operatively excised stenotic aortic valves to preoperative transvalvular peak systolic pressure gradients and to calculated aortic valve areas. *J Am Coll Cardiol*. 2004;44:1847–1855.

70. Roberts WC, Ko JM. Frequency by decades of unicuspid, bicuspid, and tricuspid aortic valves in adults having isolated aortic valve replacement for aortic stenosis, with or without associated aortic regurgitation. *Circulation*. 2005;111:920–925.

71. Roberts WC, Ko JM. Clinical and morphologic features of the congenitally unicuspid acommissural stenotic and regurgitant aortic valve. *Cardiology*. 2007;108:79–81.

72. Roberts WC, Ko JM, Filardo G. Comparison of heavier versus lighter operatively excised stenotic aortic valves in adults with aortic stenosis and implications for percutaneous aortic valve implantation without replacement. *Am J Cardiol*. 2009;104:393–405.

73. Roberts WC, Ko JM, Filardo G, Henry AC, Hebeler RF Jr, Cheung EH, Matter GJ, Hamman BL. Valve structure and survival in septuagenarians having aortic valve replacement for aortic stenosis (±aortic regurgitation) with versus without coronary artery bypass grafting at a single US medical center (1993 to 2005). *Am J Cardiol*. 2007;100:1157–1165.

74. Roberts WC, Ko JM, Filardo G, Henry AC, Hebeler RF Jr, Cheung EH, Matter GJ, Hamman BL. Valve structure and survival in sexagenarians having aortic valve replacement for aortic stenosis (±aortic regurgitation) with versus without coronary artery bypass grafting at a single US medical center (1993 to 2005). *Am J Cardiol*. 2007;100:1286–1292.

75. Roberts WC, Ko JM, Filardo G, Henry AC, Hebeler RF Jr, Cheung EH, Matter GJ, Hamman BL. Valve structure and survival in quinquagenarians having aortic valve replacement for aortic stenosis (±aortic regurgitation) with versus without coronary artery bypass grafting at a single US medical center (1993 to 2005). *Am J Cardiol*. 2007;100:1584–1591.

76. Roberts WC, Ko JM, Filardo G, Kitchens BL, Henry AC, Hebeler RF Jr, Cheung EH, Matter GJ, Hamman BL. Valve structure and survival in quadragenarians having aortic valve replacement for aortic stenosis (±aortic regurgitation) with versus without coronary artery bypass grafting at a single US medical center (1993 to 2005). *Am J Cardiol*. 2007;100:1683–1690.

77. Roberts WC, Ko JM, Garner WL, Filardo G, Henry AC, Hebeler RF Jr, Matter GJ, Hamman BL. Valve structure and survival in octogenarians having aortic valve replacement for aortic stenosis (±aortic regurgitation) with versus without coronary artery bypass grafting at a single US medical center (1993 to 2005). *Am J Cardiol*. 2007;100:489–498.

78. Roberts WC, Ko JM, Hamilton C. Comparison of valve structure, valve weight, and severity of the valve obstruction in 1849 patients having isolated aortic valve replacement for aortic valve stenosis (with or without associated aortic regurgitation) studied at 3 different medical centers in 2 different time periods. *Circulation*. 2005;112:3919–3929.

79. Roberts WC, Ko JM, Matter GJ. Aortic valve replacement for aortic stenosis in nonagenarians. *Am J Cardiol*. 2006;98:1251–1253.

80. Roberts WC, Ko JM, Moore TR, Jones WH III. Causes of pure aortic regurgitation in patients having isolated aortic valve replacement at a single US tertiary hospital (1993 to 2005). *Circulation*. 2006;114:422–429.

81. Roberts WC, Morrow AG. Congenital aortic stenosis produced by a unicommissural valve. *Br Heart J*. 1965;27:505–510.

82. Roberts WC, Morrow AG, Braunwald E. Complete interruption of the aortic arch. *Circulation*. 1962;26:39–59.

83. Roberts WC, Morrow AG, McIntosh CL, Jones M, Epstein SE. Congenitally bicuspid aortic valve causing severe, pure aortic regurgitation without superimposed infective endocarditis. Analysis of 13 patients requiring aortic valve replacement. *Am J Cardiol*. 1981;47:206–209.

84. Roberts WC, Perloff JK, Costantino T. Severe valvular aortic stenosis in patients over 65 years of age. A clinicopathologic study. *Am J Cardiol*. 1971;27:497–506.

85. Roberts WC, Perry LW, Chandra RS, Myers GE, Shapiro SR, Scott LP. Aortic valve atresia: a new classification based on necropsy study of 73 cases. *Am J Cardiol*. 1976;37:753–756.

86. Roberts CS, Roberts WC. Dissection of the aorta associated with congenital malformation of the aortic valve. *J Am Coll Cardiol*. 1991;17:712–716.

87. Roberts WC, Vowels TJ, Ko JM. Comparison of interpretations of valve structure between cardiac surgeon and cardiac pathologist among adults having isolated aortic valve replacement for aortic valve stenosis (±aortic regurgitation). *Am J Cardiol*. 2009;103:1139–1145.

88. Roberts WC, Vowels TJ, Ko JM, Filardo G, Hebeler RF Jr, Henry AC, Matter GJ, Hamman BL. Comparison of the structure of the aortic valve and ascending aorta in adults having aortic valve replacement for aortic stenosis versus for pure aortic regurgitation and resection of the ascending aorta for aneurysm. *Circulation*. 2011;123:896–903.

89. Ross J Jr, Braunwald E. Aortic stenosis. *Circulation*. 1968;38:61–67.

90. Sabet HY, Edwards WD, Tazelaar HD, Daly RC. Congenitally bicuspid aortic valves: a surgical pathology study of 542 cases (1991 through 1996) and a literature review of 2,715 additional cases. *Mayo Clin Proc*. 1999;74:14–26.

91. Sohval AR, Gross L. Calcific sclerosis of the aortic valve (Monckeberg type). *Arch Pathol*. 1936;22:477–494.

92. Smith DE, Matthews MB. Aortic valvular stenosis with coarctation of the aorta. With special reference to the development of aortic stenosis upon congenital bicuspid valves. *Br Heart J*. 1955;17:198–206.

93. Stephan PJ, Henry AC III, Hebeler RF Jr, Whiddon L, Roberts WC. Comparison of age, gender, number of aortic valve cusps, concomitant coronary artery bypass grafting, and magnitude of left ventricular-systemic arterial peak systolic gradient in adults having aortic valve replacement for isolated aortic valve stenosis. *Am J Cardiol*. 1997;79:166–172.

94. Subramanian R, Olson LJ, Edwards WD. Surgical pathology of pure aortic stenosis: a study of 374 cases. *Mayo Clin Proc*. 1984;59:683–690.

95. Tadros TM, Klein MD, Shapira OM. Ascending aortic dilatation associated with bicuspid aortic valve. Pathophysiology, molecular biology, and clinical implications. *Circulation*. 2009;119:880–890.

96. Tzemos N, Therrien J, Yip J, Thanassoulis G, Tremblay S, Jamorski MT, Webb GD, Siu SC. Outcomes in adults with bicuspid aortic valves. *JAMA*. 2008;300:1317–1325.

97. Vallely MP, Semsarian C, Bannon PG. Management of the ascending aorta in patients with bicuspid aortic valve disease. *Heart Lung Circ*. 2008;17:357–363.

98. Vaslef SN, Roberts WC. Early descriptions of aortic valve stenosis. *Am Heart J*. 1993;125:1465–1474.

99. Vaslef SN, Roberts WC. Early descriptions of aortic regurgitation. *Am Heart J*. 1993;125:1475–1483.

100. Wauchope GM. The clinical importance of variations in the number of cusps forming the aortic and pulmonary valves. *Q J Med*. 1928;21:383–406.

101. White PD. *Heart Disease*. 4th ed. New York: MacMillan; 1951.

102. Wilson W, Taubert KA, Gewitz M, Lockhart PB, Baddour LM, Levison M, Bolger A, Cabell CH, Takahashi M, Baltimore RS, Newburger JW, Strom BL, Tani LY, Gerber M, Bonow RO, Pallasch T, Shulman ST, Rowley AH, Burns JC, Ferrieri P, Gardner T, Goff D, Durack DT. Prevention of infective endocarditis: guidelines from the American Heart Association: a guideline from the American Heart Association Rheumatic Fever, Endocarditis, and Kawasaki Disease Committee, Council on Cardiovascular Disease in the Young, and the Council on Clinical Cardiology, Council on Cardiovascular Surgery and Anesthesia, and the Quality of Care and Outcomes Research Interdisciplinary Working Group. *Circulation*. 2007;116:1736–1754.

103. Wood P. *Diseases of the Heart and Circulation*. 3rd ed. London: Eyre & Spottiswoode; 1968.

104. Yasuda H, Nakatani S, Stugaard M, Tsujita-Kuroda Y, Bando K, Kobayashi J, Yamagishi M, Kitakaze M, Kitamura S, Miyatake K. Failure to prevent progressive dilatation of ascending aorta by aortic valve replacement in patients with bicuspid aortic valve: comparison with tricuspid aortic valve. *Circulation*. 2003;108(Suppl 1):II291–II294.

Morphological features of temporal arteritis

William C. Roberts, MD, Saleha Zafar, MD, and Jo Mi Ko, BA

Although it varies from center to center, the frequency of temporal artery biopsy in patients suspected of having temporal arteritis (TA) is relatively small. Most commonly, patients suspected of having TA are placed on prednisone for varying periods of time, and if symptoms disappear or lessen the diagnosis is made. During a recent 13-year period at Baylor University Medical Center at Dallas, 15 patients with TA had the diagnosis of TA confirmed by histological examination of a biopsy of one temporal artery. The length of the biopsied artery varied from 0.7 to 5.5 cm (mean 2.7). The 15 patients ranged in age from 68 to 94 years (mean 82, median 85), and 11 (73%) were women. In 13 of the 15 patients (87%), the lumen of the temporal artery was narrowed >95% in cross-sectional area by the panarteritis, and the temporal artery was associated with giant cells in 11 patients (73%). Large collections of erythrocytes were present in the inflamed arterial walls in 5 patients (33%). All 15 patients were treated with varying doses of prednisone with favorable response in each. Eight patients (53%) died from 1 to 105 months (mean 52, median 57) after biopsy of the temporal artery. We have neither positive nor negative evidence that the TA played a role in the patients' death. Despite the present study and numerous others in the last 70 years, the cause of TA remains a mystery.

In 1932 and in 1934, Bayard T. Horton, a vascular specialist at the Mayo Clinic, and others (1, 2) reported two patients with headache, scalp tenderness, weight loss, fever, and night sweats, and histologic examination of one biopsied temporal artery disclosed granulomatous panarteritis. Thereafter, the condition was called *temporal arteritis* (TA) by some and *Horton's disease* by others. In 1937, Horton and Magath (3) described visual loss, jaw claudication, and elevated erythrocyte sedimentation rates in several additional patients with the disease. According to Boes (4), Horton in 1942 was the first to give a patient with TA Kendall's adrenocorticoid extract (nonpure), but apparently it had no effect on the patient's disease. Shick and colleagues (5), in 1950, also at the Mayo Clinic, reported clinical improvement in two patients with TA using a pure form of cortisone. The present study summarizes findings in 15 patients with TA seen at Baylor University Medical Center at Dallas (BUMC) in the last 13 years and describes in detail the various histological features in the temporal artery in these patients.

METHODS

Cases coded as TA by the surgical pathology division of the Department of Pathology of BUMC from 1997 through 2012 were retrieved. Fifteen such cases having biopsy of one temporal artery were found. The paraffin blocks of the temporal artery in each patient were retrieved and recut. The resulting 6-micron-thick sections were stained by both the hematoxylin-eosin method and by the Movat method, and the sections were examined. The clinical records in each patient were retrieved and examined in the BUMC record room, and pertinent findings were tabulated in each patient. Finally, the Social Security Death Index was searched to determine how many of the 15 patients had died.

RESULTS

Pertinent findings in the 15 patients are summarized in *Tables 1 and 2*. The 15 patients ranged in age from 68 to 94 years (mean 82) at the time of the temporal artery biopsy; 11 were women and 4 were men. The age at biopsy in all 15 patients corresponded to the age at which symptoms and/or signs of TA appeared. The symptoms at the time of temporal artery biopsy are displayed for each patient in Table 1: headache in 12, visual disturbance in 10, mastication pain in 7, and temporal artery tenderness in 6. At the time of biopsy, the indirect systemic arterial pressure was ≥140 mm Hg systolic and/or ≥90 mm Hg diastolic in 11 patients (73%). The body mass index was >25 kg/m^2 in 8 of the 15 patients, but in none was it ≥30 kg/m^2. Anemia (hematocrit <35%) was present in 8 (57%) of the 14 patients in which the result of this test was available. The platelet count was >250 mm^3 in 9 of the 11 patients in whom it was performed. The erythrocyte sedimentation rates were elevated (>20 mm/hour) in all 10 patients where the results were available. The serum C-reactive protein was elevated in all 5 patients in which it was done. One patient (#2) had an aortic aneurysm, and one patient (#8) had had a stroke a few months before

From the Baylor Heart and Vascular Institute (Roberts, Zafar, Ko) and the Departments of Pathology and Internal Medicine (Division of Cardiology) (Roberts), Baylor University Medical Center at Dallas.

Corresponding author: William C. Roberts, MD, Baylor Heart and Vascular Institute, 621 North Hall Street, Dallas, TX 75226 (e-mail: wc.roberts@BaylorHealth.edu).

Table 1. Clinical and laboratory findings in the 15 patients with temporal arteritis confirmed by biopsy and treated with prednisone

Patient	Date of biopsy	Age at biopsy (years)	Sex	Interval from biopsy to death (mo)	Age at death (yr)	Age at symptom onset (yr)	Symptoms at time of biopsy: H	MP	VD	CS	PR	LC	Temporal artery tenderness	BP s/d (mm Hg)	Hgb (g/dL)	HCT (%)	Platelet count (mm³)	ESR (mm/hr)	CRP (mg/dL)	BMI (kg/m²)	Minimal time on prednisone (mo)	Maximal dose of prednisone (mg)
1	8/6/1998	75	F	–	–	75	+	+	+	0	0	+	0	130/80	11.7	35.2		–	–	20.8	73	70
2	8/3/2001	75	F	50	79	75	+	+	+	+	0	+	+	170/75	8.5	26.9	331	–	–	20.0	26	60
3	6/25/1997	77	F	–	–	77	+	0	+	0	0	0	0	140/80	11.5	37.0		76	–	27.1	–	60
4	10/23/2001	77	F	105	85	77	+	0	0	+	0	0	0	180/90	13.3	40.1	470	–	–	26.2	17	40
5	11/21/2002	80	F	65	85	80	+	+	0	+	+	+	+	130/60	10.5	32.0	347	121	–	24.6	–	60
6	1/29/2002	82	F	87	90	82	+	0	+	0	0	0	0	130/90	12.4	38.2	379	–	–	23.0	73	60
7	3/22/2001	85	F	1	85	85	+	+	+	0	+	+	0	140/80	10.6	32.2	245	92	26	24.3	0.5	60
8	11/22/2010	86	F	–	–	86	0	0	+	0	0	0	0	150/55	12.1	35.8	230	↑	↑	26.0	0.25	60
9	3/26/2002	86	F	–	–	86	+	0	0	0	0	0	+	140/60	11.2	33.5	269	↑	–	20.8	11	60
10	9/8/2004	89	F	74	96	89	+	+	+	0	0	0	+	220/80	9.8	29.9	565	130	28	29.1	14	60
11	2/10/2000	90	F	28	92	90	+	0	0	0	0	0	0	175/80	13.6	32.4		↑	–	21.8	24	60
12	9/9/2010	68	M	3	68	68	0	+	0	0	0	+	0	110/70	11.0	32.0	258	57	–	25.1	4	60
13	4/25/1998	81	M	–	–	81	+	0	+	+	0	+	+	155/95	–	–	–	–	–	29.8	–	60
14	8/22/2008	83	M	–	–	83	0	0	+	0	0	0	0	115/70	9.9	29.5	369	103	19	25.4	3	50
15	4/13/2009	94	M	–	–	94	+	+	+	0	+	+	+	160/90	14.3	40.0	281	41	6	26.2	19	60

BMI indicates body mass index; BP, blood pressure; CRP, C-reactive protein; CS, cigarette smokers; ESR, erythrocyte sedimentation rate; H, headache; HCT, hematocrit; Hgb, hemoglobin; LC, leg claudication; MP, mastication pain; PR, polymyalgia rheumatica; S/D, peak systole/end diastole; VD, visual disturbance; –, not done, not applicable, or no information.

biopsy. The length of the temporal artery biopsied ranged from 0.7 to 5.5 cm (mean 2.7); sample images and descriptions appear in *Figures 1 to 9*. In 13 of the 15 patients (87%), the lumen of the temporal artery was narrowed >95% in cross-sectional area. The temporal artery was associated with giant cells in 11 patients (73%). All 15 patients received prednisone (maximal dose 40–70 mg) for 0.25 to 73 months (mean 22), and all had symptomatic improvement, including 5 with loss or virtual loss of symptoms.

DISCUSSION

It might seem a bit inappropriate in 2013 to report a series of only 15 patients with biopsy-proven TA when others have reported such large series of patients with biopsy-proven TA (6–35). Gonzalez-Gay and colleagues (13, 19, 20, 25, 26, 28, 31), for example, in 7 articles from 1998 to 2011 described anywhere from 161 to 255 patients with biopsy-proven TA (called "giant cell arteritis" by the authors), but none contained a photomicrograph of a temporal artery. Indeed, of the 30 studies presented in *Table 3* (6–35), only two included a photomicrograph of a temporal artery, and in both only hematoxylin-eosin–stained sections had been used. It is not possible to demonstrate the locations of the panarteritis, i.e., how much of the process involved the intima, media, and adventitia, without an elastic tissue stain that readily identifies the internal and external elastic membranes allowing clear demonstration of media, thus separating it from the intima and adventitia. We employed the Movat stain for this purpose in our study (36).

We prefer the phrase "temporal arteritis" to the phrase "giant cell arteritis" because giant cells are not seen in all TA patients having biopsies of the temporal arteries. Among our 15 patients, we found giant cells in only 11. Mahr and colleagues (37) suggested that finding giant cells in patients with TA is determined in part by the lengths of the temporal arteries examined. These authors examined surgical

Table 2. Morphological findings in the 15 patients with biopsy-proven temporal arteritis

Patient	Length (cm) of excised TA	Number of histological cross-sections	Maximal diameter (mm) of cross-sections	Cross-sectional narrowing	Collection of red blood cells in intima	Lympho-cytes	Giant cells
1	4.2	8	3	>95%	0	+++	++
2	4.7	11	2	>95%	+	+++	++
3	2.4	8	2	>95%	0	+++	++
4	2.0	8	2	>95%	+	+++	++
5	2.4	12	2	>95%	+	+++	++
6	0.7	3	2	>95%	0	+	0
7	2.6	8	2	51%–75%	+	+	0
8	2.2	4	2	>95%	0	+++	++
9	5.5	19	6	>95%	0	+++	++
10	3.0	8	4	>95%	0	+++	+
11	0.7	2	2	>95%	0	+	+
12	1.9	4	2	>95%	+	+++	++
13	2.1	6	3	>95%	0	+++	++
14	3.5	7	4	>95%	0	+++	0
15	3.0	7	3	51%–75%	0	+++	0

TA indicates temporal arteritis.

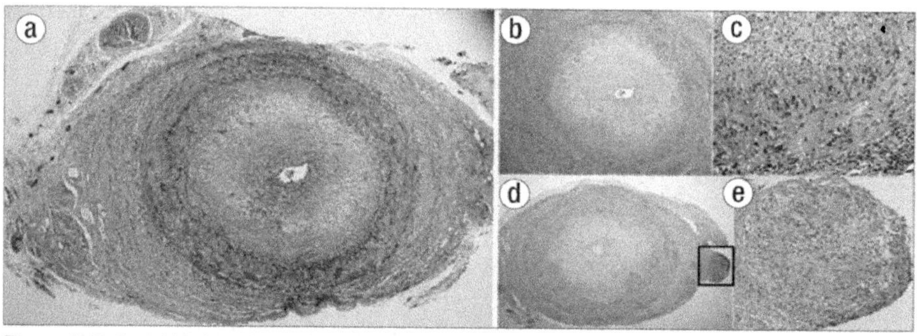

Figure 1. *Patient 1.* Various views of the temporal artery. **(a)** Movat-stained section (×40) showing relatively intact media *(pink)*, very thickened intima *(green)* with severe luminal narrowing, and severely thickened fibrous tissue of the adventitia *(tan)*. **(b)** Hematoxylin-eosin (H&E)–stained section showing numerous inflammatory cells involving the outer intima, media, and inner adventitia (×100). **(c)** A close-up showing intimal granulomatous-type cells adjacent to the media with penetration of the media (H&E, ×400). **(d)** Another view showing an inflamed nodule in brackets in the adventitia (H&E, ×40). **(e)** A close-up of that nodule (H&E, ×400).

reports of temporal artery biopsies in 223 patients with TA and found that 164 (74%) of the reports mentioned the presence of giant cells. These authors also mentioned that a temporal artery length of at least 0.5 cm was sufficient for diagnosis of TA. Our smallest length among the patients was 0.7 cm. Among the four patients in whom we did not see giant cells, the lengths of the temporal artery biopsied were 0.7, 2.6, 3.0, and 3.5 cm; the latter three lengths were among the longest in the patients we studied.

Although the present study focuses on the histologic features of TA, one might reasonably ask if biopsy of this artery is a useful routine endeavor. A near universal observation in TA is a rapid, sometimes dramatic, diminution or loss of symptoms after corticosteroid therapy has been initiated. If there is not a quick symptomatic response, biopsy can then be performed. There appears to be little change in the histologic features of the TA before corticosteroid therapy and up to about 6 weeks after initiation of therapy (10). A report by Guevara et al described a positive biopsy after 6 months of prednisone treatment (38). If a patient with suspected TA has a negative biopsy of the temporal artery, is it useful then to biopsy the contralateral temporal artery? According to a study by Boyev and colleagues (18), biopsy of one temporal artery in a patient with TA provides a 97% chance that the same findings would be present in the contralateral temporal artery, so that the additional biopsy would rarely be useful diagnostically.

On occasion, TA resolves without corticosteroid therapy. Horton et al, in their original two patients, described temporary remissions with relapses (1), and they later described seven additional patients in whom remission occurred without drug therapy months after diagnosis (3). Patients have been described where headaches and local symptoms have disappeared simply by removal of a portion of the temporal artery for diagnostic purposes (39, 40).

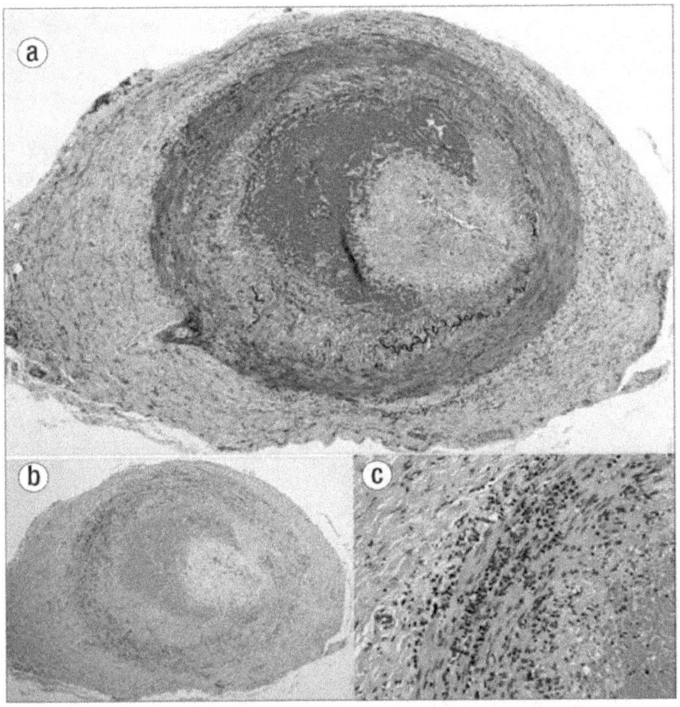

Figure 2. *Patient 2.* **(a)** A Movat-stained section (×100) of temporal artery with severely narrowed lumen *(within the green portion)* of the intima with blood *(red)* within the intimal plaque and marked disruption of the internal elastic membrane *(black)*. The adventitia is thickened by dense fibrous tissue *(tan)*. **(b)** The same section stained by hematoxylin-eosin (×100). **(c)** A close up of a portion of the media showing numerous mononuclear cells (×400).

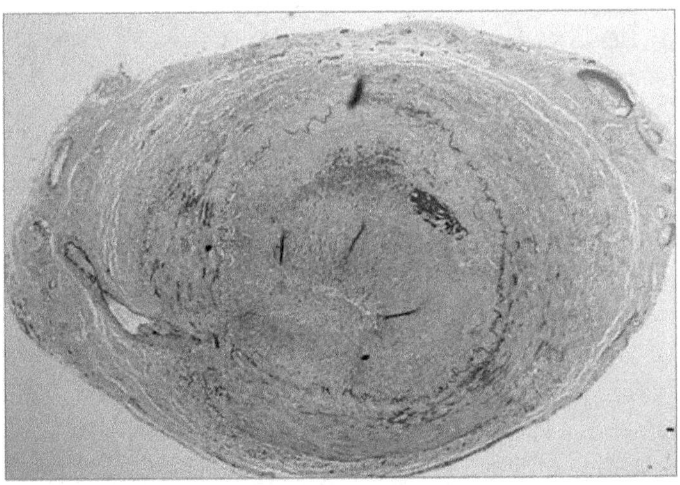

Figure 3. *Patient 4.* Movat-stained section (×40) of the temporal artery showing near-total occlusion of the lumen, blood *(red)* within the intimal plaque, disruption of the internal elastic membrane *(black)*, and severely thickened adventitia by dense fibrous tissue *(tan)*. The absence of much lumen and the marked thickening of the adventitia by dense fibrous tissue makes these arteries, by external palpation, quite firm and nodular.

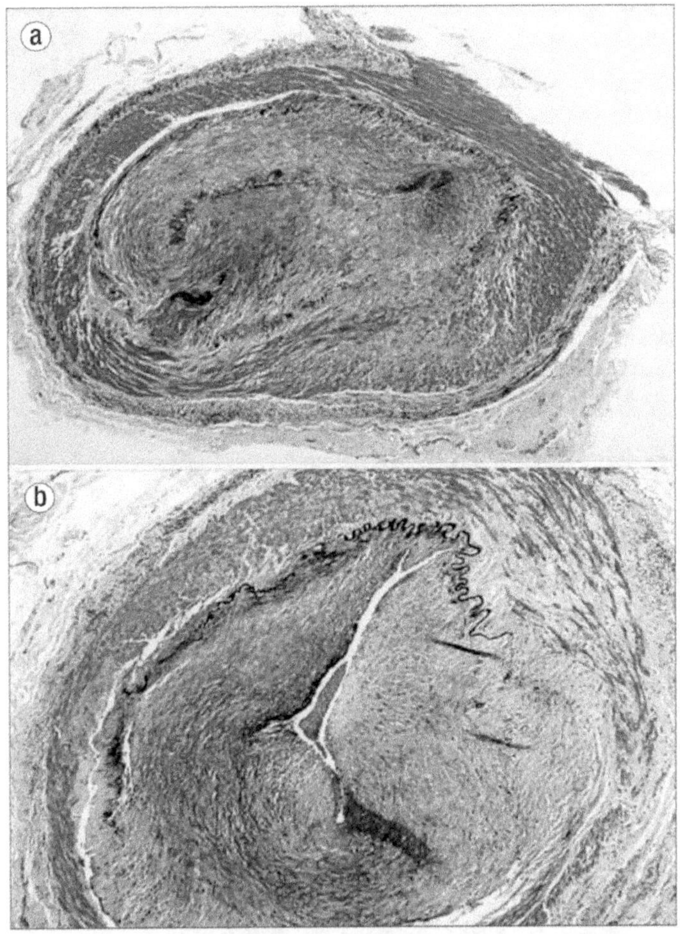

Figure 4. *Patient 6.* Two views of Movat-stained sections of the temporal artery showing **(a)** virtual occlusion (×100) and **(b)** severe narrowing (×100). The internal elastic membrane *(black)* is interrupted and the quantity of fibrous tissue in the adventitia is considerably less than in previously illustrated cases.

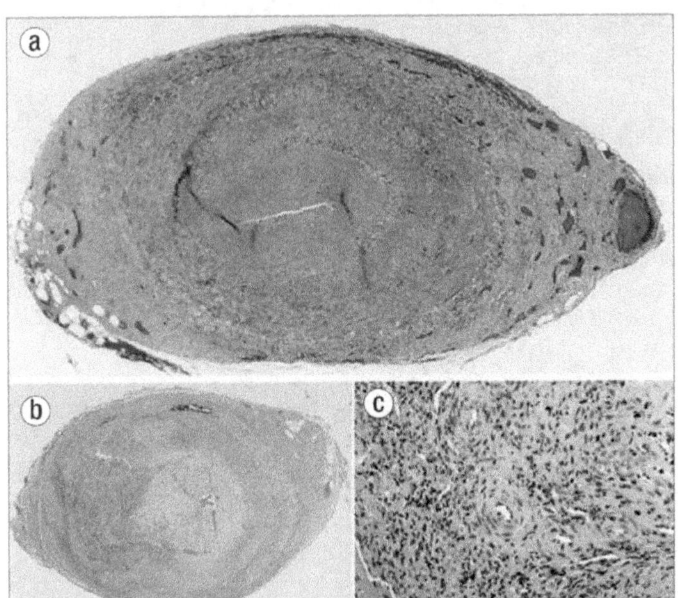

Figure 5. *Patient 8.* **(a)** A Movat-stained section of the temporal artery showing near occlusion of the lumen by fibrous tissue and mucopolysaccharide material *(green)* and dense fibrous tissue causing considerable thickening of the adventitia. **(b)** Hematoxylin-eosin stain (×40) of another section of the same artery showing numerous inflammatory cells between the 8:00 and 11:00 positions. **(c)** Close-up (×400) of a portion of the inflammatory cells.

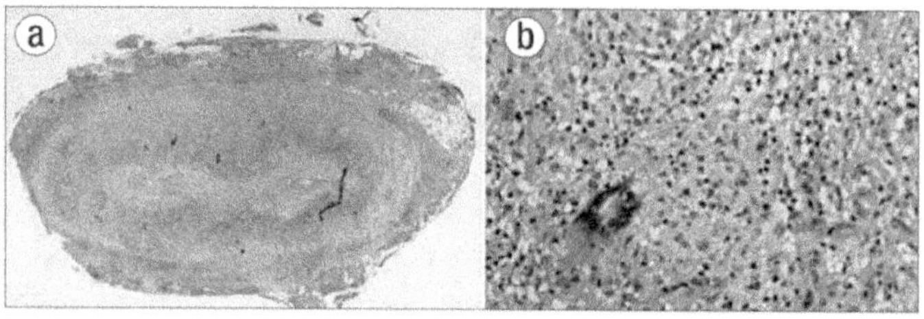

Figure 6. *Patient 9.* **(a)** View of a hematoxylin-eosin–stained section (×20) of the temporal artery with virtual total occlusion of its lumen. The darkened area represents collections of inflammatory cells. The adventitia is thickened by fibrous tissue. **(b)** A close-up (×400) of a minute portion of the inflammatory infiltrates. Granulomatous-type cells and a giant cell are visible.

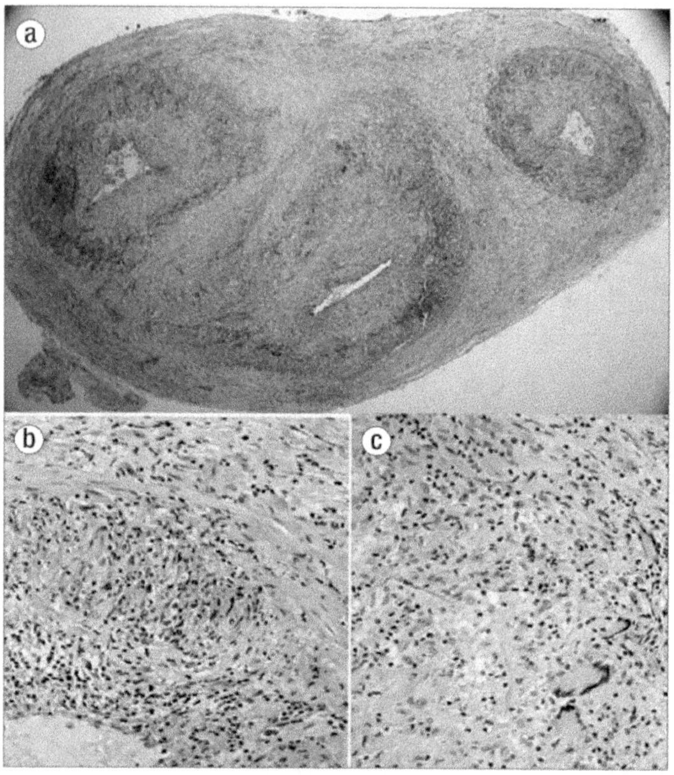

Figure 7. *Patient 9.* **(a)** A Movat-stained section (×40) of three branches of a temporal artery with narrowing of each branch, marked disruption of the media in two of the branches, and dense fibrous tissue in the adventitia. **(b)** A close-up of a hematoxylin-eosin–stained section (×400) of a portion of the inflammatory cells in the media. **(c)** Another hematoxylin-eosin stained section (×400) showing giant cells among the collection of cells.

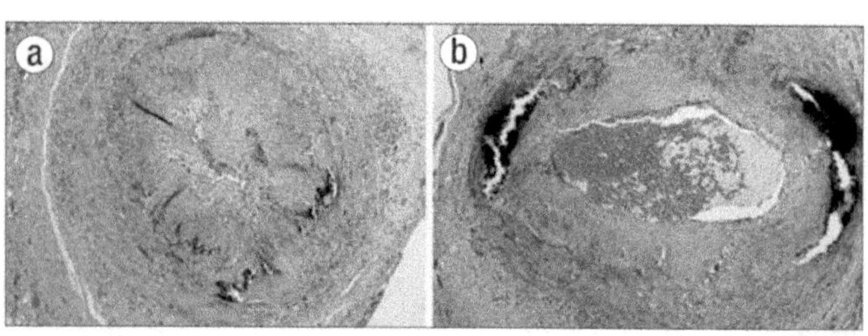

Figure 8. *Patient 10.* A Movat-stained section of the temporal artery showing **(a)** severe narrowing of the lumen (×100) and **(b)** less narrowing (×100). The amount of adventitial fibrous tissue is considerable. Inflammatory cells are present in the intima, media, and adventitia. The dark staining in the medial wall in part b represents calcific deposits.

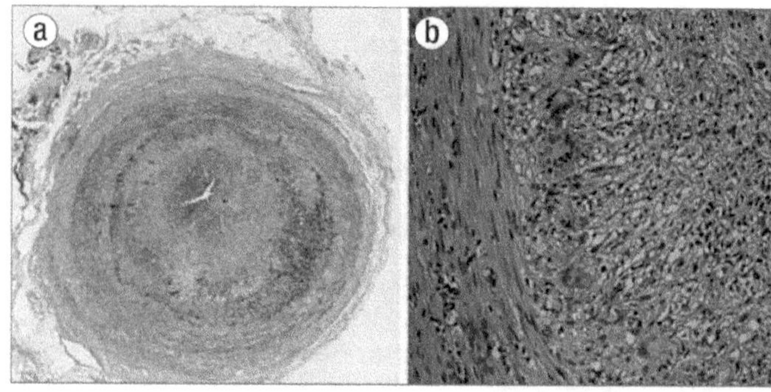

Figure 9. *Patient 13.* **(a)** A Movat-stained section of the temporal artery (×40) with severe luminal narrowing. The lumen in all sections in temporal arteritis tends to be in the more central portion of the artery and not on the periphery, as it is in typical atherosclerosis. **(b)** A close-up hematoxylin-eosin–stained section (×400) shows several giant cells in the outer intima adjacent to the media. These cells are lined up perpendicular to the smooth muscle cells in the media.

1. Horton BT, Magath TB, Brown GE. An undescribed form of arteritis of the temporal vessels. *Proc Staff Meet Mayo Clinic* 1932;7:700–701.
2. Horton BT, Magath TB, Brown GE. Arteritis of the temporal vessels: a previously undescribed form. *Arch Intern Med* 1934;53:400–409.
3. Horton BT, Magath TB. Arteritis of the temporal vessels: report of seven cases. *Proc Staff Meet Mayo Clinic* 1937;12:548–553.
4. Boes CJ. Bayard Horton's clinicopathological description of giant cell (temporal) arteritis. *Cephalalgia* 2007;27(1):68–75.
5. Shick RM, Baggenstoss AH, Fuller BF, Polley HF. Effects of cortisone and ACTH on periarteritis nodosa and cranial arteritis. *Proc Staff Meet Mayo Clin* 1950;25(17):492–494.
6. Birkhead NC, Wagener HP, Shick RM. Treatment of temporal arteritis with adrenal corticosteroids; results in fifty-five cases in which lesion was proved at biopsy. *J Am Med Assoc* 1957;163(10):821–827.
7. Huston KA, Hunder GG, Lie JT, Kennedy RH, Elveback LR. Temporal arteritis: a 25-year epidemiologic, clinical, and pathologic study. *Ann Intern Med* 1978;88(2):162–167.
8. Graham E, Holland A, Avery A, Russell RW. Prognosis in giant-cell arteritis. *Br Med J (Clin Res Ed)* 1981;282(6260):269–271.
9. Nordborg E, Bengtsson BA. Death rates and causes of death in 284 consecutive patients with giant cell arteritis confirmed by biopsy. *BMJ* 1989;299(6698):549–550.
10. Achkar AA, Lie JT, Hunder GG, O'Fallon WM, Gabriel SE. How does previous corticosteroid treatment affect the biopsy findings in giant cell (temporal) arteritis? *Ann Intern Med* 1994;120(12):987–992.
11. Lie JT. Aortic and extracranial large vessel giant cell arteritis: a review of 72 cases with histopathologic documentation. *Semin Arthritis Rheum* 1995;24(6):422–431.
12. Salvarani C, Gabriel SE, O'Fallon WM, Hunder GG. The incidence of giant cell arteritis in Olmsted County, Minnesota: apparent fluctuations in a cyclic pattern. *Ann Intern Med* 1995;123(3):192–194.
13. González-Gay MA, Blanco R, Rodríguez-Valverde V, Martínez-Taboada VM, Delgado-Rodriguez M, Figueroa M, Uriarte E. Permanent visual loss and cerebrovascular accidents in giant cell arteritis: predictors and response to treatment. *Arthritis Rheum* 1998;41(8):1497–1504.
14. Cid MC, Font C, Oristrell J, de la Sierra A, Coll-Vinent B, López-Soto A, Vilaseca J, Urbano-Márquez A, Grau JM. Association between strong inflammatory response and low risk of developing visual loss and other cranial ischemic complications in giant cell (temporal) arteritis. *Arthritis Rheum* 1998;41(1):26–32.
15. Duhaut P, Pinede L, Demolombe-Rague S, Loire R, Seydoux D, Ninet J, Pasquier J; Groupe de Recherche sur l'Artérite à Cellules Géantes. Giant cell arteritis and cardiovascular risk factors: a multicenter, prospective case-control study. *Arthritis Rheum* 1998;41(11):1960–1965.
16. Duhaut P, Pinède L, Bornet H, Demolombe-Ragué S, Dumontet C, Ninet J, Loire R, Pasquier J; Groupe de Recherche sur l'Artérite à Cellules Géantes. Biopsy proven and biopsy negative temporal arteritis:

Table 3. Reported studies of patients with temporal arteritis confirmed by biopsy of the temporal artery

First author, year of publication	Patients (n)	Biopsy-proven TA (n)	M/F	Age range (mean)	Length of study (yr)	Follow-up (yr)	Deaths (n)	Deaths attributed to TA	Mean ESR values (mm/hr)	Median hemo-globin values (g/dl)	Median platelet count (mm^3)	Visual loss (n)	Received cortico-steroids (n)	Maximal length of treatment (mo)	Patients that relapsed (n)	Tem-poral artery photo mics	Giant cell histol-ogy (n)
Birkhead, 1957	55	55	28/27	60–83	6	–	–	–	–	–	–	21	55	15	–	0	–
Huston, 1978	42	38	9/33	56–92 (75)	25	19	21	1	96	11.5	–	17	42	77	11	0	–
Graham, 1981	90	90	26/64	55–88	10	11	32	3	81	–	–	55	90	84	18	0	–
Nordborg, 1989	284	284	–	–	10	1	82	7	–	–	–	–	–	–	–	0	–
Achkar, 1994	535	175	190/345	31–93 (71.7)	3	–	–	–	63	–	–	–	249	–	–	0	–
Lie, 1995	72	67	21/51	54–96 (69)	25	–	–	–	96	–	–	–	–	–	–	0	–
Salvarani, 1995	125	115	22/103	50–80+	42	–	–	–	–	–	–	–	–	–	–	0	–
Gonzalez-Gay, 1998	239	239	106/133	50+ (73.5)	21	–	–	–	94	–	–	64	239	–	–	0	–
Cid, 1998	200	200	59/141	57–92 (74.5)	16	–	–	–	82.7	12.2	337,000	28	–	–	–	0	–
Duhaut, 1998	400	207	118/282	50+ (74)	6	–	–	–	–	–	–	–	–	–	–	0	–
Duhaut, 1999	292	207	50/157	50+ (74.5)	6	36	38	1	88	15.6	424,000	20	292	36	–	0	–
Brack, 1999	148	74	16/58	50+ (72)	36	–	–	–	–	–	–	18	74	–	–	0	–
Boyev, 1999	756	722	–	–	28	–	–	–	–	–	–	–	–	–	–	0	–
Gonzalez-Gay, 2000	190	161	79/82	50–80+ (75)	18	–	–	–	93	11.8	412,816	42	–	–	–	0	–
Gonzalez-Gay, 2001	190	161	79/82	50–80+ (75)	18	–	–	–	93	11.8	412,816	–	–	–	–	0	–
Liozon, 2001	174	147	38/109	– (75)	22	–	–	–	90	11.3	419,000	58	174	–	–	0	–
Ray-Chaudhur, 2002	11	9	3/8	65–90 (75)	–	–	–	–	66	–	–	5	11	1.5	–	0	7
Hall, 2003	181	74	–	–	11	2	–	–	–	–	–	–	–	–	–	0	–
Salvarani, 2004	173	151	36/137	50–80+	50	6.8	–	–	–	–	–	–	–	–	–	0	–
Gonzalez-Gay, 2005	240	240	110/130	50–80+ (74)	23	–	–	–	93	11.7	397,000	21	–	–	–	0	–
Larsson, 2006	49	49	0/49	50–69 (64.1)	9	3	–	–	–	–	–	–	–	–	–	0	–
Gonzalez-Gay, 2007	255	255	116/139	55–94 (75)	25	–	–	–	–	–	–	89	–	–	–	0	–
Narvaez, 2007	78	57	28/50	56–89 (74.6)	18	–	–	–	94.4	11.4	340,000	16	78	1	–	0	–
Makkuni, 2008	30	30	10/20	– (77.5)	6	–	–	–	78.5	–	–	12	–	–	–	+	–
Gonzalez-Gay, 2009	287	287	132/155	50–80+	27	–	–	–	–	–	–	138	–	–	–	0	–
Zhou, 2009	107	26	–	–	19	–	–	–	–	–	–	–	–	–	–	+	26
Martinez-Lado, 2011	207	174	80/94	(74.2)	14	3.5	0	0	92.7	11.7	392,000	36	174	44.1	71	0	–
Walvick, 2011	3001	459	–	–	9	–	–	–	81	–	391,000	–	–	–	–	0	–
Ninan, 2011	225	225	62/163	(78.2)	14	5.5	71	12	–	–	–	–	–	–	–	0	–

ESR indicates erythrocyte sedimentation rate; F, female; M, male; TA, temporal arteritis; –, no information.

differences in clinical spectrum at the onset of the disease. *Ann Rheum Dis* 1999;58(6):335–341.

17. Brack A, Martinez-Taboada V, Stanson A, Goronzy JJ, Weyand CM. Disease pattern in cranial and large-vessel giant cell arteritis. *Arthritis Rheum* 1999;42(2):311–317.
18. Boyev LR, Miller NR, Green WR. Efficacy of unilateral versus bilateral temporal artery biopsies for the diagnosis of giant cell arteritis. *Am J Ophthalmol* 1999;128(2):211–215.
19. González-Gay MA, García-Porrúa C, Llorca J, Hajeer AH, Brañas F, Dababneh A, González-Louzao C, Rodriguez-Gil E, Rodríguez-Ledo P, Ollier WE. Visual manifestations of giant cell arteritis. Trends and clinical spectrum in 161 patients. *Medicine (Baltimore)* 2000;79(5):283–292.
20. González-Gay MA, Garcia-Porrua C, Rivas MJ, Rodriguez-Ledo P, Llorca J. Epidemiology of biopsy proven giant cell arteritis in northwestern Spain: trend over an 18 year period. *Ann Rheum Dis* 2001;60(4):367–371.
21. Liozon E, Herrmann F, Ly K, Robert PY, Loustaud V, Soria P, Vidal E. Risk factors for visual loss in giant cell (temporal) arteritis: a prospective study of 174 patients. *Am J Med* 2001;111(3):211–217.
22. Ray-Chaudhuri N, Kiné DA, Tijani SO, Parums DV, Cartlidge N, Strong NP, Dayan MR. Effect of prior steroid treatment on temporal artery biopsy findings in giant cell arteritis. *Br J Ophthalmol* 2002;86(5):530–532.
23. Hall JK, Volpe NJ, Galetta SL, Liu GT, Syed NA, Balcer LJ. The role of unilateral temporal artery biopsy. *Ophthalmology* 2003;110(3):543–548.
24. Salvarani C, Crowson CS, O'Fallon WM, Hunder GG, Gabriel SE. Reappraisal of the epidemiology of giant cell arteritis in Olmsted County, Minnesota, over a fifty-year period. *Arthritis Rheum* 2004;51(2):264–268.
25. Gonzalez-Gay MA, Lopez-Diaz MJ, Barros S, Garcia-Porrua C, Sanchez-Andrade A, Paz-Carreira J, Martin J, Llorca J. Giant cell arteritis: laboratory tests at the time of diagnosis in a series of 240 patients. *Medicine (Baltimore)* 2005;84(5):277–290.
26. Gonzalez-Gay MA, Barros S, Lopez-Diaz MJ, Garcia-Porrua C, Sanchez-Andrade A, Llorca J. Giant cell arteritis: disease patterns of clinical presentation in a series of 240 patients. *Medicine (Baltimore)* 2005;84(5):269–276.
27. Larsson K, Mellström D, Nordborg E, Odén A, Nordborg E. Early menopause, low body mass index, and smoking are independent risk factors for developing giant cell arteritis. *Ann Rheum Dis* 2006;65(4):529–532.
28. Gonzalez-Gay MA, Miranda-Filloy JA, Lopez-Diaz MJ, Perez-Alvarez R, Gonzalez-Juanatey C, Sanchez-Andrade A, Martin J, Llorca J. Giant cell arteritis in northwestern Spain: a 25-year epidemiologic study. *Medicine (Baltimore)* 2007;86(2):61–68.
29. Narváez J, Bernad B, Roig-Vilaseca D, García-Gómez C, Gómez-Vaquero C, Juanola X, Rodriguez-Moreno J, Nolla JM, Valverde J. Influence of previous corticosteroid therapy on temporal artery biopsy yield in giant cell arteritis. *Semin Arthritis Rheum* 2007;37(1):13–19.
30. Makkuni D, Bharadwaj A, Wolfe K, Payne S, Hutchings A, Dasgupta B. Is intimal hyperplasia a marker of neuro-ophthalmic complications of giant cell arteritis? *Rheumatology (Oxford)* 2008;47(4):488–490.
31. Gonzalez-Gay MA, Vazquez-Rodriguez TR, Gomez-Acebo I, Pego-Reigosa R, Lopez-Diaz MJ, Vazquez-Triñanes MC, Miranda-Filloy JA, Blanco R, Dierssen T, Gonzalez-Juanatey C, Llorca J. Strokes at time of disease diagnosis in a series of 287 patients with biopsy-proven giant cell arteritis. *Medicine (Baltimore)* 2009;88(4):227–235.
32. Zhou L, Luneau K, Weyand CM, Biousse V, Newman NJ, Grossniklaus HE. Clinicopathologic correlations in giant cell arteritis: a retrospective study of 107 cases. *Ophthalmology* 2009;116(8):1574–1580.
33. Martinez-Lado L, Calviño-Díaz C, Piñeiro A, Dierssen T, Vazquez-Rodriguez TR, Miranda-Filloy JA, Lopez-Diaz MJ, Blanco R, Llorca J, Gonzalez-Gay MA. Relapses and recurrences in giant cell arteritis: a population-based study of patients with biopsy-proven disease from northwestern Spain. *Medicine (Baltimore)* 2011;90(3):186–193.
34. Walvick MD, Walvick MP. Giant cell arteritis: laboratory predictors of a positive temporal artery biopsy. *Ophthalmology* 2011;118(6):1201–1204.
35. Ninan J, Nguyen AM, Cole A, Rischmueller M, Dodd T, Roberts-Thomson P, Hill CL. Mortality in patients with biopsy-proven giant cell arteritis: a south Australian population-based study. *J Rheumatol* 2011;38(10):2215–2217.
36. Movat HZ. Demonstration of all connective tissue elements in a single stain: pentochrome stains. *Arch Pathol* 1955;60:289–295.
37. Mahr A, Saba M, Kambouchner M, Polivka M, Baudrimont M, Brochériou I, Coste J, Guillevin L. Temporal artery biopsy for diagnosing giant cell arteritis: the longer, the better? *Ann Rheum Dis* 2006;65(6):826–828.
38. Guevara RA, Newman NJ, Grossniklaus HE. Positive temporal artery biopsy 6 months after prednisone treatment. *Arch Ophthalmol* 1998;116(9):1252–1253.
39. Bowers JM. Arteritis of the temporal vessels: report of a case. *Arch Intern Med* 1940;66:384–392.
40. Harrison CV. Giant-cell or temporal arteritis: a review. *J Clin Pathol* 1948;1:197–211.

Dramatically Different Phenotypic Expressions of Hypertrophic Cardiomyopathy in Male Cousins Undergoing Cardiac Transplantation With Identical Disease-Causing Gene Mutation

William C. Roberts, MD[a,b,d,*], Carey Camille Roberts[d], Jong Mi Ko, BA[d], Paul A. Grayburn, MD[b,d], Anumeha Tandon, MD[b], Johannes J. Kuiper, MD[b], John E. Capehart, MD[c], and Shelley A. Hall, MD[b]

Described herein are certain findings in 2 male cousins who underwent cardiac transplantation for severe heart failure (HF), one of the diastolic type (ejection fraction ≈65%), and one of the systolic type (ejection fraction ≈20%), both the consequence of hypertrophic cardiomyopathy (HC), and each had identical disease-causing gene mutations. The implanted heart in one had normal-sized ventricular cavities and no grossly visible ventricular wall lesions (except in one papillary muscle) and the other patient had severely dilated ventricular cavities and multiple extensive ventricular wall scars. The heart mass and the age of onset of symptoms was similar in each patient. A number of other family members had evidence of HC. **(Am J Cardiol 2013;111:1818–1822)**

Hypertrophic cardiomyopathy (HC) is a genetically transmitted cardiac disease with a diverse variety of clinical and morphologic manifestations. Its frequency of 1 in 500 persons is similar to that of familial hypercholesterolemia.[1] Some patients with HC remain asymptomatic or nearly so throughout a long life; others die suddenly, usually prematurely; many have symptoms related to left ventricular outflow obstruction and once the obstruction is relieved the symptoms vanish or at least decrease in frequency, and some patients develop end-stage HF that can be relieved only by cardiac transplantation (CT).[2–4] Recently, we encountered 2 male cousins with HC, both of whom underwent CT, and examination of the recipient heart disclosed nearly opposite morphologic features of the disease although both had identical disease-causing gene mutations. A description of certain findings in them is the purpose of this report.

Patient Descriptions

Pertinent clinical and morphologic findings in the 2 patients are tabulated in Table 1. The pedigrees of the family are illustrated in Figure 1. Both were African American men, one had CT at age 45 and the other, at age 48 years. One became symptomatic from HF about 6 years before CT, the other 7 years, before CT. Both had class IV HF. Each also had one or more episodes of syncope, atrial fibrillation, and runs of ventricular tachycardia. Neither had a precordial murmur. Neither had obstruction to outflow from either the right or left ventricle. Both had normal epicardial coronary arteries. The left ventricular ejection fractions were strikingly different. In case #1 it was ≈65%, and in case #2, ≈20%. Both patients had elevated pulmonary arterial pressures. Both had cardiac defibrillators implanted several years before CT. Patient #2 had a left ventricular assist device. Echocardiograms before CT are shown in Figures 2–4.

Table 1
Certain clinical and morphologic findings in the 2 African American male cousins who underwent cardiac transplantation for end-stage heart failure secondary to hypertrophic cardiomyopathy

Variable	Case #1	Case #2
Age (yrs) at cardiac transplantation	45	48
Age (yrs) onset symptoms	39	41
Heart failure class IV	+	+
Chest pain	0	+
Syncope	+	+
Precordial murmur	0	0
Atrial fibrillation	+	+
Ventricular tachycardia	+	+
Body mass index (Kg/m^2)	26.5	30.6
Left ventricular ejection fraction	65%	20%
Cardiac index (l/min/m^2)	1.3	1.8
Pulmonary artery peak systolic pressure (mm Hg)	82	56
Coronary narrowing by angiogram	0	0
Left ventricular assist device inserted	0	+
Heart weight (g)	410	410
Scars (0-4+), left ventricular wall and ventricular septum	0*	+(4+)
Dilated right ventricle	0	+
Dilated left ventricle	0	+
Mitral valve	normal	normal
Mural endocardial thickening in the left ventricular outflow tract in apposition to anterior mitral leaflet	0	0
Mitral annular calcium	3+/4+	0
Abnormal intramural coronary arteries	0	+

* Scarring in one left ventricular papillary muscles.

[a]Department of Pathology, [b]Department of Internal Medicine, Division of Cardiology, [c]Department of Cardiothoracic Surgery, and [d]Baylor Heart and Vascular Institute, Baylor University Medical Center, Dallas, Texas. Manuscript received September 19, 2012; revised manuscript received and accepted February 6, 2013.

See page 1822 for disclosure information.

*Corresponding author: Tel: 214-820-7911; fax: 214-820-7533.
E-mail address: wc.roberts@baylorhealth.edu (W.C. Roberts).

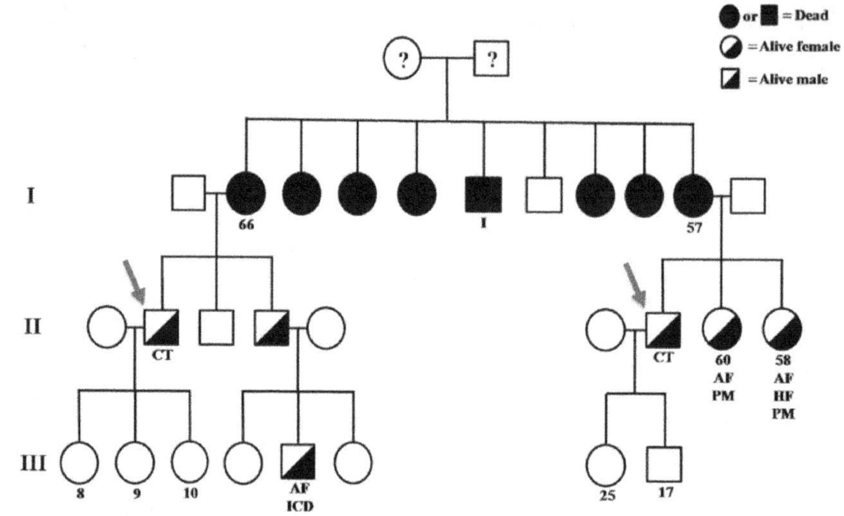

Figure 1. Pedigree of the family of case #1 *(left)* and case #2 *(right)*. Whether or not the grand parents had heart disease is unclear but 8 of their 9 children died of heart disease, several of them suddenly and prematurely, and others from heart failure of varying durations. The *arrows* designate the 2 patients described herein. The numbers represent the ages at death or presently (2012). AF = atrial fibrillation; CT = cardiac transplantation; HF = heart failure; I = stillbirth; ICD = intracardiac defibrillator; PM = pacemaker.

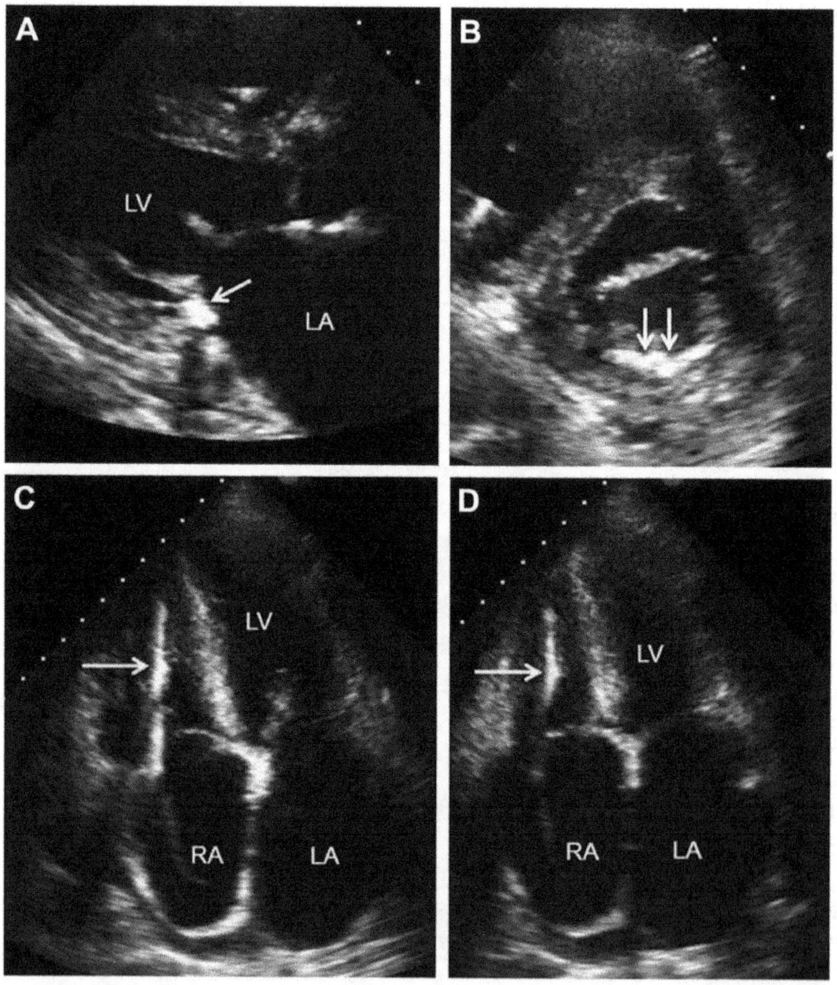

Figure 2. Echocardiogram in patient #1. *(A)* Parasternal long-axis view showing a very dilated left atrium (LA) and a non-dilated left ventricle (LV). The *arrow* points to calcium in the mitral annular area. *(B)* Parasternal short-axis view of the ventricles. The *arrows* again point to calcium deposits in the mitral valve area. *(C)* Four-chamber view during ventricular diastole. The *arrow* points to the intracardiac defibrillator catheter. *(D)* Four-chamber view in ventricular systole. Cavity size is much smaller than in diastole, consistent with a left ventricular ejection fraction of ≈65%.

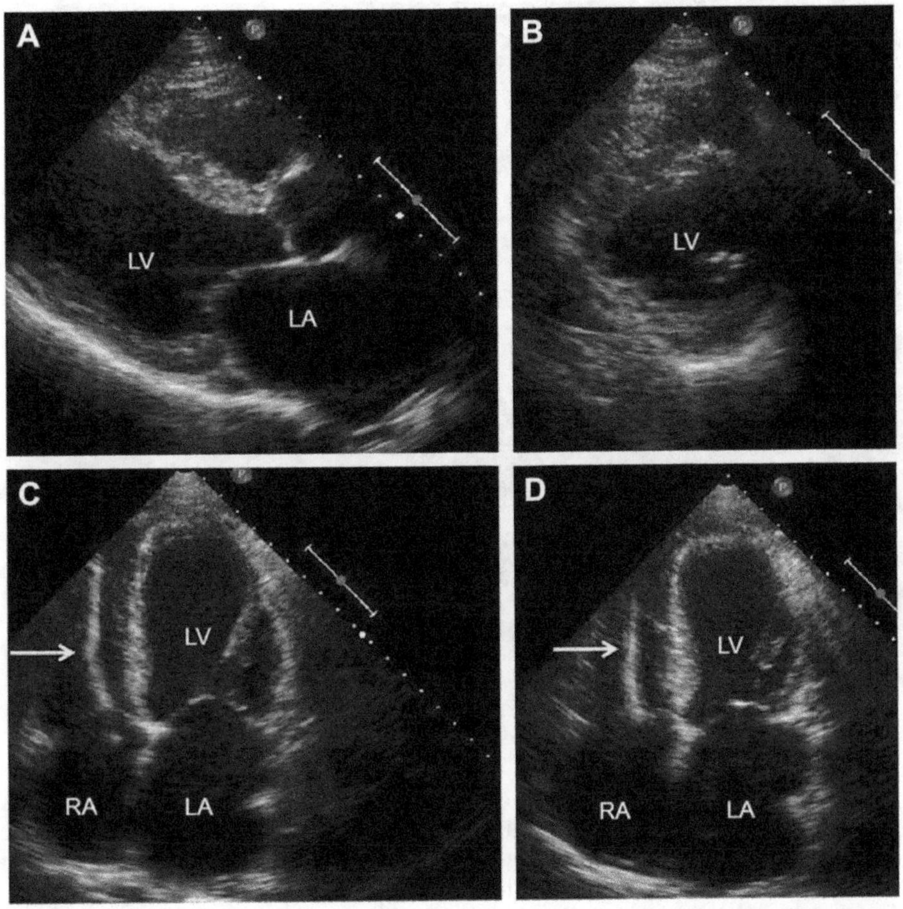

Figure 3. Echocardiogram is patient #2. *(A)* Parasternal long-axis view showing very dilated left ventricle (LV) and left atrium (LA). *(B)* Parasternal short-axis view of the left ventricle. *(C)* Four-chamber view showing the very dilated left ventricles in ventricular diastole with its thin walls. The *arrow* points to the implanted intracardiac defibrillator catheter. RA = right atrium. *(D)* Same view in ventricular systole, with minimal change in ventricular size and wall thickness indicative of markedly depressed systolic function.

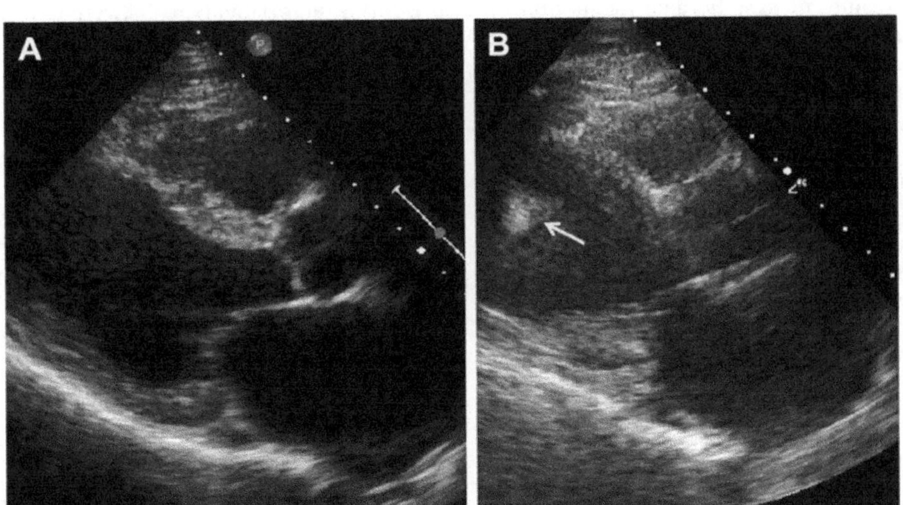

Figure 4. Echocardiogram in patient #2 before *(A)* and after *(B)* insertion of a left ventricular assist device *(arrow)*. The size of the left ventricular cavity is larger before than after insertion of the device.

The explanted heart in each patient weighed 410 g (portions of the atrial walls are not included in the weight) (Figures 5 and 6). Both hearts contained excessive subepicardial adipose tissue. In case #1, neither cardiac ventricles was dilated. Except for one left ventricular papillary muscle, no grossly visible myocardial scars were

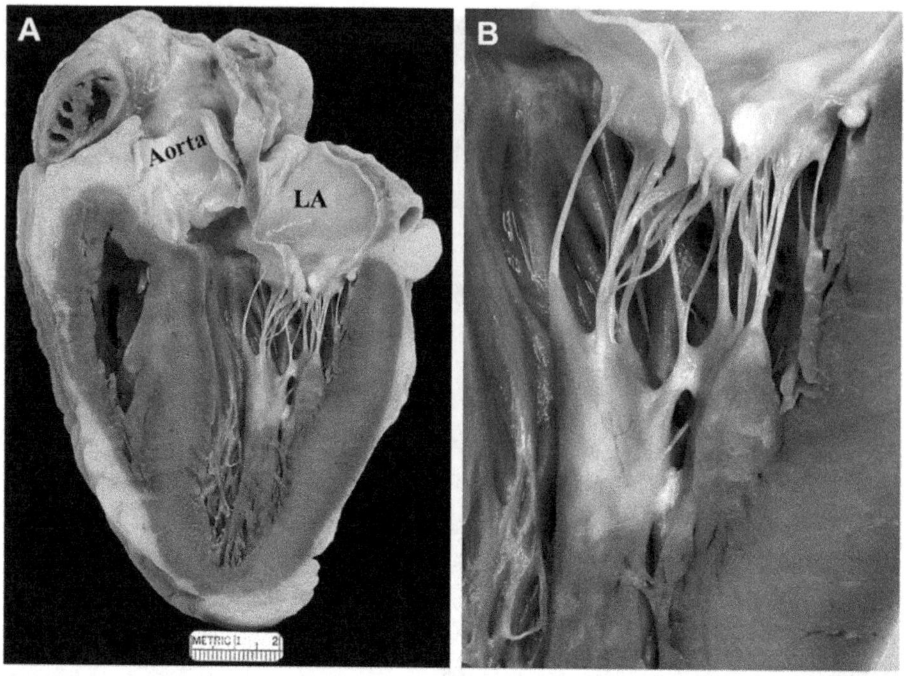

Figure 5. Case #1. *(A)* Longitudinal view of the left ventricle, right ventricular outflow tract, aortic valve, mitral valve, and left atrium. The thickness of the ventricular septum is a bit greater than that of the left ventricular free wall. The apical portion of the posteromedial papillary muscle is scarred. Calcium is present in the mitral annular region. *(B)* Close-up of the scarred papillary muscle.

present. In case #2, in contrast, there was extensive, usually transmural, scarring of the left ventricular free wall and ventricular septum with some scarring also in the right ventricular free wall. The ventricular cavities were dilated in case #2 but not as dilated as would have occurred had not a left ventricular assist device been inserted 29 months earlier. Neither patient had mural endocardial thickening in the ventricular septum in apposition to the anterior mitral leaflet, the anatomic feature of systolic anterior motion of the anterior mitral leaflet with septal contact. Patient #1, but not patient #2, had calcium in the mitral annular region.[5] Histologic study demonstrated considerable enlargement of the myocardial fibers in both patients. The intramural coronary arteries in patient #2 were increased in number and size and the lumens in many were narrowed. The quantity of interstitial fibrous tissue between myofibers was increased in both patients.

Several months after CT, both patients had blood samples (in EDTA) sent to Gene Dx (207 Perry Parkway, Gaithersburg, Maryland 20877) for "hypertrophic cardiomyopathy panel" analysis. Both patients had the p.Arg 186Gln (CGG>GAG)(R186Q) mutation in exon 8 of the troponin I (TNN13) gene (NM_000363.4), confirming that both patients had the identical disease-causing gene mutation despite strikingly different phenotypic expressions.

Discussion

Although HC is a genetically transmitted disease with an autosomal dominant trait, the penetrance into the family of the 2 cousins described herein is particularly striking. Some family members died suddenly, usually prematurely, others developed severe heart failure, and others developed various arrhythmias and conduction disturbances with intracardiac pacemakers and implantable intracardiac defibrillators implanted.

Cardiac transplantation for patients with HC is relatively infrequent, and most patients with HC having CT have severe systolic heart failure and no obstruction to either left or right ventricular outflow. Warren and colleagues[6] in 1988 appear to have been the first to describe CT for HC. Both of their patients had severe diastolic heart failure with normal sized ventricular cavities, apparently similar to our patient #1. Shirani and colleagues[7] in 1993 described 10 patients with HC who had CT and all of them had severe systolic heart failure with severe left ventricular and ventricular septal scarring, similar to that in our patient #2. Hecht and associates[8] in the same year described 2 patients with end-stage systolic heart failure who underwent CT. Contu and colleagues[9] in 2004 described 14 patients with HC who underwent CT, 13 of whom underwent CT for severe heart failure, presumably systolic in type, and 1 for malignant ventricular arrhythmias. Biagini and associates[10] in 2008 described 18 patients with HC who underwent CT, 17 of whom had severe systolic heart failure and severely dilated ventricular cavities and 1 of whom had severe diastolic heart failure with normal sized ventricular cavities. Maron and colleagues[11] in 2010 acquired data from the United Network of Organ-Sharing Registry and found among 26, 706 patients $\geq$18 years of age having CT that 303 (1%) had CT for HC. Among those 303 patients it is unclear how many had systolic or diastolic HF. They found that survival after CT was at least similar to that in non-HC patients having CT and maybe better. And finally, Kato and colleagues[12] in 2012 described 41 patients with HC who underwent CT, 39 (95%) for "refractory heart failure" and 2

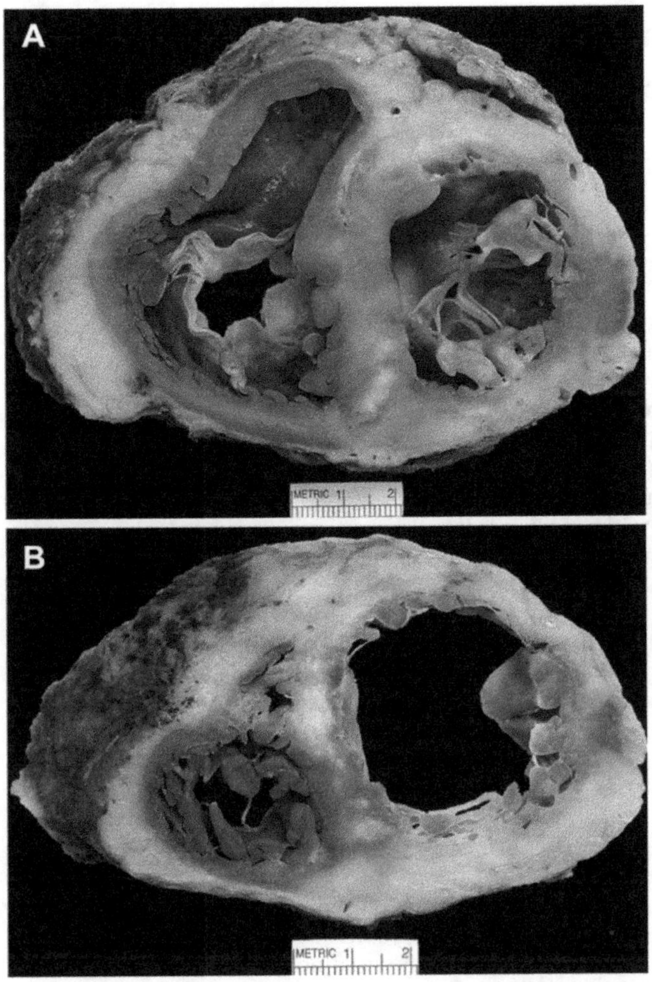

Figure 6. Case #2. Basal portion of the heart *(A)* and more caudal portion *(B)* showing extensive scarring in the left ventricular free wall and ventricular septum and scarring in the moderator band of the right ventricle. Both ventricular cavities dilated.

from "recurrent ventricular arrhythmias." Prior to CT only 14 (34%) of the 41 patients had a dilated left ventricular cavity (left ventricular end-diastolic dimension >55 mm) and 27 patients (66%) had smaller left ventricular cavities. Survival of their 41 HC patients after CT was better than that for their 771 non-HC patients. Thus, CT is a useful procedure for the relatively small percentage of patients with HC who develop end-stage HF or refractory ventricular arrhythmias unassociated with left or right ventricular outflow obstruction.

Acknowledgment: We thank Ms. Carolyn Q. Alexander, RN, BSN, for arranging the acquisition of the genetic tests in each of the 2 patients.

Disclosures

The authors have no conflicts of interest to disclose.

1. Maron BJ, Gardin JM, Flack JM, Gidding SS, Kurosaki TT, Bild DE. Prevalence of hypertrophic cardiomyopathy in a general population of young adults: echocardiographic analysis of 4111 subjects in the CARDIA study. *Circulation* 1995;92:785–789.
2. Maron BJ. Hypertrophic cardiomyopathy. *Lancet* 1997;350:127–133.
3. Spirito P, Seidman CE, McKenna WJ, Maron BJ. The management of hypertrophic cardiomyopathy. *New Eng J Med* 1997;366:775–785.
4. Maron BJ, Maron MS, Wigle ED, Bruanwald E. The 50-year history, controversy, and clinical implication of left ventricular outflow tract obstruction in hypertrophic cardiomyopathy. From idiopathic cardiomyopathy subaortic stenosis to hypertrophic cardiomyopathy. *J Am Coll Cardiol* 2009;54:191–200.
5. Motamed HE, Roberts WC. Frequency and significance of mitral anular calcium in hypertrophic cardiomyopathy: analysis of 200 necropsy patients. *Am J Cardiol* 1987;60:877–884.
6. Warren SE, Cohn LH, Schoen FJ, Mudge GH Jr, Lorell BH. Advanced diastolic heart failure in familial hypertrophic cardiomyopathy managed with cardiac transplantation. *J Appl Cardiol* 1988;3:415–422.
7. Shirani J, Maron BJ, Cannon RO III, Shahin S, Roberts WC. Clinicopathologic features of hypertrophic cardiomyopathy managed by cardiac transplantation. *Am J Cardiol* 1993;72:434–440.
8. Hecht GM, Heinrich GK, Roberts WC, Maron BJ. Coexistence of sudden cardiac death and end-stage heart failure in familial hypertrophic cardiomyopathy. *J Am Coll Cardiol* 1993;22:489–497.
9. Coutu M, Parrault LP, White M, Pelletier GB, Racine N, Poirier NC, Carrier M. Cardiac transplantation for hypertrophic cardiomyopathy: a valid therapeutic option. *J Heart Lung Transplant* 2004;43:413–417.
10. Biagini E, Spirito P, Leone O, Piccio FM, Coccolo F, Ragni L, Lofiego C, Grigioni F, Potena L, Rocchi G, Bacchi-Reggiani L, Boriani G, Prandstraller D, Arbustini E, Branzi A, Rapezzi C. Heart transplantation in hypertrophic cardiomyopathy. *Am J Cardiol* 2008;101:387–392.
11. Maron MS, Kalsmith BM, Udelson JE, Li W, DeNofrio D. Survival after cardiac transplantation in patients with hypertrophic cardiomyopathy. *Circ Heart Fail* 2010;3:574–579.
12. Kato TS, Takayama H, Yoshizawa S, Morboe C, Schulze PS, Farr M, Naka Y, Mancini D, Maurer MS. Cardiac transplantation in patients with hypertrophic cardiomyopathy. *Am J Cardiol* 2012;110:568–574.

Natural History of Unoperated Aortic Stenosis During a 50-Year Period of Cardiac Valve Replacement

William C. Roberts, MD[a,b,c,d,*], Travis J. Vowels, BBA[a], Giovanni Filardo, PhD, MPH[e,f], Jong M. Ko, BA[a], Raj P. Mathur, MD[d], and Jamshid Shirani, MD[d]

Although a number of publications have described the natural history of patients with aortic stenosis (AS), the definition of "natural history" varies widely. Those describing a large number of patients with AS without operative therapy with necropsy findings are rare. Two hundred sixty patients >15 years of age with AS were studied at necropsy over a 50-year period by the same investigator. Of the 260 patients, the valve in 37 (14%) was congenitally unicuspid, in 123 (47%), congenitally bicuspid, and in 100 (38%), tricuspid. Aortic valve structure varied with age of death (in years; unicuspid 52 ± 17, bicuspid 63 ± 12, and tricuspid 70 ± 14 years); gender (men/women: unicuspid 95%/5%, bicuspid 78%/22%, and tricuspid 63%/37%), and frequency of calcium in the mitral valve annulus and epicardial coronary arteries. The patients with cardiac-related symptoms compared with those without were more likely to have a congenitally malformed valve (unicuspid 17% vs 12%; bicuspid 51% vs 29%; tricuspid 31% vs 60%; unadjusted p = 0.013), to die from cardiac disease (86% vs 54%; unadjusted p = 0.001), and to have larger hearts (mean cardiac weight 606 ± 138 g vs 523 ± 121 g; unadjusted p = 0.009) and a larger quantity of calcium in the aortic valve cusps. In conclusion, the length of survival in adults with AS is related to valve structure, gender, presence of cardiac-related symptoms, cardiac mass, and quantity of calcium in the aortic valve cusps. **(Am J Cardiol 2013;112:541–553)**

During the past 80 years or so, a number of reports describing the natural history of patients with valvular aortic stenosis (AS) have been published. Before 1970, most focused on patients with AS studied at necropsy, and most centered on the cause of the AS.[1] After predictably successful aortic valve replacement became a reality in the early 1960s, more reports appeared on the natural history of AS, but "natural history" meant something different in most studies. In some studies, it meant what happened when patients were followed for a specified period of time. In others, the term focused on the survival duration of symptomatic or asymptomatic patients until either an aortic valve operation was performed or death. A few included only subjects who had cardiac catheterization or echocardiography performed such that the severity of the AS was accurately known. No study in the past 50 years has focused on a large group of adults with AS studied at necropsy in whom an aortic valve operation during life had never been performed. Such is the purpose of this report.

Methods

From January 1956 until July 2012, 260 patients with AS unassociated with mitral stenosis were studied at necropsy either at the National Institutes of Health (Pathology Branch, National Heart, Lung, and Blood Institute, Bethesda, Maryland) or at Baylor University Medical Center, Dallas, Texas; they are the subject of this study. All hearts were examined and classified by one of us (WCR). Many hearts had been submitted from other hospitals, particularly those in the Washington, DC, and surrounding areas. To be included in this study, at the time of necropsy, patients had to be >15 years of age, have a nonstenotic mitral valve, and had no operative procedure at any time on any cardiac valve. The aortic valve morphologically had to be clearly stenotic, that is, contain enough calcific deposits such that mobility of the aortic valve cusp or cusps was clearly diminished. The underlying structure of the stenotic aortic valve (i.e., unicuspid, bicuspid, or tricuspid) was determined in all cases by the same observer (WCR). The major epicardial coronary arteries were examined for obstructions, and the left ventricular walls were examined for foci of necrosis and fibrosis. Myocardial necrosis/fibrosis was confirmed by study of histologic sections of these areas. The medical records were sought and received from the hospitals submitting the heart

[a]Baylor Heart and Vascular Institute, [b]Department of Internal Medicine, Division of Cardiology, and [c]Department of Pathology, Baylor University Medical Center, Dallas, Texas; [d]Pathology Branch, National Heart, Lung, and Blood Institute, National Institutes of Health, Bethesda, Maryland; [e]Institute for Health Care Research and Improvement, Baylor University Medical Center; and [f]Department of Statistical Science, Southern Methodist University, Dallas, Texas. Manuscript received March 21, 2013; revised manuscript received and accepted April 3, 2013.

TJV is a first year medical student at the University of Texas Medical School at Houston, TX.

Present address (RPM): 106 Irving NW St Suite 218, Washington, DC 20010.

Present address (JS): St. Luke's University Health Network Cardiology, 801 Ostrum Street, Bethlehem, PA 18015.

This work was supported by grants from the Baylor Heart and Vascular Institute Cardiovascular Research Review Committee and Baylor Health Care System Foundation.

See page 552 for disclosure information.

*Corresponding author: Tel: (214) 820-7911; fax: (214) 820-7533.

E-mail address: wc.roberts@baylorhealth.edu (W.C. Roberts).

Table 1
Morphologic and clinical variables, and modes of death in 260 patients with valvular aortic stenosis according to aortic valve structure

Variable	Unicuspid	Bicuspid	Tricuspid	Unadjusted* p Value
	n = 37 (14%)	n = 123 (47%)	n = 100 (38%)	
Age in years: range (n = 254)	16–87	23–89	36–99	0.001
(Mean ± SD)	(52 ± 17)	(63 ± 12)	(70 ± 14)	
95% CI	47,56	60,65	67,72	
Men/Women (n = 257)	35/2	93/27	63/37	0.005
	95%/5%	78%/22%	63%/37%	
Symptoms† (n = 260)				0.013
Symptomatic	30 (81%)	89 (72%)	54 (54%)	
Asymptomatic	6 (16%)	15 (12%)	31 (31%)	
Unknown	1 (3%)	19 (16%)	15 (15%)	
Mode of death (n = 260)				0.511
Cardiac				
Sudden	6 (16%)	29 (24%)	26 (26%)	
Non-sudden	28 (76%)	66 (54%)	47 (47%)	
Vascular	1 (3%)	5 (4%)	2 (2%)	
Noncardiac, nonvascular	2 (5%)	20 (16%)	25 (25%)	
Unknown	0	3 (2%)	0	
Heart weight (g): range (n = 231)	320–880	340–1,050	305–960	0.127‡
(Mean ± SD)	(633 ± 136)	(591 ± 148)	(552 ± 132)	
95% CI	585,681	564,618	523,581	
Men	320–880	385–1,050	380–960	
	(637 ± 137)	(620 ± 147)	(603 ± 115)	
Women	510	340–730	305–710	
	—	(496 ± 119)	(458 ± 108)	
Number of enlarged hearts§ (n = 215 of 231)	31 of 33 (94%)	100 of 106 (94%)	84 of 92 (91%)	0.689
Narrowing of ≥1 major coronary arteries >75% (n = 96/234)	6 (17%)	43 (41%)	47 (51%)	0.018
Left ventricular (n = 260)				0.513
Necrosis only	1 (3%)	8 (7%)	6 (6%)	
Fibrosis only	15 (41%)	44 (36%)	25 (25%)	
Both	2 (5%)	7 (6%)	5 (5%)	
Neither	19 (51%)	64 (52%)	64 (64%)	
Calcium				
Aortic valve (n = 251)				0.404
0	1 (3%)	1 (1%)	1 (1%)	
1+	5 (14%)	9 (8%)	7 (7%)	
2+	2 (5%)	15 (13%)	18 (18%)	
3+	10 (27%)	27 (23%)	30 (31%)	
4+	19 (51%)	64 (55%)	42 (43%)	
Mitral annulus (n = 89 of 245)	7 (19%)	22 (20%)	60 (61%)	0.001
Coronary arteries (n = 121 of 232)	11 (31%)	43 (41%)	67 (73%)	0.001

* Multiplicity accounted for.
† Symptoms include heart failure, angina pectoris, and syncope, or any combination of the 3.
‡ Unicuspid versus tricuspid p value = 0.051.
§ Hearts weighing >350 g in women and >400 g in men.

specimens. Most stenotic aortic valves were photographed at either the Pathology Branch, National Heart, Lung, and Blood Institute, or in the Cardiovascular Laboratory at Baylor University Medical Center.

Means, SDs, and percentages were calculated to describe the study cohort (n = 260). Differences in demographic, clinical, and morphologic details were tested with a Wilcoxon (for continuous factors) or a chi-square (for categorical factors) test. Unadjusted p values and 95% confidence intervals (CIs) were also estimated. A Bonferroni correction was used to account for multiplicity. A multivariable logistic regression model was used to assess the adjusted-association between patients having symptoms (heart failure, angina pectoris, and/or syncope) and cause of death (e.g., cardiac or vascular).[2] Covariates included gender, valve structure, heart weight (in grams), degree of coronary narrowing, foci of left ventricular necrosis and/or fibrosis, presence of calcium in the coronary arteries (in ≥1 coronary arteries). Likewise, 2 multivariable logistic regression models were used to assess the adjusted-association between age and (1) congenital valve disease and (2) presence of calcium in the coronary arteries. Covariates included patient having symptoms (heart failure, angina pectoris, and/or syncope), gender, valve structure (for calcium model only), heart weight (in grams), degree of coronary narrowing, foci of left ventricular necrosis and/or fibrosis, and presence of calcium in the coronary arteries (congenital valve model only). Restricted cubic splines were used for all continuous variables, and multiple imputation via

Table 2
Morphologic and clinical variables, and modes of death in 257 patients with valvular aortic stenosis according to gender

Variable	Men	Women	Unadjusted* p Value
	n = 191 (74%)	n = 66 (26%)	
Age in years: range (n = 254)	16–99	32–90	0.001
(Mean ± SD)	(61 ± 15)	(70 ± 13)	
95% CI	59,64	66,73	
Aortic valve structure (n = 257)			0.005
Unicuspid	35 (18%)	2 (3%)	
Bicuspid	93 (49%)	27 (41%)	
Tricuspid	63 (33%)	37 (56%)	
Symptoms† (n = 257)			0.973
Symptomatic	129 (68%)	44 (67%)	
Asymptomatic	38 (20%)	14 (21%)	
Unknown	24 (12%)	8 (12%)	
Mode of death (n = 257)			0.558
Cardiac			
Sudden	45 (24%)	16 (24%)	
Non-sudden	109 (57%)	32 (48%)	
Vascular	6 (3%)	2 (3%)	
Noncardiac, nonvascular	30 (16%)	16 (24%)	
Unknown	1 (1%)	0	
Heart weight (g): range (n = 231)	320–1,050	305–730	0.001
(Mean ± SD)	(617 ± 135)	(474 ± 112)	
95% CI	598,636	440,509	
Number of enlarged hearts‡ (n = 215 of 231)	167 of 175 (95%)	48 of 56 (86%)	0.129
Coronary narrowing >75%§ (n = 95 of 233)	74 (43%)	21 (35%)	0.292
Left ventricular (n = 257)			0.829
Necrosis only	11 (6%)	4 (6%)	
Fibrosis only	69 (36%)	14 (21%)	
Both	11 (6%)	2 (3%)	
Neither	100 (52%)	46 (70%)	
Calcium			
Aortic valve (n = 249)			0.385
0	3 (2%)	0	
1+	17 (9%)	4 (6%)	
2+	27 (15%)	8 (12%)	
3+	51 (28%)	14 (22%)	
4+	86 (47%)	39 (60%)	
Mitral annulus (n = 88 of 243)	51 (28%)	37 (59%)	0.001
Coronary arteries (n = 120 of 231)	85 (49%)	35 (61%)	0.100

* Multiplicity accounted for.
† Symptoms include heart failure, angina pectoris, and syncope, or any combination of the 3.
‡ Hearts weighing >350 g in women and >400 g in men.
§ In cross-sectional area.

predictive mean matching was used to account for missing data regarding the independent variables in this model. The adjusted p values, odds ratios, and 95% CIs were also estimated.[2,3]

The study protocol was approved by the Institutional Review Board of Baylor University Medical Center.

Results

The findings in the present study are summarized in Tables 1 through 7. Table 1 displays data according to aortic valve structure, Table 2 according to gender, Table 3 according to symptomatic status, Table 4 according to age group at death, Table 5 according to heart weight, and Table 6 according to degree of coronary narrowing. Table 7 provides findings in the 37 patients who had left-sided cardiac catheterization. Table 8 lists findings in the 29 patients whose stenotic aortic valves are illustrated in Figures 1 through 4. Figure 5 illustrates the length of survival after onset of symptoms: angina pectoris, heart failure, syncope, and various combinations of these. Figure 6 shows the length of survival after onset of any cardiac symptom: angina pectoris, heart failure, syncope, or any combination of these. Figure 7 displays the relation of age to the probability of having a congenitally malformed aortic valve (unicuspid or bicuspid) and calcium in ≥1 coronary arteries.

Of the 260 patients, the aortic valve was *unicuspid* in 37 (14%; Figure 1), *bicuspid* in 123 (47%; Figures 2 and 3), and *tricuspid* in 100 (38%; Figure 4; Table 1). The fewer the number of aortic valve cusps, the higher the frequency of males (95% with unicuspid valves, 78% with bicuspid valves, and 63% with tricuspid valves, unadjusted p = 0.005). The

Table 3
Morphologic and clinical variables, and modes of death in 260 patients with valvular aortic stenosis according to the presence or absence of symptoms*

Variable	Symptomatic n = 173 (67%)	Asymptomatic n = 52 (20%)	Unknown n = 35 (13%)	Unadjusted† p Value
Age in years: range (n = 254)	16–92	23–89	37–99	0.854
(Mean ± SD)	(64 ± 14)	(64 ± 17)	(62 ± 15)	
95% CI	62,66	60,68	57,68	
Men/Women (n = 257)	129/44	38/14	24/8	0.973
	75%/25%	73%/27%	75%/25%	
Aortic valve structure (n = 260)				0.013
Unicuspid	30 (17%)	6 (12%)	1 (3%)	
Bicuspid	89 (51%)	15 (29%)	19 (54%)	
Tricuspid	54 (31%)	31 (60%)	15 (43%)	
Mode of death (n = 260)				0.001
Cardiac				
Sudden	38 (22%)	14 (27%)	9 (26%)	
Non-sudden	111 (64%)	14 (27%)	16 (46%)	
Vascular	4 (2%)	4 (8%)	0	
Noncardiac, nonvascular	20 (12%)	20 (38%)	7 (20%)	
Unknown	0	0	3 (9%)	
Heart weight (g): range (n = 231)	320–1,050	305–920	310–1,000	0.009
(Mean ± SD)	(606 ± 138)	(523 ± 121)	(563 ± 173)	
95% CI	584,628	484,561	511,608	
Men	320–1,050	340–920	420–1,000	
	(638 ± 131)	(543 ± 115)	(633 ± 147)	
Women	370–730	305–650	310–500	
	(499 ± 106)	(465 ± 123)	(381 ± 72)	
Number of enlarged hearts‡ (n = 215 of 231)	148 of 152 (97%)	43 of 50 (86%)	24 of 29 (83%)	0.015
Narrowing of ≥1 major coronary arteries >75% (n = 96 of 234)	67 (41%)	15 (33%)	14 (56%)	0.161
Left ventricular (n = 260)				0.449
Necrosis only	9 (5%)	4 (8%)	2 (6%)	
Fibrosis only	64 (37%)	9 (17%)	11 (31%)	
Both	12 (7%)	0	2 (6%)	
Neither	88 (51%)	39 (75%)	20 (57%)	
Calcium				
Aortic valve (n = 251)				0.038
0	2 (1%)	1 (2%)	0	
1+	10 (6%)	6 (12%)	5 (17%)	
2+	19 (11%)	13 (25%)	3 (10%)	
3+	40 (23%)	15 (29%)	12 (41%)	
4+	100 (58%)	16 (31%)	9 (31%)	
Mitral annulus (n = 89 of 245)	59 (35%)	18 (36%)	12 (43%)	0.745
Coronary arteries (n = 121 of 232)	80 (49%)	24 (52%)	17 (71%)	0.147

* Symptoms include heart failure, angina pectoris, and syncope, or any combination of the 3.
† Multiplicity accounted for.
‡ Hearts weighing >350 g in women and >400 g in men.

frequency of angina pectoris, heart failure, and/or syncope was similar in patients with unicuspid and bicuspid valves and less in those with tricuspid valves (83% vs 86% vs 64%, unadjusted p = 0.013). Men had mean heart weights larger than women in all 3 valve-structure groups; the patients with unicuspid valves had larger hearts than those with tricuspid aortic valves (633 vs 552 g, unadjusted p = 0.051). Calcific deposits in the coronary arteries and in the mitral annulus were less frequent in those with unicuspid and bicuspid valves than in those with tricuspid valves (19% vs 20% vs 61%, unadjusted p = 0.001, and 31% vs 41% vs 73%, unadjusted p = 0.001, respectively). Coronary narrowing >75% in cross-sectional area by atherosclerotic plaques was less the fewer the number of aortic valve cusps (17% vs 41% vs 51%, unadjusted p = 0.018). No significant differences were observed in modes of death, frequency of foci of left ventricular wall necrosis or fibrosis, or both or neither.

Differences among the 8 variables analyzed between *men* and *women* are summarized in Table 2. The mean ages, number of aortic valve cusps, heart weight, and calcium in the mitral annular region were significantly different between genders. No significant differences were observed between men and women in the frequency of cardiac symptoms, mode of death, frequency of severe (>75%) coronary narrowing or foci of left ventricular necrosis and/or fibrosis, and quantity of calcium in the aortic valve and in the coronary arteries.

Table 3 summarizes differences in the various variables in the *symptomatic versus the asymptomatic patients*. Of the symptomatic patients, 69% had a unicuspid or bicuspid valve and 31%, a tricuspid valve; of the asymptomatic patients, 40%

Table 4
Morphologic and clinical variables, and modes of death in 254 patients with valvular aortic stenosis according to age group

Variable	Age Groups (years)			Unadjusted* p Value
	16–35	36–65	>65	
	n = 11 (4%)	n = 119 (47%)	n = 124 (49%)	
Men/Women (n = 254)	10/1 91%/9%	97/22 82%/18%	81/43 65%/35%	0.069
Aortic valve structure (n = 254)				0.001
Unicuspid	9 (82%)	22 (18%)	6 (5%)	
Bicuspid	2 (18%)	64 (54%)	52 (42%)	
Tricuspid	0	33 (28%)	66 (53%)	
Symptoms[†] (n = 254)				0.229
Symptomatic	6 (55%)	83 (70%)	84 (68%)	
Asymptomatic	5 (45%)	17 (14%)	30 (24%)	
Unknown	0	19 (16%)	10 (8%)	
Mode of death (n = 254)				0.380
Cardiac				
Sudden	3 (27%)	32 (27%)	26 (21%)	
Non-sudden	6 (55%)	68 (57%)	64 (52%)	
Vascular	1 (9%)	2 (2%)	5 (4%)	
Noncardiac, nonvascular	1 (9%)	16 (13%)	29 (23%)	
Unknown	0	1 (1%)	0	
Heart weight (g): range (n = 230)	480–880	305–1,050	310–860	0.107[‡]
(Mean ± SD)	(622 ± 116)	(609 ± 157)	(554 ± 126)	
95% CI	538,706	582,636	527,580	
Men	480–880 (633 ± 116)	320–1,050 (638 ± 148)	380–860 (593 ± 117)	
Women	510	305–730 (483 ± 133)	310–710 (468 ± 103)	
Number of enlarged hearts[§] (214 of 230)	11 of 11 (100%)	99 of 108 (92%)	104 of 111 (94%)	0.547
Narrowing of ≥1 major coronary arteries >75% (n = 95/232)	0	41 (37%)	54 (48%)	0.069
Left ventricular (n = 254)				0.502
Necrosis only	2 (18%)	5 (4%)	7 (6%)	
Fibrosis only	4 (36%)	38 (32%)	41 (33%)	
Both	0	8 (7%)	5 (4%)	
Neither	5 (45%)	68 (57%)	71 (57%)	
Calcium				
Aortic valve (n = 248)				0.101
0	1 (9%)	1 (1%)	1 (1%)	
1+	0	11 (9%)	10 (8%)	
2+	3 (27%)	18 (16%)	14 (12%)	
3+	5 (45%)	27 (23%)	33 (27%)	
4+	2 (18%)	59 (51%)	63 (52%)	
Mitral annulus (n = 88 of 242)	0	36 (32%)	52 (44%)	0.059
Coronary arteries (n = 119 of 230)	1 (10%)	34 (33%)	84 (71%)	0.001

* Multiplicity accounted for.
† Symptoms include heart failure, angina pectoris, and syncope, or any combination of the 3.
‡ Age groups 36 to 65 versus >65 p value = 0.042.
§ Hearts weighing >350 g in women and >400 g in men.

had either a unicuspid or bicuspid valve and 60%, a tricuspid valve (unadjusted p = 0.013). The symptomatic patients had larger hearts than the asymptomatic ones (606 vs 523 g, unadjusted p = 0.009), more left ventricular wall scarring (46% vs 18%), and a larger quantity of calcific deposits in the aortic valve cusps (unadjusted p = 0.038). No significant differences were observed between the symptomatic and asymptomatic groups in age, gender, frequency of severe coronary narrowing, frequency of foci of left ventricular necrosis, or the frequency of calcific deposits in the mitral annulus or coronary arteries. However, the adjusted analysis showed that patients having symptoms (heart failure, angina pectoris, and/or syncope) were more likely to die from cardiac causes than asymptomatic patients (adjusted odds ratio = 3.61; 95% CI: 1.85, 7.05, p <0.001).

Findings according to *age group* (16 to 35, 36 to 65, and >65 years) are summarized in Table 4. All 11 patients aged 16 to 35 had unicuspid (n = 9) or bicuspid (n = 2) valves; 72% of the 119 patients aged 36 to 65 had unicuspid (n = 22) or bicuspid (n = 64) valves, and 47% of the 124 patients aged >65 years had unicuspid (n = 6) or bicuspid (n = 52) valves (unadjusted p = 0.001; Figure 6). The frequency of calcium in either the coronary arteries or mitral annulus was least in the younger age group and greatest in

Table 5
Morphologic and clinical variables, and modes of death in 234 patients with valvular aortic stenosis according to heart weight

Variable	Heart Weight (g)			Unadjusted* p Value
	≤400	401–600	>600	
	n = 26 (11%)	n = 108 (46%)	n = 100 (43%)	
Age in years: range (n = 230)	47–90	23–99	16–89	0.021
(Mean ± SD)	67 ± 11	66 ± 15	59 ± 15	
Men/Women (n = 231)	8/18	76/29	91/9	0.001
	31%/69%	72%/28%	91%/9%	
Aortic valve structure (n = 234)				0.202
Unicuspid	2 (8%)	11 (10%)	20 (20%)	
Bicuspid	11 (42%)	53 (49%)	45 (45%)	
Tricuspid	13 (50%)	44 (41%)	35 (35%)	
Symptoms† (n = 234)				0.031
Symptomatic	12 (46%)	62 (57%)	78 (78%)	
Asymptomatic	8 (31%)	31 (29%)	11 (11%)	
Unknown	6 (23%)	15 (14%)	11 (11%)	
Mode of death (n = 234)				0.659
Cardiac				
Sudden	9 (35%)	21 (19%)	23 (23%)	
Non-sudden	8 (31%)	57 (53%)	62 (62%)	
Vascular	2 (8%)	2 (2%)	3 (3%)	
Noncardiac, nonvascular	7 (27%)	26 (24%)	11 (11%)	
Unknown	0	2 (2%)	1 (1%)	
Narrowing of ≥1 major coronary arteries >75% (n = 92/213)	11 (42%)	43 (40%)	38 (38%)	0.922
Left ventricular (n = 234)				0.729
Necrosis only	1 (4%)	10 (9%)	3 (3%)	
Fibrosis only	9 (35%)	28 (26%)	42 (42%)	
Both	0	6 (6%)	8 (8%)	
Neither	16 (62%)	64 (59%)	47 (47%)	
Calcium				
Aortic valve (n = 229)				0.261
0	0	0	3 (3%)	
1+	4 (15%)	8 (8%)	6 (6%)	
2+	3 (12%)	20 (19%)	10 (10%)	
3+	7 (27%)	29 (28%)	27 (27%)	
4+	12 (46%)	47 (45%)	53 (54%)	
Mitral annulus (n = 80/223)	11 (42%)	35 (32%)	34 (34%)	0.558
Coronary arteries (n = 110/211)	16 (62%)	55 (51%)	39 (39%)	0.578

* Multiplicity accounted for.
† Symptoms include heart failure, angina pectoris, and syncope, or any combination of the 3.

the oldest age group (0% vs 32% vs 44%, p = 0.059, and 10% vs 33% vs 71%, unadjusted p = 0.001) (Figure 6). No significant differences were observed among the 3 age groups in gender, symptomatic status, mode of death, heart weight, frequency of severe coronary narrowing, or left ventricular necrosis or fibrosis.

Findings according to 3 *heart weight* groups are summarized in Table 5. Women had smaller hearts than men, and 69% of the smaller hearts (≤400 g) belonged to women; of the 100 hearts weighing >600 g, 91 (91%) belonged to men (unadjusted p = 0.001). Of the 33 patients with unicuspid aortic valves, 31 (94%) weighed >400 g and 20 (61%) weighed >600 g, and of the 92 patients with tricuspid aortic valves, 79 (86%) weighed >400 g, but only 35 (38%) weighed >600 g. No significant differences were observed in the 3 age groups in aortic valve structure, mode of death, percent with severe (>75%) coronary narrowing or left ventricular necrosis or fibrosis, or presence of calcium in the aortic valve, mitral annulus, or coronary arteries.

Findings according to whether *coronary narrowing* >75% in cross-sectional area occurred is summarized in Table 6. Those with severe coronary narrowing were more likely to be older, to have a tricuspid aortic valve, to have calcific deposits in the coronary arteries and foci of left ventricular necrosis and/or fibrosis than those with lesser degrees of coronary narrowing (unadjusted p = 0.001).

Pertinent findings in the 37 patients who underwent *left-sided cardiac catheterization* are summarized in Table 7.

Discussion

This study of 260 adult patients with unoperated AS followed to death and autopsy demonstrated that patients with unicuspid or bicuspid valves (congenital origin) as

Table 6
Morphologic and clinical variables, and modes of death in 234 patients with valvular aortic stenosis according to coronary artery narrowing

Variable	Coronary Narrowing (Cross-Sectional Area)		Unadjusted* p Value
	>75%	<75%	
	n = 96 (41%)	n = 138 (59%)	
Age in years: range (n = 232)	42–99	16–90	0.001
(Mean ± SD)	68 ± 12	61 ± 15	
Men/Women (n = 233)	74/21	99/39	0.292
	78%/22%	72%/28%	
Aortic valve structure (n = 234)			0.018
Unicuspid	6 (6%)	30 (22%)	
Bicuspid	43 (45%)	63 (46%)	
Tricuspid	47 (48%)	45 (33%)	
Symptoms† (n = 234)			0.161
Symptomatic	67 (69%)	96 (70%)	
Asymptomatic	15 (16%)	31 (22%)	
Unknown	14 (15%)	11 (8%)	
Mode of death (n = 234)			0.245
Cardiac			
Sudden	26 (27%)	31 (22%)	
Non-sudden	47 (49%)	80 (58%)	
Vascular	5 (5%)	2 (1%)	
Noncardiac, nonvascular	17 (18%)	25 (18%)	
Unknown	1 (1%)	0	
Heart weight (g): range (n = 212)	305–1,050	310–960	0.222
(Mean ± SD)	566 ± 137	590 ± 142	
Men	320–1,050	380–960	
	593 ± 132	630 ± 130	
Women	305–730	310–710	
	472 ± 118	473 ± 105	
Number of enlarged hearts‡ (n = 197 of 212)	85 of 91 (93%)	112 of 121 (93%)	0.813
Left ventricular (n = 234)			0.001
Necrosis only	7 (7%)	5 (4%)	
Fibrosis only	49 (51%)	28 (20%)	
Both	8 (8%)	4 (3%)	
Neither	32 (33%)	101 (73%)	
Calcium			
Aortic valve (n = 234)			0.464
0	0	3 (2%)	
1+	10 (10%)	9 (7%)	
2+	13 (14%)	22 (16%)	
3+	22 (23%)	35 (25%)	
4+	51 (53%)	69 (50%)	
Mitral annulus (n = 81/231)	39 (41%)	42 (30%)	0.112
Coronary arteries (n = 111/221)	64 (67%)	47 (34%)	0.001

* Multiplicity accounted for.
† Symptoms include heart failure, angina pectoris, and syncope, or any combination of the 3.
‡ Hearts weighing >350 g in women and >400 g in men.

opposed to those with tricuspid valves (acquired origin) had a younger age of death, a greater likelihood of being male, a higher likelihood of having cardiac-related symptoms, heavier hearts, larger quantities of calcium in the aortic valve cusps, but a lower frequency of calcium in the epicardial coronary arteries and in the mitral annulus.

Although a number of reports before 1960 described clinical and/or necropsy findings in patients with AS, the structure of the aortic valve and the severity of AS were infrequently mentioned.[1] The morphologic data in most studies were garnered from autopsy protocols prepared by a number of prosectors with varying expertise in cardiovascular disease. Additionally, few contained photographs of the stenotic valves, or the number was quite limited, preventing the reader's being assured of the severity of the AS. Moreover, some studies of patients with AS also included patients with mitral stenosis, highly prevalent before World War II. Indeed, many of the morphologic studies concluded that rheumatic heart disease was the origin of AS in most patients.[1] The present study excluded patients with mitral stenosis in an attempt to exclude rheumatic heart disease as a cause of the AS in any of our 260 patients.[4]

Table 7
Clinical and morphologic findings in 37 patients seen at necropsy having valvular aortic stenosis and a left heart catheterization within 2 years of death

Patient	Age (Years)	Gender	Number of AV Cusps	AV Calcium	Interval from Cath to Death (Days)	Left Ventricle		Aorta		PSG (mm Hg)	Heart Weight (g)
						Systolic (mm Hg)	Diastolic (mm Hg)	Systolic (mm Hg)	Diastolic (mm Hg)		
1	32	F	1	4+	34	172	26	82	66	90	510
2	33	M	1	3+	24	135	50	120	60	15	880
3	34	M	1	3+	37	184	36	92	68	92	570
4	39	M	1	4+	40	162	25	96	66	66	750
5	57	M	1	4+	670	202	18	122	72	80	630
6	60	M	1	1+	30	—	—	—	—	60	—
7	16	M	2	3+	11	230	8	105	75	125	680
8	37	M	2	4+	365	146	37	96	74	50	750
9	42	F	2	2+	10	240	12	115	65	125	420
10	52	M	2	3+	30	—	—	—	—	80	630
11	52	F	2	4+	1	230	30	100	70	130	700
12	54	M	2	4+	30	238	37	90	70	148	850
13	54	M	2	4+	2	192	10	63	34	129	700
14	56	M	2	3+	30	191	24	104	61	87	—
15	58	M	2	1+	60	—	—	—	—	20	—
16	59	M	2	4+	720	200	12	155	60	45	580
17	59	M	2	2+	1	—	—	—	—	35	470
18	60	F	2	4+	15	—	—	—	—	110	680
19	61	M	2	4+	2	165	40	111	—	54	630
20	67	M	2	2+	730	202	7	175	95	27	—
21	67	M	2	4+	30	—	35	—	—	55	740
22	67	M	2	4+	90	—	8	—	—	72	680
23	68	M	2	1+	522	123	20	112	59	11	550
24	75	F	2	4+	1	—	—	—	—	125	—
25	77	M	2	4+	2	—	—	—	—	50	570
26	44	M	3	4+	9	—	—	—	—	82	590
27	49	M	3	4+	12	188	20	114	48	74	710
28	51	M	3	2+	720	—	—	—	—	20	960
29	62	M	3	3+	1	—	—	—	—	15	500
30	66	M	3	4+	30	182	40	120	60	62	655
31	71	M	3	2+	570	—	—	—	—	20	800
32	76	F	3	4+	1	—	—	—	—	60	—
33	77	F	3	3+	90	180	4	115	—	65	380
34	79	M	3	3+	8	150	10	120	80	30	505
35	61	M	2	4+	90	—	—	—	—	100	530
36	60	M	2	—	180	197	12	186	72	11	540
37	70	M	2	—	92	—	—	—	—	93	—

AV = aortic valve; Cath = catheterization; F = female; M = male; PSG = peak systolic pressure gradient; — = no information available.

Beginning in approximately 1960, a number of clinical studies focused on the "natural history" of patients with AS.[5–20] Early on the focus was mainly in children and young adults with congenital AS and, by the 1980s, most studies centered on older adults. An early article by Ross and Braunwald[21] delineated the average length of survival in patients with AS after onset of symptoms (angina pectoris, heart failure, and/or syncope) based on earlier studies, and their predictions have subsequently proven to be quite accurate. Cohen and colleagues[2] in 1972 reported on 15 initially asymptomatic children with congenital AS studied at cardiac catheterization at an average age of 8.5 years and then again at an average age of 15.1 years and showed that there was in general a poor correlation among the presence of symptoms, the electrocardiographic and radiographic findings, and the severity of the AS. Frank and colleagues[8] in 1973 studied 15 adults with the degree of AS documented hemodynamically and no aortic valve operation performed. During follow-up of 10 years, 13 of the 15 had died. Subsequently, many reports of "natural history" of symptomatic and asymptomatic AS have appeared with the severity of AS documented by cardiac catheterization or by echocardiogram with the patients followed for a specific period of time after hemodynamic or echocardiographic documentation or until death or aortic valve operation. Most confirmed the dire predictions of Ross and Braunwald. None of the reports of "natural history" of AS in the past 50 years have focused on adults with AS studied at necropsy.

The strong point of the present study is that it includes a large group of patients with AS unassociated with mitral stenosis and each case at necropsy was studied by a single individual over a period of more than 50 years. No patient had an aortic valve operation, and all were followed to death with subsequent autopsy. All attempts were made in this

Table 8
Clinical and morphologic findings in 29 patients whose stenotic aortic valves are illustrated in Figures 1 through 4

Figure	Age (Years)	Gender	Number of AV Cusps	Year of Death	AS Diagnosed During Life	Cause of Death	Symptomatic			Duration of Symptoms (Months)	Left Ventricular		CAD	MAC	PSG (mm Hg)	Heart Weight (g)
							Heart Failure	Syncope	Angina Pectoris		Necrosis	Fibrosis				
1A	68	M	1	1963	—	NC	0	0	+	—	+	+	0	0	—	750
1B	77	M	1	1971	+	C (NS)	+	0	0	1	0	0	0	0	—	495
1C	83	M	1	1978	—	C (NS)	+	0	0	48	0	0	0	0	—	805
1D	54	M	1	1961	+	C (NS)	+	0	0	108	0	+	0	0	129	700
1E	54	M	1	1966	—	C (NS)	+	0	0	36	0	0	0	0	—	—
1F	59	M	1	1969	+	C (NS)	+	+	0	11	0	0	0	0	—	650
1G	34	M	1	1966	+	C (NS)	+	0	+	180	0	+	0	+	92	570
1H	48	M	1	1968	+	C (NS)	+	0	0	132	0	+	0	+	—	750
1I	60	M	1	1971	+	C (NS)	+	0	0	12	0	+	0	+	—	700
2A	49	M	2	1985	+	C (NS)	+	0	+	96	0	+	+	0	—	525
2B	59	M	2	1964	+	C (NS)	+	0	0	42	0	0	0	0	45	580
2C	77	M	2	1989	+	C (NS)	+	0	0	1	0	0	+	0	50	570
2D	56	F	2	1970	+	C (NS)	—	—	—	—	0	+	+	0	—	375
2E	66	M	2	1984	—	C (NS)	+	0	0	11	0	+	+	0	—	500
2F	81	F	2	1980	—	C (NS)	+	0	0	12	0	0	0	0	—	550
2G	66	M	2	1968	—	C (NS)	+	0	0	336	0	+	0	+	—	800
2H	71	M	2	1969	—	C (NS)	+	0	0	36	0	+	+	+	—	650
2I	87	M	2	1970	—	C (NS)	+	0	+	1	0	+	+	0	—	625
2J	52	F	2	1968	+	C (NS)	+	0	0	36	0	0	0	+	130	700
2K	59	M	2	1984	0	C (S)	0	+	0	2	0	+	+	0	—	575
2L	65	F	2	1991	0	NC	+	0	0	3	0	0	0	0	—	440
3A, A′	54	F	2	1969	—	C (S)	+	0	0	48	0	0	0	+	—	430
3B–B‴	60	M	2	1971	—	C (NS)	+	0	+	8	+	+	+	+	—	1,050
4A	75	F	3	1980	—	C (NS)	+	0	0	48	0	+	+	+	—	520
4B	77	F	3	1969	—	C (NS)	0	+	0	12	+	0	+	+	—	380
4C	79	M	3	1988	+	NC	0	0	0	—	0	0	0	+	30	505
4D	81	F	3	1970	—	C (S)	0	0	+	12	0	0	0	0	—	400
4E	87	F	3	1970	—	C (S)	+	0	+	72	0	0	0	0	—	430
4F	90	F	3	1981	—	C (NS)	—	—	—	—	0	0	0	+	—	345

AS = aortic stenosis; AV = aortic valve; C = cardiac; CAD = coronary artery disease; Cath = catheterization; F = female; M = male; MAC = mitral annular calcium; NC = noncardiac; NS = non-sudden; PSG = peak systolic pressure gradient; S = sudden; — = no information available/not applicable.

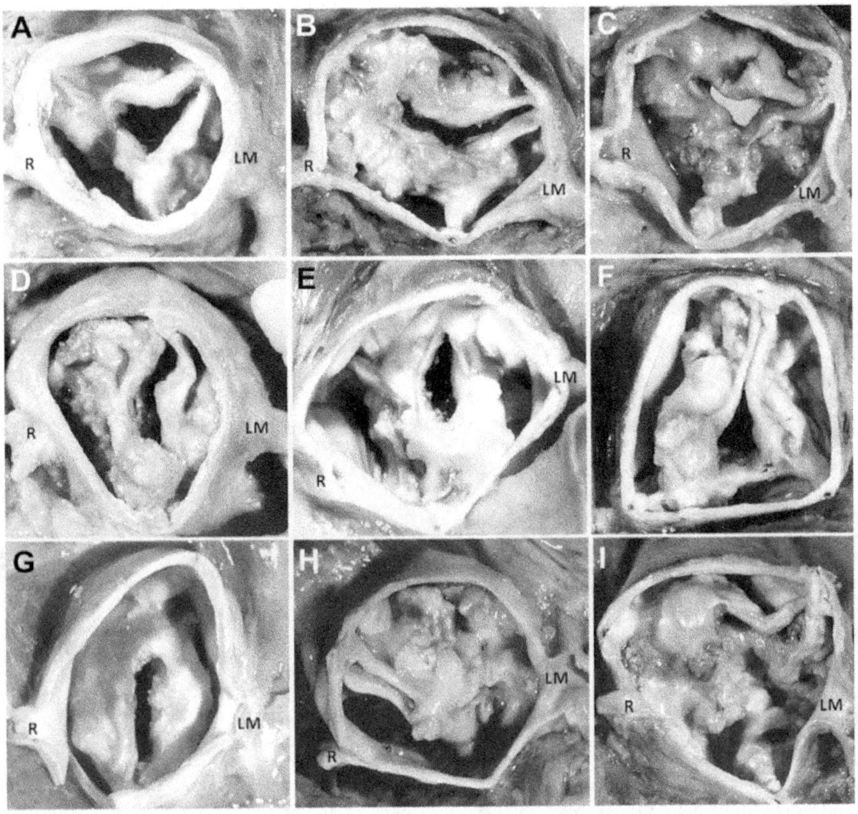

Figure 1. Unicuspid stenotic aortic valves from above. See Table 8 for clinical data on each patient. LM = left main coronary artery; R = right coronary artery. (Figure 1H was reproduced with permission from Roberts WC, Vowels TJ, Ko JM. Natural history of adults with congenitally malformed aortic valves (unicuspid or bicuspid). *Medicine* 2012;91:287–308.)

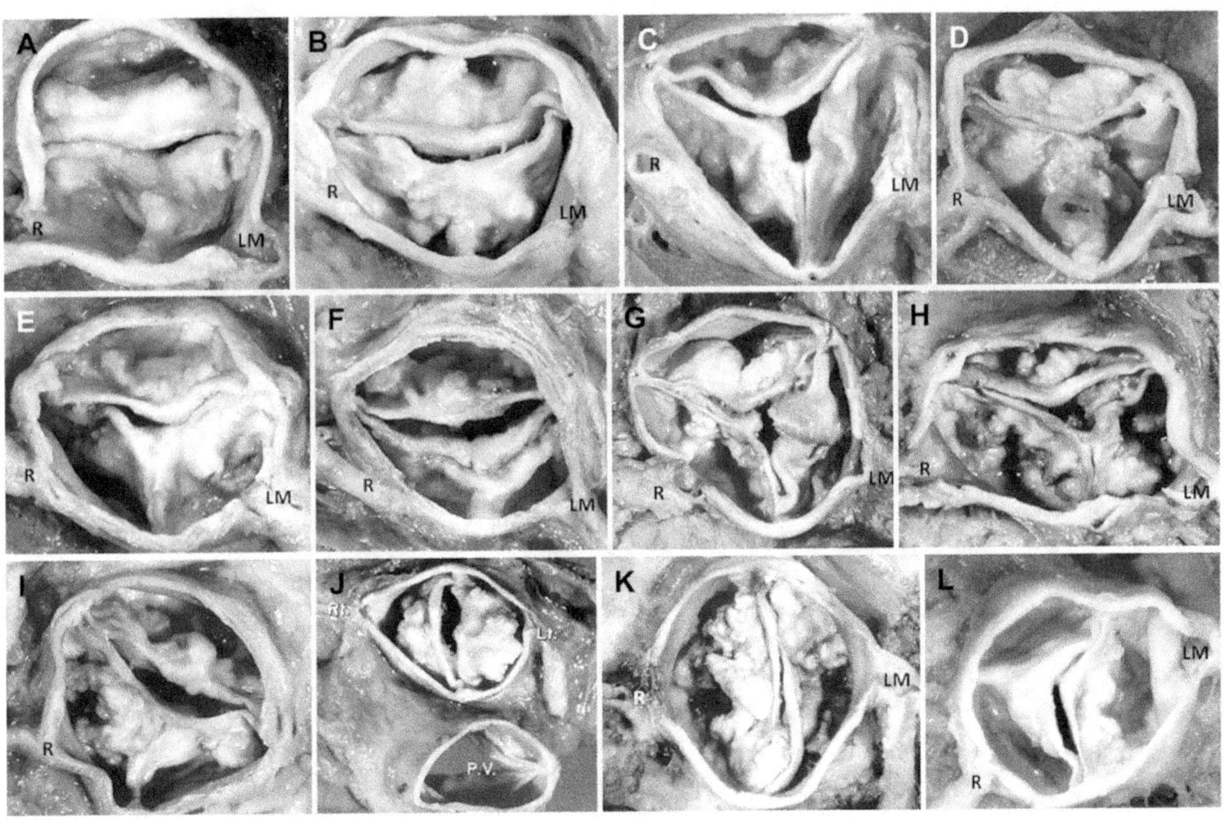

Figure 2. Bicuspid stenotic aortic valves from above orientated anterior-posterior *(A–F, H, I)* such that both coronary ostia arise from behind the anterior cusp, and right-left *(G, J–L)* such that each coronary ostium arises from behind a separate cusp. See Table 8 for clinical data on each patient. LM = left main coronary artery; PV = pulmonic valve; R = right coronary artery. (Figure 2C and 2I were reproduced with permission from Roberts WC, Vowels TJ, Ko JM. Natural history of adults with congenitally malformed aortic valves (unicuspid or bicuspid). *Medicine* 2012;91:287-308.)

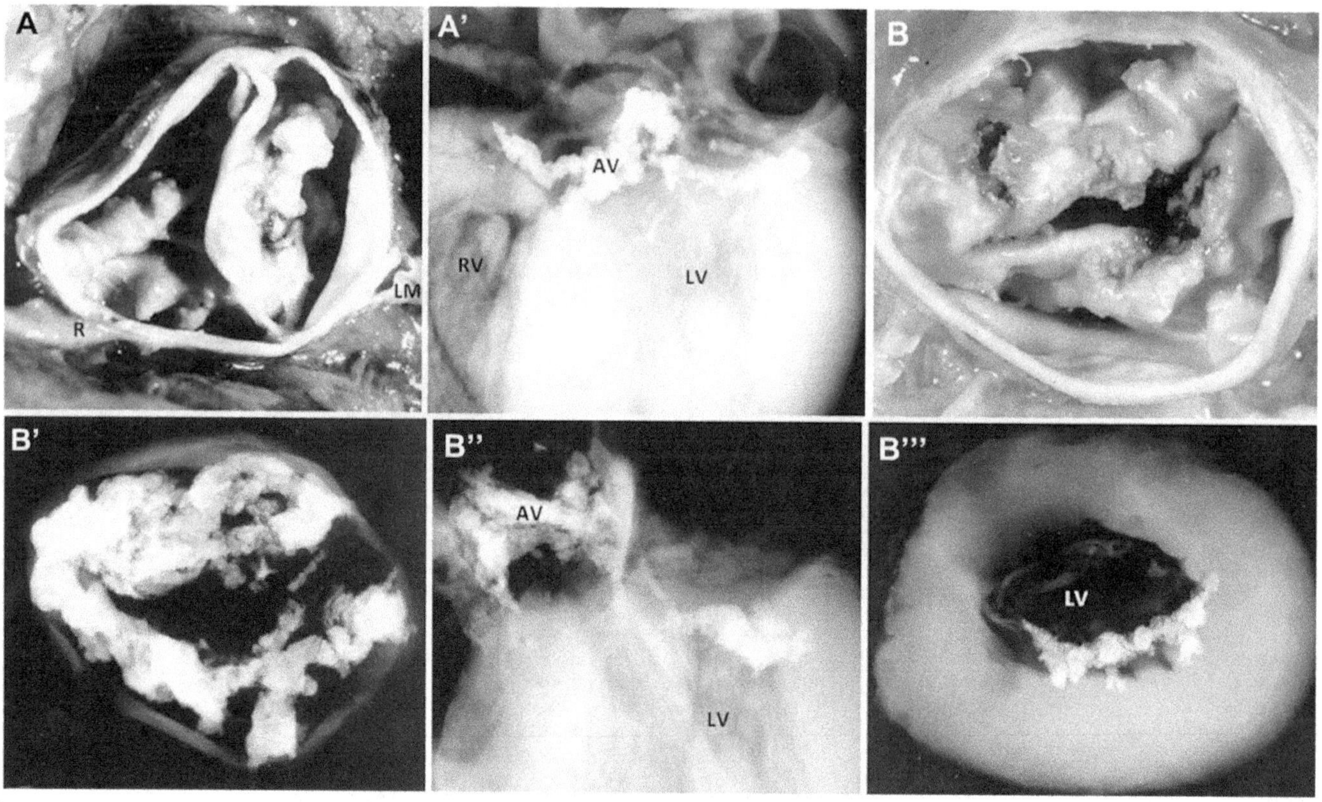

Figure 3. Bicuspid stenotic aortic valves from above (*A* and *B*) and radiographs showing calcific deposits on the aortic valve and mitral annulus (A', $B'-B'''$). See Table 8 for clinical data on each patient. AV = aortic valve; LM = left main coronary artery; LV = left ventricle; R = right coronary artery; RV = right ventricle.

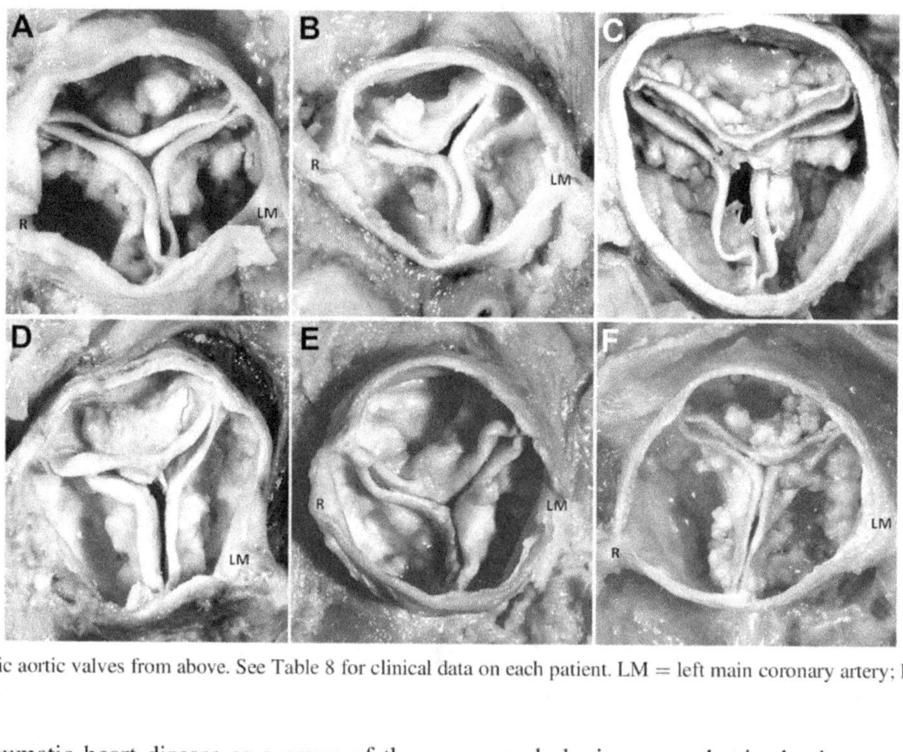

Figure 4. Tricuspid stenotic aortic valves from above. See Table 8 for clinical data on each patient. LM = left main coronary artery; R = right coronary artery.

study to exclude rheumatic heart disease as a cause of the AS by excluding any patient with associated mitral stenosis.

The present study, like virtually all studies, has limitations. The severity of the AS was determined mainly by morphologic means, that is, the degree of rigidity of the aortic valve cusps as a result of calcific deposits, and not by hemodynamic or echocardiographic means. Only 37 patients (14%) had left-sided cardiac catheterization or at least had that data

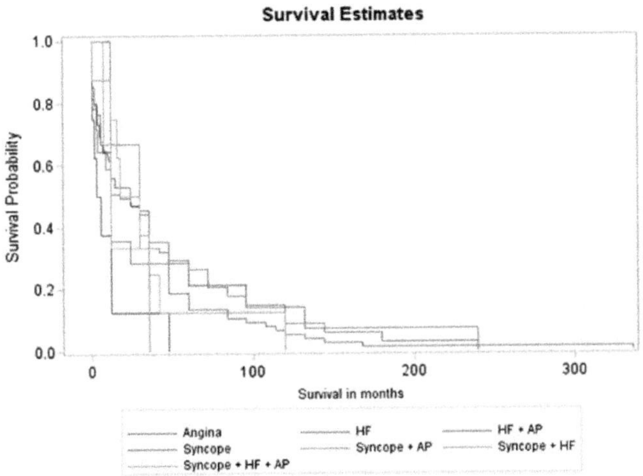

Figure 5. This graph displays survival from the onset of symptoms (heart failure, angina pectoris, and/or syncope) in patients having aortic valve stenosis.

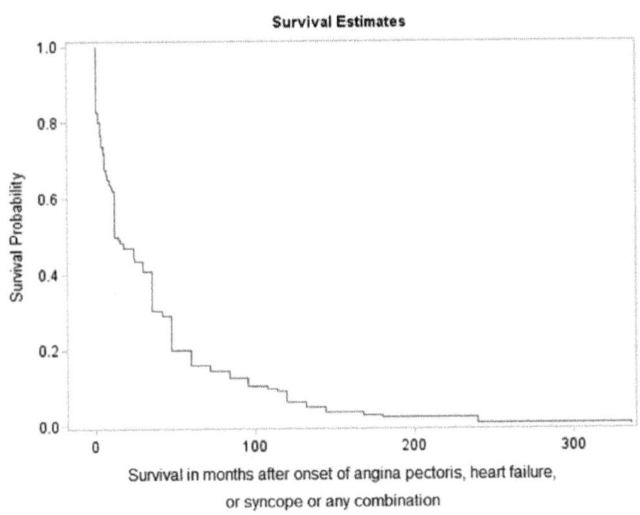

Figure 6. This graph displays survival from onset of symptoms (heart failure, angina pectoris, or syncope or any combination) in patients having aortic valve stenosis.

available to us. Four of these 37 patients had peak systolic pressure gradients between left ventricle and aorta in the teens, but all 4 had rather rigid aortic valve cusps at autopsy, and all 4 had hearts weighing ≥500 g. The interval from catheterization to death was relatively long in 2 of the 4 patients. The appearance of the aortic valves at necropsy in the patients who did not have left-sided cardiac catheterization were similar to those who did undergo cardiac catheterization. Most patients included died between 1960 and 1980, a period when the echocardiogram was unavailable or rarely used, but it was also a period when autopsies were more commonly performed than in the past 3 decades.

The causes of death in the older patients were complicated by their higher frequency of associated coronary arterial narrowing compared with the younger patients. The older patients (>65 years of age) had high frequencies of tricuspid aortic valves, and the etiology of the AS in them

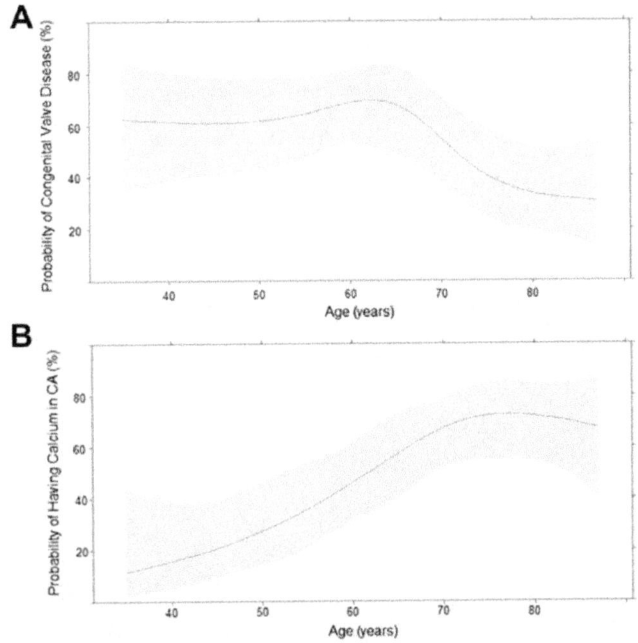

Figure 7. These graphs display the propensity-adjusted probability of having a unicuspid or bicuspid aortic valve *(A)* (p = 0.007) or calcium in ≥1 coronary arteries *(B)* (p = 0.001) by age. The propensity models were adjusted for patient having symptoms (heart failure, angina pectoris, and/or syncope), gender, valve structure (for calcium model only), heart weight (g), degree of coronary narrowing, foci of left ventricular necrosis and/or fibrosis, and presence of calcium in the coronary arteries (congenital valve model only).

was attributed to atherosclerosis. Most patients ≤65 years of age had congenitally malformed valves.

Disclosures

The authors have no conflicts of interest to disclose.

1. Roberts WC, Vowels TJ, Ko JM. Natural history of adults with congenitally malformed aortic valves (unicuspid or bicuspid). *Medicine* 2012;91:287–308.
2. Harrell FE Jr. Regression Modeling Strategies: With Application to Linear Models, Logistic Regression, and Survival Analysis. New York: Springer-Verlag, 2001.
3. Filardo G, Hamilton C, Hamman B, Ng HK, Grayburn P. Categorizing BMI may lead to biased results in studies investigating in-hospital mortality after isolated CABG. *J Clin Epidemiol* 2007;60:1132–1139.
4. Roberts WC. Anatomically isolated aortic valvular disease: the case against its being of rheumatic etiology. *Am J Med* 1970;49:151–159.
5. Peckham GB, Keith JD, Evans JR. Congenital aortic stenosis: some observations on the natural history and clinical assessment. *Can Med Assoc J* 1964;91:639–643.
6. Campbell M. The natural history of congenital aortic stenosis. *Br Heart J* 1968;30:514–526.
7. Cohen LS, Friedman WF, Braunwald E. Natural history of mild congenital aortic stenosis elucidated by serial hemodynamic studies. *Am J Cardiol* 1972;30:1–5.
8. Frank S, Johnson A, Ross J Jr. Natural history of valvular aortic stenosis. *Br Heart J* 1973;35:41–46.
9. Mills P, Leech G, Davies M, Leatham A. The natural history of a non-stenotic bicuspid aortic valve. *Br Heart J* 1978;40:951–957.
10. Hossack KF, Neutze JM, Lowe JB, Barratt-Boyes BG. Congenital valvar aortic stenosis: natural history and assessment for operation. *Br Heart J* 1980;43:561–573.
11. Chizner MA, Peale DL, deLeon AC Jr. The natural history of aortic stenosis in adults. *Am Heart J* 1980;99:419–424.

12. Horstkotte D, Loogen F. The natural history of aortic valve stenosis. *Eur Heart J* 1988;9(Suppl E):57–64.
13. Pellikka PA, Nishimura RA, Bailey KR, Tajik AJ. The natural history of adults with asymptomatic, hemodynamically significant aortic stenosis. *J Am Coll Cardiol* 1990;15:1012–1017.
14. Kennedy KD, Nishimura RA, Holmes DR Jr, Bailey KR. Natural history of moderate aortic stenosis. *J Am Coll Cardiol* 1991;17:313–319.
15. Livanainen AM, Lindroos M, Rilvis R, Heikkilä J, Kupari M. Natural history of aortic valve stenosis of varying severity in the elderly. *Am J Cardiol* 1996;78:97–101.
16. Christensen KL, Ivarsen HR, Thuesen L, Kristensen BO, Egeblad H. Aortic valve stenosis: fatal natural history despite normal left ventricular function and low invasive peak-to-peak pressure gradients. *Cardiology* 2004;102:147–151.
17. Rosenhek R, Klaar U, Schemper M, Scholten C, Heger M, Gabriel H, Binder T, Maurer G, Baumgartner H. Mild and moderate aortic stenosis: natural history and risk stratification by echo-cardiography. *Eur Heart J* 2004;25:199–205.
18. Pai RG, Kapoor N, Bansal RC, Varadarajan P. Malignant natural history of asymptomatic severe aortic stenosis: benefit of aortic valve replacement. *Ann Thorac Surg* 2006;82:2116–2122.
19. Michaelena HI, Desjardins VA, Avierinos JF, Russo A, Nkomo VT, Sundt TM, Pellikka PA, Tajik AJ, Enriquez-Sarano M. Natural history of asymptomatic patients with normally functioning or minimally dysfunctional bicuspid aortic valve in the community. *Circulation* 2008;117:2776–2784.
20. Rosenhek R, Zilberszac R, Schemper M, Czerny M, Mundigler G, Graf S, Bergler-Klein J, Grimm M, Gabriel H, Maurer G. Natural history of very severe aortic stenosis. *Circulation* 2010;121: 151–156.
21. Ross J Jr, Braunwald E. Aortic stenosis. *Circulation* 1968;38: V61–V67.

Comparison of Total 12-Lead QRS Voltage in a Variety of Cardiac Conditions and Its Usefulness in Predicting Increased Cardiac Mass

William C. Roberts, MD[a,b,*], Giovanni Filardo, PhD[c,d,e,f], Jong Mi Ko, BA[b], Robert J. Siegel, MD[g], Allen L. Dollar, MD[g], Elizabeth M. Ross, MD[g], and Jamshid Shirani, MD[g]

Echocardiography provides a more accurate method to determine increased cardiac mass than does electrocardiography. Nevertheless, most offices of physicians do not possess echocardiographic machines, but many possess electrocardiographic machines. Many electrocardiographic criteria have been used to determine increased cardiac mass, but few of the criteria have been measured against cardiac weight determined at necropsy or after cardiac transplantation. Such was the purpose of the present study. Cardiac weight at necropsy or after transplantation was determined in 359 patients with 11 different cardiac conditions, and total 12-lead electrocardiographic QRS voltage (from the peak of the R wave to the nadir of either the Q or the S wave, whichever was deeper) was measured in each patient. Even in hearts with massively increased cardiac mass (>1,000 g), the total 12-lead QRS voltage was clearly increased (>175 mm) in only 94%, but this criterion was superior to that of previously described electrocardiographic criteria for "left ventricular hypertrophy." Hearts with excessive adipose tissue infrequently had increased total 12-lead QRS voltage despite increased cardiac weight. Likewise, patients with fatal cardiac amyloidosis had hearts of increased weight but quite low total 12-lead QRS voltage. In conclusion, 12-lead QRS voltage is useful in predicting increased cardiac mass, but that predictability is dependent in part on the cause of the increased cardiac mass. **(Am J Cardiol 2013;112:904–909)**

Various electrocardiographic criteria have been used to predict left ventricular hypertrophy (LVH), but few have been compared with the actual weight of the heart at necropsy or after cardiac transplantation. Exceptions are the studies by Griep[1] in 1959, and by Allenstein and Hiroyoshi[2] in 1960. The most common criterion used in the past 60 years is that recommended in 1949 by Sokolow and Lyon,[3] who studied 12-lead electrocardiograms in patients who were believed to have LVH on the basis of "a cardiac disorder capable of producing increased strain on the left ventricle (such as hypertension, aortic valve lesions, coarctation of the aorta, patent ductus arteriosus)." These investigators produced a variety of electrocardiographic criteria for LVH, including among others R in lead V_5 + S_1 in lead V_1 $\geq$35 mm. A number of other criteria have been suggested subsequently (Table 1).[4–11] Siegel and Roberts[12] in 1982 proposed that measuring the total amplitude (from the peak of the R wave to the nadir of either the Q or the S wave, whichever was deeper) of the QRS complex in all 12 electrocardiographic leads was a better determinant of cardiac mass than the previously reported criteria (Figure 1). Subsequently, several investigators from the same laboratory measured total 12-lead QRS voltage in a variety of cardiac conditions and in each compared it with the heart weight determined by the same investigators.[13–22] Here, we review their findings in 11 different cardiac conditions.

[a]Departments of Internal Medicine and Pathology; [b]Baylor Heart and Vascular Institute, Dallas, Texas; [c]Institute for Health Care Research and Improvement, Baylor Health Care System; [d]Cardiovascular Epidemiology, Baylor University Medical Center, Dallas, Texas; [e]Cardiovascular Epidemiology, The Heart Hospital Baylor, Plano, Texas; [f]Southern Methodist University, Dallas, Texas; and [g]Pathology Branch, National Heart, Lung, and Blood Institute, National Institutes of Health, Bethesda, Maryland. Manuscript received April 3, 2013; revised manuscript received and accepted April 23, 2013.

Present address (RJS): Cedars-Sinai Medical Center, Division of Cardiology, 8700 Beverly Boulevard, Suite 5623, Los Angeles, CA 90048.

Present address (ALD): Emory University School of Medicine (Cardiology), 49 Jesse Hill Drive, Atlanta, GA 30303.

Present address (EMR): 2021 K Street, NW, Suite 315, Washington, DC 20006.

Present address (JS): St. Luke's University Health Network Cardiology, 801 Ostrum Street, Bethlehem, PA 18015.

This work was supported by grants from Baylor Health Care System Foundation.

See page 909 for disclosure information.

*Corresponding author: Tel: (214) 820-7911; fax: (214) 820-7533.

E-mail address: wc.roberts@baylorhealth.edu (W.C. Roberts).

Methods

To be included in this study, a heart had to be studied in the Pathology Branch of the National Heart, Lung, and Blood Institute of the National Institutes of Health (Bethesda, Maryland). An accurate heart weight and a 12-lead electrocardiogram had to be available in all cases to be included in this study. The patients were divided into 11 groups (Table 2). The electrocardiographic QRS voltage was measured in each of the 12 leads, as demonstrated in Figure 1. In patients with >1 twelve-lead electrocardiogram available, the one measured was the one recorded closest to the patient's death or closest to cardiac transplantation. The medical records were reviewed in all cases to provide pertinent clinical information. All hearts were examined and classified morphologically by one investigator (WCR). The QRS measurements were

Table 1
Recommended or modified electrocardiographic criteria for determining left ventricular hypertrophy as to 17 patients with hearts at necropsy weighing >1,000 grams*

No.	QRS Complex Measured	Value Considered Upper Limit of Normal (mm)	No. (%) of 17 Patients Above Normal Limit
1a	$SV_1 + RV_5$ or V_6 (larger)	35	12 (71%)
1b	$SV_1 + RV_5$ or V_6 (larger)	40	11 (65%)
2a	SV_1 or V_2 (larger) + RV_5 or V_6 (larger)	35	15 (88%)
2b	SV_1 or V_2 (larger) + RV_5 or V_6 (larger)	40	14 (82%)
3a	SV_1 or V_2 (larger) + RV_6	35	15 (88%)
3b	SV_1 or V_2 (larger) + RV_6	40	13 (76%)
4a	$SV_2 + RV_5$	35	14 (82%)
4b	$SV_2 + RV_5$	40	14 (82%)
5a	Deepest $SV_1 - V_3$ + tallest $RV_4 - V_6$	35	14 (82%)
5b	Deepest $SV_1 - V_3$ + tallest $RV_4 - V_6$	40	13 (76%)
5c	Deepest $SV_1 - V_3$ + tallest $RV_4 - V_6$	45	13 (76%)
5d	Deepest $SV_1 - V_3$ + tallest $RV_4 - V_6$	50	13 (76%)
6a	Tallest R + deepest S in any V lead	35	14 (82%)
6b	Tallest R + deepest S in any V lead	40	14 (82%)
7a	Deepest $SV_1 - V_3$	25	14 (82%)
7b	Deepest $SV_1 - V_3$	30	12 (71%)
8a	Tallest $RV_4 - V_6$	25	9 (53%)
8b	Tallest $RV_4 - V_6$	30	8 (27%)
9a	Deepest $SV_1 - V_2$	25	14 (82%)
9b	Deepest $SV_1 - V_2$	30	12 (71%)
10a	Tallest RV_5 or V_6	25	9 (53%)
10b	Tallest RV_5 or V_6	30	8 (27%)
11	$RV_6 > RV_5$	≤1	13 (76%)
12a	Tallest limb-lead R + deepest limb-lead S	15	15 (88%)
12b	Tallest limb-lead R + deepest limb-lead S	20	12 (71%)
13a	$R_1 + S_3$	15	12 (71%)
13b	$R_1 + S_3$	20	10 (59%)
14a	Tallest limb-lead R	10	14 (82%)
14b	Tallest limb-lead R	15	6 (35%)
15a	Deepest limb-lead S	10	10 (59%)
15b	Deepest limb-lead S	15	6 (35%)
16	R_1	10	11 (65%)
17	S_3	10	7 (41%)
18a	Total 12-lead QRS voltage	175	16 (94%)
18b	Total 12-lead QRS voltage	200	15 (88%)
18c	Total 12-lead QRS voltage	225	13 (76%)
18d	Total 12-lead QRS voltage	250	13 (76%)

* From Roberts and Podolak.[13]

performed by the first author of each study and "spot checked" by WCR when not the first author.

Means, SDs, and percentages were calculated to describe the study cohort (n = 359). A multivariate linear regression model was used to assess the adjusted association between patients' heart weight (grams) and 12-lead QRS voltage (millimeters).[23] Covariates included gender, age, and cardiac condition. Restricted cubic splines were used for all continuous variables.[24] Adjusted p values and plots of the association between patient's heart weight and 12-lead QRS voltage were also estimated.

Results

A total of 359 patients, 208 men (58%) and 151 women (42%), were included and divided into 11 groups (Table 2). Their ages ranged from 14 to 85 years; of the 359 patients, 8 (2%) were aged ≤20 years, including 1 aged 20 years, 5 aged 19 years, 1 aged 16 years, and 1 aged 14 years. The heart weights in the 359 patients ranged from 150 to 1,360 g, and the mean heart weights were of increased mass (heart weight >350 g in women and >400 g in men) in 8 of the 11 groups in men and in 10 of the 11 groups in women. Total 12-lead QRS voltage (measured with normal [10 mm] standardization [10 mm = 1 mV]) ranged from 58 to 601 mm. In 8 of the 11 groups, the mean total 12-lead QRS voltage was lower in male than in female patients; in contrast, the mean heart weight was higher in male than in female patients in 9 of the 11 groups. Additionally, the ratio of total 12-lead QRS voltage (millimeters) to heart weight (grams) was lower in male than in female patients in all 11 groups. Figure 2 depicts the adjusted (by age and gender) association between heart weight and total 12-lead QRS voltage in the 10 patient groups and in the normal group. (Individual patient-level data in the aortic stenosis patient group were not available.) The electrocardiograms obtained in the patients who underwent

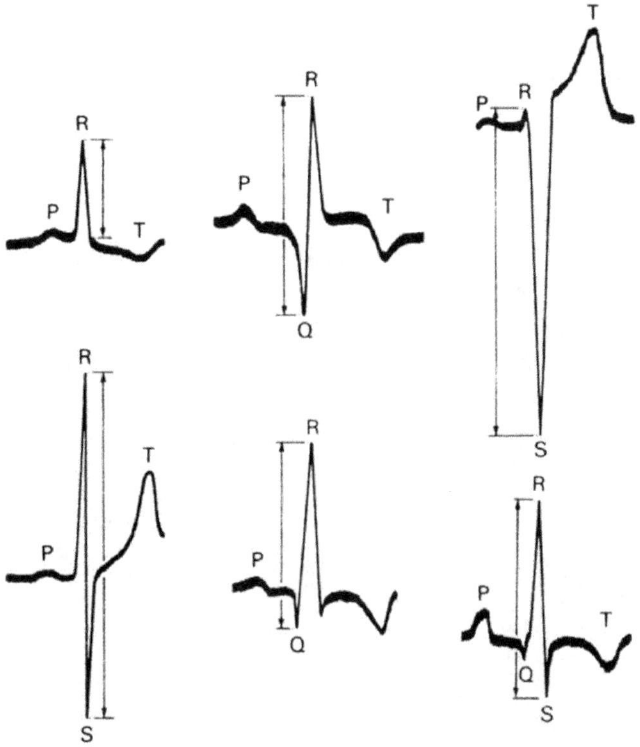

Figure 1. Various QRS complexes showing how each was measured. Reproduced from Siegel and Roberts[12] with permission of the publisher.

cardiac operations were the ones recorded immediately preoperatively.

Hearts weighing >1,000 g[13]: Of these 17 patients, 16 (94%) were men aged 29 to 64 years (mean 42). The one woman's heart weighed 1,250 g (3.6 times the upper limit of normal), and her total 12-lead QRS voltage, 601 mm, was the largest of any of the 359 patients. The cause of the massive cardiomegaly in these 17 patients was isolated pure aortic regurgitation (5 patients), combined pure aortic regurgitation and pure mitral regurgitation (4 patients), pure aortic regurgitation plus ventricular septal defect (2 patients), aortic stenosis and regurgitation (2 patients), aortic regurgitation plus mitral stenosis with regurgitation (1 patient), hypertrophic cardiomyopathy (2 patients), and ventricular septal defect with mitral stenosis (1 patient). The total 12-lead QRS voltage was highest in this group than in any of the others.

Aortic valve stenosis[12]: These 50 patients, aged 16 to 65 years (mean 48), had peak systolic transvalvular pressure gradients ranging from 52 to 180 mm Hg (mean 98) and peak left ventricular systolic pressures ranging from 149 to 270 mm Hg (average 210). All had anatomically normal mitral valves. Aortic valve replacement had been done in 38 patients (76%), and all died <6 weeks after the operation; 2 others died during anesthesia induction. The aortic valve was unicuspid unicommissural in 5 patients (12%), congenitally bicuspid in 29 patients (58%), and tricuspid in 15 patients (30%). Because the total 12-lead QRS amplitude (millimeters) roughly equaled the peak left ventricular systolic pressure (millimeters of mercury), Siegel and Roberts[13] suggested that the total 12-lead QRS voltage (millimeters) minus the systemic arterial systolic pressure (millimeters of mercury) roughly equaled the peak systolic pressure gradient (millimeters of mercury) between the left ventricle and the systemic artery.

Aortic regurgitation[14]: These 30 patients, aged 19 to 65 years (mean 45), all had chronic pure (no element of aortic stenosis) severe aortic regurgitation secondary to infective endocarditis that had healed (8 patients), syphilis (6 patients), ankylosing spondylitis (5 patients), Marfan syndrome (5 patients), and uncertain or other causes (6 patients). Nineteen patients (63%) had undergone aortic valve replacement, and all died <60 days after the operation. Only 2 of these 30 hearts weighed >1,000 g (1,010 and 1,100 g).

Mitral regurgitation[15]: These 24 patients, aged 21 to 84 years (mean 42), all had chronic isolated severe pure (no element of stenosis) mitral regurgitation. The cause of the regurgitation was attributed to rheumatic disease (14 patients), mitral valve prolapse (7 patients), and infective endocarditis that had healed (3 patients). Nine patients (30%) had undergone mitral valve replacement.

Hypertrophic cardiomyopathy (studied at necropsy)[16]: These 57 patients ranged in age from 14 to 87 years (mean 49). Cardiac catheterization data within 2 years of death were available in 42 patients: left ventricular to systemic arterial peak pressure gradient at rest >10 mm Hg was present in 32 patients (77%) and with provocation in 35 patients (85%). The resting peak systolic gradients ranged from 12 to 162 mm Hg (mean 79) and the provoked gradients, from 40 to 190 mm Hg (mean 104). There were no differences between patients with and without outflow pressure gradients with regard to heart weight, ventricular septal thickness, total 12-lead QRS amplitude, and Romhilt-Estes score.[6] The mean Sokolow-Lyon index was insignificantly different: 37 in the obstructive group and 28 in the nonobstructive group.

Hypertrophic cardiomyopathy (studied after cardiac transplantation)[17]: These 10 patients, aged 19 to 46 years (mean 35), all had severe chronic heart failure, and only 1 had left ventricular outflow obstruction. Nine had dilated left ventricular cavities, and 8 had extensive left ventricular wall scarring without narrowing of the epicardial coronary arteries. Six of the 9 had left ventricular ejection fractions <50%.

Idiopathic dilated cardiomyopathy[18]: These 49 patients, aged 19 to 75 years (mean 45), had typical clinical and morphologic cardiac features of this condition.

Lipomatous hypertrophy of the atrial septum[19]: The thickness of the atrial septum cephalad to the fossa ovalis is these 28 patients ranged from 2.0 to 5.0 cm (mean 2.8). The 12 men ranged in age from 48 to 84 years (mean 67) and the 16 women, from 59 to 83 years (mean 74). The total 12-lead QRS voltage in the men ranged from 93 to 241 mm (mean 140) and in the women from 59 to 266 mm (mean 124). The heart weights in the men averaged 576 g and in the women, 502 g.

Carcinoid syndrome[20]: Of these 36 patients, 21 (57%) had carcinoid heart disease and 15 (43%) did not. The 2 groups were similar in mean age (54 vs 55 years), duration of clinical illness (4.7 vs 6.3 years), body weight (50 vs 52 kg), and systemic blood pressure (117/77 vs 128/77 mm Hg). The 2 groups were different in the frequency of the presence

Table 2
Total 12-lead QRS voltage, heart weight, and age of groups of 331 patients with various cardiac conditions

Condition	Gender	Number of Cases	Ages (yrs), Range (Mean)	Total 12-Lead QRS Voltage (mm), Mean	Patients With 12-Lead QRS Voltage >175 mm	Heart Weight (g), Range (Mean)	Total 12-Lead QRS Voltage (mm)/Heart Weight (g)	Year of Publication	Authors (Reference Number)
Hearts weighing >1,000 g	M	16	29–64 (42)	140–414 (306)	16	1,005–1,360 (1,102)	0.28	1985	Roberts and Podolak[13]
	F	1	20	601	(94%)	1,250	0.48		
Aortic valve stenosis	M	36	16–64 (48)	144–417 (249)	47	440–880 (639)	0.39	1982	Siegel and Roberts[12]
	F	14	16–65 (47)	193–376 (277)	(94%)	380–700 (521)	0.53		
Aortic regurgitation	M	22	19–59 (44)	109–428 (271)	27	430–1,100 (717)	0.38	1985	Roberts and Day[14]
	F	8	35–56 (48)	169–384 (275)	(90%)	375–950 (638)	0.43		
Mitral regurgitation	M	11	24–84 (47)	111–364 (245)	17	400–775 (629)	0.39	1992	Glick and Roberts[15]
	F	13	21–64 (37)	114–290 (199)	(71%)	350–675 (472)	0.42		
Hypertrophic cardiomyopathy without cardiac transplantation	M	21	14–68 (46)	107–339 (190)	30	325–1,070 (671)	0.28	1989	Dollar and Roberts[16]
	F	36	19–87 (51)	68–327 (201)	(53%)	290–1,230 (547)	0.38		
Hypertrophic cardiomyopathy with cardiac transplantation	M	6	19–46 (35)	109–201 (142)	4	310–480 (393)	0.36	1993	Shirani et al[17]
	F	4	24–45 (35)	172–378 (241)	(40%)	290–650 (408)	0.59		
Idiopathic dilated cardiomyopathy	M	35	19–73 (46)	74–281 (147)	20	400–940 (620)	0.24	1987	Roberts et al[18]
	F	14	22–75 (54)	75–243 (167)	(41%)	400–860 (602)	0.28		
Lipomatous hypertrophy of the atrial septum	M	12	48–84 (67)	93–24 (140)	3	410–795 (576)	0.24	1993	Shirani and Roberts[19]
	F	16	59–83 (74)	59–266 (124)	(11%)	330–680 (502)	0.25		
Carcinoid syndrome									
With carcinoid heart disease	M	11	39–72 (56)	58–227 (120)	2	220–480 (350)	0.34	1985	Ross and Roberts[20]
	F	8	28–64 (54)	58–128 (84)	(11%)	200–290 (245)	0.34		
Without carcinoid heart disease	M	10	42–75 (55)	89–129 (137)	2	240–570 (350)	0.39		
	F	5	28–67 (50)	102–135 (121)	(13%)	150–270 (230)	0.53		
Cardiac amyloidosis	M	15	32–69 (52)	60–197 (99)	2	410–850 (570)	0.17	1983	Roberts and Waller[21]
	F	15	21–93 (69)	58–199 (109)	(7%)	370–900 (494)	0.22		
Cardiac adiposity	M	13	51–73 (64)	73–159 (114)	1	320–795 (485)	0.24	1995	Shirani et al[22]
	F	17	40–85 (70)	77–210 (124)	(3%)	250–575 (395)	0.31		

of precordial murmurs consistent with tricuspid regurgitation and/or pulmonary stenosis (95% vs 13%), cardiomegaly by chest x-ray (38% vs 0%), low voltage on electrocardiography (47% vs 0%), and location of the primary carcinoid neoplasm. Total 12-lead QRS voltage was similar in each group (105 vs 132 mm; 10 mm = 1 mV). Of those with carcinoid heart disease, 43% died of cardiac causes, whereas in those without carcinoid heart disease, none died of a cardiac cause.

Cardiac amyloidosis[21]: All 30 patients, aged 32 to 92 years (mean 59), died from amyloidosis that involved the heart extensively and also multiple other organs. The peak systemic arterial systolic pressure in the 9 patients with hemodynamic studies was ≤110 mm Hg.

Cardiac adiposity (cor adiposum)[22]: These 30 patients died from noncardiac causes. The heart weights ranged from 250 to 795 g (mean 435) and were increased (>350 g in women, >400 g in men) in 17 (57%). Adipose tissue constituted 4% to 52% (mean 22%) of the total heart weight (mean weight of adipose tissue = 105 g). No heart had grossly visible evidence of myocardial fibrosis or necrosis. Total 12-lead QRS voltage decreased significantly as the quantity of cardiac adipose tissue increased. As the ratio of adipose tissue to heart weight × 100 increased from 12 ± 3 to 20 ± 4 to 32 ± 9 mm/100 g, the ratio of total 12-lead QRS voltage to heart weight × 100 decreased significantly from 36 ± 9 to 34 ± 9 to 21 ± 6 mm/100 g. The amount of subepicardial fat increased with increasing body weight. Simple visual assessment of the extent of cardiac adiposity and the degree of buoyancy of the heart when placed in a container of water estimated well the amounts of subepicardial fat. If the amount of subepicardial fat was considered normal by visual

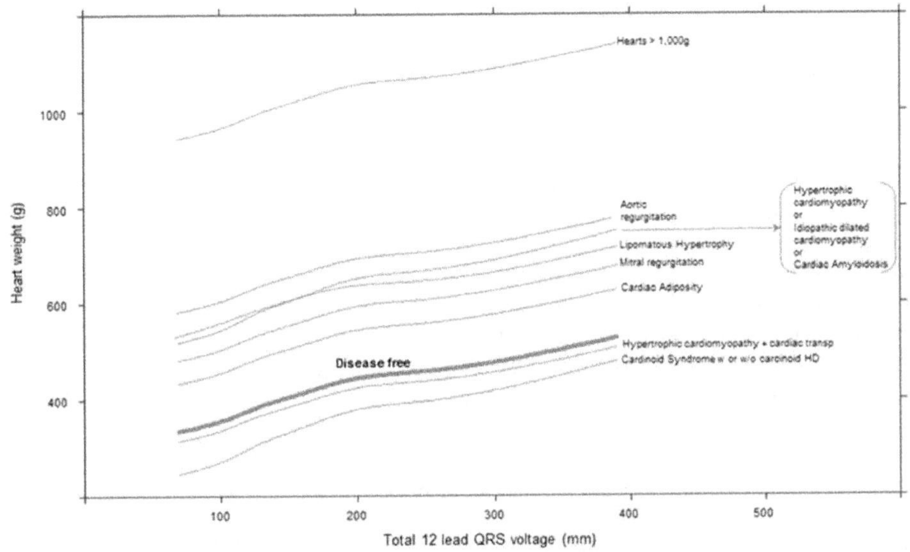

Figure 2. Adjusted (by gender and age) association between patient's heart weight and 12-lead QRS voltage by cardiac condition. HD = heart disease; transp = transplantation.

inspection, then the adipose tissue constituted a mean of 12% (range 4% to 14%) of the heart weight; if the subepicardial tissue was increased but the heart did not float in water, then fat constituted a mean of 20% (range 15% to 28%) of the heart weight; in the 12 hearts that floated in water, a mean of 32% (range 21% to 52%) of the heart weight was composed of adipose tissue.

Discussion

This study summarizes 11 previously published studies on total 12-lead QRS voltage in 11 different cardiac conditions and compares that voltage with heart weight. The best cut-off point for total 12-lead QRS voltage separating hearts with increased weight compared with those of normal weight has not been fully established. Odom et al[25] determined heart weight in 30 men free of cardiopulmonary disease and found that total 12-lead QRS voltage ranged from 80 to 185 mm (mean 127; 10 mm = 1 mV). These authors considered 175 mm as the best upper range of normal 12-lead QRS voltage. Rodríguez Padial[26] studied M-mode and 2-dimensional echocardiograms and 12-lead electrocardiograms in 74 consecutive patients with systemic hypertension and calculated left ventricular mass. This author found a total 12-lead QRS voltage >120 mm to be a good electrocardiographic criterion and "better than those most frequently used."[27] Yang et al[28] studied total 12-lead QRS voltage in 120 adults free of cardiopulmonary disease and 114 patients with LVH by echocardiography. They found >190 mm to be a good criterion for LVH, with sensitivity of 77%, specificity of 96%, and accuracy of 87%, and suggested that total 12-lead QRS voltage had a relatively high reliability for diagnosing LVH. Pelliccia et al[29] studied total 12-lead QRS voltage in 67 patients with idiopathic dilated cardiomyopathy and found that total 12-lead QRS voltage (also the sum of T/R wave ratios) was the only independent predictor of left ventricular mass determined by either angiography or echocardiography.

In the present study of patients with clear increased cardiac mass at autopsy (>350 g in women, >400 g in men) total 12-lead QRS voltage in 118 men averaged 239 mm (range 107 to 428). These 118 men included 16 with hearts weighing >1,000 g, 36 with aortic stenosis, 22 with pure aortic regurgitation, 11 with pure mitral regurgitation, and 21 with hypertrophic cardiomyopathy (without cardiac transplantation). The upper limit for total 12-lead QRS voltage in women without cardiopulmonary disease has not been established. As listed in Table 2, 12-lead QRS voltage generally was slightly higher in women than men with the same cardiac condition, although heart weight on average was lower in the women than in the men. Clearly, total 12-lead QRS voltage is not perfect in diagnosing increased cardiac mass, but as listed in Table 1, it is more reliable in predicting increased cardiac mass than are previously recommended electrocardiographic criteria for LVH.

There is some variation in the relation of total 12-lead QRS voltage to heart weight depending on the underlying cardiac condition. As listed in Table 2, all 49 patients with idiopathic dilated cardiomyopathy had hearts weighing ≥400 g, and yet the mean total 12-lead QRS voltage in men and women was relatively low (147 and 167 mm, respectively). Wilensky et al[30] showed that QRS voltage in patients with this condition diminishes with time, and therefore, electrocardiograms recorded shortly before death show lower QRS voltages than those recorded at earlier times. Additionally, all 30 patients with fatal cardiac amyloidosis had hearts of increased mass, but mean total 12-lead QRS voltage in them averaged only 104 mm. Possibly as much as half or more of their cardiac mass, however, was contributed by the amyloid deposits in the heart and not by cardiac myocardium. The patients with excessive cardiac adiposity, with or without lipomatous hypertrophy of the atrial septum, also usually had hearts of increased mass with relatively low total 12-lead QRS voltages.

Lanti et al[31] studied electrocardiograms in 154 men without clinical evidence of heart disease and compared electrocardiographic findings in 67 who died suddenly to the 87 who had nonsudden death. They found that 12-lead QRS voltage had a significant and independent relation to sudden death and helped identify subjects at increased risk for sudden coronary death. These investigators also found that the Sokolow-Lyon index was inversely related to nonsudden death.

The strong features of the present study are the following: (1) the 12-lead QRS voltage was determined in a variety of cardiac conditions, and (2) heart weights in all patients studied were available and accurately determined. Relatively few previous studies on electrocardiographic determination of LVH actually compared the electrocardiographic criteria with actual heart weight, and those that did acquired those data from autopsy protocols produced by a variety of prosecutors with varying expertise in cardiovascular disease.

Disclosures

The authors have no conflicts of interest to disclose.

1. Griep AH. Pitfalls in the electrocardiographic diagnosis of left ventricular hypertrophy: a correlative study of 200 autopsied patients. *Circulation* 1959;20:30–34.
2. Allenstein BJ, Hiroyoshi M. Evaluation of electrocardiographic diagnosis of ventricular hypertrophy based on autopsy comparison. *Circulation* 1960;21:401–412.
3. Sokolow M, Lyon TP. The ventricular complex in left ventricular hypertrophy as obtained by unipolar precordial and limb leads. *Am Heart J* 1949;37:161–186.
4. Holt DH, Spodick DH. The Rv_6:Rv_5 voltage ratio in left ventricular hypertrophy. *Am Heart J* 1962;63:65–66.
5. Carter WA, Estes EH Jr. Electrocardiographic manifestations of ventricular hypertrophy; a computer study of ECG-anatomic correlations in 319 cases. *Am Heart J* 1964;68:173–182.
6. Romhilt DW, Estes WH Jr. A point-score system for the ECG diagnosis of left ventricular hypertrophy. *Am Heart J* 1968;75: 752–758.
7. Romhilt DW, Bove KE, Norris RJ, Conyers E, Conradi S, Rowlands DT, Scott RC. A critical appraisal of the electrocardiographic criteria for the diagnosis of left ventricular hypertrophy. *Circulation* 1969;40: 185–195.
8. Bennett DH, Evans DW. Correlation of left ventricular mass determined by echocardiography with vectorcardiographic and electrocardiographic voltage measurements. *Br Heart J* 1974;36:981–987.
9. Casale PN, Devereux RB, Alonso DR, Camp E, Kligfield P. Improved sex-specific criteria of left ventricular hypertrophy for clinical and computer interpretation of electrocardiograms: validation with autopsy findings. *Circulation* 1987;3:565–572.
10. Koito H, Spokick DH. Accuracy of the RV_6:RV_5 voltage ratio for increased left ventricular mass. *Am J Cardiol* 1988;62:985–987.
11. Velury S, Spodick DH. Increased left ventricular mass in patients with lateral low voltage electrocardiograms. *Am J Cardiol* 1992;69: 707–708.
12. Siegel RJ, Roberts WC. Electrocardiographic observations in severe aortic valve stenosis: correlative necropsy study to clinical, hemodynamic, and ECG variables demonstrating relation of 12-lead QRS amplitude to peak systolic transaortic pressure gradient. *Am Heart J* 1982;103:210–221.
13. Roberts WC, Podolak MJ. The king of hearts: analysis of 23 patients with hearts weighing 1000 grams or more. *Am J Cardiol* 1985;55: 485–494.
14. Roberts WC, Day PJ. Electrocardiographic observations in clinically isolated, pure, chronic, severe aortic regurgitation: analysis of 30 necropsy patients aged 19 to 65 years. *Am J Cardiol* 1985;55:431–438.
15. Glick BN, Roberts WC. Usefulness of total 12-lead QRS voltage in diagnosing left ventricular hypertrophy in clinically isolated, pure, chronic, severe mitral regurgitation. *Am J Cardiol* 1992;70:1088–1092.
16. Dollar AL, Roberts WC. Usefulness of total 12-lead QRS voltage compared with other criteria for determining left ventricular hypertrophy in hypertrophic cardiomyopathy: analysis of 57 patients studied at necropsy. *Am J Med* 1989;87:377–381.
17. Shirani J, Maron BJ, Cannon RO III, Shahin S, Roberts WC. Clinicopathologic features of hypertrophic cardiomyopathy managed by cardiac transplantation. *Am J Cardiol* 1993;72:434–440.
18. Roberts WC, Siegel RJ, McManus BM. Idiopathic dilated cardiomyopathy: analysis of 152 necropsy patients. *Am J Cardiol* 1987;60:1340–1355.
19. Shirani J, Roberts WC. Clinical, electrocardiographic and morphologic features of massive fatty deposits ("lipomatous hypertrophy") in the atrial septum. *J Am Coll Cardiol* 1993;22:226–238.
20. Ross EM, Roberts WC. The carcinoid syndrome: comparison of 21 necropsy subjects with carcinoid heart disease to 15 necropsy subjects without carcinoid heart disease. *Am J Heart* 1985;79:339–354.
21. Roberts WC, Waller BF. Cardiac amyloidosis causing cardiac dysfunction: analysis of 54 necropsy patients. *Am J Cardiol* 1983;52:137–146.
22. Shirani J, Berezowski K, Roberts WC. Quantitative measurement of normal and excessive (cor adiposum) subepicardial adipose tissue, its clinical significance, and its effect on electrocardographic QRS voltage. *Am J Cardiol* 1995;76:414–418.
23. Harrell FE Jr. Regression Modeling Strategies: With Application to Linear Models, Logistic Regression, and Survival Analysis. New York: Springer-Verlag, 2001.
24. Filardo G, Hamilton C, Hamman B, Ng HK, Grayburn P. Categorizing BMI may lead to biased results in studies investigating in-hospital mortality after isolated CABG. *J Clin Epidemiol* 2007;60:1132–1139.
25. Odom H II, Davis JL, Dinh H, Baker BJ, Roberts WC, Murphy ML. QRS voltage measurements in autopsied men free of cardiopulmonary disease: a basis for evaluating total QRS voltage as a index of left ventricular hypertrophy. *Am J Cardiol* 1986;58:801–804.
26. Rodríguez Padial L. Usefulness of total 12-lead QRS voltage for determining the presence of left ventricular hypertrophy in systemic hypertension. *Am J Cardiol* 1991;68:261–262.
27. Rodríguez Padial L, Navarro A, Sánchez J. RVG: RV_5 voltage ratio in systemic hypertension. *Am J Cardiol* 1990;66:869–871.
28. Yang TH, Deng SY, Cai YC. The normal values of total 12-lead QRS voltage and its significance in diagnosing left ventricular hypertrophy. *Chinese J Cardiol* 1988;16:353–355.
29. Pelliccia F, Critelli G, Cianfrocca C, Nigri A, Reale A. Electrocardiographic correlates with left ventricular morphology in idiopathic dilated cardiomyopathy. *Am J Cardiol* 1991;68:642–647.
30. Wilensky RL, Yudelman P, Cohen A, Fletcher RD, Atkinson J, Virmani R, Roberts WC. Serial electrocardiographic changes in idiopathic dilated cardiomyopathy confirmed at necropsy. *Am J Cardiol* 1988;62:276–283.
31. Lanti M, Puddu PE, Menotti A. Voltage criteria of left ventricular hypertrophy in sudden and nonsudden coronary artery disease mortality: the Italian section of the seven countries study. *Am J Cardiol* 1990;66:1181–1185.

Anomalous Cord From the Raphe of a Congenitally Bicuspid Aortic Valve to the Aortic Wall Producing Either Acute or Chronic Aortic Regurgitation

Travis J. Vowels, BBA,* Gonzalo V. Gonzalez-Stawinski, MD,† Jong M. Ko, BA,* Gregory D. Trachiotis, MD,‡ Brad J. Roberts, BS, RCS,* Charles S. Roberts, MD,§ William C. Roberts, MD*||¶

Dallas, Texas; Washington, DC; and Charleston, South Carolina

Objectives This report calls attention to an unappreciated cause of both acute and chronic aortic regurgitation (AR).

Background Although stenosis develops in most patients with a congenitally bicuspid aortic valve (BAV), in others with this anomaly, pure AR (no element of stenosis) develops, some in the absence of infection or other clear etiology.

Methods We describe 5 men who underwent aortic valve replacement for pure AR associated with a BAV containing an anomalous cord attaching the raphe of the conjoined cusp near its free margin to the wall of the ascending aorta cephalad to the sinotubular junction.

Results Three of these 5 patients had a history of progressive dyspnea, and the anomalous cord, which was intact at operation, appeared to cause chronic AR by preventing proper coaptation of the 2 aortic valve cusps. The other 2 patients heard a "pop" during physical exertion and immediately became dyspneic, and at operation, the anomalous cord was found to have ruptured. Prolapse of the conjoined aortic valve cusp toward the left ventricular cavity resulted in severe acute AR.

Conclusions This variant of the purely regurgitant BAV may cause either chronic AR (when the anomalous cord does not rupture) or acute severe AR (when the cord ruptures). (J Am Coll Cardiol 2014;63:153–7)

The congenitally bicuspid aortic valve (BAV) occurs in an estimated 1% of the population, such that in the United States, an estimated 3 million individuals have this malformation (1). Although in some individuals the BAV functions normally for an entire lifetime, stenosis develops in most, superimposed infection (infective endocarditis) develops in some, and pure aortic regurgitation (AR) unassociated with infective endocarditis or its consequences develops in some (2). A subgroup of those with pure AR unassociated with infection have an anomalous cord extending from the raphe of 1 of the 2 cusps to the wall of the aorta, and the cord serves to keep the raphe cusp from prolapsing toward the left ventricle (Table 1). During a 50-year period, we examined 5 operatively excised purely regurgitant BAVs with an anomalous cord from the raphe to the wall of the aorta. A brief description of these 5 cases is the purpose of this report.

Methods

During a nearly 50-year period, we examined 5 operatively excised aortic valves that were congenitally bicuspid and had a cord attached from the margin of the raphe cusp to the wall of the aorta. The clinical records in all 5 patients were subsequently examined, and all 5 valves were photographed.

From the *Baylor Heart and Vascular Institute, Baylor University Medical Center, Dallas, Texas; †Department of Cardiothoracic Surgery, Baylor University Medical Center, Dallas, Texas; ‡Division of Cardiothoracic Surgery, The George Washington University Medical Center and Veterans Affairs Medical Center, Washington, DC; §Palmetto Cardiovascular and Thoracic Associates, Trident Medical Center, Charleston, South Carolina; ||Department of Internal Medicine (Division of Cardiology), Baylor University Medical Center, Dallas, Texas; and the ¶Department of Pathology, Baylor University Medical Center, Dallas, Texas. The study was funded by the Baylor Health Care System Foundation, Dallas, Texas. Mr. Vowels is a second-year medical student at the University of Texas Medical School at Houston. The authors have reported that they have no relationships relevant to the contents of this paper to disclose.

Manuscript received July 27, 2013; revised manuscript received August 30, 2013, accepted September 10, 2013.

Abbreviations and Acronyms

AR = aortic regurgitation

BAV = bicuspid aortic valve

Results

Pertinent findings in the 5 patients are summarized in Table 2; all patients were men. Three (Patients #1, #2, and #5) had chronic AR and 2 had acute AR. The latter 2 were asymptomatic until 1 or 2 days before aortic valve replacement: both heard a popping noise in his chest, 1 patient while working in his yard and 1 while working on his car beneath the hood. Both became suddenly dyspneic, and the dyspnea progressed rather rapidly, prompting pulmonary edema and hospitalization. A median sternotomy was emergently performed in each for severe AR. The cord extending from the raphe to the wall of the aorta had ruptured, causing the raphe cusp to prolapse toward the left ventricular cavity (Fig. 1). Each of the other 3 patients had chronic AR, and in none of them had the anomalous cord ruptured. Photographs of the operatively excised BAVs are shown in Figures 2 to 5.

Discussion

This report describes 5 men with a BAV and pure AR with an anomalous cord extending from the raphe of the conjoined cusp to the wall of the ascending aorta cephalad to the sinotubular junction. In the 3 patients who presented with chronic AR, the cord appeared to prevent complete coaptation of the 2 aortic valve cusps by pinning the raphe of the conjoined cusp to the aortic wall. In the 2 patients who presented with acute AR, the cord had ruptured, resulting in the conjoined cusp prolapsing toward the left ventricular cavity and the acute onset of symptoms.

This variant of the BAV has been previously described (Table 1), and its association with AR has been well documented (1,3–13). Of the 33 previously published cases, 25

Table 1 Previous Publications of Patients Having an Anomalous Cord Extending From the Raphe of a Congenitally BAV to the Wall of the Aorta Causing Either Acute or Chronic Pure Aortic Regurgitation

Year of Publication	First Author (Ref. #)	No. of Patients With a BAV Containing an Anomalous Cord	No. With Cord Rupture	Mean Age, yrs (Range)	No. of Men	Severity of AR (No. of Patients) 1+	2+	3+	4+
1970	Roberts (1)	1*	0	27	1	0	0	0	1
1971	Carter et al. (3)	1	1	59	1	NA	NA	NA	NA
1977	Becker and Düren (4)	1	1	45	1	0	0	0	1
1984	Olson et al. (5)	11†	1	NA	NA	NA	NA	NA	NA
1986	Yamagishi et al. (6)	1	0	32	1	0	0	0	1
1990	Waller et al. (7)	2	0	53	2	0	0	0	2
1990	Arikawa et al. (8)	2	NA	NA	NA	NA	NA	NA	NA
1992	Hamada et al. (9)	2	1	53	NA	NA	NA	1	NA
1993	Misawa et al. (10)	1	NA	NA	NA	NA	NA	NA	NA
1994	Walley et al. (11)	9	2	61 (46-73)	7	1	1	1	6
2000	Akiyama et al. (12)	1	1	57	1	0	0	1	0
2011	Journigan and Clements (13)	1	1	48	1	0	0	0	1
Total		33	8 (24%)		15/17 (88%)				12/16 (75%)

*Patient is included in the present study (Patient #1). †The author described the bicuspid aortic valves as containing "either a fenestrated raphe or a raphal cord."
BAV = bicuspid aortic valve; NA = not available.

Table 2 Clinical Data for 6 Men Having AVR for a Purely Regurgitant (4+/4+) Congenitally Bicuspid Aortic Valve With an Anomalous Cord Extending From the Raphe of One Cusp to the Wall of the Aorta

Patient #	Age, yrs	Age, yrs: Precordial Murmur First Heard	Age, yrs: S/S of Heart Failure First Appeared	SH	LVEF, %*	Rupture of Anomalous Cord	AVR (yr)	Type of Valve Implanted
1†‡	27	17	25	0	NA	–	1966	Mechanical
2	45	NA	NA	+	50	–	2013	Mechanical
3	49	49	49	0	55	+§	2012	Bioprosthesis
4	55	55	55	0	NA	+§	2012	Bioprosthesis
5	71	70	70	+	50	–	2012	Bioprosthesis

*LVEF was measured by echocardiography in Patients #2 and #3 and by cardiac catheterization in patient 5. †Patient was previously reported by Roberts (1) in 1970. ‡Patient's aorta coursed over his right main bronchus (right aortic arch). §Producing acute aortic regurgitation.
AVR = aortic valve replacement; LVEF = left ventricular ejection fraction; NA = not available; SH = systemic hypertension; S/S = signs and symptoms; + = positive or present; – = negative or absent.

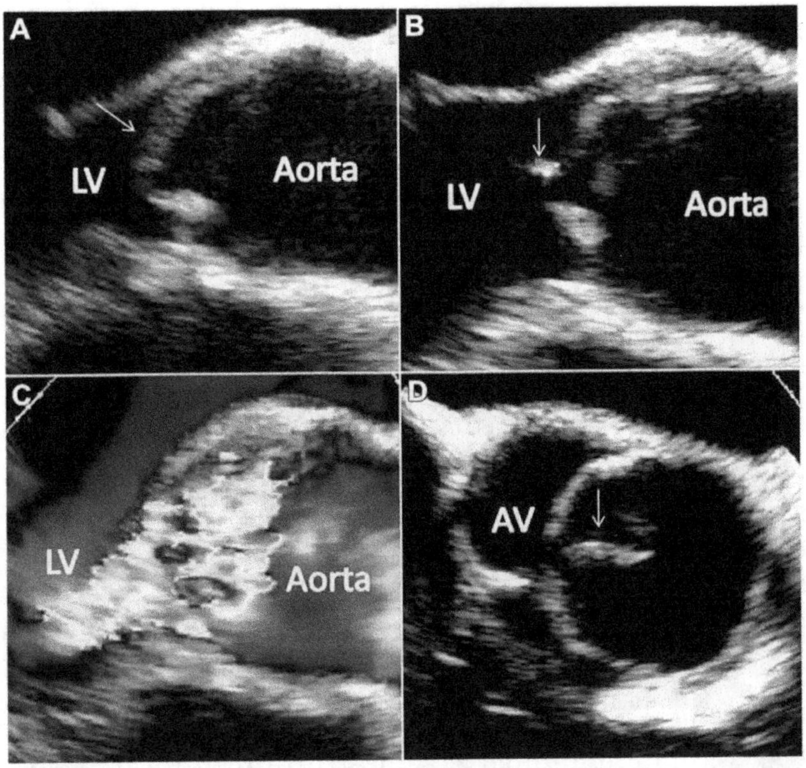

Figure 1 **Patient #3: Pre-Operative Transesophageal Echocardiogram Showing a Congenitally Bicuspid Aortic Valve**

(A) Long-axis view showing the conjoined cusp **(arrow)** prolapsing toward the left ventricular cavity during diastole. **(B)** Long-axis view showing the anomalous cord **(arrow)** prolapsing toward the left ventricular cavity during diastole. **(C)** Long-axis color Doppler view showing aortic regurgitation. **(D)** Short-axis view showing the flail cord **(arrow)**. AV = aortic valve; LV = left ventricle.

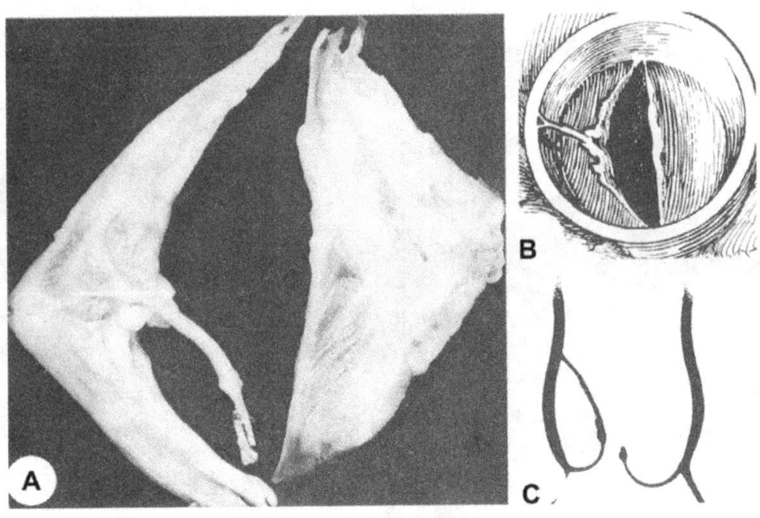

Figure 2 **Patient #1**

(A) A congenitally bicuspid aortic valve devoid of calcific deposits containing an anomalous cord attached to the conjoined cusp in a 27-year-old man who was found to have a murmur consistent with aortic regurgitation at age 17 years. He remained asymptomatic until age 25 years when exertional dyspnea appeared. On pre-operative cardiac catheterization, the left ventricular pressure was 125/35 mm Hg, the brachial arterial pressure was 125/55 mm Hg, and the cardiac index (Fick method) was 2.2 l/min/m^2. The patient underwent aortic valve replacement with a mechanical aortic valve prosthesis for chronic aortic regurgitation and died 13 months later. His heart weighed 800 g. **(B)** Diagram of a short-axis view of the aortic aspect of the bicuspid aortic valve before aortic valve replacement showing the attachment of the anomalous cord from the raphe to the wall of the aorta. **(C)** Diagram of a long-axis view of the same valve. Reproduced with permission from Roberts (1).

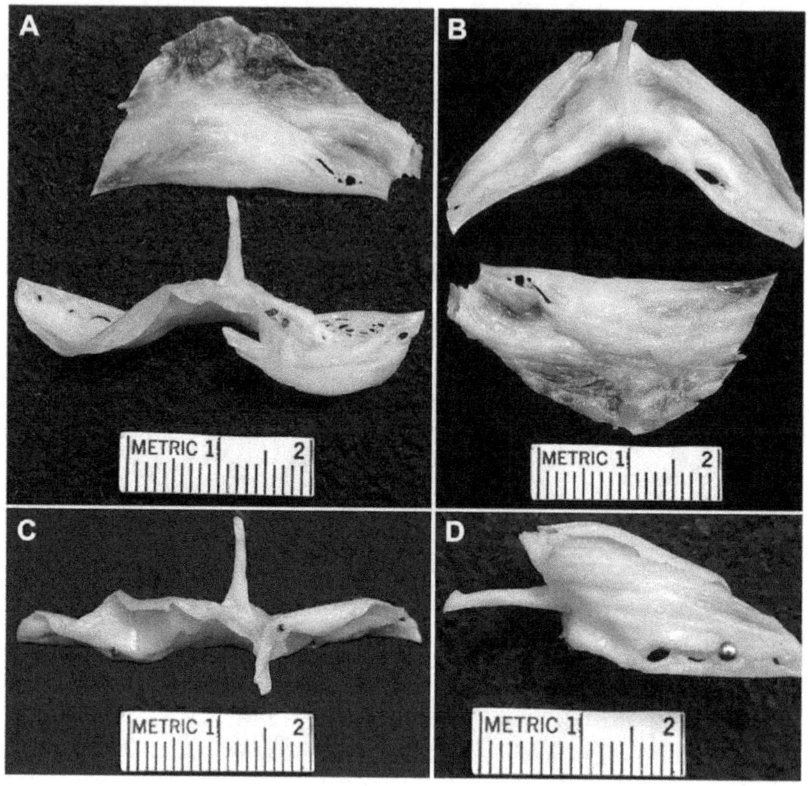

Figure 3 **Patient #2**

A congenitally bicuspid aortic valve with an anomalous cord extending from the raphe of the conjoined right and left coronary cusps in a 45-year-old man with a history of dyspnea. Pre-operative echocardiogram revealed 4+/4+ aortic regurgitation and a 50% left ventricular ejection fraction. He underwent successful aortic valve replacement with a 27 mm St. Jude Medical Regent mechanical aortic valve (St. Jude Medical Inc., St. Paul, Minnesota). **(A)** View of valve from ventricular aspect. **(B)** View from aortic aspect. **(C)** Lateral view showing the length of the anomalous cord. **(D)** Similar to **C**.

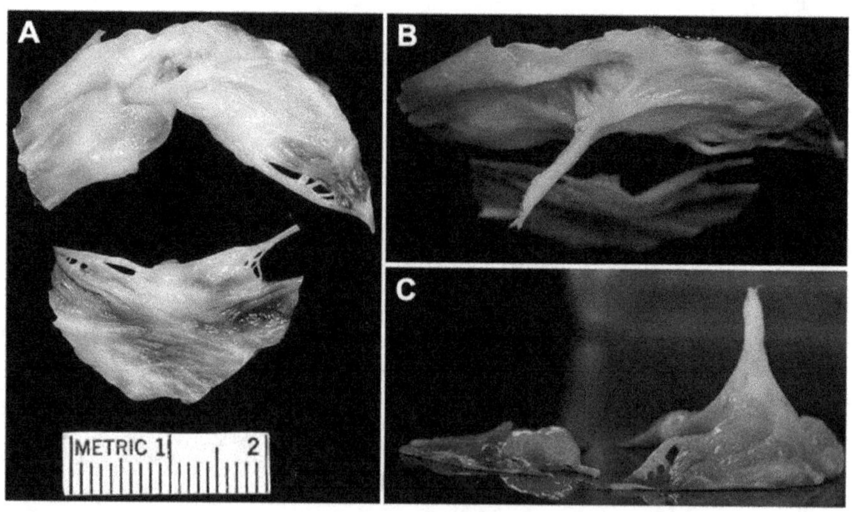

Figure 4 **Patient #3**

(A) The aortic aspect of a congenitally bicuspid aortic valve with an anomalous cord extending from the raphe in a 49-year-old man who heard a loud "pop" while working in his yard with subsequent chest pain and dyspnea. Two days later, he presented to the emergency department with severe dyspnea, and a chest radiograph revealed bilateral pulmonary edema. A precordial murmur was later heard, and echocardiography revealed a "flail" aortic valve cusp causing severe aortic regurgitation. The left ventricular ejection fraction was 55%. Aortotomy disclosed an anomalous cord attached to his bicuspid aortic valve, and it had ruptured. The valve was replaced with a 23-mm Carpentier-Edwards PERIMOUNT pericardial bioprosthesis (Edward Lifesciences Inc., Irvine, California). **(B)** The torn edge of the anomalous cord. **(C)** From the side of the same valve.

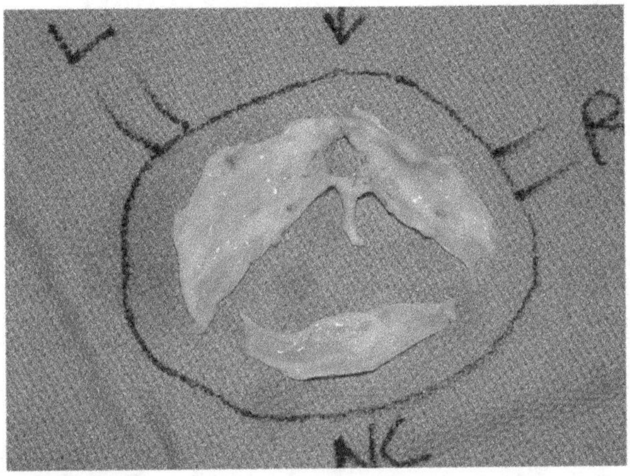

Figure 5 **Patient #4**

A congenitally bicuspid aortic valve with an anomalous cord attached at 1 end to the raphe near the free margin in a 55-year-old man who heard a loud "pop" while working on his car and suddenly became dyspneic. He underwent emergent aortic valve replacement with a bioprosthesis for severe acute aortic regurgitation caused by rupture of the anomalous cord where it attached to the wall of the aorta.

(76%) had evidence of chronic AR as a result of having an intact anomalous cord, and 8 (24%) patients presented with acute AR due to rupture of the anomalous cord. Waller et al. (14) in 1973 described 2 other patients, not included in Table 2, with similar BAVs: 1 was an 8-year-old boy with coarctation of the aorta, and 1 was an 81-year-old man with no other associated congenital anomalies. There was no mention of function of the BAV in these 2 patients. In 1994, Walley et al. (11) described 8 patients with this anomalous cord attached to a stenotic BAV in addition to the 9 patients with a purely regurgitant BAV included in Table 1. The presence of an anomalous cord extending to the wall of the aorta from the raphe of a BAV thus may be associated with stenosis but far more commonly with pure AR.

In none of the 5 men included in the present study was the diagnosis of this variant of the purely regurgitant BAV made pre-operatively. Most symptomatic patients with this congenital anomaly present with chronic AR and slowly progressing symptoms. Rupture of an anomalous cord should be considered as a possible etiology of pure acute AR when infection, aortic dissection, and trauma have been ruled out.

Reprint requests and correspondence: Dr. William C. Roberts, Baylor Heart and Vascular Institute, Baylor University Medical Center at Dallas, 3500 Gaston Avenue, Dallas, Texas 75246. E-mail: wc.roberts@baylorhealth.edu.

REFERENCES

1. Roberts WC. The congenitally bicuspid aortic valve. A study of 85 autopsy cases. Am J Cardiol 1970;26:72–83.
2. Roberts WC, Vowels TJ, Ko JM. Natural history of adults with congenitally malformed aortic valves (unicuspid and bicuspid). Medicine 2012;91:287–308.
3. Carter JB, Sethi S, Lee GB, Edwards JE. Prolapse of semilunar cusps as causes of aortic insufficiency. Circulation 1971;43:922–32.
4. Becker AE, Düren DR. Spontaneous rupture of bicuspid aortic valve. An unusual cause of aortic insufficiency. Chest 1977;72:361–2.
5. Olson LJ, Subramanian R, Edwards WD. Surgical pathology of pure aortic insufficiency: a study of 225 cases. Mayo Clin Proc 1984;59:835–41.
6. Yamagishi M, Anzai N, Yamada M. An exceptional form of congenitally bicuspid aortic valve resulting in pure aortic regurgitation. Jpn Heart J 1986;27:267–71.
7. Waller BF, Taliercio CP, Dickos DK, Howard J, Adlam JH, Jolly W. Rare or unusual causes of chronic, isolated, pure aortic regurgitation. Clin Cardiol 1990;13:577–81.
8. Arikawa K, Chosa N, Kinjoh T, et al. Pure aortic valve regurgitation due to congenital bicuspid valve. Analysis of 7 cases and a report of 2 rare cases. Nihon Kyobu Geka Gakkai Zasshi 1990;38:2401–3.
9. Hamada Y, Iijima T, Yoshida I, et al. Bicuspid aortic valve with sudden onset of aortic insufficiency due to rare causes: report of two cases. Kyobugeka 1992;45:519–21.
10. Misawa Y, Hasegawa T, Oyama H, Sudo H, Hasegawa N, Kamisawa O. Congenital bicuspid aortic valve with regurgitation. A rare case showing a fibrous band between the conjoined cusp and the ascending aorta. Nihon Kyobu Geka Gakkai Zasshi 1993;41:2156–9.
11. Walley VM, Antecol DH, Kyrollos AG, Chan KL. Congenitally bicuspid aortic valves: study of a variant with fenestrated raphe. Can J Cardiol 1994;10:535–42.
12. Akiyama K, Taniyasu N, Iba Y, Hirota J, Asano S. Sudden deterioration of aortic regurgitation due to rupture of a raphal cord on the conjoined cusp. Jpn Circ J 2000;64:477–80.
13. Journigan JG, Clements SD Jr. Case study: acute aortic regurgitation due to spontaneous rupture of a congenitally malformed bicuspid valve. J Med Assoc Ga 2011;100:26–7.
14. Waller BF, Carter JB, Williams HJ Jr., Wang K, Edwards JE. Bicuspid aortic valve: comparison of congenital and acquired types. Circulation 1973;48:1140–50.

Key Words: aortic regurgitation ▪ bicuspid aortic valve ▪ congenital heart disease.

Gross and Histological Features of Excised Portions of Posterior Mitral Leaflet in Patients Having Operative Repair of Mitral Valve Prolapse and Comments on the Concept of Missing (= Ruptured) Chordae Tendineae

William C. Roberts, MD,*†‡ Travis J. Vowels, BBA,* Jong M. Ko, BA,* Robert F. Hebeler, Jr, MD§

Dallas, Texas

Objectives The aim of the study is to describe gross and histological features of operatively excised portions of mitral valves in patients with mitral valve prolapse (MVP).

Background Although numerous articles on MVP (myxomatous or myxoid degeneration, billowing or floppy mitral valve) have appeared, 2 virtually constant histological features have been underemphasized or overlooked: 1) the presence of superimposed fibrous tissue on both surfaces of the leaflets and surrounding many chordae tendineae; and 2) the absence of many chordae tendineae on the ventricular surfaces of the leaflets as the result of their being hidden (i.e., covered up) by the superimposed fibrous tissue.

Methods We examined operatively excised portions of prolapsed posterior mitral leaflets in 37 patients having operative repair.

Results Histological study of elastic-tissue stained sections disclosed that the leaflet thickening was primarily due to the superimposed fibrous tissue. All leaflets had variable increases in the spongiosa element within the leaflet itself with some disruption and/or loss of the fibrosa element and occasionally complete separation of it from the spongiosa element. Both the leaflet and chordae were separated from the superimposed fibrous tissue by their black-staining elastic membranes.

Conclusions These findings demonstrate that the posterior leaflet thickening in MVP is mainly due to the superimposed fibrous tissue rather than to an increased volume of the spongiosa element of the leaflet itself. The superimposed fibrous tissue on both leaflet and chordae is likely the result of subsequent abnormal contact of the leaflets and chordae with one another. Chordal rupture (i.e., missing chordae) occurred in all 37 patients, but finding individual ruptured chords was rare. (J Am Coll Cardiol 2014;63:1667–74) © 2014 by the American College of Cardiology Foundation

Although numerous publications have appeared describing auscultory, angiographic, echocardiographic, and morphological features of mitral valve prolapse (MVP) (myxomatous or myxoid degeneration), surprisingly, none have reproduced the various histological features of the operatively excised mitral valves or parts thereof in color after staining for elastic fibers, an absolute necessity for proper evaluation, because a black-staining elastic membrane separates the leaflet and chordae from the superimposed fibrous tissue, a constant feature of MVP. In this report, we focus on the contribution of the superimposed fibrous tissue to the leaflet and chordal thickening, and second, we introduce the concept that missing or hidden chords (those lying beneath the superimposed fibrous tissue) are equivalent to ruptured chords.

From the *Baylor Heart and Vascular Institute, Baylor University Medical Center, Dallas, Texas; †Department of Internal Medicine (Division of Cardiology), Baylor University Medical Center, Dallas, Texas; ‡Department of Pathology, Baylor University Medical Center, Dallas, Texas; and the §Department of Cardiothoracic Surgery, Baylor University Medical Center, Dallas, Texas. The study was funded by the Baylor Health Care System Foundation, Dallas, Texas. The authors have reported that they have no relationships relevant to the contents of this paper to disclose.

Manuscript received August 31, 2013; revised manuscript received November 7, 2013, accepted November 12, 2013.

Methods

Since March 1993, all specimens excised at operation by cardiac surgeons at Baylor University Medical Center at

Abbreviations and Acronyms

MR = mitral regurgitation

MVP = mitral valve prolapse

Dallas have been submitted to the surgical pathology division of the pathology department, and all such specimens have been described by one of us (W.C.R.) who submitted the pathology report. Most gross specimens were photographed. After describing the submitted specimen, clinical, echocardiographic, and hemodynamic data were retrieved online via the Baylor University Medical Center at the Dallas Electronic Medical Records and the Apollo Cardiovascular Database. A total of 500 mitral valves or portions thereof were received from January 2005 through June 2013 (Fig. 1). Of this number, 140 patients underwent mitral valve repair or replacement for severe mitral regurgitation (MR) secondary to MVP. After excluding those patients where preoperative echocardiograms (n = 71) were not available to us or histological sections of the excised valves were not prepared or retrievable (n = 14) or the patients had chronic renal failure (n = 4), 51 patients were available for study: 14 had mitral valve replacement and were then excluded from the present study; 37 had mitral valve repair, and in each, portions of the posterior leaflet were studied. Sections of the posterior leaflets were cut from the margin of attachment to the free margin and submitted for histological preparation. After processing in alcohol and xylene, 2 sections were cut from each paraffin block: one was stained by hematoxylin/eosin, and the other, by elastic van Geison.

Results

Pertinent data from the 37 patients are summarized in Table 1. (Data on the 14 patients having mitral valve replacement for MVP are shown in the table simply for comparison.) The operative report in all 37 patients indicated "prolapse" of a portion of posterior mitral leaflet and that the prolapsed segment was the one almost always excised. None of the 37 had calcific deposits in the operatively excised specimens. All 37 patients also had an annular ring inserted.

Examination of the posterior mitral leaflet in the 37 patients disclosed several consistent features (Figs. 2 to 9, Table 2). All 37 operatively excised portions of posterior mitral leaflet had "missing" (i.e., ruptured) chordae tendineae on gross examination. Histologically, the leaflet itself and the chordae tendineae were clearly demarcated by an elastic membrane (elastic van Geison stain). Both atrial and ventricular aspects of the leaflet in all 37 patients contained superimposed fibrous tissue, thicker on the atrial side than on the ventricular side. Additionally, numerous elastic fibers were present in the superimposed fibrous tissue on the atrial aspect, whereas few if any were present in the superimposed fibrous tissue on the

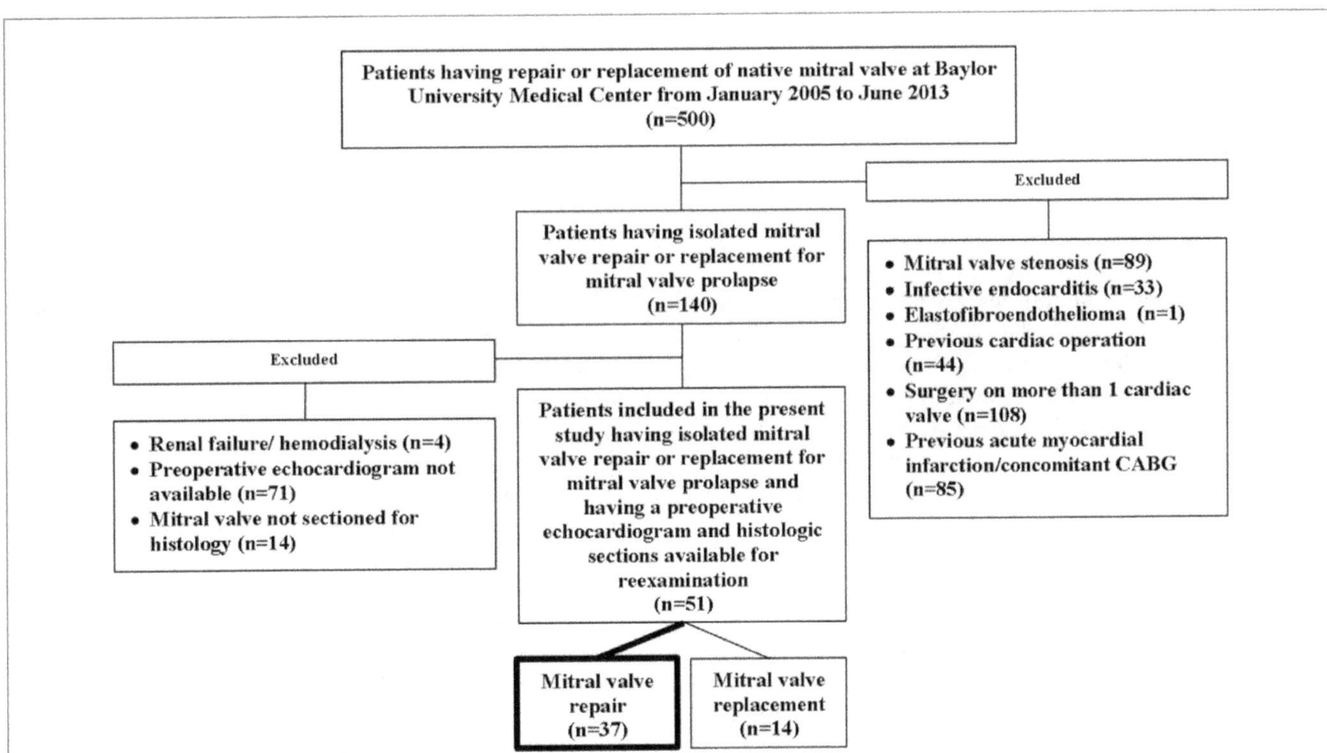

Figure 1 Flow Chart

Chart showing the origin of the 37 patients included in the present study. CABG = coronary artery bypass grafting.

Table 1 Comparison of Various Variables Among Patients Having Isolated MV Repair or Replacement for Mitral Valve Prolapse

Variable	MV Repair (n = 37) (73%)	MV Replacement* (n = 14) (27%)
Age (yrs)	56 ± 13 [59] (31-78)	59 ± 15 [56] (34-79)
Sex		
M	31 (84%)	7 (50%)
F	6 (16%)	7 (50%)
Ethnicity		
W	32 (86%)	11 (79%)
B	2 (5%)	3 (21%)
H	2 (5%)	0
A	1 (3%)	0
Atrial fibrillation	13 (35%)	7 (50%)
Pressures (mm Hg)		
Pulmonary arterial wedge (n = 29)	15 ± 5 [15] (7-27)	21 ± 10 [21] (6-39)
RV		
Peak systole (n = 32)	39 ± 13 [34] (16-70)	44 ± 15 [41] (18-66)
End diastole (n = 32)	11 ± 4 [11] (2-19)	14 ± 6 [14] (3-23)
Right atrial mean (n = 31)	7 ± 4 [5] (0-16)	11 ± 8 [11] (0-21)
LV		
Peak systole (n = 34)	120 ± 19 [118] (90-162)	115 ± 16 [111] (99-144)
End diastole (n = 36)	18 ± 6 [18] (6-31)	19 ± 8 [16] (12-35)
Aorta		
Peak systole (n = 34)	117 ± 19 [115] (79-147)	121 ± 19 [120] (95-155)
End diastole (n = 34)	66 ± 15 [69] (19-93)	73 ± 15 [69] (56-101)
Cardiac index (l/min/m^2) (n = 27)	2.66 ± 0.48 [2.63] (1.97-3.71)	2.25 ± 0.68 [2.34] (1.38-3.35)
EF (%) (n = 30) (by catheterization)	60 ± 10 [65] (30-75)	55 ± 20 [60] (25-80)
MV regurgitation		
3+	3 (8%)	2 (14%)
4+	34 (92%)	12 (86%)
MV weight (g)	0.70 ± 0.46 [0.51] (0.20-1.94)	1.52 ± 1.18 [1.50] (0.04-4.07)
MV size (mm)		
Ring	31 ± 3	—
Prosthesis	—	29 ± 3

Values are mean ± SD, [median], (range), or n (%). *These cases are included here simply for quick comparison with the patients having mitral valve (MV) repair.

A = Asian; B = black; EF = ejection fraction; H = Hispanic; LV = left ventricle; RV = right ventricle; W = white; + = positive or present; 0 = negative or absent.

ventricular aspect. The fibrous tissue surrounding the chordae tendineae was similar to that on the ventricular aspect of the leaflet. Within the mitral leaflet itself—enclosed by the elastic membrane—the spongiosa element seemed increased in quantity in all patients, more so in the distal one-half than in the proximal one-half of the leaflet; and the fibrosa element was interrupted focally and/or decreased in quantity or both.

Discussion

Examination of operatively excised portions of posterior mitral leaflet in each of the 37 patients having mitral repair for MVP produced 2 major findings: 1) the leaflet and chordal thickening in patients with MVP is due in large part to superimposed fibrous tissue on both the atrial and ventricular surfaces of the leaflets and surrounding the chordae tendineae; and 2) rupture of posterior leaflet chordae tendineae is a nearly universal finding in patients with MVP, and MR is severe enough to warrant operative repair but that seeing 1 or more ruptured chordae is infrequent, because they are covered ("hidden") by the superimposed fibrous tissue on the ventricular surface of the leaflet. In essence, the absence of chordae (missing chordae) is synonymous with earlier rupture of chordae.

We surmise that the superimposed fibrous tissue on both leaflet and chordae is entirely due to abnormal contact of the leaflets with one another over many years or decades. That the underlying leaflet and chordae are essentially intact suggests that the basic process in MVP is a slow, gradual loss and/or interruption of collagen fibers (in the fibrosa element of the leaflet and in the chordae tendineae, which are devoid of a spongiosa element). The loss and/or interruption of collagen fibers within the leaflet and chordae seems to be responsible for the gradual elongation of the leaflets and chordae in MVP, which in turn leads to inappropriate leaflet contact and to the superimposed fibrous tissue ("callus" formation) (Fig. 10).

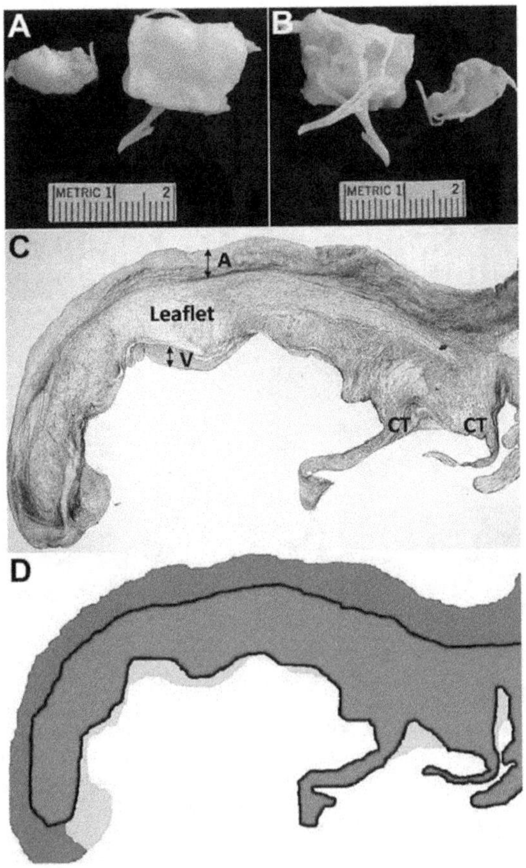

Figure 2 Patient #1 in Table 2

Photographs of the atrial (A) surface **(A)** and ventricular (V) surface **(B)** of a portion of excised posterior mitral valve leaflet. Most chordae are missing from the V surface shown in **B. (C)** Photomicrograph showing superimposed fibrous tissue on both the A and V surfaces and increased spongiosa element within the leaflet itself outlined by its black-staining elastic membrane (elastic van Geison, 20×). **(D)** Rendering of the same valve with **red** representing the leaflet itself, **green** representing the superimposed fibrous tissue on the A surface, and **yellow** representing the superimposed fibrous tissue on the V surface. CT = chordae tendineae.

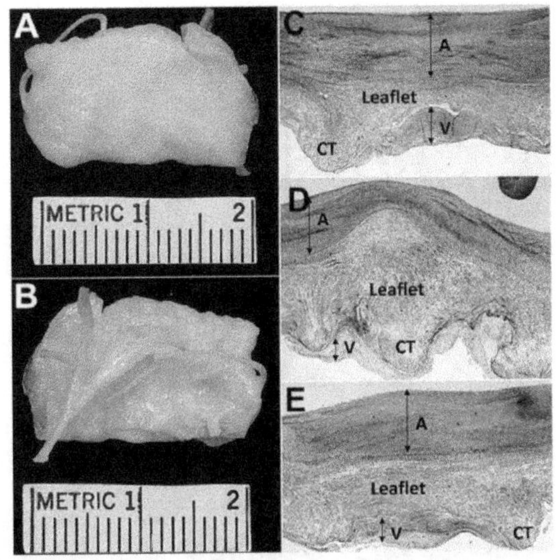

Figure 3 Patient #2 in Table 2

Photographs of the A surface **(A)** and V surface **(B)** of a portion of excised posterior leaflet. Most chordae are missing from the V surface shown in **B. (C to E)** Photomicrographs showing superimposed fibrous tissue on both the A and V surfaces and increased spongiosa element within the leaflet itself outlined by its black-staining elastic membrane (elastic van Geison, 40×). Abbreviations as in Figure 2.

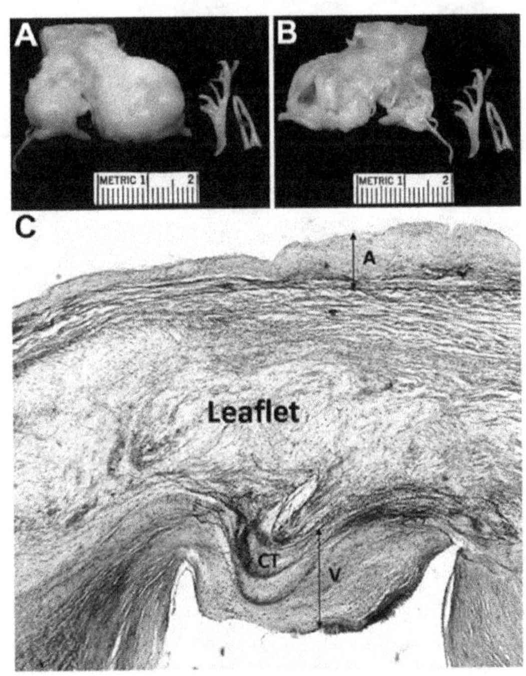

Figure 4 Patient #3 in Table 2

Photographs of the A surface **(A)** and V surface **(B)** of a portion of posterior leaflet. Most chordae are missing from the V surface shown in **B. (C)** Photomicrograph showing superimposed fibrous tissue on both the A and V surfaces and severely increased spongiosa element within the leaflet itself outlined by its black-staining elastic membrane (elastic van Geison, 40×). Abbreviations as in Figure 2.

The superimposed fibrous tissue on the atrial and ventricular aspects of the posterior mitral leaflet is quite different histologically. On the atrial aspect, the surface is usually smooth, and the fibrous tissue is dense and contains numerous parallel-lying elastic fibers, simulating in a way the media of an elastic artery. By contrast, the superimposed fibrous tissue on the ventricular surface and surrounding the chordae tends to have an irregular surface, the collagen is less dense, and it contains few, if any, elastic fibers. The atrial surfaces, of course, are the ones making abnormal leaflet contact; the ventricular surfaces are receiving the impact of the left ventricular systolic pressure. The reason for the structural difference between the 2 surfaces is unclear.

That the identification of a ruptured chord is infrequent but that covered (by fibrous tissue) chordae are nearly

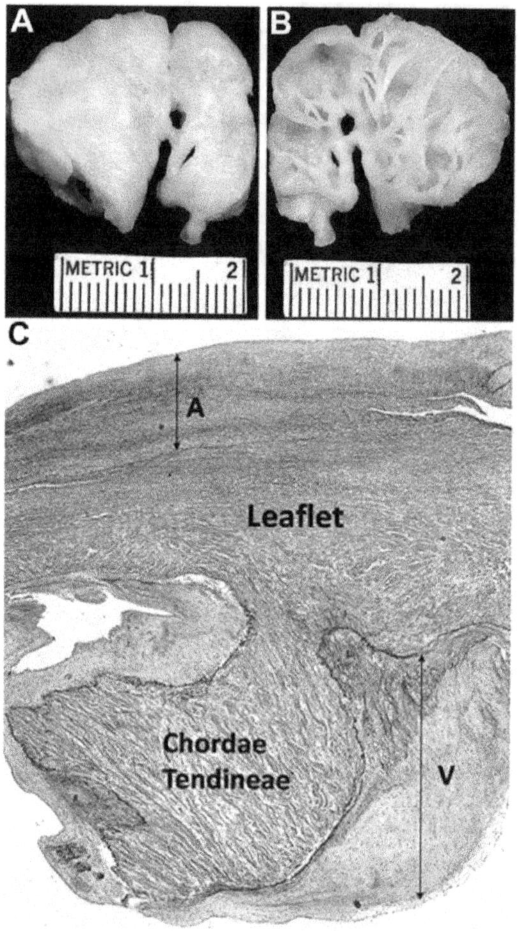

Figure 5 **Patient #4 in Table 2**

Photographs of the A surface **(A)** and V surface **(B)** of a portion of excised posterior leaflet. Most chordae are missing from or tangled on the V surface shown in **B**. **(C)** Photomicrograph showing superimposed fibrous tissue on both the A and V surfaces and no or minimal increase in the spongiosa element within the leaflet itself, which is outlined by its black-staining elastic membrane (elastic van Geison, 40×). Abbreviations as in Figure 2.

universal in patients with MVP and MR severe enough to warrant operative repair strongly suggest that most chordal ruptures are clinically silent and occur possibly multiple times through the years. Also, the patients having acute heart failure might have ruptured a primary chord (i.e., one arising from a papillary muscle itself and not one actually attached to the mitral leaflet, as would be the case with a tertiary chord, which would unlikely lead to MR or to a sudden worsening of MR).

This article, of course, follows numerous ones discussing gross and histological features of prolapsed mitral valves examined at either necropsy or after operative excision (1–20). Few, however, mentioned the superimposed fibrous tissue on the leaflet and chordae, probably because elastic-tissue stains were not used, a requirement to see the outline of the underlying leaflet and chordae. Additionally, none mentioned hidden—previously ruptured—chordae by the overlying fibrous tissue. Thus, chordal rupture in MVP is far more common than previously appreciated (10,13,14,16,21–23).

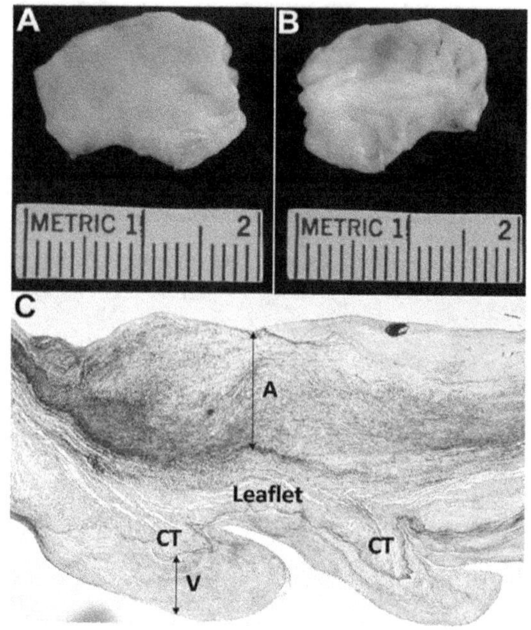

Figure 6 **Patient #5 in Table 2**

Photographs of the A surface **(A)** and V surface **(B)** of a portion of excised posterior leaflet. All chordae are missing from the V surface shown in **B**. **(C)** Photomicrograph showing superimposed fibrous tissue on both the A and V surfaces and only mildly increased spongiosa element within the leaflet itself, outlined by its black-staining elastic membrane (elastic van Geison, 40×). Abbreviations as in Figure 2.

Elastic-tissue stains were prepared on all histological sections of the operatively excised posterior mitral leaflets, a requirement to separate the superimposed fibrous tissue from the underlying leaflet itself. In all cases, the operative specimen and histological sections of it were studied and described by the same individual (namely, W.C.R.) and not by a variety of persons with varying knowledge of and interest in cardiovascular disease. All patients included had pre-operative echocardiograms described by the reader to be characteristic of MVP. The present report excluded all patients with angiographic evidence of significant coronary narrowing and any patient having coronary artery bypass grafting; all patients with a dysfunctioning aortic valve or aortic valve repair or replacement and all patients with associated mitral stenosis or prior infective endocarditis at any time were also excluded. All these exclusions were an attempt to make certain the patients included herein were a group with "pure" MVP.

Study limitations. We studied only patients with MVP who had MR severe enough to warrant mitral valve repair. Whether our observations hold true for younger patients

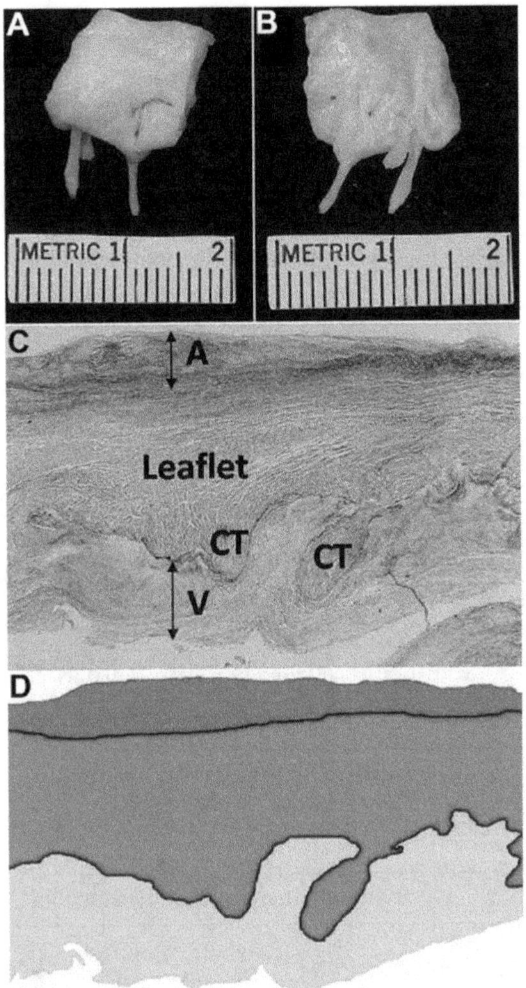

Figure 7 Patient #6 in Table 2

Photographs of the A surface **(A)** and V surface **(B)** of a portion of excised posterior leaflet. Most chordae are missing from the V surface. **(C)** Photomicrograph showing superimposed fibrous tissue on both the A and V surfaces and mildly increased spongiosa element within the leaflet itself, which is outlined by its black-staining elastic membrane (elastic van Geison, 40×). **(D)** Rendering of the same valve with **red** representing the leaflet itself, **green** representing the superimposed fibrous tissue on the A surface, and **yellow** representing the superimposed fibrous tissue on the V surface. Abbreviations as in Figure 2.

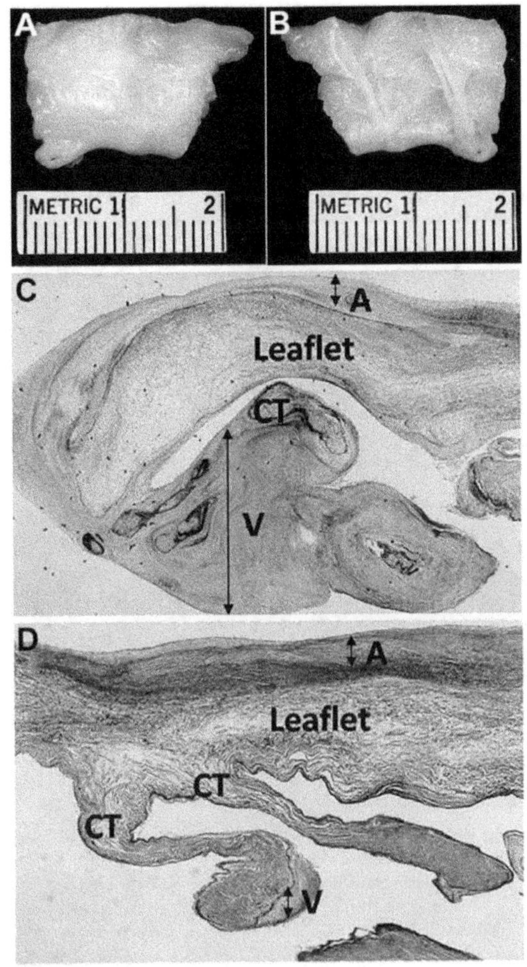

Figure 8 Patient #7 in Table 2

Photographs of the A surface **(A)** and V surface **(B)** of a portion of excised posterior leaflet. Most chordae are missing from the V surface shown in **B**. **(C)** Photomicrograph distally at the free margin showing a large amount of superimposed fibrous tissue on both the A and V surfaces and almost complete replacement of the fibrosa element by the spongiosa element within the leaflet itself outlined by its black-staining elastic membrane (elastic van Geison, 40×). **(D)** Photomicrograph of the same valve to the annulus showing less superimposed fibrous tissue on the A and V surfaces and only a moderate increase in the spongiosa element within the leaflet (elastic van Geison, 40×). Abbreviations as in Figure 2.

(e.g., with mild MR from MVP) is unclear. Additionally, the amount of mitral leaflet tissue available to examine varied from patient to patient. Although all 37 patients had precordial systolic murmurs recorded in the medical record, whether the murmur was pansystolic or late systolic only or accompanied by 1 or more systolic clicks was not recorded. The echocardiograms were interpreted by a number of different echocardiographers. Details of the thickness of the mitral leaflets were not recorded in any echocardiographic report and not by any surgeon at operation.

Conclusions

This study of operatively-excised posterior mitral leaflets in patients with MR secondary to MVP indicates that the leaflet thickening is the result primarily of superimposed fibrous tissue on both surfaces of the leaflet and that previously ruptured chordae, nearly universal, are usually covered by the superimposed fibrous tissue on the ventricular surface by the time of operative intervention.

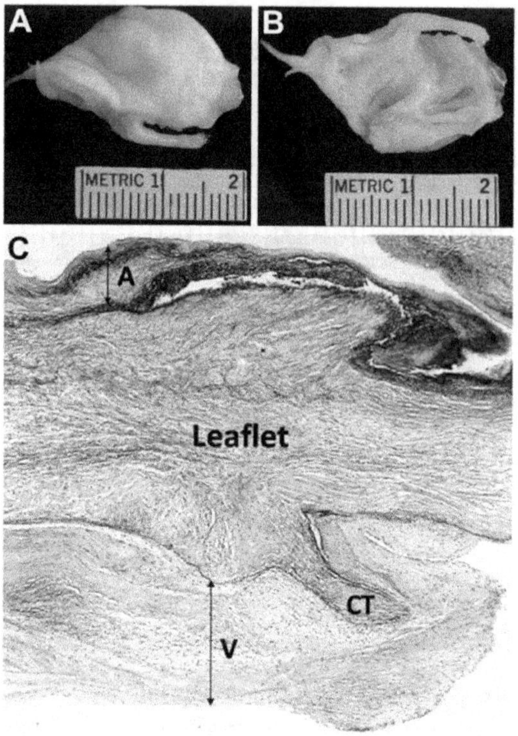

Figure 9 Patient #8 in Table 2

Photographs of the A surface **(A)** and V surface **(B)** of a portion of excised posterior leaflet. Most chordae are missing from the V surface. **(C)** Photomicrograph showing superimposed fibrous tissue on both the A and V surfaces and increased spongiosa element within the valve leaflet itself, outlined by its black-staining elastic membrane (elastic van Geison, 40×). Abbreviations as in Figure 2.

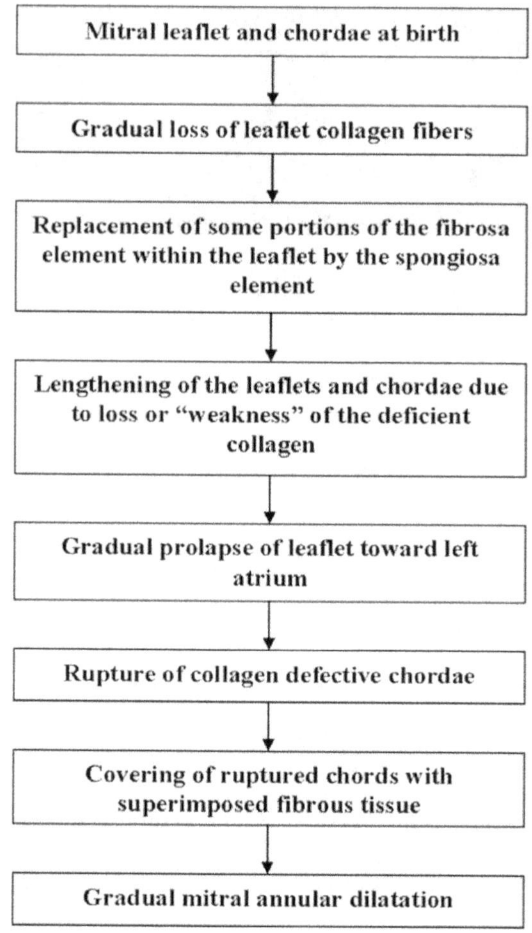

Figure 10 Chart Showing Likely Mechanism of Mitral Valve Prolapse

Mitral valve prolapse going from initial loss of collagen, to partial replacement by the spongiosa element, to leaflet elongation and chordal rupture with focal leaflet prolapse, and gradual thickening due to superimposed fibrous tissue.

Table 2 Comparison of Various Variables Among 8 Patients Having Isolated MV Repair for MV Prolapse Whose Valves Are Illustrated Both Grossly and Histologically

					Pressures (mm Hg)				
Patient #	Figure #	Age (yrs)	Sex	Race	RV (s/d)	LV (s/d)	Aorta (s/d)	EF (%)	MV Weight (g)
1	2	43	M	W	34/15	112/12	111/74	70	1.02
2	3	46	F	W	26/10	101/13	104/55	40	0.64
3	4	48	M	W	38/14	102/23	106/67	65	1.94
4	5	54	M	W	31/11	—	120/55*	65	1.61
5	6	54	F	W	—	—	100/55*	—	0.33
6	7	55	M	W	34/10	137/19	135/80	70	0.31
7	8	59	M	A	41/9	116/14	121/85	30	0.47
8	9	66	M	W	16/2	92/6	96/69	—	0.81

*Indirect blood pressure measurement.
s/d = systole/diastole; other abbreviations as in Table 1.

Reprint requests and correspondence: Dr. William C. Roberts, Baylor Heart and Vascular Institute, Baylor University Medical Center at Dallas, 3500 Gaston Avenue, Dallas, Texas 75246. E-mail: wc.roberts@baylorhealth.edu.

REFERENCES

1. Fernex M, Fernex C. Mucoid degenerescence of the mitral valve; functional repercussions. Helv Med Acta 1958;25:694–705.
2. Read RC, Thal AP, Wendt VE. Symptomatic valvular myxomatous transformation (the floppy valve syndrome). A possible forme frusta of the Marfan syndrome. Circulation 1965;32:897–910.
3. Bittar N, Sosa JA. The billowing mitral valve leaflet. Report on fourteen patients. Circulation 1968;38:763–70.
4. Trent JK, Adelman AG, Wigle ED, Silver MD. Morphology of a prolapsed posterior mitral valve leaflet. Am Heart J 1970;79:539–43.
5. McCarthy LJ, Wolf PL. Mucoid degeneration of heart valves: "blue valve syndrome". Am J Clin Pathol 1970;54:852–6.
6. Shappell SD, Marshall CE. Ballooning posterior leaflet syndrome. Syncope and sudden death. Arch Intern Med 1975;135:664–7.
7. Davies MJ, Moore BP, Braimbridge MV. The floppy mitral valve. Study of incidence, pathology, and complications in surgical, necropsy, and forensic material. Br Heart J 1978;40:468–81.
8. Olsen EGJ, Al-Rufaie HK. The floppy mitral valve. Study on pathogenesis. Br Heart J 1980;44:674–83.
9. Rippe J, Fishbein MC, Carabello B, et al. Primary myxomatous degeneration of cardiac valves. Clinical, pathological, haemodynamic, and echocardiographic profile. Br Heart J 1980;44:621–9.
10. Hickey AJ, Wilcken DEL, Wright JS, Warren BS. Primary (spontaneous) chordal rupture: relation to myxomatous valve disease and mitral valve prolapse. J Am Coll Cardiol 1985;5:1341–6.
11. van der Bel-Kahn J, Duren DR, Becker AE. Isolated mitral valve prolapse: chordal architecture as an anatomic basis in older patients. J Am Coll Cardiol 1985;5:1335–40.
12. Hanson TP, Edwards BS, Edwards JE. Pathology of surgically excised mitral valves. Arch Pathol Lab Med 1985;109:823–8.
13. Olson LJ, Subramanian R, Ackermann DM, Orszulak TA, Edwards WD. Surgical pathology of the mitral valve: a study of 712 cases spanning 21 years. Mayo Clin Proc 1987;62:22–34.
14. Roberts WC, McIntosh CL, Wallace RB. Mechanisms of severe mitral regurgitation in mitral valve prolapse determined from analysis of operatively excised valves. Am Heart J 1987;113:1316–23.
15. Virmani R, Atkinson JB, Forman MB. The pathology of mitral valve prolapse. Herz 1988;13:215–26.
16. Turri M, Thiene G, Bortolotti U, Mazzucco A, Gallucci V. Surgical pathology of disease of the mitral valve, with special reference to lesions promoting valvular incompetence. Int J Cardiol 1989;22:213–9.
17. Dollar AL, Roberts WC. Morphologic comparison of patients with mitral valve prolapse who died suddenly with patients who died from severe valvular dysfunction or other conditions. J Am Coll Cardiol 1991;17:921–31.
18. Agozzino L, Falco A, de Vivo F, de Vinventiis C, de Luca L, Esposito S, Cotrufo M. Surgical pathology of the mitral valve: gross and histological study of 1288 surgically excised valves. Int J Cardiol 1992;37:79–89.
19. Shirani J, Roberts WC. Clinical and morphologic features of mitral valve prolapse in octogenarians. Am J Cardiol 1993;72:1316–9.
20. Butany J, Privitera S, David TE. Mitral valve prolapse: an atypical variation of the anatomy. Can J Cardiol 2003;19:1367–73.
21. Cooley DA, Gerami S, Hallman GL, Wukasch DC, Hall RJ. Mitral insufficiency due to myxomatous transformation: "floppy valve syndrome". J Cardiovasc Surg 1972;13:346–9.
22. Chadraratna PA, Aronow WS. Incidence of ruptured chordae tendineae in mitral valve prolapse syndrome. An echocardiographic study. Chest 1979;75:334–9.
23. Grenadier E, Alpan G, Keidar S, Palant A. The prevalence of ruptured chordae tendineae in the mitral valve prolapse syndrome. Am Heart J 1983;105:603–10.

Key Words: mitral regurgitation ▪ mitral valve prolapse ▪ mitral valve repair.

Morphologic Features of the Recipient Heart in Patients Having Cardiac Transplantation and Analysis of the Congruence or Incongruence Between the Clinical and Morphologic Diagnoses

William C. Roberts, MD, Carey Camille Roberts, BS, Jong Mi Ko, BA, Giovanni Filardo, PhD, John Edward Capehart, MD, and Shelley Anne Hall, MD

Abstract: Cardiac transplantation (CT) has been one of the great medical advances of the last nearly 50 years. We studied the explanted hearts of 314 patients having CT at Baylor University Medical Center Dallas from 1993 to 2012, and compared the morphologic diagnoses to the clinical diagnoses before CT. Among the 314 patients the morphologic and clinical diagnoses were congruent in 272 (87%) and incongruent in 42 (13%). Most of the incongruity occurred among the 166 patients with non-ischemic cardiomyopathy (non-IC) (36/166 [22%]), and of that group the major incongruity occurred among the patients with hypertrophic cardiomyopathy (7/17 [41%]), non-compaction left ventricular cardiomyopathy (NCLVC) (3/3 [100%]), mononuclear myocarditis (3/3 [100%]), arrhythmogenic right ventricular cardiomyopathy (ARVC) (4/4 [100%]), and cardiac sarcoidosis (8/8 [100%]). The phrase "non-IC" is a general term that includes several subsets of cardiac diseases and simply means "insignificant narrowing of 1 or more of the epicardial coronary arteries," but it does not specify the specific cause of the heart failure leading to CT. A number of cardiac illustrations are provided to demonstrate the morphologic variability occurring among the patients with IC and non-IC.

(*Medicine* 2014;93: 211–235)

Abbreviations: ARVC = arrhythmogenic right ventricular cardiomyopathy, CT = cardiac transplantation, HC = hypertrophic cardiomyopathy, IC = ischemic cardiomyopathy, IDC = idiopathic dilated cardiomyopathy, NCLVC = non-compaction left ventricular cardiomyopathy.

INTRODUCTION

The first cardiac transplantation (CT) procedure was done in Capetown, South Africa, by Christiaan Barnard in 1967.[3] From that time through 2012, more than 90,000 CT procedures were performed worldwide, approximately 3500 a year with about 2200 of that number being performed in the United States.[30] The immediate pre-op care, the operation, and the first 6-month post-operative care cost about $1,000,000. Although most have been performed in patients with idiopathic dilated cardiomyopathy (IDC) or ischemic cardiomyopathy (IC), CT is also performed, albeit less frequently, for a variety of other cardiac conditions. In 1998 Waller and colleagues reported clinical and morphologic findings in 92 patients who had had CT for IDC, IC, or hypertrophic cardiomyopathy (HC).[71] Of them, 57 had CT at Baylor University Medical Center (BUMC) Dallas from March 1993 through June 1997. (The remaining 35 patients had CT at other institutions and are not included in the present analysis.) Surprisingly, that clinico-pathologic study appears to have been the first to report morphologic findings in a systematic fashion in the recipient hearts in those 3 conditions. The present report was prompted by finding incongruity between the clinical and morphologic diagnoses in some patients having CT, and that incongruity led to a thorough analysis of that frequency in 314 patients who had had CT at BUMC in the past 20 years.

METHODS

The recipient hearts in each of the 314 patients were submitted to the surgical pathology division of the department of pathology of BUMC Dallas. The patients included had undergone CT at BUMC from March 1993 through June 2012. All hearts during this period were described and classified by 1 of the authors (WCR). Figure 1 displays the number of CTs done at BUMC during each of those 20 years and the 3 major reasons for CT among the 314 patients. Each heart after formalin fixation and "cleaning" was weighed carefully by WCR, opened by him, and photographed (most by JMK). Although some were opened by parasagittal cuts, especially in those patients with HC, the cardiac ventricles in most were incised by transverse cuts parallel to the posterior atrioventricular sulcus. The resulting "bread-loaf" slices were approximately 1 cm in thickness except for the most apical portion, which was about 3 cm thick. The heart was weighed after these cuts and after all extraneous tissues were removed. The left ventricular cavity was measured both from anterior to posterior and from right to left dimensions, and the largest of these cavity numbers were used as the maximal cavity dimension. The right ventricular cavity dimension was the length from the right ventricular aspect of the ventricular septum to the endocardial lining of the right ventricular free wall along the posterior wall of this chamber.

From the Departments of Internal Medicine (Division of Cardiology) (WCR, SAH), Pathology (WCR), and Cardiothoracic Surgery (JEC), and the Baylor Heart and Vascular Institute (WCR, CCR, JMK), Baylor University Medical Center, Dallas, Texas. Carey Camille Roberts is currently a freshman at Georgetown University School of Medicine, Washington, DC.

Correspondence: Dr. William C. Roberts, Baylor Heart and Vascular Institute, Baylor University Medical Center, 3500 Gaston Avenue, Dallas, TX (e-mail: wc.roberts@baylorhealth.edu).

Financial support and conflicts of interest: Support for this investigation was provided by the Baylor Health Care System Foundation. The authors have no conflicts of interest to disclose.

ISSN: 0025-7974

DOI: 10.1097/MD.0000000000000038

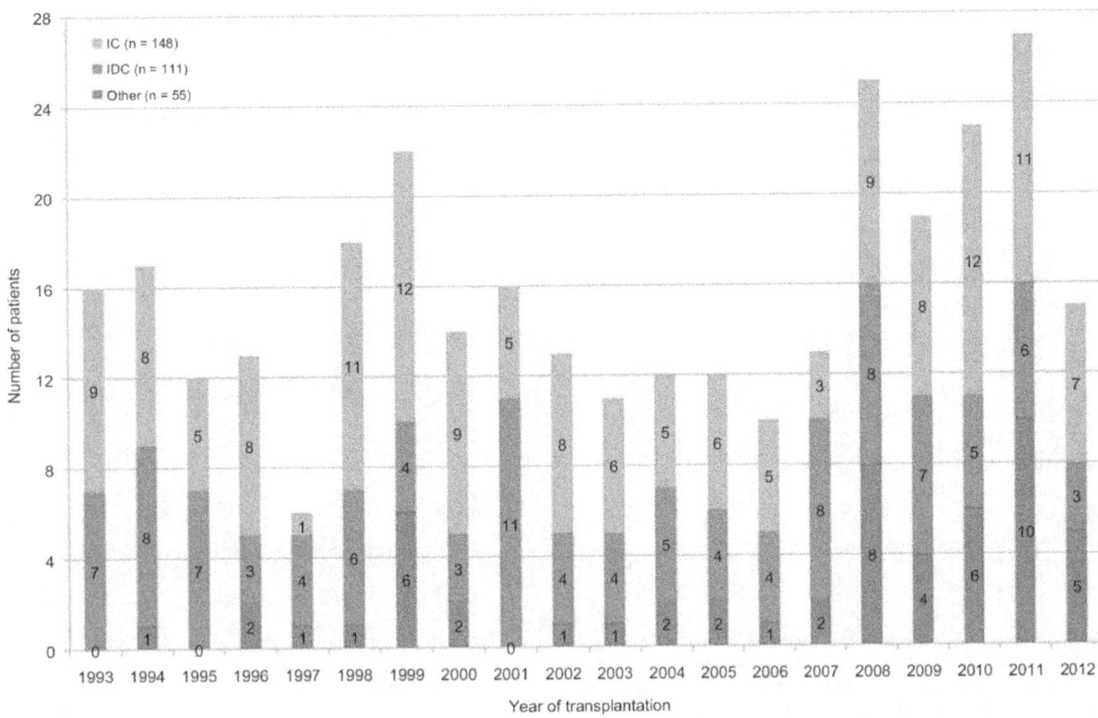

FIGURE 1. Bar graph showing the number of cardiac transplantation procedures done each year at Baylor University Medical Center 1993–2012 (through June 2012), and the 3 major reasons for the transplant (IC = ischemic cardiomyopathy [green]; IDC = idiopathic dilated cardiomyopathy [red], and other [blue]).

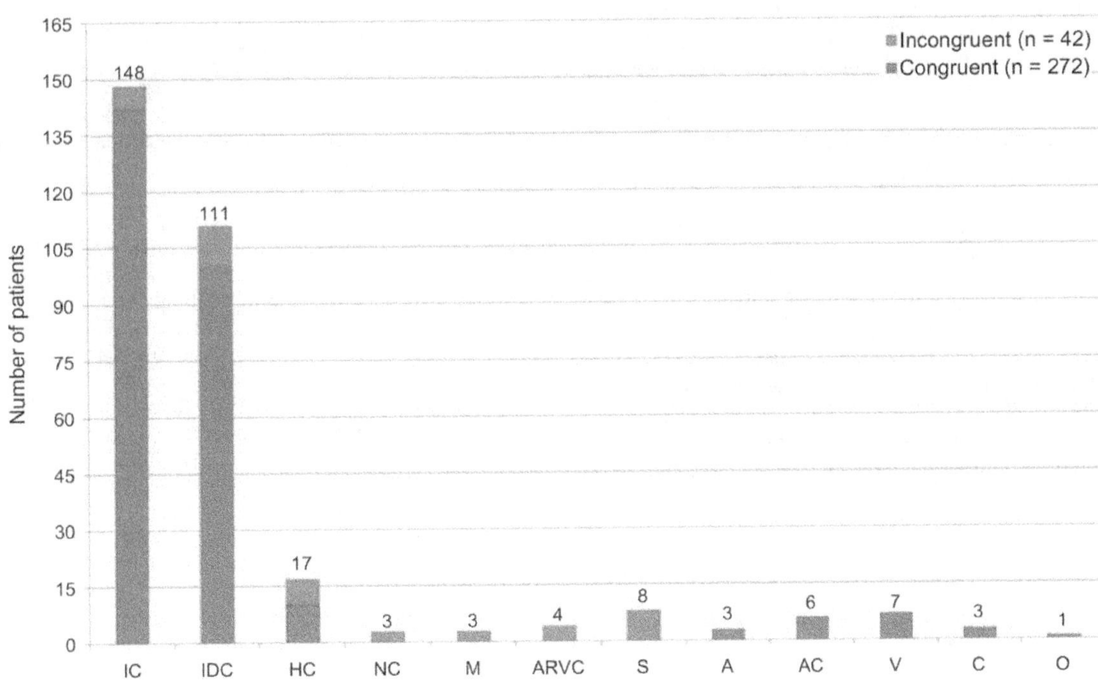

FIGURE 2. Bar graph showing frequency of congruence and incongruence among the various conditions cardiac transplantation among the 314 patients. IC = ischemic cardiomyopathy; IDC = idiopathic dilated cardiomyopathy; HC = hypertrophic cardiomyopathy; NC = non-compaction left ventricular cardiomyopathy; M = mononuclear myocarditis; ARVC = arrhythmogenic right ventricular cardiomyopathy; S = sarcoidosis; A = amyloidosis; V = valvular heart disease; C = congenital heart disease; O = other.

TABLE 1. Clinical and Morphologic Diagnoses of the 2 Basic Conditions Leading to Cardiac Transplantation: Ischemic Cardiomyopathy and Non-Ischemic Cardiomyopathy, and Incongruence Found Between the Diagnoses (Number of Patients in Each Category With the Clinical and Morphologic Diagnoses)

Condition	Clinical Diagnosis	Morphologic Diagnosis	Incongruence Between Clinical and Morphologic Diagnosis
Ischemic cardiomyopathy	142 (96%)	148	6 (4%)*
Non-ischemic cardiomyopathy	130 (78%)	166	36 (22%)
Idiopathic dilated	100	111	11†
Hypertrophic	10	17	7‡
Non-compaction left ventricular	0	3	3‡
Mononuclear myocarditis	0	3	3‡
Arrhythmogenic right ventricular	0	4	4‡
Cardiac sarcoidosis	0	8	8‡
Cardiac amyloidosis	3	3	0
Adriamycin cardiomyopathy	6	6	0
Valvular heart disease	7	7	0
Cyanotic congenital heart disease	3	3	0
Other	1	1	0
Total	272 (87%)	314	42 (13%)

*All 6 morphologically had normal or near normal coronary arteries.
†All 11 had severe narrowing of 1 or more epicardial coronary arteries by atherosclerotic plaques.
‡All 25 were diagnosed clinically as "non-ischemic cardiomyopathy."

The orifices of the right and left main coronary arteries in the aorta were carefully examined for proper location and degrees of narrowing, if any. Random cuts were made in the 4 major (right, left main, left anterior descending, and left circumflex) coronary arteries, and the arteries were probed (1.5 mm diameter probe) both anterograde and retrograde. The 2 coronary orifices in the aorta were probed to determine any resistance to movement of the probe. Additionally, all incisions into the major coronary arteries were carefully explored for atherosclerotic plaques and luminal narrowing.

Each of the 4 cardiac valves was examined for abnormality.

At least 6 sections of each heart were submitted for preparation of histology slides. They included at least 2 sections of the left ventricular free wall, 1 of ventricular septum, 1 of right ventricular free wall, and 1 each of the walls of left and right atria. If coronary artery bypass grafts were present, sections of them were also prepared. Both hematoxylin-eosin and Masson stains were prepared on all myocardial sections and Movat stains were prepared on all sections of coronary bypass conduits and/or native coronary arteries. If heavy calcific deposits were palpated in the epicardial coronary arteries or in other areas of the heart, usually a radiograph was made of the recipient heart.

The clinical, echocardiographic, hemodynamic, and operative records were sought from the patients' medical records and/or the BUMC Apollo cardiovascular database. Information regarding death of any patient was obtained from the medical records in deaths during hospitalization at the time of CT and from the Social Security Death Index for post-hospitalization deaths. Survival was assessed as March 31, 2013.

Means, standard deviations (SDs), and percentages were calculated to describe the study cohort. The Kaplan-Meier method was used to construct the survival curve for the whole population. The log-rank test statistic was computed to compare unadjusted survival curves between men and women.

The study was approved by the institutional review board at BUMC.

RESULTS

The main findings in the 314 patients are summarized in Tables 1 and 2. All patients at the time of CT were aged >18 years of age: 230 (73%) were men, and 84 (27%) were women. The patients included had CT only; there were no patients having heart/lung, heart/liver, or heart/bone marrow transplantation. Clinically, the patients were divided into 2 major groups: 1) *ischemic cardiomyopathy* (IC), 148 patients (47%); and 2) *non-ischemic cardiomyopathy* (N-IC), 166 patients (53%). The N-IC patients were subdivided into 11 groups, the 2 largest being IDC, 111 patients (66%), and HC, 17 patients (10%). The remaining 9 groups under N-IC consisted of 38 patients (23% of 166).

The frequency of congruity between the clinical and morphologic diagnoses is summarized in Table 1 and in Figure 2. Both the clinical and morphologic diagnoses were congruous in 272 (87%) of the 314 patients: in 142 (96%) of the 148 patients with IC and in 130 (78%) of the 166 patients with N-IC. Incongruity between the clinical and morphologic diagnoses was most glaring among the patients with HC (10 of 17 [59%]), non-compaction left ventricular cardiomyopathy (0 of 3); arrhythmogenic right ventricular cardiomyopathy (0 of 4), and cardiac sarcoidosis (0 of 8). Details of individual patients in the non-IC subgroups (excluding IDC) are tabulated in Tables 3–10.

Ischemic Cardiomyopathy

The 148 IC patients had hearts with dilated left ventricular cavities (>3.5 cm: range, 3.5–8.5 cm [mean 5.9]);

TABLE 2. Morphologic Findings in Patients Having Cardiac Transplantation, by Cardiac Condition (n = 314)

Variable	IC (n = 148)	IDC (n = 111)	HC (n = 17)	NCLVC (n = 3)	M (n = 3)	ARVC (n = 4)	S (n = 8)	A (n = 3)	AC (n = 6)	V (n = 7)	C (n = 3)	O (n = 1*)
Age (mean), yr												
Men	38–70 (58)	24–69 (51)	19–68 (51)	45	24, 56	21–44 (30)	50–54 (52)	57–61 (58)	30, 55	30–65 (50)	40	62
Women	30–66 (55)	26–67 (51)	35–56 (46)	36, 49	46	NA	50–59 (55)	NA	49–69 (62)	43–64 (56)	28,38	NA
Sex												
Male	129 (87%)	66 (59%)	13 (76%)	1 (33%)	2 (67%)	4 (100%)	3 (38%)	3 (100%)	2 (30%)	5 (71%)	1 (33%)	1 (100%)
Female	19 (13%)	45 (41%)	4 (24%)	2 (67%)	1 (33%)	0	5 (62%)	0	4 (60%)	2 (29%)	2 (67%)	0
Heart weight (mean), g												
Men	324–839 (531)	285–940 (544)	355–780 (547)	438	443, 545	314–686 (521)	440–604 (518)	420–550 (494)	366, 526	605–732 (651)	653	707
Women	255–726 (451)	232–660 (444)	220–424 (358)	380, 422	356	NA	371–562 (453)	NA	326–558 (446)	258–635 (388)	460,573	NA
Number of major coronary arteries narrowed >50% in cross-sectioned area												
0	0	100	13	3	2	4	7	1	5	5	3	1
1	25	5	3	0	1	0	0	2	1	0	0	0
2	30	6	0	0	0	0	1	0	0	1	0	0
3	51	0	1	0	0	0	0	0	0	0	0	0
4	42	0	0	0	0	0	0	0	0	1	0	0
LV cavity size (mean), cm	3.5–8.5 (5.9)	3–10 (6.3)	3.0–7.5 (5.5)	7.5–8 (7.5)	7–9 (8)	4.5–11 (6.6)	5–9 (6.3)	3.0–4.5 (3.8)	6–8 (6.7)	3.4–7.5 (5.4)	5.5–7 (6.1)	6
RV cavity size (mean), cm	1.0–5.0 (2.8)	0.7–9 (3.1)	1.0–4.5 (2.6)	2.5–4 (3.2)	2–2.5 (2.3)	3–6 (4.6)	2–9 (4.4)	3.0–4.0 (3.5)	2–3 (2.5)	2–5 (3.3)	3	5.5
Grossly visible LV scarring	147	5	13	1	3	1	8	0	0	5	2	1
Grossly visible foci of necrosis	2	0	0	0	0	0	0	0	0	1	0	0
Died postoperatively												
≤60 d	6	1	0	0	0	0	0	0	1	1	0	0
>60 d	25	20	3	0	1	0	1	1	0	0	0	1
Previous major cardiac operation												
Coronary artery bypass grafting	52	2	2	0	0	0	0	0	0	1	0	0

LVAD insertion	22	10	6	0	0	0	3	0	0	1	1	0
Valve operation	2[†]	1	0	0	0	0	0	0	0	7	3	0
Body mass index (kg/m^2)	n = 118	n = 86	n = 15	n = 3	n = 3	n = 4	n = 8	n = 3	n = 6	n = 6	n = 3	n = 1
<25.0	33 (28%)	33 (38%)	6 (40%)	2 (67%)	3 (100%)	2 (50%)	3 (38%)	1 (33%)	2 (33%)	2 (33%)	2 (66%)	0
≥25.0–30.0	62 (53%)	39 (45%)	7 (47%)	1 (33%)	0	2 (50%)	5 (62%)	0	2 (33%)	3 (50%)	1 (33%)	1 (100%)
>30.0–35.0	21 (18%)	12 (14%)	2 (13%)	0	0	0	0	2 (66%)	2 (33%)	1 (17%)	0	0
>35.0–40.0	2 (1%)	2 (2%)	0	0	0	0	0	0	0	0	0	0
>40.0	0	0	0	0	0	0	0	0	0	0	0	0

Abbreviations: A = cardiac amyloidosis, AC = Adriamycin cardiomyopathy, C = congenital heart disease, LV = left ventricular, LVAD = left ventricular assist device, M = myocarditis, NA = not applicable, O = other, RV = right ventricular, S = cardiac sarcoidosis, V = valvular heart disease.
*Previously reported.[48]
[†]Mitral valve repairs.

1 or more major epicardial coronary arteries narrowed >75% in cross-sectional area by atherosclerotic plaque; 1 or more grossly visible transmural (>50% of wall thickness) scars in the left ventricular free wall with or without similar scars in the ventricular septum and right ventricular free wall; normal or nearly normal cardiac valves; and absent inflammatory, giant, neoplastic cell or non-fibrous infiltrates (such as amyloid).[56] Additionally, the intramural coronary arteries were normal. Of the total 314 patients, 148 (47%) morphologically fulfilled these criteria. Of these 148 patients, 52 (35%) had had a coronary artery bypass grafting procedure previously and 22 (15%) had a left ventricular assist device. Of these 148 patients, 142 (96%) before CT were diagnosed as IC; the remaining 6 patients were diagnosed clinically as IDC because coronary angiograms, some performed several years earlier, had indicated no significant luminal narrowing, although all 6 had transmural left ventricular scars and severe (>75% cross-sectional area) narrowing of 1 or more major coronary arteries. Examples of IC are shown in Figures 3–13.

Idiopathic Dilated Cardiomyopathy

The 111 IDC patients had dilated left ventricular cavities (4.0–10.0 cm [mean 6.3]); normal or nearly normal cardiac valves; normal epicardium; no inflammatory, giant, neoplastic cells or non-fibrous interstitial infiltrates (such as amyloid) in the cardiac walls; and usually normal epicardial coronary arteries (Figures 14–17).[20,51,54,71] A few patients had some atherosclerotic plaques but the plaques had narrowed the lumen ≤50% in cross-sectional area in 1 or more of the 4 major epicardial coronary arteries. Eleven patients had narrowing of 1 or more major epicardial coronary arteries >75% in cross-sectional area by plaques, but none of them had grossly visible left ventricular or ventricular septal scars. These 11 patients do not fulfill our definition of IDC because of the coronary narrowing, but none of the 11 had 1 or more grossly visible left ventricular scars. In these patients the coronary angiogram appeared to simply underestimate the degree of coronary narrowing. Their lack of myocardial scarring prevents them from being placed in the IC group. It is likely that these 11 patients actually had IDC, but because they lived in a high-cholesterol environment (United States), their coronary arteries developed significant plaque.[55] Five patients with normal epicardial coronary arteries had grossly visible left ventricular free wall and/or ventricular septal scars. The 5 patients were diagnosed morphologically and clinically as IDC.[23]

Hypertrophic Cardiomyopathy

The 17 HC patients (Table 3) had either normal sized (<4 cm) (5 patients) or dilated (>4 cm) (12 patients) left ventricular cavities and past clinical evidence of non-dilated left ventricular cavities (Figures 18–21).[5,13,21,24,33,36,37,42,49,61] Transmural scarring involved the ventricular septum and left ventricular free walls in 13 patients (76%) with or without grossly visible scarring of portions of the right ventricular free wall. The ventricular septum at sometime in the past or presently was thicker than the left ventricular free wall; typical myofiber disorganization was present in the ventricular septum, and the intramural coronary arteries on histologic study were abnormal in all 13 patients with ventricular wall scarring.[35] None of the 17 HC patients had clinical or hemodynamic evidence of left

TABLE 3. Pertinent Data in 17 Patients Having Cardiac Transplantation for Hypertrophic Cardiomyopathy

Patient	Age at CT (yr)	Sex	Clinical Diagnosis	BMI (kg/m^2)	Lowest LVEF (%)	Year of CT	HW (g)	LV Diameter (cm)	Narrowed Coronary Arteries	Grossly Visible LV Scar*	LVAD
1	35	F	Non-IC	26.9	15	2010	367	5.0	0	+	+
2	43	F	HC	–	60	1994	220	3.7	0	+	0
3	50	F	HC	21.7	–	1999	422	3.7	0	+	0
4	56	F	Non-IC	18.4	10	2012	424	7.0	0	+	0
5	19	M	HC	16.8	58	1999	451	3.5	0	0	0
6	35	M	HC	35.5	5	2011	705	6.0	0	+	+
7	41	M	HC	27.6	27	2009	566	6.5	0	+	0
8	45	M	Non-IC	25.7	65	2010	411	3.0	0	0	0
9	48	M	Non-IC	30.6	25	2012	442	4.5	+	+	+
10	50	M	HC	–	10	1999	674	7.5	0	0	0
11	54	M	Non-IC	28.7	20	1997	637	5.5	0	+	0
12	55	M	IC†	27.3	25	1998	506	4.5	+	+	+
13	58	M	HC	–	15	1996	355	6.9	+	+	0
14	58	M	HC & IC†	29.4	35	1999	374	7.0	+	+	+
15	63	M	HC	21.7	–	2011	625	7.4	0	0	0
16	68	M	Non-IC	32.4	10	2009	780	7.5	0	+	+
17	68	M	HC	25.4	35	2010	580	3.5	0	+	0

Abbreviations: See previous tables. BMI = body mass index, CT = cardiac transplantation, HW = heart weight, LVEF = left ventricular ejection fraction.

*Excludes papillary muscles.

†Each also had coronary artery bypass grafting.

TABLE 4. Pertinent Data in 3 Patients Having Cardiac Transplantation for Non-Compaction Left Ventricular Cardiomyopathy*

Patient	Age at CT (yr)	Sex	Clinical Diagnosis	BMI (kg/m^2)	Lowest LVEF (%)	Year of CT	HW (g)	Diameter (cm)		LV Scar
								LV	RV	
1	36	F	Non-IC	22.6	15	2008	422	7.0	4.0	0
2	49	F	Non-IC	22.5	5	2011	380	7.5	3.0	0
3	45	M	Non-IC	26.1	10	2011	438	8.0	2.5	+

*None had narrowed coronary arteries or coronary artery bypass grafting or a left ventricular assist device.

TABLE 5. Pertinent Data in 3 Patients Having Cardiac Transplantation for Active or Healed Mononuclear Myocarditis*

Patient	Age at CT (yr)	Sex	Clinical Diagnosis	BMI (kg/m^2)	Lowest LVEF (%)	Year of CT	HW (g)	Diameter (cm)		Narrowed Coronary Arteries	LV Scar
								LV	RV		
1	46	F	Non-IC	24.6	20	2008	356	7.0	2.5	0	+
2	24	M	Non-IC	19.8	5	2011	545	9.0	2.0	0	+
3	56	M	IC	18.4	10	2008	443	8.0	2.5	+	+

Abbreviations: See previous tables.

*None had coronary artery bypass grafting or a left ventricular assist device.

TABLE 6. Pertinent Data in 4 Men Having Cardiac Transplantation for Arrhythmogenic Right Ventricular Cardiomyopathy*

Patient	Age at CT (yr)	Clinical Diagnosis	BMI (kg/m^2)	Lowest LVEF (%)	Year of CT	HW (g)	Diameter (cm) LV	Diameter (cm) RV	LV Scar	RV Scar
1	21	Non-IC	26.5	10	2012	489	4.5	6	0	+
2	26	Non-IC	24.8	10	2009	594	6.0	5.5	0	+
3	30	Non-IC	27.6	10	2008	686	11.0	3.0	+	+
4	44	Non-IC	22.5	25	2008	314	5.0	4.0	0	+

Abbreviations: See previous tables.
*None had narrowed coronary arteries or coronary artery bypass grafting or a left ventricular assist device.

TABLE 7. Pertinent Data in 8 Patients Having Cardiac Transplantation for Cardiac Sarcoidosis*

Patient	Age at CT (yr)	Sex	Clinical Diagnosis	BMI (kg/m^2)	Lowest LVEF (%)	Year of CT	HW (g)	Diameter (cm) LV	Diameter (cm) RV	Narrowed Coronary Arteries	LV Scar	LVAD
1	50	F	Non-IC	27.0	20	2012	442	7.5	4.0	0	+	0
2	52	F	Non-IC	28.7	20	2010	441	5.5	2.0	0	+	0
3	56	F	Non-IC	25.7	15	2009	447	5.5	3.5	0	+	0
4	58	F	Non-IC	26.4	20	2012	562	5.0	2.5	0	+	0
5	59	F	Non-IC	20.8	20	2006	371	5.0	7.5	+	+	+
6	50	M	Non-IC†	24.7	10	2005	604	7.0	2.5	0	+	+
7	52	M	Non-IC†	21.6	20	2005	440	—	—	0	+	+
8	54	M	Non-IC†	27.5	10	1999	511	9.0	9.0	0	+	0

Abbreviations: See previous tables.
*None had coronary artery bypass grafting.
†Diagnosis of cardiac sarcoid made from histologic study of "left ventricular core" excised for insertion of a left ventricular assist device.

TABLE 8. Pertinent Data in 3 Men Having Cardiac Transplantation for Cardiac Amyloidosis*

Patient	Age at CT (yr)	Clinical Diagnosis	BMI (kg/m^2)	Lowest LVEF (%)	Year of CT	HW (g)	Diameter (cm) LV	Diameter (cm) RV	Narrowed Coronary Arteries	LV Scar
1	57	Amyloidosis	20.2	30	2004	550	4.0	3.5	0	0
2	57	Amyloidosis	32.0	20	2010	420	4.5	3.0	+†	0
3	61	Amyloidosis	30.6	46	2008	513	3.0	4.0	+	0

Abbreviations: See previous tables.
*None had coronary artery bypass grafting or a left ventricular assist device.
†Stent to the right coronary artery in October 2009.

TABLE 9. Pertinent Data in 6 Patients Having Cardiac Transplantation for Adriamycin Cardiomyopathy*

Patient	Age at CT (yr)	Sex	Clinical Diagnosis	BMI (kg/m^2)	Lowest LVEF (%)	Year of CT	HW (g)	Diameter (cm) LV	Diameter (cm) RV	Narrowed Coronary Arteries	LV Scar
1	49	F	AC	—	—	2007	404	8.0	2.5	0	0
2	64	F	AC	24.6	10	2004	326	6.5	3.0	+	0
3	65	F	AC	25.7	—	2011	558	6.5	2.5	0	0
4	69	F	AC	34.3	25	2011	497	6.0	3.0	0	0
5	30	M	AC	25.9	35	2008	366	7.0	2.0	0	0
6	55	M	AC	31.6	15	2011	526	6.0	2.2	0	0

Abbreviations: See previous tables. AC = Adriamycin cardiomyopathy.
*None had coronary artery bypass grafting or a left ventricular assist device.

TABLE 10. Pertinent Data in 6 Patients Having Cardiac Transplantation for Valvular Disease

Patient	Age at CT (yr)	Sex	Clinical Valve Dysfunction	Valve Replaced	Interval (yr) AVR → CT	BMI (kg/m^2)	Lowest LVEF (%)	Year of CT	HW (g)	Diameter (cm) LV	Diameter (cm) RV	Narrowed Coronary Arteries	LV Scar	CABG	LVAD
1	30	M	AS (BAV)	Aortic	8	25	10	1999	650	5.5	2.8	0	+	0	0
2	47	M	AS (BAV)	Aortic*	–	–	–	1996	605	–	–	0	+	0	0
3	56	M	AS (BAV)	Aortic	4.7	28.3	5	2007	732	6.0	4.0	0	0	0	+
4	65	M	AS (BAV)	Aortic	5.2	18.4	20	2003	616	7.5	3.0	+	+	+[†]	0
5	43	F	AR[‡], MR[‡]	Aortic, mitral	–	–	30	2002	258	3.4	2.0	0	0	0	0
6	64	F	MS, MR	Mitral (x2)	–	31.8	25	2010	635	5.5	5.0	0	+	0	0
7	60	F	MR[‡]	0[§]	–	27.1	35	2011	271	4.5	3.0	+	+	0	0

Abbreviations: See previous tables. AR = aortic regurgitation, AS = aortic stenosis, AVR = aortic valve replacement, BAV = bicuspid aortic valve, CABG = coronary artery bypass grafting, MR = mitral regurgitation, MS = mitral stenosis.

*Procedure at another hospital (non-BUMC).

[†]CABG done 6 yr before AVR.

[‡]Radiation therapy for Hodgkin disease.

[§]Mitral valve repair twice.

TABLE 11. Pertinent Data in 3 Patients Having Cardiac Transplantation for Congenital Heart Disease*

Patient	Age at CT (yr)	Sex	Clinical Diagnosis	BMI (kg/m^2)	Lowest LVEF (%)	Year of CT	HW (g)	LV Diameter (cm)	LV Scar	LVAD
1	28	F	TGA	19.4	10	2008	460	7.0	+	0
2	38	F	RV hypoplasia	19.6	10	2011	573	5.9	0	+
3	40	M	T of F	27.3	10	2010	653	5.5	+	0

Abbreviations: See previous tables. TGA = transposition of great arteries, T of F = tetralogy of Fallot.

*None had narrowed coronary arteries or coronary artery bypass grafting.

TABLE 12. Previously Reported Data on Congruity vs Incongruity Among 296 Patients Having Cardiac Transplantation (From Luk et al[29])

Cardiac Condition	Clinical Diagnosis (No.)	Morphologic Diagnosis (No.)
Ischemic cardiomyopathy	140	144
Idiopathic dilated cardiomyopathy	96	54
Hypertrophic cardiomyopathy	15	17
Myocarditis	8*	25†
Valvular "cardiomyopathy"	6	5
Infiltrative	5‡	4‡
Congenital	18	18
Doxorubicin	6	6
Becker's muscular dystrophy	1	1
Fabry's	1	2
Arrhythmogenic RV cardiomyopathy	0	12
Cardiac sarcoid	0	6
Mitochondrial myopathy	0	1
Iron cardiomyopathy	0	1
TOTAL	296	296

Modified and reprinted with permission from Elsevier.[29]
*"Viral myocarditis" in 6, hypersensitive/eosinophilic in 2.
†"Viral myocarditis" in 20, hypersensitive/eosinophilic in 4, and giant cell in 1.
‡Amyloid in 3.

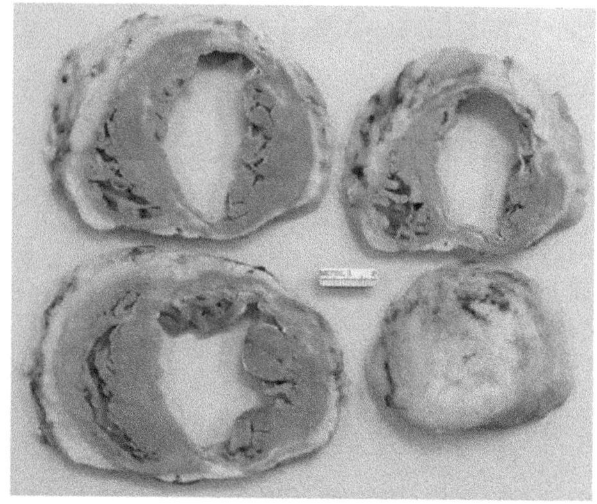

FIGURE 4. Ischemic cardiomyopathy. Photographs of sections of the cardiac ventricles caudal to the mitral valve in a 54-year-old woman who had an acute myocardial infarction when she was 33 years of age and underwent percutaneous coronary intervention at that time. At age 39 years, she had another acute myocardial infarct and underwent coronary artery bypass grafting. Cardiac catheterization 2 years later disclosed that all bypass conduits were closed. At age 42 years, she had another percutaneous coronary intervention. The left ventricular ejection fraction shortly before cardiac transplantation was 10%. These views show a healed myocardial infarct in the anterior wall of left ventricle and another in the posterior wall opposite one another. The quantity of subepicardial adipose tissue is clearly increased. The left ventricular cavity is quite dilated.

ventricular outflow obstruction just prior to CT. Four (24%) of the 17 patients also had severe narrowing of 1 or more epicardial coronary arteries, and all 4 had grossly visible left ventricular and ventricular septal scars. Nine other HC patients had left ventricular or ventricular septal scar without narrowing of the epicardial coronary arteries. The clinical diagnosis in 6 of the 17 patients was "non-IC," in 1 patient IC, and in 1 patient both HC and IC. Each of the latter 2 patients had coronary bypass grafting in the remote past before CT. Thus, the clinical and morphologic diagnosis were incongruous in 7 (41%) of these 17 patients.

Non-Compaction Left Ventricular Cardiomyopathy

Three patients had NCLVC (Table 4, Figures 22 and 23). Each had very dilated ventricular cavities with the non-compacted portion of left ventricular free wall in 1 or

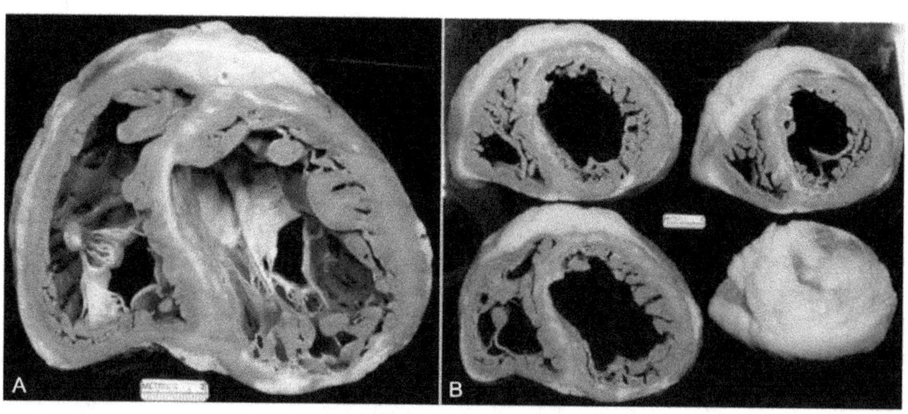

FIGURE 3. Ischemic cardiomyopathy. The heart in a 48-year-old man who had had at least 2 acute myocardial infarcts in the past. One is located posteriorly and the other anteriorly. The left ventricular ejection fraction was about 5%. (a) View of the heart showing both tricuspid and mitral valves. Both ventricles are greatly dilated. The 2 healed myocardial infarcts are clearly seen, and they are opposite one another. The left ventricular cavity measures up to 8 cm. (b) Views of the cardiac ventricles caudal to the picture shown on the left. These views show both the anterior and posterior scars are present from apex to base.

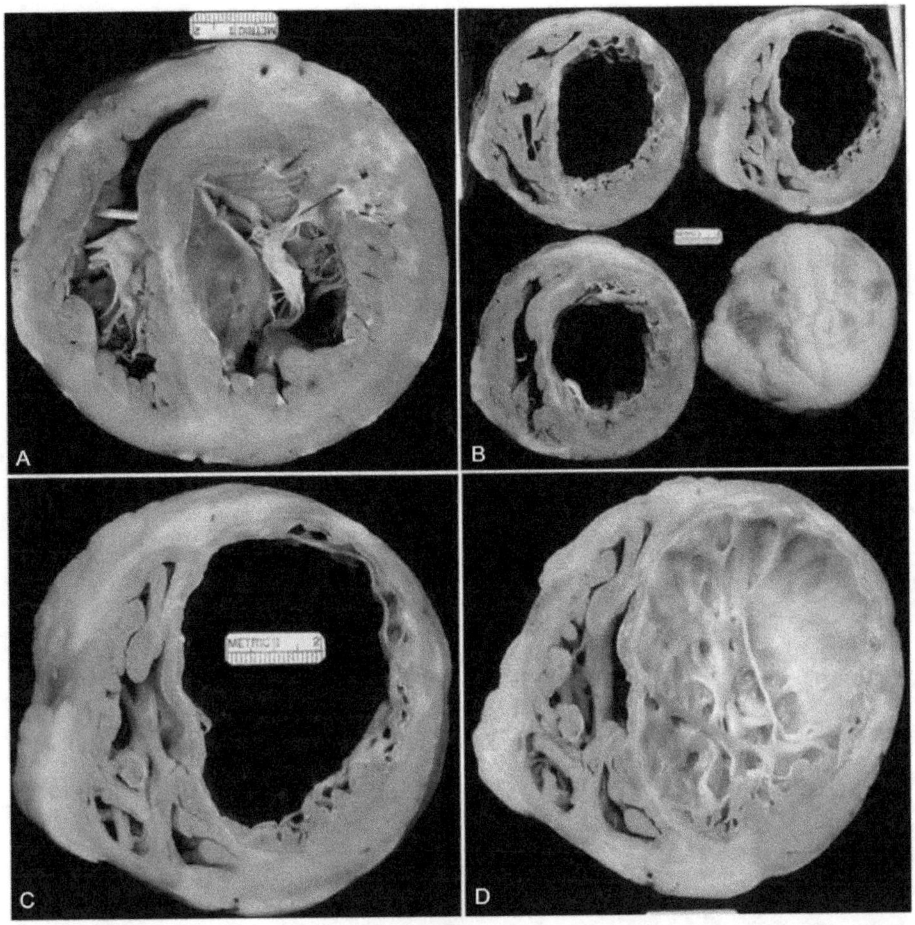

FIGURE 5. Ischemic cardiomyopathy. Heart in a 56-year-old man who had a large anterior wall acute myocardial infarct at age 46 years. Subsequently, a stent was inserted into the left anterior descending and left circumflex coronary arteries. His left ventricular ejection fraction shortly before cardiac transplantation was 10%. (a) View of the ventricular cavities at the base showing both tricuspid and mitral valves. A scar is present in the central portion of the ventricular septum and in the anterior left ventricular free wall. (b) Views of the cardiac ventricles caudal to the base showing a huge amount of scaring in the anterior wall of left ventricle with scaring of the entire ventricular septum. Less than half of the left ventricular free wall is devoid of scars. (c) A close-up view of a portion of ventricular walls showing full thickness scarring of the ventricular septum and anterior lateral left ventricular free wall. (d) View of the interior of the left ventricular apex showing the extensive septal and free wall left ventricular scaring.

more areas being >2 times the thickness of the underlying compacted portion of the wall and unassociated with narrowing of the epicardial coronary arteries.[11,45,68] Clinically, each of the 3 patients were diagnosed as "non-IC." One of the 3 patients had a small grossly visible left ventricular scar.

Mononuclear Myocarditis

Three patients had active or healed mononuclear myocarditis (Table 5, Figures 24 and 25). The key identifying mark of this condition was focal subepicardial left ventricular wall lesions.[19,25,58,60,62,65] Each had mononuclear -cell infiltrates–mainly lymphocytes–in the left ventricular free wall or subepicardial scars with or without mononuclear-cell infiltrates and without granulomas. The hearts were of increased weight (>350 g in women; >400 g in men), and the ventricular cavities were very dilated. One of the 3 patients had significant narrowing by atherosclerotic plaque of 1 or more epicardial coronary arteries. This patient clinically was diagnosed as IC, the other 2 as "non-IC."

Arrhythmogenic Right Ventricular Cardiomyopathy

Four patients had ARVC; pertinent findings for them are summarized in Table 6 and illustrated in Figure 26.[2,4,8,12,14,28,31,32,46,64,66,70,72,73] All 4 during life were diagnosed as "non-IC." All 4 had thinning of the right ventricular free wall with replacement of the myocardial wall focally by adipose tissue and/or scar tissue without focal thinning (except in 1 patient) of the left ventricular free wall. All 4 had very dilated ventricular chambers. Before CT all 4 had documented runs of ventricular tachycardia. Three had other family members with a similar cardiac disease.

Cardiac Sarcoidosis

Pertinent findings in the 8 cardiac sarcoidosis patients are summarized in Table 7 and illustrated in Figure 27.[9,15,43,47,52,62,67] All 8 were diagnosed clinically as "non-IC." Six had focal but extensive scars in the free walls of both right and left ventricles and in the ventricular septum

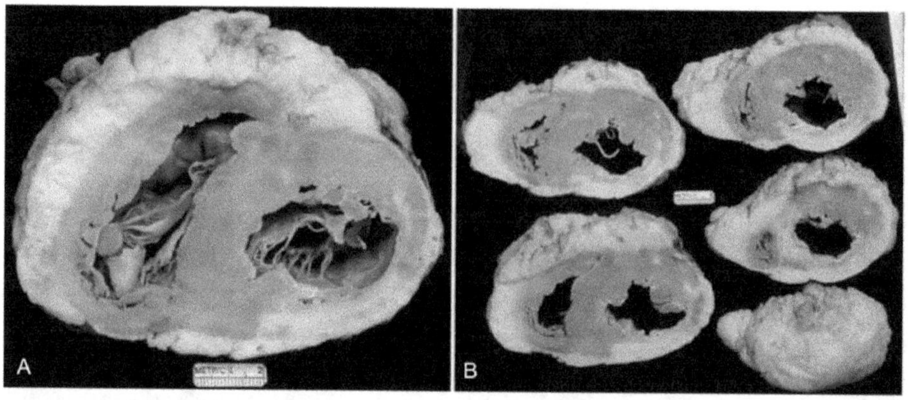

FIGURE 6. Ischemic cardiomyopathy. Heart in a 56-year-old man who at age 49 years had an acute myocardial infarction, and percutaneous coronary intervention with multiple stents was performed. Six months later he underwent coronary artery bypass grafting. Heart failure gradually progressed thereafter such that the left ventricular ejection fraction fell to 25%. (a) View of the basal portion of the heart exposing both tricuspid and mitral valves. The posterior wall of left ventricular is transmurally scarred resulting in the ventricular septum's being thicker than the left ventricular free wall. The quantity of subepicardial adipose tissue is enormous, such that the heart floated in a container of formaldehyde. (b) Views of the ventricles more caudally showing that the posterior wall infarct extends from apex to base.

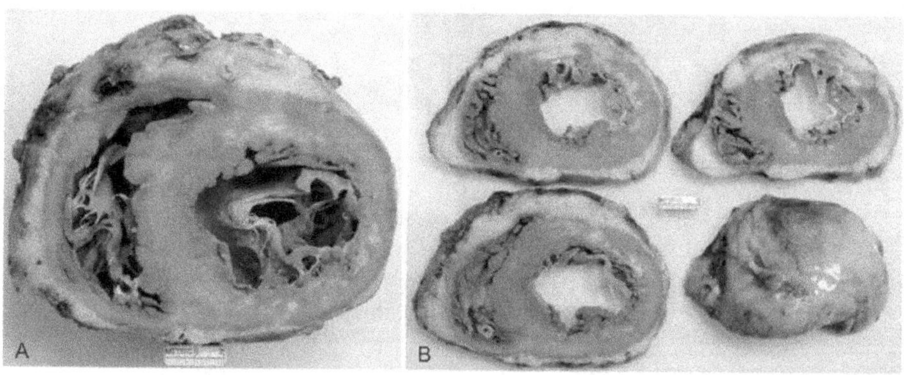

FIGURE 7. Ischemic cardiomyopathy. Views of the heart showing a transmural left ventricular scar from apex to base and a lateral and posterior walls scar which is probably not transmural in a 57-year-old man who had an acute myocardial infarct at age 48 years followed later by a coronary bypass grafting. Heart failure gradually progressed through the years, and his lowest left ventricular ejection fraction was 30%. (a) View of the base of the heart exposing both tricuspid and mitral valves. There is scarring in the anterior wall and in the posterior lateral wall. The lateral wall is much thinner than the ventricular septum. (b) Views of the ventricles more caudally showing extensive transmural anterior wall scarring. The quantity of subepicardial adipose tissue is increased.

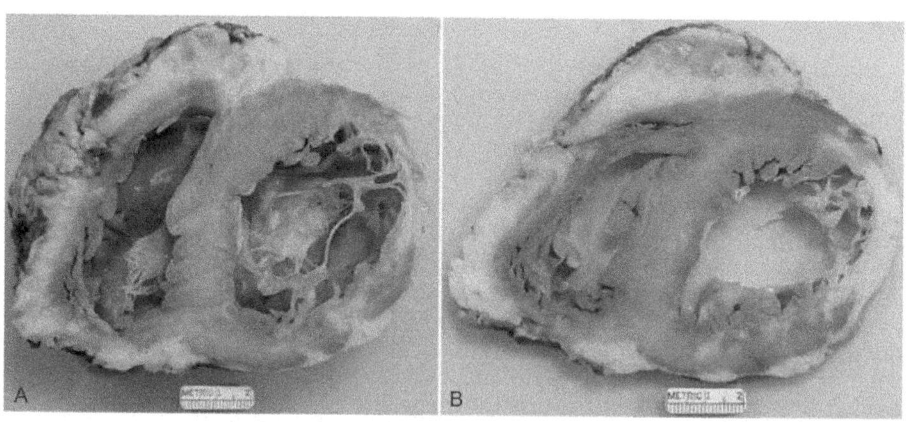

FIGURE 8. Ischemic cardiomyopathy. Heart in a 58-year-old man who had an acute myocardial infarct at age 29 years. A sibling and a parent had had myocardial infarcts at age 42 years. He clearly had heterozygous familial hypercholesterolemia. At age 30 years, he had coronary bypass grafting. His lowest left ventricular ejection fraction was 20%. (a) View of the basal portion of the heart exposing both tricuspid and mitral valves. The anterolateral wall is transmurally scarred such that the ventricular septum is thicker than the left ventricular free wall. (b) A more caudal view of the left ventricular wall showing the severe degree of scarring in the lateral wall with lesser degrees of scarring in the anterior and posterior walls. The quantity of subepicardial adipose tissue is increased.

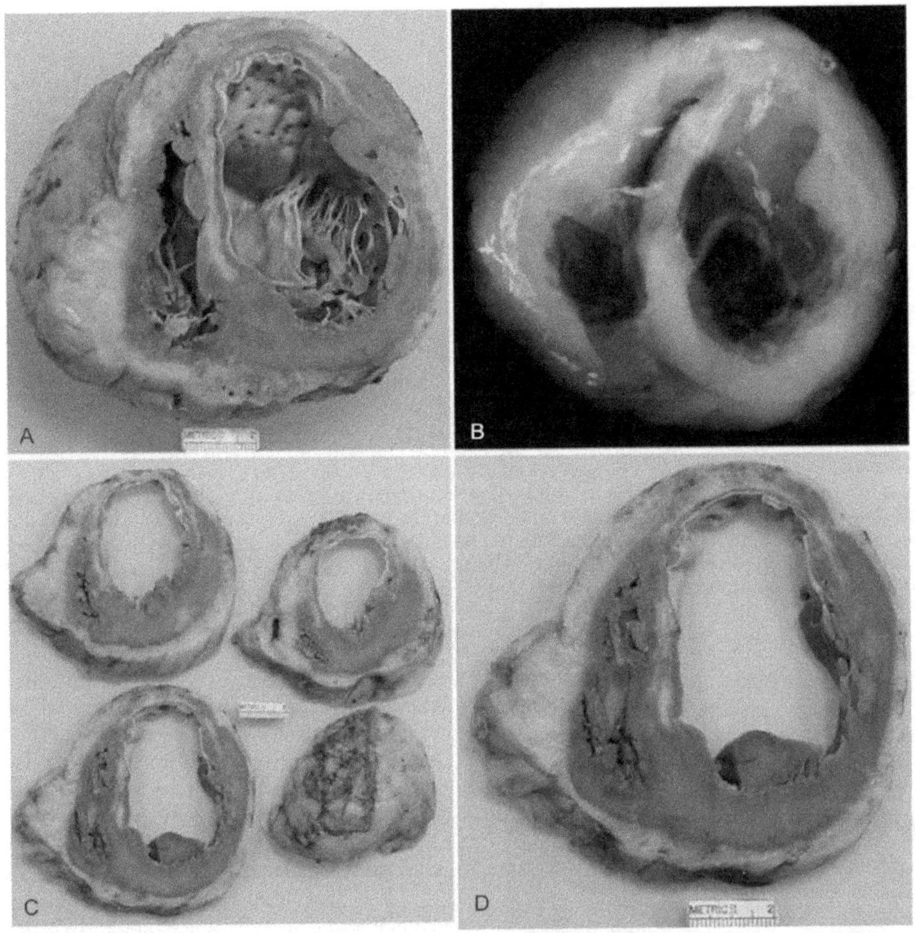

FIGURE 9. Ischemic cardiomyopathy. Heart in a 63-year-old man who had an acute myocardial infarct when he was 51 years of age. Subsequently, he underwent coronary artery bypass grafting. Percutaneous coronary intervention followed the bypass operation, and at age 58 years an implantable cardioverter defibrillator was inserted. Not long before cardiac transplantation his ejection fraction was 15%. At age 61 years, he had a stroke, and also during that year he underwent bilateral iliac stent implantation. (a) View of the basal portion of the heart exposing both tricuspid and mitral valves. Nearly the entire septum is scarred as is the anterior left ventricular free wall. The left ventricular cavity is greatly dilated. The quantity of subepicardial adipose tissue is considerably increased. (b) Radiograph of the basal portion of the heart showing a metallic stent in the right coronary artery with considerable scarring of the right and left anterior descending coronary arteries. (c) These more basal portions of the ventricular wall show that the large infarct extends to the cardiac apex. (d) View of 1 of the slices of left ventricular free wall showing marked thinning due to scar of the anterior wall.

without associated narrowing of the epicardial coronary arteries (except for 1 patient), and the scarring tended to be subepicardial. The ventricular chambers were very dilated in all 8 patients. Non-caseating giant cell granulomas were present in the ventricular walls in 7 of the 8 patients. In 1 patient the typical "hard" granulomas were present in the portion of left ventricular free wall excised to insert a left ventricular assist device but not in the recipient heart sometime later. Another patient had right and left ventricular free wall and ventricular septal scarring typical of cardiac sarcoidosis but no granulomas were found in the histologic sections of left ventricular free wall. This case we believe is an example of "burnt out" sarcoidosis.[43]

Cardiac Amyloidosis

Pertinent findings in the 3 cardiac amyloidosis patients are summarized in Table 8, and the hearts are illustrated in Figure 28.[7,10,16–18,40,53,69] The clinical and morphologic diagnoses were congruous in all 3 patients. The ventricular cavities were either not dilated or dilated to a small degree. The patients had firm—actually rubbery—myocardium, no grossly visible focal myocardial lesions but focal endocardial lesions in either the right atrium or left atrium or both and in the tricuspid valve leaflets. The presence of amyloid was confirmed by Congo-red stains of sections of the heart. Two of the 3 patients had narrowing >75% in cross-sectional area by atherosclerotic plaque, but none had grossly visible ventricular wall scars.

Adriamycin Cardiomyopathy

Pertinent findings in the 6 patients with Adriamycin cardiomyopathy are summarized in Table 9 and illustrated in Figure 29.[22,26,27,41,44] The clinical and morphologic diagnoses were congruous in each. All 6 had severely dilated ventricular chambers. All had received Adriamycin for cancer treatment.

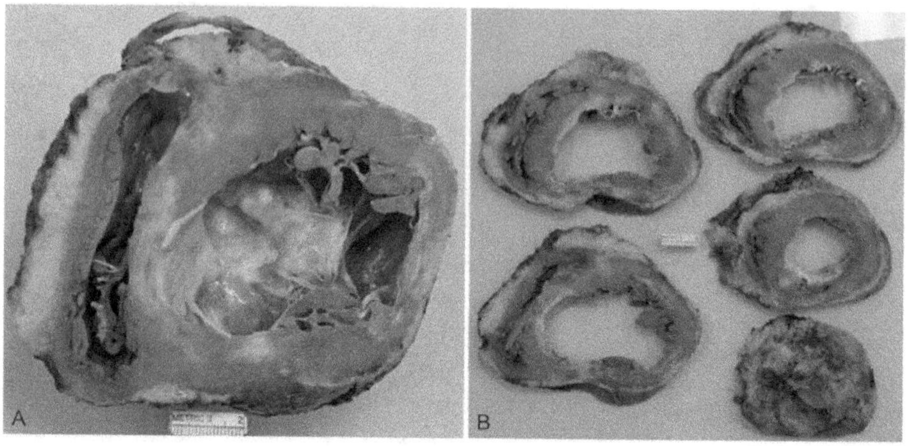

FIGURE 10. Ischemic cardiomyopathy. Heart in a 61-year-old man who had a acute myocardial infarct at age 53 years followed by a coronary artery bypass grafting. By age 59 years, his left ventricular ejection fraction was as low as 15%. An intracardiac defibrillator had been inserted also at age 54 years. (a) View of the basal portion of the heart showing a portion of tricuspid valve and a good bit of the anterior mitral leaflet. A large transmural scar is present in the lateral wall between the 2 left ventricular papillary muscles and in the ventricular septum in apposition to the lateral wall infarct. The left ventricular cavity is greatly dilated. (b) View of the more caudal portions of the ventricular wall again showing the 2 infarcts extending almost to the apex of the heart.

Valvular Heart Disease

Pertinent findings in the 7 patients with valvular heart disease are summarized in Table 10.[39,50,57] Four had aortic valve stenosis initially and repeated valve replacements; 1 had mitral valve replacements for mitral stenosis in 1 and for pure mitral regurgitation in the other. The latter patient also had severe tricuspid valve regurgitation, which had not been approached at a previous operation. The clinical and morphologic diagnoses were congruous in all 7 patients.

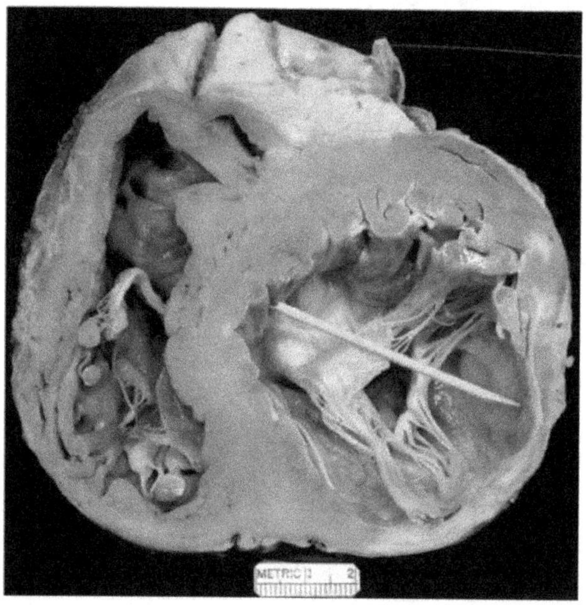

FIGURE 11. Ischemic cardiomyopathy. Heart in a 67-year-old man who had a large acute myocardial infarction at age 53 followed by coronary artery bypass grafting. At age 60, he had another bypass grafting operation. Heart failure progressed and was accompanied by several mitral regurgitation. His ejection fraction not long before cardiac transplantation was 10%. The view of the heart shows its basal portion exposing both mitral and tricuspid valves. The posterior and lateral walls of the heart are extremely thin from the extensive scarring. The posteromedial papillary muscle is flattened from the scarring and the anterolateral 1 is atrophied. The ventricular septum as a consequence is much thicker than the left ventricular free wall.

Cyanotic Congenital Heart Disease

Pertinent findings in the 3 patients with cyanotic congenital heart disease are summarized in Table 11.[38,63] One had complex complete transposition of the great arteries, 1 severe right ventricular hypoplasia, and 1 tetralogy of Fallot. All 3 had had more than 1 previous cardiac operation. The clinical and morphologic diagnosis were congruous in all 3.

Other

One patient had CT for ventricular septal defect resulting from a stab wound to the heart many years earlier. Details of this patient are described elsewhere.[48]

Outcomes

The survival probabilities for all 257 patients are shown in Figure 30. Of the 257 (of 314) patients in whom survival data are available, 66 (26%) have died: 8 (12%) within 60 days of CT and 58 (88%) at later periods. The log-rank test show no significant survival differences between men and women (log-rank = 0.479, p value = 0.4926) (Figure 30).

DISCUSSION

The present study serves 2 major functions: 1) it illustrates by gross photographs of the hearts the variability that occurs morphologically in each of the etiologic categories, and 2) it determines the frequency among the 314 patients of discrepancies between the clinical and morphologic diagnoses. Just like clinical presentations and courses are quite variable among patients with various types of cardiac diseases, the morphologic features in each type of cardiac

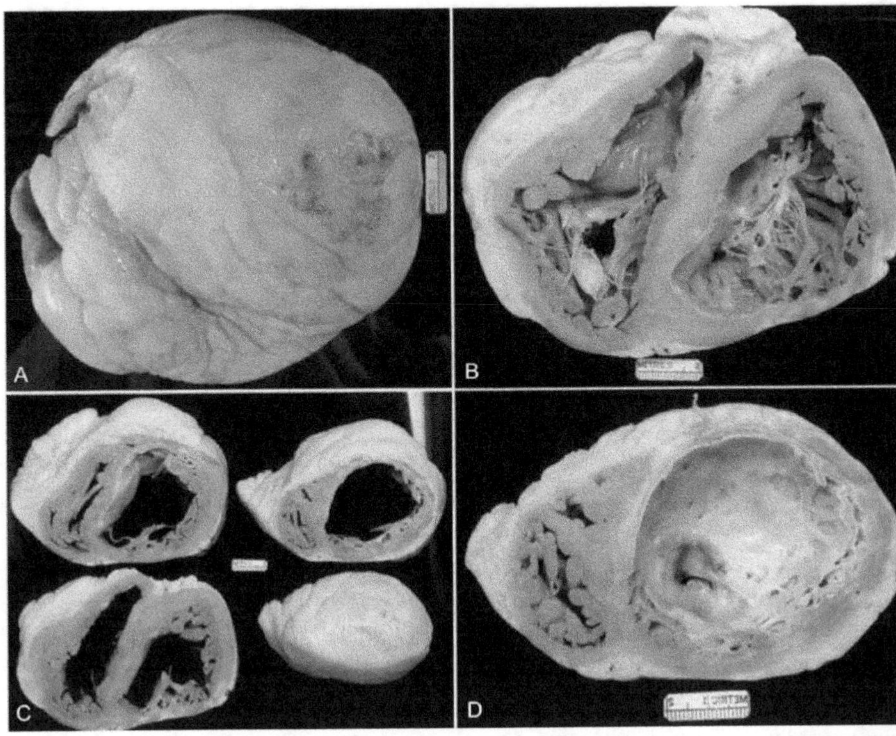

FIGURE 12. Ischemic cardiomyopathy. Heart in a 67-year-old man who had a large anterior wall infarct and another posterior wall infarct in the distant past. The exact dates of the infarcts are unclear, but radiograph of the excised heart showed calcium in the wall of the apex of the left ventricle indicating that the infarct was probably at least 10 years earlier. Heart failure had been a problem for many years. The left ventricular ejection fraction not long before cardiac transplantation was as low as 5%. (a) View of the exterior of the heart showing that most of the myocardial walls are covered by adipose tissue. (b) View of the base of the heart exposing both tricuspid and mitral valves. The posterior left ventricular free wall is thinned by scar tissue. (c) Views of the ventricles more caudally now showing both anterior and posterior wall infarcts. (d) View of the apex showing scarring in probably 300° of the 360° left ventricular wall. The heart contained so much adipose tissue that it floated in formaldehyde.

disease are also quite variable. To properly illustrate that variability a number of photographs of recipient hearts are presented.

As part of the second purpose of this report, we determined the frequency of congruity or incongruity between the clinical and morphologic diagnoses among the 314 patients. As shown in Table 1, most (96%) of the patients with IC at morphologic study had been diagnosed with that condition clinically. The discrepancy occurred when 6 patients with IC anatomically had insignificant coronary narrowing by angiography before CT, but nevertheless severe narrowing of 1 or more major epicardial coronary arteries morphologically and extensive left ventricular wall scarring. We defined IC as the presence of severe

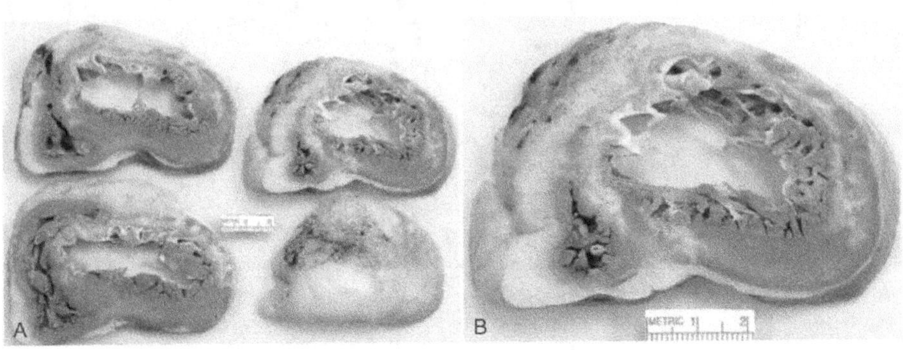

FIGURE 13. Ischemic cardiomyopathy. Heart in a 69-year-old man who had a large myocardial infarct, involving the anterior, septal, and lateral walls of the left ventricle only 4 months earlier with severe heart failure thereafter. (a) Sections of the ventricular walls caudal to the atrioventricular valves show a healed septal, anterior, and lateral wall infarct from apex to base. (b) A close-up of 1 of the slices showing the extensive scarring.

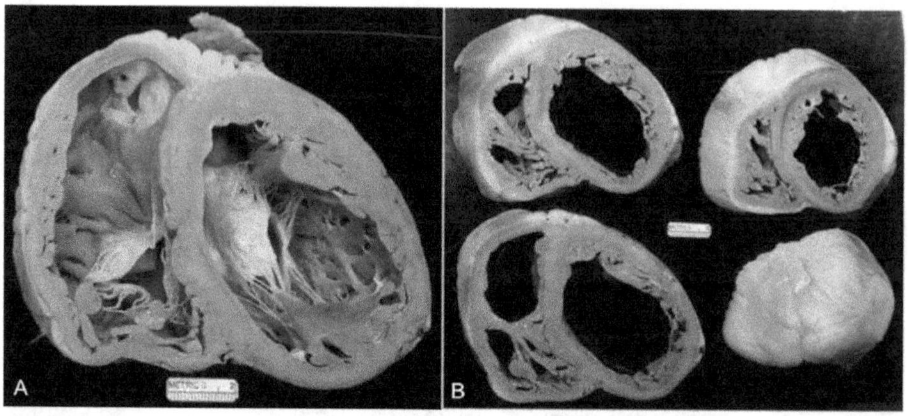

FIGURE 14. Idiopathic dilated cardiomyopathy. Heart of a 68-year-old man who had had evidence of heart failure since age 54 years. He was known to have severe hypothyroidism and was treated appropriately. He had never had chest pain. He did however have evidence of chronic obstructive lung disease and at 1 time was a habitual alcoholic. He also was known to have a fatty liver. The lowest left ventricular ejection fraction before transplantation was 5%. (a) View of the cardiac ventricles at the base exposing the tricuspid, mitral, and pulmonic valves. Both ventricular cavities are enormously dilated, and the walls of the left ventricle, ventricular septum, and right ventricle are free of foci of fibrosis and necrosis. (b) Views of the ventricles caudal to the atrioventricular valves. The moderator band is prominent in the right ventricle. The right coronary artery wall was quite calcified, and the lumen was quite narrowed. Nevertheless, the patient was classified as having idiopathic dilated cardiomyopathy because there were no lesions in the myocardial walls. It appears that this happened to be a patient who had both a narrowed coronary artery and idiopathic dilated cardiomyopathy.

(>75% in cross-sectional area) coronary narrowing accompanied by 1 or more transmural left ventricular wall scars. The reverse occurred in the case of IDC. Of the 111 patients with IDC anatomically (no left ventricular wall lesion grossly), 11 had severe narrowing of 1 or more major epicardial coronary arteries such that these patients in actuality did not fulfill our definitions for either IC or IDC. We suspect, however, that these 11 patients actually had IDC but resided in a high-cholesterol environment (United States), where coronary atherosclerosis is so prevalent.

Most of the incongruity between clinical and morphologic diagnoses occurred in the non-IC subgroups other than IDC. Thus, among the 56 patients with non-IC, excluding the patients with IDC, only 31 (55%) had congruity between the clinical and morphologic diagnoses. Specifically, among the 17 patients with HC, the 3 with NCLVC, the 3 with

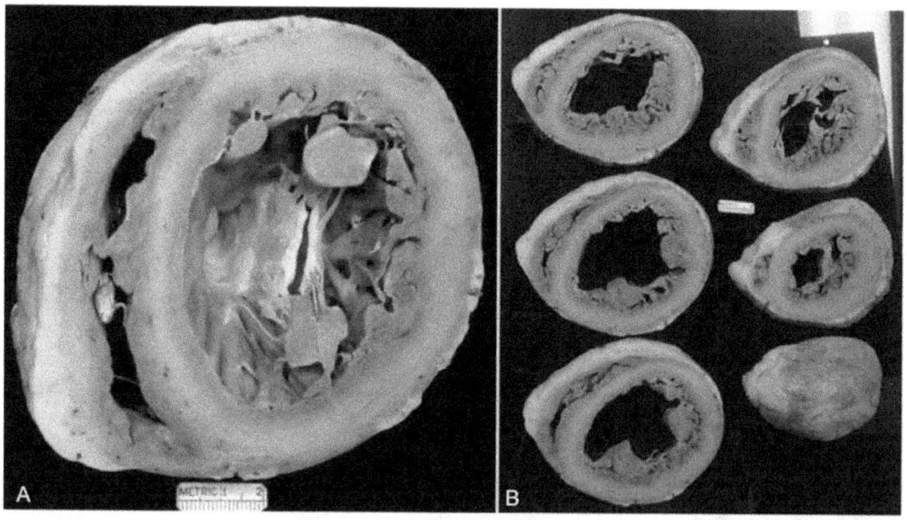

FIGURE 15. Idiopathic dilated cardiomyopathy. Views of the heart in a 61-year-old woman who had had evidence of chronic heart failure since age 51 years. She did reasonably well on medical therapy until age 59 years, when the heart failure worsened considerably and an implantable cardiac defibrillator was inserted. During the 2 years before transplant, the heart failure progressively worsened, and the left ventricular ejection fraction fell to a low of approximately 10%. She never had chest pain. Earlier in life she had had several children. (a) Basal portion of heart exposing well the mitral valve. The left ventricle is greatly enlarged measuring up to 7.5 cm. No foci of fibrosis or necrosis are seen in the ventricular walls. (b) Views of the ventricles caudal to the mitral valve, again showing considerable left ventricular cavity dilatation.

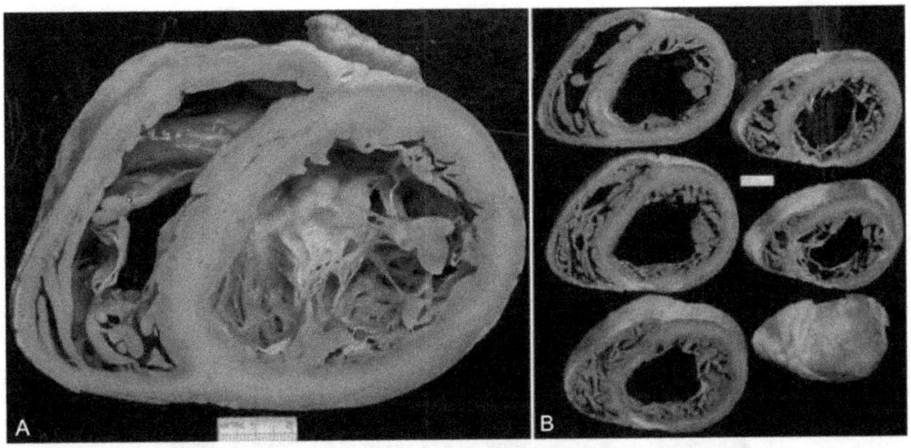

FIGURE 16. Idiopathic dilated cardiomyopathy. Heart in a 62-year-old woman who developed evidence of heart failure at age 55 years, which progressed thereafter. During the 7 months before cardiac transplant, the heart failure worsened considerably. Coronary angiography showed the major epicardial coronary arteries to be wide open. (a) Basal portion of heart exposing both tricuspid and mitral valves. Both ventricular cavities are considerably dilated. No foci of fibrosis or necrosis were noted in this portion of the ventricular walls. (b) Views of the ventricles caudal to the atrioventricular valves. In this view the posterior wall is thinned by scar tissue as is the most posterior portion of ventricular septum. The right coronary artery, as well as the others, was wide open. The focal scar may have been due to a coronary embolus many years earlier.

mononuclear myocarditis, the 4 with ARVC, and the 8 with cardiac sarcoidosis, a total of 35 patients, only 11 (31%) had the specific diagnosis made clinically. One could argue that including the single case without cardiac granulomas in the sarcoid group is improper. The type and distribution of the myocardial scarring, however, is absolutely typical of the other cases of cardiac sarcoidosis, a type of scarring not seen by us in any other condition.[43] Additionally, documented sarcoid granulomas in the lungs have been shown to disappear as the scarring increases.[59] Obviously, it is not sufficient to stop clinically with the diagnosis of non-IC cardiomyopathy. Ideally, of course, the specific subgroup needs to be sought even though therapy and outcome might not be altered by that knowledge.

The present study is not the first to compare the frequencies of discrepancies between the clinical and morphologic diagnoses in patients having CT. Bortman and colleagues[6] in 1994 examined the congruity-incongruity issue in 112 patients who underwent their first orthotopic CT at the authors' institution (University of Texas Southwestern

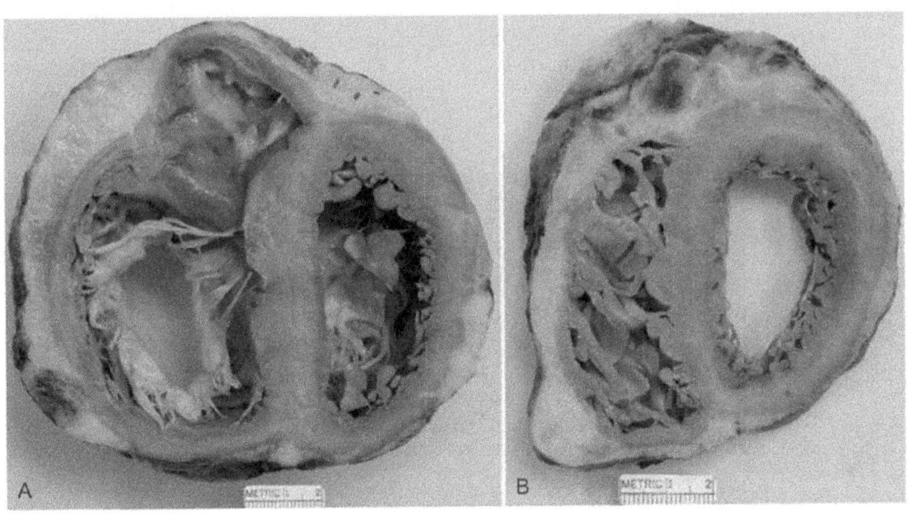

FIGURE 17. Idiopathic dilated cardiomyopathy. Heart of a 68-year-old man who was found to have heart failure at age 50 years, and, at the time, also to have severe mitral regurgitation. Coronary angiogram showed the coronary arteries to be wide open. At age 50 years, the patient underwent repair of the mitral valve including the insertion of an annular ring. The mitral regurgitation was reduced from severe to mild, but the heart failure continued and progressed. A left ventricular assist device was inserted before the cardiac transplantation. (a) View of the basal portion of the heart showing dilatation of both right and left ventricular cavities. The tricuspid annulus is quite dilated. No lesions are noted in the ventricular walls although the ventricular septum is thicker than the left ventricular free wall. (b) View more caudal showing impressive pectinate muscles within the right ventricular cavity. Again, no myocardial lesions are noted. The quantity of subepicardial adipose tissue is considerably increased.

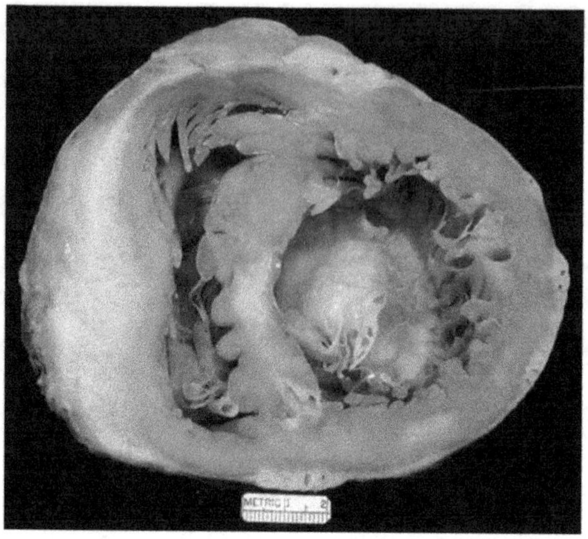

FIGURE 18. Hypertrophic cardiomyopathy. Heart in a 41-year-old man in whom hypertrophic cardiomyopathy was diagnosed when he was 6 years of age. At age 26 years, atrial fibrillation appeared and during the next 15 years he was cardioverted 98 times. He eventually developed complete heart block, and a pacemaker was inserted. At age 30 years, an intracardiac defibrillator was implanted, and at the same time an alcohol septal ablation procedure was performed. Nevertheless, evidence of heart failure persisted and a heart transplant was performed. View of the basal portion exposing both tricuspid and mitral valves. The left ventricular cavity is quite dilated. The focal scar in the ventricular septum may be the result of the alcohol septal ablation. Another small scar is present in the posterior wall of left ventricle. The thickness of the ventricular septum is greater than that of the left ventricular free wall.

Medical Center at Dallas). Among their 64 patients diagnosed with IC clinically, all had severe coronary narrowing morphologically; of their 48 patients with IDC clinically, 12 (25%) morphologically had severe coronary disease, and 3 had acute myocarditis. Thus, of their 112 patients a discrepancy between pre- and post-transplant diagnosis occurred in 15 (13%). Neither gross photographs nor definitions of the entities were provided.

In 1999, Angelini and colleagues[1] from Padua, Italy, studied the agreement or lack thereof between pre- and post-CT diagnoses in 257 patients having CT, and found a discrepancy between clinical and pathologic diagnoses in 20 patients (8%). Among their 87 patients with a clinical diagnoses of IC, 3 had IDC and 1 granulomatous myocarditis; among their 126 patients whose clinical diagnosis was non-IC, 7 morphologically had IC, 5 myocarditis, 1 ARVC, and 1 with NCLVC; among their 10 patients with a clinical diagnosis of HC, 1 had ARVC, and 1 had a cardiac fibroma.[1] No gross photographs of the heart or definitions of the conditions were provided.

In 2009, Luk and colleagues[29] from Toronto, Canada, studied the problem in 296 patients who had had CT from

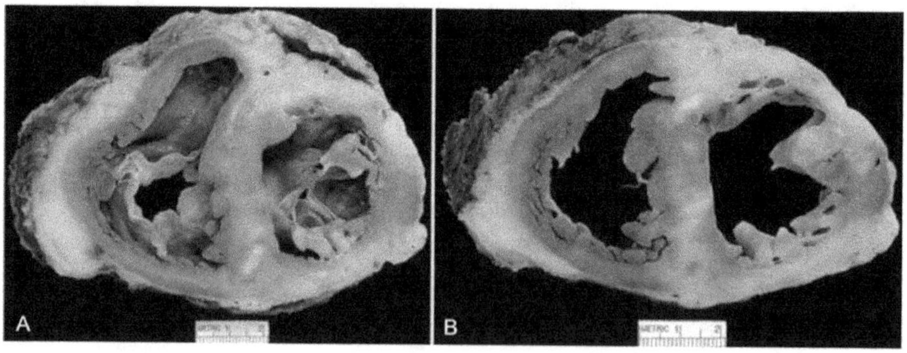

FIGURE 19. Hypertrophic cardiomyopathy. The heart in a 48-year-old man who developed heart failure at age 41 years and had an intracardiac defibrillator inserted shortly thereafter. A left ventricular assist device was inserted 2.3 years before cardiac transplantation. At age 45 years, he developed atrial fibrillation and had several cardioversion procedures performed. A parent and several cousins had heart disease of unclear type and were either asymptomatic or had died from it. (a) View of the base of the heart exposing both tricuspid and mitral valves. There is considerable scarring in the left ventricular and ventricular septal walls and in both papillary muscles. Both cavities are quite dilated. The thickness of the ventricular septum is greater than that of the left ventricular free wall. (b) Another view more caudal showing extensive scarring. The left anterior descending coronary artery is narrowed on this slice, probably the result of extensive scaring surrounding it. (Figure 19a is reprinted with permission from Elsevier.[49])

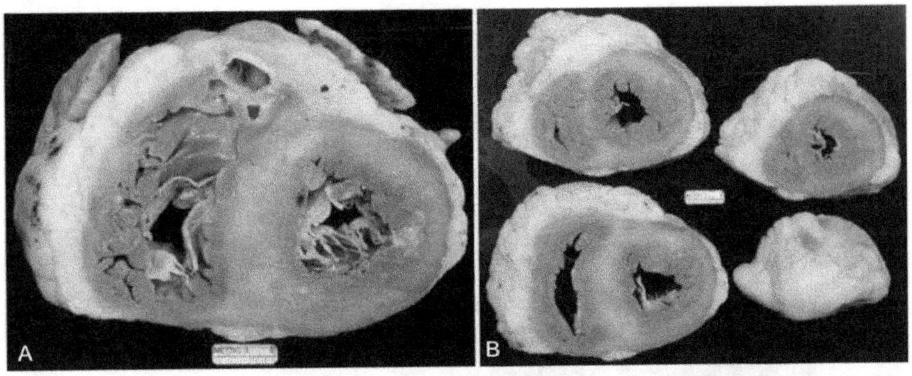

FIGURE 20. Hypertrophic cardiomyopathy. This 68-year-old man was diagnosed with hypertrophic cardiomyopathy many years earlier. His major problem was recurrent episodes of ventricular tachycardia, and he underwent an ablation procedure for that. He also had atrial fibrillation and other atrial arrhythmias. An implantable cardiac defibrillator was inserted. He also was obese, had obstructive sleep apnea, and chronic renal disease, stage 3. (a) View of the cardiac base exposing tricuspid, pulmonic, and mitral valves. The thickness of the ventricular septum is greater than that of the left ventricular free wall. The 2 ventricular cavities are only mildly dilated. Calcium was present in the mitral annular area. (b) Views of the ventricles caudal to the views shown on the left.

1987 to 2006 (Table 12). The frequency of the diagnosis made clinically and after examination of the recipient heart is shown in Table 12. It is apparent that the incongruity between the clinical and morphologic diagnoses was relatively frequent. Three gross photographs of the heart were presented. Definitions of the various conditions were not provided.

It is apparent from the present and previous studies that the largest incongruity between clinical and morphologic diagnosis in patients having CT is among the non-IC subtypes, particularly the dilated (end-stage) form of HC, mononuclear myocarditis, cardiac sarcoidosis, ARVC, and NCLVC. Would the use of additional diagnostic "instruments of precision" have allowed more precise pre-CT diagnosis among the non-IC group? Possibly so, particularly more use of magnetic resonance imaging among the patients with HC and sarcoidosis.[35] Would a more

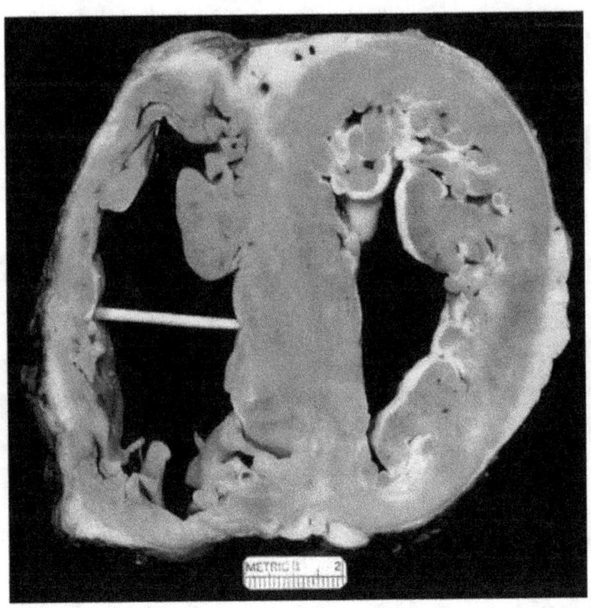

FIGURE 21. Hypertrophic cardiomyopathy. View of the heart in a 68-year-old man who was known to have some form of heart disease since age 38 years. The problem during the 30 years was various degrees of heart failure which began progressing about age 55 years. In the 2 years before cardiac transplantation he had multiple hospitalizations for decompensated heart failure. He had an intracardiac defibrillator in place for several years. Because of the severity of the heart failure, a left ventricular assist device was inserted 7 months before cardiac transplantation. The heart failure severity, however, continued, and before heart transplantation the left ventricular ejection fraction was approximately 10%. Both cardiac ventricles are dilated, the right more than the left. The ventricular septum is thicker than the left ventricular free wall. The mural endocardium of the left ventricle is thickened by white fibrous tissue. A scar is present in the posterior portion of the left ventricular free wall and also in the posterior portion of the ventricular septum.

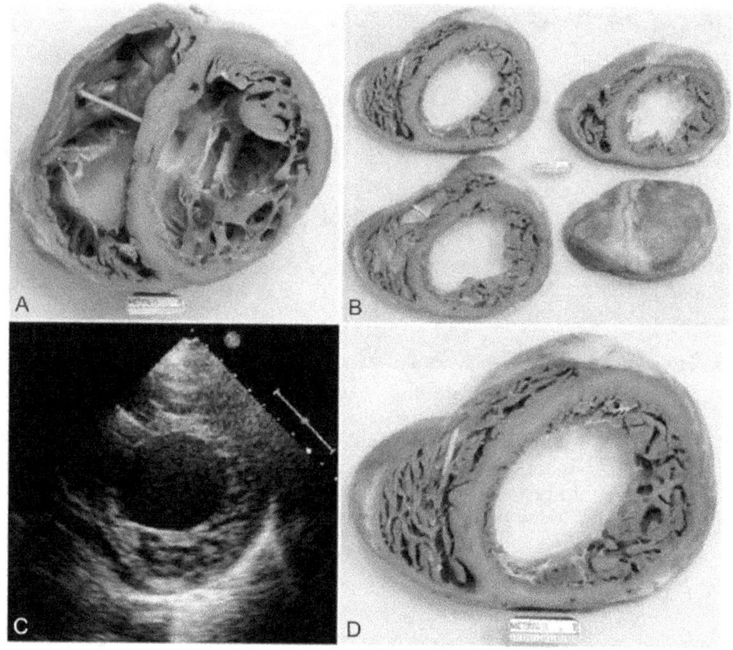

FIGURE 22. Left ventricular non-compaction cardiomyopathy. Heart in a 49-year-old man who had been well until age 33 years when symptoms of heart failure appeared. At the time, echocardiogram showed both ventricles to be dilated and the left ventricular systolic function to be severely depressed. A defibrillator was inserted at age 39 years, and cardiac resynchronization therapy at age 43 years. He underwent ablation therapy for multiple episodes of ventricular tachycardia. His left ventricular ejection fraction just before cardiac transplantation was 15%. (a) View of both ventricles just caudal to the tricuspid and mitral valves. The thickness of the ventricular septum is much greater than that of the left ventricular free wall. The compacted portion of left ventricular free wall is much thinner than the non-compacted portion. Both ventricular cavities are greatly dilated. The left ventricular free wall posteriorly is focally scarred. (a) View of the basal portion of the heart exposing the tricuspid and mitral valves. Both ventricles are greatly dilated. The posterolateral wall is focally scarred. The compacted portion of left ventricular free wall is much thinner than the trabeculated portion. (b) Views of sections of the ventricular walls caudal to the view shown in the upper left. (c) Echocardiogram showing hypertrabeculation of the left ventricular free wall. (d) Section of the left ventricular free wall corresponding to the echocardiogram. (Reprinted with permission from Elsevier.[45]).

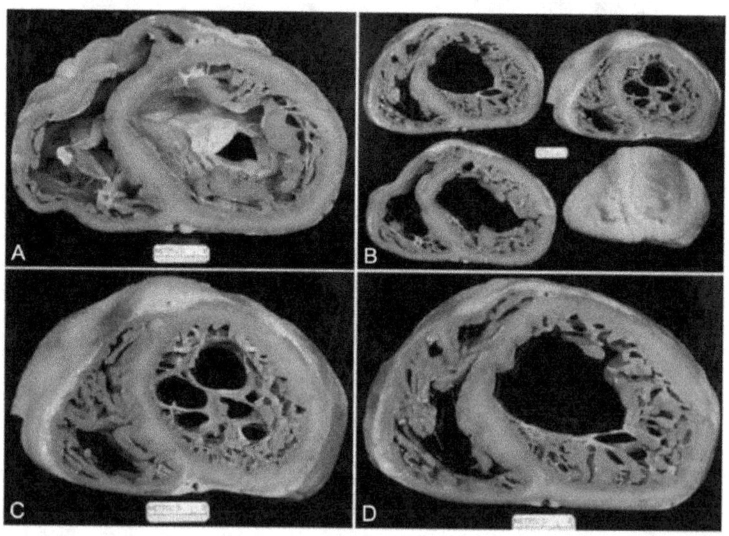

FIGURE 23. Left ventricular non-compaction cardiomyopathy. Heart of a 36-year-old woman who was well until approximately age 35 years when she developed evidence of heart failure, which slowly but gradually progressed thereafter such that when she was aged 34 years her left ventricular ejection fraction had fallen to 20% and she was in chronic atrial fibrillation. She also developed runs of ventricular tachycardia for which a defibrillator was inserted. (a) View of the heart showing both tricuspid and mitral valves. Both ventricular cavities are enormously dilated, and the ventricular walls are free of foci of fibrosis and necrosis. (b) Views of the ventricles caudal to the view shown in upper left. (c) Close-up view of 1 of the slices in upper right. (d) View showing the hypertrabeculated or non-compacted portion of the left ventricular wall to be much thicker than the compacted portion. (Reprinted with permission from Elsevier.[45]).

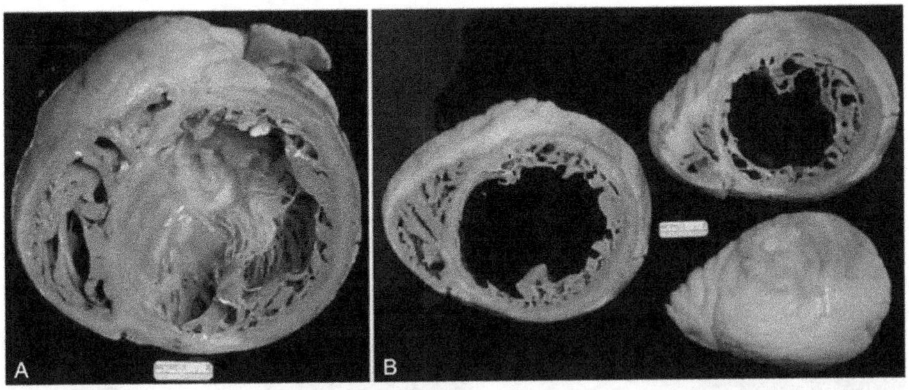

FIGURE 24. Mononuclear myocarditis. The heart in a 56-year-old man who had been well until age 48 years, when he had a cardiac event that resulted in the appearance of heart failure, which progressed thereafter. He also smoked heavily and had evidence of chronic obstructive lung disease. A defibrillator was inserted when he was 53 years old. (a) Basal portion of the heart showing severe dilatation of the left ventricular cavity with transmural scarring in the posterior and anterior left ventricular free wall and in the anterior portion of the ventricular septum. (b) Sections of the ventricular cavities caudal to the view shown on the left. The ventricular septum in 2 of the slices is completely scarred. Histologic section showed focal collections of mononuclear cells in the walls of left ventricle and ventricular septum. The coronary arteries at necropsy were wide open.

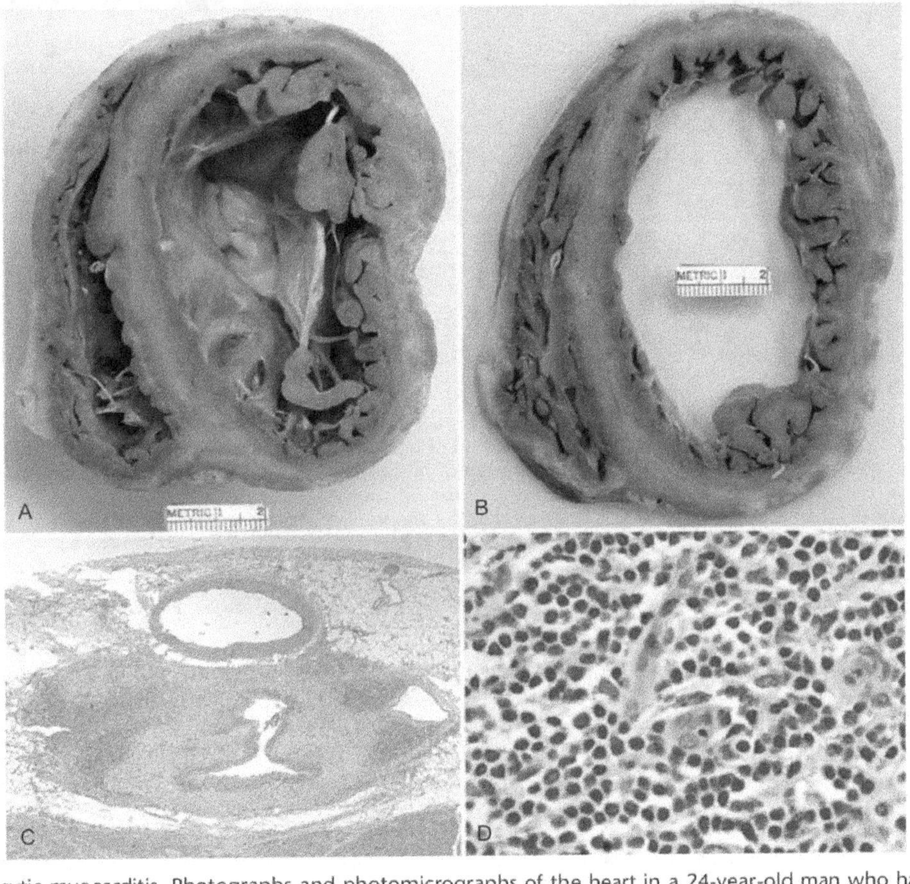

FIGURE 25. Monocytic myocarditis. Photographs and photomicrographs of the heart in a 24-year-old man who had been well until approximately 2.5 years earlier when evidence of heart failure appeared and not long thereafter his left ventricular ejection fraction was approximately 15%. A defibrillator was implanted. Progressive worsening of the heart failure prompted the CT. The echocardiogram 15 months before cardiac transplantation showed his left ventricular ejection fraction to be as low as 5%. (a) View of the cardiac base exposing the mitral valve. (b) Slice of the ventricles more caudal. The scarring and inflammatory cell infiltrates are mainly subepicardial in location. (c) Inflammatory cell collection in the subepicardial adipose tissue (Movat stain ×20). (d) Close-up of the lymphocytes (hematoxylin/eosin stain, ×100).

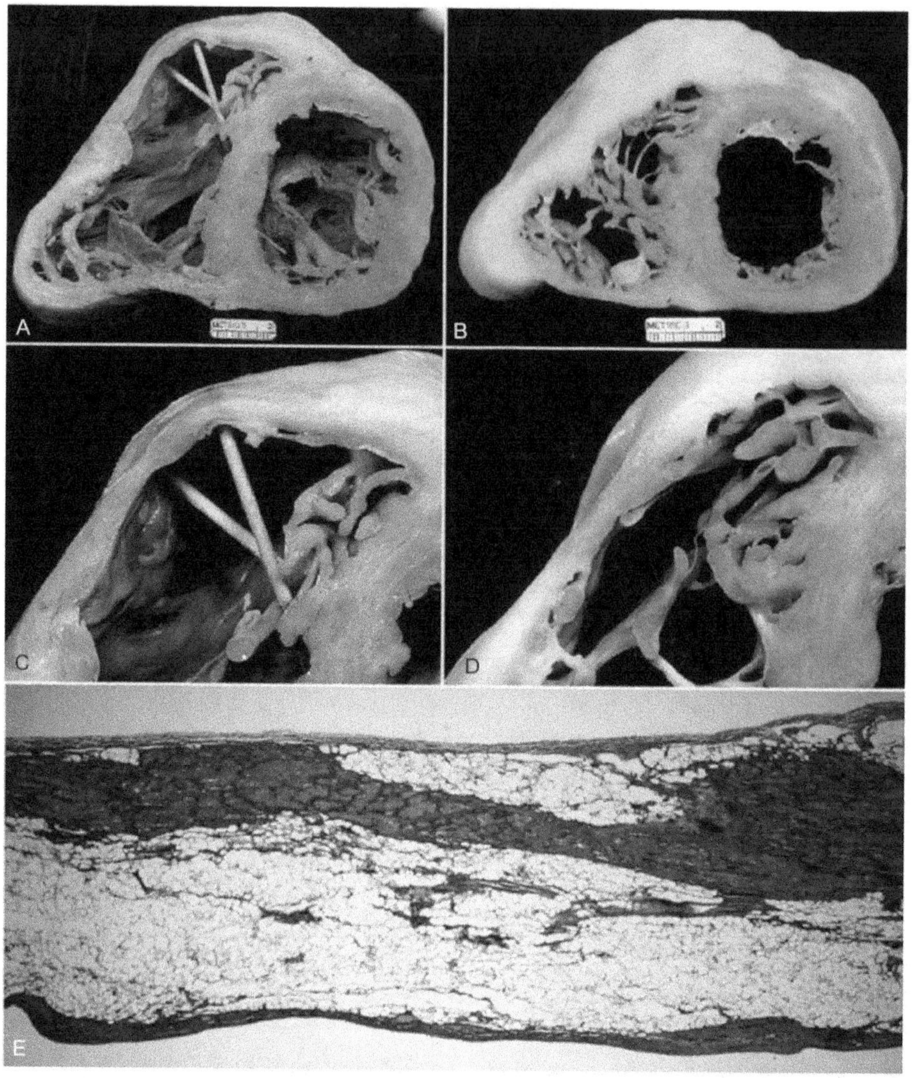

FIGURE 26. Arrhythmogenic right ventricular cardiomyopathy. The heart in a 26-year-old man who developed symptoms of heart failure at age 12 years, followed later by ventricular arrhythmias and bundle branch block. His left ventricular ejection fraction fell to 15%. (a) View of the base of the heart showing marked dilatation of both ventricles. The right ventricular wall in its outflow tract is thin (b, c, d). (e) Photomicrograph of the right ventricular wall in the right ventricular outflow tract, which consists of adipose tissue, fibrous tissue, and a few myocardial cells (Masson stain, ×20). (Reprinted with permission from Elsevier.[46]).

accurate pre-CT diagnosis among the non-IC group have led to a re-evaluation of the need for CT in the first place? Or, if clinicians had actually known the specific non-IC diagnosis, would treatment have been different and might CT have been avoided? Among the 314 patients included in this study, the morphologic and clinical diagnoses were incongruent in 42 (13%), including 7 of 17 patients with HC, 3 of 3 with NCLVC, 3 of 3 with mononuclear myocarditis, 4 of 4 with ARVC, and 8 of 8 with cardiac sarcoidosis. This incongruity certainly leaves open the possibility that, if immunosuppressive or immunomodulatory treatment had been used in certain cases, such as specific antiarrhythmic agents for ARVC or intracardiac defibrillator for non-obstructive HC with normal or near-normal left ventricular ejection fraction, this therapy might have made a difference with respect to treatment, outcome, and even potentially the need for CT.

The positive features of the present study include the fact that all hearts were examined and described and all morphologic diagnoses were provided by the same person (WCR), who has been studying cardiovascular diseases for several decades. Had many of the non-IC cases been "grossed" by a first or second year trainee, which is the modus of operation in the surgical pathology laboratory at BUMC—except for the cardiovascular cases—it is unlikely that the cases of burnt-out or end-stage HC, or ARVC, or NCLVC would have been recognized grossly, and histologic examination in these cases would unlikely have provided the proper morphologic diagnoses.

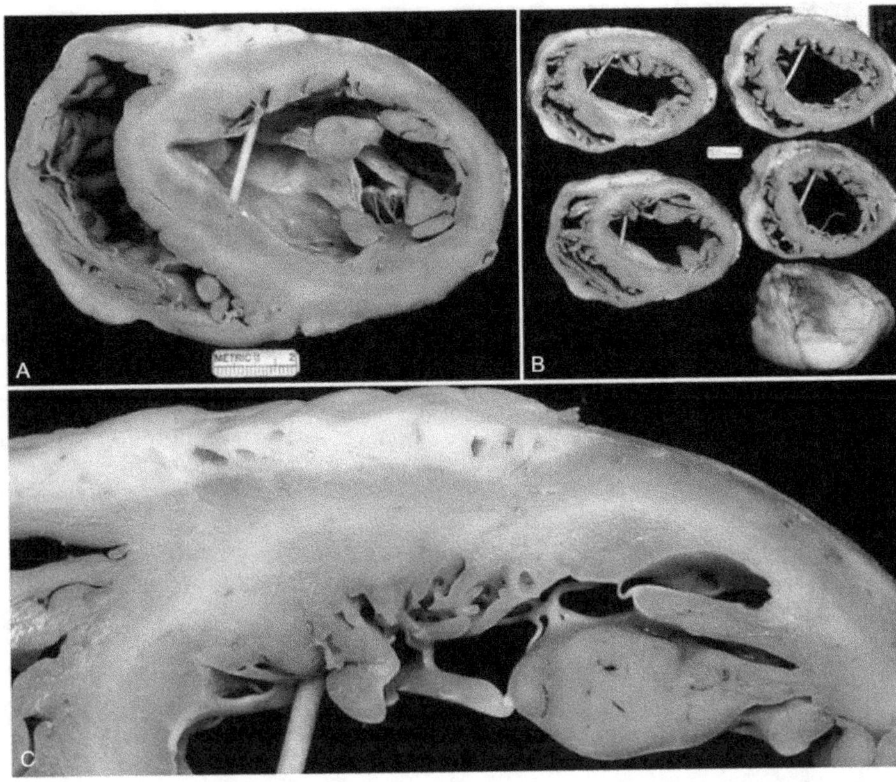

FIGURE 27. Cardiac sarcoidosis. Heart in a 52-year-old black woman who had developed evidence of heart failure beginning at age 48 years. It progressed, and an implantable cardiac defibrillator/pacemaker was placed. Runs of ventricular tachycardia occasionally were seen. Cardiac catheterization 8 months before cardiac transplantation disclosed normal coronary arteries, severe global left ventricular hypokinesis, and an estimated ejection fraction of 10%. The pressures in mm Hg were as follows: left ventricle, 115/34; right ventricle, 59/15; pulmonary artery wedge a wave 20, v wave 20, mean 18; right atrium a wave 12, v wave 10, mean 9. The cardiac index was 1.7 L/min per m2. A diagnosis of cardiac sarcoidosis was never entertained clinically. (a) Heart at the base showing the greatly dilated ventricular cavities and scarring in the ventricular septum and left ventricular free wall anteriorly. (b) Cross-section of the ventricles showing the extent of the scarring. (c) Close-up of the left ventricular free wall and ventricular septum showing the scarring. (Reprinted with permission from Elsevier.[43]).

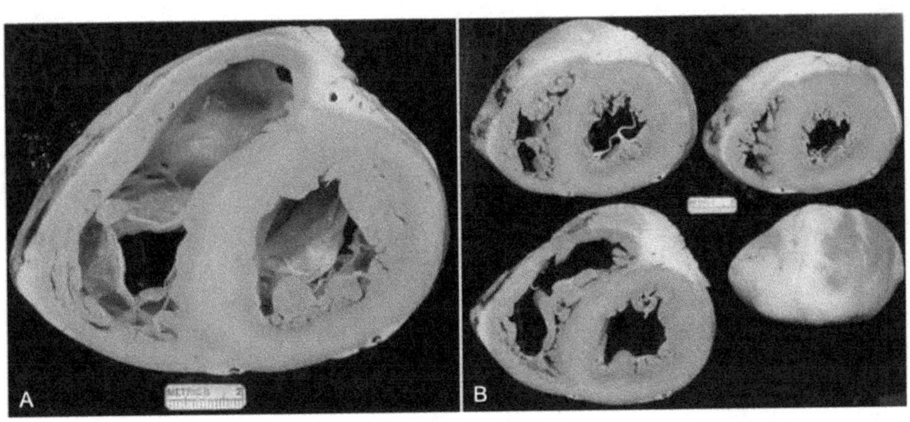

FIGURE 28. Cardiac amyloidosis. Heart in a 57-year-old man who had been well until 1 year before cardiac transplantation, when evidence of heart failure appeared. On examination 2 months later he was noted to have periorbital ecchymoses and a biopsy of an abdominal fat pad disclosed amyloidosis. During the year before CT, he lost 40 pounds, and the dyspnea and exercise intolerance progressively worsened. Echocardiogram 5 months before CT disclosed an ejection fraction of 55%, a restrictive diastolic filling pattern, and an "ineffective atrial kick." The heart weighed 420 g and amyloid deposits were extensively present in the walls of all 4 cardiac chambers. The right ventricular cavity was larger than the left ventricular cavity. The epicardial coronary arteries were wide open. Amyloid deposits were extensive in the walls of all 4 cardiac chambers. (a) View of the cardiac base. (b) Views of the more caudal portions of the heart.

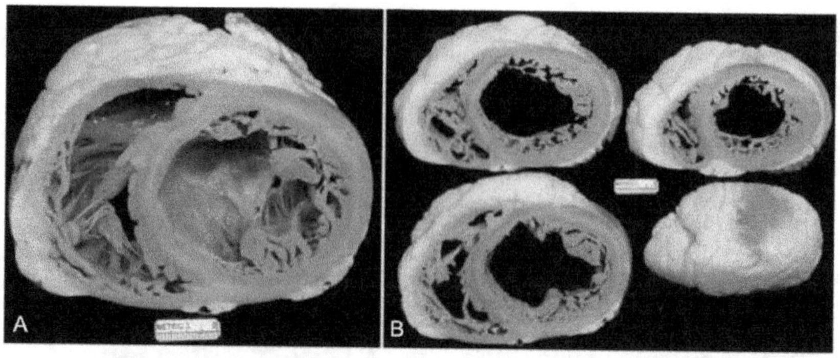

FIGURE 29. Adriamycin-induced cardiomyopathy. Heart in a 50-year-old woman who had received Adriamycin at age 38 years (12 years earlier) for cancer of the right breast with total mastectomy. She had evidence of heart failure only a couple of months before CT with rapid progression thereafter such that 1 month before CT her left ventricular ejection fraction was only 10%. The pressures in mm Hg were left ventricle 85/23; aorta 85/50. The cardiac output was 1.2L/min, the ventricular cavities were severely dilated, and the epicardial coronary arteries were wide open. The heart weighed 405g and the ventricles were dilated. Histologically, no specific cardiac lesions are present. (a) View of the cardiac base. (b) View of the more caudal cardiac slices.

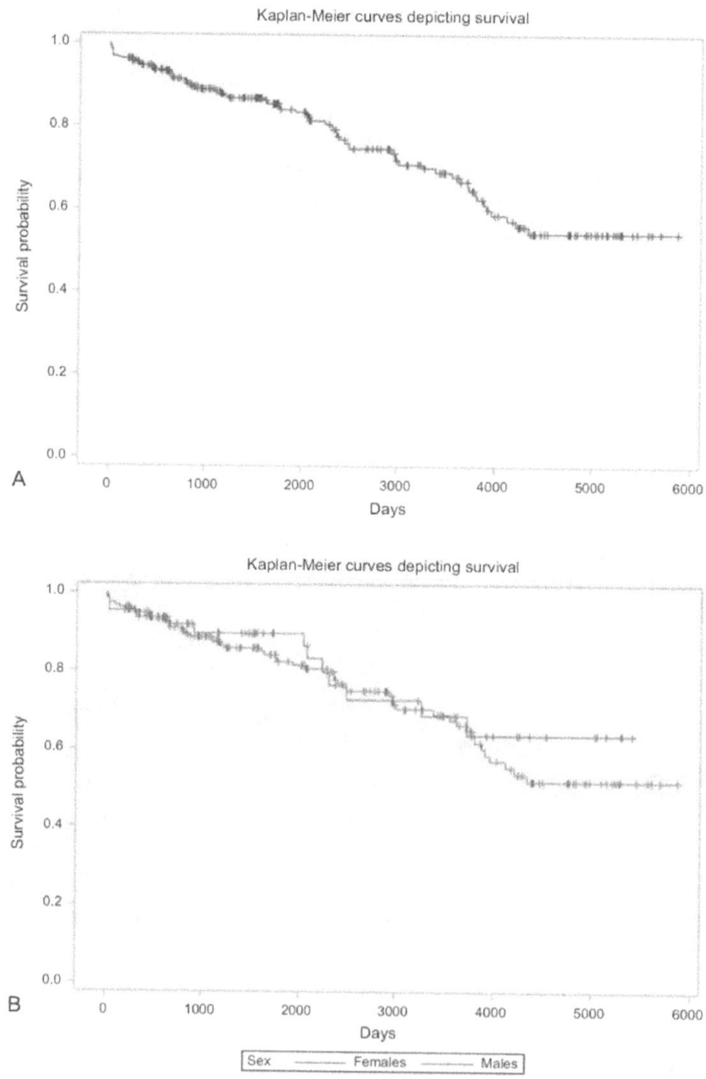

FIGURE 30. Kaplan-Meier survival curves for 257 patients whose survival data were available. (a) The unadjusted survival curve. (b) The unadjusted survival curves by sex.

REFERENCES

1. Angelini A, Boffa GM, Livi U, et al. Discordance between pre and post cardiac transplant diagnosis: implications for pre- and postoperative decision making. *Cardiovasc Pathol.* 1999; 8:17–23.
2. Avella A, d'Amati G, Zachara E, et al. Comparison between electro-anatomic and pathologic findings in a patient with arrhythmogenic right ventricular cardiomyopathy/dysplasia treated with orthotopic cardiac transplant. *Heart Rhythm.* 2010; 7:828–831.
3. Barnard CN. The Operation. A human heart transplant: an interim report of a successful operation performed at Groote Schuur Hospital, Cape Town. *S AFr Med J.* 1967; 41:1271–1274.
4. Basso C, Corrado D, Marcus FI, et al. Arrhythmogenic right ventricular cardiomyopathy. *Lancet.* 2009; 373:1289–1300.
5. Biagini E, Spirito P, Leone O, et al. Heart transplantation in hypertrophic cardiomyopathy. *Am J Cardiol.* 2008; 101:387–392.
6. Bortman G, Sellanes M, Odell DS, et al. Discrepancy between pre- and post-transplant diagnosis of end-stage dilated cardiomyopathy. *Am J Cardiol.* 1994; 74:921–924.
7. Bradshaw SH, Veinot JP. Cardiac amyloidosis: what are the indications for transplant?. *Curr Opin Cardiol.* 2012; 27:143–147.
8. Burke AP, Farb A, Tashko G, et al. Arrhythmogenic right ventricular cardiomyopathy and fatty replacement of the right ventricular myocardium: are they different diseases?. *Circulation.* 1998; 97:1571–1580.
9. Chang TI, Chi NH, Chou NK, et al. Isolated cardiac sarcoidosis in heart transplantation. *Transplant Proc.* 2012; 44:903–906.
10. Conner R, Hosenpud JD, Norman DJ, et al. Heart transplantation for cardiac amyloidosis: successful one-year outcome despite recurrence of the disease. *J Heart Transplant.* 1988; 7:165–167.
11. Conraads V, Paelinck B, Vorlat A, et al. Isolated non- compaction of the left ventricle: A rare indication for transplantation. *J Heart Lung Transplant.* 2001; 20:904–907.
12. Corrado D, Basso C, Thiene G, et al. Spectrum of clinicopathologic manifestations of arrhythmogenic right ventricular cardiomyopathy/dysplasia: a multicenter study. *J Am Coll Cardiol.* 1997; 30: 1512–1520.
13. Coutu M, Perrault LP, White M, et al. Cardiac transplantation for hypertrophic cardiomyopathy: a valid therapeutic option. *J Heart Lung Transplant.* 2004; 23:413–417.
14. Dalal D, Nasir K, Bomma C, et al. Arrhythmogenic right ventricular dysplasia: a United States experience. *Circulation.* 2005; 112:3823–3832.
15. Donsky AS, Escobar J, Capehart J, et al. Heart Transplantation for undiagnosed cardiac sarcoidosis. *Am J Cardiol.* 2002; 89:1447–1450.
16. Dubrey SW, Burke MM, Hawkins PN, et al. Cardiac transplantation for amyloid heart disease: the United Kingdom experience. *J Heart Lung Transplant.* 2004; 23:1142–1153.
17. Dubrey SW, Burke MM, Khaghani A, et al. Long term results of heart transplantation in patients with amyloid heart disease. *Heart.* 2001; 85:202–207.
18. Falk RH. Cardiac amyloidosis: a treatable disease, often overlooked. *Circulation.* 2011; 124:1079–1085.
19. Garner WL, Starling C, Kuiper JJ, et al. Lymphocytic myocarditis as a cause of fulminant fatal heart failure. *Proc (Bayl Univ Med Cent).* 2006; 19:122–123.
20. Gungor H, Oguz E, Ayik MF, et al. Comparison of heart transplantation patients with ischemic and idiopathic dilated cardiomyopathy. *Transplant Proc.* 2011; 43:3847–3850.
21. Hamada T, Kubo T, Kitaoka H, et al. Clinical features of the dilated phase of hypertrophic cardiomyopathy in comparison with those of dilated cardiomyopathy. *Clin Cardiol.* 2010; 33:E24–E28.
22. Isner JM, Ferrans VJ, Cohen SR, et al. Clinical and morphologic cardiac findings after anthracycline chemotherapy. Analysis of 64 patients studied at necropsy. *Am J Cardiol.* 1983; 51:1167–1174.
23. Isner JM, Virmani R, Itscoitz SB, et al. Left and right ventricular myocardial infarction in idiopathic dilated cardiomyopathy. *Am Heart J.* 1980; 9:235–242.
24. Kato TS, Takayama H, Yoshizawa S, et al. Cardiac transplantation in patients with hypertrophic cardiomyopathy. *Am J Cardiol.* 2012; 110:568–574.
25. Kindermann I, Barth C, Mahfoud F, et al. Update on myocarditis. *J Am Coll Cardiol.* 2012; 59:779–792.
26. Kumar S, Marfatia R, Tannenbaum S, et al. Doxorubicin-induced cardiomyopathy 17 years after chemotherapy. *Tex Heart Inst J.* 2012; 39:424–427.
27. Lennenman AJ, Wang L, Wigger M, et al. Heart transplant survival outcomes for adriamycin-dilated cardiomyopathy. *Am J Cardiol.* 2013; 111:609–612.
28. Lobo FV, Silver MD, Butany J, et al. Left ventricular involvement in right ventricular dysplasia/cardiomyopathy. *Can J Cardiol.* 1999; 15:1239–1247.
29. Luk A, Metawee M, Ahn E, et al. Do clinical diagnoses correlate with pathological diagnoses in cardiac transplant patients? The importance of endomyocardial biopsy. *Can J Cardiol.* 2009; 25:e48–e54.
30. Mancini D, Lietz K. Selection of cardiac transplantation candidates in 2010. *Circulation.* 2010; 122:173–183.
31. Marcus FI, Zareba W, Calkins H, et al. Arrhythmogenic right ventricular cardiomyopathy/dysplasia clinical presentation and diagnostic evaluation: results from the North American Multidisciplinary Study. *Heart Rhythm.* 2009; 6:984–992.
32. Marcus GM, Glidden DV, Polonsky B, et al. Multidisciplinary Study of Right Ventricular Dysplasia Investigators. Efficacy of antiarrhythmic drugs in arrhythmogenic right ventricular cardiomyopathy: a report from the North American ARVC Registry. *J Am Coll Cardiol.* 2009; 54:609–615.
33. Maron BJ, Maron MS, Wigle ED, et al. The 50-year history, controversy, and clinical implications of left ventricular outflow tract obstruction in hypertrophic cardiomyopathy. *J Am Coll Cardiol.* 2009; 54:191–200.
34. Maron BJ, Maron MS. Hypertrophic cardiomyopathy. *Lancet.* 2013; 381:242–255.
35. Maron BJ, Wolfson JK, Epstein SE, et al. Intramural ("small vessel") coronary artery disease in hypertrophic cardiomyopathy. *J Am Coll Cardiol.* 1986; 8:545–557.
36. Maron BJ. Hypertrophic cardiomyopathy. *Lancet.* 1997; 350:127–133.
37. Maron MS, Kalsmith BM, Udelson JE, et al. Survival after cardiac transplantation in patients with hypertrophic cardiomyopathy. *Circ Heart Fail.* 2010; 3:574–579.
38. Parisi F. Heart transplantation in congenital heart disease. *Curr Cardiol Rev.* 2011; 7:50.
39. Pavie A. Heart transplantation for end-stage valvular disease: indications and results. *Curr Opin Cardiol.* 2006; 21:100–105.
40. Pelosi F, Capehart JE, Roberts WC. Effectiveness of cardiac transplantation for primary (AL) cardiac amyloidosis. *Am J Cardiol.* 1997; 79:532–535.
41. Ried M, Rupprecht L, Hirt S, et al. Sequential therapy of primary cardiac lymphoma with cardiectomy, total artificial heart support, and cardiac transplantation. *J Heart Lung Transplant.* 2010; 29: 707–709.
42. Roberts CS, Roberts WC. Morphologic features (of hypertrophic cardiomyopathy). *Progress in Cardiology 2/2.* In: Zipes DP, Rowlands DJ, editor Philadelphia: Lea & Febiger, 1989; pp. 3–32.

43. Roberts WC, Chung MS, Ko JM, et al. Morphologic features of cardiac sarcoidosis in native hearts of patients having cardiac transplantation. *Am J Cardiol.* 2014; 113:706–712.

44. Roberts WC, Glancy DL, DeVita VT. Heart in malignant lymphoma (Hodgkin's disease, lymphosarcoma, reticulum cell sarcoma and mycosis fungoides). A study of 196 autopsy cases. *Am J Cardiol.* 1968; 22:85–107.

45. Roberts WC, Karia SJ, Ko JM, et al. Examination of isolated ventricular non-compaction (hypertrabeculation) as a distinct entity in adults. *Am J Cardiol.* 2011; 108:747–752.

46. Roberts WC, Ko JM, Kuiper JJ, et al. Some previously neglected examples of arrhythmogenic right ventricular dysplasia /cardiomyopathy and frequency of its various reported manifestations. *Am J Cardiol.* 2010; 106:268–274.

47. Roberts WC, McAllister HA, Ferrans VJ. Sarcoidosis of the Heart. A clinicopathologic study of 35 necropsy patients (Group I) and review of 78 previously described necropsy patients (Group II). *Am J Med.* 1977; 63:86–108.

48. Roberts WC, Phillips SD, Escobar JM, et al. Cardiac transplantation 40 years after a stab wound to the heart. *Proc (Bayl Univ Med Cent).* 2001; 14:241–242.

49. Roberts WC, Roberts CC, Ko JM, et al. Dramatically different phenotypic expressions of hypertrophic cardiomyopathy in male cousins undergoing cardiac transplantation with identical disease-causing gene mutation. *Am J Cardiol.* 2013; 111:1818–1822.

50. Roberts WC, Roberts CC, Ko JM, et al. Cardiac transplantation in adults with aortic valve disease with focus on the bicuspid aortic valve. *Am J Cardiol.* 2012; 109:1212–1214.

51. Roberts WC, Siegel RJ, McManus BM. Idiopathic dilated cardiomyopathy: Analysis of 152 necropsy patients. *Am J Cardiol.* 1987; 60:1340–1355.

52. Roberts WC, Vowels TJ, Ko JM, et al. Cardiac transplantation for cardiac sarcoidosis with initial diagnosis by examination of the left ventricular apical "core" excised for insertion of a left ventricular assist device for severe chronic heart failure. *Am J Cardiol.* 2009; 103:110–114.

53. Roberts WC, Waller BF. Cardiac amyloidosis causing cardiac dysfunction: analysis of 54 necropsy patients. *Am J Cardiol.* 1983; 52:137–146.

54. Roberts WC. Defining idiopathic dilated cardiomyopathy: A courtroom discussion. *Am J Cardiol.* 1989; 63:893–896.

55. Ross EM, Roberts WC. Severe atherosclerotic coronary arterial narrowing and chronic congestive heart failure without myocardial infarction; analysis of 18 patients studied at necropsy. *Am J Cardiol.* 1986; 57:51–56.

56. Ross EM, Roberts WC. Severe atherosclerotic coronary artery disease, healed myocardial infarction and chronic congestive heart failure; analysis of 81 patients studied at necropsy. *Am J Cardiol.* 1986; 57:44–50.

57. Rotela Samaniego JA, Castells E, Manito N, et al. Clinical evolution of heart transplantation in patients with previous valvular cardiomyopathy. *Transplant Proc.* 2007; 39:2355–2356.

58. Sagar S, Liu PP, Cooper LT. Myocarditis. *Lancet.* 2012; 379:738–747.

59. Scadding JG. A 'burnt-out' case of sarcoidosis. *Postgrad Med J.* 1968; 4:105–108.

60. Shirani J, Freant LJ, Roberts WC. Gross and semiquantitative histologic findings in mononuclear cell myocarditis causing sudden death, and implications for endomyocardial biopsy. *Am J Cardiol.* 1993; 72:952–957.

61. Shirani J, Maron BJ, Cannon RO, et al. Clinicopathologic features of hypertrophic cardiomyopathy managed by cardiac transplantation. *Am J Cardiol.* 1993; 72:434–440.

62. Shirani J. Subepicardial myocardial lesions. *Am Heart J.* 1993; 125:1346–1352.

63. Siân Pincott E, Burch M. Indications for heart transplantation in congenital heart disease. *Curr Cardiol Rev.* 2011; 7:51–58.

64. Tedford RJ, James C, Judge DP, et al. Cardiac transplantation in arrhythmogenic right ventricular dysplasia/cardiomyopathy. *J Am Coll Cardiol.* 2012; 9:289–290.

65. Theleman KP, Kuiper JJ, Roberts WC. Acute myocarditis (predominately lymphocytic) causing sudden death without heart failure. *Am J Cardiol.* 2001; 88:1078–1083.

66. Tops LF, Prakasa K, Tandri H, et al. Prevalence and pathophysiologic attributes of ventricular dyssynchrony in arrhythmogenic right ventricular dysplasia/cardiomyopathy. *J Am Coll Cardiol.* 2009; 54:445–451.

67. Valantine HA, Tazelaar HD, Macoviak J, et al. Cardiac sarcoidosis: response to steroids and transplantation. *J Heart Transplant.* 1987; 6:244–250.

68. Val-Bernal JF, Nistal JF, Martino M, et al. Isolated non-compaction of the left ventricular myocardium in an adult treated with heart transplantation. *Pathol Int.* 2006; 56:35–39.

69. Varr BC, Liedtke M, Arai S, et al. Heart transplantation and cardiac amyloidosis: approach to screening and novel management strategies. *J Heart Lung Transplant.* 2012; 31:325–331.

70. Waller BF, Smith ER, Blackbourne BD, et al. Congenital hypoplasia of portions of both right and left ventricular myocardial walls. Clinical and necropsy observations in two patients with parchment heart syndrome. *Am J Cardiol.* 1980; 46:885–891.

71. Waller TA, Hiser WL, Capehart JE, et al. Comparison of clinical and morphologic cardiac findings in patients having cardiac transplantation for ischemic cardiomyopathy, idiopathic dilated cardiomyopathy, and dilated hypertrophic cardiomyopathy. *Am J Cardiol.* 1998; 81:884–894.

72. Xu T, Yang Z, Vatta M, et al. Multidisciplinary Study of Right Ventricular Dysplasia Investigators. Compound and digenic heterozygosity contributes to arrhythmogenic right ventricular cardiomyopathy. *J Am Coll Cardiol.* 2010; 55:587–597.

73. Yoda M, Minami K, Fritzsche D, et al. Three cases of orthotopic heart transplantation for arrhythmogenic right ventricular cardiomyopathy. *Ann Thorac Surg.* 2005; 80:2358–2360.

Commonalities of Cardiac Rupture (Left Ventricular Free Wall or Ventricular Septum or Papillary Muscle) During Acute Myocardial Infarction Secondary to Atherosclerotic Coronary Artery Disease

William C. Roberts, MD[a,b,c,*], Kendall H. Burks[a,1], Jong Mi Ko, BA[a], Giovanni Filardo, PhD[d], and Joseph M. Guileyardo, MD[c]

Although mortality rates during acute myocardial infarction (AMI) continue to drop, cardiac rupture (left ventricular free wall [LVFW] or ventricular septum [VS] or papillary muscle [PM] or combination) remains relatively common. The aim was to identify commonalities among patients with AMI complicated by cardiac rupture. During a 22-year period (1993-2014) 64 patients hospitalized for AMI were studied and clinical and morphologic variables in those with (25 patients) – vs – those without (39 patients) cardiac rupture were compared, and previous reports on this topic were reviewed. Compared to the non-rupture cases, the rupture group was significantly older (71 years – vs – 60 years); had a much higher frequency of huge deposits of adipose tissue in the heart (floated in formaldehyde) (88% – vs – 20%) but a lower mean body mass index (28.2 Kg/m^2 – vs – 33.2 Kg/m^2); a much lower frequency of healed myocardial infarct (scar) (4% – vs – 28%); a lower frequency of diabetes mellitus (24% – vs – 47%), and a higher frequency of thrombolytic therapy during the fatal AMI (32% – vs – 10%). None of the rupture cases had evidence of dilated left ventricular cavities or evidence of heart failure before the AMI complicated by rupture. In conclusion, cardiac rupture appears to account for a high percent of deaths during a first AMI. It most commonly occurs in patients with extremely fatty hearts and in those without evidence of prior heart failure. (Am J Cardiol 2015;115:125–140)

During the last 80 years many publications on cardiac rupture complicating acute myocardial infarction (AMI) have appeared (Table 1).[1–29] Some have compared findings at necropsy in fatal AMI with – vs – without rupture of either the left ventricular free wall (LVFW) or ventricular septum (VS),[2,16,21,23,26–28] and others have described only the rupture cases.[8,13,19,26] Many previous publications provided no photographs of the ruptured hearts. One of us (WCR) has been involved since 1967 in a number of studies on cardiac rupture secondary to AMI,[25,30–42] including an examination at necropsy of 204 such patients with rupture of the LVFW or VS or papillary muscle (PM) studied from 1968 to 1989.[25] Despite these previous studies commonalities among these 3 types of cardiac rupture during AMI have not been clearly delineated. The present study attempts to fill that void by examining a new series of 25 patients with cardiac rupture studied at necropsy from 1993 to 2014, compares clinical and necropsy findings in them to 37 patients with fatal AMI without rupture, and focuses on commonalities observed in these patients and in previously reported ones.

Methods

The 64 patients with fatal AMI were seen at Baylor University Medical Center during a 22-year period (1993-2014). With 3 exceptions (gross photographs studied), all hearts were examined and described by WCR. At necropsy, the presence or absence of hemopericardium was determined by the prosector, most commonly under the supervision of JMG. At necropsy, the hearts were placed unopened in a container of formaldehyde, and after fixation for usually 3 to 5 days the hearts were opened and described by WCR, the specimens were photographed, (usually by JMK), and sections were cut by WCR for histologic study. After excising extraneous (non-cardiac) tissues, all hearts were placed in a container of 10% formaldehyde to see if they floated to the surface after removing any air inside of the cardiac chambers. Nearly all hearts were opened by cutting the ventricular walls parallel to the posterior atrioventricular sulcus at about 1 cm intervals, except for the most apical cut which was about 3 cm in thickness. All hearts were superficially dried with paper towels and weighed on an very accurate scale (to ± 1 g). The atria were incised by a cut about midway between the atrioventricular valve annulae and the most cephalad extension of the atrial walls. The pulmonary trunk was excised about 2 cm cephalad to its sinotubular junction and the ascending aorta about 3 cm cephalad to its sino-tubular junction. At least 4 histologic sections were

[a]Baylor Heart and Vascular Institute, Departments of [b]Internal Medicine (Division of Cardiology), and [c]Pathology, Baylor University Medical Center at Dallas, Texas; and [d]Department of Epidemiology, Office of Chief Quality Officer, Baylor Scott & White Health, Dallas, Texas. Manuscript received October 2, 2014; accepted October 4, 2014.

Funding: The study was funded by the Cardiovascular Research Review Committee of the Baylor Health Care System Foundation, Dallas, Texas.

See page 139 for disclosure information.

*Corresponding author: Tel: 214-820-7911; fax: 214-820-7533.
E-mail address: wc.roberts@baylorhealth.edu (W.C. Roberts).

[1] K.H.B is a sophomore, Rice University, Houston, TX 77005.

Table 1
Reported Frequency 1938-1968 of Rupture of the Left Ventricular Free Wall or Ventricular Septum in 12,984 Necropsy Patients with Fatal Acute Myocardial Infarction

Author (Year) [Reference]	No. Patients With Fatal AMI	Rupture Cases				
		Number Ruptured	Location		M/F	Ages (Years) Range (Mean)
			LV	VS		
BEFORE CORONARY CARE UNITS						
Bean (1938) [1]	300	17 (6%)	16	1	8/9	-
Edmonson and Hoxie (1942) [2]	865	72 (8%)	59	13	40/32	30-90 (-)
Friedman & White (1944) [3]	105	10 (10%)	10	0	7/3	51-80 (66)
Diaz-River & Miller (1948) [4]	53	5 (9%)	4	1	1/4	-
Wang et al (1948) [5]	267	23 (9%)	22	1	-	-
Selzer (1948) [6]	95	8 (8%)	7	1	-	-
Zinn& Cosby (1950) [7]	430	34 (8%)	34	0	12/22	54-82 (71)
Oblath et al (1952) [8]	1,026	80 (9%)	80	0	47/33	60-80 (-)
Wessler et al (1952) [9]	124	20 (16%)	15	5	-	-
Waldron et al (1954) [10]	545	40 (8%)	40	0	-	-
Goetz & Gropper (1954) [11]	145	14 (10%)	11	3	-	56-76 (-)
Maher et al (1956) [12]	183	21 (12%)	19	2	10/11	54-92 (69)
Griffith et al (1961) [13]	1,212	52 (4%)	44	8	-	-
Spiekerman et al (1962) [14]	87	21 (24%)	18	3	10/11	-
Ross & Young (1963) [15]	606	43 (7%)	43	0	27/16	35-90 (-)
London & London (1965) [16]	1,001	47 (5%)	42	5	27/20	- (69)
Sievers (1966) [17]	811	104 (13%)	104	0	52/52	- (69)
Sugiura et al (1968) [18]	50	8 (16%)	6	2	5/3	68-88 (77)
Lewis (1969) [19]	1,228	106 (9%)	106	0	52/54	42-92 (71)
Subtotal	9,133	725 (8%)	680 (94%)	45 (6%)	298/270 (52%)/(48%)	30-92 (-)
AFTER CORONARY CARE UNITS						
Hammer et al (1972) [20]	47	10 (21%)	7	3	6/4	55-80 (64)
Rasmussen et al (1979) [21]	401	64 (16%)	61	3	42/30	46-90 (-)
Dellborg et al (1985) [22]	329	56 (17%)	51	5	28/28	- (71)
Hiramori (1987) [23]	143	26 (18%)	20	6	-	23-92 (62)
Herlitz (1988) [24]	76	32 (42%)*	32	0	-	- (67)†
Reddy & Roberts (1989) [25]	648	204 (31%)‡	137	53	112/92	43-94 (68)
Batts et al (1990) [26]	1,251	100 (8%)	100	0	51/49	- (74)†
Pollak et al (1994) [27]	533	105 (20%)§	105	0	-	-
Hutchins et al (2002) [28]	153	47 (31%)‖	47	0	22/25	46-97 (70)
Markowicz-Pawlus et al (2012) [29]	270	49 (18%)	49	0	12/37	- (70)
Subtotal	3,851	693 (18%)	609 (90%)	70 (10%)	273/265 (51%)/(49%)	23-97 (-)

AMI = acute myocardial infarction; LV = left ventricular free wall; VS = ventricular septum; - = no information available.
* Study does not specify location of rupture.
† Mean age calculated as a weighted average of ages reported by the authors in separate patient groups.
‡ Five of these patients also had rupture of a left ventricular papillary muscle.
§ One case of rupture diagnosed intraoperatively.
‖ Includes one reported case of right ventricular free wall rupture.

prepared in each heart. Each was stained by hematoxylin-eosin and by the trichrome method and all sections were examined by WCR and frequently by JMG.

The medical records were obtained in all 64 patients and data in each of the variables listed in Tables 2 and 3 were sought.

Inclusion into this study required the presence at necropsy of AMI and the onset of the AMI *before* admission to BUMC. Patients who developed an AMI after admission to the hospital were not included. The later patients, for example, were those who developed an AMI after a percutaneous coronary intervention or after coronary bypass or cardiac valve replacement or ascending aorta resection or hepatic or renal or cardiac transplantation or during or shortly after hemodialysis (for chronic renal disease). Additionally, patients who developed a coronary embolus during active infective endocarditis were excluded. The attempt was to collect a non-rupture group of AMI patients as similar as possible to the rupture group of AMI patients.

Means, standard deviations (SDs) and percentages were calculated to describe the study cohort (n=64). Differences in demographic and clinical details were tested with a Wilcoxon (for continuous factors) or a chi-square (for categorical factors) test. Unadjusted p-values were also

Table 2
Clinical and Morphologic Findings in 25 Patients with Fatal Rupture of Left Ventricular Free Wall, Ventricular Septum, and/or Papillary Muscle Secondary to Acute Myocardial Infarction and Studied at Baylor University Medical Center from July 1993 through July 2014

Patient Number	Age	Race	Sex	BMI (kg/m²)	DM	SH	BP Rx	CABG	TT	PCI	LV Scar	Rupture Site	Location of AMI	Interval of Onset MI to Death (Days)	RV Infarct	HW (g)	Float	H	Figure Number
1	68	W	F	24.2	+	0	0	0	+	+	0	LVFW	A	2	0	375	+	+	-
2	70	B	F	-	+	+	-	0	0	0	0	LVFW	L	3	0	405	0	+	3
3	72	B	F	-	0	+	-	0	+	0	0	LVFW	Apical	1	0	415	-	+	-
4	72	W	F	28.2	0	+	0	0	+	+	0	LVFW	P	6	0	555	+	+	4
5*	78	W	F	23.9	0	+	0	+	+	+	0	LVFW	A	1	0	325	-	+	-
6	83	W	F	41.3	0	0	0	0	0	+	0	LVFW	P	4	+	415	+	+	5
7	47	W	M	28.3	0	0	0	0	0	+	0	LVFW	A	45	0	435	+	+	6
8	57	W	M	27.2	0	+	+	+	+	0	0	LVFW	A	15	0	640	+	+	-
9*	66	W	M	25.8	0	+	0	+	0	0	+	LVFW	A	2	0	430	+	+	-
10	67	W	M	28.4	0	+	0	0	0	+	0	LVFW	A	3	0	390	+	+	7
11	67	W	M	29.4	+	+	+	0	0	0	0	LVFW	P	3	0	660	+	+	8
12	70	W	M	24.3	+	+	+	0	0	+	0	LVFW	P	5	0	395	+	0	-
13	70	W	M	30.4	0	+	0	0	0	0	0	LVFW	P	4	0	530	+	+	-
14	75	W	M	30.1	0	+	0	0	0	+	0	LVFW	L	2	0	450	+	+	9
15	75	W	M	25.2	+	+	+	0	0	0	0	LVFW	P	3	+	575	+	+	-
16	78	W	M	26.8	0	+	+	0	+	0	0	LVFW	A	1	0	415	+	+	10
17	81	W	M	-	0	+	-	0	0	0	0	VS	A	1	0	500	+	0	-
18	80	W	F	27.4	0	-	-	0	0	+	0	PM[‡]	P	3	+	380	0	0	11
19	62	W	M	31.6	0	+	+	+[§]	0	0	0	PM[‡]	A	3	0	570	+	0[†]	-
20*	63	W	M	27.1	0	+	+	0	0	0	0	PM[‡]	P	2	0	740	+	0	-
21	72	W	F	25.1	0	+	+	0	+	0	0	LVFW & VS	P	3	+	310	+	+	12
22	67	W	M	26.1	+	+	0	+	0	+	0	LVFW & VS	P	7	+	480	+	0[†]	13
23	67	W	M	26.9	0	+	0	0	0	0	0	LVFW & VS	P	1	+	530	0	+	-
24	81	W	M	32.3	0	+	0	0	+	+	0	LVFW & VS	P	4	+	565	0	+	14
25	77	W	F	30.2	0	+	0	+	0	0	0	LVFW & PM	L	7	0	525	+	+	15

Abbreviations: A = anterior; AMI = acute myocardial infarct; B = black; BMI = body mass index; BP = blood pressure; C = circumferential; CABG = coronary artery bypass graft; DM = diabetes mellitus; F = female; HW = heart weight; H=hemopericardium; Hx = history; L = lateral; LV = left ventricular; LVFW = left ventricular free wall; M = male; P = posterior; PCI = percutaneous coronary intervention; PM = papillary muscle; RV = right ventricular; Rx = therapy; SH = systemic hypertension; TT=thrombolytic therapy; VS = ventricular septum; W = white; 0 = absent or negative; + = present or positive; - = no information available.

* Heart specimen was not examined by WCR, but photographs taken at autopsy were available.

† No hemopericardium due to earlier CABG causing absence of pericardial space (diffuse adherence of parietal and epicardial surface).

‡ Partial rupture.

§ Redo CABG performed.

estimated. A Bonferroni correction was employed to account for multiplicity.

The study protocol was approved by the Institutional Review Board of Baylor University Medical Center.

Results

Findings in each of the 25 patients with cardiac rupture secondary to AMI are detailed in Table 2 and the findings in them are compared to the 39 non-rupture patients in Table 3. The number of cases observed during each of the 22 years are shown in Figure 1. Of the 25 rupture cases, 16 (64%) had isolated rupture of the LVFW; 1 (4%), isolated rupture of the VS; 3 (12%), isolated rupture of a single PM, and 6 (24%) patients had combined rupture (both LVFW and VS in 4 and rupture of the LVFW plus PM [anterolateral] in 1.) (Figures 2-15).The interval from AMI to death varied from 1 to 45 days (median 3). Eight (32%) rupture patients received thrombolysis during the AMI, and 11 (44%) had percutaneous coronary intervention after admission for AMI. Five patients (20%) underwent coronary artery bypass grafting after onset of the AMI, all 5 within 5 days of death. An additional patient had coronary artery bypass grafting 6 years before the fatal AMI.

In the 21 patients with LVFW rupture, the rupture site was at the junction of the LVFW and VS in 18 patients (82%): anterior in 7 and posterior in 10; in 3 others in the lateral wall, and in 1 at the apex (Figure 2). Of the 5 patients with rupture of the VS, 1 was anterior, and the other 4, all of whom also had LVFW rupture, was posterior. Of the latter 4 patients the rupture of the VS was partial, not complete. Of the 4 patients with PM rupture, all partial, the posteromedial muscle was involved in 2 and the anterolateral muscle in 2.

The unadjusted comparison of floating heart, left ventricular scar, diabetes mellitus, body mass index, age, and presence of hemopericardium between non-rupture and rupture patients were statistically significant (Table 3).

Discussion

The present study examines certain clinical and necropsy findings in 64 patients admitted to a single hospital during a 22-year period because of AMI, and compares the 25 (39%) with rupture of the LVFW or VS or PM or combinations to the

Table 3
Clinical and Necropsy Findings in 64 Patients with Fatal Acute Myocardial Infarction: 25 Patients with Cardiac Rupture and 39 without Rupture

Variable	Rupture		P Value*
	Yes (n=25)	No (n=39)	
Men : Women	16 (64%) : 9 (36%)	23 (59%) : 16 (41%)	0.690
Ages (years) range (mean)			0.001
Men	47-81 (68)	33-83 (56)	
Women	68-83 (75)	42-88 (65)	
Black : white	2 (8%) : 23 (92%)	10 (28%) : 26 (72%)†	0.060
Body mass index (kg/m^2)			0.048
Men	15/16	12/23	
Range (mean)	24.3-32.3 (28.0)	26.0-64.6 (35.3)	
Women	7/9	13/16	
Range (mean)	23.9-41.3 (28.6)	18.7-49.5 (31.2)	
Diabetes mellitus			0.034
Men	4 (25%)	6/19 (32%)	
Women	2 (22%)	12 (75%)	
Systemic hypertension (by history)			0.162
Men	15/16 (94%)	17/20 (85%)	
Women	6/8 (75%)	9 (56%)	
Coronary bypass	6 (24%)	11/35 (31%)	0.532
Thrombolytic therapy	8 (32%)	4 (10%)	0.031
Percutaneous coronary intervention	11 (44%)	17/38 (45%)	0.954
Left ventricular Scar	1 (4%)	11 (28%)	0.016
Location of AMI			0.470
Posterior	12 (48%)	22 (56%)	
Anterior	9 (36%)	10 (26%)	
Lateral	3 (12%)	5 (13%)	
Circumferential	0	2 (5%)	
Apical	1 (4%)	0	
Right ventricular Infarct	7 (28%)	5 (13%)	0.132
Heart weight (g) range (mean)			0.929
Men	390-740 (519)	375-1060 (565)	
Women	310-555 (412)	310-660 (402)	
Floating Heart	19/23 (83%)	6/30 (20%)	<0.001
Hemopericardium	19 (76%)	0	<0.0001

AMI=acute myocardial infarction.
* P-values account for multiple comparisons.
† Data missing in 3 patients.

39 patients (61%) studied in the same hospital and during the same time frame without cardiac rupture. Patients developing an AMI after admission to the hospital were excluded. Compared to the non-rupture cases, the rupture cases were significantly older (71 years – vs – 60 years); had a much higher frequency of huge deposits of adipose tissue in the heart (floated in formaldehyde) (88% – vs – 20%); a much lower frequency of having a healed myocardial infarct (scar) (4% – vs – 28%); a lower frequency of diabetes mellitus (24% – vs – 47%); a lower body mass index (28.2 kg/m^2– vs – 33.2 kg/m^2), and a higher frequency of thrombolytic therapy during the AMI (32% – vs – 10%).

Although the present report indicated a significant difference in age (mean 71 – vs – 60 years) between the rupture and none rupture groups, that has not been the case uniformly. Mann and Roberts (40), for example, found no significant difference in mean ages among men – vs – women in 138 necropsy patients with –vs – 50 without LVFW rupture (men: 63 years – vs – 63 years; women: 73 years – vs – 71 years) or a difference in 38 unoperated necropsy patients with – vs – without rupture of the VS (men: 65 years – vs – 63 years; women: 74 years – vs – 71 years) (39). Of the 22 patients with rupture of the PM secondary to AMI reported by Barbour and Roberts,[36] the mean ages of the 15 men was 60 years (non-rupture mean age 63 years) and that in the 7 women, 75 years (non-rupture mean age 71 years). The mean ages of the women were significantly higher than that of the men in both the rupture and non-rupture groups in all these studies.

Because AMI is more common in men than women, the proportion of men in most published studies of rupture secondary to AMI is slightly higher in men but the percentage of men is less than in the AMI group without rupture. Of the 444 non-rupture cases of AMI studied at necropsy by Reddy and Roberts,[25] 70% were men and 30% were women; of the 204 rupture cases (LVFW or VS) studied by the same authors, 55% were men and 45% were women. Of the 22 cases of rupture of the PM reported by Barbour and Roberts,[36] 15 were men (68%) and 7 (32%) were women.

Although most patients with AMI have a body mass index ≥ 25 Kg/m^2, the mean BMI in the present study was significantly *lower* in the rupture group than in the non-rupture

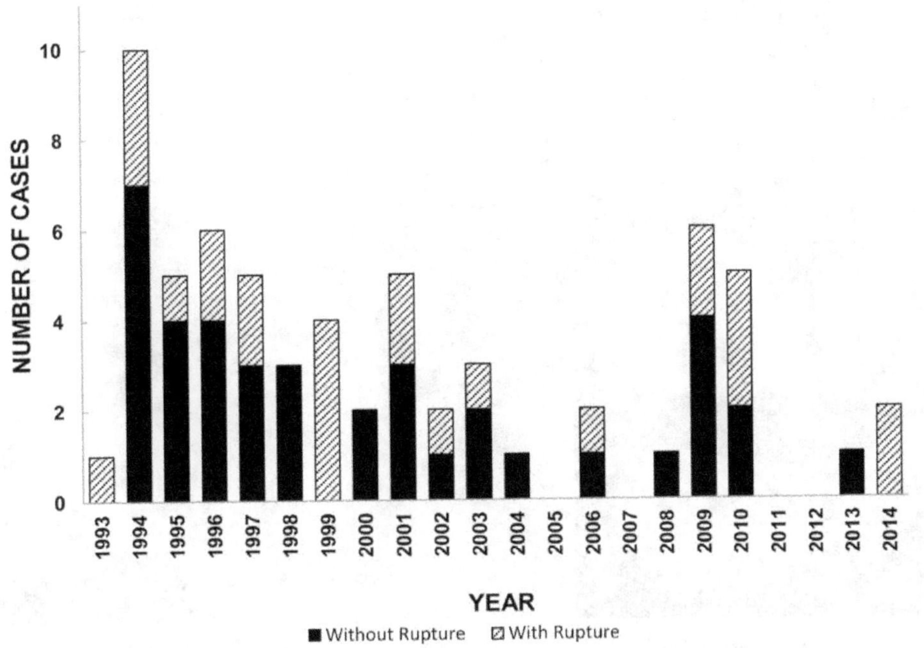

Figure 1. Bar graph Comparing the number of patients with fatal acute myocardial infarction at Baylor University Medical Center from 1993 through June 2014 showing the patients with acute myocardial infarction without rupture in black and those with rupture in gray. Of the total 64 patients studied both clinically and at necropsy, 25 had rupture of the left ventricular free wall or ventricular septum or left ventricular papillary muscle or combinations and 39 had fatal acute myocardial infarction without rupture.

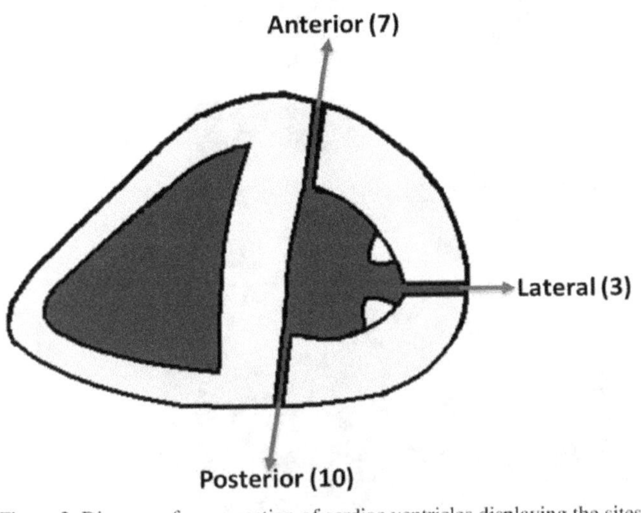

Figure 2. Diagram of cross-section of cardiac ventricles displaying the sites of the 21 left ventricular free wall ruptures. The left ventricular free wall ruptures were anterior in 7 patients, posterior in 10, and lateral (roughly between the 2 papillary muscles) in 3 patients. The left and right ventricular cavities are shown in red and the myocardium in yellow.

group. This finding is surprising because the quantity of adipose was significantly *greater* in the rupture – vs – the non-rupture groups. This finding was also observed in a previous LVFW rupture and VS rupture studies by Mann and Roberts.[37,38] The PM rupture study by Barbour and Roberts,[36] also disclosed a high frequency of cardiac adiposity, specifically a higher frequency of those with floating hearts among the PM rupture than the non-rupture cases. The greater the quantity of cardiac fat the greater the likelihood that the heart will float in a container of formaldehyde.[43] In the present study, 83% of the rupture hearts floated compared to only 20% of the non-rupture hearts. Because adipose tissue is lighter than formaldehyde (or water), hearts with enormous quantities of fat usually float except when the myocardial mass is particularly large. Shirani and colleagues[44] in a necropsy study of cardiac adiposity demonstrated that in the floating hearts the subepicardial adipose tissue constituted a mean of 32 ± 9% (range 21% to 52%) of the cardiac weight. Thus, irrespective of the rupture site, the quantity of cardiac adipose tissue in these patients is nearly always increased.

What does cardiac adipose tissue have to do with cardiac rupture? The cardiac adipose tissue is mainly in the subepicardial regions, particularly over the right ventricle, and around the epicardial coronary arteries particularly those in the atrioventricular sulci, and also in the atrial septa (lipomatous hypertrophy of the atrial septum), but not in the wall of the left ventricle or VS or in the left ventricular PM, the sites where rupture secondary to AMI occur. Although when excessive it usually penetrates the myocardial wall of the right ventricle, subepicardial adipose tissue does not infiltrate the left ventricular free wall, with the exception of sites of healed myocardial infarcts, an infrequent occurrence in patients with non-traumatic cardiac rupture. Cardiac adiposity can be viewed as a reflection of excessive adipose tissue in non-cardiac structures. One might assume from this observation that non-obese people infrequently have cardiac rupture as a consequence of AMI, but most individuals with AMI with or without subsequent rupture are overweight or obese.

Although a few patients with rupture during AMI have preexisting angina pectoris, the AMI complicated by rupture is nearly always the first AMI and virtually always the first clinically recognized AMI. This observation is confirmed by the infrequency of a grossly-visible scar in the left ventricular

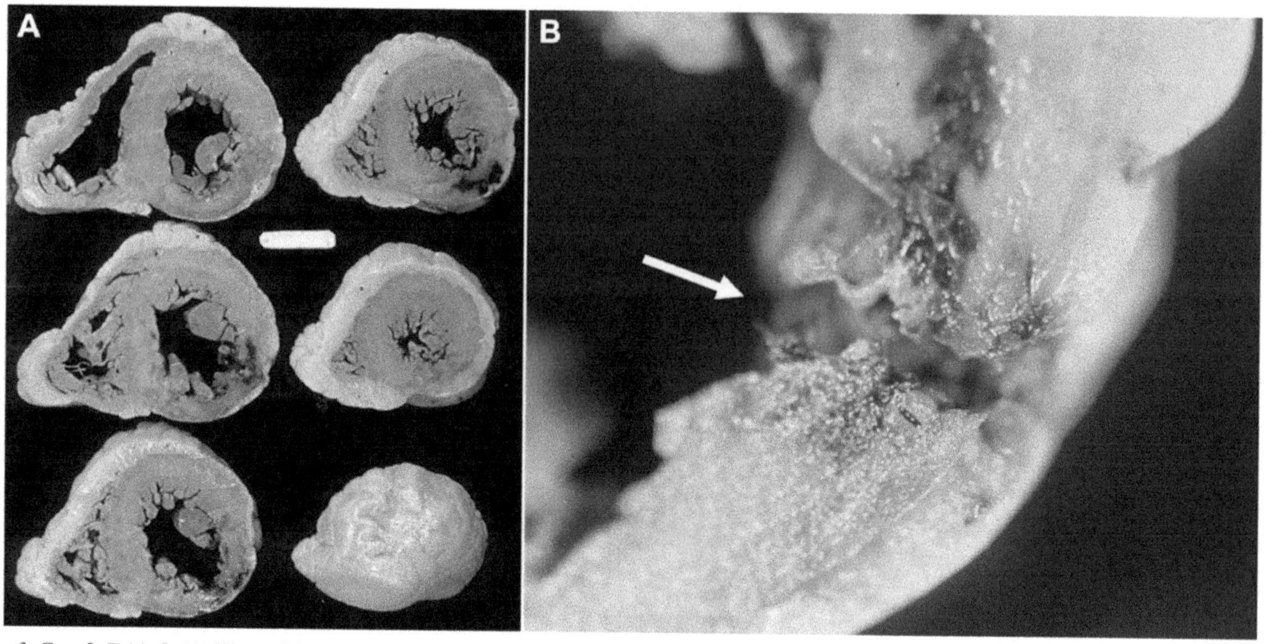

Figure 3. Case 2, Table 2. *(A)* Slices of the cardiac ventricles showing the infarct in the lateral wall and a great deal of subepicardial adipose tissue. *(B)* close-up of the lateral wall rupture showing the rupture site *(arrow)*.

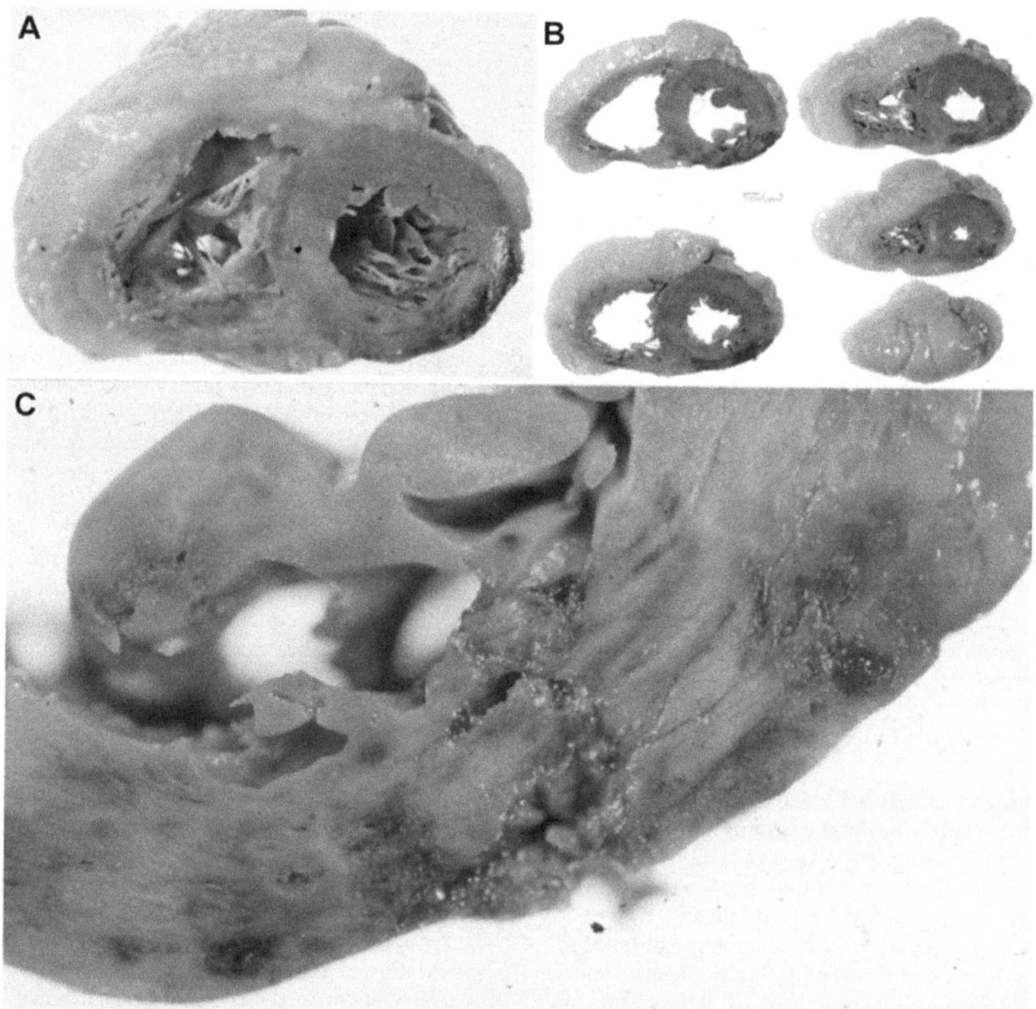

Figure 4. Case 4, Table 2. *(A)* View of both ventricles near the base of the heart. The infarct involves the left ventricular free wall just beneath the posteromedial papillary muscle. The quantity of subepicardial adipose tissue is huge. *(B)* Views of the ventricular cavities and walls caudal to the views shown in *(C)*. *Lower*: Close-up view of the ruptured site.

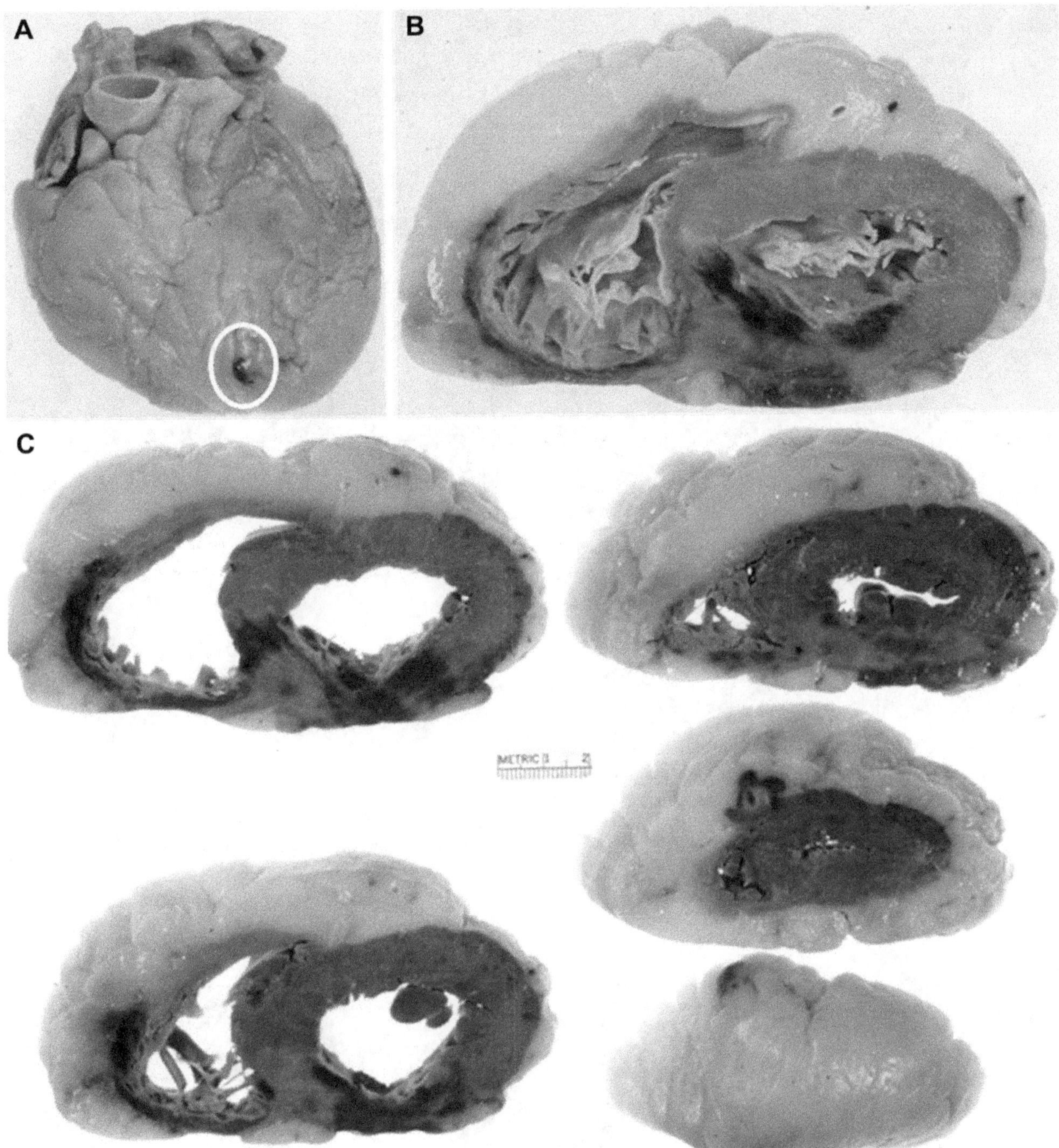

Figure 5. Case 6, Table 2. *(A)* View of the exterior of the heart anteriorly showing an enormous amount of subepicardial adipose tissue and the rupture site near the cardiac apex *(circle)*. *(B)* View of the more basal portion of the ventricles showing the tricuspid and mitral valves, an acute infarction involving the left ventricular free wall posteriorly, the ventricular septum, and a large portion of the right ventricular free wall. *(C)* Views of the ventricles caudal to the view shown in the *(B)*. The basal portions are quite dilated. The amount of infarction of the right ventricular free wall is enormous. The quantity of subepicardial adipose tissue is such that in some of these cross-sections no myocardium is visible exteriorly.

wall in the patients with rupture during AMI. In the present study, only 1 (4%) of the 25 rupture cases compared to 11 (28%) of the 39 non-rupture cases had a scar in the LVFW. In the necropsy study by Reddy and Roberts[25] of 648 cases of AMI, 29 (13%) of the 204 patients with rupture compared to 188 (42%) of 444 non-rupture cases had a preexisting left ventricular scar before the fatal AMI. The infrequency of preexisting left ventricular scar strongly indicates that before the AMI which ruptured that systolic heart failure was absent. Indeed, examination of the hearts with LVFW rupture typically show a non-dilated left ventricular cavity; in contrast, those with rupture of the VS or a PM are usually dilated but the absence of left ventricular scar indicates that the dilatation occurred after the AMI which ruptured not before the event.

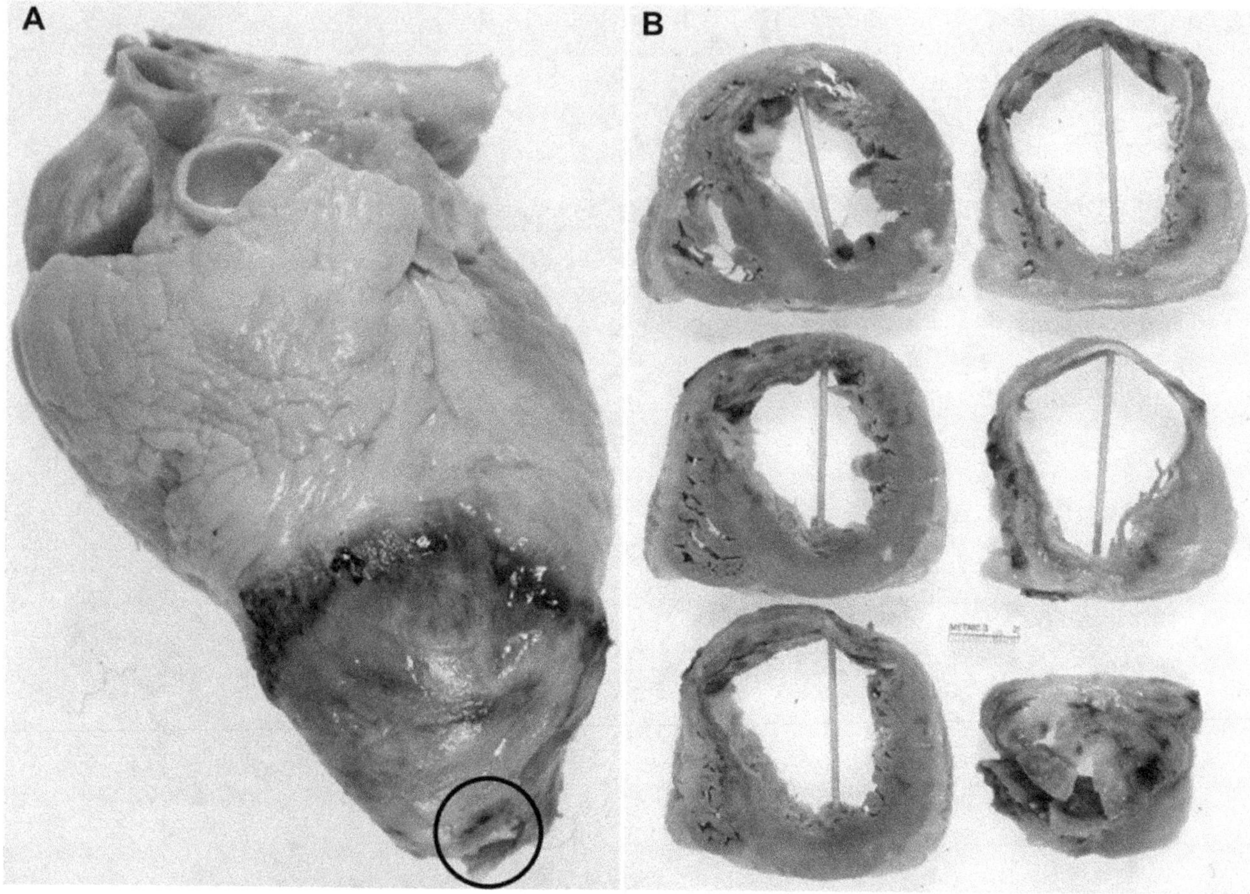

Figure 6. Case 7, Table 2. *(A)* Exterior of the heart, anterior view showing a large apical aneurysm which ruptured at the most apical portion *(circle)*. *(B)* Views of the ventricles showing severe dilatation of the left ventricular cavity, marked thinning of its wall, and, in some sections, nearly circumferential infarction). The rupture site is at the thinnest point shown best in *(B)*. The interval from onset of the acute myocardial infarction to rupture was 45 days, the longest of any of the 26 patients. This long interval allowed the free wall to thin considerably such that the rupture site was not between viable muscle and nonviable muscle but at the most central portion of the large myocardial infarct. Additionally, this was the largest infarct of any of the 25 patients with rupture.

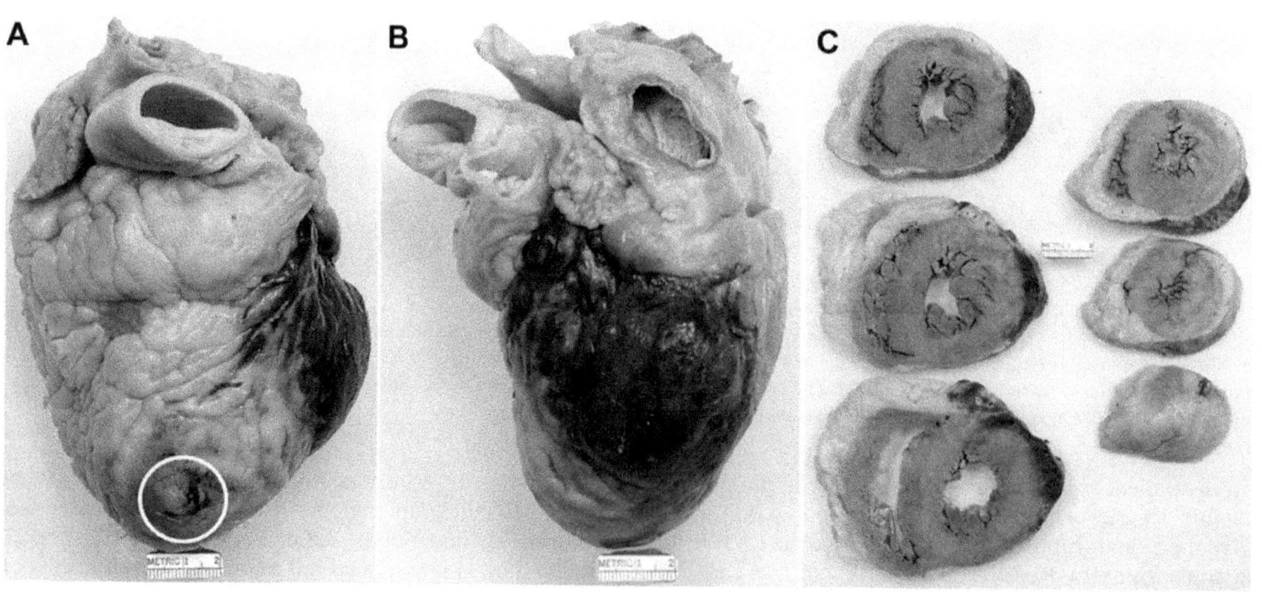

Figure 7. Case 10, Table 2. *(A)* View of the anterior wall of the heart showing hemorrhage into the subepicardial adipose tissue, which is excessive. The rupture site is circled. *(B)* View of the heart from the left lateral aspect showing the extent of the hemorrhage into the subepicardial adipose tissue. *(C)* Cross-sections of the cardiac ventricles showing the rupture site at the junction of the anterior freewall and ventricular septum.

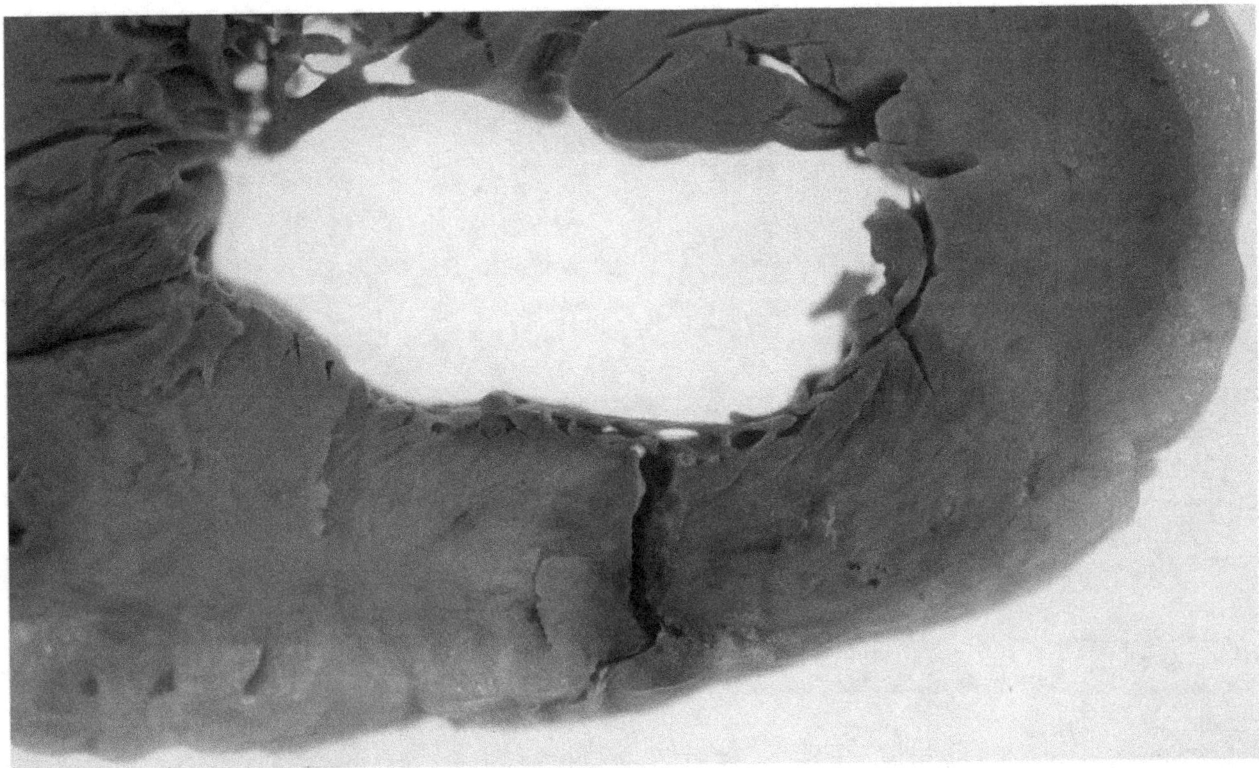

Figure 8. Case 11, Table 2. View of left ventricular freewall showing the rupture site. The size of the acute infarct was relatively small. The quantity of subepicardial adipose tissue is increased.

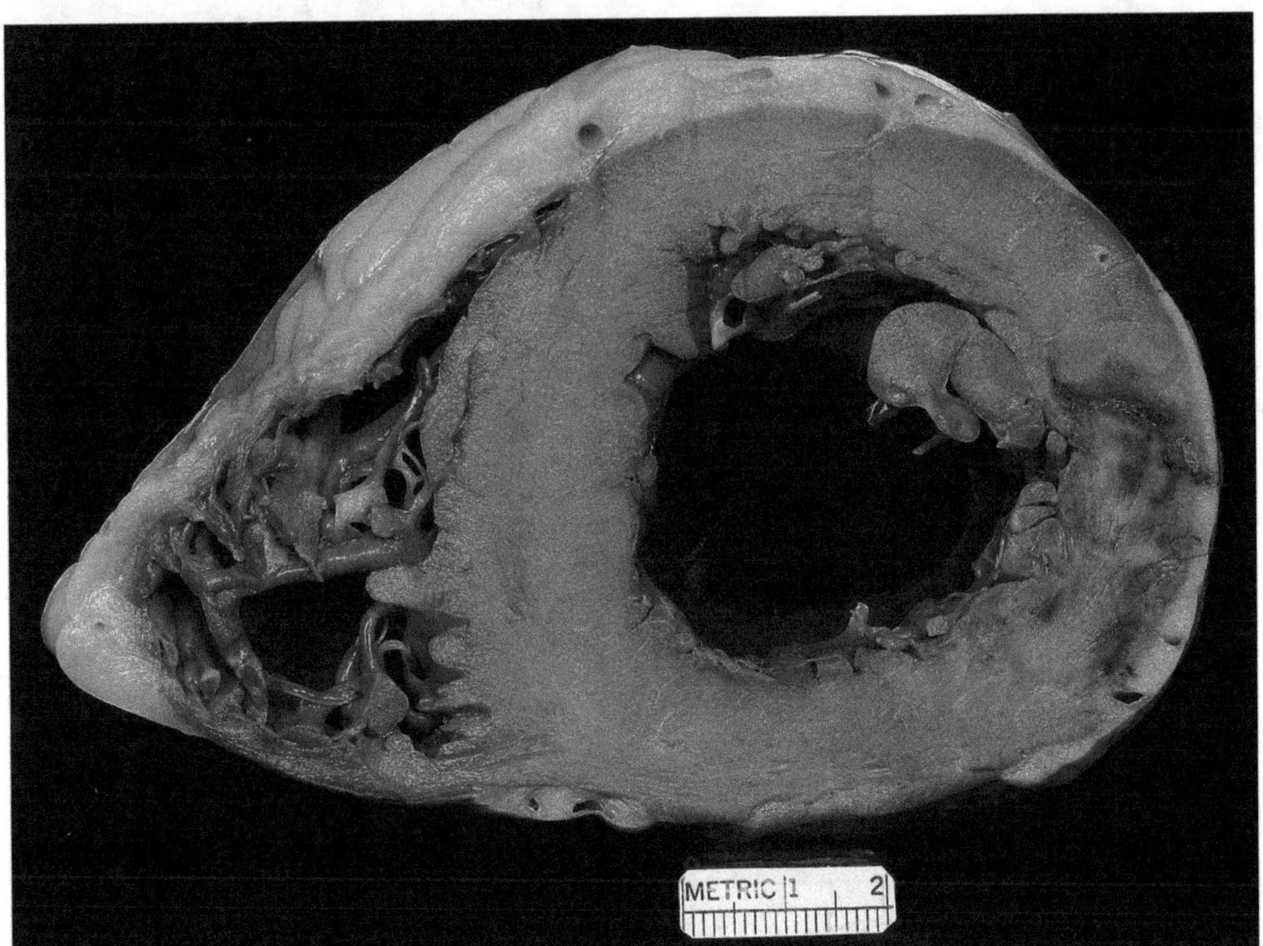

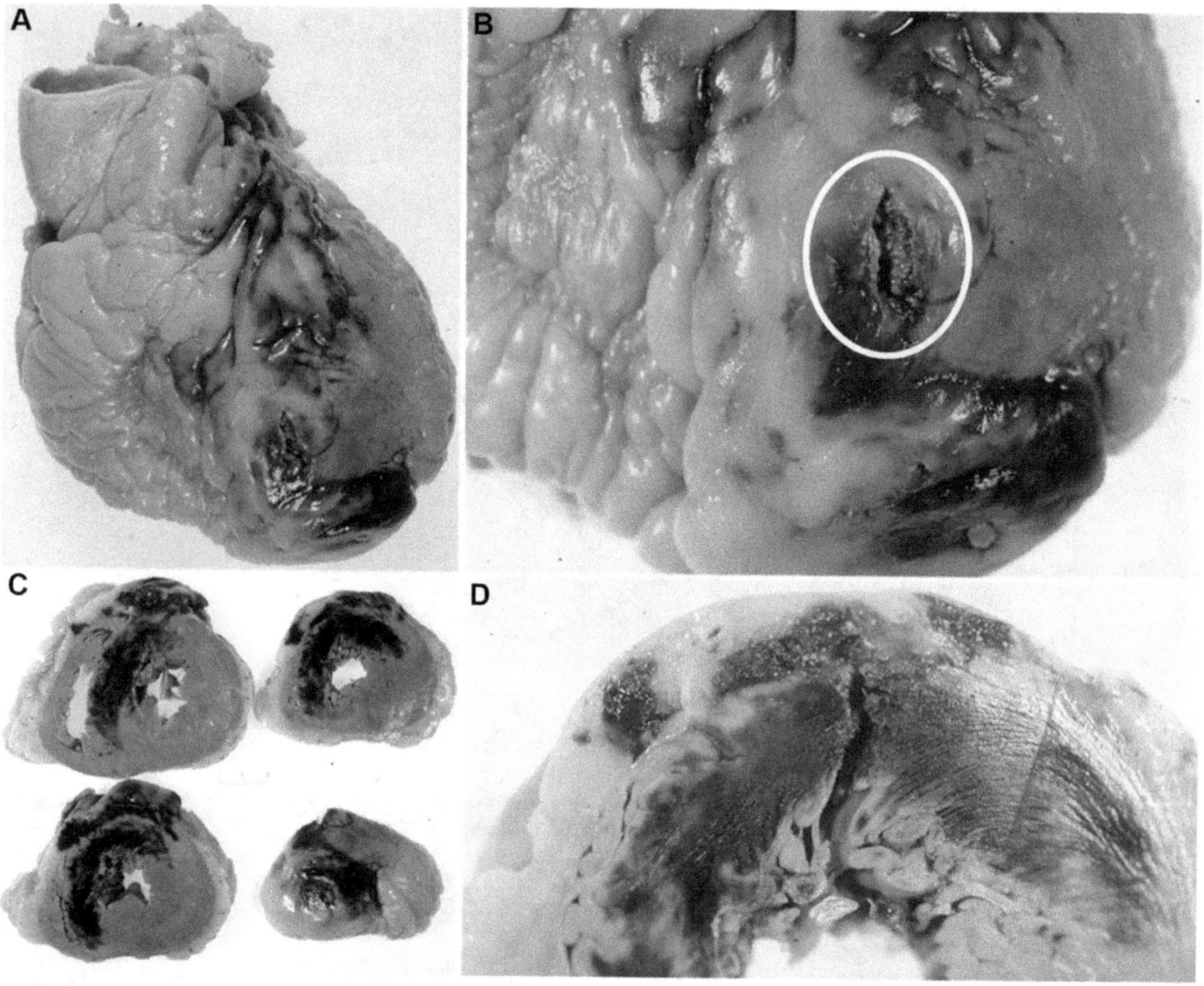

Figure 10. Case 16, Table 2. *(A)* View of the heart anteriorly showing patchy subepicardial hemorrhages. *(B)* View of the rupture site exteriorly *(circle)*. *(C)* Cross-section of the cardiac ventricles showing a large hemorrhagic infarct involving the anteroseptal walls. *(D)* Close up view of the rupture site. The patient received thrombolytic therapy.

Thus, the patient with preexisting heart failure from a previous AMI which healed is very unlikely to rupture with a subsequent AMI. Rupture during AMI generally indicates a good functioning left ventricle before the rupture event and usually up to the actual rupture event in the LVFW rupture cases. Furthermore and not surprisingly, the size of the acute infarct in the rupture cases is usually smaller than in the non-rupture cases. Saffitz and associates[45] compared at necropsy the size of the acute infarct in AMI patients in whom death was caused by cardiogenic shock, arrhythmia, or cardiac rupture, and found that the patients dying from cardiogenic shock had the largest acute infarcts ($37 \pm 11\%$ of the total left ventricular mass), and those who died of cardiac rupture had the smallest infarcts ($15 \pm 9\%$).

Much has been written on the relation of systemic hypertension *before* the AMI which ruptured but the results are conflicting. Although it appears logical that elevation of the peak left ventricular systolic pressure persisting *after* AMI would more likely lead to rupture compared to patients in whom the peak left ventricular systolic pressure fell to normal or lower levels, such evidence is speculative at best. The frequency of systemic hypertension before the AMI was insignificantly different in the present study and in the previous Reddy and Roberts study between the rupture and non-rupture groups.[25] Additionally, heart weights were insignificantly different between the rupture and non-rupture cases in the present and in the previous Reddy and Roberts[25] study. Preexisting hypertension of course may cause thickening of the LVFW, VS, and PMs. One could reason that the thicker these structures the less likely they might rupture. In only 3 (12%) of the 25 rupture cases in the present study did the heart weigh > 600 g.

One might be surprised by the high frequency of rupture in the present study (39% of the total AMI cases). All of the patients included herein were studied in the last 2 decades, a period of improved medicines to manage patients with AMI and of course hospitalization in the coronary care units where now fatal arrhythmias are relatively infrequent. Reddy and Roberts[25] reviewed published reports of the frequency of rupture of the LVFW or VS among necropsy cases of AMI *before* and *after* the widespread use of coronary care units (Table 1): the frequency of rupture ranged

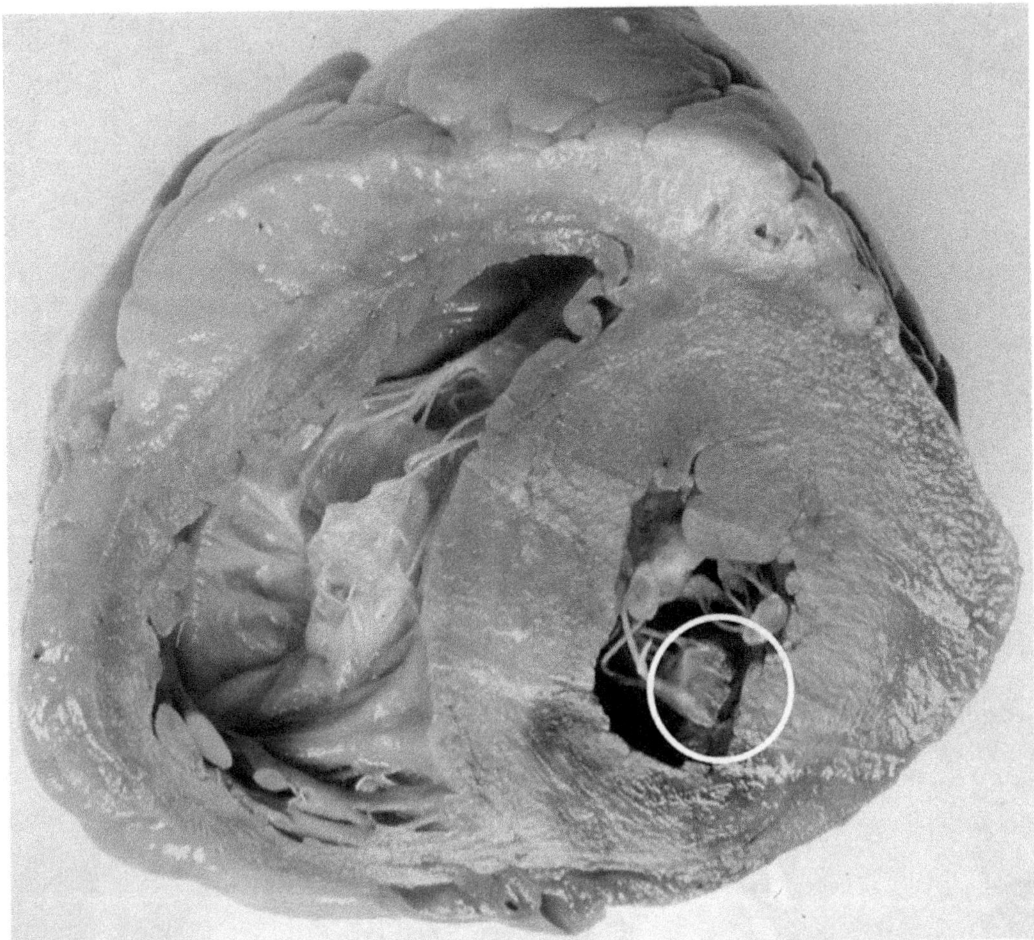

Figure 11. Case 18, Table 2. View of the base of the heart showing a ruptured posteromedial papillary muscle with an acute infarct involving the posterior wall and a portion of the ventricular septum. The ruptured muscle is circled.

from 4% to 24% (mean 8%) (680 of 9,133 cases); of the 3,851 necropsy patients reported by them *after* the common use of coronary care units, 693 (18%) ruptured the LVFW or VS (Table 1). Of the cases studied by Reddy and Roberts, however, 204 (31%) of the 648 necropsy patients with AMI ruptured.[25] Although the rupture cases are probably more likely to have an autopsy, the frequency of rupture of the LVFW or VS as a cause of death during AMI appears to have increased substantially since the widespread use of coronary care units, even though the total mortality from AMI has decreased dramatically (from roughly 35% to the present 5%).

The relation of thrombolysis therapy during AMI to the frequency of cardiac rupture remains unclear. Thrombolysis tends to convert an ischemic (pale) infarct into a hemorrhagic infarct. Roberts and colleagues[46] demonstrated experimentally in dogs that ischemic and hemorrhagic infarcts healed at the same rates. In the present study the frequency of thrombolysis therapy was significantly higher in the rupture cases compared to the non-rupture cases (32% – vs – 10%). Among the 648 AMI cases studied by Reddy and Roberts,[25] 56 (9%) had received streptokinase or recombinant tissue-type plasminogen activator during the first hours after onset of AMI: 18 (32%) had rupture of the LVFW or VS, a percentage similar to that in the group who had not received thrombolytic therapy (186 of 592 [31%]). Pollak et al[27] found LVFW rupture during AMI in 3 (0.7%) of 447 patients treated with thrombolysis and in 102 (4%) of 2,403 patients not treated with thrombolysis (84% autopsy rate). Yusuf and colleagues[47] pooled the results of 33 randomized trials of thrombolytic agents for AMI, and found similar frequencies of cardiac rupture in patients and in control subjects. Honan et al[48] pooled the results of 4 randomized trials involving 1,638 patients, and observed that the risk of rupture (58 cases, autopsy rate $\geq$ 50%) was directly correlated with time to treatment.

Few studies have reported on the degrees of narrowing of the major epicardial coronary arteries in patients with cardiac rupture secondary to AMI. Mann and Roberts[39,40] compared the number of major (right, left anterior descending, and left circumflex) epicardial coronary arteries narrowed > 75% in cross-sectional area by atherosclerotic plaque alone and found that the rupture cases (LVFW or VS) had significantly less narrowing than did the non-rupture cases. As shown in Table 4, both the LVFW and the VS rupture cases had a lower percent of patients with all of these 3 major coronary arteries narrowed > 75% in cross-sectional area by plaque and also a lower percent of major

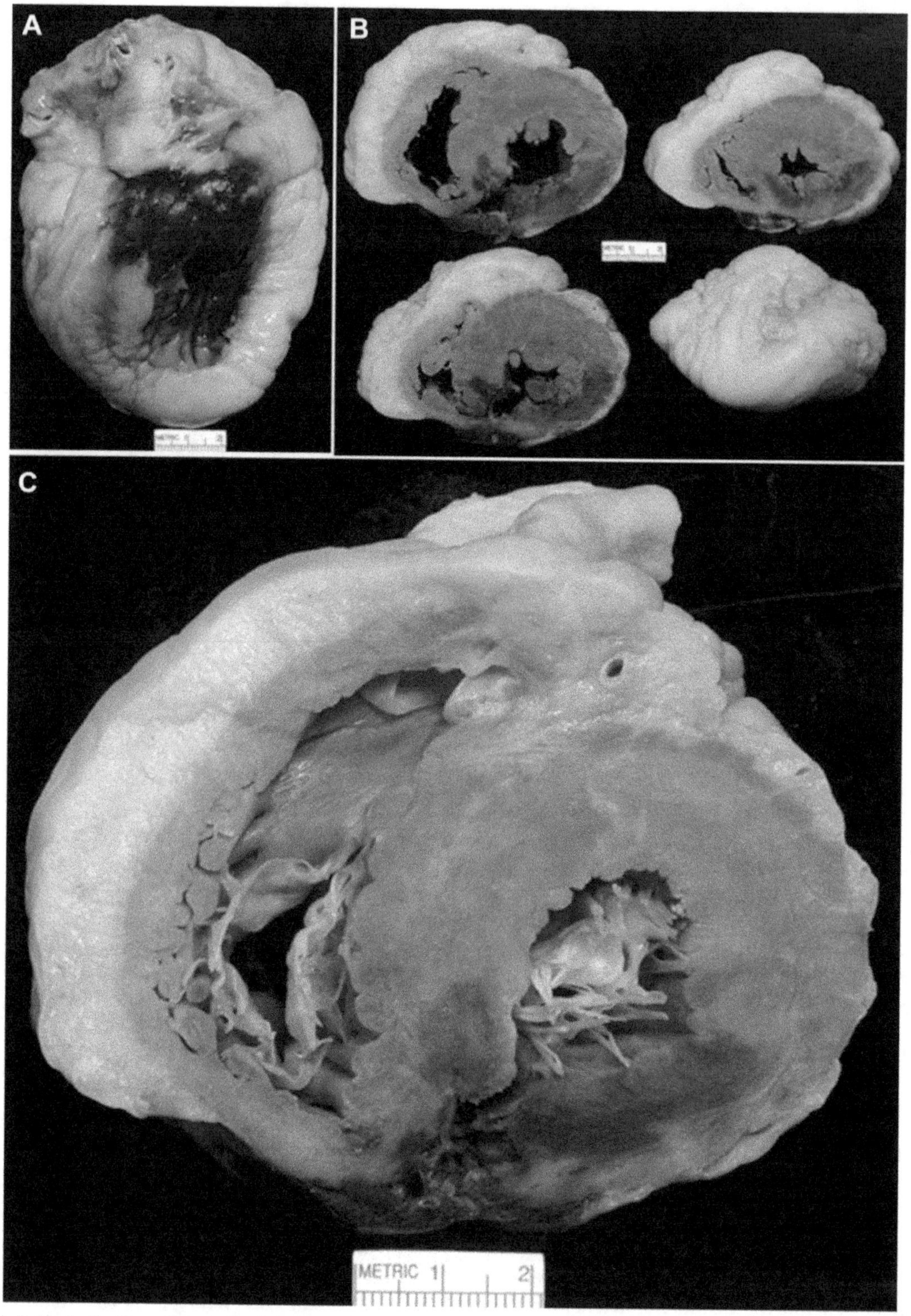

Figure 12. Case 21, Table 2. *(A)* View of the back of the heart showing a great deal of blood in the subepicardial adipose tissue. *(B)* View of the ventricles showing the rupture site involving both ventricular septum and left ventricular free wall. The quantity of subepicardial adipose tissue is enormous. *(C)* Close-up view of the rupture site. The infarct is hemorrhagic. The patient received thrombolytic therapy.

arteries narrowed insignificantly (≤25%) by plaque. Additionally, these authors[39,40] also studied the extent of the atherosclerotic process in these patients by examining each 5-mm long segment histologically of the 4 (includes left main) major epicardial coronary arteries. As shown in Table 5, the LVFW and VS rupture cases had 50% fewer 5-mm segments narrowed > 75% by atherosclerotic plaque and also about double the percent of segments narrowed ≤ 25% in cross-sectional area. The Mann and Roberts[39,40] studies were the first to examine carefully the status of the epicardial coronary arteries in rupture – vs – non-rupture cases. Barbour and Roberts[36] also studied the status of the

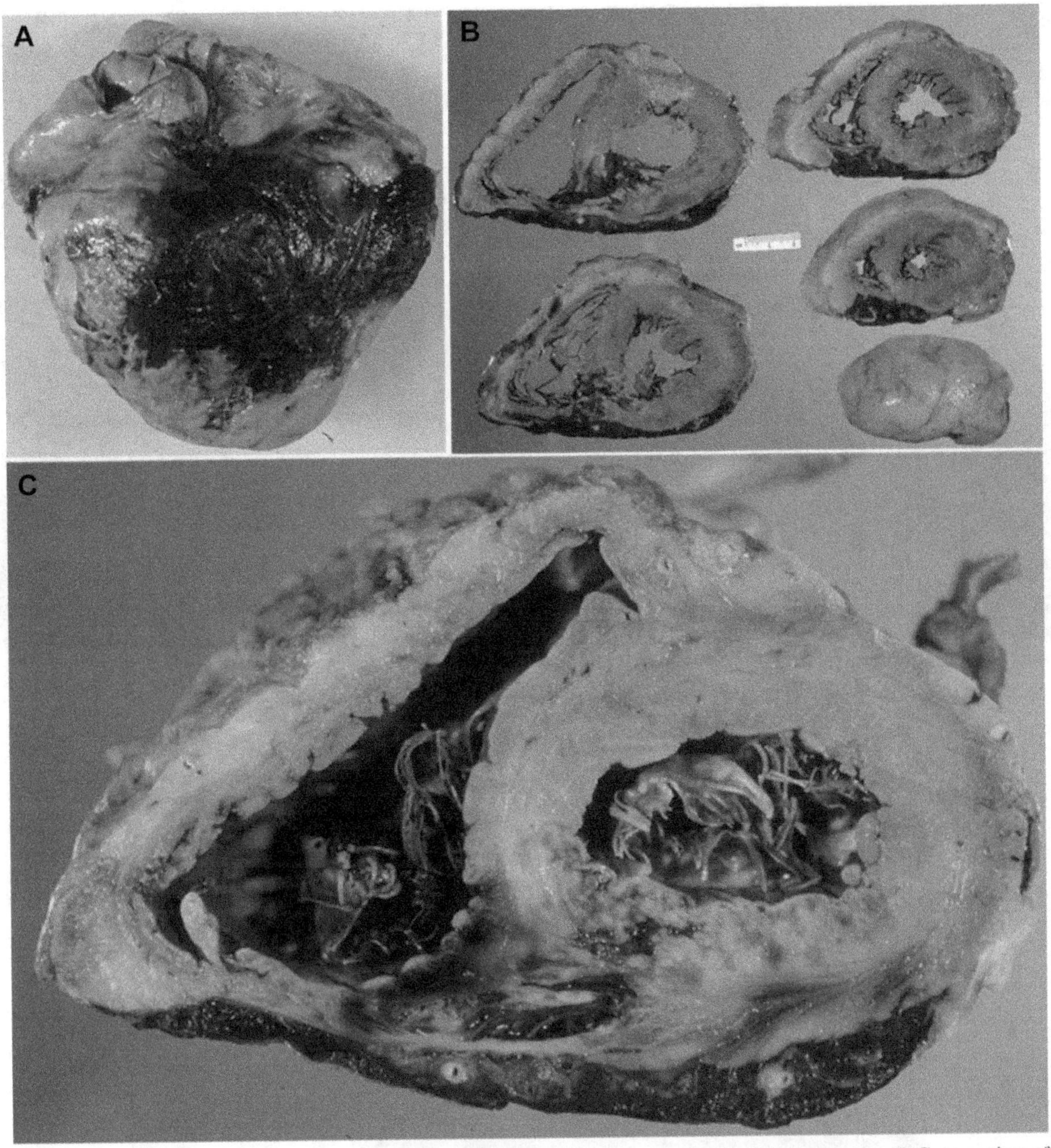

Figure 13. Case 22, Table 2. *(A)* Back of the heart showing a huge amount of hemorrhage into the subepicardial adipose tissue. *(B)* Cross-sections of the cardiac ventricles showing rupture of the ventricular septum and of the left ventricular free wall just posterior to the septum. *(C)* Close-up view of the ruptured site through the left ventricular free wall and ventricular septum show the ventricular septal rupture and also its exit from the right ventricular free wall.

epicardial coronary arteries in necropsy patients with PM rupture and also found significantly less coronary narrowing in the PM rupture group than in their non-rupture control group. A different control group was used than used in the LVFW and VS Mann and Roberts studies. In the LVFW and VS studies both patients and controls had no left ventricular scars (These cases were excluded.), whereas in the PM studies nearly half of the control group had left ventricular scars (a previously healed myocardial infarct).

Some features of the present study make it a bit different from previously reported ones on cardiac rupture. With the exception of 3 cases, all 64 hearts were studied at necropsy by the same individual (WCR) and described, weighed, and sectioned by him. The information as a consequence would appear to be more reliable than that obtained simply by examining autopsy records produced by many different individuals with varying degrees of expertise in cardiovascular disease. A limitation of course of the present study is the number of cases studied in a 22-year-period at a very large tertiary hospital with an autopsy rate of approximately 4% among hospital deaths. As shown in Figure 1 the number of patients with onset of AMI before hospitalization with later autopsy ranged from none in 4 years to as high as 10 in one year; in 2 years all AMI cases coming to autopsy had rupture. There is likely a greater tendency among clinicians to get an autopsy if

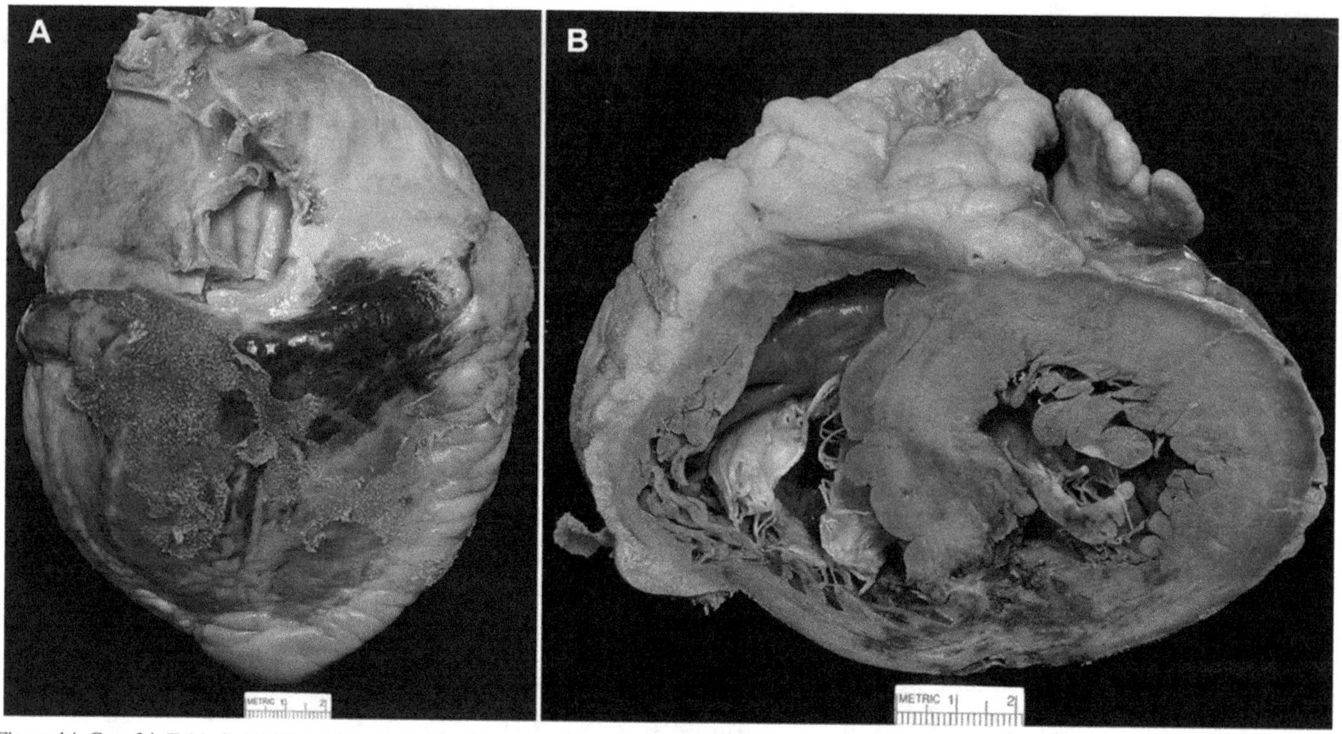

Figure 14. Case 24, Table 2. *(A)* View of the back of the heart showing extravasated blood in and around the right atrioventricular sulcus. *(B)* View of the base of the ventricles showing rupture of the ventricular septum and of the left ventricular free wall. The quantity of subepicardial adipose tissue is considerable.

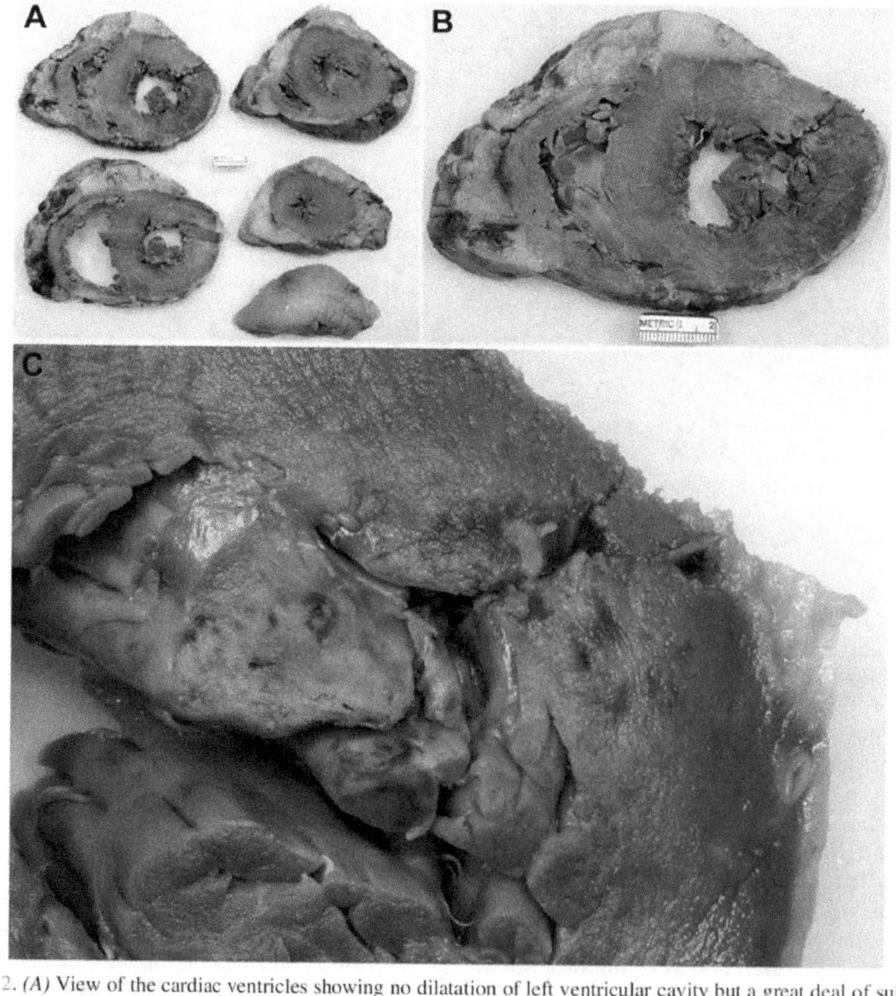

Figure 15. Case 25, Table 2. *(A)* View of the cardiac ventricles showing no dilatation of left ventricular cavity but a great deal of subepicardial adipose tissue. *(B)* View of the rupture site behind the anterolateral papillary muscle. *(C)* Close-up of the rupture site.

Table 4
Number of 3 Major Coronary Arteries (Right, Left Anterior Descending and Left Circumflex) Narrowed > 75% in Cross-Sectional Area by Atherosclerotic Plaque Alone in Patients with Rupture of the Left Ventricular Free Wall — vs — Rupture of the Ventricular Septum — vs — Non-Rupture Controls. All with Fatal First Acute Myocardial Infarction

Number of 3 major (R, LAD, LC) coronary arteries narrowed > 75% in CSA by plaque	Rupture		Non-rupture control (n=50)*
	LVFW (n=117)*	VS (n=33)*	
0	7 (8%)†	1 (3%)†	1 (22%)†
1	25 (28%)	8 (24%)	7 (15%)
2	24 (27%)	9 (27%)	12 (25%)
3	33 (37%)	15 (45%)	28 (58%)

CSA=cross-sectional area; LAD=left anterior descending; LC=left circumflex; LVFW=left ventricular free wall; R=right; VS=ventricular septum.

* Excludes patients with a left ventricular scar (healed myocardial infarct), in other words, all patients included in this table had only a first and only acute myocardial infarction.

† Of these 9 patients, 8 had total occlusion of the coronary artery by thrombus superimposed on atherosclerotic plaque.

Table 5
Analysis of the Extent of Atherosclerotic Plaque in the 4 Major (Right, Left Main, Left Anterior Descending and Left Circumflex) Epicardial Coronary Arteries in Patients with Rupture of the Left Ventricular Free Wall — vs — Rupture of the Ventricular Septum — vs — Non-Rupture Controls with Fatal First Acute Myocardial Infarction

Four categories of cross-sectional area narrowing (%)	Number of 5-mm long 5-mm segments of the 4 major coronary arteries		
	Rupture		Non-rupture Group (Patients=50) (Five-mm segments=1848)
	LVFW (Patients=66) (Five-mm segments=3287)	VS (Patients=18) (Five-mm segments=825)	
0-25	571 (17%)	118 (14%)	132 (7%)
26-50	1186 (31%)	287 (35%)	632 (34%)
51-75	1018 (14%)	319 (39%)	576 (31%)
76-100	513 (15%)	101 (13%)	508 (28%)

LVFW=left ventricular free wall; VS=ventricular septum.

the immediate cause of death is unclear or if rupture is suspected. This likely bias needs to be kept in mind when determining frequency of this particular event. In any study involving cardiac rupture, an autopsy is mandatory to achieve diagnostic accuracy.

Conclusion

Cardiac rupture is an increasingly more frequent cause of death during AMI. It complicates a first AMI, occurs in hearts which contain an enormous quantity of adipose tissue, the left ventricular cavity is usually of normal size until the rupture occurs, and the area of the infarct is usually relatively small.

Disclosures

There are no conflicts of interest and no author has any relation with industry.

1. Bean WB. Infarction of heart: III. Clinical course and morphological findings. *Ann Intern Med* 1938;12:71–94.
2. Edmondson HA, Hoxie HJ. Hypertension and cardiac rupture: A clinical and pathologic study of seventy-two cases, in thirteen of which rupture of the interventricular septum occurred. *Am Heart J* 1942;24: 719–733.
3. Friedman S, White PD. Rupture of the heart in myocardial infarction. *Ann Intern Med* 1944;21:778–782.
4. Diaz-Rivera RS, Miller AJ. Rupture of heart following acute myocardial infarction: incidence in public hospital, with five illustrative cases including one of perforation of interventricular septum diagnosed ante mortem. *Am Heart J* 1948;35:126–133.
5. Wang CH, Bland EF, White PD. Note on coronary occlusion and myocardial infarction found post mortem at Massachusetts General Hospital during twenty year period from 1926 to 1945 inclusive. *Ann Intern Med* 1948;29:601–606.
6. Selzer A. Immediate sequelae of myocardial infarction: their relation to prognosis. *Am J Med Sci* 1948;216:172–178.
7. Zinn WJ, Cosby RS. Myocardial infarction: Statistical study of 679 autopsy-proven cases. *Am J Med* 1950;8:169–176.
8. Oblath RW, Levinson DC, Griffith GC. Factors influencing rupture of the heart after myocardial infarction. *JAMA* 1952;149: 1276–1281.
9. Wessler S, Zoll PM, Schlesinger MI. The pathogenesis of spontaneous cardiac rupture. *Circulation* 1952;6:334–351.
10. Waldron BR, Fennell RH, Castleman B, Bland EF. Myocardial rupture and hemopericardium associated with anticoagulant therapy. *N Engl J Med* 1954;251:829–894.
11. Goetz AA, Gropper AN. Perforation of the interventricular septum. Report of three cases with ante-mortem diagnosis. *Am Heart J* 1954;48: 103–140.
12. Maher JF, Mallory GK, Laurenz GA. Rupture of the heart after myocardial infarction. *N Engl J Med* 1956;255:1–10.
13. Griffith GC, Hedge B, Oblath RW. Factors in myocardial rupture: An analysis of 204 cases at Los Angeles County Hospital between 1924-1959. *Am J Cardiol* 1961;8:792–798.

14. Spiekerman RE, Brandeburg JT, Anchor RWP, Edwards JE. The spectrum of coronary heart disease in a community of 30,000. A clinicopathologic study. *Circulation* 1962;35:57–65.
15. Ross RM, Young JA. Clinical and necropsy findings in rupture of the myocardium. A review of 43 cases. *Scott Med J* 1963;8:222–226.
16. London RE, London SB. Rupture of the heart: A critical analysis of 47 consecutive autopsy cases. *Circulation* 1965;31:202–208.
17. Sievers J. Cardiac rupture in acute myocardial infarction. *Geriatrics* 1966;21:125–130.
18. Sugiura M, Okada R, Morii T, Hiraoka K, Shimada H, Nakanishi A. A clinicopathological study on the cardiac rupture following myocardial infarction in the aged. *Jpn Heart J* 1968;9:265–280.
19. Lewis AJ, Burchell HB, Titus JL. Clinical and pathologic features of postinfarction cardiac rupture. *Am J Cardiol* 1969;23:43–53.
20. Hammer J, Fabian J, Pavlovic J, Smid J. Myocardial rupture in acute myocardial infarction. *Cor Vasa* 1972;14:180–187.
21. Rasmussen S, Leth A, Kjoller E, Pedersen A. Cardiac rupture in acute myocardial infarction. *Acta Med Scand* 1979;205:11–16.
22. Dellborg M, Held P, Swedberg K, Vedin A. Rupture of the myocardium: Occurrence and risk factors. *Br Heart J* 1985;54:11–16.
23. Hiramori K. Major causes of death from acute myocardial infarction in a coronary care unit. *Jpn Circ J* 1987;51:1041–1047.
24. Herlitz J, Samuelsson SO, Richter A, Hjalmarson A. Prediction of rupture in acute myocardial infarction. *Clin Cardiol* 1988;11:63–69.
25. Reddy WG, Roberts WC. Frequency of rupture of the left ventricular free wall or ventricular septum among necropsy cases of fatal acute myocardial infarction since introduction of coronary care unit. *Am J Cardiol* 1989;63:906–911.
26. Batts KP, Ackermann DM, Edwards WD. Postinfarction rupture of the left ventricular free wall: Clinicopathologic correlates in 100 consecutive autopsy cases. *Hum Pathol* 1990;21:530–535.
27. Pollak H, Nobis H, Miczoch J. Frequency of left ventricular free wall rupture complicating acute myocardial infarction since the advent of thrombolysis. *Am J Cardiol* 1994;74:184–186.
28. Hutchins KD, Skurnick J, Lavenhar M, Natarajan GA. Cardiac rupture in acute myocardial infarction: A reassessment. *Am J Forensic Med Pathol* 2002;23:78–82.
29. Markowicz-Pawlus E, Nożyński J, Duszańska A, Hawranek M, Jarski P, Kalarus Z. The impact of a previous history of ischaemic episodes on the occurrence of left ventricular free wall rupture in the setting of myocardial infarction. *Kardiol Pol* 2012;70:713–717.
30. Roberts WC, Morrow AG. Pseudoaneurysm of the left ventricle: An unusual sequel of myocardial infarction and rupture of the heart. *Am J Med* 1967;43:639–644.
31. Morrow AG, Cohen LS, Roberts WC, Braundwald NS, Braunwald E. Severe mitral regurgitation following acute myocardial infarction and ruptured papillary muscle: Hemodynamic findings and results of operative treatment in 4 patients. *Circulation* 1968;37 (Suppl II):II-124–II-132.
32. Glancy DL, Stinson EB, Shepherd RL, Itscoitz SB, Roberts WC, Epstein SE, Morrow AG. Results of valve replacement for severe mitral regurgitation due to papillary muscle rupture or fibrosis. *Am J Cardiol* 1973;32:313–321.
33. Nagel MR, Ronan JA Jr, Roberts WC. Left-to-right shunt at atrial level after rupture of papillary muscle from acute myocardial infarction. *Am Heart J* 1973;86:112–116.
34. Hammer WJ, Ferrans VJ, Roberts WC. Myocardial embolus to coronary artery. *Chest* 1975;66:843–844.
35. Roberts WC. Cardiac rupture, abdominal aneurysmal rupture and dissecting aortic rupture. *Am J Cardiol* 1986;57:892–893.
36. Barbour DJ, Roberts WC. Rupture of a left ventricular papillary muscle during acute myocardial infarction: Analysis of 22 necropsy patients. *J Am Coll Cardiol* 1986;8:558–565.
37. Mann JM, Roberts WC. Fatal rupture of both left ventricular free wall and ventricular septum (double rupture) during acute myocardial infarction: analysis of seven patients studied at necropsy. *Am J Cardiol* 1987;60:722–724.
38. Mann JA, Kalan JM, Wallace RB, Roberts WC. Rupture of the ventricular septum or left ventricular free wall from acute myocardial infarction early after coronary artery bypass grafting. *Am J Cardiol* 1987;60:374–375.
39. Mann JM, Roberts WC. Acquired ventricular septal defect during acute myocardial infarction: Analysis of 38 unoperated necropsy patients and comparison with 50 unoperated necropsy patients without rupture. *Am J Cardiol* 1988;62:8–19.
40. Mann JM, Roberts WC. Rupture of the left ventricular free wall during acute myocardial infarction: Analysis of 138 necropsy patients and comparison with 50 necropsy patients with acute myocardial infarction without rupture. *Am J Cardiol* 1988;62:847–859.
41. Roberts WC. Rupture of the left ventricular free wall during acute myocardial infarction without hemopericardium. *Am J Cardiol* 1990;65:1033–1034.
42. Shirani J, Berezowski K, Roberts WC. Out-of-hospital sudden death from left ventricular free wall rupture during acute myocardial infarction as the first and only manifestation of atherosclerotic coronary artery disease. *Am J Cardiol* 1994;73:88–92.
43. Roberts WC, Roberts JD. The floating heart or the heart too fat to sink: Analysis of 55 necropsy patients. *Am J Cardiol* 1983;52:1286–1289.
44. Shirani J, Berezowski K, Roberts WC. Quantitative measurement of normal and excessive (cor adiposum) subepicardial adipose tissue, its clinical significance, and its effect on electrocardiographic QRS voltage. *Am J Cardiol* 1995;76:414–418.
45. Saffitz JE, Fredrickson RC, Roberts WC. Relation of size of transmural acute myocardial infarct to mode of death, interval between infarction and death and frequency of coronary arterial thrombus. *Am J Cardiol* 1986;57:1249–1254.
46. Roberts CS, Schoen FJ, Kloner RA. Effect of coronary reperfusion on myocardial hemorrhage and infarct healing. *Am J Cardiol* 1983;52:610–614.
47. Yusuf S, Collins R, Peto R, Furberg C, Stampfer MJ, Goldhaber SZ, Hennekens CH. Intravenous and intracoronary fibrinolytic therapy in acute myocardial infarction: overview of results on mortality, reinfarction and side-effects from 33 randomized controlled trials. *Eur Heart J* 1985;6:556–585.
48. Honan MB, Harrell FE, Reimer KA, Califf RM, Mark DB, Pryor DB, Hlatky MA. Cardiac rupture, mortality and the timing of thrombolytic therapy: a meta-analysis. *J Am Coll Cardiol* 1990;16:359–367.

Clinical and Morphologic Features of Acute, Subacute and Chronic Cor Pulmonale (Pulmonary Heart Disease)

William Clifford Roberts, MD[a,b,c,*], Alexis E. Shafii, MD[d], Paul A. Grayburn, MD[a,b], Jong Mi Ko, BS[a], Matthew R. Weissenborn, MD[e], Randall L. Rosenblatt, MD[b], and Joseph M. Guileyardo, MD[c]

Described are certain clinical and morphologic features of one patient with *acute*, another with *subacute*, and one with *chronic* cor pulmonale. All 3 had evidence of severe pulmonary hypertension. The patient with acute cor pulmonale 4 days after coronary bypass for unstable angina pectoris suddenly developed severe breathlessness with cyanosis and had fatal cardiac arrest and necropsy disclosed massive pulmonary embolism. The patient with subacute cor pulmonale had severe right-sided heart failure for 5 weeks and necropsy disclosed microscopic-sized neoplastic pulmonary emboli from a gastric carcinoma without parenchymal pulmonary metastases. The patient with chronic cor pulmonale had evidence of right-sided heart failure for years, the result of primary or idiopathic pulmonary hypertension almost certainly present from birth because the pattern of elastic fibers in the pulmonary trunk was that seen in newborns where the pressure in the pulmonary trunk and ascending aorta are similar. The patient with chronic cor pulmonale had plexiform pulmonary lesions indicative of irreversible pulmonary hypertension. Neither the acute nor the subacute patient had chronic pulmonary vascular changes. All 3 patients had dilated right ventricular cavities and non-dilated left ventricular cavities and only the patient with chronic cor pulmonale had right ventricular hypertrophy. (Am J Cardiol 2015;115:697−703)

In Paul Dudley White's third edition of his *Heart Disease* published in 1951, sixteen pages were devoted to acute and chronic cor pulmonale.[1] In Braunwald's ninth edition of *Heart Disease* published in 2012, cor pulmonale was not mentioned in the index, although many pages were devoted to pulmonary hypertension,[2] the common denominator of acute, subacute, and chronic cor pulmonale. Cor pulmonale may be defined as dilatation of the right ventricular cavity without hypertrophy of its wall (*acute* and *subacute* cor pulmonale) or both dilatation of the right ventricular cavity and hypertrophy of its wall (*chronic* cor pulmonale), secondary to pulmonary hypertension not caused by a condition involving the left side of the heart. Although chronic cor pulmonale appears to have been recognized by Laennec by 1821,[3] acute cor pulmonale was not described until 1935 by McGinn and White[4] and the subacute form was described initially by Brill and Robertson in 1937.[5] Although the echocardiographic or computed tomographic features of acute cor pulmonale have been well described, we were unable to find any published reports describing clinical and morphologic features in patients with all 3 forms of cor pulmonale. Our purpose herein is simply to illustrate these characteristic features in 3 patients, 1 each with the acute, the subacute, and the chronic forms of cor pulmonale.

Table 1
Clinical and Morphologic Findings in the 3 Patients with Cor Pulmonale

Variable	Acute	Subacute	Chronic
Age (Years)	67	52	33
Sex	Man	Woman	Woman
Duration of symptoms of heart failure	< 1 hour	5 weeks	20 years
Cause of pulmonary hypertension	Massive PE	PE (Neoplastic)	PPH
Echocardiogram			
Dilated right ventricular cavity	-*	3+/4+	3+/4+
Dilated right atrial cavity	-*	0/4+	2+/4+
Thickened right ventricular wall	-*	0/4+	4+/4+
Left ventricular ejection fraction (%)	65	55	55
Pressures (mm Hg)			
Pulmonary artery wedge (a/v/mean)	-	6/10/6	16/18/14†
Pulmonary artery (s/d)	-	70/30	94/45†
Right ventricle (s/d)	-	70/14	94/31†
Right atrium (a/v/mean)	-	13/10/8	19/15/15†
Systemic artery (s/d)	-	115/70	90/50
Cardiac index (L/min/m^2)	-	1.7	-
Hematocrit (%)	43	37	41
Body mass index (Kg/m^2)	43	32	21
Children	1	3	0
Heart and lung transplant	0	0	+
Heart weight (g)	570	385	430
Floating heart‡	+	+	+

a = a wave; PE = pulmonary embolism; PPH = primary pulmonary hypertension; s/d = peak systolic/end diastolic; v = v wave.
* Unable to access because of severe obesity.
† At age 27 years.
‡ Indicative of severe cardiac adiposity.

[a]Baylor Heart and Vascular Institute, Departments of [b]Internal Medicine, [c]Pathology, [d]Cardiothoracic Surgery, and [e]Radiology, Baylor University Medical Center, Dallas, Texas. Manuscript received November 6, 2014; revised manuscript received and accepted December 5, 2014.

Support for this investigation was provided by the Baylor Health Care System Foundation.

See page 703 for disclosure information.

*Corresponding author: Tel: (214) 820-7911; fax: (214) 820-7533.
E-mail address: wc.roberts@baylorhealth.edu (W.C. Roberts).

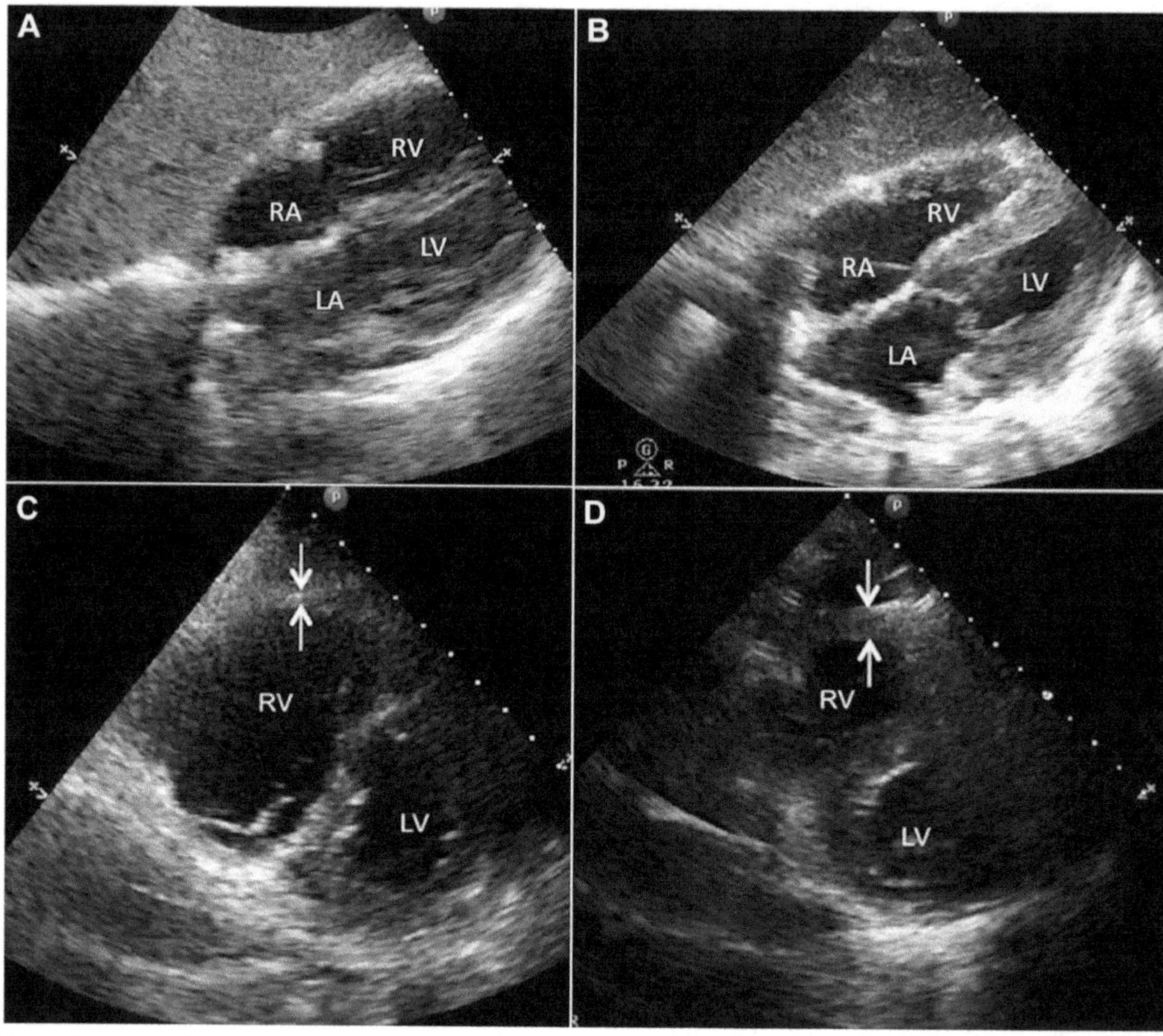

Figure 1. Echocardiograms in the patients with subacute *(A* and *C)* and chronic *(B* and *D)* cor pulmonale. *A* and *B* represent 4-chamber views and *C* and *D* represent cross-sectional views. The right ventricular (RV) cavity is dilated in both patients and the left ventricular (LV) cavity is not dilated in either patient. The RV wall is very thick in the patient with chronic cor pulmonale *(B* and *D)* but not in the patient with subacute cor pulmonale *(A* and *C)*. LA = left atrium; RA = right atrium. The arrows indicate normal RV wall thickness in *C* and abnormally thick RV in *D*.

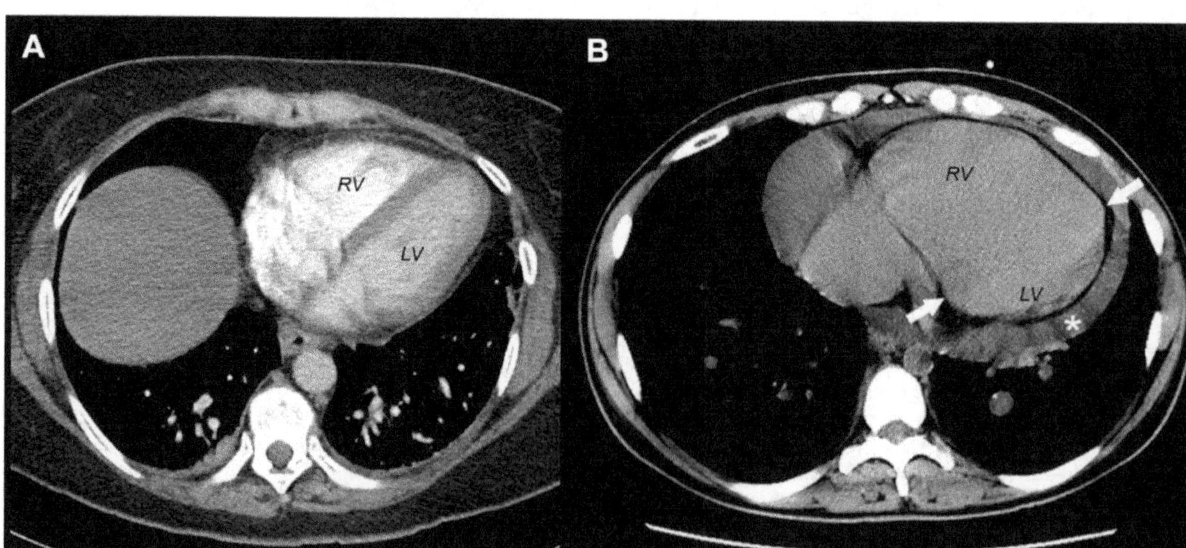

Figure 2. Computed tomographic pictures in the subacute patient *(A)* and in the chronic patient *(B)*. The right ventricular cavity is greatly dilated. A pericardial effusion is present in *B*. The left ventricular cavity in *B* is minute. The arrows point to the ventricular septum. LV = left ventricle; RV = right ventricle; * = pericardial effusion.

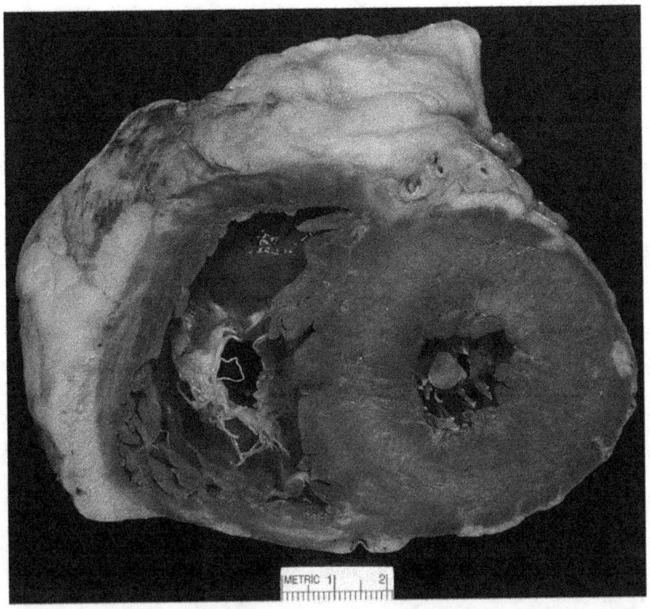

Figure 3. Acute cor pulmonale. Cross sections of the cardiac ventricles showing a dilated right ventricle and a normal size left ventricular cavity. The right ventricular wall is not thickened. The quantity of subepicardial adipose tissue is so extensive that the heart floated in a container of formaldehyde (body mass index 43 Kg/m^2).

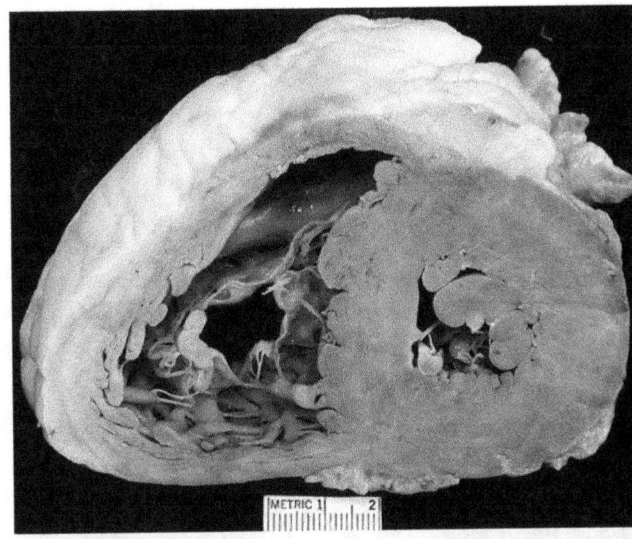

Figure 4. Subacute cor pulmonale. Transverse view of the ventricles showing the tricuspid valve and mitral valve. The right ventricular cavity is greatly dilated but the left ventricular cavity is not. The right ventricular wall is not thickened. The quantity of subepicardial adipose tissue is greatly increased such that the heart floated in a container of formaldehyde.

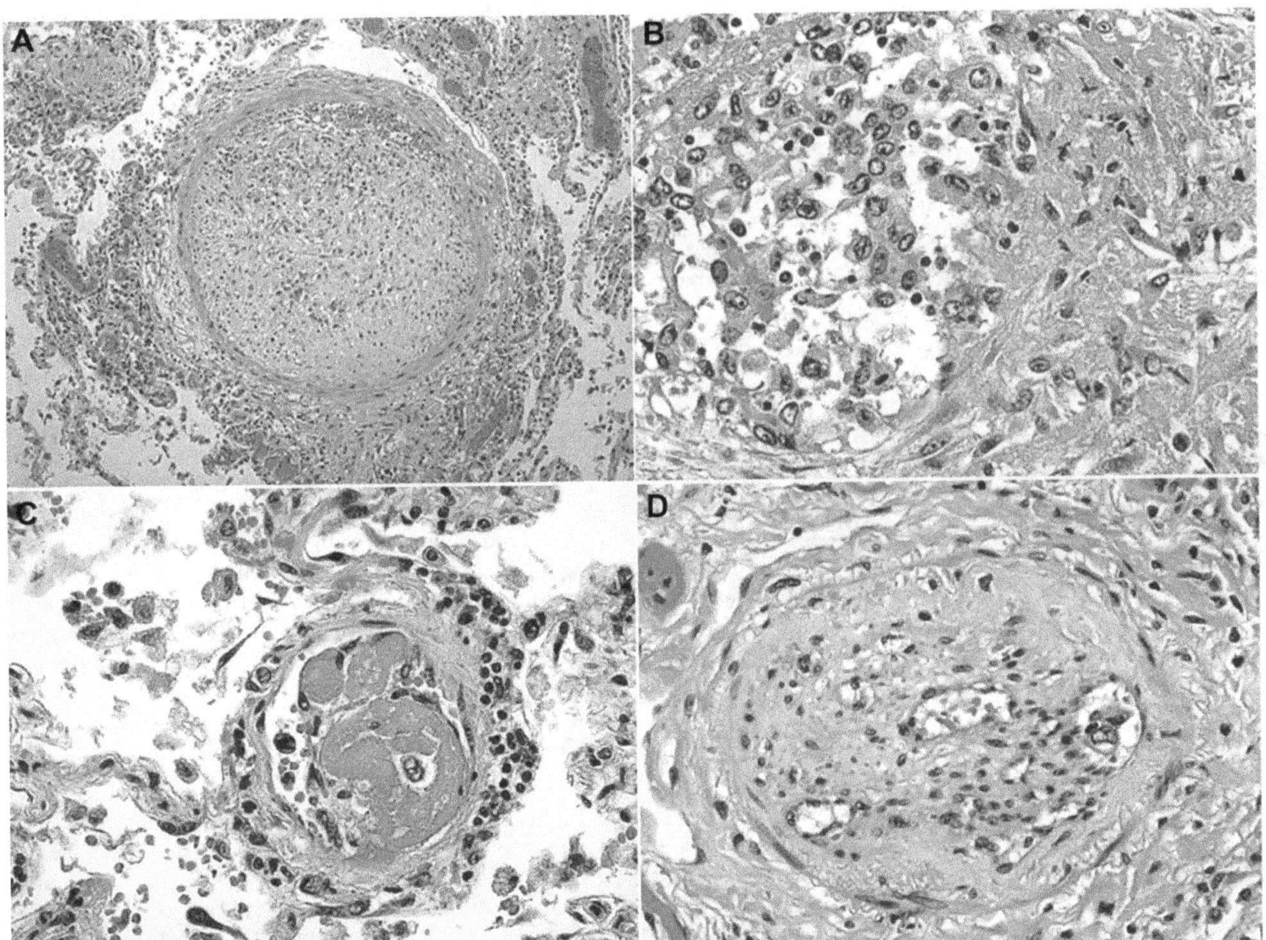

Figure 5. Subacute cor pulmonale. Photomicrographs of intrapulmonary arteries occluded or narrowed by metastatic cells within the lumen and with superimposed thrombus. The artery in *A* is virtually occluded. The gastric cancer cells are easily seen in the pulmonary artery illustrated in *B* and there is also some fibrin deposits within the lumen. *C* This small pulmonary artery is narrowed mainly by fibrin but a few gastric carcinoma cells are present. *D* This pulmonary artery contains organized thrombus and 4 small recanalized channels indicating that the emboli to the lungs probably occurred during the 5 symptomatic last weeks of this patient's life. Hematoxylin-eosin stains: X 100 *(A)*; X 400 *(B, C* and *D)*.

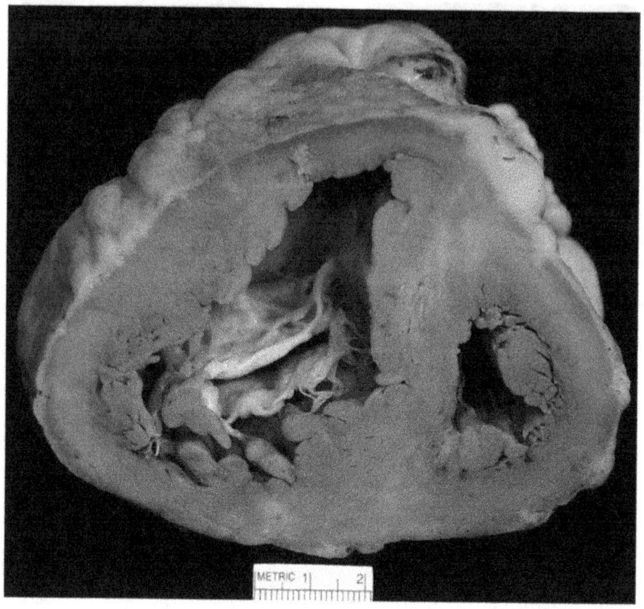

Figure 6. Chronic cor pulmonale. Transverse section of the ventricles in the patient with primary pulmonary hypertension. The right ventricular cavity is considerably dilated and the left ventricular is not. The right ventricular wall is about as thick as the left ventricular wall. The margins of the tricuspid valve leaflets are thickened, presumably the result of the very high closing pressure (peak right ventricular systolic pressure). The ventricular septum is thicker than either the right or left ventricular free walls.

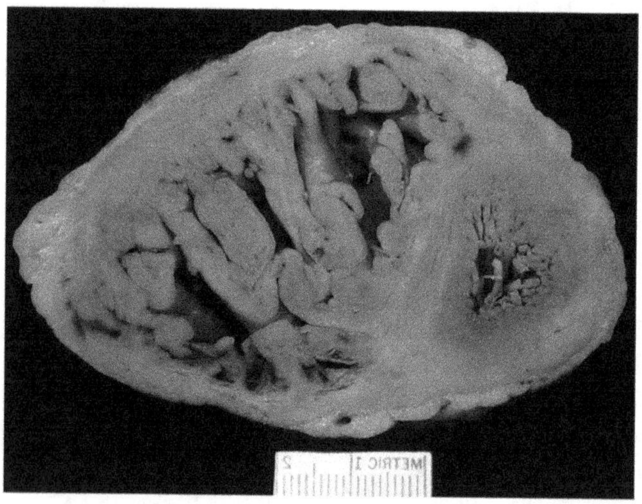

Figure 7. Chronic cor pulmonale. This view is a transverse cut in the apical half of the cardiac ventricles and it is shown to show how thick the pectinate muscles are in the right ventricular cavity. In this view the anterior and posterior right ventricular walls are really not thickened but the pectinate muscles are enormously thickened. Thickening of the pectinate muscles is one of the best signs of right ventricular hypertrophy, better than wall thickness. The left ventricular cavity is minute.

Patient Descriptions

Pertinent features of each of the 3 patients are summarized in Table 1. Echocardiographic and computed tomographic features in the subacute and chronic cases are shown in Figures 1 and 2. The acute patient, aged 67, had symptoms

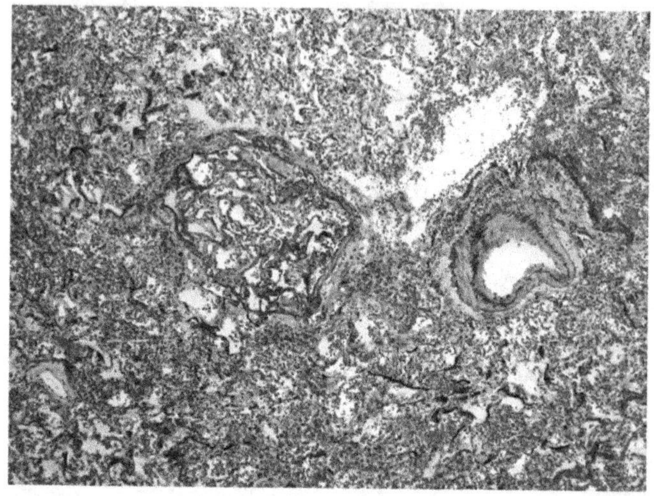

Figure 8. Chronic Cor pulmonale. Photomicrograph of a portion of lung showing a large plexiform lesion and a muscular pulmonary artery with thickening of its media and of its intima. Erythrocytes have entered most of the alveolar spaces. Movat stain, x100.

suggesting a respiratory catastrophe for only several minutes and necropsy disclosed massive pulmonary emboli (Figure 3); the subacute patient, aged 52, had symptoms for 5 weeks, determined at necropsy to be the result of multiple microscopic-sized pulmonary neoplastic emboli without parenchymal lung metastases from carcinoma of the stomach (Figures 4 and 5), and the chronic patient, only 33 years old, had symptoms of right-sided heart failure and periodic substernal chest pain for about 20 years (Figures 6–8). All 3 had very dilated right ventricular cavities, the acute and subacute patients without right ventricular wall thickening, and the chronic patient with both right ventricular dilatation and severe right ventricular wall thickening. The subacute and chronic patients had documented severely elevated right ventricular and pulmonary arterial peak systolic pressures (70 and 94 mm Hg, respectively), and the acute patient almost certainly did as well. Neither the acute nor the subacute patients had thickened walls of the pulmonary arteries and neither had plexiform lesions. The chronic patient, in contrast, had classic findings of primary pulmonary hypertension (medial and intimal thickening of the pulmonary arteries and numerous pulmonary plexiform lesions) (Figure 8). Sections of the pulmonary trunk in the acute and subacute patient disclosed a typical adult pattern of the medial elastic fibers whereas in the chronic patient the pattern was that present at birth and similar to the medial elastic fiber pattern of the aorta (Figures 9 and 10).

Discussion

Each of the 3 patients described herein fulfilled a definition of acute, subacute, and chronic cor pulmonale. The causes of the pulmonary hypertension in them, however, were quite different. The acute patient had a massive pulmonary embolus and died within a few minutes. The patient with the subacute syndrome had extensive neoplastic emboli to the small pulmonary arteries without emboli to the major pulmonary arteries or metastases from her gastric cancer to the pulmonary parenchyma and had symptoms of right-sided heart failure for

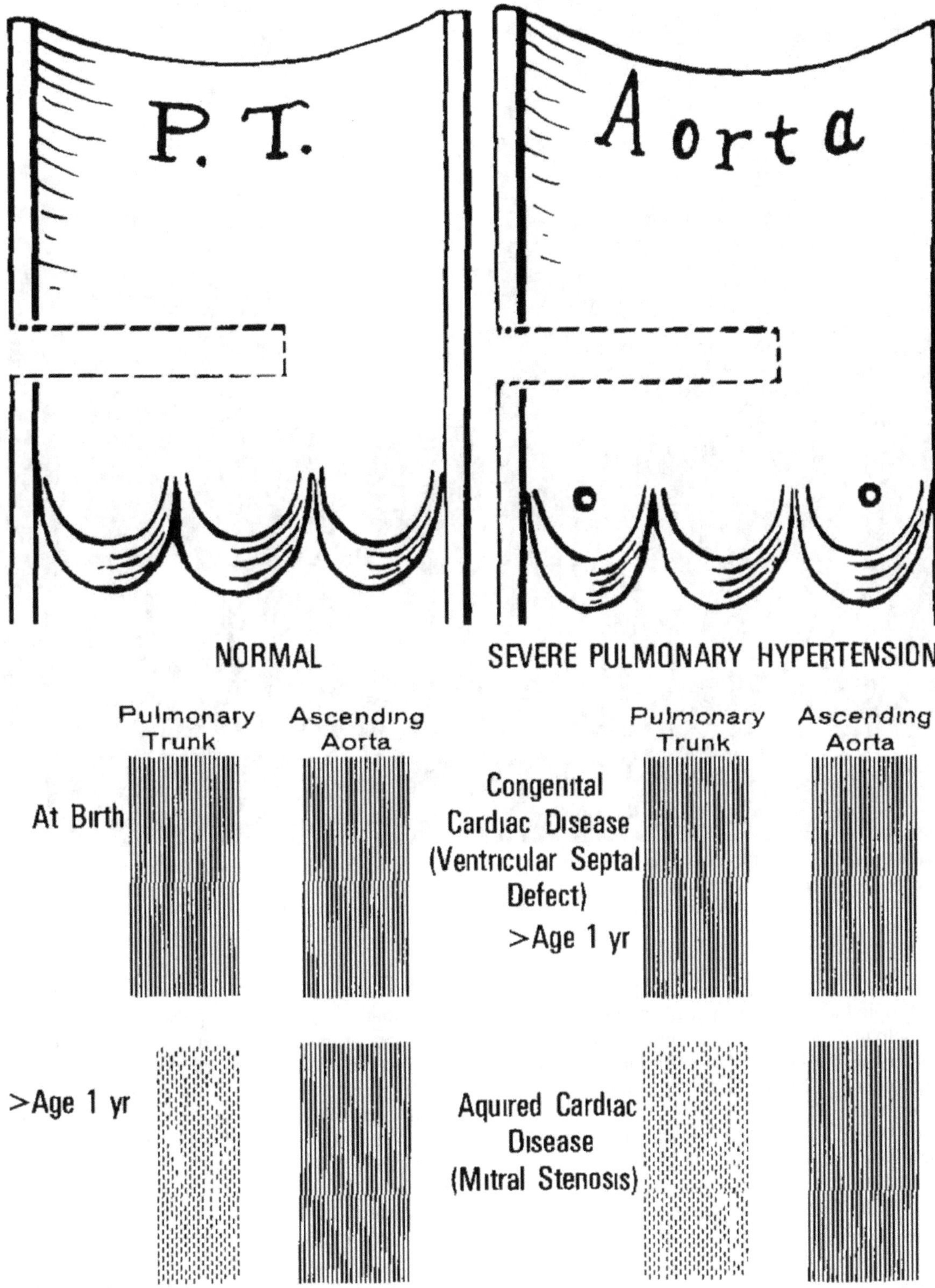

Figure 9. Configuration of elastic fibers in the pulmonary trunk at birth, after 1 year of age, with pulmonary *hypertension from birth* (VSD), and with an acquired condition (*mitral stenosis*). The sketch (*top*) shows the sites in the pulmonary trunk (PT) and aorta at which the sections for histologic examination were taken. At birth the configuration of the elastic fibers in both the pulmonary trunk and ascending aorta are identical and wall thicknesses are similar. Normally, after a year of age the number of elastic fibers in the pulmonary trunk diminishes considerably to reach an "adult configuration," and the thickness of the wall also diminishes. If a large ventricular septal defect or a aorticopulmonary defect is present from birth, both the configuration of the elastic fibers and wall thickness of the pulmonary trunk remains similar to that of the normal aorta. The information on the configuration of elastic fibers in the pulmonary trunk is based on original work by Heath and associates.[9,10]

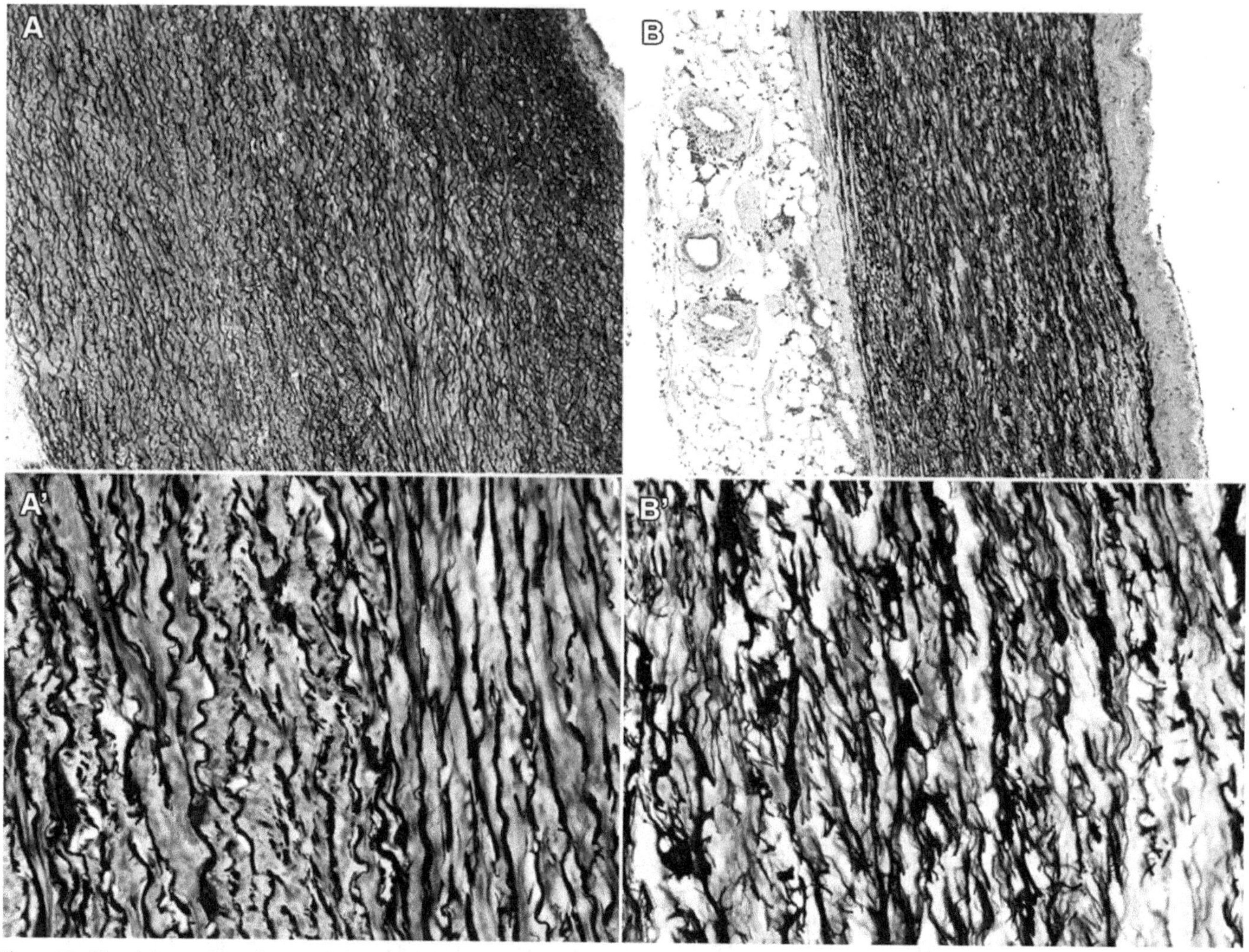

Figure 10. Chronic cor pulmonale. *A* and *A'* are sections of the ascending aorta stained for elastic fibers, and *B* and *B'* are sections of the pulmonary trunk stained for elastic fibers. The aorta is much thicker than is the pulmonary trunk but the configuration of the elastic fibers in the aorta and pulmonary trunk are similar, indicating that the pulmonary hypertension was almost certainly present from the time of birth. Movat stains X 100 *(A* and *B)*; X 400 *(A'* and *B')*.

5 weeks. Microscopic pulmonary neoplastic emboli without pulmonary parenchymal metastases was originally described by Brill and Robertson[5] in 1937 and they termed the condition "subacute cor pulmonale." Subsequently, a number of such cases has been reported.[6–8]

The patient with chronic cor pulmonale had primary or idiopathic pulmonary hypertension.[9] The unusual feature is that pulmonary hypertension appears to have been present from the time of birth. The evidence comes from studies by Heath and colleagues[10] and Heath and Edwards[11] who examined histologic sections of the pulmonary trunk and ascending aorta and found from study of patients with large left-to-right shunts (ventricular septal defect or patent ductus arteriosus) that the configuration of the elastic fibers in each of these arteries was similar when the pulmonary hypertension was present from birth, whereas in the patients who acquired pulmonary hypertension later in life (for example, from mitral stenosis) the pulmonary trunk had few elastic fibers and those present were disrupted (The aorta retains its fetal pattern of medial elastic fibers throughout life.). At birth, peak systolic pressures in the pulmonary trunk and ascending aorta are similar and therefore the configuration of elastic fibers in both pulmonary trunk and ascending aorta are similar. By one year of age, the peak systolic pressure in the pulmonary trunk has fallen to about one fifth of the peak systolic pressure in the ascending aorta and the elastic fibers have also decreased by approximately 80%, proportional to the reduction in peak systolic pressure.

Heath and Edwards[11] also found that some patients with primary pulmonary hypertension retain the fetal elastic pattern in the pulmonary trunk suggesting that the high pressure in the pulmonary circuit persisted from birth. A similar study by Roberts[12] in 1963 found the classic fetal pattern of elastic fibers in the pulmonary trunk in 1 and probably in 2 of 5 adults with primary pulmonary hypertension studied by him, again strongly suggesting that the high pulmonary pressure present at birth was retained into adulthood.

Neither our acute nor subacute cor pulmonale patient had medial or intimal thickening of the intrapulmonary

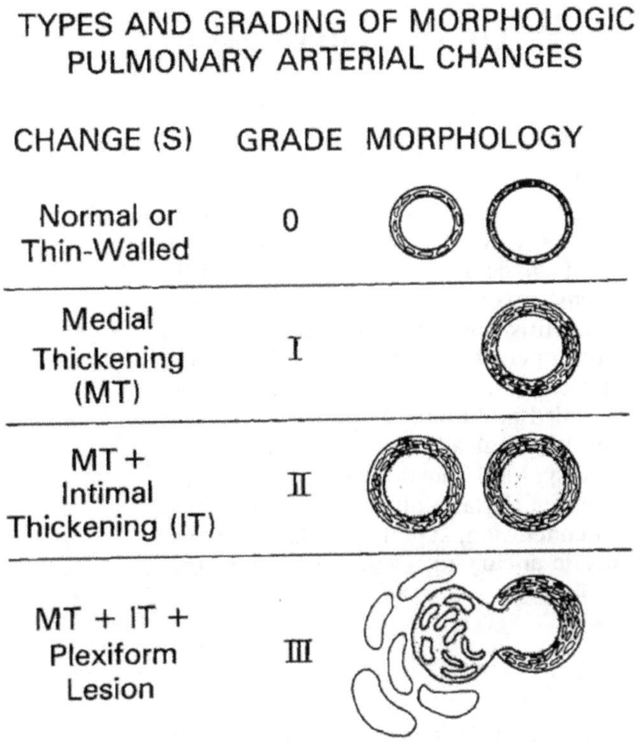

Figure 11. Diagram showing the types and grading of morphologic arterial changes in the lungs. Any elevation of pulmonary arterial pressure can cause medial thickening and if the pressure persists also intimal thickening. Plexiform lesions have occurred only in patients with severe pulmonary hypertension, usually pulmonary artery systolic pressures equivalent to aortic peak systolic pressures and indicate that the pulmonary hypertension is irreversible.

pulmonary arteries or plexiform lesion, whereas our chronic cor pulmonale patient had intrapulmonary arteries with thickened intima and media and numerous plexiform lesions (Figure 11). The plexiform lesions are indicative of irreversible pulmonary hypertension.[13]

Disclosures

The authors have no conflicts of interest to disclose.

1. White PD. Heart Disease. Fourth Edition. New York: The McMillan Company, 1951:1015.
2. Bonow RO, Mann DL, Zipes DP, Libby P, eds. Braunwald's HEART DISEASE. A Textbook of Cardiovascular Medicine. Ninth Edition. Philadelphia: Elsevier Saunders, 2012:1961.
3. Laennec RTH, Forbes J. A Treatise on the Diseases of the Chest and on Mediate Auscultation. London: Thomas & George Underwood, 1829: 736.
4. McGinn S, White PD. Acute cor pulmonale resulting from pulmonary embolism: its clinical recognition. *JAMA* 1935;104:1473–1480.
5. Brill IC, Robertson TD. Subacute cor pulmonale. *Arch Intern Med* 1937;60:1043–1057.
6. Mason DG. Subacute cor pulmonale. *Arch Intern Med* 1940;40: 1221–1229.
7. Schriner RW, Ryu JH, Edwards WD. Microscopic pulmonary tumor embolism causing subacute cor pulmonale: A difficult antemortem diagnosis. *Mayo Clin Proc* 1991;66:143–148.
8. Domanski MJ, Cunnion RE, Fernicola DJ, Roberts WC. Fatal cor pulmonale caused by extensive tumor emboli in the small pulmonary arteries without emboli in the major pulmonary arteries or metastases in the pulmonary parenchyma. *Am J Cardiol* 1993;72:233–234.
9. Simonneau G, Gatzoulis MA, Adatia I, Celermajer D, Denton C, Ghofrani A, Gomez Sanchez MA, Krishna Kumar R, Landzberg M, Machado RF, Olschewski H, Robbins IM, Souza R. Updated clinical classification of pulmonary hypertension. *J Am Coll Cardiol* 2013;62:D34–41.
10. Heath D, DeShane JW, Wood EH, Edwards JE. The structure of the pulmonary trunk at different ages and in case of pulmonary hypertension and pulmonary stenosis. *J Pathol Bacteriol* 1959;77:443.
11. Heath D, Edwards JE. Configuration of elastic tissue of pulmonary trunk in idiopathic pulmonary hypertension. *Circulation* 1960;21:59.
12. Roberts WC. The histologic structure of the pulmonary trunk in patients with "primary" pulmonary hypertension. *Am Heart J* 1963;65:230–236.
13. Roberts WC. A simple histologic classification of pulmonary arterial hypertension. *Am J Cardiol* 1986;58:385–386.

Syphilis as a Cause of Thoracic Aortic Aneurysm

William C. Roberts, MD[a,b,c,*], Clay M. Barbin, MD[a], Matthew R. Weissenborn, MD[d], Jong M. Ko, BA[c], and A. Carl Henry, MD[c]

In 2009, we described morphologic findings in 22 patients having resection of an ascending aortic aneurysm in the previous 11 years at the Baylor University Medical Center, and histologic examination of the aneurysmal wall disclosed classic findings of syphilitic aortitis. The major purpose of that extensively illustrated report was to describe the characteristic gross features of the aneurysm such that syphilitic aortitis might be better recognized at operation and appropriate antibiotics administered postoperatively. The aim of the present study was to emphasize that syphilis remains a major cause of ascending aortic aneurysm. From January 1, 2009, to December 31, 2014, we studied additional 23 patients who had resection of an ascending aortic aneurysm that again histologically had classic features of syphilitic aortitis. All 23 patients were found to have syphilitic aortitis grossly and histologically. The aneurysm involved the ascending portion of aorta in all 23, the arch portion in 12, and the descending thoracic portion in 10. In conclusion, syphilis has far from disappeared. It remains a major cause of ascending aortic aneurysm. **(Am J Cardiol 2015;116:1298−1303)**

In 2009, we described finding in 22 patients who underwent operative resection of an ascending aortic aneurysm at the Baylor University Medical Center (BUMC) from 1998 to 2008, and histologic examination of the aneurysmal wall was typical of syphilitic aortitis.[1] The emphasis of that report was the describing of the morphologic features of syphilitic aortitis so that the condition could be more readily diagnosed at operation and also to emphasize that syphilis as a cause of thoracic aortic aneurysm had not disappeared. The present study was prompted by studying an additional 23 patients who underwent resection of an ascending aortic aneurysm caused by syphilitic aortitis at the same institution during the subsequent 6 years, again to emphasize that this condition has far from disappeared.

Methods

Since March 1993, all operatively excised specimens excised by cardiovascular surgeons at the BUMC have been described grossly and histologically by WCR and photographed mainly by JMK, and since 2003, the clinical records were available online. From January 1, 2009, to December 31, 2014, 23 patients were found to have diffuse panaortitis of the tubular portion of ascending aorta. The diffuseness of the involvement of the ascending aorta was determined by gross examination and the panaortitis by histologic examination. Takayasu's arteritis was ruled out by the absence of giant cells in any layer of the aneurysmal wall.[2,3] Ankylosing spondylitis was ruled out by the absence of arthritic disease, by the minimal involvement of the tubular portion of ascending aorta, by extension of the process into the walls of the sinus portion of aorta and onto the bases of the aortic valve cusps, and by the extension of the process onto the anterior mitral leaflet and into the membranous ventricular septum.[4,5]

All 23 patients at operation were stated to have 3-cuspid aortic valves that were free of calcific deposits. The free margins, mainly their central portions, were described as being mildly thickened in some patients. The sinus portion of aorta was not dilated or described as being abnormal.

A positive or reactive serologic test for syphilis (STS) was not considered a criterion for inclusion in the present study because the test was never done in most patients, or, if performed, the results were unavailable.

Results

Pertinent findings in each of the 23 patients are listed in Table 1. The 11 men ranged in age from 33 to 84 years (mean 61), and the 12 women from 58 to 83 years (mean 70). Eighteen were white; 4, black; and 1, Asian. The body mass index ranged from 16 to 47 kg/m^2 (mean 28); it was >25 in 15 (65%).

The aneurysm involved the ascending portion of aorta in all 23 patients, the arch portion in 12, and the descending thoracic portion in 10. In all patients, the aneurysm was fusiform, that is, the entire aortic wall was part of the aneurysmal wall. Additionally, at least 5 patients had saccular aneurysms projecting from the fusiform

Departments of [a]Internal Medicine, [b]Pathology, [d]Radiology, [c]Cardiothoracic Surgery, and [e]The Baylor Heart and Vascular Institute, Baylor University Medical Center, Dallas, Texas. Manuscript received June 30, 2015; revised manuscript received and accepted July 3, 2015.

The study was funded by the Baylor Health Care System Foundation, 3600 Gaston Avenue, Barnett Tower, Suite 100 Dallas, TX 75246.

See page 1303 for disclosure information.

*Corresponding author: Tel: (214) 820-7911; fax: (214) 820-7533.

E-mail address: wc.roberts@baylorhealth.edu (W.C. Roberts).

Table 1
Surgical cases of syphilitic aortitis at Baylor University Medical Center from January 1, 2009 to December 31, 2014

Patient	Age (years)	Race	BMI (Kg/m^2)	Pressures (mmHg) (s/d)		Aneurysm					AVR	Weight of AV (g)	STS	Result	CABG
						Location			Type						
				LV	SA	Asc	Arch	DT	Saccular	Fusiform					
MEN															
1	33	W	24.7	118/27	132/72	+	0	0	0	+	+	0.47	—	—	0
2	45	B	23.0	—	180/100	+	0	0	+	+	0	—	+	Ab, RPR 1:128	0
3	48	B	27.9	—	106/65	+	+	0	+	+	0	—	—	—	0
4	51	W	28.1	148/20	131/60	+	0	0	0	+	0	—	0	—	0
5	59	A	28.4	—	170/80	+	+	+	+	+	0	—	0	—	0
6	59	B	34.4	—	120/70	+	+	0	0	+	+	0.83	0	—	0
7	60	W	28.9	120/7	140/90	+	+	0	0	+	0	—	0	—	0
8	70	W	37.7	190/40	190/90	+	+	+	0	+	0	—	0	—	+
9	80	W	28.0	123/5	145/85	+	+	+	0	+	0	—	0	—	+
10	83	W	24.4	130/10	150/80	+	0	0	0	+	+	0.91	0	—	+
11	84	W	26.5	120/20	120/70	+	+	+	0	+	+	0.86	0	—	+
	33-84 (61±17)		23.0-37.7 (28.4±4.3)												
WOMEN															
1	58	B	31.7	126/30	140/90	+	0	0	0	+	0	—	0	—	0
2	59	W	28.9	0	160/90	+	+	+	0	+	0	—	0	—	0
3	62	W	45.6	155/25	170/65	+	0	+	+	+	+	0.78	+	NR (Ab)	0
4	65	W	46.5	114/16	120/65	+	0	+	0	+	0	—	0	—	0
5	65	W	28.9	142/10	130/75	+	+	+	0	+	0	—	0	—	0
6	67	W	26.2	124/4	135/60	+	0	0	0	+	0	—	+	NR (Ab)	0
7	69	W	15.8	101/3	100/60	+	0	+	0	+	0	—	0	—	+
8	70	W	21.6	—	170/80	+	0	0	0	+	0	—	+	NR (RPR)	0
9	79	W	24.8	—	140/55	+	+	+	+	+	0	—	0	—	+
10	80	W	28.6	145/30	145/60	+	0	0	0	+	0	—	+	NR (RPR)	0
11	83	W	18.6	175/20	175/70	+	0	0	0	+	+	0.55	0	—	0
12	83	W	22.3	120/10	120/40	+	0	0	0	+	0	—	0	—	0
	58-83 (70±9)		15.8-46.5 (28.3±9.5)												

A = Asian; Ab = antibody; Asc = ascending; AV = aortic valve; AVR = aortic valve replacement; B = black; BMI = body mass index; CABG = coronary artery bypass grafting; DT = descending thoracic; LV = left ventricle; NR = non-reactive; RPR = rapid plasma reagin; SA = systemic artery; STS = serologic test for syphilis; W = white; — = not available.

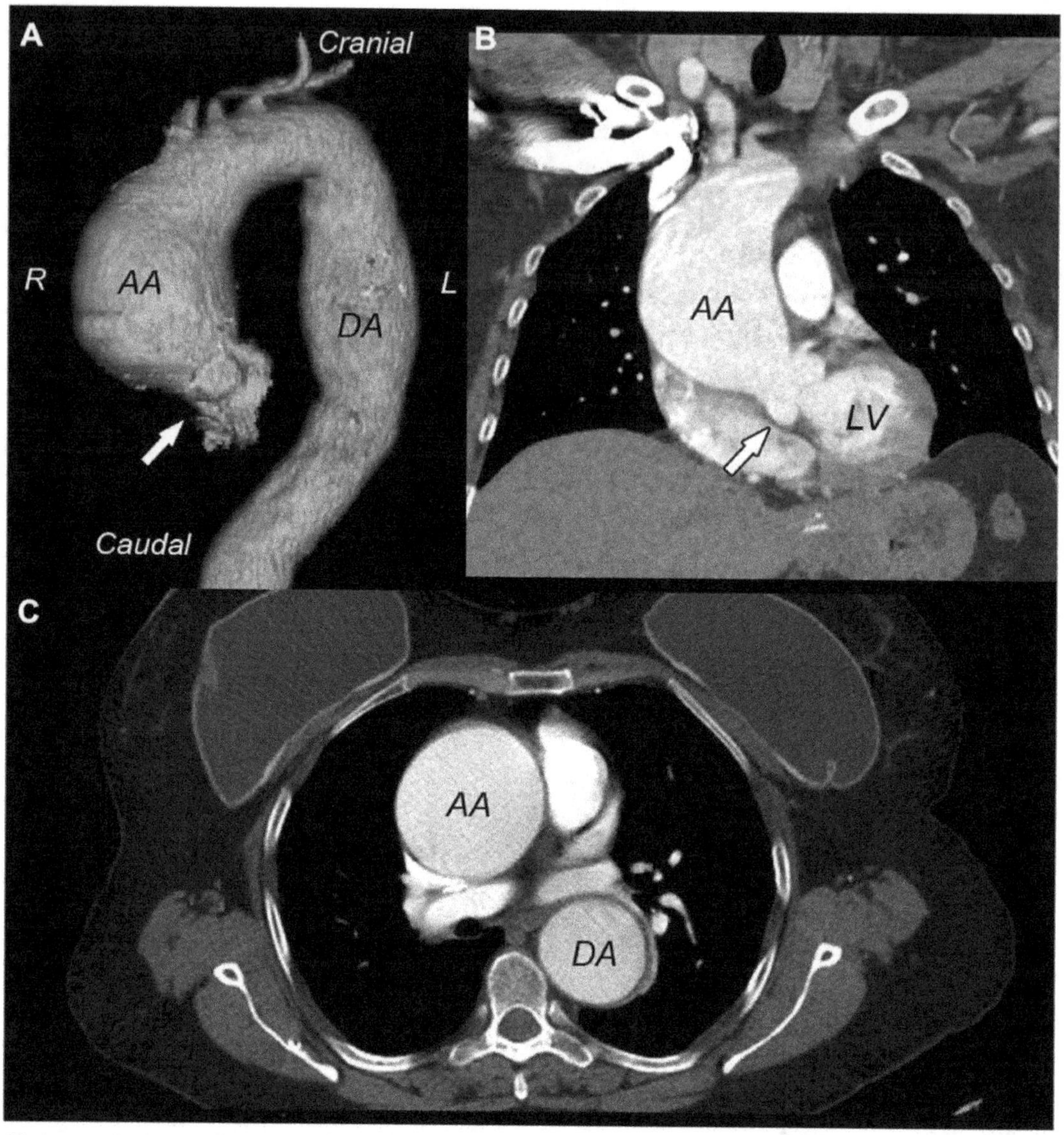

Figure 1. Patient #2, woman (Table 1). *(A)* Volume-rendered 3-dimensional reconstruction and *(B)* contrast-enhanced coronal and *(C)* axial CT images show a fusiform aneurysm of the AA and DA. The aortic sinuses are unaffected *(white arrows)*. The distal descending thoracic aorta is normal in caliber. AA = ascending aorta; DA = descending aorta; LV = left ventricular.

aneurysm. The aortic specimen in the 11 men ranged in weight from 14 to 46 g (mean 29) and in 11 of the 12 women from 11 to 27 g (mean 20). The 1 case not included in the weight of the aorta was a woman who had only a biopsy rather than resection of the aorta. Six patients also had aortic valve replacement because of pure aortic regurgitation. Their excised 3-cuspid valves weighed from 0.47 to 0.91 (mean 0.73, the normal aortic valve weighs ~0.50[6]). Coronary bypass also was performed at the time of ascending aortic resection in 6 patients (26%), and all 6 were ≥70 years of age.

An STS preoperatively was performed in 5 patients, and in only 1, the test result was positive. Some representative preoperative computed tomographic images and photographs of operatively excised ascending aortas are illustrated in Figures 1 to 4.

Histologic sections of the wall of the ascending aorta were similar in all 23 patients. All sections were stained by hematoxylin/eosin and by Movat methods, the latter to delineate the internal and external elastic membranes and the medial elastic fibers so that the intima, media, and adventitia could be clearly separated from one another.

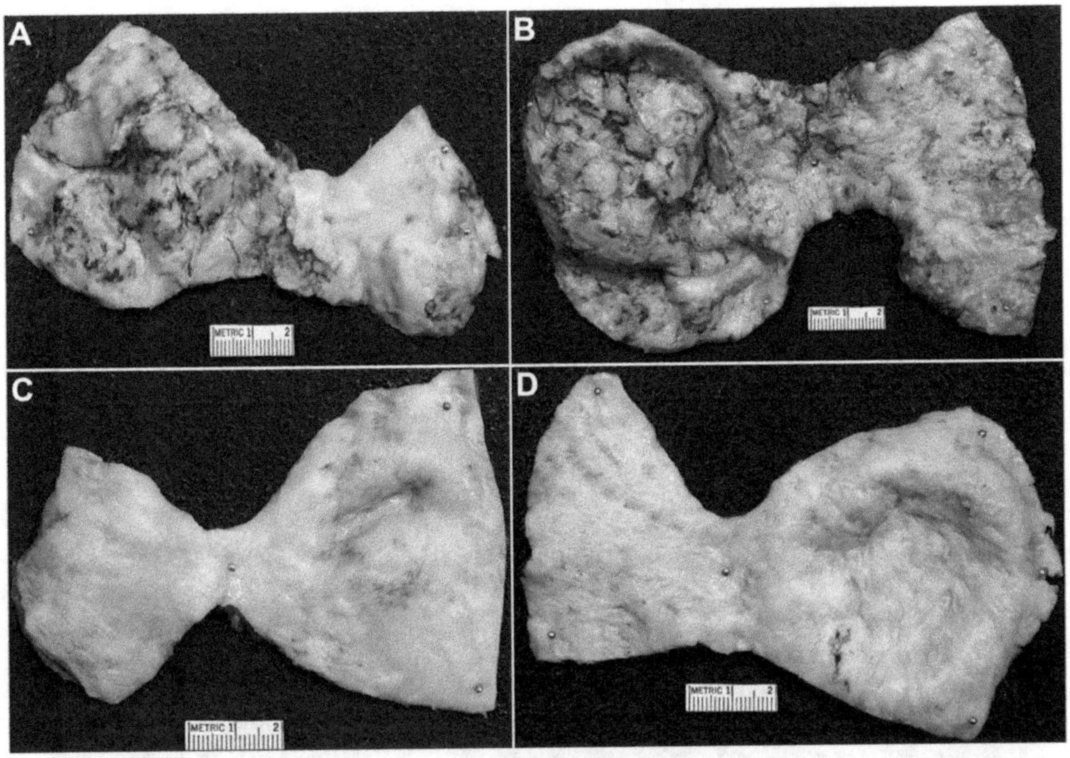

Figure 2. Excised ascending aortas in 4 patients, and arch is diffusely involved with the syphilitic process. *(A)* Case #1, man; *(B)* case #4, man; *(C)* case #8, man; *(D)* case #10, woman. *(A)* and *(B)* have extensive intimal calcific deposits, whereas *(C)* and *(D)* have no calcific deposits.

The wall of the aorta was thickened in all 23 patients because of thickening of the intima, mainly by fibrous tissue with or without calcific deposits, and by thickening of the adventitia by fibrous tissue within which were clumps of mononuclear cells (lymphocytes and plasmacytes). The vasa vasora in the adventitia were thickened, and the lumens of many were narrowed. The media was not thickened, but its elastic fibers were focally but extensively replaced by fibrous tissue. Occasionally, a few mononuclear cells were present in the media. Giant cells were absent.

Comments

The major purpose of this report is to emphasize that syphilis remains a major cause of aneurysm of the ascending aorta with or without similar involvement of the arch and descending thoracic aorta. The 23 cases described here were seen in just over a 6-year period such that nearly 4 cases of syphilitic aortic aneurysms were resected at BUMC yearly.

Several decades ago, an STS was a requirement for admission to any US hospital. Today, an STS is infrequently performed in hospitalized patients in the United States. In 2004, the US Preventative Services Task Force found that there was no benefit in morbidity or mortality of screening for syphilis in asymptomatic adults or patients with high risk.[7] There are no studies, however, that evaluate the risks associated with screening and treating asymptomatic adult patients with syphilis. Given the morbidity associated with cardiovascular and neurologic syphilis, it is reasonable to do an STS in any patient with a 3-cuspid aortic valve and aneurysmal dilation of the ascending aorta with or without associated aortic regurgitation. Although there is a lack of randomized controlled trials, there is general consensus among the infectious disease community to treat patients with tertiary syphilis in an effort to prevent progression of the disease process. Unfortunately, the serologic test result for syphilis is often negative or nonreactive in patients with syphilitic aortitis, and thus, a negative result does not exclude this entity.[8]

Superimposition of a saccular aneurysm on a fusiform aneurysm of ascending aorta is virtually diagnostic of syphilitic aortitis. The syphilitic process begins at the sinotubular junction and spares the sinus portion of aorta, which, for example, is always involved in patients with the Marfan's syndrome or forme fruste varieties of that syndrome.[9,10]

Syphilis only involves the heart in a secondary manner. Aortic regurgitation in this entity is the consequence of the aortic dilation and not because of direct involvement of the

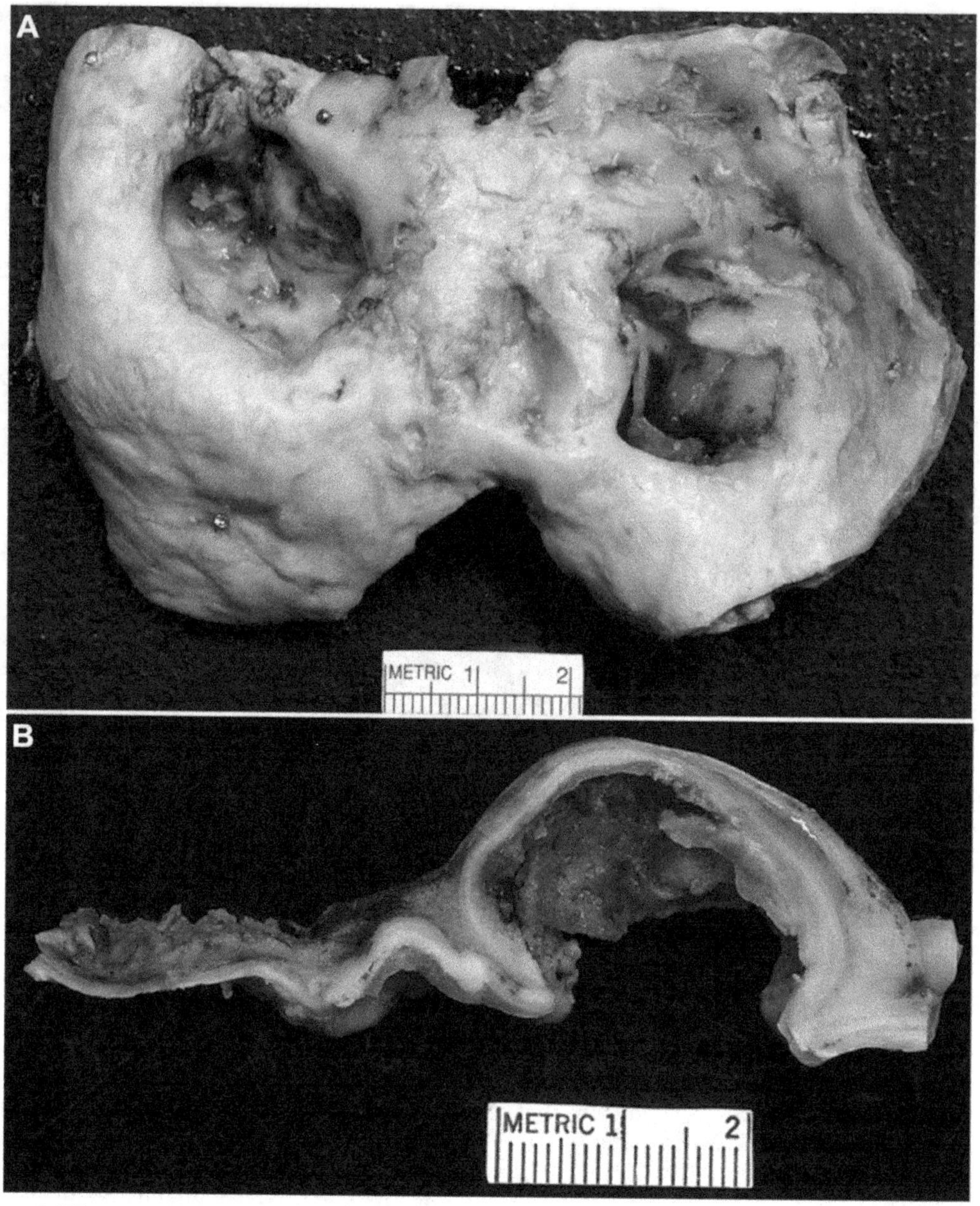

Figure 3. Case #3, man. *(A)* This resected ascending aorta contains 2 large saccular aneurysms arising from the fusiform aneurysm. *(B)* Cross-section of one of the saccular aneurysm partially filled with thrombus.

aortic valve cusps, the situation, for example, in ankylosing spondylitis that histologically is similar to syphilis, but this arthritic condition extends below (caudal to) the aortic valve, something syphilis never does. Additionally, syphilis never involves an epicardial coronary artery directly. Syphilis affects only the coronary ostia, nearly always the right one, and the narrowing is the result of the syphilitic process affecting the aorta, not the coronary artery directly. Consequently, it seems better to use the phrase "syphilitic aortitis" or "vascular syphilis" rather than the phrase "cardiovascular syphilis."

Syphilis is limited to the thoracic aorta and never involves the abdominal aorta.[11,12] The reason apparently is that vasa vasora are present only in the thoracic aorta, and they are absent in the abdominal aorta, and syphilis basically appears to be a disease of the vasa vasora, at least initially. Thus, when a fusiform abdominal aneurysm accompanies an ascending aortic aneurysm—in the

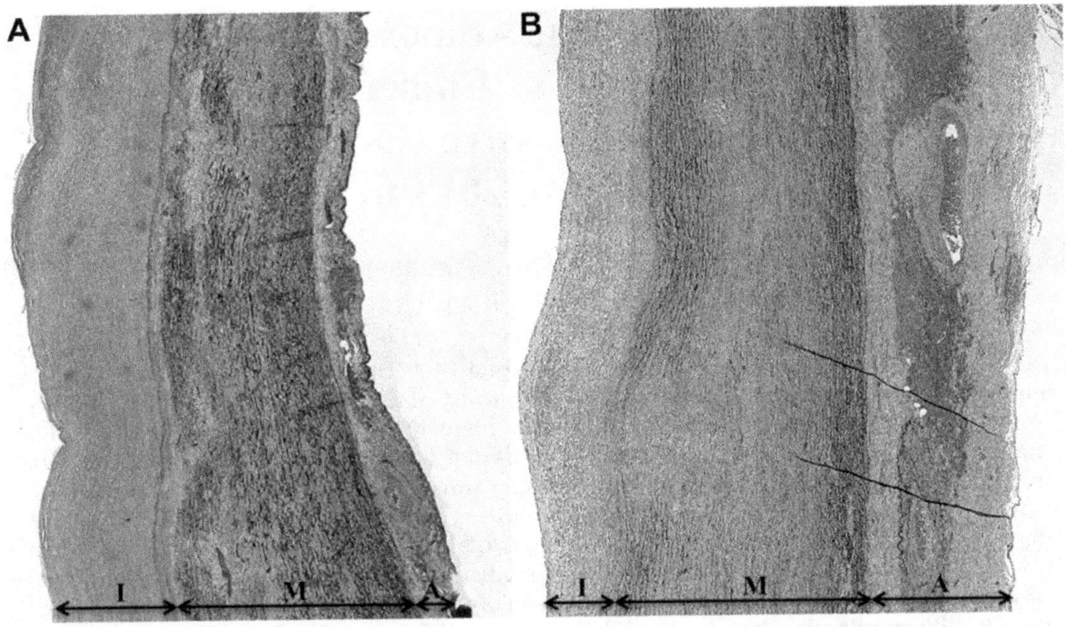

Figure 4. Photomicrographs of portions of ascending aorta in 2 patients. *(A)* Case #8, woman (Table 1). *(B)* Case #11, woman (Table 1). In each, the intima (I) and adventitia (A) are thickened, mainly by fibrous tissue. The adventitia contains large collections of lymphocytes and plasmacytes, shown best in *(B)*. The cells stain purple. The media (M) is not thickened, but many elastic fibers have been lost and replaced by fibrous tissue. Movat stains, ×40 *(A)*; ×40 *(B)*.

absence of aortic dissection—2 different processes are at work.

Disclosures

The authors have no conflicts of interest to disclose.

1. Roberts WC, Bose R, Ko JM, Henry AC, Hamman BL. Identifying cardiovascular syphilis at operation. *Am J Cardiol* 2009;104:1588–1594.
2. Roberts WC, Wibin EA. Idiopathic panaortitis, supraaortic arteritis, granulomatous myocarditis and pericarditis. A cause of pulseless disease and possibly left ventricular aneurysm in the African. *Am J Med* 1966;41:453–461.
3. Roberts WC, Zafar S, Ko JM. Morphological features of temporal arteritis. *Proc (Bayl Univ Med Cent)* 2013;26:109–115.
4. Bulkley BH, Roberts WC. Ankylosing spondylitis and aortic regurgitation: description of the characteristic cardiovascular lesion from study of eight necropsy patients. *Circulation* 1973;48:1014–1027.
5. Roberts WC, Hollingsworth JF, Bulkley BH, Jaffe RB, Epstein SE, Stinson EB. Combined mitral and aortic regurgitation in ankylosing spondylitis: angiographic and anatomic features. *Am J Med* 1974;56:237–243.
6. Silver MA, Roberts WC. Detailed anatomy of the normally functioning aortic valve in hearts of normal and increased weight. *Am J Cardiol* 1985;55:454–461.
7. Calonge N; U.S. Preventive Services Task Force. Screening for syphilis infection: recommendation statement. *Ann Fam Med* 2004;2:362–365.
8. Hart G. Syphilis tests in diagnostic and therapeutic decision making. *Ann Intern Med* 1986;104:368–376.
9. Waller BF, Reis RL, McIntosh CL, Epstein SE, Roberts WC. Marfan cardiovascular disease without the Marfan syndrome. *Chest* 1980;77:533–540.
10. Roberts WC, Honig HS. The spectrum of cardiovascular disease in the Marfan syndrome: a clinico-morphologic study of 18 necropsy patients and comparison to 151 previously reported necropsy patients. *Am Heart J* 1982;104:115–135.
11. Roberts WC, Lensing FD, Kourlis H Jr, Ko JM, Newberry JW, Smerud MJ, Burton EC, Hebeler RF Jr. Full blown cardiovascular syphilis with aneurysm of the innominate artery. *Am J Cardiol* 2009;104:1595–1600.
12. Wolinsky H, Glagov S. Nature of species differences in the medial distribution of aortic vasa vasorum in mammals. *Circ Res* 1967;20:409–421.

Frequency of Massive Cardiac Adiposity (Floating Heart) at Necropsy and Comparison of Clinical and Morphologic Variables With Cases With Nonmassive Cardiac Adiposity at a Single Texas Hospital, 2013 to 2014

William C. Roberts, MD[a,b,c,*], Vera S. Won, BS[a], Anupama Vasudevan, BDS, MPH, PhD[a], Jong Mi Ko, BA[a], and Joseph M. Guileyardo, MD[b]

Body weight continues to increase worldwide primarily because of the increase in body fat. This study analyzes the frequency of massive adiposity at autopsy determined by the ability of the heart to float in a container of 10% formaldehyde (because adipose tissue is lighter than myocardium) and compares certain findings in the patients with floating to those with nonfloating hearts. The hearts studied at necropsy during a 2-year period (2013 to 2014) at Baylor University Medical Center were carefully "cleaned" and weighed by the same person and tested as to their ability to float in a container of formaldehyde, an indication of severe cardiac adiposity. Of the 146 hearts studied, 76 (52%) floated in a container of formaldehyde and 70 (48%) did not. Comparison of the 76 patients with floating hearts with the 70 with nonfloating hearts showed significant differences in ages (62 ± 13 vs 58 ± 14 years). No significant differences between the 2 groups were found in gender, body mass index, frequency of systemic hypertension or diabetes mellitus, either acute or healed myocardial infarction, or whether death was due to a coronary or a noncoronary condition. A weak correlation was found between body mass index and heart weight in both men and women and in both floating and nonfloating hearts. The massive quantity of cardiac adipose tissue (floating heart) appears to have increased enormously in recent decades in the United States. **(Am J Cardiol 2016;117:1006−1013)**

Overweightness including obesity is now a worldwide problem. One commercial airline (Samoa Air) now bases ticket costs on body weight plus luggage.[1] Although the fattest major US cities seem to vary each year, Houston, San Antonio, El Paso, and Dallas rank high in virtually every annual survey.[2,3] Houston has more fast food outlets than any city in the United States.[4] We studied the frequency of massive fatty deposits in the heart at necropsy during a 2-year period (2013 to 2014) in a single hospital located in Dallas and also compared various clinical variables in the floating versus nonfloating hearts studied during the same period.

Methods

Because adipose tissue is lighter than cardiac muscle, hearts with enormous quantities of fat tend to float in containers of 10% formaldehyde and often in water.

During 2013 and 2014, Dr. Joseph M. Guileyardo, head of the autopsy service at Baylor University Medical Center, performed a total of 165 autopsies on adults. In 8, the autopsy permit did not allow examination of the heart; in 3 others, the autopsy was in patients who had previous cardiac transplantation. Of the remaining 154 autopsies in adults, WCR examined and described the hearts in 146 (95%). This study is limited to these 146 cases.

The hearts were "cleaned" of extraneous tissues, such as parietal pericardium, and then placed in a container of 10% fresh formaldehyde to determine if the heart floated to the surface after carefully removing any residual air from each chamber by compressing the heart several times when it was submerged. The heart was incised in various fashions depending on the perceived cardiac condition present (or absent) and weighed after gently "patting" all exposed surfaces by paper towels to remove extraneous water or formaldehyde. The scales used were accurate to 0.1 g (Ohaus Scott Pro Scale, Parsippany, New Jersey) or to 1.0 g (Acculab Vicon Digital Scale, Arvada, Colorado). All hearts were weighted by WCR.

The anterior surfaces of many of the 146 hearts were photographed, and, after opening, all hearts were photographed (by JMK). The clinical records were then obtained on each of the 146 patients through Baylor Health Care System's electronic medical record (Allscripts Sunrise Enterprise, Chicago, Illinois).

Statistical analysis was done using STATA 14.0.[5] The baseline characteristics of patients with floating and

[a]Baylor Heart and Vascular Institute, [b]Department of Pathology, and [c]Department of Internal Medicine, Baylor University Medical Center, Dallas, Texas. Manuscript received October 22, 2015; revised manuscript received and accepted December 16, 2015.

This study was funded by the Baylor Health Care System Foundation through the Cardiovascular Research Review Committee and in co-operation with the Baylor Heart and Vascular Institute.

See page 1012 for disclosure information.

*Corresponding author: Tel: (214) 820-7911; fax: (214) 820-7533.

E-mail address: wc.roberts@baylorhealth.edu (W.C. Roberts).

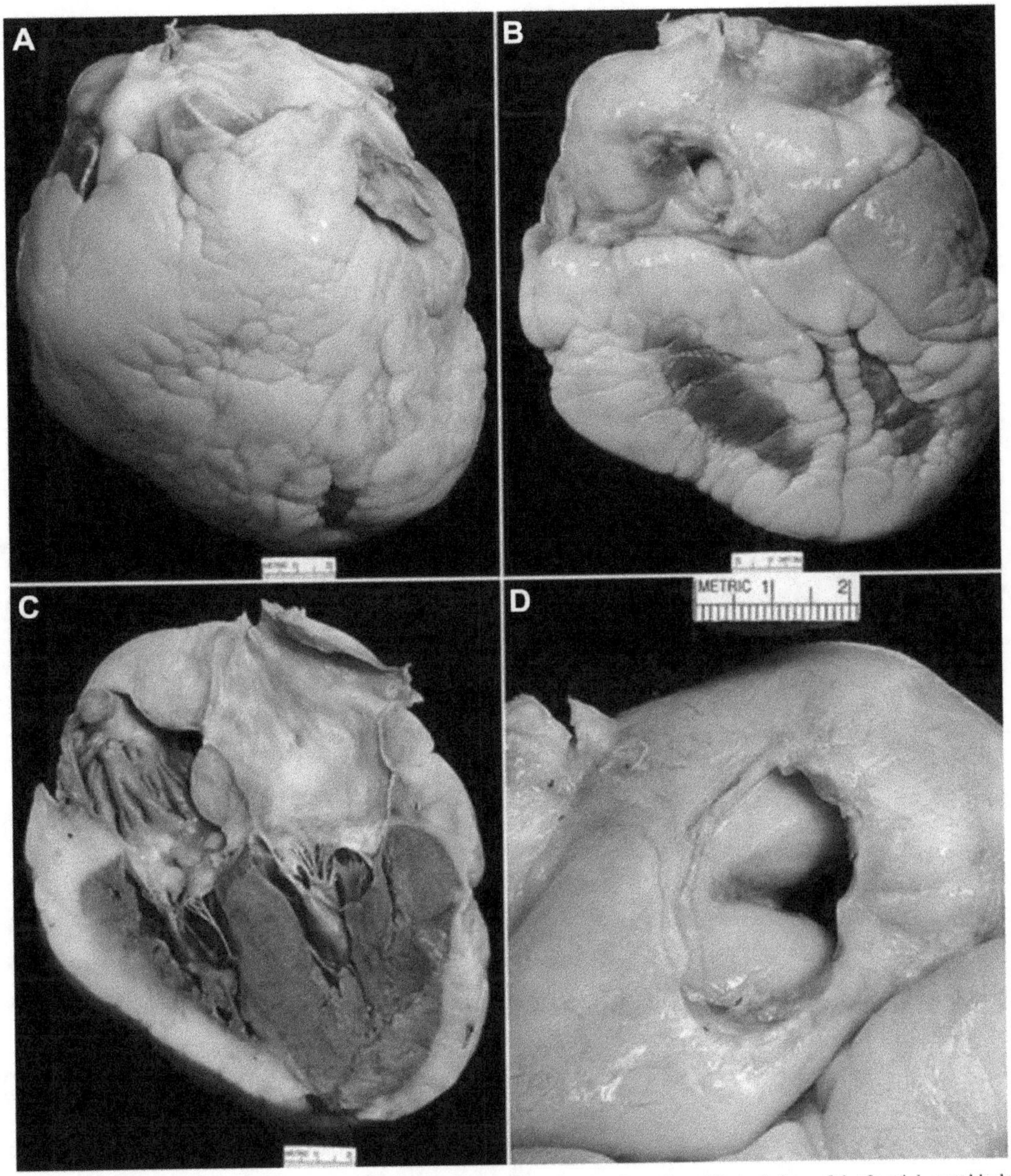

Figure 1. Shown here is a 780-g floating heart—anterior view *(A)*, posterior view *(B)*, 4-chamber view *(C)*, and view of the 2 atrial septal bulges from the orifice of the inferior vena cava *(D)* are shown. The quantity of subepicardial adipose tissue is massive and from the anterior aspect both right and left ventricles are covered by adipose tissue except for an extremely small portion of left ventricle at the apex. The photograph in *(B)* not only shows the huge quantities of fat on the posterior surface of the ventricles but also in the walls of the atria. The 4-chamber view *(C)* shows severe fatty infiltration of the atrial septum except for the fossa ovale region (lipomatous hypertrophy of the atrial septum). The coronary system in this patient was co-dominant: the lumens of the right and left circumflex coronary arteries are wide open. The adipose tissue covering the right ventricular wall is thicker than its muscular wall. Neither ventricular cavity is dilated. The 2 bulges shown in *(D)* are of the atrial septum toward the right atrium. The indentation is the area of the fossa ovale region, which is devoid of adipose tissue. This 64-year-old black woman had undergone sleeve gastrectomy 4 months before death and her BMI just before operation was >50 kg/m^2. Eighteen days after the operation, the BMI was 52 kg/m^2. The patient had diabetes mellitus, systemic hypertension, obstructive sleep apnea, chronic obstructive pulmonary disease, and rheumatoid arthritis.

nonfloating hearts were compared using the chi-square or Fisher's exact tests for proportions and *t* test/Wilcoxon's rank-sum test for continuous variables where applicable. In addition, comparisons were conducted separately for men and women. Correlations among heart weight, age, and body mass index (BMI) were evaluated using Pearson's correlation analysis. For correlation analyses, the data were rendered normal by removing any outliers.

Results

The major finding in this study was the high frequency of massive cardiac adiposity (as determined by whether the heart floated in a container of formaldehyde) at necropsy (Figures 1 to 3). Of the 146 hearts, 76 (52%) contained such large quantities of adipose tissue that they floated and 70 (48%) did not float.

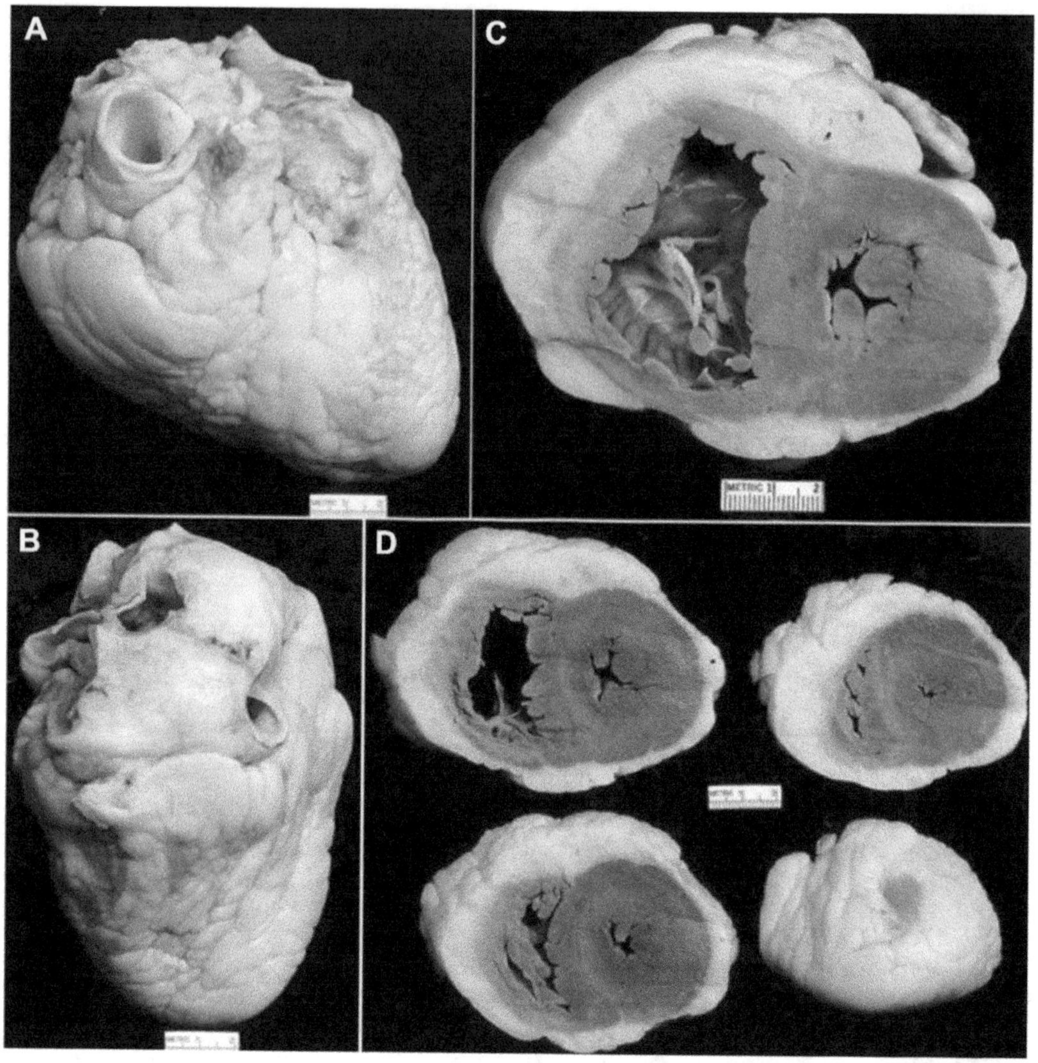

Figure 2. Shown here is the 490-g floating heart of a 55-year-old white woman who had a laparoscopic Nissen fundoplication operation 6 months before death because of a BMI >40 kg/m^2 postoperatively multiple gastrointestinal complications followed. At necropsy, the heart weighed 490 g and floated in a container of 10% formaldehyde. Shown here is the anterior view *(A)*, posterior view *(B)*, base of the heart after cutting the cardiac ventricles in several slices parallel to the posterior atrioventricular sulcus *(C)*, and 4 views of the ventricles *(D)* caudal to the view shown in *(C)*. From the anterior aspect, myocardium cannot be seen. The thickness of the adipose tissue covering the right ventricular free wall is thicker than its muscular wall. The left ventricular cavity is not dilated. The right ventricular cavity is dilated.

The second finding was comparison of various clinical and morphologic variables in the patients with floating versus nonfloating hearts (Table 1). As shown in the accompanying table, age was the only variable that was significantly different between the 76 patients with floating hearts (62 ± 13 years) and the 70 patients with nonfloating hearts (58 ± 14 years). Women with floating hearts were older (62 ± 13 years) compared with those with nonfloating hearts (52 ± 15 years), whereas no difference in age was noted among men. Comparison of the patients with floating hearts versus nonfloating hearts showed no significant differences in gender, BMI, frequency of systemic hypertension or diabetes mellitus, heart weight, either acute or healed myocardial infarcts or both at necropsy, or whether death was due to coronary or noncoronary disease (Table 1). The mean heart weights were larger in the men than in the women whether the heart floated or did not float.

Figure 4 graphically shows the relation between BMI and heart weight in both floating and nonfloating hearts in both men and women. A weak positive correlation was found. Most hearts were of increased weight (>350 g in women and >400 g in men). Figure 5 graphically shows the relation of heart weight to age in both men and women and also the relation of the 2 variations to whether the heart floated. These relations were negative.

Of the 146 patients, 37 (25%) died from consequences of coronary heart disease and 109 (75%) from noncoronary causes. There was no significant difference in the frequency of floating hearts in the 37 patients dying of coronary heart disease compared with the 109 patients dying from noncoronary cases (p = 0.51). Of the 146 patients, 19 had

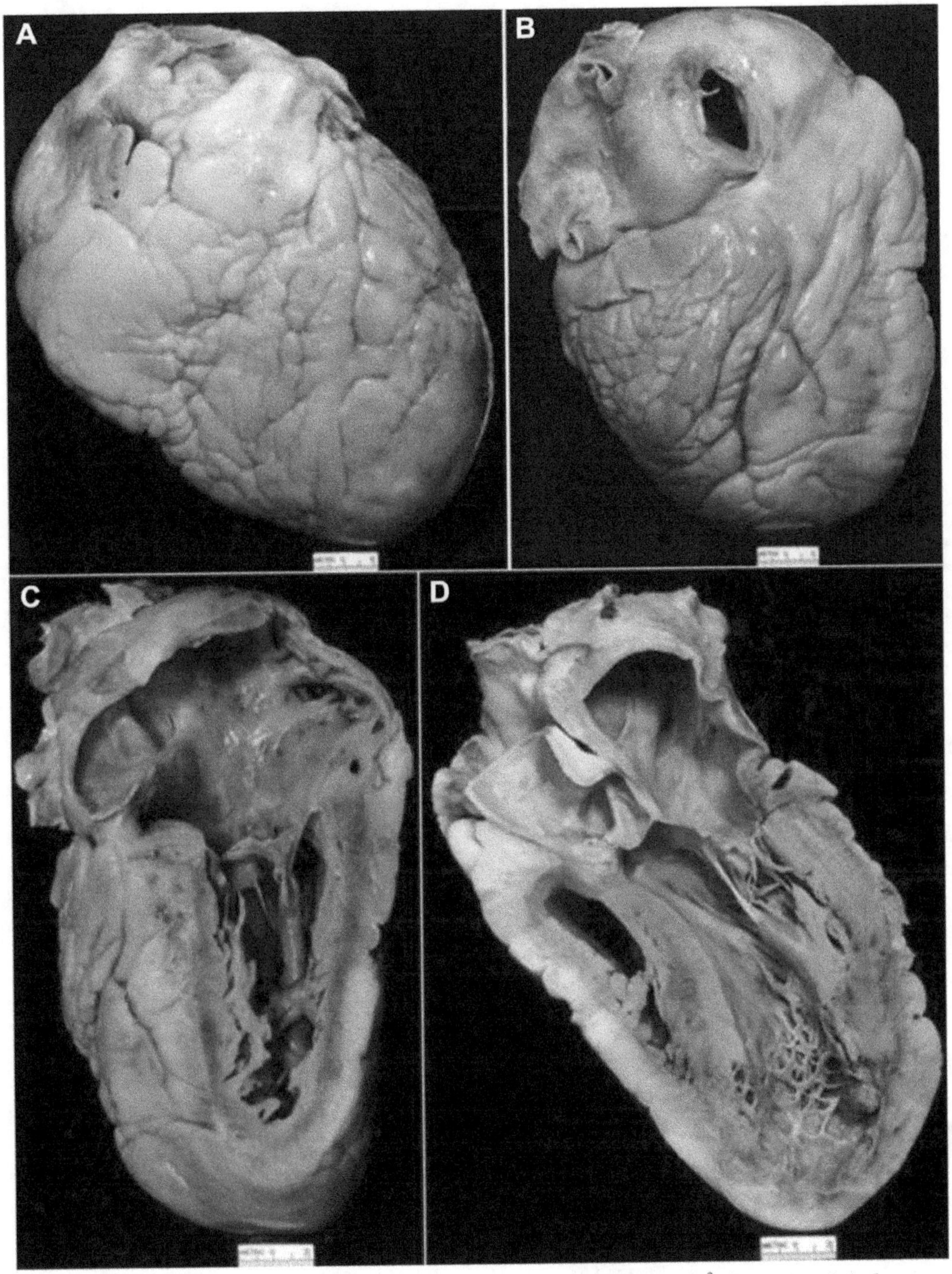

Figure 3. Shown here is the 830-g floating heart of a 64-year-old white woman whose BMI was 57 kg/m^2. This patient died of acute myocardial infarction involving the apical half of left ventricle and was in severe heart failure for some time. A thrombus developed in the apex of left ventricle. The left ventricular ejection fraction by echocardiogram was 33%. She had severe narrowing of the left anterior descending and left circumflex coronary arteries and stents were placed in both. The anterior surface of the heart *(A)*, the posterior portion of the heart *(B)*, a parasagittal view of the right side of the heart showing the right atrium, tricuspid valve, and right ventricular inflow tract *(C)*, and left parasagittal cut *(D)* showing the infarct in the apical half of the left ventricular free wall are shown. The quantity of subepicardial adipose tissue is massive. The entire walls of both right and left ventricles are covered by adipose tissue. The right coronary artery shown in *(C)* is wide open. The thickness of the subepicardial adipose tissue over the right ventricle is thicker than then the right ventricular myocardial wall.

received chronic prednisone therapy and the hearts in 10 (53%) of them floated in a container of formaldehyde; of the 127 patients who were never on chronic prednisone or other corticosteroid therapy, 66 (52%) floated in a container of formaldehyde (p = ns).

Discussion

The concept of "floating heart" was presented initially in an article by Roberts and Roberts in 1983 who described 5% frequency of floating hearts in 55 necropsy patients included in a 2.5-year period in the early 1980s.[6] The most

Table 1
Clinical and morphologic data in the 146 patients comparing various variables in those with floating and nonfloating hearts

Variable	Total (N=146)	Float (n=76)	Nonfloat (n=70)	p Value
Age (years) (Mean±SD)	60±13	62±13	58±14	0.03
Range [median]	23-90 [60]	30-87 [62]	23-90 [58]	
Men				
Mean±SD	62±13	63±14	61±12	0.39
Range [median]	30-90 [63]	30-87 [65]	42-90 [59]	
21-40	3/81 (4%)	3/3 (100%)	0/3 (0%)	
41-60	35/81 (43%)	12/35 (34%)	23/35 (66%)	
61-80	34/81 (42%)	17/34 (50%)	17/34 (50%)	
81-100	9/81 (11%)	5/9 (56%)	4/9 (44%)	0.11
Women				
Mean±SD	58±14	62±13	52±15	0.009
Range [median]	23-86 [58]	37-86 [60]	23-81 [52]	
21-40	9/65 (14%)	2/9 (22%)	7/9 (78%)	
41-60	31/65 (48%)	20/31 (65%)	11/31 (35%)	
61-80	20/65 (31%)	13/20 (65%)	7/20 (35%)	
81-100	5/65 (8%)	4/5 (80%)	1/5 (20%)	0.08
Sex				
Men	81/146 (55%)	37/81 (46%)	44/81 (54%)	0.09
Women	65/146 (45%)	39/65 (60%)	26/65 (40%)	
Body Mass Index (kg/m^2) (Mean±SD)	31±9	32±8	30±9	
Range [median]	15-72 [29]	18-55 [30]	15-72 [29]	0.19
Men				
Mean±SD	31±9	32±8	31±10	
Range [median]	16-72 [29]	21-48 [30]	16-72 [29]	0.52
≤25	19/81 (23%)	7/19 (37%)	12/19 (63%)	
>25-30	26/81 (32%)	12/26 (46%)	14/26 (54%)	
>30	36/81 (44%)	18/36 (50%)	18/36 (50%)	0.65
Women				
Mean±SD	31±9	32±8	28±7	
Range [median]	15-55 [30]	18-54 [30]	15-42 [30]	0.11
≤25	21/65 (32%)	10/21 (48%)	11/21 (52%)	
>25-30	13/65 (20%)	10/13 (77%)	3/13 (23%)	
>30	31/65 (48%)	19/31 (61%)	12/31 (39%)	0.23
Coronary Artery Disease	53 (36%)	29/53 (55%)	24/53 (45%)	0.63
Healed myocardial infarct	29 (20%)	12/29 (41%)	17/29 (59%)	0.20
Acute myocardial infarct	16 (11%)	11/16 (69%)	5/16 (31%)	0.19
Both	3 (2%)	2/3 (67%)	1/3 (33%)	1.00
Neither	13 (9%)	8/13 (62%)	5/13 (38%)	0.57
Diabetes Mellitus	54 (37%)	29/54 (54%)	25/54 (46%)	0.76
Hypertension	95 (65%)	48/95 (51%)	47/95 (49%)	0.61
Heart Weight (g) Mean±SD	490±143	469±124	512±160	0.07
Range [median]	142-1070 [475]	208-830 [455]	142-1070 [488]	
Men				
Mean±SD	548±135	519±108	572±151	0.08
Range [median]	335-1070 [515]	335-720 [505]	375-1070 [547.5]	
>400g	72/81 (89%)	32/72 (44%)	40/72 (56%)	0.53
Women				
Mean±SD	417±119	422±121	410±118	0.68
Range [median]	142-830 [410]	208-830 [395]	142-735 [410]	
>350g	45/65 (69%)	27/45 (60%)	18/45 (40%)	1.00

important finding in this study was the high frequency (52%) of massive cardiac adiposity (floating heart) at autopsy. Comparison of the patients with floating versus nonfloating hearts showed only significant differences in age and that was entirely because of a 10-year mean difference in the ages of the women (floating hearts, age 62; nonfloating, age 52 years; Table 1). There also was a significant but weak correlation between BMI and heart weight in both women and men and in both the floating and the nonfloating hearts.

The contribution of fat to heart weight can be enormous. Shirani and colleagues[7] in 1995 excised subepicardial adipose tissue and fatty atrial septa in 30 patients at necropsy and found that adipose tissue in the heart contributed up to 50% of the cardiac weight. Of the 30 cases studied by them, the heart floated in 12 and in them the adipose tissue

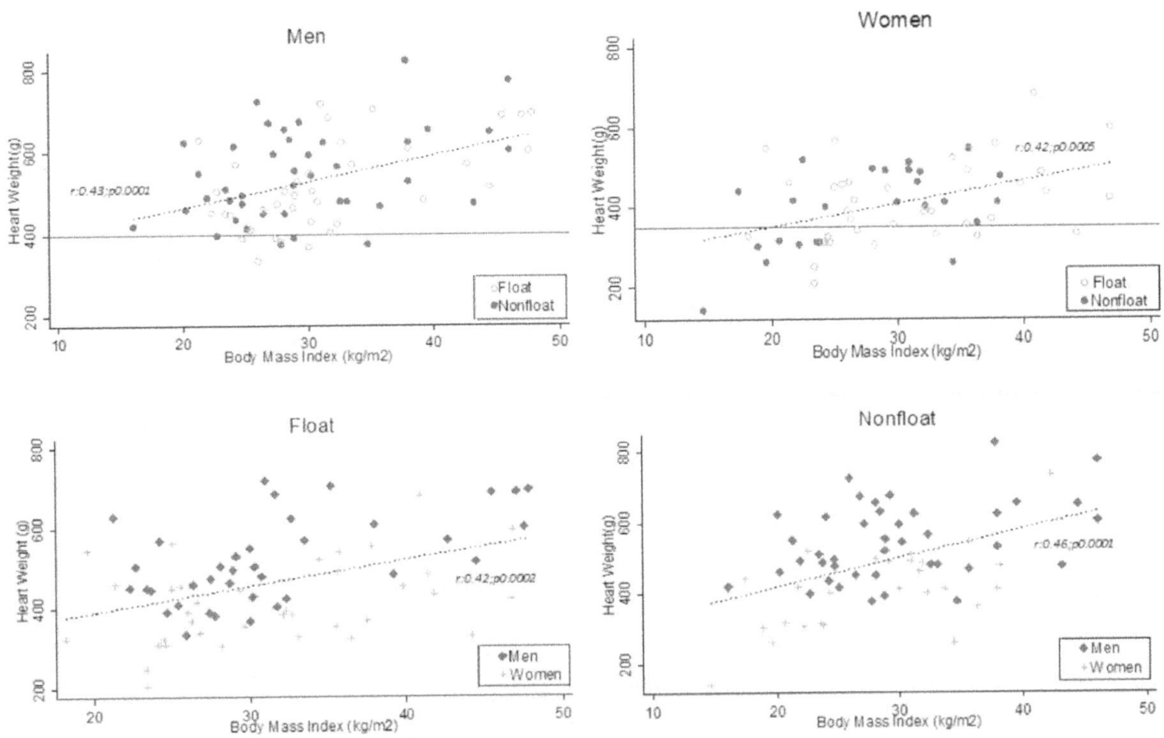

Figure 4. This graph shows the relation between BMI and heart weight in both men and women in both the hearts which floated and those which did not. There was a weak but significant correlation between BMI and heart weight in both groups. The *horizontal line* in the 2 upper graphs show the upper limits for normal heart weight in men (400 g) and women (350 g). The men are represented by *diamond* signs and the women by *plus* signs. Three men, who were outliers, were excluded from top left graph and also from the bottom right graph; 2 women, also outliers, were excluded from top right graph and 1 woman from bottom left graph.

comprised a mean of 32 ± 9% (range 21% to 52%) of the total cardiac weight at necropsy.

The occurrence of such large fatty deposits in the heart in a single Texas hospital in the second decade of the twenty-first century is astounding. It is unlikely that such huge cardiac fatty deposits were as frequent at necropsy in the United States 30, 40, or 50 years ago. Indeed, Roberts and Roberts[6] in a report in 1983 found that only 5% of hearts studied at necropsy in patients >40 years in a 2.5-year period in the early 1980s floated. Certainly, overweightness including obesity has skyrocketed in the last 30 years, and the present study did show a correlation between BMI and heart weight in both the floating and nonfloating hearts.

Osler, in his 1892, *The Principles and Practice of Medicine*[8] described "fatty overgrowth," which he defined as "...a single excess of the normal subepicardial fat, to which the term *cor adiposum* was given by older writers. In other instances, the fat infiltrates the muscular substance and, separating the strands, may reach even to the endocardium. In corpulent persons, there is always much pericardial fat. It forms part of the general obesity ...The entire heart may be enveloped in a thick sheeting of fat through which not a trace of muscle substance can be seen. On section, the fat infiltrates the muscle, separating the fibres, and in extreme cases—particularly in the right ventricle—reaches the endocardium. In some places, there may be even complete substitution of fat for the muscle substance ..." In contrast to Osler's textbook appearing 123 years ago, modern cardiologic textbooks generally fail to mention "cardiac adiposity," or "fatty heart" or "cor adiposum!".

In recent times, the quantity of subepicardial adipose tissue has received increasing attention but that attention almost entirely has been through echocardiographic,[9–16] computed tomographic,[17–25] and magnetic resonance imaging[26–28] and not from morphologic studies.[29,30] The findings in their studies, of course, were not completely uniform but most showed that the quantity (thickness of fat over the right ventricular free wall or total epicardial fat volume) correlated significantly with the quantity of visceral adipose tissue, left ventricular mass, left atrial cavity size, left ventricular diastolic function, systolic and diastolic systemic arterial pressures, the presence of and the severity of coronary atherosclerosis, the quantity of coronary arterial calcium, carotid arterial intimal-medial thickness, the level of serum triglycerides, high-density lipoprotein cholesterol, and fasting blood glucose, and the presence of the metabolic syndrome and diabetes mellitus. The cardiac adipose tissue was an independent risk factor for cardiovascular disease and even a useful predictor of recurrence of atrial fibrillation after ablation.[21]

The present study of course has strengths and limitations. The major strength is the large percent of floating hearts, namely 52%, at a single institution in a recent 2-year period. The demonstration, in 3 different views of hearts, containing enough adipose tissue to float also has not been illustrated previously. That a heart floats in formaldehyde or water indicates that the heart contains a huge quantity of adipose

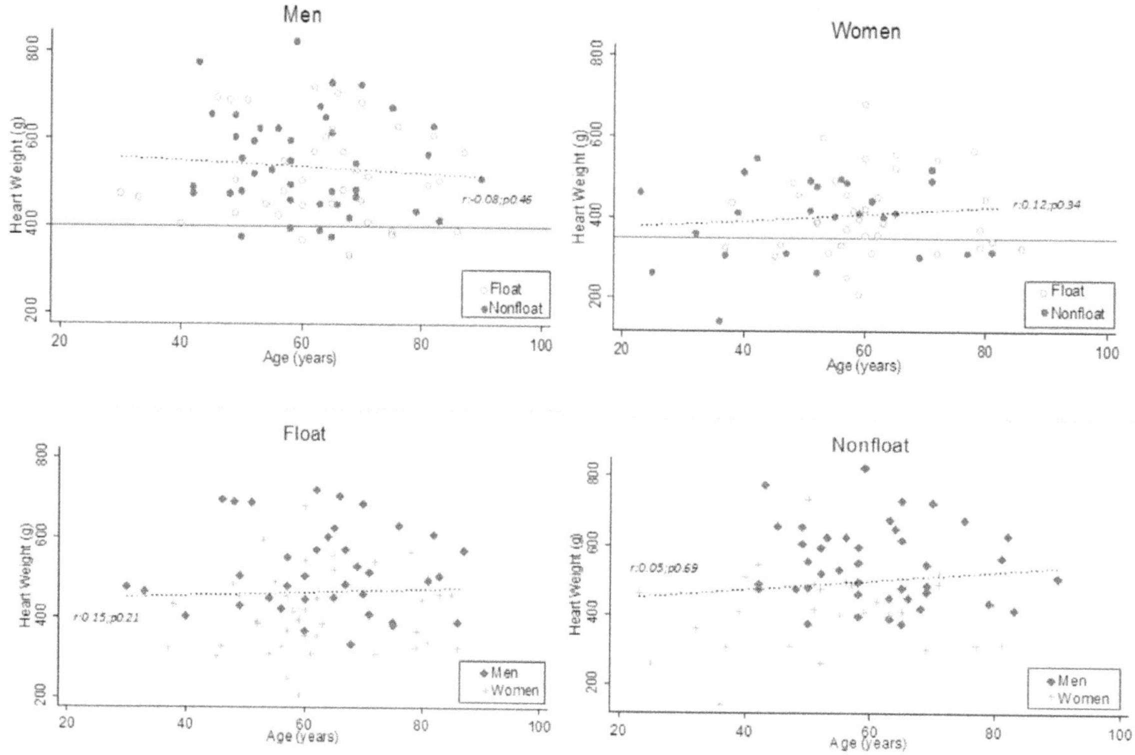

Figure 5. This diagram shows the lack of correlation of heart weight to age in hearts that floated and those that did not. In each diagram, the men and women are designated by a different symbol. The floating hearts are represented by the *"open" circles* and the nonfloating by the *"closed" circles*. The *solid line* in the women separates the hearts that weighed >350g from those that did not. The *solid line* in the men separates the hearts that weighed >400g from those that did not. Two men, who were outliers, were excluded from the top left graph and also from the bottom right graph; 2 women, who were outliers, were excluded from the top right graph and 1 woman from the bottom left graph.

tissue. If, however, the myocardial mass is considerable although the quantity of adipose is also considerable the heart may not float because the myocardial mass, by weighing more than the fatty mass, prevents the heart from floating. Although the present study focuses primarily on necropsy patients with floating hearts, indicating massive cardiac adiposity, the nonfloating hearts, with few exceptions, also had a considerably increased quantity of cardiac adipose tissue, just not quite enough to allow the heart to float. The latter fact may explain the lack of more significant clinical differences between the floating and nonfloating cases.

Disclosures

The authors have no conflicts of interest to disclose.

1. Craymer L. Weigh more, pay more: Samoa Air pegs ticket prices to passenger pounds. *Wall Street J* 2013.
2. Millado, Nate. "The fittest and fattest cities in America." Men's Fitness. Available at: *http://www.mensfitness.com/weight-loss/burn-fat-fast/the-fittest-and-fattest-cities-in-america*. Accessed on August 18, 2015.
3. Sauter MB, McIntyre DA, Weigley S. "America's fattest cities". 24/7 Wall St 2013. Available at: *http://247wallst.com/special-report/2013/04/12/americas-fattest-cities/*. Accessed on August 18, 2015.
4. Cohen J. Houston is America's fattest city. *Texas Monthly* 2013. Available at: *http://www.texasmonthly.com/articles/houston-is-americas-fattest-city/*. Accessed on August 18, 2015.
5. StataCorp. *Stata Statistical Software: Release 14*. College Station, TX: StataCorp LP, 2015.
6. Roberts WC, Roberts JD. The floating heart or the heart too fat to sink: analysis of 55 necropsy patients. *Am J Cardiol* 1983;52:1286–1289.
7. Shirani J, Berezowski K, Roberts WC. Quantitative measurement of normal and excessive (cor adiposum) subepicardial adipose tissue, its clinical significance, and its effect on electrocardiographic QRS voltage. *Am J Cardiol* 1995;76:414–418.
8. Osler W. The Principles and Practice of Medicine. Designed for the Use of Practitioners and Students of Medicine. New York: D. Appleton and Company, 1892:642–643.
9. Iacobellis G, Ribaudo MC, Leto G, Zappaterreno A, Vecci E, Di Mario U, Leonetti F. Influence of excess fat on cardiac morphology and function: study in uncomplicated obesity. *Obes Res* 2002;10:767–773.
10. Iacobellis G, Ribaudo MC, Assael F, Vecci E, Tiberti C, Zappaterreno A, Di Mario U, Leonetti F. Echocardiographic epicardial adipose tissue is related to anthropometric and clinical parameters of metabolic syndrome: a new indicator of cardiovascular risk. *J Clin Endocrinol Metab* 2003;88:5163–5168.
11. Iacobellis G, Pond CM, Sharma AM. Different "weight" of cardiac and general adiposity in predicting left ventricle morphology. *Obesity* 2006;14:1679–1684.
12. Chaowalit N, Somers VK, Pellikka PA, Rihal CS, Lopez-Jimenez F. Subepicardial adipose tissue and the presence and severity of coronary artery disease. *Atherosclerosis* 2006;186:354–359.
13. Willens HJ, Byers P, Chirinos JA, Labrador E, Hare JM, de Marchena E. Effects of weight loss after bariatric surgery on epicardial fat measured using echocardiography. *Am J Cardiol* 2007;99:1242–1245.
14. Willens HJ, Gómez-Marín O, Chirinos JA, Goldberg R, Lowery MH, Iacobellis G. Comparison of epicardial and pericardial fat thickness assessed by echocardiography in African American and non-hispanic white men: a pilot study. *Ethn Dis* 2008;18:311–316.
15. Iacobellis G, Willens HJ. Echocardiographic epicardial fat: a review of research and clinical applications. *J Am Soc Echocardiogr* 2009;22:1311–1319.

16. Liu J, Fox CS, Hickson DA, May WL, Ding J, Carr JJ, Taylor HA. Pericardial fat and echocardiographic measures of cardiac abnormalities: the Jackson Heart Study. *Diabetes Care* 2011;34:341–346.
17. Gorter PM, de Vos AM, van der Graaf Y, Stella PR, Doevendans PA, Meijs MFL, Prokop M, Visseren FLJ. Relation of epicardial and pericoronary fat to coronary atherosclerosis and coronary artery calcium in patients undergoing coronary angiography. *Am J Cardiol* 2008;102:380–385.
18. Sarin S, Wenger C, Marwaha A, Qureshi A, Go BDM, Woomert CA, Clark K, Nassef LA, Shirani J. Clinical significance of epicardial fat measured using cardiac multislice computed tomography. *Am J Cardiol* 2008;102:767–771.
19. de Vos AM, Prokop M, Roos CJ, Meijs MFL, van Der Schouw YT, Rutten A, Gorter PM, Cramer MJ, Doevendans PA, Rensing BJ, Bartelink ML, Velthuis BK, Mosterd A, Bots ML. Peri-coronary epicardial adipose tissue is related to cardiovascular risk factors and coronary artery calcification in post-menopausal women. *Eur Heart J* 2008;29:777–783.
20. Djaberi R, Schuijf JD, van Werkhoven JM, Nucifora G, Jukema JW, Bax JJ. Relation of epicardial adipose tissue to coronary atherosclerosis. *Am J Cardiol* 2008;102:1602–1607.
21. Lee YJ, Wang CP, Hsu HL, Hung WC, Yu TH, Chen YH, Chiu CA, Lu LF, Chung FM, Shin SJ. Increased epicardial adipose tissue (EAT) volume in type 2 diabetes mellitus and association with metabolic syndrome and severity of coronary atherosclerosis. *Clin Endocrinol (Oxf)* 2009;70:876–882.
22. Mahabadi AA, Massaro JM, Rosito GA, Levy D, Murabito JM, Wolf PA, O'Donnell CJ, Fox CS, Hoffmann U. Association of pericardial fat, intrathoracic fat, and visceral abdominal fat with cardiovascular disease burden: the Framingham Heart Study. *Eur Heart J* 2009;30:850–856.
23. Wang TD, Lee WJ, Shih FY, Huang CH, Chang YC, Chen WJ, Lee YT, Chen MF. Relations of epicardial adipose tissue measured by multidetector computed tomography to components of the metabolic syndrome are region-specific and independent of anthropometric indexes and intraabdominal visceral fat. *J Clin Endocrinol Metab* 2009;94:662–669.
24. Ding J, Hsu FC, Harris TB, Liu Y, Kritchevsky SB, Szklo M, Ouyang P, Espeland MA, Lohman KK, Criqui MH, Allison M, Bluemke DA, Carr JJ. The association of pericardial fat with incident coronary heart disease: the multi-ethnic study of atherosclerosis (MESA). *Am J Clin Nutr* 2009;90:499–504.
25. Greif M, Becker A, Von Ziegler F, Lebherz C, Lehrke M, Broedl UC, Tittus J, Parhofer K, Becker C, Reiser M, Knez A, Leber AW. Pericardial adipose tissue determined by dual source CT is a risk factor for coronary atherosclerosis. *Arterioscler Thromb Vasc Biol* 2009;29:781–786.
26. Staten MA, Totty WG, Kohrt WM. Measurement of fat distribution by magnetic resonance imaging. *Invest Radiol* 1989;24:345–349.
27. Iacobellis G, Sharma AM. Epicardial adipose tissue as new cardio-metabolic risk marker and potential therapeutic target in the metabolic syndrome. *Curr Pharm Des* 2007;13:2180–2184.
28. Fox CS, Gona P, Hoffmann U, Porter SA, Salton CJ, Massaro JM, Levy D, Larson MG, Agostino RBD, O'onnell CJ, Manning WJ. Pericardial fat, intrathoracic fat, and measures of left ventricular structure and function. *Circulation* 2009;119:1586–1591.
29. Reiner L, Mazzoleni A, Rodriguez F. Statistical analysis of the epicardial fat weight in human hearts. *AMA Arch Pathol* 1955;60:369–373.
30. Domenico C, Roberta M, Sergio C, Paolo P, Matteo G, Tu VL, Cesare B. The ventricular epicardial fat is related to the myocardial mass in normal, ischemic and hypertrophic hearts. *Cardiovasc Pathol* 2004;13:313–316.

Frequency of Massive Cardiac Adiposity (Floating Heart) in the Native Hearts of Patients Having Heart Transplantation at a Single Texas Hospital (2013 to 2015) and Comparison of Various Clinical and Morphologic Variables in the Patients With Massive Versus Nonmassive Cardiac Adiposity

William C. Roberts, MD[a,b,c,*], Vera S. Won, BS[a], Anupama Vasudevan, BDS, MPH, PhD[a], Jong Mi Ko, BA[a], Shelley A. Hall, MD[b], and Gonzalo V. Gonzalez-Stawinski, MD[d]

Body weight continues to increase worldwide due primarily to the increase in body fat. This study analyzes the frequency of massive adiposity at hearts of patients who underwent heart transplantation (HT) determined by the ability of the heart to float in a container of 10% formaldehyde (because adipose tissue is lighter than myocardium) and compares certain characteristics of those patients with and without floating hearts. The hearts studied at HT during a 3-year period (2013 to 2015) at Baylor University Medical Center were carefully "cleaned" and weighed by the same individual and tested as to their ability to float in a container of formaldehyde, an indication of severe cardiac adiposity. Of the 220 hearts studied, 84 (38%) floated in a container of formaldehyde and 136 (62%) did not. Comparison of the 84 patients with floating hearts to the 136 with nonfloating hearts showed a significant difference in ages, but a nonsignificant difference in gender, body mass index, frequency of systemic hypertension, or diabetes mellitus. The odds of a heart being a floating one was increased in patients with a diagnosis of ischemic cardiomyopathy (unadjusted odds ratio 2.12, 95% CI 1.21 to 3.70). The frequency of massive cardiac adiposity in the native hearts of patients having HT (38%) is striking and appears to have increased in frequency in the recent decades. **(Am J Cardiol 2016;117:1375−1380)**

Because overweightness including obesity is now a worldwide problem, it is reasonable to believe that hearts of patients who underwent heart transplantation (HT) would possess considerable quantities of adipose tissues. We studied the native hearts of 220 patients having HT at Baylor University Medical Center in a 3-year period (2013 to 2015) and compared various clinical and morphologic variables in those with massive (floating hearts) versus nonmassive quantities of cardiac adipose tissue.

Methods

All cardiovascular specimens removed at operation at the Baylor University Medical Center since April 1993 have been described by one of us (W.C.R.) and most have been photographed by one of us (J.M.K.). After removing all extraneous tissues after fixation for 2 to 4 days, the hearts were tested for floating in a container of 10% formaldehyde. If the heart floated in the container after asserting that all air had been removed from the cardiac chambers, it was considered "a floating heart," which indicated that the heart contained a "massive" amount of adipose tissue[1] because adipose tissue is lighter than myocardial tissue. If the heart did not float in the container, it was considered "a nonfloating heart," which indicates that the quantity of cardiac adipose tissue is usually less than that present in the floating heart. After excising all extraneous tissues, the hearts were weighed (by W.C.R.) after opening the cardiac chambers, removing all intrachamber clot and gently drying all exposed portions of the heart with paper towels. The scales used were accurate to 0.1 g (Ohaus Scout Pro Scale) or to 1.0 g (Acculab Vicon Digital Scale).

The clinical records were then obtained on all 220 patients through the Baylor Health Care System's electronic medical record (Allscripts Sunrise Enterprise).

Statistical analysis was done using STATA 14.0 (StataCorp. 2015. Stata Statistical Software: Release 14, College Station, TX: StataCorp LP). The baseline characteristics of patients with floating and nonfloating hearts were compared using chi-square/Fisher's exact tests for proportions and *t*-test/Wilcoxon rank-sum test for continuous variables

[a]Department of Baylor Heart and Vascular Institute, [b]Division of Cardiology, Department of Internal Medicine, [c]Department of Pathology, and [d]Department of Cardiothoracic Surgery, Baylor University Medical Center, Dallas, Texas. Manuscript received January 15, 2016; revised manuscript received and accepted January 20, 2016.

This study was funded by the Baylor Health Care System Foundation through the Cardiovascular Research Review Committee and in cooperation with the Baylor Heart and Vascular Institute.

See page 1380 for disclosure information.

*Corresponding author: Tel: +(214) 820-7911; fax: +(214) 820-7533.
E-mail address: wc.roberts@baylorhealth.edu (W.C. Roberts).

Table 1
Clinical and morphologic finding in the 220 patients who underwent cardiac transplantation at Baylor University Medical Center from January 2013 to November 2015 comparing the finding in the patients with floating and nonfloating hearts

Variable	Total (n = 220)	Transplant (n = 220)		p-Value	Unadjusted OR (95%CI)
		Float (n = 84 [38%])	Nonfloat (n = 136 [62%])		
Sex					
Men	160 (73%)	66 (41%)	94 (59%)		
Women	60 (27%)	18 (30%)	42 (70%)	0.13	0.61 (0.32-1.15)
Age (years) (Mean±SD)	56±11	59±9	54±12		
Range [median]	20-76 [58]	32-76 [62]	20-71 [57]	0.01	1.03 (1.01-1.07)
Men					
Mean±SD	57±11	59±9	56±12		
Range [median]	20-76 [60]	32-76 [62]	20-71 [59]	0.1	
20-40	14 (9%)	3 (21%)	11 (79%)		
41-60	70 (44%)	26 (37%)	44 (63%)		
61-80	76 (48%)	37 (49%)	39 (51%)	0.11	
Women					
Mean±SD	53±11	57±10	51±12		
Range [median]	26-69 [55]	34-69 [56]	26-69 [54]	0.09	
20-40	10 (17%)	1 (10%)	9 (90%)		
41-60	31 (51%)	9 (29%)	22 (71%)		
61-80	19 (32%)	8 (42%)	11 (58%)		
Coronary Artery Disease	93 (42%)	40 (43%)	53 (57%)	0.21	1.42 (0.82-2.47)
Healed myocardial infarct	73 (33%)	35 (48%)	38 (52%)	0.04	1.84 (1.04-3.27)
Acute myocardial infarct	1 (0.5%)	1 (100%)	0	0.38	NA
Both	2 (1%)	1 (50%)	1 (50%)		
Neither	17 (8%)	3 (18%)	14 (82%)		
Diabetes Mellitus	82 (37%)	32 (39%)	50 (61%)	0.84	1.05 (0.60-1.86)
Hypertension (by history)	132 (60%)	47 (36%)	85 (64%)	0.34	0.76 (0.44-1.33)
Body Mass Index (kg/m^2) (Mean±SD)	29.1±5	29.6±5	28.9±5		
Range [median]	17.8-42.3 [28.9]	20.3-39.1 [29.8]	17.8-42.3 [28.4]	0.18	1.03 (0.97-1.08)
16-20	5 (2%)	0	5 (100%)		
21-25	48 (22%)	15 (31%)	33 (69%)		
26-30	78 (36%)	32 (41%)	46 (59%)		
31-35	60 (27%)	27 (45%)	33 (55%)		
36-40	26 (12%)	10 (38%)	16 (62%)		
41-45	3 (1%)	0	3 (100%)	0.23	
Men					
Mean±SD	29.1±5	29.5±4	28.9±5		
BMI Range [median]	19-41.4 [28.8]	20.7-37.8 [29.7]	19-41.4 [28.4]	0.25	
Women					
Mean±SD	29.2±6	29.9±5	28.9±6		
BMI Range [median]	17.8-42.3 [29.0]	20.3-39.1 [30.6]	17.8-42.3 [28.5]	0.46	
Diagnosis					
Ischemic Cardiomyopathy	88 (40%)	43 (49%)	45 (51%)	0.008	2.12 (1.21-3.70)
Men	74 (47%)	39 (53%)	35 (47%)	0.006	
Women	14 (24%)	4 (29%)	10 (71%)	1.00	
Idiopathic Dilated Cardiomyopathy	88 (40%)	29 (33%)	59 (67%)	0.19	0.69 (0.39-1.21)
Men	53 (33%)	17 (32%)	36 (68%)	0.13	
Women	35 (58%)	12 (34%)	23 (66%)	0.57	
Other*	44 (20%)	12 (27%)	32 (73%)	0.09	0.54 (0.26-1.12)
Men	33 (21%)	10 (30%)	23 (70%)	0.15	
Women	11 (19%)	2 (18%)	9 (82%)	0.48	
Heart Weight (g)(Mean±SD)†	486±119	490±103	483±128		
Range [median]	215-883 [480]	285-755 [490]	215-883 [478]	0.47	1.004 (0.99-1.003)
Men					
Mean±SD	509±119	508±94	509±135		
Range [median]	215-883 [502]	285-695 [508]	215-883 [494]	0.71	
>400g	130 (82%)	53 (41%)	77 (59%)	0.95	
Women					
Mean±SD	423±93	420±107	425±88		
Range [median]	235-755 [425]	290-755 [420]	235-599 [429]	0.49	
>350g	46 (78%)	12 (26%)	34 (74%)	0.38	
Left Ventricular Assist Device	43 (20%)	16 (37%)	27 (63%)	0.88	0.95 (0.48-1.89)

Table 2
Cardiac condition included in the category labeled "other" in Table 1

Cardiac Condition	Number of Patients	Age (years) mean ± SD	BMI (kg/m2) mean ± SD	M/F	Floating/ Nonfloating
Amyloidosis	8	56±13	27.4±4	7/1	2/6
Hypertrophic cardiomyopathy	6	48±10	29±5	4/2	3/3
Congential heart disease	8	53±11	29±7	7/1	4/4
Sarcoidosis	6	58±4	27.3±5	5/1	2/4
Arrhythmogenic right ventricular cardiomyopathy	3	46±12	27.4±5	2/1	0/3
Valvular heart disease	3	55±9	32.4±5	2/1	0/3
Radiation heart disease	3	50±13	30±6	2/1	0/3
Pericardial heart disease (constriction)*	1	55	22.3	1/0	0/1
Primary pulmonary hypertension	1	33	24.0	0/1	0/1
Chagas disease	1	28	19.2	0/1	0/1
Toxic cardiomyopathy (adriamycin)	1	27	26.3	1/0	0/1
Ehlers-Danlos Syndrome	1	31	17.8	0/1	0/1
Anthracycline cardiomyopathy	1	57	26	1/0	1/0
Multivessel disease	1	66	31.1	1/0	0/1
Totals	44	52±12	27.9±5	33/11	12/32 (38%)

BMI = body mass index; F = female; M = male.
* Two previous operations for relief of calcific pericardial constriction of uncertain cause had been performed.

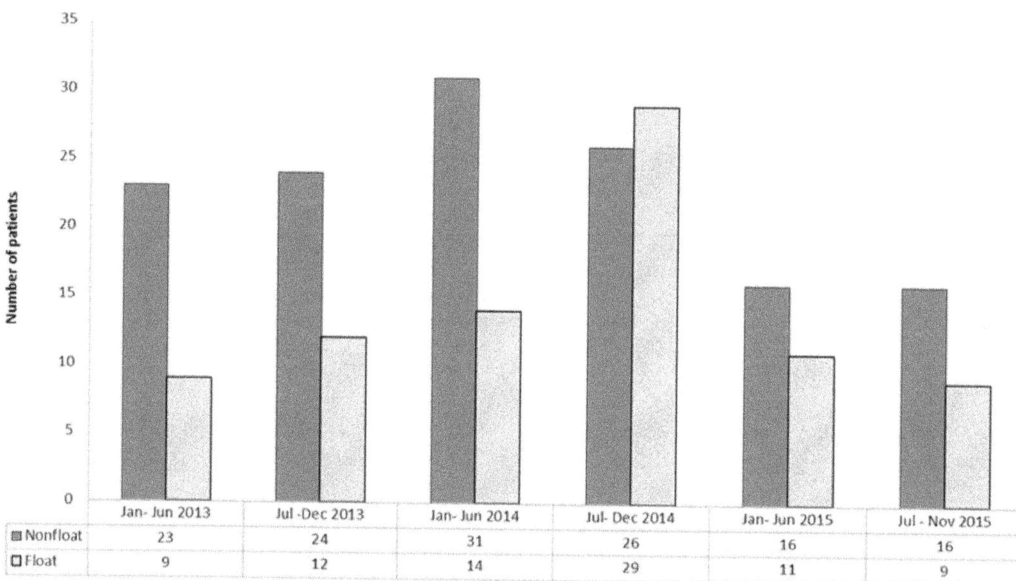

Figure 1. Distribution of floating and nonfloating hearts during the study period (2013 to 2015).

where applicable. In addition, comparisons were repeated separately for men and women. Unadjusted odds ratios with 95% CI were obtained for these variables of interest by logistic regression analysis.

The study was approved by an institutional review board.

Results

The major findings are summarized in Tables 1 and 2. Of the 220 hearts, 84 (38%) contained such a large quantity of adipose tissue that they floated in a container of 10% formaldehyde, and 136 (62%) did not float. The proportion of the hearts that floated in the container increased from 30% in 2013 to 40% in 2014 (Figure 1). The distribution of age, body mass index, and heart weight in the patients with floating and nonfloating hearts are shown in Figure 2. Comparison of the 84 patients with floating hearts to the 136 with nonfloating hearts showed a significant difference in mean ages, but a nonsignificanct difference in gender, body mass index, frequency of systemic hypertension, and diabetes mellitus. The odds of a heart floating in formaldehyde increased with age (unadjusted odds ratio 1.04, 95% CI 1.01 to 1.07) and ischemic cardiomyopathy (unadjusted odds ratio 2.12, 95% CI 1.21 to 3.70). The median body mass index increased over the years in those with floating hearts, whereas it decreased in those patients with nonfloating hearts (Figure 3). Photographs of 2 floating hearts are shown in Figures 4 and 5.

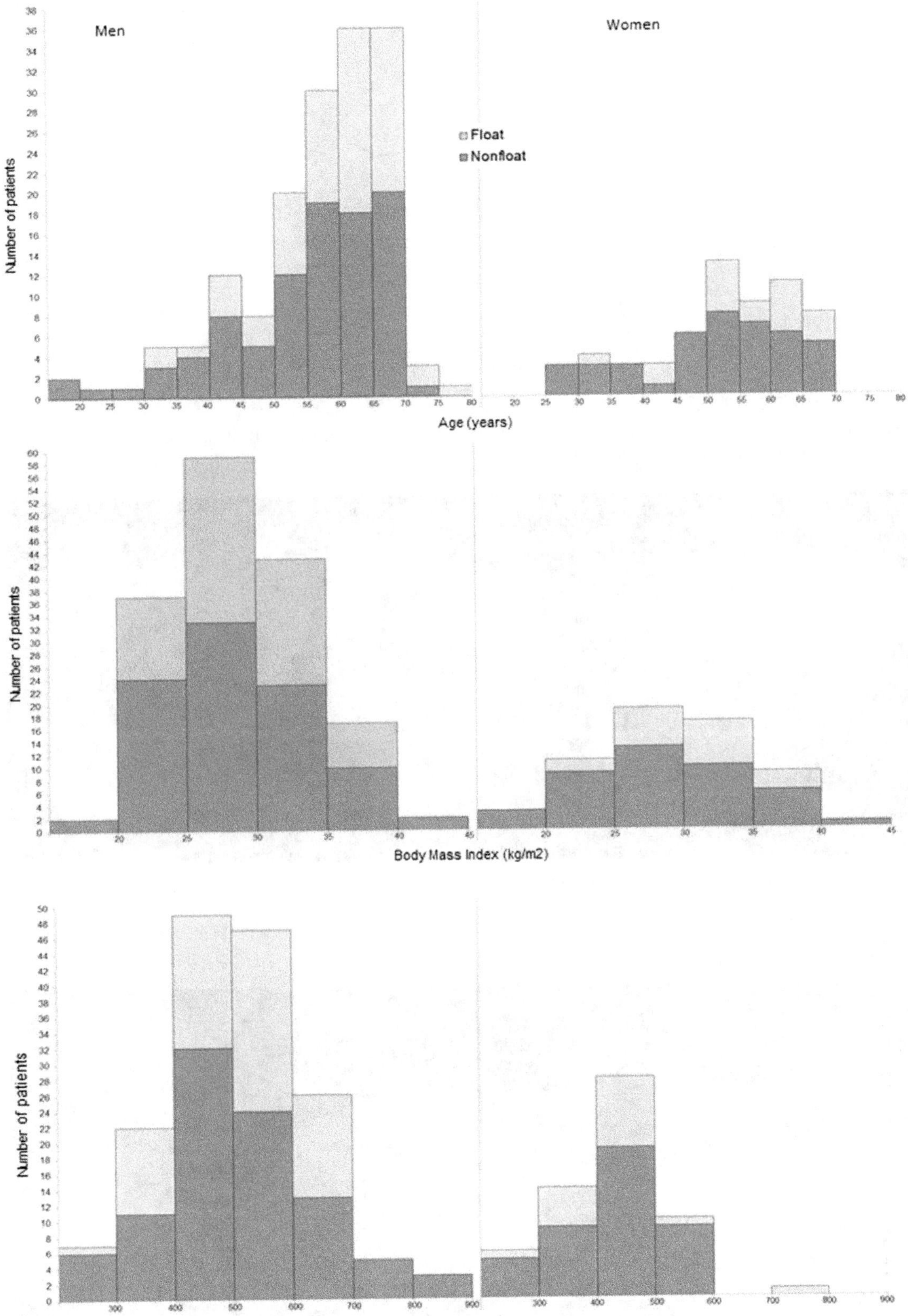

Figure 2. Stacked bar graphs showing ages, body mass indexes, and heart weight of the men and women sorted by numbers of those with and without floating hearts.

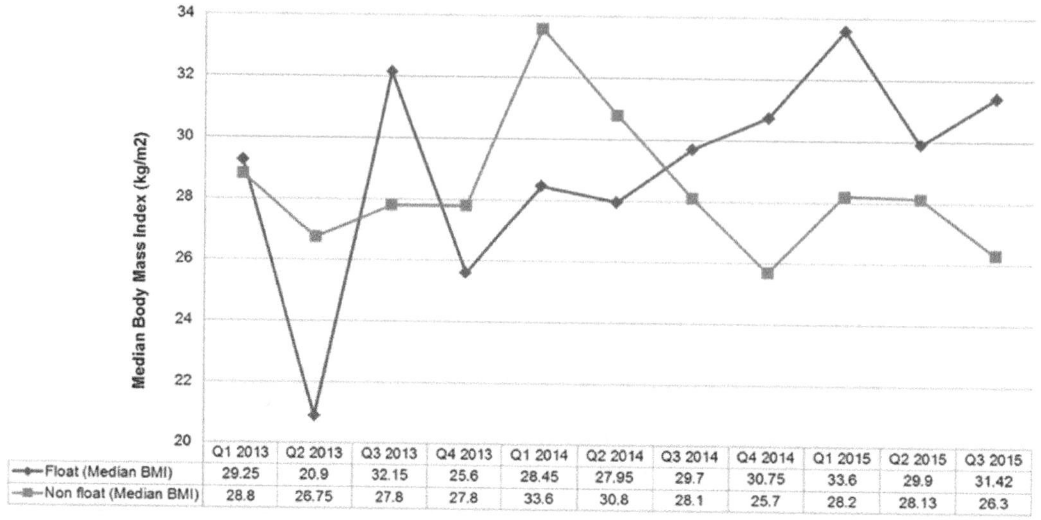

	Q1 2013	Q2 2013	Q3 2013	Q4 2013	Q1 2014	Q2 2014	Q3 2014	Q4 2014	Q1 2015	Q2 2015	Q3 2015
Float (Median BMI)	29.25	20.9	32.15	25.6	28.45	27.95	29.7	30.75	33.6	29.9	31.42
Non float (Median BMI)	28.8	26.75	27.8	27.8	33.6	30.8	28.1	25.7	28.2	28.13	26.3

Figure 3. Body mass index (BMI) in floating and nonfloating patients during the study period. The median BMI increased over the years in those with floating hearts, whereas it decreased in those patients with nonfloating hearts.

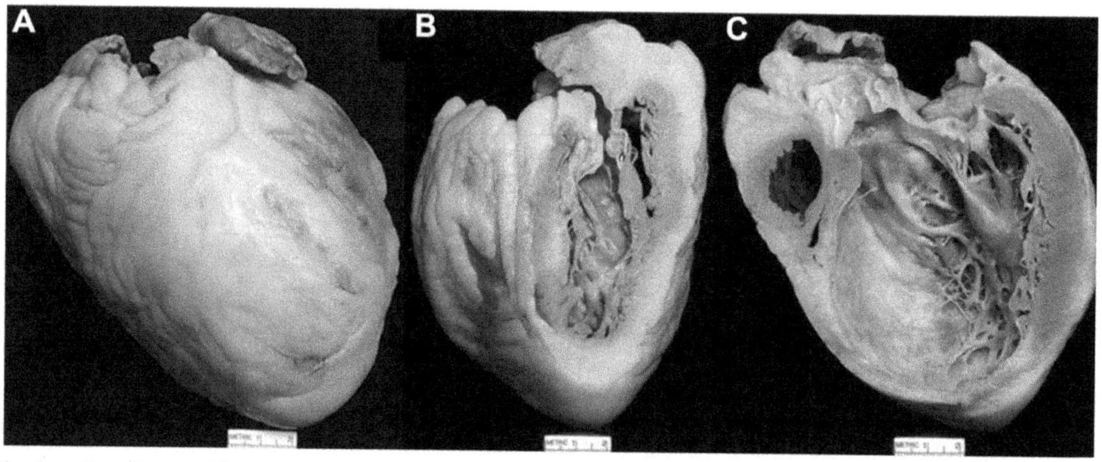

Figure 4. Floating heart in a 59-year-old woman who had had a large acute myocardial infarction at age 37 years and heart failure and periodic ventricular tachycardia subsequently shown here in the external view of the 405-g heart nearly covered with adipose tissue *(A)*; a left parasagittal view showing a huge anteroseptal scar and marked left ventricular dilation *(B)*; and a right parasagittal view exposing the tricuspid valve and right ventricular inflow portion and the excessive subepicardial adipose tissue.

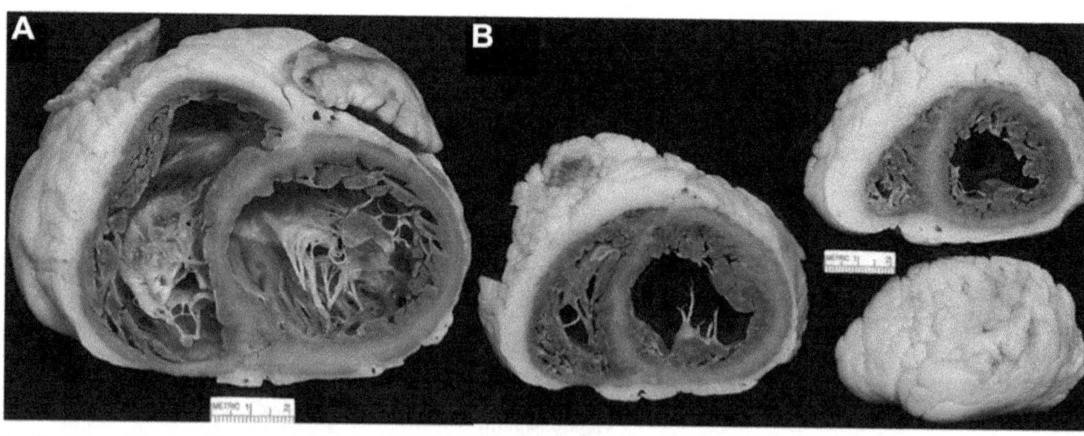

Figure 5. Floating heart in a 63-year-old woman with heart failure some age 43 years. Angiography disclosed no luminal narrowing, and examination of the heart conformed the diagnosis of idiopathic dilated cardiomyopathy shown in *(A)* is the basal portion of the heart exposing the extremely dilated ventricle, the tricuspid and mitral valves, the wide-open coronary artery, the absence of grossly visible myocardial lesion, and the excess subepicardial adipose tissue. Shown in *(B)* are more apical cuts of the ventricular wall, nearly all of which are covered by adipose tissue.

Discussion

The major finding in this study is the high frequency (38%) of massive cardiac adiposity (floating hearts) in the patients having HT, an observation not reported previously. The second important finding was the lack of significant differences between the patients with floating versus those with nonfloating hearts in age, gender, body mass index, and use of a left ventricular assist device.

The concept of "floating heart" was presented initially in an article by Roberts and Roberts[1] in 1983 who described a 5% frequency of floating hearts in 55 necropsy patients included in a 2.5-year period in the early 1980s. A more recent study by Roberts et al[2] at a single Texas hospital in 2013 to 2014 showed a 52% frequency of floating hearts in 146 "necropsy" patients. Thus, a dramatic increase in the frequency of the floating heart, that is, massive cardiac adiposity, during the 32-year interval.

The present study of course has limitations. That a heart floats in formaldehyde or water indicates that the heart contains a huge quantity of adipose tissue. If, however, the myocardial mass is considerable and even though the quantity of adipose tissue is also considerable, the heart may not float because the myocardial mass, by weighing more than the fatty mass, prevents the heart from floating. Although the present study focuses on HT patients with floating hearts, indicating massive cardiac adiposity, the nonfloating hearts, with few exceptions, also had a considerably increased quantity of cardiac adipose tissue, just not quite enough to allow the heart to float. The latter fact may explain the lack of significant clinical differences between the floating and nonfloating cases.

Disclosures

The authors have no conflicts of interest to disclose.

1. Roberts WC, Roberts JD. The floating heart or the heart too fat to sink: analysis of 55 necropsy patients. *Am J Cardiol* 1983;52:1286–1289.
2. Roberts WC, Won VS, Vasudevan A, Ko JM, Guileyardo JM. Frequency of massive cardiac adiposity (floating heart) at necropsy and comparison of clinical and morphologic variables with nonmassive cardiac adiposity at a single Texas hospital, 2013 to 2014. *Am J Cardiol*, http://dx.doi.org/10.1016/j.amjcard.2015.12.039, 2016;117.

Quantitative Extent of Atherosclerotic Plaque in the Major Epicardial Coronary Arteries in Patients with Fatal Coronary Heart Disease, in Coronary Endarterectomy Specimens, in Aorta-Coronary Saphenous Venous Conduits, and Means to Prevent the Plaques: A Review after Studying the Coronary Arteries for 50 Years

William C. Roberts, MD

This review tries to answer the following 15 questions: Is atherosclerosis a systemic or a regional disease? Is atherosclerosis in any particular region focal or diffuse? What is the quantity of atherosclerotic plaques in endarterectomy specimens of the right coronary artery in patients undergoing coronary artery bypass grafting (CABG) compared to that in the right coronary artery in patients with fatal coronary artery disease? How do the units used for measuring arterial narrowing by angiography compare to the units used for measuring arterial narrowing at necropsy? What do atherosclerotic plaques consist of in coronary arteries in patients with fatal coronary disease? What is the quantity of atherosclerotic plaque in bypassed -vs- non-bypassed native coronary arteries in patients dying early (<60 days) or late (>60 days) after coronary artery bypass grafting? What is the frequency of acute coronary lesions and multi-luminal channels at necropsy in patients with unstable angina pectoris, sudden coronary death, and acute myocardial infarction? What is the mechanism of luminal widening by angioplasty in the coronary arteries? What observations suggest that atherosclerotic plaques are the result at least in part of organization of thrombi? Is atherosclerosis a multifactoral or a unifactoral disease? What characteristics distinguish carnivores and herbivores? What are reasonable guidelines for whom to treat with lipid-altering agents? What is the rule of 5 and the rule of 7 in statin therapy? What is the effect of lipid lowering drug therapy on coronary luminal narrowing? What are some requisites for a healthy life?
(Am J Cardiol 2018;121:1413–1435)

Most studies describing the severity of coronary artery disease (CAD) refer to it as one, two, or three vessel diseases or "left main disease." That classification usually designates the number of major (right, left main, left anterior descending, and left circumflex) epicardial coronary arteries narrowed to a certain degree, often 70% diameter reduction, by angiogram or >75% cross-sectional narrowing by intra-arterial ultrasonic imaging or when studied at necropsy. This type of classification obviously has proven to be useful from both therapeutic and prognostic standpoints. This classification, however, does not describe the extent of the narrowing or the extent (quantity, burden) of the atherosclerotic plaques in the full lengths of each of the 4 major epicardial coronary arteries. This review summarizes a number of studies describing the amounts of luminal narrowing not at a single point in any of these 4 coronary arteries but in each 5-mm segment of each of the 4 major epicardial coronary arteries in a large number of patients with fatal CAD studied at necropsy or in those with non-fatal CAD who had coronary endarterectomy specimens available for study. Since the lengths of the 4 major epicardial coronary arteries in adults generally add up to about 27 cm (right = 10; left main = 2; left anterior descending = 10; left circumflex [quite variable] = 6), a total of about 54 five-mm segments of coronary artery are generally available for examination in each patient (Figure 1). One histologic section of each 5-mm segment was

Baylor Heart and Vascular Institute and the Department of Internal Medicine, Division of Cardiology, Baylor University Medical Center at Dallas, Baylor Scott & White Health, Dallas, Texas. Manuscript received February 8, 2018; accepted February 12, 2018.

Abbreviations

AMI	acute myocardial infarction
CABG	coronary artery bypass grafting
CAD	coronary artery disease
LDL	low-density lipoprotein
RCA	right coronary artery

See page 1433 for disclosure information.

E-mail address: William.Roberts1@bswhealth.org.

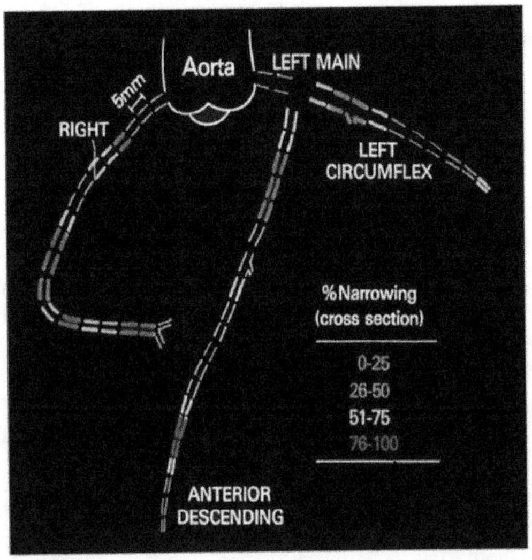

Figure 1. This diagram shows each of the 4 major epicardial coronary arteries and shows how each 5-mm segment is graded in cross-sectional area.

stained for elastic tissue (so that the internal elastic membranes would clearly be discernable for baseline demarcation purposes), usually a Movat stain, and examined from each patient. Before cutting the 5-mm long segments, each major epicardial coronary artery was carefully excised from the heart and decalcified, if necessary. This method is both time consuming and expensive, and both reasons probably account for the absence of this type study by nearly all investigators. The studies described herein were carried out over several decades and with few exceptions before statin therapy was available. I like to refer to this 5-mm segment approach as a *quantitative* one and the 1-, 2-, 3-vessel disease approach as a *qualitative* one.

Is Atherosclerosis a Systemic or a Regional Disease?

A systemic disease. A high percentage of patients with claudication, abdominal aortic aneurysm or obstruction, and carotid arterial narrowing die from atherosclerotic CAD. Mautner and associates[1] reported at necropsy the status of each 5-mm long segment of each of the 4 major coronary arteries in patients with an abdominal aortic aneurysm ≥5.0 cm in its widest transverse diameter. During life, 12 of the 27 patients (44%) had symptoms of myocardial ischemia and 10 (37%) died from its consequences. Grossly visible left ventricular foci of necrosis or fibrosis, or both, was present in 15 patients (56%). Of the 27 patients, 23 (85%) at necropsy had narrowing 76% to 100% in cross-sectional area of ≥1 major coronary artery by atherosclerotic plaque. Of the 1,475 five-mm segments of the major coronary arteries in the 27 patients, 17% were narrowed 0 to 25% in cross-sectional area; 37%, 26% to 50%; 28%, 51% to 75%; 15%, 76% to 95%, and 3%, 96% to 100%. The percentages of these 5-mm segments narrowed >75% in cross-sectional areas were similar in the right, left anterior descending, and left circumflex coronary arteries. The authors concluded that patients with abdominal aortic aneurysm nearly always have diffuse and severe coronary atherosclerosis.

Mautner et al[2] also determined the amounts of coronary arterial narrowing by atherosclerotic plaque at necropsy in patients who had had lower extremity amputation secondary to peripheral arterial atherosclerosis. During life, 15 of the 26 patients (58%) had symptoms of myocardial ischemia and 12 of the 26 (42%) died from it. Grossly visible foci of left ventricular necrosis or fibrosis, or both, was present in 21 patients (81%), and 24 (92%) of the 26 patients had narrowing 76 to 100% in cross-sectional area of ≥1 major epicardial coronary arteries by atherosclerotic plaque (mean 2.3 ± 1.0/4.0). Of the 104 major coronary arteries in the 26 patients (4 per patient), 60 (58%) were narrowed >75% in cross-sectional area by plaque. The 4 major coronary arteries were divided into 5-mm segments and the mean percentages of the resulting 1,322 segments narrowed in cross-sectional area were the following: 17%, 0 to 25%; 20%, 26 to 50%; 35%, 51 to 75%; 19%, 76 to 95%, and 9%, >95%. The percentages of the segments narrowed >75% in cross-sectional area were similar in the right, left anterior descending and left circumflex coronary arteries. Thus, patients with peripheral arterial atherosclerosis severe enough to warrant amputation nearly always have diffuse and severe coronary atherosclerosis at the time of necropsy.

Is Atherosclerosis in Any Specific Region Focal or Diffuse? a Look at the Coronary Arteries

Table 1 shows the modes of death in fatal CAD in 1,889 patients' ≥30 years of age studied at necropsy by Roberts and colleagues[3] from 1960 to 1990. Table 2 shows the various coronary events in a number of patients studied at necropsy in which each 5-mm segment of the 4 major coronary arteries was studied histologically.[4-34] Several of these studies were summarized by Roberts in 1989.[35] A summary of the findings in one group, namely acute myocardial infarction (AMI), is summarized in Figures 2 and 3.[8] The 4 major coronary arteries in all of these coronary subsets were excised intact from the heart, decalcified (if necessary) and divided into 5-mm segments and a histologic section was prepared from each and stained by an elastic tissue stain (Movat) and then examined histologically. The average number of 5-mm segments per patient was 54. Of the patients with AMI studied at autopsy, 34% of the 5-mm segments of the 4 major coronary arteries were narrowed 76 to 100% by atherosclerotic plaque alone (excludes thrombus); 38% were narrowed 51 to 75%; 23%,

Table 1
MODES of death in fatal coronary artery disease, (889 Necropsy Patients ≥30 Years of Age)

Modes of Death	Numbers
I. Acute Myocardial Infarct (MI)	426 (48%)
(Healed MI = 119 [28%])	
II. Sudden Out-of-Hospital Death	239 (27%)
(Healed MI = 118 [49%])	
III. Chronic HF + Healed MI	170 (19%)
(LV aneurysm = 33 [19%])	
IV. Sudden In-Hospital Death	55 (6%)
(Unstable angina = 35 [67%])	
(Healed MI = 30 [55%])	
TOTALS	**889 (100%)**

HF = heart failure; LV = left ventricular.

Table 2

Quantitative studies (Five-mm segments of all 4 major epicardial coronary arteries) on amounts of coronary narrowing in patients with coronary events

Subgroup (Reference)	Year Published	No. Pts	Men	Mean Age (Yrs)	No.5-mm Segments	No. (%) of 5-mm Segments Narrowed			
						0 - 25%	26 - 50%	51 - 75%	76 - 100%
I. SUDDEN CORONARY DEATH									
A. All sudden coronary deaths	1984	60	60	51	2,995	546 (18)	604 (20)	995 (33)	850 (28)
B. With -vs- without coronary thrombus									
With	1984		12	43	639	173 (27%)	115 (18%)	179 (28%)	173 (27%)
Without	1984	57	45	57	2,845	541 (19%)	569 (20%)	939 (33%)	768 (27%)
C. Cath Lab death with angina pectoris	1981	10	7	47	354	23 (6%)	45 (13%)	83 (23%)	203 (58%)
D. With -vs- without previous cardiac event	1984	70	63	50					
Previously symptomatic		31			1,493	223 (15%)	328 (22%)	493 (33%)	448 (30%)
Previously asymptomatic		39			1,991	498 (25%)	358 (18%)	637 (32%)	498 (25%)
II. ACUTE MYOCARDIAL INFARCTION (MI)—ALL	1980	27	21	50	1,403	285 (28%)	319 (23%)	528 (38%)	484 (34%)
III. HEALED MYOCARDIAL INFARCTION	1982	56	52	62	2,424	212 (9%)	381 (16%)	837 (34%)	994 (41%)
A. Ischemic cardiomyopathy	1986	56	53	62	2,999	804 (27%)	911 (30%	584 (20%)	700 (23%)
B. LV aneurysm after healed MI	1980	22	19	62	992	40 (4%)	210 (21%)	419 (42%)	323 (33%)
C. Healed MI and non-cardiovascular death	1981	18	15	66	924	101 (11%)	210 (23%)	321 (35%)	292 (32%)
D. Anterior -vs- Posterior MI	1985	59							
Anterior wall	1982	22	15		895	79 (9%)	173 (19%)	303 (34%)	340 (38%)
Posterior wall	1982	37	27		1,713	134 (8%)	229 (13%)	560 (33%)	790 (46%)
E. Clinically recognized -vs- unrecognized MI	1982	61							
Clinically recognized	1982	33			1,443	84 (6%)	230 (16%)	519 (36%)	611 (42%)
Clinically silent	1982	28			1,262	139 (11%)	197 (16%)	374 (30%)	552 (43%)
F. Small -vs- large healed MI	1982								
Small	1982	28	21	62	1,260	136 (11%)	195 (15%)	394 (31%)	535 (42%)
Large	1982	28	21	62	1,229	76 (6%)	186 (15%)	443 (36%)	524 (43%)
IV. UNSTABLE ANGINA PECTORIS WITH DEATH AFTER CORONARY BYPASS		22	13	48	1,049	119 (11%)	454 (48%)	305 (29%)	497 (47%)
V. JUVENILE DIABETES MELLITUS	1978	9	6	29	382	116 (31%)	85 (22%)	123 (32%)	58 (15%)

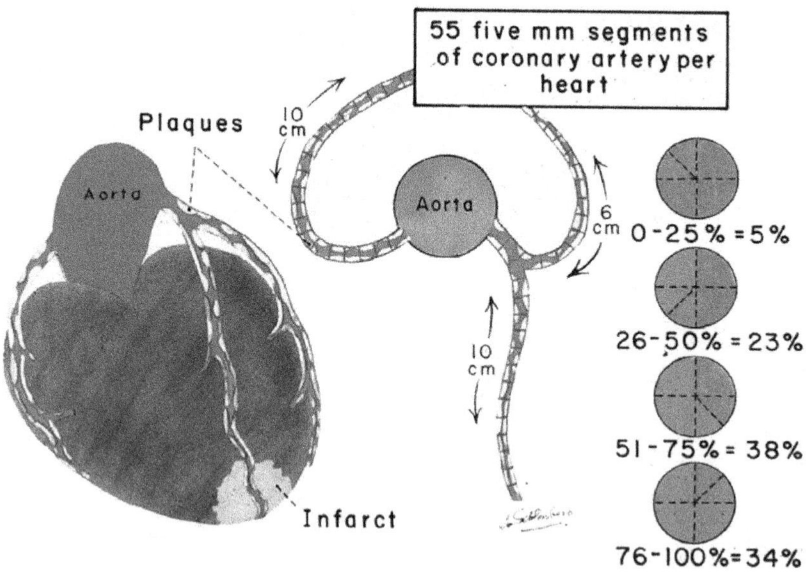

Figure 2. This diagram shows the quantity of cross-sectional area narrowing in each 5-mm segment in 27 patients with acute myocardial infarction studied at autopsy. As shown in the bottom right, 34% of the 5-mm segments were narrowed 76–100% in cross-sectional area and only 5% 25% or less, and not a single 5-mm segment was devoid of plaque.

26 to 50%, and 5%, 0 to 25%, and not a single segment was devoid of plaque (Figure 2). The quantity of narrowing, and this was typical of all the coronary subsets studied, in each of the 4 major coronary arteries was similar (Figure 3). In the 27 patients, 1,403 five-mm segments were examined. The amounts of narrowing at each of the 4 categories of narrowing in the right, left anterior descending, and left circumflex were similar. The percent of patients with severe narrowing (76 to 100%) of the left main coronary artery was approximately 10%.

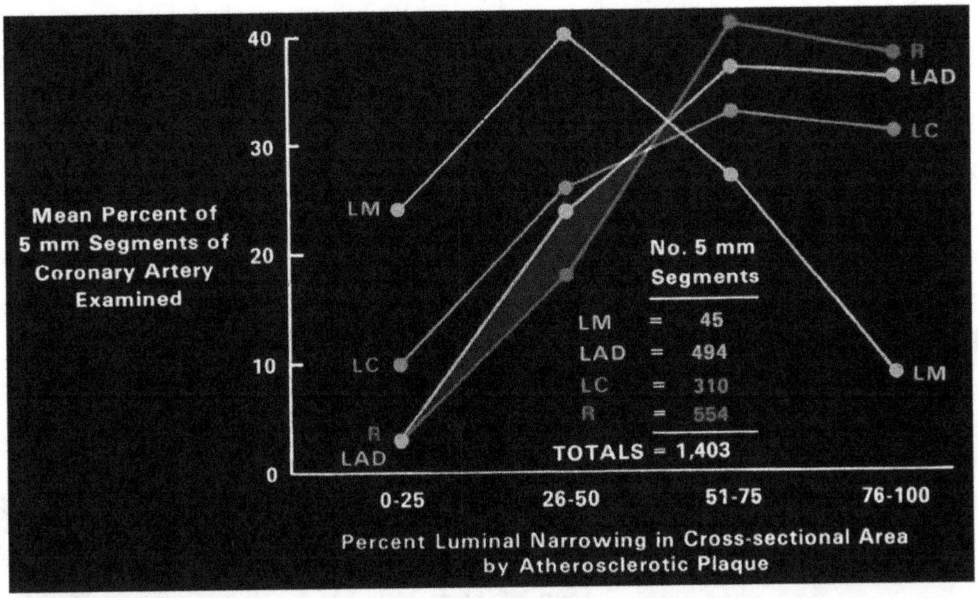

Figure 3. This diagram shows the mean percent of 5-mm segments of each of the 4 major epicardial coronary arteries narrowed to various degrees in acute myocardial infarction: 27 patients and 1,403 5-mm segments were studied. The horizontal axis shows the 4 categories of cross-sectional area narrowing and the vertical axis shows the mean percent of 5-mm segments of coronary artery examined in the 4 coronary arteries: left main (LM); left anterior descending (LAD); left circumflex (LC), and right (R). This diagram shows that the LAD, R, and LC coronary arteries have similar degrees of narrowing at each of the 4 categories of narrowing; the LM in contrast had only 10% of the 5-mm segments narrowed >75% in cross-sectional area. *Reproduced with permission from* Roberts WC, Jones AA. Quantification of coronary arterial narrowing at necropsy in acute transmural myocardial infarction. Analysis and comparison of findings in 27 patients and 22 controls. *Circulation* 1980; 61:786–790.

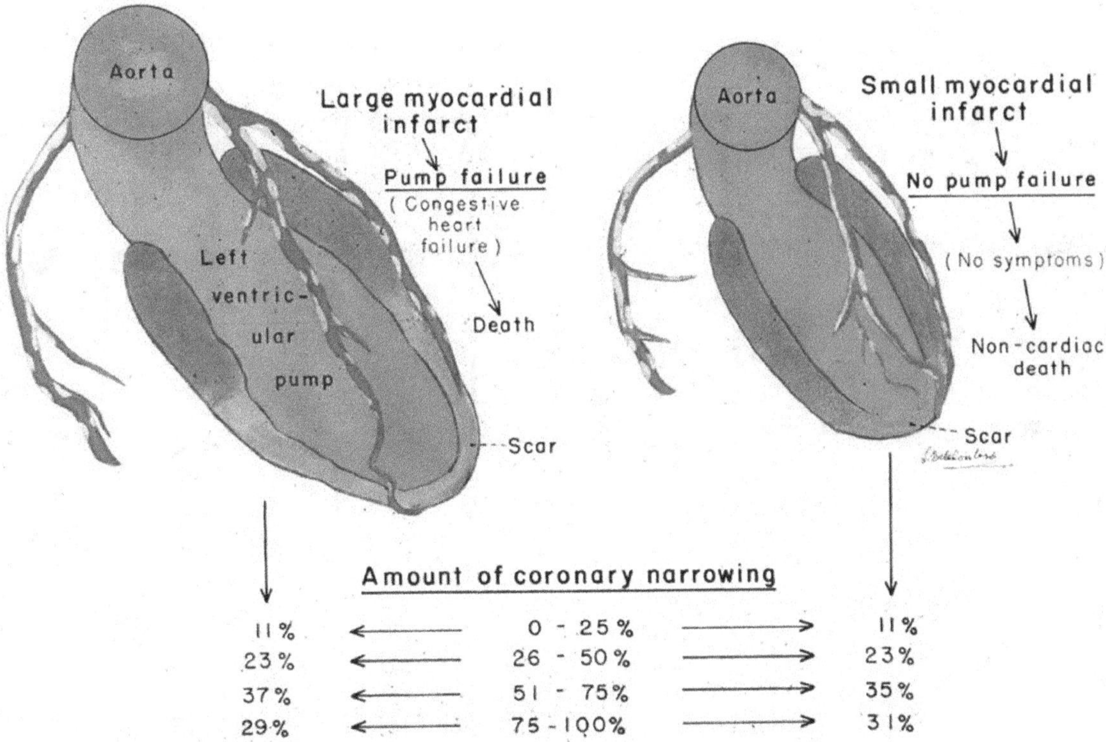

Figure 4. This diagram contrasts the quantity of coronary narrowing in a group of patients who had healed myocardial infarcts. The diagram on the left represents patients who had very large myocardial infarcts which healed and the left ventricular cavity was quite dilated. This feature is typical of course of ischemic cardiomyopathy. The diagram on the right represents a group of patients who had a myocardial infarct which healed but thereafter there was never clinical evidence of myocardial ischemia and these patients died from a non-coronary events. As shown on the bottom right the quantity of atherosclerotic plaque was similar in each of these 2 groups of patients showing that the size of a healed infarct is not helpful in determining the quantity of atherosclerotic burden.

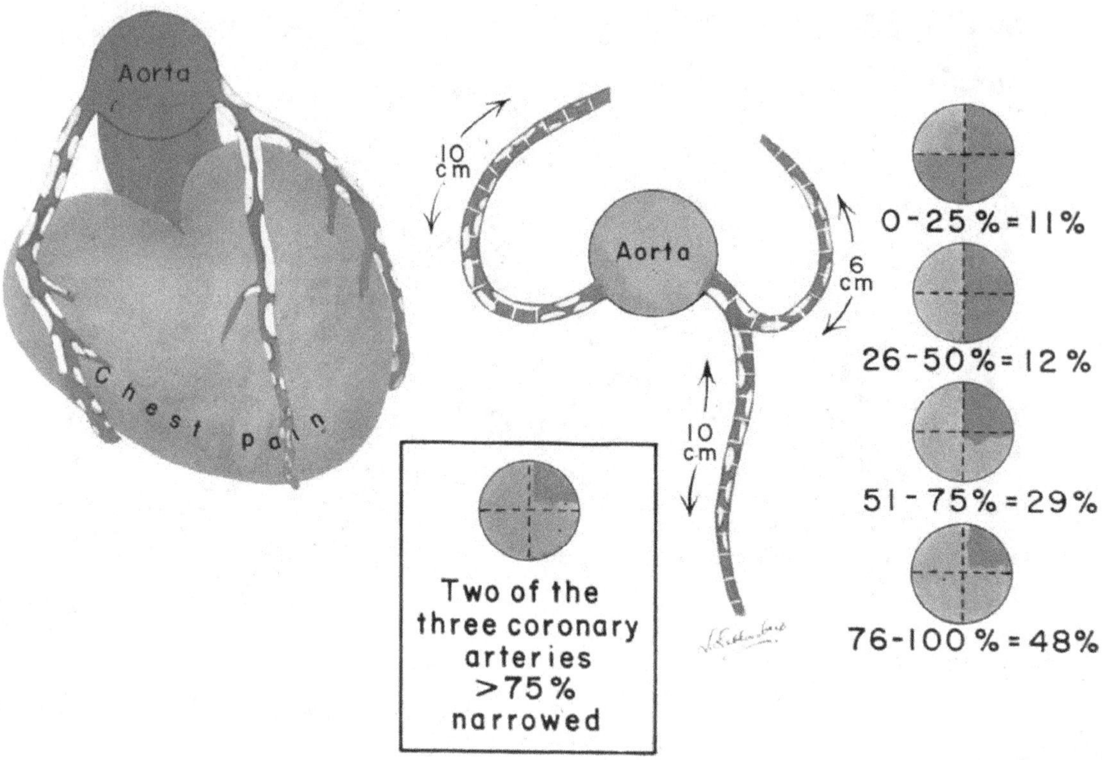

Figure 5. This diagram shows the quantity of narrowing in each 5-mm segment in a group of patients with unstable angina pectoris who underwent coronary bypass grafting and died shortly thereafter. Although the cardiac output in these patients was entirely normal and the left ventricular cavity was of normal size and there were no myocardial scars the quantity of coronary narrowing was greater than any of the other subsets, namely 48% of the 5-mm segments were narrowed 76–100% and 29% were narrowed 51–75% in cross-sectional area.

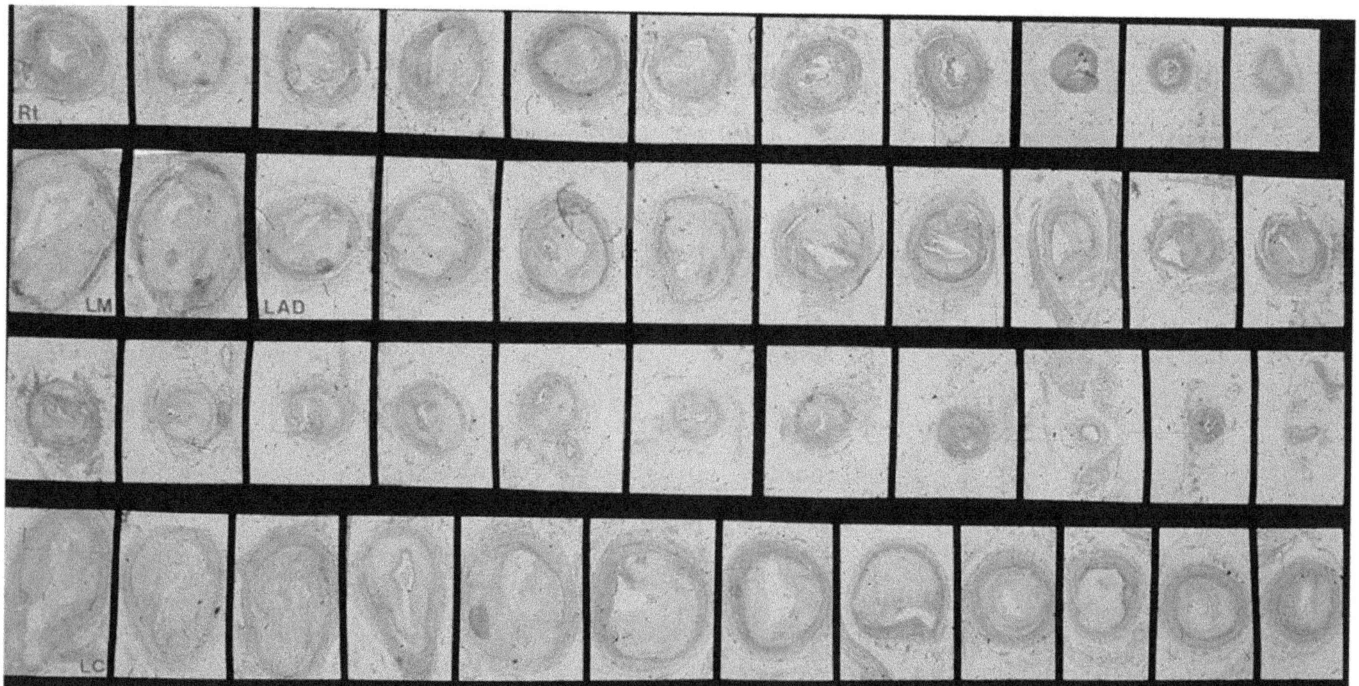

Figure 6. This montage of Movat stained sections in each 5-mm segment of the coronary tree in a single patient with unstable angina shows severe narrowing most of the 5-mm segments including considerable narrowing of the left main (LM) coronary artery. LAD = left anterior descending; LC = left circumflex, and RT = right. Reproduced with permission from Roberts WC, Virmani R. Quantification of coronary arterial narrowing in clinically-isolated unstable angina pectoris. An analysis of 22 necropsy patients. *Am J Med* 1979; 67:792–799.

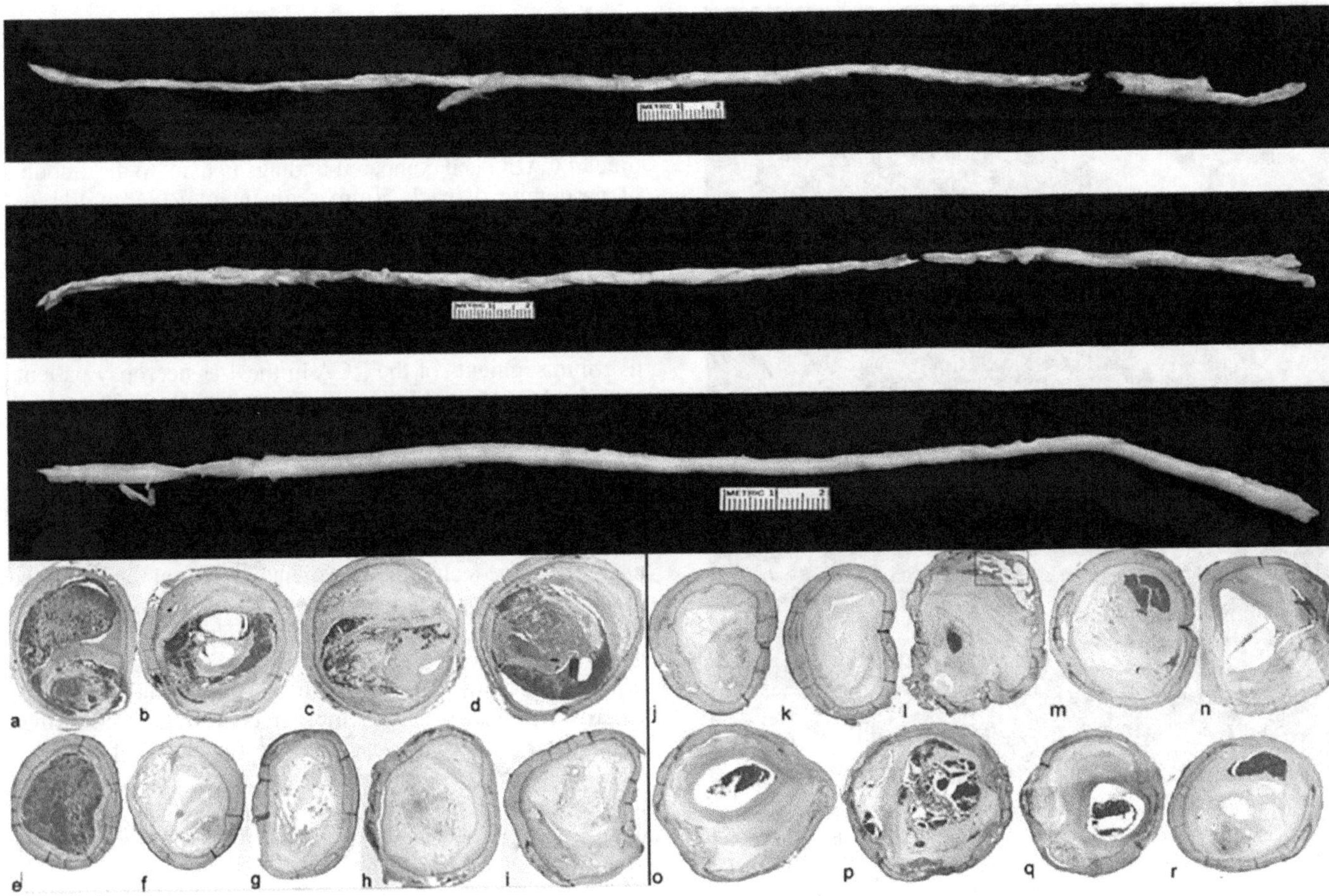

Figure 7. Shown here are endarterectomy specimens of the superficial femoral artery in 3 patients with severe peripheral vascular disease. Each of these endarterectomy specimens is about 25 cm in length. What is shown is the atherosclerotic plaque within the lumen. There are no areas where plaque is not present. These are examples of the diffuse nature of atherosclerosis in any region in patients with either symptomatic or fatal atherosclerotic events. These 3 endarterectomy specimens were excised by Dr. Gregory Pearl of Baylor University Medical Center. The lower panel contains photomicrographs in 18 of the 28 five-mm sections prepared from the superficial femoral artery shown at the bottom of the 3 upper specimens. The cross-sections proximally are represented by the earlier alphabetic letter and those more distally by the later letters. Thrombus with ruptured plaque is seen in *a* through *d*. Additional thrombus without underlying plaque rupture is seen in *e*. In *j* and *k*, the lumen is totally occluded mainly by fibrous plaque. Media is present circumferentially on all sections, indicating that the operative dissection plaque was in the media. All sections contain plaque. Movat stains, X 100. The patient was a 60-year-old man who had debilitating claudication. At age 44 he had had percutaneous coronary intervention because of angina pectoris and at age 58 he had coronary bypass because of recurrence of angina. The bottom endarterectomy specimen and the photomicrographs are reproduced with permission from Roberts WC, Ko MK, and Pearl GP. *Am J Geriatric Cardiol* 2008; 17:50–52.

The quantity of myocardial scar in patients with a healed AMI is not proportional to the quantity of plaque in the coronary arteries. No differences in the quantity of coronary plaque was observed in patients with large healed -vs- small healed infarcts (Figure 4).

The quantity of coronary plaque was found to be greater in patients with unstable angina pectoris than in any other coronary subset (Figure 5).[5] Although the left ventricular ejection fractions were normal in each patient, nearly half of the 5-mm coronary segments were narrowed >75% in cross-sectioned area by atherosclerotic plaque alone. A montage of photomicrographs from the 5-mm cross sections in one of these patients is shown in Figure 6. No segment was devoid of atherosclerotic plaque.

The coronary arteries are not the only arterial system in which the atherosclerotic process is diffuse in patients with symptomatic or fatal atherosclerotic events. Vascular surgeons have observed that the atherosclerotic process in the legs is diffuse in patients with femoral arterial occlusive disease.[36] Shown in Figure 7 are endarterectomy specimens of superficial femoral arteries from 3 patients. The entire endarterectomy specimen in each patient is >15 cm in length. The lumen of each artery was filled with plaque. There were no normal areas, i.e., areas devoid of plaque.

What is the Quantity of Atherosclerotic Plaque in Endarterectomy Specimens of the Right Coronary Artery in Patients Undergoing Coronary Artery Bypass Grafting (CABG) Compared to That in the Right Coronary Artery in Patients with Fatal Coronary Artery Disease?

Roberts and colleagues[37] compared the amounts of cross-sectional area narrowing of the right coronary artery (RCA)

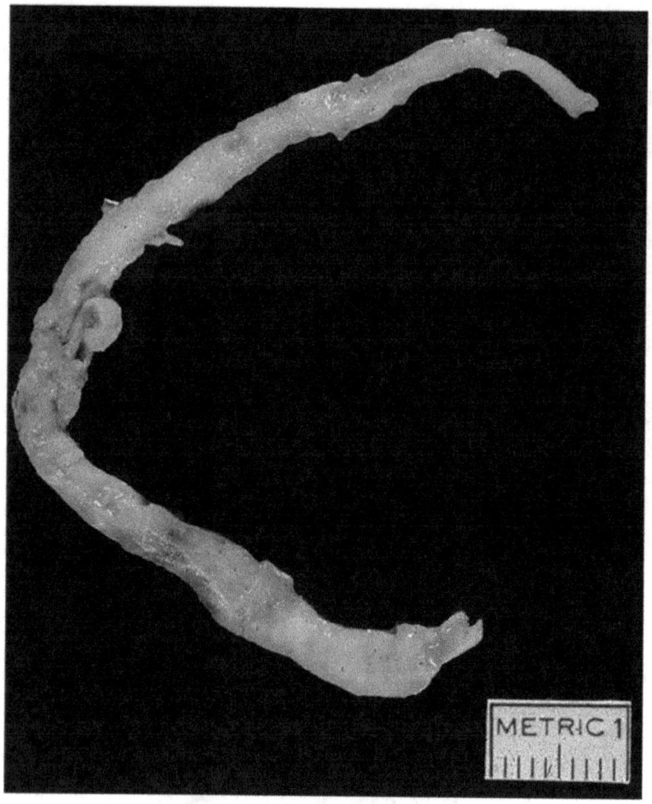

Figure 8. Shown here is an endarterectomy specimen of the entire right coronary artery in a patient who had severe narrowing not only of the right but also of the left anterior descending and left circumflex coronary arteries. The ostium of the right coronary artery is shown at the bottom and at the top is a little posterior descending branch. This endarterectomy specimen shows that the atherosclerotic process is continuous and there are not areas where plaque is not present. Reproduced with permission from Roberts WC, Turnage TA II, Whiddon LL. Quantitative comparison of amounts of cross-sectional area narrowing in coronary endarterectomy specimens in patients having coronary artery bypass grafting to amounts of narrowing in the same artery in patients with fatal coronary artery disease studied at necropsy. *Am J Cardiol* 2007; 99:588–592.

in patients having endarterectomy of this artery at the time of CABG (live patients) to the amounts of narrowing of the same artery at necropsy in patients with fatal CAD (Figure 8). They examined each 5-mm segment of endarterectomy specimens of the RCA in 39 patients having this procedure at the time of CABG and compared findings in them to the amounts of narrowing of each 5-mm segment of RCA in 141 patients with fatal CAD studied at necropsy. Of the 564 five mm RCA segments in the endarterectomy specimens, 371 (66%) were narrowed >75% in cross-sectional area by atherosclerotic plaque: another 112 (20%), 51 to 75%; 64 (11%) 26 to 50%; and 17 (3%) 1 to 25%. In contrast, of the 2,699 five-mm segments of the RCA in the 141 necropsy patients with fatal CAD, 1,217 (45%) were narrowed >75% in cross-sectional area; another 966 (36%), 51 to 75%; 405 (15%), 26 to 50%, and 114 (4%), 1 to 25% by plaque. These authors concluded that the amount of severe narrowing found in coronary endarterectomy specimens excised at the time of CABG in live patients is at least as great as that found using the same technique in patients with fatal CAD studied at necropsy. The event which prompted the CABG in many of these patients was their first event. This observation suggests that an even greater emphasis should be placed on primary prevention of atherosclerotic events and, indeed, of atherosclerotic plaques. A more recent study[38] confirmed these observations and described the frequency of coronary endarterectomy at the time of coronary bypass by several different cardiac surgeons. Some cardiac surgeons frequently perform coronary endarterectomy and others rarely at the time of CABG.

An endarterectomy specimen (a continuous plaque) of the RCA is shown in Figure 8. ("Endarterectomy" is a misnomer because the "endarterectomy" specimen virtually always also includes a portion of media. The split is in the media, not at the junction of intima and media such that the internal elastic membrane is incorporated into the endarterectomy specimen.)

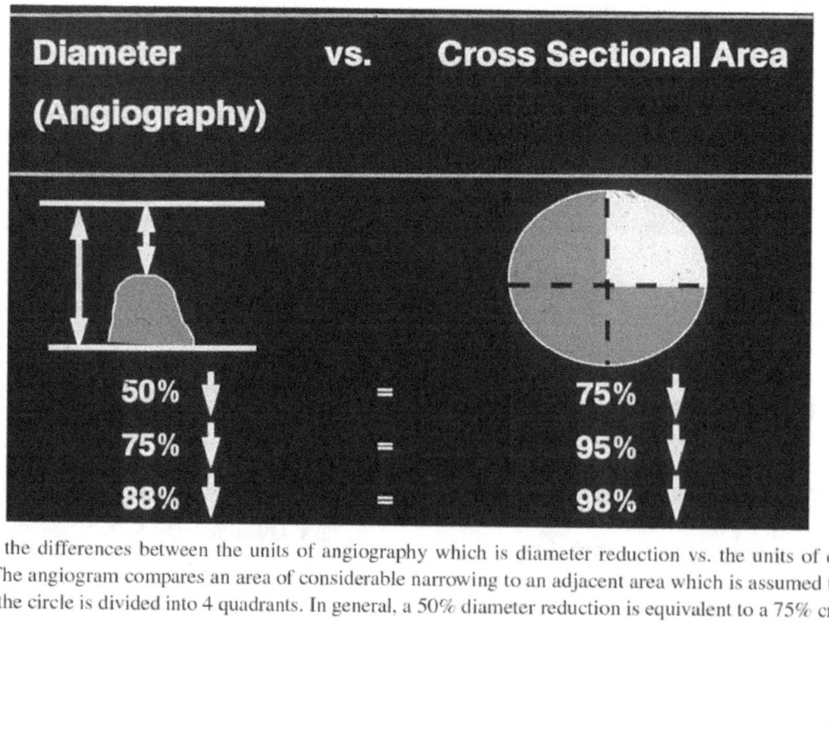

Figure 9. This diagram shows the differences between the units of angiography which is diameter reduction vs. the units of echocardiography or autopsy which is cross-sectional area. The angiogram compares an area of considerable narrowing to an adjacent area which is assumed to be normal. Cross-sectional area is most easily measured if the circle is divided into 4 quadrants. In general, a 50% diameter reduction is equivalent to a 75% cross-sectional area narrowing.

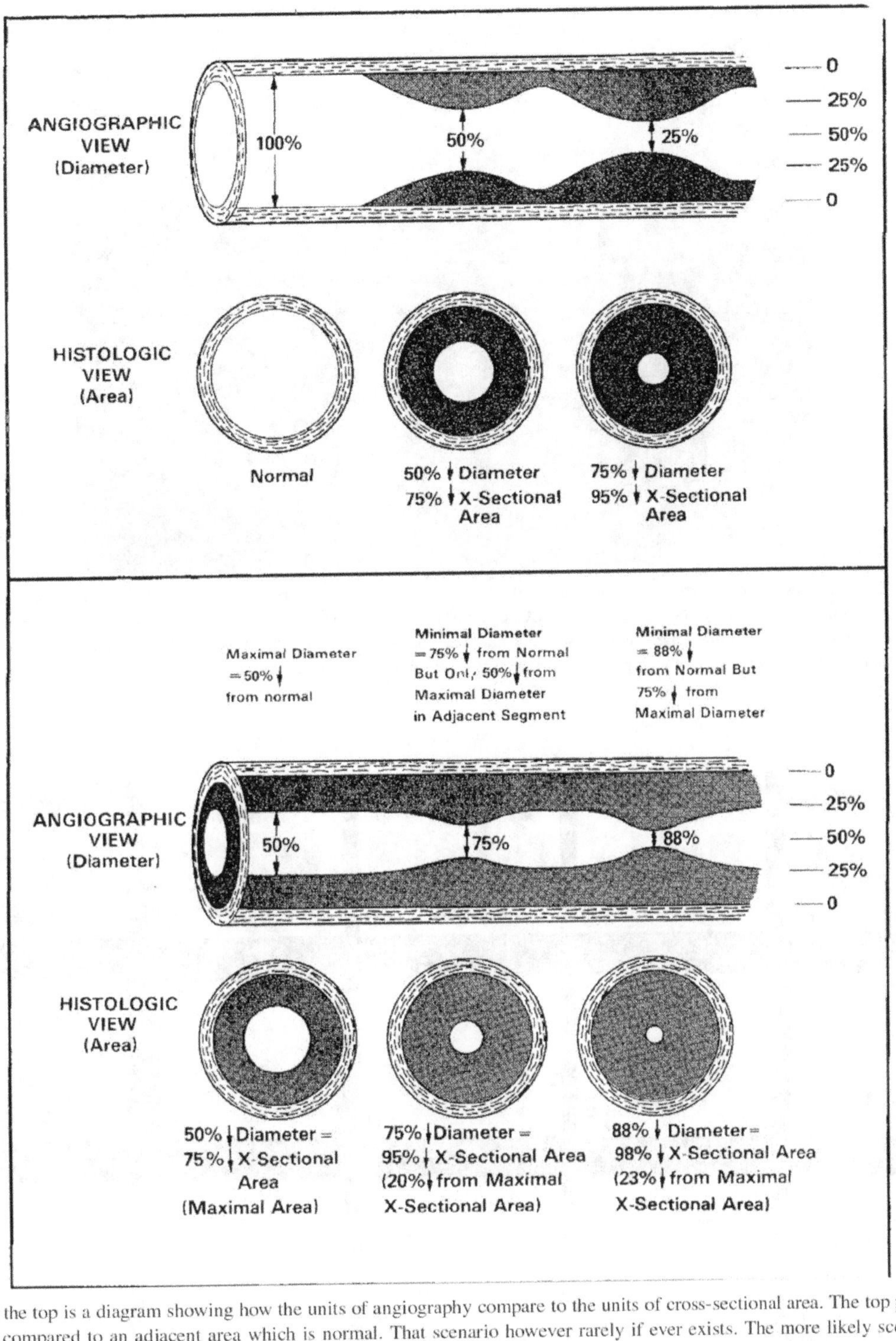

Figure 10. Shown at the top is a diagram showing how the units of angiography compare to the units of cross-sectional area. The top panel assumes that the area of narrowing is compared to an adjacent area which is normal. That scenario however rarely if ever exists. The more likely scenario is shown in the bottom diagram such that an area of severe narrowing is simply compared to an adjacent area which is less narrowed but not normal. Reproduced with permission from Arnett EN, Isner JM, Redwood DR, Kent KM, Baker WP, Ackerstein H, Roberts WC. Coronary artery narrowing in coronary heart disease: Comparison of cineangiographic and necropsy findings. *Ann Intern Med* 1979; 91:350–356.

How Do the Units Used for Measuring Arterial Narrowing by Angiography Compare to the Units Used for Measuring Arterial Narrowing at Necropsy?

The unit of measurement of angiography is *diameter reduction*: the area of maximal narrowing is compared to an adjacent area which is assumed to be normal such that if the narrowed area is half that of the adjacent area it is considered a "50% lesion" (Figure 9 and 10).[39] *Cross-sectional area* narrowing is the unit used at necropsy and by echocardiography. The circle is divided into 4 quadrants, and the severity of narrowing is determined by how many of these quadrants are obliterated by plaque. In general, a 75% cross-sectional area

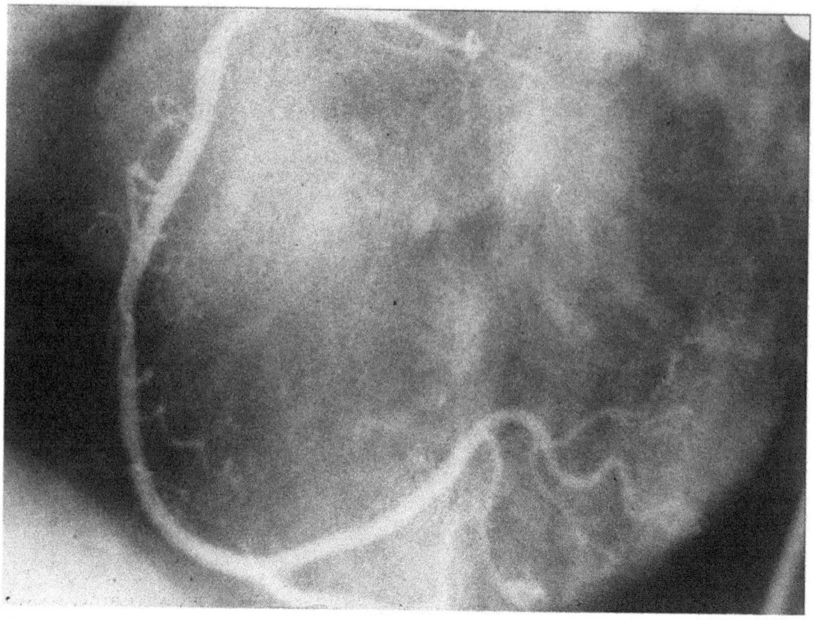

Figure 11. Shown here is an angiogram of the right coronary artery in a patient who has severe narrowing of the LAD and LC coronary arteries. A coronary bypass operation was planned with conduits to be inserted in the LC system and in the LAD coronary artery. The right coronary artery was preoperatively judged to have some irregularity but not enough narrowing to warrant the insertion of a conduit. Unfortunately, this patient died 3 days after the bypass operation and 5-mm segments were prepared from that right coronary artery at autopsy and they are shown in Figure 12.

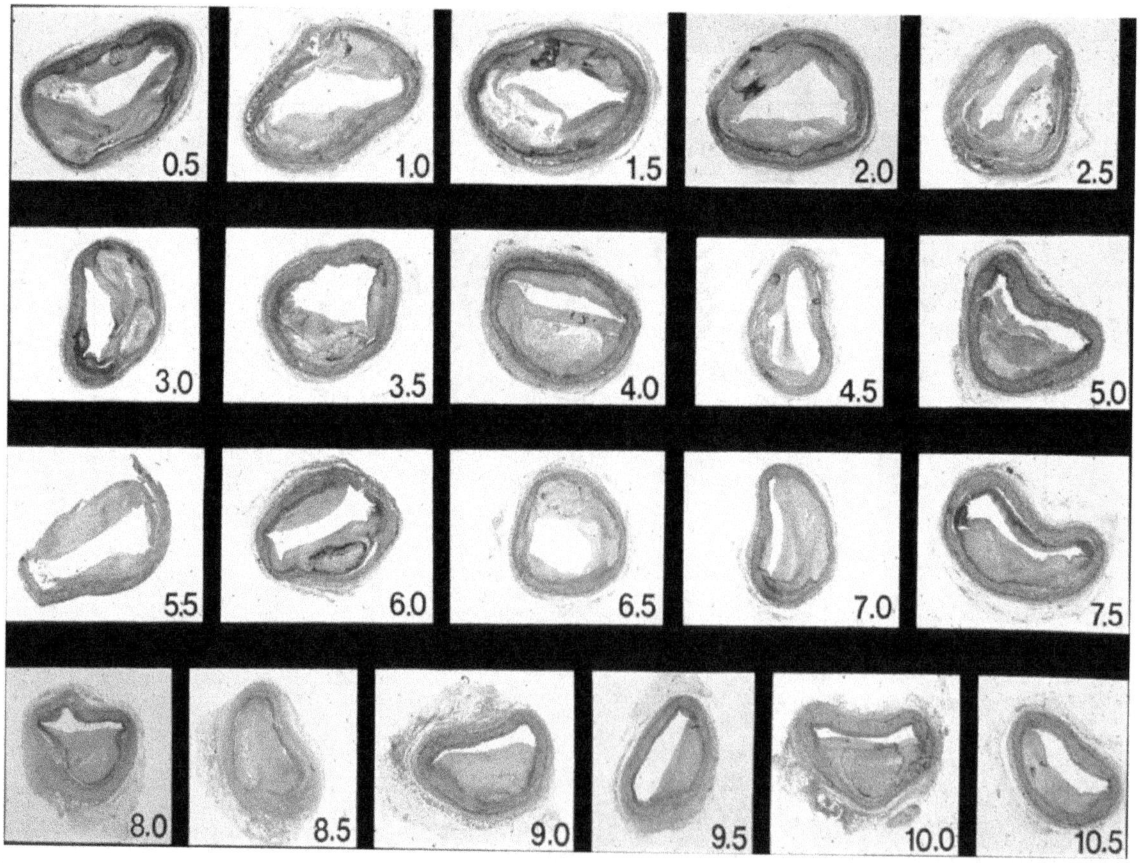

Figure 12. Shown here are Movat-stained cross-sections of each 5-mm segment of the right coronary artery whose angiogram is shown in Figure 11. The numbers are centimeters from the ostium of the right coronary artery. Each of these 5-mm segments contains plaque but most of the lumens extend from one wall of the aorta to the opposite wall and the contrast material is in the lumen and if the diameter of the lumen is roughly normal the angiogram can appear to be free or relatively free of underlying plaque. Segment 8.5 cm from the ostium is relatively narrowed.

narrowing is equivalent to a 50% diameter reduction. Also, in general, an artery (or valve orifice) has to be narrowed >75% in cross-sectional area for flow to be diminished. If the 4 major epicardial coronary arteries have diffuse plaque in them (as in patients with symptomatic or fatal CAD) there is no area in the artery that is completely normal. Thus, an area of maximal narrowing is simply compared to an adjacent area which is assumed to be normal but in actuality is simply less narrowed (Figure 10). There is a built-in under-reading by coronary angiography because of the absence of totally normal segments to compare to the narrowed segments. Intra-luminal echocardiography, in contrast to angiography, compares quite favorably to cross-sectional area examination of endarterectomy or necropsy specimens because it too uses cross-sectional area narrowing as the unit of measurement.

Shown in Figure 11 is an angiogram of a RCA in a patient with unstable angina pectoris who was scheduled for coronary bypass because of severe narrowing of the left anterior descending and the left circumflex coronary systems. The judgment was made that, although there was a bit of irregularity of this RCA, it did not need the insertion of a conduit. Figure 12, however, shows photomicrographs of each 5-mm segments of that RCA because the patient died 3 days after CABG and was studied at necropsy. Every 5-mm segment contains plaque. The purpose of these photomicrographs is not to suggest that the clinical judgment was wrong but simply to demonstrate that each of the 5-mm segments contained plaque. Many of the lumens stretched from one side of the artery to the other and that is why the angiogram appeared to be relatively devoid of significant narrowing. Angiograms, of course, are luminograms and they do not demonstrate the quantity of underlying atherosclerotic plaques. The amount of narrowing shown by angiography is the tip of the iceberg; most of the iceberg (plaque) is below the surface of the water (Figure 13).

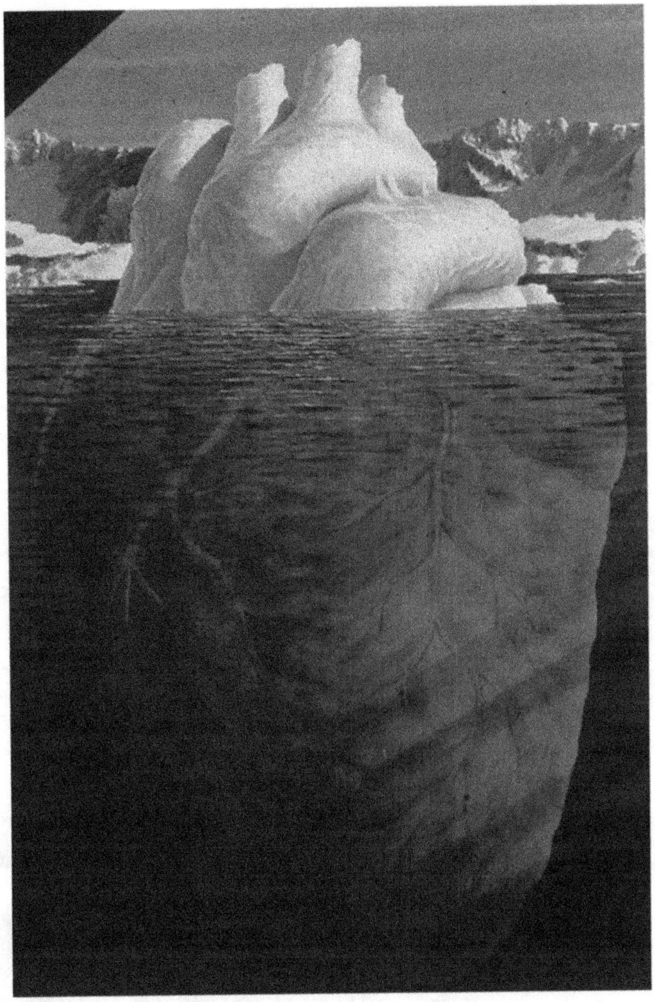

Figure 13. This diagram shows a heart under the surface of the water with the great arteries protruding above the surface. The point of this picture is to emphasize that most of the atherosclerotic plaque in the coronary arteries is not seen well by angiography.

What Do Atherosclerotic Plaques Consist of in Coronary Arteries of Patients with Fatal Coronary Disease?

There appears to be a general belief that coronary atherosclerotic plaques consist mainly of lipids, but multiple studies of all 5-mm segments of the 4 major coronary arteries in a variety of patients show that fibrous tissue in the dominant component of coronary plaques,[30,40–45] including the young as well as the old,[31,32] those with extremely high serum cholesterol levels (homozygous familial hypercholesterolemia),[30] inflammatory coronary disease—Buerger's disease,[45] and cocaine addicts.[27] Of the various components of coronary atherosclerotic plaques in patients with fatal coronary events, irrespective of the amounts of luminal narrowing, *fibrous tissue* is the dominant component, be it dense or be it cellular (Figure 14). In the segments that are minimally narrowed (1 to 25%) cellular fibrous tissue still is the dominant component whereas in those segments causing luminal narrowing 96 to 100% in cross-sectional area, dense fibrous tissue is the dominant component. *Calcium* occurred only in those segments narrowed >50% in cross-sectional area and progressively increased as the quantity of narrowing increased. *Foam cells* are rare in severely narrowed coronary segments.

Fibrous tissue appears to be is the dominant component of coronary plaques in both the young and the old.[31,32] The various components of coronary plaques in a group of patients with *juvenile diabetes mellitus* is shown in Figure 15.[43,45] The average age of onset was 9 years, and the average age of death was 29. Shown in the figure are the combined findings in the patients. In the 5-mm segments narrowed 1 to 25%, cellular fibrous tissue was the dominant component whereas in the segments narrowed 96 to 100% dense fibrous tissue was the dominant component. Calcific deposits were infrequent. The quantity of extracellular lipid was relatively small. Fibrous tissue appears to be the dominant component of plaques of both young and old people.

The composition of plaques in saphenous vein conduits is similar to that of the *native coronary arteries* after a period of several years as shown in Figure 16.[41,42] Cellular fibrous tissue was the dominant component in the 5-mm segments of the saphenous vein grafts that were minimally narrowed (1 to 25%) and dense fibrous tissue was the dominant component in the grafts which were narrowed 96 to

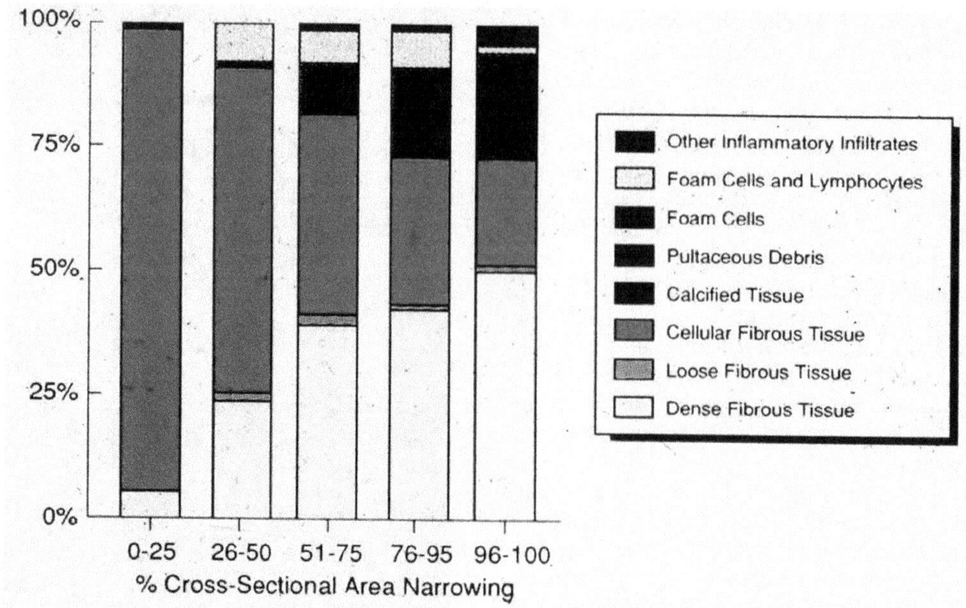

Figure 14. Shown on this bar graph showing various components of the atherosclerotic plaque in a number of patients with fatal coronary artery disease. The horizontal axis shows the degrees of cross-sectional area narrowing and the vertical axis shows the percent of the 5-mm segments narrowed to each of these 5 categories. The combination of dense, loose, and cellular fibrous tissue is by far the dominant component of the coronary plaques irrespective of the degree of cross-sectional area narrowing. Pultaceous debris and calcified fragments were not observed unless the lumen was narrowed >50% in cross-sectional areas.

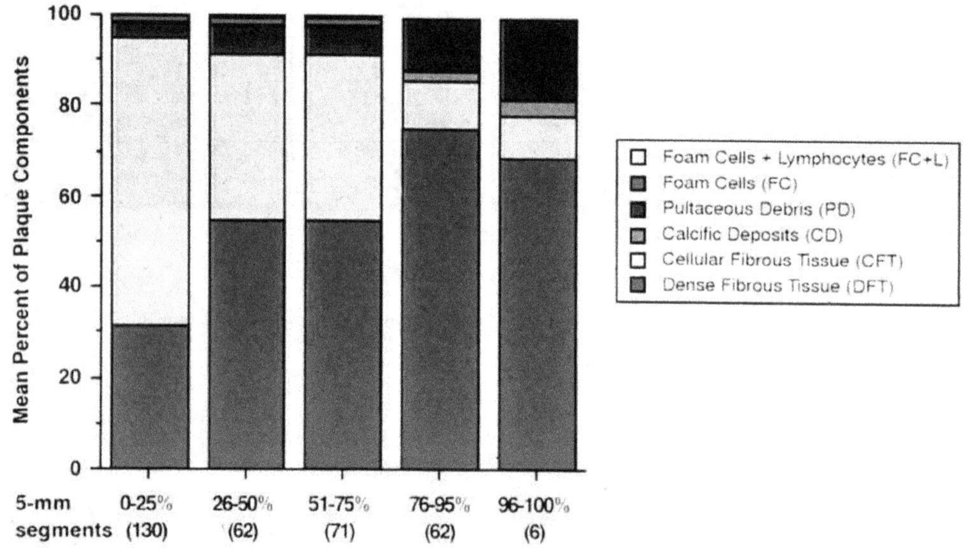

Figure 15. Shown in this bar graph are coronary arteries in 9 patients with fatal juvenile diabetes. The average age of onset in these 9 patients was 9 years and the average age of death was 29 years. The code in this diagram is different from that in Figure 14. The red represents dense fibrous tissue and the yellow represents cellular fibrous tissue and the diagram shows that irrespective of the quantity of cross-sectional area narrowing fibrous tissue is the dominant component of the atherosclerotic plaque. Pultaceous debris (extracellular lipid) was excessive only in the patients in whom the luminal narrowing was extremely severe (>75% in cross-sectional areas). Reproduced with permission from Crall FV Jr, Roberts WC. The extramural and intramural coronary arteries in juvenile diabetes mellitus: analysis of nine necropsy patients aged 19 to 38 years with onset of diabetes before age 15 years. *Am J Med* 1978;64:221–230.

100% in cross-sectional area. In the native coronary arteries, irrespective of the degrees of luminal narrowing, dense fibrous tissue was the dominant component. Cellular fibrous tissue was the next most frequent component. The composition of plaque in 'native' coronary arteries and in saphenous venous grafts varies a bit among men -vs- women as shown in Figure 17.[43]

What is the Quantity of Atherosclerotic Plaque in Bypassed -vs- Non-Bypassed Native Coronary Arteries in Patients Dying Early (<60 Days) or Late (>60 Days) after Coronary Artery Bypass Grafting?

If CAD is so diffuse, as described in earlier portions of this review, is it logical to put conduits in some native

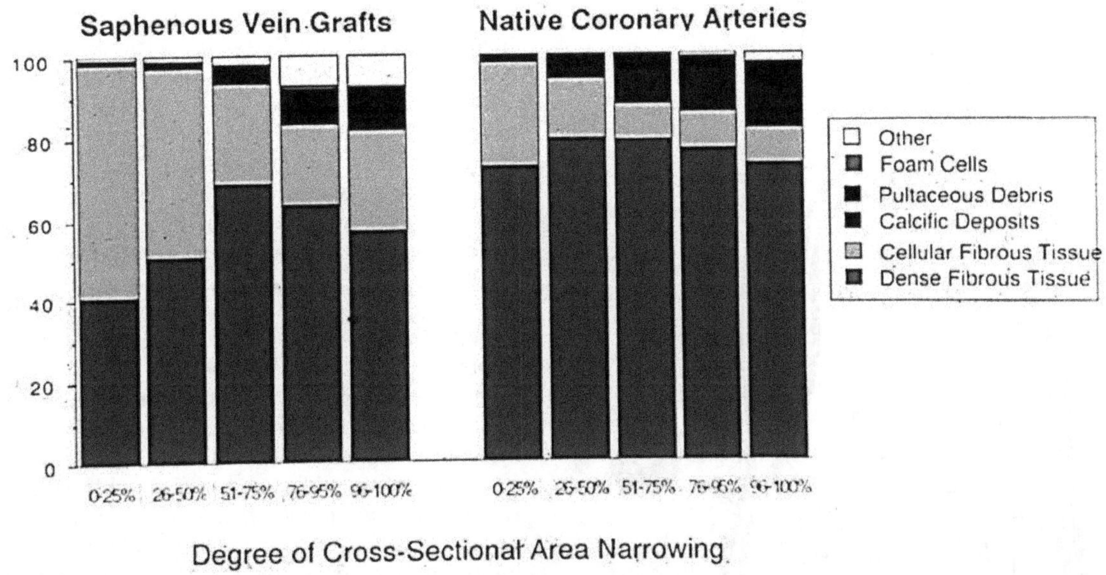

Figure 16. This diagram shows the relation of plaque composition relative to the degrees of cross-sectional area of luminal narrowing. Shown on the left are bars at various degrees of cross-sectional area narrowing in saphenous venous conduits studied at autopsy compared to the cross-sectional area narrowing and composition of the plaques in the native coronary arteries. The plaques in the saphenous venous grafts again show that fibrous tissue is the dominant component whether it is cellular or dense. It took approximately 80 months for the atherosclerotic plaques in the saphenous venous grafts to look like the plaques in the native coronary arteries. Reproduced with permission from Mautner SL, Mautner GC, Hunsberger SA, Roberts WC. Comparison of composition of atherosclerotic plaques in saphenous veins used as aortocoronary bypass conduits with plaques in native coronary arteries in the same men. *Am J Cardiol* 1992; 70:1380–1387.

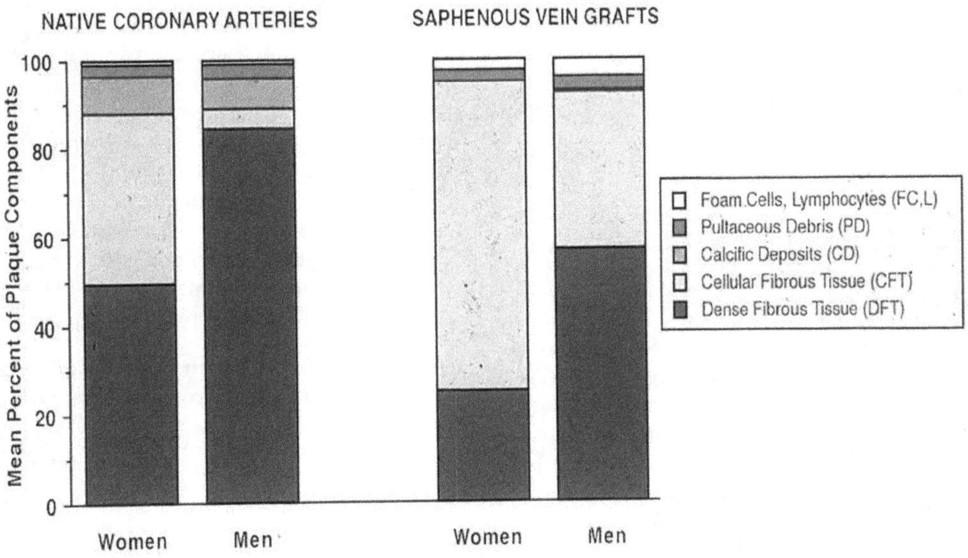

Figure 17. This diagram compares the composition of the atherosclerotic plaques in women versus men in native coronary arteries and in saphenous venous grafts. It shows that the quantity of dense fibrous tissue in women in both native coronary arteries and in saphenous venous graft is less than in the men. Reproduced with permission from Mautner SL, Lin F, Mautner GC, Roberts WC. Comparison in women versus men of composition of atherosclerotic plaques in native coronary arteries and in saphenous veins used as aortocoronary conduits. *J Am Coll Cardiol* 1993; 21:1312–1318.

arteries and no conduits in others? This question was examined by Waller and Roberts[10] who compared the quantity of narrowing in the native coronary arteries that were bypassed versus those not bypassed in patients dying early (<60 days) and later after CABG (Figure 18). The percent of the 5-mm segments narrowed >75% in cross-sectional areas was similar in the bypassed and non-bypassed native coronary arteries whether the patient died early or late (Figure 19). This is another example of the diffuseness of coronary atherosclerotic plaques in patients with symptomatic CAD.

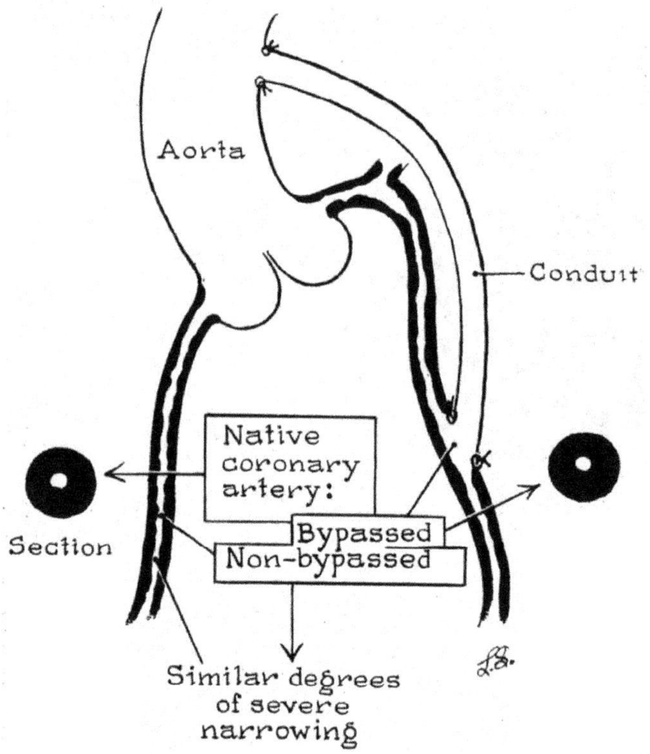

Figure 18. This diagram shows how the study to be described in Figure 19 was carried out. The study involved studying the native coronary arteries by the 5-mm segment approach in native arteries which were bypassed and in native arteries which were not bypassed to ask if there was differences in the degrees of cross-sectional area narrowing. Reproduced with permission from Waller BF, Roberts WC. Amount of narrowing by atherosclerotic plaque in 44 nonbypassed and 52 bypassed major epicardial coronary arteries in 32 necropsy patients who died within 1 month of aortocoronary bypass grafting. *Am J Cardiol* 1980; 46:956–962.

What is the Frequency of Acute Coronary Lesions and Multi-Luminal Channels at Necropsy in Patients with Unstable Angina Pectoris, Sudden Coronary Death, and Acute Myocardial Infarction?

Kragel and colleagues[33] examined this question by studying 5-mm sections of each of the 4 major coronary arteries in a group of patients who had a single isolated coronary event (Table 3). They studied 14 patients at necropsy with *unstable angina pectoris* and these individuals had no foci of left ventricular necrosis or fibrosis, indicating that they never had either an acute or healed myocardial infarct and none of them died suddenly. They studied another 21 patients who *died suddenly outside the hospital* and these individuals likewise had never had either an acute or healed myocardial infarct and their records indicated that angina pectoris was absent. They also studied 32 patients who had had a *fatal first AMI*. The authors knew that it was their first and only coronary event because there were no scars in the left ventricular wall. These patients died in the hospital and they did not at any time have angina pectoris. Thrombi were present in a coronary artery in some patients in all 3 groups, but their frequency and size varied enormously: thrombi occurred in 73% of the AMI patients and it completely occupied the lumen overlying an atherosclerotic plaque. Nearly 30% of those with unstable angina pectoris and sudden coronary death had thrombi but these were minute (<10% of the residual lumen), located over a plaque, and they did not interfere with blood flow. *Plaque rupture* occurred predominately in the patients with acute infarcts but it was not universal in that 25% of these patients did not have evidence of ruptured plaque even though every 5-mm sections of the 4 major epicardial coronary arteries were studied histologically. *Plaque hemorrhage* was seen far more frequently in the AMI group but the hemorrhage did not appear to further narrow the lumen of the coronary artery at the site of the hemorrhage. *Multi-luminal channels* occurred in one or more 5-mm segments in all patients, most prominent in the patients with unstable angina pectoris.

Brosius and Roberts[46] described among patients with their first AMI the amount of narrowing at the site of the thrombus due to underlying atherosclerotic plaque versus the amount by overlying thrombus. They found that at the site of the thrombus the lumen was narrowed in cross-sectional area by underlying plaque from 33 to 98% (mean 81%), indicating that the amount of lumen occupied by thrombus varied from 67% to 2% (mean 19%). This finding supports the observation that primary angioplasty produces better results early after AMI than does thrombolysis: the latter simply lysis the clot whereas angioplasty both disrupts the clot and cracks the underlying plaque resulting in a wider lumen. Just proximal and just distal to the thrombus, the amount of lumen occupied by plaque averaged 76% proximally and 81% distally.

What is the Mechanism of Luminal Widening by Angioplasty in the Coronary Arteries?

Potkin and Roberts[23] examined 5-mm segments of the 4 major epicardial coronary arteries in patients who had undergone coronary angioplasty and found that the mechanism

Table 3
Frequency of acute coronary lesions and of multiliminal channels at *In Patients* with unstable angina pectoris (UAP), Sudden coronary death (SCD) and acute myocardial infarction (AMI)

Coronary Subset	Number of Patients	Coronary Arteries			
		Thrombi	Plaque Rupture	Plaque Hemorrhage	Multiluminal Channels
UAP	**14**	**4 (29%)***	**5 (36%)***	**3 (21%)***	**14 (100%)**
SCD	**21**	**6 (29%)***	**4 (19%)***	**4 (19%)***	**17 (81%)**
AMI	**32**	**22 (69%)****	**24 (75%)****	**20 (63%)****	**29 (90%)**
Totals	**67**	**32 (48%)**	**33 (49%)**	**27 (40%)**	**60 (90%)**

*, ** = p < .02.

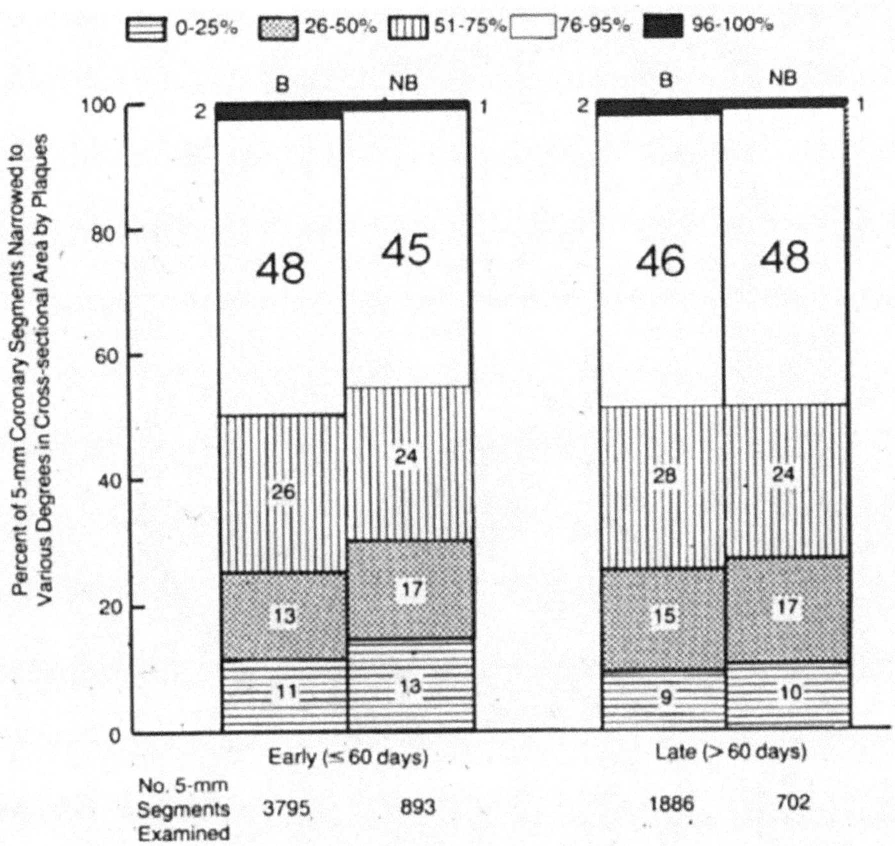

Figure 19. This bar graph compares the quantity of narrowing in 5-mm segments by plaque in bypassed (B) (226 coronary arteries) and non-bypassed (NB) (80 coronary arteries) in 102 patients dying early (65 patients) or late (37 patients) after aorto-coronary bypass grafting. Whether the patients died early (≤60 days) or later the quantity of plaque in the 5-mm segments of both native bypassed and non-bypassed arteries were similar. Reproduced with permission from Waller BF, Roberts WC. Amount of narrowing by atherosclerotic plaque in 44 nonbypassed and 52 bypassed major epicardial coronary arteries in 32 necropsy patients who died within 1 month of aortocoronary bypass grafting. *Am J Cardiol* 1980; 46:956–962.

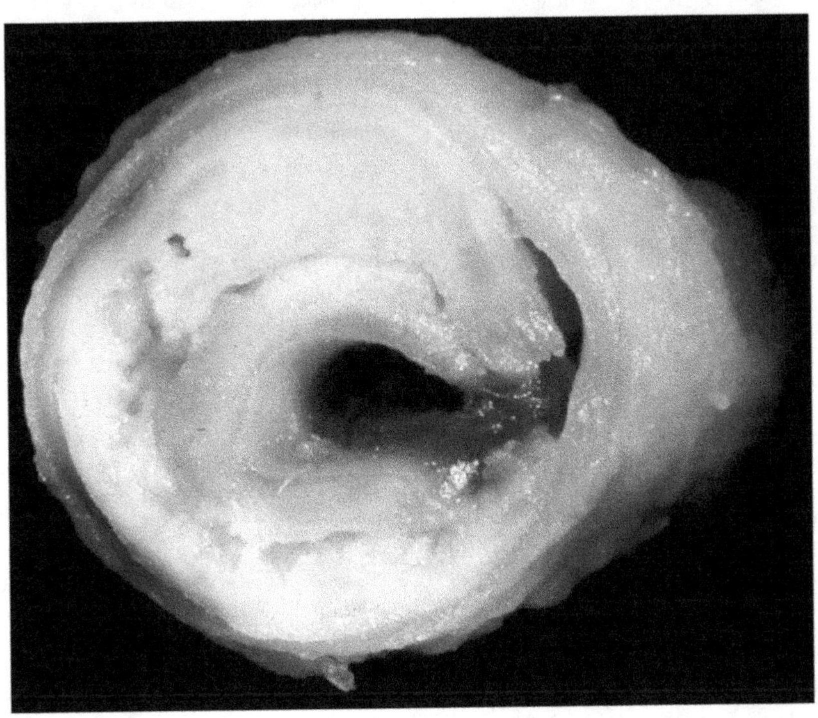

Figure 20. This is a photograph of a coronary artery which had undergone coronary angioplasty at this site. The plaque is cracked and a small dissection is apparent.

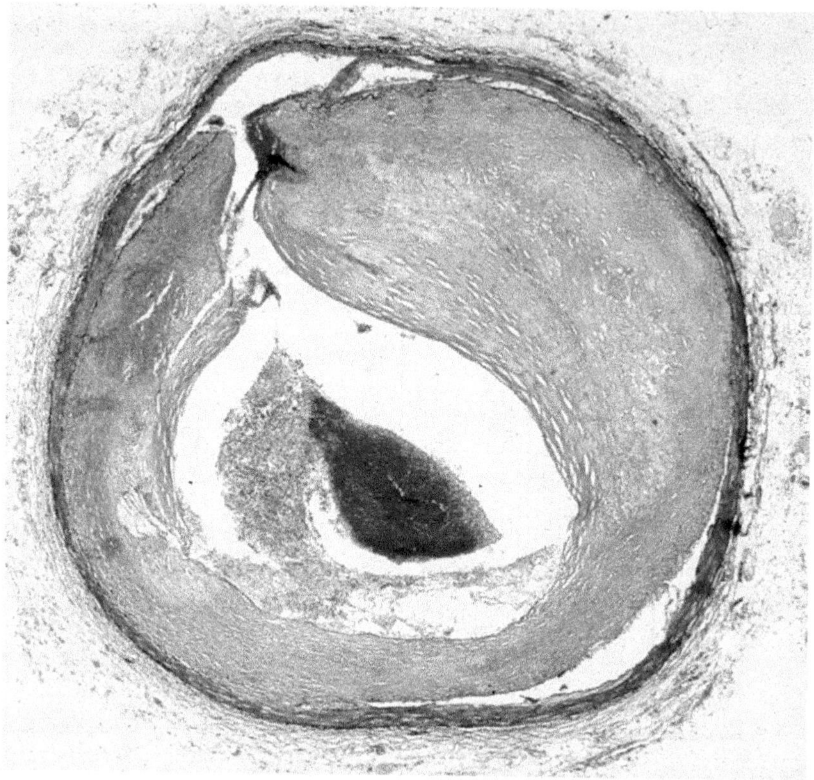

Figure 21. Shown here is a photomicrograph of a coronary artery at the site of coronary angioplasty. The atherosclerotic plaque is cracked and a dissection is created between the internal elastic membrane and overlying intimal plaque. Movat stain, X 40.

Table 4
Statin therapy—rule of 5 and 7

Statin therapy—rule of 5 and 7									
mg equivalent dose						⑤ ↓ TC	⑦ ↓ LDL	E 10 mg ↓ LDL	Total LDL ↓
R	A	S	P	L	F				
1.25	5	10	20	20	40	22%	27%	18%	45%
2.5	10	20	40	40	80	27%	34%	18%	52%
5	20	40	80	80	-	32%	41%	14%	55%
10	40	80	-	-	-	37%	48%	12%	60%
20	80	-	-	-	-	42%	55%	10%	65%
40	-	-	-	-	-	45%	62%	10%	72%

A = atorvastatin; E = ezetimibe; F = fluvastatin; L = lovastatin; LDL = low-density lipoprotein cholesterol; P = pravastatin; R = rosuvastatin; S = simvastatin; TC = total cholesterol.

by which the procedure works is by cracking the underlying atherosclerotic plaque. It is not by compressing the plaque. Figure 20 shows a gross photograph with partial cracking of the plaque and a small dissection. Figures 21 and 22 show photomicrographs of plaques cracked by angioplasty with dissection of a portion of the coronary media in several. Both mechanisms serve to widen the lumen. Figure 23 shows what may happen late after coronary angioplasty: cellular fibrous tissue has filled in a portion of the lumen present after the previous angioplasty. It appears that the initial angioplasty opened the artery considerably and probably ruptured it into the pultaceous debris shown at approximately 9:00. The fact that coronary plaques consist mainly of fibrous tissue may

Table 5
Differences in carnivores and herbivores

Characteristics	Carnivores	Herbivores
Appendages	**Claws**	**Hands or hoofs**
Teeth	**Sharp**	**Flat**
Intestines	**Short**	**Long**
Body cooling	**Pant**	**Sweat**
Drinking water	**Lap it**	**Sip it**
Vitamin C	**Make it themselves**	**Obtained solely from diet**

explain in part why angioplasty is generally successful (Figure 24).

What Observations Suggest That Atherosclerotic Plaques are the Result at Least in Part of Organization of Thrombi?

There are 4 observations that suggest that atherosclerotic plaques are the result, at least in part, of organization of thrombi[47]: 1) The dominant component of coronary plaques is fibrous tissue, commonly the result of organization of thrombus; 2) The presence of known components of thrombi —namely fibrin and platelets —within atherosclerotic plaques; 3) The occurrence of known components of atherosclerotic plaques—namely fibrous tissue, foam cells, cholesterol clefts, pultaceous debris, calcium—in organized hematomas or known thrombi wherever they might occur in the body (for example, in left atrial thrombi in mitral stenosis), and 4) The presence

Table 6
Shown in this diagram are guidelines for who to treat with lipid-altering drugs at various times. These guidelines are an attempt to decrease risk of an atherosclerotic event, not to prevent atherosclerotic plaques from forming. Much lower levels of low-density lipoproteins (LDL) will be necessary to prevent plaques

Drug guidelines (To decrease risk)		
LDL (mg/dL)	Other RF	Goal
>190	**≤1**	**<160**
>160	**>1**	**<130**
>130	**HA**	<100 (<70)

HA = heart attack; RF = risk factor.

of multiple channels in lumens, a recognized consequence of organization of pulmonary arterial emboli.

Figures 25 shows a coronary artery stained for fibrin and bands of fibrin deposits are located more or less parallel to the margins of the lumen. A close-up of the fibrin deposits is shown in the same figure. Figure 26 is a photomicrograph of a coronary artery showing lines of demarcation (arrows) between what might be considered plaques formed at different times from organization of thrombi. The demarcation lines consist of elastic tissue which makes the separation relatively easy. Figure 27 shows a coronary artery with at least 4 revascularization channels. If one injects thrombi into a systemic vein, for example the femoral vein, these clots go into the lungs and organize and they often organize into multiluminal channels, a finding extremely common in coronary arteries, suggesting that thrombi do play a role in their organization. Figure 28 is a picture of the interior lining of the left atrium in a patient who died after mitral valve replacement.[48] This patient underwent planned mitral commissurotomy without cardiopulmonary bypass about 20 years earlier but the body of the left atrium as well as its appendage was filled with thrombus and therefore the commissurotomy was not performed. At mitral valve replacement 20 years later, the thrombus in left atrial body was absent and now the lining of the free wall consisted of typical atherosclerotic plaque containing cholesterol clefts, pultaceous debris, and dense fibrous tissue, suggesting that these "atherosclerotic plaques" resulted entirely from organization of thrombi.

Another study supporting the view that atherosclerotic plaques are formed at least in part by organization of thrombi was provided by Virmani and Roberts[48] who examined 1,290

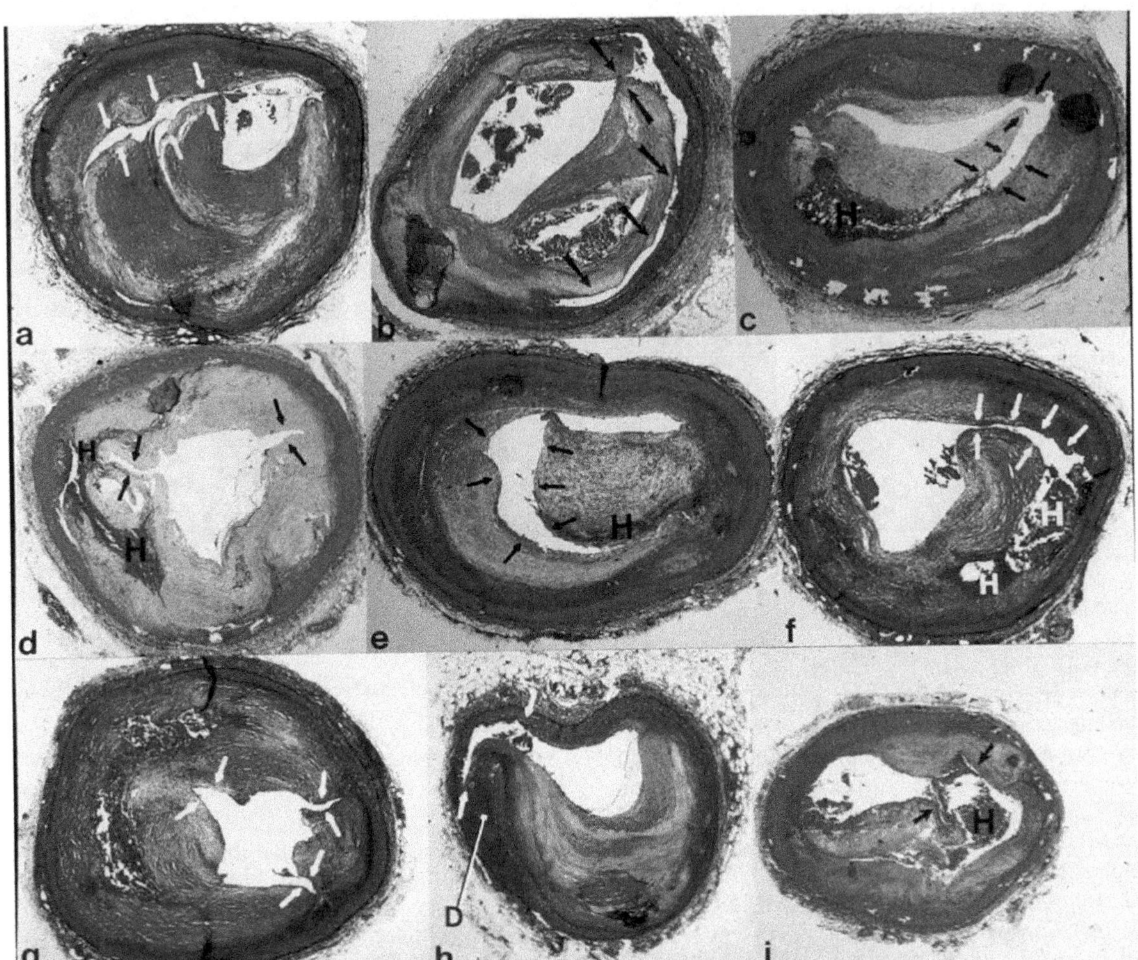

Figure 22. Shown here are photomicrographs of cross-sectional areas at sites of previous coronary angioplasty in 6 different patients. The arrows show where cracks in plaque occurred. Movat stains, X 20 (a, b); X 27 (c, d); X14 (e, f); X22 (g, h). Reproduced with permission from Potkin BN, Roberts WC. Effects of percutaneous transluminal coronary angioplasty on atherosclerotic plaques and relation of plaque composition and arterial size to outcome. *Am J Cardiol* 1988; 62:41–50.

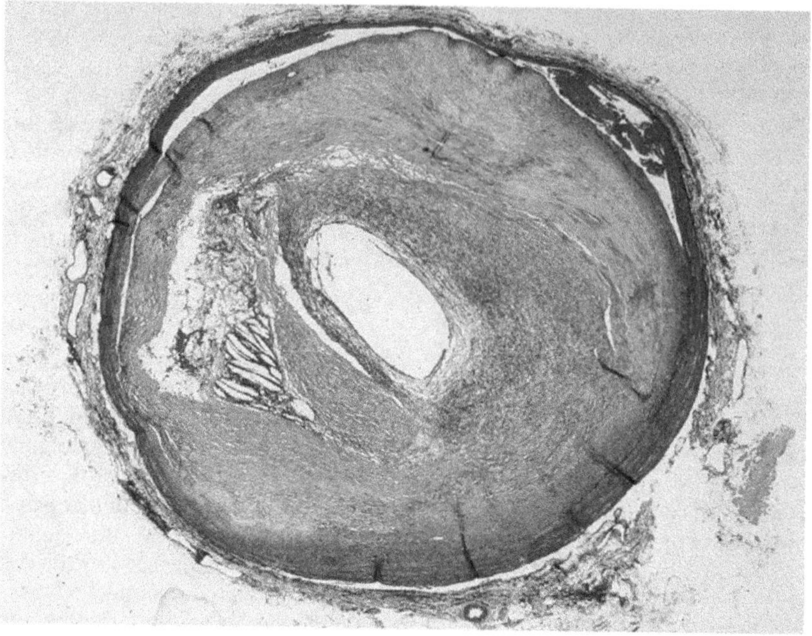

Figure 23. Shown is a photomicrograph of a coronary artery which had coronary angioplasty several months earlier. Surrounding the lumen is fibromuscular tissue which is quite different from the underlying dense fibrous tissue shown closer to the media. The angioplasty procedure appeared to have ruptured the plaque into the area of pultaceous debris located at approximately 11:00 and another plaque shown at approximately 6:00. The introduction of stents may prevent or lessen this neo-intimal fibromuscular proliferation.

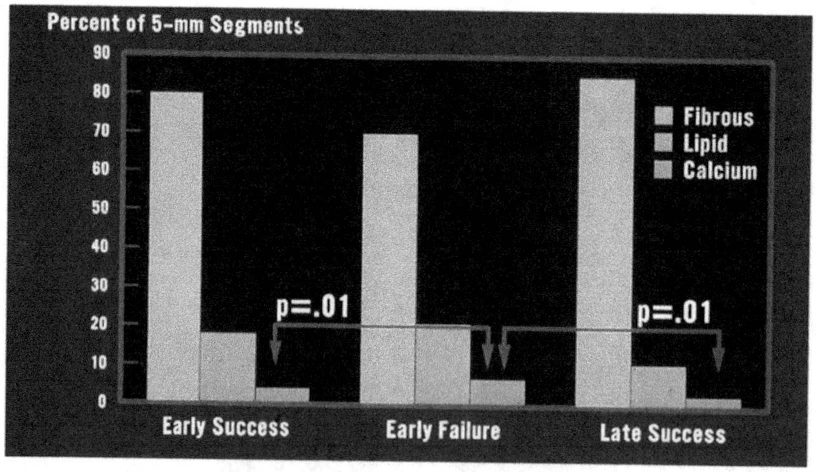

Figure 24. Shown here is a diagram of plaque composition in patients having coronary angioplasty and the 5-mm segments at sites of angioplasty were determined for composition. The green represents fibrous tissue, the blue, extracellular lipid, and the pink, calcium. Whether there was early or late success or early failure, fibrous tissue was the dominant component at the site of the angioplasty.

histologic sections (1 per 5-mm segment) from 224 major epicardial coronary arteries in 57 patients with fatal CAD and compared findings with those in 27 controls: *intraplaque fibrin deposits* were present in 2% of the segments (controls <1%), in 17% of the arteries (c = 3%), and in 63% of the patients (c = 7%); *intraluminal thrombus*, present only in the patients with AMI and in none of the controls, occurred in 3% of the segments, in 8% of the arteries and in 26% of the patients (in 42 of the 57 patients [74%] with AMI); *intraplaque extravasated erythrocytes* were present in 10% of the segments (c = 1%), in 35% of the arteries (c = 4%), and in 84% of the patients (c = 19%); *iron* was present in 4% of the segments (c = < 1%), in 14% of the arteries (c = 4%), and in 57% of the patients (c = 22%).

Is Atherosclerosis a Multifactoral or a Unifactoral Disease?

Figure 29 shows 10 "atherosclerotic risk factors" and asks the question of each factor: Is this factor required to form atherosclerotic plaques? And the answer to the first 9 is "No".[49] One does not have to have the atherosclerotic gene to have atherosclerotic plaques. According to Brown and Goldstein,[50] the atherosclerotic gene is present in only 1 of 500 persons. Recent studies suggest that the frequency may be half that.[50] When I was in medical school I was taught that atherosclerosis was a degenerative disease, the consequence of living on planet Earth. I have had the opportunity to examine 6 hearts in patients who died when ≥100 years of age and 3 had wide open

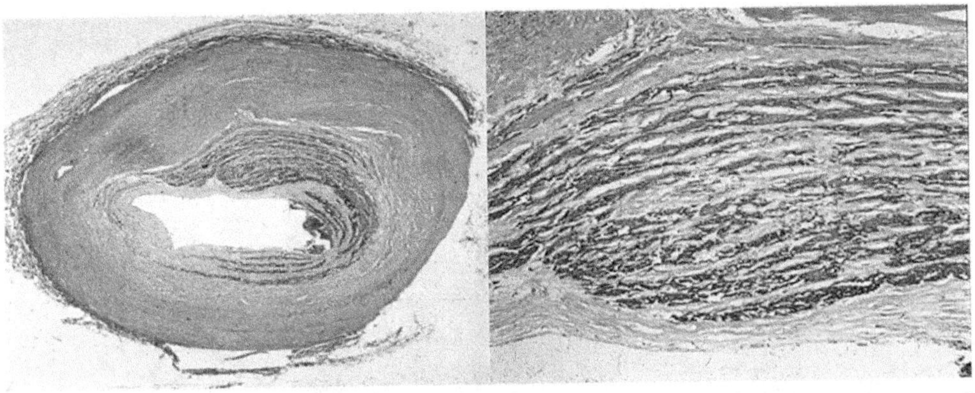

Figure 25. Shown on the *left* is a section of coronary artery showing some purple lines parallel to one another and near the lumen of the artery and a more peripheral portion of the artery consisting of dense fibrous tissue. Shown on the *right* is a close up of one area in the left diagram showing fibrous tissue, fibrin, fibrous tissue, fibrin, suggesting that the fibrous tissue at least in part was the result of organization of fibrin by far the dominant component of thrombus. Reproduced with permission from Roberts WC. Does thrombosis play a major role in the development of symptom-producing atherosclerotic plaques? *Circulation* 1973; 48:1161–1166.

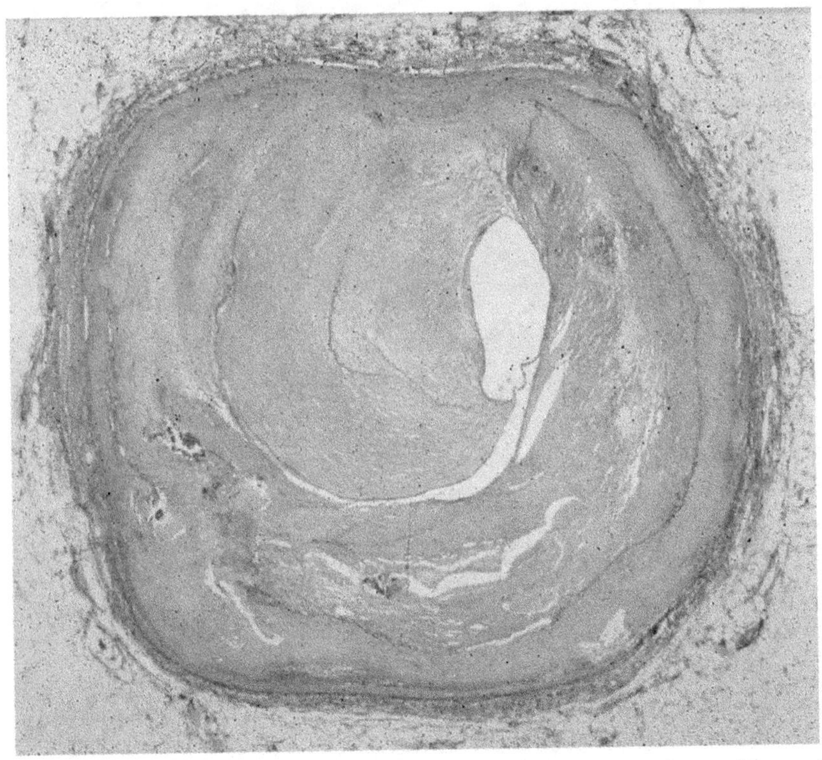

Figure 26. Shown here is a cross-section of a coronary artery showing various lines of demarcation separating possibly one plaque from another plaque suggesting that possibly thrombus was laid down and then organized and then laid down again and then organized. Reproduced with permission from Roberts WC. Does thrombosis play a major role in the development of symptom-producing atherosclerotic plaques? *Circulation* 1973; 48:1161–1166.

lumens and only minimal plaques. Russell Ross[51] in an article in 1986 declared that atherosclerosis was an inflammatory disease and much study has been done, particularly by the Harvard group, subsequently examining that thesis.[52] If one asks, however, if an elevated C-reactive protein or another cytokine is necessary to have atherosclerosis, the answer is "No". Certainly, cigarette smoking is not healthy but cigarette smoking in and of itself does not cause atherosclerotic plaques. Although systemic hypertension and diabetes mellitus may worsen the burden, neither by itself causes plaques. One does not have to be overweight to have atherosclerotic disease. There is no evidence that exercise prevents plaques, particularly if one stops at a McDonald's on the way home from the run. What is stressful to one person is not necessarily stressful to another; it is very difficult to put a number on stress. In my view, atherosclerosis is a consequence of abnormal cholesterol levels.[53–66]

What is the evidence that atherosclerosis is a cholesterol problem? There are 4 factors: 1) *Experimental evidence*. Atherosclerosis is one of the easiest diseases to produce

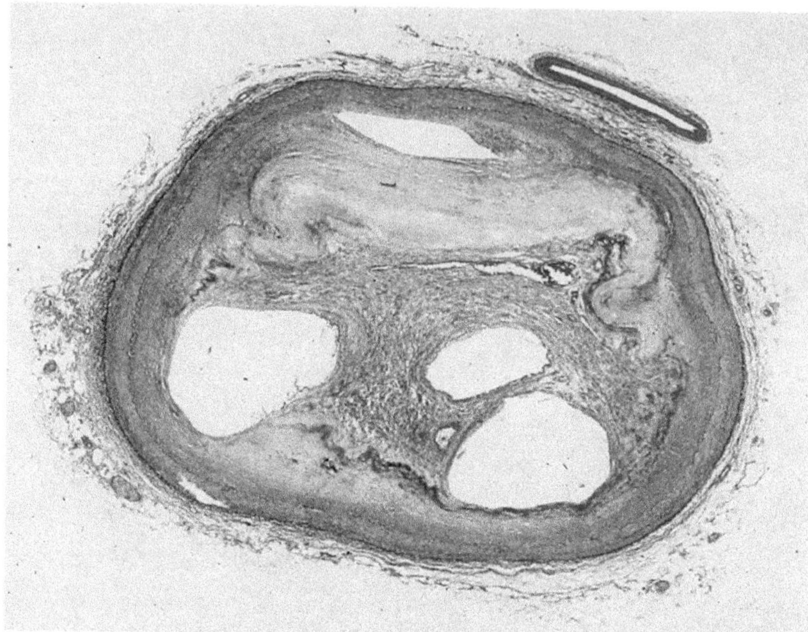

Figure 27. Shown here is a coronary artery with 4 revascularized channels, something commonly seen when thrombus organizes in various arterial systems. These multi-luminal channels are seen in about 5% of coronary trees when studied by the 5-mm segment approach.

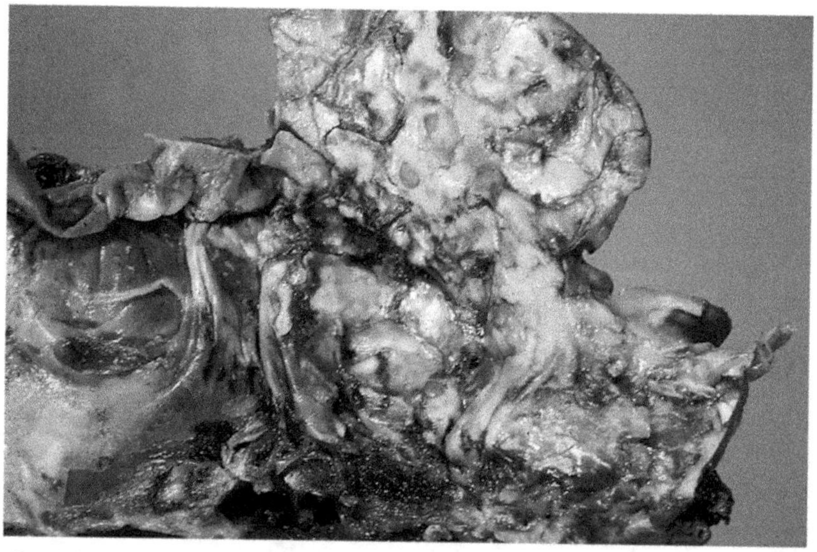

Figure 28. Shown here is the wall of left atrium in a patient who had severe mitral stenosis and underwent planned mitral commissurotomy 20 years earlier. When the surgeon entered the pericardial space he found that the entire left atrial body and appendage was filled with thrombus and since there was no cardiopulmonary bypass available at the time, the thoracotomy was closed. Twenty years later the same patient returned for a mitral valve replacement and now there was no thrombus in the left atrial cavity but the left atrial wall contained classic heavily calcified atherosclerotic plaques, a bit of evidence that one can start with a thrombus and end with a plaque. Reproduced with permission from Roberts WC. Does thrombosis play a major role in the development of symptom-producing atherosclerotic plaques? *Circulation* 1973; 48:1161–1166.

experimentally. If one gives herbivores (rabbits, monkeys) a diet high in cholesterol and/or saturated fat, atherosclerotic plaques are produced and they are similar to those occurring in human beings. 2) *Morphologic evidence*. There is cholesterol in the plaques. 3) *Epidemiologic evidence*. The best study in my view is the Seven Countries Study headed by Ancel Keys and colleagues.[67] They studied portions of populations in 7 countries and found that those populations with high levels of total cholesterol (Finland, for example) had a very high frequency of atherosclerotic events whereas those with much lower total cholesterol levels (for example, Japan) had far fewer atherosclerotic events. 4) *Therapeutic evidence*. Numerous statin trials have shown that when cholesterol levels are lowered atherosclerotic events decrease considerably (Table 4), and the lower the better.[64,68]

Although some investigators have considered cholesterol the cause of atherosclerosis for several decades, 26 authors mainly from Europe, in April 2017, published an article titled

Atherosclerotic Risk Factors

Risk factor	Is this factor necessary to form plaques?
1. Genetic (1/500) 2. Degenerative 3. Inflammatory 4. Cigarette smoking 5. Systemic hypertension 6. Diabetes mellitus 7. Overweight 8. Inactivity 9. Stress	NO
10. Cholesterol problem	YES

Figure 29. Shown here are various atherosclerotic risk factors and the question is asked, "Is each necessary to form plaques?" The only one where the answer is "Yes" is an elevated cholesterol level. Reproduced with permission from Roberts WC. Atherosclerotic risk factors: are there ten or is there only one? *Am J Cardiol* 1989; 64:552–554.

"Low-density lipoproteins cause atherosclerotic cardiovascular disease…" a consensus statement from the European Atherosclerosis Society Consensus Panel.[66] I was glad to see the article that soundly supports the view that cholesterol is the cause of atherosclerosis.

Another very important article also appeared in March 2017, namely *"Long-term safety and efficacy in achieving very low levels of low-density lipoprotein cholesterol…"* in *JAMA Cardiology* authored by 11 prominent authors who studied 15,281 patients to determine whether achieving an LDL-cholesterol level <30 mg/dL was safe.[68] The study was carried out over a 6-year period. The patients with these low levels were compared to those with higher levels. The data provides reassurance regarding the longer-term safety in patients achieving LDL-cholesterol levels <30 mg/dl. I have been on a statin (plus ezetimibe most years) for nearly 3 decades and my most recent lipid values in mg/dL were as follows: total cholesterol 102; LDL cholesterol 27; high-density lipoprotein cholesterol 68, and triglycerides 34. Some physicians worry that these very low levers are dangerous but this recent study is indeed reassuring that they are not dangerous. It appears that LDL-cholesterol levels have to be <50 mg/dL to prevent the formation of atherosclerotic plaques.

These two studies are very important in heart disease and provide clear evidence that cholesterol is the villain.

What Characteristics Distinguish Carnivores and Herbivores?

Carnivores and herbivores have different characteristics (Table 5).[69] Humans of course fit far better into the herbivore category than the carnivore category. Atherosclerosis does not occur in carnivores and cannot be produced experimentally in carnivores unless they are previously made hypothyroid.

What are Reasonable Guidelines for Whom to Treat with Lipid-Altering Agents?

The National Cholesterol Education Program in 1988, 1993, 2001, with revisions in 2004, and now the American Heart Association/American College of Cardiology 2013 guidelines have provided advice as to who to treat with cholesterol-lowering agents (Table 6). These treatment guidelines focus exclusively on decreasing the risk of having atherosclerotic events. They are not designed to prevent the formation of atherosclerosis plaques or to shrink those already present. My guideline is to prevent the formation of atherosclerotic plaques and to do so the LDL cholesterol needs to be <50 mg/dl, and the other risk factors must be worked on: an elevated blood pressure must be lowered, body weight must be reduced if elevated, exercise must be increased if presently avoided, and all cigarettes must be eliminated. The goal is not to decrease risk but to prevent atherosclerotic plaques! If atherosclerotic plaques are prevented, atherosclerotic consequences do not occur.

What is the Rule of 5 and the Rule of 7 in Statin Therapy?

The statin drugs, in my view, are the finest cardiovascular drugs ever created. The statin drugs are to atherosclerosis what penicillin was to infectious disease.[57] Table 4 shows a list of 6 statin drugs and what their milligram equivalent doses are and what average reductions in total cholesterol and LDL cholesterol can be expected from those doses.[58] Each time the statin dose is doubled an average of 5% additional reduction in total cholesterol occurs and an average of 7% additional reduction of LDL cholesterol occurs. The initial dose of the statin drug provides the greatest reduction in total and LDL cholesterol. With the lowest Federal Drug Administration's approved dose of any of the statin drugs there is a 22% average reduction in total cholesterol and a 27% average reduction in LDL cholesterol. Thus, the maximal dose of the most powerful statin (rosuvastatin; 40 mg) provides a 45% average total cholesterol reduction and an average 62% LDL-cholesterol reduction. That dose, however, is equivalent to 160 mg of atorvastatin and 320 mg of simvastatin. The addition of ezetimibe 10 mg to the lower levels of statin doses lower LDL cholesterol an additional 18 to 25% so that the combination of ezetimibe with the lowest doses of the statin drugs leads to a 45% average LDL-cholesterol reduction. With the first doubling of the statin dose the combination leads to a 52% LDL reduction. To get that degree of LDL reduction by statin monotherapy alone it would be necessary to triple the statin dose. It is for that reason that I like the combination, statin + ezetimibe. It is well recognized that one drug rarely does the job in treating patients with systemic hypertension. That same principle, in my view, needs to be more frequently applied to lipid-lowering therapy.

What is the Effect of Lipid Lowering Drug Therapy on Coronary Luminal Narrowing?

It is never too late to begin lipid-lowering therapy. Several angiographic studies and several intracoronary ultrasound studies have shown that lumens of coronary and carotid arteries can become wider after periods of lipid-lowering therapy.[64] Assuming that an individual has to have >75% cross-sectional narrowing in one or more major epicardial coronary arteries to have a coronary event, if the lumen can be widened such that it becomes <75% narrowed in cross-sectional area theoretically the flow through that widened artery is normal.

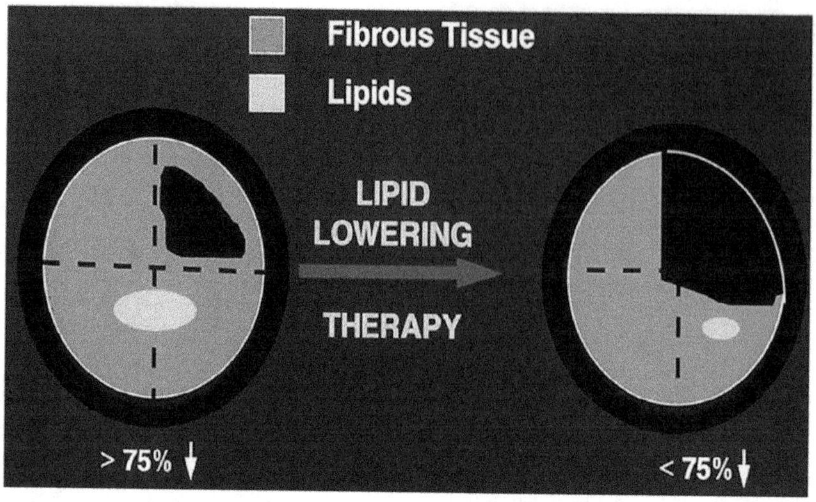

Figure 30. This diagram shows the theoretical situation if one lowers one's LDL cholesterol considerably. It appears that the lipid portion of plaques is reversible if the LDL cholesterol levels are severely lowered. If an atherosclerotic plaque narrows a lumen >75% in cross-sectional area flow through that artery is limited. If the plaque can be reduced such that the lumen is <75% narrowed in cross-sectional area, flow through that lumen theoretically is relatively normal.

There is good evidence that the lipid portion of atherosclerotic plaques can be shrunk and diminishing the quantity of lipid results in widening of the lumens. Figure 30 attempts to display that thesis graphically.

What are Some Requisites for a Healthy Life?

An LDL cholesterol <50 mg/dL; a blood pressure <115/75 mm/Hg; a body mass index <25 kg/m^2; an empty colon (orlistat 120 mg/day is useful) or better (vegetarian-fruit diet); a non-smoking and limited alcohol lifestyle, and a bit of luck.

Conclusion

In patients with symptomatic or fatal CAD, the atherosclerotic process involves every 5-mm segment of all major (right, left main, left anterior descending, and left circumflex) epicardial coronary arteries. Likewise, when involving symptomatic or fatal aortic or peripheral arterial atherosclerosis, the process is also diffuse in those regions. Fibrous tissue is the dominant component of coronary plaques. Angioplasty works by cracking plaques. Atherosclerosis is caused by cholesterol. Four factors support the cholesterol cause of atherosclerosis. Humans fundamentally are herbivores, not carnivores. The rule of 5 and 7 is useful in statin therapy. There are at least 6 requisites for a long healthy life: an LDL cholesterol <50 mg/dl; a blood pressure <115/75 mm Hg; a body mass index <25 kg/m^2; a rapid colonic transit time (vegetarian and fruit diet and/or orlistat); no smoking or excessive alcohol, and a bit of luck.

Disclosures

The authors have no conflicts of interest to disclose.

1. Mautner GC, Berezowski K, Mautner SL, Roberts WC. Degrees of coronary arterial narrowing at necropsy in men with large fusiform abdominal aortic aneurysm. *Am J Cardiol* 1992;70:1143–1146.
2. Mautner GC, Mautner SL, Roberts WC. Amounts of coronary arterial narrowing by atherosclerotic plaque at necropsy in patients with lower extremity amputation. *Am J Cardiol* 1992;70:1147–1151.
3. Roberts WC, Potkin BN, Solus DE, Reddy SG. Mode of death, frequency of healed and acute myocardial infarction, number of major epicardial coronary arteries severely narrowed by atherosclerotic plaque, and heart weight in fatal atherosclerotic coronary artery disease: Analysis of 889 patients studied at necropsy. *J Am Coll Cardiol* 1990;15:196–203.
4. Roberts WC, Jones AA. Quantitation of coronary arterial narrowing at necropsy in sudden coronary death. Analysis of 31 patients and comparison with 25 control subjects. *Am J Cardiol* 1979;44:39–45.
5. Roberts WC, Virmani R. Quantification of coronary arterial narrowing in clinically-isolated unstable angina pectoris. An analysis of 22 necropsy patients. *Am J Med* 1979;67:792–799.
6. Virmani R, Roberts WC. Quantification of coronary arterial narrowing and of left ventricular myocardial scarring in healed myocardial infarction with chronic eventually fatal, congestive cardiac failure. *Am J Med* 1980;68:831–838.
7. Cabin HS, Roberts WC. True left ventricular aneurysm and healed myocardial infarction. Clinical and necropsy observations including quantification of degrees of coronary arterial narrowing. *Am J Cardiol* 1980;46:754–763.
8. Roberts WC, Jones AA. Quantification of coronary arterial narrowing at necropsy in acute transmural myocardial infarction. Analysis and comparison of findings in 27 patients and 22 controls. *Circulation* 1980;61:786–790.
9. Isner JM, Wu M, Virmani R, Jones AA, Roberts WC. Comparison of degrees of coronary arterial luminal narrowing determined by visual inspection of histologic sections under magnification among three independent observers and comparison to that obtained by video planimetry. An analysis of 559 five-millimeter segments of 61 coronary arteries from eleven patients. *Lab Invest* 1980;42:566–570.
10. Waller BF, Roberts WC. Amount of narrowing by atherosclerotic plaque in 44 nonbypassed and 52 bypassed major epicardial coronary arteries in 32 necropsy patients who died within 1 month of aortocoronary bypass grafting. *Am J Cardiol* 1980;46:956–962.
11. Cabin HS, Roberts WC. Quantification of amounts of coronary arterial narrowing in patients with types II and IV hyperlipoproteinemia and in those with known normal lipoprotein patterns. *Am Heart J* 1981;101:52–58.
12. Cabin HS, Schwartz DE, Virmani R, Brewer HB Jr, Roberts WC. Type III hyperlipoproteinemia; quantification, distribution, and nature of atherosclerotic coronary arterial narrowing in five necropsy patients. *Am Heart J* 1981;102:830–835.

13. Cabin HS, Roberts WC. Comparison of amount and extent of coronary narrowing by atherosclerotic plaque and of myocardial scarring at necropsy in anterior and posterior healed transmural myocardial infarction. *Circulation* 1982;66:93–99.
14. Cabin HS, Roberts WC. Relation of healed transmural myocardial infarct size to length of survival after acute myocardial infarction, age at death, and amount and extent of coronary arterial narrowing by atherosclerotic plaques; analysis of 70 necropsy patients. *Am Heart J* 1982;104:216–220.
15. Cabin HS, Roberts WC. Relation of serum total cholesterol and triglyceride levels to the amount and extent of coronary arterial narrowing by atherosclerotic plaque in coronary heart disease. Quantitative analysis of 2,037 five-mm segments of 160 major epicardial coronary arteries in 40 necropsy patients. *Am J Med* 1982;73:227–234.
16. Cabin HS, Roberts WC. Quantitative comparison of extent of coronary narrowing and size of healed myocardial infarct in 33 necropsy patients with clinically recognized and in 28 with clinically unrecognized ("silent") previous acute myocardial infarction. *Am J Cardiol* 1982;50:677–681.
17. Warnes CA, Roberts WC. Sudden coronary death; relation of amount and distribution of coronary narrowing at necropsy to previous symptoms of myocardial ischemia, left ventricular scarring and heart weight. *Am J Cardiol* 1984;54:65–73.
18. Warnes CA, Roberts WC. Comparison at necropsy by age group of amount and distribution of narrowing by atherosclerotic plaque in 2995 five-mm long segments of 240 major coronary arteries in 60 men aged 31 to 70 years with sudden coronary death. *Am Heart J* 1984;108:431–435.
19. Ross EM, Roberts WC. Severe atherosclerotic coronary artery disease, healed myocardial infarction and chronic congestive heart failure; analysis of 81 patients studied at necropsy. *Am J Cardiol* 1986;57:44–50.
20. Ross EM, Roberts WC. Severe atherosclerotic coronary arterial narrowing and chronic congestive heart failure without myocardial infarction; analysis of 18 patients studied at necropsy. *Am J Cardiol* 1986;57:51–56.
21. Warnes CA, Roberts WC. Morphologic findings in sudden coronary death; a comparison of those with and those without previous symptoms of myocardial ischemia. *Cardiovasc Clin* 1986;4:607–615.
22. Barbour DJ, Warnes CA, Roberts WC. Cardiac findings associated with sudden death secondary to atherosclerotic coronary artery disease; comparison of patients with and those without previous angina pectoris and/or healed myocardial infarction. *Circulation* 1987;75:II9–II11.
23. Potkin BN, Roberts WC. Effects of percutaneous transluminal coronary angioplasty on atherosclerotic plaques and relation of plaque composition and arterial size to outcome. *Am J Cardiol* 1988;62:41–50.
24. Kalan JM, Roberts WC. Morphologic findings in patients undergoing coronary artery bypass grafting for acute myocardial infarction. *Am J Cardiol* 1988;62:144–147.
25. Kragel AH, Reddy SG, Wittes JT, Roberts WC. Morphometric analysis of the composition of atherosclerotic plaques in the four major epicardial coronary arteries in acute myocardial infarction and in sudden coronary death. *Circulation* 1989;80:1747–1756.
26. Kragel AH, Reddy SG, Wittes JT, Roberts WC. Morphometric analysis of the composition of coronary arterial plaques in isolated unstable angina pectoris with pain at rest. *Am J Cardiol* 1990;66:562–567.
27. Dressler FA, Malekzadeh S, Roberts WC. Quantitative analysis of amounts of coronary arterial narrowing in cocaine addicts. *Am J Cardiol* 1990;65:536–537.
28. Kalan JM, Roberts WC. Morphologic findings in saphenous veins used as coronary arterial bypass conduits for longer than 1 year: necropsy analysis of 53 patients, 123 saphenous veins and 1865 five-millimeter segments of veins. *Am Heart J* 1990;119:1164–1184.
29. Gertz SD, Kragel AH, Kalan JM, Braunwald E, Roberts WC, TIMI Investigators. Comparison of coronary and myocardial morphologic findings in patients with and without thrombolytic therapy during fatal first acute myocardial infarction. *Am J Cardiol* 1990;66:904–909.
30. Kragel AH, Roberts WC. Composition of atherosclerotic plaques in the coronary arteries in homozygous familial hypercholesterolemia. *Am Heart J* 1991;121:210–211.
31. Gertz SD, Malekzadeh S, Dollar AL, Kragel AH, Roberts WC. Composition of atherosclerotic plaques in the four major epicardial coronary arteries in patients ≥90 years of age. *Am J Cardiol* 1991;67:1228–1233.
32. Dollar AL, Kragel AH, Fernicola DJ, Waclawiw MA, Roberts WC. Composition of atherosclerotic plaques in coronary arteries in women <40 years of age with fatal coronary artery disease and implications for plaque reversibility. *Am J Cardiol* 1991;67:1223–1227.
33. Kragel AH, Gertz SD, Roberts WC. Morphologic comparison of frequency and types of acute lesions in the major epicardial coronary arteries in unstable angina pectoris, sudden coronary death and acute myocardial infarction. *J Am Coll Cardiol* 1991;18:801–808.
34. Roberts WC, Kragel AH, Gertz SD, Roberts CS, Kalan JM. The heart in fatal unstable angina pectoris. *Am J Cardiol* 1991;68:22B–27B.
35. Roberts WC. Qualitative and quantitative comparison of amounts of narrowing by atherosclerotic plaques in the major epicardial coronary arteries at necropsy in sudden coronary death, transmural acute myocardial infarction, transmural healed myocardial infarction and unstable angina pectoris. *Am J Cardiol* 1989;64:324–328.
36. Roberts WC, Ko JM, Pearl GJ. Morphologic features of atherosclerotic plaque in occlusive femoral artery disease treated by endarterectomy. *Am J Geriatr Cardiol* 2008;17:50–52.
37. Roberts WC, Turnage TA II, Whiddon LL. Quantitative comparison of amounts of cross-sectional area narrowing in coronary endarterectomy specimens in patients having coronary artery bypass grafting to amounts of narrowing in the same artery in patients with fatal coronary artery disease studied at necropsy. *Am J Cardiol* 2007;99:588–592.
38. Roberts WC, Barry AE. Frequency of coronary endarterectomy in patients undergoing coronary artery bypass grafting at a single tertiary Texas Hospital 2010–2016 with morphologic studies of the operatively excised specimens. *Am J Cardiol* 2017;120:2164–2169.
39. Arnett EN, Isner JM, Redwood DR, Kent KM, Baker WP, Ackerstein H, Roberts WC. Coronary artery narrowing in coronary heart disease: Comparison of cineangiographic and necropsy findings. *Ann Intern Med* 1979;91:350–356.
40. Gertz SD, Kalan JM, Kragel AH, Roberts WC, Braunwald E, TIMI Investigators. Cardiac morphologic finds in patients with acute myocardial infarction treated with recombinant tissue plasminogen activator. *Am J Cardiol* 1990;65:953–961.
41. Crall FV Jr, Roberts WC. The extramural and intramural coronary arteries in juvenile diabetes mellitus: Analysis of nine necropsy patients aged 19 to 38 years with onset of diabetes before age 15 years. *Am J Med* 1978;64:221–230.
42. Mautner SL, Mautner GC, Hunsberger SA, Roberts WC. Comparison of composition of atherosclerotic plaques in saphenous veins used as aortocoronary bypass conduits with plaques in native coronary arteries in the same men. *Am J Cardiol* 1992;70:1380–1387.
43. Mautner SL, Lin F, Mautner GC, Roberts WC. Comparison in women versus men of composition of atherosclerotic plaques in native coronary arteries and in saphenous veins used as aortocoronary conduits. *J Am Coll Cardiol* 1993;21:1312–1318.
44. Mautner GC, Mautner SL, Roberts WC. Composition of atherosclerotic plaques in the epicardial coronary arteries in juvenile (Type I) diabetes mellitus. *Am J Cardiol* 1992;70:1264–1268.
45. Mautner GC, Mautner SL, Lin F, Roggin GM, Roberts WC. Amounts of coronary arterial luminal narrowing and composition of the material causing the narrowing in Buerger's disease. *Am J Cardiol* 1993;71:486–490.
46. Brosius FC III, Roberts WC. Significance of coronary arterial thrombus in transmural acute myocardial infarction: A study of 54 necropsy patients. *Circulation* 1981;63:810–816.
47. Roberts WC. Does thrombosis play a major role in the development of symptom-producing atherosclerotic plaques? *Circulation* 1973;48:1161–1166.
48. Virmani R, Roberts WC. Extravasated erythrocytes, iron, and fibrin in atherosclerotic plaques of coronary arteries in fatal coronary heart disease and their relation to luminal thrombus: Frequency and significance in 57 necropsy patients and in 2958 five-mm segments of 224 major epicardial coronary arteries. *Am Heart J* 1983;105:788–797.
49. Roberts WC. Atherosclerotic risk factors: are there ten or is there only one? *Am J Cardiol* 1989;64:552–554.
50. Brown MS, Goldstein JL. How LDL receptors influence cholesterol and atherosclerosis. *Sci Am* 1984;251:58–66.
51. Ross R. The pathogenesis of atherosclerosis—an update. *New England J Med* 1986;314:488–500.

52. Ridker PM, Everett BM, Thuren T, MacFadyen JG, Chang WH, Ballantyne C, Fonseca F, Nicolau J, Koenig W, Anker SD, Kastelein JJP, Cornel JH, Pais P, Pella D, Genest J, Cifkova R, Lorenzatti A, Forster T, Kobalava Z, Vida-Simiti L, Flather M, Shimokawa H, Ogawa H, Dellborg M, Rossi PRF, Troquay RPT, Libby P, Glynn RJ, CANTOS Trial Group. Antiinflammatory Therapy with Canakinumab for Atherosclerotic Disease. *N Engl J Med* 2017;377:1119–1131.
53. Roberts WC. Extreme hypercholesterolemia = malignant atherosclerosis. *Am J Cardiol* 1984;54:242–243.
54. Roberts WC. Lipid-lowering therapy after an atherosclerotic event. *Am J Cardiol* 1989;64:693–695.
55. Roberts WC. Getting cardiologists interested in lipids. *Am J Cardiol* 1993;72:744–745.
56. Roberts WC. Preventing and arresting coronary atherosclerosis. *Am Heart J* 1995;130:580–600.
57. Roberts WC. The underused miracle drugs: The statin drugs are to atherosclerosis what penicillin was to infectious disease. *Am J Cardiol* 1996;78:377–378.
58. Roberts WC. The rule of 5 and the rule of 7 in lipid-lowering by statin drugs. *Am J Cardiol* 1997;80:106–107.
59. Roberts WC. Shifting from decreasing risk to actually preventing and arresting atherosclerosis. *Am J Cardiol* 1999;83:816–817.
60. Roberts WC. Twenty questions on atherosclerosis. *Proc (Bayl Univ Med Cen)* 2000;13:139–143.
61. Roberts WC. Getting more people on statins. *Am J Cardiol* 2002;90:683–685.
62. Roberts WC. Atherosclerosis: its cause and it's prevention. *Am J Cardiol* 2006;98:1550–1555.
63. Roberts WC. The cause of atherosclerosis. *Nutr Clin Pract* 2008;23:464–467.
64. Roberts WC. Evaluating lipid-lowering trials in the twenty-first century. *Am J Cardiol* 2009;103:1325–1328.
65. Roberts WC. It's the cholesterol, stupid! *Am J Cardiol* 2010;106:1364–1366.
66. Ference BA, Ginsberg HN, Graham I, Ray KK, Packard CJ, Bruckert E, Hegele RA, Krauss RM, Raal FJ, Schunkert H, Watts GF, Borén J, Fazio S, Horton JD, Masana L, Nicholls SJ, Nordestgaard BJ, van de Sluis B, Taskinen MJ, Tokgözoğlu L, Landmesser U, Laufs U, Wiklund O, Stock JK, Chapman MJ, Catapano AL. Low-density lipoproteins cause atherosclerotic cardiovascular disease. 1. Evidence from genetic, epidemiologic, and clinical studies. A consensus statement from the European Atherosclerosis Society Consensus Panel. *Eur Heart J* 2017;0:1–14.
67. Keys A. Coronary heart disease in seven countries. *Circulation* 1970;41(suppl):1–211.
68. Giugliano RP, Wiviott SD, Blazing MA, De Ferrari GM, Park J, Murphy SA, White JA, Tershakovec AM, Cannon CP, Braunwald E. Long-term safety and efficacy of achieving very low levels of low-density lipoprotein cholesterol: a pre-specified analysis of the IMPROVE-IT Trial. *JAMA Cardiol* 2017;2:598–607. Jun 1.
69. Roberts WC. We think we are one, we act as if we are one, but we are not one. *Am J Cardiol* 1990;66:896.

Hazards of Mitral Valve Replacement for Mitral Stenosis Caused by Massive Mitral Annular Calcium With or Without Aortic Valve Replacement for Aortic Stenosis

William C. Roberts, MD*

Mitral annular calcium (MAC) is common in older adults in the Western World and if extensive may cause mitral stenosis . The purpose of this report is to describe outcomes of 12 patients having mitral valve replacement for mitral stenosis secondary to massive MAC. Operatively excised deposits of calcium removed from the mitral annular area and the accompanying stenotic mitral valves were examined and then the patients' medical records were examined to confirm the diagnosis and the degree of valvular dysfunction. A total of 12 patients with massive MAC causing mitral stenosis and receiving mitral valve replacement with or without aortic valve replacement for aortic stenosis were observed in 2013 to 2015. Of the 12 patients, 7 died from 5 to 44 days (mean 19) after the valve operation and all had "stormy" postoperative courses; one survived 150 days and another, 600 days; the remaining 3 were improved by the operation and are alive 22, 27, and 59 months postoperatively. In conclusion, the high mortality in these patients suggests that mitral valve replacement in the setting of massive MAC be considered with caution. **(Am J Cardiol 2019;123:650−657)**

Deposits of calcium beneath the posterior mitral leaflet and especially near its attachment to the left atrial and left ventricular junctional regions, so called *mitral annular calcium* (MAC), is relatively common in older patients, especially in women, in patients with chronic renal disease, in those with left ventricular outflow obstruction (aortic stenosis [AS] and hypertrophic cardiomyopathy), and in younger persons with mitral valve prolapse, mucopolysaccharidosis and the Marfan syndrome.[1−8] In older patients MAC is usually accompanied by calcific deposits in the epicardial coronary arteries and in the aortic valve cusps, producing what has been termed "the senile cardiac calcification syndrome"[9] (Figure 1). The quantity of calcium in the mitral annular region varies from minimal to massive and when the latter is the case the result may be mitral stenosis (MS), especially in the setting of associated AS.[10−15] We have encountered through the years many patients who have had aortic valve replacement for AS and who had massive MAC but no operative procedure was carried out on the mitral valve (Figure 2). In recent times in patients with combined AS and massive MAC causing MS there has been a tendency among some surgeons to replace the mitral valve as well as the aortic valve in this scenario.[16−25] This report describes certain clinical and morphologic findings in 12 patients with massive MAC causing MS and leading to isolated mitral valve replacement or to combined mitral and aortic valve replacement, the latter for AS.

Methods

Since March 1993, I have examined, described, and submitted the report on all surgical specimens excised from the heart or aorta at Baylor University Medical Center (BUMC). During a recent 3-year period—2013, 2014, and 2015—portions of the mitral valve in 130 patients were submitted to the surgical pathology unit of the department of pathology at BUMC (Figure 3). Of the 130 patients, 58 (45%) had mitral valve repair for pure mitral regurgitation (no element of stenosis), and 73 (56%) had mitral valve replacement. Of the latter 72 patients, 53 (74%) had isolated mitral valve replacement (only the mitral valve was replaced) and 19 (26%) had replacement of both the mitral and aortic valves. Of the 53 patients with isolated mitral valve replacement; 16 (30%) had mitral stenosis resulting from massive MAC in 6 and from rheumatic heart disease in 10. Of the 19 patients having combined mitral and aortic valve replacements, 10 had combined mitral stenosis and aortic stenosis, the result of rheumatic heart disease, and in 6 from massive MAC. This report focuses on the 6 patients having MS and isolated mitral replacement from massive MAC, and on the 4 patients who had both mitral and aortic valve replacement for combined MS resulting from massive MAC and aortic valve stenosis. Additionally, 2 other patients with massive MAC causing MS and associated with AS and operated on at another Dallas hospital also were included in this study.

The medical records in all of the 130 patients were examined.

Departments of Internal Medicine (Division of Cardiology) and Pathology, and the Baylor Scott & White Heart and Vascular Institute, Baylor University Medical Center, a part of Baylor Scott & White Health, Dallas, Texas. Manuscript received October 3, 2018; revised manuscript received November 12, 2018; revised manuscript received and accepted November 12, 2018.

See page 656 for disclosure information.

*Corresponding author: Tel: (214) 820-7911; fax: (214) 820-7533.

E-mail address: william.roberts1@bswhealth.org

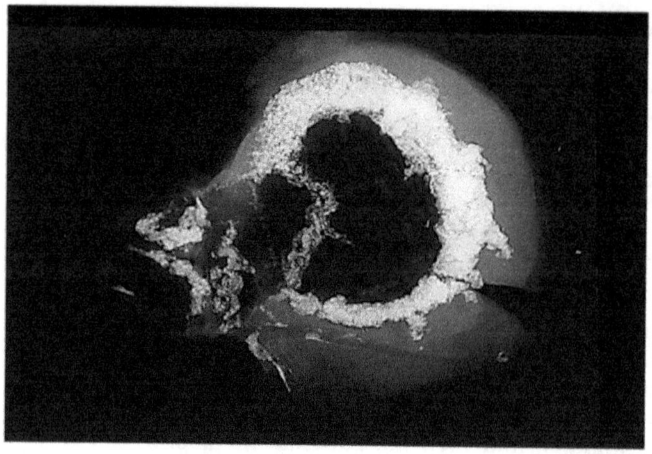

Figure 1. Shown here is a radiograph of the heart specimen at autopsy in an 82-year-old woman who died of volvulus of the colon. She never had symptoms of cardiac dysfunction. The amount of calcium in the mitral annular area is enormous. The calcium behind posterior mitral leaflet forms a beautiful "C" and the bar of calcium below the aortic valve is that on the ventricular aspect of anterior leaflet. Calcific deposits also are present in each of the three valve cusps causing some degree of aortic stenosis. Additionally, calcium is present focally in the left circumflex and left anterior descending coronary arteries. (Figure reproduced from Roberts WC, Perloff JK. Mitral valvular disease: A clinicopathologic survey of the conditions causing the mitral valve to function abnormally. *Ann Intern Med* 1972 Dec; 77:939–975.)

"Massive MAC" was defined by the presence of a huge quantity of calcium underlying the posterior mitral leaflet forming a circle C and extending across all or nearly all of the ventricular aspect of the anterior mitral leaflet to "close" the "C" forming a circle O. Examples of massive MAC forming a circle O are shown in Figures 1 and 2.

The present study includes all patients having mitral valve replacement for massive MAC encountered at BUMC during the 3-year period (2013 to 2015). Several other patients having mitral valve replacement for mitral valve prolapse causing mitral regurgitation had small focal deposits of calcium behind posterior mitral leaflet but in no patients were the deposits behind mitral leaflet large and in none did calcium extend across the ventricular aspect of anterior mitral leaflet.

Results

Pertinent clinical and morphologic data in these 12 patients were sought and the findings are summarized in Table 1. The 12 patients ranged in age from 25 to 82 years (median 59); 8 were women and 4 were men. Six patients had isolated mitral valve replacement and 6 had combined mitral and aortic valve replacement.

Preoperatively, the peak systolic pulmonary pressures ranged from 50 to 117 mm Hg (average 79); the pulmonary artery wedge-left ventricular mean diastolic gradients at rest ranged from 6 to 23 mm Hg (average 11) and the peak systolic left ventricular to systemic artery peak pressure gradients ranged from 20 to 28 mm Hg. Four patients had considerable coronary arterial narrowing by angiogram, 3 of whom had coronary bypass performed. Preoperatively, 8 patients had atrial fibrillation, 1 had complete heart block, and 1 had right bundle branch block. Six patients had diabetes mellitus. The body mass index (11 patients) ranged from 21 to 52 kg/m^2 including 8 patients (73%) in whom the value was ≥30 kg/m^2. The 12 patients were operated on by 5 different surgeons.

Of the 12 patients, 7 died from 5 to 44 days after valve replacement, 1 at 150 days and 1 other at 600 days after the valve replacement. The remaining 3 were improved by the operation and are alive 22, 27, and 59 months after the valve operation. The operatively-excised mitral specimens ranged in weight from 1.92 to 7.20 g. The operatively excised aortic valves (3 patients) weighed 0.49, 1.20, and 2.95 g, respectively.

Several of the operatively excised mitral and aortic specimens are illustrated in Figures 4 to 8. Autopsies were performed in 2 patients: in each considerable quantities of calcium remained in the mitral annular area. Periannular mitral disruptions were present in each of the 2 autopsied patients.

Discussion

It is apparent from study of these hitherto described 12 patients that mitral valve replacement in the setting of *massive* MAC is hazardous. Nine of the 12 patients have died, 7 within 45 days of the operation and 2 others 150 and 600 days, respectively, postoperatively. The postoperative courses in the 7 early deaths were complicated by stroke; excessive bleeding (requiring return to the operating room); parabasilar mitral regurgitation; long periods of intubation, and usually evidence of inadequate cardiac output ("multiorgan failure").

In the early days of cardiac valve replacement (1960s and 1970s), combined mitral and aortic valve replacement was a frequent procedure and was usually because of rheumatic heart disease, most commonly resulting in stenosis of both valves, occasionally causing pure regurgitation of both valves, and rarely producing 1 stenotic and 1 purely regurgitant valve. Today in the Western World, rheumatic heart disease, of course, is far less frequent than in the past, and now both isolated MS and that combined with AS may commonly be the result of massive MAC. Replacement of both left-sided cardiac valves at the same operation is a formidable operation, especially when both valves are stenotic.[26] In this latter setting, usually the left ventricular free wall is thickened, the left ventricular cavity is not dilated, and the ascending aorta is not dilated. When the mitral dysfunction is caused by massive MAC the operation is even more formidable. At least in the patients with combined rheumatic MS and AS the patients are usually relatively young, and the mitral annulus is not calcified. In the patients with MAC of sufficient quantity to obstruct the mitral orifice, the patients are usually in the older age group.

The Tiron E. David group[16,18] in Toronto has written extensively on methods and results for replacing and/or repairing the mitral valve in the setting of "extensive" MAC. In one of their reports the operative mortality was 6.2 times that occurring in patients having mitral valve

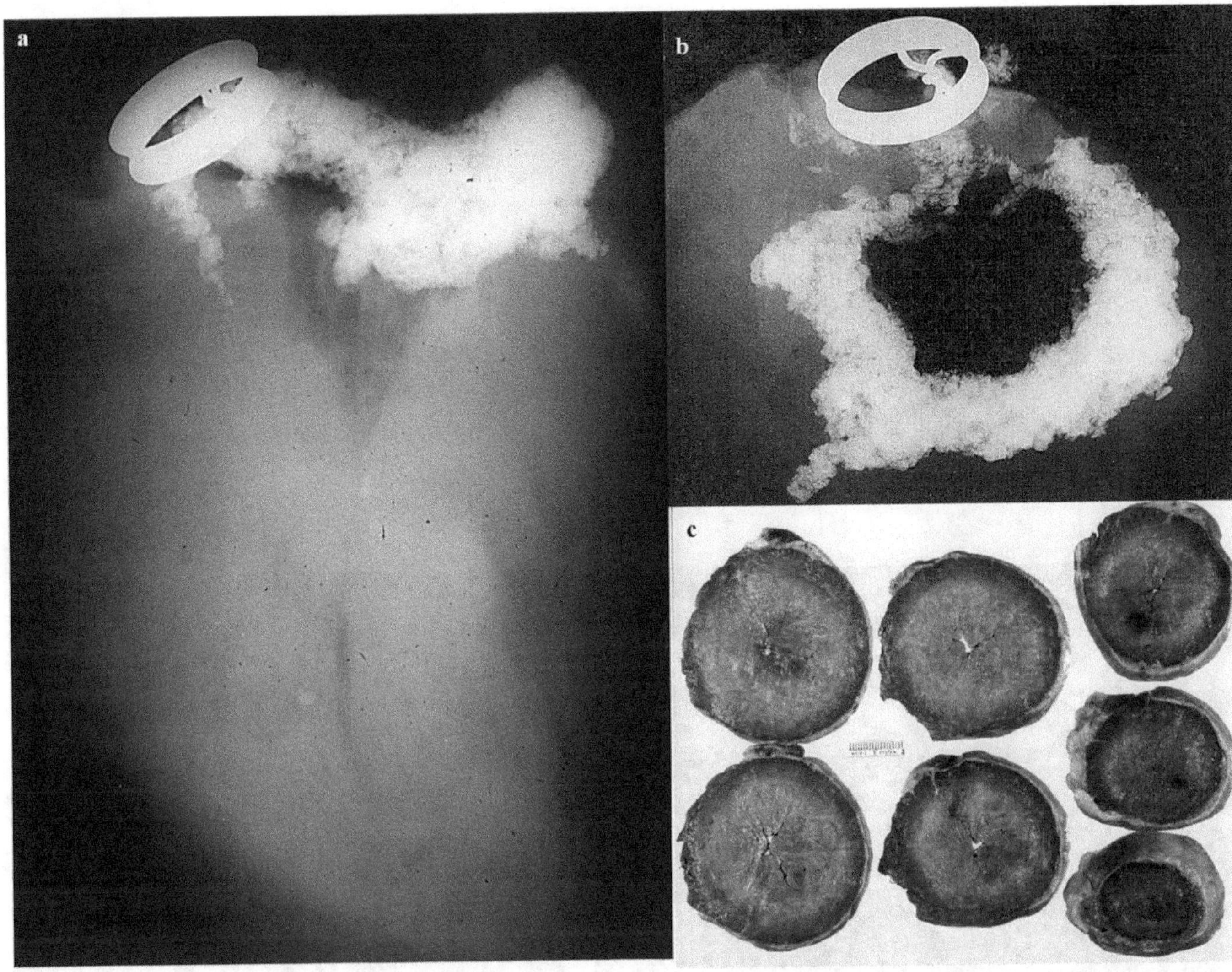

Figure 2. Shown here in *a*, *b*, and *c* views are radiographs of the heart at necropsy. There is massive mitral annular calcium which forms nearly a "C" as shown in *b*. The aortic valve was replaced with a Bjork-Shailey prosthesis. No replacement of the mitral valve was attempted even though the mitral orifice was stenotic. *c* shows transverse sections of the left ventricle to illustrate its small cavity. Death occurs in peak systole, so the left ventricular cavity would be larger during ventricular diastole.

procedures at their institution without MAC. Early postoperative complications in their 54 MAC patients included re-exploration for bleeding (9%), permanent heart block requiring a pacemaker (20%), reoperation later related to valve complications (7%), late postoperative thromboembolic events (9%), and late major hemorrhagic complications (5%). Their series of 54 patients having mitral operations—combined with aortic valve replacement for AS in 23 (43%)—appear to be the best from anywhere in the setting of extensive MAC. Possibly, most of their patients had smaller quantities of MAC than the patients described herein. In 31 (57%) of their 54 patients the MAC was located only behind the posterior mitral leaflet and did not extend across the ventricular aspect of anterior mitral leaflet as it did in the 12 patients described herein. These investigators emphasize the difficulty of the operation and state the following:

> "Extensive calcification of the mitral annulus may present a formidable surgical challenge during mitral valve surgery. The patient is at risk from such potentially fatal complications as intractable hemorrhage, atrioventricular disruption, and ventricular rupture...Although we recommend removal of the calcium bar, this is a major undertaking and should not be considered lightly..."

Another unemphasized difficulty of mitral replacement in the setting of massive MAC and associated AS is the lack of dilatation of the left ventricular cavity in most of these patients including all 12 described herein.[26] Shown in Figure 2 is the heart of a 70-year-old woman who died shortly after replacement of a severely stenotic congenitally bicuspid aortic valve (peak transvalvular gradient = 153 mm Hg). A 15-mm Hg mean diastolic pressure gradient was present between left atrium

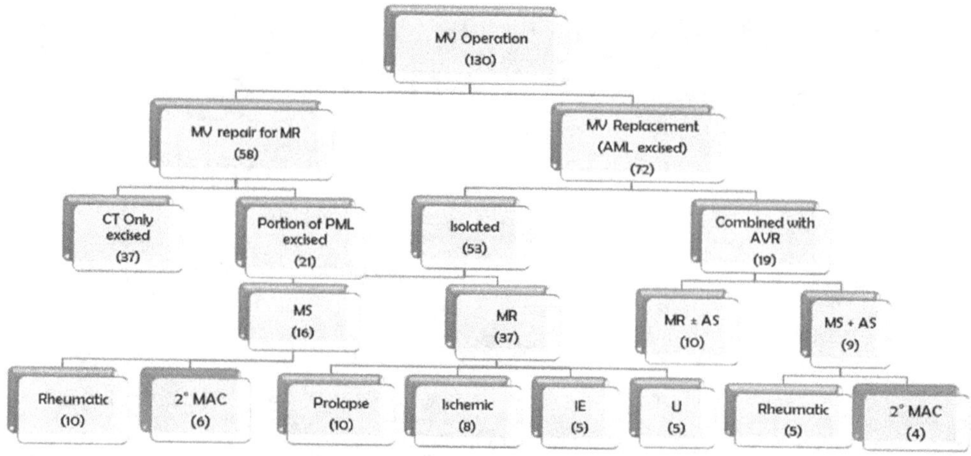

Figure 3. Reason for mitral valve operations at Baylor University Medical Center at Dallas during the 3 years: 2013, 2014, and 2015. Abbreviations: AML = anterior mitral leaflet; AS = aortic stenosis; AVR = aortic valve replacement; CT = chordae tendineae; IE = infective endocarditis; MAC = mitral annular calcium; MR = mitral regurgitation; MV = mitral valve; PML = posterior mitral leaflet; U = unknown.

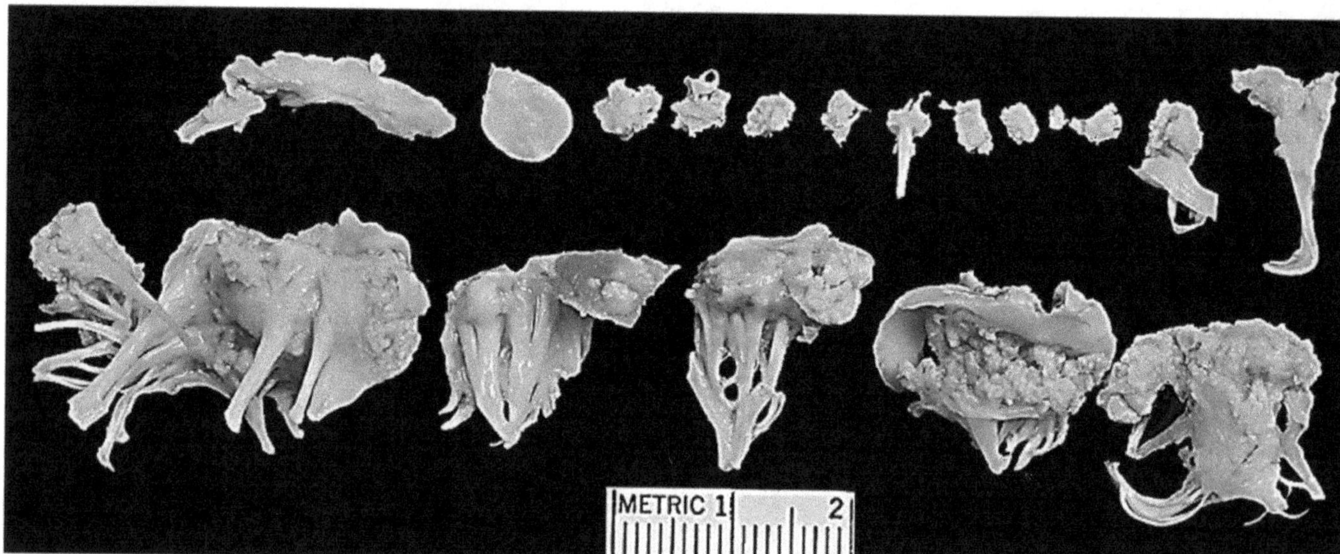

Figure 4. Case #1, Table 1. Portions of the posterior and anterior leaflets of the mitral valve and fragments of calcium excised from the mitral annular region. Calcium extends across the ventricular aspect of the anterior mitral leaflet.

and left ventricle. The mitral valve, however, was not replaced. The reason for showing these photos is to emphasize the small size of the left ventricular cavity in the setting of combined MS and AS. The small sized ventricular cavity makes it especially difficult to insert a prosthesis or a bioprosthesis in the mitral position in addition to the difficulty in excising the massive MAC in this scenario.

There has been recent interest in transcatheter mitral valve implantation in patients with MS caused by MAC.[27,28] Sud and colleagues[27] reviewed 10 previously-reported case studies of patients having transcatheter mitral valve implantation and 44 patients in a global registry having the percutaneous procedure. In the individual case studies, no deaths were reported. In the series of 44 patients, the 1-year all-cause mortality was 36%. The transvalvular gradients were reduced in most patients although nonfatal complications were frequent. Guerrero and associates[28] updated the MAC Global Registry multicenter data to include 106 patients followed >1 year. One and 12-month all-cause mortality was 25% and 54%, respectively. Of the 77 patients who were alive 30 days after the procedure, 49 (64%) were alive at 1 year. The mean transmitral pressure gradient by echocardiogram, available in 34 patients, at 1 year was 6±2 mm Hg. Examination of hearts with massive MAC causing MS as shown in Figures 1 and 2 suggest why both the surgical and the percutaneous approach for treatment of MS secondary to massive MAC is fraught with difficulty.

One of the reviewers of this manuscript asked why the results of the present study were so much worse than those described by Ng and colleagues[20] in 2000. Study of the Na report suggests that their 37 patients had far less mitral annular calcium than the patients described herein. None of Ng's

Table 1

Pertinent findings in the 12 patients with massive mitral annular calcium and mitral valve replacement for mitral stenosis with or without aortic valve replacement for aortic stenosis

Case	Age (years)	Sex	MS	MVR	Mitral valve weight (g)	Substitute mitral valve (mm)	AS	AVR	Aortic valve weight (g)	Substitute aortic valve (mm)	CKD	Narrowed coronary arteries	AF	BMI (Kg/m^2)	DM	Interval VR $\rightarrow$ D (days)
1	39	F	+	+	6.0	SJM (25)	0	0	–	–	+(H)	0	0	21	0	8
2	52	F	+	+	3.9	Bioprosthesis (29)	0	0	–	–	0	0	0	40	+	Alive [‡]
3	58	M	+	+	3.2	Bioprosthesis (27)	0	0	–	–	+ (RT)	+ (CABG)	0	30	+	Alive [§]
4	61	F	+	+	1.5	SJM (33)	0	0	–	–	0	0	+	38	0	Alive [¶]
5	62	F	+	+	5.7	SJM (27)	0	0	–	–	0	0	+	28	0	5
6	76	M	+	+	1.9	Bicor (29)	0	0	–	–	0	+ (CABG)	+	36	+	44
7	40	M	+	+	3.3	$O_2 - X$ (25)	+ [*]	+	3.0	Carbomedius (21)	+(P)	0	+	34	0	600
8	42	F	+	+	1.9	SJM (27)	+	+ [†]	–	SJM (21)	+(H)	0	+	–	0	150
9	71	F	+	+	–	St. Jude Epic (–)	+	+	–	Magna Ease (21)	0	+ (CABG)	+	31	+	32
10	74	F	+	+	7.2	ATS Mech (24)	+	+	1.2	ATS Mech (20)	+	0	+	36	+	12
11	76	F	+	+	4.7	Bicor (25)	+	+	0.5	CE (19)	+	0	0	52	+	25
12	82	M	+	+	–	Edwards Magna (27)	+	+	–	–	0	+	+	–	0	11

Abbreviations: AF = atrial fibrillation; AS = aortic stenosis; AVR = aortic valve replacement; BMI = body mass index; CABG = coronary artery bypass grafting; CKD = chronic kidney disease; D = death; DM = diabetes mellitus; F = female; H = hemodialysis initiated months or years before MVR; LV = left ventricle; M = male; MS = mitral stenosis; MVR = mitral valve replacement; P = peritoneal dialysis; RT = renal transplant earlier; VR = valve replacement.

* BAV;

† AVR 22 months before excision of the bioprosthesis in the aortic valve position and replacement of the MV;

‡ Alive 36 months postoperatively. Improved, less breathlessness, twenty pounds less (250→230);

§ Alive 59 months postoperatively. Much improved. Little breathlessness;

¶ Alive 27 months postoperatively. Greatly improved. Nearly no breathlessness. Thirty pounds weight loss (240→210).

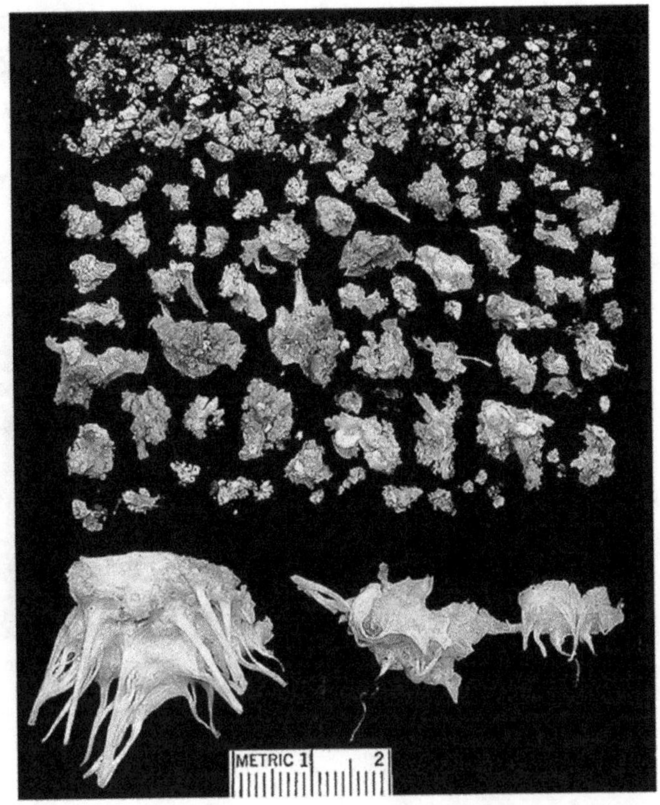

Figure 5. Case 5, Table 1. Shown here are large deposits of calcium excised from the mitral annular region and the anterior mitral leaflet with a bar of calcium across its ventricular aspect and two fragments of posterior leaflet. The quantity of calcium in the mitral annular area was obviously enormous.

patients had mitral stenosis, only mitral regurgitation and it is likely that much heavier deposits of calcium are required to obstruct the mitral orifice by annular calcium than to produce only regurgitation. It is unlikely that the annular calcium behind posterior leaflet extended across the ventricular surface of anterior mitral leaflet in Ng's patients as it did in the patients described herein. Indeed Ng et al wrote: "Five patients were excluded from (their) study due to severe calcification of nearly the entire annulus..." None of Ng's patients had associated aortic stenosis, a feature in half of the patients in the present study and something that tends to make the left ventricular cavity smaller and probably the mitral orifice smaller. Finally, none of Ng's patients had mitral valve replacement as did all the patients in the present study.

The mechanism of development of MAC and its commonly associated AS is not entirely clear but most likely is a consequence of atherosclerosis, although that word would have to be redefined to include MAC and AS under that heading. Most young people living in the Western World have yellow deposits on the undersurface of the posterior mitral leaflet and fewer such deposits on the ventricular surface of anterior mitral leaflet. Additionally, similar deposits occur on the aortic aspects of the aortic valve cusps, whether its structure is tricuspid or bicuspid. In later life the lipid deposits may transform into calcific deposits, and, depending on the quantity of those deposits in the 2 valves, may or may not

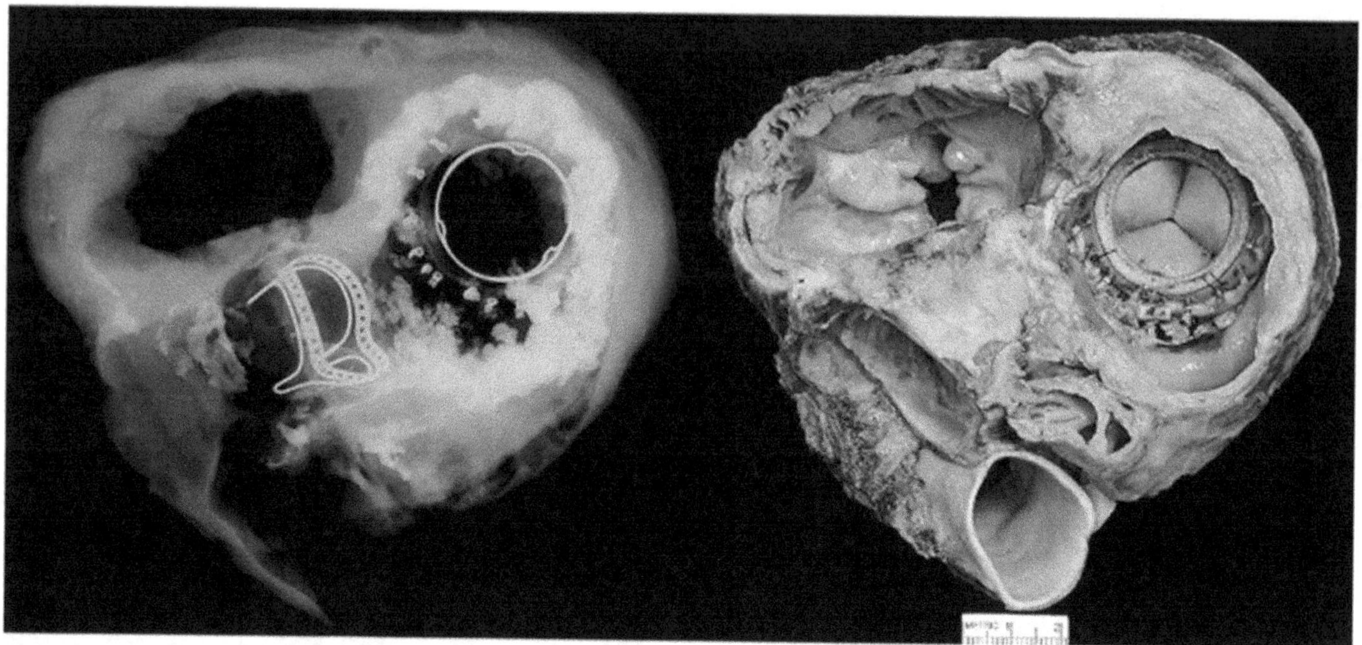

Figure 6. Case #9, Table 1. Shown here is a radiograph of the heart specimen at necropsy on the *left* and the actual specimen shown on the *right*. Both the mitral and aortic valves were replaced because of stenosis. A large amount of calcium was removed from the mitral annular region at operation but there is still a great deal of calcium left in that area. The more anterolateral portion of the mitral annulus had a communication between the cloth ring and the annulus so there was a para-annular leak. Heavy calcific deposits are also seen in the epicardial coronary arteries.

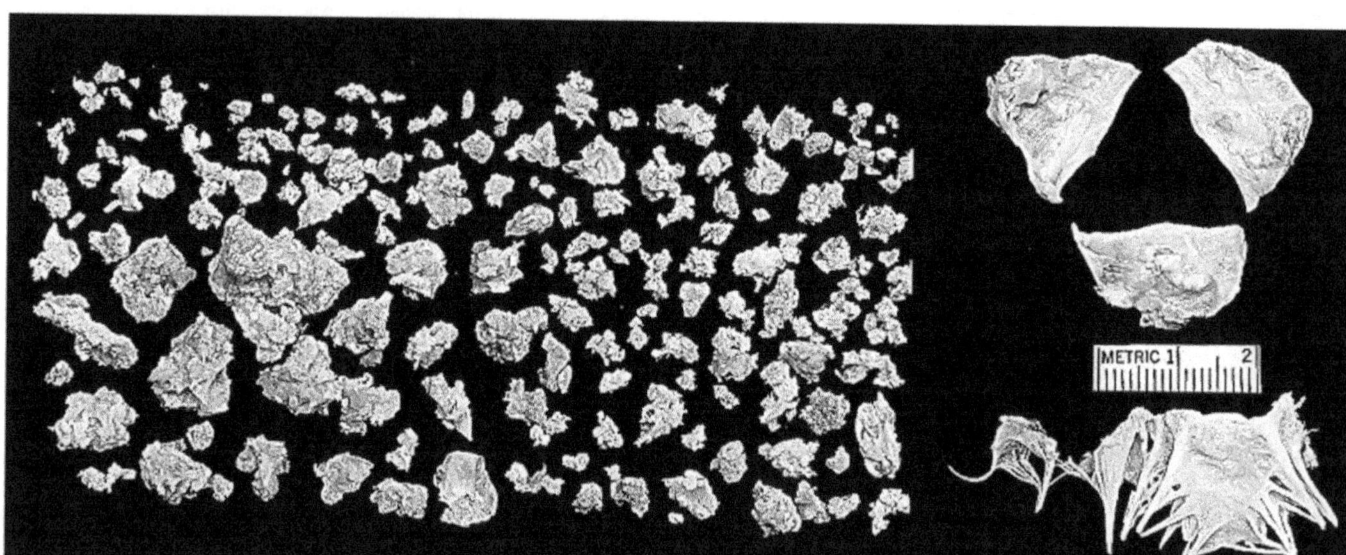

Figure 7. Case 10, Table 1. Shown here are huge calcific fragments excised from the mitral annular region (*left*), the operatively excised aortic valve cusps containing calcific fragments (*top right*), and the ventricular aspect of anterior mitral leaflet (*bottom right*). About half of the anterior leaflet has a bar of calcium extending across its ventricular aspect.

lead to symptoms of cardiac dysfunction. Because "atherosclerosis" preferentially affects the systemic arteries, associated coronary narrowing in these patients is common.

In conclusion, performing mitral valve replacement in the setting of *massive* MAC is both difficult and hazardous, even more so when the aortic valve is also stenotic.

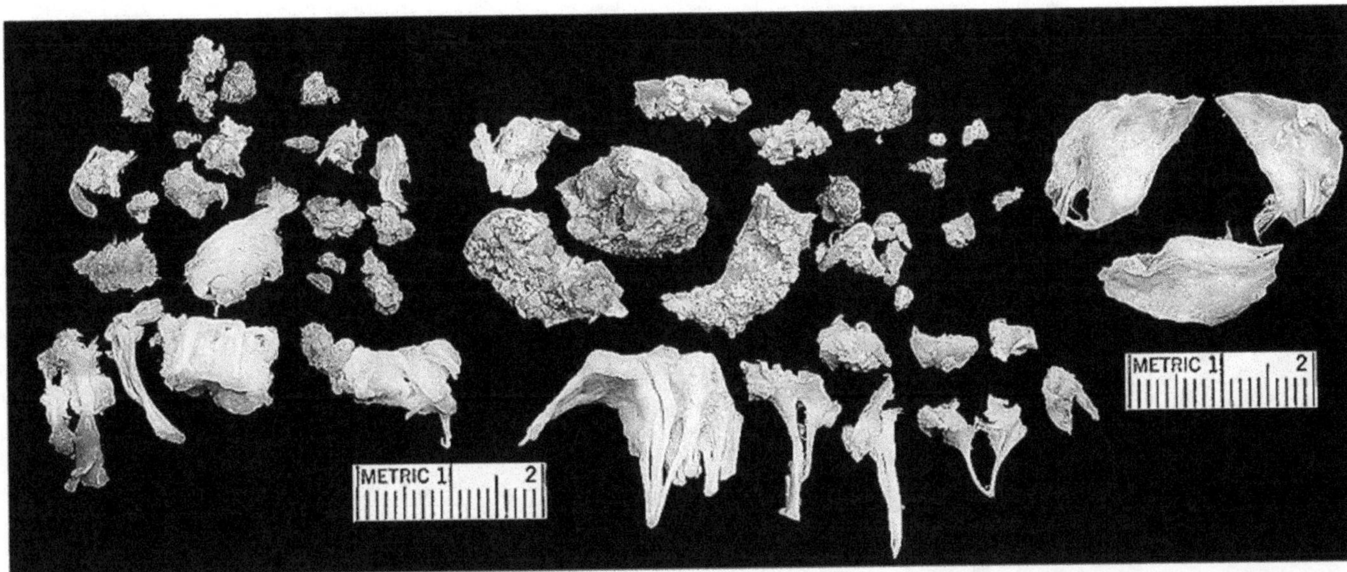

Figure 8. Case 11, Table 1. Shown here is both the operatively excised mitral valve and the 3-cuspid aortic valve plus the numerous calcific fragments excised from the mitral annular region. These fragments together weighed 4.72 g. Of course, not all the calcium in the mitral annular region was excised.

Disclosures

The author has no conflict of interests to disclose.

1. Korn D, DeSanctis RW, Sell S. Massive calcification of the mitral annulus. A clinicopathological study of fourteen cases. *N Engl J Med* 1962;267:900–908.
2. Roberts WC, Shirani J. Comparison of cardiac findings at necropsy in octogenarians, nonagenarians, and centenarians. *Am J Cardiol* 1998;82:627–631.
3. Roberts WC, Taylor MA, Shirani J. Cardiac findings at necropsy in patients with chronic kidney disease maintained on chronic hemodialysis. *Medicine* 2012;91:165–178.
4. Roberts WC, Vowels TJ, Filardo G, Ko JM, Mathur RP, Shirani J. Natural history of unoperated aortic stenosis during a 50-year period of cardiac valve replacement. *Am J Cardiol* 2013;112:541–553.
5. Motamed HE, Roberts WC. Frequency and significance of mitral annular calcium in hypertrophic cardiomyopathy: analysis of 200 necropsy patients. *Am J Cardiol* 1987;60:877–884.
6. Roberts WC, McIntosh CL, Wallace RB. Mechanisms of severe mitral regurgitation in mitral valve prolapse determined from analysis of operatively excised valves. *Am Heart J* 1987;113:1316–1323.
7. Renteria VG, Ferrans VJ, Roberts WC. The heart in the Hurler Syndrome: gross, histologic and ultrastructural observations in five necropsy cases. *Am J Cardiol* 1976;38:487–501.
8. Roberts WC. Morphologic aspects of cardiac valve dysfunction. *Am Heart J* 1992;123:1610–1632.
9. Roberts WC. The senile cardiac calcification syndrome. *Am J Cardiol* 1986;58:572–574.
10. Roberts WC, Waller BF. Mitral valve "anular" calcium forming a complete circle of "O" configuration: clinical and necropsy observations. *Am Heart J* 1981;101:619–621.
11. Theleman KP, Grayburn PA, Roberts WC. Mitral "annular" calcium forming a complete circle "O" causing mitral stenosis in association with a stenotic congenitally bicuspid aortic valve and severe coronary artery disease. *Am J Geriatr Cardiol* 2006;15:58–61.
12. Hammer WJ, Roberts WC, deLeon AC Jr. "Mitral stenosis" secondary to combined "massive" mitral annular calcific deposits and small, hypertrophied left ventricles: hemodynamic documentation in four patients. *Am J Med* 1978;64:371–376.
13. Ramirez J, Flowers NC. Severe mitral stenosis secondary to massive calcification of the mitral annulus with unusual echocardiographic manifestations. *Clin Cardiol* 1980;3:284–287.
14. Osterberger LE, Goldstein S, Khaja F, Lakier JB. Functional mitral stenosis in patients with massive mitral annular calcification. *Circulation* 1981;64:472–476.
15. Pressman GS, Agarwal A, Braitman LE, Muddassir SM. Mitral annular calcium causing mitral stenosis. *Am J Cardiol* 2010;105:389–391.
16. David TE, Feindel CM, Armstrong S, Sun Z. Reconstruction of the mitral annulus: a ten-year experience. *J Thorac Cardiovasc Surg* 1995;110:1323–1332.
17. Carpenter AF, Pellerin M, Fuzellier JF, Relland JYM. Extensive calcification of the mitral valve annulus: pathology and surgical management. *J Thorac Cardiovasc Surg* 1996;111:718–729.
18. David TE, Kuo J, Armstrong S. Aortic and mitral valve replacement with reconstruction of the intervalvular fibrous body. *J Thorac Cardiovasc Surg* 1997;114:766–772.
19. Lin PY, Kan CD, Luo CY, Yang YJ. Mitral valve replacement in the presence of massive posterior annular calcification. *J Card Surg* 1999;14:266–269.
20. Ng CK, Punzengruber C, Pachinger O, Nesser J, Auer H, Franke H, Hartl P. Valve repair in mitral regurgitation complicated by severe annulus calcification. *Ann Thorac Surg* 2000;70:53–58.
21. Fasol R, Mahdjoobian K, Joubert-Hubner E. Mitral repair in patients with severely calcified annulus: feasibility, surgery and results. *J Heart Valve Dis* 2002;11:153–159.
22. Feindel CM, Tufail Z, David TE, Ivanov J, Armstrong S. Mitral valve surgery in patients with extensive calcification of the mitral annulus. *J Thorac Cardiovasc Surg* 2003;126:777–782.
23. DiStefano S, Lopez J, Flórez S, Rey J, Arevalo A, San Román A. Building a new annulus: a technique for mitral valve replacement in heavily calcified annulus. *Ann Thorac Surg* 2009;87:1625–1627.
24. Atoui R, Lash V, Mohammadi S, Cecere R. Intra-atrial implantation of a mitral valve prosthesis in a heavily calcified mitral annulus. *Eur J Cardiothorac Surg* 2009;36. 776-768.
25. Nomura A, Fukuda I, Daitoku K, Fukui K. Enucleation of calcium core and in-situ valve replacement for massive posterior mitral annular calcification. *Interact Cardiovasc Thorac Surg* 2011;12:652–654.
26. Roberts WC, Sullivan MF. Clinical and necropsy observations early after simultaneous replacement of the mitral and aortic valves. *Am J Cardiol* 1986;58:1067–1084.
27. Sud K, Agarwal S, Parashar A, Raza MQ, Patel K, Min D, Rodriguez LL, Krishnaswamy A, Mick SL, Gillinov AM, Tuzcu M, Kapadia SR. Degenerative mitral stenosis: unmet need for percutaneous interventions. *Circulation* 2016;133:1594–1604.
28. Guerrero M, Urena M, Himbert D, Wang DD4, Eleid M5, Kodali S, George I, Chakravarty T, Mathur M, Holzhey D, Pershad A, Fang HK, O'Hair D, Jones N, Mahadevan VS, Dumonteil N, Rodés-Cabau J, Piazza N, Ferrari E, Ciaburri D, Nejjari M, DeLago A, Sorajja P, Zahr

F, Rajagopal V, Whisenant B, Shah PB, Sinning JM, Witkowski A, Eltchaninoff H, Dvir D, Martin B, Attizzani GF, Gaia D, Nunes NSV, Fassa AA, Kerendi F, Pavlides G, Iyer V, Kaddissi G, Witzke C, Wudel J, Mishkel, Raybuck B, Wang C, Waksman R, Palacios I, Cribier A, Webb J, Bapat V, Reisman M, Makkar R, Leon M, Rihal C, Vahanian A, O'Neill W, Feldman T. 1-year outcomes of transcatheter mitral valve replacement in patients with severe mitral annular calcification. *J Am Coll Cardiol* 2018;71:1841–1853.

From the Editor
Pellagra, Osler, Roberts, Goldberger, the Atherosclerotic Diet, Niacin, the Beginning of the Atherosclerotic Epidemic, and the First Lipid-Altering Drug

William Osler (1849 to 1919) in 1892 published *The Principles and Practice of Medicine* (1). Under the heading "grain poisoning" Osler devoted just over one-half page in the 1,079-page book to Pellagra. He described it this way:

> "This is a nutritional disturbance due to the use of altered maize. The disease occurs extensively in parts of Italy, in the south of France, and in Spain. It has not been observed in this country. It prevails extensively among the poorer classes, particularly in the country districts and appears to be associated in some way with the use of maize which...is fermented or diseased. In the early stage the symptoms are indefinite, characterized by debility, pains in the spine, insomnia, digestive disturbances, more rarely diarrhea. The first clear manifestation of the disease is the pellagral erythema, which almost invariably appears in the spring. This is followed by desiccation and exfoliation of the epidermis, which becomes very rough and dry and occasionally crusts form...with these cutaneous manifestations there are digestive troubles – salivation, dyspepsia and diarrhea – which may be of a dysenteric nature. After lasting for a few months, improvement occurs in milder cases and convalescence is gradually established. In the more severe and chronic forms there are "pronounced nervous symptoms – headache, backache, spasms, and finally paralysis and mental disturbances..."

In 1912, my father, Stewart R. Roberts (1878 to 1941), published a 272-page book entitled "Pellagra: History, Distribution, Diagnosis, Prognosis, Treatment, and Etiology" (2). The book was dedicated as follows:

> "To that long line of physicians and scientists from Casals, through Lombroso to Sambon, and those who shall come after them who have been and are and shall be students of pellagra, with the hope that the day is not far distant when there shall arise from among them one to whom shall be revealed with clear and certain proof the true cause of the Mal de la Rosa."

Because the disease was so common in Italy, Dr. Roberts spent some time seeing patients and touring institutions in Italy in preparation of his book. In Chapter 10, he reviewed the various theories as to the cause of pellagra and he emphasized that its cause at that time was unknown. He reviewed the intoxication and infectious theories, the 2 major hypotheses at the time. The chapter on Cause was the last one in his book and the chapter on Treatment of Pellagra was chapter 9. He wrote:

> "The first step to the treatment of pellagra is to ascertain whether any other disease is present...pellagra is disease enough for any patient to have at one time. Its draining and resistance-lowering powers increase the capacity of any associated infection or disease to do greater damage. Pellagra affords fight enough to test the strength of the patient and the skill of the physician. Any other disease increases the danger and lessens the chance of improvement from treatment. Pellagra acts as an alarm clock to awaken a sleeping infection. The pellagrin should be examined for tuberculosis, intestinal parasites, and malaria, and syphilis is not to be forgotten. The feces should be examined for amebae and especially for hookworm ova, and occasionally other ova...In the South a latent malaria or hookworm infection is chiefly to be expected and associated infection...there is no drug which cures pellagra."

> "The pellagrin should be on as generous and as nutritious a diet as is compatible with his powers of digestion and the condition of his alimentary tract. His strength is to be conserved and his diet is to him both a food and a stimulant. When the attack is at its height, the mouth raw and sore, solid food cannot be taken. Even acid liquids–as orange juice, orange and lemon albumen, and grape juice–give pain and are to be avoided. At this time soups or broths of the ordinary kind, milk, strained oatmeal, coffee, tea, malted milk, may be used...As convalescence begins, the liquid diet may be changed to a light diet, with the addition of mashed Irish potatoes, mashed sweet potatoes, boiled or scrambled eggs, butter, toast, scraped beef, rice with milk, and fruits...With continued improvement, the change from the light diet to a general diet may be made, with a continuance, so far as possible, of the nourishment between meals and bedtime. Added the articles already mentioned are meats, as broiled steak, roast beef, chicken, and fish. Hog meat is to be avoided...there is a demand on the part of his system for protein containing foods. In addition to the meat, eggs can be freely given and the lighter variety of cheese. Rice, hominy, the more easily digested vegetables–especially potatoes, English peas, Boston baked beans–are favorites at this time...Butter and fats are to be given in large quantities, and, as a rule, will be found to be digested easily. The pellagrin and his tissues demand proteins, carbohydrates, and fats, and his diet is to be as generous as his condition permits and as his digestion is good."

Two years after my father's book appeared, Dr. Joseph Goldberger (1874 to 1929), an ingenious epidemiologist and a fearless epidemic fighter, with the rank of surgeon in the US Public Health and Marine Hospital Service (USMHS) (later called Public Health Service) was assigned in February 1914 by Surgeon General Rupert Blue to take

WILLIAM C. ROBERTS, MD

over the pellagra studies from Dr. Claude Lavinder, who had requested reassignment. The story of Goldberger's war against pellagra is beautifully described in a book entitled *Goldberger's War: The Life and Work of a Public Health Crusader* by Alan M. Kraut (3). The remainder of this piece comes from Kraut's wonderful book.

When 9 years of age, Joseph Goldberger immigrated with his family to the United States and settled in New York City in 1883. His father, Samuel Goldberger became a proprietor of a mom-and-pop grocery store in Manhattan. The family lived in the East Side tenements such that young Joseph grew up smelling the stench of urban poverty. The Goldbergers' saw education as the port of entry to American life and Joseph entered the College of the City of New York at the age of 18 (later named City College). He intended initially to become an engineer but after 2 years he left to become a student at Bellevue Hospital Medical College of New York University. A popular lecturer was Dr. Austin Flint, Jr., who had a reputation for exciting his classes. Goldberger received his MD degree in 1895, a month before his 21st birthday. He had scored high on his hospital examination and by October 1897, he had completed his 2-year internship at Bellevue Hospital. He then went into private practice, initially in New York City, and then in Wilkes-Barre, Pennsylvania. Goldberger found being a family doctor in a small city intellectually unfulfilling. In 1898, he tried to join the US Navy at the outbreak of the Spanish-American War, but the Navy rejected him. He then joined the USMHS (later changed to the US Public Health and USMHS and then to US Public Health Service). Between 1902 and 1914, Goldberger was a public health physician becoming an expert epidemic fighter. He battled yellow fever in Mexico, Puerto Rico, Mississippi, and Louisiana. He fought typhoid in Washington, D.C., dengue fever in Texas, and typhus in Mexico City. On 3 occasions Goldberger contracted the disease he was studying: yellow fever, dengue fever, and typhus. Later, he did research on measles and battled diphtheria. In 1914, Surgeon General Rupert Blue assigned him to supervise the federal government's pellagra investigation.

After being assigned to the pellagra mission in February 1914, Goldberger initially went to the library of the Hygienic Laboratory (later called the National Institutes of Health) and read everything he could about pellagra. The library closed at 10:00 pm and he was unable to remove books so on many occasions he brought a cot to the library so he could stay the night. By the time he had finished reading about the disease he believed it was not an infectious disease but was somehow related to diet. Rather than believing that there was some toxic substance in the food he was the first to believe that there was an essential substance absent from the food the pellagrin was eating.

The notion that eating certain foods prevented specific illnesses was known to Goldberger. As early as 1753, well before scurvy was fully understood as a deficiency disease, James Lynn had discovered that citrus fruit could prevent the condition. Similarly, beriberi was being successfully treated from extract of rice bran before anyone understood why it worked. As Goldberger pondered the relation of diet to pellagra others were wondering if the malformities of Rickets were not the result of a dietary deficiency also.

His homework completed, Goldberger boarded the train, one of the many he would be riding across the South in the months and years ahead. It had prepared himself to examine the telltale signs of pellagra on the bodies of the victims. He was anxious to visit institutions housing large numbers of pellagrins to observe how they lived and what they ate. Only then could he test his hypothesis that the pellagrin germ was a myth, that corn was not the culprit, and that the root cause of the scourge was in the diet. Goldberger now 40 years old, first stopped in Stanton, Virginia, where he visited several insane asylums in that state. From Virginia he went to Georgia, Alabama, Florida, and Kentucky, then back East to Columbia, South Carolina, and Atlanta, and on to New Orleans, and again to Alabama and then to Mississippi visiting asylums, orphanages, and prisons—places where pellagra frequently appeared. Everywhere he went he asked institution superintendents for data on the pellagra incidence, diets of inmates and staff, especially corn consumption, and permission to inspect sanitary conditions. As he had done in the alleys of Puerto Rico, Mexico, and Brownsville, Texas, he hunted for insects that might be carrying the disease from victim to victim. What struck Goldberger most was that in all the institutions he visited not a single staff member had pellagra. (No infectious disease selects victims by status!) In May 1914, he visited Jackson, Mississippi, and there encountered the orphanages that would become crucial sites for his studies. With his usual meticulous work habits, Goldberger wrote in his small notebook all that he knew up to that point about the orphans' home and what the youngsters ate at each meal.

In June 1914, Goldberger, for the first time, told the public health community what he believed about pellagra. In an article titled "The Etiology of Pellagra," he concluded that pellagra was not a contagious disease. This message came home when not in a single institution he had visited had a staff member who had gotten pellagra. The staff ate different diets than did the residents. He agreed with certain previous investigators that pellagra was generally a rural disease and one associated with poverty. He asked, however, what important difference there was between poverty in urban slums and those in rural areas? He believed that the very poor in cities had a more varied diet than the poor in rural sections. His suggestion for therapy was to improve the diet of the afflicted. Specifically, he called for a reduction in cereals, vegetables, and canned foods, and an increase in the fresh animal food component, such as fresh meat, eggs, and milk. Goldberger knew that he needed to test humans for his dietary hypothesis and that started in September 1914. To one group of orphans, he gave fresh meat, milk, and eggs, and to the other group, the diet of the institution. Although the orphan experiment was still in progress, Goldberger, confident that he knew the answer for pellagra, published another report entitled "The Treatment and Prevention of Pellagra" emphasizing his 3 preliminary conclusions: (1) that pellagra was not an infectious disease but a disease of dietary origin; (2) that is, was dependent on a still unknown fault in the diet in which the animal or leguminous protein component was disproportionately small and the nonleguminous vegetable component was disproportionately high; and (3) that no pellagra developed in those eating a mixed well-balanced and varied diet. He emphasized that no pellagra was seen among the enlisted men—Army, Navy, and Marine Corps—for the World War I conflict. Based on these conclusions, Goldberger and his colleagues recommended that as long as clinical evidence of pellagra manifested, the patient should be given and urged to eat an abundance of fresh milk, eggs, fresh lean meat, beans, and peas. Milk, he described, as the most valuable single food. He urged adults to drink not less than a pint and a half to 2 pints each 24-hour. He recommended 4 eggs per day and fresh lean meat. He encouraged adults to take at least a half-pound of lean meat a day in addition to the milk, eggs, and legumes. He also recommended excluding corn. Not only did his diet offer a cure, a well-balanced varied diet rich in animal protein also was the best preventative of pellagra.

In December 1914, Goldberger was invited to Cambridge, Massachusetts, to give the prestigious Cutter Lecture on Preventive Medicine. He titled it "Diet and Pellagra." He began his presentation by explaining the enormity of the pellagra problem citing "not less than 50,000 cases" for 1914 with 11,000 in the state of Mississippi alone. He emphasized that "pellagra is essentially a rural disease and a disease of poverty." His data revealed that women were at a greater risk than men and that blacks at a greater risk than whites. In Mississippi in 1913, 56/100,000 blacks and 26/100,000 whites had died of pellagra. He emphasized that a pellagrin's diet was missing a substance, which could be found in animal protein foods—meat or milk or both. Goldberger emphasized that pellagra was due to a lack or deficiency of an animal-protein food, "a fault" brought about in some yet undetermined way in diets of a certain type (largely corn or other cereal or starchy food or combination of them) and that this fault was corrected or prevented by including in such diets a suitable portion of animal-protein foods. He also emphasized that the common legumes (beans and peas) were of value in this respect.

After returning to the field, Goldberger produced pamphlets describing how to prevent and to treat pellagra, and he distributed them in churches and stores and by mail. In Georgia alone, 80,000 pamphlets were circulated.

The orphanage experiences were coming to fruition. They began by treating the orphans under 12 years of age with a 7-ounce cup of milk twice a day and at least 1 egg a day. For those under 6 years, milk was prescribed 3 times a day. Meat was prescribed 3 to 4 times a week rather than once a week. Beans and peas were made part of every meal. Because Goldberger regarded the corn theory of pellagra as highly suspect he chose not to eliminate corn from the orphan's diets altogether. Cornbread was served once a week and grits were allowed for those over 12, once or twice a week. At one orphanage, 67 of the 79 pellagrins after 1 year of using the Goldberger diet had no signs of recurrence of pellagra. At the other orphanage, 105 of the 130 pellagrins had no evidence of a recurrence of pellagra at 1 year.

Nevertheless, Goldberger had to prove that the poor diet could produce pellagra. Together with the Governor of Mississippi and the Rankin State Prison Farm, a facility for white convicts about 8 miles from Jackson, Mississippi, Goldberger screened with the governor's permission and with full permission from each state prisoner, permission to give the deficient diet to produce the disease. Earl Brewer, the Governor of Mississippi, and Goldberger dangled the promise of pardons before approximately 80 inmates. The requirement was that the prisoner volunteer for 6 months eating the deficient diet. Among the 80 prisoners, Goldberger selected 12, half of them murderers serving life terms. The 12 convict volunteers were housed in what was commonly called "the new hospital building"—a small-screened one-story cottage away from "the cage" where the other inmates lived. Goldberger's volunteers were strictly separated from the other convicts to ensure they were not contaminated by personal contact with other inmates who might have pellagra or who might supply them with some foods. A typical breakfast included what Goldberger often saw in the asylum inmate: biscuits, fried mush, grits, brown gravy, cane syrup, and coffee with sugar. Lunch included cornbread, collards, sweet potatoes, grits, and syrup. Supper included biscuits, mush, rice, gravy, syrup, and coffee with sugar. This was the typical diet of cotton mill workers, sharecroppers, and tenant farmers. The entire inmate population of the "camp" was considered the control group and they all ate meat, drank milk, and, ate good vegetables daily, and none had any symptoms of pellagra. The diet started February 1, 1915, and ended October 30, 1915. The results of the Rankin Prison experiment were announced November 1, 1915. Six of the 11 men who finished the experiment showed clear evidence of pellagra. The evidence was confirmed by a number of outside physicians who examined the prisoners. Newspapers all over the country trumpeted Goldberger's demonstration that he could induce pellagra in strong healthy men by depriving them of fresh milk, lean meat, and vegetables. Although Goldberger could not yet identify the pellagra preventive, he knew what kind of foods contained it and what the dire results were when they were absent. Like beriberi and scurvy, pellagra was the result of a nutritional deficiency and not an errant microbe. All the 11 men at the end of the experiment were pale, weak, and emaciated. All were pardoned and released.

The final piece of the pellagra puzzle was set in place by researchers at the University of Wisconsin and announced modestly 22 years later and 8 years after Goldberger had died. Dr. Conrad A. Elvehjem and his colleagues reported their breakthrough in a letter to the editor of the September 1937 issue of the *Journal of the American Chemical Society*. Elvehjem stated that they had found it "most interesting" that "black tongue" was caused by a deficiency of nicotinic acid (niacin). Physicians by now were curing pellagra with liver extract. They learned that rats on a diet deficient in the "P-P factor," as Goldberger had understood it, were stimulated to grow with nicotinamide and nicotinic acid, both substances synthesized from liver extract. Because there was no rodent equivalent of pellagra, the scientists began working with dogs. After inducing black-tongue disease using a diet developed by Goldberger—yellow corn, casing, cottonseed oil, and mineral supplements—Elvehjem and Koehn in the Department of Agricultural Chemistry at the University of Wisconsin confirmed that nicotinic acid affected the canines dramatically. Dogs that got a single dose were hungry and with their improved appetite grew and the black-tongue lesions disappeared.

In 1938, Tom Spies, at the University of Cincinnati, College of Medicine, started giving humans small doses of nicotinic acid, none of whom had pellagra. They developed flushing and tingling of the skin but no serious side effects when the drug was given intravenously. After establishing that healthy subjects and a few nonpellagrins tolerated nicotinic acid well, Spies gave a selected group of pellagrins both oral and injections of nicotinic acid but not the Goldberger diet. Evidences of pellagra improved, confirming that nicotinic acid was the deficient product. Another study at the University of Wisconsin demonstrated that corn consumption depressed the level of nicotinic acid in the body. White corn, the kind favored in the South, was even more deleterious that yellow corn. Later, it was learned that tryptophan could be converted into nicotinic acid under certain conditions. Thus, pellagra was a deficiency of both tryptophan and nicotinic acid. Other B-vitamins, pyridoxine, and riboflavin, are involved in the metabolism of tryptophan and pyridoxine is required to synthesize niacin from tryptophan. Biochemistry was such a new field that Goldberger lacked the tools to analyze fully the ramifications of his research observations.

In the early 1960s, it was demonstrated that niacin was a good cholesterol-altering drug and indeed it was the first cholesterol lowering drug. Thus, the deficiency which produced pellagra, which was cured by an atherogenic diet, namely milk, meat, butter, and eggs resulted in elevating the blood cholesterol values leading to an increase in the frequency of atherosclerotic events. Niacin preceded both the acid resins and the statins as cholesterol-altering agents. A full circle so to speak.

Disclosures

The authors have no conflicts of interest to disclose.

William Clifford Roberts, MD*
Baylor Scott & White Heart and Vascular Institute, Baylor University Medical Center, Baylor Scott & White Health, Dallas, Texas
* Corresponding author: Tel: (214) 820-7911; fax: (214) 820-7533. (William.Roberts1@bswhealth.org).

Comparison of Clinical and Morphologic Findings in Patients With Cardiac Sarcoidosis Severe Enough to Warrant Heart Transplantation in Those With -vs- Those Without Non-Caseating Granulomas in the Explanted Heart (Burnt-Out Sarcoid)

Samreen Fathima, MBBS[a,b], and William C. Roberts, MD[a,b,*]

Can cardiac sarcoidosis with heart failure severe enough to warrant orthotopic heart transplantation (OHT) be present without non-caseating granulomas in the explanted heart? The objective is to compare clinical and morphological features in patients with cardiac sarcoidosis severe enough to warrant OHT with -vs-without non-caseating granulomas in the explanted heart. The study was conducted at Baylor University Medical Center in Dallas, Texas. From a total of 671 explanted hearts examined from 1993 to 2018, twenty-five (4%) had gross morphologic features characteristic of cardiac sarcoidosis. At the time of OHT, the patients ranged in age from 50 to 69 years [mean 57]. Cardiac sarcoidosis was diagnosed before OHT in 3 (12%) patients, by percutaneous biopsy of the heart in 2 patients and by histologic examination of the "left ventricular core" in 1 patient who had a left ventricular assist device inserted, and, by examination of the native heart after OHT in the remaining 22 (88%) patients. Of the 25 patients, 16 (64%) had typical sarcoid non-caseating granulomas in the explanted heart, and 9 (36%) had no granulomas in the explanted heart. Comparison of certain clinical and morphologic features in the group with -vs- the group without cardiac granulomas showed no significant differences. In conclusion, of patients with cardiac sarcoidosis severe enough to warrant OHT, some have typical non-caseating granulomas in the explanted heart and some do not. The clinical and gross morphologic features of those with and those without cardiac granulomas are similar. **(Am J Cardiol 2019;124:599−603)**

Sarcoidosis has usually been defined by the presence of non-caseating granulomas containing multinucleated giant cells, epithelioid cells and lymphocytes in one or more body organs. When sarcoidosis attacks an organ, scar tissue develops in the areas of the granulomas and eventually it appears that the scar tissue can obliterate all evidence of previous inflammation, including the giant cells. This scenario appears to occur in cardiac sarcoidosis. Herein, we describe certain clinical and cardiac morphologic findings in 25 patients who had orthotopic heart transplant (OHT) for what proved to be cardiac sarcoidosis. We compared clinical and morphologic features of the cases with to those without non-caseating granulomas in the explanted hearts.

Methods

Since March 1993 one of us (WCR) has examined all specimens excised by cardiac surgeons at Baylor University Medical Center (BUMC) and submitted the report on each. From March 1993 through December 2018, we examined 671 native hearts excised at the time of OHT at BUMC. All hearts were opened and sections made by WCR. The weights of the hearts were all done by the same investigator after opening the chambers, removing any excess tissue (parietal pericardium for example), and incising the aorta and pulmonary trunk about 2 cm cephalad to the sino-tubular junction. The hearts were weighed within one week after their fixation in formaldehyde. Photographs were prepared on virtually all the explanted hearts, all of which have been retained. Of these 671 native hearts examined since 1993, twenty-five (4%) had gross morphologic features characteristic of cardiac sarcoidosis. Histologic sections were prepared in each heart, and stained by both hematoxylin/eosin and trichrome. At least 5 sections of myocardium were prepared in each case: 4 from the ventricles and 1 from the atria. All sections were examined by WCR. Photomicrographs were prepared from many of the cases. After examination of the heart and before submitting the final pathology report, the medical records in each case were examined.

Results

Of the 25 cases, 16 (64%) had typical sarcoid non-caseating granulomas in the explanted heart, and 9 (36%) had no granulomas in the explanted heart. Comparison of

[a]Division of Cardiology, Departments of Internal Medicine, Baylor Scott & White Heart and Vascular Institute, Baylor University Medical Center, Baylor Scott & White Health, Dallas, Texas; and [b]Department of Pathology, Baylor Scott & White Heart and Vascular Institute, Baylor University Medical Center, Baylor Scott & White Health, Dallas, Texas. Manuscript received April 19, 2019; revised manuscript received and accepted May 7, 2019.

*Corresponding author: Tel: (214) 820-7911.

E-mail address: William.Roberts1@bswhealth.org (W.C. Roberts).

certain clinical and gross morphologic features in the group with -vs- the group without cardiac granulomas showed no significant differences (Table 1). Pertinent data in each of the 25 patients is tabulated in Table 2. Three patients (cases #2, #11 and #18 Table 2) had left ventricular assist devices inserted before OHT and all 3 had granulomas in the excised "left ventricular core", including one (case #18, Table 2) who did not have granulomas in the explanted heart. Of the 9 patients without granulomas in the explanted heart, 3 previously had morphologic proof of cardiac sarcoidosis (2 by percutaneous biopsies of the heart [cases #19 and #22, Table 2] and one by examination of the portion of left ventricular free wall excised to insert a left ventricular assist device [case #18, Table 2].) Each of these 3 patients in whom cardiac sarcoidosis was proven by tissue examination before OHT were treated with corticosteroid therapy (cases #18, #19, and #22, Table 2). Additionally, two of the remaining 22 patients in whom the diagnosis of cardiac sarcoidosis was not proven before OHT also were treated with corticosteroid drugs because of biopsy proved pulmonary sarcoidosis (Cases #2 and #24, Table 2). Two patients (case #4 and #7, Table 2) had significant coronary narrowing, one (case #4, Table 2) of whom had coronary artery bypass grafting. Electrocardiographic features before OHT in each of the 25 patients are tabulated in table 3.

Table 1

Comparison in patients with clinical and morphologic findings of cardiac sarcoidosis severe enough to warrant heart transplantation in those with -vs- those without non-caseating granulomas in the explanted heart

Variable	Total (n = 25)	Cardiac granulomas		p Value
		No (n = 9)	Yes (n = 16)	
Age (years)	57 ± 6	56 ± 9	57 ± 5	0.81
Men	13 (52%)	6 (67%)	7 (44%)	0.41
Women	12 (48%)	3 (33%)	9 (56%)	
White	19 (76%)	6 (67%)	13 (81%)	0.63
Black	6 (24%)	3 (33%)	3 (19%)	
Duration (months), symptoms	72 ± 53	76 ± 65	70 ± 48	0.79
Atrial arrhythmias	7 (28%)	4 (44%)	3 (20%)	0.36
Ventricular arrhythmias	8 (32%)	1 (11%)	7 (47%)	0.18
Bundle branch block				0.28
Left	4 (16%)	1 (11%)	3 (19%)	
Right	10 (40%)	3 (33%)	7 (44%)	
Indeterminate	3 (12%)	0	3 (19%)	
Total 12-lead QRS Voltage (mm)	88 ± 36	99 ± 20	82 ± 41	0.30
Total cholesterol (mg/dl)	150 ± 42	160 ± 47	145 ± 40	0.44
LDL cholesterol (mg/dl)	90 ± 29	96 ± 27	87 ± 30	0.48
Body mass index (Kg/m^2)	28 ± 5	29 ± 7	28 ± 3	0.70
Prior LVAD	3 (12%)	2 (22%)	1 (6%)	0.60
Corticosteroid therapy	5 (24%)	4 (44%)	1 (6%)	0.097
Heart weight (g)				
Men	490 ± 58	491 ± 80	492 ± 51	0.91
Women	423 ± 86	438 ± 141	418 ± 71	0.75
Floating heart	12 (48%)	4 (44%)	8 (53%)	1.00

LDL = low density lipoprotein; LVAD =left ventricular assist device.

Discussion

The present report describes 25 patients who underwent OHT because of chronic severe heart failure resulting from cardiac sarcoidosis: 16 of the patients had classic non-caseating granulomas in the operatively-excised native hearts and 9 had no granulomas in the explanted hearts, although 3 of them had typical granulomas in percutaneous biopsies of heart or in the "left ventricular core" excised at the time of insertion of left ventricular assist device. Comparison of various clinical and gross morphologic features of the 16 patients with granulomas in the explanted hearts to the 9 patients without disclosed no significant differences.

Typical gross and histologic features of cardiac sarcoidosis severe enough to warrant OHT include focal but extensive scars in the walls of both left and right ventricles and ventricular septum.[1–8] Scars in the atrial walls are infrequent.[5] The focal scars in the right ventricular wall are usually transmural; those involving the left ventricular wall may also be transmural but often they are only subepicardial, the opposite of what occurs in hearts of patients with coronary heart disease, which is subendocardial or transmural or both but not subepicardial.[9] The ventricular walls are more often thinner than normal rather than thicker than normal. The ventricular cavities are severely dilated (unless a left ventricular assist device had been inserted earlier). Histologically, the non-caseating granulomas are typically located within the scars and numerous ones are present in some scars. In most patients some ventricular wall scars contain granulomas and others do not. The numbers of nuclei present in the giant cells may exceed 50. Lymphocytes also are present.

How can we be certain that the 9 patients without non-caseating granulomas in the explanted hearts have cardiac sarcoidosis? In 3 of these 9 patients an earlier percutaneous biopsy (in 2) or examination of the portion of left ventricular wall excised to insert a left ventricular assist device (in 1) did indeed contain non-caseating granulomas. The interval from this tissue examination to the OHT in these 3 patients was 0.1, 7, and 53 months, respectively. Another supporting factor was that many of the ventricular wall scars in the 16 patients with granulomas present in the explanted heart also had ventricular-wall scars without any granulomas. The latter observation suggests it would not be a "stretch" for all the scars to eventually be devoid of granulomas. Three of the 9 patients without granulomas in the explanted hearts were treated with cortico-steroid therapy, a known cause of converting non-caseating granulomas into scars without granulomas.[1] (Each of the 3 patients in whom the diagnosis was made by examination of cardiac tissue some time before the OHT were treated with prednisone.)

The positive features of this report are the following: (1) no previous report has emphasized that cardiac sarcoidosis may be present without non-caseating granulomas being present in the heart. (2) No previous study has compared clinical and gross morphologic findings in the patients with to those without non-caseating granulomas in the heart.

Limitations of the present study include the following: (1) perhaps not enough histologic sections of myocardium were studied. (We examined at least 4 large

Table 2
Pertinent clinical and morphological findings in 25 patients who had orthotopic heart transplantation for cardiac sarcoidosis

Case	Age (years)	Sex	Race	Duration of symptoms before OHT (months)	BMI l(Kg/m^2)	TC (mg/dl)	LDL (mg/dl)	CI (l/min/m^2)	P-Rx	Clinical cardiac diagnosis	ICD	HW (g)	Heart floats	G	Location of granulomas		
															RV	VS	LV
1	50	F	B	132	25	124	74	–	0	IDC	+	440	0	+	1+	3+	3+
2	52	M	W	192	28	172	108	1.6	+	IDC*	0	440	0	+	1+	2+	1+
3	52	F	B	50	31	166	64	2.3	0	IDC	+	440	0	+	1+	3+	3+
4	53	M	W	12	27	188	112	1.6	0	IDC	0	555	+	+	3+	3+	3+
5	54	F	W	46	26	74	46	1.8	0	IDC	0	425	0	+	3+	3+	3+
6	54	M	W	108	30	210	134	-	0	IDC	0	511	-	+	3+	3+	3+
7	56	F	W	11	26	143	118	–	0	IDC	0	450	+	+	1+	3+	3+
8	57	F	W	46	30	138	94	1.4	0	IDC	0	380	0	+	3+	3+	3+
9	58	F	W	60	27	229	147	2.2	0	IDC	+	560	+	+	3+	3+	3+
10	58	M	W	48	25	114	64	1.2	0	IDC	0	420	0	+	3+	3+	3+
11	59	F	B	72	26	134	69	1.3	0	IDC	+	370	0	+	1+	2+	1+
12	60	F	W	36	28	130	93	1.2	0	IDC	0	401	+	+	1+	3+	3+
13	61	F	W	120	25	119	60	1.2	0	IDC	0	300	+	+	3+	3+	3+
14	63	M	W	84	33	109	52	1.6	0	IDC	+	470	+	+	3+	3+	3+
15	63	M	W	48	24	157	86	1.7	0	IDC	0	540	+	+	3+	3+	3+
16	67	M	W	48	30	116	70	1.6	0	IDC	0	510	+	+	3+	3+	3+
17	40	F	W	11	45	107	78	1.4	0	IDC	0	370	0	0	0	0	0
18	50	M	W	36	28	185	119	1.7	+	CS	+	605	0	0	0	0	0
19	53	M	W	60	31	233	120	1.9	+	CS	0	535	0	0	0	0	0
20	54	F	B	100	24	191	108	1.8	0	IDC	0	345	0	0	0	0	0
21	57	M	W	36	30	119	82	1.2	0	IDC	0	420	+	0	0	0	0
22	59	M	W	48	28	–	–	–	+	CS	+	420	+	0	0	0	0
23	62	F	B	216	19	182	129	1.5	0	IDC	+	600	0	0	0	0	0
24	65	M	B	139	29	160	82	–	+	IDC	+	475	+	0	0	0	0
25	69	M	W	36	23	101	50	1.3	0	IDC	0	475	+	0	0	0	0

AB = black; BMI = body mass index; CI = cardiac index; CS = cardiac sarcoidosis; F = female; G = granuloma; HW = heart weight; I = indirect; ICD = intracardiac defibrillator; IDC = ischemic dilated cardiomyopathy; L = left; LDL = low-density lipoprotein; LV = left ventricle; M = male; OHT = orthotopic heart transplant; P = prednisone Rx; R = right; RV = right ventricle; TC = total cholesterol; VS = ventricular septum; W = white.

* Because the patient had biopsy-proven pulmonary sarcoid, the patient clinically was considered to have cardiac sarcoid as well, but a cardiac biopsy done before the OHT was negative for sarcoid.

Table 3
Electrocardiographic findings before orthotopic heart transplantation in 25 patients with cardiac sarcoidosis

Case	Paced	QRS amplitude in each electrocardiographic lead (mm)												Total 12-lead QRS voltage (mm)	Arrhythmias		BBB (Type)	CHB	Prolonged QT Interval
		I	II	III	aVR	aVL	aVF	V1	V2	V3	V4	V5	V6		A (Type)	V (Type)			
	0	0	0	0	0	0	0	0	0	0	0	0	0	0	0	0			
1	+	2	23	13	6	7	28	4	12	16	20	18	12	161	0	0	+ (NS)	+	0
2	0	14	12	8	13	11	7	12	8	8	18	22	22	155	0	0	+ (R)	0	0
3	+	5	5	5	5	2	8	6	7	7	5	5	7	67	0	+ (VPC)	+ (L)	0	0
4	+	4	12	9	6	3	9	7	7	3	7	10	9	86	0	+ (VPC)	+ (R)	+	0
5	+	4	4	5	2	8	4	–	–	–	–	–	–	–	0	0	0	+	0
6	–	–	–	–	–	–	–	–	–	–	–	–	–	–	–	–	–	-	-
7	+	4	7	8	5	6	8	4	8	4	5	7	7	73	0	+ (VT)	0	0	0
8	0	5	1	6	3	6	4	5	9	5	4	2	2	52	+ (AT)	0	+ (R)	0	0
9	0	8	8	15	3	11	12	5	7	4	4	6	6	89	0	0			
	+	3	3	4	2	3	3	3	7	3	3	4	4	69	0	0	+ (R)	0	0
10	+	9	9	6	4	4	6	5	3	8	8	8	7	77	0	0	+ (L)	0	0
11	0	11	11	17	8	14	13	9	5	9	12	16	19	144	0	0			
	+	10	12	19	8	14	15	8	9	10	13	15	14	147	0	0	+ (R)	+	0
12	0	5	3	4	5	7	3	3	7	4	6	2	5	54	+ (AF)	+ (VPC)	0	0	0
13	+	4	4	5	3	6	4	4	10	5	7	7	8	72	0	0	+ (R)	+	+
14	+	5	12	8	8	5	10	8	9	14	10	9	5	103	0	+ (VPC)	+ (L)	+	0
15	0	8	6	3	6	6	4	9	10	13	18	22	29	134					
	+	5	8	11	5	6	11	2	4	12	17	11	3	95	+ (AF)	+ (VPC)	+ (R)	0	0
16	+	4	5	7	2	5	5	2	2	6	5	3	1	47	0	+ (VT)	+ (NS)	+	0
17	0	18	6	13	6	13	7	6	6	6	6	5	6	98	+ (APC)	+ (VPC)	0	0	0
18	0	7	11	14	5	9	12	6	14	19	7	10	7	121	+ (APC)	0	+ (L)	0	0
19	+	7	7	10	4	8	9	5	7	5	6	7	6	81	0	0	0	+	0
20	0	3	7	7	4	4	6	4	8	11	9	12	14	89	0	0	0	0	+
21	0	5	8	4	5	4	6	7	10	28	26	22	6	131	+ (APC)	0	+ (R)	0	+
22	0	4	1	5	4	3	4	–	–	–	–	–	–	–	0	0	0	0	0
23	0	10	11	10	7	7	7	10	9	7	9	10	10	107	0	0	+ (R)	0	0
24	0	5	7	5	6	4	5	5	4	5	7	10	11	74	+ (AF)	0	+ (R)	0	0
25	0	10	5	6	6	11	12	11	6	4	4	12	4	91	0	0	0	0	0

A = atrial; AF = atrial fibrillation; APC = atrial premature complexes; AT= atrial tachycardia; BBB = bundle branch block; CHB = complete heart block; L = left; NS = non-specific; R = right; V= ventricular; VPC = ventricular premature complexes; VT = ventricular tachycardia.

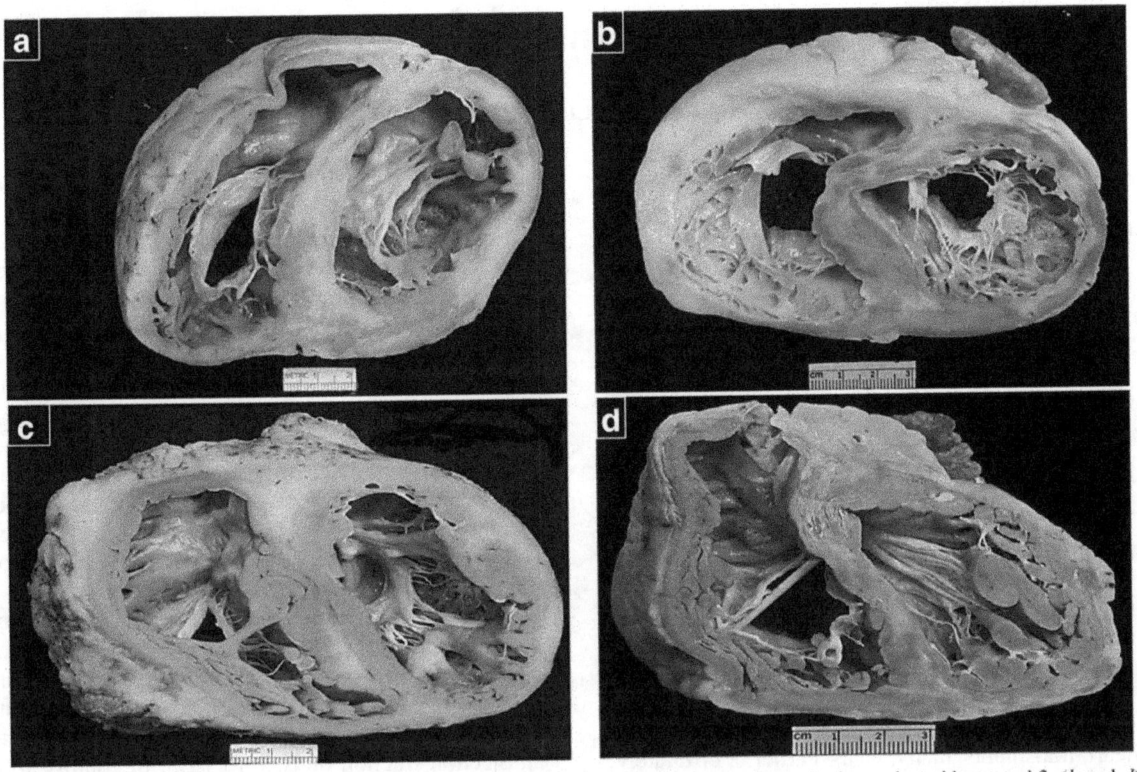

Figure 1. Shown here are basal portions of the heart in 4 patients, 2 of whom (*a* and *c*) had granulomas in the explanted heart and 2, (*b* and *d*) did not. (*a*) patient #5 (Table 2); (*b*) patient #23 (Table 2); (*c*) patient #12 (Table 2); *d*) patient #20 (Table 2). Both ventricles are dilated in each of these 4 patients. Portions of the tricuspid and mitral valves are visible in all 4 patients. The white areas of right ventricular free wall, ventricular septum and left ventricular free wall represent sites of scarring, some of which contained non-caseating granulomas and some of which did not.

[endocardium-to-epicardium] sections of the ventricular walls in all 25 patients and far more [up to 20] in a few patients.); (2) perhaps the 9 patients without tissue proof of cardiac sarcoidosis *in the explanted hearts*, namely the presence of non-caseating granulomas, did not have cardiac sarcoidosis. We believe this scenario to be highly unlikely because 3 of the 9 patients had earlier proof of cardiac sarcoidosis (biopsy or left ventricular "core" examination), and, additionally, we know of no other cardiac condition that even remotely resembles the full-blown morphologic features of cardiac sarcoidosis (Figures 1 and 2).

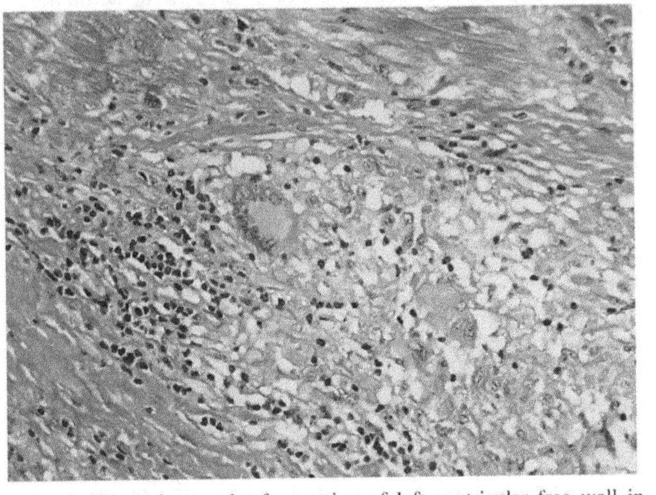

Figure 2. Photomicrograph of a portion of left ventricular free wall in patient #16 (Table 2). The myocardial wall is partially replaced by a dense fibrous tissue which stains blue within which is a sarcoid granuloma. Trichrome stain, original magnification × 40.

1. Roberts WC, McAllister HA Jr, Ferrans VJ. Sarcoidosis of the heart. A clinicopathologic study of 35 necropsy patients (Group I) and review of 78 previously described necropsy patients (Group II). *Am J Med* 1977;63:86–108.
2. Virmani R, Bures JC, Roberts WC. Cardiac sarcoidosis: a major cause of sudden death in young individuals. *Chest* 1980;77:423–428.
3. Donsky AS, Escobar J, Capehart J, Roberts WC. Heart transplantation for undiagnosed cardiac sarcoidosis. *Am J Cardiol* 2002;89:1447–1450.
4. Roberts WC, Vowels TJ, Ko JM, Capehart JE, Hall SA. Cardiac transplantation for cardiac sarcoidosis with initial diagnosis by examination of the left ventricular apical "core" excised for insertion of a left ventricular assist device for severe chronic heart failure. *Am J Cardiol* 2009;103:110–114.
5. Sharma PS, Lubahn JG, Donsky AS, Yoon ADH, Carry MM, Grayburn PA, Wood PB, Ko JM, Burton EC, Roberts WC. Diagnosing cardiac sarcoidosis clinically without tissue confirmation. *Proc (Bayl Univ Med Cent)* 2009;22:236–238.
6. Roberts WC, Chung MS, Ko JM, Capehart JE, Hall SA. Morphologic features of cardiac sarcoidosis in native hearts of patients having cardiac transplantation. *Am J Cardiol* 2014;113:706–712.
7. Armstrong D, Gonzalez-Stawinski GV, Ko JM, Hall SA, Roberts WC. The two extremes of cardiac sarcoidosis and the effect of prednisone therapy. *Am J Cardiol* 2015;115:150–153.
8. Roberts WC, Becker TM, Hall SA. Usefulness of total 12-lead QRS voltage as a clue to diagnosis of patients with cardiac sarcoidosis severe enough to warrant orthotopic heart transplant. *JAMA Cardiol* 2018;3:64–68.
9. Shirani J, Roberts WC. Subepicardial myocardial lesions. *Am Heart J* 1993;125:1346–1352.

Examining One's Own Heart

William C. Roberts, MD[a,b,*], and Saba Ilyas, BS[a]

Although billions of people have inhabited planet Earth, few have examined their own heart. Cardiac transplantation, which began December 3, 1967, is the procedure that made self-examination possible.

At Baylor University Medical Center (BUMC) in Dallas, we began showing heart transplantation recipients their hearts in 2010. Since that time, we have shown 157 patients their own hearts (through March 2020). The exercise was initiated not by me or another physician but by a heart transplant recipient, Mr. Marvin Jones. I was walking in the corridor near the cardiac catheterization waiting room and next to me was Mr. Jones. He leaned over and asked if I was Dr. Roberts. "Yes," I answered. He said, "I understand that you have my heart." I invited him to our weekly cardiovascular pathology conference so that several physicians could observe a person examining their own heart.[1] Subsequently, the heart transplant cardiologists, surgeons, their nurses and coordinators have gotten on board to encourage their heart transplant patients to "Call Dr. Roberts" to make the arrangements to view their own hearts. Some of the patients had their heart transplants many years earlier. Fortunately, BUMC has provided us with a heart storage facility and all transplant and autopsy hearts have resided there since 1993. Thus, all heart transplant recipients who want to see their hearts since that time can have their requests fulfilled.

How does the procedure to view their own heart work? One of us (SI) meets the recipient at a designed location and brings him/her to the cardiovascular laboratory. Most recipients do not come alone. They bring their family – spouses, offspring, grandchildren and friends. We sit around a table and I ask the recipient a few questions. I usually begin by discussing their cardiac illness. When did the cardiac illness start? What were the initial symptoms and signs? What diagnosis did your physician indicate that you had? Did other family members have a similar cardiac condition? What type of work do (did) you do? Are you still working? How did you get to BUMC? Who told you that you could see your own heart? During this questioning section the heart is laid out before me on the table (covered by a towel) and the transplant recipient is sitting to my right. I usually ask if they are ready to see their own heart. I prewarn them that their heart is no longer reddish brown but tan because it has resided in formaldehyde for some time. The blue towel is then pulled away. I always look at their face as the towel is removed. Nearly always there is no change in facial expression. Of the 157 recipients to whom I have shown their heart, only one turned his head as the towel was being removed. Only one recipient cried. He, however, was the youngest (age 21) who only 2 months earlier had developed a fulminating myocarditis. The shock of suddenly becoming terribly ill from a previously healthy life and then confronted with his own heart certainly made his crying understandable.

The hearts, of course, had been incised before their showing and a few sections had been prepared for histologic study. We discuss the anatomic location of the cardiac chambers, the valves, and how the blood flows through the heart. The most striking finding to most recipients is the yellow covering of portions of the heart due to the subepicardial adipose tissue. The patients with ischemic cardiomyopathy, obviously, have one or more left ventricular scars and those are pointed out and their origins discussed. Nearly all of the patients who had heart transplants have dilated ventricles and the more dilated the ventricle the lower the ejection fraction. Nearly all recipients are familiar with the concept of ejection fraction. I show with my hand how poorly a dilated ventricle contracts in contrast to a normal-sized ventricle. The recipients are usually shocked by the size of the normal ventricle with an ejection fraction of 60% to 70% in contrast to their left ventricle with an ejection fraction of 10% to 15%. In contrast to the hearts with ischemic cardiomyopathy the recipients with idiopathic dilated cardiomyopathy are disappointed to learn that we have no idea what caused their condition.

After the viewing of the heart, I give the recipient and their families a little "sermon" on heart transplantation in general to help them understand how lucky they are to have received a new heart. With the use of a flip chart I point out the present US population (≈330 million), the number >20 years of age (≈240 million) and then ask how many of the latter 240 million have chronic heart failure. The response is usually in the multiple decades. The answer, of course, is approximately 6.5 million. Then we discuss the number of those 6.5 million who each year in the US have a heart transplant. Their answers are usually astronomical compared to the actual number (approximately 3,000). This revelation is usually a shock to the recipients and to their families. The point of this exercise is to emphasize how lucky they are and that now it is their responsibility to take care of the new heart. We discuss what they eat for breakfast, lunch and dinner and what snacks are eaten in between meals and at bedtime. The first food mentioned for all meals usually is the flesh consumed (bovine muscle [beef], porcine muscle [pork], chicken, etc.). Most of the transplant recipients are overweight (body mass index ≥30 kg/m^2) so we discuss reducing the number of calories consumed daily.[2] We discuss whether they exercise and if so, how much, and its importance for them. The nonrecipient family members also hear these discussions and I have heard later that some of them have changed "their ways."

A surprise for me has been how few of the transplant recipients know the actual name of their cardiac diagnosis. When I ask, "What cardiac diagnosis did your cardiologist say you had?" The answer is usually "heart failure." Whether ischemic cardiomyopathy or idiopathic cardiomyopathy is usually unclear. Those with cardiac amyloidosis or hypertrophic cardiomyopathy or cardiac sarcoidosis, or arrhythmogenic right

[a]Baylor Scott & White Heart and Vascular Institute, Dallas Texas; and [b]Division of Cardiology, Department of Internal Medicine, Baylor University Medical Center, Baylor Scott & White Health, Dallas Texas. Manuscript received March 20, 2020; revised manuscript received and accepted April 14, 2020.

See page 51 for disclosure information.

*Corresponding author: Tel: (214) 820-7911; fax: (214) 820-7933.
E-mail address: William.Roberts1@bswhealth.org (W.C. Roberts).

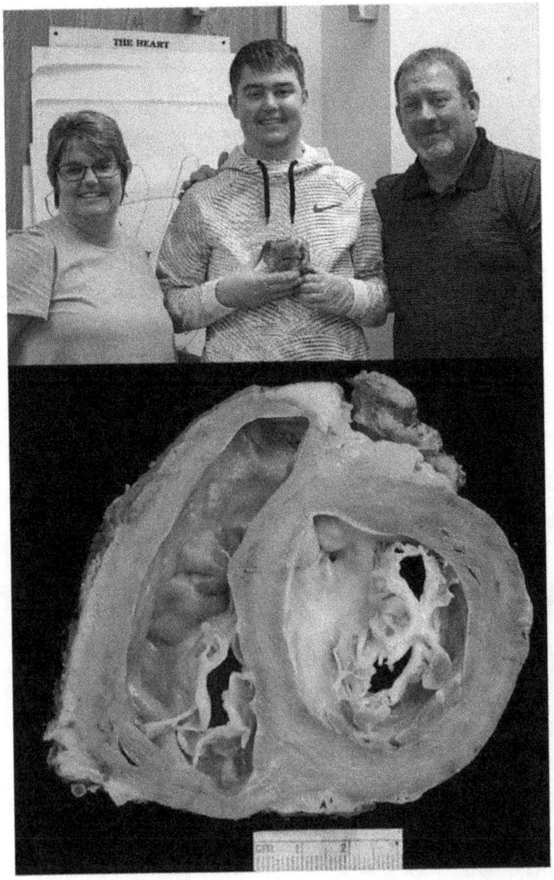

Figure 1. Grant J. Kepheart, a 19-year-old man, had a heart transplant in October 2017 for heart failure secondary to idiopathic dilated cardiomyopathy and the heart viewing was 75 days later. At age 16, a left ventricular assist device was inserted because of severe right sided heart failure, and an Alfieri stitch procedure was performed because of severe functional mitral regurgitation. Since the heart transplant he has been asymptomatic. His heart weighed 330 g.

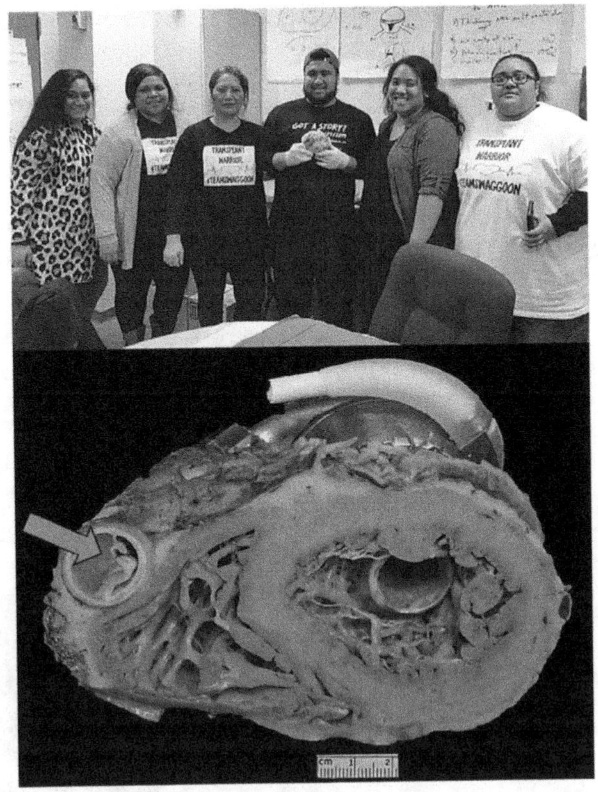

Figure 2. Kennedy Ngungutau, a 24-year-old Polynesian man, had a left ventricular assist device (LVAD) inserted in March 2018, and a heart transplant in April 2019, and his heart viewing was in February 2020. His excised heart weighed 420 g. His previous body weight was up to 290 lbs. His family came with him to observe the heart viewing. *Bottom:* The lumen of the canula from his LVAD is severely narrowed by thrombus (arrow). In his letter granting us permission to show the family picture, he wrote: "*...It was a great experience. I have lost 14 lbs. in the last month because I started to stay healthy with eating, and the times I eat and everything and I thank you all for it.*"

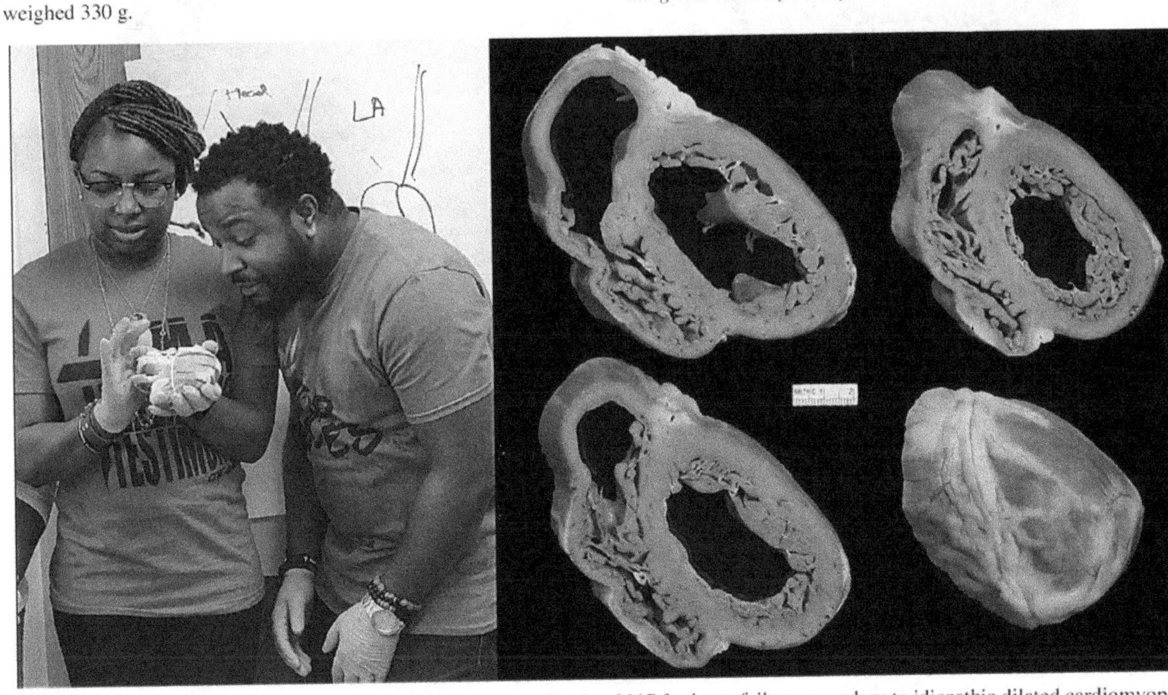

Figure 3. Erica P. Wilcox, a 33-year-old woman, had a heart transplant in May 2017 for heart failure secondary to idiopathic dilated cardiomyopathy and her heart viewing was in September 2019. At 25 years of age she weighed 260 pounds and subsequently lost to a body weight of 130 lbs. Her heart weighed 390 g. Her husband is quite curious about his wife's heart.

ventricular cardiomyopathy or valvular heart disease is usually known. I write their proper diagnosis in bold letters on the flip chart paper and give it to them to take home.

And finally, photos of the recipients standing up holding their hearts just in front of their sternum (Figures 1-21) are made routinely by SI. While the recipients continue to hold their hearts, they are photographed with their family members. Finally, while still holding their heart they are usually photographed with me. The pictures of their hearts and pictures holding their hearts are sent to the recipients. The exercise usually takes 45 to 60 minutes. My impression is that the activity is useful to both recipients and families.

A sidelight: The media, both television and print, have been fascinated by the idea of a person seeing his/her own heart. Consequently, several local and national networks have aired these activities. One recipient learned of the possibility of seeing her own heart by reading a piece in *Reader's Digest*, which described one of these Heart-to-Heart sessions at BUMC.

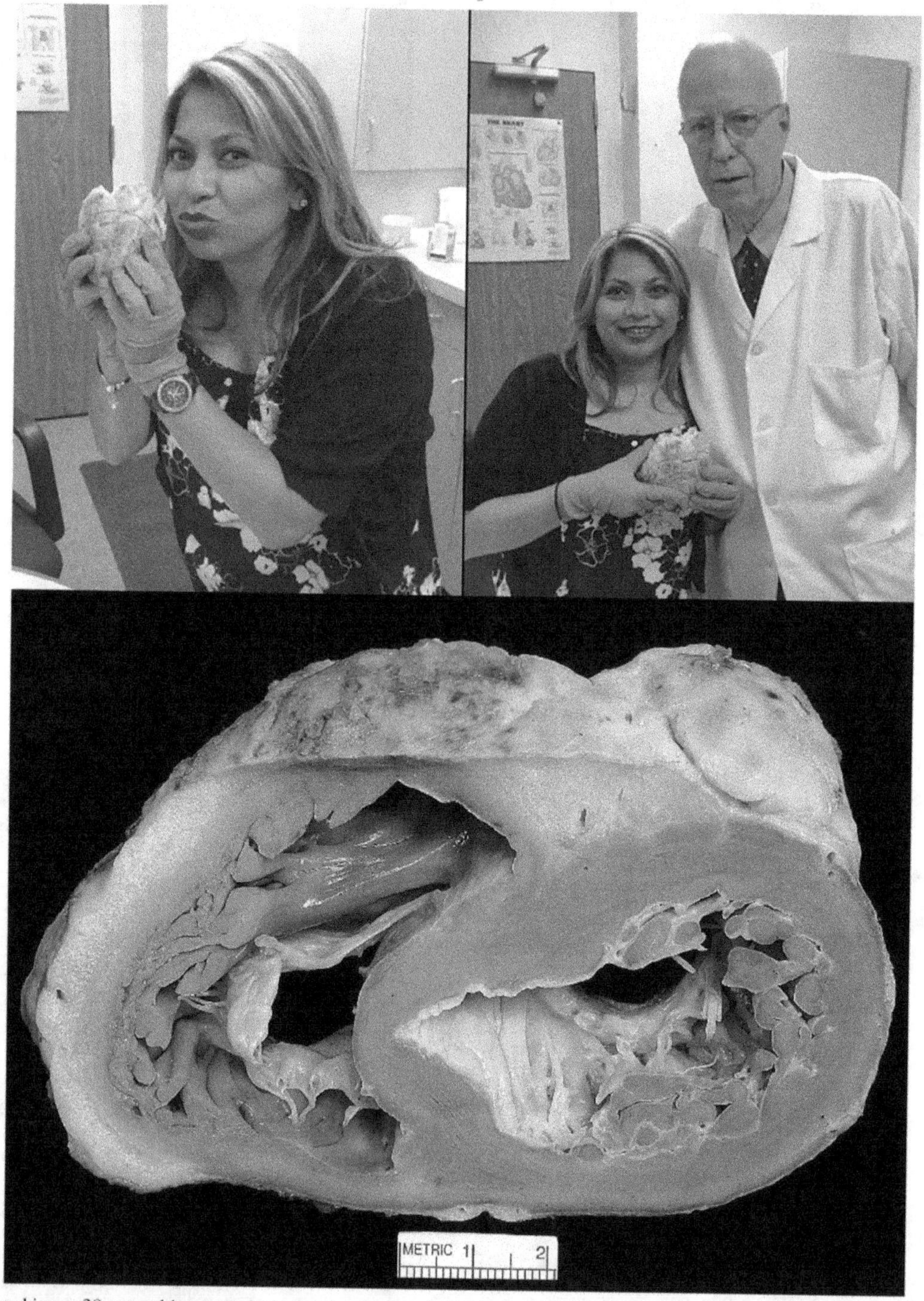

Figure 4. Manuela Arechiga, a 39-year-old woman, had a heart transplant in February 2015 and her heart viewing in July 2015. She had had a mitral valve replacement with a mechanical prosthesis in July 2014 for pure mitral regurgitation. In retrospect, the mitral valve replacement likely had been done for secondary mitral regurgitation, the consequence of idiopathic dilated cardiomyopathy. The cause of the endocardial thickening focally within the left ventricle is unclear. Her heart weighed 255 g.

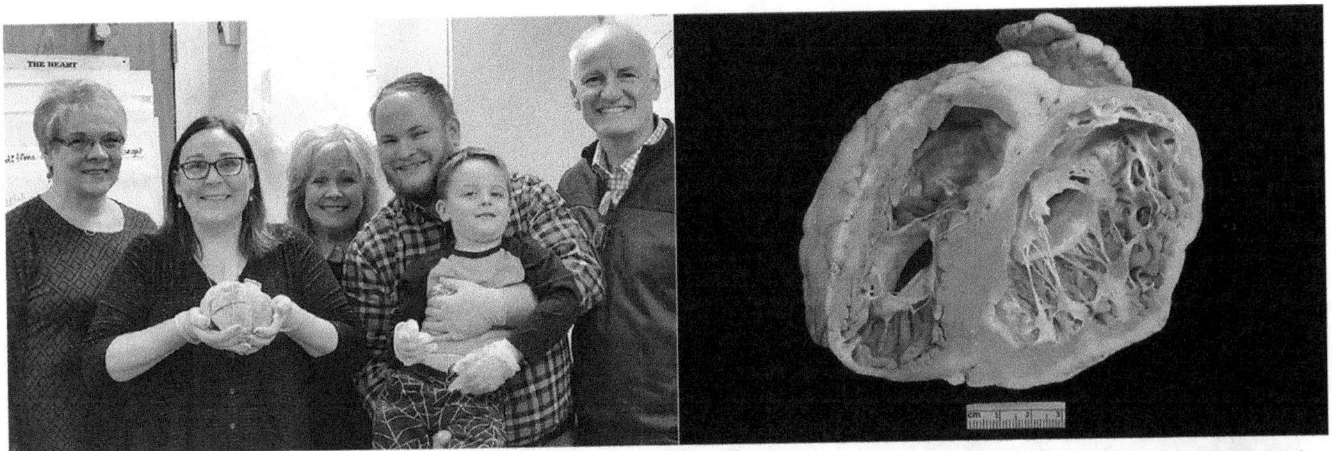

Figure 5. Marley Sterns, a 41-year-old woman, had a heart transplant in July 2019 because of severe heart failure from cardiac sarcoidosis and her heart viewing in October 2019. She developed heart failure about 8 years before her heart transplant. *Left*: Shown with her are members of her family. *Right*: The left ventricular wall is severely thin and typical sarcoid granulomas are present in the scarred areas. In her letter giving us permission to show the family picture, she wrote: "*...That experience meant so much to me and my family.*"

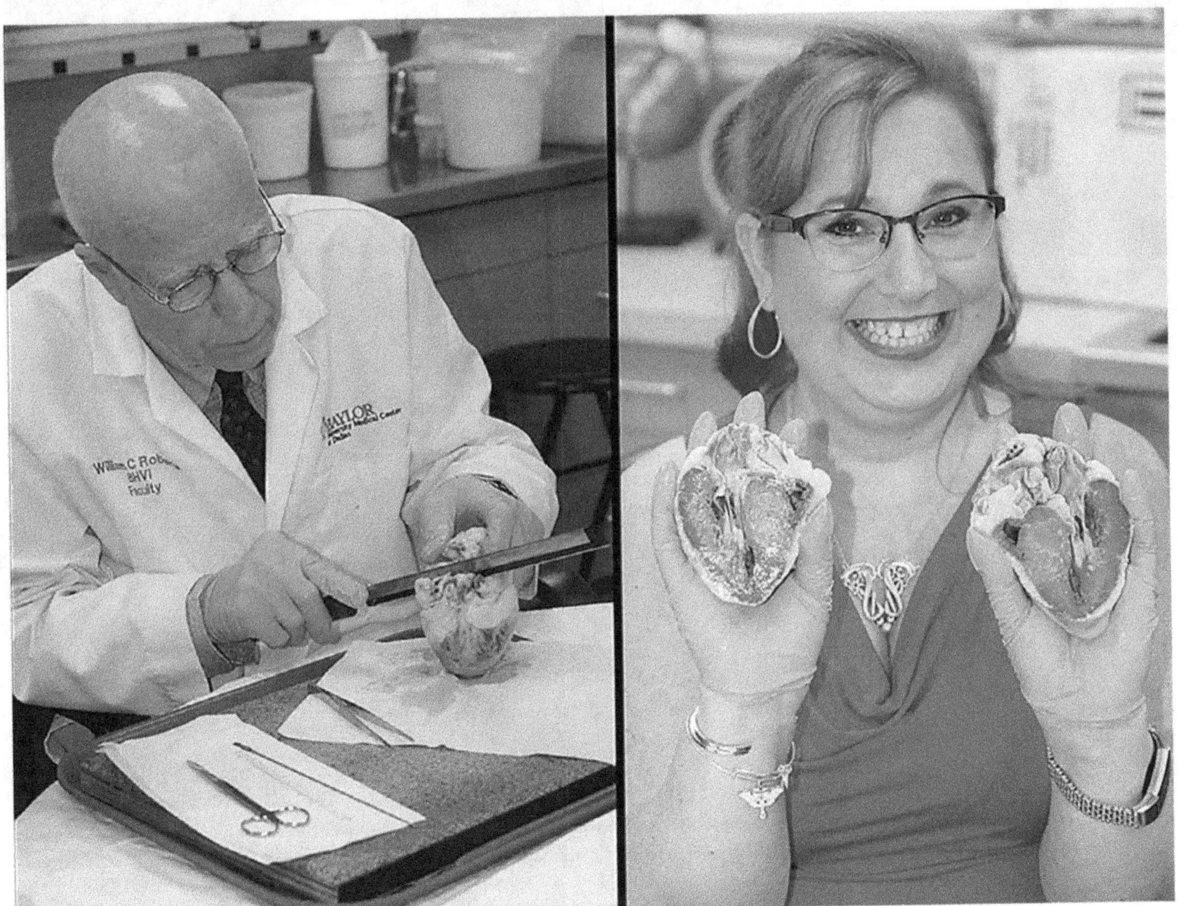

Figure 6. Lisa Salberg, a 48-year-old woman, had a heart transplant in April 2017 for hypertrophic cardiomyopathy and her heart viewing in August 2019. She brought her heart to WCR to open. She then had it plasticized so that she could keep it and show it to anyone interested. Her heart weighed 340 g. Ms. Salberg is the Founder and CEO of the Hypertrophic Cardiomyopathy Association located in Danville, New Jersey. She is a lovely lady who has done much for patients with hypertrophic cardiomyopathy.

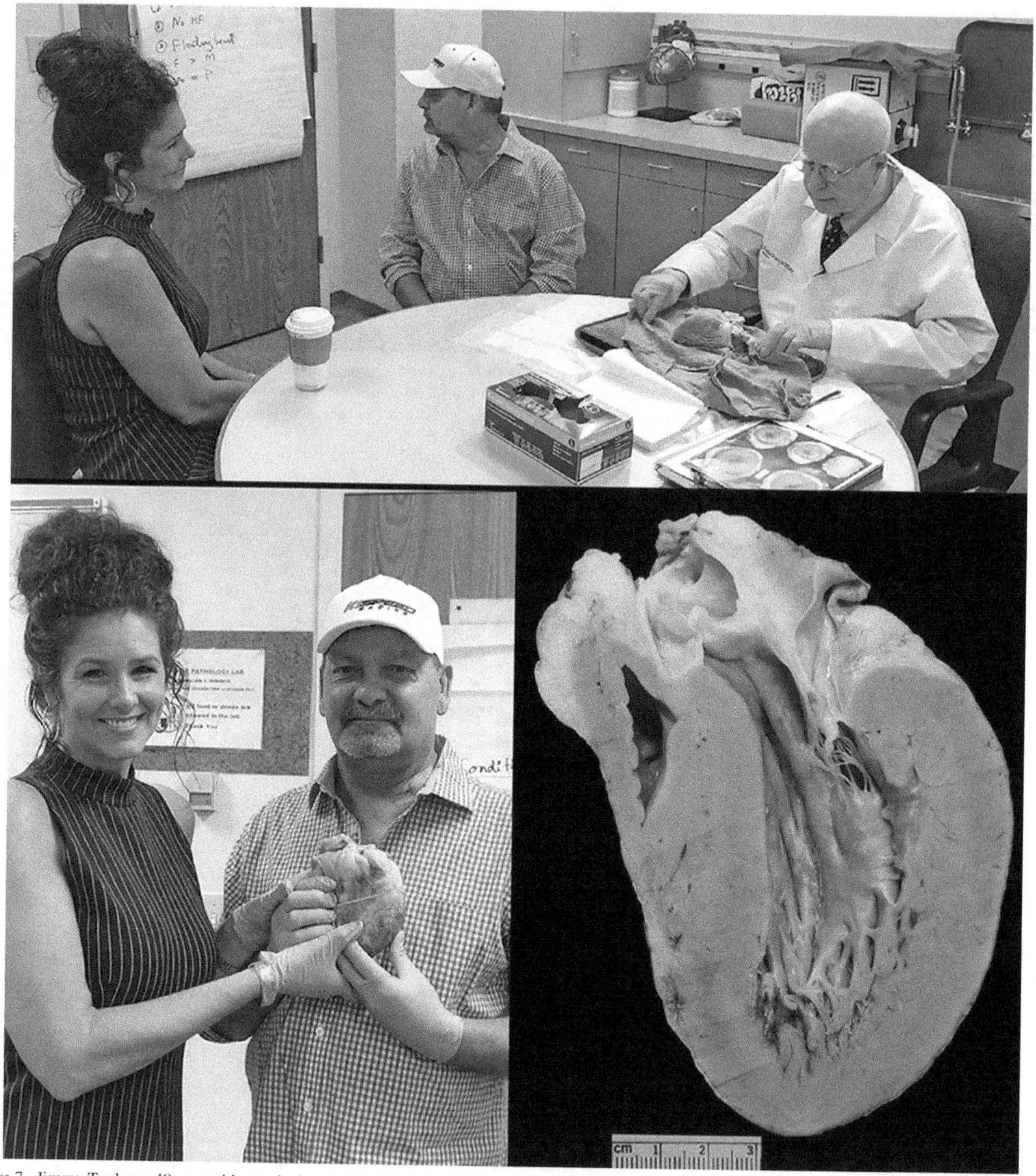

Figure 7. Jimmy Taylor, a 48-year-old man, had a combined heart and kidney transplant in May 2018 and his heart viewing in August 2019. The cause of the heart transplant was unclear clinically, but study of the actual heart showed classic features of ankylosing spondylitis. The heart weighed 675 g. While at the round table, I asked him if he was ready to see his heart? He replied, "Yes." But as I took the towel off his heart, he turned his head to the right and didn't look for a few minutes. Later he smiled. His wife Kelli is to his right. In his consent letter he wrote: *"We are so very blessed, and we hope that our journey is an inspiration to others who may have lost hope and a useful tool to those who help people like us."*

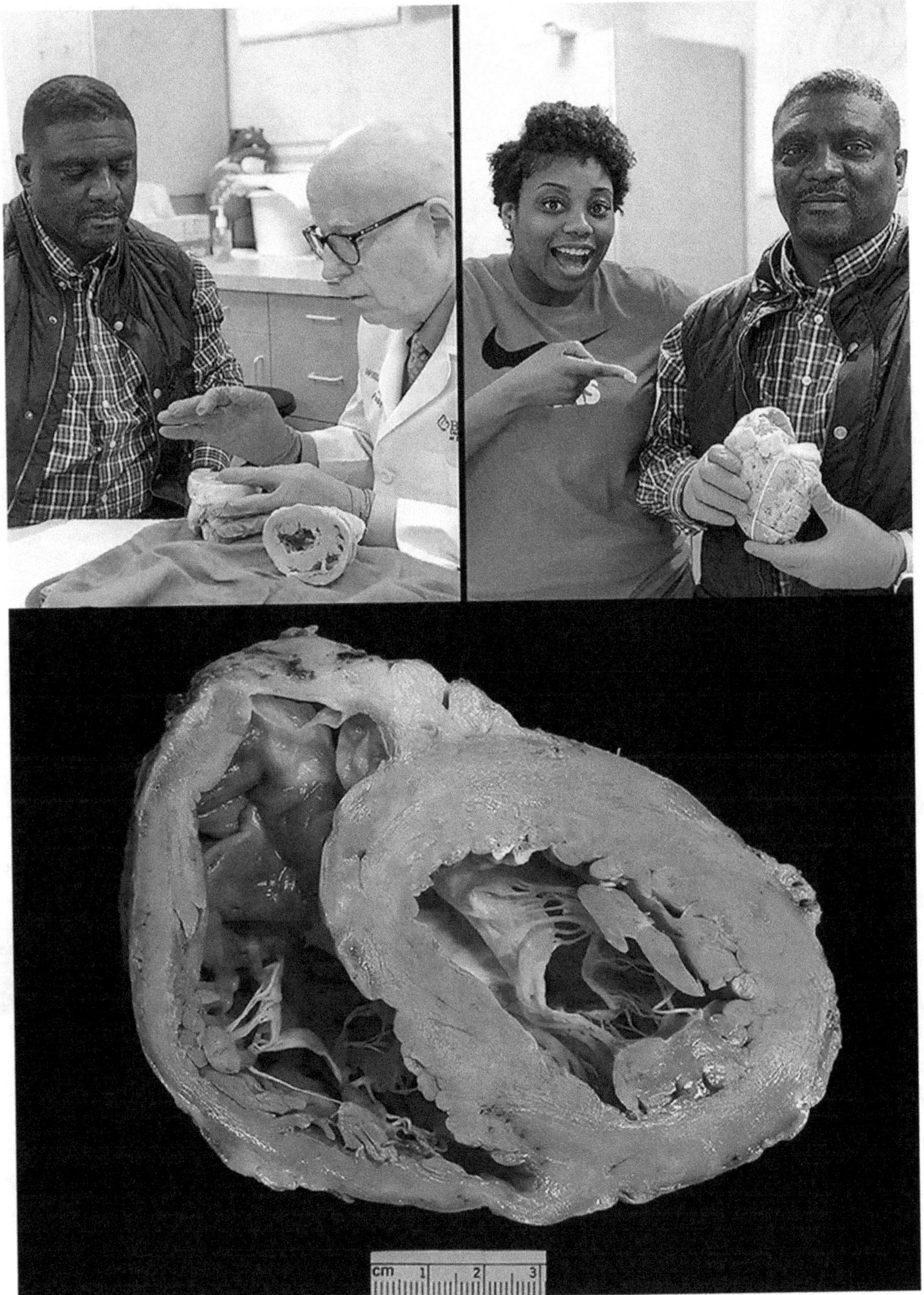

Figure 8. Todd Hickman, a 50-year-old man, had a heart transplant in December 2017 because of severe heart failure secondary to idiopathic dilated cardiomyopathy and his heart viewing in February 2020. At one time he weighed 290 lbs. He had had heart failure since age 41. Both of his paternal grandparents died of heart disease and a paternal uncle had a heart transplant at another hospital in 2016. *Top right*: His wife is obviously pointing at his heart. His heart weighed 565 g.

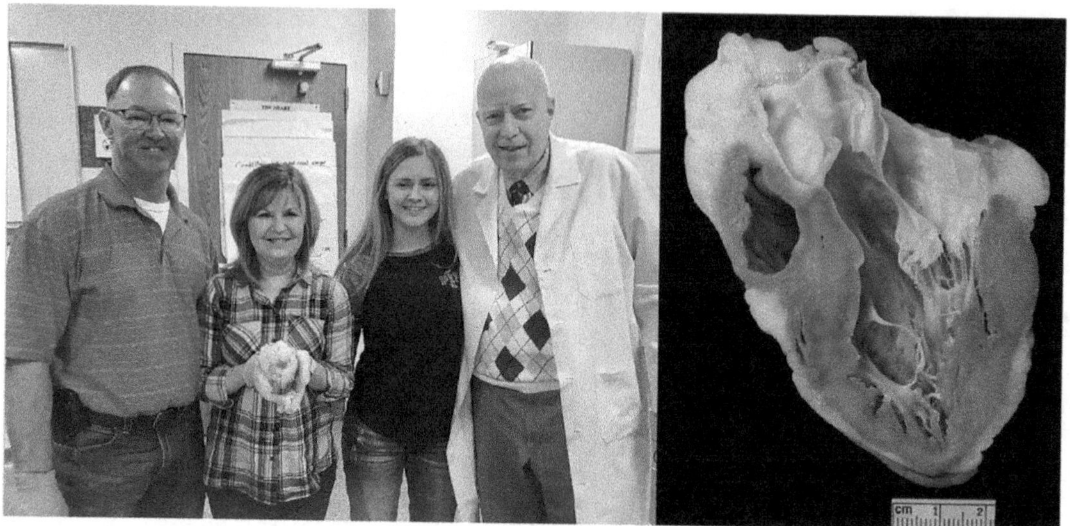

Figure 9. Vickie Coker, a 55-year-old, five-foot-tall woman, with her husband and 21-year-old daughter had a heart transplant for hypertrophic cardiomyopathy in January 2020 and the heart viewing in February 2020. Both mother and daughter had hypertrophic cardiomyopathy. The daughter (shown here) had a heart transplant at age 13. A son had died of hypertrophic cardiomyopathy in his teenage years. One of Mrs. Coker's sisters had ablation for atrial fibrillation at age 42, and later a heart transplant due to hypertrophic cardiomyopathy. The same sister had 2 daughters, both of whom had hypertrophic cardiomyopathy. Another sister died suddenly with heart failure and she too probably had the same condition. *Left*: Her husband and daughter with WCR. Ms. Coker's heart weighed only 255 g. The heart is unusual for hypertrophic cardiomyopathy in that there is no evidence of left ventricular outflow obstruction, no scarring in the ventricular walls, and the ventricular septum is only minimally thicker than the left ventricular free wall. In her consent letter she stated: *"I hope and pray that my story helps people see the importance of organ donation."*

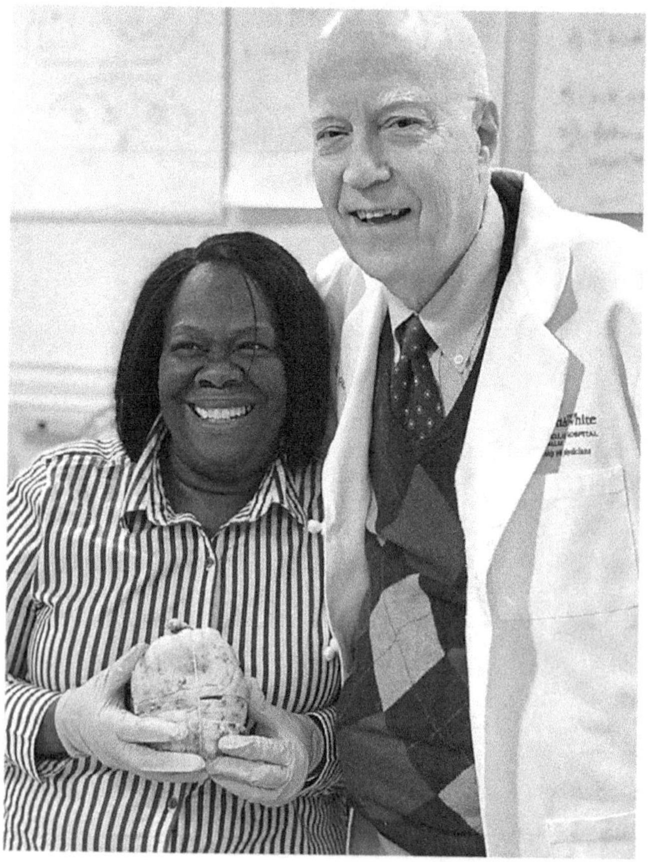

Figure 10. Debra R. Bruce, a 57-year-old woman, had a heart transplant in January 2018 because of severe heart failure secondary to idiopathic dilated cardiomyopathy and the heart viewing in January 2020. She had a son who had died of heart failure probably also from idiopathic dilated cardiomyopathy. Her heart weighed 425 g. In her consent letter she indicated that showing her heart was *"...one of the best days of my life."*

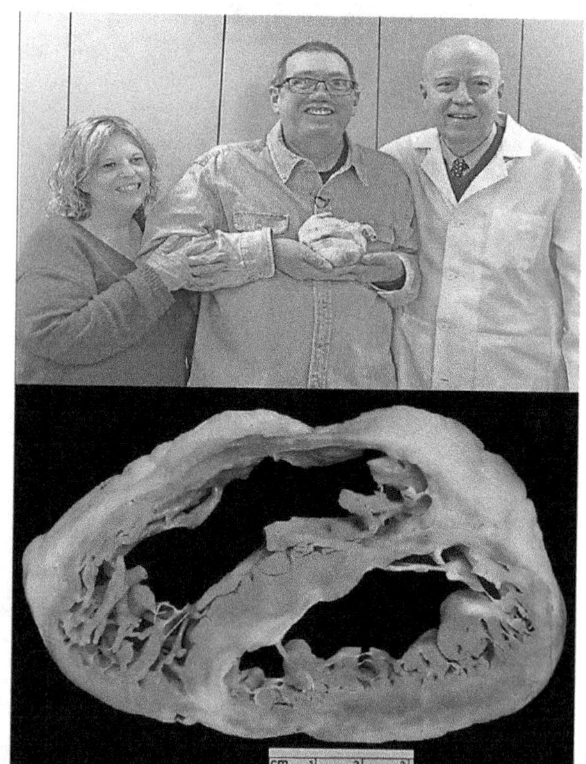

Figure 11. Darryl Glen Moore, a 58-year-old man, had a heart transplant in November 2019 for burnt-out cardiac sarcoidosis and the heart viewing in February 2020. He had classic gross features of cardiac sarcoidosis, but no granulomas were found in the heart. The white areas displayed in the photograph are scarred areas, but no granulomas were found within them. The coronary arteries were wide open. The heart weighed 440 g and he weighed 170 lbs. He had received immunosuppression with Imuran for 5 years prior to the transplant because of autoimmune hepatitis. Possibly this drug (Azathioprine) wiped out the granulomas.

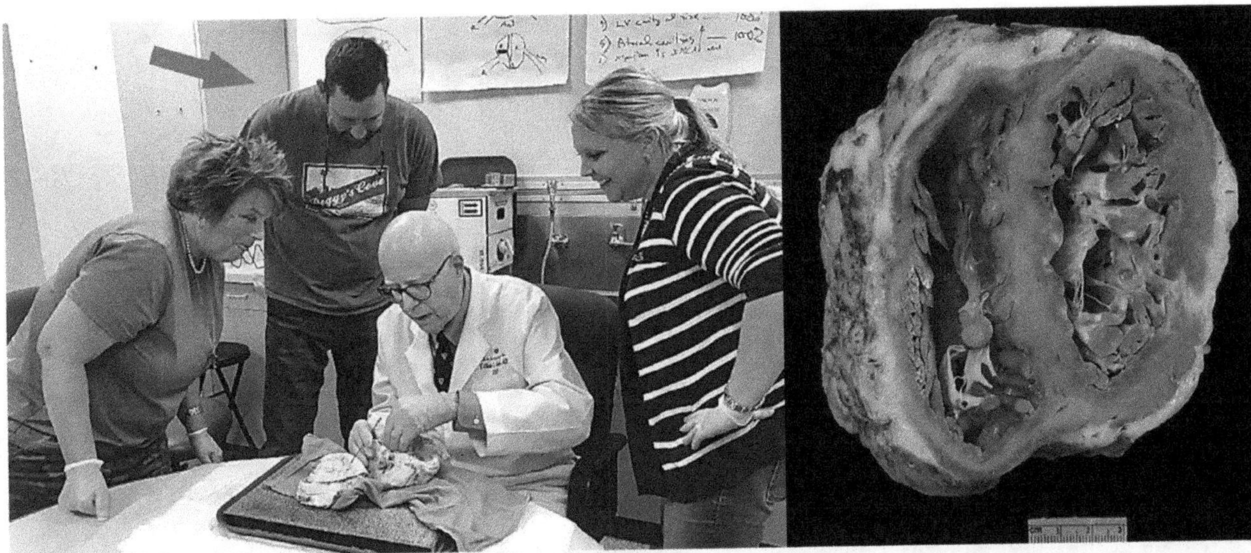

Figure 12. Robert J. Kraus (arrow), a 58-year-old man, had a heart transplant in March 2019 and the heart viewing in October 2019. His congenitally bicuspid aortic valve had been replaced when he was 21 years of age because of severe aortic regurgitation secondary to infective endocarditis. The mechanical prothesis worked well for 35 years. His resected heart weighed 915 g. Six years earlier he weighed 275 lbs. The heart is nearly surrounded by adipose tissue.

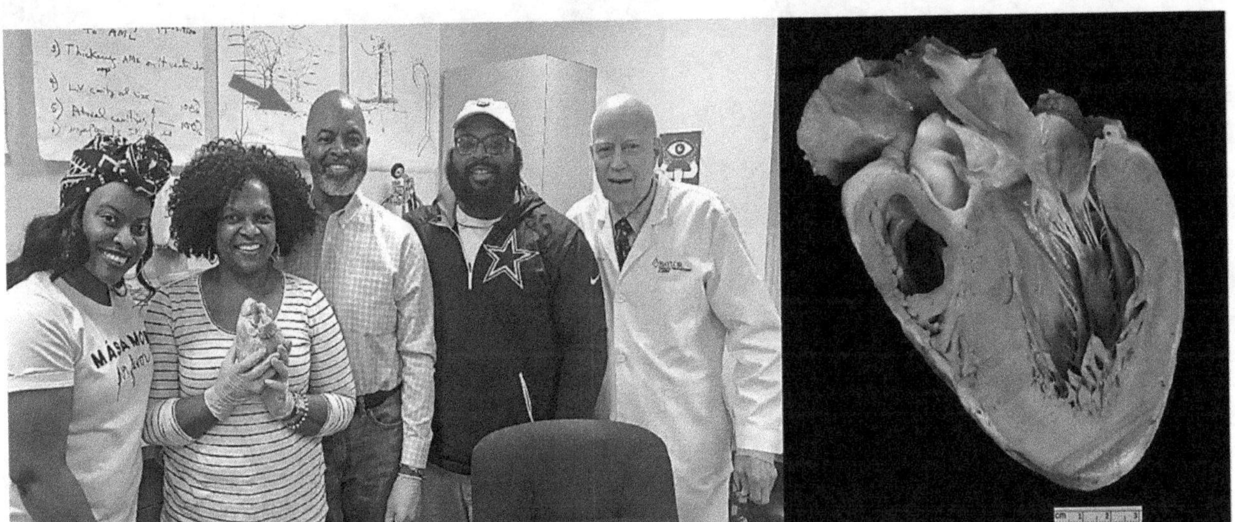

Figure 13. Ellis Robert Mayberry (arrow), a 61-year-old man, had a heart transplant in February 2019 because of amyloidosis and the heart viewing in February 2020. He has been asymptomatic subsequently. His wife, adjacent to her husband, is holding his heart. His amyloid-infiltrated heart is shown, and it weighed 580 g. He also had a renal transplant at the time of his heart transplant.

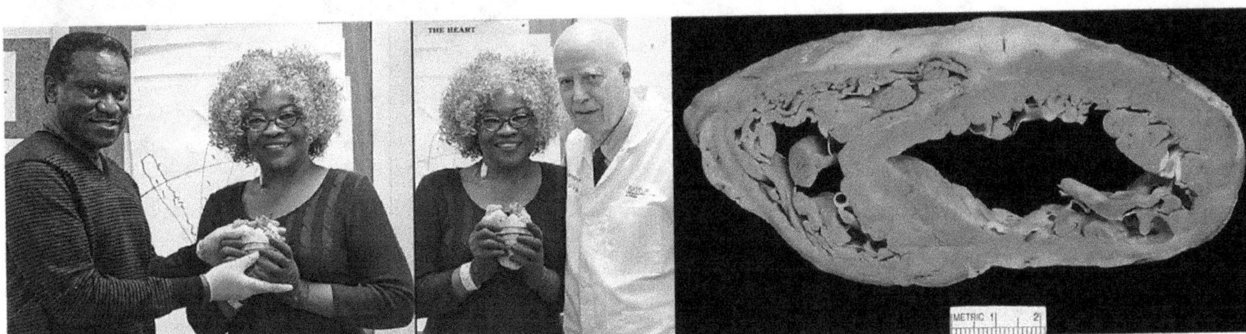

Figure 14. Sandra Jean Harvey, a 62-year-old woman, had a heart transplant in April 2017 because of idiopathic dilated cardiomyopathy and the heart viewing in January 2018. Her heart was relatively small (320 g) even though she had weighed 230 lbs. at one time. *Left*: Both she and her husband are holding her heart. *Center*: Photograph with WCR. *Right*: A cross-section of her cardiac ventricles. In her consent letter she wrote: *"I still talk about the conversation with Dr. Roberts and seeing my heart is still enlightening to me and other to do the right things for our health."*

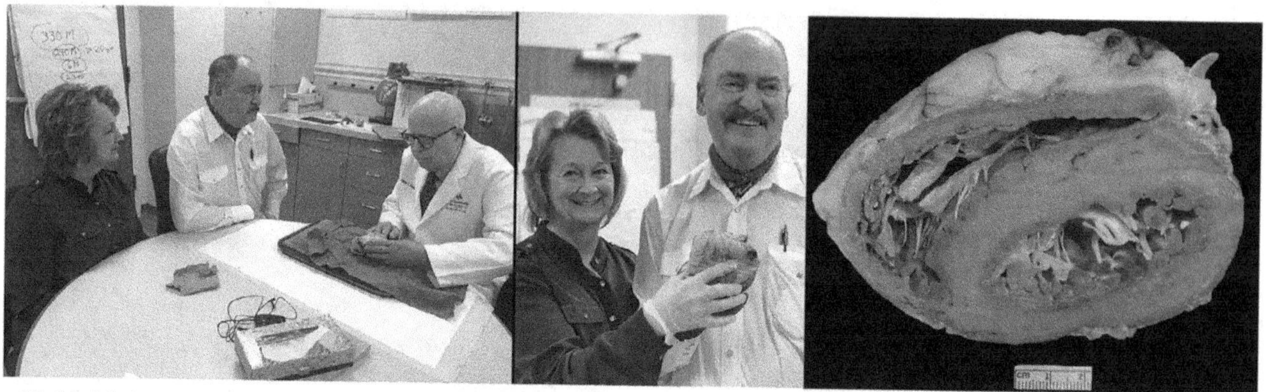

Figure 15. Mark Lehman, a 62-year-old man, had a heart transplant because of severe heart failure resulting from severe mitral regurgitation secondary to mitral valve prolapse in December 2019 and the heart viewing in January 2020. He also had severe coronary arterial narrowing but no myocardial lesions. His heart weighed 455 g.

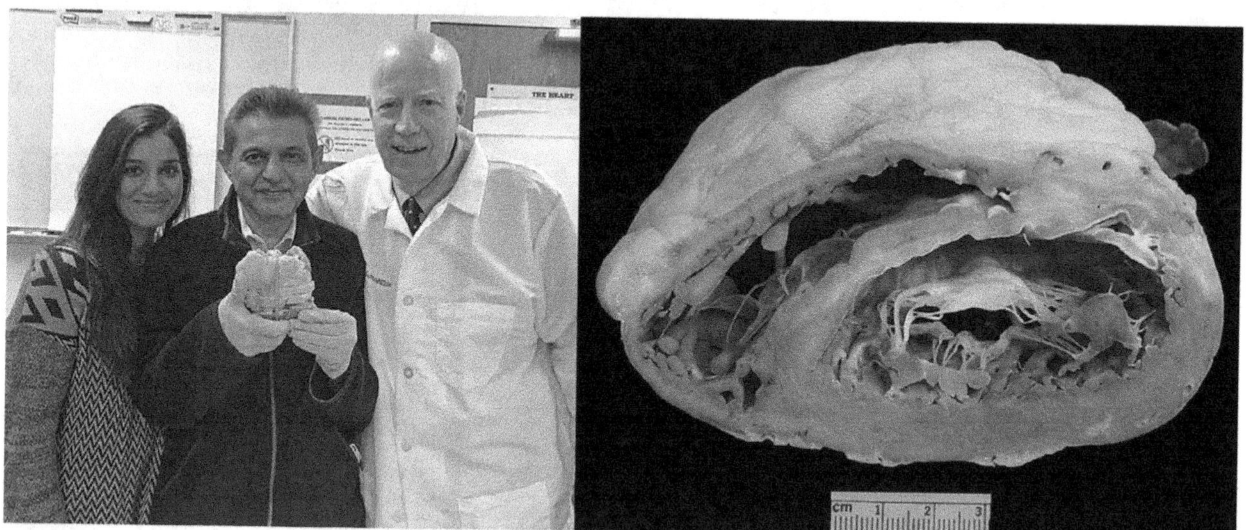

Figure 16. Habib Nooruddin, a 64-year-old man, had a heart transplant in September 2017 for ischemic cardiomyopathy and the heart viewing in November 2017. His heart weighed 302 g and he weighed 143 lbs. There is considerable scarring in the anteroseptal and anterolateral portions of his left ventricular wall. The cavity is quite dilated. The epicardial coronary arteries are severely narrowed by atherosclerotic plaque. In his consent letter he wrote: *"It's an honor to be included in your article, continuing to educate people about organ donation and how it impacts the lives of families. One donation can positively change the lives of so many individuals."*

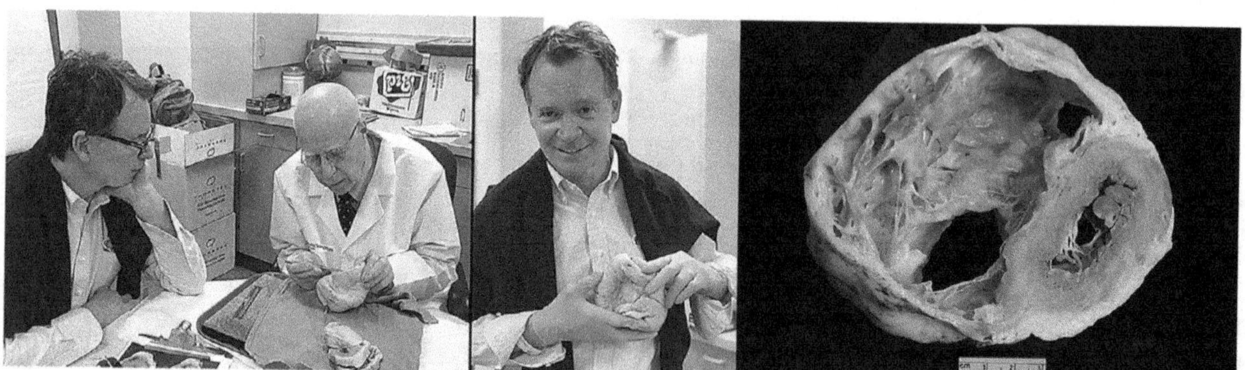

Figure 17. Zack Bacon, a 65-year-old man, had a heart transplant in July 2018 for heart failure secondary to arrhythmogenic right ventricular cardiomyopathy and the heart viewing in September 2018. *Left*: WCR explaining his heart disease to him. *Center*: Mr. Bacon is holding his own heart. *Right*: A picture of his heart showing a huge right ventricular cavity, a much smaller left ventricular cavity, and much of the right ventricular free wall replaced by adipose tissue. His heart weighed 485 g.

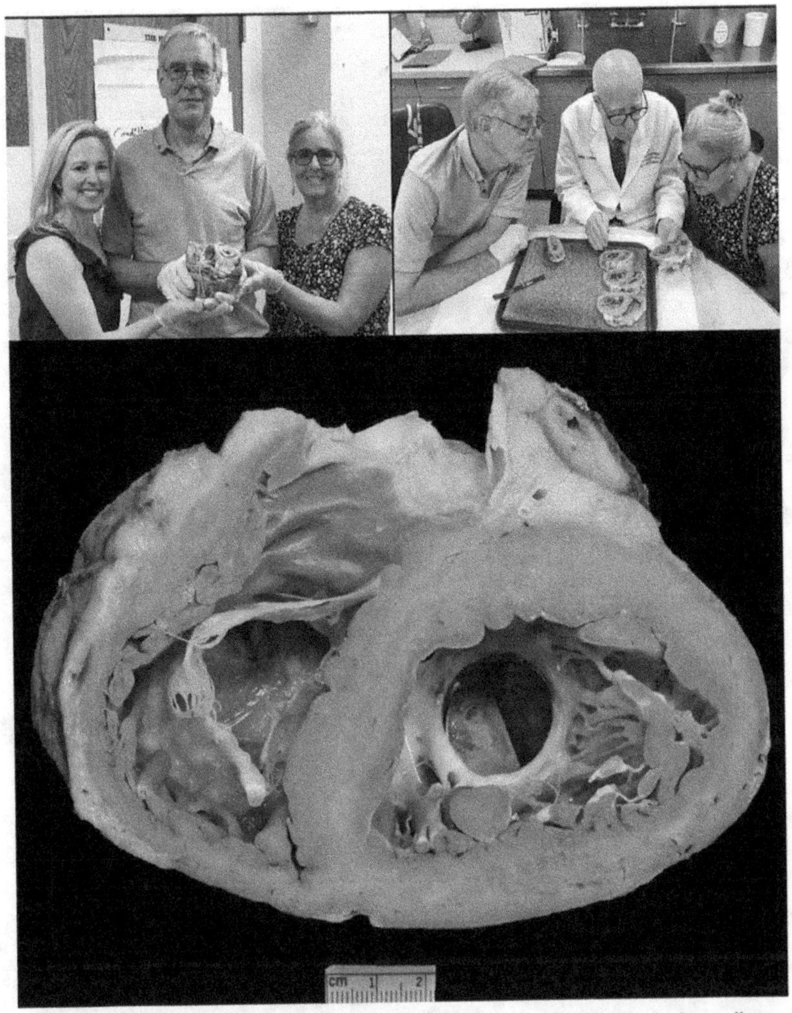

Figure 18. Mark Francis Gengler, a 66-year-old man, had a heart transplant in May 2019 for probable valvular heart disease and the heart viewing in September 2019. At age 46, both mitral and aortic valves were replaced, and his ascending aorta was resected and replaced. His heart weighed 620 g. He has done well since the transplant.

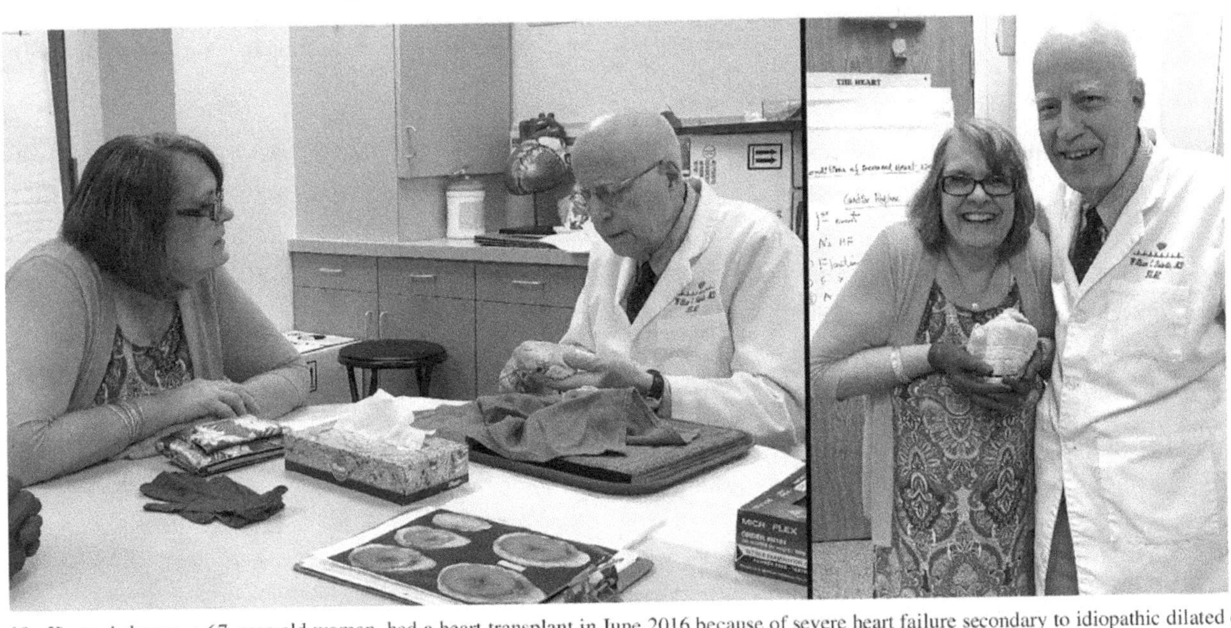

Figure 19. Karen Acheson, a 67-year-old woman, had a heart transplant in June 2016 because of severe heart failure secondary to idiopathic dilated cardiomyopathy and the heart viewing in August 2018. She has been asymptomatic ever since. Her heart weighed 460 g.

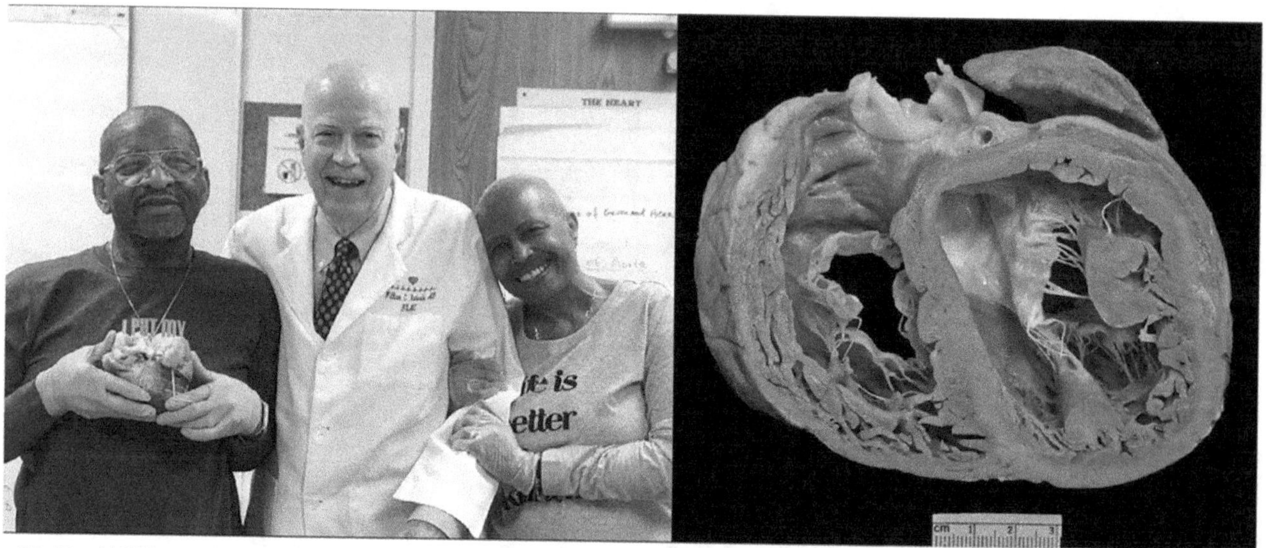

Figure 20. Harold Wilson, a 68-year-old man, had a heart transplant in April 2019 for heart failure secondary to idiopathic dilated cardiomyopathy and the heart viewing in September 2019. He has been asymptomatic subsequently. His heart weighed 385 g. At one time he weighed 270 lbs. He weighed 199 lbs. at the time of the transplant. In his consent letter he wrote: "*...thank you guys for all you've done in my life.*"

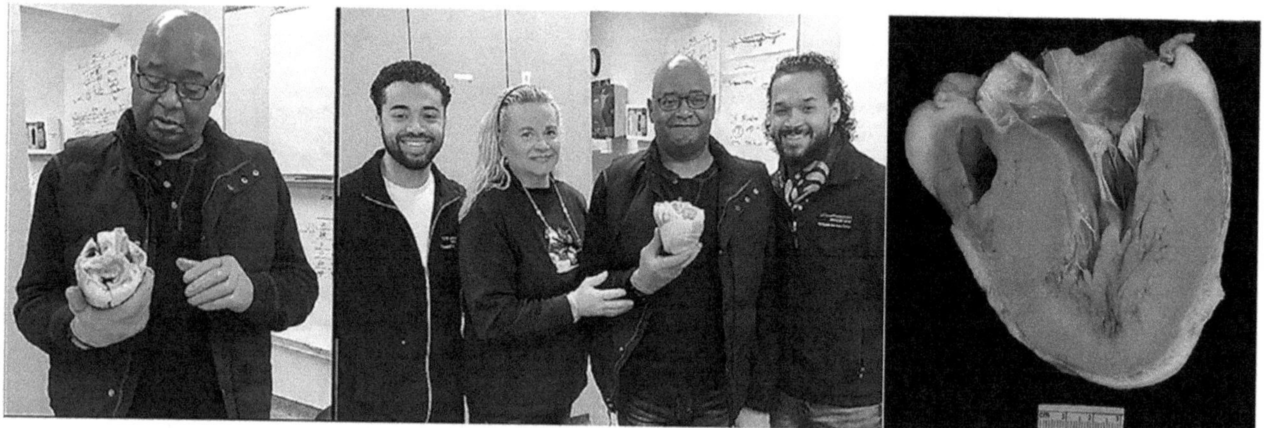

Figure 21. Alphonso Robinson, a 69-year-old man, had a heart transplant in August 2019 because of heart failure secondary to cardiac amyloidosis and the heart viewing in December 2019. He has been asymptomatic subsequently. *Left:* Mr. Robinson looking at his heart. *Center*: Mr. Robinson holding his heart with his wife and two children. *Right*: His amyloid-infiltrated heart weighed 580 g.

Author credit statement

None.

Disclosures

The authors have no conflicts of interest to disclose.

1. Roberts WC. So you want to see your heart. *Am J Cardiol* 2010;106:1520.
2. Roberts WC, Won VS, Vasudevan A, Kapoor P, Ko JM, Meyer DM, Hall SA, Gonzalez-Stawinski G. Comparison of characteristics of patients undergoing heart transplantation in the same hospital in two different time periods (1997 – 2012 and 2013-2015). *Am J Cardiol* 2016;118:288–291.

The Importance of Acquiring Financial Security for Physicians

William C. Roberts, MD

Baylor Scott & White Heart and Vascular Institute, Baylor University Medical Center, Dallas, Texas.

ABSTRACT

This review tries to make the case that physicians should be adequately rewarded financially so that they can have a clear fiduciary responsibility to do only what is best for their patients without unseemly personal financial gain. To develop financial security, physicians need to save a portion of their income regularly to invest. The stock market is the best place to increase one's monetary worth over a long period.

 • *The American Journal of Medicine (2020) 133:1403–1405*

KEYWORDS: Avoid debt; Avoid divorce; Conservative; Diversification; Dividends; Finance; Frugality; Long-term investor; Save; Stay healthy; Stock market

Herb Shriner (1918-1970) (American humorist, radio and television personality, and famous harmonica player) once said "Our doctor would never really operate unless it was necessary. He was just that way. If he didn't need the money, he wouldn't lay a hand on you."

A Punch cartoon in 1925:

Doctor: What did you operate on Jones for?
Surgeon: A hundred pounds.
Doctor: No, I mean what had he got?
Surgeon: A hundred pounds.

Physicians are often faced with dilemmas: one may provide a nice financial reward to the physician and the other, none or little personal financial benefit. Physicians, of course, have a fiduciary responsibility to do only what is best for the patient. Financially insecure physicians might be less prone to obey this fiduciary principle than financially secure physicians. Physicians, in my view, should always have an income where a decision for a patient is never influenced by personal financial reward! This type of thinking prompted this piece about physicians' acquiring financial security. It is based on investing in the stock market over a 50-year period.

1) Save. Saving is the key to building wealth. Be frugal. Small sums saved regularly add up to large sums over time. Learn to get as much pleasure out of saving a dollar as spending a dollar. Never buy a house or an automobile that you cannot afford. Prior to purchasing anything, ask yourself if you really need this item. Forget the $4 cup of coffee. Don't smoke (a pack of cigarettes [n = 20] now costs $10). Eat out less. Vegetarianism is not only a healthy lifestyle but also an inexpensive one. Trade babysitting with friends instead of hiring a babysitter. Check for unnecessary charges on monthly bills. Learn to do routine maintenance projects around the house.
2) Invest in the stock market. Despite what is going on presently (COVID-19 pandemic), the stock market is the best place to increase one's monetary worth over a long period.
3) Acquire a certain amount (ideally >$10,000 or the equivalent of 4 to 6 months' income) to respond to emergencies (eg, getting fired, medical bills, the Coronavirus) prior to investing in stocks. A low-fee Standard and Poor's Stock Index Fund might be considered. This fund provides ready diversity, but it also includes purchasing the bad stocks as well as the good ones. It is also probably better than buying individual stocks for one not really interested in spending

Funding: None.
Conflict of Interest: None.
Authorship: As sole author, I am responsible for all content.

Requests for reprints should be addressed to William C. Roberts, MD, Baylor Scott & White Heart and Vascular Institute, 621 N. Hall Street, Suite H-030, Dallas, Texas 75226.

E-mail address: William.Roberts1@bswhealth.org

the time necessary to become relatively savvy with stocks. A preferable alternative might be Warren Buffett's Berkshire Hathaway, a collection of about 80 companies plus shares in a variety of companies not managed by Berkshire Hathaway. In contrast to the Standard & Poor's collection of stocks, Buffett has few bad stocks!

4) Learn patience. The market always swings: goes up and down. Do not panic. Most stock owners buy stocks when they are too high and sell them when they are too low. Doing the opposite is the way to make money. If price swings are too much for your nervous system, stay out of the market.
5) Diversify. Do not overweigh any one area: technology, financials, industrials, transportation, utilities, health care, telecommunications, oil and gas, basic materials. One area is usually up when another is down. Those who invested predominately in technology in the 1990s lost a fortune. Try to buy stocks in the area that is down for the moment.
6) Favor stocks that pay dividends. If a stock goes down and it pays a dividend, one still earns money during its down cycle. One potentially loses money only when the stock is sold.
7) Recognize the beauty of compound interest, which Einstein called "the greatest invention."
8) Put a "limit" on the price you will pay for a stock. Never indicate buy "at market."
9) Have an investment goal and stick to it.
10) Beware of stock tips from friends and neighbors. No one has a monopoly on successful stock picking. Have a good reason for purchasing or selling a particular stock.
11) Avoid mutual funds and annuities. The fees are too high. There are no fees now for buying or selling a stock online!
12) Never buy or sell all at once. Start buying slowly. If the price falls, buy more; if the price rises, do not feel obligated to chase it.
13) Have a list of stocks to watch so when the price falls sufficiently, jump on it.
14) Avoid shorting stocks unless you become a knowledgeable pro. Be a long-term investor.
15) Never borrow money to buy stocks. "Margin accounts" are dangerous.
16) Survey your stocks daily. It takes only a few minutes. The correct number of stocks to own varies with one's interest in keeping up with them. Always be on the lookout for good buys. Know why you purchased or sold a particular stock.
17) Be more conservative as you get older. Take more risks when young.
18) Beware of bonds. They are for old people. With stocks you buy shares of the company—a part ownership. Bonds represent loans to companies.
19) Beware of trying to time the market—when it will rise or fall. Always keep some cash available for purchasing stocks when their prices are low.
20) Invest for the long term. Frequent trading rarely pays.
21) Prior to buying a stock, know its price/earnings (P/E) ratio (its price compared with its earnings); dividend; debt; percent of its net used to pay its dividend; range of its stock price, at least in the last year; views of various analysts; and whether it presently has legal issues. I tend to avoid stocks with high P/E ratios. But, be cautious when the P/E ratio falls considerably because the price of the stock may have fallen considerably. Check on the number of years that the stock has paid a dividend, and whether the dividend increased or decreased through the years.
22) Look favorably at stocks that Warren Buffett owns. Consider purchase as soon as you learn what companies or stocks he has recently purchased. (He does not have to announce his purchases until he has had them for 6 months.) Buffet is not perfect, however. He has lost big on airlines recently, for example.
23) Listen to business channels. Nearly every stock has its proponents and detractors. Learn if your instincts are good and if so, go with them.
24) Buy stocks in companies you believe in. Refrain from buying stocks in companies that produce products not good for your health, tobacco companies or fast-food chains, for example.
25) Subscribe to *The Wall Street Journal* and *Barron's*. You can deduct their subscription costs from your taxes. Barron's, particularly, provides many ideas for stock market investors.
26) Do not ignore recent trends and try to get out early: retail stores, particularly those located in malls (the overwhelming power of Amazon), one-product companies (upstart pharmaceutical or technology companies.)
27) Stay out of debt. One can never make much money in the stock market or elsewhere if the buyer is in debt. Never have credit card debt! The interest rate is too high, nearly 20%. Try to make mortgage loans a 15-year proposition,

CLINICAL SIGNIFICANCE

- Physicians need to develop financial security so that their patient decisions are free of inappropriate financial reward.
- That requires becoming financially secure, which requires regular savings and appropriate spending.
- The best way to become financially secure is to invest in the stock market regularly over a long period of time.
- Buying and holding is not ideal, but it is better than frequent buying and selling.
- Stay out of debt.
- Stay healthy and live long. Good health is better than gold.

not a 30-year one. Do not make a loan where paying it off early produces a penalty. Try to obtain a mortgage loan that allows the paying of next month's principle with the present month's principle plus interest. Then, the next month's interest is nullified. Try to save for the next car during the years between car purchases so that a car loan will not be necessary. Unless you plan to keep your vehicle for 10 or more years, consider a used car. Leasing is more expensive than buying.

28) Try not to divorce. Get a prenuptial agreement. Marry a frugal person!
29) Beware of sales. Although, of course, sales save the buyer money, many of us buy things we do not need when they are on sale.
30) Do not let the price of a stock be confused with its value. Fallen stocks are certainly worth investigating, as their problems may be temporary, but they also may be facing insurmountable challenges that will sink them further. Think twice about selling a stock near its 52-week high. The best stocks tend to keep hitting new highs over decades, rewarding patient investors. Beware of purchasing very low-priced stocks (<$5.00).
31) Have a monthly budget. Know where your money is going. Start with recording any fixed monthly payments: rent or mortgage, loan repayments, cable bills, cell phone charges, gym membership fees, prescription drugs. Next, record variable monthly expenses: groceries, restaurant meals, clothing, recreation, transportation, electricity. Next, record infrequent or nonrecurring expenses: insurance, vacation travel, dental work, tuition payments, etc. Finally, subtract your total spending from your total income. Ideally, cover one's monthly expenses and still manage to save 10% of the income for savings and investments. Find ways to shrink spending, a requirement if spending exceeds income. Call your credit card company at year's end for a summary of your year's spending.
32) Avoid retiring early. Start saving early for retirement. Do not procrastinate. Wasting less time usually leads to wasting less money.
33) Calculate stock profits and losses annually. If you buy a stock for $40 and it rises to $80, that is a 100% gain ("a 2-bagger"). If it goes from $40 to $44, that is a 10% gain. But, if the $40 stock at purchase falls to $20, to get back to $40 it will need a 100% gain; if it falls to $10, to return to $40 the stock would need to quadruple in price.
34) Don't be fooled by the splitting of a stock. If you own, let's say, 100 shares of a company at $10 each, a forward split might increase the number of shares to 200, but each share would be worth $5. Thus, there is no financial gain. Unfortunately, there is the reverse split (a red flag), whereby the stock price is increased, and the number of shares is decreased. Let's say you own 100 shares of a $4 stock and the company executes a 1-for-10 reverse split. You will then end up with a $40 stock but own only 10 shares of it. Citigroup did this a few years back. Occasionally, a company will pay its dividend by providing shares of its stock.
35) Study the 1929 US stock market crash, the worst event that ever happened to the US stock market. In October 1929, in 2 days (28th and 29th) the Dow Jones Industrial Average ("Dow") fell 25%. (In the COVID-19 crash in 2020, the Dow fell 30% in 30 days! The 1929 crash in today's terms would mean more than a 6000-point drop in 2 days.) The Dow peaked at 381 on September 3, 1929, and finally hit "bedrock" at 41 on July 8, 1932, a 90% decline in 35 months. That does not include reinvested dividends, but most investors in those days took their dividends in cash. That fall is equivalent to investing $1 in the stock market and its shrinking to 10 cents. No one foresaw how long and how terrible that bear market would be. The Dow did not surpass its 1929 high until November 23, 1954, 25 years later! The exact reason(s) for the 1929 crash remain unclear.
36) Own some gold in your portfolio, ideally about 5% to 10% of your investments. Buy gold coins and put them in your bank safety deposit box.
37) Stay healthy and live long. Good health is better than gold, advised Mahatma Gandhi.

P.S. A side benefit to picking individual stocks is that the picker learns a great deal about himself/herself: whether one is basically conservative or a risk taker, the degree of one's patience, one's worry level, one's reasoning and analytical ability, whether one finds buying and selling stocks pleasant and educational or an unpleasant activity, and finally, how one handles "the winning hand," "the losing hand," and the uncertainty in general. I have found the decision to buy a stock to be far easier than the decision to sell a stock.

Aortic Intimal-Medial Tear Without Dissection, the Marfan Syndrome, and Its Forme Fruste Variety

William C. Roberts, MD[1,2,3,*], Minseob Jeong, MD[1], and Charles S. Roberts, MD[4]

Acute aortic dissection is a relatively common disease involving the aorta. All aortic dissections start with an intimal-medial tear prior to the medial dissection. Several cases of aortic intimal-medial tear without dissection have been reported previously, but only one article presented a photograph of the intimal-medial tear. Herein, we describe 16 patients whose ascending aortas were operatively excised because of what clinically was believed to be acute aortic dissection. Of the 16 patients, 14 had aortic intimal-medial tears without dissection and the other 2 had acute medial dissection of the aorta adjacent to a healed aortic intimal-medial tear without dissection. These aortic intimal-medial tears have been seen in the Marfan syndrome, but none of our 16 patients had the Marfan syndrome. At least 9 of the 16 patients, however, had had aortas similar to those seen in the Marfan syndrome (forme fruste variety). Although the 8 surgeons who operated on these 16 patients described the intimal-medial tears as "aortic dissection", only 2 had acute dissection adjacent to a healed intimal-medial tear without dissection. In conclusion, although the aortic intimal-medial tear is the initiator of aortic dissection, some patients with intimal-medial tears have no accompanying dissection. **(Am J Cardiol 2022;184:31−40)**

Introduction

Acute aortic dissection is the most common primary disease of the ascending aorta.[1] Aortic dissection begins with an intimal-medial tear and the dissection usually propagates in the outer media. On rare occasion an intimal-medial tear occurs in the ascending aorta without leading to medial dissection. Although previously seen in the ascending aorta in the Marfan syndrome,[2] the present study describes 16 patients seen in a 12-year period with classic intimal-medial tear in the ascending aorta unaccompanied by medial dissection. A description of these cases is the purpose of this report.

Patients studied

From January 2010 to March 2022, sixteen operatively resected ascending aortas with intimal-medial tears without dissection were submitted to the Surgical Pathology division of the Department of Pathology at Baylor University Medical Center. All specimens were examined and the official reports submitted by WCR. Later, all specimens were examined by MJ. All specimens were photographed by Ms. Saba Ilyas. All specimens had sections of aorta prepared for histologic study and all sections were stained by both hematoxylin-eosin and by the Movat method.[3] The clinical records were examined by both WCR and MJ.

[1]Baylor Scott & White Heart and Vascular Institute; [2]the Departments of Internal Medicine; [3]Pathology; and [4]Cardiac Surgery Baylor University Medical Center, Baylor Scott & White Health, Dallas, Texas. Manuscript received June 23, 2022; revised manuscript received and accepted August 9, 2022.

*Corresponding Author: William C. Roberts, MD, Baylor Scott & White Heart and Vascular Institute, 621 N. Hall Street, Suite H-030, Dallas, Texas 75226. (214) 820-7911 Office; (214) 820-7533 Fax

E-mail address: william.roberts1@bswhealth.org (W.C. Roberts).

Results

Clinical and morphologic findings in the 16 patients are summarized in Table 1. Their ages ranged from 27 to 86 years (mean 54); 12 (75%) were men, 4 (25%) were women. Eleven (69%) had a body mass index > 25 kg/m^2. Although no patient was diagnosed clinically as having characteristic features of the Marfan syndrome, 9 (56%) had major loss of aortic medial elastic fibers (4+/4+) as these patients almost certainly had the forme fruste variety of the Marfan syndrome (Figure 1). Eight had an indirect blood pressure of > 140 mmHg systolic or > 90 mmHg diastolic or both. The sinus portion of aorta (11 patients) ranged from 34 to 70 mm in diameter (mean 52), and the tubular portion of aorta (15 patients) ranged from 33 to 63 mm (mean 52). The aortic valve was 3 cuspid in 12 patients (75%) and congenitally bicuspid in 4 (25%). The aortic valve was stenotic in 1 of the 12 patients with three-cuspid aortic valves and in 1 of the 4 patients with bicuspid valves. Some degree of aortic regurgitation was present in 15 patients (94%). The aortic valve was replaced in 9 (56%) of the 16 patients. Examination of the ascending aorta disclosed severe loss of medial elastic fibers (4+/4+) in 9 patients, 1+/4+ in 2, and normal number of medial elastic fibers (0/4+) in 5 patients. The aorta is illustrated in 11 of the 16 patients (Figures 2 − 12).

Discussion

Described herein are 16 patients whose dilated ascending aorta was excised because clinically each was believed to have aortic medial dissection. Examination, however, of the operatively resected aorta disclosed an intimal-medial healed tear in 14 without medial dissection, and in the other 2 patients a healed intimal-medial tear with dissection adjacent to an acute intimal-medial tear leading to an acute

Table 1

Clinical and morphologic findings in 16 patients who underwent resection of the ascending aorta and had intimal-medial tear without dissection at Baylor University Medical Center from January 2010 to March 2022

Variable	Case #1	Case #2	Case #3	Case #4	Case #5	Case #6	Case #7	Case #8	Case #9[b]	Case #10	Case #11	Case #12	Case #13	Case #14[d]	Case #15	Case #16
Age at operation (years)	27	31	36	39	39	47	53	54	61	62	68	71	77	77	78	86
Race	B	B	W	B	A	B	N	W	W	W	W	B	W	W	W	W
Sex	M	M	M	F	F	M	M	M	M	M	F	M	F	M	M	M
Body weight (lbs)	201	168	180	288	93	179	234	205	146	221	114	253	164	196	190	215
Height (in)	72	75	70	65	60	74	72	75	73	71	65	70	63	72	70	67
Body mass index (kg/m2)	27.2	21.2	25.8	47.9	18.2	23.0	31.7	25.6	19.3	30.8	19.0	36.4	29.1	26.6	27.3	33.7
Forme Fruste variety of the Marfan syndrome	+	+	0	+	+	0	0	+	0	0	0	+	+	+	+	0
Systemic hypertension																
by history	0	0	+	+	0	+	+	0	+	+	+	+	+	+	+	+
by antihypertensive medication	0	0	+	+	+	0	+	+	+	+	+	+	+	+	+	+
by indirect blood pressure recording (mmHg)	110/60	110/70	125/65	130/60	110/75	130/60	115/60	105/55	95/60	105/60	130/60	120/75	120/60	125/65	120/75	110/80
highest recorded blood pressure (mmHg)	110/60	130/80	165/95	130/60	130/80	140/80	130/75	140/80	155/60	155/70	145/70	155/85	150/70	145/70	155/75	110/80
Acute type A aortic dissection with previously healed aortic intimal medial tear	0	0	+	0	0	0	0	0	0[c]	0	0	0[c]	0	+	0	0
Preoperative arrhythmias	0	0	0	0	0	0	0	+ (AF)	0	0	0	0	0	+ (AF)	+ (SVT)	0
Number of narrowed (>75%) major coronary arteries	0	0	0	+[a]	0	+ (3)	0	0	0	0	+ (1)	0	0	0	0	0
Coronary artery bypass grafting	0	0	0	0	0	+	0	0	0	0	0	0	0	0	0	0
Bentall procedure	+	+	0	+	0	+	+	+	+	0	0	0	0	0	+	0
Renal replacement therapy	0	0	+	0	0	0	0	0	0	0	0	0	0	0	0	0
Left ventricular ejection fraction (%)	50	50	50	30	50	40	60	20	60	60	55	65	55	55	70	50
Diameter of the left ventricle (cm)																
at diastole	5.2	"normal"	"normal"	"dilated"	"normal"	6.4	"normal"	"normal"	4.2	7.0	-	-	"normal"	"dilated"	4.8	5.9
at systole	3.9	-	-	-	-	5.1	-	-	2.5	5.2	-	-	-	-	2.8	4.3
Diameter of ascending aorta (mm)																
sinus portion	↑↑↑	61 [E]	-	50 [E]	51 [E]	50 [E]	60 [E]	38 [E]	34 [E]	72 [E]	-	50 [CT]	-	-	-	53 [E]
tubular portion	56 [E]	63 [E]	45 [E]	-	33 [E]	52 [E]	56 [E]	52 [E]	53 [E]	50 [E]	53 [CT]	55 [CT]	44 [E]	63 [E]	51 [CT]	52 [E]
Aortic valve function																
stenosis	0	0	0	0	0	0	0	0	+	0	0	0	0	0	+	0
regurgitation	+	+	+	+	+	+	+	+	+	+	0	+	+	+	+	+
Number of aortic valve cusps	3	3	3	3	3	3	2	2	2	3	2	3	3	3	3	3
Aortic valve replacement (weight [g])	+ (0.59)	+ (0.33)	0	+ (0.50)	0	+ (0.60)	+ (0.52)	+ (1.28)	+ (2.35)	0	0	0	0	0	+ (2.16)	+ (0.72)
Weight of ascending aorta excised (g)	13.8	13.6	10.5	0.8	3.6	18.8	17.9	8.1	14.3	17.0	10.5	11.4	11.0	14	11.2	23.1
Medial elastic fiber loss (0 - 4+)	4+	4+	0	4+	4+	0	1+	4+	0	0	0	4+	4+	4+	4+	1+

A = Asian; AF = atrial fibrillation; B = Black; CT = computed tomography; E = echocardiogram; F = female; M = male; N = native American; SVT = supraventricular tachycardia; W = White

[a] CAD involving multiple major coronary arteries associated with Kawasaki disease that prompted the patient to undergo coronary artery bypass grafting 7 years prior to resection of the aneurysmal ascending aorta

[b] The patient died 38 days postoperatively

[c] Aortic intimal-medial tear without dissection associated with healed chronic type B aortic dissection

[d] Brother of the patient had acute type A aortic dissection

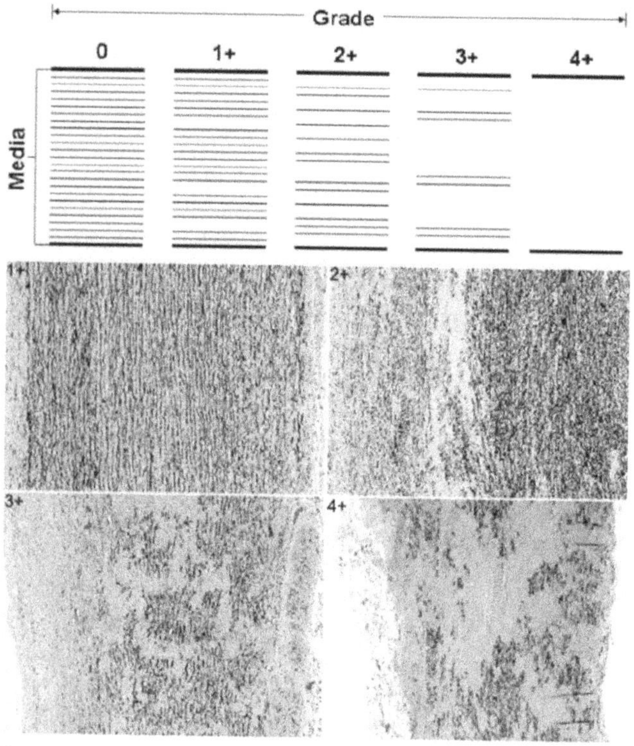

Figure 1. Diagram showing the grading system used in this study. (Top) Diagram showing 0 to 4+ loss of medial elastic fibers. The internal (top dark line) and external (bottom dark line) elastic membranes and elastic fibers in the media (lighter lines) are represented. (Bottom) The photomicrographs show loss of the medial elastic fibers from 1+ (middle left) to 4+ (lower right) (Movat stain X 100). (Reproduced with permission from W. C. Roberts and the publisher of Circulation 2011;123:896-903.)

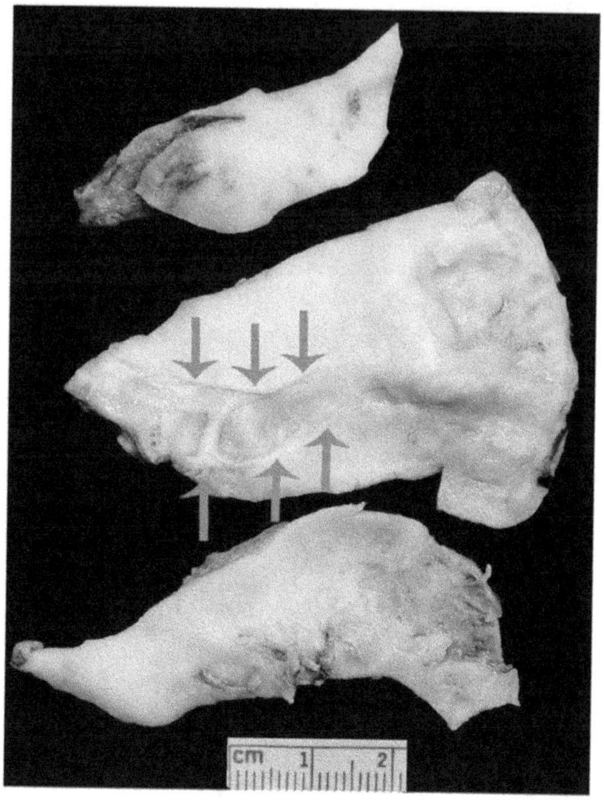

Figure 2. Table 1, **Case #1.** Shown here are three operatively excised portions of ascending aorta in a 27-year-old man who had almost certainly the forme fruste form of the Marfan Syndrome. Shown in the larger fragments are 2 intimal medial tears between the arrows. Histologic examination of the aorta disclosed 4+/4+ loss of medial elastic fibers. There was no aortic dissection.

medial dissection. Two of the 14 patients without acute type A medial dissection had a healed medial dissection involving the descending thoracic aorta with a healed intimal-medial tear at the aortic isthmus. Some degree of aortic regurgitation occurred in 15 (94%) of the 16 patients. Each of the 8 surgeons who operated on the 16 patients included in this study all described "aortic dissection" as the diagnosis from examination of the excised ascending aorta.

It seems reasonable to believe that healed intimal-medial tear without medial dissection described herein are related to the Marfan syndrome. Indeed, Roberts and Honig[2] in 1982 described 18 patients at necropsy with classic clinical features of the Marfan syndrome: 13 had dilated ascending aortas including both sinus and tubular portions, and 8 of them had healed intimal-medial tears in the ascending aorta without medial dissection, identical lesions to those found in the present 16 patients. All 13 patients had severe loss of medial elastic fibers; 3 other patients with the Marfan syndrome described by Roberts and Honig had typical acute aortic dissection with an intimal-medial tear in ascending aorta but histologic examination of the wall of the aorta disclosed no loss of medial elastic fibers, i.e., normal aorta except for the acute dissection. It appears that the media of an aortic wall is difficult to dissect if it is extensively replaced by a great deal of fibrous tissue (grade 4+/4+) (Figure 1).

None of the 16 patients in the present study had the Marfan syndrome but 13 had severe dilatation of the ascending and 9 of them had severe loss of medial elastic fiber loss (4 +/4+) (Figure 1), both being typical findings of the Marfan syndrome.[2,4] The aortic findings typical of the Marfan but without the typical skeleton and ocular finding of the syndrome generally go by the name "forme fruste" variety of the syndrome.

Four of the patients included herein had congenitally bicuspid aortic valves, stenotic in 1, purely regurgitant in 2, and functionally normal in 1. One of the patients (#8, Table 1) with a purely regurgitant aortic valve had 4+/4+ loss of medial elastic fibers and the other 3 had no significant loss.

Aortic intimal-medial tears without dissection has gone by a variety of names,[2,5-11] shown in Table 2. We believe that this entity is not a part of the condition referred to as "intramural hematoma." Only one of those previously described articles illustrated a healed tear.[6]

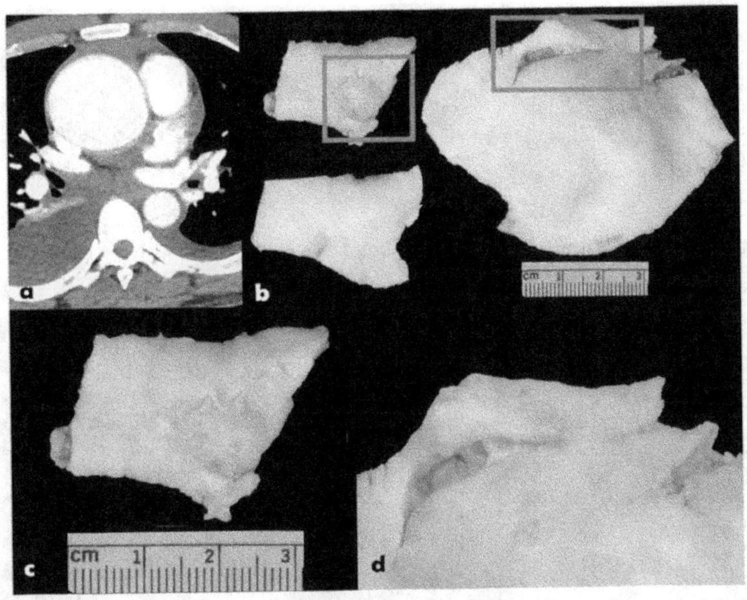

Figure 3. Table 1, **Case #2.** Shown here is the computed tomographic image of the very dilated ascending aorta (a) and portions of the aorta which were operatively excised showing at least 2 intimal medial tears. The one on the bottom left is a healed tear and the one on the bottom right a is a more recent tear, neither of which led to aortic dissection.

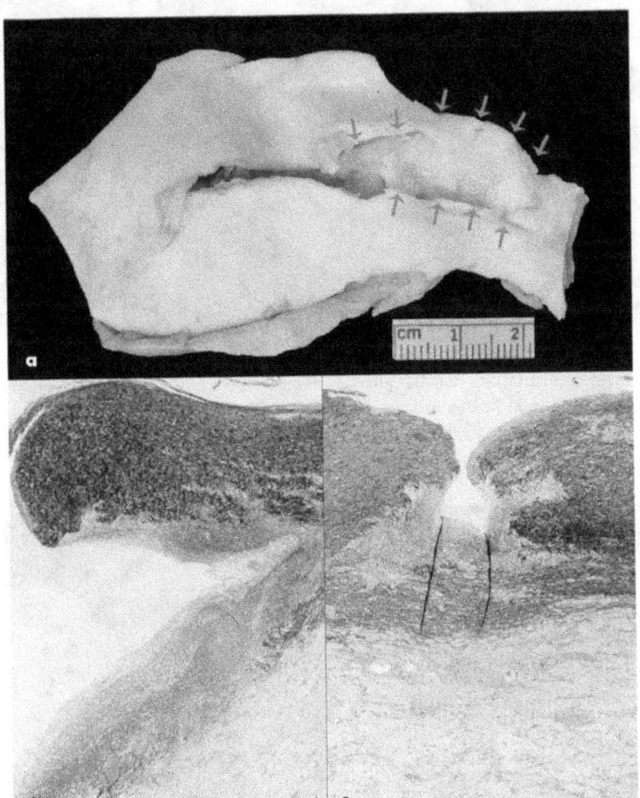

Figure 4. Table 1, **Case # 3.** Shown here is an open ascending aorta showing a healed tear between the arrows without dissection adjacent to an acute tear leading to type A aortic dissection. b, a histologic section of a portion of the healed tear showing the tear to the left of the protrusion and that tear went through 90% of the wall of the aorta but it did not lead to dissection. With time the tear stretched out but nearly all of the elastic fibers in the media are gone from the base of the tear. It appears that the number of elastic fibers in the media before the initial tear or the second tear were normal. Shown in c is another intimal medial tear without dissection which extended about 75% through the wall of the aorta, again the elastic fibers are essentially normal. The base of the tear has some loss of elastic fibers with replacement by nonelastic fibrous tissue. This patient was only 36 years of age. The patient had a Bentall procedure performed. It also appears that there were no symptoms resulting from the intimal medial tear which healed but acute symptoms resulting from the acute tear adjacent to the previous healed tear.

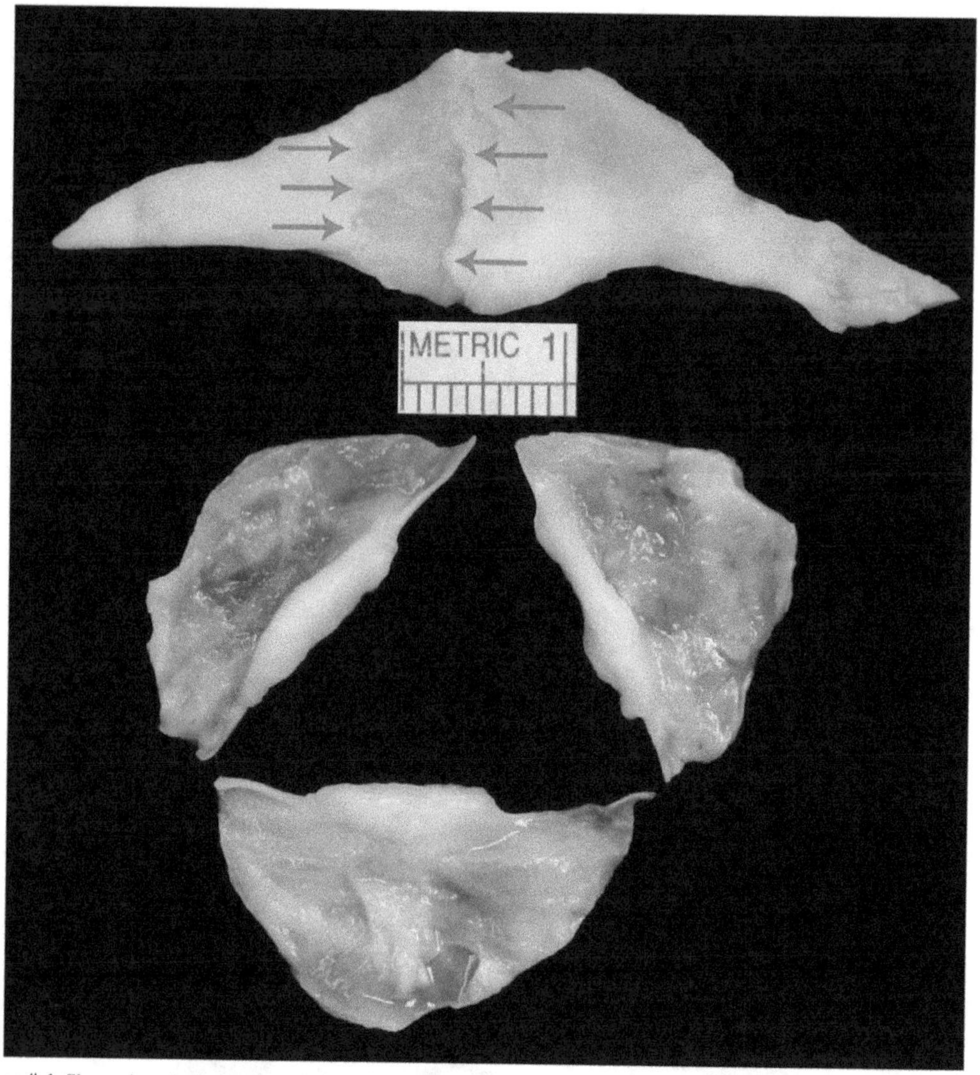

Figure 5. Table 1, **Case # 4.** Shown here is the portion of ascending aorta that was operatively excised with a healed tear, not leading to dissection, between the arrows. The patient had considerable aortic regurgitation, and the aortic valve was consequently operatively excised. The fibrous thickening of the free margin, particularly in the central portion of each cusp, indicates that there was chronic aortic regurgitation.

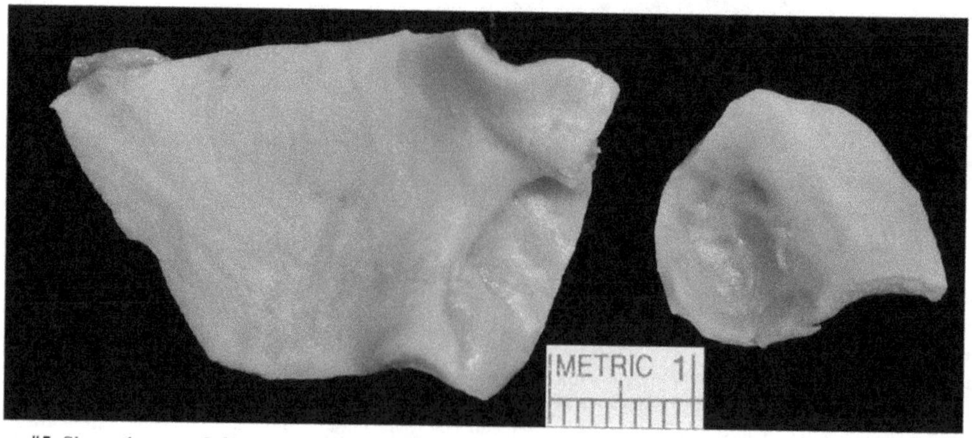

Figure 6. Table 1, **Case #5.** Shown here are 2 fragments of the ascending aorta that were operatively excised. Each shows an intimal medial tear unassociated with a dissection.

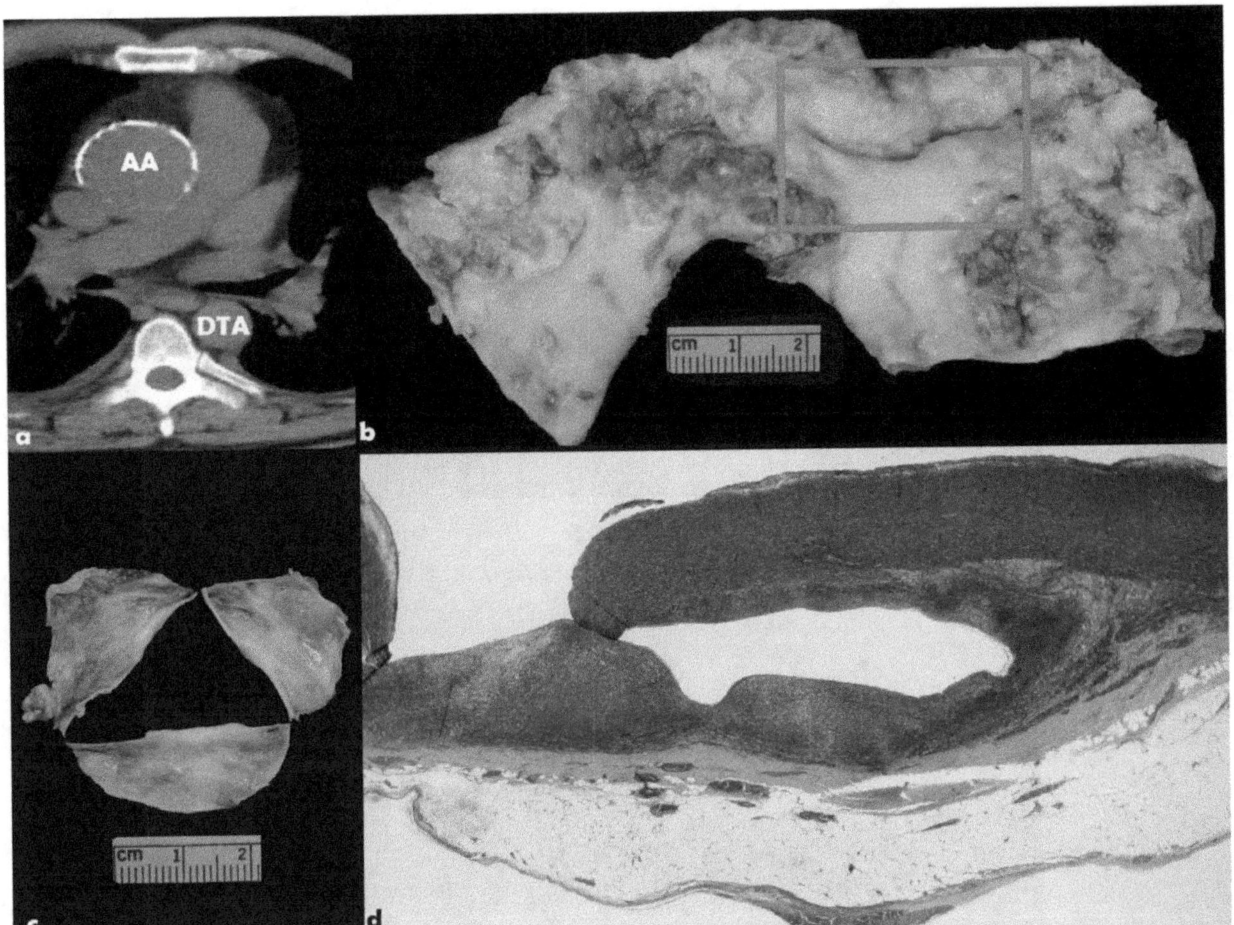

Figure 7. Table 1, **Case #6.** Shown here in a is an aortogram showing the dilated ascending aorta (AA) with calcific deposits in much of the aortic wall. The red arrow points to a saccular aneurysm which is probably the healed tear. The descending thoracic aorta (DTA) is much smaller than the ascending aorta. In b the healed intimal medial tear is enclosed in the red box. The unusual feature of this case is the presence of large calcific deposits in the aortic intima. The aortic valve was excised in this case and it is normal except for small calcific deposit near one commissure. Shown in d is the intimal medial tear which spread out as it healed. The more intimal portion of the medial wall contacts the outer wall of the healed intimal medial tear. Most of the elastic fibers in the wall of the stretched tear are devoid of elastic fibers but in the normal portion of aorta the quantity of elastic fibers appears to be normal. The unusual feature here is the large calcific deposits. The intimal medial tear is between these calcific deposits. This patient was only 47 years of age and underwent a Bentall procedure.

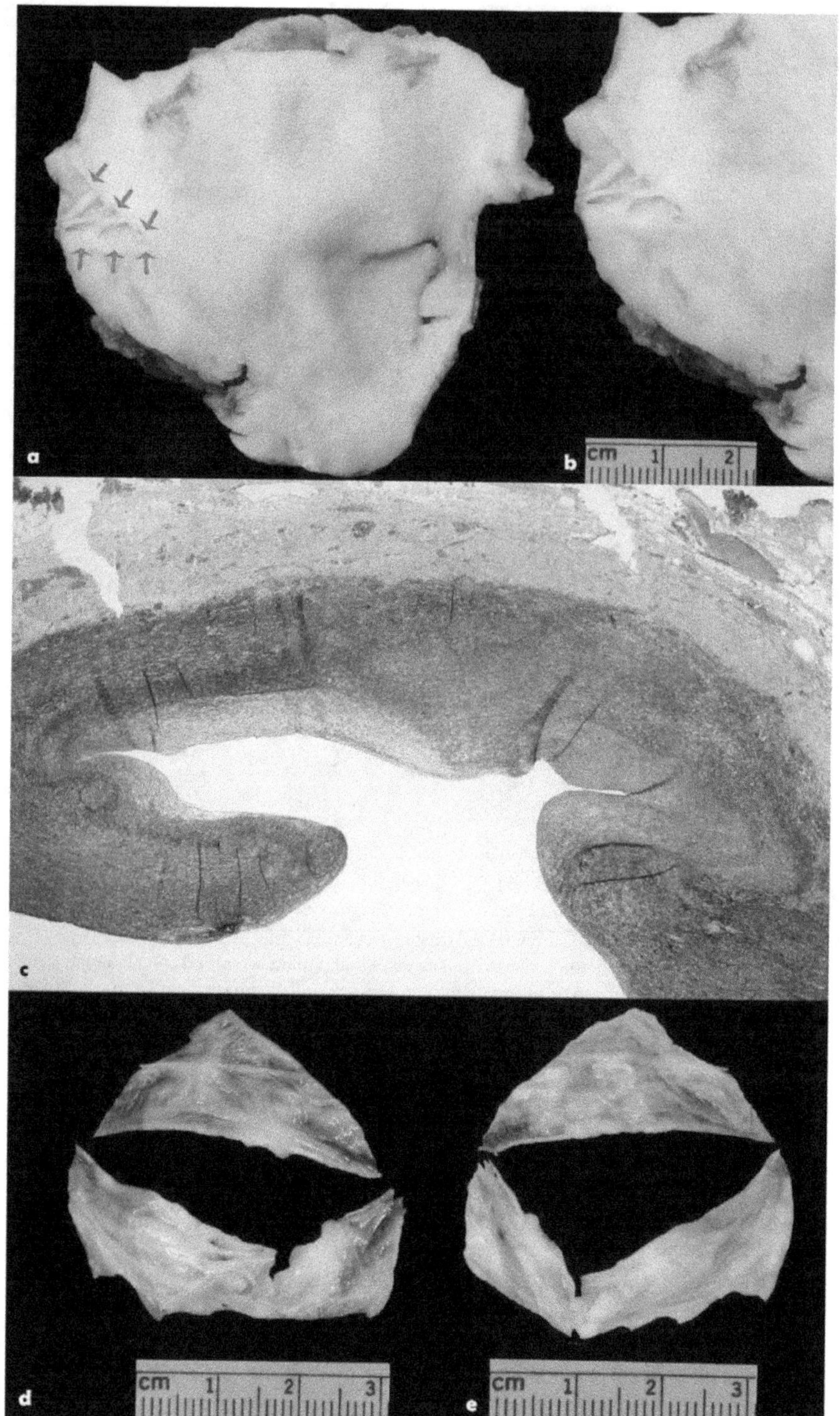

Figure 8. Table 1, **Case #7.** Shown here in a is a healed intimal medial tear surrounded by the red arrows. There was no associated dissection. This healed intimal medial tear was later associated with an acute aortic dissection, type A, but the new tear was not adjacent to the old tear. Shown in c is a histologic section of the intimal medial tear. It looks like a healed peptic ulcer but there was no dissection associated with this intimal medial tear. The number of elastic fibers in the aorta appears to be only slightly reduced. Shown in d is the aortic valve excised and it appears to be a congenitally bicuspid one which was torn at operation, slightly at the raphe. This valve apparently functioned entirely normally. Again, a Bentall procedure was performed. The patient was 53 years of age.

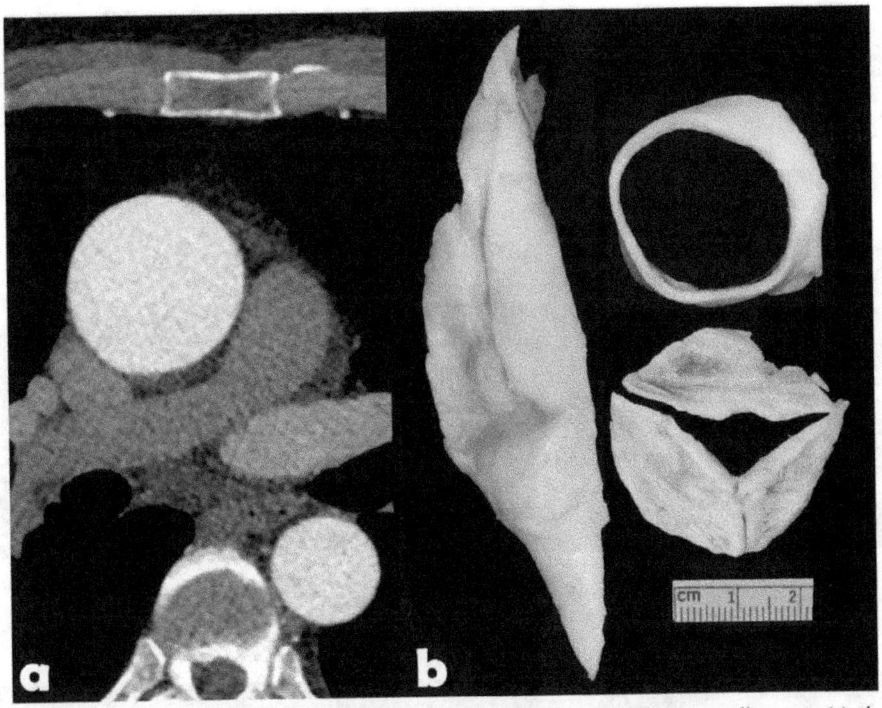

Figure 9. Table 1, **Case # 8.** Shown here is the computerized tomographic image showing a very dilated ascending aorta (a), the portion of ascending aorta excised operatively showing a very large intimal medial tear without dissection, and the congenitally malformed aortic valve (b).

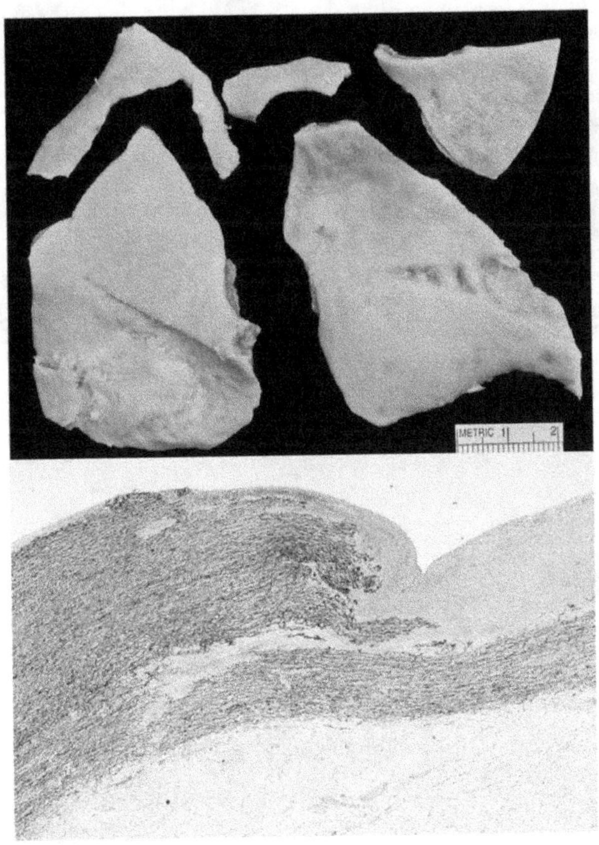

Figure 10. Table 1, **Case # 10.** Shown in the upper panel are five fragments of ascending aorta excised at operation. The two larger portions show intimal-medial tears without dissection. The tears in some areas are "stretched out" and the surfaces of the resulting gaps are irregular and gray in color in contrast with the slightly yellow covered surfaces of the normal portions of aorta. Shown in the lower panel is a photomicrograph at the side of one tear. The black staining elastic fibers are torn and the resulting stretched portion at the sight of that tear is now covered by fibromuscular connective tissue (MOVAT stain x 40).

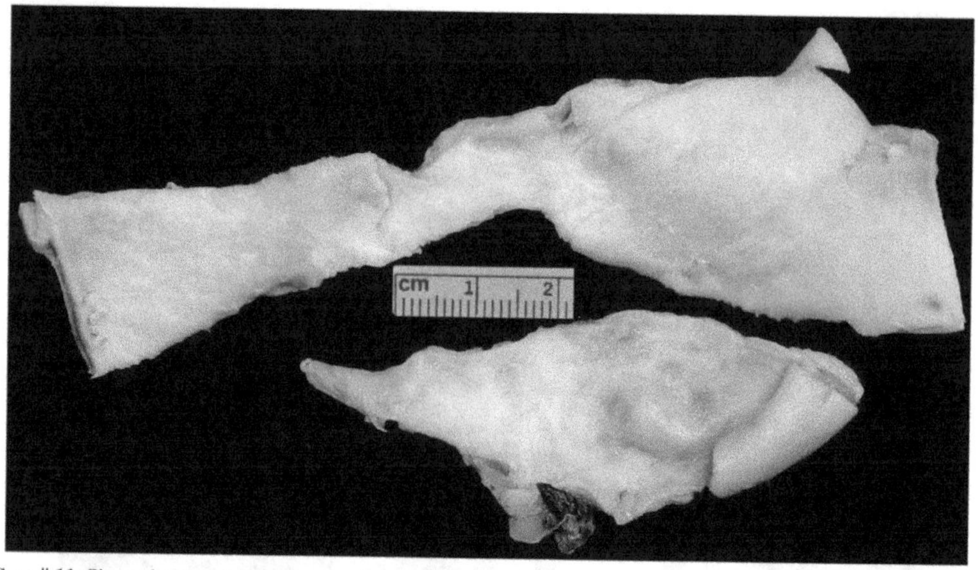

Figure 11. Table 1, **Case # 11.** Shown here are two fragments of ascending aorta excised at operation. Very large intimal medial tears are seen in both specimens. There was no medial dissection.

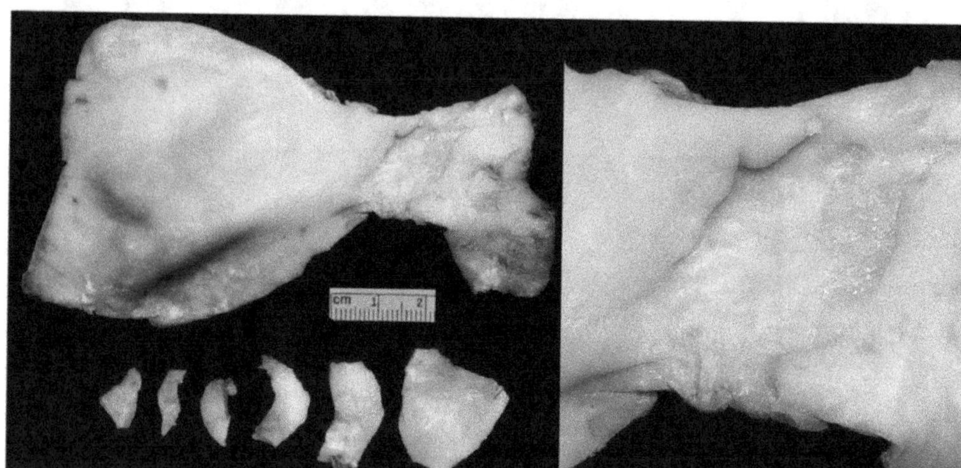

Figure 12. Table 1, **Case # 12.** Shown here are portions of the ascending aorta operatively excised. In the larger fragment a rather large intimal medial tear is present and it is blown up in the right figure. There was no associated medial dissection.

Table 2
Different names of the aortic intimal-medial tear without dissection used by others

Number	First author (reference)	Year of publication	Name
1	Murray[5]	1973	"Incomplete dissecting aneurysm"
2	Roberts[2]	1982	"Nontransmural tear"
3	Silver[6]	1997	"Healed and sealed aortic intimomedial tear"
4	Svensson[7]	1998	"Limited intimal tear"
5	Morimoto[8]	2006	"Localized intimomedial defect"
6	Chirillo[9]	2007	"Subtle-discrete aortic dissection"
7	Mitsomoy[10]	2015	"Intimal tear without medial hematoma"
8	Velasco[11]	2017	"Intimal-medial tear unassociated with aortic dissection"
9	Chin[12]	2018	"Mushroom caps" "Stretch marks" "Focal flaps"

Chin and colleagues[12] described "acute limited intimal tears of the thoracic aorta" in 24 (5%) of 497 patients admitted for "acute aortic syndrome" at their single center (Stanford) over a 10-year period. The 2 most common "acute aortic syndromes" were classic aortic dissection [279 (56%)] and intramural hematoma [121 (24%)]. The most common associated condition in the patients with limited intimal-medial tears was systemic hypertension (22 of 24 patients [92%]). Most of the acute intimal-medial tears affected the ascending aorta (17 [72%]). Most (20 [83%]) were aneurysmal (> 40 mm). The location of these tears was parallel to the long axis of the aorta (10 [42%]) or perpendicular to the long axis (14 [58%]). The article by Chin and associates[12] is a superb contribution to the aortic field but their study is limited to acute intimal-medial tears, not healed ones as described in the present study.

1. Roberts WC. Aortic dissection: anatomy, consequences, and causes. *Am Heart J* 1981;101:195–214.
2. Roberts WC, Honig HS. The spectrum of cardiovascular disease in the Marfan syndrome: a clinico-morphologic study of 18 necropsy patients and comparison to 151 previously reported necropsy patients. *Am Heart J* 1982;104:115–135.
3. Movat HZ. Demonstration of all connective tissue elements in a single section; pentachrome stains. *AMA Arch Pathol* 1955;60:289–295.
4. Waller BF, Reis RL, McIntosh CL, Epstein SE, Roberts WC. Marfan cardiovascular disease without the Marfan syndrome. Fusiform ascending aortic aneurysm with aortic and mitral valve regurgitation. *Chest* 1980;77:533–540.
5. Murray C, Edwards JE. Spontaneous laceration of ascending aorta. *Circulation* 1973;47:848–858.
6. Silver MD. The healed and sealed aortic intimomedial tear. *Cardiovasc Pathol* 1997;6:315–320.
7. Svensson LG, Labib SB, Eisenhauer AC, Butterly JR. Intimal tear without hematoma: an important variant of aortic dissection that can elude current imaging techniques. *Circulation* 1999;99:1331–1336.
8. Morimoto N, Okita Y, Okada K, Yamashita T, Nakagiri K, Maruo A, Kawanishi Y, Matsumori M, Asano M. A localized intimomedial defect resulted in aortic regurgitation. *J Thorac Cardiovasc Surg* 2006;131:232–233.
9. Chirillo F, Salvador L, Bacchion F, Grisolia EF, Valfrè C, Olivari Z. Clinical and anatomical characteristics of subtle-discrete dissection of the ascending aorta. *Am J Cardiol* 2007;100:1314–1319.
10. Mitsomoy MF, Alexoiu V, Kirsch M. Svensson class IV ascending aortic dissection, often confused with penetrating ulcer. *J Cardiovasc Thorac Res* 2015;7:41–42.
11. Velasco CE, Hashemi H, Roullard CP, Machannaford J, Roberts WC. Asymptomatic ascending aorta aneurysm with severe aortic regurgitation caused by multiple intimal-medial tears unassociated with aortic dissection. *Am J Cardiol* 2018;121:668–669.
12. Chin AS, Willemink MJ, Kino A, Hinostroza V, Sailer AM, Fischbein MP, Mitchell RS, Berry GJ, Miller DC, Fleischmann D. Acute limited intimal tears of the thoracic aorta. *J Am Coll Cardiol* 2018;71 (24):2773–2785.

www.ingramcontent.com/pod-product-compliance
Lightning Source LLC
LaVergne TN
LVHW080416220926
848484LV00007BC/1799